OTHER PMIC TITLES OF INTEREST

RISK MANAGEMENT TITLES
Malpractice Depositions
Medical Risk Management
Preparing for Your Deposition
Preventing Emergency Malpractice
Testifying in Court

FINANCIAL MANAGEMENT TITLES
A Physician's Guide to Financial Independence
Business Ventures for Physicians
Financial Valuation of Your Practice
Personal Money Management for Physicians
Personal Pension Plan Strategies for Physicians
Securing Your Assets

DICTIONARIES AND OTHER REFERENCE TITLES
Drugs of Abuse
Health and Medicine on the Internet
Medical Acronyms and Abbreviations
Medical Phrase Index
Medical Word Building
Medico Mnemonica
Medico-Legal Glossary
Spanish/English Handbook for Medical Professionals

MEDICAL REFERENCE AND CLINICAL TITLES
Advance Medical Directives
Clinical Research Opportunities
Gastroenterology: Problems in Primary Care
Manual of IV Therapy
Medical Care of the Adolescent Athlete
Medical Procedures for Referral
Neurology: Problems in Primary Care
Orthopaedics: Problems in Primary Care
Patient Care Emergency Handbook
Patient Care Flowchart Manual
Patient Care Procedures for Your Practice
Physician's Office Laboratory
Pulmonary Medicine: Problems in Primary Care
Questions and Answers on AIDS

**AVAILABLE FROM YOUR LOCAL MEDICAL
BOOK STORE OR CALL 1-800-MED-SHOP**

OTHER PMIC TITLES OF INTEREST

CODING AND REIMBURSEMENT TITLES
Collections Made Easy!
CPT Coders Choice®, Thumb Indexed
CPT & HCPCS Coding Made Easy!
CPT Easy Links
CPT Plus!
DRG Plus!
E/M Coding Made Easy!
Getting Paid for What You Do
HCPCS Coders Choice®, Color Coded, Thumb Indexed
Health Insurance Carrier Directory
HIPAA Compliance Manual
ICD-9-CM, Coders Choice®, Thumb Indexed
ICD-9-CM Coding for Physicians' Offices
ICD-9-CM Coding Made Easy!
ICD-9-CM, Home Health Edition
Medical Fees in the United States
Medicare Compliance Manual
Medicare Rules & Regulations
Physicians Fee Guide
Reimbursement Manual for the Medical Office

PRACTICE MANAGEMENT TITLES
Accounts Receivable Management for the Medical Practice
Achieving Profitability With a Medical Office System
Encyclopedia of Practice and Financial Management
Managed Care Organizations
Managing Medical Office Personnel
Marketing Strategies for Physicians
Medical Marketing Handbook
Medical Office Policy Manual
Medical Practice Forms
Medical Practice Handbook
Medical Staff Privileges
Negotiating Managed Care Contracts
Patient Satisfaction
Performance Standards for the Laboratory
Professional and Practice Development
Promoting Your Medical Practice
Starting in Medical Practice
Working With Insurance and Managed Care Plans

**AVAILABLE FROM YOUR LOCAL MEDICAL
BOOK STORE OR CALL 1-800-MED-SHOP**

ICD·9·CM

International Classification of Diseases
9th Revision

Clinical Modification
Sixth Edition

Color Coded
2008

Volumes 1 & 2

ISBN 978-1-57066-449-6 (Coder's Choice® Soft cover)
ISBN 978-1-57066-452-6 (Spiral)

Volumes 1, 2, & 3

ISBN 978-1-57066-451-9 (Coder's Choice® Soft cover)
ISBN 978-1-57066-453-3 (Spiral)
ISBN 978-1-57066-454-0 (Home Health Edition)

Non-indexed versions

ISBN 978-1-57066-448-9 (Volumes 1 & 2)
ISBN 978-1-57066-450-2 (Volumes 1, 2, & 3)

Practice Management Information Corporation [PMIC]
4727 Wilshire Boulevard, Suite 300
Los Angeles, California 90010
1-800-MED-SHOP
http://www.pmiconline.com

Printed in China

Copyright© 2007 under the Uniform Copyright Convention. All rights reserved. This book is protected by copyright. No part of it may be reproduced, stored in a retrieval system, or transmitted in any form or by any means, electronic, mechanical, photocopying, recording, or otherwise, without written permission from the publisher.

Preface

Health care professionals have long used coding systems to describe procedures, services, and supplies. However, most described the reason for the procedure, service or supply with a diagnostic statement. Of those health care professionals who do code the diagnosis, either due to a requirement for a computer billing system and/or electronic claims filing, many do not code completely or accurately. With the passage of the Medicare Catastrophic Coverage Act of 1988, diagnostic coding using *ICD-9-CM* became mandatory for Medicare claims. In the area of health care reimbursement rules and regulations, the typical progression is that changes required for Medicare are followed shortly by similar changes for Medicaid and private insurance carriers.

To some professionals, the requirement to use diagnostic coding may have seemed like a burden or simply another excuse for Medicare intermediaries to delay or deny payment. However, it is important to understand that the proper use of coding systems for both procedures and diagnoses gives the professional absolute control over his or her billing and reimbursement. Accurate diagnosis coding is not easy. It requires a good working knowledge of medical terminology and a fundamental understanding of *ICD-9-CM*. In addition, the coder must know the rules and regulations required to comply with Medicare requirements for coding.

This edition of the *International Classification of Diseases, 9th Revision, Clinical Modification (ICD-9-CM)* is published by Practice Management Information Corporation in recognition of its responsibility to promulgate this classification throughout the United States for morbidity coding and billing purposes. *The International Classification of Diseases, 9th Revision*, originally published by the World Health Organization (WHO) is the foundation of the *ICD-9-CM* and continues to be the classification employed in cause-of-death coding in the United States.

The *ICD-9-CM* is recommended for use in all clinical settings, but is required for reporting diagnoses and diseases to all U.S. Public Health Service and Department of Health and Human Services programs, such as Medicare and Medicaid. This version faithfully follows and contains the same information found in the official U.S. government version of the *ICD-9-CM*.

All official authorized addenda effective October 1, 2007, have been included in this edition. A new revision will be available approximately September 15th of each year. Revised editions may be purchased from:

Practice Management Information Corporation
4727 Wilshire Boulevard, Suite 300
Los Angeles, California 90010
1-800-MED-SHOP

Or by contacting our web site at http://www.pmiconline.com.

Disclaimer

This publication includes all official ICD-9-CM codes, descriptions, annotations and guidelines as maintained by the U.S. Department of Health and Human Services with the exception that this publication includes special symbols to indicate additions and revisions from the previous edition and special symbols to facilitate identification of diagnostic codes that require 4th or 5th digit specificity, the use of color coding to alert the user to special coding considerations, and thumb indexing to make locating codes easier. This publication is revised annually so that we may present the most current information possible. Though all of the information is carefully researched and checked for accuracy and completeness, the publisher accepts no responsibility with regard to errors, omissions, misuse or misinterpretation.

Table of Contents

PREFACE iii
DISCLAIMER iv
INTRODUCTION 1
  Historical Perspective 1
    ICD-9-CM Background 2
    Use of ICD-9-CM Codes for Professional Billing 2
  Terminology 3
  Format of ICD-9-CM 5
    The Tabular List (Volume 1) 5
      Classification of Diseases and Injuries 5
      Supplementary Classifications 6
      Appendices 6
      Specifications for the Tabular List 6
    The Alphabetic Index (Volume 2) 7
      Supplementary Sections 8
      Special Tables 8
      Specifications for the Alphabetic Index 8
    Procedures: Tabular List and Alphabetic Index (Volume 3) 8
      Tabular List of Procedures 8
      Alphabetic Index to Procedures 9
      Specifications for the Procedure Classification 9
  Conventions Used in the Tabular List 9
    Abbreviations 9
    Punctuation 10
    Symbols 10
    Other Conventions 10
    Instructional Notations 11
    Related Terms 11
  Color Coding 12
    Volume 1 12
    Volume 3 12
  Medicare Requirements for ICD-9-CM Coding 13
    CMS Guidelines for Using ICD-9-CM Codes 13
    Completing the CMS1500 Claim Form 15
    Medicare Penalties for Non-compliance 16
  Coding and Billing Issues 17
    Diagnosis Codes Must Support Procedure Codes 17
    Place (Location) of Service 17
    Level of Service Provided 17
    Frequency of Services 17
    Concurrent Care 17
  ICD-10 18
    Implementation of ICD-10 in the United States 18
  Where to Get Answers to Questions About ICD-9-CM 19

TABLE OF CONTENTS

ICD-9-CM CODING FUNDAMENTALS ... 21
Nine Steps for Accurate ICD-9-CM Coding ... 21
Italicized Entries ... 22
Other and Unspecified Codes ... 22
Acute and Chronic Coding ... 24
Coding Suspected Conditions ... 24
Combination Codes ... 24
Multiple Coding ... 25
Coding Late Effects ... 26
Coding Impending or Threatened Conditions ... 28
Coding Injuries ... 29
Coding Traumatic Fractures ... 29
Coding Burns ... 30
Poisoning and Adverse Effects of Drugs ... 32
Poisoning ... 32
Adverse Reaction in Spite of Proper Administration of Correct Substance ... 32
How Do You Identify Poisoning By Drugs? ... 33
Adverse Effects of Drugs ... 33
Locating the Proper E Code ... 34
Drug Interactions Between Two or More Drugs ... 35
Coding Complications of Medical and Surgical Care ... 36
Complications from Mechanical Devices ... 37
Cardiac Complications ... 37
Special Coding Situations ... 38
Coding Diseases of Blood and Blood Forming Organs ... 38
Coding Circulatory Diseases ... 39
Diseases of Mitral and Aortic Valves ... 39
Ischemic Heart Disease ... 40
Myocardial Infarction ... 41
Arteriosclerotic Cardiovascular Disease (ASCVD) ... 41
Cerebrovascular Disease ... 42
Hypertensive Disease ... 43
High Blood Pressure Versus Elevated Blood Pressure ... 46
Diseases of the Respiratory System ... 46
COPD and Asthma ... 46
COPD and Bronchitis ... 47
Diabetes Mellitus Coding (250) ... 47
Coding Mental Disorders ... 48
Infectious and Parasitic Diseases ... 49
Human Immunodeficiency Virus (HIV) Disease ... 50
Septicemia, SIRS, Sepsis, Severe Sepsis and Septic Shock ... 51
Manifestations ... 53
Etiology/Manifestation Convention ... 53
Coding of Neoplasms ... 54
Table of Neoplasms ... 56
Definitions of Site and Behaviors of Neoplasms ... 57
Steps to Coding Neoplasms ... 57

TABLE OF CONTENTS

Chronic Kidney Disease 62
Pregnancy, Childbirth and the Puerperium.................... 62
    General Rules for Obstetrics Cases 63
    Selection of OB Principal or First-Listed Diagnosis.................... 63
    Fetal Conditions Affecting the Management of the Mother.................... 64
    HIV Infection in Pregnancy, Childbirth and the Puerperium 64
    Current Conditions 64
    Diabetes Mellitis 64
    Gestational Diabetes 64
    Normal Delivery.................... 65
    The Postpartum Period 65
    Late Effect of Complication of Pregnancy, Childbirth
        and the Puerperium.................... 66
    Abortions 66
Newborn (Perinatal) Guidelines.................... 67
    Use of Codes V30-V39.................... 68
    Use of Category V29 68
    Use of Other V Codes on Perinatal Record.................... 68
    Maternal Causes of Perinatal Morbidity 69
    Congenital Anomalies 69
    Coding of Additional Perinatal Diagnoses 69
    Prematurity and Fetal Growth Retardation 69
    Newborn Sepsis.................... 70
V Codes: Classification of Factors Influencing Health Status
    and Contact With Health Service.................... 70
    Categories of V Codes 71
        Contact/Exposure 71
        Inoculations and Vaccinations 71
        Status.................... 71
        History (of).................... 73
        Screening 74
        Observation.................... 75
        Aftercare.................... 75
        Follow-Up.................... 76
        Donor 77
        Counseling 77
        Obstetrics and Related Conditions 77
        Newborn, Infant and Child.................... 78
        Routine and Administrative Examinations 78
        Miscellaneous V Codes 79
        Nonspecific V Codes.................... 79
    V Code Table 81
E Codes: Supplemental Classification of External Causes
    of Injury and Poisoning 85
    General E Code Coding Guidelines 86
    Place of Occurrence Guideline 86
    Adverse Effects of Drugs, Medicinal and Biological Substances
        Guidelines.................... 86
    Multiple Cause Coding Guidelines.................... 87

TABLE OF CONETENTS

    Child and Adult Abuse Guidelines........................... 87
    Unknown or Suspected Intent Guidelines 88
    Undetermined Cause Guidelines 88
    Late Effects of External Cause Guidelines.................... 88
    Misadventures and Complications of Care Guidelines 88
    Terrorism Guidelines..................................... 88
    Examples Using E Codes.................................. 89
    Principal and Additional Diagnosis(es): Guidelines for Inpatient,
        Short-Term, Acute Care Hospital Records 90
        Selecting Principal Diagnoses 90
        Rules for Reporting Additional Diagnoses...................... 92
    Diagnostic Coding and Reporting Guidelines for Outpatient Services 93

ANATOMICAL ILLUSTRATIONS............................. 97

DISEASES: TABULAR LIST VOLUME 1....................... 147
    1. Infectious and Parasitic Diseases........................ 149
    2. Neoplasms 189
    3. Endocrine, Nutritional, and Metabolic Diseases,
       and Immunity Disorders 225
    4. Diseases of the Blood and Blood-Forming Organs 243
    5. Mental Disorders................................... 253
    6. Diseases of the Nervous System and Sense Organs 277
    7. Diseases of the Circulatory System 333
    8. Diseases of the Respiratory System...................... 361
    9. Diseases of the Digestive System 377
    10. Diseases of the Genitourinary System 407
    11. Complications of Pregnancy, Childbirth, and the Puerperium 431
    12. Diseases of the Skin and Subcutaneous Tissue 453
    13. Diseases of the Musculoskeletal System and Connective Tissue 467
    14. Congenital Anomalies............................... 491
    15. Certain Conditions Originating in the Perinatal Period 515
    16. Symptoms, Signs, and Ill-Defined Conditions 529
    17. Injury and Poisoning 547

Supplementary Classifications
    V CODES: Classification of Factors Influencing Health Status and
       Contact With Health Services 619
    E CODES: Classification of External Causes of Injury and Poisoning.... 653

Appendices
    A. Morphology of Neoplasms.............................. 711
    B. Glossary of Mental Disorders (Removed from FY2005 ICD-9-CM) .. 725
    C. Classification of Drugs by American Hospital Formulary Service List
       Number and Their ICD-9-CM Equivalents 727
    D. Classification of Industrial Accidents According to Agency 733
    E. List of Three-Digit Categories........................... 737

DISEASES: ALPHABETIC INDEX VOLUME 2 761
    Hypertension Chart 1083
    Neoplasm Chart 1184
    Table of Drugs and Chemicals............................ 1415

TABLE OF CONTENTS

Index to External Causes 1497
Summary of Additions, Deletions and Revisions to Volume 1 1539
PROCEDURES: TABULAR LIST VOLUME 3 [1] 1543
    1. Operations on the Nervous System (01-05) 1545
    2. Operations on the Endocrine System (06-07) 1561
    3. Operations on the Eye (08-16) 1565
    4. Operations on the Ear (18-20) 1575
    5. Operations on the Nose, Mouth and Pharynx (21-29) 1579
    6. Operations on the Respiratory System (30-34) 1589
    7. Operations on the Cardiovascular System (35-39) 1597
    8. Operations on the Hemic and Lymphatic Systems (40-41) 1619
    9. Operations on the Digestive System (42-54) 1623
    10. Operations on the Urinary System (55-59) 1649
    11. Operations on the Male Genital Organs (60-64) 1659
    12. Operations on the Female Genital Organs (65-71) 1665
    13. Obstetrical Procedures (72-75) 1675
    14. Operations on the Musculoskeletal System (76-84) 1679
    15. Operations on the Integumentary System (85-86) 1701
    16. Miscellaneous Diagnostic and Therapeutic Procedures (87-99) 1709
PROCEDURES: ALPHABETIC INDEX VOLUME 3 [1] 1737
Summary of Additions, Deletions and Revisions to Volume 3 [1] 1905

---

[1] These listings appear only in the three volume edition

INTRODUCTION

Introduction to ICD-9-CM

ICD-9-CM is an acronym for *International Classification of Diseases, 9th Revision, Clinical Modification*, published under different names since 1900. *ICD-9-CM* is a statistical classification system that arranges diseases and injuries into groups according to established criteria. Most *ICD-9-CM* codes are numeric and consist of three, four or five numbers and a description. The codes are revised approximately every 10 years by the World Health Organization and annual updates are published by Center for Medicare and Medicaid Services (CMS).

HISTORICAL PERSPECTIVE

The *International Classification of Diseases, 9th Revision, Clinical Modification (ICD-9-CM)* is based on the official version of the *World Health Organization's (WHO) 9th Revision, International Classification of Diseases (ICD-9)*. ICD-9 is designed for the classification of morbidity and mortality information for statistical purposes, and for the indexing of medical records by disease and operations, and for data storage and retrieval. *ICD-9-CM* replaced the Eighth Revision International Classification of Diseases, Adapted for Use in the United States commonly referred to as *ICDA*.

The concept of extending the International Classification of Diseases for use in hospital indexing was originally developed in response to a need for a more efficient basis for storage and retrieval of diagnostic data. In 1950, the U.S. Public Health Service and the Veterans Administration began independent tests of the International Classification of Diseases for hospital indexing purposes. In the following year, the Columbia Presbyterian Medical Center in New York City adopted the International Classification of Diseases, 6th Revision for use in its medical record department. A few years later, the Commission on Professional and Hospital Activities adopted the International Classification of Diseases for use in hospitals participating in the Professional Activity Study (PAS).

In view of the growing interest in the use of the International Classification of Diseases for hospital indexing, a study was undertaken in 1956 by the American Medical Association and the American Medical Record Association of the relative efficiencies of coding systems for diagnostic indexing. Following this study, the major uses of the International Classification of Diseases for hospital indexing purposes consolidated their experiences and an adaptation was published in December 1959. A revision containing the first "Classification of Operations and Treatments" was published in 1962.

In 1968, following a study by the American Hospital Association, the United States Public Health Service published the Eighth Revision International Classification of Diseases, Adapted for Use in the United States. This publication became commonly known as ICDA, and served as the basis for coding diagnostic data for official morbidity and mortality statistics in the United States.

ICD-9-CM Background

In February 1977, a committee was convened by the National Center for Health Statistics to provide advice and counsel for the development of clinical modification of the ICD-9. The organizations represented on the committee included:

    American Association of Health Data Systems
    American Hospital Association
    American Medical Record Association
    Association for Health Records
    Commission on Professional and Hospital Activities
    Council on Clinical Classifications, sponsored by:

        American Academy of Pediatrics
        American College of Obstetricians and Gynecologists
        American College of Physicians
        American College of Surgeons
        American Psychiatric Association

    Health Care Financing Administration
    WHO Center for Classification of Diseases

The resulting *ICD-9-CM* is a clinical modification of the *World Health Organization's International Classification of Diseases, 9th Revision (ICD-9)*. The term "clinical" is used to emphasize the modifications intent; namely, to serve as a useful tool in the area of classification of morbidity data for indexing of medical records, medical care review, ambulatory and other medical care programs, as well as for basic health statistics.

In use since January 1979, *ICD-9-CM* provides a diagnostic coding system that is more precise than those needed only for statistical groupings and trend analysis. Official addenda (updates) to *ICD-9-CM* are issued in October each year by the National Center for Health Statistics (NCHS), part of the Centers for Disease Control (CDC).

Use of ICD-9-CM Codes for Professional Billing

Until passage of the Medicare Catastrophic Coverage Act of 1988, health care professionals were not required to report *ICD-9-CM* codes when billing government or private insurance carriers for reimbursement. The exception to this requirement was for those health care professionals who filed insurance claims electronically and those who used "code driven" computer billing services or computer systems.

Most health care professionals simply included the text or description of the injury, illness, sign or symptom that was the reason for the encounter. Insurance carriers who used *ICD-9-CM* coding had to code the diagnostic statements prior to input into their computer systems for reimbursement processing.

A specific requirement of the Medicare Catastrophic Coverage Act of 1988 required health care professionals to include *ICD-9-CM* codes on their Medicare claim forms effective April 1, 1989. A two-month grace period, to June 1, 1989, was allowed at the request of the American Medical Association, to allow health care professionals additional time to develop the knowledge and systems necessary to implement the requirement.

TERMINOLOGY

There are terms used throughout this publication that are important for a proper understanding of *ICD-9-CM*. The following terms are defined specifically as they are used for *ICD-9-CM* with the knowledge that some terms may have other definitions and meanings.

acute	refers to the condition that is the primary reason for the current encounter.
addenda	official updates to ICD-9-CM published continuously since 1986, that become effective on October 1st of each year.
adverse	any response to a drug that is noxious and unintended and occurs with proper dosage.
aftercare	an encounter for something planned in advance, for example, cast removal.
AHFS	American Hospital Formulary Service.
alphabetic index	the portion of ICD-9-CM that lists definitions and codes in alphabetic order. Also called Volume 2.
category	refers to diagnoses codes listed within a specific three-digit category, for example category 250, Diabetes Mellitus.
cause	that which brings about any condition or produces any effect.
chronic	continuing over a long period of time or recurring frequently.
coding	the process of transferring written or verbal descriptions of diseases, injuries and procedures into numerical designations.
combination	a code that combines a diagnosis with an associated secondary process or complication.
complication	the occurrence of two or more diseases in the same patient at the same time.
concurrent	when a patient is being treated by more than one provider for different care conditions at the same time.
conventions	refers to the use of certain abbreviations, punctuation, symbols, type faces, and other instructions that must be clearly understood in order to use ICD-9-CM.
CPT	Current Procedural Terminology. Listing of codes and descriptions for procedures, services and supplies published by the American Medical Association. Used to bill insurance carriers.
diagnosis	a written description of the reason(s) for the procedure, service, supply or encounter.
down coding	the process where insurance carriers reduce the value of a procedure, and the resulting reimbursement, due to either 1) a mismatch of CPT code and description or 2) ICD-9-CM code does not justify the procedure or level of service.
E codes	specific ICD-9-CM codes used to identify the cause of injury, poisoning and other adverse effects.
eponyms	medical procedures or conditions named after a person or a place.
etiology	the cause(s) or origin of a disease.

INTRODUCTION

HCFA1500	Uniform health insurance claim form used for billing services to Medicare and other insurance carriers.
hierarchy	a system that ranks items one above another.
ICD-9-CM	International Classification of Diseases, 9th Revision, Clinical Modification.
ICD-10	International Classification of Diseases, 10th Revision
late effect	a residual effect (condition produced) after the acute phase of an illness or injury has ended.
main term	refers to listings in the Alphabetic Index appearing **BOLDFACE** type.
manifestation	characteristic signs or symptoms of an illness.
multiple	refers to the need to use more than one ICD-9-CM code to fully identify coding a condition.
primary code	the ICD-9-CM code that defines the main reason for the current encounter.
residual	the long-term condition(s) resulting from a previous acute illness or injury.
rule out	refers to a method used to indicate that a condition is probable, suspected, or questionable but unconfirmed. ICD-9-CM has no provisions for the use of this term.
secondary	code(s) listed after the primary code that further indicate the cause(s) code for the current encounter or define the need for higher levels of care.
sections	refers to portions of the Tabular List that are organized in groups of three-digit code numbers. For example, Malignant Neoplasm of Lip, Oral Cavity and Pharynx (140-149).
sequencing	the process of listing ICD-9-CM codes in the proper order.
specificity	refers to the requirement to code to the highest number of digits possible, 3, 4 or 5, when choosing an ICD-9-CM code.
sub term	refers to listings appearing in the Alphabetic Index under MAIN TERMS and always indented two spaces to the right.
subcategories	refers to groupings of four-digit codes listed under three-digit categories.
Tabular List	the portion of ICD-9-CM that lists codes and definitions in numeric order. Also referred to as Volume 1.
V codes	specific ICD-9-CM codes used to identify encounters for reasons other than illness or injury, for example, immunization.
Volume 1	see TABULAR LIST
Volume 2	see ALPHABETIC INDEX
Volume 3	procedure codes used only for hospital coding. Volume 3 contains both a numeric listing and an alphabetic index.

FORMAT OF ICD-9-CM

The *International Classification of Diseases, 9th Revision, Clinical Modification* was originally published as a three volume set (2nd edition). Newer versions of *ICD-9-CM* are available as two separate books containing Volume 1 and Volume 2 in one book and Volumes 1, 2 and 3 in the other. It is also now available on CD-ROM from the U.S. Government.

This edition of *ICD-9-CM* includes all official addenda from October 1986 through October 2007.

The Tabular List (Volume 1)

The Tabular List (Volume 1) is a *numeric* listing of diagnosis codes and descriptions consisting of 17 chapters that classify diseases and injuries, two sections containing supplementary codes (V codes and E codes) and six appendices.

Classification of Diseases and Injuries

The Classification of Diseases and Injuries includes the following 17 chapters:

Chapter 1	Infectious and Parasitic Diseases (001-139)
Chapter 2	Neoplasms (140-239)
Chapter 3	Endocrine, Nutritional and Metabolic Diseases, and Immunity Disorders (240-279)
Chapter 4	Diseases of the Blood and Blood-Forming Organs (280-289)
Chapter 5	Mental Disorders (290-319)
Chapter 6	Diseases of the Nervous System and Sense Organs (320-389)
Chapter 7	Diseases of the Circulatory System (390-459)
Chapter 8	Diseases of the Respiratory System (460-519)
Chapter 9	Diseases of the Digestive System (520-579)
Chapter 10	Diseases of the Genitourinary System (580-629)
Chapter 11	Complications of Pregnancy, Childbirth, and the Puerperium (630-677)
Chapter 12	Diseases of the Skin and Subcutaneous Tissue (680-709)
Chapter 13	Diseases of the Musculoskeletal System and Connective Tissue (710-739)
Chapter 14	Congenital Anomalies (740-759)
Chapter 15	Certain Conditions Originating in the Perinatal Period (760-779)
Chapter 16	Symptoms, Signs and Ill-defined Conditions (780-799)
Chapter 17	Injury and Poisoning (800-999)

INTRODUCTION

Each chapter of the Tabular List (Volume 1) is structured into four components, namely:

    Sections: groups of three-digit code numbers

    Categories: three-digit code numbers

    Subcategories: four-digit code numbers

    Fifth-Digit Subclassifications: five-digit code numbers

Supplementary Classifications

There are two supplementary classifications included in the Tabular List (Volume 1). These are:

V Codes	Supplementary Classification of Factors Influencing Health Status and Contact with Health Services (V01-V86)
E Codes	Supplementary Classification of External Causes of Injury and Poisoning (E800-E999)

Appendices

The Tabular List (Volume 1) includes four appendices. These are:

Appendix A Morphology of Neoplasms

Appendix C Classification of Drugs by American Hospital Formulary Service List Number and Their ICD-9-CM Equivalents

Appendix D Classification of Industrial Accidents According to Agency

Appendix E List of Three-Digit Categories

Specifications for the Tabular List

1. Three-digit rubrics and their contents are unchanged from *ICD-9*.

2. The sequence of three-digit rubrics is unchanged from *ICD-9*.

3. Three-digit rubrics are not added to the main body of the classification.

4. Unsubdivided three-digit rubrics are subdivided where necessary to:

   a) Add clinical detail

   b) Isolate terms for clinical accuracy

5. The modification in *ICD-9-CM* is accomplished by the addition of a fifth digit to existing *ICD-9* rubrics, except as noted under number 7 below.

6. Four-digit rubrics are added to subdivided three-digit codes only when there is no other means of achieving desired detail. These codes, unique to *ICD-9-CM* (28 three-digit categories) are marked with the symbol in the Tabular List.

7. The optional dual classification in *ICD-9* is modified.

   a) Duplicate rubrics are deleted:

      1) Four-digit manifestation categories duplicating etiology entries.

      2) Manifestation inclusion terms duplicating etiology entries.

   b) Manifestations of diseases are identified, to the extent possible, by creating five digit codes in the etiology rubrics.

   c) When the manifestation of a disease cannot be included in the etiology rubrics, provision for its identification is made by retaining the *ICD-9* rubrics used for classifying manifestations of disease.

8. The format of *ICD-9-CM* is revised from that used in *ICD-9*.

   a) American spelling of medical terms is used.

   b) Inclusion terms are indented beneath the titles of codes.

   c) Codes not to be used for primary tabulation of disease are printed in italics with the notation, "code also underlying disease."

The Alphabetic Index (Volume 2)

The Alphabetic Index (Volume 2) of *ICD-9-CM* consists of an alphabetic list of terms and codes, two supplementary Sections following the alphabetic listing, plus two special tables found within the alphabetic listing. The Alphabetic Index (Volume 2) is structured as follows:

MAIN TERMS: appear in **BOLDFACE** type

SUBTERMS: are always indented two spaces to the right under main terms

CARRY-OVER
LINES: are always indented more than two spaces from the level of the preceding line

Supplementary Sections

The supplementary sections following the Alphabetic Index are:

TABLE OF DRUGS AND CHEMICALS

>This table contains a classification of drugs and other chemical substances to identify poisoning states and external causes of adverse effects.

INDEX TO EXTERNAL CAUSES OF INJURIES & POISONINGS (E-CODES)

>This section contains the index to the codes that classify environmental events, circumstances, and other conditions as the cause of injury and other adverse effects.

Special Tables

The two special tables, located within the Alphabetic Index, and found under the main terms as underlined below, are:

HYPERTENSION TABLE

NEOPLASM TABLE

Specifications for the Alphabetic Index

1. Format of the Alphabetic Index follows the format of the ICD-9.

2. Main terms in the Alphabetic Index are printed in bold face type.

3. When two codes are required to indicate etiology and manifestation, the optional manifestation code appears in brackets, e.g., diabetic cataract 250.5 *[366.41]*.

Procedures: Tabular List and Alphabetic Index (Volume 3)

Volume 3 consists of two sections, a Tabular List of codes and an alphabetic index. These codes define procedures instead of diagnoses. Frequently used incorrectly by health care professionals, codes from Volume 3 are intended only for use by hospitals. The Fourth Edition of ICD-9-CM printed by the U.S. Government Printing Office did not include Volume 3. The Fifth and subsequent Editions of ICD-9-CM issued by the U.S. Government included Volume 3 on a CD-ROM.

The ICD-9-CM Procedure Classification is a modification of WHO's *Fascicle V, Surgical Procedures*, and is published as Volume 3 of ICD-9-CM. It contains both a Tabular List and an Alphabetic Index. Greater detail has been added to the ICD-9-CM Procedure Classification necessitating expansion of the codes from three to four digits. Approximately 90% of the rubrics refer to surgical procedures with the remaining 10% accounting for other investigative and therapeutic procedures.

Tabular List of Procedures

The Tabular List includes 16 chapters containing codes and descriptions for surgical procedures and miscellaneous diagnostic and therapeutic procedures.

Alphabetic Index to Procedures

The Alphabetic Index provides an alphabetic index to the Tabular List of Volume 3

Specifications for the Procedure Classification

1. The ICD-9-CM Procedure Classification is published in its own volume containing both a Tabular List and an Alphabetic Index.

2. The classification is a modification of *Fascicle V Surgical Procedures* of the ICD-9 Classification of Procedures in Medicine, working from the draft dated Geneva, 30 September-6 October 1975, and labeled WHO/ICD-9/Rev. Conf. 75.4.

3. All three-digit rubrics in the range 01-86 are maintained as they appear in *Fascicle V*, whenever feasible.

4. Nonsurgical procedures are segregated from the surgical procedures and confined to the rubrics 87-99, whenever feasible.

5. Selected detail contained in the remaining fascicles of the *ICD-9 Classification of Procedures in Medicine* is accommodated where possible.

6. The structure of the classification is based on anatomy rather than surgical specialty.

7. The *ICD-9-CM* Procedure Classification is numeric only, i.e., no alphabetic characters are used.

8. The classification is based on a two-digit structure with two decimal digits where necessary.

9. Compatibility with the *ICD-9 Classification of Procedures in Medicine* was not maintained when a different axis was deemed more clinically appropriate.

CONVENTIONS USED IN THE TABULAR LIST

The *ICD-9-CM* Tabular List (Volume 1) makes use of certain abbreviations, punctuation, symbols, and other conventions that must be clearly understood. The purpose of these conventions is to first, provide special coding instructions, and second, to conserve space.

Abbreviations

NOS — Not Otherwise Specified. Equivalent to Unspecified. This abbreviation refers to a lack of sufficient detail in the statement of diagnosis to be able to assign it to a more specific sub division within the classification.

NEC — Not Elsewhere Classified. Used with ill-defined terms to alert the coder that a specified form of the condition is classified differently. The category number for the term including NEC is to be used only when the coder lacks the information necessary to code the term to a more specific category.

Punctuation

( )   PARENTHESES are used to enclose supplementary words that may be present or absent in a statement of disease without affecting the code assignment.

[ ]   SQUARE BRACKETS are used to enclose synonyms, alternate wordings or explanatory phrases.

:   COLONS are used after an incomplete phrase or term that requires one or more of the modifiers indented under it to make it assignable to a given category. EXCEPTION to this rule pertains to the abbreviation NOS.

Symbols

●   A filled BLACK CIRCLE preceding a code indicates that the code is new to this revision of ICD-9-CM. A symbol key appears on all left-hand pages of the Tabular List, Volume 1 and Volume 3.

▲   A filled BLACK TRIANGLE preceding a code indicates that there is a revision to the text of an existing code. A symbol key appears on all left-hand pages of the Tabular List, Volume 1 and Volume 3.

④ ⑤   A circle containing the number 4 or the number 5 preceding a code indicates that a fourth or fifth digit is required for coding to the highest level of specificity. Valid digits are in [brackets] under each code if the fourth- and fifth-digit codes themselves are not listed. Definitions of valid fifth digits are found under the major category.

Other conventions

Type Face:

       BOLD: Bold type face is used for all codes and titles in the Tabular List.

       Italics: Italicized type face is used for all exclusion notes and to identify those rubrics that are not to be used for primary tabulations of disease.

Format: ICD-9-CM uses an indented format for ease in reference.

Instructional Notations

Instructional terms define what is, or what is not, included in a given subdivision. This is accomplished by using both inclusion and exclusion terms.

INCLUDES: Indicates separate terms, such as, modifying adjectives, sites and conditions, entered under a subdivision, such as a category, to further define or give examples of, the content of the category.

Excludes: Exclusion terms are enclosed in a box and are printed in italics to draw attention to their presence. The importance of this instructional term is its use as a guideline to direct the coder to the proper code assignment. In other words, all terms following the word EXCLUDES: are to be coded elsewhere as indicated in each instance.

NOTES These are used to define terms and give coding instructions. Often used to list the fifth-digit subclassifications for certain categories.

SEE The "see" instruction following a main term in the index indicates that another term should be referenced. It is necessary to go to the main term referenced with the "see" note to locate the correct code.

SEE CATEGORY A variation of the instructional term SEE. This refers the coder to a specific category. You must *always* follow this instructional term.

SEE ALSO A "see also" instruction following a main term in the index instructs that there is another main term that may also be referenced that may provide additional index entries that may be useful. It is not necessary to follow the "see also" note when the original main term provides the necessary code.

CODE FIRST This instructional note is used for those codes not intended to be used as a principal diagnosis, or not to be sequenced before the underlying disease. The note requires that the underlying disease (etiology) be coded first with the code the note is applied to being coded second. This note appears only in the Tabular List (Vol. 1).

USE ADDITIONAL CODE This instruction is placed in the Tabular List in those categories where the coder may wish to add further information, by using an additional code, to give a more complete picture of the diagnosis or procedure.

Related terms

AND The word "and" should be interpreted to mean either "and" or "or" when it appears in a title.

WITH The word "with" in the alphabetic index is sequenced immediately following the main term, not in alphabetical order.

INTRODUCTION

COLOR CODING

A PMIC versions of ICD-9-CM include color-coding to alert the user to special coding situations or conditions that require additional attention. The use of color-coding is found in the Tabular List of Volume 1 and the Tabular List of Volume 3. The color is applied as solid rectangular bars over the codes only so that the descriptions remain clear and legible. The color codes and definitions are printed at the bottom of all right-sided pages of Volume 1 and Volume 3.

Volume 1

Three digit codes. Coding to fourth or fifth digit specificity is required.

Unspecified code. Descriptions include the term "unspecified." Use only if a more specific diagnosis is not known or available.

Nonspecific code. Descriptions include the term "nonspecific, unspecified, other specified or other." A report *may* be required by insurance carriers.

Manifestation codes. Used only to code the manifestation of an underlying disease. Code the underlying disease first.

Medicare secondary payer (MSP) alert. Diagnoses that may trigger a post-payment review by Medicare. Medicare is usually the secondary payer for these diagnoses.

Secondary diagnosis only. V codes that may only be used as additional codes, not as first-listed codes.

Primary diagnosis only. V codes which are only acceptable as first listed codes.

Volume 3*

Noncovered operating room procedure. An operating room procedure that is not covered by Medicare.

Non-operating room procedure. A procedure that is not performed in the operating room that affects DRG assignment.

Bilateral procedure.

Valid operating room procedure. Prompts a change in DRG assignment.

Nonspecific operating room procedure. Choose a more precise code if possible.

*These colors appear only in the three-volume edition

INTRODUCTION

MEDICARE REQUIREMENTS FOR ICD-9-CM CODING

The Medicare Catastrophic Coverage Act of 1988 (PL 100-330) requires that health care professionals submit an appropriate diagnosis code, using the *International Classification of Diseases, 9th Revision, Clinical Modification* (*ICD-9-CM*) for each procedure, service, or supply billed under Medicare Part B.

To comply with the regulations, health care professionals must convert the reason(s) for the procedures, services or supplies, performed or issued, from written diagnostic statements that may include specific diagnoses, signs, symptoms and/or complaints, into ICD-9-CM diagnosis codes. The Health Care Financing Administration (now CMS) originally set the implementation date for this requirement as April 1, 1989, however, it was subsequently delayed until June 1, 1989, at the request of the American Medical Association, to give health care providers additional time to prepare for the change.

CMS Guidelines for Using ICD-9-CM Codes

The Center for Medicare and Medicaid Services (CMS, formerly HCFA) has prepared guidelines for using ICD-9-CM codes and instructions on how to report them on claim forms. In addition, CMS has directed your medicare intermediary to provide you with a written copy of these instructions. The basic CMS guidelines are summarized below, however, it is very important that you obtain a copy of the guidelines from your Medicare intermediary as implementation of CMS requirements varies from one intermediary to another.

These guidelines are a set of rules that have been developed to accompany and complement the official conventions and instructions provided within the ICD-9-CM itself. These guidelines are based on the coding and sequencing instructions in Volumes 1, 2 and 3 of ICD-9-CM, but provide additional instruction. Adherence to these guidelines when assigning ICD-9-CM diagnosis and procedure codes is required under the Health Insurance Portability and Accountability Act (HIPAA). The diagnosis codes (Volumes 1-2) have been adopted under HIPAA for all healthcare settings. Volume 3 procedure codes have been adopted for inpatient procedures reported by hospitals.

A joint effort between the healthcare provider and the coder is essential to achieve complete and accurate documentation, code assignment, and reporting of diagnoses and procedures. These guidelines have been developed to assist both the healthcare provider and the coder in identifying those diagnoses and procedures that are to be reported. The importance of consistent, complete documentation in the medical record cannot be overemphasized. Without such documentation, accurate coding cannot be achieved.

The entire record should be reviewed to determine the specific reason for the encounter and the conditions treated.

The term encounter is used for all settings, including hospital admissions. In the context of these guidelines, the term provider is used throughout the guidelines to mean physician or any qualified health care practitioner who is legally accountable for establishing the patient's diagnosis. Only this set of guidelines, approved by the Cooperating Parties, is official.

INTRODUCTION

1. Indicate on the claim form or itemized statement the appropriate code(s) from the ICD-9-CM code range 001.0 through V86 to identify diagnoses, symptoms, conditions, problems, complaints or other reason(s) for the procedure, service or supply provided.

    A. In choosing codes to describe the reason for the encounter, the health care professional will frequently be using codes within the range from 001.0 through 999.9, the section of ICD-9-CM for the classification of diseases and injuries (e.g. infectious and parasitic diseases; neoplasms; signs, symptoms and ill-defined conditions). Codes that describe symptoms as opposed to diagnoses are acceptable if this is the highest level of certainty documented by the physician.

    B. ICD-9-CM also provides codes to deal with visits for circumstances other than a disease or injury, such as an encounter for a laboratory test only. These codes are found in the V-code section and range from V01.0 through V86.

2. The ICD-9-CM code for the diagnosis, condition, problem, or other reason for the encounter documented in the medical record as the main reason for the procedure, service or supply provided should be listed first. Additional ICD-9-CM codes that describe any current coexisting conditions are then listed. Do not include codes for conditions that were previously treated and no longer exist.

3. ICD-9-CM codes should be used at their highest level of specificity.

    A. Assign three digit codes only if there are no four digit codes within the coding category.

    B. Assign four digit codes only if there is no fifth digit subclassification for that category.

    C. Assign the fifth digit subclassification code for those categories where it exists.

    Claims submitted with three or four digit codes where four and five digit codes are available may be returned to you by the Medicare intermediary for proper coding. It is recognized that a very specific diagnosis may not be known at the time of the initial encounter. However, that is not an acceptable reason to submit a three digit code when four or five digits are available.

    For example, if the patient has chronic bronchitis, ICD-9-CM code 491, and the physician has not yet documented whether the bronchitis is simple, mucopurulent, or obstructive, the code for unspecified chronic bronchitis, ICD-9-CM code 491.9, should be listed.

4. Diagnoses documented as "probable," "suspected," "questionable," or "rule out" should not be coded as if the diagnosis is confirmed. The condition(s) should be coded to the highest degree of certainty for the encounter, such as describing symptoms, signs, abnormal test results, or other reasons for the encounter.

5. Chronic disease(s) treated on an ongoing basis may be coded and reported as many times as the patient receives treatment and care for the condition(s).

INTRODUCTION

6. When patients receive ancillary diagnostic services only during an encounter, the appropriate "V code" for the service should be listed first, and the diagnosis or problem for which the diagnostic procedures are being performed should be listed second.

   A. V codes will be used frequently by radiologists who perform radiological examinations on referrals. For example, ICD-9-CM code V72.5, Radiological examination, not elsewhere classified, describes the reason for the encounter and should be listed first on the claim form or statement. If the reason for the referral is known, a second ICD-9-CM code that describes the signs or symptoms for which the examination was ordered should be listed.

   B. Failure to list a second ICD-9-CM code in addition to the V code may result in claim delays or denials. The ICD-9-CM code V72.5, Radiological examination, not elsewhere classified, includes referrals for routine chest x-rays that are not covered by the Medicare program. Medicare intermediaries may establish screening programs to verify that the referrals were not for routine chest x-rays. By supplying a second ICD-9-CM code to describe the reason for the referral, these claims can be clearly identified by the Medicare intermediary as referrals to evaluate symptoms, signs or diagnoses. The mission of a second ICD-9-CM code may lead to requests for additional information from Medicare intermediaries prior to processing the claim.

7. For patients receiving only ancillary therapeutic services during an encounter, list the appropriate V code first, followed by the ICD-9-CM code for the diagnosis or problem for which the services are being performed. For example, a patient with multiple sclerosis presenting for rehabilitation services would be coded using either V57.1 Other physical therapy, or V57.89 Other care involving use of rehabilitation procedures, followed by code 340 Multiple sclerosis.

8. For surgical procedures, use the ICD-9-CM code for the diagnosis for which the surgery was performed. If the postoperative diagnosis is known to be different at the time the claim is filed, use the ICD-9-CM code for the post-operative diagnosis.

9. Code all documented conditions that coexist at the time of the visit that require or affect patient care, treatment or management. Do not code conditions that were previously treated and no longer exist.

Completing the UB-92 (CMS1450) Claim Form

Home Health Agencies report services using the UB-92 health insurance claim form. The UB-92 (also known as the CMS1450) is a uniform institutional provider bill suitable for use in billing multiple third party payers. Because it serves the needs of many payers, a particular payer may not need some data elements. The UB-92 may be filed as a Request for Anticipated Payment (RAP) or as a Home Health PPS claim. Reporting of diagnostic coding is as follows:

INTRODUCTION

Completing the CMS1500 Claim Form

Health care professionals using the Uniform Health Insurance Claim Form, CMS1500, to file claims for services provided to Medicare beneficiaries must list a minimum of one ICD-9-CM code and may list up to four total ICD-9-CM codes on the claim form.

The ICD-9-CM code for the diagnosis, condition, problem or other reason for the encounter is listed first, followed by up to three additional codes that describe any coexisting conditions. At times, there may be several conditions that equally resulted in the encounter. In these cases, the health care professional is free to select the one that will be listed first.

The ICD-9-CM codes are listed in Box 23 of the "old" HCFA1500 (10/84) claim form and Box 21 of the "new" CMS1500 (12/90) claim form (see example). In addition, in Box 24 D of both versions of the form, you must indicate by a number from 1 to 4, or combination of numbers, which diagnoses from Box 23 support the procedure, service or supply listed in Box 24 C.

Due to space limitations on the claim form you may use only up to four ICD-9-CM codes for diagnoses, conditions, or signs and symptoms. Frequently the patient may have more than four conditions present at the time of the encounter, however, you must choose only four codes to be listed on the claim form.

If you strongly believe that additional diagnostic information is needed by the Medicare intermediary for proper claim processing you may attach additional supporting documentation to your manual claim. Keep in mind that in most cases the additional documentation will be ignored by the claims examiners, and, in other cases will result in reimbursement delay while someone reviews your documentation.

Medicare Penalties for Non-compliance

The Medicare Catastrophic Coverage Act of 1988 mandates submission of an appropriate ICD-9-CM diagnosis code or codes for each procedure, service, or supply furnished by the health care professional to Medicare Part B beneficiaries. The Act further specifies that compliance is mandatory and that penalties may be assessed for noncompliance.

The penalties for noncompliance differ depending upon whether or not the health care professional has agreed to accept assignment or not.

1. For health care professionals who accept assignment on a Medicare claim and who fail to include ICD-9-CM codes as required will have their claim(s) returned for proper coding and may be subject to post-payment review by the Medicare intermediary, as well as payment denials.

2. For health care professionals who do not accept assignment, the penalties are more severe.

    A. If the original claim form does not include ICD-9-CM codes as required, and the health care professional refuses to provide the codes promptly on request to the Medicare intermediary, the professional may be subject to a civil monetary penalty in an amount not to exceed $2,000, per claim.

B. If the health care professional continuously fails to provide ICD-9-CM codes as requested, the professional may be subject to the sanction process described in section 1842 (j) (2) (A), that mandates that the professional may be barred from participation in the Medicare program for a period not to exceed five years.

CODING AND BILLING ISSUES

Diagnosis Codes Must Support Procedure Codes

Each service or procedure performed for a patient should be represented by a diagnosis that would substantiate those particular services or procedures as necessary in the investigation or treatment of their condition based on currently accepted standards of practice by the medical profession.

Place (Location) of Service

The actual setting that the services are rendered in for particular diagnoses plays an important part in reimbursement. Many people became accustomed to using emergency rooms for any type of illness or injury. By utilizing highly specialized places of service for conditions that were not true emergencies, third party payer were being billed with CPT codes indicating emergency services were rendered. Since the cost of services rendered on an emergency basis is considerably more expensive than those services in an non-emergency situation, third party payers began watching for those claims with diagnoses that did not indicate that a true emergency existed. Payment then was based on what the cost would have been had the patient been treated in the proper setting.

Level of Service Provided

The patient's condition and the treatment of that condition must be billed according to the criteria, as published by the AMA, for each level of service (i.e., minimal, brief, limited, intermediate, extended, comprehensive). Many practices bill the office visit level that they know will pay better rather than to consider the criteria that must be met to use a particular level of service. Again, the patient's diagnosis enters into this concept as well as it is often the diagnosis that indicates the complexity of the level of service to be used.

Frequency of Services

Many times claims are submitted for a patient with the same diagnosis and the same procedure(s) time after time. When the diagnosis indicates a chronic condition and the claims do not indicate any change in the patient's treatment or, give any indication that the patient's condition has been altered (i.e., exacerbated, other symptomology) the third party payer may deny payment based on the frequency of services for the reported condition.

Concurrent Care

Reimbursement problems often arise when a patient is being treated by different professionals, within the same billing entity (medical group or clinic), for different problems at the same time. This is known as concurrent care. For example, a patient may be hospitalized by a clinic's general surgeon for an operation and may also be seen while hospitalized by the group's cardiologist for an unrelated cardiac condition.

If you submit claims for daily hospital visits by both of the above professionals without explanation, most third-party payers will reject one daily visit as an apparent "duplication of service." The proper selection of ICD-9-CM diagnosis codes to justify multiple visits on the same date of service by physicians of different medical specialties should resolve the problem.

ICD-10

Since 1948, the World Health Organization has revised the *International Classification of Diseases* approximately every 10 years, with a modified version appearing in the United States about one to three years following the WHO publication. Based on the regular schedule, *ICD-10* should have been released in 1987. However, due to difficulties in coordinating the international committees, the first volume of *ICD-10*, the Tabular List, was not published until June of 1992.

Implementation of ICD-10 in the United States

Prior to being implemented in the United States, *ICD-10* must be converted to "American" English and pass through a variety of private and government committees, agencies, associations and organizations. As of this printing, the official position of the CMS is that *ICD-10* will not be mandated for Medicare claims for several years.

WHERE TO GET ANSWERS TO QUESTIONS ABOUT ICD-9-CM

Questions regarding the use and interpretation of the *International Classification of Diseases, 9th Revision, Clinical Modification* should be directed in writing to any of the organizations listed below.

Coding Advice/Central Office on ICD-9-CM
American Hospital Association
One North Franklin
Chicago, Illinois 60606
Vols. 1 and 2: kayala@aha.org

World Health Organization Collaborating Center
for Classification of Diseases in North America
National Center for Health Statistics
Department of Health and Human Services
6525 Belcrest Road
Hyattsville, Maryland 20782

Morbidity Classification Branch
National Center for Health Statistics
Department of Health and Human Services
6525 Belcrest Road, Room 1100
Hyattsville, Maryland 20782

Center for Medicare and Medicaid Services (CMS)
Division of Prospective Payment
Mail Stop C5-06-27
7500 Security Blvd.
Baltimore, MD 21244-1850
Vol. 3: pbrooks@cms.hhs.gov

Comments, questions or suggestions regarding the PMIC version of ICD-9-CM should be directed in writing to:

Managing Editor
Practice Management Information Corporation
4727 Wilshire Boulevard, Suite 300
Los Angeles, California 90010
http://www.pmiconline.com

ICD-9-CM Coding Fundamentals

Learning and following the basic steps of coding will increase your chances of better and faster reimbursement from third party payers, as well as establish meaningful profiles for future reimbursement rates. To become a proficient coder, two basic principles always must be considered.

First, it is imperative that you use both the Alphabetic Index (Volume 2) and the Tabular List (Volume 1) when locating and assigning codes. Coding only from the Alphabetic Index will cause you to miss any additional information provided only in the Tabular List, such as exclusions, instructions to use additional codes or the need for a fifth-digit.

Second, the level of specificity is important in all coding situations. A three-digit code that has subdivisions indicates you must use the appropriate subdivision code. Also, any time a fifth-digit subclassification is provided, you must use the fifth-digit code.

NINE STEPS FOR ACCURATE ICD-9-CM CODING

1. Locate the main term within the diagnostic statement.

2. Locate that main term in the Alphabetic Index (Volume 2). Keep in mind that the primary arrangement for main terms is by condition in the Alphabetic Index (Volume 2); main terms can be referred to in outmoded, ill-defined and lay terms as well as proper medical terms; main terms can be expressed in broad or specific terms, as nouns, adjectives or eponyms and can be with or without modifiers. Certain conditions may be listed under more than one main term.

3. Remember to refer to all notes under the main term. Be guided by the instructions in any notes appearing in a box immediately after the main term.

4. Examine any modifiers appearing in parentheses next to the main term. See if any of these modifiers apply to any of the qualifying terms used in the diagnostic statement.

5. Take note of the subterms indented beneath the main term. Subterms differ from main terms in that they provide greater specificity, becoming more specific the further they are indented to the right of the main term in 2-space increments; also, they provide the anatomical sites affected by the disease or injury.

6. Be sure to follow any cross reference instructions. These instructional terms ("see" or "see also") must be followed to locate the correct code.

7. Confirm the code selection in the Tabular List (Volume 1). Make certain you have selected the appropriate classification in accordance with the diagnosis.

8. Follow instructional terms in the Tabular List (Volume 1). Watch for exclusion terms, notes and fifth-digit instructions that apply to the code number you are verifying. It is necessary to search not only the selected code number for instructions but also the category, section and chapter in which the code number is collapsible. Many times the instructional information is located one or more pages preceding the actual page you find the code number on.

9. Finally, assign the code number you have determined to be correct.

ITALICIZED ENTRIES

During the process of designating a code to identify a principal diagnosis it is important to remember that italicized entries or codes in slanted brackets cannot be used. In these instances, it is required that the etiology code be sequenced first and the manifestation code be listed second even if the physician recorded them in the opposite order.

OTHER AND UNSPECIFIED CODES

Subcategories for diagnoses listed as "Other" and "Unspecified" are referred to as residual subcategories. Remember, the subdivisions are arranged in a hierarchy starting with the more specific and ending with the least specific. In the Tabular List (Volume 1), in most instances, the four-digit subcategory ".8" has been reserved for "Other" specified conditions not classifiable elsewhere and the four-digit subcategory ".9" has been reserved for "Unspecified" conditions. Following is an example demonstrating this principle.

005 Other food poisoning (bacterial)

Excludes: salmonella infections (003.0-003.9)
toxic effect of:
food contaminants (989.7)
noxious foodstuffs (988-0-988.9)

005.0 Staphylococcal food poisoning
Staphylococcal toxemia specified as due to food

005.1 Botulism food poisoning
Botulism NOS
Food poisoning due to Clostridium botulinum
Excludes: infant botulism 040.41
wound botulism 040.42

005.2 Food poisoning due to Clostridium perfringens [C. welchii]
Enteritis necroticans

005.3 Food poisoning due to other Clostridia

005.4 Food poisoning due to Vibrio parahaemolyticus

005.8 Other bacterial food poisoning
Excludes: salmonella food poisoning (003.0-003.9)

005.81 Food poisoning due to Vibrio vulnificus

005.89 Other bacterial food poisoning
Food poisoning due to Bacillus cereus

005.9 Food poisoning, unspecified

ICD-9-CM CODING FUNDAMENTALS

As you look at Category 005, note that codes 005.0-005.4 indicate that the food poisoning is related to specific types of organisms. Therefore, subcategories 005.0-005.4 are regarded as more specific than subcategory 005.9. Fifth-digit subclassification 005.89 *Other bacterial food poisoning* would include other specific types of bacterial food poisoning not classified elsewhere, as well as bacterial food poisoning NOS. Whereas subcategory 005.9 *Food poisoning unspecified* would be used for a diagnostic statement of "Food poisoning NOS" where the causative organism is not mentioned.

The hierarchy from more specific to less specific is not consistently maintained at the fifth-digit level. The level of specificity at the fifth-digit level is usually (not always) indicated by the use of 0 and 9. The digit 9 identifies the entry for "Other specified" while the digit 0 identifies the "Unspecified" entry. Below is an example.

279 Disorders involving the immune mechanism

    279.0 Deficiency of humoral immunity

        279.00 Hypogammaglobulinemia, unspecified
                Agammaglobulinemia NOS

        279.01 Selective IgA immunodeficiency

        279.02 Selective IgM immunodeficiency

        279.03 Other selective immunoglobulin deficiencies
                Selective deficiency of IgG

        279.04 Congenital hypogammaglobulinemia
                Agammaglobulinemia:
                    Bruton's type
                    X-linked

        279.05 Immunodeficiency with increased IgM
                Immunodeficiency with hyper-IgM:
                  autosomal recessive
                  X-linked

        279.06 Common variable immunodeficiency
                Dysgammaglobulinemia (acquired)
                  (congenital) (primary)
                Hypogammaglobulinemia:
                  acquired primary
                  congenital non-sex-linked
                  sporadic

        279.09 Other
                Transient hypogammaglobulinemia of infancy

Notice that the fifth-digit 0 identifies "Unspecified" and the fifth-digit 9 identifies "Other specified."

ACUTE AND CHRONIC CODING

Whenever a particular condition is described as both acute and chronic, code according to the subentries in the Alphabetic Index (Volume 2) for the stated condition. The following directions should be considered:

1. If there are separate subentries listed for acute, subacute and chronic, then use both codes, sequencing the code for the acute condition first.

2. If there are no subentries to identify acute, subacute or chronic, ignore these adjectives when selecting the code for the particular condition.

3. If a certain condition is described as a subacute condition and the index does not provide a subentry designating subacute, then code the condition as if it were acute.

CODING SUSPECTED CONDITIONS

Whenever the diagnosis is stated as "questionable," "probable," "likely," or "rule out," it is advisable to code documented symptoms or complaints by the patient. The reason for this is that you do not want an insurance carrier to include a disease code in the patient's history if in fact the "suspected" condition is never proven.

Keep in mind that there are no "rule out" codes per se in the ICD-9-CM coding system. If your diagnostic statement is "Rule out Breast Carcinoma" and you use code 174.9 *Malignant neoplasm of female breast, unspecified*, the code definition does not state "rule out." Therefore, the insurance carrier processes the code 174.9 as is, which results in the patient having an insurance history of breast cancer.

To avoid what could become a problem for you and your patient (including the potential of litigation), you should use codes for signs and symptoms in these cases. For example, use code 611.72 *Lump or mass in breast*, or 611.71 *Mastodynia (breast pain)* if these symptoms exist and this is the highest degree of certainty you can code to.

If the patient is asymptomatic but there is a family history of breast cancer then you should consider using a V-code, such as V16.3 *Family history of malignant neoplasm, breast* as your diagnosis code. There are also V-codes to indicate screening for a particular illness or disease. In the above example, code V76.1 *Special screening for malignant neoplasm, breast* could also have been used.

It is important to note that when you use a screening code from the V-code section you should also code signs or symptoms. The reason for doing so is because most health insurance carriers do not provide coverage for routine screening procedures or preventive medicine.

COMBINATION CODES

A combination code is used to fully identify an instance where two diagnoses or a diagnosis with an associated secondary process (manifestation) or complication is included in the description of a single code number. These combination codes are identified by referring to the subterms in the Alphabetic Index (Volume 2) and the inclusion and exclusion terms in the Tabular List (Volume 1).

Examples of commonly used combination codes include 034.0 *Streptococcal sore throat* and 404 *Hypertensive heart and chronic kidney disease.* Code 034.0 exists because the throat is often infected with Streptococcus and code 404 must be used whenever a patient has both heart and chronic kidney disease instead of assigning codes from categories 402 and 403.

Two main terms may be joined together by combination terms listed in the Alphabetic Index (Volume 2) as subterms such as:

associated with   *in*
complicated (by)   *secondary to*
due to   *with*
during   *without*
following

The listing for the above terms advises the coder to use one or two codes depending on the condition.

MULTIPLE CODING

There are single conditions that require more than one code. "Use additional code" notes are found in the Tabular List at codes that are not part of an etiology/manifestation pair where a secondary code is useful to fully describe a condition. The sequencing rule is the same: "use additional code" indicates that a secondary code should be added.

For example, for infections that are not included in Chapter 1, a secondary code from category 041, *Bacterial infection in conditions classified elsewhere and of unspecified site,* may be required to identify the bacterial organism causing the infection. A "use additional code" note will normally be found at the infection code and indicates a need for the organism code to be added as the secondary code.

There are also "code first" notes under certain codes that are not specifically manifestation codes but may be due to an underlying cause. When a "code first" note is present and an underlying condition is present, the underlying condition should be sequenced first.

"Code, if applicable, any causal condition first" notes indicate that this code may be assigned as a principal diagnosis when the causal condition is unknown or not applicable. If a causal condition is known, then the code for that condition should be sequenced as the principal or first-listed diagnosis.

Multiple codes may be needed for late effects, complication codes and obstetric codes to more fully describe a condition. See the specific guidelines for these sections for further instruction.

When is multiple coding mandatory? Only if the instructional term "code also" appears in italics under an italicized subdivision in the Tabular List (Volume 1). In this instance, you should interpret mandatory as: "requires the use of both codes, and these codes must be sequenced with the code for the etiology being listed first and the code identifying the manifestation listed second." You will recognize mandatory multiple coding situations by instructional terms used in the Tabular List (Volume 1). Terms to watch for are: "Code also....," "Use additional code...," and "Note:..."

If you turn to Category 330 in the Tabular List (Volume 1), you will notice the instructional term cited: "Use additional code, if desired, to identify associated mental retardation." The phrase "...identify associated mental retardation" should be interpreted as "...identify associated mental retardation, if stated to be present in the diagnostic statement." With this understood, these diagnostic statements would be coded as below.

Coding Examples

Cerebral degeneration in childhood with mental retardation

    330.9   **Unspecified cerebral degeneration in childhood**

    319   **Unspecified mental retardation**

Cerebral degeneration in childhood

    330.9   **Unspecified cerebral degeneration in childhood**

In the Alphabetic Index (Volume 2), if two codes are listed, the first should be sequenced first with the code in italicized brackets listed second to indicate the additional code. However, the fact that two codes appear after a subterm in the Alphabetic Index does not automatically indicate mandatory multiple coding. It is necessary to verify both code numbers in the Tabular List. If, in the Tabular List, the code number is also in italics as in the Alphabetical Index and, the instructional term "Code also" appears in italics, then both criteria have been met for mandatory multiple coding.

Coding Example

Diabetic neuropathy

    250.60   **Diabetes with neurological manifestations**

    357.2   **Polyneuropathy in diabetes**

In the Alphabetic Index (Volume 2) under "Diabetes," you will find "Neuropathy" listed followed by the codes 250.6 and *[357.2]* in brackets.

It should also be noted at this point, that even though mandatory multiple coding is always indicated by the presence of the instructional term "Code first" in italics beneath the italicized code number and title for the manifestation, this does not always hold true under the code number for the etiology. Multiple coding is not to be used in those instances when a combination code accurately identifies all of the elements within the diagnostic statement.

CODING LATE EFFECTS

A late effect is the residual effect (condition produced) after the acute phase of an illness or injury has terminated. There is no time limit on when a late effect code can be used. The residual may be apparent early, such as in cerebrovascular accident cases, or it may occur months or years later, such as that due to a previous injury. Coding of late effects generally requires two codes sequenced in the following order: The condition or nature of the late effect first; the late effect code second.

An exception to the above guideline is when the code for late effect is followed by a manifestation code identified in the Tabular List and title, or when the late effect code has been expanded (at the fourth and fifth-digit levels) to include the manifestation(s). The code for the acute phase of an illness or injury that led to the late effect is never used with a code for the late effect.

Coding Example

Hemiplegia due to previous cerebral vascular accident

    342.90   **Hemiplegia, unspecified, affecting unspecified side**

    438.20   **Late effects of cerebrovascular disease, Hemiplegia affecting unspecified side**

The *residual* for this statement is "Hemiplegia" as it is the long term condition that resulted from a previous acute illness. The *cause* for this statement is "Cerebral vascular accident" as it is the original illness no longer in its acute phase but which did cause the long term residual condition now present.

How do you recognize when to use late effects coding and when not to? Often, the diagnostic statement will contain key words to help identify a late effects situation. Key words used in defining late effects include:

> *late*
> *due to an old injury*
> *due to a previous illness/injury*
> *due to an illness/injury occurring one year or more ago*

In cases where these key words (phrases) are not included within the diagnostic statement, an effect is considered to be late if sufficient time has elapsed between the occurrence of the acute illness/injury and the development of the residual effect.

Coding Example

Excessive scar tissue due to third degree burn, right leg

    709.2   **Scar conditions and fibrosis of skin**

    906.7   **Late effect of burn of other extremities**

The previous diagnostic statement does not indicate the time element with any modifying terms as "old" or "previous." The fact that enough time has elapsed for the development of scar tissue indicates that the acute phase of the injury has subsided and the scarring should be coded as a late effect.

If a diagnostic statement only specifies the cause of the late effect and does not indicate the residual, then use the code number for the cause.

Coding Example

Residuals of tuberculosis

    137.0   **Late effects of respiratory or unspecified tuberculosis**

The above statement does not identify the actual residuals, so you would use the code for the cause.

To find the code for such a statement in the Alphabetic Index (Volume 2), refer to the main term "LATE" and the subterm "EFFECTS OF." The only codes available for causes of late effects are:

137	Late effects of tuberculosis
138	Late effects of acute poliomyelitis
139	Late effects of other infectious and parasitic diseases
268.1	Rickets, late effect
326	Late effects of intracranial abscess or pyogenic infection
438	Late effects of cerebrovascular disease
677	Late effect of complication of pregnancy, childbirth and the puerperium
905	Late effects of musculoskeletal and connective tissue injuries
906	Late effects of injuries to skin and subcutaneous tissues
907	Late effects of injuries to the nervous system
908	Late effects of other and unspecified injuries
909	Late effects of other and unspecified external causes

Be sure to distinguish between a late effect and a historical statement in a diagnosis. Whenever the statement uses the terms "effects of old...," "sequela of...," or "residuals of...," then code as late effects. If the diagnosis is expressed in terms as "history of...," these are coded to personal history of the illness or injury and are coded to the V-Codes (V-10 to V-15).

CODING IMPENDING OR THREATENED CONDITIONS

Code any condition described at the time of discharge as impending or threatened as follows:

1. If it did occur, code as confirmed diagnosis.

2. If it did not occur, reference the Alphabetic Index to determine if the condition has a subentry term for impending or threatened and also reference main term entries for Impending and for Threatened.

3. If the subterms are listed, assign the given code.

4. If the subterms are not listed, code the existing underlying condition(s) and not the condition described as impending or threatened.

CODING INJURIES

Injuries comprise a major section of ICD-9-CM. Categories 800-959 include fractures, dislocations, sprains and various other types of injuries. Injuries are classified first according to the general type of injury and within each type there is a further breakdown by anatomical site.

When coding injuries, assign separate codes for each injury unless a combination code is provided, in which case the combination code is assigned. Multiple injury codes are provided in ICD-9-CM, but should not be assigned unless information for a more specific code is not available. These codes are not to be used for normal, healing surgical wounds or to identify complications of surgical wounds.

The code for the most serious injury, as determined by the physician, is sequenced first.

1. Superficial injuries such as abrasions or contusions are not coded when associated with more severe injuries of the same site.

2. When a primary injury results in minor damage to peripheral nerves or blood vessels, the primary injury is sequenced first with additional code(s) from categories 950-957, *Injury to nerves and spinal cord*, and/ or 900-904, *Injury to blood vessels*. When the primary injury is to the blood vessels or nerves, that injury should be sequenced first.

In cases where a patient has multiple injuries, the most severe injury is the principal diagnosis. Where multiple sites of injury are specified in the diagnosis, you should interpret the term "with" as indicating involvement of both sites, and interpret the term "and" as indicating involvement of either or both sites. You will also note that fifth-digits are commonly used when coding injuries to provide information regarding level of consciousness, specific anatomical sites and severity of injuries.

Coding Traumatic Fractures

The principles of multiple coding of injuries should be followed in coding fractures. Fractures of specified sites are coded individually by site in accordance with both the provisions within categories 800-829 and the level of detail furnished by medical record content. Combination categories for multiple fractures are provided for use when there is insufficient detail in the medical record (such as trauma cases transferred to another hospital), when the reporting form limits the number of codes that can be used in reporting pertinent clinical data, or when there is insufficient specificity at the fourth-digit or fifth-digit level. More specific guidelines are as follows:

1. Multiple fractures of same limb classifiable to the same three-digit or four-digit category are coded to that category.

2. Multiple unilateral or bilateral fractures of same bone(s) but classified to different fourth-digit subdivisions (bone part) within the same three-digit category are coded individually by site.

3. Multiple fracture categories 819 and 828 classify bilateral fractures of both upper limbs (819) and both lower limbs (828), but without any detail at the fourth-digit level other than open and closed type of fractures.

4. Multiple fractures are sequenced in accordance with the severity of the fracture and the physician should be asked to list the fracture diagnoses in the order of severity.

Some general rules to apply when coding fractures follow. Fractures can either be "open" or "closed." An "open" fracture is when the skin has been broken and there is communication with the bone and the outside of the body. Whereas, with a "closed" fracture the bone does not have contact with the outside of the body.

Note the following descriptions as set forth in the ICD-9-CM at the four-digit subdivision level to help distinguish between an "open" and "closed" fracture.

Closed Fractures

comminuted *simple*
linear *greenstick*
fissured *depressed*
spiral *march*
impacted *fractured NOS*
elevated *slipped epiphysis*

Open Fractures

compound *with foreign body*
missile *infected*
puncture

Anytime that it is not indicated whether a fracture is open or closed, code it as if it were closed. Fracture-dislocations are classified as fractures. Pathological fractures are classified to the condition causing the fracture (i.e. osteoporosis) with the use of an additional code to identify the *Pathologic fracture* (733.1).

Coding Burns

Current burns (940-949) are classified by depth, extent and by agent (E code). Burns are classified by depth as first degree (erythema), second degree (blistering), and third degree (full-thickness involvement).

1. Sequence first the code that reflects the highest degree of burn when more than one burn is present.

    A. When the reason for the admission or encounter is for treatment of external multiple burns, sequence first the code that reflects the burn of the highest degree.

    B. When a patient has both internal and external burns, the circumstances of admission govern the selection of the principal diagnosis or first-listed diagnosis.

    C. When a patient is admitted for burn injuries and other related conditions such as smoke inhalation and/or respiratory failure, the circumstances of admission govern the selection of the principal or first-listed diagnosis.

2. Classify burns of the same local site (three-digit category level, 940-947) but of different degrees to the subcategory identifying the highest degree recorded in the diagnosis.

ICD-9-CM CODING FUNDAMENTALS

3. Non-healing burns are coded as acute burns. Necrosis of burned skin should be coded as a non-healed burn.

4. Assign code 958.3, *Posttraumatic wound infection, not elsewhere classified*, as an additional code for any documented infected burn site.

5. When coding burns, assign separate codes for each burn site. Category 946 *Burns of Multiple specified sites,* should only be used if the location of the burns are not documented. Category 949, *Burn, unspecified*, is extremely vague and should rarely be used.

6. Assign codes from category 948, *Burns classified according to extent of body surface involved*, when the site of the burn is not specified or when there is a need for additional data. It is advisable to use category 948 as additional coding when needed to provide data for evaluating burn mortality, such as that needed by burn units. It is also advisable to use category 948 as an additional code for reporting purposes when there is mention of a third-degree burn involving 20 percent or more of the body surface.

   In assigning a code from category 948:

   A. Fourth-digit codes are used to identify the percentage of total body surface involved in a burn (all degree).

   B. Fifth-digits are assigned to identify the percentage of body surface involved in third-degree burn.

   C. Fifth-digit zero (0) is assigned when less than 10 percent or when no body surface is involved in a third-degree burn.

   Category 948 is based on the classic rule of nines in estimating body surface involved: head and neck are assigned nine percent, each arm nine percent, each leg 18 percent, the anterior trunk 18 percent, posterior trunk 18 percent, and genitalia one percent. Physicians may change these percentage assignments where necessary to accommodate infants and children who have proportionately larger heads than adults and patients who have large buttocks, thighs, or abdomen that involve burns.

7. Encounters for the treatment of the late effects of burns (i.e., scars or joint contractures) should be coded to the residual condition (sequelae) followed by the appropriate late effect code (906.5-906.9). A late effect E code may also be used, if desired.

8. When appropriate, both a sequelae with a late effect code, and a current burn code may be assigned on the same record.

9. Excisional debridement involves an excisional debridement (surgical removal or cutting away), as opposed to a mechanical (brushing, scrubbing, washing) debridement. For coding purposes, excisional debridement is assigned to code 86.22.

   Nonexcisional debridement is assigned to code 86.28.

Remember when coding burns, code only the most severe degree of burns when the burns are of the same site but of different degrees. In cases of burns where it is noted that there is an infection, assign the code for the burn and also the code for the infection (958.3 *Posttraumatic wound infection NEC*).

POISONING AND ADVERSE EFFECTS OF DRUGS

There are two different sets of code numbers to use to differentiate between poisoning and adverse reactions to the correct substances properly administered. First, you must make the distinction between poisoning and adverse reaction. Poisoning by drugs includes:

Poisoning

Accidental

1. Given in error during diagnostic or therapeutic procedures.

2. Given in error by one person to another (for example, mother to child).

3. Taken in error by self.

Purposeful

1. Suicide attempt.

2. Homicide attempt.

Adverse Reaction in Spite of Proper Administration of Correct Substance

1. In therapeutic of diagnostic procedure.

2. Taken by self or given to another as prescribed.

3. Accumulative effect (intoxication due to....).

4. Interaction of prescribed drugs.

5. Synergistic reaction (enhancing the effect of another drug).

6. Allergic reaction.

7. Hypersensitivity.

To code poisoning by drugs, use the Alphabetic Index (Volume 2) which contains the Table of Drugs and Chemicals. This table includes one column to identify the poisoning code (960-989) and four columns of External Cause Codes to classify whether the poisoning was an accident, suicide, assault or undetermined.

The column labeled "Therapeutic Use" is not used for poisonings but in coding adverse reactions to correct substances properly administered. The External Cause Codes are optional but may be used if a facility's coding policy requires their use.

Note that in the Alphabetic Index (Volume 2) that the subterm entry "Drug" under the main term of "Poisoning" refers the coder to the Table of Drugs and Chemicals for the code assignment. Because the Table of Drugs and Chemicals is so extensive, it is acceptable to code directly from the Table without verifying the code obtained in Volume 1.

What if the drug which caused the poisoning is not listed in the Table of Drugs and Chemicals?

1. Refer to Appendix C in Volume 1 (American Hospital Formulary Service) and locate the name of the drug.

2. Note the AHFS category number listed.

3. Turn to the Table of Drugs and Chemicals in the Alphabetic Index (Volume 2) of ICD-9-CM.

4. Locate the term "Drug."

5. Refer to the subterm "AHFS List."

6. Look through the list until you find the AHFS Category Number determined in step 2 above. The AHFS Category Numbers are listed in numeric order.

7. Assign the code.

How Do You Identify Poisoning by Drugs?

The statement of diagnosis will usually have descriptive terms that would indicate poisoning. Look for terms such as:

Intoxication   *Toxic effect*
Overdose   *Wrong drug given/taken in error*
Poisoning   *Wrong dosage given/taken in error*

Adverse effects of a medicine taken in combination with alcohol or from taking a prescribed drug in combination with a drug the patient took on his/her own initiative (for example antihistamines) are coded as poisonings. If you wish to code a manifestation of the poisoning as well, this code is always listed second, after listing the code identifying the poison first.

Adverse Effects of Drugs

The World Health Organization (WHO) defines adverse drug reaction as any response to a drug "which is noxious and unintended and which occurs at doses used in man for prophylaxis, diagnosis or therapy." Notice that this definition does not include the terms "overdose" or "poisoning."

Why does ICD-9-CM differentiate between poisoning and adverse drug reaction? Tabulation of statistical data indicates how often a drug reaction occurred because of the drug itself versus how often the drug was either not given or taken properly. Two codes are required when coding adverse drug reactions to the correct substance properly administered. One code is used to identify the manifestation or the nature of the adverse reaction such as urticaria, vertigo, gastritis, etc. This code is assigned from Categories 001-799 in Volume 1.

Refer to the main term identifying the manifestation in the Alphabetic Index (Volume 2). But remember that the Table of Drugs and Chemicals is not used to locate the code for the manifestation, and the code used to identify the manifestation does not identify the drug responsible for the adverse reaction.

A second code is required to identify the drug causing the adverse reaction. In ICD-9-CM, the only codes provided to identify the drug causing an adverse reaction to a substance properly administered are E930 through E949. Anytime a code is selected from the E930-E949 range, it can never be sequenced first or be a solo code.

When the drug was correctly prescribed and properly administered, code the reaction plus the appropriate code from the E930-E949 series. Codes from the E930-E949 series must be used to identify the causative substance for an adverse effect of drug, medicinal and biological substances, correctly prescribed and properly administered. The effect, such as tachycardia, delirium, gastrointestinal hemorrhaging, vomiting, hypokalemia, hepatitis, renal failure, or respiratory failure, is coded and followed by the appropriate code from the E930-E949 series.

Adverse effects of therapeutic substances correctly prescribed and properly administered (toxicity, synergistic reaction, side effect, and idiosyncratic reaction) may be due to (1) differences among patients, such as age, sex, disease, and genetic factors, and (2) drug-related factors, such as type of drug, route of administration, duration of therapy, dosage, and bioavailability.

Poisoning

1. Errors made in drug prescription or in the administration of the drug by provider, nurse, patient, or other person, use the appropriate poisoning code from the 960-979 series.

2. If an overdose of a drug was intentionally taken or administered and resulted in drug toxicity, it would be coded as a poisoning (960-979 series).

3. If a nonprescribed drug or medicinal agent was taken in combination with a correctly prescribed and properly administered drug, any drug toxicity or other reaction resulting from the interaction of the two drugs would be classified as a poisoning.

4. When coding a poisoning or reaction to the improper use of a medication (e.g., wrong dose, wrong substance, wrong route of administration), the poisoning code is sequenced first, followed by a code for the manifestation. If there is also a diagnosis of drug abuse or dependence to the substance, the abuse or dependence is coded as an additional code.

Toxic Effects

1. When a harmful substance is ingested or comes in contact with a person, this is classified as a toxic effect. The toxic effect codes are in categories 980-989.

2. A toxic effect code should be sequenced first, followed by the code(s) that identify the result of the toxic effect.

3. An external cause code from categories E860-E869 for accidental exposure, codes E950.6 or E950.7 for intentional self-harm, category E962 for assault, or categories E980-E982 (undetermined), should also be assigned to indicate intent.

Locating the Proper E Code

How do you locate the proper E code to identify the drug which was responsible for causing an adverse reaction to a correct substance properly administered? Turn to the Table of Drugs and Chemicals in the Alphabetic Index (Volume 2). Earlier we noted that the column labeled "Therapeutic Use" was not used for coding instances involving poisoning. However, for adverse drug reactions to a correct substance properly administered, the "Therapeutic Use" column is used to find the proper code within the range E930 through E949 to identify the drug.

Drug Interactions Between Two or More Drugs

Drug interactions between two or more prescribed drugs are classified as adverse drug reactions to a correct substance properly administered. This holds true regardless of whether the drugs were prescribed by the same physician or different physicians.

Two types of drug interactions should be noted:

1. Synergistic interaction. One drug enhances the action of another drug so that the combined effect is greater than the sum of the effects of each used alone.

2. Antagonistic interaction. One drug represses the action of another drug.

To properly code drug interactions, first code the manifestation. Then code each drug involved in the interaction using the E codes from the column labeled "Therapeutic Use" from the Table of Drugs and Chemicals.

Coding Example

Gastritis due to interaction between Motrin and Procainamide

535.50   Unspecified gastritis and gastroduodenitis

List the manifestation first

E935.8   Other specified analgesics and antipyretics

E942.0   Cardiac rhythm regulators

Coding Example

When a diagnostic statement does not state specifically the manifestation or nature of the adverse reaction, you should use the code provided to identify an adverse drug reaction of unspecified nature, 995.2 *Unspecified adverse effect of drug, medicinal and biological substance.* For example:

Allergic reaction to Motrin, proper dose

995.2   Unspecified adverse effect of drug, medicinal and biological substance

E935.8   Other specified analgesics and antipyretics

Note in the above example that the code indicating the manifestation, although unspecified as to the nature, is listed first followed by the E code to identify the drug. When the drug causing an adverse effect is unknown or unspecified, use code E947.9 *Unspecified drug or medicinal substance.*

It is very important to remember that codes in the range 960 through 979 are never used in combination with codes in the range E930 through E949 because codes in the range 960-979 identify poisonings and codes in the range E930-E949 identify the external cause of adverse reactions to the correct substance properly administered.

CODING COMPLICATIONS OF MEDICAL AND SURGICAL CARE

A complication is when you have the occurrence of two or more diseases in the same patient. Recent studies have revealed serious deficiencies in properly coding complications for insurance claims processing. Often the complication is never mentioned. Complications are responsible for many of the procedures that are ordered for patients, therefore the complication should be coded and submitted on your insurance claims.

Postoperative complications that affect a specific anatomical site or body system are classified to the appropriate Chapter 1 through 16 of the Tabular Index (Volume 1). Postoperative complications affecting more than one anatomical site or body system are classified in the chapter on injury and poisoning (Chapter 17, Categories 996-999). If the Alphabetic Index (Volume 2) does not provide a specific main term and subterm to identify a postoperative complication, classify the complication to categories 996-999.

Coding Example

Postcholecystectomy syndrome

    576.0   Postcholecystectomy syndrome

The Alphabetic Index (Volume 2) specifically classifies the postoperative condition to one of the categories from 001 through 799. See main term "Complication," subterms "surgical procedure" and "postcholecystectomy syndrome."

Coding Examples

Postoperative wound infection

    998.59   Postoperative infection

The Alphabetic Index (Volume 2) has a main term "Infection" and subterms "wound, postoperative" for this condition. Note that this code appears in Chapter 17 within categories 996-999.

Postoperative atelectasis

    997.3   Respiratory complications

Refer to the main term "Atelectasis" in the Alphabetic Index (Volume 2). Note there is no subterm for postoperative beneath this main term. Therefore, you must presume this complication is classified to one of the categories in the range 969-999. You may also code 518.0 *Pulmonary collapse*, to identify the nature of the respiratory complication for statistical purposes; however, the code for the complication must be listed first.

Complications From Mechanical Devices

Subcategories in the range 996.0 through 996.5 are used to identify mechanical complications of devices. Mechanical complications are the result of a malfunction on the part of the internal prosthetic implant or device. What indicates a mechanical complication? Breakdown or obstruction, displacement, leakage, perforation or protrusion of the devices are all forms of mechanical complications.

Coding Example

Displacement of cardiac pacemaker electrode

> 996.01 Mechanical complication of cardiac device, implant, and graft due to cardiac pacemaker (electrode)

Other complications of devices, such as infection or hemorrhage, are due to an abnormal reaction of the body to an otherwise properly functioning device. All complications involving infection are coded to category 996.7 *Other complications of internal prosthetic device, implant and graft.*

Coding Examples

Infected arteriovenous shunt

> 996.62 Infection and inflammatory reaction due to internal prosthetic device, implant, and graft

Anterior chamber hemorrhage due to displaced prosthetic lens

> 996.72 Other complications of internal (biological) (synthetic) prosthetic device, implant, and graft

Cardiac Complications

In the case of cardiac complications, ICD-9-CM defines the "immediate postoperative period" as "the period between surgery and the time of discharge from the hospital." This definition is the basis of whether to code cardiac complications under subcategory 997.1 *Cardiac complications affecting specified body systems, not elsewhere classified*, or under subcategory 429.4 *Functional disturbances following cardiac surgery.*

Use 997.1 for a cardiac complication that occurs anytime between surgery and hospital discharge from any type of procedure performed. Use subcategory 429.4 to code long-term cardiac complications resulting from cardiac surgery.

It is important to distinguish between complications and aftercare. Aftercare is usually an encounter for something planned in advance (example, removal of Kirshner wire). Aftercare is classified using codes in the range of V51-V58. An encounter for a complication occurs from unforeseen circumstances, such as wound infection, resulting in complication of the patient's condition.

Transplant Complications

1. **Transplant complications other than kidney:** Codes under subcategory 996.8, *Complications of transplanted organ,* are for use for both complications and rejection of transplanted organs. A transplant complication code is only assigned if the complication affects the function of the transplanted organ. Two codes are required to fully describe a transplant complication, the appropriate code from subcategory 996.8 and a secondary code that identifies the complication.

   Pre-existing conditions or conditions that develop after the transplant are not coded as complications unless they affect the function of the transplanted organs.

   Post-transplants surgical complications that do not relate to the function of the transplanted organ are classified to the specific complication. For example, a surgical wound dehiscence would be coded to the wound dehiscence, not as a transplant complication.

   Post-transplant patients who are seen for treatment unrelated to the transplanted organ should be assigned a code from category V42, *Organ or tissue replaced by transplant*, to identify the transplant status of the patient. A code from category V42 should never be used with a code from subcategory 996.8.

2. **Kidney transplant complication:** Code 996.81, *Complications of tranplanted organs, kidney,* should be assigned for documented complications such as transplant failure or rejection. It should not be assigned for post kidney transplant patients who have chronic kidney disease (CKD) unless a transplant complication is documented in the medical record.

SPECIAL CODING SITUATIONS

As you become an experienced coder you will encounter situations where the standard rules do not seem to apply, or which require a special understanding in order to code properly. These situations include coding of circulatory diseases, diabetes, mental disorders, infectious diseases, manifestations, neoplasms, and pregnancy and childbirth. The following sections address these specific special coding situations.

CODING DISEASES OF BLOOD AND BLOOD FORMING ORGANS

Subcategory 285.2, *Anemia in chronic illness,* has codes for anemia in chronic kidney disease, code 285.21; anemia in neoplastic disease, code 285.22; and anemia in other chronic illness, code 285.29. These codes can be used as the principal/first listed code if the reason for the encounter is to treat the anemia. They may also be used as secondary codes if treatment of the anemia is a component of an encounter, but not the primary reason for the encounter. When using a code from subcategory 285, it is also necessary to use the code for the chronic condition causing the anemia.

1. When assigning code 285.21, *Anemia in chronic kidney disease,* it is also necessary to assign a code from category 585, *Chronic kidney disease*, to indicate the stage of chronic kidney disease.

2. When assigning code 285.22, *Anemia in neoplastic disease*, it is also necessary to assign the neoplasm code that is responsible for the anemia. Code 285.22 is for use for anemia that is due to the malignancy, not for anemia due to antineoplastic chemotherapy drugs, which is an adverse effect.

CODING CIRCULATORY DISEASES

Because of the variety of terms and phrases used by physicians to identify diseases of the circulatory system, you will often experience difficulty in coding. To accurately code disorders of the circulatory system, it is imperative that the coder carefully read all inclusion, exclusion and "use additional code" notations contained in the Tabular List (Volume 1).

Fifth digit subclassifications are also frequently used to code combination disorders or to provide further specificity in this section. Even those in specialties other than cardiology will frequently find themselves coding circulatory system diagnoses due to the prevalence of circulatory disorders in this country.

Chapter 7 of the Tabular List (Volume 1), titled Diseases of the Circulatory System, contains the following major sections:

Acute Rheumatic Fever (390-392)

Chronic Rheumatic Heart Disease (393-398)

Hypertensive Disease (401-405)

Ischemic Heart Disease (410-414)

Diseases of Pulmonary Circulation (415-417)

Other Forms of Heart Disease (420-429)

Cerebrovascular Disease (430-438)

Diseases of Arteries, Arterioles, and Capillaries (440-449)

Diseases of Veins, Lymphatics, and Other Diseases of the Circulatory System (451-459)

Diseases of Mitral and Aortic Valves

Certain diseases of the mitral valve of unspecified etiology are presumed to be of rheumatic origin and others are not. None of the disorders of the aortic valve of unspecified etiology are presumed to be of rheumatic origin. When you have disorders involving both the mitral and aortic valves of unspecified etiology, then they are presumed to be of rheumatic origin.

Coding Examples

Mitral valve insufficiency

    424.0   Mitral valve disorders

Refer to the main term "Insufficiency" in the Alphabetic Index (Volume 2). Note the subterm "mitral (valve)."

Mitral valve stenosis

    394.0   Mitral stenosis

Refer to the main term "Stenosis" and the sub-term "mitral (valve)" in the Alphabetic Index (Volume 2).

Aortic valve insufficiency

    424.1   Aortic valve disorders

Aortic valve stenosis

    424.1   Aortic valve disorders

Look up the main term "Stenosis" and the subterm "aortic" in the Alphabetic Index (Volume 2). Remember that aortic valve disorders of unspecified etiology are not considered rheumatic in nature or origin.

Insufficiency of mitral and aortic valves

    396.3   Mitral valve insufficiency and aortic valve insufficiency

Under the main term "Insufficiency" in the Alphabetic Index (Volume 2) you will find the subterm "aortic." Further review will locate "with," "mitral valve disease," "insufficiency, incompetence or regurgitation" which directs you to code 396.3.

Ischemic Heart Disease

In ischemic heart disease, the manifestations are due to a lack of blood flow to the heart rather than to the anatomical lesion of the coronary arteries. The most common cause of coronary heart disease is coronary atherosclerosis. However, ischemic heart disease can be due to non-coronary disease, such as aortic valvular stenosis, as well. There are many synonyms used to indicate ischemic heart disease such as: coronary artery heart disease, ASHD, and coronary ischemia. Categories in the range 410-414, Ischemic Heart Disease, includes that with mention of hypertension. Use an additional code to identify the presence of hypertension.

Coding Examples

Angina pectoris

    413.9   Other and unspecified angina pectoris

As no mention of hypertension is made in the diagnostic statement, a single code is all that is required.

Angina pectoris with essential hypertension

    413.9   Other and unspecified angina pectoris

    401.9   Essential hypertension, unspecified

In this example, the mention of hypertension in the diagnostic statement requires the use of a second code.

Myocardial Infarction

A myocardial infarction is classified as acute if it is either specified as "acute" in the diagnostic statement or with a stated duration of eight weeks or less. When a myocardial infarction is specified as "chronic" or with symptoms after eight weeks from the date of the onset, it should be coded to subcategory 414.8 *Other specified forms of chronic ischemic heart disease.* If a myocardial infarction is specified as old or healed or has been diagnosed by special investigation (EKG) but is currently not presenting any symptoms, code using category 412 *Old myocardial infarction.*

1. The ICD-9-CM codes for acute myocardial infarction (AMI) identify the site, such as anterolateral wall or true posterior wall. Subcategories 410.0-410.6 and 410.8 are used for ST elevation myocardial infarction (STEMI). Subcategory 410.7, *Subendocardial infarction,* is used for non-ST elevation myocardial infarction (NSTEMI) and nontransmural MIs.

2. Subcategory 410.9 is the default for the unspecified term acute myocardial infarction. If only STEMI or transmural MI without the site is documented, query the provider as to the site, or assign a code from subcategory 410.9.

3. If an AMI is documented as nontransmural or subendocardial, but the site is provided, it is still coded as a subendocardial AMI. If NSTEMI evolves to STEMI, assign the STEMI code. If STEMI converts to NSTEMI due to thrombolytic therapy, it is still coded as STEMI.

Coding Examples

Myocardial infarction three weeks ago

    410.92   Acute myocardial infarction, unspecified site

Chronic myocardial infarction with angina

    414.8   Other specified forms of chronic ischemic heart disease

    413.9   Other and unspecified angina pectoris

Myocardial infarction diagnoses by EKG, symptomatic

    412   Old myocardial infarction

Arteriosclerotic Cardiovascular Disease (ASCVD)

Arteriosclerotic cardiovascular disease (ASCVD) is classified to subcategory 429.2 *Cardiovascular disease, unspecified.* You should use an additional code to identify the presence of arteriosclerosis when coding ASCVD. For example, the diagnostic statement "generalized arteriosclerotic cardiovascular disease" should be coded using 429.2 followed by 440.9 *Generalized and unspecified atherosclerosis.*

"Other forms of heart disease," categories 420-429, are used for multiple coding purposes to fully identify a stated diagnosis. The exception to this rule is if the Alphabetic Index (Volume 2) or Tabular List (Volume 1) specifically instructs you otherwise.

Coding Examples

Arteriosclerotic heart disease with acute pulmonary edema

    428.1   **Left heart failure**

    414.00   **Coronary atherosclerosis, of unspecified type of vessel, native or graft**

Note that the code for ASHD (414.00) is listed second as a possible underlying cause of the acute situation.

Arteriosclerotic heart disease with congestive heart failure

    428.0   **Congestive heart failure, unspecified**

    414.00   **Coronary atherosclerosis, of unspecified type of vessel, native or graft**

Cerebrovascular Disease

When coding cerebrovascular disease (codes 430-438), you should code the component parts of the diagnostic statement identifying the cerebrovascular disease, unless specifically instructed to do otherwise in the Alphabetic Index (Volume 2) or Tabular List (Volume 1).

Coding Examples

Cerebrovascular arteriosclerosis with subarachnoid hemorrhage

    430   **Subarachnoid hemorrhage**

    437.0   **Cerebral atherosclerosis**

Cerebrovascular accident secondary to thrombosis

    434.00   **Cerebral thrombosis, without mention of cerebral infarction**

In this example, you use only one code because of the instructions in the Alphabetic Index (Volume 2). When you look up the main term "Accident" with subterm "cerebrovascular," you are instructed to "(see also Disease, cerebrovascular, acute) 436." When you locate the main term "Disease" and subterms "cerebrovascular," "acute" and "thrombotic," you are further instructed to "see Thrombosis, brain." This is where you finally locate the single code for this diagnosis, 434.0. When you look up the code in the Tabular List (Volume 1), you are instructed to add a fifth digit "0" if it is without mention of cerebral infarction, and "1" if it is with cerebral infarction.

Whenever there are conditions resulting from the acute cerebrovascular disease, code them if they are stated to be residual(s). If the resulting condition is stated to be transient, do not code them.

Coding Examples

Cerebrovascular accident with residual aphasia

    434.91   **Cerebral artery occlusion, unspecified, with cerebral infarction**

    784.3   **Aphasia**

Cerebrovascular accident with transient hemiparesis

    434.91   **Cerebral artery occlusion, unspecified, with cerebral infarction**

Cerebral Infarction/Stroke/Cerebrovascular Accident (CVA)

The terms stroke and CVA are often used interchangeably to refer to a cerebral infarction. The terms stroke, CVA, and cerebral infarction NOS are all indexed to the default code 434.91, *Cerebral artery occlusion, unspecified, with infarction*. Code 436, *Acute, but ill-defined, cerebrovascular disease*, should not be used when the documentation states stroke or CVA.

A cerebrovascular hemorrhage or infarction that occurs as a result of medical intervention is coded to 997.02, *Iatrogenic cerebrovascular infarction or hemorrhage*. Medical record documentation should clearly specify the cause-and-effect relationship between the medical intervention and the cerebrovascular accident in order to assign this code. A secondary code from the code range 430-432 or from a code from subcategories 433 or 434 with a fifth digit of "1" should also be used to identify the type of hemorrhage or infarct.

This guideline conforms to the use additional code note instruction at category 997. Code 436, *Acute, but ill-defined, cerebrovascular disease*, should not be used as a secondary code with code 997.02.

Late Effects of Cerebrovascular Disease

Category 438 is used to indicate conditions classifiable to categories 430-437 as the causes of late effects (neurologic deficits), themselves classified elsewhere. These late effects include neurologic deficits that persist after initial onset of conditions classifiable to 430-437. The neurologic deficits caused by cerebrovascular disease may be present from the onset or may arise at any time after the onset of the condition classifiable to 430-437.

Codes from category 438 may be assigned on a health care record with codes from 430-437, if the patient has a current cerebrovascular accident (CVA) and deficits from an old CVA. Assign code V12.59 (and not a code from category 438) as an additional code for history of cerebrovascular disease when no neurologic deficits are present.

Hypertensive Disease

As demonstrated earlier with ischemic heart disease, conditions that are classified to cerebrovascular disease (codes 430-438) include that with mention of hypertension, but you must identify the hypertension with another code (401-405) and list it second.

ICD-9-CM CODING FUNDAMENTALS

Hypertension is frequently the cause of various forms of heart and vascular disease. However, the mention of hypertension with some heart conditions should not be interpreted as a combination resulting in hypertensive heart disease. The combination is only to be made if there is a cause-and-effect relationship between hypertension and a heart condition classified to subcategories 425.8, 428.0-428.9, 429.0-429.3 and 429.8-429.9.

Hypertensive disease is classified to the categories 401-405. The Table of Hypertension is located in the Alphabetic Index (Volume 2) under the main term "Hypertension." This Table contains subterms to identify types of hypertension and complications. It contains a complete listing of all conditions due to or associated with hypertension and classifies them according to malignant, benign, and unspecified.

1. Hypertension, Essential or NOS

    Assign hypertension (arterial) (essential) (primary) (systemic) (NOS) to category code 401 with the appropriate fourth digit to indicate malignant (.0), benign (.1), or unspecified (.9). Do not use either .0 malignant or .1 benign unless medical record documentation supports such a designation.

2. Hypertension with Heart Disease

    Heart conditions (425.8, 429.0-429.3, 429.8, 429.9) are assigned to a code from category 402 when a causal relationship is stated (due to hypertension) or implied (hypertensive). Use an additional code from category 428 to identify the type of heart failure in those patients with heart failure. More than one code from category 428 may be assigned if the patient has systolic or diastolic failure and congestive heart failure.

    The same heart conditions (425.8, 429.0-429.3, 429.8, 429.9) with hypertension, but without a stated causal relationship, are coded separately. Sequence according to the circumstances of the admission/encounter.

3. Hypertensive Kidney Disease

    Assign codes from category 403, *Hypertensive chronic kidney disease*, when conditions classified to categories 585-587 are present. Unlike hypertension with heart disease, ICD-9-CM presumes a cause-and-effect relationship and classifies renal failure with hypertension as hypertensive kidney disease.

4. Hypertensive Heart and Kidney Disease

    Assign codes from combination category 404, *Hypertensive heart and chronic kidney disease*, when both hypertensive kidney disease and hypertensive heart disease are stated in the diagnosis. Assume a relationship between the hypertension and the kidney disease, whether or not the condition is so designated. Assign an additional code from category 428, to identify the type of heart failure. More than one code from category 428 may be assigned if the patient has systolic or diastolic failure and congestive heart failure.

5. Hypertensive Cerebrovascular Disease

    First assign codes from 430-438, *Cerebrovascular disease*, then the appropriate hypertension code from categories 401-405.

6. Hypertensive Retinopathy

   Two codes are necessary to identify the condition. First assign the code from subcategory 362.11, *Hypertensive retinopathy*, then the appropriate code from categories 401-405 to indicate the type of hypertension.

7. Hypertension, Secondary

   Two codes are required: one to identify the underlying etiology and one from category 405 to identify the hypertension. Sequencing of codes is determined by the reason for admission/encounter.

8. Hypertension, Transient

   Assign code 796.2, *Elevated blood pressure reading without diagnosis of hypertension*, unless patient has an established diagnosis of hypertension. Assign code 642.3x for transient hypertension of pregnancy.

9. Hypertension, Controlled

   Assign appropriate code from categories 401-405. This diagnostic statement usually refers to an existing state of hypertension under control by therapy.

10. Hypertension, Uncontrolled

    Uncontrolled hypertension may refer to untreated hypertension or hypertension not responding to current therapeutic regimen. In either case, assign the appropriate code from categories 401-405 to designate the stage and type of hypertension. Code to the type of hypertension.

11. Elevated Blood Pressure

    For a statement of elevated blood pressure without further specificity, assign code 796.2, *Elevated blood pressure reading without diagnosis of hypertension*, rather than a code from category 401.

First you need to be able to make a distinction between conditions specified as "due to" or "with" hypertension. Keep in mind that the phrase "due to hypertension" and the word "hypertensive" are considered synonymous.

Coding Examples

Hypertensive heart disease

402.90   Hypertensive heart disease, unspecified, without heart failure

Heart disease due to hypertension

402.90   Hypertensive heart disease, unspecified, without heart failure

Each of the above diagnostic statements indicate clearly a cause-and-effect relationship between hypertension and the condition by specifying that the condition is "due to." Therefore, both statements are coded using 402.90.

If the phrase "with hypertension" is stated or, the diagnostic statement mentions the conditions separately, then you code the conditions separately.

Coding Example

Myocarditis with hypertension

429.0 Myocarditis, unspecified

401.9 Essential hypertension, unspecified

As a cause-and-effect relationship is not indicated in the diagnostic statement, the conditions are coded separately.

High Blood Pressure Versus Elevated Blood Pressure

With the ICD-9-CM coding system there is a differentiation made between high blood pressure (hypertension) and elevated blood pressure without a diagnosis of hypertension. If the diagnostic statement indicates elevated blood pressure without the diagnosis of hypertension, it is coded to subcategory 796.2 *Elevated blood pressure reading without diagnosis of hypertension*. If the diagnostic statement indicates high blood pressure or hypertension, it is coded to category 401 *Essential hypertension*.

DISEASES OF THE RESPIRATORY SYSTEM

Chronic Obstructive Pulmonary Disease [COPD] and Asthma

1. Conditions that comprise COPD and asthma

    The conditions that comprise COPD are obstructive chronic bronchitis, subcategory 491.2, and emphysema, category 492. All asthma codes are under category 493, *Asthma*. Code 496, *Chronic airway obstruction, not elsewhere classified*, is a nonspecific code that should be used only when the documentation in a medical record does not specify the type of COPD being treated.

2. Acute exacerbation of chronic obstructive bronchitis and asthma

    The codes for chronic obstructive bronchitis and asthma distinguish between uncomplicated cases and those in acute exacerbation. An acute exacerbation is a worsening or a decompensation of a chronic condition. An acute exacerbation is not equivalent to an infection superimposed on a chronic condition, though an exacerbation may be triggered by an infection.

3. Overlapping nature of the conditions that comprise COPD and asthma

    Due to the overlapping nature of the conditions that make up COPD and asthma, there are many variations in the way these conditions are documented. Code selection must be based on the terms as documented. When selecting the correct code for the documented type of COPD and asthma, it is essential to first review the index and then verify the code in the tabular list. There are many instructional notes under the different COPD subcategories and codes. It is important that all such notes be reviewed to assure correct code assignment.

4. Acute exacerbation of asthma and status asthmaticus

An acute exacerbation of asthma is an increased severity of the asthma symptoms, such as wheezing and shortness of breath. Status asthmaticus refers to a patient's failure to respond to therapy administered during an asthmatic episode and is a life-threatening complication that requires emergency care. If status asthmaticus is documented by the provider with any type of COPD or with acute bronchitis, the status asthmaticus should be sequenced first. It supersedes any type of COPD including that with acute exacerbation or acute bronchitis. It is inappropriate to assign an asthma code with fifth-digit 2, with acute exacerbation, together with an asthma code with fifth-digit 1, with status asthmatics. Only the fifth-digit 1 should be assigned.

Chronic Obstructive Pulmonary Disease [COPD] and Bronchitis

Acute bronchitis, code 466.0, is due to an infectious organism. When acute bronchitis is documented with COPD, code 491.22, *Obstructive chronic bronchitis with acute bronchitis,* should be assigned. It is not necessary to also assign code 466.0. If a medical record documents acute bronchitis with COPD with acute exacerbation, only code 491.22 should be assigned. The acute bronchitis included in code 491.22 supersedes the acute exacerbation. If a medical record documents COPD with acute exacerbation without mention of acute bronchitis, only code 491.21 should be assigned.

DIABETES MELLITUS CODING (250)

Diabetes mellitus codes under category 250, *Diabetes mellitus,* identify complications/manifestations associated with diabetes mellitus. A fifth digit is required for all category 250 codes to identify the type of diabetes mellitus and whether the diabetes is controlled or uncontrolled.

1. The following are the fifth digits for the codes under category 250:

    0   type II or unspecified type, not stated as uncontrolled

    1   type I, [juvenile type], not stated as uncontrolled

    2   type II or unspecified type, uncontrolled

    3   type I, [juvenile type], uncontrolled

    The age of a patient is not the sole determining factor, though most type I diabetics develop the condition before reaching puberty. For this reason type I diabetes mellitus is also referred to as juvenile diabetes.

2. If the type of diabetes mellitus is not documented in the medical record, the default is type II.

3. All type I diabetics must use insulin to replace what their bodies do not produce. However, the use of insulin does not mean that a patient is a type I diabetic. Some patients with type II diabetes mellitus are unable to control their blood sugar through diet and oral medication alone and do require insulin. If the documentation in a medical record does not indicate the type of diabetes but does indicate that the patient uses insulin, the appropriate fifth digit for type II must be used. For type II patients who routinely use insulin, code V58.67, *Long-term (current) use of insulin,* should also be assigned to

ICD-9-CM CODING FUNDAMENTALS

indicate that the patient uses insulin. Code V58.67 should not be assigned if insulin is given temporarily to bring a type II patient's blood sugar under control during an encounter.

4. When assigning codes for diabetes and its associated conditions, the code(s) from category 250 must be sequenced before the codes for the associated conditions. The diabetes codes and the secondary codes that correspond to them are paired codes that follow the etiology/manifestation convention of the classification (see Section I.A.6., Etiology/manifestation convention). Assign as many codes from category 250 as needed to identify all of the associated conditions that the patient has. The corresponding secondary codes are listed under each of the diabetes codes.

   A. Diabetic retinopathy/diabetic macular edema

   Diabetic macular edema, code 362.07, is only present with diabetic retinopathy. Another code from subcategory 362.0, *Diabetic retinopathy*, must be used with code 362.07. Codes under subcategory 362.0 are diabetes manifestation codes, so they must be used following the appropriate diabetes codes.

5. Insulin pump malfunction is handled as follows:

   A. Underdose of insulin due to insulin pump failure

   An underdose of insulin due to an insulin pump failure should be assigned 996.57, *Mechanical complication due to insulin pump*, as the principal or first listed code, followed by the appropriate diabetes mellitus code based on documentation.

   B. Overdose of insulin due to insulin pump failure

   The principal or first listed code for an encounter due to an insulin pump malfunction resulting in an overdose of insulin should also be 996.57, *Mechanical complication due to insulin pump*, followed by code 962.3, *Poisoning by insulins and antidiabetic agents*, and the appropriate diabetes mellitus code based on documentation.

Do not assume a patient has insulin-dependent diabetes simply because the patient is receiving insulin, as some non-dependent diabetics may require temporary use when they encounter stressful situations such as surgery or physical or mental illness.

Anytime diabetes is described as "brittle" or "uncontrolled" you should interpret it as diabetes mellitus complicated and assign code 250.9 with the appropriate fifth-digit, 0, 1, 2 or 3. However, if there is also a specific complication present, then assign the code identifying that specific complication, for example, Diabetes mellitus, brittle, with ketoacidosis would be 250.13.

CODING MENTAL DISORDERS

You should be aware of the existence of the glossary of mental disorders in Appendix B of the Tabular List (Volume 1). This glossary is not used for coding purposes but rather as a guide to provide a common frame of reference for statistical comparisons. It is simply an alphabetized listing of mental disorders with definitions.

The coder should choose code assignments based on the terminology used by the physician or psychiatrist and not by the coder's impression of the content of the categories and subcategories. The chapter on mental disorders has many fifth digit subclassifications to watch for when selecting your code.

INFECTIOUS AND PARASITIC DISEASES

There are two categories for identifying the organism causing diseases classified elsewhere. These codes may be used as either additional codes, or as solo codes depending on the diagnostic statement.

041 Bacterial infection in conditions classified elsewhere and of unspecified site

079 Viral and chlamydial infection in conditions classified elsewhere and of unspecified site

Coding Examples

Acute UTI due to Escherichia coli

599.0 Urinary tract infection, site not specified

041.4 Escherichia coli [E. coli]

Staphylococcus infection

041.11 Staphylococcus aureus

Bacterial infection

041.9 Bacterial infection, unspecified

The basic coding principles regarding combination codes (one code accurately identifies the components of the condition) applies throughout the chapter on Infectious and Parasitic Diseases.

In the Alphabetic Index (Volume 2), a subterm that identifies an infectious organism takes precedence in code assignment over a subterm at the same indentation level that identifies a site or other descriptive term.

Coding Example

Chronic syphilitic cystitis

095.8 Other specified forms of late symptomatic syphilis

Using the Alphabetic Index (Volume 2) to look up the main term "Cystitis (bacillary)," you will note the subterms "chronic 595.2" and "syphilitic 095.8" at the same indentation level under the main term. Therefore, code 095.8 is assigned to this diagnostic statement, as the organism has precedence over other descriptive terms or anatomical sites.

Human Immunodeficiency Virus (HIV) Disease

1. Code only confirmed cases of HIV infection/illness. This is an exception to the hospital inpatient guideline Section II, H.

   In this context, confirmation does not require documentation of positive serology or culture for HIV; the physician's diagnostic statement that the patient is HIV positive, or has an HIV-related illness is sufficient.

2. Selection and sequencing

   A. If a patient is admitted for an HIV-related condition, the principal diagnosis should be 042, followed by additional diagnosis codes for all reported HIV-related conditions.

   B. If a patient with HIV disease is admitted for an unrelated condition (such as a traumatic injury), the code for the unrelated condition (e.g., the nature of injury code) should be the principal diagnosis. Other diagnoses would be 042 followed by additional diagnosis codes for all reported HIV-related conditions.

   C. Whether the patient is newly diagnosed or has had previous admissions/ encounters for HIV conditions is irrelevant to the sequencing decision.

   D. V08 *Asymptomatic human immunodeficiency virus [HIV] infection status*, is to be applied when the patient without any documentation of symptoms is listed as being HIV positive, known HIV, HIV test positive, or similar terminology. Do not use this code if the term AIDS is used or if the patient is treated for any HIV-related illness or is described as having any condition(s) resulting from his/her HIV positive status; use 042 instead.

   E. Patients with inconclusive HIV serology, but no definitive diagnosis or manifestations of the illness, may be assigned code 795.71, *Nonspecific serologic evidence of human immunodeficiency virus [HIV]*.

   F. Previously diagnosed HIV-related illness: Patients with any known prior diagnosis of an HIV-related illness should be coded to 042. Once a patient had developed an HIV-related illness, the patient should always be assigned code 042 on every subsequent admission/encounter. Patients previously diagnosed with any HIV illness (042) should never be assigned to 795.71 or V08.

   G. HIV Infection in Pregnancy, Childbirth and the Puerperium: During pregnancy, childbirth or the puerperium, a patient admitted (or presenting for a health care encounter) because of an HIV-related illness should receive a principal diagnosis of 647.6X, *Other viral diseases in the mother classifiable elsewhere, but complicating the pregnancy, childbirth or the puerperium*, followed by 042 and the code(s) for the HIV-related illness(es). Codes from Chapter 11 *Pregnancy, Childbirth and the Puerperium* always take sequencing priority.

   Patients with asymptomatic HIV infection status admitted (or presenting for a health care encounter) during pregnancy, childbirth, or the puerperium should receive codes of 647.6X and V08.

H. Encounters for Testing for HIV: If a patient is being seen to determine his/her HIV status, use code V73.89, *Screening for other specified viral disease*. Use code V69.8, *Other problems related to lifestyle*, as a secondary code if an asymptomatic patient is in a known high risk group for HIV. Should a patient with signs or symptoms or illness, or a confirmed HIV related diagnosis be tested for HIV, code the signs and symptoms or the diagnosis. An additional code V65.44 *HIV counseling* may be used if counseling is provided during the encounter for the test.

When a patient returns to be informed of his/her HIV test results use code V65.44, *HIV counseling*, if the results of the test are negative.

If the results are positive but the patient is asymptomatic use code V08, *Asymptomatic HIV infection*. If the results are positive and the patient is symptomatic use code 042, *HIV disease*, with codes for the HIV related symptoms or diagnosis. The HIV counseling code may also be used if counseling is provided for patients with positive test results.

Septicemia, Systemic Inflammatory Response Syndrome (SIRS), Sepsis, Severe Sepsis and Septic Shock

The coding of SIRS, sepsis and severe sepsis requires a minimum of two codes: first a code for the underlying cause (i.e., infection or trauma); and then a code from subcategory 995.9, *Systemic Inflammatory Response Syndromes (SIRS)*.

1. Sequencing sepsis and severe sepsis

    A. Sepsis as primary diagnosis: If sepsis or severe sepsis is present on admission and meets the definition of principal diagnosis, the systemic infection code (e.g., 038.xx, 112.5, etc) should be assigned as the principal diagnosis, followed by code 995.91, *Sepsis*, or 995.92, *Severe sepsis*, as required by the sequencing rules in the Tabular List. Codes from subcategory 995.9 can never be assigned as a principal diagnosis. A code should also be assigned for any localized infection, if present.

    B. Sepsis and severe sepsis as secondary diagnoses: When sepsis or severe sepsis develops during the encounter (it was not present on admission), the systemic infection code and code 995.91 or 995.92 should be assigned as secondary diagnoses.

    C. If the documentation is not clear whether the sepsis was present on admission, the provider should be queried. Sepsis or severe sepsis may be present on admission but the diagnosis may not be confirmed until after admission.

2. In most cases, it will be a code from category 038 *Septicemia* that will be used in conjunction with a code from subcategory 995.9.

    A. If the documentation in the record states streptococcal sepsis, codes 038.0 and code 995.91 should be used, in that sequence.

    B. If the documentation states streptococcal septicemia, only code 038.0 should be assigned, however, the physician should be queried whether the patient has sepsis, and infection with SIRS.

3. If the reason for admission is both sepsis, severe sepsis, or SIRS and a localized infection such as pneumonia or cellulitis, a code for the systemic infection (038.xx, 112.5, etc.) should be assigned first, then code 995.91 or 995.92, followed by the code for the initial infection.

Note: The term urosepsis is a nonspecific term. If that is the only term documented then only code 599.0 should be assigned based on the default for the term in the ICD-9-CM index, in addition to the code for the causal organism if known.

4. If a patient has sepsis and an acute organ dysfunction, but the medical record documentation indicates that the acute organ dysfunction is related to a medical condition other than the sepsis, do not assign code 995.92, Severe sepsis. An acute organ dysfunction must be associated with the sepsis in order to assign the severe sepsis code. If the documentation is not clear as to whether an acute organ dysfunction is related to the sepsis or another medical condition, query the provider.

5. Documentation of septic shock is handled as follows:

   A. Septic shock generally refers to circulatory failure associated with severe sepsis, and therefore it represents a type of acute organ dysfunction. For all cases of septic shock, the code for the systemic infection should be sequenced first, followed by codes 995.92 and 785.52. Any additional codes for other acute organ dysfunctions should also be assigned. As noted in the sequencing instructions in the Tabular List, the code for septic shock cannot be assigned as a principal diagnosis.

   B. Septic shock indicates the presence of severe sepsis. Code 995.92, *Severe sepsis*, must be assigned with 785.52, *Septic shock* even if the term "severe sepsis" is not documented in the medical record.

6. Sepsis and septic shock complicating abortion, ectopic pregnancy, and molar pregnancy are classified to category codes in Chapter 11 (630-639).

7. Negative or inconclusive blood cultures do not preclude a diagnosis of septicemia or sepsis in patients with clinical evidence of the condition, however, the physician should be queried.

8. Sepsis resulting from a postprocedural infection is a complication of care. For such cases code 998.59, *Other postoperative infections*, or 674.3X, *Other complication of obstetrical surgical wound*, should be coded first followed by the appropriate sepsis codes. The other guidelines for coding sepsis should then be followed for the assignment of additional codes.

9. In some cases, a non-infectious process, such as trauma, injury or burn, may lead to an infection which can result in sepsis or severe sepsis. If sepsis or severe sepsis is documented as associated with a non-infectious condition, and this condition meets the definition for principal diagnosis, the code for the non-infectious condition should be sequenced first, followed by the code for the systemic infection and either code 995.91 or 995.92. Additional codes for any associated acute organ dysfunction(s) should also be assigned for cases of severe sepsis. If the sepsis or severe sepsis meets the definition of principal diagnosis, the systemic infection and sepsis codes should be sequenced before the non-infectious condition.

MANIFESTATIONS

Manifestations are characteristic signs or symptoms of an illness. Signs and symptoms that point rather definitely to a given diagnosis are assigned to the appropriate chapter of ICD-9-CM. For example, hematuria is assigned to the Genitourinary System chapter. However, Chapter 16 *Symptoms, Signs and Ill-Defined Conditions* (780-799), includes ill-defined conditions and symptoms that may suggest two or more diseases or may point to two or more systems of the body, and are used in cases lacking the necessary study to make a final diagnosis. Conditions allocated to Chapter 16 include:

1. Cases for which no more specific diagnosis can be made even after all facts bearing on the case have been investigated; for example code 784.0 *Headache*.

2. Signs or symptoms existing at the time of initial encounter that proved to be transient and whose cause could not be determined; for example code 780.2 *Syncope and collapse*.

3. Provisional diagnoses in a patient who failed to return for further investigation or care; for example code 782.4 *Jaundice, unspecified, not of newborn*.

4. Cases referred elsewhere for investigation or treatment before the diagnosis was made; for example code 782.5 *Cyanosis*.

5. Cases in which a more precise diagnosis was not available for any other reason; for example code 780.4 *Dizziness and giddiness*.

6. Certain symptoms which represent important problems in medical care and which it might be desired to classify in addition to a known cause; for example, code 780.01 *Coma*.

In the last case, if the cause of a symptom or sign is stated in the diagnosis, assign the code identifying the cause. An additional code may be assigned to further identify this symptom or sign if there is a need to further identify the symptom or sign. In such cases, the code identifying the cause will ordinarily be listed as the principal diagnosis.

Etiology/Manifestation Convention

Certain conditions have both an underlying etiology and multiple body system manifestations. For such conditions, the ICD-9-CM has a coding convention that requires the underlying condition be sequenced first followed by the manifestation. Wherever such a combination exists there is a "Use additional code" note at the etiology code, and a "Code first" note at the manifestation code. These instructional notes indicate the proper sequencing order of the codes, etiology followed by manifestation.

In most cases, the manifestation codes will have "in diseases classified elsewhere" in the code title. Such codes are a component of the etiology/manifestation convention. The code title indicates that it is a manifestation code. The "diseases classified elsewhere" codes are never permitted to be used as first listed or principal diagnosis codes. They must be used in conjunction with an underlying condition code and they must be listed following the underlying condition.

There are manifestation codes that do not have "in diseases classified elsewhere" in their title. For such codes a "Use additional code" note will still be present and the rules for sequencing apply. In addition to the notes in the Tabular Listing, these conditions also have a specific index entry structure. In the alphabetical index, both conditions are listed together with the etiology code first followed by the manifestation codes in [brackets]. The code in brackets is always to be sequenced second.

The most commonly used etiology/manifestation combinations are the codes for *Diabetes mellitus,* category 250. For each code under category 250 there is a "Use additional code" note for the manifestation that is specific for that particular diabetic manifestation. Should a patient have more than one manifestation of diabetes, more than one code from category 250 may be used with as many manifestation codes as are needed to fully describe the patient's complete diabetic condition. The diabetes category 250 codes should be sequenced first, followed by the manifestation codes.

"Code first" and "Use additional code" notes are also used as sequencing rules in the classification for certain codes that are not part of an etiology/manifestation combination.

CODING OF NEOPLASMS

General Guidelines

Chapter 2 of the ICD-9-CM contains the codes for most benign and all malignant neoplasms. Certain benign neoplasms, such as prostatic adenomas, may be found in the specific body system chapters. To properly code a neoplasm it is necessary to determine from the record if the neoplasm is benign, in-situ, malignant, or of uncertain histologic behavior. If malignant, any secondary (metastatic) sites should also be determined.

The Neoplasm Table in the Alphabetic Index should be referenced first. However, if the histological term is documented, that term should be referenced first, rather than going immediately to the Neoplasm Table, in order to determine which column in the Neoplasm Table is appropriate. For example, if the documentation indicates "adenoma," refer to the term in the Alphabetic Index to review the entries under this term and the instructional note to "see also neoplasm, by site, benign." The table provides the proper code based on the type of neoplasm and the site. It is important to select the proper column in the table that corresponds to the type of neoplasm. The tabular should then be referenced to verify that the correct code has been selected from the table and that a more specific site code does not exist.

1. If the treatment is directed at the malignancy, designate the malignancy as the principal diagnosis.

2. When a patient is admitted because of a primary neoplasm with metastasis and treatment is directed toward the secondary site only, the secondary neoplasm is designated as the principal diagnosis even though the primary malignancy is still present.

3. Coding and sequencing of complications associated with the malignancies or with the therapy thereof are subject to the following guidelines:

    A. When admission/encounter is for management of an anemia associated with the malignancy, and the treatment is only for anemia, the appropriate anemia code (such as code 285.22, *Anemia in neoplastic disease*) is designated at the principal diagnosis and is followed by the appropriate code(s) for the malignancy. Code 285.22 may also be used as a secondary code if the patient suffers from anemia and is being treated for the malignancy.

ICD-9-CM CODING FUNDAMENTALS

    B. When the admission/encounter is for management of an anemia associated with chemotherapy, immunotherapy or radiotherapy and the only treatment is for the anemia, the anemia is sequenced first followed by code E933.1. The appropriate neoplasm code should be assigned as an additional code.

    C. When the admission/encounter is for management of dehydration due to the malignancy or the therapy, or a combination of both, and only the dehydration is being treated (intravenous rehydration), the dehydration is sequenced first, followed by the code(s) for the malignancy.

    D. When the admission/encounter is for treatment of a complication resulting from a surgical procedure, designate the complication as the principal or first-listed diagnosis if treatment is directed at resolving the complication.

4. When a primary malignancy has been previously excised or eradicated from its site and there is no further treatment directed to that site and there is no evidence of any existing primary malignancy, a code from category V10, *Personal history of malignant neoplasm*, should be used to indicate the former site of the malignancy. Any mention of extension, invasion, or metastasis to another site is coded as a secondary malignant neoplasm to that site. The secondary site may be the principal or first-listed with the V10 code used as a secondary code.

5. Admissions/encounters involving chemotherapy, immunotherapy and radiation therapy are handled as follows:

    A. When an episode of care involves the surgical removal of a neoplasm, primary or secondary site, followed by adjunct chemotherapy or radiation treatment during the same episode of care, the neoplasm code should be assigned as principal or first-listed diagnosis, using codes in the 140-198 series or where appropriate in the 200-203 series.

    B. If a patient admission/encounter is solely for the administration of chemotherapy, immunotherapy or radiation therapy, assign code V58.0, *Encounter for radiation therapy*, or V58.11, *Encounter for antineoplastic chemotherapy*, or V58.12, *Encounter for antineoplastic immunotherapy*, as the first-listed or principal diagnosis. If a patient receives more than one of these therapies during the same admission, more than one of these codes may be assigned, in any sequence.

    C. When a patient is admitted for the purpose of radiotherapy, immunotherapy or chemotherapy and develops complications such as uncontrolled nausea and vomiting or dehydration, the principal or first-listed diagnosis is V58.0, *Encounter for radiotherapy*, or V58.11, *Encounter for antineoplastic chemotherapy*, or V58.12, *Encounter for antineoplastic immunotherapy*, followed by any codes for the complications.

6. When the reason for admission/encounter is to determine the extent of the malignancy, or for a procedure such as paracentesis or thoracentesis, the primary malignancy or appropriate metastatic site is designated as the principal or first-listed diagnosis, even though chemotherapy or radiotherapy is administered.

7. Symptoms, signs, and ill-defined conditions listed in Chapter 16 characteristic of, or associated with, an existing primary or secondary site malignancy cannot be used to replace the malignancy as principal or first-listed diagnosis, regardless of the number of admissions or encounters for treatment and care of the neoplasm.

8. For encounters specifically for prophylactic removal of breasts, ovaries, or another organ due to a genetic susceptibility to cancer or a family history of cancer, the principal or first-listed code should be a code from subcategory V50.4, *Prophylactic organ removal,* followed by the appropriate genetic susceptibility code and the appropriate family history code.

If the patient has a malignancy of one site and is having prophylactic removal of another site to prevent either a new primary malignancy or metastatic disease, a code for the malignancy should also be assigned in addition to a code from subcategory V50.4. A V50.4 code should not be assigned if the patient is having organ removal for treatment of a malignancy, such as the removal of the testes for the treatment of prostate cancer.

The coding of neoplasms requires a good understanding of medical terminology. All neoplasms are classified in the Tabular List (Volume 1) in Chapter 2 *Neoplasms* 140-239 which contains the following broad groups:

140-195	Malignant neoplasms, stated or presumed to be primary, of specified sites, except of lymphatic and hematopoietic tissue
196-198	Malignant neoplasms, stated or presumed to be secondary, of specified sites
199	Malignant neoplasms, without specification of site
200-208	Malignant neoplasms, stated or presumed to be primary of lymphatic and hematopoietic tissue
210-229	Benign neoplasms
230-234	Carcinoma in situ
235-238	Neoplasms of uncertain behavior
239	Neoplasms of unspecified nature

Table of Neoplasms

The Table of Neoplasms appears in the Alphabetic Index (Volume 2) under the main term "Neoplasms." This table gives the code numbers for neoplasms of anatomical site. For each anatomical site there are six possible code numbers according to whether the neoplasm in questions is either:

Malignant:
    Primary
    Secondary
    Ca in situ
Benign
Of uncertain behavior
Of unspecified nature

Definitions of Site and Behaviors of Neoplasms

Primary — Identifies the stated or presumed site of origin.

Secondary — Identifies site(s) to which the primary site has spread (direct extension) or metastasized by lymphatic spread, invading local blood vessels, or by implantation as tumor cells shed into body cavities.

In-situ — Tumor cells that are undergoing malignant changes but are still confined to the point of origin without invasion of surrounding normal tissue (non-infiltrating, non-invasive or pre-invasive carcinoma).

Benign — Tumor does not invade adjacent structures or spread to distant sites but may displace or exert pressure on adjacent structures.

Of Uncertain Behavior — The pathologist is not able to determine whether the tumor is benign or malignant because some features of each are present.

Of Unspecified Nature — Neither the behavior nor the histological type of tumors are specified in the diagnostic statement. This type of diagnosis may be encountered when the patient has been treated elsewhere and comes in terminally ill without accompanying information, is referred elsewhere for work-up, or no work-up is performed because of advanced age or poor condition of the patient.

Steps to Coding Neoplasms

1. ICD-9-CM disregards classification of neoplasms by histological type (according to tissue origin) with the exception of lymphatic and hematopoietic neoplasms, malignant melanoma of skin, lipoma, and a few common tumors of bone, uterus, ovary, etc. All other tumors are classified by system, organ or site. The existence of these exceptions makes it necessary to first consult the Alphabetic Index (Volume 2) to determine whether a specific code has been assigned to a specified histological type. For example, *Malignant melanoma of skin of scalp* is coded 172.4 although the code specified in the "Malignant: Primary Column" of the Neoplasm Table for skin of scalp is 173.4.

2. The General Alphabetical Index (Volume 2) also provides guidance to the appropriate column for neoplasms which are not assigned a specific code by histological type. For example, if you look up *Lipomyoma, specified site* in the Alphabetic Index (Volume 2), you will find "see Neoplasm, connective tissue, benign."

   The guidance in the Alphabetic Index (Volume 2) can be over-ridden if a descriptor is present. For example, *Malignant adenoma of colon* is coded as 153.9 and not as 211.3 because the adjective "malignant" overrides the entry "adenoma — *see also* Neoplasm, benign."

3. The Neoplasm Table may be consulted directly if a specific neoplasm diagnosis indicates which column of the table is appropriate but does not delineate a specific type of tumor.

ICD-9-CM CODING FUNDAMENTALS

4. Sites marked with an asterisk (*), such as buttock NEC* or calf*, should be classified to malignant neoplasm of skin of these sites if the variety of neoplasm is a squamous cell carcinoma or an epidermoid carcinoma and to benign neoplasm of skin of these sites if the variety of neoplasm is a papilloma (of any type).

5. Primary malignant neoplasms are classified to the site of origin of the neoplasm. In some cases, it may not be possible to identify the site of origin, such as malignant neoplasms originating from contiguous sites.

    Neoplasms with overlapping site boundaries are classified to the fourth-digit subcategory .8 "other." For example, code 151.8 *Malignant neoplasm of contiguous or overlapping sites of stomach* whose point of origin cannot be determined.

6. Neoplasms which demonstrate functional activity require an additional code to identify the functional activity.

    Coding Example

    Cushing's syndrome due to malignant pheochromocytoma

    > 194.0   Malignant neoplasm of adrenal gland
    >
    > 255.0   Disorders of adrenal glands; Cushing's syndrome

    Code sequencing depends on the circumstances of the encounter.

7. Two categories in the malignant neoplasm section represent departures from the usual principles of classification in that the fourth-digit subdivisions in each case are not mutually exclusive. These categories are 150 *Malignant neoplasm of esophagus* and 201 *Hodgkin's disease.* The dual axis is provided to account for differing terminology, for there is no uniform international agreement on the use of these terms.

    Coding Example

    Malignant neoplasm of the esophagus

    > 150.0   Cervical esophagus
    >
    > 150.1   Thoracic esophagus
    >
    > 150.2   Abdominal esophagus

    or using alternate coding

    > 150.3   Upper third of esophagus
    >
    > 150.4   Middle third of esophagus
    >
    > 150.5   Lower third of esophagus

8. When the treatment is directed at the primary site of the malignancy, designate the primary site as the principal diagnosis, except when the encounter or hospital admission is solely for *Radiotherapy* (V58.0) or, for *Chemotherapy* (V58.1).

9. When surgical intervention for removal of a primary site or secondary site malignancy is followed by adjunct chemotherapy or radiotherapy, code the malignancy using codes in the 140-198 series, or, where appropriate, in the 200-203 series as long as chemotherapy or radiotherapy is being actively administered. If the admission is for chemotherapy or radiotherapy, the malignancy code is listed second.

10. When the primary malignancy has been previously excised or eradicated from its site and there is no adjunct treatment directed to that site, and there is no evidence of any remaining malignancy at the primary site, use the appropriate code from the V10 series to indicate the site of the primary malignancy. Any mention of extension, invasion or metastasis to a nearby structure or organ, or to a distant site, is coded as a secondary malignant neoplasm to that site and may be the principal diagnosis in the absence of the primary site.

11. If the patient has no secondary malignancy and if the reason for admission or for the visit is follow-up of the malignancy, two codes are used and sequenced.

Coding Example

Follow-up of breast cancer treated with chemotherapy. No evidence of recurrence.

V67.2   **Follow-up examination following chemotherapy**

V10.3   **Personal history of carcinoma of breast**

12. Malignancies of hematopoietic and lymphatic tissue are always coded to the 200.0-208.9 series unless specified as "in remission." If they are in remission, they are coded as V10.60-V10.79.

13. If the primary malignant neoplasm previously excised or eradicated has recurred, code it as primary malignancy of the stated site unless the Alphabetic Index (Volume 2) directs you to do otherwise.

Coding Examples

Recurrence of prostate carcinoma

185   **Malignant neoplasm of prostate**

Recurrence of breast carcinoma in mastectomy site

198.2   **Secondary malignant neoplasm of other specified sites, skin of breast**

Make sure to code any mention of secondary site(s).

14. Terminology referring to metastatic cancer is often ambiguous, so when there is doubt as to the meaning intended, the following rules should be used:

   A. Cancer described as metastatic "from" a site should be interpreted as primary of that site.

   B. Cancer described as metastatic "to" a site should be interpreted as secondary of that site.

ICD-9-CM CODING FUNDAMENTALS

Coding Examples

Carcinoma in axillary lymph nodes and lungs metastatic from breast

    174.9   **Malignant neoplasm of breast (female), unspecified**

    196.3   **Secondary and unspecified malignant neoplasm of lymph nodes of axilla and upper limb**

    197.0   **Secondary malignant neoplasm of lung**

Adenocarcinoma of colon with extension to peritoneum

    153.9   **Malignant neoplasm of colon, unspecified**

    197.6   **Secondary malignant neoplasm of retroperitoneum and peritoneum**

15. Diagnostic statements when only one site is identified as metastatic:

    A. Code to the category for "primary of unspecified site" for the morphological type concerned UNLESS the code thus obtained is either 199.0 or 199.1.

    B. If the code obtained in the above step is 199.0 or 199.1, then code the site qualified as "metastatic" as for a primary malignant neoplasm of the stated site EXCEPT for the sites listed below, which should always be coded as secondary neoplasm of the state site:

        Bone   *Mediastinum*
        Brain   *Meninges*
        Diaphragm   *Peritoneum*
        Heart   *Pleura*
        Liver   *Retroperitoneum*
        Lymph nodes *Spinal cord*

    Sites classifiable to 195

    C. Also assign the appropriate code for primary or secondary malignant neoplasm of specified or unspecified site, depending on the diagnostic statement you are coding.

Coding Examples

Metastatic renal cell carcinoma of lung

    189.0   **Malignant neoplasm of kidney, except pelvis**

    197.0   **Secondary malignant neoplasm of lung**

Metastatic carcinoma of lung

    162.9   **Malignant neoplasm of bronchus and lung, unspecified**

    199.1   **Malignant neoplasm without specification of site, other**

ICD-9-CM CODING FUNDAMENTALS

This code is assigned to identify "secondary neoplasm of unspecified site" per the instructions in step C above.

Metastatic carcinoma of brain

198.3 **Secondary malignant neoplasm of other specified sites, brain and spinal cord**

199.1 **Malignant neoplasm without specification of site, other**

In this case, the brain is one of the sites listed in Step B as an exception. So for this diagnostic statement, the code assignment is for secondary neoplasm of the brain and primary malignant neoplasm of unspecified site.

16. When two or more sites are stated in the diagnostic statement and all are qualified to be "metastatic," you should code as for "primary site unknown" and code the stated sites as secondary neoplasms of those sites.

Coding Example

Metastatic melanoma of lung and liver

172.9 **Malignant melanoma of skin, site unspecified**

197.0 **Secondary malignant neoplasm of lung**

197.7 **Secondary malignant neoplasm of liver, specified as secondary**

17. When there is no site specified in the diagnostic statement, but the morphological type is qualified as "metastatic," code as for "primary site unknown." Then assign the code for secondary neoplasms of unspecified site.

Coding Example

Metastatic apocrine adenocarcinoma

173.9 **Other malignant neoplasms of skin, site unspecified**

199.1 **Malignant neoplasm without specification of site, other**

18. When two or more sites are stated in the diagnosis and only some are qualified as "metastatic" while others are not, code as for "primary site unknown." However, you should interpret the following sites as secondary neoplasms:

Bone	*Meninges*
Brain	*Peritoneum*
Diaphragm	*Pleura*
Heart	*Retroperitoneum*
Liver	*Spinal Cord*

Sites classifiable to category 195

Coding Example

Carcinoma of lung, metastatic, and brain

198.3   Secondary malignant neoplasm of brain and spinal cord

197.0   Secondary malignant neoplasm of lung

199.1   Malignant neoplasm without specification of site, other

CHRONIC KIDNEY DISEASE

Stages of Chronic Kidney Disease (CKD)

The ICD-9-CM classifies CKD based on severity. The severity of CKD is designated by stages I-V. Stage II, code 585.2, equates to mild CKD; stage III, code 585.3, equates to moderate CKD; and stage IV, code 585.4, equates to severe CKD. Code 585.6, *End stage renal disease (ESRD)*, is assigned when the provider has documented end-stage renal disease (ESRD).

If both a stage of CKD and ESRD are documented, assign code 585.6 only.

Chronic Kidney Disease and Kidney Transplant Status

Patients who have undergone kidney transplant may still have some form of CKD because the kidney transplant may not fully restore kidney function. Code V42.0 may be assigned with the appropriate CKD code for patients who are status post-kidney transplant, based on the patient's post-transplant stage. The *use additional code* note under category 585 provides this instruction.

Use of a 585 code with V42.0 does not necessarily indicate transplant rejection or failure. Patients with mild or moderate CKD following a transplant should not be coded as having transplant failure, unless it is documented in the medical record. For patients with severe CKD or ESRD it is appropriate to assign code 996.81, *Complications of transplanted organ, kidney transplant,* when kidney transplant failure is documented. If a post kidney transplant patient has CKD and it is unclear from the documentation whether there is transplant failure or rejection, it is necessary to query the provider.

Chronic Kidney Disease With Other Conditions

Patients with CKD may also suffer from other serious conditions, most commonly diabetes mellitus and hypertension. The sequencing of the CKD code in relationship to codes for other contributing conditions is based on the conventions in the tabular list.

PREGNANCY, CHILDBIRTH, AND THE PUERPERIUM

Chapter 11 of the Tabular List (Volume 1) uses fifth-digit subclassifications extensively. In general, the fifth digit is not given in the Alphabetic Index (Volume 2), so each code must be verified in the Tabular List (Volume 1).

ICD-9-CM CODING FUNDAMENTALS

General Rules for Obstetrics Cases

1. Obstetric cases require codes from Chapter 11, codes in the range 630-677, *Complications of Pregnancy, Childbirth, and the Puerperium*. Should the physician document that the pregnancy is incidental to the encounter, then code V22.2 should be used in place of any Chapter 11 codes. It is the physician's responsibility to state that the condition being treated is not affecting the pregnancy.

2. Chapter 11 codes have sequencing priority over codes from other chapters. Additional codes from other chapters may be used in conjunction with Chapter 11 codes to further specify conditions. For example, sepsis and septic shock associated with abortion, ectopic pregnancy, and molar pregnancy are classified to category codes in Chapter 11 (630-639).

3. Chapter 11 codes are to be used only on the maternal record, never on the record of the newborn.

4. Categories 640-648 and 651-676 have required fifth-digits, which indicate whether the encounter is antepartum or postpartum, and whether a delivery has also occurred.

5. The fifth-digits that are appropriate for each code number, are listed in brackets under each code. The fifth-digits on each code should all be consistent with each other. That is, should a delivery occur, all of the fifth-digits should indicate that the delivery occurred.

Selection of OB Principal or First-Listed Diagnosis

1. For routine outpatient prenatal visits when no complications are present, codes V22.0, *Supervision of normal first pregnancy*, and V22.1, *Supervision of other normal pregnancy*, should be used as the first-listed diagnoses. These codes should not be used in conjunction with Chapter 11 codes.

2. For prenatal outpatient visits for patients with high-risk pregnancies, a code from category V23, *Supervision of high-risk pregnancy*, should be used as the principal or first-listed diagnosis. Secondary Chapter 11 codes may be used in conjunction with these codes if appropriate.

3. In episodes when no delivery occurs, the principal diagnosis should correspond to the principal complication of the pregnancy that necessitated the encounter. Should more than one complication exist, all of which are treated or monitored, any of the complications codes may be sequenced first.

4. When a delivery occurs, the principal diagnosis should correspond to the main circumstances or complication of the delivery. In cases of cesarean delivery, the selection of the principal diagnosis should correspond to the reason the cesarean delivery was performed unless the reason for admission/encounter was unrelated to the condition resulting in the cesarean delivery.

5. An outcome of delivery code, V27.0-V27.9, should be included on every maternal record when a delivery has occurred. These codes are not to be used on subsequent records or on the newborn record.

Fetal Conditions Affecting the Management of the Mother

Codes from category 655, *Known or suspected fetal abnormality affecting management of the mother*, and category 656, *Other fetal and placental problems affecting the management of the mother*, are assigned only when the fetal condition is actually responsible for modifying the management of the mother, i.e., by requiring diagnostic studies, additional observation, special care, or termination of pregnancy. The fact that the fetal condition exists does not justify assigning a code from this series to the mother's record.

In cases when surgery is performed on the fetus, a diagnosis code from category 655, *Known or suspected fetal abnormalities affecting management of the mother*, should be assigned identifying the fetal condition. Procedure code 75.36, *Correction of fetal defect*, should be assigned on the hospital inpatient record.

No code from Chapter 15, the perinatal codes, should be used on the mother's record to identify fetal conditions. Surgery performed in utero on a fetus is still to be coded as an obstetric encounter.

HIV Infection in Pregnancy, Childbirth and the Puerperium

During pregnancy, childbirth or the puerperium, a patient admitted because of an HIV-related illness should receive a principal diagnosis of 647.6x, *Other viral diseases in the mother classifiable elsewhere, but complicating the pregnancy, childbirth or the puerperium*, followed by 042 *HIV disease*, and the code(s) for the HIV-related illness(es). This is an exception to the sequencing rule found in above.

Patients with asymptomatic HIV infection status admitted during pregnancy, childbirth, or the puerperium should receive codes of 647.6x and V08.

Current Conditions Complicating Pregnancy

Assign a code from subcategory 648.x for patients that have current conditions when the condition affects the management of the pregnancy, childbirth, or the puerperium. Use additional secondary codes from other chapters to identify the conditions, as appropriate.

Diabetes Mellitus in Pregnancy

Diabetes mellitus is a significant complicating factor in pregnancy. Pregnant women who are diabetic should be assigned code 648.0x, *Diabetes mellitus complicating pregnancy*, and a secondary code from category 250, *Diabetes mellitus*, to identify the type of diabetes. Code V58.67, *Long-term (current) use of insulin*, should also be assigned if the diabetes mellitus is being treated with insulin.

Gestational Diabetes

Gestational diabetes can occur during the second and third trimester of pregnancy in women who were not diabetic prior to pregnancy. Gestational diabetes can cause complications in the pregnancy similar to those of pre-existing diabetes mellitus. It also puts the woman at greater risk of developing diabetes after the pregnancy. Gestational diabetes is coded to 648.8x, *Abnormal glucose tolerance*. Codes 648.0x and 648.8x should never be used together on the same record.

Code V58.67, *Long-term (current) use of insulin*, should also be assigned if the gestational diabetes is being treated with insulin.

Normal Delivery

1. Code 650, *Normal delivery*, is for use in cases when a woman is admitted for a full-term normal delivery and delivers a single, healthy infant without any complications antepartum, during the delivery, or postpartum during the delivery episode. Code 650 is always a principal diagnosis. It is not to be used if any other code from Chapter 11 is needed to describe a current complication of the antenatal, delivery, or perinatal period. Additional codes from other chapters may be used with code 650 if they are not related to or are in any way complicating the pregnancy.

2. Code 650 may be used if the patient had a complication at some point during her pregnancy but the complication is not present at the time of the admission for delivery.

3. Code 650 is always a principal diagnosis. It is not to be used if any other code from Chapter 11 is needed to describe a current complication of the antenatal, delivery, or perinatal period. Additional codes from other chapters may be used with code 650 if they are not related to or are in any way complicating the pregnancy.

4. V27.0, *Single liveborn*, is the only outcome of delivery code appropriate for use with 650.

The Postpartum Period

1. The postpartum period begins immediately after delivery and continues for six weeks following delivery.

2. A postpartum complication is any complication occurring within the six-week period.

3. Chapter 11 codes may also be used to describe pregnancy-related complications after the six-week period should the physician document that a condition is pregnancy related.

4. Postpartum complications that occur during the same admission as the delivery are identified with a fifth-digit of subsequent admissions/encounters for postpartum complications, should identified with a fifth-digit of "4.".

5. When the mother delivers outside the hospital prior to admission and is admitted for routine postpartum care and no complications are noted, code V24.0, *Postpartum care and examination immediately after delivery*, should be assigned as the principal diagnosis.

6. A delivery diagnosis code should not be used for a woman who has delivered prior to admission to the hospital. Any postpartum procedures should be coded.

Late Effect of Complication of Pregnancy, Childbirth, and the Puerperium

1. Code 677, *Late effect of complication of pregnancy, childbirth, and the puerperium* is for use in those cases when an initial complication of a pregnancy develops a sequelae requiring care or treatment at a future date.

2. This code may be used at any time after the initial postpartum period.

3. This code, like all late effect codes, is to be sequenced following the code describing the sequelae of the complication.

Abortions

1. Fifth-digits are required for abortion categories 634-637. Fifth-digit 1, *Incomplete*, indicates that all of the products of conception have not been expelled from the uterus. Fifth-digit 2, *Complete*, indicates that all products of conception have been expelled from the uterus prior to the episode of care.

2. A code from categories 640-648 and 651-657 may be used as additional codes with an abortion code to indicate the complication leading to the abortion.

    Fifth-digit 3 is assigned with codes from these categories when used with an abortion code because the other fifth-digits will not apply. Codes from the 660-669 series are not to be used for complications of abortion.

3. Code 639, *Complications following abortion and ectopic and molar pregnancies*, is to be used for all complications following abortion. Code 639 cannot be assigned with codes from categories 634-638.

4. When an attempted termination of pregnancy results in a liveborn fetus, assign code 644.21, *Early onset of delivery*, with an appropriate code from category V27, *Outcome of delivery*. The procedure code for the attempted termination of pregnancy should also be assigned.

5. Subsequent admissions for retained products of conception following a spontaneous or legally induced abortion are assigned the appropriate code from category 634, *Abortion*, or 635, *Legally induced abortion*, with a fifth digit of 1, *Incomplete*. This advice is appropriate even when the patient was discharged previously with a discharge diagnosis of "complete abortion."

Pregnancy Coding Examples

Pregnancy, 3 months gestation complicated by benign essential hypertension

642.03 **Benign essential hypertension complicating pregnancy, childbirth, and the puerperium, antepartum condition or complication**

Categories 647 and 648 are used for conditions that are usually classified elsewhere, but which have been classified here because they are complications of pregnancy. The interaction of certain conditions with the pregnant state complicates the pregnancy and/or aggravates the non-obstetrical condition (i.e., diabetes mellitus, drug dependence, thyroid dysfunction) and are the main reasons for the obstetrical care provided.

Coding Example

Rubella in woman, 7 months gestation

> 647.53   Infectious and parasitic conditions in the mother classifiable elsewhere, but complicating pregnancy, childbirth or the puerperium, rubella, antepartum condition or complication

Pregnancy with diabetes mellitus

> 648.03   Other current conditions in the mother classifiable elsewhere, but complicating pregnancy, childbirth or the puerperium, diabetes mellitus, antepartum condition or complication

If greater detail is needed for the complication, use an additional code to identify the complication more completely.

Coding Example

Pregnancy with pernicious anemia

> 648.23   Other current conditions in the mother classifiable elsewhere, but complicating pregnancy, childbirth or the puerperium, anemia, antepartum condition or complication
>
> 281.0   Pernicious anemia

NEWBORN (PERINATAL) GUIDELINES

For coding and reporting purposes, the perinatal period is defined as birth through the 28th day following birth. The following guidelines are provided for reporting purposes. Hospitals may record other diagnoses as needed for internal data use.

General Perinatal Rules

1. Chapter 15 codes are *never* for use on the maternal record. Codes from Chapter 11, the obstetric chapter, are never permitted on the newborn record. Chapter 15 code may be used throughout the life of the patient if the condition is still present.

2. Generally, codes from Chapter 15 should be sequenced as the principal/first-listed diagnosis on the newborn record, with the exception of the appropriate V30 code for the birth episode, followed by codes from any other chapter that provide additional detail. The "use additional code" note at the beginning of the chapter supports this guideline. If the index does not provide a specific code for a perinatal condition, assign code 779.89, *Other specified conditions originating in the perinatal period*, followed by the code from another chapter that specifies the condition. Codes for signs and symptoms may be assigned when a definitive diagnosis has not been established.

3. If a newborn has a condition that may be either due to the birth process or community-acquired and the documentation does not indicate which it is, the default is due to the birth process and the code from Chapter 15 should be used. If the condition is community-acquired, a code from Chapter 15 should not be assigned.

4. All clinically significant conditions noted on routine newborn examination should be coded. A condition is clinically significant if it requires:

- clinical evaluation; or
- therapeutic treatment; or
- diagnostic procedures; or
- extended length of hospital stay; or
- increased nursing care and/or monitoring; or
- has implications for future health care needs

Note: The perinatal guidelines listed above are the same as the general coding guidelines for "additional diagnoses," except for the final point regarding implications for future health care needs. Codes should be assigned for conditions that have been specified by the provider as having implications for future health care needs. Codes from the perinatal chapter should not be assigned unless the provider has established a definitive diagnosis.

Use of Codes V30-V39

When coding the birth of an infant, assign a code from categories V30-V39, according to the type of birth. A code from this series is assigned as a principal diagnosis and assigned only once to a newborn at the time of birth.

Newborn Transfers

If the newborn is transferred to another institution, the V30 series is not used at the receiving hospital.

Use of Category V29

1. Assign a code from category V29, *Observation and evaluation of newborns and infants for suspected conditions not found*, to identify those instances when a healthy newborn is evaluated for a suspected condition that is determined after study not to be present. Do not use a code from category V29 when the patient has identified signs or symptoms of a suspected problem; in such cases, code the sign or symptom.

    A code from category V29 may also be assigned as a principal code for readmissions or encounters when the V30 code no longer applies. Codes from category V29 are for use only for healthy newborns and infants for which no condition after study is found to be present.

2. A V29 code is to be used as a secondary code after the V30, *Outcome of delivery*, code.

Use of Other V Codes on Perinatal Records

V codes other than V30 and V29 may be assigned on a perinatal or newborn record code. The codes may be used as a principal or first-listed diagnosis for specific types of encounters or for readmissions or encounters when the V30 code no longer applies.

Maternal Causes of Perinatal Morbidity

Codes from categories 760-763, *Maternal causes of perinatal morbidity and mortality,* are assigned only when the maternal condition has actually affected the fetus or newborn. The fact that the mother has an associated medical condition or experiences some complication of pregnancy, labor or delivery does not justify the routine assignment of codes from these categories to the newborn record.

Congenital Anomalies

For the birth admission, the appropriate code from category V30, *Liveborn infants according to type of birth,* should be sequenced as the principal diagnosis, followed by any congenital anomaly codes, categories 740-759. Use additional secondary codes from other chapters to specify conditions associated with the anomaly, if applicable. Assign an appropriate code(s) from categories 740-759, *Congenital Anomalies,* when an anomaly is documented.

When a congenital anomaly does not have a unique code assignment, assign additional code(s) for any manifestations that may be present. When the code assignment specifically identifies the congenital anomaly, manifestations that are an inherent component of the anomaly should not be coded separately. Additional codes should be assigned for manifestations that are not an inherent component.

A congenital anomaly may be the principal/first-listed diagnosis on a record or a secondary diagnosis. Use additional secondary codes from other chapters to specify conditions associated with the anomaly, if applicable. Codes from Chapter 14 may be used throughout the life of the patient. If a congenital anomaly has been corrected, a personal history code should be used to identify the history of the anomaly. Although present at birth, a congenital anomaly may not be identified until later in life. Whenever the condition is diagnosed by the physician, it is appropriate to assign a code from codes 740-759.

Coding of Additional Perinatal Diagnoses

1. Assign codes for conditions that require treatment or further investigation, prolong the length of stay, or require resource utilization.

2. Assign codes for conditions that have been specified by the physician as having implications for future health care needs.

    Note: This guideline should not be used for adult patients.

3. Assign a code for *Newborn conditions originating in the perinatal period* (categories 760-779), as well as complications arising during the current episode of care classified in other chapters, only if the diagnoses have been documented by the responsible physician at the time of transfer or discharge as having affected the fetus or newborn.

Prematurity and Fetal Growth Retardation

Codes from category 764, *Slow fetal growth and fetal malnutrition,* and subcategories 765.0, *Extreme immaturity,* and 765.1, *Other preterm infant,* should not be assigned based solely on recorded birthweight or estimated gestational age, but on the attending physician's clinical assessment of maturity of the infant. Note: since physicians may utilize different criteria in determining prematurity, do not code the diagnosis of prematurity unless the physician documents this condition.

A code from subcategory 765.2x, *Weeks of gestation,* should be assigned as an additional code with category 764 and codes 765.0 and 765.1 in order to specify weeks of gestation as documented by the physician.

Newborn Sepsis

Code 771.81, *Septicemia [sepsis] of newborn,* should be assigned with a secondary code from category 041, *Bacterial infections in conditions classified elsewhere and of unspecified site,* to identify the organism. It is not necessary to use a code from subcategory 995.9, *Systemic inflammatory response syndrome (SIRS),* on a newborn record. A code from category 038, *Septicemia,* should not be used on a newborn record. Code 771.81 describes the sepsis.

V CODES: CLASSIFICATION OF FACTORS INFLUENCING HEALTH STATUS AND CONTACT WITH HEALTH SERVICE

ICD-9-CM provides codes to deal with encounters for circumstances other than a disease or injury. *The Supplementary Classification of Factors Influencing Health Status and Contact with Health Services* (V01.0-V84.8) is provided to deal with occasions when circumstances other than a disease or injury (codes 001-999) are recorded as a diagnosis or problem.

V codes are used for four primary circumstances:

1. When a person who is not currently sick encounters the health services for some specific reason, such as to act as an organ donor, to receive prophylactic care such as inoculations or health screenings, or to receive counseling on health related issue.

2. When a person with a resolving disease or injury, or a chronic, long-term condition requiring continuous care, encounters the health care system for specific aftercare of that disease or injury (e.g., dialysis for renal disease, chemotherapy for malignancy, or a cast change). Note: A diagnosis/symptom code should be used whenever a current/acute diagnosis is being treated or a sign or symptom is being studied.

3. When circumstances or problems influence a person's health status but are not in themselves a current illness or injury.

4. For newborns, to indicate birth status.

V codes are for use in both the inpatient and outpatient setting but are generally more applicable to the outpatient setting. V codes may be used as either a first listed (principal diagnosis code in the inpatient setting) or secondary code depending on the circumstances of the encounter. Certain V codes may only be used as first listed, and others only as secondary codes.

V codes indicate a reason for an encounter. They are not procedure codes. A corresponding procedure code must accompany a V code to describe the procedure performed. Key words found in diagnostic statements which may result in selection of a V code include:

Admission for	Health or healthy
Aftercare	History (of)
Attention to	Maintenance
Care (of)	Maladjustment
Carrier	Observation
Checking/checkup	Problem (with)
Contact	Prophylactic
Contraception	Replacement (by)(of)
Counseling	Screening
Dialysis	Status
Donor	Supervision (of)
Examination	Test
Fitting of	Transplant
Follow up	Vaccination

Categories of V Codes

Contact/Exposure

Category V01 indicates *Contact with or exposure to communicable diseases*. These codes are for patients who do not show any sign or symptom of a disease but have been exposed to it by close personal contact with an infected individual or are in an area where a disease is epidemic. These codes may be used as a first-listed code to explain an encounter for testing, or, more commonly, as a secondary code to identify a potential risk.

Inoculations and Vaccinations

Categories V03-V06 are used for encounters for inoculations and vaccinations. These codes indicate that a patient is being seen to receive a prophylactic inoculation against a disease. The injection itself must be represented by the appropriate procedure code. A code from V03-V06 may be used as a secondary code if the inoculation is given as a routine part of preventive health care, such as well-baby visit.

Status

Status codes indicate that a patient is either a carrier of a disease or has the sequelae or residual of a past disease or condition. This includes such things as the presence of prosthetic or mechanical devices resulting from past treatment. A status code is informative because the status may affect the current course of treatment and its outcome. A status code is distinct from a history code. The history code indicates that the patient no longer has the condition.

Status V codes/categories

V02   Carrier or suspected carrier of infectious diseases

Carrier status indicates that a person harbors the specific organisms of a disease without manifest symptoms and is capable of transmitting the infection.

V08   Asymptomatic HIV infection status

This code indicates that a patient has tested positive for HIV but has manifested no signs or symptoms of the disease.

V09   *Infection with drug-resistant microorganisms*

        This category indicates that a patient has an infection which is resistant to drug treatment. Sequence the infection code first.

V21   *Constitutional states in development*

V22.2   *Pregnant state, incidental*

        This code is a secondary code only for use when the pregnancy is in no way complicating the reason for visit. Otherwise, a code from the obstetric chapter is required.

V26.5X   *Sterilization status*

V42   *Organ or tissue replaced by transplant*

V43   *Organ or tissue replaced by other means*

V44   *Artificial opening status*

V45   *Other postprocedural states*

V46   *Other dependence on machines*

V49.6   *Upper limb amputation status*

V49.7   *Lower limb amputation status*

V49.81   *Asymptomatic menopausal status (age-related) (natural)*

V49.82   *Dental sealant status*

V49.83   *Awaiting organ transplant status*

V58.6   *Long-term (current) drug use*

        This subcategory indicates a patient's continuous use of a prescribed drug (including such things as aspirin therapy) for the long-term treatment of a condition or for prophylactic use. It is not for use for patients who have addictions to drugs.

        Assign a code from subcategory V58.6, *Long-term (current) drug use,* if the patient is receiving a medication for an extended period as a prophylactic measure (such as for the prevention of deep vein thrombosis) or as treatment of a chronic condition (i.e., arthritis) or a disease requiring a lengthy course of treatment (such as cancer). Do not assign a code from subcategory V58.6 for medication being administered for a brief period of time to treat an acute illness or injury (such as a course of antibiotics to treat acute bronchitis).

V83   *Genetic carrier status*

        Genetic carrier status indicates that a person carries a gene, associated with a particular disease, which may be passed to offspring who may develop that disease. The person does not have the disease and is not at risk of developing the disease.

V84   *Genetic susceptibility status*

                Genetic susceptibility indicates that a person has a gene that increases the risk of that person developing the disease.

                Codes from category V84, *Genetic susceptibility to disease*, should not be used as principal or first-listed codes. If the patient has the condition to which he/she is susceptible, and that condition is the reason for the encounter, the code for the current condition should be sequenced first. If the patient is being seen for follow-up after completed treatment for this condition, and the condition no longer exists, a follow-up code should be sequenced first, followed by the appropriate personal history and genetic susceptibility codes. If the purpose of the encounter is genetic counseling associated with procreative management, a code from subcategory V26.3, *Genetic counseling and testing*, should be assigned as the first-listed code, followed by a code from category V84. Additional codes should be assigned for any applicable family or personal history.

V86   *Estrogen receptor status*

Note: Categories V42-V46 and subcategories V49.6, V49.7 are for use only if there are no complications or malfunctions of the organ or tissue replaced, the amputation site or the equipment on which the patient is dependent.

History (of)

There are two types of history V codes: personal and family. Personal history codes explain a patient's past medical condition that no longer exists and is not receiving any treatment, but that has the potential for recurrence and, therefore, may require continued monitoring. The exceptions to this general rule are category V14, *Personal history of allergy to medicinal agents* and subcategory V15.0, *Allergy, other than to medicinal agents*. A person who has had an allergic episode to a substance or food in the past should always be considered allergic to the substance.

Family history codes are used when a patient has a family member(s) who has had a particular disease that causes the patient to be at higher risk of also contracting the disease.

Personal history codes may be used in conjunction with follow-up codes and family history codes may be used in conjunction with screening codes to explain the need for a test or procedure. History codes are also acceptable on any medical record regardless of the reason for visit. A history of an illness, even if no longer present, is important information that may alter the type of treatment ordered.

History V codes/categories:

V10   Personal history of malignant neoplasm

V12   Personal history of certain other diseases

V13   Personal history of other diseases

                Except: V13.4, *Personal history of arthritis*, and V13.6, *Personal history of congenital malformations*. These are lifelong conditions so are not true history codes.

V14   *Personal history of allergy to medicinal agents*

V15   *Other personal history presenting hazards to health*

        Except: V15.7, *Personal history of contraception.*

V16   *Family history of malignant neoplasm*

V17   *Family history of certain chronic disabling diseases*

V18   *Family history of certain other specific conditions*

V19   *Family history of other conditions*

Screening

Screening is the testing for disease or disease precursors in seemingly well individuals so that early detection and treatment can be provided for those who test positive for the disease. Screenings that are recommended for many subgroups in a population include: routine mammograms for women over 40 or a fecal occult blood test for everyone over 50, because the incidence of breast cancer and colon cancer in these subgroups is higher than in the general population; or an amniocentesis to rule out a fetal anomaly for pregnant women over 35, because the incidence of Down's syndrome is higher in older mothers.

The testing of a person to rule out or confirm a suspected diagnosis because the patient has some sign or symptom is a diagnostic examination, not a screening. In these cases, the sign or symptom is used to explain the reason for the test.

A screening code may be a first-listed code if the reason for the visit is specifically the screening exam. It may also be used as an additional code if the screening is done during an office visit for other health problems. A screening code is not necessary if the screening is inherent to a routine examination, such as a pap smear done during a routine pelvic examination.

Should a condition be discovered during the screening then the code for the condition may be assigned as an additional diagnosis.

The V code indicates that a screening exam is planned. A procedure code is required to confirm that the screening was performed.

Screening V codes/categories:

V28   *Antenatal screening*

V73-V82   *Special screening examinations*

Observation

There are two observation V code categories. They are for use in very limited circumstances when a person is being observed for a suspected condition that is ruled out. The observation codes are not for use if an injury or illness or any signs or symptoms related to the suspected condition are present. In such cases the diagnosis/symptom code is used with the corresponding E code to identify any external cause.

The observation codes are to be used as principal diagnosis only. The only exception to this is when the principal diagnosis is required to be a code from category V30, *Live born infant*. Then the V29 observation code is sequenced after the V30 code. Additional codes may be used in addition to the observation code but only if they are unrelated to the suspected condition being observed.

Observation V codes/categories:

V29   Observation and evaluation of newborns for suspected condition not found

> For the birth encounter, a code from category V30 should be sequenced before the V29 code.

V71   Observation and evaluation for suspected conditions not found

Aftercare

Aftercare visit codes cover situations when the initial treatment of a disease or injury has been performed and the patient requires continued care during the healing or recovery phase, or for the long-term consequences of the disease. The aftercare V code should not be used if treatment is directed at a current, acute disease or injury. The diagnosis code is to be used in these cases. Exceptions to this rule are codes V58.0, *Radiotherapy*, and codes from subcategory V58.1, *Encounter for chemotherapy and immunotherapy for neoplastic conditions*. These codes are to be first listed, followed by the diagnosis code when a patient's encounter is solely to receive radiation therapy or chemotherapy for the treatment of a neoplasm. Should a patient receive both chemotherapy and radiation therapy during the same encounter, codes V58.0 and V58.1 may be used together with either one being sequenced first.

The aftercare codes are generally first listed to explain the specific reason for the encounter. An aftercare code may be used as an additional code when some type of aftercare is provided in addition to the reason for admission and no diagnosis code is applicable. An example of this would be the closure of a colostomy during an encounter for treatment of another condition.

Certain aftercare V code categories need a secondary diagnosis code to describe the resolving condition or sequelae. For others, the condition is inherent in the code title. Additional V code aftercare category terms include, "fitting and adjustment," and "attention to artificial openings."

Status V codes may be used with aftercare V codes to indicate the nature of the aftercare. For example, code V45.81, *Aortocoronary bypass status*, may be used with code V58.73, *Aftercare following surgery of the circulatory system, NEC*, to indicate the surgery for which the aftercare is being performed. Also, a transplant status code may be used following code V58.44, *Aftercare following organ transplant*, to identify the organ transplanted. A status code should not be used when the aftercare code indicates the type of status, such as using V55.0, *Attention to tracheostomy* with V44.0, *Tracheostomy status*.

Aftercare V codes/categories:

V52	Fitting and adjustment of prosthetic device and implant
V53	Fitting and adjustment of other device
V54	Other orthopedic aftercare
V55	Attention to artificial openings
V56	Encounter for dialysis and dialysis catheter care
V57	Care involving the use of rehabilitation procedures
V58.0	Radiotherapy
V58.11	Encounter for antineoplastic chemotherapy
V58.12	Encounter for antineoplastic immunotherapy
V58.3X	Attention to surgical dressings and sutures
V58.41	Encounter for planned post-operative wound closure
V58.42	Aftercare following surgery for neoplasm
V58.43	Aftercare following surgery for injury and trauma
V58.44	Aftercare following organ transplant
V58.49	Other specified aftercare following surgery
V58.7X	Aftercare following surgery to specified body systems NEC
V58.81	Fitting and adjustment of vascular catheter
V58.82	Fitting and adjustment of non-vascular catheter NEC
V58.83	Encounter for therapeutic drug monitoring
V58.89	Other specified aftercare

Follow-Up

The follow-up codes are for use to explain continuing surveillance following completed treatment of a disease, condition, or injury. They infer that the condition has been fully treated and no longer exists. They should not be confused with aftercare codes which explain current treatment for a healing condition or its sequelae.

Follow-up codes may be used in conjunction with history codes to provide the full picture of the healed condition and its treatment. The follow-up code is sequenced first, followed by the history code.

A follow-up code may be used to explain repeated visits. Should a condition be found to have recurred on the follow-up visit, then the diagnosis code should be used in place of the follow-up code.

ICD-9-CM CODING FUNDAMENTALS

Follow-up V codes/categories:

V24   Postpartum care and evaluation

V67   Follow-up examination

Donor

Category V59 is the donor codes. They are for use for living individuals who are donating blood or other body tissue. These codes are only for individuals donating for others, not for self donations. They are not to identify cadaveric donations.

Counseling

Counseling V codes are for use for when a patient or family member receives assistance in the aftermath of an illness or injury, or when support is required in coping with family or social problems. They are not necessary for use in conjunction with a diagnosis code when the counseling component of care is considered integral to standard treatment.

Counseling V codes/categories:

V25.0   General counseling and advice for contraceptive management

V26.3   Genetic counseling and testing

V26.4   General counseling and advice for procreative management

V61   Other family circumstances

V65.1   Person consulting on behalf of another person

V65.3   Dietary surveillance and counseling

V65.4   Other counseling, not elsewhere classified

Obstetrics and Related Conditions

See the Obstetrics guidelines for further instruction on the use of these codes. V codes for pregnancy are for use in those circumstances when none of the problems or complications included in the codes from the Obstetrics chapter exist, such as a routine prenatal visit or postpartum care. V22.0, *Supervision of normal first pregnancy*, and V22.1, *Supervision of other normal pregnancy*, are always first listed and are not to be used with any other code from the Obstetrics chapter.

Category V27, *Outcome of delivery*, should be included on all maternal delivery records. It is always a secondary code. V codes for family planning (contraceptive) or procreative management and counseling should be included on an obstetric record either during the pregnancy or the postpartum stage, if applicable.

Obstetrics and related conditions V codes/categories:

V22   Normal pregnancy

V23	*Supervision of high-risk pregnancy*

> Except: V23.2, *Pregnancy with history of abortion.* Code 646.3, *Habitual aborter,* from the OB chapter is required to indicate a history of abortion during a pregnancy.

V24	*Postpartum care and evaluation*
V25	*Encounter for contraceptive management*

> Except: V25.0X (See counseling above)

V26	*Procreative management*

> Except: V26.5x, *Sterilization status,* V26.3 and V26.4 *(Counseling)*

V27	*Outcome of delivery*
V28	*Antenatal screening*

Newborn, Infant and Child

See the Newborn Guidelines for further instruction on the use of these codes.

Newborn V codes/categories:

V20	*Health supervision of infant or child*
V29	*Observation and evaluation of newborns for suspected condition not found*
V30-V39	*Liveborn infant according to type of birth*

Routine and Administrative Examinations

The V codes allow for the description of encounters for routine examinations, such as a general check-up, or examinations for administrative purposes, such as a pre-employment physical. The codes are for use as first-listed codes only and are not to be used if the examination is for diagnosis of a suspected condition or for treatment purposes. In such cases the diagnosis code is used. During a routine exam, should a diagnosis or condition be discovered, it should be coded as an additional code. Pre-existing and chronic conditions, and history codes may also be included as additional codes as long as the examination is for administrative purposes and not focused on any particular condition.

Pre-operative examination V codes are for use only in those situations when a patient is being cleared for surgery and no treatment is given.

Routine and administrative examinations V codes/categories:

V20.2	*Routine infant or child health check*

> Any injections given should have a corresponding procedure code.

V70	*General medical examination*
V72	*Special investigations and examinations* Except V72.5 and V72.6

Miscellaneous V Codes

The miscellaneous V codes capture a number of other health care encounters that do not fall into one of the other categories. Certain of these codes identify the reason for the encounter, others are for use as additional codes which provide useful information on circumstances which may affect a patient's care and treatment.

For encounters specifically for prophylactic removal of breasts, ovaries, or another organ due to a genetic susceptibility to cancer or a family history of cancer, the principal or first listed code should be a code from subcategory V50.4, *Prophylactic organ removal*, followed by the appropriate genetic susceptibility code and the appropriate family history code.

If the patient has a malignancy of one site and is having prophylactic removal at another site to prevent either a new primary malignancy or metastatic disease, a code for the malignancy should also be assigned in addition to a code from subcategory V50.4. A V50.4 code should not be assigned if the patient is having organ removal for treatment of a malignancy, such as the removal of the testes for the treatment of prostate cancer.

Miscellaneous V codes/categories:

V07	Need for isolation and other prophylactic measures
V50	Elective surgery for purposes other than remedying health states
V58.5	Orthodontics
V60	Housing, household, and economic circumstances
V62	Other psychosocial circumstances
V63	Unavailability of other medical facilities for care
V64	Persons encountering health services for specific procedures, not carried out
V66	Convalescence and palliative care
V68	Encounters for administrative purposes
V69	Problems related to lifestyle
V85	Body mass index

Nonspecific V Codes

Certain V codes are so non-specific, or potentially redundant with other codes in the classification, that there can be little justification for their use in the inpatient setting. Their use in the outpatient setting should be limited to those instances when there is no further documentation to permit more precise coding. Otherwise, any sign or symptom, or any other reason for the visit which is captured in another code, should be used instead.

ICD-9-CM CODING FUNDAMENTALS

Nonspecific V codes/categories:

V11   Personal history of mental disorder

                A code from the mental disorders chapter, with an in remission fifth-digit, should be used.

V13.4	Personal history of arthritis
V13.69	Personal history of congenital malformations
V13.9	Personal history of unspecified disease
V15.7	Personal history of contraception
V40	Mental and behavioral problems
V41	Problems with special senses and other special functions
V46.9	Unspecified machine dependence
V47	Other problems with internal organs
V48	Problems with head, neck, and trunk
V49.0	Deficiencies of limbs
V49.1	Mechanical problems with limbs
V49.2	Motor problems with limbs
V49.3	Sensory problems with limbs
V49.4	Disfigurements in limbs
V49.5	Other problems with limbs
V49.9	Unspecified condition influencing health status
V51	Aftercare involving the use of plastic surgery
V58.2	Blood transfusion, without reported diagnosis
V58.5	Orthodontics
V58.9	Unspecified aftercare
V72.9	Unspecified examination

V Code Coding Example

Colostomy status with colostomy malfunction

    569.60 Colostomy and enterostomy complications, unspecified

The code V44.3 *Artificial opening status, colostomy* would not be used in this case because of the complication.

V CODE TABLE

First Listed Only

V Codes/Categories/Subcategories That Are Only Acceptable as Principal/First Listed

Codes:

V22.0	Supervision of normal first pregnancy
V22.1	Supervision of other normal pregnancy
V46.12	Encounter for respirator dependence during power failure
V46.13	Encounter for weaning from respirator [ventilator]
V56.0	Extracorporeal dialysis
V58.0	Radiotherapy

> V58.0 and V58.11 may be used together on a record with either one being sequenced first, when a patient receives both chemotherapy and radiation therapy during the same encounter.

V58.11	Encounter for antineoplastic chemotherapy

> V58.0 and V58.11 may be used together on a record with either one being sequenced first, when a patient receives both chemotherapy and radiation therapy during the same encounter.

V58.12	Encounter for antineoplastic immunotherapy

Categories/Subcategories:

V20	Health supervision of infant or child
V24	Postpartum care and examination
V29	Observation and evaluation of newborns for suspected condition not found

> Exception: A code from V30-V39 may be sequenced before V29 if it is the newborn record.

V30-V39	Liveborn infants according to type of birth
V57	Care involving use of rehabilitation procedures
V59	Donors
V66	Convalescence and palliative care

> Exception: V66.7 *Palliative care*

V68	Encounters for administrative purposes

V70	General medical examination
	Exception: V70.7 *Examination of participant in clinical trial*
V71	Observation and evaluation for suspected conditions not found

First or Additional

V Codes/Categories/Subcategories That May Be Either Principal/First-Listed or Additional Codes

Codes:

V15.88	History of fall
V43.22	Fully implantable artificial heart status
V46.14	Mechanical complication of respiratory [ventilator]
V49.81	Asymptomatic postmenopausal status (age-related) (natural)
V49.84	Bed confinement status
V49.89	Other specified conditions influencing health status
V70.7	Examination of participant in clinical trial

Categories/Subcategories:

V01	Contact with or exposure to communicable diseases
V02	Carrier or suspected carrier of infectious diseases
V03-V06	Need for prophylactic vaccination and inoculations
V07	Need for isolation and other prophylactic measures
V08	Asymptomatic HIV infection status
V10	Personal history of malignant neoplasm
V12	Personal history of certain other diseases
V13	Personal history of other diseases
	Exceptions: V13.4 *Personal history of arthritis* V13.6X *Congenital malformations* V13.9 *Personal history of unspecified disease*
V16-V19	Family history of disease
V23	Supervision of high-risk pregnancy
V25	Encounter for contraceptive management

ICD-9-CM CODING FUNDAMENTALS

V26	*Procreative management*
	Exception: V26.5 *Sterilization status*
V28	*Encounter for antenatal screening of mother*
V45.7	*Acquired absence of organ*
V49.6X	*Upper limb amputation status*
V49.7X	*Lower limb amputation status*
V50	*Elective surgery for purposes other than remedying health states*
V52	*Fitting and adjustment of prosthetic device and implant*
V53	*Fitting and adjustment of other device*
V54	*Other orthopedic aftercare*
V55	*Attention to artificial openings*
V56	*Encounter for dialysis and dialysis catheter care*
	Exception: V56.0 *Extracorporeal dialysis*
V58.3X	*Attention to dressings and sutures*
V58.4X	*Other aftercare following surgery*
V58.7X	*Aftercare following surgery to specified body systems, not elsewhere classified*
V58.8X	*Other specified procedures and aftercare*
V61	*Other family circumstances*
V63	*Unavailability of other medical facilities for care*
V65	*Other persons seeking consultation without complaint or sickness*
V67	*Follow-up examination*
V69	*Problems related to lifestyle*
V72	*Special investigations and examinations*
	Exception: V72.9 *Unspecified examination*
V73-V82	*Special screening examinations*
V83	*Genetic carrier status*

Additional Only

V Codes/Categories/Subcategories That May Only Be Used As Additional Codes, Not As Principal/First Listed

Codes:

V13.61	Personal history of hypospadias
V22.2	Pregnancy state, incidental
V46.11	Dependence on respirator, status
V49.82	Dental sealant status
V49.83	Awaiting organ transplant status
V66.7	Palliative care

Categories/Subcategories:

V09	Infection with drug-resistant microorganisms
V14	Personal history of allergy to medicinal agents
V15	Other personal history presenting hazards to health

> Exception:
> V15.7 *Personal history of contraception*
> V15.88 *History of fall*

V21	Constitutional states in development
V26.5X	Sterilization status
V27	Outcome of delivery
V42	Organ or tissue replaced by transplant
V43	Organ or tissue replaced by other means

> Exception: V43.22 *Fully implantable artificial heart status*

V44	Artificial opening status
V45	Other postsurgical states

> Exception: Subcategory V45.7 *Acquired absence of organ*

V46	Other dependence on machines

> Exceptions:
> V46.12 *Encounter for respirator dependence during power failure*
> V46.13 *Encounter for weaning from respirator [ventilator]*
> V46.14 *Mechanical complication of respirator [ventilator]*
> V46.9x *Unspecified machine dependence*

V58.6X	Long-term (current) drug use
V60	Housing, household, and economic circumstances
V62	Other psychosocial circumstances
V64	Persons encountering health services for specified procedure, not carried out
V84	Genetic susceptibility to disease
V85	Body mass index
V86	Estrogen receptor status

E CODES: SUPPLEMENTAL CLASSIFICATION OF EXTERNAL CAUSES OF INJURY AND POISONING

E-codes permit the classification of environmental events, circumstances and conditions as the cause of injury, poisoning and other adverse effects. The use of E-codes, together with the code identifying the injury or condition, provides additional information of particular concern to industrial medicine, insurance carriers, national safety programs and public health agencies. External causes of injury and poisoning codes (E codes) are intended to provide data for injury research and evaluation of injury prevention strategies. E codes capture how the injury or poisoning happened (cause), the intent (unintentional or accidental; or intentional, such as suicide or assault), and the place where the event occurred.

The following guidelines are provided for those who are currently collecting E codes in order that there will be standardization in the process. If your institution plans to begin collecting E codes, these guidelines are to be applied. The use of E codes is supplemental to the application of ICD-9-CM diagnosis codes. E codes are never to be recorded as a principal diagnosis (first-listed in non-inpatient setting) and are not required for reporting to CMS.

These guidelines apply for the coding and collection of E codes from records in hospitals, outpatient clinics, emergency departments, other ambulatory care settings and physician offices, and nonacute care settings, except when other specific guidelines apply.

Some major categories of E codes include:

- transport accidents;
- poisoning and adverse effects of drugs, medicinal substances and biologicals;
- accidental falls;
- accidents caused by fire and flames;
- accidents due to natural and environmental factors;
- late effects of accidents, assaults or self injury;
- assaults or purposely inflicted injury;
- suicide or self inflicted injury.

General E Code Coding Guidelines

1. An E code may be used with any code in the range of 001-V84.8, which indicates an injury, poisoning, or adverse effect due to an external cause.

2. Assign the appropriate E code for all initial treatments of an injury, poisoning, or adverse effect of drugs, not for subsequent treatment.

3. Use the full range of E codes to completely describe the cause, the intent and the place of occurrence, if applicable, for all injuries, poisonings and adverse effects of drugs.

4. Assign as many E codes as necessary to fully explain each cause. If only one E code can be recorded, assign the E code most related to the principal diagnosis.

5. The selection of the appropriate E code is guided by the Index to External Causes, which is located after the alphabetical index to diseases, and by "Inclusion" and "Exclusion" notes in the Tabular List.

6. An E code can never be a principal (first-listed) diagnosis.

7. An external cause code(s) is not appropriate with a code from subcategory 995.9, *Systemic inflammatory response syndrome*, unless the patient also has an injury, poisoning or adverse effect of drugs.

Place of Occurrence Guideline

Use an additional code from category E849 to indicate the *Place of Occurrence* for injuries and poisonings. This describes the place where the event occurred and not the patient's activity at the time of the event.

Note: Do not use E849.9 if the place of occurrence is not stated.

Adverse Effects of Drugs, Medicinal and Biological Substances Guidelines

1. Do not code directly from the Table of Drugs and Chemicals. Always refer back to the Tabular List.

2. Use as many codes as necessary to describe completely all drugs, medicinal or biological substances.

3. If the same E code would describe the causative agent for more than one adverse reaction, assign the code only once.

4. If two or more drugs, medicinal or biological substances are reported, code each individually unless the combination code is listed in the Table of Drugs and Chemicals. In that case, assign the E code for the combination.

5. When a reaction results from the interaction of a drug(s) and alcohol, use poisoning codes and E codes for both.

6. If the reporting format limits the number of E codes that can be used in reporting clinical data, code the one most related to the principal diagnosis. Include at least one from each category (cause, intent, place) if possible.

If there are different fourth-digit codes in the same three-digit category, use the code for *Other specified* of that category. If there is no *Other specified* code in that category, use the appropriate *Unspecified* code in that category.

If the codes are in different three-digit categories, assign the appropriate E code for other multiple drugs and medicinal substances.

7. Codes from the E930-E949 series must be used to identify the causative substance for an adverse effect of drug, medicinal and biological substances, correctly prescribed and properly administered. The effect, such as tachycardia, delirium, gastrointestinal hemorrhaging, vomiting, hypokalemia, hepatitis, renal failure, or respiratory failure, etc., is coded and followed by the appropriate code from the E930-E949 series.

Multiple Cause Coding Guidelines

If two or more events cause separate injuries, an E code should be assigned for each cause. The first-listed E code will be selected in the following order:

1. E codes for child and adult abuse take priority over all other E codes—see Child and Adult Abuse Guidelines below.

2. E codes for terrorism events take priority over all other E codes except child and adult abuse.

3. E codes for cataclysmic events take priority over all other E codes except child and adult abuse, and terrorism.

4. E codes for transport accidents take priority over all other E codes except cataclysmic events, and child and adult abuse, and terrorism.

5. The first-listed E code should correspond to the cause of the most serious diagnosis due to an assault, accident or self-harm, following the order of hierarchy listed above.

Child and Adult Abuse Guidelines

1. When the cause of an injury or neglect is intentional child or adult abuse, the first-listed E code should be assigned from categories E960-E969, *Homicide and injury purposely inflicted by other persons*, (except category E967). An E code from category E967, *Perpetrator of child and adult abuse*, should be added as an additional code to identify the perpetrator, if known.

2. In cases of neglect when the intent is determined to be accidental, E code E904.0, *Abandonment or neglect of infants and helpless persons*, should be the first listed E code.

Unknown or Suspected Intent Guidelines

1. If the intent (accident, self-harm, assault) of the cause of an injury or poisoning is unknown or unspecified, code the intent as undetermined E980-E989.

2. If the intent (accident, self-harm, assault) of the cause of an injury or poisoning is questionable, probable or suspected, code the intent as undetermined E980-E989.

Undetermined Cause Guidelines

When the intent of an injury or poisoning is known, but the cause is unknown, use codes: E928.9, *Unspecified accident*; E958.9, *Suicide and self-inflicted injury by unspecified means*; or E968.9, *Assault by unspecified means*.

These E codes should rarely be used, since the documentation in the medical record, in inpatient, outpatient and other setting, should normally provide sufficient detail to determine the cause of the injury.

Late Effects of External Cause Guidelines

1. Late effect E codes exist for injuries and poisonings but not for adverse effects of drugs, misadventures and surgical complications.

2. A late effect E code (E929, E959, E969, E977, E989, or E999.1) should be used with any report of a late effect or sequela resulting from a previous injury or poisoning (905-909).

3. A late effect E code should never be used with a related current "nature of injury" code.

4. Use a late effect E code for subsequent visits when a late effect of the initial injury or poisoning is being treated. There is no late effect E code for adverse effects of drugs. Do not use a late effect E code for subsequent visits for follow-up care (e.g., to assess healing, to receive rehabilitative therapy) of the injury or poisoning when no late effect of the injury has been documented.

Misadventures and Complications of Care Guidelines

1. Assign a code in the range of E870-E876 if misadventures are stated by the physician.

2. Assign a code in the range of E878-E879 if the physician attributes an abnormal reaction or later complication to a surgical or medical procedure, but does not mention misadventure at the time of the procedure as the cause of the reaction.

Terrorism Guidelines

1. When the cause of an injury is identified by the Federal Government (FBI) as terrorism, the first-listed E code should be from category E979, *Terrorism*. The definition of terrorism employed by the FBI is found at the inclusion note at E979. The terrorism E code is the only E code that should be assigned. Additional E codes from the assault categories should not be assigned.

2. When the cause of an injury is only *suspected* to be the result of terrorism, a code from category E979 should *not* be assigned. Assign an E code based on circumstances in the documentation of intent and mechanism.

3. Assign code E979.9, *Terrorism, secondary effects*, for conditions occurring subsequent to the terrorist event. This code should not be assigned for conditions that are due to the initial terrorist act.

4. For statistical purposes, these codes will be tabulated within the category for assault, expanding the current category from E960-E969 to include E979 and E999.1.

Examples Using E Codes

When using E-codes, search the Alphabetic Index (Volume 2) for the main term identifying the cause such as "accident," "fire," "shooting," "fall," or "collision." To find the E-code for an adverse reaction to surgical or medical treatment, use the main term "reaction."

Coding Example

Burns to right arm, occurred while burning trash

943.00 Burn of upper limb, except wrist and hand, unspecified degree

E897 Accident caused by controlled fire not in building or structure

E-codes are important for providing the details of an accident to an insurance carrier to enable them to issue faster and more accurate reimbursement. Most insurance carriers want to be sure they reimburse only for services covered under their policy and not for services covered under worker's compensation, automobile or homeowner's insurance. A clear understanding of the circumstances will eliminate questions from the insurance carrier which cause delays in reimbursements.

Coding Example

Fractured ribs due to fall from ladder at home

807.00 Fracture of ribs, closed, unspecified

E881.0 Fall from ladder

E849.0 Place of occurrence, home

Using the above E-codes to provide important information regarding the circumstances of the injury to the insurance carrier eliminates any doubt about the insurer's responsibility for coverage. When using E-codes always list the E-codes as secondary or supplemental to the code(s) describing the injury.

PRINCIPAL AND ADDITIONAL DIAGNOSIS(ES): GUIDELINES FOR INPATIENT, SHORT-TERM, ACUTE CARE HOSPITAL RECORDS

Selecting Principal Diagnoses

The circumstances of inpatient admission always govern the selection of principal diagnosis. The principal diagnosis is defined in the Uniform Hospital Discharge Data Set (UHDDS) as that condition established after study to be chiefly responsible for occasioning the admission of the patient to the hospital for care.

The UHDDS definitions are used by all non-outpatient settings including acute care, short term, long term care and psychiatric hospitals; home health agencies; rehab facilities; and nursing homes. In determining principal diagnosis, the coding conventions in the ICD-9-CM, Volumes I and II take precedence over these official coding guidelines. (See Section IA).

The importance of consistent, complete documentation in the medical record cannot be overemphasized. Without such documentation the application of all coding guidelines is a difficult, if not impossible, task.

1. Codes for symptoms, signs, and ill-defined conditions.

    Codes for symptoms, signs, and ill-defined conditions from Chapter 16 are not to be used as principal diagnosis when a related definitive diagnosis has been established.

2. Two or more interrelated conditions, each potentially meeting the definition for principal diagnosis.

    When there are two or more interrelated conditions (such as diseases in the same ICD-9-CM chapter or manifestations characteristically associated with a certain disease) potentially meeting the definition of principal diagnosis, either condition may be sequenced first, unless the circumstances of the admission, the therapy provided, the Tabular List, or the Alphabetic Index indicate otherwise.

3. Two or more diagnoses that equally meet the definition for principal diagnosis.

    In the unusual instance when two or more diagnoses equally meet the criteria for principal diagnosis as determined by the circumstances of admission, diagnostic workup and/or therapy provided, and the Alphabetic Index, Tabular List, or other coding guideline does not provide sequencing direction, any one of the diagnoses may be sequenced first.

4. Two or more comparative or contrasting conditions.

    In those rare instances when two or more contrasting or comparative diagnoses are documented as either/or (or similar terminology), they are coded as if the diagnoses were confirmed. The diagnoses are sequenced according to the circumstances of the admission. If no further determination can be made as to which diagnosis should be principal, either diagnosis may be sequenced first.

ICD-9-CM CODING FUNDAMENTALS

5. Symptom(s) followed by contrasting/comparative diagnoses.

   When a symptom(s) is followed by contrasting/comparative diagnoses, the symptom code is sequenced first. All the contrasting/comparative diagnoses should be coded as additional diagnoses.

6. Original treatment plan not carried out.

   Sequence as the principal diagnosis the condition, which after study occasioned the admission to the hospital, even though treatment may not have been carried out due to unforeseen circumstances.

7. Complications of surgery and other medical care.

   When the admission is for treatment of a complication resulting from surgery or other medical care, the complication code is sequenced as the principal diagnosis. If the complication is classified to the 996-999 series and the code lacks the necessary specificity in describing the complication, an additional code for the specific complication may be assigned.

8. Uncertain Diagnosis.

   If the diagnosis documented at the time of discharge is qualified as "probable," "possible," "suspected," "likely," "questionable," or "still to be ruled out," code the condition as if it existed or was established. The basis for these guidelines are the diagnostic workup, arrangements for further workup or observation, and initial therapeutic approach that correspond the closest to the established diagnosis. Note: This guideline is applicable only to short-term, acute, long-term care and psychiatric hospitals.

9. Admission from Observation Unit

   A. Admission Following Medical Observation

   When a patient is admitted to an observation unit for a medical condition, which either worsens or does not improve, and is subsequently admitted as an inpatient of the same hospital for this same medical condition, the principal diagnosis would be the medical condition which led to the hospital admission.

   B. Admission Following Post-Operative Observation

   When a patient is admitted to an observation unit to monitor a condition (or complication) that develops following outpatient surgery, and then is subsequently admitted as an inpatient of the same hospital, hospitals should apply the Uniform Hospital Discharge Data Set (UHDDS) definition of principal diagnosis as "that condition established after study to be chiefly responsible for occasioning the admission of the patient to the hospital for care."

10. Admission from Outpatient Surgery

    When a patient receives surgery in the hospital's outpatient surgery department and is subsequently admitted for continuing inpatient care at the same hospital, the following guidelines should be followed in selecting the principal diagnosis for the inpatient admission:

- If the reason for the inpatient admission is a complication, assign the complication as the principal diagnosis.

- If no complication or other condition is documented as the reason for the inpatient admission, assign the reason for the outpatient surgery as the principal diagnosis.

- If the reason for the inpatient admission is another condition unrelated to the surgery, assign the unrelated condition as the principal diagnosis.

Rules For Reporting Additional Diagnoses

For reporting purposes, the definition for "other diagnoses" is interpreted as additional conditions that affect patient care in terms of requiring: clinical evaluation; or therapeutic treatment; or diagnostic procedures; or extended length of hospital stay; or increased nursing care and/or monitoring.

The UHDDS item #11-b defines *Other Diagnoses* as "all conditions that coexist at the time of admission, that develop subsequently, or that affect the treatment received and/or the length of stay. Diagnoses that relate to an earlier episode which have no bearing on the current hospital stay are to be excluded."

UHDDS definitions apply to all non-outpatient settings including: acute care, short term, long term care and psychiatric hospitals; home health agencies; rehab facilities; and nursing homes. The UHDDS definitions are used by acute care short-term and long-term care hospitals to report inpatient data elements in a standardized manner.

The following guidelines are to be applied in designating other diagnoses when neither the Alphabetic Index nor the Tabular List in ICD-9-CM provide direction. The listing of the diagnoses in the patient record is the responsibility of the attending physician.

1. Previous conditions

    If the physician has included a diagnosis in the final diagnostic statement, such as the discharge summary or the face sheet, it should ordinarily be coded. Some physicians include in the diagnostic statement: resolved conditions or diagnoses and status-post procedures from previous admission that have no bearing on the current stay. Such conditions are not to be reported and are coded only if required by hospital policy.

    However, history codes (V10-V19) may be used as secondary codes if the historical condition or family history has an impact on current care or if it influences treatment.

2. Abnormal findings

    Abnormal findings (laboratory, x-ray, pathologic, and other diagnostic results) are not coded and reported unless the physician indicates their clinical significance. If the findings are outside the normal range and the attending physician has ordered other tests to evaluate the condition or prescribed treatment, it is appropriate to ask the physician whether the abnormal finding should be added.

    Note: This differs from the coding practices in the outpatient setting for coding encounters for diagnostic tests that have been interpreted by a physician.

3. Uncertain Diagnosis

   If the diagnosis documented at the time of discharge is qualified as probable, possible, suspected, likely, questionable, or still to be ruled out, code the condition as if it existed or was established. The basis for these guidelines are the diagnostic workup, arrangements for further workup or observation, and initial therapeutic approach that correspond most closely with the established diagnosis.

DIAGNOSTIC CODING AND REPORTING GUIDELINES FOR OUTPATIENT SERVICES

These coding guidelines for outpatient diagnoses have been approved for use by hospitals/physicians in coding and reporting hospital-based outpatient services and physician office visits.

Information about the use of certain abbreviations, punctuation, symbols, and other conventions used in the ICD-9-CM Tabular List (code numbers and titles), can be found under Conventions Used in the Tabular List. Information about the correct sequence to use in finding a code is also described previously in Section I.

The terms "encounter" and "visit" are often used interchangeably in describing outpatient service contacts and, therefore, appear together in these guidelines without distinguishing one from the other.

Though the conventions and general guidelines apply to all settings, coding guidelines for outpatient and physician reporting of diagnoses will vary in a number of instances from those for inpatient/hospital diagnoses, recognizing that:

   The Uniform Hospital Discharge Data Set (UHDDS) definition of "principal diagnosis" applies only to inpatients in acute, short-term, general and long-term care and psychiatric hospitals.

   Coding guidelines for inconclusive diagnoses (probable, suspected, rule out, etc.) were developed for inpatient reporting and do not apply to outpatients.

1. Selection of first-listed condition

   In the outpatient setting, the term "first-listed diagnosis" is used in lieu of "principal diagnosis."

   In determining the first-listed diagnosis, the coding conventions of ICD-9-CM —as well as the general and disease-specific guidelines—take precedence over the outpatient guidelines.

   Diagnoses often are not established at the time of the initial encounter/visit. It may take two or more visits before the diagnosis is confirmed.

   The most critical rule involves beginning the search for the correct code assignment through the Alphabetic Index. Never begin searching initially in the Tabular List as this will lead to coding errors.

2. The appropriate code or codes from 001.0 through V84.8 must be used to identify diagnoses, symptoms, conditions, problems, complaints, or other reason(s) for the encounter/visit.

ICD-9-CM CODING FUNDAMENTALS

3. For accurate reporting of ICD-9-CM diagnosis codes, the documentation should describe the patient's condition using terminology which includes specific diagnoses as well as symptoms, problems, or reasons for the encounter. There are ICD-9-CM codes to describe all of these.

4. The selection of codes 001.0 through 999.9 will frequently be used to describe the reason for the encounter. These codes are from the section of ICD-9-CM for the classification of diseases and injuries (e.g. infectious and parasitic diseases; neoplasms; symptoms, signs, and ill-defined conditions, etc.).

5. Codes that describe symptoms and signs, as opposed to diagnoses, are acceptable for reporting purposes when a diagnosis has not been established (confirmed) by the physician. Chapter 16 of ICD-9-CM, *Symptoms, Signs, and Ill-defined Conditions* (codes 780.0 to 799.9) contain many, but not all codes for symptoms.

6. ICD-9-CM provides codes to deal with encounters for circumstances other than a disease or injury. *The Supplementary Classification of Factors Influencing Health Status and Contact with Health Services* (V01.0-V83.89) is provided to deal with occasions when circumstances other than a disease or injury are recorded as diagnosis or problems.

7. Level of Detail in Coding

   a. ICD-9-CM is composed of codes with either 3, 4, or 5 digits. Codes with three digits are included in ICD-9-CM as the heading of a category of codes that may be further subdivided by the use of fourth and/or fifth digits, which provide greater specificity.

   b. A three-digit code is to be used only if it is not further subdivided. Where fourth-digit subcategories and/or fifth-digit subclassifications are provided, they must be assigned. A code is invalid if it has not been coded to the full number of digits required for that code.

8. List first the ICD-9-CM code for the diagnosis, condition, problem, or other reason for encounter/visit shown in the medical record to be chiefly responsible for the services provided. List additional codes that describe any coexisting conditions. In some cases the first-listed diagnosis may be a symptom when a diagnosis has not been established (confirmed) by the physician.

9. Do not code diagnoses documented as probable, suspected, questionable, rule out, or working diagnosis. Rather, code the condition(s) to the highest degree of certainty for that encounter/visit, such as symptoms, signs, abnormal test results, or other reason for the visit.

   Note: This differs from the coding practices used by hospital medical record departments for coding the diagnosis of acute care, short-term hospital inpatients.

10. Chronic diseases treated on an ongoing basis may be coded and reported as many times as the patient receives treatment and care for the condition(s).

11. Code all documented conditions that coexist at the time of the encounter/visit, and require or affect patient care treatment or management. Do not code conditions that were previously treated and no longer exist. However, history codes (V10-V19) may be used as secondary codes if the historical condition or family history has an impact on current care or influences treatment.

ICD-9-CM CODING FUNDAMENTALS

12. For patients receiving *diagnostic* services only during an encounter/visit, sequence first the diagnosis, condition, problem, or other reason for encounter/visit shown in the medical record to be chiefly responsible for the outpatient services provided during the encounter/visit. Codes for other diagnoses (e.g., chronic conditions) may be sequenced as additional diagnoses.

    For encounters for routine laboratory/radiology testing in the absence of any signs, symptoms, or associated diagnosis, assign V72.5 and V72.6. If routine testing is performed during the same encounter as a test to evaluate a sign, symptom, or diagnosis, it is appropriate to assign both the V code and the code describing the reason for the non-routine test.

    For outpatient encounters for diagnostic tests that have been interpreted by a physician, and the final report is available at the time of coding, code any confirmed or definitive diagnosis(es) documented in the interpretation. Do not code related signs and symptoms as additional diagnoses.

    Note: This differs from the coding practice in the hospital inpatient setting regarding abnormal findings on test results.

13. For patients receiving *therapeutic* services only during an encounter/visit, sequence first the diagnosis, condition, problem, or other reason for encounter/visit shown in the medical record to be chiefly responsible for the outpatient services provided during the encounter/visit. Codes for other diagnoses (e.g., chronic conditions) may be sequenced as additional diagnoses.

    The only exception to this rule is that when the primary reason for the admission/encounter is chemotherapy, radiation therapy, or rehabilitation, the appropriate V code for the service is listed first, and the diagnosis or problem for which the service is being performed listed second.

14. For patient's receiving preoperative evaluations only, sequence a code from category V72.8, *Other specified examinations*, to describe the pre-op consultations. Assign a code for the condition to describe the reason for the surgery as an additional diagnosis. Code also any findings related to the pre-op evaluation.

15. For ambulatory surgery, code the diagnosis for which the surgery was performed. If the postoperative diagnosis is known to be different from the preoperative diagnosis at the time the diagnosis is confirmed, select the postoperative diagnosis for coding, since it is the most definitive.

16. For routine outpatient prenatal visits when no complications are present, codes V22.0, *Supervision of normal first pregnancy*, and V22.1, *Supervision of other normal pregnancy*, should be used as principal diagnoses. These codes should not be used in conjunction with Chapter 11 *Pregnancy, Childbirth and the Puerperium* codes.

ICD-9-CM CODING FUNDAMENTALS

Anatomical Illustrations

A fundamental knowledge and understanding of basic human anatomy and physiology is a prerequisite for accurate diagnosis coding. While a comprehensive treatment of anatomy and physiology is beyond the scope of this text, the large scale, full color anatomical illustrations on the following pages are designed to facilitate the diagnosis coding process for both beginning and experienced coders.

The illustrations provide an anatomical perspective of diagnosis coding by providing a side-by-side view of the major systems of the human body and a corresponding list of the most common diagnoses categories used to support medical, surgical and diagnostic services performed on the illustrated system.

The diagnostic categories listed on the left facing page of each anatomical illustration are three-digit categories and may not be used for coding. These categories are provided as "pointers" to the appropriate section of the ICD-9-CM Volume 1 where the complete listings, including 4th and 5th digits if appropriate, may be found.

Plate	System	Page
Plate 1	Skin and subcutaneous tissue — male	99
Plate 2	Skin and subcutaneous tissue — female	101
Plate 3	Skin and subcutaneous tissue — female breast	103
Plate 4	Muscular system and connective tissue — anterior view	105
Plate 5	Muscular system and connective tissue — posterior view	107
Plate 6	Shoulder and elbow	109
Plate 7	Hand and wrist	111
Plate 8	Hip and knee	113
Plate 9	Foot and ankle	115
Plate 10	Skeletal system — anterior view	117
Plate 11	Skeletal system — posterior view	119
Plate 12	Vertebral column	121
Plate 13	Respiratory system	123
Plate 14	Heart and pericardium	125
Plate 15	Circulatory system	127
Plate 16	Digestive system	129
Plate 17	Genitourinary system	131
Plate 18	Male reproductive system	133
Plate 19	Female reproductive system	135
Plate 20	Female reproductive system — pregnancy, lateral view	137
Plate 21	Brain	139
Plate 22	Nervous system	141
Plate 23	Right eye — horizontal section	143
Plate 24	The Ear	145

PLATE 1. SKIN AND SUBCUTANEOUS TISSUE — MALE

Viral diseases accompanied by exanthem	050-057
Neoplasms	
Malignant melanoma of skin	172
Other malignant neoplasm of skin	173
Malignant neoplasm of male breast	175
Kaposi's sarcoma	176
Benign neoplasm of skin	216
Carcinoma in situ of skin	232
Infections of skin and subcutaneous tissue	
Carbuncle and furuncle	680
Cellulitis and abscess of finger and toe	681
Other cellulitis and abscess	682
Acute lymphadenitis	683
Impetigo	684
Pilonidal cyst	685
Other local infections of skin and subcutaneous tissue	686
Other inflammatory conditions of skin and subcutaneous tissue	
Erythematosquamous dermatosis	690
Atopic dermatitis and related conditions	691
Contact dermatitis and other eczema	692
Dermatitis due to substances taken internally	693
Bullous dermatoses	694
Erythematous conditions	695
Psoriasis and similar disorders	696
Lichen	697
Pruritus and related conditions	698
Other diseases of skin and subcutaneous tissue	
Corns and callosities	700
Other hypertrophic and atrophic conditions of skin	701
Diseases of nail	703
Diseases of hair and hair follicles	704
Disorders of sweat glands	705
Diseases of sebaceous glands	706
Chronic ulcer of skin	707
Urticaria	708
Other disorders of skin and subcutaneous tissue	709
Symptoms involving skin and other integumentary tissue	782
Symptoms, signs and ill-defined conditions	780-799

ANATOMICAL ILLUSTRATIONS

PLATE 2. SKIN AND SUBCUTANEOUS TISSUE — FEMALE

Viral diseases accompanied by exanthem	050-057

Neoplasms

Malignant melanoma of skin	172
Other malignant neoplasm of skin	173
Malignant neoplasm of female breast	174
Kaposi's sarcoma	176
Benign neoplasm of skin	216
Carcinoma in situ of skin	232

Infections of skin and subcutaneous tissue

Carbuncle and furuncle	680
Cellulitis and abscess of finger and toe	681
Other cellulitis and abscess	682
Acute lymphadenitis	683
Impetigo	684
Pilonidal cyst	685
Other local infections of skin and subcutaneous tissue	686

Other inflammatory conditions of skin and subcutaneous tissue

Erythematosquamous dermatosis	690
Atopic dermatitis and related conditions	691
Contact dermatitis and other eczema	692
Dermatitis due to substances taken internally	693
Bullous dermatoses	694
Erythematous conditions	695
Psoriasis and similar disorders	696
Lichen	697
Pruritus and related conditions	698

Other diseases of skin and subcutaneous tissue

Corns and callosities	700
Other hypertrophic and atrophic conditions of skin	701
Other dermatoses	702
Diseases of nail	703
Diseases of hair and hair follicles	704
Disorders of sweat glands	705
Diseases of sebaceous glands	706
Chronic ulcer of skin	707
Urticaria	708
Other disorders of skin and subcutaneous tissue	709
Symptoms involving skin and other integumentary tissue	782

Symptoms, signs and ill-defined conditions	780-799

ANATOMICAL ILLUSTRATIONS

PLATE 3. FEMALE BREAST

Malignant neoplasm of bone, connective tissue, skin, and breast
Malignant neoplasm of female breast 174
Benign neoplasm of breast 217
Carcinoma in situ of breast and genitourinary system 233

Disorders of breast
Benign mammary dysplasias 610
Other disorders of breast 611

Complications of the puerperium
Infections of the breast and nipple associated with childbirth 675
Other disorders of the breast associated with childbirth,
    and disorders of lactation 676

Symptoms, signs and ill-defined conditions 780-799

Persons without reported diagnosis encountered during examination
Observation and evaluation for suspected conditions not found V71
Special screening for malignant neoplasms V76

ANATOMICAL ILLUSTRATIONS

Female Breast

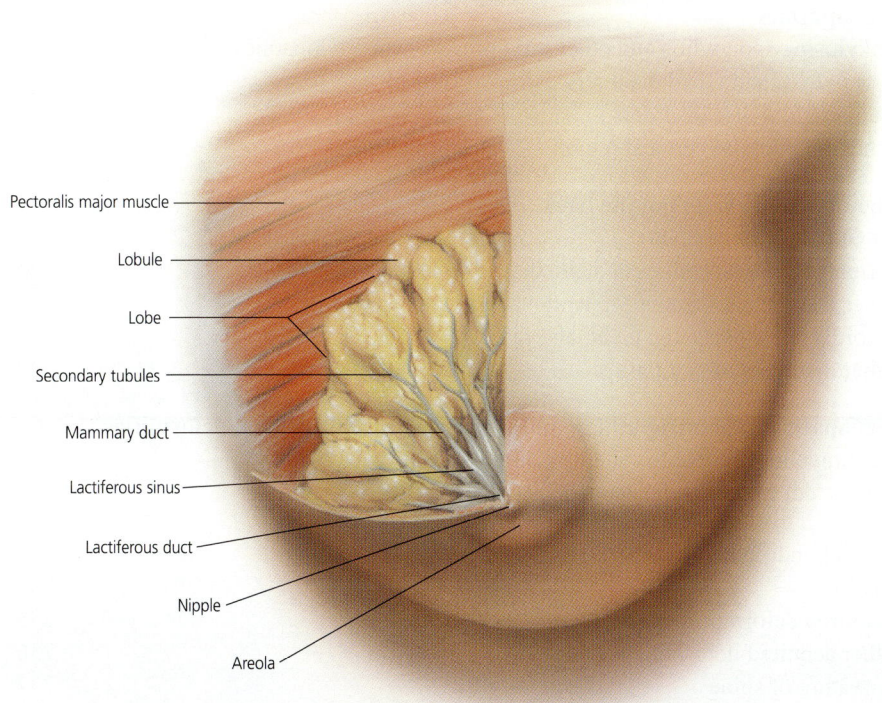

PLATE 4. MUSCULAR SYSTEM AND CONNECTIVE TISSUE — ANTERIOR VIEW

Arthropathies and related disorders
Diffuse diseases of connective tissue	710
Arthropathy associated with infections	711
Crystal arthropathies	712
Arthropathy associated with other disorders classified elsewhere	713
Rheumatoid arthritis and other inflammatory polyarthropathies	714
Osteoarthrosis and allied disorders	715
Internal derangement of knee	717
Other derangement of joint	718

Dorsopathies
Ankylosing spondylitis and other inflammatory spondylopathies	720
Spondylosis and allied disorders	721
Intervertebral disc disorders	722
Other disorders of cervical region	723

Rheumatism, excluding the back
Polymyalgia rheumatica	725
Peripheral enthesopathies and allied syndromes	726
Other disorders of synovium, tendon, and bursa	727
Disorders of muscle, ligament, and fascia	728
Other disorders of soft tissues	729

Osteopathies, chondropathies, and acquired musculoskeletal deformities
Osteomyelitis, periostitis, and other infections involving bone	730
Osteitis deformans and osteopathies associated with other disorders classified elsewhere	731
Osteochondropathies	732
Flat foot	734
Acquired deformities of toe	735
Other acquired deformities of limbs	736
Curvature of spine	737
Other acquired deformity	738
Nonallopathic lesions, not elsewhere classified	739

Symptoms, signs and ill-defined conditions 780-799

ANATOMICAL ILLUSTRATIONS

Muscular System
(Anterior View)

©Scientific Publishing Ltd., Rolling Meadows, IL

PLATE 5. MUSCULAR SYSTEM AND CONNECTIVE TISSUE — POSTERIOR VIEW

Arthropathies and related disorders
Diffuse diseases of connective tissue	710
Arthropathy associated with infections	711
Crystal arthropathies	712
Arthropathy associated with other disorders classified elsewhere	713
Rheumatoid arthritis and other inflammatory polyarthropathies	714
Osteoarthrosis and allied disorders	715
Other and unspecified arthropathies	716
Internal derangement of knee	717
Other derangement of joint	718
Other and unspecified disorders of joint	719

Dorsopathies
Ankylosing spondylitis and other inflammatory spondylopathies	720
Spondylosis and allied disorders	721
Intervertebral disc disorders	722
Other disorders of cervical region	723
Other and unspecified disorders of back	724

Rheumatism, excluding the back
Polymyalgia rheumatica	725
Peripheral enthesopathies and allied syndromes	726
Other disorders of synovium, tendon, and bursa	727
Disorders of muscle, ligament, and fascia	728
Other disorders of soft tissues	729

Osteopathies, chondropathies, and acquired musculoskeletal deformities
Osteomyelitis, periostitis, and other infections involving bone	730
Osteitis deformans and osteopathies associated with other disorders classified elsewhere	731
Osteochondropathies	732
Other disorders of bone and cartilage	733
Flat foot	734
Acquired deformities of toe	735
Other acquired deformities of limbs	736
Curvature of spine	737
Other acquired deformity	738
Nonallopathic lesions, not elsewhere classified	739

Symptoms, signs and ill-defined conditions 780-799

ANATOMICAL ILLUSTRATIONS

Muscular System
(Posterior View)

© Practice Management Information Corp., Los Angeles, CA

107

PLATE 6. MUSCULAR SYSTEM — SHOULDER AND ELBOW

Arthropathies and related disorders
Diffuse diseases of connective tissue	710
Arthropathy associated with infections	711
Crystal arthropathies	712
Arthropathy associated with other disorders classified elsewhere	713
Rheumatoid arthritis and other inflammatory polyarthropathies	714
Osteoarthrosis and allied disorders	715
Other and unspecified arthropathies	716
Internal derangement of knee	717
Other derangement of joint	718
Other and unspecified disorders of joint	719

Dorsopathies
Ankylosing spondylitis and other inflammatory spondylopathies	720
Spondylosis and allied disorders	721
Intervertebral disc disorders	722
Other disorders of cervical region	723
Other and unspecified disorders of back	724

Rheumatism, excluding the back
Polymyalgia rheumatica	725
Peripheral enthesopathies and allied syndromes	726
Other disorders of synovium, tendon, and bursa	727
Disorders of muscle, ligament, and fascia	728
Other disorders of soft tissues	729

Osteopathies, chondropathies, and acquired musculoskeletal deformities
Osteomyelitis, periostitis, and other infections involving bone	730
Osteitis deformans and osteopathies associated with other disorders classified elsewhere	731
Osteochondropathies	732
Other disorders of bone and cartilage	733
Flat foot	734
Acquired deformities of toe	735
Other acquired deformities of limbs	736
Curvature of spine	737
Other acquired deformity	738
Nonallopathic lesions, not elsewhere classified	739

Symptoms, signs and ill-defined conditions   780-799

Sprains and strains of joints and adjacent muscles
Sprains and strains of shoulder and upper arm	840
Sprains and strains of elbow and forearm	841
Other and ill-defined sprains and strains	848

ANATOMICAL ILLUSTRATIONS

Shoulder and Elbow
(Anterior View)

PLATE 7. MUSCULAR SYSTEM — HAND AND WRIST

Arthropathies and related disorders
Diffuse diseases of connective tissue	710
Arthropathy associated with infections	711
Crystal arthropathies	712
Arthropathy associated with other disorders classified elsewhere	713
Rheumatoid arthritis and other inflammatory polyarthropathies	714
Osteoarthrosis and allied disorders	715
Other and unspecified arthropathies	716
Other derangement of joint	718
Other and unspecified disorders of joint	719

Rheumatism, excluding the back
Polymyalgia rheumatica	725
Peripheral enthesopathies and allied syndromes	726
Other disorders of synovium, tendon, and bursa	727
Disorders of muscle, ligament, and fascia	728
Other disorders of soft tissues	729

Osteopathies, chondropathies, and acquired musculoskeletal deformities
Osteomyelitis, periostitis, and other infections involving bone	730
Osteitis deformans and osteopathies associated with other disorders classified elsewhere	731
Osteochondropathies	732
Other disorders of bone and cartilage	733
Other acquired deformities of limbs	736
Other acquired deformity	738
Nonallopathic lesions, not elsewhere classified	739

Symptoms, signs and ill-defined conditions 780-799

Sprains and strains of joints and adjacent muscles
Sprains and strains of wrist and hand	842
Other and ill-defined sprains and strains	848

ANATOMICAL ILLUSTRATIONS

Hand and Wrist

©Practice Management Information Corp., Los Angeles, CA

PLATE 8. MUSCULOSKELETAL SYSTEM — HIP AND KNEE

Arthropathies and related disorders
Diffuse diseases of connective tissue	710
Arthropathy associated with infections	711
Crystal arthropathies	712
Arthropathy associated with other disorders classified elsewhere	713
Rheumatoid arthritis and other inflammatory polyarthropathies	714
Osteoarthrosis and allied disorders	715
Other and unspecified arthropathies	716
Internal derangement of knee	717
Other derangement of joint	718
Other and unspecified disorders of joint	719

Rheumatism, excluding the back
Polymyalgia rheumatica	725
Peripheral enthesopathies and allied syndromes	726
Other disorders of synovium, tendon, and bursa	727
Disorders of muscle, ligament, and fascia	728
Other disorders of soft tissues	729

Osteopathies, chondropathies, and acquired musculoskeletal deformities
Osteomyelitis, periostitis, and other infections involving bone	730
Osteitis deformans and osteopathies associated with other disorders classified elsewhere	731
Osteochondropathies	732
Other disorders of bone and cartilage	733
Other acquired deformities of limbs	736
Curvature of spine	737
Other acquired deformity	738
Nonallopathic lesions, not elsewhere classified	739

Symptoms, signs and ill-defined conditions — 780-799

Sprains and strains of joints and adjacent muscles
Sprains and strains of hip and thigh	843
Sprains and strains of knee and leg	844
Other and ill-defined sprains and strains	848

PLATE 9. MUSCULOSKELETAL SYSTEM — FOOT AND ANKLE

Arthropathies and related disorders

Diffuse diseases of connective tissue	710
Arthropathy associated with infections	711
Crystal arthropathies	712
Arthropathy associated with other disorders classified elsewhere	713
Rheumatoid arthritis and other inflammatory polyarthropathies	714
Osteoarthrosis and allied disorders	715
Other and unspecified arthropathies	716
Other derangement of joint	718
Other and unspecified disorders of joint	719

Rheumatism, excluding the back

Polymyalgia rheumatica	725
Peripheral enthesopathies and allied syndromes	726
Other disorders of synovium, tendon, and bursa	727
Disorders of muscle, ligament, and fascia	728
Other disorders of soft tissues	729

Osteopathies, chondropathies, and acquired musculoskeletal deformities

Osteomyelitis, periostitis, and other infections involving bone	730
Osteitis deformans and osteopathies associated with other disorders classified elsewhere	731
Osteochondropathies	732
Other disorders of bone and cartilage	733
Flat foot	734
Acquired deformities of toe	735
Other acquired deformities of limbs	736
Other acquired deformity	738
Nonallopathic lesions, not elsewhere classified	739

Symptoms, signs and ill-defined conditions 780-799

Sprains and strains of joints and adjacent muscles

Sprains and strains of ankle and foot	845
Other and ill-defined sprains and strains	848

ANATOMICAL ILLUSTRATIONS

Foot and Ankle

ANATOMICAL ILLUSTRATIONS

PLATE 10. SKELETAL SYSTEM — ANTERIOR VIEW

Symptoms, signs and ill-defined conditions	780-799
Fracture of skull	
Fracture of vault of skull	800
Fracture of base of skull	801
Fracture of face bones	802
Multiple fractures involving skull or face with other bones	804
Fracture of neck and trunk	
Fracture of vertebral column without mention of spinal cord injury	805
Fracture of vertebral column with spinal cord injury	806
Fracture of rib(s), sternum, larynx and trachea	807
Fracture of pelvis	808
Fracture of upper limb	
Fracture of clavicle	810
Fracture of scapula	811
Fracture of humerus	812
Fracture of radius and ulna	813
Fracture of carpal bone(s)	814
Fracture of metacarpal bone(s)	815
Fracture of one or more phalanges of hand	816
Multiple fractures of hand bones	817
Fracture of lower limb	
Fracture of neck of femur	820
Fracture of other and unspecified parts of femur	821
Fracture of patella	822
Fracture of tibia and fibula	823
Fracture of ankle	824
Fracture of one or more tarsal and metatarsal bones	825
Fracture of one or more phalanges of foot	826
Dislocation	
Dislocation of jaw	830
Dislocation of shoulder	831
Dislocation of elbow	832
Dislocation of wrist	833
Dislocation of finger	834
Dislocation of hip	835
Dislocation of knee	836
Dislocation of ankle	837
Dislocation of foot	838

ANATOMICAL ILLUSTRATIONS

Skeletal System
(Anterior View)

PLATE 11. SKELETAL SYSTEM — POSTERIOR VIEW

Symptoms, signs and ill-defined conditions	780-799
Fracture of skull	
Fracture of vault of skull	800
Fracture of base of skull	801
Fracture of face bones	802
Multiple fractures involving skull or face with other bones	804
Fracture of neck and trunk	
Fracture of vertebral column without mention of spinal cord injury	805
Fracture of vertebral column with spinal cord injury	806
Fracture of rib(s), sternum, larynx and trachea	807
Fracture of pelvis	808
Fracture of upper limb	
Fracture of clavicle	810
Fracture of scapula	811
Fracture of humerus	812
Fracture of radius and ulna	813
Fracture of carpal bone(s)	814
Fracture of metacarpal bone(s)	815
Fracture of one or more phalanges of hand	816
Multiple fractures of hand bones	817
Fracture of lower limb	
Fracture of neck of femur	820
Fracture of other and unspecified parts of femur	821
Fracture of patella	822
Fracture of tibia and fibula	823
Fracture of ankle	824
Fracture of one or more tarsal and metatarsal bones	825
Fracture of one or more phalanges of foot	826
Dislocation	
Dislocation of jaw	830
Dislocation of shoulder	831
Dislocation of elbow	832
Dislocation of wrist	833
Dislocation of finger	834
Dislocation of hip	835
Dislocation of knee	836
Dislocation of ankle	837
Dislocation of foot	838

PLATE 12. SKELETAL SYSTEM — VERTEBRAL COLUMN

Arthropathies and related disorders

Diffuse diseases of connective tissue	710
Arthropathy associated with infections	711
Crystal arthropathies	712
Arthropathy associated with other disorders classified elsewhere	713
Rheumatoid arthritis and other inflammatory polyarthropathies	714
Osteoarthrosis and allied disorders	715

Dorsopathies

Ankylosing spondylitis and other inflammatory spondylopathies	720
Spondylosis and allied disorders	721
Intervertebral disc disorders	722
Other disorders of cervical region	723
Other and unspecified disorders of back	724

Osteopathies, chondropathies, and acquired musculoskeletal deformities

Osteomyelitis, periostitis, and other infections involving bone	730
Osteitis deformans and osteopathies associated with other disorders classified elsewhere	731
Osteochondropathies	732
Other disorders of bone and cartilage	733
Curvature of spine	737
Other acquired deformity	738
Nonallopathic lesions, not elsewhere classified	739

Symptoms, signs and ill-defined conditions 780-799

Fracture of neck and trunk

Fracture of vertebral column without mention of spinal cord injury	805
Fracture of vertebral column with spinal cord injury	806

ANATOMICAL ILLUSTRATIONS

Vertebral Column
(Lateral View)

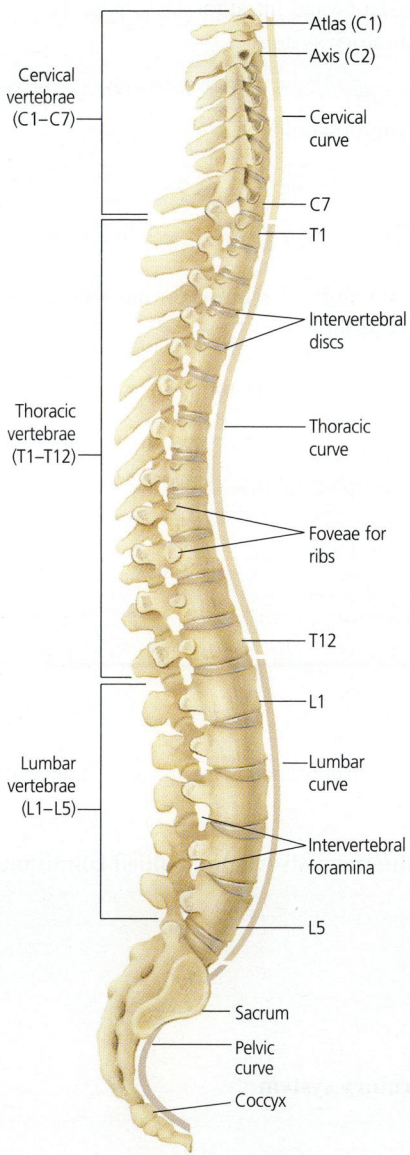

PLATE 13. RESPIRATORY SYSTEM

Malignant neoplasm of respiratory and intrathoracic organs	160-165
Malignant neoplasm of larynx	161
Malignant neoplasm of trachea, bronchus, and lung	162
Benign neoplasm of respiratory and intrathoracic organs	212
Carcinoma in situ of respiratory system	231
Acute respiratory infections	
Acute nasopharyngitis [common cold]	460
Acute sinusitis	461
Acute pharyngitis	462
Acute tonsillitis	463
Acute laryngitis and tracheitis	464
Acute upper respiratory infections of multiple or unspecified sites	465
Acute bronchitis and bronchiolitis	466
Other diseases of upper respiratory tract	
Deviated nasal septum	470
Nasal polyps	471
Chronic pharyngitis and nasopharyngitis	472
Chronic sinusitis	473
Chronic disease of tonsils and adenoids	474
Peritonsillar abscess	475
Chronic laryngitis and laryngotracheitis	476
Allergic rhinitis	477
Pneumonia and influenza	
Viral pneumonia	480
Pneumococcal pneumonia [Streptococcus pneumoniae pneumonia]	481
Influenza	487
Chronic obstructive pulmonary disease and allied conditions	
Chronic bronchitis	491
Emphysema	492
Asthma	493
Bronchiectasis	494
Extrinsic allergic alveolitis	495
Other diseases of respiratory system	
Empyema	510
Pleurisy	511
Pneumothorax	512
Abscess of lung and mediastinum	513
Pulmonary congestion and hypostasis	514
Postinflammatory pulmonary fibrosis	515

ANATOMICAL ILLUSTRATIONS

Respiratory System

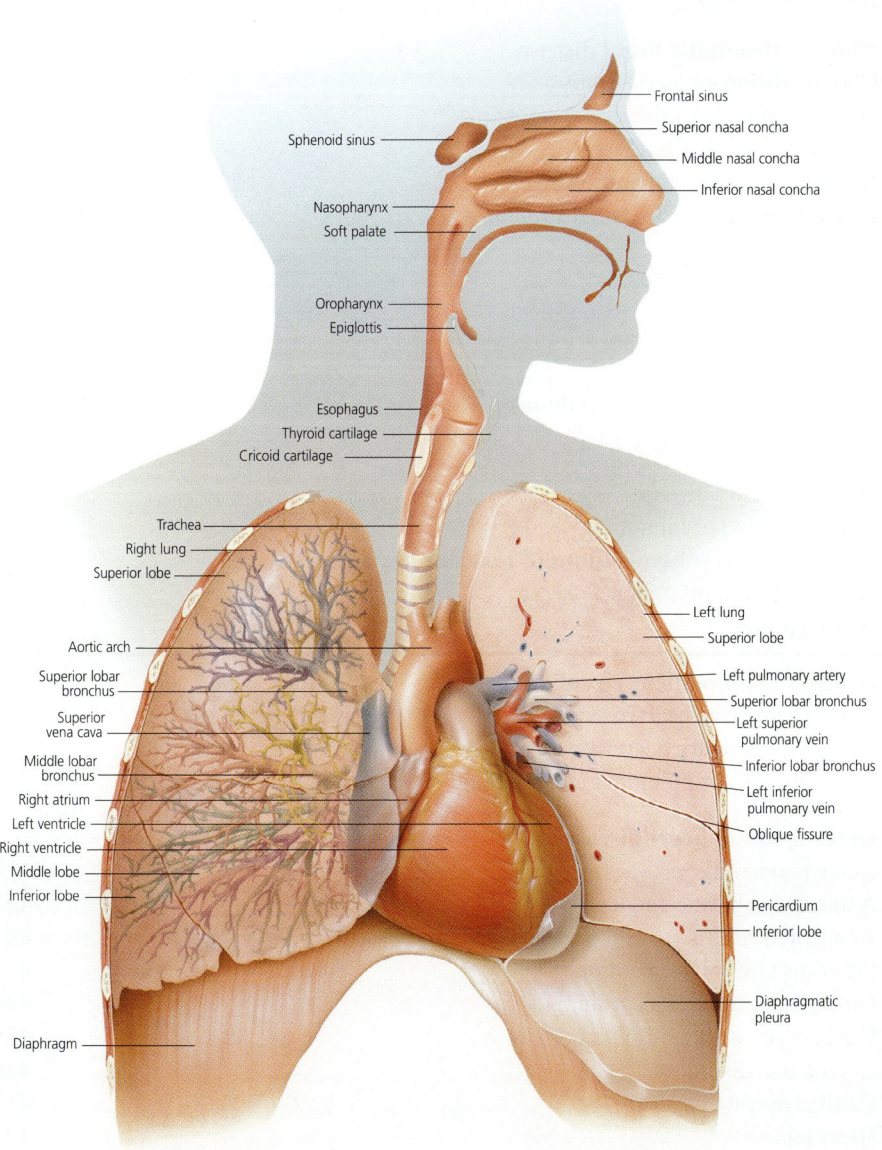

PLATE 14. HEART AND PERICARDIUM

Acute rheumatic fever
Rheumatic fever without mention of heart involvement	390
Rheumatic fever with heart involvement	391
Rheumatic chorea	392

Chronic rheumatic heart disease
Chronic rheumatic pericarditis	393
Diseases of mitral valve	394
Diseases of aortic valve	395
Diseases of mitral and aortic valves	396
Diseases of other endocardial structures	397

Hypertensive disease
Essential hypertension	401
Hypertensive heart disease	402
Hypertensive renal disease	403
Hypertensive heart and renal disease	404
Secondary hypertension	405

Ischemic heart disease
Acute myocardial infarction	410
Other acute and subacute forms of ischemic heart disease	411
Old myocardial infarction	412
Angina pectoris	413

Diseases of pulmonary circulation
Acute pulmonary heart disease	415
Chronic pulmonary heart disease	416
Other diseases of pulmonary circulation	417

Other forms of heart disease
Acute pericarditis	420
Acute and subacute endocarditis	421
Acute myocarditis	422
Other diseases of pericardium	423
Other diseases of endocardium	424
Cardiomyopathy	425
Conduction disorders	426
Cardiac dysrhythmias	427
Heart failure	428

Symptoms, signs and ill-defined conditions   780-799

ANATOMICAL ILLUSTRATIONS

PLATE 15. CIRCULATORY SYSTEM

Diseases of arteries, arterioles, and capillaries
Atherosclerosis	440
Aortic aneurysm and dissection	441
Arterial embolism and thrombosis	444
Polyarteritis nodosa and allied conditions	446
Other disorders of arteries and arterioles	447
Diseases of capillaries	448

Diseases of veins and lymphatics, and other circulatory system
Phlebitis and thrombophlebitis	451
Portal vein thrombosis	452
Varicose veins of lower extremities	454
Hemorrhoids	455
Varicose veins of other sites	456
Noninfectious disorders of lymphatic channels	457
Hypotension	458

Symptoms, signs and ill-defined conditions
780-799

Injury to blood vessels
Injury to blood vessels of head and neck	900
Injury to blood vessels of thorax	901
Injury to blood vessels of abdomen and pelvis	902
Injury to blood vessels of upper extremity	903
Injury to blood vessels of lower extremity and unspecified sites	904

ANATOMICAL ILLUSTRATIONS

PLATE 16. DIGESTIVE SYSTEM

Malignant neoplasms of digestive organs and peritoneum
Malignant neoplasm of esophagus	150
Malignant neoplasm of stomach	151
Malignant neoplasm of small intestine, including duodenum	152
Malignant neoplasm of colon	153
Malignant neoplasm of rectum, rectosigmoid junction, and anus	154
Malignant neoplasm of liver and intrahepatic bile ducts	155
Malignant neoplasm of gallbladder and extrahepatic bile ducts	156
Malignant neoplasm of pancreas	157
Benign neoplasm of other parts of digestive system	211
Carcinoma in situ of digestive organs	230

Diseases of esophagus, stomach, and duodenum
Diseases of esophagus	530
Gastric ulcer	531
Duodenal ulcer	532
Gastrojejunal ulcer	534
Gastritis and duodenitis	535

Appendicitis
Acute appendicitis	540
Appendicitis, unqualified	541

Hernia of abdominal cavity
Inguinal hernia	550
Other hernia of abdominal cavity, with gangrene	551
Other hernia of abdominal cavity, with obstruction, but without mention of gangrene	552
Other hernia of abdominal cavity without mention of obstruction or gangrene	553

Noninfectious enteritis and colitis
Regional enteritis	555
Ulcerative colitis	556
Vascular insufficiency of intestine	557

Other diseases of intestines and peritoneum
Intestinal obstruction without mention of hernia	560
Diverticula of intestine	562
Anal fissure and fistula	565
Abscess of anal and rectal regions	566
Peritonitis	567

Other diseases of digestive system
Acute and subacute necrosis of liver	570
Chronic liver disease and cirrhosis	571
Cholelithiasis	574
Diseases of pancreas	577
Gastrointestinal hemorrhage	578

ANATOMICAL ILLUSTRATIONS

Digestive System

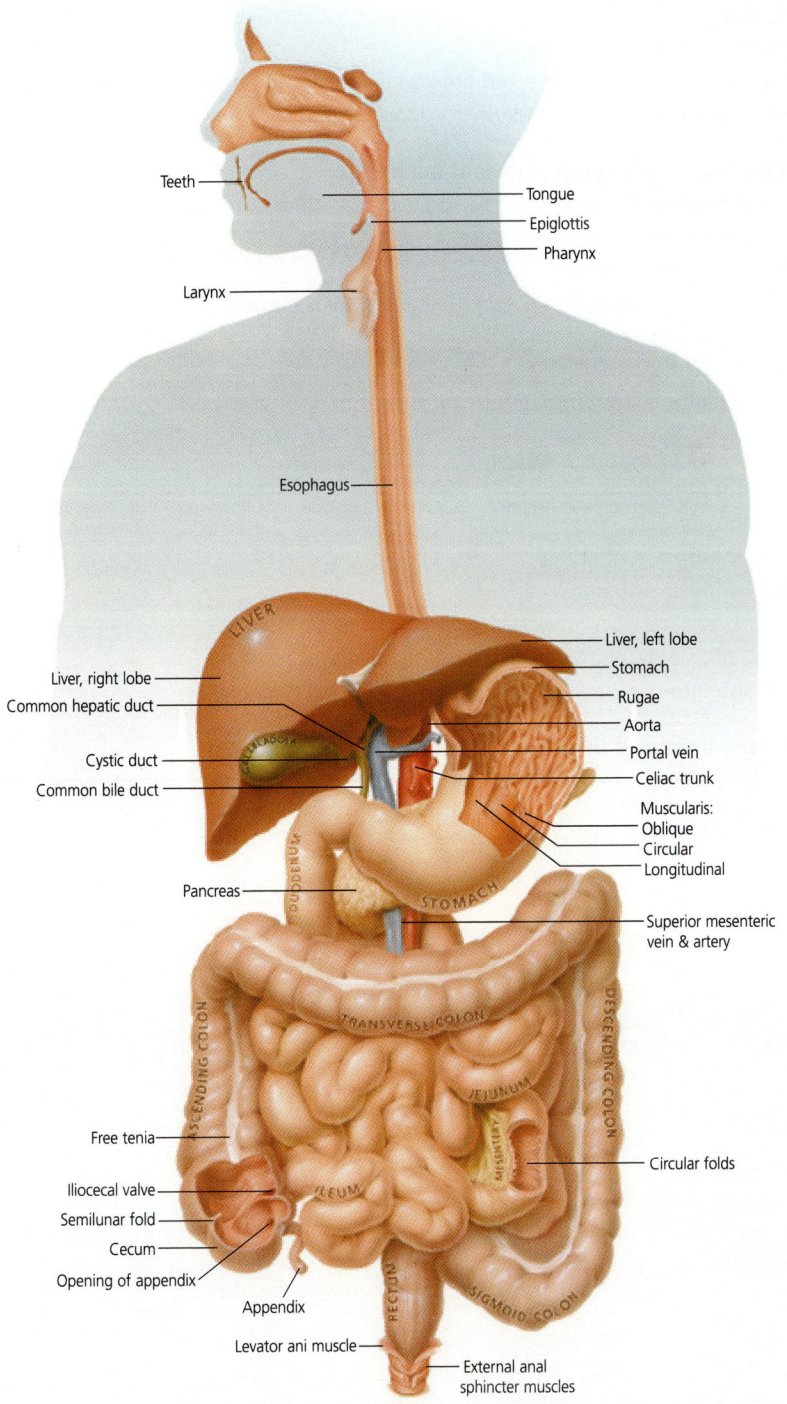

PLATE 17. GENITOURINARY SYSTEM

Neoplasms
Malignant neoplasm of bladder	188
Malignant neoplasm of kidney and other and unspecified urinary organs	189
Benign neoplasm of kidney and other urinary organs	223

Nephritis, nephrotic syndrome, and nephrosis
Acute glomerulonephritis	580
Nephrotic syndrome	581
Chronic glomerulonephritis	582
Nephritis and nephropathy, not specified as acute or chronic	583
Acute renal failure	584
Chronic renal failure	585
Disorders resulting from impaired renal function	588

Other diseases of urinary system
Infections of kidney	590
Hydronephrosis	591
Calculus of kidney and ureter	592
Calculus of lower urinary tract	594
Cystitis	595
Urethritis, not sexually transmitted, and urethral syndrome	597
Urethral stricture	598

Symptoms, signs and ill-defined conditions   780-799

ANATOMICAL ILLUSTRATIONS

Urinary System

PLATE 18. MALE REPRODUCTIVE SYSTEM

Neoplasms

Malignant neoplasm of prostate	185
Malignant neoplasm of testis	186
Malignant neoplasm of penis and other male genital organs	187
Benign neoplasm of male genital organs	222

Diseases of male genital organs

Hyperplasia of prostate	600
Inflammatory diseases of prostate	601
Hydrocele	603
Orchitis and epididymitis	604
Redundant prepuce and phimosis	605
Infertility, male	606
Disorders of penis	607

Symptoms, signs and ill-defined conditions   780-799

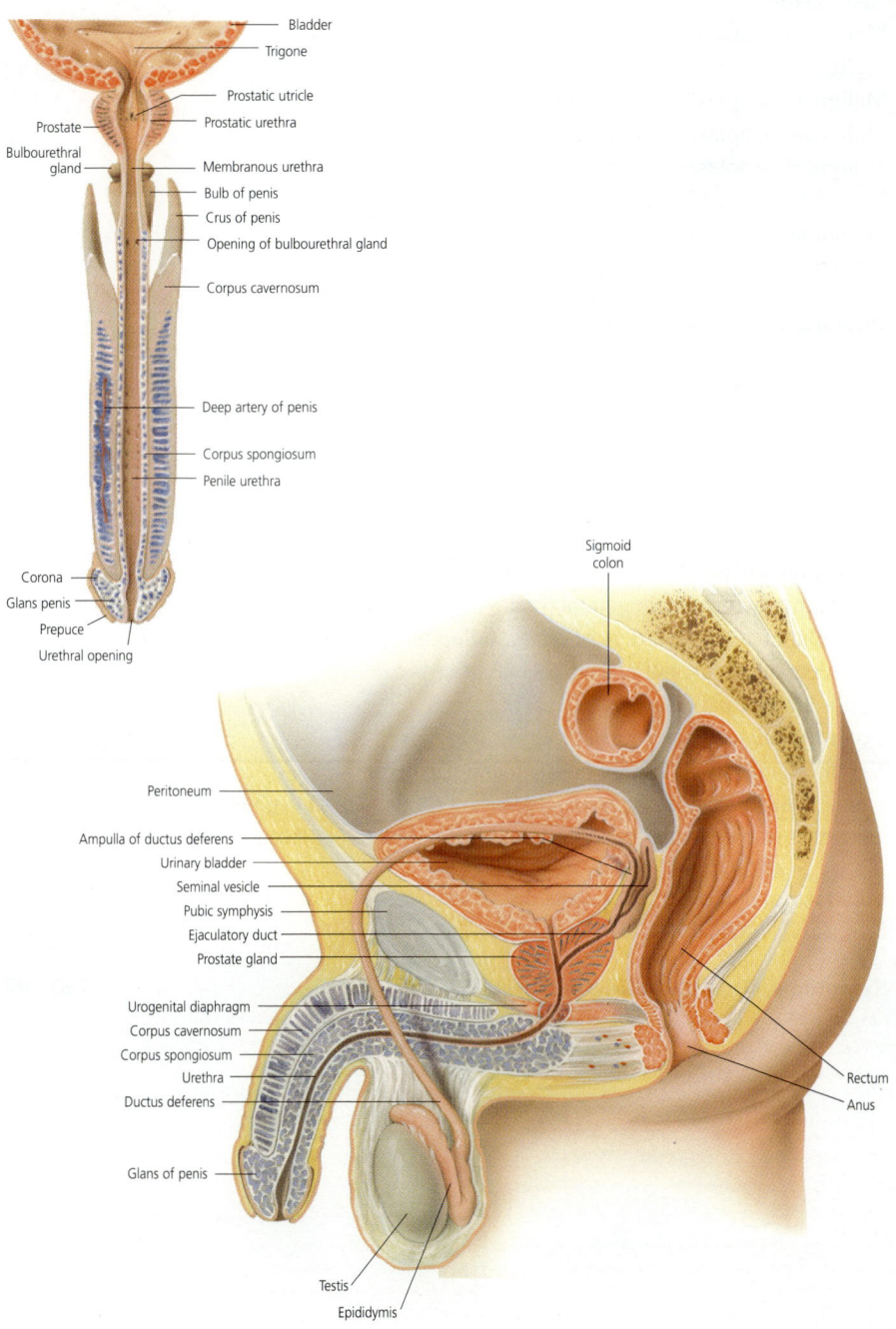

PLATE 19. FEMALE REPRODUCTIVE SYSTEM

Neoplasms

Malignant neoplasm of uterus, part unspecified	179
Malignant neoplasm of cervix uteri	180
Malignant neoplasm of placenta	181
Malignant neoplasm of body of uterus	182
Malignant neoplasm of ovary and other uterine adnexa	183
Other benign neoplasm of uterus	219
Benign neoplasm of ovary	220
Benign neoplasm of other female genital organs	221

Inflammatory disease of female pelvic organs

Inflammatory disease of ovary, fallopian tube, pelvic cellular tissue, and peritoneum	614
Inflammatory diseases of uterus, except cervix	615
Inflammatory disease of cervix, vagina, and vulva	616

Other disorders of female genital tract

Endometriosis	617
Genital prolapse	618
Fistula involving female genital tract	619
Noninflammatory disorders of ovary, fallopian tube, and broad ligament	620
Disorders of uterus, not elsewhere classified	621
Noninflammatory disorders of cervix	622
Noninflammatory disorders of vagina	623
Noninflammatory disorders of vulva and perineum	624
Pain and other symptoms associated with female genital organs	625
Disorders of menstruation and other abnormal bleeding from female genital tract	626
Menopausal and postmenopausal disorders	627
Infertility, female	628

Symptoms, signs and ill-defined conditions   780-799

ANATOMICAL ILLUSTRATIONS

Female Reproductive System

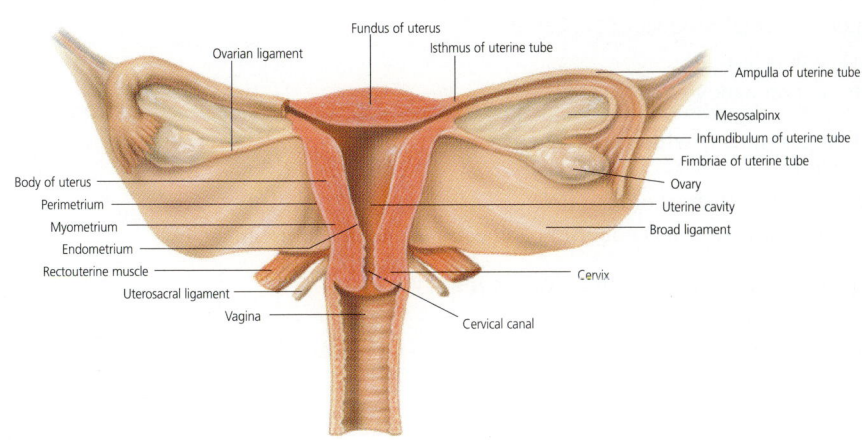

PLATE 20. PREGNANCY, CHILDBIRTH AND THE PUERPERIUM

Ectopic and molar pregnancy
Hydatidiform mole	630
Other abnormal product of conception	631
Missed abortion	632
Ectopic pregnancy	633

Other pregnancy with abortive outcome
Abortion	634
Legally induced abortion	635
Complications following abortion and ectopic and molar pregnancies	639

Complications mainly related to pregnancy
Hemorrhage in early pregnancy	640
Antepartum hemorrhage, abruptio placentae, and placenta previa	641
Hypertension complicating pregnancy, childbirth, and the puerperium	642
Excessive vomiting in pregnancy	643
Early or threatened labor	644
Late pregnancy	645

Normal delivery, other indications for care in pregnancy and delivery
Normal delivery	650
Multiple gestation	651
Malposition and malpresentation of fetus	652
Disproportion	653
Polyhydramnios	657

Complications occurring mainly in the course of labor and delivery
Obstructed labor	660
Abnormality of forces of labor	661
Long labor	662
Umbilical cord complications	663
Trauma to perineum and vulva during delivery	664
Postpartum hemorrhage	666
Retained placenta or membranes, without hemorrhage	667

Complications of the puerperium
Major puerperal infection	670
Venous complications in pregnancy and the puerperium	671
Pyrexia of unknown origin during the puerperium	672
Obstetrical pulmonary embolism	673

Persons encountering health services in circumstances related to reproduction
Normal pregnancy	V22
Supervision of high-risk pregnancy	V23
Postpartum care and examination	V24
Encounter for contraceptive management	V25
Procreative management	V26

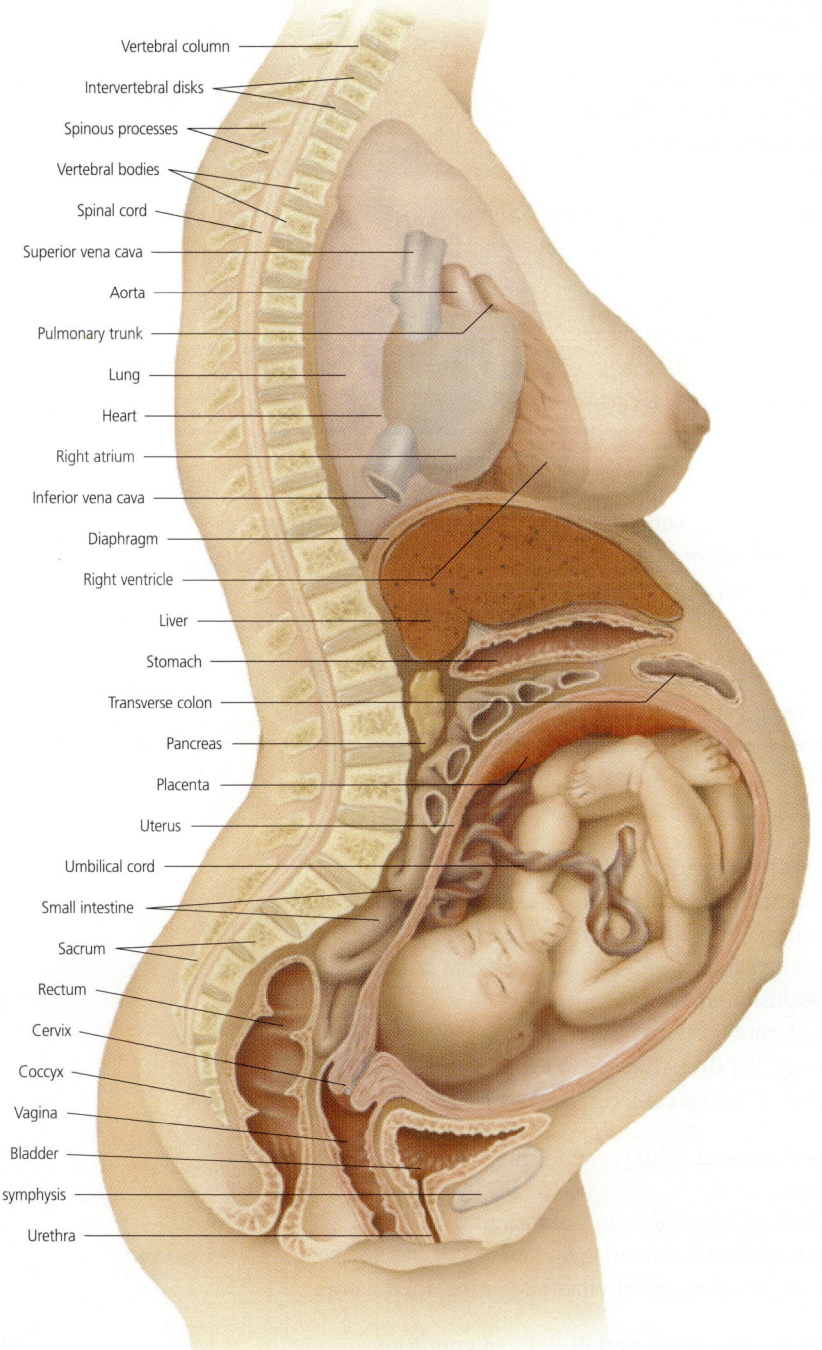

PLATE 21. NERVOUS SYSTEM — BRAIN

Neoplasms
Malignant neoplasm of brain	191

Organic psychotic conditions
Senile and presenile organic psychotic conditions	290
Alcoholic psychoses	291
Drug psychoses	292
Transient organic psychotic conditions	293
Other organic psychotic conditions (chronic)	294

Other psychoses
Schizophrenic psychoses	295
Affective psychoses	296
Paranoid states (Delusional disorders)	297
Other nonorganic psychoses	298
Psychoses with origin specific to childhood	299

Neurotic, personality, and other nonpsychotic disorders
Neurotic disorders	300
Personality disorders	301
Specific nonpsychotic mental disorders due to organic brain damage	310
Hyperkinetic syndrome of childhood	314

Mental retardation
Mild mental retardation	317
Other specified mental retardation	318
Unspecified mental retardation	319

Cerebrovascular disease
Subarachnoid hemorrhage	430
Intracerebral hemorrhage	431
Occlusion and stenosis of precerebral arteries	433
Occlusion of cerebral arteries	434
Transient cerebral ischemia	435
Acute but ill-defined cerebrovascular disease	436
Late effects of cerebrovascular disease	438

Intracranial injury, excluding those with skull fracture
Concussion	850
Cerebral laceration and contusion	851
Subarachnoid, subdural, and extradural hemorrhage, following injury	852
Intracranial injury of other and unspecified nature	854

Symptoms, signs and ill-defined conditions   780-799

ANATOMICAL ILLUSTRATIONS

Brain
(Base View)

PLATE 22. NERVOUS SYSTEM

Inflammatory diseases of the central nervous system
Bacterial meningitis	320
Meningitis due to other organisms	321
Encephalitis, myelitis, and encephalomyelitis	323
Intracranial and intraspinal abscess	324
Phlebitis and thrombophlebitis of intracranial venous sinuses	325

Hereditary and degenerative diseases of the central nervous system
Cerebral degenerations usually manifest in childhood	330
Other cerebral degenerations	331
Parkinson's disease	332
Spinocerebellar disease	334
Anterior horn cell disease	335
Other diseases of spinal cord	336
Disorders of the autonomic nervous system	337

Other disorders of the central nervous system
Multiple sclerosis	340
Other demyelinating diseases of central nervous system	341
Hemiplegia and hemiparesis	342
Infantile cerebral palsy	343
Other paralytic syndromes	344
Epilepsy	345
Migraine	346
Cataplexy and narcolepsy	347

Disorders of the peripheral nervous system
Trigeminal nerve disorders	350
Facial nerve disorders	351
Disorders of other cranial nerves	352
Nerve root and plexus disorders	353
Mononeuritis of upper limb and mononeuritis multiplex	354
Mononeuritis of lower limb and unspecified site	355
Hereditary and idiopathic peripheral neuropathy	356
Inflammatory and toxic neuropathy	357
Myoneural disorders	358
Muscular dystrophies and other myopathies	359

Injury to nerves and spinal cord
Injury to optic nerve and pathways	950
Injury to other cranial nerve(s)	951
Spinal cord injury without evidence of spinal bone injury	952
Injury to nerve roots and spinal plexus	953
Injury to other nerve(s) of trunk, excluding shoulder and pelvic girdles	954
Injury to peripheral nerve(s) of shoulder girdle and upper limb	955
Injury to peripheral nerve(s) of pelvic girdle and lower limb	956

ANATOMICAL ILLUSTRATIONS

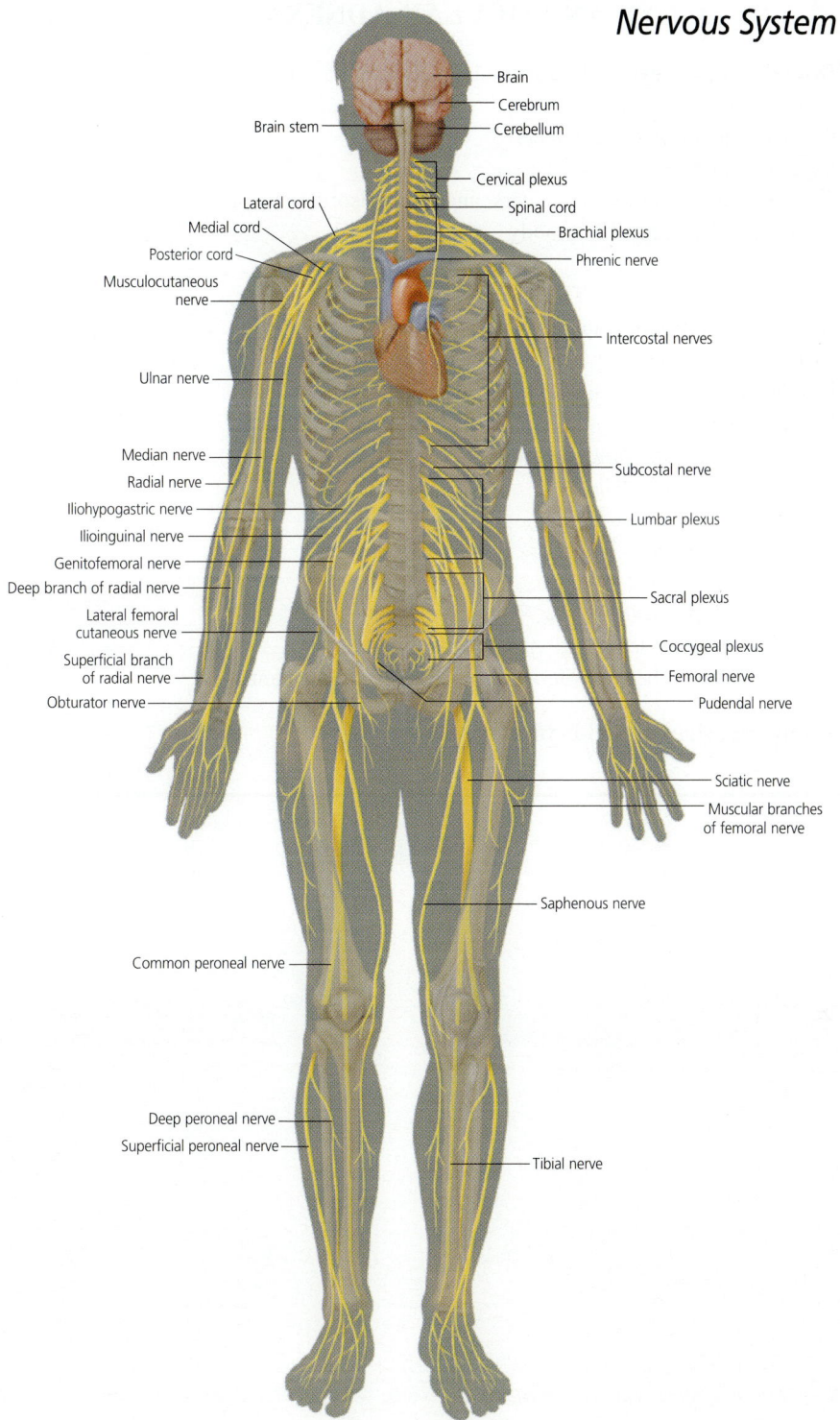

PLATE 23. EYE AND OCULAR ADNEXA

Disorders of the eye and adnexa
Disorders of the globe	360
Retinal detachments and defects	361
Other retinal disorders	362
Chorioretinal inflammations, scars, and other disorders of choroid	363
Disorders of iris and ciliary body	364
Glaucoma	365
Cataract	366
Disorders of refraction and accommodation	367
Visual disturbances	368
Blindness and low vision	369
Keratitis	370
Corneal opacity and other disorders of cornea	371
Disorders of conjunctiva	372
Inflammation of eyelids	373
Other disorders of eyelids	374
Disorders of lacrimal system	375
Disorders of the orbit	376
Disorders of optic nerve and visual pathways	377
Strabismus and other disorders of binocular eye movements	378

Symptoms, signs and ill-defined conditions   780-799

ANATOMICAL ILLUSTRATIONS

Right Eye
(Horizontal Section)

PLATE 24. AUDITORY SYSTEM

Diseases of the ear and mastoid process
Disorders of external ear 380
Nonsuppurative otitis media and Eustachian tube disorders 381
Suppurative and unspecified otitis media 382
Mastoiditis and related conditions 383
Other disorders of tympanic membrane 384
Other disorders of middle ear and mastoid 385
Vertiginous syndromes and other disorders of vestibular system 386
Otosclerosis 387
Hearing loss 389

Symptoms, signs and ill-defined conditions 780-799

ANATOMICAL ILLUSTRATIONS

The Ear

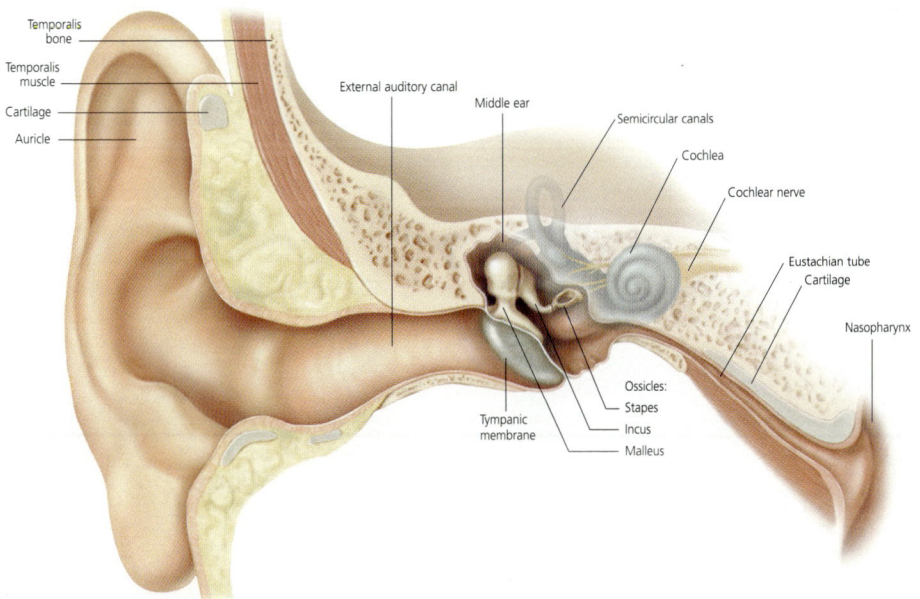

ANATOMICAL ILLUSTRATIONS

DISEASES: TABULAR LIST

VOLUME 1

INFECTIOUS AND PARASITIC DISEASES

1. INFECTIOUS AND PARASITIC DISEASES (001-139)

Note: Categories for "late effects" of infectious and parasitic diseases are to be found at 137-139.
Includes: diseases generally recognized as communicable or transmissible as well as a few diseases of unknown but possibly infectious origin

Excludes: *acute respiratory infections (460-466)*
carrier or suspected carrier of infectious organism (V02.0-V02.9)
certain localized infections
influenza (487.0-487.8, 488)

INTESTINAL INFECTIOUS DISEASES (001-009)

Excludes: *helminthiases (120.0-129)*

001 Cholera
    001.0 Due to Vibrio cholerae
    001.1 Due to Vibrio cholerae el tor
    001.9 Cholera, unspecified

002 Typhoid and paratyphoid fevers
    002.0 Typhoid fever
        Typhoid (fever) (infection) [any site]
    002.1 Paratyphoid fever A
    002.2 Paratyphoid fever B
    002.3 Paratyphoid fever C
    002.9 Paratyphoid fever, unspecified

003 Other salmonella infections
    Includes: infection or food poisoning by Salmonella [any serotype]
    003.0 Salmonella gastroenteritis
        Salmonellosis
    003.1 Salmonella septicemia
  ⑤ **003.2 Localized salmonella infections**
        003.20 Localized salmonella infection, unspecified
        003.21 Salmonella meningitis
        003.22 Salmonella pneumonia
        003.23 Salmonella arthritis
        003.24 Salmonella osteomyelitis
        003.29 Other
    003.8 Other specified salmonella infections
    003.9 Salmonella infection, unspecified

004 Shigellosis
    Includes: bacillary dysentery
    004.0 Shigella dysenteriae
        Infection by group A Shigella (Schmitz) (Shiga)
    004.1 Shigella flexneri
        Infection by group B Shigella
    004.2 Shigella boydii
        Infection by group C Shigella
    004.3 Shigella sonnei
        Infection by group D Shigella
    004.8 Other specified shigella infections
    004.9 Shigellosis, unspecified

005 Other food poisoning (bacterial)
    Excludes: *salmonella infections (003.0-003.9)*
        toxic effect of:
            food contaminants (989.7)
            noxious foodstuffs (988.0-988.9)

    005.0 Staphylococcal food poisoning
        Staphylococcal toxemia specified as due to food

149

TABULAR LIST

▲ **005.1 Botulism food poisoning**
Botulism NOS
Food poisoning due to Clostridium botulinum

Excludes: infant botulism (040.41)
wound botulism (040.42)

005.2 Food poisoning due to Clostridium perfringens [C. welchii]
Enteritis necroticans

005.3 Food poisoning due to other Clostridia

005.4 Food poisoning due to Vibrio parahaemolyticus

⑤ **005.8 Other bacterial food poisoning**

Excludes: salmonella food poisoning (003.0-003.9)

005.81 Food poisoning due to Vibrio vulnificus

005.89 Other bacterial food poisoning
Food poisoning due to Bacillus cereus

005.9 Food poisoning, unspecified

006 Amebiasis
Includes: infection due to Entamoeba histolytica

Excludes: amebiasis due to organisms other than Entamoeba histolytica (007.8)

006.0 Acute amebic dysentery without mention of abscess
Acute amebiasis

006.1 Chronic intestinal amebiasis without mention of abscess
Chronic:
amebiasis
amebic dysentery

006.2 Amebic nondysenteric colitis

006.3 Amebic liver abscess
Hepatic amebiasis

006.4 Amebic lung abscess
Amebic abscess of lung (and liver)

006.5 Amebic brain abscess
Amebic abscess of brain (and liver) (and lung)

006.6 Amebic skin ulceration
Cutaneous amebiasis

006.8 Amebic infection of other sites
Amebic: Ameboma
appendicitis
balanitis

Excludes: specific infections by free-living amebae (136.2)

006.9 Amebiasis, unspecified
Amebiasis NOS

007 Other protozoal intestinal diseases
Includes: protozoal:
colitis
diarrhea
dysentery

007.0 Balantidiasis
Infection by Balantidium coli

007.1 Giardiasis
Infection by Giardia lamblia
Lambliasis

007.2 Coccidiosis
Infection by Isospora belli and Isospora hominis
Isosporiasis

007.3 Intestinal trichomoniasis

007.4 Cryptosporidiosis

007.5 Cyclosporiasis

007.8 Other specified protozoal intestinal diseases
Amebiasis due to organisms other than Entamoeba histolytica

007.9 Unspecified protozoal intestinal disease
Flagellate diarrhea   Protozoal dysentery NOS

● Code new to this edition	▲ Revision of existing code	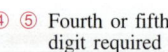 Fourth or fifth digit required

INFECTIOUS AND PARASITIC DISEASES

008 **Intestinal infections due to other organisms**
Includes: any condition classifiable to 009.0-009.3 with mention of the responsible organisms

Excludes: food poisoning by these organisms (005.0-005.9)

⑤ **008.0 Escherichia coli [E. coli]**

008.00 E. coli, unspecified
E. coli enteritis NOS

008.01 Enteropathogenic E. coli

008.02 Enterotoxigenic E. coli

008.03 Enteroinvasive E. coli

008.04 Enterohemorrhagic E. coli

008.09 Other intestinal E. coli infections

008.1 Arizona group of paracolon bacilli

008.2 Aerobacter aerogenes
Enterobacter aerogenes

008.3 Proteus (mirabilis) (morganii)

⑤ 008.4 Other specified bacteria

008.41 Staphylococcus
Staphylococcal enterocolitis

008.42 Pseudomonas

008.43 Campylobacter

008.44 Yersinia enterocolitica

008.45 Clostridium difficile
Pseudomembranous colitis

008.46 Other anaerobes
Anaerobic enteritis NOS
Bacteroides (fragilis)
Gram-negative anaerobes

008.47 Other Gram-negative bacteria
Gram-negative enteritis NOS

Excludes: Gram-negative anaerobes (008.46)

008.49 Other

008.5 **Bacterial enteritis, unspecified**

⑤ 008.6 Enteritis due to specified virus

008.61 Rotavirus

008.62 Adenovirus

008.63 Norwalk virus
Norwalk-like agent

008.64 Other small round viruses [SRV's]
Small round virus NOS

008.65 Calcivirus

008.66 Astrovirus

008.67 Enterovirus NEC
Coxsackie virus
Echovirus

Excludes: poliovirus (045.0-045.9)

008.69 Other viral enteritis
Torovirus

008.8 Other organism, not elsewhere classified
Viral:
enteritis NOS
gastroenteritis

Excludes: influenza with involvement of gastrointestinal tract (487.8)

 Add 4th or 5th digit   Nonspecific code Unspecified code 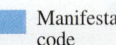 Manifestation code

151

TABULAR LIST

009 Ill-defined intestinal infections

Excludes: diarrheal disease or intestinal infection due to specified organism (001.0-008.8)
diarrhea following gastrointestinal surgery (564.4)
intestinal malabsorption (579.0-579.9)
ischemic enteritis (557.0-557.9)
other noninfectious gastroenteritis and colitis (558.1-558.9)
regional enteritis (555.0-555.9)
ulcerative colitis (556)

009.0 Infectious colitis, enteritis, and gastroenteritis
Colitis, septic
Enteritis, septic
Gastroenteritis, septic
Dysentery:
  NOS
  catarrhal
  hemorrhagic

009.1 Colitis, enteritis, and gastroenteritis of presumed infectious origin

Excludes: colitis NOS (558.9)
enteritis NOS (558.9)
gastroenteritis NOS (558.9)

009.2 Infectious diarrhea
Diarrhea:
  dysenteric
  epidemic
Infectious diarrheal disease NOS

009.3 Diarrhea of presumed infectious origin

Excludes: diarrhea NOS (787.91)

TUBERCULOSIS (010-018)

Includes: infection by Mycobacterium tuberculosis (human) (bovine)

Excludes: congenital tuberculosis (771.2)
late effects of tuberculosis (137.0-137.4)

The following fifth-digit subclassification is for use with categories 010-018:

0 unspecified
1 bacteriological or histological examination not done
2 bacteriological or histological examination unknown (at present)
3 tubercle bacilli found (in sputum) by microscopy
4 tubercle bacilli not found (in sputum) by microscopy, but found by bacterial culture
5 tubercle bacilli not found by bacteriological examination, but tuberculosis confirmed histologically
6 tubercle bacilli not found by bacteriological or histological examination but tuberculosis confirmed by other methods [inoculation of animals]

010 Primary tuberculous infection

Excludes: nonspecific reaction to tuberculin skin test without active tuberculosis (795.5)
positive PPD (795.5)
positive tuberculin skin test without active tuberculosis (795.5)

010.0 Primary tuberculous complex

010.1 Tuberculous pleurisy in primary progressive tuberculosis

010.8 Other primary progressive tuberculosis

Excludes: tuberculous erythema nodosum (017.1)

010.9 Primary tuberculous infection, unspecified

011 Pulmonary tuberculosis

Use additional code, if desired, to identify any associated silicosis (502)

011.0 Tuberculosis of lung, infiltrative

011.1 Tuberculosis of lung, nodular

011.2 Tuberculosis of lung with cavitation

011.3 Tuberculosis of bronchus

Excludes: isolated bronchial tuberculosis (012.2)

011.4 Tuberculous fibrosis of lung

011.5 Tuberculous bronchiectasis

INFECTIOUS AND PARASITIC DISEASES

- ⑤ 011.6 Tuberculous pneumonia [any form]
- ⑤ 011.7 Tuberculous pneumothorax
- ⑤ **011.8** Other specified pulmonary tuberculosis
- ⑤ **011.9** Pulmonary tuberculosis, unspecified
  Respiratory tuberculosis NOS
  Tuberculosis of lung NOS

⑤ **012** Other respiratory tuberculosis

> *Excludes:* respiratory tuberculosis, unspecified (011.9)

- ⑤ 012.0 **Tuberculous pleurisy**
  Tuberculosis of pleura   Tuberculous hydrothorax
  Tuberculous empyema

  > *Excludes:* pleurisy with effusion without mention of cause (511.9)
  > tuberculous pleurisy in primary progressive tuberculosis (010.1)

- ⑤ 012.1 **Tuberculosis of intrathoracic lymph nodes**
  Tuberculosis of lymph nodes:
   hilar
   mediastinal
   tracheobronchial
  Tuberculous tracheobronchial adenopathy

  > *Excludes:* that specified as primary (010.0-010.9)

- ⑤ 012.2 Isolated tracheal or bronchial tuberculosis
- ⑤ 012.3 **Tuberculous laryngitis**
  Tuberculosis of glottis
- ⑤ **012.8** Other specified respiratory tuberculosis
  Tuberculosis of: Tuberculosis of:
   mediastinum   nose (septum)
   nasopharynx   sinus [any nasal]

⑤ **013** Tuberculosis of meninges and central nervous system

- ⑤ 013.0 **Tuberculous meningitis**
  Tuberculosis of meninges   Tuberculous:
    (cerebral) (spinal)   leptomeningitis
                                  meningoencephalitis

  > *Excludes:* tuberculoma of meninges (013.1)

- ⑤ 013.1 Tuberculoma of meninges
- ⑤ 013.2 **Tuberculoma of brain**
  Tuberculosis of brain (current disease)
- ⑤ 013.3 Tuberculous abscess of brain
- ⑤ 013.4 Tuberculoma of spinal cord
- ⑤ 013.5 Tuberculous abscess of spinal cord
- ⑤ 013.6 Tuberculous encephalitis or myelitis
- ⑤ **013.8** Other specified tuberculosis of central nervous system
- ⑤ **013.9** Unspecified tuberculosis of central nervous system
  Tuberculosis of central nervous system NOS

⑤ **014** Tuberculosis of intestines, peritoneum, and mesenteric glands

- ⑤ 014.0 **Tuberculous peritonitis**
  Tuberculous ascites
- ⑤ **014.8** Other
  Tuberculosis (of):   Tuberculous enteritis
   anus
   intestine (large) (small)
   mesenteric glands
   rectum
   retroperitoneal (lymph nodes)

 Add 4th or 5th digit
 Nonspecific code
 Unspecified code
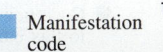 Manifestation code

153

TABULAR LIST

015 Tuberculosis of bones and joints
Use additional code, if desired, to identify manifestation, as:
tuberculous:
arthropathy (711.4)
necrosis of bone (730.8)
osteitis (730.8)
osteomyelitis (730.8)
synovitis (727.01)
tenosynovitis (727.01)

015.0 Vertebral column
Pott's disease
Use additional code, if desired, to identify manifestation, as:
curvature of spine [Pott's] (737.4)
kyphosis (737.4)
spondylitis (720.81)

015.1 Hip

015.2 Knee

015.5 Limb bones
Tuberculous dactylitis

015.6 Mastoid
Tuberculous mastoiditis

015.7 Other specified bone

015.8 Other specified joint

015.9 Tuberculosis of unspecified bones and joints

016 Tuberculosis of genitourinary system

016.0 Kidney
Renal tuberculosis
Use additional code, if desired, to identify manifestation, as:
tuberculous:
nephropathy (583.81)
pyelitis (590.81)
pyelonephritis (590.81)

016.1 Bladder

016.2 Ureter

016.3 Other urinary organs

016.4 Epididymis

016.5 Other male genital organs
Use additional code, if desired, to identify manifestation, as:
tuberculosis of:
prostate (601.4)
seminal vesicle (608.81)
testis (608.81)

016.6 Tuberculous oophoritis and salpingitis

016.7 Other female genital organs
Tuberculous:
cervicitis
endometritis

016.9 Genitourinary tuberculosis, unspecified

017 Tuberculosis of other organs

017.0 Skin and subcutaneous cellular tissue

Lupus:	Tuberculosis:
exedens	colliquativa
vulgaris	cutis
Scrofuloderma	lichenoides
	papulonecrotica
	verrucosa cutis

Excludes: lupus erythematosus (695.4)
disseminated (710.0)
lupus NOS (710.0)
nonspecific reaction to tuberculin skin test without active tuberculosis (795.5)
positive PPD (795.5)
positive tuberculin skin test without active tuberculosis (795.5)

INFECTIOUS AND PARASITIC DISEASES

⑤ **017.1 Erythema nodosum with hypersensitivity reaction in tuberculosis**
　　　Bazin's disease　　　　　　Tuberculosis indurativa
　　　Erythema:
　　　　induratum
　　　　nodosum, tuberculous

　　Excludes: erythema nodosum NOS (695.2)

⑤ **017.2 Peripheral lymph nodes**
　　　Scrofula　　　　　　　　　Tuberculous adenitis
　　　Scrofulous abscess

　　Excludes: tuberculosis of lymph nodes:
　　　　　　　　bronchial and mediastinal (012.1)
　　　　　　　　mesenteric and retroperitoneal (014.8)
　　　　　　　tuberculous tracheobronchial adenopathy (012.1)

⑤ **017.3 Eye**
　　Use additional code, if desired, to identify manifestation, as:
　　　　tuberculous:
　　　　　chorioretinitis, disseminated (363.13)
　　　　　episcleritis (379.09)
　　　　　interstitial keratitis (370.59)
　　　　　iridocyclitis, chronic (364.11)
　　　　　keratoconjunctivitis (phlyctenular) (370.31)

⑤ **017.4 Ear**
　　　Tuberculosis of ear
　　　Tuberculous otitis media

　　Excludes: tuberculous mastoiditis (015.6)

⑤ **017.5 Thyroid gland**

⑤ **017.6 Adrenal glands**
　　　Addison's disease, tuberculous

⑤ **017.7 Spleen**

⑤ **017.8 Esophagus**

⑤ **017.9 Other specified organs**
　　Use additional code, if desired, to identify manifestation, as:
　　　　tuberculosis of:
　　　　　endocardium [any valve] (424.91)
　　　　　myocardium (422.0)
　　　　　pericardium (420.0)

⑤ **018 Miliary tuberculosis**
　　Includes: tuberculosis:
　　　　　　　disseminated
　　　　　　　generalized
　　　　　　　miliary, whether of a single specified site, multiple sites, or unspecified site
　　　　　　　polyserositis

⑤ **018.0 Acute miliary tuberculosis**

⑤ **018.8 Other specified miliary tuberculosis**

⑤ **018.9 Miliary tuberculosis, unspecified**

ZOONOTIC BACTERIAL DISEASES (020-027)

020 Plague
　　Includes: infection by Yersinia [Pasteurella] pestis

　　020.0 Bubonic

　　020.1 Cellulocutaneous

　　020.2 Septicemic

　　020.3 Primary pneumonic

　　020.4 Secondary pneumonic

　　020.5 Pneumonic, unspecified

　　020.8 Other specified types of plague
　　　　Abortive plague　　　　　　Pestis minor
　　　　Ambulatory plague

　　020.9 Plague, unspecified

 Add 4th or 5th digit
 Nonspecific code
 Unspecified code
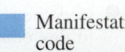 Manifestation code

TABULAR LIST

021 Tularemia
Includes: deerfly fever
infection by Francisella [Pasteurella] tularensis
rabbit fever

- **021.0 Ulceroglandular tularemia**
- **021.1 Enteric tularemia**
  Tularemia:
  cryptogenic
  intestinal
  typhoidal
- **021.2 Pulmonary tularemia**
  Bronchopneumonic tularemia
- **021.3 Oculoglandular tularemia**
- **021.8 Other specified tularemia**
  Tularemia:
  generalized or disseminated
  glandular
- **021.9 Unspecified tularemia**

022 Anthrax

- **022.0 Cutaneous anthrax**
  Malignant pustule
- **022.1 Pulmonary anthrax**
  Respiratory anthrax
  Wool-sorters' disease
- **022.2 Gastrointestinal anthrax**
- **022.3 Anthrax septicemia**
- **022.8 Other specified manifestations of anthrax**
- **022.9 Anthrax, unspecified**

023 Brucellosis
Includes: fever:
Malta
Mediterranean
undulant

- **023.0 Brucella melitensis**
- **023.1 Brucella abortus**
- **023.2 Brucella suis**
- **023.3 Brucella canis**
- **023.8 Other brucellosis**
  Infection by more than one organism
- **023.9 Brucellosis, unspecified**

024 Glanders
Infection by: Farcy
Actinobacillus mallei Malleus
Malleomyces mallei
Pseudomonas mallei

025 Melioidosis
Infection by:
Malleomyces pseudomallei
Pseudomonas pseudomallei
Whitmore's bacillus
Pseudoglanders

026 Rat-bite fever

- **026.0 Spirillary fever**
  Rat-bite fever due to Spirillum minor [S. minus]
  Sodoku
- **026.1 Streptobacillary fever**
  Epidemic arthritic erythema
  Haverhill fever
  Rat-bite fever due to Streptobacillus moniliformis
- **026.9 Unspecified rat-bite fever**

● Code new to this edition ▲ Revision of existing code ④ ⑤ Fourth or fifth digit required

INFECTIOUS AND PARASITIC DISEASES

027 Other zoonotic bacterial diseases

027.0 Listeriosis
Infection by Listeria monocytogenes
Septicemia by Listeria monocytogenes

Use additional code to identify manifestations, as meningitis (320.7)

Excludes: congenital listeriosis (771.2)

027.1 Erysipelothrix infection
Erysipeloid (of Rosenbach)
Infection by Erysipelothrix insidiosa [E. rhusiopathiae]
Septicemia by Erysipelothrix insidiosa [E. rhusiopathiae]

027.2 Pasteurellosis
Pasteurella pseudotuberculosis infection
Mesenteric adenitis by Pasteurella multocida [P. septica]
Septic infection (cat bite) (dog bite) by Pasteurella multocida [P. septica]

Excludes: infection by:
Francisella [Pasteurella] tularensis (021.0-021.9)
Yersinia [Pasteurella] pestis (020.0-020.9)

027.8 Other specified zoonotic bacterial diseases
027.9 Unspecified zoonotic bacterial disease

OTHER BACTERIAL DISEASES (030-041)

Excludes: bacterial venereal diseases (098.0-099.9)
bartonellosis (088.0)

030 Leprosy
Includes: Hansen's disease
infection by Mycobacterium leprae

030.0 Lepromatous [type L]
Lepromatous leprosy (macular) (diffuse) (infiltrated) (nodular) (neuritic)

030.1 Tuberculoid [type T]
Tuberculoid leprosy (macular) (maculoanesthetic) (major) (minor) (neuritic)

030.2 Indeterminate [group I]
Indeterminate [uncharacteristic] leprosy (macular) (neuritic)

030.3 Borderline [group B]
Borderline or dimorphous leprosy (infiltrated) (neuritic)

030.8 Other specified leprosy
030.9 Leprosy, unspecified

031 Diseases due to other mycobacteria

031.0 Pulmonary
Infection by Mycobacterium:
avium
intracellulare [Battey bacillus]
kansasii
Battey disease

031.1 Cutaneous
Buruli ulcer
Infection by Mycobacterium:
marinum [M. balnei]
ulcerans

031.2 Disseminated
Disseminated mycobacterium avium-intracellulare complex (DMAC)
Mycobacterium avium-intracellulare complex (MAC) bacteremia

031.8 Other specified mycobacterial diseases
031.9 Unspecified diseases due to mycobacteria
Atypical mycobacterium infection NOS

032 Diphtheria
Includes: infection by Corynebacterium diphtheriae

032.0 Faucial diphtheria
Membranous angina, diphtheritic

032.1 Nasopharyngeal diphtheria

032.2 Anterior nasal diphtheria

TABULAR LIST

- **032.3 Laryngeal diphtheria**
  Laryngotracheitis, diphtheritic
- ⑤ **032.8 Other specified diphtheria**
  - **032.81 Conjunctival diphtheria**
    Pseudomembranous diphtheritic conjunctivitis
  - **032.82 Diphtheritic myocarditis**
  - **032.83 Diphtheritic peritonitis**
  - **032.84 Diphtheritic cystitis**
  - **032.85 Cutaneous diphtheria**
  - **032.89 Other**
- **032.9 Diphtheria, unspecified**

033 Whooping cough
Includes: pertussis

Use additional code, if desired, to identify any associated pneumonia (484.3)

- **033.0 Bordetella pertussis [B. pertussis]**
- **033.1 Bordetella parapertussis [B. parapertussis]**
- **033.8 Whooping cough due to other specified organism**
  Bordetella bronchiseptica [B. bronchiseptica]
- **033.9 Whooping cough, unspecified organism**

034 Streptococcal sore throat and scarlet fever

- **034.0 Streptococcal sore throat**
  Septic:
    angina
    sore throat
  Streptococcal:
    angina
    laryngitis
    pharyngitis
    tonsillitis
- **034.1 Scarlet fever**
  Scarlatina
  Excludes: parascarlatina (057.8)

035 Erysipelas
Excludes: postpartum or puerperal erysipelas (670)

036 Meningococcal infection

- **036.0 Meningococcal meningitis**
  Cerebrospinal fever
    (meningococcal)
  Meningitis:
    cerebrospinal
    epidemic
- **036.1 Meningococcal encephalitis**
- **036.2 Meningococcemia**
  Meningococcal septicemia
- **036.3 Waterhouse-Friderichsen syndrome, meningococcal**
  Meningococcal hemorrhagic adrenalitis
  Meningococcic adrenal syndrome
  Waterhouse-Friderichsen syndrome NOS
- ⑤ **036.4 Meningococcal carditis**
  - **036.40 Meningococcal carditis, unspecified**
  - **036.41 Meningococcal pericarditis**
  - **036.42 Meningococcal endocarditis**
  - **036.43 Meningococcal myocarditis**
- ⑤ **036.8 Other specified meningococcal infections**
  - **036.81 Meningococcal optic neuritis**
  - **036.82 Meningococcal arthropathy**
  - **036.89 Other**
- **036.9 Meningococcal infection, unspecified**
  Meningococcal infection NOS

INFECTIOUS AND PARASITIC DISEASES

037 Tetanus
> *Excludes:* tetanus:
>> complicating:
>>> abortion (634-638 with .0, 639.0)
>>> ectopic or molar pregnancy (639.0)
>> neonatorum (771.3)
>> puerperal (670)

038 Septicemia
> *Excludes:* bacteremia (790.7)
>> during labor (659.3)
>> following ectopic or molar pregnancy (639.0)
>> following infusion, injection, transfusion, or vaccination (999.3)
>> postpartum, puerperal (670)
>> septicemia (sepsis) of newborn (771.81)
>> that complicating abortion (634-638 with .0, 639.0)

Use additional code for systemic inflammatory response syndrome (SIRS) (995.91-995.92)

- **038.0 Streptococcal septicemia**
- **038.1 Staphylococcal septicemia**
  - **038.10 Staphylococcal septicemia, unspecified**
  - **038.11 Staphylococcus aureus septicemia**
  - **038.19 Other staphylococcal septicemia**
- **038.2 Pneumococcal septicemia**
- **038.3 Septicemia due to anaerobes**
  Septicemia due to bacteroides
  > *Excludes:* gas gangrene (040.0)
  >> that due to anaerobic streptococci (038.0)
- **038.4 Septicemia due to other gram-negative organisms**
  - **038.40 Gram-negative organism, unspecified**
    Gram-negative septicemia NOS
  - **038.41 Hemophilus influenzae [H. influenzae]**
  - **038.42 Escherichia coli [E. coli]**
  - **038.43 Pseudomonas**
  - **038.44 Serratia**
  - **038.49 Other**
- **038.8 Other specified septicemias**
  > *Excludes:* septicemia (due to):
  >> anthrax (022.3)
  >> gonococcal (098.89)
  >> herpetic (054.5)
  >> meningococcal (036.2)
  >> septicemic plague (020.2)
- **038.9 Unspecified septicemia**
  Septicemia NOS
  > *Excludes:* bacteremia NOS (790.7)

039 Actinomycotic infections
> Includes: actinomycotic mycetoma
> infection by Actinomycetales, such as species of Actinomyces, Actinomadura, Nocardia, Streptomyces
> maduromycosis (actinomycotic)
> schizomycetoma (actinomycotic)

- **039.0 Cutaneous**
  Erythrasma   Trichomycosis axillaris
- **039.1 Pulmonary**
  Thoracic actinomycosis
- **039.2 Abdominal**
- **039.3 Cervicofacial**
- **039.4 Madura foot**
  > *Excludes:* madura foot due to mycotic infection (117.4)
- **039.8 Of other specified sites**

TABULAR LIST

039.9 **Of unspecified site**
  Actinomycosis NOS
  Maduromycosis NOS
  Nocardiosis NOS

040 **Other bacterial diseases**
  Excludes: bacteremia NOS (790.7)
  bacterial infection NOS (041.9)

  040.0 **Gas gangrene**
    Gas bacillus infection
      or gangrene
    Infection by Clostridium:
      histolyticum
      oedematiens
      perfringens [welchii]
      septicum
      sordellii
    Malignant edema
    Myonecrosis, clostridial
    Myositis, clostridial

  040.1 **Rhinoscleroma**

  040.2 **Whipple's disease**
    Intestinal lipodystrophy

  040.3 **Necrobacillosis**

  ● **040.4** **Other specified botulism**
    Non-foodborne intoxication due to toxins of Clostridium botulinum [C. botulinum]
    Excludes: botulism NOS (005.1)
    food poisoning due to toxins of Clostridium botulinum (005.1)

    ● **040.41** **Infant botulism**

    ● **040.42** **Wound botulism**
      Non-foodborne botulism NOS
    Use additional code to identify complicated open wound

  ⑤ **040.8** **Other specified bacterial diseases**

    040.81 **Tropical pyomyositis**

    040.82 **Toxic shock syndrome**
      Use additional code to identify the organism

    040.89 **Other**

041 **Bacterial infection in conditions classified elsewhere and of unspecified site**
  Note: This category is provided to be used as an additional code where it is desired to identify the bacterial agent in diseases classified elsewhere. This category will also be used to classify bacterial infections of unspecified nature or site.
  Excludes: septicemia (038.0-038.9)

  ⑤ **041.0** **Streptococcus**
    041.00 **Streptococcus, unspecified**
    041.01 **Group A**
    041.02 **Group B**
    041.03 **Group C**
    041.04 **Group D [Enterococcus]**
    041.05 **Group G**
    041.09 **Other Streptococcus**

  ⑤ **041.1** **Staphylococcus**
    041.10 **Staphylococcus, unspecified**
    041.11 **Staphylococcus aureus**
    041.19 **Other Staphylococcus**

  041.2 **Pneumococcus**

  041.3 **Friedländer's bacillus**
    Infection by Klebsiella pneumoniae

  041.4 **Escherichia coli [E. coli]**

  041.5 **Hemophilus influenzae [H. influenzae]**

  041.6 **Proteus (mirabilis) (morganii)**

  041.7 **Pseudomonas**

  ⑤ **041.8** **Other specified bacterial infections**

| ● Code new to this edition | ▲ Revision of existing code | ④ ⑤ Fourth or fifth digit required |

INFECTIOUS AND PARASITIC DISEASES

041.81 **Mycoplasma**
Eaton's agent
Pleuropneumonia-like organisms [PPLO]

041.82 **Bacteroides fragilis**

041.83 **Clostridium perfringens**

041.84 **Other anaerobes**
Gram-negative anaerobes

Excludes: Helicobacter pylori (041.86)

041.85 **Other Gram-negative organisms**
Aerobacter aerogenes
Gram-negative bacteria NOS
Mima polymorpha
Serratia

Excludes: Gram-negative anaerobes (041.84)

041.86 **Helicobacter pylori (H. pylori)**

041.89 **Other specified bacteria**

041.9 **Bacterial infection, unspecified**

HUMAN IMMUNODEFICIENCY VIRUS (HIV) INFECTION (042)

042 **Human immunodeficiency virus [HIV] disease**
Acquired immune deficiency syndrome
Acquired immunodeficiency syndrome
AIDS
AIDS-like syndrome
AIDS-related complex
ARC
HIV infection, symptomatic

Use additional code(s) to identify all manifestations of HIV

Use additional code, if desired, to identify HIV-2 infection (079.53)

Excludes: asymptomatic HIV infection status (V08)
exposure to HIV virus (V01.79)
nonspecific serologic evidence of HIV (795.71)

POLIOMYELITIS AND OTHER NON-ARTHROPOD-BORNE VIRAL DISEASES OF CENTRAL NERVOUS SYSTEM (045-049)

⑤ **045** **Acute poliomyelitis**

Excludes: late effects of acute poliomyelitis (138)

The following fifth-digit subclassification is for use with category 045:

0 poliovirus, unspecified type
1 poliovirus type I
2 poliovirus type II
3 poliovirus type III

⑤ **045.0** **Acute paralytic poliomyelitis specified as bulbar**
Infantile paralysis (acute) specified as bulbar
Poliomyelitis (acute) (anterior) specified as bulbar
Polioencephalitis (acute) (bulbar)
Polioencephalomyelitis (acute) (anterior) (bulbar)

⑤ **045.1** **Acute poliomyelitis with other paralysis**
Paralysis:
 acute atrophic, spinal
 infantile, paralytic
Poliomyelitis (acute):
 anterior, with paralysis except bulbar
 epidemic, with paralysis except bulbar

⑤ **045.2** **Acute nonparalytic poliomyelitis**
Poliomyelitis (acute):
 anterior, specified as nonparalytic
 epidemic, specified as nonparalytic

⑤ **045.9** **Acute poliomyelitis, unspecified**
Infantile paralysis, unspecified whether paralytic or nonparalytic
Poliomyelitis (acute):
 anterior, unspecified whether paralytic or nonparalytic
 epidemic, unspecified whether paralytic or nonparalytic

TABULAR LIST

046 **Slow virus infection of central nervous system**

046.0 **Kuru**

046.1 **Jakob-Creutzfeldt disease**
Subacute spongiform encephalopathy

046.2 **Subacute sclerosing panencephalitis**
Dawson's inclusion body encephalitis
Van Bogaert's sclerosing leukoencephalitis

046.3 **Progressive multifocal leukoencephalopathy**
Multifocal leukoencephalopathy NOS

046.8 **Other specified slow virus infection of central nervous system**

046.9 **Unspecified slow virus infection of central nervous system**

047 **Meningitis due to enterovirus**
Includes: meningitis:
abacterial
aseptic
viral

Excludes: meningitis due to:
adenovirus (049.1)
arthropod-borne virus (060.0-066.9)
leptospira (100.81)
virus of:
herpes simplex (054.72)
herpes zoster (053.0)
lymphocytic choriomeningitis (049.0)
mumps (072.1)
poliomyelitis (045.0-045.9)
any other infection specifically classified elsewhere

047.0 **Coxsackie virus**

047.1 **ECHO virus**
Meningo-eruptive syndrome

047.8 **Other specified viral meningitis**

047.9 **Unspecified viral meningitis**
Viral meningitis NOS

048 **Other enterovirus diseases of central nervous system**
Boston exanthem

049 **Other non-arthropod-borne viral diseases of central nervous system**

Excludes: late effects of viral encephalitis (139.0)

049.0 **Lymphocytic choriomeningitis**
Lymphocytic:
meningitis (serous) (benign)
meningoencephalitis (serous) (benign)

049.1 **Meningitis due to adenovirus**

049.8 **Other specified non-arthropod-borne viral diseases of central nervous system**
Encephalitis: Encephalitis:
  acute: lethargica
    inclusion body   Rio Bravo
    necrotizing   von Economo's disease
  epidemic

Excludes: human herpesvirus 6 encephalitis (058.21)
other human herpesvirus encephalitis (058.29)

049.9 **Unspecified non-arthropod-borne viral diseases of central nervous system**
Viral encephalitis NOS

VIRAL DISEASES ACCOMPANIED BY EXANTHEM (050-057)

Excludes: arthropod-borne viral diseases (060.0-066.9)
Boston exanthem (048)

050 **Smallpox**

050.0 **Variola major**
Hemorrhagic (pustular)   Malignant smallpox
smallpox   Purpura variolosa

050.1 **Alastrim**
Variola minor

INFECTIOUS AND PARASITIC DISEASES

- **050.2** Modified smallpox
  Varioloid
- **050.9** Smallpox, unspecified

051 Cowpox and paravaccinia
- **051.0** Cowpox
  Vaccinia not from vaccination
  Excludes: vaccinia (generalized) (from vaccination) (999.0)
- **051.1** Pseudocowpox
  Milkers' node
- **051.2** Contagious pustular dermatitis
  Ecthyma contagiosum   Orf
- **051.9** Paravaccinia, unspecified

052 Chickenpox
- **052.0** Postvaricella encephalitis
  Postchickenpox encephalitis
- **052.1** Varicella (hemorrhagic) pneumonitis
- **052.2** Postvaricella myelitis
  Postchickenpox myelitis
- **052.7** With other specified complications
- **052.8** With unspecified complication
- **052.9** Varicella without mention of complication
  Chickenpox NOS
  Varicella NOS

053 Herpes zoster
  Includes: shingles
             zona
- **053.0** With meningitis
- ⑤ **053.1** With other nervous system complications
  - **053.10** With unspecified nervous system complication
  - **053.11** Geniculate herpes zoster
    Herpetic geniculate ganglionitis
  - **053.12** Postherpetic trigeminal neuralgia
  - **053.13** Postherpetic polyneuropathy
  - **053.14** Herpes zoster myelitis
  - **053.19** Other
- ⑤ **053.2** With ophthalmic complications
  - **053.20** Herpes zoster dermatitis of eyelid
    Herpes zoster ophthalmicus
  - **053.21** Herpes zoster keratoconjunctivitis
  - **053.22** Herpes zoster iridocyclitis
  - **053.29** Other
- ⑤ **053.7** With other specified complications
  - **053.71** Otitis externa due to herpes zoster
  - **053.79** Other
- **053.8** With unspecified complication
- **053.9** Herpes zoster without mention of complication
  Herpes zoster NOS

054 Herpes simplex
  Excludes: congenital herpes simplex (771.2)
- **054.0** Eczema herpeticum
  Kaposi's varicelliform eruption
- ⑤ **054.1** Genital herpes
  - **054.10** Genital herpes, unspecified
    Herpes progenitalis
  - **054.11** Herpetic vulvovaginitis
  - **054.12** Herpetic ulceration of vulva

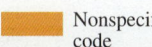 Add 4th or 5th digit   Nonspecific code   Unspecified code   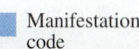 Manifestation code

163

TABULAR LIST

   054.13 Herpetic infection of penis
   054.19 Other
  054.2 Herpetic gingivostomatitis
  054.3 Herpetic meningoencephalitis
    Herpes encephalitis
    Simian B disease
   Excludes: human herpesvirus 6 encephalitis (058.21)
       other human herpesvirus encephalitis (058.29)
⑤ 054.4 With ophthalmic complications
   054.40 With unspecified ophthalmic complication
   054.41 Herpes simplex dermatitis of eyelid
   054.42 Dendritic keratitis
   054.43 Herpes simplex disciform keratitis
   054.44 Herpes simplex iridocyclitis
   054.49 Other
  054.5 Herpetic septicemia
  054.6 Herpetic whitlow
    Herpetic felon
⑤ 054.7 With other specified complications
   054.71 Visceral herpes simplex
   054.72 Herpes simplex meningitis
   054.73 Herpes simplex otitis externa
   054.74 Herpes simplex myelitis
   054.79 Other
  054.8 With unspecified complication
  054.9 Herpes simplex without mention of complication

055 **Measles**
   Includes: morbilli
       rubeola
  055.0 Postmeasles encephalitis
  055.1 Postmeasles pneumonia
  055.2 Postmeasles otitis media
⑤ 055.7 With other specified complications
   055.71 Measles keratoconjunctivitis
     Measles keratitis
   055.79 Other
  055.8 With unspecified complication
  055.9 Measles without mention of complication

056 **Rubella**
   Includes: German measles
   Excludes: congenital rubella (771.0)
⑤ 056.0 With neurological complications
   056.00 With unspecified neurological complication
   056.01 Encephalomyelitis due to rubella
     Encephalitis due to rubella
     Meningoencephalitis due to rubella
   056.09 Other
⑤ 056.7 With other specified complications
   056.71 Arthritis due to rubella
   056.79 Other
  056.8 With unspecified complications
  056.9 Rubella without mention of complication

057 **Other viral exanthemata**
  057.0 Erythema infectiosum [fifth disease]

INFECTIOUS AND PARASITIC DISEASES

057.8 **Other specified viral exanthemata**
Dukes (-Filatow) disease   Parascarlatina
Fourth disease   Pseudoscarlatina
Excludes: exanthema subitum [sixth disease] (058.10-058.12)
roseola infantum (058.10-058.12)

057.9 **Viral exanthem, unspecified**

OTHER HUMAN HERPESVIRUSES (058)

● **058** **Other human herpesvirus**
Excludes: congenital herpes (771.2)
cytomegalovirus (078.5)
Epstein-Barr virus (075)
herpes NOS (054.0-054.9)
herpes simplex (054.0-054.9)
herpes zoster (053.0-053.9)
human herpesvirus NOS (054.0-054.9)
human herpesvirus 1 (054.0-054.9)
human herpesvirus 2 (054.0-054.9)
human herpesvirus 3 (052.0-053.9)
human herpesvirus 4 (075)
human herpesvirus 5 (078.5)
varicella (052.0-052.9)
varicella-zoster virus (052.0-053.9)

● **058.1** **Roseola infantum**
Exanthema subitum [sixth disease]

● **058.10** **Roseola infantum, unspecified**
Exanthema subitum [sixth disease], unspecified

● **058.11** **Roseola infantum due to human herpesvirus 6**
Exanthema subitum [sixth disease] due to human herpesvirus 6

● **058.12** **Roseola infantum due to human herpesvirus 7**
Exanthema subitum [sixth disease] due to human herpesvirus 7

● **058.2** **Other human herpesvirus encephalitis**
Excludes: herpes encephalitis NOS (054.3)
herpes simplex encephalitis (054.3)
human herpesvirus encephalitis NOS (054.3)
simian B herpes virus encephalitis (054.3)

● **058.21** **Human herpesvirus 6 encephalitis**

● **058.29** **Other human herpesvirus encephalitis**
Human herpesvirus 7 encephalitis

● **058.8** **Other human herpesvirus infections**

● **058.81** **Human herpesvirus 6 infection**

● **058.82** **Human herpesvirus 7 infection**

● **058.89** **Other human herpesvirus infection**
Human herpesvirus 8 infection
Kaposi's sarcoma-associated herpesvirus infection

ARTHROPOD-BORNE VIRAL DISEASES (060-066)

Use additional code, if desired, to identify any associated meningitis (321.2)
Excludes: late effects of viral encephalitis (139.0)

060 **Yellow fever**

060.0 **Sylvatic**
Yellow fever:
jungle
sylvan

060.1 **Urban**

060.9 **Yellow fever, unspecified**

061 **Dengue**
Breakbone fever
Excludes: hemorrhagic fever caused by dengue virus (065.4)

062 **Mosquito-borne viral encephalitis**

062.0 **Japanese encephalitis**

 Nonspecific code
 Unspecified code
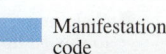 Manifestation code

TABULAR LIST

        Japanese B encephalitis

062.1 Western equine encephalitis

062.2 Eastern equine encephalitis

> *Excludes:* *Venezuelan equine encephalitis (066.2)*

062.3 St. Louis encephalitis

062.4 Australian encephalitis
    Australian arboencephalitis
    Australian X disease
    Murray Valley encephalitis

062.5 California virus encephalitis
    Encephalitis: Tahyna fever
      California
      La Crosse

062.8 Other specified mosquito-borne viral encephalitis
    Encephalitis by Ilheus virus

> *Excludes:* *West Nile virus (066.40-066.49)*

062.9 Mosquito-borne viral encephalitis, unspecified

063 Tick-borne viral encephalitis
    Includes: diphasic meningoencephalitis

063.0 Russian spring-summer [taiga] encephalitis

063.1 Louping ill

063.2 Central European encephalitis

063.8 Other specified tick-borne viral encephalitis
    Langat encephalitis
    Powassan encephalitis

063.9 Tick-borne viral encephalitis, unspecified

064 Viral encephalitis transmitted by other and unspecified arthropods
    Arthropod-borne viral encephalitis, vector unknown
    Negishi virus encephalitis

> *Excludes:* *viral encephalitis NOS (049.9)*

065 Arthropod-borne hemorrhagic fever

065.0 Crimean hemorrhagic fever [CHF Congo virus]
    Central Asian hemorrhagic fever

065.1 Omsk hemorrhagic fever

065.2 Kyasanur Forest disease

065.3 Other tick-borne hemorrhagic fever

065.4 Mosquito-borne hemorrhagic fever
    Chikungunya hemorrhagic fever
    Dengue hemorrhagic fever

> *Excludes:* *Chikungunya fever (066.3)*
>   *dengue (061)*
>   *yellow fever (060.0-060.9)*

065.8 Other specified arthropod-borne hemorrhagic fever
    Mite-borne hemorrhagic fever

065.9 Arthropod-borne hemorrhagic fever, unspecified
    Arbovirus hemorrhagic fever NOS

066 Other arthropod-borne viral diseases

066.0 Phlebotomus fever
    Changuinola fever
    Sandfly fever

066.1 Tick-borne fever
    Nairobi sheep disease   Tick fever:
    Tick fever: Kemerovo
      American mountain Quaranfil
      Colorado

066.2 Venezuelan equine fever
    Venezuelan equine encephalitis

INFECTIOUS AND PARASITIC DISEASES

066.3 Other mosquito-borne fever
Fever (viral):
 Bunyamwera
 Bwamba
 Chikungunya
 GuamaR Mayaro
 Mucambo
 O'nyong-nyong
Fever (viral):
 Oropouche
 Pixuna
 Rift valley
 Ross river
 Wesselsbron
 Zika

Excludes: dengue (061)
 yellow fever (060.0-060.9)

⑤ **066.4 West Nile fever**

066.40 West Nile fever, unspecified
West Nile fever NOS
West Nile fever without complications
West Nile virus NOS

066.41 **West Nile fever with encephalitis**
West Nile encephalitis
West Nile encephalomyelitis

066.42 West Nile fever with other neurologic manifestation
Use additional code to specify the neurologic manifestation

066.49 West Nile fever with other complications
Use additional code to specify the other conditions

066.8 Other specified arthropod-borne viral diseases
Chandipura fever
Piry fever

066.9 Arthropod-borne viral disease, unspecified
Arbovirus infection NOS

OTHER DISEASES DUE TO VIRUSES AND CHLAMYDIAE (070-079)

070 **Viral hepatitis**
Includes: viral hepatitis (acute) (chronic)

Excludes: cytomegalic inclusion virus hepatitis (078.5)

The following fifth-digit subclassification is for use with categories 070.2 and 070.3:

0 acute or unspecified, without mention of hepatitis delta
1 acute or unspecified, with hepatitis delta
2 chronic, without mention of hepatitis delta
3 chronic, with hepatitis delta

070.0 **Viral hepatitis A with hepatic coma**

070.1 **Viral hepatitis A without mention of hepatic coma**
Infectious hepatitis

⑤ 070.2 **Viral hepatitis B with hepatic coma**

⑤ 070.3 **Viral hepatitis B without mention of hepatic coma**
Serum hepatitis

⑤ 070.4 **Other specified viral hepatitis with hepatic coma**

070.41 Acute hepatitis C with hepatic coma

070.42 Hepatitis delta without mention of active hepatitis B disease with hepatic coma
Hepatitis delta with hepatitis B carrier state

070.43 Hepatitis E with hepatic coma

070.44 Chronic hepatitis C with hepatic coma

070.49 Other specified viral hepatitis with hepatic coma

⑤ 070.5 **Other specified viral hepatitis without mention of hepatic coma**

070.51 Acute hepatitis C without mention of hepatic coma

070.52 Hepatitis delta without mention of active hepatitis B disease or hepatic coma

070.53 Hepatitis E without mention of hepatic coma

070.54 Chronic hepatitis C without mention of hepatic coma

070.59 Other specified viral hepatitis without mention of hepatic coma

 Add 4th or 5th digit
 Nonspecific code
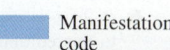 Unspecified code
Manifestation code

TABULAR LIST

070.6 **Unspecified viral hepatitis with hepatic coma**

Excludes: unspecified viral hepatitis C with hepatic coma (070.71)

⑤ 070.7 **Unspecified viral hepatitis C**

070.70 **Unspecified viral hepatitis C without hepatic coma**
Unspecified viral hepatitis C NOS

070.71 **Unspecified viral hepatitis C with hepatic coma**

070.9 **Unspecified viral hepatitis without mention of hepatic coma**
Viral hepatitis NOS

Excludes: unspecified viral hepatitis C without hepatic coma (070.70)

071 Rabies
Hydrophobia   Lyssa

072 Mumps

072.0 **Mumps orchitis**

072.1 **Mumps meningitis**

072.2 **Mumps encephalitis**
Mumps meningoencephalitis

072.3 **Mumps pancreatitis**

⑤ 072.7 **Mumps with other specified complications**

072.71 **Mumps hepatitis**

072.72 **Mumps polyneuropathy**

072.79 **Other**

072.8 **Mumps with unspecified complication**

072.9 **Mumps without mention of complication**
Epidemic parotitis
Infectious parotitis

073 Ornithosis
Includes: parrot fever
psittacosis

073.0 **With pneumonia**
Lobular pneumonitis due to ornithosis

073.7 **With other specified complications**

073.8 **With unspecified complication**

073.9 **Ornithosis, unspecified**

074 Specific diseases due to Coxsackie virus

Excludes: Coxsackie virus:
infection NOS (079.2)
meningitis (047.0)

074.0 **Herpangina**
Vesicular pharyngitis

074.1 **Epidemic pleurodynia**
Bornholm disease   Epidemic:
Devil's grip   myalgia
                                          myositis

⑤ 074.2 **Coxsackie carditis**

074.20 **Coxsackie carditis, unspecified**

074.21 **Coxsackie pericarditis**

074.22 **Coxsackie endocarditis**

074.23 **Coxsackie myocarditis**
Aseptic myocarditis of newborn

074.3 **Hand, foot, and mouth disease**
Vesicular stomatitis and exanthem

074.8 **Other specified diseases due to Coxsackie virus**
Acute lymphonodular pharyngitis

075 Infectious mononucleosis
Glandular fever   Pfeiffer's disease
Monocytic angina

● Code new to this edition   ▲ Revision of existing code   ④ ⑤ Fourth or fifth digit required

INFECTIOUS AND PARASITIC DISEASES

076 Trachoma

> *Excludes:* late effect of trachoma (139.1)

- **076.0 Initial stage**
  Trachoma dubium
- **076.1 Active stage**
  Granular conjunctivitis (trachomatous)
  Trachomatous:
    follicular conjunctivitis
    pannus
- **076.9 Trachoma, unspecified**
  Trachoma NOS

077 Other diseases of conjunctiva due to viruses and Chlamydiae

> *Excludes:* ophthalmic complications of viral diseases classified elsewhere

- **077.0 Inclusion conjunctivitis**
  Paratrachoma
  Swimming pool conjunctivitis
  > *Excludes:* inclusion blennorrhea (neonatal) (771.6)
- **077.1 Epidemic keratoconjunctivitis**
  Shipyard eye
- **077.2 Pharyngoconjunctival fever**
  Viral pharyngoconjunctivitis
- **077.3 Other adenoviral conjunctivitis**
  Acute adenoviral follicular conjunctivitis
- **077.4 Epidemic hemorrhagic conjunctivitis**
  Apollo:
    conjunctivitis
    disease
  Conjunctivitis due to enterovirus type 70
  Hemorrhagic conjunctivitis (acute) (epidemic)
- **077.8 Other viral conjunctivitis**
  Newcastle conjunctivitis
- ⑤ **077.9 Unspecified diseases of conjunctiva due to viruses and Chlamydiae**
  - **077.98 Due to Chlamydiae**
  - **077.99 Due to viruses**
    Viral conjunctivitis NOS

078 Other diseases due to viruses and Chlamydiae

> *Excludes:* viral infection NOS (079.0-079.9)
>   viremia NOS (790.8)

- **078.0 Molluscum contagiosum**
- ⑤ **078.1 Viral warts**
  Viral warts due to Human papillomavirus
  - **078.10 Viral warts, unspecified**
    Condyloma NOS
    Verruca:
      NOS
      vulgaris
    Warts (infectious)
  - **078.11 Condyloma acuminatum**
  - **078.19 Other specified viral warts**
    Genital warts NOS
    Verruca:
      plana
      plantaris
- **078.2 Sweating fever**
  Miliary fever
  Sweating disease
- **078.3 Cat-scratch disease**
  Benign lymphoreticulosis (of inoculation)
  Cat-scratch fever

TABULAR LIST

078.4 Foot and mouth disease
Aphthous fever
Epizootic:
aphthae
stomatitis

078.5 Cytomegaloviral disease
Cytomegalic inclusion disease
Salivary gland virus disease
Use additional code, if desired, to identify manifestation, as:
cytomegalic inclusion virus:
hepatitis (573.1)
pneumonia (484.1)

> *Excludes:* congenital cytomegalovirus infection (771.1)

078.6 Hemorrhagic nephrosonephritis
Hemorrhagic fever: Hemorrhagic fever:
epidemic   Russian
Korean   with renal syndrome

078.7 Arenaviral hemorrhagic fever
Hemorrhagic fever: Hemorrhagic fever:
Argentine   Junin virus
Bolivian   Machupo virus

⑤ **078.8 Other specified diseases due to viruses and Chlamydiae**

> *Excludes:* epidemic diarrhea (009.2)
> lymphogranuloma venereum (099.1)

078.81 Epidemic vertigo

078.82 Epidemic vomiting syndrome
Winter vomiting disease

078.88 Other specified diseases due to Chlamydiae

078.89 Other specified diseases due to viruses
Epidemic cervical myalgia
Marburg disease
Tanapox

079 Viral and Chlamydial infection in conditions classified elsewhere and of unspecified site
Note: This category is provided to be used as an additional code where it is desired to identify the viral agent in diseases classifiable elsewhere. This category will also be used to classify virus infection of unspecified nature or site.

079.0 Adenovirus

079.1 ECHO virus

079.2 Coxsackievirus

079.3 Rhinovirus

079.4 Human papillomavirus

⑤ **079.5 Retrovirus**

> *Excludes:* human immunodeficiency virus, type 1 [HIV-1] (042)
> human T-cell lymphotrophic virus, type III [HTLV-III] (042)
> lymphadenopathy-associated virus [LAV] (042)

079.50 Retrovirus, unspecified

079.51 Human T-cell lymphotrophic virus, type I [HTLV-I]

079.52 Human T-cell lymphotrophic virus, type II [HTLV-II]

079.53 Human immunodeficiency virus, type 2 [HIV-2]

079.59 Other specified retrovirus

079.6 Respiratory syncytial virus (RSV)

⑤ **079.8 Other specified viral and chlamydial infections**

079.81 Hantavirus

079.82 SARS-associated coronavirus

● **079.83 Parvovirus B19**
Human parvovirus
Parvovirus NOS

> *Excludes:* erythema infectiosum [fifth disease] (057.0)

079.88 Other specified chlamydial infection

---

170   ● Code new to this edition   ▲ Revision of existing code   ④ ⑤ Fourth or fifth digit required

INFECTIOUS AND PARASITIC DISEASES

079.89 Other specified viral infection

⑤ 079.9 **Unspecified viral and chlamydial infections**
Excludes: viremia NOS (790.8)

079.98 Unspecified chlamydial infection
Chlamydial infection NOS

079.99 Unspecified viral infection
Viral infection NOS

RICKETTSIOSES AND OTHER ARTHROPOD-BORNE DISEASES (080-088)

Excludes: arthropod-borne viral diseases (060.0-066.9)

080 Louse-borne [epidemic] typhus
Typhus (fever):
  classical
  epidemic
Typhus (fever):
  exanthematic NOS
  louse-borne

081 Other typhus

081.0 Murine [endemic] typhus
Typhus (fever):
  endemic
  flea-borne

081.1 Brill's disease
Brill-Zinsser disease
Recrudescent typhus (fever)

081.2 Scrub typhus
Japanese river fever
Kedani fever
Mite-borne typhus
Tsutsugamushi

081.9 Typhus, unspecified
Typhus (fever) NOS

082 Tick-borne rickettsioses

082.0 Spotted fevers
Rocky mountain spotted fever
São Paulo fever

082.1 Boutonneuse fever
African tick typhus
India tick typhus
Kenya tick typhus
Marseilles fever
Mediterranean tick fever

082.2 North Asian tick fever
Siberian tick typhus

082.3 Queensland tick typhus

⑤ **082.4 Ehrlichiosis**

082.40 Ehrlichiosis, unspecified

082.41 Ehrlichiosis chafeensis (E. chafeensis)

082.49 Other ehrlichiosis

082.8 Other specified tick-borne rickettsioses
Lone star fever

082.9 Tick-borne rickettsiosis, unspecified
Tick-borne typhus NOS

083 Other rickettsioses

083.0 Q fever

083.1 Trench fever
Quintan fever
Wolhynian fever

083.2 Rickettsialpox
Vesicular rickettsiosis

083.8 Other specified rickettsioses

083.9 Rickettsiosis, unspecified

084 Malaria
Note: Subcategories 084.0-084.6 exclude the listed conditions with mention of pernicious complications (084.8-084.9).
Excludes: congenital malaria (771.2)

 Nonspecific code
 Unspecified code
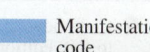 Manifestation code

171

TABULAR LIST

084.0 Falciparum malaria [malignant tertian]
Malaria (fever):
by Plasmodium falciparum
subtertian

084.1 Vivax malaria [benign tertian]
Malaria (fever) by Plasmodium vivax

084.2 Quartan malaria
Malaria (fever) by Plasmodium malariae
Malariae malaria

084.3 Ovale malaria
Malaria (fever) by Plasmodium ovale

084.4 Other malaria
Monkey malaria

084.5 Mixed malaria
Malaria (fever) by more than one parasite

084.6 Malaria, unspecified
Malaria (fever) NOS

084.7 Induced malaria
Therapeutically induced malaria

Excludes: *accidental infection from syringe, blood transfusion, etc. (084.0-084.6, above, according to parasite species)*
transmission from mother to child during delivery (771.2)

084.8 Blackwater fever
Hemoglobinuric: Malarial hemoglobinuria
fever (bilious)
malaria

084.9 Other pernicious complications of malaria
Algid malaria
Cerebral malaria
Use additional code, if desired, to identify complication, as:
malarial:
hepatitis (573.2)
nephrosis (581.81)

085 Leishmaniasis

085.0 Visceral [kala-azar]
Dumdum fever   Leishmaniasis:
Infection by Leishmania: dermal, post-kala-azar
donovani   Mediterranean
infantum   visceral (Indian)

085.1 Cutaneous, urban
Aleppo boil   Leishmaniasis, cutaneous:
Baghdad boil   dry form
Delhi boil   late
Infection by Leishmania   recurrent
tropica (minor)   ulcerating
                                Oriental sore

085.2 Cutaneous, Asian desert
Infection by Leishmania tropica major
Leishmaniasis, cutaneous:
acute necrotizing
rural
wet form
zoonotic form

085.3 Cutaneous, Ethiopian
Infection by Leishmania ethiopica
Leishmaniasis, cutaneous:
diffuse
lepromatous

085.4 Cutaneous, American
Chiclero ulcer
Infection by Leishmania mexicana
Leishmaniasis tegumentaria diffusa

INFECTIOUS AND PARASITIC DISEASES

085.5 **Mucocutaneous (American)**
  Espundia
  Infection by Leishmania braziliensis
  Uta

085.9 Leishmaniasis, unspecified

086 Trypanosomiasis
Use additional code, if desired, to identify manifestations, as:
  trypanosomiasis:
    encephalitis (323.2)
    meningitis (321.3)

086.0 **Chagas' disease with heart involvement**
  American trypanosomiasis with heart involvement
  Infection by Trypanosoma cruzi with heart involvement
  Any condition classifiable to 086.2 with heart involvement

086.1 **Chagas' disease with other organ involvement**
  American trypanosomiasis with involvement of organ other than heart
  Infection by Trypanosoma cruzi with involvement of organ other than heart
  Any condition classifiable to 086.2 with involvement of organ other than heart

086.2 **Chagas' disease without mention of organ involvement**
  American trypanosomiasis
  Infection by Trypanosoma cruzi

086.3 **Gambian trypanosomiasis**
  Gambian sleeping sickness
  Infection by Trypanosoma gambiense

086.4 **Rhodesian trypanosomiasis**
  Infection by Trypanosoma rhodesiense
  Rhodesian sleeping sickness

086.5 African trypanosomiasis, unspecified
  Sleeping sickness NOS

086.9 Trypanosomiasis, unspecified

087 Relapsing fever
Includes: recurrent fever

087.0 **Louse-borne**

087.1 **Tick-borne**

087.9 Relapsing fever, unspecified

088 Other arthropod-borne diseases

088.0 **Bartonellosis**
  Carrión's disease   Verruga peruana
  Oroya fever

⑤ 088.8 **Other specified arthropod-borne diseases**

  088.81 **Lyme Disease**
    Erythema chronicum migrans

  088.82 **Babesiosis**
    Babesiasis

  088.89 Other

088.9 Arthropod-borne disease, unspecified

SYPHILIS AND OTHER VENEREAL DISEASES (090-099)

Excludes: nonvenereal endemic syphilis (104.0)
  urogenital trichomoniasis (131.0)

090 Congenital syphilis

090.0 **Early congenital syphilis, symptomatic**
  Congenital syphilitic: Syphilitic (congenital):
    choroiditis   epiphysitis
    coryza (chronic)   osteochondritis
    hepatomegaly   pemphigus
    mucous patches   Any congenital syphilitic condition specified as early or
    periostitis   manifest less than two years after birth
    splenomegaly

090.1 **Early congenital syphilis, latent**
  Congenital syphilis without clinical manifestations, with positive serological reaction
    and negative spinal fluid test, less than two years after birth

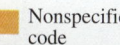

173

TABULAR LIST

090.2 Early congenital syphilis, unspecified
Congenital syphilis NOS, less than two years after birth

090.3 Syphilitic interstitial keratitis
Syphilitic keratitis:
  parenchymatous
  punctata profunda
Excludes: interstitial keratitis NOS (370.50)

⑤ **090.4 Juvenile neurosyphilis**
Use additional code, if desired, to identify any associated mental disorder

    090.40 Juvenile neurosyphilis, unspecified
      Congenital neurosyphilis
      Dementia paralytica juvenilis
      Juvenile:
        general paresis
        tabes
        taboparesis

    090.41 Congenital syphilitic encephalitis

    090.42 Congenital syphilitic meningitis

    090.49 Other

090.5 Other late congenital syphilis, symptomatic
Gumma due to congenital syphilis
Hutchinson's teeth
Syphilitic saddle nose
Any congenital syphilitic condition specified as late or manifest two years or more after birth

090.6 Late congenital syphilis, latent
Congenital syphilis without clinical manifestations, with positive serological reaction and negative spinal fluid test, two years or more after birth

090.7 Late congenital syphilis, unspecified
Congenital syphilis NOS, two years or more after birth

090.9 Congenital syphilis, unspecified

091 Early syphilis, symptomatic
Excludes: early cardiovascular syphilis (093.0-093.9)
         early neurosyphilis (094.0-094.9)

  091.0 Genital syphilis (primary)
    Genital chancre

  091.1 Primary anal syphilis

  091.2 Other primary syphilis
    Primary syphilis of: Primary syphilis of:
      breast   lip
      fingers   tonsils

  091.3 Secondary syphilis of skin or mucous membranes
    Condyloma latum   Secondary syphilis of:
    Secondary syphilis of: skin
      anus   tonsils
      mouth   vulva
      pharynx

  091.4 Adenopathy due to secondary syphilis
    Syphilitic adenopathy (secondary)
    Syphilitic lymphadenitis (secondary)

⑤ **091.5 Uveitis due to secondary syphilis**

    091.50 Syphilitic uveitis, unspecified

    091.51 Syphilitic chorioretinitis (secondary)

    091.52 Syphilitic iridocyclitis (secondary)

⑤ **091.6 Secondary syphilis of viscera and bone**

    091.61 Secondary syphilitic periostitis

    091.62 Secondary syphilitic hepatitis
      Secondary syphilis of liver

    091.69 Other viscera

  091.7 Secondary syphilis, relapse
    Secondary syphilis, relapse (treated) (untreated)

● Code new to this edition   ▲ Revision of existing code   ④ ⑤ Fourth or fifth digit required

INFECTIOUS AND PARASITIC DISEASES

- ⑤ **091.8 Other forms of secondary syphilis**
    - 091.81 Acute syphilitic meningitis (secondary)
    - 091.82 Syphilitic alopecia
    - 091.89 Other
- **091.9 Unspecified secondary syphilis**
- **092 Early syphilis, latent**
  Includes: syphilis (acquired) without clinical manifestations, with positive serological reaction and negative spinal fluid test, less than two years after infection
    - **092.0 Early syphilis, latent, serological relapse after treatment**
    - **092.9 Early syphilis, latent, unspecified**
- **093 Cardiovascular syphilis**
    - **093.0 Aneurysm of aorta, specified as syphilitic**
      Dilatation of aorta, specified as syphilitic
    - **093.1 Syphilitic aortitis**
    - ⑤ **093.2 Syphilitic endocarditis**
        - 093.20 Valve, unspecified
          Syphilitic ostial coronary disease
        - 093.21 Mitral valve
        - 093.22 Aortic valve
          Syphilitic aortic incompetence or stenosis
        - 093.23 Tricuspid valve
        - 093.24 Pulmonary valve
    - ⑤ **093.8 Other specified cardiovascular syphilis**
        - 093.81 Syphilitic pericarditis
        - 093.82 Syphilitic myocarditis
        - 093.89 Other
    - **093.9 Cardiovascular syphilis, unspecified**
- **094 Neurosyphilis**
  Use additional code, if desired, to identify any associated mental disorder
    - **094.0 Tabes dorsalis**
      Locomotor ataxia (progressive)
      Posterior spinal sclerosis (syphilitic)
      Tabetic neurosyphilis
      Use additional code, if desired, to identify manifestation, as:
        neurogenic arthropathy [Charcot's joint disease] (713.5)
    - **094.1 General paresis**
      Dementia paralytica   Paretic neurosyphilis
      General paralysis (of the   Taboparesis
        insane) (progressive)
    - **094.2 Syphilitic meningitis**
      Meningovascular syphilis
      Excludes: acute syphilitic meningitis (secondary) (091.81)
    - **094.3 Asymptomatic neurosyphilis**
    - ⑤ **094.8 Other specified neurosyphilis**
        - 094.81 Syphilitic encephalitis
        - 094.82 Syphilitic Parkinsonism
        - 094.83 Syphilitic disseminated retinochoroiditis
        - 094.84 Syphilitic optic atrophy
        - 094.85 Syphilitic retrobulbar neuritis
        - 094.86 Syphilitic acoustic neuritis
        - 094.87 Syphilitic ruptured cerebral aneurysm
        - 094.89 Other
    - **094.9 Neurosyphilis, unspecified**
      Gumma (syphilitic) of central nervous system NOS
      Syphilis (early) (late) of central nervous system NOS
      Syphiloma of central nervous system NOS

TABULAR LIST

095 Other forms of late syphilis, with symptoms
   Includes: gumma (syphilitic)
              syphilis, late, tertiary, or unspecified stage

  095.0 Syphilitic episcleritis
  095.1 Syphilis of lung
  095.2 Syphilitic peritonitis
  095.3 Syphilis of liver
  095.4 Syphilis of kidney
  095.5 Syphilis of bone
  095.6 Syphilis of muscle
             Syphilitic myositis
  095.7 Syphilis of synovium, tendon, and bursa
             Syphilitic:
               bursitis
               synovitis
  095.8 Other specified forms of late symptomatic syphilis
     Excludes: cardiovascular syphilis (093.0-093.9)
               neurosyphilis (094.0-094.9)
  095.9 Late symptomatic syphilis, unspecified

096 Late syphilis, latent
     Syphilis (acquired) without clinical manifestations, with positive serological reaction and negative spinal fluid test, two years or more after infection

097 Other and unspecified syphilis
  097.0 Late syphilis, unspecified
  097.1 Latent syphilis, unspecified
             Positive serological reaction for syphilis
  097.9 Syphilis, unspecified
             Syphilis (acquired) NOS
     Excludes: syphilis NOS causing death under two years of age (090.9)

098 Gonococcal infections
  098.0 Acute, of lower genitourinary tract
             Gonococcal: Gonorrhea (acute):
               Bartholinitis (acute)   NOS
               urethritis (acute)   genitourinary (tract) NOS
               vulvovaginitis (acute)

  ⑤ **098.1** Acute, of upper genitourinary tract
       098.10 Gonococcal infection (acute) of upper genitourinary tract, site unspecified
       098.11 Gonococcal cystitis (acute)
                   Gonorrhea (acute) of bladder
       098.12 Gonococcal prostatitis (acute)
       098.13 Gonococcal epididymo-orchitis (acute)
                   Gonococcal orchitis (acute)
       098.14 Gonococcal seminal vesiculitis (acute)
                   Gonorrhea (acute) of seminal vesicle
       098.15 Gonococcal cervicitis (acute)
                   Gonorrhea (acute) of cervix
       098.16 Gonococcal endometritis (acute)
                   Gonorrhea (acute) of uterus
       098.17 Gonococcal salpingitis, specified as acute
       098.19 Other
  098.2 Chronic, of lower genitourinary tract
             Gonococcal:
               Bartholinitis specified as chronic or with duration of two months or more
               urethritis specified as chronic or with duration of two months or more
               vulvovaginitis specified as chronic or with duration of two months or more
             Gonorrhea:
               NOS specified as chronic or with duration of two months or more
               genitourinary (tract) specified as chronic or with duration of two months or more
             Any condition classifiable to 098.0 specified as chronic or with duration of two months or more

INFECTIOUS AND PARASITIC DISEASES

⑤ **098.3 Chronic, of upper genitourinary tract**
  Includes: any condition classifiable to 098.1 stated as chronic or with a duration of two months or more

  098.30 Chronic gonococcal infection of upper genitourinary tract, site unspecified

  098.31 Gonococcal cystitis, chronic
  Any condition classifiable to 098.11, specified as chronic
  Gonorrhea of bladder, chronic

  098.32 Gonococcal prostatitis, chronic
  Any condition classifiable to 098.12, specified as chronic

  098.33 Gonococcal epididymo-orchitis, chronic
  Any condition classifiable to 098.13, specified as chronic
  Chronic gonococcal orchitis

  098.34 Gonococcal seminal vesiculitis, chronic
  Any condition classifiable to 098.14, specified as chronic
  Gonorrhea of seminal vesicle, chronic

  098.35 Gonococcal cervicitis, chronic
  Any condition classifiable to 098.15, specified as chronic
  Gonorrhea of cervix, chronic

  098.36 Gonococcal endometritis, chronic
  Any condition classifiable to 098.16, specified as chronic

  098.37 Gonococcal salpingitis (chronic)

  098.39 Other

⑤ **098.4 Gonococcal infection of eye**

  098.40 Gonococcal conjunctivitis (neonatorum)
  Gonococcal ophthalmia (neonatorum)

  098.41 Gonococcal iridocyclitis

  098.42 Gonococcal endophthalmia

  098.43 Gonococcal keratitis

  098.49 Other

⑤ **098.5 Gonococcal infection of joint**

  098.50 Gonococcal arthritis
  Gonococcal infection of joint NOS

  098.51 Gonococcal synovitis and tenosynovitis

  098.52 Gonococcal bursitis

  098.53 Gonococcal spondylitis

  098.59 Other
  Gonococcal rheumatism

098.6 Gonococcal infection of pharynx

098.7 Gonococcal infection of anus and rectum
  Gonococcal proctitis

⑤ **098.8 Gonococcal infection of other specified sites**

  098.81 Gonococcal keratosis (blennorrhagica)

  098.82 Gonococcal meningitis

  098.83 Gonococcal pericarditis

  098.84 Gonococcal endocarditis

  098.85 Other gonococcal heart disease

  098.86 Gonococcal peritonitis

  098.89 Other
  Gonococcemia

099 Other venereal diseases

  099.0 Chancroid
  Bubo (inguinal):   Chancre:
    chancroidal   Ducrey's
    due to Hemophilus ducreyi   simple
                       soft
  Ulcus molle (cutis) (skin)

  099.1 Lymphogranuloma venereum
  Climatic or tropical bubo   Esthiomene
  (Durand-) Nicolas- Favre   Lymphogranuloma inguinale
    disease

TABULAR LIST

099.2 Granuloma inguinale
- Donovanosis
- Granuloma pudendi (ulcerating)
- Granuloma venereum
- Pudendal ulcer

099.3 Reiter's disease
- Reiter's syndrome
- Use additional code for associated:
    - arthropathy (711.1)
    - conjunctivitis (372.33)

⑤ **099.4 Other nongonococcal urethritis [NGU]**

- **099.40 Unspecified**
    - Nonspecific urethritis
- **099.41 Chlamydia trachomatis**
- **099.49 Other specified organism**

⑤ **099.5 Other venereal diseases due to Chlamydia trachomatis**

Excludes: Chlamydia trachomatis infection of conjunctiva (076.0-076.9, 077.0, 077.9)
Lymphogranuloma venereum (099.1)

- **099.50 Unspecified site**
- **099.51 Pharynx**
- **099.52 Anus and rectum**
- **099.53 Lower genitourinary sites**

Excludes: urethra (099.41)
Use additional code, if desired, to specify site of infection, such as:
- bladder (595.4)
- cervix (616.0)
- vagina and vulva (616.11)

- **099.54 Other genitourinary sites**

Use additional code, if desired, to specify site of infection, such as:
- pelvic inflammatory disease NOS (614.9)
- testis and epididymis (604.91)

- **099.55 Unspecified genitourinary site**
- **099.56 Peritoneum**
    - Perihepatitis
- **099.59 Other specified site**

099.8 Other specified venereal diseases

099.9 Venereal disease, unspecified

OTHER SPIROCHETAL DISEASES (100-104)

100 Leptospirosis

100.0 Leptospirosis icterohemorrhagica
- Leptospiral or spirochetal jaundice (hemorrhagic)
- Weil's disease

⑤ **100.8 Other specified leptospiral infections**

- **100.81 Leptospiral meningitis (aseptic)**
- **100.89 Other**
    - Fever:
        - Fort Bragg
        - pretibial
        - swamp
    - Infection by Leptospira:
        - australis
        - bataviae
        - pyrogenes

100.9 Leptospirosis, unspecified

101 Vincent's angina
- Acute necrotizing ulcerative:
    - gingivitis
    - stomatitis
- Fusospirochetal pharyngitis
- Spirochetal stomatitis
- Trench mouth
- Vincent's:
    - gingivitis
    - infection [any site]

102 Yaws
- Includes: frambesia
- pian

INFECTIOUS AND PARASITIC DISEASES

102.0 Initial lesions
Chancre of yaws
Frambesia, initial or primary
Initial frambesial ulcer
Mother yaw

102.1 Multiple papillomata and wet crab yaws
Butter yaws
Frambesioma
Pianoma
Planter or palmer papilloma of yaws

102.2 Other early skin lesions
Early yaws (cutaneous) (macular) (papular) (maculopapular) (micropapular)
Frambeside of early yaws
Cutaneous yaws, less than five years after infection

102.3 Hyperkeratosis
Ghoul hand
Hyperkeratosis, palmer or plantar (early) (late) due to yaws
Worm-eaten soles

102.4 Gummata and ulcers
Nodular late yaws (ulcerated)
Gummatous frambeside

102.5 Gangosa
Rhinopharyngitis mutilans

102.6 Bone and joint lesions
Goundou, of yaws (late)
Gumma, bone, of yaws (late)
Gummatous osteitis or periostitis, of yaws (late)
Hydrarthrosis, of yaws (early) (late)
Osteitis, of yaws (early) (late)
Periostitis (hypertrophic), of yaws (early) (late)

102.7 Other manifestations
Juxta-articular nodules of yaws
Mucosal yaws

102.8 Latent yaws
Yaws without clinical manifestations, with positive serology

102.9 Yaws, unspecified

103 Pinta

103.0 Primary lesions
Chancre (primary) of pinta [carate]
Papule (primary) of pinta [carate]
Pintid of pinta [carate]

103.1 Intermediate lesions
Erythematous plaques of pinta [carate]
Hyperchromic lesions of pinta [carate]
Hyperkeratosis of pinta [carate]

103.2 Late lesions
Cardiovascular lesions, of pinta [carate]
Skin lesions:
  achromic of pinta [carate]
  cicatricial of pinta [carate]
  dyschromic of pinta [carate]
Vitiligo of pinta [carate]

103.3 Mixed lesions
Achromic and hyperchromic skin lesions of pinta [carate]

103.9 Pinta, unspecified

104 Other spirochetal infection

104.0 Nonvenereal endemic syphilis
Bejel
Njovera

104.8 Other specified spirochetal infections
Excludes: relapsing fever (087.0-087.9)
syphilis (090.0-097.9)

104.9 Spirochetal infection, unspecified

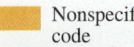 Add 4th or 5th digit
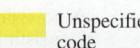 Nonspecific code / Unspecified code
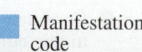 Manifestation code

TABULAR LIST

MYCOSES (110-118)

Use additional code, if desired, to identify manifestation, as:
arthropathy (711.6)
meningitis (321.0-321.1)
otitis externa (380.15)

Excludes: infection by Actinomycetales, such as species of Actinomyces, Actinomadura, Nocardia, Streptomyces (039.0-039.9)

110 Dermatophytosis
Includes: infection by species of Epidermophyton, Microsporum, and Trichophyton
tinea, any type except those in 111

110.0 Of scalp and beard
Kerion
Sycosis, mycotic
Trichophytic tinea [black dot tinea], scalp

110.1 Of nail
Dermatophytic onychia   Tinea unguium
Onychomycosis

110.2 Of hand
Tinea manuum

110.3 Of groin and perianal area
Dhobie itch   Tinea cruris
Eczema marginatum

110.4 Of foot
Athlete's foot   Tinea pedis

110.5 Of the body
Herpes circinatus
Tinea imbricata [Tokelau]

110.6 Deep seated dermatophytosis
Granuloma trichophyticum
Majocchi's granuloma

110.8 Of other specified sites

110.9 Of unspecified site
Favus NOS   Ringworm NOS
Microsporic tinea NOS

111 Dermatomycosis, other and unspecified

111.0 Pityriasis versicolor
Infection by Malassezia [Pityrosporum] furfur
Tinea flava
Tinea versicolor

111.1 Tinea nigra
Infection by   Microsporosis nigra
    Cladosporium species   Pityriasis nigra
Keratomycosis nigricans   Tinea palmaris nigra

111.2 Tinea blanca
Infection by Trichosporon (beigelii) cutaneum
White piedra

111.3 Black piedra
Infection by Piedraia hortai

111.8 Other specified dermatomycoses

111.9 Dermatomycosis, unspecified

112 Candidiasis
Includes: infection by Candida species
moniliasis

Excludes: neonatal monilial infection (771.7)

112.0 Of mouth
Thrush (oral)

112.1 Of vulva and vagina
Candidal vulvovaginitis   Monilial vulvovaginitis

112.2 Of other urogenital sites
Candidal balanitis

● Code new to this edition   ▲ Revision of existing code   ④ ⑤ Fourth or fifth digit required

INFECTIOUS AND PARASITIC DISEASES

112.3 Of skin and nails
Candidal intertrigo
Candidal onychia
Candidal perionyxis [paronychia]

112.4 Of lung
Candidal pneumonia

112.5 Disseminated
Systemic candidiasis

⑤ **112.8 Of other specified sites**

112.81 Candidal endocarditis

112.82 Candidal otitis externa
Otomycosis in moniliasis

112.83 Candidal meningitis

112.84 Candidal esophagitis

112.85 Candidal enteritis

112.89 Other

112.9 Of unspecified site

114 Coccidioidomycosis
Includes: infection by Coccidioides (immitis)
Posada-Wernicke disease

114.0 Primary coccidioidomycosis (pulmonary)
Acute pulmonary coccidioidomycosis
Coccidioidomycotic pneumonitis
Desert rheumatism
Pulmonary coccidioidomycosis
San Joaquin Valley fever

114.1 Primary extrapulmonary coccidioidomycosis
Chancriform syndrome
Primary cutaneous coccidioidomycosis

114.2 Coccidioidal meningitis

114.3 Other forms of progressive coccidioidomycosis
Coccidioidal granuloma
Disseminated coccidioidomycosis

114.4 Chronic pulmonary coccidioidomycosis

114.5 Pulmonary coccidioidomycosis, unspecified

114.9 Coccidioidomycosis, unspecified

⑤ **115 Histoplasmosis**
The following fifth-digit subclassification is for use with category 115:

    0 without mention of manifestation

    1 meningitis

    2 retinitis

    3 pericarditis

    4 endocarditis

    5 pneumonia

    9 other

⑤ **115.0 Infection by Histoplasma capsulatum**
American histoplasmosis
Darling's disease
Reticuloendothelial cytomycosis
Small form histoplasmosis

⑤ **115.1 Infection by Histoplasma duboisii**
African histoplasmosis
Large form histoplasmosis

⑤ **115.9 Histoplasmosis, unspecified**
Histoplasmosis NOS

TABULAR LIST

116 Blastomycotic infection

116.0 Blastomycosis
Blastomycotic dermatitis
Chicago disease
Cutaneous blastomycosis
Disseminated blastomycosis
Gilchrist's disease
Infection by Blastomyces [Ajellomyces] dermatitidis
North American blastomycosis
Primary pulmonary blastomycosis

116.1 Paracoccidioidomycosis
Brazilian blastomycosis
Infection by Paracoccidioides [Blastomyces] brasiliensis
Lutz-Splendore-Almeida disease
Mucocutaneous-lymphangitic paracoccidioidomycosis
Pulmonary paracoccidioidomycosis
South American blastomycosis
Visceral paracoccidioidomycosis

116.2 Lobomycosis
Infections by Loboa [Blastomyces] loboi
Keloidal blastomycosis
Lobo's disease

117 Other mycoses

117.0 Rhinosporidiosis
Infection by Rhinosporidium seeberi

117.1 Sporotrichosis
Cutaneous sporotrichosis
Disseminated sporotrichosis
Infection by Sporothrix [Sporotrichum] schenckii
Lymphocutaneous sporotrichosis
Pulmonary sporotrichosis
Sporotrichosis of the bones

117.2 Chromoblastomycosis
Chromomycosis
Infection by Cladosporidium carrionii, Fonsecaea compactum, Fonsecaea pedrosoi, Phialophora verrucosa

117.3 Aspergillosis
Infection by Aspergillus species, mainly A. fumigatus, A. flavus group, A. terreus group

117.4 Mycotic mycetomas
Infection by various genera and species of Ascomycetes and Deuteromycetes, such as Acremonium [Cephalosporium] falciforme, Neotestudina rosatii, Madurella grisea, Madurella mycetomii, Pyrenochaeta romeroi, Zopfia [Leptosphaeria] senegalensis
Madura foot, mycotic
Maduromycosis, mycotic

Excludes: actinomycotic mycetomas (039.0-039.9)

117.5 Cryptococcosis
Busse-Buschke's disease
European cryptococcosis
Infection by Cryptococcus neoformans
Pulmonary cryptococcosis
Systemic cryptococcosis
Torula

117.6 Allescheriosis [Petriellidosis]
Infections by Allescheria [Petriellidium] boydii [Monosporium apiospermum]

Excludes: mycotic mycetoma (117.4)

117.7 Zygomycosis [Phycomycosis or Mucormycosis]
Infection by species of Absidia, Basidiobolus, Conidiobolus, Cunninghamella, Entomophthora, Mucor, Rhizopus, Saksenaea

117.8 Infection by dematiacious fungi, [Phaehyphomycosis]
Infection by dematiacious fungi, such as Cladosporium trichoides [bantianum], Dreschlera hawaiiensis, Phialophora gougerotii, Phialophora jeanselmi

117.9 Other and unspecified mycoses

INFECTIOUS AND PARASITIC DISEASES

118 Opportunistic mycoses
Infection of skin, subcutaneous tissues, and/or organs by a wide variety of fungi generally considered to be pathogenic to compromised hosts only (e.g., infection by species of Alternaria, Dreschlera, Fusarium)

HELMINTHIASES (120-129)

120 Schistosomiasis [bilharziasis]

120.0 Schistosoma haematobium
Vesical schistosomiasis NOS

120.1 Schistosoma mansoni
Intestinal schistosomiasis NOS

120.2 Schistosoma japonicum
Asiatic schistosomiasis NOS
Katayama disease or fever

120.3 Cutaneous
Cercarial dermatitis
Infection by cercariae
  of Schistosoma
Schistosome dermatitis
Swimmers' itch

120.8 Other specified schistosomiasis
Infection by Schistosoma:
  bovis
  intercalatum
  mattheii
Infection by Schistosoma spindale
Schistosomiasis chestermani

120.9 Schistosomiasis, unspecified
Blood flukes NOS
Hemic distomiasis

121 Other trematode infections

121.0 Opisthorchiasis
Infection by:
  cat liver fluke
  Opisthorchis (felineus) (tenuicollis) (viverrini)

121.1 Clonorchiasis
Biliary cirrhosis due to clonorchiasis
Chinese liver fluke disease
Hepatic distomiasis due to Clonorchis sinensis
Oriental liver fluke disease

121.2 Paragonimiasis
Infection by Paragonimus
Lung fluke disease (oriental)
Pulmonary distomiasis

121.3 Fascioliasis
Infection by Fasciola:
  gigantica
  hepatica
Liver flukes NOS
Sheep liver fluke infection

121.4 Fasciolopsiasis
Infection by Fasciolopsis [buski]
Intestinal distomiasis

121.5 Metagonimiasis
Infection by Metagonimus yokogawai

121.6 Heterophyiasis
Infection by:
  Heterophyes heterophyes
  Stellantchasmus falcatus

121.8 Other specified trematode infections
Infection by:
  Dicrocoelium dendriticum
  Echinostoma ilocanum
  Gastrodiscoides hominis

121.9 Trematode infection, unspecified
Distomiasis NOS
Fluke disease NOS

122 Echinococcosis
Includes: echinococciasis
  hydatid disease
  hydatidosis

122.0 Echinococcus granulosus infection of liver

122.1 Echinococcus granulosus infection of lung

TABULAR LIST

- **122.2** Echinococcus granulosus infection of thyroid
- **122.3** Echinococcus granulosus infection, other
- **122.4** Echinococcus granulosus infection, unspecified
- **122.5** Echinococcus multilocularis infection of liver
- **122.6** Echinococcus multilocularis infection, other
- **122.7** Echinococcus multilocularis infection, unspecified
- **122.8** Echinococcosis, unspecified, of liver
- **122.9** Echinococcosis, other and unspecified

123 Other cestode infection

- **123.0** Taenia solium infection, intestinal form
  Pork tapeworm (adult) (infection)
- **123.1** Cysticercosis
  Cysticerciasis
  Infection by Cysticercus cellulosae [larval form of Taenia solium]
- **123.2** Taenia saginata infection
  Beef tapeworm (infection)
  Infection by Taeniarhynchus saginatus
- **123.3** Taeniasis, unspecified
- **123.4** Diphyllobothriasis, intestinal
  Diphyllobothrium (adult) (latum) (pacificum) infection
  Fish tapeworm (infection)
- **123.5** Sparganosis [larval diphyllobothriasis]
  Infection by:
    Diphyllobothrium larvae
    Sparganum (mansoni) (proliferum)
    Spirometra larvae
- **123.6** Hymenolepiasis
  Dwarf tapeworm (infection)
  Hymenolepis (diminuta) (nana) infection
  Rat tapeworm (infection)
- **123.8** Other specified cestode infection
  Diplogonoporus (grandis) infection
  Dipylidium (caninum) infection
  Dog tapeworm (infection) infection
- **123.9** Cestode infection, unspecified
  Tapeworm (infection) NOS

124 Trichinosis
Trichinella spiralis infection
Trichinellosis
Trichiniasis

125 Filarial infection and dracontiasis

- **125.0** Bancroftian filariasis
  Chyluria due to Wuchereria bancrofti
  Elephantiasis due to Wuchereria bancrofti
  Infection due to Wuchereria bancrofti
  Lymphadenitis due to Wuchereria bancrofti
  Lymphangitis due to Wuchereria bancrofti
  Wuchereriasis
- **125.1** Malayan filariasis
  Brugia filariasis due to Brugia [Wuchereria] malayi
  Chyluria due to Brugia [Wuchereria] malayi
  Elephantiasis due to Brugia [Wuchereria] malayi
  Infection due to Brugia [Wuchereria] malayi
  Lymphadenitis due to Brugia [Wuchereria] malayi
  Lymphangitis due to Brugia [Wuchereria] malayi
- **125.2** Loiasis
  Eyeworm disease of Africa
  Loa loa infection
- **125.3** Onchocerciasis
  Onchocerca volvulus infection
  Onchocercosis

● Code new to this edition ▲ Revision of existing code ④ ⑤ Fourth or fifth digit required

INFECTIOUS AND PARASITIC DISEASES

- **125.4 Dipetalonemiasis**
  Infection by:
  Acanthocheilonema perstans
  Dipetalonema perstans

- **125.5 Mansonella ozzardi infection**
  Filariasis ozzardi

- **125.6 Other specified filariasis**
  Dirofilaria infection
  Infection by:
  Acanthocheilonema streptocerca
  Dipetalonema streptocerca

- **125.7 Dracontiasis**
  Guinea-worm infection
  Infection by Dracunculus medinensis

- **125.9 Unspecified filariasis**

126 Ancylostomiasis and necatoriasis
Includes: cutaneous larva migrans due to Ancylostoma
hookworm (disease) (infection)
uncinariasis

- **126.0 Ancylostoma duodenale**
- **126.1 Necator americanus**
- **126.2 Ancylostoma braziliense**
- **126.3 Ancylostoma ceylanicum**
- **126.8 Other specified Ancylostoma**
- **126.9 Ancylostomiasis and necatoriasis, unspecified**
  Creeping eruption NOS
  Cutaneous larva migrans NOS

127 Other intestinal helminthiases

- **127.0 Ascariasis**
  Ascaridiasis
  Infection by Ascaris lumbricoides
  Roundworm infection

- **127.1 Anisakiasis**
  Infection by Anisakis larva

- **127.2 Strongyloidiasis**
  Infection by Strongyloides stercoralis
  Excludes: trichostrongyliasis (127.6)

- **127.3 Trichuriasis**
  Infection by Trichuris trichiuria
  Trichocephaliasis
  Whipworm (disease) (infection)

- **127.4 Enterobiasis**
  Infection by Enterobius vermicularis
  Oxyuriasis
  Oxyuris vermicularis infection
  Pinworm (disease) (infection)
  Threadworm infection

- **127.5 Capillariasis**
  Infection by Capillaria philippinensis
  Excludes: infection by Capillaria hepatica (128.8)

- **127.6 Trichostrongyliasis**
  Infection by Trichostrongylus species

- **127.7 Other specified intestinal helminthiasis**
  Infection by:
  Oesophagostomum apiostomum and related species
  Ternidens diminutus
  other specified intestinal helminth
  Physalopteriasis

- **127.8 Mixed intestinal helminthiasis**
  Infection by intestinal helminths classified to more than one of the categories 120.0-127.7
  Mixed helminthiasis NOS

TABULAR LIST

127.9 Intestinal helminthiasis, unspecified

128 Other and unspecified helminthiases

- **128.0** Toxocariasis
  - Larva migrans visceralis
  - Toxocara (canis) (cati) infection
  - Visceral larva migrans syndrome

- **128.1** Gnathostomiasis
  - Infection by Gnathostoma spinigerum and related species

- **128.8** Other specified helminthiasis
  - Infection by:
    - Angiostrongylus cantonensis
    - Capillaria hepatica
    - other specified helminth

- **128.9** Helminth infection, unspecified
  - Helminthiasis NOS
  - Worms NOS

129 Intestinal parasitism, unspecified

OTHER INFECTIOUS AND PARASITIC DISEASES (130-136)

130 Toxoplasmosis
  - Includes: infection by toxoplasma gondii
    - toxoplasmosis (acquired)
  - Excludes: congenital toxoplasmosis (771.2)

- **130.0** Meningoencephalitis due to toxoplasmosis
  - Encephalitis due to acquired toxoplasmosis

- **130.1** Conjunctivitis due to toxoplasmosis

- **130.2** Chorioretinitis due to toxoplasmosis
  - Focal retinochoroiditis due to acquired toxoplasmosis

- **130.3** Myocarditis due to toxoplasmosis
- **130.4** Pneumonitis due to toxoplasmosis
- **130.5** Hepatitis due to toxoplasmosis
- **130.7** Toxoplasmosis of other specified sites
- **130.8** Multisystemic disseminated toxoplasmosis
  - Toxoplasmosis of multiple sites
- **130.9** Toxoplasmosis, unspecified

131 Trichomoniasis
  - Includes: infection due to Trichomonas (vaginalis)

- ⑤ **131.0** Urogenital trichomoniasis
  - **131.00** Urogenital trichomoniasis, unspecified
    - Fluor (vaginalis) trichomonal or due to Trichomonas (vaginalis)
    - Leukorrhea (vaginalis) trichomonal or due to Trichomonas (vaginalis)
  - **131.01** Trichomonal vulvovaginitis
    - Vaginitis, trichomonal or due to Trichomonas (vaginalis)
  - **131.02** Trichomonal urethritis
  - **131.03** Trichomonal prostatitis
  - **131.09** Other

- **131.8** Other specified sites
  - Excludes: intestinal (007.3)

- **131.9** Trichomoniasis, unspecified

132 Pediculosis and phthirus infestation

- **132.0** Pediculus capitis [head louse]
- **132.1** Pediculus corporis [body louse]
- **132.2** Phthirus pubis [pubic louse]
  - Pediculus pubis
- **132.3** Mixed infestation
  - Infestation classifiable to more than one of the categories 132.0-132.2
- **132.9** Pediculosis, unspecified

133 Acariasis

INFECTIOUS AND PARASITIC DISEASES

- **133.0 Scabies**
  Infestation by Sarcoptes scabiei
  Norwegian scabies
  Sarcoptic itch
- **133.8 Other acariasis**
  Chiggers
  Infestation by:
  Demodex folliculorum
  Trombicula
- **133.9 Acariasis, unspecified**
  Infestation by mites NOS

134 Other infestation
- **134.0 Myiasis**
  Infestation by: Infestation by:
  Dermatobia (hominis)   maggots
  fly larvae   Oestrus ovis
  Gasterophilus (intestinalis)
- **134.1 Other arthropod infestation**
  Infestation by: Jigger disease
  chigoe   Scarabiasis
  sand flea   Tungiasis
  Tunga penetrans
- **134.2 Hirudiniasis**
  Hirudiniasis (external) (internal)
  Leeches (aquatic) (land)
- **134.8 Other specified infestations**
- **134.9 Infestation, unspecified**
  Infestation (skin) NOS
  Skin parasites NOS

135 Sarcoidosis
Besnier-Boeck- Schaumann disease   Sarcoid (any site):
Lupoid (miliary) of Boeck   NOS
Lupus pernio (Besnier)   Boeck
Lymphogranulomatosis, benign   Darier-Roussy
(Schaumann's)   Uveoparotid fever

136 Other and unspecified infectious and parasitic diseases
- **136.0 Ainhum**
  Dactylolysis spontanea
- **136.1 Behçet's syndrome**
- **136.2 Specific infections by free-living amebae**
  Meningoencephalitis due to Naegleria
- **136.3 Pneumocystosis**
  Pneumonia due to Pneumocystis carinii
  Pneumonia due to Pneumocystis jiroveci
- **136.4 Psorospermiasis**
- **136.5 Sarcosporidiosis**
  Infection by Sarcocystis lindemanni
- **136.8 Other specified infectious and parasitic diseases**
  Candiru infestation
- **136.9 Unspecified infectious and parasitic diseases**
  Infectious disease NOS
  Parasitic disease NOS

LATE EFFECTS OF INFECTIOUS AND PARASITIC DISEASES (137-139)

137 Late effects of tuberculosis
Note: This category is to be used to indicate conditions classifiable to 010-018 as the cause of late effects, which are themselves classified elsewhere. The "late effects" include those specified as such, as sequelae, or as due to old or inactive tuberculosis, without evidence of active disease.

- **137.0 Late effects of respiratory or unspecified tuberculosis**
- **137.1 Late effects of central nervous system tuberculosis**
- **137.2 Late effects of genitourinary tuberculosis**
- **137.3 Late effects of tuberculosis of bones and joints**

 Nonspecific code
 Unspecified code
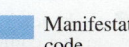 Manifestation code

TABULAR LIST

137.4 **Late effects of tuberculosis of other specified organs**

138 **Late effects of acute poliomyelitis**
> Note: This category is to be used to indicate conditions classifiable to 045 as the cause of late effects, which are themselves classified elsewhere. The "late effects" include conditions specified as such, or as sequelae, or as due to old or inactive poliomyelitis, without evidence of active disease.

139 **Late effects of other infectious and parasitic diseases**
> Note: This category is to be used to indicate conditions classifiable to categories 001-009, 020-041, 046-136 as the cause of late effects, which are themselves classified elsewhere. The "late effects" include conditions specified as such; they also include sequela of diseases classifiable to the above categories if there is evidence that the disease itself is no longer present.

139.0 **Late effects of viral encephalitis**
Late effects of conditions classifiable to 049.8-049.9, 062-064

139.1 **Late effects of trachoma**
Late effects of conditions classifiable to 076

139.8 **Late effects of other and unspecified infectious and parasitic diseases**

NEOPLASMS

2. NEOPLASMS (140-239)

Notes:

1. Content
This chapter contains the following broad groups:

140-195	Malignant neoplasms, stated or presumed to be primary, of specified sites, except of lymphatic and hematopoietic tissue
196-198	Malignant neoplasms, stated or presumed to be secondary, of specified sites
199	Malignant neoplasms, without specification of site
200-208	Malignant neoplasms, stated or presumed to be primary, of lymphatic and hematopoietic tissue
210-229	Benign neoplasms
230-234	Carcinoma in situ
235-238	Neoplasms of uncertain behavior
239	Neoplasms of unspecified nature

2. Functional activity
All neoplasms are classified in this chapter, whether or not functionally active. An additional code from Chapter 3 may be used, if desired, to identify such functional activity associated with any neoplasm, e.g.:
  catecholamine-producing malignant pheochromocytoma of adrenal:
    code 194.0, additional code 255.6
  basophil adenoma of pituitary with Cushing's syndrome:
    code 227.3, additional code 255.0

3. Morphology [Histology]
For those wishing to identify the histological type of neoplasms, a comprehensive coded nomenclature, which comprises the morphology rubrics of the ICD-Oncology, is given in Appendix A.

4. Malignant neoplasms overlapping site boundaries
Categories 140-195 are for the classification of primary malignant neoplasms according to their point of origin. A malignant neoplasm that overlaps two or more subcategories within a three-digit rubric and whose point of origin cannot be determined should be classified to the subcategory .8 "Other." For example, "carcinoma involving tip and ventral surface of tongue" should be assigned to 141.8. On the other hand, "carcinoma of tip of tongue, extending to involve the ventral surface" should be coded to 141.2, as the point of origin, the tip, is known. Three subcategories (149.8, 159.8, 165.8) have been provided for malignant neoplasms that overlap the boundaries of three-digit rubrics within certain systems. Overlapping malignant neoplasms that cannot be classified as indicated above should be assigned to the appropriate subdivision of category 195 (Malignant neoplasm of other and ill-defined sites).

MALIGNANT NEOPLASM OF LIP, ORAL CAVITY, AND PHARYNX (140-149)

Excludes: carcinoma in situ (230.0)

140 Malignant neoplasm of lip
Excludes: skin of lip (173.0)

140.0 Upper lip, vermilion border
Upper lip:
  NOS
  external
  lipstick area

140.1 Lower lip, vermilion border
Lower lip:
  NOS
  external
  lipstick area

140.3 Upper lip, inner aspect
Upper lip: Upper lip:
  buccal aspect   mucosa
  frenulum   oral aspect

140.4 Lower lip, inner aspect
Lower lip: Lower lip:
  buccal aspect   mucosa
  frenulum   oral aspect

140.5 Lip, unspecified, inner aspect
Lip, not specified whether upper or lower:
  buccal aspect   frenulum
  mucosa   oral aspect

140.6 Commissure of lip
Labial commissure

Add 4th or 5th digit | Nonspecific code | Unspecified code | Manifestation code

189

TABULAR LIST

140.8 Other sites of lip
Malignant neoplasm of contiguous or overlapping sites of lip whose point of origin cannot be determined

140.9 Lip, unspecified, vermilion border
Lip, not specified as upper or lower:
NOS
external
lipstick area

141 Malignant neoplasm of tongue

141.0 Base of tongue
Dorsal surface of base of tongue
Fixed part of tongue NOS

141.1 Dorsal surface of tongue
Anterior two-thirds of tongue, dorsal surface
Dorsal tongue NOS
Midline of tongue
Excludes: dorsal surface of base of tongue (141.0)

141.2 Tip and lateral border of tongue

141.3 Ventral surface of tongue
Anterior two-thirds of tongue, ventral surface
Frenulum linguae

141.4 Anterior two-thirds of tongue, part unspecified
Mobile part of tongue NOS

141.5 Junctional zone
Border of tongue at junction of fixed and mobile parts at insertion of anterior tonsillar pillar

141.6 Lingual tonsil

141.8 Other sites of tongue
Malignant neoplasm of contiguous or overlapping sites of tongue whose point of origin cannot be determined

141.9 Tongue, unspecified
Tongue NOS

142 Malignant neoplasm of major salivary glands
Includes: salivary ducts

Excludes: malignant neoplasm of minor salivary glands:
NOS (145.9)
buccal mucosa (145.0)
soft palate (145.3)
tongue (141.0-141.9)
tonsil, palatine (146.0)

142.0 Parotid gland

142.1 Submandibular gland
Submaxillary gland

142.2 Sublingual gland

142.8 Other major salivary glands
Malignant neoplasm of contiguous or overlapping sites of salivary glands and ducts whose point of origin cannot be determined

142.9 Salivary gland, unspecified
Salivary gland (major) NOS

143 Malignant neoplasm of gum
Includes: alveolar (ridge) mucosa
gingiva (alveolar) (marginal)
interdental papillae

Excludes: malignant odontogenic neoplasms (170.0-170.1)

143.0 Upper gum

143.1 Lower gum

143.8 Other sites of gum
Malignant neoplasm of contiguous or overlapping sites of gum whose point of origin cannot be determined

143.9 Gum, unspecified

144 Malignant neoplasm of floor of mouth

● Code new to this edition ▲ Revision of existing code ④ ⑤ Fourth or fifth digit required

NEOPLASMS

- **144.0 Anterior portion**
  Anterior to the premolar-canine junction
- **144.1 Lateral portion**
- **144.8 Other sites of floor of mouth**
  Malignant neoplasm of contiguous or overlapping sites of floor of mouth whose point of origin cannot be determined
- **144.9 Floor of mouth, part unspecified**

145 Malignant neoplasm of other and unspecified parts of mouth

Excludes: mucosa of lips (140.0-140.9)

- **145.0 Cheek mucosa**
  Buccal mucosa   Cheek, inner aspect
- **145.1 Vestibule of mouth**
  Buccal sulcus (upper) (lower)
  Labial sulcus (upper) (lower)
- **145.2 Hard palate**
- **145.3 Soft palate**
  Excludes: nasopharyngeal [posterior] [superior] surface of soft palate (147.3)
- **145.4 Uvula**
- **145.5 Palate, unspecified**
  Junction of hard and soft palate
  Roof of mouth
- **145.6 Retromolar area**
- **145.8 Other specified parts of mouth**
  Malignant neoplasm of contiguous or overlapping sites of mouth whose point of origin cannot be determined
- **145.9 Mouth, unspecified**
  Buccal cavity NOS
  Minor salivary gland, unspecified site
  Oral cavity NOS

146 Malignant neoplasm of oropharynx

- **146.0 Tonsil**
  Tonsil:
    NOS
    faucial
    palatine
  Excludes: lingual tonsil (141.6)
            pharyngeal tonsil (147.1)
- **146.1 Tonsillar fossa**
- **146.2 Tonsillar pillars (anterior) (posterior)**
  Faucial pillar   Palatoglossal arch
  Glossopalatine fold   Palatopharyngeal arch
- **146.3 Vallecula**
  Anterior and medial surface of the pharyngoepiglottic fold
- **146.4 Anterior aspect of epiglottis**
  Epiglottis, free border [margin]
  Glossoepiglottic fold(s)
  Excludes: epiglottis:
              NOS (161.1)
              suprahyoid portion (161.1)
- **146.5 Junctional region**
  Junction of the free margin of the epiglottis, the aryepiglottic fold, and the pharyngoepiglottic fold
- **146.6 Lateral wall of oropharynx**
- **146.7 Posterior wall of oropharynx**
- **146.8 Other specified sites of oropharynx**
  Branchial cleft
  Malignant neoplasm of contiguous or overlapping sites of oropharynx whose point of origin cannot be determined
- **146.9 Oropharynx, unspecified**

Add 4th or 5th digit	Nonspecific code	Unspecified code	Manifestation code

TABULAR LIST

147 Malignant neoplasm of nasopharynx

147.0 Superior wall
Roof of nasopharynx

147.1 Posterior wall
Adenoid   Pharyngeal tonsil

147.2 Lateral wall
Fossa of Rosenmüller   Pharyngeal recess
Opening of auditory tube

147.3 Anterior wall
Floor of nasopharynx
Nasopharyngeal [posterior] [superior] surface of soft palate
Posterior margin of nasal septum and choanae

147.8 Other specified sites of nasopharynx
Malignant neoplasm of contiguous or overlapping sites of nasopharynx whose point of origin cannot be determined

147.9 Nasopharynx, unspecified
Nasopharyngeal wall NOS

148 Malignant neoplasm of hypopharynx

148.0 Postcricoid region

148.1 Pyriform sinus
Pyriform fossa

148.2 Aryepiglottic fold, hypopharyngeal aspect
Aryepiglottic fold or interarytenoid fold:
   NOS
   marginal zone

Excludes: aryepiglottic fold or interarytenoid fold, laryngeal aspect (161.1)

148.3 Posterior hypopharyngeal wall

148.8 Other specified sites of hypopharynx
Malignant neoplasm of contiguous or overlapping sites of hypopharynx whose point of origin cannot be determined

148.9 Hypopharynx, unspecified
Hypopharyngeal wall NOS   Hypopharynx NOS

149 Malignant neoplasm of other and ill-defined sites within the lip, oral cavity, and pharynx

149.0 Pharynx, unspecified

149.1 Waldeyer's ring

149.8 Other
Malignant neoplasms of lip, oral cavity, and pharynx whose point of origin cannot be assigned to any one of the categories 140-148

Excludes: "book leaf" neoplasm [ventral surface of tongue and floor of mouth] (145.8)

149.9 Ill-defined

MALIGNANT NEOPLASM OF DIGESTIVE ORGANS AND PERITONEUM (150-159)

Excludes: carcinoma in situ (230.1-230.9)

150 Malignant neoplasm of esophagus

150.0 Cervical esophagus

150.1 Thoracic esophagus

150.2 Abdominal esophagus
Excludes: adenocarcinoma (151.0)
         cardio-esophageal junction (151.0)

150.3 Upper third of esophagus
Proximal third of esophagus

150.4 Middle third of esophagus

150.5 Lower third of esophagus
Distal third of esophagus

Excludes: adenocarcinoma (151.0)
         cardio-esophageal junction (151.0)

150.8 Other specified part
Malignant neoplasm of contiguous or overlapping sites of esophagus whose point of origin cannot be determined

● Code new to this edition   ▲ Revision of existing code   ④ ⑤ Fourth or fifth digit required

NEOPLASMS

150.9 Esophagus, unspecified

151 Malignant neoplasm of stomach

Excludes: malignant stromal tumor of stomach (171.5)

- **151.0 Cardia**
  Cardiac orifice   Cardio-esophageal junction
  Excludes: squamous cell carcinoma (150.2, 150.5)

- **151.1 Pylorus**
  Prepylorus   Pyloric canal

- **151.2 Pyloric antrum**
  Antrum of stomach NOS

- **151.3 Fundus of stomach**

- **151.4 Body of stomach**

- **151.5 Lesser curvature, unspecified**
  Lesser curvature, not classifiable to 151.1-151.4

- **151.6 Greater curvature, unspecified**
  Greater curvature, not classifiable to 151.0-151.4

- **151.8 Other specified sites of stomach**
  Anterior wall, not classifiable to 151.0-151.4
  Posterior wall, not classifiable to 151.0-151.4
  Malignant neoplasm of contiguous or overlapping sites of stomach whose point of origin cannot be determined

- **151.9 Stomach, unspecified**
  Carcinoma ventriculi   Gastric cancer

152 Malignant neoplasm of small intestine, including duodenum

Excludes: malignant stromal tumor of small intestine (171.5)

- **152.0 Duodenum**
- **152.1 Jejunum**
- **152.2 Ileum**
  Excludes: ileocecal valve (153.4)
- **152.3 Meckel's diverticulum**
- **152.8 Other specified sites of small intestine**
  Duodenojejunal junction
  Malignant neoplasm of contiguous or overlapping sites of small intestine whose point of origin cannot be determined
- **152.9 Small intestine, unspecified**

153 Malignant neoplasm of colon

- **153.0 Hepatic flexure**
- **153.1 Transverse colon**
- **153.2 Descending colon**
  Left colon
- **153.3 Sigmoid colon**
  Sigmoid (flexure)
  Excludes: rectosigmoid junction (154.0)
- **153.4 Cecum**
  Ileocecal valve
- **153.5 Appendix**
- **153.6 Ascending colon**
  Right colon
- **153.7 Splenic flexure**
- **153.8 Other specified sites of large intestine**
  Malignant neoplasm of contiguous or overlapping sites of colon whose point of origin cannot be determined
  Excludes: ileocecal valve (153.4)
  rectosigmoid junction (154.0)
- **153.9 Colon, unspecified**
  Large intestine NOS

154 Malignant neoplasm of rectum, rectosigmoid junction, and anus

Add 4th or 5th digit | Nonspecific code | Unspecified code | Manifestation code

TABULAR LIST

154.0 Rectosigmoid junction
Colon with rectum   Rectosigmoid (colon)

154.1 Rectum
Rectal ampulla

154.2 Anal canal
Anal sphincter
> Excludes: skin of anus (172.5, 173.5)

154.3 Anus, unspecified
> Excludes: anus:
>   margin (172.5, 173.5)
>   skin (172.5, 173.5)
>   perianal skin (172.5, 173.5)

154.8 Other
Anorectum
Cloacogenic zone
Malignant neoplasm of contiguous or overlapping sites of rectum, rectosigmoid junction, and anus whose point of origin cannot be determined

155 Malignant neoplasm of liver and intrahepatic bile ducts

155.0 Liver, primary
Carcinoma:
    liver, specified as primary
    hepatocellular
    liver cell
Hepatoblastoma

155.1 Intrahepatic bile ducts
Canaliculi biliferi   Intrahepatic:
Interlobular: biliary passages
    bile ducts   canaliculi
    biliary canals   gall duct
> Excludes: hepatic duct (156.1)

155.2 Liver, not specified as primary or secondary

156 Malignant neoplasm of gallbladder and extrahepatic bile ducts

156.0 Gallbladder

156.1 Extrahepatic bile ducts
Biliary duct or passage NOS   Cystic duct
Common bile duct   Hepatic duct
                               Sphincter of Oddi

156.2 Ampulla of Vater

156.8 Other specified sites of gallbladder and extrahepatic bile ducts
Malignant neoplasm of contiguous or overlapping sites of gallbladder and extrahepatic bile ducts whose point of origin cannot be determined

156.9 Biliary tract, part unspecified
Malignant neoplasm involving both intrahepatic and extrahepatic bile ducts

157 Malignant neoplasm of pancreas

157.0 Head of pancreas

157.1 Body of pancreas

157.2 Tail of pancreas

157.3 Pancreatic duct
Duct of:
    Santorini
    Wirsung

157.4 Islets of Langerhans
Islets of Langerhans, any part of pancreas
Use additional code, if desired, to identify any functional activity

157.8 Other specified sites of pancreas
Ectopic pancreatic tissue
Malignant neoplasm of contiguous or overlapping sites of pancreas whose point of origin cannot be determined

157.9 Pancreas, part unspecified

158 Malignant neoplasm of retroperitoneum and peritoneum

● Code new to this edition   ▲ Revision of existing code   Fourth or fifth digit required

NEOPLASMS

158.0 Retroperitoneum
Periadrenal tissue
Perinephric tissue
Perirenal tissue
Retrocecal tissue

158.8 Specified parts of peritoneum
Cul-de-sac (of Douglas)
Mesentery
Mesocolon
Omentum
Peritoneum:
  parietal
  pelvic
Rectouterine pouch
Malignant neoplasm of contiguous or overlapping sites of retroperitoneum and peritoneum whose point of origin cannot be determined

158.9 Peritoneum, unspecified

159 Malignant neoplasm of other and ill-defined sites within the digestive organs and peritoneum

159.0 Intestinal tract, part unspecified
Intestine NOS

159.1 Spleen, not elsewhere classified
Angiosarcoma of spleen
Fibrosarcoma of spleen

Excludes: *Hodgkin's disease (201.0-201.9)*
lymphosarcoma (200.1)
reticulosarcoma (200.0)

159.8 Other sites of digestive system and intra-abdominal organs
Malignant neoplasm of digestive organs and peritoneum whose point of origin cannot be assigned to any one of the categories 150-158

Excludes: *anus and rectum (154.8)*
cardio-esophageal junction (151.0)
colon and rectum ORANGE (154.0)

159.9 Ill-defined
Alimentary canal or tract NOS
Gastrointestinal tract NOS

Excludes: *abdominal NOS (195.2)*
intra-abdominal NOS (195.2)

MALIGNANT NEOPLASM OF RESPIRATORY AND INTRATHORACIC ORGANS (160-165)

Excludes: *carcinoma in situ (231.0-231.9)*

160 Malignant neoplasm of nasal cavities, middle ear, and accessory sinuses

160.0 Nasal cavities
Cartilage of nose
Conchae, nasal
Internal nose
Septum of nose
Vestibule of nose

Excludes: *nasal bone (170.0)*
nose NOS (195.0)
olfactory bulb (192.0)
posterior margin of septum and choanae (147.3)
skin of nose (172.3, 173.3)
turbinates (170.0)

160.1 Auditory tube, middle ear, and mastoid air cells
Antrum tympanicum
Eustachian tube
Tympanic cavity

Excludes: *auditory canal (external) (172.2, 173.2)*
bone of ear (meatus) (170.0)
cartilage of ear (171.0)
ear (external) (skin) (172.2, 173.2)

160.2 Maxillary sinus
Antrum (Highmore) (maxillary)

160.3 Ethmoidal sinus

160.4 Frontal sinus

160.5 Sphenoidal sinus

TABULAR LIST

160.8 Other
Malignant neoplasm of contiguous or overlapping sites of nasal cavities, middle ear, and accessory sinuses whose point of origin cannot be determined

160.9 Accessory sinus, unspecified

161 Malignant neoplasm of larynx

161.0 Glottis
Intrinsic larynx
Laryngeal commissure (anterior) (posterior)
True vocal cord
Vocal cord NOS

161.1 Supraglottis
Aryepiglottic fold or interarytenoid fold, laryngeal aspect
Epiglottis (suprahyoid portion) NOS
Extrinsic larynx
False vocal cords
Posterior (laryngeal) surface of epiglottis
Ventricular bands

Excludes: anterior aspect of epiglottis (146.4)
aryepiglottic fold or interarytenoid fold:
  NOS (148.2)
  hypopharyngeal aspect (148.2)
  marginal zone (148.2)

161.2 Subglottis

161.3 Laryngeal cartilages
Cartilage:
  arytenoid
  cricoid
Cartilage:
  cuneiform
  thyroid

161.8 Other specified sites of larynx
Malignant neoplasm of contiguous or overlapping sites of larynx whose point of origin cannot be determined

161.9 Larynx, unspecified

162 Malignant neoplasm of trachea, bronchus, and lung

162.0 Trachea
Cartilage of trachea
Mucosa of trachea

162.2 Main bronchus
Carina
Hilus of lung

162.3 Upper lobe, bronchus or lung

162.4 Middle lobe, bronchus or lung

162.5 Lower lobe, bronchus or lung

162.8 Other parts of bronchus or lung
Malignant neoplasm of contiguous or overlapping sites of bronchus or lung whose point of origin cannot be determined

162.9 Bronchus and lung, unspecified

163 Malignant neoplasm of pleura

163.0 Parietal pleura

163.1 Visceral pleura

163.8 Other specified sites of pleura
Malignant neoplasm of contiguous or overlapping sites of pleura whose point of origin cannot be determined

163.9 Pleura, unspecified

164 Malignant neoplasm of thymus, heart, and mediastinum

164.0 Thymus

164.1 Heart
Endocardium
Epicardium
Myocardium
Pericardium

Excludes: great vessels (171.4)

164.2 Anterior mediastinum

164.3 Posterior mediastinum

NEOPLASMS

164.8 Other
　　Malignant neoplasm of contiguous or overlapping sites of thymus, heart, and mediastinum whose point of origin cannot be determined

164.9 Mediastinum, part unspecified

165 Malignant neoplasm of other and ill-defined sites within the respiratory system and intrathoracic organs

165.0 Upper respiratory trace, part unspecified

165.8 Other
　　Malignant neoplasm of respiratory and intrathoracic organs whose point of origin cannot be assigned to any one of the categories 160-164

165.9 Ill-defined sites within the respiratory system
　　Respiratory tract NOS

　　Excludes: intrathoracic NOS (195.1)
　　　　　　thoracic NOS (195.1)

MALIGNANT NEOPLASM OF BONE, CONNECTIVE TISSUE, SKIN, AND BREAST (170-176)

Excludes: carcinoma in situ:
　　　breast (233.0)
　　　skin (232.0-232.9)

170 Malignant neoplasm of bone and articular cartilage
　Includes: cartilage (articular) (joint)
　　　　　　periosteum

　Excludes: bone marrow NOS (202.9)
　　　cartilage:
　　　　ear (171.0)
　　　　eyelid (171.0)
　　　　larynx (161.3)
　　　　nose (160.0)
　　　synovia (171.0-171.9)

170.0 Bones of skull and face, except mandible

Bone:	Bone:
ethmoid	sphenoid
frontal	temporal
malar	zygomatic
nasal	Maxilla (superior)
occipital	Turbinate
orbital	Upper jaw bone
parietal	Vomer

　Excludes: carcinoma, any type except intraosseous or odontogenic:
　　　maxilla, maxillary (sinus) (160.2)
　　　upper jaw bone (143.0)
　　　jaw bone (lower) (170.1)

170.1 Mandible
　　Inferior maxilla　　　　　Lower jaw bone
　　Jaw bone NOS

　Excludes: carcinoma, any type except intraosseous or odontogenic:
　　　jaw bone NOS (143.9)
　　　　lower (143.1)
　　　upper jaw bone (170.0)

170.2 Vertebral column, excluding sacrum and coccyx
　　Spinal column　　　　Vertebra
　　Spine

　Excludes: sacrum and coccyx (170.6)

170.3 Ribs, sternum, and clavicle
　　Costal cartilage　　　　Xiphoid process
　　Costovertebral joint

170.4 Scapula and long bones of upper limb
　　Acromion　　　　　　　Radius
　　Bones NOS of upper limb　Ulna
　　Humerus

TABULAR LIST

170.5 Short bones of upper limb
- Carpal
- Cuneiform, wrist
- Metacarpal
- Navicular, of hand
- Phalanges of hand
- Pisiform
- Scaphoid (of hand)
- Semilunar or lunate
- Trapezium
- Trapezoid
- Unciform

170.6 Pelvic bones, sacrum, and coccyx
- Coccygeal vertebra
- Ilium
- Ischium
- Pubic bone
- Sacral vertebra

170.7 Long bones of lower limb
- Bones NOS of lower limb
- Femur
- Fibula
- Tibia

170.8 Short bones of lower limb
- Astragalus [talus]
- Calcaneus
- Cuboid
- Cuneiform, ankle
- Metatarsal
- Navicular (of ankle)
- Patella
- Phalanges of foot
- Tarsal

170.9 Bone and articular cartilage, site unspecified

171 Malignant neoplasm of connective and other soft tissue

Includes:
- blood vessel
- bursa
- fascia
- fat
- ligament, except uterine
- malignant stromal tumors
- muscle
- peripheral, sympathetic, and parasympathetic nerves and ganglia
- synovia
- tendon (sheath)

Excludes: cartilage (of):
- articular (170.0-170.9)
- larynx (161.3)
- nose (160.0)

connective tissue:
- breast (174.0-175.9)
- internal organs (except stromal tumors)—code to malignant neoplasm of the site [e.g., leiomyosarcoma of stomach, 151.9]
- heart (164.1)
- uterine ligament (183.4)

171.0 Head, face, and neck
Cartilage of:
- ear
- eyelid

171.2 Upper limb, including shoulder
- Arm
- Finger
- Forearm
- Hand

171.3 Lower limb, including hip
- Foot
- Leg
- Popliteal space
- Thigh
- Toe

171.4 Thorax
- Axilla
- Diaphragm
- Great vessels

Excludes: heart (164.1)
- mediastinum (164.2-164.9)
- thymus (164.0)

171.5 Abdomen
- Abdominal wall
- Hypochondrium

Excludes: peritoneum (158.8)
- retroperitoneum (158.0)

NEOPLASMS

171.6 Pelvis
- Buttock
- Groin
- Inguinal region
- Perineum

Excludes: pelvic peritoneum (158.8)
retroperitoneum (158.0)
uterine ligament, any (183.3-183.5)

171.7 Trunk, unspecified
- Back NOS
- Flank NOS

171.8 Other specified sites of connective and other soft tissue
Malignant neoplasm of contiguous or overlapping sites of connective tissue whose point of origin cannot be determined

171.9 Connective and other soft tissue, site unspecified

172 Malignant melanoma of skin
Includes: melanocarcinoma
melanoma (skin) NOS

Excludes: skin of genital organs (184.0-184.9, 187.1-187.9)
sites other than skin—code to malignant neoplasm of the site

172.0 Lip

Excludes: vermilion border of lip (140.0-140.1, 140.9)

172.1 Eyelid, including canthus

172.2 Ear and external auditory canal
- Auricle (ear)
- Auricular canal, external
- External [acoustic] meatus
- Pinna

172.3 Other and unspecified parts of face
- Cheek (external)
- Chin
- Eyebrow
- Forehead
- Nose, external
- Temple

172.4 Scalp and neck

172.5 Trunk, except scrotum
- Axilla
- Breast
- Buttock
- Groin
- Perianal skin
- Perineum
- Umbilicus

Excludes: anal canal (154.2)
anus NOS (154.3)
scrotum (187.7)

172.6 Upper limb, including shoulder
- Arm
- Finger
- Forearm
- Hand

172.7 Lower limb, including hip
- Ankle
- Foot
- Heel
- Knee
- Leg
- Popliteal area
- Thigh
- Toe

172.8 Other specified sites of skin
Malignant melanoma of contiguous or overlapping sites of skin whose point of origin cannot be determined

172.9 Melanoma of skin, site unspecified

173 Other malignant neoplasm of skin
Includes: malignant neoplasm of:
sebaceous glands
sudoriferous, sudoriparous glands
sweat glands

Excludes: Kaposi's sarcoma (176.0-176.9)
malignant melanoma of skin (172.0-172.9)
skin of genital organs (184.0-184.9, 187.1-187.9)

173.0 Skin of lip

Excludes: vermilion border of lip (140.0-140.1, 140.9)

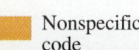 Add 4th or 5th digit
 Nonspecific code
Unspecified code
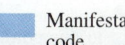 Manifestation code

TABULAR LIST

173.1 Eyelid, including canthus
  Excludes: cartilage of eyelid (171.0)

173.2 Skin of ear and external auditory canal
  Auricle (ear)   External meatus
  Auricular canal, external   Pinna
  Excludes: cartilage of ear (171.0)

173.3 Skin of other and unspecified parts of face
  Cheek, external   Forehead
  Chin   Nose, external
  Eyebrow   Temple

173.4 Scalp and skin of neck

173.5 Skin of trunk, except scrotum
  Axillary fold   Skin of:
  Perianal skin   buttock
  Skin of: chest wall
    abdominal wall   groin
    anus   perineum
    back   Umbilicus
    breast
  Excludes: anal canal (154.2)
            anus NOS (154.3)
            skin of scrotum (187.7)

173.6 Skin of upper limb, including shoulder
  Arm   Forearm
  Finger   Hand

173.7 Skin of lower limb, including hip
  Ankle   Leg
  Foot   Popliteal area
  Heel   Thigh
  Knee   Toe

173.8 Other specified sites of skin
  Malignant neoplasm of contiguous or overlapping sites of skin whose point of origin cannot be determined

173.9 Skin, site unspecified

174 Malignant neoplasm of female breast

Use additional code to identify estrogen receptor status (V86.0, V86.1)
  Includes: breast (female)
             connective tissue
             soft parts
             Paget's disease of:
               breast
               nipple
  Excludes: skin of breast (172.5, 173.5)

174.0 Nipple and areola

174.1 Central portion

174.2 Upper-inner quadrant

174.3 Lower-inner quadrant

174.4 Upper-outer quadrant

174.5 Lower-outer quadrant

174.6 Axillary tail

174.8 Other specified sites of female breast
  Ectopic sites
  Inner breast
  Lower breast
  Midline of breast
  Outer breast
  Upper breast
  Malignant neoplasm of contiguous or overlapping sites of breast whose point of origin cannot be determined

174.9 Breast (female), unspecified

● Code new to this edition   ▲ Revision of existing code   ④ ⑤ Fourth or fifth digit required

NEOPLASMS

175 Malignant neoplasm of male breast
Use additional code to identify estrogen receptor status (V86.0,V86.1)
Excludes: skin of breast (172.5, 173.5)

175.0 Nipple and areola

175.9 Other and unspecified sites of male breast
Ectopic breast tissue, male

176 Kaposi's sarcoma

176.0 Skin

176.1 Soft tissue
Includes: Blood vessel
Connective tissue
Fascia
Ligament
Lymphatic(s) NEC
Muscle

Excludes: lymph glands and nodes (176.5)

176.2 Palate

176.3 Gastrointestinal sites

176.4 Lung

176.5 Lymph nodes

176.8 Other specified sites
Includes: Oral cavity NEC

176.9 Unspecified
Viscera NOS

MALIGNANT NEOPLASM OF GENITOURINARY ORGANS (179-189)

Excludes: carcinoma in situ (233.1-233.9)

179 Malignant neoplasm of uterus, part unspecified

180 Malignant neoplasm of cervix uteri
Includes: invasive malignancy [carcinoma]

Excludes: carcinoma in situ (233.1)

180.0 Endocervix
Cervical canal NOS   Endocervical gland
Endocervical canal

180.1 Exocervix

180.8 Other specified sites of cervix
Cervical stump
Squamocolumnar junction of cervix
Malignant neoplasm of contiguous or overlapping sites of cervix uteri whose point of origin cannot be determined

180.9 Cervix uteri, unspecified

181 Malignant neoplasm of placenta
Choriocarcinoma NOS
Chorioepithelioma NOS

Excludes: chorioadenoma (destruens) (236.1)
hydatidiform mole (630)
  malignant (236.1)
invasive mole (236.1)
male choriocarcinoma NOS (186.0-186.9)

182 Malignant neoplasm of body of uterus

Excludes: carcinoma in situ (233.2)

182.0 Corpus uteri, except isthmus
Cornu   Fundus
Endometrium   Myometrium

182.1 Isthmus
Lower uterine segment

 Add 4th or 5th digit
 Nonspecific code
 Unspecified code
 Manifestation code

TABULAR LIST

182.8 Other specified sites of body of uterus
Malignant neoplasm of contiguous or overlapping sites of body of uterus whose point of origin cannot be determined
Excludes: uterus NOS (179)

183 Malignant neoplasm of ovary and other uterine adnexa
Excludes: Douglas' cul-de-sac (158.8)

183.0 Ovary
Use additional code, if desired, to identify any functional activity

183.2 Fallopian tube
Oviduct
Uterine tube

183.3 Broad ligament
Mesovarium
Parovarian region

183.4 Parametrium
Uterine ligament NOS
Uterosacral ligament

183.5 Round ligament

183.8 Other specified sites of uterine adnexa
Tubo-ovarian
Utero-ovarian
Malignant neoplasm of contiguous or overlapping sites of ovary and other uterine adnexa whose point of origin cannot be determined

183.9 Uterine adnexa, unspecified

184 Malignant neoplasm of other and unspecified female genital organs
Excludes: carcinoma in situ (233.30-233.39)

184.0 Vagina
Gartner's duct
Vaginal vault

184.1 Labia majora
Greater vestibular [Bartholin's] gland

184.2 Labia minora

184.3 Clitoris

184.4 Vulva, unspecified
External female genitalia NOS
Pudendum

184.8 Other specified sites of female genital organs
Malignant neoplasm of contiguous or overlapping sites of female genital organs whose point of origin cannot be determined

184.9 Female genital organ, site unspecified
Female genitourinary tract NOS

185 Malignant neoplasm of prostate
Excludes: seminal vesicles (187.8)

186 Malignant neoplasm of testis
Use additional code, if desired, to identify any functional activity

186.0 Undescended testis
Ectopic testis
Retained testis

186.9 Other and unspecified testis
Testis:
  NOS
  descended
  scrotal

187 Malignant neoplasm of penis and other male genital organs

187.1 Prepuce
Foreskin

187.2 Glans penis

187.3 Body of penis
Corpus cavernosum

NEOPLASMS

187.4 Penis, part unspecified
Skin of penis NOS

187.5 Epididymis

187.6 Spermatic cord
Vas deferens

187.7 Scrotum
Skin of scrotum

187.8 Other specified sites of male genital organs
Seminal vesicle
Tunica vaginalis
Malignant neoplasm of contiguous or overlapping sites of penis and other male genital organs whose point of origin cannot be determined

187.9 Male genital organ, site unspecified
Male genital organ or tract NOS

188 Malignant neoplasm of bladder
Excludes: carcinoma in situ (233.7)

188.0 Trigone of urinary bladder

188.1 Dome of urinary bladder

188.2 Lateral wall of urinary bladder

188.3 Anterior wall of urinary bladder

188.4 Posterior wall of urinary bladder

188.5 Bladder neck
Internal urethral orifice

188.6 Ureteric orifice

188.7 Urachus

188.8 Other specified sites of bladder
Malignant neoplasm of contiguous or overlapping sites of bladder whose point of origin cannot be determined

188.9 Bladder, part unspecified
Bladder wall NOS

189 Malignant neoplasm of kidney and other and unspecified urinary organs

189.0 Kidney, except pelvis
Kidney NOS
Kidney parenchyma

189.1 Renal pelvis
Renal calyces
Ureteropelvic junction

189.2 Ureter
Excludes: ureteric orifice of bladder (188.6)

189.3 Urethra
Excludes: urethral orifice of bladder (188.5)

189.4 Paraurethral glands

189.8 Other specified sites of urinary organs
Malignant neoplasm of contiguous or overlapping sites of kidney and other urinary organs whose point of origin cannot be determined

189.9 Urinary organ, site unspecified
Urinary system NOS

MALIGNANT NEOPLASM OF OTHER AND UNSPECIFIED SITES (190-199)

Excludes: carcinoma in situ (234.0-234.9)

190 Malignant neoplasm of eye
Excludes: carcinoma in situ (234.0)
eyelid (skin) (172.1, 173.1)
cartilage (171.0)
optic nerve (192.0)
orbital bone (170.0)

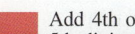 Add 4th or 5th digit

 Nonspecific code

Unspecified code

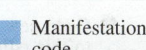 Manifestation code

TABULAR LIST

190.0 Eyeball, except conjunctiva, cornea, retina, and choroid
    Ciliary body   Sclera
    Crystalline lens   Uveal tract
    Iris

190.1 Orbit
    Connective tissue of orbit
    Extraocular muscle
    Retrobulbar

    Excludes: bone of orbit (170.0)

190.2 Lacrimal gland

190.3 Conjunctiva

190.4 Cornea

190.5 Retina

190.6 Choroid

190.7 Lacrimal duct
    Lacrimal sac
    Nasolacrimal duct

190.8 Other specified sites of eye
    Malignant neoplasm of contiguous or overlapping sites of eye whose point of origin cannot be determined

190.9 Eye, part unspecified

191 Malignant neoplasm of brain

    Excludes: cranial nerves (192.0)
                   retrobulbar area (190.1)

191.0 Cerebrum, except lobes and ventricles
    Basal ganglia   Globus pallidus
    Cerebral cortex   Hypothalamus
    Corpus striatum   Thalamus

191.1 Frontal lobe

191.2 Temporal lobe
    Hippocampus
    Uncus

191.3 Parietal lobe

191.4 Occipital lobe

191.5 Ventricles
    Choroid plexus
    Floor of ventricle

191.6 Cerebellum NOS
    Cerebellopontine angle

191.7 Brain stem
    Cerebral peduncle   Midbrain
    Medulla oblongata   Pons

191.8 Other parts of brain
    Corpus callosum
    Tapetum
    Malignant neoplasm of contiguous or overlapping sites of brain whose point of origin cannot be determined

191.9 Brain, unspecified
    Cranial fossa NOS

192 Malignant neoplasm of other and unspecified parts of nervous system

    Excludes: peripheral, sympathetic, and parasympathetic nerves and ganglia (171.0-171.9)

192.0 Cranial nerves
    Olfactory bulb

192.1 Cerebral meninges
    Dura (mater)   Meninges NOS
    Falx (cerebelli) (cerebri)   Tentorium

192.2 Spinal cord
    Cauda equina

192.3 Spinal meninges

NEOPLASMS

192.8 Other specified sites of nervous system
Malignant neoplasm of contiguous or overlapping sites of other parts of nervous system whose point of origin cannot be determined

192.9 Nervous system, part unspecified
Nervous system (central) NOS

Excludes: *meninges NOS (192.1)*

193 Malignant neoplasm of thyroid gland
Thyroglossal duct

Use additional code, if desired, to identify any functional activity

194 Malignant neoplasm of other endocrine glands and related structures
Use additional code, if desired, to identify any functional activity

Excludes: *islets of Langerhans (157.4)*
ovary (183.0)
testis (186.0-186.9)
thymus (164.0)

194.0 Adrenal gland
Adrenal cortex   Suprarenal gland
Adrenal medulla

194.1 Parathyroid gland

194.3 Pituitary gland and craniopharyngeal duct
Craniobuccal pouch   Rathke's pouch
Hypophysis   Sella turcica

194.4 Pineal gland

194.5 Carotid body

194.6 Aortic body and other paraganglia
Coccygeal body   Para-aortic body
Glomus jugulare

194.8 Other
Pluriglandular involvement NOS

Note: If the sites of multiple involvements are known, they should be coded separately.

194.9 Endocrine gland, site unspecified

195 Malignant neoplasm of other and ill-defined sites
Includes: malignant neoplasms of contiguous sites, not elsewhere classified, whose point of origin cannot be determined

Excludes: *malignant neoplasm:*
lymphatic and hematopoietic tissue (200.0-208.9)
secondary sites (196.0-198.8)
unspecified site (199.0-199.1)

195.0 Head, face, and neck
Cheek NOS   Nose NOS
Jaw NOS   Supraclavicular region NOS

195.1 Thorax
Axilla   Intrathoracic NOS
Chest (wall) NOS

195.2 Abdomen
Intra-abdominal NOS

195.3 Pelvis
Groin
Inguinal region NOS
Presacral region
Sacrococcygeal region
Sites overlapping systems within pelvis, as:
rectovaginal (septum)
rectovesical (septum)

195.4 Upper limb

195.5 Lower limb

195.8 Other specified sites
Back NOS   Trunk NOS
Flank NOS

205

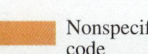 Add 4th or 5th digit
 Nonspecific code
Unspecified code
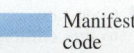 Manifestation code

TABULAR LIST

196 Secondary and unspecified malignant neoplasm of lymph nodes

Excludes: any malignant neoplasm of lymph nodes, specified as primary (200.0-202.9)
Hodgkin's disease (201.0-201.9)
lymphosarcoma (200.1)
reticulosarcoma (200.0)
other forms of lymphoma (202.0-202.9)

196.0 Lymph nodes of head, face, and neck
Cervical
Cervicofacial
Scalene
Supraclavicular

196.1 Intrathoracic lymph nodes
Bronchopulmonary
Intercostal
Mediastinal
Tracheobronchial

196.2 Intra-abdominal lymph nodes
Intestinal
Mesenteric
Retroperitoneal

196.3 Lymph nodes of axilla and upper limb
Brachial
Epitrochlear
Infraclavicular
Pectoral

196.5 Lymph nodes of inguinal region and lower limb
Femoral
Groin
Popliteal
Tibial

196.6 Intrapelvic lymph nodes
Hypogastric
Iliac
Obturator
Parametrial

196.8 Lymph nodes of multiple sites

196.9 Site unspecified
Lymph nodes NOS

197 Secondary malignant neoplasm of respiratory and digestive systems

Excludes: lymph node metastasis (196.0-196.9)

197.0 Lung
Bronchus

197.1 Mediastinum

197.2 Pleura

197.3 Other respiratory organs
Trachea

197.4 Small intestine, including duodenum

197.5 Large intestine and rectum

197.6 Retroperitoneum and peritoneum

197.7 Liver, specified as secondary

197.8 Other digestive organs and spleen

198 Secondary malignant neoplasm of other specified sites

Excludes: lymph node metastasis (196.0-196.9)

198.0 Kidney

198.1 Other urinary organs

198.2 Skin
Skin of breast

198.3 Brain and spinal cord

198.4 Other parts of nervous system
Meninges (cerebral) (spinal)

198.5 Bone and bone marrow

198.6 Ovary

198.7 Adrenal gland
Suprarenal gland

⑤ **198.8 Other specified sites**

198.81 Breast

Excludes: skin of breast (198.2)

198.82 Genital organs

● Code new to this edition   ▲ Revision of existing code   ④ ⑤ Fourth or fifth digit required

NEOPLASMS

198.89 Other

Excludes: retroperitoneal lymph nodes (196.2)

199 **Malignant neoplasm without specification of site**

199.0 Disseminated
Carcinomatosis unspecified site (primary) (secondary)
Generalized:
cancer unspecified site (primary) (secondary)
malignancy unspecified site (primary) (secondary)
Multiple cancer unspecified site (primary) (secondary)

199.1 Other
Cancer unspecified site (primary) (secondary)
Carcinoma unspecified site (primary) (secondary)
Malignancy unspecified site (primary) (secondary)

MALIGNANT NEOPLASM OF LYMPHATIC AND HEMATOPOIETIC TISSUE (200-208)

Excludes: secondary neoplasm of:
bone marrow (198.5)
spleen (197.8)
secondary and unspecified neoplasm of lymph nodes (196.0-196.9)

The following fifth-digit subclassification is for use with categories 200-202:

0 unspecified site, extranodal and solid organ sites
1 lymph nodes of head, face, and neck
2 intrathoracic lymph nodes
3 intra-abdominal lymph nodes
4 lymph nodes of axilla and upper limb
5 lymph nodes of inguinal region and lower limb
6 intrapelvic lymph nodes
7 spleen
8 lymph nodes of multiple sites

▲ **200** Lymphosarcoma and reticulosarcoma and other specified malignant tumors of lymphatic tissue

⑤ **200.0** Reticulosarcoma
Lymphoma (malignant):
histiocytic (diffuse):
nodular
pleomorphic cell type
reticulum cell type
Reticulum cell sarcoma:
NOS
pleomorphic cell type

⑤ **200.1** Lymphosarcoma
Lymphoblastoma (diffuse)   Lymphosarcoma:
Lymphoma (malignant):   NOS
  lymphoblastic (diffuse)   diffuse NOS
  lymphocytic (cell type)   lymphoblastic (diffuse)
    (diffuse)   lymphocytic (diffuse)
  lymphosarcoma type   prolymphocytic

Excludes: lymphosarcoma:
follicular or nodular (202.0)
mixed cell type (200.8)
lymphosarcoma cell leukemia (207.8)

⑤ **200.2** Burkitt's tumor or lymphoma
Malignant lymphoma, Burkitt's type

● **200.3** Marginal zone lymphoma
Extranodal marginal zone B-cell lymphoma
Mucosa associated lymphoid tissue [MALT]
Nodal marginal zone B-cell lymphoma
Splenic marginal zone B-cell lymphoma

● **200.4** Mantle cell lymphoma

● **200.5** Primary central nervous system lymphoma

● **200.6** Anaplastic large cell lymphoma

● **200.7** Large cell lymphoma

 Add 4th or 5th digit
 Nonspecific code
 Unspecified code
 Manifestation code

TABULAR LIST

- ⑤ **200.8** **Other named variants**
    Lymphoma (malignant):
        lymphoplasmacytoid type
        mixed lymphocytic-histiocytic (diffuse)
    Lymphosarcoma, mixed cell type (diffuse)
    Reticulolymphosarcoma (diffuse)

- ⑤ **201** **Hodgkin's disease**
  - ⑤ **201.0** **Hodgkin's paragranuloma**
  - ⑤ **201.1** **Hodgkin's granuloma**
  - ⑤ **201.2** **Hodgkin's sarcoma**
  - ⑤ **201.4** **Lymphocytic-histiocytic predominance**
  - ⑤ **201.5** **Nodular sclerosis**
        Hodgkin's disease, nodular sclerosis:
            NOS
            cellular phase
  - ⑤ **201.6** **Mixed cellularity**
  - ⑤ **201.7** **Lymphocytic depletion**
        Hodgkin's disease, lymphocytic depletion:
            NOS
            diffuse fibrosis
            reticular type
  - ⑤ **201.9** **Hodgkin's disease, unspecified**
        Hodgkin's: Malignant:
            disease NOS   lymphogranuloma
            lymphoma NOS   lymphogranulomatosis

- ⑤ **202** **Other malignant neoplasms of lymphoid and histiocytic tissue**
  - ⑤ **202.0** **Nodular lymphoma**
        Brill-Symmers disease   Lymphosarcoma:
        Lymphoma: follicular (giant)
            follicular (giant)   nodular
            lymphocytic, nodular
  - ⑤ **202.1** **Mycosis fungoides**
  - ⑤ **202.2** **Sézary's disease**
  - ⑤ **202.3** **Malignant histiocytosis**
        Histiocytic medullary reticulosis
        Malignant:
            reticuloendotheliosis
            reticulosis
  - ⑤ **202.4** **Leukemic reticuloendotheliosis**
        Hairy-cell leukemia
  - ⑤ **202.5** **Letterer-Siwe disease**
        Acute:
            differentiated progressive histiocytosis
            histiocytosis X (progressive)
            infantile reticuloendotheliosis
            reticulosis of infancy

        Excludes: *Hand-Schüller-Christian disease (277.89)*
            histiocytosis (acute) (chronic) (277.89)
            histiocytosis X (chronic) (277.89)

  - ⑤ **202.6** **Malignant mast cell tumors**
        Malignant: Mast cell sarcoma
            mastocytoma   Systemic tissue mast cell disease
            mastocytosis

        Excludes: *mast cell leukemia (207.8)*

  - ● **202.7** **Peripheral T-cell lymphoma**
  - ⑤ **202.8** **Other lymphomas**
        Lymphoma (malignant):
            NOS
            diffuse

        Excludes: *benign lymphoma (229.0)*

---

208   ● Code new to this edition   ▲ Revision of existing code   ④ ⑤ Fourth or fifth digit required

NEOPLASMS

⑤ **202.9** Other and unspecified malignant neoplasms of lymphoid and histiocytic tissue
  Follicular dendritic cell sarcoma
  Interdigitating dendritic cell sarcoma
  Langerhans cell sarcoma
  Malignant neoplasm of bone marrow NOS

⑤ **203** Multiple myeloma and immunoproliferative neoplasms
  The following fifth-digit subclassification is for use with category 203
      0 without mention of remission
      1 in remission

⑤ **203.0** Multiple myeloma
  Kahler's disease
  Myelomatosis
  Excludes: solitary myeloma (238.6)

⑤ **203.1** Plasma cell leukemia
  Plasmacytic leukemia

⑤ **203.8** Other immunoproliferative neoplasms

⑤ **204** Lymphoid leukemia
  Includes: leukemia:
    lymphatic
    lymphoblastic
    lymphocytic
    lymphogenous
  The following fifth-digit subclassification is for use with category 204
      0 without mention of remission
      1 in remission

⑤ **204.0** Acute
  Excludes: acute exacerbation of chronic lymphoid leukemia (204.1)

⑤ **204.1** Chronic

⑤ **204.2** Subacute

⑤ **204.8** Other lymphoid leukemia
  Aleukemic leukemia:
    lymphatic
    lymphocytic
    lymphoid

⑤ **204.9** Unspecified lymphoid leukemia

⑤ **205** Myeloid leukemia
  Includes: leukemia:
    granulocytic   myelomonocytic
    myeloblastic   myelosclerotic
    myelocytic   myelosis
    myelogenous
  The following fifth-digit subclassification is for use with category 205
      0 without mention of remission
      1 in remission

⑤ **205.0** Acute
  Acute promyelocytic leukemia
  Excludes: acute exacerbation of chronic myeloid leukemia (205.1)

⑤ **205.1** Chronic
  Eosinophilic leukemia   Neutrophilic leukemia

⑤ **205.2** Subacute

⑤ **205.3** Myeloid sarcoma
  Chloroma
  Granulocytic sarcoma

⑤ **205.8** Other myeloid leukemia
  Aleukemic leukemia:
    granulocytic
    myelogenous
    myeloid
  Aleukemic myelosis

⑤ **205.9** Unspecified myeloid leukemia

| Add 4th or 5th digit | Nonspecific code | Unspecified code | 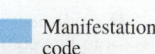 Manifestation code |

TABULAR LIST

206 Monocytic leukemia
Includes: leukemia:
histiocytic
monoblastic
monocytoid

The following fifth-digit subclassification is for use with category 206

    0 without mention of remission
    1 in remission

206.0 Acute
Excludes: acute exacerbation of chronic monocytic leukemia (206.1)

206.1 Chronic

206.2 Subacute

206.8 Other monocytic leukemia
Aleukemic:
  monocytic leukemia
  monocytoid leukemia

206.9 Unspecified monocytic leukemia

207 Other specified leukemia
Excludes: leukemic reticuloendotheliosis (202.4)
         plasma cell leukemia (203.1)

The following fifth-digit subclassification is for use with category 207

    0 without mention of remission
    1 in remission

207.0 Acute erythremia and erythroleukemia
Acute erythremic myelosis   Erythremic myelosis
Di Guglielmo's disease

207.1 Chronic erythremia
Heilmeyer-Schöner disease

207.2 Megakaryocytic leukemia
Megakaryocytic myelosis   Thrombocytic leukemia

207.8 Other specified leukemia
Lymphosarcoma cell leukemia

208 Leukemia of unspecified cell type
The following fifth-digit subclassification is for use with category 208

    0 without mention of remission
    1 in remission

208.0 Acute
Acute leukemia NOS   Stem cell leukemia
Blast cell leukemia
Excludes: acute exacerbation of chronic unspecified leukemia (208.1)

208.1 Chronic
Chronic leukemia NOS

208.2 Subacute
Subacute leukemia NOS

208.8 Other leukemia of unspecified cell type

208.9 Unspecified leukemia
Leukemia NOS

BENIGN NEOPLASMS (210-229)

210 Benign neoplasm of lip, oral cavity, and pharynx
Excludes: cyst (of):
    jaw (526.0-526.2, 526.89)
    oral soft tissue (528.4)
    radicular (522.8)

210.0 Lip
Frenulum labii
Lip (inner aspect) (mucosa) (vermilion border)
Excludes: labial commissure (210.4)
        skin of lip (216.0)

NEOPLASMS

210.1 Tongue
Lingual tonsil

210.2 Major salivary glands
Gland:
  parotid
  sublingual
  submandibular

Excludes: benign neoplasms of minor salivary glands:
  NOS (210.4)
  buccal mucosa (210.4)
  lips (210.0)
  palate (hard) (soft) (210.4)
  tongue (210.1)
  tonsil, palatine (210.5)

210.3 Floor of mouth

210.4 Other and unspecified parts of mouth
Gingiva
Gum (upper) (lower)
Labial commissure
Oral cavity NOS
Oral mucosa
Palate (hard) (soft)
Uvula

Excludes: benign odontogenic neoplasms of bone (213.0-213.1)
  developmental odontogenic cysts (526.0)
  mucosa of lips (210.0)
  nasopharyngeal [posterior] [superior] surface of soft palate (210.7)

210.5 Tonsil
Tonsil (faucial) (palatine)

Excludes: lingual tonsil (210.1)
  pharyngeal tonsil (210.7)
  tonsillar:
    fossa (210.6)
    pillars (210.6)

210.6 Other parts of oropharynx
Branchial cleft or vestiges
Epiglottis, anterior aspect
Fauces NOS
Mesopharynx NOS
Tonsillar:
  fossa
  pillars
Vallecula

Excludes: epiglottis:
  NOS (212.1)
  suprahyoid portion (212.1)

210.7 Nasopharynx
Adenoid tissue
Lymphadenoid tissue
Pharyngeal tonsil
Posterior nasal septum

210.8 Hypopharynx
Arytenoid fold
Laryngopharynx
Postcricoid region
Pyriform fossa

210.9 Pharynx, unspecified
Throat NOS

211 Benign neoplasm of other parts of digestive system

Excludes: benign stromal tumors of digestive system (215.5)

211.0 Esophagus

211.1 Stomach
Body of stomach
Cardia of stomach
Fundus of stomach
Cardiac orifice
Pylorus

211.2 Duodenum, jejunum, and ileum
Small intestine NOS

Excludes: ampulla of Vater (211.5)
  ileocecal valve (211.3)

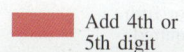 Add 4th or 5th digit
 Nonspecific code
 Unspecified code
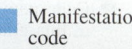 Manifestation code

TABULAR LIST

211.3 Colon
    Appendix   Ileocecal valve
    Cecum   Large intestine NOS
    Excludes: rectosigmoid junction (211.4)

211.4 Rectum and anal canal
    Anal canal or sphincter   Rectosigmoid junction
    Anus NOS
    Excludes: anus:
            margin (216.5)
            skin (216.5)
            perianal skin (216.5)

211.5 Liver and biliary passages
    Ampulla of Vater   Gallbladder
    Common bile duct   Hepatic duct
    Cystic duct   Sphincter of Oddi

211.6 Pancreas, except islets of Langerhans

211.7 Islets of Langerhans
    Islet cell tumor
Use additional code, if desired, to identify any functional activity

211.8 Retroperitoneum and peritoneum
    Mesentery   Omentum
    Mesocolon   Retroperitoneal tissue

211.9 Other and unspecified site
    Alimentary tract NOS   Intestinal tract NOS
    Digestive system NOS   Intestine NOS
    Gastrointestinal tract NOS   Spleen, not elsewhere classified

212 Benign neoplasm of respiratory and intrathoracic organs

212.0 Nasal cavities, middle ear, and accessory sinuses
    Cartilage of nose   Sinus:
    Eustachian tube   ethmoidal
    Nares   frontal
    Septum of nose   maxillary
                                   sphenoidal
    Excludes: auditory canal (external) (216.2)
                bone of:
                   ear (213.0)
                   nose [turbinates] (213.0)
                cartilage of ear (215.0)
                ear (external) (skin) (216.2)
                nose NOS (229.8)
                skin (216.3)
                olfactory bulb (225.1)
                polyp of:
                   accessory sinus (471.8)
                   ear (385.30-385.35)
                   nasal cavity (471.0)
                posterior margin of septum and choanae (210.7)

212.1 Larynx
    Cartilage: Epiglottis (suprahyoid portion) NOS
         arytenoid   Glottis
         cricoid   Vocal cords (false) (true)
         cuneiform
         thyroid
    Excludes: epiglottis, anterior aspect (210.6)
                polyp of vocal cord or larynx (478.4)

212.2 Trachea

212.3 Bronchus and lung
    Carina   Hilus of lung

212.4 Pleura

212.5 Mediastinum

212.6 Thymus

212.7 Heart
    Excludes: great vessels (215.4)

● Code new to this edition   ▲ Revision of existing code   ④ ⑤ Fourth or fifth digit required

NEOPLASMS

212.8 Other specified sites

212.9 Site unspecified
　　Respiratory organ NOS
　　Upper respiratory tract NOS

　　Excludes: intrathoracic NOS (229.8)
　　　　　　 thoracic NOS (229.8)

213 Benign neoplasm of bone and articular cartilage
　Includes: cartilage (articular) (joint)
　　　　　　periosteum

　　Excludes: cartilage of:
　　　　　　　ear (215.0)
　　　　　　　eyelid (215.0)
　　　　　　　larynx (212.1)
　　　　　　　nose (212.0)
　　　　　　exostosis NOS (726.91)
　　　　　　synovia (215.0-215.9)

213.0 Bones of skull and face
　　Excludes: lower jaw bone (213.1)

213.1 Lower jaw bone

213.2 Vertebral column, excluding sacrum and coccyx

213.3 Ribs, sternum, and clavicle

213.4 Scapula and long bones of upper limb

213.5 Short bones of upper limb

213.6 Pelvic bones, sacrum, and coccyx

213.7 Long bones of lower limb

213.8 Short bones of lower limb

213.9 Bone and articular cartilage, site unspecified

214 Lipoma
　Includes: angiolipoma
　　　　　　fibrolipoma
　　　　　　hibernoma
　　　　　　lipoma (fetal) (infiltrating) (intramuscular)
　　　　　　myelolipoma
　　　　　　myxolipoma

214.0 Skin and subcutaneous tissue of face

214.1 Other skin and subcutaneous tissue

214.2 Intrathoracic organs

214.3 Intra-abdominal organs

214.4 Spermatic cord

214.8 Other specified sites

214.9 Lipoma, unspecified site

215 Other benign neoplasm of connective and other soft tissue
　Includes: blood vessel
　　　　　　bursa
　　　　　　fascia
　　　　　　ligament
　　　　　　muscle
　　　　　　peripheral, sympathetic, and parasympathetic nerves and ganglia
　　　　　　synovia
　　　　　　tendon (sheath)

　　Excludes: cartilage:
　　　　　　　articular (213.0-213.9)
　　　　　　　larynx (212.1)
　　　　　　　nose (212.0)
　　　　　　connective tissue of:
　　　　　　　breast (217)
　　　　　　　internal organ, except lipoma and hemangioma — code to benign neoplasm of the site
　　　　　　lipoma (214.0-214.9)

215.0 Head, face, and neck

215.2 Upper limb, including shoulder

TABULAR LIST

215.3 Lower limb, including hip

215.4 Thorax

> Excludes: heart (212.7)
> mediastinum (212.5)
> thymus (212.6)

215.5 Abdomen
Abdominal wall
Benign stromal tumors of abdomen
Hypochondrium

215.6 Pelvis
Buttock
Groin
Inguinal region
Perineum

> Excludes: uterine:
> leiomyoma (218.0-218.9)
> ligament, any (221.0)

215.7 Trunk, unspecified
Back NOS
Flank NOS

215.8 Other specified sites

215.9 Site unspecified

216 Benign neoplasm of skin
Includes: blue nevus
dermatofibroma
hydrocystoma
pigmented nevus
syringoadenoma
syringoma

> Excludes: skin of genital organs (221.0-222.9)

216.0 Skin of lip

> Excludes: vermilion border of lip (210.0)

216.1 Eyelid, including canthus

> Excludes: cartilage of eyelid (215.0)

216.2 Ear and external auditory canal
Auricle (ear)
Auricular canal, external
External meatus
Pinna

> Excludes: cartilage of ear (215.0)

216.3 Skin of other and unspecified parts of face
Cheek, external
Eyebrow
Nose, external
Temple

216.4 Scalp and skin of neck

216.5 Skin of trunk, except scrotum
Axillary fold
Perianal skin
Skin of:
  abdominal wall
  anus
  back
  breast
Skin of:
  buttock
  chest wall
  groin
  perineum
Umbilicus

> Excludes: anal canal (211.4)
> anus NOS (211.4)
> skin of scrotum (222.4)

216.6 Skin of upper limb, including shoulder

216.7 Skin of lower limb, including hip

216.8 Other specified sites of skin

216.9 Skin, site unspecified

NEOPLASMS

217 Benign neoplasm of breast
Breast (male) (female)
  connective tissue
  glandular tissue
  soft parts
  > *Excludes:* adenofibrosis (610.2)
  >   benign cyst of breast (610.0)
  >   fibrocystic disease (610.1)
  >   skin of breast (216.5)

218 Uterine leiomyoma
Includes: fibroid (bleeding) (uterine)
  uterine:
    fibromyoma
    myoma

    218.0 Submucous leiomyoma of uterus

    218.1 Intramural leiomyoma of uterus
        Interstitial leiomyoma of uterus

    218.2 Subserous leiomyoma of uterus
        Subperitoneal leiomyoma of uterus

    218.9 Leiomyoma of uterus, unspecified

219 Other benign neoplasm of uterus

    219.0 Cervix uteri

    219.1 Corpus uteri
        Endometrium   Myometrium
        Fundus

    219.8 Other specified parts of uterus

    219.9 Uterus, part unspecified

220 Benign neoplasm of ovary
Use additional code, if desired, to identify any functional activity (256.0-256.1)
  > *Excludes:* cyst:
  >   corpus albicans (620.2)
  >   corpus luteum (620.1)
  >   endometrial (617.1)
  >   follicular (atretic) (620.0)
  >   graafian follicle (620.0)
  >   ovarian NOS (620.2)
  >   retention (620.2)

221 Benign neoplasm of other female genital organs
Includes: adenomatous polyp
  benign teratoma
  > *Excludes:* cyst:
  >   epoophoron (752.11)
  >   fimbrial (752.11)
  >   Gartner's duct (752.11)
  >   parovarian (752.11)

    221.0 Fallopian tube and uterine ligaments
        Oviduct   Uterine ligament (broad) (round) (uterosacral)
        Parametrium   Uterine tube

    221.1 Vagina

    221.2 Vulva
        Clitoris
        External female genitalia NOS
        Greater vestibular [Bartholin's] gland
        Labia (majora) (minora)
        Pudendum
        > *Excludes:* Bartholin's (duct) (gland) cyst (616.2)

    221.8 Other specified sites of female genital organs

    221.9 Female genital organ, site unspecified
        Female genitourinary tract NOS

222 Benign neoplasm of male genital organs

    222.0 Testis
Use additional code, if desired, to identify any functional activity

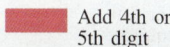 Add 4th or 5th digit   Nonspecific code   Unspecified code   Manifestation code

TABULAR LIST

222.1 Penis
 Corpus cavernosum   Prepuce
 Glans penis

222.2 Prostate
 Excludes: adenomatous hyperplasia of prostate (600.20-600.21)
  prostatic:
   adenoma (600.20-600.21)
   enlargement (600.00-600.01)
   hypertrophy (600.00-600.01)

222.3 Epididymis

222.4 Scrotum
 Skin of scrotum

222.8 Other specified sites of male genital organs
 Seminal vesicle
 Spermatic cord

222.9 Male genital organ, site unspecified
 Male genitourinary tract NOS

223 Benign neoplasm of kidney and other urinary organs

223.0 Kidney, except pelvis
 Kidney NOS
 Excludes: renal:
  calyces (223.1)
  pelvis (223.1)

223.1 Renal pelvis

223.2 Ureter
 Excludes: ureteric orifice of bladder (223.3)

223.3 Bladder

223.8 Other specified sites of urinary organs
 223.81 Urethra
  Excludes: urethral orifice of bladder (223.3)
 223.89 Other
  Paraurethral glands

223.9 Urinary organ, site unspecified
 Urinary system NOS

224 Benign neoplasm of eye

 Excludes: cartilage of eyelid (215.0)
  eyelid (skin) (216.1)
  optic nerve (225.1)
  orbital bone (213.0)

224.0 Eyeball, except conjunctiva, cornea, retina, and choroid
 Ciliary body   Sclera
 Iris   Uveal tract

224.1 Orbit
 Excludes: bone of orbit (213.0)

224.2 Lacrimal gland

224.3 Conjunctiva

224.4 Cornea

224.5 Retina
 Excludes: hemangioma of retina (228.03)

224.6 Choroid

224.7 Lacrimal duct
 Lacrimal sac
 Nasolacrimal duct

224.8 Other specified parts of eye

224.9 Eye, part unspecified

NEOPLASMS

225 **Benign neoplasm of brain and other parts of nervous system**
Excludes: hemangioma (228.02)
neurofibromatosis (237.7)
peripheral, sympathetic, and parasympathetic nerves and ganglia (215.0-215.9)
retrobulbar (224.1)

225.0 Brain

225.1 Cranial nerves

225.2 Cerebral meninges
Meninges NOS
Meningioma (cerebral)

225.3 Spinal cord
Cauda equina

225.4 Spinal meninges
Spinal meningioma

225.8 Other specified sites of nervous system

225.9 Nervous system, part unspecified
Nervous system (central) NOS
Excludes: meninges NOS (225.2)

226 Benign neoplasm of thyroid glands
Use additional code, if desired, to identify any functional activity

227 Benign neoplasm of other endocrine glands and related structures
Use additional code, if desired, to identify any functional activity
Excludes: ovary (220)
pancreas (211.6)
testis (222.0)

227.0 Adrenal gland
Suprarenal gland

227.1 Parathyroid gland

227.3 Pituitary gland and craniopharyngeal duct (pouch)
Craniobuccal pouch   Rathke's pouch
Hypophysis   Sella turcica

227.4 Pineal gland
Pineal body

227.5 Carotid body

227.6 Aortic body and other paraganglia
Coccygeal body   Para-aortic body
Glomus jugulare

227.8 Other

227.9 Endocrine gland, site unspecified

228 Hemangioma and lymphangioma, any site
Includes: angioma (benign) (cavernous) (congenital) NOS
cavernous nevus
glomus tumor
hemangioma (benign) (congenital)

Excludes: benign neoplasm of spleen, except hemangioma and lymphangioma (211.9)
glomus jugulare (227.6)
nevus:
  NOS (216.0-216.9)
  blue or pigmented (216.0-216.9)
  vascular (757.32)

⑤ **228.0 Hemangioma, any site**

    228.00 Of unspecified site

    228.01 Of skin and subcutaneous tissue

    228.02 Of intracranial structures

    228.03 Of retina

    228.04 Of intra-abdominal structures
        Peritoneum
        Retroperitoneal tissue

    228.09 Of other sites
        Systemic angiomatosis

Add 4th or 5th digit	Nonspecific code	Unspecified code	Manifestation code

TABULAR LIST

228.1 Lymphangioma, any site
Congenital lymphangioma
Lymphatic nevus

229 Benign neoplasm of other and unspecified sites

229.0 Lymph nodes
Excludes: lymphangioma (228.1)

229.8 Other specified sites
Intrathoracic NOS
Thoracic NOS

229.9 Site unspecified

CARCINOMA IN SITU (230-234)

Includes: Bowen's disease
erythroplasia
Queyrat's erythroplasia

Excludes: leukoplakia—see Alphabetic Index

230 Carcinoma in situ of digestive organs

230.0 Lip, oral cavity, and pharynx
Gingiva
Hypopharynx
Mouth [any part]
Nasopharynx
Oropharynx
Salivary gland or duct
Tongue

Excludes: aryepiglottic fold or interarytenoid fold, laryngeal aspect (231.0)
epiglottis:
NOS (231.0)
suprahyoid portion (231.0)
skin of lip (232.0)

230.1 Esophagus

230.2 Stomach
Body of stomach
Cardia of stomach
Fundus of stomach
Cardiac orifice
Pylorus

230.3 Colon
Appendix
Cecum
Ileocecal valve
Large intestine NOS

Excludes: rectosigmoid junction (230.4)

230.4 Rectum
Rectosigmoid junction

230.5 Anal canal
Anal sphincter

230.6 Anus, unspecified

Excludes: anus:
margin (232.5)
skin (232.5)
perianal skin (232.5)

230.7 Other and unspecified parts of intestine
Duodenum
Ileum
Jejunum
Small intestine NOS

Excludes: ampulla of Vater (230.8)

230.8 Liver and biliary system
Ampulla of Vater
Common bile duct
Cystic duct
Gallbladder
Hepatic duct
Sphincter of Oddi

230.9 Other and unspecified digestive organs
Digestive organ NOS
Gastrointestinal tract NOS
Pancreas
Spleen

NEOPLASMS

231 **Carcinoma in situ of respiratory system**

231.0 Larynx
Cartilage:
  arytenoid
  cricoid
  cuneiform
  thyroid

Epiglottis:
  NOS
  posterior surface
  suprahyoid portion
  Vocal cords (false) (true)

Excludes: aryepiglottic fold or interarytenoid fold:
  NOS (230.0)
  hypopharyngeal aspect (230.0)
  marginal zone (230.0)

231.1 Trachea

231.2 Bronchus and lung
Carina
Hilus of lung

231.8 Other specified parts of respiratory system
Accessory sinuses   Nasal cavities
Middle ear   Pleura

Excludes: ear (external) (skin) (232.2)
  nose NOS (234.8)
  skin (232.3)

231.9 Respiratory system, part unspecified
Respiratory organ NOS

232 **Carcinoma in situ of skin**
Includes: pigment cells

232.0 Skin of lip
Excludes: vermilion border of lip (230.0)

232.1 Eyelid, including canthus

232.2 Ear and external auditory canal

232.3 Skin of other and unspecified parts of face

232.4 Scalp and skin of neck

232.5 Skin of trunk, except scrotum
Anus, margin   Skin of:
Axillary fold   breast
Perianal skin   buttock
Skin of: chest wall
  abdominal wall groin
  anus   perineum
  back   Umbilicus

Excludes: anal canal (230.5)
  anus NOS (230.6)
  skin of genital organs (233.30-233.39, 233.5-233.6)

232.6 Skin of upper limb, including shoulder

232.7 Skin of lower limb, including hip

232.8 Other specified sites of skin

232.9 Skin, site unspecified

233 **Carcinoma in situ of breast and genitourinary system**

233.0 Breast
Excludes: Paget's disease (174.0-174.9)
  skin of breast (232.5)

233.1 Cervix uteri
Adenocarcinoma in situ of cervix
Cervical intraepithelial glandular neoplasia
Cervical intraepithelial neoplasia III [CIN III]
Severe dysplasia of cervix

Excludes: cervical intraepithelial neoplasia II [CIN II] (622.12)
  cytologic evidence of malignancy without histologic confirmation (795.06)
  high grade squamous intraepithelial lesion (HGSIL) (795.04)
  moderate dysplasia of cervix (622.12)

233.2 Other and unspecified parts of uterus

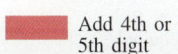 Add 4th or 5th digit
 Nonspecific code
 Unspecified code
 Manifestation code

TABULAR LIST

⑤ **233.3 Other and unspecified female genital organs**
- **233.30 Unspecified female genital organ**
- **233.31 Vagina**
  Severe dysplasia of vagina
  Vaginal intraepithelial neoplasia III [VAIN III]
- **233.32 Vulva**
  Severe dysplasia of vulva
  Vulvar intraepithelial neoplasia III [VIN III]
- **233.39 Other female genital organ**

233.4 Prostate

233.5 Penis

233.6 Other and unspecified male genital organs

233.7 Bladder

233.9 Other and unspecified urinary organs

234 Carcinoma in situ of other and unspecified sites

234.0 Eye
Excludes: cartilage of eyelid (234.8)
eyelid (skin) (232.1)
optic nerve (234.8)
orbital bone (234.8)

234.8 Other specified sites
Endocrine gland [any]

234.9 Site unspecified
Carcinoma in situ NOS

NEOPLASMS OF UNCERTAIN BEHAVIOR (235-238)

Note: Categories 235-238 classify by site certain histo-morphologically well-defined neoplasms, the subsequent behavior of which cannot be predicted from the present appearance.

235 Neoplasm of uncertain behavior of digestive and respiratory systems
Excludes: stromal tumors of uncertain behavior of digestive system (238.1)

235.0 Major salivary glands
Gland:
 parotid
 sublingual
 submandibular
Excludes: minor salivary glands (235.1)

235.1 Lip, oral cavity, and pharynx
Gingiva   Nasopharynx
Hypopharynx   Oropharynx
Minor salivary glands   Tongue
Mouth
Excludes: aryepiglottic fold or interarytenoid fold, laryngeal aspect (235.6)
epiglottis:
 NOS (235.6)
 suprahyoid portion (235.6)
skin of lip (238.2)

235.2 Stomach, intestines, and rectum

235.3 Liver and biliary passages
Ampulla of Vater   Gallbladder
Bile ducts [any]   Liver

235.4 Retroperitoneum and peritoneum

235.5 Other and unspecified digestive organs
Anal: Esophagus
 canal   Pancreas
 sphincter   Spleen
Anus NOS
Excludes: anus:
 margin (238.2)
 skin (238.2)
 perianal skin (238.2)

NEOPLASMS

235.6 Larynx

Excludes: aryepiglottic fold or interarytenoid fold:
 NOS (235.1)
 hypopharyngeal aspect (235.1)
 marginal zone (235.1)

235.7 Trachea, bronchus, and lung

235.8 Pleura, thymus, and mediastinum

235.9 Other and unspecified respiratory organs
 Accessory sinuses   Nasal cavities
 Middle ear   Respiratory organ NOS

Excludes: ear (external) (skin) (238.2)
 nose (238.8)
 skin (238.2)

236 Neoplasm of uncertain behavior of genitourinary organs

236.0 Uterus

236.1 Placenta
 Chorioadenoma (destruens)
 Invasive mole
 Malignant hydatid(iform) mole

236.2 Ovary
Use additional code, if desired, to identify any functional activity

236.3 Other and unspecified female genital organs

236.4 Testis
Use additional code, if desired, to identify any functional activity

236.5 Prostate

236.6 Other and unspecified male genital organs

236.7 Bladder

⑤ **236.9 Other and unspecified urinary organs**

 236.90 Urinary organ, unspecified

 236.91 Kidney and ureter

 236.99 Other

237 Neoplasm of uncertain behavior of endocrine glands and nervous system

237.0 Pituitary gland and craniopharyngeal duct
Use additional code, if desired, to identify any functional activity

237.1 Pineal gland

237.2 Adrenal gland
 Suprarenal gland

Use additional code, if desired, to identify any functional activity

237.3 Paraganglia
 Aortic body
 Carotid body
 Coccygeal body
 Glomus jugulare

237.4 Other and unspecified endocrine glands
 Parathyroid gland
 Thyroid gland

237.5 Brain and spinal cord

237.6 Meninges
 Meninges:
  NOS
  cerebral
  spinal

⑤ **237.7 Neurofibromatosis**
 von Recklinghausen's disease

 237.70 Neurofibromatosis, unspecified

 237.71 Neurofibromatosis, Type I [von Recklinghausen's disease]

 237.72 Neurofibromatosis, Type II [acoustic neurofibromatosis]

| Add 4th or 5th digit | Nonspecific code | Unspecified code | Manifestation code |

TABULAR LIST

237.9 Other and unspecified parts of nervous system
Cranial nerves
Excludes: peripheral, sympathetic, and parasympathetic nerves and ganglia (238.1)

238 Neoplasm of uncertain behavior of other and unspecified sites and tissues

238.0 Bone and articular cartilage
Excludes: cartilage:
   ear (238.1)
   eyelid (238.1)
   larynx (235.6)
   nose (235.9)
   synovia (238.1)

238.1 Connective and other soft tissue
Peripheral, sympathetic, and parasympathetic nerves and ganglia
Stromal tumors of digestive system
Excludes: cartilage (of):
   articular (238.0)
   larynx (235.6)
   nose (235.9)
   connective tissue of breast (238.3)

238.2 Skin
Excludes: anus NOS (235.5)
   skin of genital organs (236.3, 236.6)
   vermilion border of lip (235.1)

238.3 Breast
Excludes: skin of breast (238.2)

238.4 Polycythemia vera

238.5 Histiocytic and mast cells
Mast cell tumor NOS
Mastocytoma NOS

238.6 Plasma cells
Plasmacytoma NOS
Solitary myeloma

⑤ 238.7 Other lymphatic and hematopoietic tissues
Excludes: acute myelogenous leukemia (205.0)
   chronic myelomonocytic leukemia (205.1)
   myelofibrosis (289.83)
   myelosclerosis NOS (289.89)
   myelosis:
      NOS (205.9)
      megakaryocytic (207.2)

   238.71 Essential thrombocythemia
   Essential hemorrhagic thrombocythemia
   Essential thrombocytosis
   Idiopathic (hemorrhagic) thrombocythemia
   Primary thrombocytosis

   238.72 Low grade myelodysplastic syndrome lesions
   Refractory anemia (RA)
   Refractory anemia with ringed sideroblasts (RARS)
   Refractory cytopenia with multilineage dysplasia (RCMD)
   Refractory cytopenia with multilineage dysplasia and ringed sideroblasts (RCMD-RS)

   238.73 High grade myelodysplastic syndrome lesions
   Refractory anemia with excess blasts-1 (RAEB-1)
   Refractory anemia with excess blasts-2 (RAEB-2)

   238.74 Myelodysplastic syndrome with 5q deletion
   5q minus syndrome NOS
   Excludes: constitutional 5q deletion (758.39)
      high grade myelodysplastic syndrome with 5q deletion (238.73)

   238.75 Myelodysplastic syndrome, unspecified

NEOPLASMS

238.76 **Myelofibrosis with myeloid metaplasia**
Agnogenic myeloid metaplasia
Idiopathic myelofibrosis (chronic)
Myelosclerosis with myeloid metaplasia
Primary myelofibrosis

Excludes: myelofibrosis NOS (289.83)
myelophthisic anemia (284.2)
myelophthisis (284.2)
secondary myelofibrosis (289.83)

238.79 **Other lymphatic and hematopoietic tissues**
Lymphoproliferative disease (chronic) NOS
Megakaryocytic myelosclerosis
Myeloproliferative disease (chronic) NOS
Panmyelosis (acute)

238.8 **Other specified sites**
Eye
Heart

Excludes: eyelid (skin) (238.2)
cartilage (238.1)

238.9 **Site unspecified**

NEOPLASMS OF UNSPECIFIED NATURE (239)

239 **Neoplasms of unspecified nature**
Note: Category 239 classifies by site neoplasms of unspecified morphology and behavior. The term "mass," unless otherwise stated, is not to be regarded as a neoplastic growth.
Includes: "growth" NOS
neoplasm NOS
new growth NOS
tumor NOS

239.0 **Digestive system**
Excludes: anus:
margin (239.2)
skin (239.2)
perianal skin (239.2)

239.1 **Respiratory system**

239.2 **Bone, soft tissue, and skin**
Excludes: anal canal (239.0)
anus NOS (239.0)
bone marrow (202.9)
cartilage:
larynx (239.1)
nose (239.1)
connective tissue of breast (239.3)
skin of genital organs (239.5)
vermilion border of lip (239.0)

239.3 **Breast**
Excludes: skin of breast (239.2)

239.4 **Bladder**

239.5 **Other genitourinary organs**

239.6 **Brain**
Excludes: cerebral meninges (239.7)
cranial nerves (239.7)

239.7 **Endocrine glands and other parts of nervous system**
Excludes: peripheral, sympathetic, and parasympathetic nerves and ganglia (239.2)

239.8 **Other specified sites**
Excludes: eyelids (skin) (239.2)
cartilage (239.2)
great vessels (239.2)
optic nerve (239.7)

239.9 **Site unspecified**

ENDOCRINE, NUTRITIONAL, METABOLIC, IMMUNITY

3. ENDOCRINE, NUTRITIONAL AND METABOLIC DISEASES, AND IMMUNITY DISORDERS (240-279)

> Excludes: endocrine and metabolic disturbances specific to the fetus and newborn (775.0-775.9)

Note: All neoplasms, whether functionally active or not, are classified in Chapter 2. Codes in Chapter 3 (i.e., 242.8, 246.0, 251-253, 255-259) may be used, if desired, to identify such functional activity associated with any neoplasm, or by ectopic endocrine tissue.

DISORDERS OF THYROID GLAND (240-246)

240 Simple and unspecified goiter

240.0 Goiter, specified as simple
Any condition classifiable to 240.9, specified as simple

240.9 Goiter, unspecified
Enlargement of thyroid
Goiter or struma:
  NOS
  diffuse colloid
  endemic
Goiter or struma:
  hyperplastic
  nontoxic (diffuse)
  parenchymatous
  sporadic

> Excludes: congenital (dyshormonogenic) goiter (246.1)

241 Nontoxic nodular goiter

> Excludes: adenoma of thyroid (226)
> cystadenoma of thyroid (226)

241.0 Nontoxic uninodular goiter
Thyroid nodule
Uninodular goiter (nontoxic)

241.1 Nontoxic multinodular goiter
Multinodular goiter (nontoxic)

241.9 Unspecified nontoxic nodular goiter
Adenomatous goiter
Nodular goiter (nontoxic) NOS
Struma nodosa (simplex)

⑤ 242 Thyrotoxicosis with or without goiter

> Excludes: neonatal thyrotoxicosis (775.3)

The following fifth-digit subclassification is for use with category 242:

  0 without mention of thyrotoxic crisis or storm
  1 with mention of thyrotoxic crisis or storm

⑤ 242.0 Toxic diffuse goiter
Basedow's disease
Exophthalmic or toxic goiter NOS
Graves' disease
Primary thyroid hyperplasia

⑤ 242.1 Toxic uninodular goiter
Thyroid nodule, toxic or with hyperthyroidism
Uninodular goiter, toxic or with hyperthyroidism

⑤ 242.2 Toxic multinodular goiter
Secondary thyroid hyperplasia

⑤ 242.3 Toxic nodular goiter, unspecified
Adenomatous goiter, toxic or with hyperthyroidism
Nodular goiter, toxic or with hyperthyroidism
Struma nodosa, toxic or with hyperthyroidism
Any condition classifiable to 241.9 specified as toxic or with hyperthyroidism

⑤ 242.4 Thyrotoxicosis from ectopic thyroid nodule

⑤ 242.8 Thyrotoxicosis of other specified origin
Overproduction of thyroid-stimulating hormone [TSH]
Thyrotoxicosis:
  factitia
  from ingestion of excessive thyroid material

Use additional E code to identify cause, if drug-induced

⑤ 242.9 Thyrotoxicosis without mention of goiter or other cause
Hyperthyroidism NOS
Thyrotoxicosis NOS

Add 4th or 5th digit | Nonspecific code | Unspecified code | Manifestation code

TABULAR LIST

243 Congenital hypothyroidism
Congenital thyroid insufficiency
Cretinism (athyrotic) (endemic)

Use additional code to identify associated mental retardation

Excludes: *congenital (dyshormonogenic) goiter (246.1)*

244 Acquired hypothyroidism
Includes: athyroidism (acquired)
hypothyroidism (acquired)
myxedema (adult) (juvenile)
thyroid (gland) insufficiency (acquired)

244.0 Postsurgical hypothyroidism

244.1 Other postablative hypothyroidism
Hypothyroidism following therapy, such as irradiation

244.2 Iodine hypothyroidism
Hypothyroidism resulting from administration or ingestion of iodide

Use additional E code to identify drug

244.3 Other iatrogenic hypothyroidism
Hypothyroidism resulting from:
P-aminosalicylic acid [PAS]
Phenylbutazone
Resorcinol
Iatrogenic hypothyroidism NOS

Use additional E code to identify drug

244.8 Other specified acquired hypothyroidism
Secondary hypothyroidism NEC

244.9 Unspecified hypothyroidism
Hypothyroidism, primary or NOS
Myxedema, primary or NOS

245 Thyroiditis

245.0 Acute thyroiditis
Abscess of thyroid
Thyroiditis:
nonsuppurative, acute
pyogenic
suppurative

Use additional code to identify organism

245.1 Subacute thyroiditis
Thyroiditis:
de Quervain's
giant cell

Thyroiditis:
granulomatous
viral

245.2 Chronic lymphocytic thyroiditis
Hashimoto's disease
Struma lymphomatosa

Thyroiditis:
autoimmune
lymphocytic (chronic)

245.3 Chronic fibrous thyroiditis
Struma fibrosa
Thyroiditis:
invasive (fibrous)
ligneous
Riedel's

245.4 Iatrogenic thyroiditis
Use additional code to identify cause

245.8 Other and unspecified chronic thyroiditis
Chronic thyroiditis:
NOS
nonspecific

245.9 Thyroiditis, unspecified
Thyroiditis NOS

246 Other disorders of thyroid

246.0 Disorders of thyrocalcitonin secretion
Hypersecretion of calcitonin or thyrocalcitonin

ENDOCRINE, NUTRITIONAL, METABOLIC, IMMUNITY

246.1 Dyshormonogenic goiter
  Congenital (dyshormonogenic) goiter
  Goiter due to enzyme defect in synthesis of thyroid hormone
  Goitrous cretinism (sporadic)

246.2 Cyst of thyroid
  Excludes: cystadenoma of thyroid (226)

246.3 Hemorrhage and infarction of thyroid

246.8 Other specified disorders of thyroid
  Abnormality of   Hyper-TBG-nemia
  thyroid-binding globulin   Hypo-TBG-nemia
  Atrophy of thyroid

246.9 Unspecified disorder of thyroid

DISEASES OF OTHER ENDOCRINE GLANDS (250-259)

250 Diabetes mellitus
  Excludes: gestational diabetes (648.8)
    hyperglycemia NOS (790.29)
    neonatal diabetes mellitus (775.1)
    nonclinical diabetes (790.29)

The following fifth-digit subclassification is for use with category 250:

  0 type II or unspecified type, not stated as uncontrolled
  Fifth-digit 0 is for use with type II patients, even if the patient requires insulin
  Use additional code, if applicable, for associated long-term (current) insulin use V58.67

  1 type I [juvenile type], not stated as uncontrolled

  2 type II or unspecified type, uncontrolled
  Fifth-digit 2 is for use with type II patients, even if the patient requires insulin
  Use additional code, if applicable, for associated long-term (current) insulin use V58.67

  3 type I [juvenile type], uncontrolled

250.0 Diabetes mellitus without mention of complication
  Diabetes mellitus without mention of complication or manifestation classifiable to 250.1-250.9
  Diabetes (mellitus) NOS

250.1 Diabetes with ketoacidosis
  Diabetic:
    acidosis without mention of coma
    ketosis without mention of coma

250.2 Diabetes with hyperosmolarity
  Hyperosmolar (nonketotic) coma

250.3 Diabetes with other coma
  Diabetic coma (with ketoacidosis)
  Diabetic hypoglycemic coma
  Insulin coma NOS
  Excludes: diabetes with hyperosmolar coma (250.2)

250.4 Diabetes with renal manifestations
Use additional code to identify manifestation, as:
    chronic kidney disease (585.1-585.9)
    diabetic:
      nephropathy NOS (583.81)
      nephrosis (581.81)
      intercapillary glomerulosclerosis (581.81)
      Kimmelstiel-Wilson syndrome (581.81)

250.5 Diabetes with ophthalmic manifestations
Use additional code to identify manifestation, as:
    diabetic:
      blindness (369.00-369.9)
      cataract (366.41)
      glaucoma (365.44)
      macular edema (362.07)
      retinal edema (362.07)
      retinopathy (362.01-362.07)

TABULAR LIST

⑤ **250.6 Diabetes with neurological manifestations**
Use additional code to identify manifestation, as:
> diabetic:
> > amyotrophy (353.1)
> > gastroparalysis (536.3)
> > gastroparesis (536.3)
> > mononeuropathy (354.0-355.9)
> > neurogenic arthropathy (713.5)
> > peripheral autonomic neuropathy (337.1)
> > polyneuropathy (357.2)

⑤ **250.7 Diabetes with peripheral circulatory disorders**
Use additional code to identify manifestation, as:
> diabetic:
> > gangrene (785.4)
> > peripheral angiopathy (443.81)

⑤ **250.8 Diabetes with other specified manifestations**
> Diabetic hypoglycemia
> Hypoglycemic shock

Use additional code to identify manifestation, as:
> any associated ulceration (707.10-707.9)
> diabetic bone changes (731.8)

Use additional E code to identify cause, if drug-induced

⑤ **250.9 Diabetes with unspecified complication**

251 Other disorders of pancreatic internal secretion

251.0 Hypoglycemic coma
> Iatrogenic hyperinsulinism
> Non-diabetic insulin coma

Use additional E code to identify cause, if drug-induced

> Excludes: hypoglycemic coma in diabetes mellitus (250.3)

251.1 Other specified hypoglycemia
> Hyperinsulinism:
> > NOS
> > ectopic
> > functional
> Hyperplasia of pancreatic islet beta cells NOS

> Excludes: hypoglycemia in diabetes mellitus (250.8)
> > hypoglycemia in infant of diabetic mother (775.0)
> > hypoglycemic coma (251.0)
> > neonatal hypoglycemia (775.6)

Use additional E code to identify cause, if drug-induced

251.2 Hypoglycemia, unspecified
> Hypoglycemia:
> > NOS
> > reactive
> > spontaneous

> Excludes: hypoglycemia:
> > with coma (251.0)
> > in diabetes mellitus (250.8)
> > leucine-induced (270.3)

251.3 Postsurgical hypoinsulinemia
> Hypoinsulinemia following complete or partial pancreatectomy
> Postpancreatectomy hyperglycemia

251.4 Abnormality of secretion of glucagon
> Hyperplasia of pancreatic islet alpha cells with glucagon excess

251.5 Abnormality of secretion of gastrin
> Hyperplasia of pancreatic alpha cells with gastrin excess
> Zollinger-Ellison syndrome

251.8 Other specified disorders of pancreatic internal secretion

251.9 Unspecified disorder of pancreatic internal secretion
> Islet cell hyperplasia NOS

228 ● Code new to this edition   ▲ Revision of existing code   ④ ⑤ Fourth or fifth digit required

ENDOCRINE, NUTRITIONAL, METABOLIC, IMMUNITY

252 Disorders of parathyroid gland

⑤ **252.0 Hyperparathyroidism**

Excludes: ectopic hyperparathyroidism (259.3)

252.00 Hyperparathyroidism, unspecified

252.01 Primary hyperparathyroidism
Hyperplasia of parathyroid

252.02 Secondary hyperparathyroidism, non-renal

Excludes: secondary hyperparathyroidism (of renal origin) (588.81)

252.08 Other hyperparathyroidism
Tertiary hyperparathyroidism

252.1 Hypoparathyroidism
Parathyroiditis (autoimmune)
Tetany:
  parathyroid
  parathyroprival

Excludes: pseudohypoparathyroidism (275.4)
pseudo-pseudohypoparathyroidism (275.4)
tetany NOS (781.7)
transitory neonatal hypoparathyroidism (775.4)

252.8 Other specified disorders of parathyroid gland
Cyst of parathyroid gland
Hemorrhage of parathyroid gland

252.9 Unspecified disorder of parathyroid gland

253 Disorders of the pituitary gland and its hypothalamic control
Includes: the listed conditions whether the disorder is in the pituitary or the hypothalamus

Excludes: Cushing's syndrome (255.0)

253.0 Acromegaly and gigantism
Overproduction of growth hormone

253.1 Other and unspecified anterior pituitary hyperfunction
Forbes-Albright syndrome

Excludes: overproduction of:
  ACTH (255.3)
  thyroid-stimulating hormone [TSH] (242.8)

253.2 Panhypopituitarism
Cachexia, pituitary   Sheehan's syndrome
Necrosis of pituitary   Simmonds' disease
  (postpartum)
Pituitary insufficiency NOS

Excludes: iatrogenic hypopituitarism (253.7)

253.3 Pituitary dwarfism
Isolated deficiency of (human) growth hormone [HGH]
Lorain-Levi dwarfism

253.4 Other anterior pituitary disorders
Isolated or partial deficiency of an anterior pituitary hormone, other than growth hormone
Prolactin deficiency

253.5 Diabetes insipidus
Vasopressin deficiency

Excludes: nephrogenic diabetes insipidus (588.1)

253.6 Other disorders of neurohypophysis
Syndrome of inappropriate secretion of antidiuretic hormone [ADH]

Excludes: ectopic antidiuretic hormone secretion (259.3)

253.7 Iatrogenic pituitary disorders
Hypopituitarism:
  hormone-induced
  hypophysectomy-induced
  postablative
  radiotherapy-induced

Use additional E code to identify cause

TABULAR LIST

253.8 Other disorders of the pituitary and other syndromes of diencephalohypophyseal origin
Abscess of pituitary
Adiposogenital dystrophy
Cyst of Rathke's pouch
Fröhlich's syndrome

Excludes: craniopharyngioma (237.0)

253.9 Unspecified
Dyspituitarism

254 Diseases of thymus gland

Excludes: aplasia or dysplasia with immunodeficiency (279.2)
hypoplasia with immunodeficiency (279.2)
myasthenia gravis (358.00-358.01)

254.0 Persistent hyperplasia of thymus
Hypertrophy of thymus

254.1 Abscess of thymus

254.8 Other specified diseases of thymus gland
Atrophy of thymus
Cyst of thymus

Excludes thymoma (212.6)

254.9 Unspecified disease of thymus gland

255 Disorders of adrenal glands
Includes: the listed conditions whether the basic disorder is in the adrenals or is pituitary-induced

255.0 Cushing's syndrome
Adrenal hyperplasia due to excess ACTH
Cushing's syndrome:
  NOS
  iatrogenic
  idiopathic
  pituitary-dependent
Ectopic ACTH syndrome
Iatrogenic syndrome of excess cortisol
Overproduction of cortisol

Excludes: congenital adrenal hyperplasia (255.2)
Use additional E code to identify cause, if drug-induced

255.1 Hyperaldosteronism

255.10 Hyperaldosteronism, unspecified
Aldosteronism NOS
Primary aldosteronism, unspecified

Excludes: Conn's syndrome (255.12)

255.11 Glucocorticoid-remediable aldosteronism
Familial aldosteronism type I

Excludes: Conn's syndrome (255.12)

255.12 Conn's syndrome

255.13 Bartter's syndrome

255.14 Other secondary aldosteronism

255.2 Adrenogenital disorders
Adrenogenital syndromes, virilizing or feminizing, whether acquired or associated with congenital adrenal hyperplasia consequent on inborn enzyme defects in hormone synthesis
Achard-Thiers syndrome
Congenital adrenal hyperplasia
Female adrenal pseudohermaphroditism
Male:
  macrogenitosomia praecox
  sexual precocity with adrenal hyperplasia
Virilization (female) (suprarenal)

Excludes: adrenal hyperplasia due to excess ACTH (255.0)
isosexual virilization (256.4)

255.3 Other corticoadrenal overactivity
Acquired benign adrenal androgenic overactivity
Overproduction of ACTH

ENDOCRINE, NUTRITIONAL, METABOLIC, IMMUNITY

⑤ **255.4 Corticoadrenal insufficiency**

Excludes: tuberculous Addison's disease (017.6)

● **255.41 Glucocorticoid deficiency**
Addisonian crisis
Addison's disease NOS
Adrenal atrophy (autoimmune)
Adrenal calcification
Adrenal crisis
Adrenal hemorrhage
Adrenal infarction
Adrenal insufficiency NOS
Combined glucocorticoid and mineralocorticoid deficiency
Corticoadrenal insufficiency NOS

● **255.42 Mineralocorticoid deficiency**
Hypoaldosteronism

Excludes: combined glucocorticoid and mineralocorticoid deficiency (255.41)

255.5 Other adrenal hypofunction
Adrenal medullary insufficiency

Excludes: Waterhouse-Friderichsen syndrome (meningococcal) (036.3)

255.6 Medulloadrenal hyperfunction
Catecholamine secretion by pheochromocytoma

255.8 Other specified disorders of adrenal glands
Abnormality of cortisol-binding globulin

255.9 Unspecified disorder of adrenal glands

256 Ovarian dysfunction

256.0 Hyperestrogenism

256.1 Other ovarian hyperfunction
Hypersecretion of ovarian androgens

256.2 Postablative ovarian failure
Use additional code for states associated with artifical menopause (627.4)
Ovarian failure:
iatrogenic
postirradiation
postsurgical

Excludes: asymptomatic age-related (natural) postmenopausal status (V49.81)
acquired absence of ovary (V45.77)

⑤ **256.3 Other ovarian failure**
Use additional code for states associated with natural menopause (627.2)

Excludes: asymptomatic age-related (natural) postmenopausal status (V49.81)

256.31 Premature menopause

256.39 Other ovarian failure
Delayed menarche
Ovarian hypofunction
Primary ovarian failure NOS

256.4 Polycystic ovaries
Isosexual virilization
Stein-Leventhal syndrome

256.8 Other ovarian dysfunction

256.9 Unspecified ovarian dysfunction

257 Testicular dysfunction

257.0 Testicular hyperfunction
Hypersecretion of testicular hormones

257.1 Postablative testicular hypofunction
Testicular hypofunction:
iatrogenic
postirradiation
postsurgical

| Add 4th or 5th digit | Nonspecific code | Unspecified code | Manifestation code |

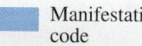

TABULAR LIST

257.2 **Other testicular hypofunction**
Defective biosynthesis of testicular androgen
Eunuchoidism:
  NOS
  hypogonadotropic
Failure:
  Leydig's cell, adult
  seminiferous tubule, adult
Testicular hypogonadism
Excludes: azoospermia (606.0)

257.8 **Other testicular dysfunction**
Excludes: androgen insensitivity syndrome (259.5)

257.9 **Unspecified testicular dysfunction**

258 **Polyglandular dysfunction and related disorders**

⑤ 258.0 **Polyglandular activity in multiple endocrine adenomatosis**
Multiple endocrine neoplasia [MEN] syndromes

Use additional codes to identify any malignancies and other conditions associated with the syndromes

- 258.01 **Multiple endocrine neoplasia [MEN] type I**
  Wermer's syndrome

- 258.02 **Multiple endocrine neoplasia [MEN] type IIA**
  Sipple's syndrome

- 258.03 **Multiple endocrine neoplasia [MEN] type IIB**

258.1 **Other combinations of endocrine dysfunction**
Lloyd's syndrome   Schmidt's syndrome

258.8 **Other specified polyglandular dysfunction**

258.9 **Polyglandular dysfunction, unspecified**

259 **Other endocrine disorders**

259.0 **Delay in sexual development and puberty, not elsewhere classified**
Delayed puberty

259.1 **Precocious sexual development and puberty, not elsewhere classified**
Sexual precocity:
  NOS
  constitutional
  cryptogenic
  idiopathic

259.2 **Carcinoid syndrome**
Hormone secretion by carcinoid tumors

259.3 **Ectopic hormone secretion, not elsewhere classified**
Ectopic:
  antidiuretic hormone secretion [ADH]
  hyperparathyroidism
Excludes: ectopic ACTH syndrome (255.0)

259.4 **Dwarfism, not elsewhere classified**
Dwarfism:
  NOS
  constitutional
Excludes: dwarfism:
  achondroplastic (756.4)
  intrauterine (759.7)
  nutritional (263.2)
  pituitary (253.3)
  renal (588.0)
  progeria (259.8)

259.5 **Androgen insensitivity syndrome**
Partial androgen insensitivity
Reifenstein syndrome

259.8 **Other specified endocrine disorders**
Pineal gland dysfunction
Progeria

ENDOCRINE, NUTRITIONAL, METABOLIC, IMMUNITY

259.9 Unspecified endocrine disorder
Disturbance:
  endocrine NOS
  hormone NOS
Infantilism NOS

NUTRITIONAL DEFICIENCIES (260-269)

Excludes: deficiency anemias (280.0-281.9)

260 Kwashiorkor
Nutritional edema with dyspigmentation of skin and hair

261 Nutritional marasmus
Nutritional atrophy
Severe calorie deficiency
Severe malnutrition NOS

262 Other severe protein-calorie malnutrition
Nutritional edema without mention of dyspigmentation of skin and hair

263 Other and unspecified protein-calorie malnutrition

263.0 Malnutrition of moderate degree

263.1 Malnutrition of mild degree

263.2 Arrested development following protein-calorie malnutrition
Nutritional dwarfism   Physical retardation due to malnutrition

263.8 Other protein-calorie malnutrition

263.9 Unspecified protein-calorie malnutrition
Dystrophy due to malnutrition
Malnutrition (calorie) NOS

Excludes: nutritional deficiency NOS (269.9)

264 Vitamin A deficiency

264.0 With conjunctival xerosis

264.1 With conjunctival xerosis and Bitot's spot
Bitot's spot in the young child

264.2 With corneal xerosis

264.3 With corneal ulceration and xerosis

264.4 With keratomalacia

264.5 With night blindness

264.6 With xerophthalmic scars of cornea

264.7 Other ocular manifestations of vitamin A deficiency
Xerophthalmia due to vitamin A deficiency

264.8 Other manifestations of vitamin A deficiency
Follicular keratosis due to vitamin A deficiency
Xeroderma due to vitamin A deficiency

264.9 Unspecified vitamin A deficiency
Hypovitaminosis A NOS

265 Thiamine and niacin deficiency states

265.0 Beriberi

265.1 Other and unspecified manifestations of thiamine deficiency
Other vitamin B_1 deficiency states

265.2 Pellagra
Deficiency:
  niacin (-tryptophan)
  nicotinamide
  nicotinic acid
  vitamin PP
Pellagra (alcoholic)

266 Deficiency of B-complex components

266.0 Ariboflavinosis
Riboflavin [vitamin B_2] deficiency

266.1 Vitamin B_6 deficiency
Deficiency:
  pyridoxal
  pyridoxamine
  pyridoxine
Vitamin B_6 deficiency syndrome

Excludes: vitamin B_6-responsive sideroblastic anemia (285.0)

Add 4th or 5th digit | Nonspecific code | Unspecified code | Manifestation code

TABULAR LIST

266.2 **Other B-complex deficiencies**
Deficiency:
cyanocobalamin
folic acid
vitamin B_{12}

Excludes: combined system disease with anemia (281.0-281.1)
deficiency anemias (281.0-281.9)
subacute degeneration of spinal cord with anemia (281.0-281.1)

266.9 **Unspecified vitamin B deficiency**

267 **Ascorbic acid deficiency**
Deficiency of vitamin C
Scurvy

Excludes: scorbutic anemia (281.8)

268 **Vitamin D deficiency**

Excludes: vitamin D-resistant:
osteomalacia (275.3)
rickets (275.3)

268.0 **Rickets, active**

Excludes: celiac rickets (579.0)
renal rickets (588.0)

268.1 **Rickets, late effect**
Any condition specified as due to rickets and stated to be a late effect or sequela of rickets
Code first the nature of late effect

268.2 **Osteomalacia, unspecified**

268.9 **Unspecified vitamin D deficiency**
Avitaminosis D

269 **Other nutritional deficiencies**

269.0 **Deficiency of vitamin K**

Excludes: deficiency of coagulation factor due to vitamin K deficiency (286.7)
vitamin K deficiency of newborn (776.0)

269.1 **Deficiency of other vitamins**
Deficiency:
vitamin E
vitamin P

269.2 **Unspecified vitamin deficiency**
Multiple vitamin deficiency NOS

269.3 **Mineral deficiency, not elsewhere classified**
Deficiency:
calcium, dietary
iodine

Excludes: deficiency:
calcium NOS (275.4)
potassium (276.8)
sodium (276.1)

269.8 **Other nutritional deficiency**

Excludes: adult failure to thrive (783.7)
failure to thrive in childhood (783.41)
feeding problems (783.3)
newborn (779.3)

269.9 **Unspecified nutritional deficiency**

OTHER METABOLIC AND IMMUNITY DISORDERS (270-279)

Use additional code to identify any associated mental retardation

270 **Disorders of amino-acid transport and metabolism**

Excludes: abnormal findings without manifest disease (790.0-796.9)
disorders of purine and pyrimidine metabolism (277.1-277.2)
gout (274.0-274.9)

234   ● Code new to this edition   ▲ Revision of existing code   ④ ⑤ Fourth or fifth digit required

ENDOCRINE, NUTRITIONAL, METABOLIC, IMMUNITY

270.0 Disturbances of amino-acid transport
Cystinosis
Cystinuria
Fanconi (-de Toni) (-Debré) syndrome
Glycinuria (renal)
Hartnup disease

270.1 Phenylketonuria [PKU]
Hyperphenylalaninemia

270.2 Other disturbances of aromatic amino-acid metabolism
Albinism
Alkaptonuria
Alkaptonuric ochronosis
Disturbances of metabolism of tyrosine and tryptophan
Homogentisic acid defects
Hydroxykynureninuria
Hypertyrosinemia
Indicanuria
Kynureninase defects
Oasthouse urine disease
Ochronosis
Tyrosinosis
Tyrosinuria
Waardenburg syndrome

Excludes: vitamin B_6-deficiency syndrome (266.1)

270.3 Disturbances of branched-chain amino-acid metabolism
Disturbances of metabolism of leucine, isoleucine, and valine
Hypervalinemia
Intermittent branched-chain ketonuria
Leucine-induced hypoglycemia
Leucinosis
Maple syrup urine disease

270.4 Disturbances of sulphur-bearing amino-acid metabolism
Cystathioninemia
Cystathioninuria
Disturbances of metabolism of methionine, homocystine, and cystathionine
Homocystinuria
Hypermethioninemia
Methioninemia

270.5 Disturbances of histidine metabolism
Carnosinemia
Histidinemia
Hyperhistidinemia
Imidazole aminoaciduria

270.6 Disorders of urea cycle metabolism
Argininosuccinic aciduria
Citrullinemia
Disorders of metabolism of ornithine, citrulline, argininosuccinic acid, arginine, and ammonia
Hyperammonemia
Hyperornithinemia

270.7 Other disturbances of straight-chain amino-acid metabolism
Glucoglycinuria
Glycinemia (with methylmalonic acidemia)
Hyperglycinemia
Hyperlysinemia
Pipecolic acidemia
Saccharopinuria
Other disturbances of metabolism of glycine, threonine, serine, glutamine, and lysine

270.8 Other specified disorders of amino-acid metabolism
Alaninemia
Ethanolaminuria
Glycoprolinuria
Hydroxyprolinemia
Hyperprolinemia
Iminoacidopathy
Prolinemia
Prolinuria
Sarcosinemia

270.9 Unspecified disorder of amino-acid metabolism

271 Disorders of carbohydrate transport and metabolism
Excludes: abnormality of secretion of glucagon (251.4)
diabetes mellitus (250.0-250.9)
hypoglycemia NOS (251.2)
mucopolysaccharidosis (277.5)

235

Add 4th or 5th digit	Nonspecific code	Unspecified code	Manifestation code

TABULAR LIST

271.0 Glycogenosis
Amylopectinosis
Glucose-6-phosphatase
  deficiency
Glycogen storage disease
McArdle's disease
Pompe's disease
von Gierke's disease

271.1 Galactosemia
Galactose-1-phosphate uridyl transferase deficiency
Galactosuria

271.2 Hereditary fructose intolerance
Essential benign fructosuria
Fructosemia

271.3 Intestinal disaccharidase deficiencies and disaccharide malabsorption
Intolerance or malabsorption (congenital) (of):
  glucose-galactose
  lactose
  sucrose-isomaltose

271.4 Renal glycosuria
Renal diabetes

271.8 Other specified disorders of carbohydrate transport and metabolism
Essential benign pentosuria
Fucosidosis
Glycolic aciduria
Hyperoxaluria (primary)
Mannosidosis
Oxalosis
Xylosuria
Xylulosuria

271.9 Unspecified disorder of carbohydrate transport and metabolism

272 Disorders of lipoid metabolism
Excludes: *localized cerebral lipidoses (330.1)*

272.0 Pure hypercholesterolemia
Familial hypercholesterolemia
Fredrickson Type IIa hyperlipoproteinemia
Hyperbetalipoproteinemia
Hyperlipidemia, Group A
Low-density-lipoid-type [LDL] hyperlipoproteinemia

272.1 Pure hyperglyceridemia
Endogenous hyperglyceridemia
Frederickson Type IV hyperlipoproteinemia
Hyperlipidemia, Group B
Hyperprebetalipoproteinemia
Hypertriglyceridemia, essential
Very-low-density-lipoid-type [VLDL] hyperlipoproteinemia

272.2 Mixed hyperlipidemia
Broad- or floating-betalipoproteinemia
Fredrickson Type IIb or III hyperlipoproteinemia
Hypercholesterolemia with endogenous hyperglyceridemia
Hyperbetalipoproteinemia with prebetalipoproteinemia
Tubo-eruptive xanthoma
Xanthoma tuberosum

272.3 Hyperchylomicronemia
Bürger-Grütz syndrome
Fredrickson type I or V hyperlipoproteinemia
Hyperlipidemia, Group D
Mixed hyperglyceridemia

272.4 Other and unspecified hyperlipidemia
Alpha-lipoproteinemia
Combined hyperlipidemia
Hyperlipidemia NOS
Hyperlipoproteinemia NOS

272.5 Lipoprotein deficiencies
Abetalipoproteinemia
Bassen-Kornzweig syndrome
High-density lipoid deficiency
Hypoalphalipoproteinemia
Hypobetalipoproteinemia (familial)

ENDOCRINE, NUTRITIONAL, METABOLIC, IMMUNITY

272.6 Lipodystrophy
Barraquer-Simons disease
Progressive lipodystrophy
Use additional E code to identify cause, if iatrogenic
Excludes: *intestinal lipodystrophy (040.2)*

272.7 Lipidoses
Chemically-induced lipidosis
Disease:
  Anderson's
  Fabry's
  Gaucher's
  I cell [mucolipidosis I]
  lipoid storage NOS
  Neimann-Pick
  pseudo-Hurler's or mucolipidosis III
Disease:
  triglyceride storage, Type I or II
  Wolman's or triglyceride storage, Type III
Mucolipidosis II
Primary familial xanthomatosis

Excludes: *cerebral lipidoses (330.1)*
Tay-Sachs disease (330.1)

272.8 Other disorders of lipid metabolism
Hoffa's disease or liposynovitis prepatellaris
Launois-Bensaude's lipomatosis
Lipoid dermatoarthritis

272.9 Unspecified disorder of lipid metabolism

273 Disorders of plasma protein metabolism
Excludes: *agammaglobulinemia and hypogammaglobulinemia (279.0 -279.2)*
coagulation defects (286.0-286.9)
hereditary hemolytic anemias (282.0-282.9)

273.0 Polyclonal hypergammaglobulinemia
Hypergammaglobulinemic purpura:
  benign primary
  Waldenström's

273.1 Monoclonal paraproteinemia
Benign monoclonal hypergammaglobulinemia [BMH]
Monoclonal gammopathy:
  NOS
  associated with lymphoplasmacytic dyscrasias
  benign
Paraproteinemia:
  benign (familial)
  secondary to malignant or inflammatory disease

273.2 Other paraproteinemias
Cryoglobulinemic:
  purpura
  vasculitis
Mixed cryoglobulinemia

273.3 Macroglobulinemia
Macroglobulinemia (idiopathic) (primary)
Waldenström's macroglobulinemia

273.4 Alpha-1-antitrypsin deficiency
AAT deficiency

273.8 Other disorders of plasma protein metabolism
Abnormality of transport protein
Bisalbuminemia

273.9 Unspecified disorder of plasma protein metabolism

274 Gout
Excludes: *lead gout (984.0-984.9)*

274.0 Gouty arthropathy

⑤ **274.1 Gouty nephropathy**
  274.10 Gouty nephropathy, unspecified
  274.11 Uric acid nephrolithiasis
  274.19 Other

⑤ **274.8 Gout with other specified manifestations**
  274.81 Gouty tophi of ear

TABULAR LIST

- **274.82 Gouty tophi of other sites**
  Gouty tophi of heart
- **274.89 Other**
  Use additional code to identify manifestations, as:
  gouty:
  iritis (364.11)
  neuritis (357.4)
- **274.9 Gout, unspecified**

275 Disorders of mineral metabolism
Excludes: abnormal findings without manifest disease (790.0-796.9)

- **275.0 Disorders of iron metabolism**
  Bronzed diabetes   Pigmentary cirrhosis (of liver)
  Hemochromatosis
  Excludes: anemia:
  iron deficiency (280.0-280.9)
  sideroblastic (285.0)

- **275.1 Disorders of copper metabolism**
  Hepatolenticular degeneration
  Wilson's disease

- **275.2 Disorders of magnesium metabolism**
  Hypermagnesemia
  Hypomagnesemia

- **275.3 Disorders of phosphorus metabolism**
  Familial hypophosphatemia
  Hypophosphatasia
  Vitamin D-resistant:
  osteomalacia
  rickets

- **275.4 Disorders of calcium metabolism**
  Excludes: parathyroid disorders (252.00-252.9)
  vitamin D deficiency (268.0-268.9)
  - **275.40 Unspecified disorder of calcium metabolism**
  - **275.41 Hypocalcemia**
  - **275.42 Hypercalcemia**
  - **275.49 Other disorders of calcium metabolism**
    Nephrocalcinosis
    Pseudohypoparathyroidism
    Pseudopseudohypoparathyroidism

- **275.8 Other specified disorders of mineral metabolism**
- **275.9 Unspecified disorder of mineral metabolism**

276 Disorders of fluid, electrolyte, and acid-base balance
Excludes: diabetes insipidus (253.5)
familial periodic paralysis (359.3)

- **276.0 Hyperosmolality and/or hypernatremia**
  Sodium [Na] excess
  Sodium [Na] overload

- **276.1 Hyposmolality and/or hyponatremia**
  Sodium [Na] deficiency

- **276.2 Acidosis**
  Acidosis:
  NOS
  lactic
  metabolic
  respiratory
  Excludes: diabetic acidosis (250.1)

- **276.3 Alkalosis**
  Alkalosis:
  NOS
  metabolic
  respiratory

ENDOCRINE, NUTRITIONAL, METABOLIC, IMMUNITY

276.4 Mixed acid-base balance disorder
Hypercapnia with mixed acid-base disorder

⑤ 276.5 Volume depletion

276.50 Volume depletion, unspecified

276.51 Dehydration

276.52 Hypovolemia
Depletion of volume of plasma

276.6 Fluid overload
Fluid retention

Excludes: ascites (789.51-789.59)
localized edema (782.3)

276.7 Hyperpotassemia
Hyperkalemia
Potassium [K]:
  excess
  intoxication
  overload

276.8 Hypopotassemia
Hypokalemia
Potassium [K] deficiency

276.9 Electrolyte and fluid disorders not elsewhere classified
Electrolyte imbalance
Hyperchloremia
Hypochloremia

Excludes: electrolyte imbalance:
  associated with hyperemesis gravidarum (643.1)
  complicating labor and delivery (669.0)
  following abortion and ectopic or molar pregnancy (634-638 with .4, 639.4)

277 Other and unspecified disorders of metabolism

⑤ 277.0 Cystic fibrosis
Fibrocystic disease of the pancreas
Mucoviscidosis

277.00 Without mention of meconium ileus
Cystic fibrosis NOS

277.01 With meconium ileus
Meconium:
  ileus (of newborn)
  obstruction of intestine in mucoviscidosis

277.02 With pulmonary manifestations
Cystic fibrosis with pulmonary exacerbation

Use additional code to identify any infectious organism present, such as:
  pseudomonas (041.7)

277.03 With gastrointestinal manifestations

Excludes: with meconium ileus (277.01)

277.09 With other manifestations

277.1 Disorders of porphyrin metabolism
Hematoporphyria   Porphyrinuria
Hematoporphyrinuria   Protocoproporphyria
Hereditary coproporphyria Protoporphyria
Porphyria   Pyrroloporphyria

277.2 Other disorders of purine and pyrimidine metabolism
Hypoxanthine-guanine-phosphoribosyltransferase deficiency [HG-PRT deficiency]
Lesch-Nyhan syndrome
Xanthinuria

Excludes: gout (274.0-274.9)
orotic aciduric anemia (281.4)

⑤ 277.3 Amyloidosis

277.30 Amyloidosis, unspecified
Amyloidosis NOS

Add 4th or 5th digit	Nonspecific code	Unspecified code	Manifestation code

239

TABULAR LIST

277.31 Familial Mediterranean fever
Benign paroxysmal peritonitis
Hereditary amyloid nephropathy
Periodic familial polyserositis
Recurrent polyserositis

277.39 Other amyloidosis
Hereditary cardiac amyloidosis
Inherited systemic amyloidosis
Neuropathic (Portuguese) (Swiss) amyloidosis
Secondary amyloidosis

277.4 Disorders of bilirubin excretion
Hyperbilirubinemia:
  congenital
  constitutional
Syndrome:
  Crigler-Najjar
  Dubin-Johnson
  Gilbert's
  Rotor's

Excludes: hyperbilirubinemias specific to the perinatal period (774.0-774.7)

277.5 Mucopolysaccharidosis
Gargoylism
Hunter's syndrome
Hurler's syndrome
Lipochondrodystrophy
Maroteaux-Lamy syndrome
Morquio-Brailsford disease
Osteochondrodystrophy
Sanfilippo's syndrome
Scheie's syndrome

277.6 Other deficiencies of circulating enzymes
Hereditary angioedema

277.7 Dysmetabolic syndrome X
Use additional code for associated manifestation, such as:
  cardiovascular disease (414.00-414.07)
  obesity (278.00-278.01)

⑤ **277.8 Other specified disorders of metabolism**

277.81 Primary carnitine deficiency

277.82 Carnitine deficiency due to inborn errors of metabolism

277.83 Iatrogenic carnitine deficiency
Carnitine deficiency due to:
  hemodialysis
  valproic acid therapy

277.84 Other secondary carnitine deficiency

277.85 Disorders of fatty acid oxidation
Carnitine palmitoyltransferase deficiencies (CPT1, CPT2)
Glutaric aciduria type II (type IIA, IIB, IIC)
Long chain 3-hydroxyacyl CoA dehydrogenase deficiency (LCHAD)
Long chain/very long chain acyl CoA dehydrogenase deficiency (LCAD, VLCAD)
Medium chain acyl CoA dehydrogenase deficiency (MCAD)
Short chain acyl CoA dehydrogenase deficiency (SCAD)

Excludes: primary carnitine deficiency (277.81)

277.86 Peroxisomal disorders
Adrenomyeloneuropathy
Neonatal adrenoleukodystrophy
Rhizomelic chrondrodysplasia punctata
X-linked adrenoleukodystrophy
Zellweger syndrome

Excludes: infantile Refsum disease (356.3)

ENDOCRINE, NUTRITIONAL, METABOLIC, IMMUNITY

- **277.87 Disorders of mitochondrial metabolism**
  Kearns-Sayre syndrome
  Mitochondrial Encephalopathy, Lactic Acidosis and Stroke-like episodes (MELAS syndrome)
  Mitochondrial Neurogastrointestinal Encephalopathy syndrome (MNGIE)
  Myoclonus with Epilepsy and with Ragged Red Fibers (MERRF syndrome)
  Neuropathy, Ataxia and Retinitis Pigmentosa (NARP syndrome)
  Use additional code for associated conditions

  Excludes: *disorders of pyruvate metabolism (271.8)*
  Leber's optic atrophy (377.16)
  Leigh's subacute necrotizing encephalopathy (330.8)
  Reye's syndrome (331.81)

- **277.89 Other specified disorders of metabolism**
  Hand-Schuller-Christian disease
  Histiocytosis (acute) (chronic)
  Histiocytosis X (chronic)

  Excludes: *histiocytosis:*
  acute differentiatied progressive (202.5)
  X, acute (progressive) (202.5)

- **277.9 Unspecified disorder of metabolism**
  Enzymopathy NOS

278 Overweight, obesity and other hyperalimentation

Excludes: *hyperalimentation NOS (783.6)*
poisoning by vitamins NOS (963.5)
polyphagia (783.6)

Use additional code to identify Body Mass Index (BMI), if known (V85.21-V85.25, V85.30-V85.39, V85.4, V85.53, V85.54)

- ⑤ **278.0 Overweight and obesity**
  Use additional code to identify Body Mass Index (BMI), if known (V85.0-V85.54)

  Excludes: *adiposogenital dystrophy (253.8)*
  obesity of endocrine origin NOS (259.9)

  - **278.00 Obesity, unspecified**
    Obesity NOS
  - 278.01 Morbid obesity
    Severe obesity
  - 278.02 Overweight

- 278.1 Localized adiposity
  Fat pad
- 278.2 Hypervitaminosis A
- 278.3 Hypercarotinemia
- 278.4 Hypervitaminosis D
- **278.8 Other hyperalimentation**

279 Disorders involving the immune mechanism

- ⑤ 279.0 Deficiency of humoral immunity
  - **279.00 Hypogammaglobulinemia, unspecified**
    Agammaglobulinemia NOS
  - 279.01 Selective IgA immunodeficiency
  - 279.02 Selective IgM immunodeficiency
  - **279.03 Other selective immunoglobulin deficiencies**
    Selective deficiency of IgG
  - 279.04 Congenital hypogammaglobulinemia
    Agammaglobulinemia:
      Bruton's type
      X-linked
  - 279.05 Immunodeficiency with increased IgM
    Immunodeficiency with hyper-IgM:
      autosomal recessive
      X-linked

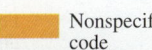 Add 4th or 5th digit   Nonspecific code   Unspecified code   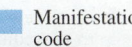 Manifestation code

TABULAR LIST

- **279.06 Common variable immunodeficiency**
  Dysgammaglobulinemia (acquired) (congenital) (primary)
  Hypogammaglobulinemia:
  acquired primary
  congenital non-sex-linked
  sporadic

- **279.09 Other**
  Transient hypogammaglobulinemia of infancy

⑤ **279.1 Deficiency of cell-mediated immunity**

- **279.10 Immunodeficiency with predominant T-cell defect, unspecified**

- **279.11 DiGeorge's syndrome**
  Pharyngeal pouch syndrome
  Thymic hypoplasia

- **279.12 Wiskott-Aldrich syndrome**

- **279.13 Nezelof's syndrome**
  Cellular immunodeficiency with abnormal immunoglobulin deficiency

- **279.19 Other**

Excludes: ataxia-telangiectasia (334.8)

279.2 Combined immunity deficiency
  Agammaglobulinemia:
  autosomal recessive
  Swiss-type
  x-linked recessive
  Severe combined immunodeficiency [SCID]
  Thymic:
  alymphoplasia
  aplasia or dysplasia with immunodeficiency

Excludes: thymic hypoplasia (279.11)

279.3 Unspecified immunity deficiency

279.4 Autoimmune disease, not elsewhere classified
  Autoimmune disease NOS

Excludes: transplant failure or rejection (996.80-996.89)

279.8 Other specified disorders involving the immune mechanism
  Single complement [C_1-C_9] deficiency or dysfunction

279.9 Unspecified disorder of immune mechanism

● Code new to this edition   ▲ Revision of existing code   ④ ⑤ Fourth or fifth digit required

BLOOD AND BLOOD-FORMING ORGANS

4. DISEASES OF THE BLOOD AND BLOOD-FORMING ORGANS (280-289)

Excludes: anemia complicating pregnancy or the puerperium (648.2)

280 Iron deficiency anemias
Includes: anemia:
  asiderotic
  hypochromic-microcytic
  sideropenic

Excludes: familial microcytic anemia (282.49)

280.0 Secondary to blood loss (chronic)
Normocytic anemia due to blood loss

Excludes: acute posthemorrhagic anemia (285.1)

280.1 Secondary to inadequate dietary iron intake

280.8 Other specified iron deficiency anemias
Paterson-Kelly syndrome
Plummer-Vinson syndrome
Sideropenic dysphagia

280.9 Iron deficiency anemia, unspecified
Anemia:
  achlorhydric
  chlorotic
  idiopathic hypochromic
  iron [Fe] deficiency NOS

281 Other deficiency anemias

281.0 Pernicious anemia
Anemia:
  Addison's
  Biermer's
  congenital pernicious
Congenital intrinsic factor [Castle's] deficiency

Excludes: combined system disease without mention of anemia (266.2)
  subacute degeneration of spinal cord without mention of anemia (266.2)

281.1 Other vitamin B_{12} deficiency anemia
Anemia:
  vegan's
  vitamin B_{12} deficiency (dietary)
  due to selective vitamin B_{12} malabsorption with proteinuria
Syndrome:
  Imerslund's
  Imerslund-Gräsbeck

Excludes: combined system disease without mention of anemia (266.2)
  subacute degeneration of spinal cord without mention of anemia (266.2)

281.2 Folate-deficiency anemia
Congenital folate malabsorption
Folate or folic acid deficiency anemia:
  NOS
  dietary
  drug-induced
Goat's milk anemia
Nutritional megaloblastic anemia (of infancy)

Use additional E code, if desired, to identify drug

281.3 Other specified megaloblastic anemias not elsewhere classified
Combined B_{12} and folate-deficiency anemia
Refractory megaloblastic anemia

281.4 Protein-deficiency anemia
Amino-acid-deficiency anemia

281.8 Anemia associated with other specified nutritional deficiency
Scorbutic anemia

281.9 Unspecified deficiency anemia
Anemia:
  dimorphic
  macrocytic
  megaloblastic NOS
Anemia:
  nutritional NOS
  simple chronic

 Add 4th or 5th digit
 Nonspecific code
 Unspecified code
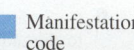 Manifestation code

243

TABULAR LIST

282 Hereditary hemolytic anemias

282.0 Hereditary spherocytosis
Acholuric (familial) jaundice
Congenital hemolytic anemia (spherocytic)
Congenital spherocytosis
Minkowski-Chauffard syndrome
Spherocytosis (familial)

Excludes: hemolytic anemia of newborn (773.0-773.5)

282.1 Hereditary elliptocytosis
Elliptocytosis (congenital)
Ovalocytosis (congenital) (hereditary)

282.2 Anemias due to disorders of glutathione metabolism
Anemia:
   6-phosphogluconic dehydrogenase deficiency
   enzyme deficiency, drug-induced
   erythrocytic glutathione deficiency
   glucose-6-phosphate dehydrogenase [G-6-PD] deficiency
   glutathione-reductase deficiency
   hemolytic nonspherocytic (hereditary), type I
Disorder of pentose phosphate pathway
Favism

282.3 Other hemolytic anemias due to enzyme deficiency
Anemia:
   hemolytic nonspherocytic (hereditary), type II
   hexokinase deficiency
   pyruvate kinase [PK] deficiency
   triosephosphate isomerase deficiency

282.4 Thalassemias

Excludes: sickle-cell:
   disease (282.60-282.69)
   trait (282.5)

282.41 Sickle-cell thalassemia without crisis
Sickle-cell thalassemia NOS
Thalassemia Hb-S disease without crisis

282.42 Sickle-cell thalassemia with crisis
Sickle-cell thalassemia with vaso-occlusive pain
Thalassemia Hb-S disease with crisis

Use additional code for types of crisis, such as:
   acute chest syndrome (517.3)
   splenic sequestration (289.52)

282.49 Other thalassemia
Cooley's anemia
Hb-Bart's disease
Hereditary leptocytosis
Mediterranean anemia (with other hemoglobinopathy)
Microdrepanocytosis
Thalassemia (alpha) (beta) (intermedia) (major) (minima) (minor) (mixed)
   (trait) (with other hemoglobinopathy)
Thalassemia NOS

282.5 Sickle-cell trait
Hb-AS genotype
Hemoglobin S [Hb-S] trait
Heterozygous:
   hemoglobin S
   Hb-S

Excludes: that with other hemoglobinopathy (282.60-282.69)
   that with thalassemia (282.49)

282.6 Sickle-cell disease
Sickle-cell anemia

Excludes: sickle-cell thalassemia (282.41-282.42)
   sickle-cell trait (282.5)

282.60 Sickle-cell disease, unspecified
Sickle-cell anemia NOS

282.61 Hb-SS disease without crisis

BLOOD AND BLOOD-FORMING ORGANS

282.62 Hb-SS disease with crisis
Hb-SS disease with vaso-occlusive pain
Sickle-cell crisis NOS

Use additional code for type of crisis, such as:
acute chest syndrome (517.3)
splenic sequestration (289.52)

282.63 Sickle-cell/Hb-C disease without crisis
Hb-S/Hb-C disease without crisis

282.64 Sickle-cell/Hb-C disease with crisis
Hb-S/Hb-C disease with crisis
Sickle-cell/Hb-C disease with vaso-occlusive pain

Use additional code for type of crisis, such as:
acute chest syndrome (517.3)
splenic sequestration (289.52)

282.68 Other sickle-cell disease without crisis
Hb-S/Hb-D disease without crisis
Hb-S/Hb-E disease without crisis
Sickle-cell/Hb-D disease without crisis
Sickle-cell/Hb-E disease without crisis

282.69 Other sickle-cell disease with crisis
Hb-S/Hb-D disease with crisis
Hb-S/Hb-E disease with crisis
Other sickle-cell disease with vaso-occlusive pain
Sickle-cell/Hb-D disease with crisis
Sickle-cell/Hb-E disease with crisis

Use additional code for type of crisis, such as:
acute chest syndrome (517.3)
splenic sequestration (289.52)

282.7 Other hemoglobinopathies
Abnormal hemoglobin NOS
Congenital Heinz-body anemia
Disease:
hemoglobin C [Hb-C]
hemoglobin D [Hb-D]
hemoglobin E [Hb-E]
hemoglobin Zurich [Hb-Zurich]
Hemoglobinopathy NOS
Hereditary persistence of fetal hemoglobin [HPFH]
Unstable hemoglobin hemolytic disease

Excludes: familial polycythemia (289.6)
hemoglobin M [Hb-M] disease (289.7)
high-oxygen-affinity hemoglobin (289.0)

282.8 Other specified hereditary hemolytic anemias
Stomatocytosis

282.9 Hereditary hemolytic anemia, unspecified
Hereditary hemolytic anemia NOS

283 Acquired hemolytic anemias

283.0 Autoimmune hemolytic anemias
Autoimmune hemolytic anemias (cold type) (warm type)
Chronic cold hemagglutinin disease
Cold agglutinin disease or hemoglobinuria
Hemolytic anemia:
cold type (secondary) (symptomatic)
drug-induced
warm type (secondary) (symptomatic)

Use additional E code, if desired, to identify cause, if drug-induced

Excludes: Evans' syndrome (287.32)
hemolytic disease of newborn (773.0-773.5)

⑤ **283.1 Non-autoimmune hemolytic anemias**
283.10 Non-autoimmune hemolytic anemia, unspecified
283.11 Hemolytic-uremic syndrome

245

TABULAR LIST

283.19 **Other non-autoimmune hemolytic anemias**
Hemolytic anemia:
mechanical
microangiopathic
toxic

Use additional E code, if desired, to identify cause

283.2 Hemoglobinuria due to hemolysis from external causes
Acute intravascular hemolysis
Hemoglobinuria:
from exertion
march
paroxysmal (cold) (nocturnal)
due to other hemolysis
Marchiafava-Micheli syndrome

Use additional E code, if desired, to identify cause

283.9 Acquired hemolytic anemia, unspecified
Acquired hemolytic anemia NOS
Chronic idiopathic hemolytic anemia

284 Aplastic anemia and other bone marrow failure syndromes

⑤ **284.0 Constitutional aplastic anemia**

284.01 Constitutional red blood cell aplasia
Aplasia, (pure) red cell:
congenital
of infants
primary
Blackfan-Diamond syndrome
Familial hypoplastic anemia

284.09 **Other constitutional aplastic anemia**
Fanconi's anemia
Pancytopenia with malformations

284.1 Pancytopenia

Excludes: *pancytopenia (due to) (with):*
aplastic anemia NOS (284.9)
bone marrow infiltration (284.2)
constitutional red blood cell aplasia (284.01)
drug induced (284.89)
hairy cell leukemia (202.4)
human immunodeficiency virus disease (042)
leukoerythroblastic anemia (284.2)
malformations (284.09)
myelodysplastic syndromes (238.72-238.75)
myeloproliferative disease (238.79)
other constitutional aplastic anemia (284.09)

284.2 Myelophthisis
Leukoerythroblastic anemia
Myelophthisic anemia

Code first the underlying disorder, such as:
malignant neoplasm of breast (174.0-174.9, 175.0-175.9)
tuberculosis (015.0-015.9)

Excludes: *idiopathic myelofibrosis (238.76)*
myelofibrosis NOS (289.83)
myelofibrosis with myeloid metaplasia (238.76)
primary myelofibrosis (238.76)
secondary myelofibrosis (289.83)

⑤ **284.8 Other specified aplastic anemias**

● **284.81 Red cell aplasia (acquired) (adult) (with thymoma)**
Red cell aplasia NOS

● **284.89** **Other specified aplastic anemias**
Aplastic anemia (due to):
chronic systemic disease
drugs
infection
radiation
toxic (paralytic)

Use additional E code to identify cause

---

246   ● Code new to this edition   ▲ Revision of existing code   ④ ⑤ Fourth or fifth digit required

BLOOD AND BLOOD-FORMING ORGANS

284.9 Aplastic anemia, unspecified
Anemia:
   aplastic (idiopathic) NOS
   aregenerative
   hypoplastic NOS
Anemia:
   nonregenerative
Medullary hypoplasia

Excludes: refractory anemia (238.72)

285 Other and unspecified anemias

285.0 Sideroblastic anemia
Anemia:
   hypochromic with iron loading
   sideroachrestic
   sideroblastic:
      acquired
      congenital
      hereditary
      primary
      secondary (drug-induced) (due to disease)
      sex-linked hypochromic
      vitamin B_6-responsive
   Pyridoxine-responsive (hypochromic) anemia

Use additional E code, if desired, to identify cause, if drug induced

Excludes: refractory sideroblastic anemia (238.72)

285.1 Acute posthemorrhagic anemia
Anemia due to acute blood loss

Excludes: anemia due to chronic blood loss (280.0)
           blood loss anemia NOS (280.0)

⑤ **285.2 Anemia of chronic disease**
Anemia in chronic illness

  285.21 Anemia in chronic kidney disease
  Anemia in end stage renal disease
  Erythropoietin-resistant anemia (EPO resistant anemia)

  285.22 Anemia in neoplastic disease

  285.29 Anemia of other chronic disease
  Anemia in other chronic illness

285.8 Other specified anemias
Anemia:
   dyserythropoietic (congenital)
   dyshematopoietic (congenital)
   von Jaksch's
Infantile pseudoleukemia

285.9 Anemia, unspecified
Anemia:
   NOS
   essential
   normocytic, not due to blood
      loss
Anemia:
   profound
   progressive
   secondary
Oligocythemia

Excludes: anemia (due to):
           blood loss:
              acute (285.1)
              chronic or unspecified (280.0)
           iron deficiency (280.0-280.9)

286 Coagulation defects

286.0 Congenital factor VIII disorder
Antihemophilic globulin [AHG] deficiency
Factor VIII (functional) deficiency
Hemophilia:
   NOS
   A
   classical
   familial
   hereditary
Subhemophilia

Excludes: factor VIII deficiency with vascular defect (286.4)

247

TABULAR LIST

286.1 Congenital factor IX disorder
Christmas disease
Deficiency:
    factor IX (functional)
    plasma thromboplastin component [PTC]
Hemophilia B

286.2 Congenital factor XI deficiency
Hemophilia C
Plasma thromboplastin antecedent [PTA] deficiency
Rosenthal's disease

286.3 Congenital deficiency of other clotting factors
Congenital afibrinogenemia
Deficiency:
    AC globulin factor:
        I [fibrinogen]
        II [prothrombin]
        V [labile]
        VII [stable]
        X [Stuart-Prower]
        XII [Hageman]
        XIII [fibrin stabilizing]
Deficiency:
    Laki-Lorand factor
    proaccelerin
Disease:
    Owren's
    Stuart-Prower
Dysfibrinogenemia (congenital)
Dysprothrombinemia (constitutional)
Hypoproconvertinemia
Hypoprothrombinemia (hereditary)
Parahemophilia

286.4 von Willebrand's disease
Angiohemophilia (A) (B)
Constitutional thrombopathy
Factor VIII deficiency with vascular defect
Pseudohemophilia type B
Vascular hemophilia
von Willebrand's (-Jürgens') disease

   Excludes: factor VIII deficiency:
        NOS (286.0)
        with functional defect (286.0)
        hereditary capillary fragility (287.8)

286.5 Hemorrhagic disorder due to intrinsic circulating anticoagulants
Antithrombinemia
Antithromboplastinemia
Antithromboplastinogenemia
Hyperheparinemia
Increase in:
    anti-VIIIa
    anti-IXa
Increase in:
    anti-Xa
    anti-XIa
    antithrombin
Secondary hemophilia

Systemic lupus erythematosus [SLE] inhibitor

286.6 Defibrination syndrome
Afibrinogenemia, acquired
Consumption coagulopathy
Diffuse or disseminated intravascular coagulation [DIC syndrome]
Fibrinolytic hemorrhage, acquired
Hemorrhagic fibrinogenolysis
Pathologic fibrinolysis
Purpura:
    fibrinolytic
    fulminans

   Excludes: that complicating:
        abortion (634-638 with .1, 639.1)
        pregnancy or the puerperium (641.3, 666.3)
        disseminated intravascular coagulation in newborn (776.2)

286.7 Acquired coagulation factor deficiency
Deficiency of coagulation factor due to:
    liver disease
    vitamin K deficiency
Hypoprothrombinemia, acquired

   Excludes: vitamin K deficiency of newborn (776.0)
Use additional E-code, if desired, to identify cause, if drug induced

BLOOD AND BLOOD-FORMING ORGANS

286.9 Other and unspecified coagulation defects
Defective coagulation NOS
Deficiency, coagulation factor NOS
Delay, coagulation
Disorder:
  coagulation
  hemostasis

Excludes: abnormal coagulation profile (790.92)
  hemorrhagic disease of newborn (776.0)
  that complicating:
    abortion (634-638 with .1, 639.1)
    pregnancy or the puerperium (641.3, 666.3)

287 Purpura and other hemorrhagic conditions

Excludes: hemorrhagic thrombocythemia (238.79)
  purpura fulminans (286.6)

287.0 Allergic purpura
Peliosis rheumatica
Purpura:
  anaphylactoid
  autoimmune
  Henoch's
Purpura:
  nonthrombocytopenic:
    hemorrhagic
    idiopathic
    rheumatica
  Schönlein-Henoch
  vascular
Vasculitis, allergic

Excludes: hemorrhagic purpura (287.39)
  purpura annularis telangiectodes (709.1)

287.1 Qualitative platelet defects
Thrombasthenia (hemorrhagic) (hereditary)
Thrombocytasthenia
Thrombocytopathy (dystrophic)
Thrombopathy (Bernard-Soulier)

Excludes: von Willebrand's disease (286.4)

287.2 Other nonthrombocytopenic purpuras
Purpura:
  NOS
  senile
  simplex

287.3 Primary thrombocytopenia

287.30 Primary thrombocytopenia, unspecified
Megakaryocytic hypoplasia

287.31 Immune thrombocytopenic purpura
Idiopathic thrombocytopenic purpura
Tidal platelet dysgenesis

287.32 Evans' syndrome

287.33 Congenital and hereditary thrombocytopenic purpura
Congenital and hereditary thrombocytopenia
Thrombocytopenia with absent radii (TAR) syndrome

Excludes: Wiskott-Aldrich syndrome (279.12)

287.39 Other primary thrombocytopenia

287.4 Secondary thrombocytopenia
Posttransfusion purpura
Thrombocytopenia (due to):
  dilutional
  drugs
  extracorporeal circulation of blood
  massive blood transfusion
  platelet alloimmunization

Use additional E code, if desired, to identify cause

Excludes: transient thrombocytopenia of newborn (776.1)

287.5 Thrombocytopenia, unspecified

287.8 Other specified hemorrhagic conditions
Capillary fragility (hereditary)
Vascular pseudohemophilia

TABULAR LIST

287.9 **Unspecified hemorrhagic conditions**
Hemorrhagic diathesis (familial)

288 **Diseases of white blood cells**
Excludes: leukemia (204.0-208.9)

⑤ **288.0** **Neutropenia**
Decreased Absolute Neutrophil Count (ANC)
Use additional code for any associated:
  fever (780.6)
  mucositis (478.11, 528.00-528.09, 538, 616.81)
Excludes: neutropenic splenomegaly (289.53)
  transitory neonatal neutropenia (776.7)

288.00 **Neutropenia, unspecified**

288.01 **Congenital neutropenia**
Congenital agranulocytosis
Infantile genetic agranulocytosis
Kostmann's syndrome

288.02 **Cyclic neutropenia**
Cyclic hematopoiesis
Periodic neutropenia

288.03 **Drug induced neutropenia**
Use additional E code to identify drug

288.04 **Neutropenia due to infection**

288.09 **Other neutropenia**
Agranulocytosis
Neutropenia:
  immune
  toxic

288.1 **Functional disorders of polymorphonuclear neutrophils**
Chronic (childhood) granulomatous disease
Congenital dysphagocytosis
Job's syndrome
Lipochrome histiocytosis (familial)
Progressive septic granulomatosis

288.2 **Genetic anomalies of leukocytes**
Anomaly (granulation) (granulocyte) or syndrome:
  Alder's (-Reilly)
  Chédiak-Steinbrinck (-Higashi)
  Jordan's
  May-Hegglin
  Pelger-Huet
Hereditary:
  hypersegmentation
  hyposegmentation
  leukomelanopathy

288.3 **Eosinophilia**
Eosinophilia
  allergic
  hereditary
  idiopathic
  secondary
Eosinophilic leukocytosis
Excludes: Löffler's syndrome (518.3)
  pulmonary eosinophilia (518.3)

288.4 **Hemophagocytic syndromes**
Familial hemophagocytic lymphohistiocytosis
Familial hemophagocytic reticulosis
Hemophagocytic syndrome, infection-associated
Histiocytic syndromes
Macrophage activation syndrome

BLOOD AND BLOOD-FORMING ORGANS

⑤ **288.5 Decreased white blood cell count**
Excludes: neutropenia (288.01-288.09)

288.50 Leukocytopenia, unspecified
Decreased leukocytes, unspecified
Decreased white blood cell count, unspecified
Leukopenia NOS

288.51 **Lymphocytopenia**
Decreased lymphocytes

288.59 Other decreased white blood cell count
Basophilic leukopenia
Eosinophilic leukopenia
Monocytopenia
Plasmacytopenia

⑤ **288.6 Elevated white blood cell count**
Excludes: eosinophilia (288.3)

288.60 Leukocytosis, unspecified
Elevated leukocytes, unspecified
Elevated white blood cell count, unspecified

288.61 **Lymphocytosis (symptomatic)**
Elevated lymphocytes

288.62 **Leukemoid reaction**
Basophilic leukemoid reaction
Lymphocytic leukemoid reaction
Monocytic leukemoid reaction
Myelocytic leukemoid reaction
Neutrophilic leukemoid reaction

288.63 **Monocytosis (symptomatic)**
Excludes: infectious mononucleosis (075)

288.64 **Plasmacytosis**

288.65 **Basophilia**

● 288.66 **Bandemia**
Bandemia without diagnosis of specific infection
Excludes: confirmed infection – code to infection leukemia (204.00-208.9)

288.69 Other elevated white blood cell count

288.8 Other specified disease of white blood cells
Excludes: decreased white blood cell counts (288.50-288.59)
elevated white blood cell counts (288.60-288.69)
immunity disorders (279.0-279.9)

288.9 Unspecified disease of white blood cells

289 Other diseases of blood and blood-forming organs

289.0 **Polycythemia, secondary**
High-oxygen-affinity hemoglobin
Polycythemia:
 acquired
 benign
 due to:
  fall in plasma volume
  high altitude
Polycythemia:
 emotional
 erythropoietin
 hypoxemic
 nephrogenous
 relative
 spurious
 stress

Excludes: polycythemia:
 neonatal (776.4)
 primary (238.4)
 vera (238.4)

289.1 **Chronic lymphadenitis**
Chronic:
 adenitis, any lymph node except mesenteric
 lymphadenitis, any lymph node except mesenteric

Excludes: acute lymphadenitis (683)
 mesenteric (289.2)
 enlarged glands NOS (785.6)

251

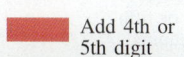 Add 4th or 5th digit
 Nonspecific code
 Unspecified code
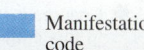 Manifestation code

TABULAR LIST

289.2　Nonspecific mesenteric lymphadenitis
　　Mesenteric lymphadenitis (acute) (chronic)

289.3　Lymphadenitis, unspecified, except mesenteric

289.4　Hypersplenism
　　"Big spleen" syndrome　　Hypersplenia
　　Dyssplenism

　　Excludes: *primary splenic neutropenia (289.53)*

⑤ **289.5　Other diseases of spleen**

　　289.50　Disease of spleen, unspecified

　　289.51　Chronic congestive splenomegaly

　　289.52　Splenic sequestration
　　　　Code first sickle-cell disease in crisis (282.42, 282.62, 282.64, 282.69)

　　289.53　Neutropenic splenomegaly

　　289.59　Other
　　　　Lien migrans　　　　　Splenic:
　　　　Perisplenitis　　　　　　fibrosis
　　　　Splenic:　　　　　　　　infarction
　　　　　abscess　　　　　　　rupture, nontraumatic
　　　　　atrophy　　　　　　Splenitis
　　　　　cyst　　　　　　　　Wandering spleen

　　　　Excludes: *bilharzial splenic fibrosis (120.0-120.9)*
　　　　　　　　hepatolienal fibrosis (571.5)
　　　　　　　　splenomegaly NOS (789.2)

289.6　Familial polycythemia
　　Familial benign polycythemia
　　Familial erythrocytosis

289.7　Methemoglobinemia
　　Congenital NADH [DPNH]-methemoglobin-reductase deficiency
　　Hemoglobin M [Hb-M] disease
　　Methemoglobinemia:
　　　NOS
　　　acquired (with sulfhemoglobinemia)
　　　hereditary
　　　toxic
　　Stokvis' disease
　　Sulfhemoglobinemia

Use additional E code, if desired, to identify cause

⑤ **289.8　Other specified diseases of blood and blood-forming organs**

　　289.81　Primary hypercoagulable state
　　　　Activated protein C resistance
　　　　Antithrombin III deficiency
　　　　Factor V Leiden mutation
　　　　Lupus anticoagulant
　　　　Protein C deficiency
　　　　Protein S deficiency
　　　　Prothrombin gene mutation

　　289.82　Secondary hypercoagulable state

　　289.83　Myelofibrosis
　　　　Myelofibrosis NOS
　　　　Secondary myelofibrosis

　　Code first the underlying disorder, such as:
　　　malignant neoplasm of breast (174.0-174.9, 175.0-175.9)

　　　Excludes: *idiopathic myelofibrosis (238.76)*
　　　　　　　　leukoerythroblastic anemia (284.2)
　　　　　　　　myelofibrosis with myeloid metaplasia (238.76)
　　　　　　　　myelophthisic anemia (284.2)
　　　　　　　　myelophthisis (284.2)
　　　　　　　　primary myelofibrosis (238.76)

　　289.89　Other specified diseases of blood and blood-forming organs
　　　　Hypergammaglobulinemia
　　　　Pseudocholinesterase deficiency

289.9　Unspecified diseases of blood and blood-forming organs
　　Blood dyscrasia NOS
　　Erythroid hyperplasia

MENTAL DISORDERS

5. MENTAL DISORDERS (290-319)

PSYCHOSES (290-299)

> *Excludes:* mental retardation (317-319)

ORGANIC PSYCHOTIC CONDITIONS (290-294)

Includes: psychotic organic brain syndrome

> *Excludes:* nonpsychotic syndromes of organic etiology (310.0-310.9)
> psychoses classifiable to 295-298 and without impairment of orientation, comprehension, calculation, learning capacity, and judgement, but associated with physical disease, injury, or condition affecting the brain [e.g., following childbirth] (295.0-298.8)

290 Dementias
Code first the associated neurological condition

> *Excludes:* dementia due to alcohol (291.0-291.2)
> dementia due to drugs (292.82)
> dementia not classified as senile, presenile, or arteriosclerotic (294.10-294.11)
> psychoses classifiable to 295-298 occurring in the senium without dementia or delirium (295.0-298.8)
> senility with mental changes of nonpsychotic severity (310.1)
> transient organic psychotic conditions (293.0-293.9)

290.0 Senile dementia, uncomplicated
Senile dementia:
  NOS
  simple type

> *Excludes:* mild memory disturbances, not amounting to dementia, associated with senile brain disease (310.1)
> senile dementia with:
>   delirium or confusion (290.3)
>   delusional [paranoid] features (290.20)
>   depressive features (290.21)

⑤ 290.1 Presenile dementia
Brain syndrome with presenile brain disease

> *Excludes:* arteriosclerotic dementia (290.40-290.43)
> dementia associated with other cerebral conditions (294.10-294.11)

290.10 Presenile dementia, uncomplicated
Presenile dementia:
  NOS
  simple type

290.11 Presenile dementia with delirium
Presenile dementia with acute confusional state

290.12 Presenile dementia with delusional features
Presenile dementia, paranoid type

290.13 Presenile dementia with depressive features
Presenile dementia, depressed type

⑤ 290.2 Senile dementia with delusional or depressive features

> *Excludes:* senile dementia:
>   NOS (290.0)
>   with delirium and/or confusion (290.3)

290.20 Senile dementia with delusional features
Senile dementia, paranoid type
Senile psychosis NOS

290.21 Senile dementia with depressive features

290.3 Senile dementia with delirium
Senile dementia with acute confusional state

> *Excludes:* senile:
>   dementia NOS (290.0)
>   psychosis NOS (290.20)

⑤ 290.4 Vascular dementia
Multi-infarct dementia or psychosis
Use additional code to identify cerebral atherosclerosis (437.0)

> *Excludes:* suspected cases with no clear evidence of arteriosclerosis (290.9)

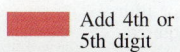 Add 4th or 5th digit
 Nonspecific code
 Unspecified code
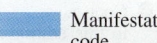 Manifestation code

253

TABULAR LIST

290.40 Vascular dementia, uncomplicated
Arteriosclerotic dementia:
NOS
simple type

290.41 Vascular dementia with delirium
Arteriosclerotic dementia with acute confusional state

290.42 Vascular dementia with delusions
Arteriosclerotic dementia, paranoid type

290.43 Vascular dementia with depressed mood
Arteriosclerotic dementia, depressed type

290.8 Other specified senile psychotic conditions
Presbyophrenic psychosis

290.9 Unspecified senile psychotic condition

291 Alcohol-induced mental disorders

Excludes: alcoholism without psychosis (303.0-303.9)

291.0 Alcohol withdrawal delirium
Alcoholic delirium
Delirium tremens

Excludes: alcohol withdrawal (291.81)

291.1 Alcohol-induced persisting amnestic disorder
Alcoholic polyneuritic psychosis
Korsakoff's psychosis, alcoholic
Wernicke-Korsakoff syndrome (alcoholic)

291.2 Alcohol-induced persisting dementia
Alcoholic dementia NOS
Alcoholism associated with dementia NOS
Chronic alcoholic brain syndrome

291.3 Alcohol-induced psychotic disorder with hallucinations
Alcoholic:
hallucinosis (acute)
psychosis with hallucinosis

Excludes: alcohol withdrawal with delirium (291.0)
schizophrenia (295.0-295.9) and paranoid states (297.0-297.9) taking the form of chronic hallucinosis with clear consciousness in an alcoholic

291.4 Idiosyncratic alcohol intoxication
Pathologic:
alcohol intoxication
drunkenness

Excludes: acute alcohol intoxication (305.0)
in alcoholism (303.0)
simple drunkenness (305.0)

291.5 Alcohol-induced psychotic disorder with delusions
Alcoholic:
paranoia
psychosis, paranoid type

Excludes: nonalcoholic paranoid states (297.0-297.9)
schizophrenia, paranoid type (295.3)

291.8 Other specified alcohol induced mental disorders

291.81 Alcohol withdrawal
Alcohol:
withdrawal syndrome or symptoms
abstinence syndrome or symptoms

Excludes: alcohol withdrawal:
delirium (291.0)
hallucinosis (291.3)
delirium tremens (291.0)

291.82 Alcohol induced sleep disorders
Alcohol induced circadian rhythm sleep disorders
Alcohol induced hypersomnia
Alcohol induced insomnia
Alcohol induced parasomnia

MENTAL DISORDERS

291.89 **Other**
Alcohol induced anxiety disorder
Alcohol induced mood disorder
Alcohol induced sexual dysfunction

291.9 **Unspecified alcohol-induced mental disorders**
Alcohol-related disorder NOS
Alcoholic:
  mania NOS
  psychosis NOS
Alcoholism (chronic) with psychosis

292 Drug induced mental disorders
Includes: organic brain syndrome associated with consumption of drugs
Use additional code for any associated drug dependence (304.0-304.9)
Use additional E code, if desired, to identify drug

292.0 Drug withdrawal
Drug:
  abstinence syndrome or symptoms
  withdrawal syndrome or symptoms

⑤ **292.1 Drug-induced psychotic disorders**

292.11 Drug-induced psychotic disorder with delusions
Paranoid state induced by drugs

292.12 Drug-induced psychotic disorder with hallucinations
Hallucinatory state induced by drugs

Excludes: states following LSD or other hallucinogens, lasting only a few days or less ["bad trips"] (305.3)

292.2 Pathological drug intoxication
Drug reaction:
  NOS resulting in brief psychotic states
  idiosyncratic resulting in brief psychotic states
  pathologic resulting in brief psychotic states

Excludes: expected brief psychotic reactions to hallucinogens ["bad trips"] (305.3)
  physiological side-effects of drugs (e.g., dystonias)

⑤ **292.8 Other specified drug induced mental disorders**

292.81 Drug induced delirium

292.82 Drug induced persisting dementia

292.83 Drug induced persisting amnestic disorder

292.84 Drug induced mood disorder
Depressive state induced by drugs

292.85 Drug induced sleep disorders
Drug induced circadian rhythm sleep disorder
Drug induced hypersomnia
Drug induced insomnia
Drug induced parasomnia

292.89 **Other**
Drug induced anxiety disorder
Drug induced organic personality syndrome
Drug induced sexual dysfunction
Drug intoxication

292.9 **Unspecified drug-induced mental disorder**
Drug-related disorder NOS
Organic psychosis NOS due to or associated with drugs

293 Transient mental disorders due to conditions classified elsewhere
Includes: transient organic mental disorders not associated with alcohol or drugs
Code first the associated physical or neurological condition

Excludes: confusional state or delirium superimposed on senile dementia (290.3)
  dementia due to:
    alcohol (291.0-291.9)
    arteriosclerosis (290.40-290.43)
    drugs (292.82)
    senility (290.0)

TABULAR LIST

293.0 Delirium due to conditions classified elsewhere
Acute:
  confusional state
  infective psychosis
  organic reaction
  posttraumatic organic psychosis
  psycho-organic syndrome
Acute psychosis associated with endocrine, metabolic, or cerebrovascular disorder
Epileptic:
  confusional state
  twilight state

293.1 Subacute delirium
Subacute:
  confusional state
  infective psychosis
  organic reaction
  posttraumatic organic psychosis
  psycho-organic syndrome
  psychosis associated with endocrine or metabolic disorder

⑤ **293.8 Other specified transient mental disorders due to conditions classified elsewhere**

293.81 Psychotic disorder with delusions in conditions classified elsewhere
Transient organic psychotic condition, paranoid type

293.82 Psychotic disorder with hallucinations in conditions classified elsewhere
Transient organic psychotic condition, hallucinatory type

293.83 Mood disorder in conditions classified elsewhere
Transient organic psychotic condition, depressive type

293.84 Anxiety disorder in conditions classified elsewhere

293.89 Other
Catatonic disorder in conditions classified elsewhere

293.9 Unspecified transient mental disorder in conditions classified elsewhere
Organic psychosis:
  infective NOS
  posttraumatic NOS
  transient NOS
Psycho-organic syndrome

294 Persistent mental disorders due to conditions classified elsewhere
Includes: organic psychotic brain syndromes (chronic), not elsewhere classified

294.0 Amnestic disorder in conditions classified elsewhere
Code first underlying condition
Korsakoff's psychosis or syndrome (nonalcoholic)

Excludes: alcoholic:
  amnestic syndrome (291.1)
  Korsakoff's psychosis (291.1)

⑤ **294.1 Dementia in conditions classified elsewhere**
Dementia of the Alzheimer's type
Code first any underlying physical condition, as:
  dementia in:
    Alzheimer's disease (331.0)
    cerebral lipidoses (330.1)
    dementia with Lewy bodies (331.82)
    dementia with Parkinsonism (331.82)
    epilepsy (345.0-345.9)
    frontal dementia (331.19)
    frontotemporal dementia (331.19)
    general paresis [syphilis] (094.1)
    hepatolenticular degeneration (275.1)
    Huntington's chorea (333.4)
    Jakob-Creutzfeldt disease (046.1)
    multiple sclerosis (340)
    Pick's disease of the brain (331.11)
    polyarteritis nodosa (446.0)
    syphilis (094.1)

Excludes: dementia:
  arteriosclerotic (290.40-290.43)
  presenile (290.10-290.13)
  senile (290.0)
  epileptic psychosis NOS (294.8)

MENTAL DISORDERS

294.10 **Dementia in conditions classified elsewhere without behavioral disturbance**
Dementia in conditions classified elsewhere NOS

294.11 **Dementia in conditions classified elsewhere with behavioral disturbance**
Aggressive behavior
Combative behavior
Violent behavior
Wandering off

294.8 **Other persistent mental disorders due to conditions classified elsewhere**
Amnestic disorder NOS
Dementia NOS
Epileptic psychosis NOS
Mixed paranoid and affective organic psychotic states

Use additional code for associated epilepsy (345.0-345.9)

Excludes: mild memory disturbances, not amounting to dementia (310.1)

294.9 **Unspecified persistent mental disorders due to conditions classified elsewhere**
Cognitive disorder NOS
Organic psychosis (chronic)

OTHER PSYCHOSES (295-299)

Use additional code to identify any associated physical disease, injury, or condition affecting the brain with psychoses classifiable to 295-298

295 Schizophrenic disorders
Includes: schizophrenia of the types described in 295.0-295.9 occurring in children

Excludes: childhood type schizophrenia (299.9)
infantile autism (299.0)

The following fifth-digit subclassification is for use with category 295:

0 unspecified
1 subchronic
2 chronic
3 subchronic with acute exacerbation
4 chronic with acute exacerbation
5 in remission

295.0 Simple type
Schizophrenia simplex

Excludes: latent schizophrenia (295.5)

295.1 Disorganized type
Hebephrenia
Hebephrenic type schizophrenia

295.2 Catatonic type
Catatonic (schizophrenia):
   agitation
   excitation
   excited type
   stupor
   withdrawn type

Schizophrenic:
   catalepsy
   catatonia
   flexibilitas cerea

295.3 Paranoid type
Paraphrenic schizophrenia

Excludes: involutional paranoid state (297.2)
paranoia (297.1)
paraphrenia (297.2)

295.4 Schizophreniform disorder
Oneirophrenia
Schizophreniform:
   attack
   psychosis, confusional type

Excludes: acute forms of schizophrenia of:
catatonic type (295.2)
hebephrenic type (295.1)
paranoid type (295.3)
simple type (295.0)
undifferentiated type (295.8)

257

TABULAR LIST

⑤ **295.5 Latent schizophrenia**
Latent schizophrenic reaction
Schizophrenia:
  borderline
  incipient
Schizophrenia:
  prepsychotic
  prodromal
  pseudoneurotic
  pseudopsychopathic

Excludes: schizoid personality (301.20-301.22)

⑤ **295.6 Residual type**
Chronic undifferentiated schizophrenia
Restzustand (schizophrenic)
Schizophrenic residual state

⑤ **295.7 Schizoaffective disorder**
Cyclic schizophrenia
Mixed schizophrenic and affective psychosis
Schizoaffective psychosis
Schizophreniform psychosis, affective type

⑤ **295.8 Other specified types of schizophrenia**
Acute (undifferentiated) schizophrenia
Atypical schizophrenia
Cenesthopathic schizophrenia

Excludes: infantile autism (299.0)

⑤ **295.9 Unspecified schizophrenia**
Schizophrenia:
  NOS
  mixed NOS
  undifferentiated NOS
  undifferentiated type
Schizophrenic reaction NOS
Schizophreniform psychosis NOS

296 Episodic mood disorders
Includes: episodic affective disorders

Excludes: neurotic depression (300.4)
         reactive depressive psychosis (298.0)
         reactive excitation (298.1)

The following fifth-digit subclassification is for use with categories 296.0-296.6:

0 unspecified
1 mild
2 moderate
3 severe, without mention of psychotic behavior
4 severe, specified as with psychotic behavior
5 in partial or unspecified remission
6 in full remission

⑤ **296.0 Bipolar I disorder, single manic episode**
Hypomania (mild) NOS, single episode or unspecified
Hypomanic psychosis, single episode or unspecified
Mania (monopolar) NOS, single episode or unspecified
Manic-depressive psychosis or reaction:
  hypomanic, single episode or unspecified
  manic, single episode or unspecified

Excludes: circular type, if there was a previous attack of depression (296.4)

⑤ **296.1 Manic disorder, recurrent episode**
Any condition classifiable to 296.0, stated to be recurrent

Excludes: circular type, if there was a previous attack of depression (296.4)

MENTAL DISORDERS

⑤ **296.2 Major depressive disorder, single episode**
Depressive psychosis, single episode or unspecified
Endogenous depression, single episode or unspecified
Involutional melancholia, single episode or unspecified
Manic-depressive psychosis or reaction, depressed type, single episode or unspecified
Monopolar depression, single episode or unspecified
Psychotic depression, single episode or unspecified

Excludes: circular type, if previous attack was of manic type (296.5)
depression NOS (311)
reactive depression (neurotic) (300.4)
psychotic (298.0)

⑤ **296.3 Major depressive disorder, recurrent episode**
Any condition classifiable to 296.2, stated to be recurrent

Excludes: circular type, if previous attack was of manic type (296.5)
depression NOS (311)
reactive depression (neurotic) (300.4)
psychotic (298.0)

⑤ **296.4 Bipolar I disorder, most recent episode (or current) manic**
Bipolar disorder, now manic
Manic-depressive psychosis, circular type but currently manic

Excludes: brief compensatory or rebound mood swings (296.99)

⑤ **296.5 Bipolar I disorder, most recent episode (or current) depressed**
Bipolar disorder, now depressed
Manic-depressive psychosis, circular type but currently depressed

Excludes: brief compensatory or rebound mood swings (296.99)

⑤ **296.6 Bipolar I disorder, most recent episode (or current) mixed**
Manic-depressive psychosis, circular type, mixed

296.7 Bipolar I disorder, most recent episode (or current) unspecified
Atypical bipolar affective disorder NOS
Manic-depressive psychosis, circular type, current condition not specified as either manic or depressive

⑤ **296.8 Other and unspecified bipolar disorders**

296.80 Bipolar disorder, unspecified
Bipolar disorder NOS
Manic-depressive:
reaction NOS
syndrome NOS

296.81 Atypical manic disorder

296.82 Atypical depressive disorder

296.89 Other
Bipolar II disorder
Manic-depressive psychosis, mixed type

⑤ **296.9 Other and unspecified episodic mood disorder**

Excludes: psychogenic affective psychoses (298.0-298.8)

296.90 Unspecified episodic mood disorder
Affective psychosis NOS
Melancholia NOS
Mood disorder NOS

296.99 Other specified episodic mood disorder
Mood swings:
brief compensatory
rebound

297 Delusional disorders
Includes: paranoid disorders

Excludes: acute paranoid reaction (298.3)
alcoholic jealousy or paranoid state (291.5)
paranoid schizophrenia (295.3)

297.0 Paranoid state, simple

 Add 4th or 5th digit
 Nonspecific code
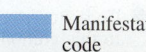 Unspecified code
Manifestation code

TABULAR LIST

297.1 Delusional disorder
Chronic paranoid psychosis
Sander's disease
Systematized delusions

Excludes: paranoid personality disorder (301.0)

297.2 Paraphrenia
Involutional paranoid state
Late paraphrenia
Paraphrenia (involutional)

297.3 Shared psychotic disorder
Folie à deux
Induced psychosis or paranoid disorder

297.8 Other specified paranoid states
Paranoia querulans
Sensitiver Beziehungswahn

Excludes: acute paranoid reaction or state (298.3)
senile paranoid state (290.20)

297.9 Unspecified paranoid state
Paranoid:
  disorder NOS
  psychosis
Paranoid:
  reaction NOS
  state NOS

298 Other nonorganic psychoses
Includes: psychotic conditions due to or provoked by:
emotional stress
environmental factors as major part of etiology

298.0 Depressive type psychosis
Psychogenic depressive psychosis
Psychotic reactive depression
Reactive depressive psychosis

Excludes: manic-depressive psychosis, depressed type (296.2-296.3)
neurotic depression (300.4)
reactive depression NOS (300.4)

298.1 Excitative type psychosis
Acute hysterical psychosis   Reactive excitation
Psychogenic excitation

Excludes: manic-depressive psychosis, manic type (296.0-296.1)

298.2 Reactive confusion
Psychogenic confusion
Psychogenic twilight state

Excludes: acute confusional state (293.0)

298.3 Acute paranoid reaction
Acute psychogenic paranoid psychosis
Bouffée délirante

Excludes: paranoid states (297.0-297.9)

298.4 Psychogenic paranoid psychosis
Protracted reactive paranoid psychosis

298.8 Other and unspecified reactive psychosis
Brief psychotic disorder
Brief reactive psychosis NOS
Hysterical psychosis
Psychogenic psychosis NOS
Psychogenic stupor

Excludes: acute hysterical psychosis (298.1)

298.9 Unspecified psychosis
Atypical psychosis
Psychosis NOS
Psychotic disorder NOS

MENTAL DISORDERS

⑤ **299 Pervasive developmental disorders**

Excludes: adult type psychoses occurring in childhood, as:
   affective disorders (296.0-296.9)
   manic-depressive disorders (296.0-296.9)
   schizophrenia (295.0-295.9)

The following fifth-digit subclassification is for use with category 299:
  0 current or active state
  1 residual state

⑤ **299.0 Autistic disorder**
   Childhood autism   Kanner's syndrome
   Infantile psychosis

Excludes: disintegrative psychosis (299.1)
    Heller's syndrome (299.1)
    schizophrenic syndrome of childhood (299.9)

⑤ **299.1 Childhood disintegrative disorder**
   Heller's syndrome

Use additional code to identify any associated neurological disorder

Excludes: infantile autism (299.0)
    schizophrenic syndrome of childhood (299.9)

⑤ **299.8 Other specified pervasive developmental disorders**
   Asperger's disorder
   Atypical childhood psychosis
   Borderline psychosis of childhood

Excludes: simple stereotypies without psychotic disturbance (307.3)

⑤ **299.9 Unspecified pervasive developmental disorder**
   Child psychosis NOS
   Pervasive developmental disorder NOS
   Schizophrenia, childhood type NOS
   Schizophrenic syndrome of childhood NOS

Excludes: schizophrenia of adult type occurring in childhood (295.0-295.9)

NEUROTIC DISORDERS, PERSONALITY DISORDERS, AND OTHER NONPSYCHOTIC MENTAL DISORDERS (300-316)

300 Anxiety, dissociative and somatoform disorders

⑤ **300.0 Anxiety states**

Excludes: anxiety in:
     acute stress reaction (308.0)
     transient adjustment reaction (309.24)
    neurasthenia (300.5)
    psychophysiological disorders (306.0-306.9)
    separation anxiety (309.21)

300.00 Anxiety state, unspecified
   Anxiety:
     neurosis
     reaction
     state (neurotic)
   Atypical anxiety disorder

300.01 Panic disorder without agoraphobia
   Panic:
     attack
     state

Excludes: panic disorder with agoraphobia (300.21)

300.02 Generalized anxiety disorder

300.09 Other

⑤ **300.1 Dissociative, conversion and factitious disorders**

Excludes: adjustment reaction (309.0-309.9)
    anorexia nervosa (307.1)
    gross stress reaction (308.0-308.9)
    hysterical personality (301.50-301.59)
    psychophysiologic disorders (306.0-306.9)

300.10 Hysteria, unspecified

 Add 4th or 5th digit
 Nonspecific code
 Unspecified code
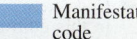 Manifestation code

TABULAR LIST

300.11 Conversion disorder
Astasia-abasia, hysterical
Conversion hysteria or reaction
Hysterical:
  blindness
  deafness
  paralysis

300.12 Dissociative amnesia
Hysterical amnesia

300.13 Dissociative fugue
Hysterical fugue

300.14 Dissociative identity disorder

300.15 Dissociative disorder or reaction, unspecified

300.16 Factitious disorder with predominantly psychological signs and symptoms
Compensation neurosis
Ganser's syndrome, hysterical

300.19 Other and unspecified factitious illness
Factitious disorder (with combined psychological and physical signs and symptoms) (with predominantly physical signs and symptoms) NOS

Excludes: multiple operations or hospital addiction syndrome (301.51)

⑤ **300.2 Phobic disorders**

Excludes: anxiety state not associated with a specific situation or object (300.0-300.09)
obsessional phobias (300.3)

300.20 Phobia, unspecified
Anxiety-hysteria NOS
Phobia NOS

300.21 Agoraphobia with panic disorder
Fear of:
  open spaces with panic attacks
  streets with panic attacks
  travel with panic attacks
Panic disorder with agoraphobia

Excludes: agoraphobia without panic disorder (300.22)
panic disorder without agoraphobia (300.01)

300.22 Agoraphobia without mention of panic attacks
Any condition classifiable to 300.21 without mention of panic attacks

300.23 Social phobia
Fear of:
  eating in public
  public speaking
  washing in public

300.29 Other isolated or specific phobias
Acrophobia   Claustrophobia
Animal phobias   Fear of crowds

300.3 Obsessive-compulsive disorders
Anancastic neurosis   Obsessional phobia [any]
Compulsive neurosis

Excludes: obsessive-compulsive symptoms occurring in:
  endogenous depression (296.2-296.3)
  organic states (e.g., encephalitis)
  schizophrenia (295.0-295.9)

300.4 Dysthymic disorder
Anxiety depression   Neurotic depressive state
Depression with anxiety   Reactive depression
Depressive reaction

Excludes: adjustment reaction with depressive symptoms (309.0-309.1)
depression NOS (311)
manic-depressive psychosis, depressed type (296.2-296.3)
reactive depressive psychosis (298.0)

MENTAL DISORDERS

300.5 Neurasthenia
Fatigue neurosis
Nervous debility
Psychogenic:
  asthenia
  general fatigue
Use additional code to identify any associated physical disorder

Excludes: anxiety state (300.00-300.09)
  neurotic depression (300.4)
  psychophysiological disorders (306.0-306.9)
  specific nonpsychotic mental disorders following organic brain damage (310.0-310.9)

300.6 Depersonalization disorder
Derealization (neurotic)
Neurotic state with depersonalization episode

Excludes: depersonalization associated with:
  anxiety (300.00-300.09)
  depression (300.4)
  manic-depressive disorder or psychosis (296.0-296.9)
  schizophrenia (295.0-295.9)

300.7 Hypochondriasis
Body dysmorphic disorder

Excludes: hypochondriasis in:
  hysteria (300.10-300.19)
  manic-depressive psychosis, depressed type (296.2-296.3)
  neurasthenia (300.5)
  obsessional disorder (300.3)
  schizophrenia (295.0-295.9)

⑤ **300.8 Somatoform disorders**

300.81 Somatization disorder
Briquet's disorder
Severe somatoform disorder

300.82 Undifferentiated somatoform disorder
Atypical somatoform disorder
Somatoform disorder NOS

300.89 Other somatoform disorders
Occupational neurosis, including writers' cramp
Psychasthenia
Psychasthenic neurosis

300.9 Unspecified nonpsychotic mental disorder
Psychoneurosis NOS

301 Personality disorders
Includes: character neurosis
Use additional code to identify any associated neurosis or psychosis, or physical condition

Excludes: nonpsychotic personality disorder associated with organic brain syndromes (310.0-310.9)

301.0 Paranoid personality disorder
Fanatic personality
Paranoid personality (disorder)
Paranoid traits

Excludes: acute paranoid reaction (298.3)
  alcoholic paranoia (291.5)
  paranoid schizophrenia (295.3)
  paranoid states (297.0-297.9)

⑤ **301.1 Affective personality disorder**

Excludes: affective psychotic disorders (296.0-296.9)
  neurasthenia (300.5)
  neurotic depression (300.4)

301.10 Affective personality disorder, unspecified

301.11 Chronic hypomanic personality disorder
Chronic hypomanic disorder
Hypomanic personality

 Add 4th or 5th digit
 Nonspecific code
 Unspecified code
 Manifestation code

TABULAR LIST

301.12 Chronic depressive personality disorder
Chronic depressive disorder
Depressive character or personality

301.13 Cyclothymic disorder
Cycloid personality
Cyclothymia
Cyclothymic personality

⑤ **301.2 Schizoid personality disorder**

Excludes: schizophrenia (295.0-295.9)

301.20 Schizoid personality disorder, unspecified

301.21 Introverted personality

301.22 Schizotypal personality disorder

301.3 Explosive personality disorder
Aggressive:
  personality
  reaction
Aggressiveness
Emotional instability (excessive)
Pathological emotionality
Quarrelsomeness

Excludes: dyssocial personality (301.7)
hysterical neurosis (300.10-300.19)

301.4 Obsessive-compulsive personality disorder
Anancastic personality
Obsessional personality

Excludes: obsessive-compulsive disorder (300.3)
phobic state (300.20-300.29)

⑤ **301.5 Histrionic personality disorder**

Excludes: hysterical neurosis (300.10-300.19)

301.50 Histrionic personality disorder, unspecified
Hysterical personality NOS

301.51 Chronic factitious illness with physical symptoms
Hospital addiction syndrome
Multiple operations syndrome
Munchausen syndrome

301.59 Other histrionic personality disorder
Personality:
  emotionally unstable
  labile
  psychoinfantile

301.6 Dependent personality disorder
Asthenic personality
Inadequate personality
Passive personality

Excludes: neurasthenia (300.5)
passive-aggressive personality (301.84)

301.7 Antisocial personality disorder
Amoral personality
Asocial personality
Dyssocial personality
Personality disorder with predominantly sociopathic or asocial manifestation

Excludes: disturbance of conduct without specifiable personality disorder (312.0-312.9)
explosive personality (301.3)

⑤ **301.8 Other personality disorders**

301.81 Narcissistic personality disorder

301.82 Avoidant personality disorder

301.83 Borderline personality disorder

301.84 Passive-aggressive personality

301.89 Other
Personality:
  eccentric
  "haltlose" type
  immature
Personality:
  masochistic
  psychoneurotic

Excludes: psychoinfantile personality (301.59)

MENTAL DISORDERS

301.9 Unspecified personality disorder
Pathological personality NOS
Personality disorder NOS
Psychopathic:
constitutional state
personality (disorder)

302 Sexual and gender identity disorders

Excludes: sexual disorder manifest in:
organic brain syndrome (290.0-294.9, 310.0-310.9)
psychosis (295.0-298.9)

302.0 Ego-dystonic sexual orientation
Ego-dystonic lesbianism
Sexual orientation conflict disorder

Excludes: homosexual pedophilia (302.2)

302.1 Zoophilia
Bestiality

302.2 Pedophilia

302.3 Transvestic fetishism

Excludes: trans-sexualism (302.5)

302.4 Exhibitionism

302.5 Trans-sexualism
Sex reassignment surgery status

Excludes: transvestism (302.3)

302.50 With unspecified sexual history

302.51 With asexual history

302.52 With homosexual history

302.53 With heterosexual history

302.6 Gender identity disorder in children
Feminism in boys
Gender identity disorder NOS

Excludes: gender identity disorder in adult (302.85)
trans-sexualism (302.50-302.53)
transvestism (302.3)

302.7 Psychosexual dysfunction

Excludes: impotence of organic origin (607.84)
normal transient symptoms from ruptured hymen
transient or occasional failures of erection due to fatigue, anxiety, alcohol, or drugs

302.70 Psychosexual dysfunction, unspecified
Sexual dysfunction NOS

302.71 Hypoactive sexual desire disorder

Excludes: decreased sexual desire NOS (799.81)

302.72 With inhibited sexual excitement
Female sexual arousal disorder
Frigidity
Impotence
Male erectile disorder

302.73 Female orgasmic disorder

302.74 Male orgasmic disorder

302.75 Premature ejaculation

302.76 Dyspareunia, psychogenic

302.79 With other specified psychosexual dysfunctions
Sexual aversion disorder

302.8 Other specified psychosexual disorders

302.81 Fetishism

302.82 Voyeurism

302.83 Sexual masochism

302.84 Sexual sadism

265

TABULAR LIST

302.85 Gender identity disorder in adolescents or adults
Use additional code to identify sex reassignment surgery status (302.5)

Excludes: gender identity disorder NOS (302.6)
gender identity disorder in children (302.6)

302.89 Other
Frotteurism
Nymphomania
Satyriasis

302.9 Unspecified psychosexual disorder
Paraphilia NOS
Pathologic sexuality NOS
Sexual deviation NOS
Sexual disorder NOS

⑤ **303 Alcohol dependence syndrome**
Use additional code to identify any associated condition, as:
  alcoholic psychoses (291.0-291.9)
  drug dependence (304.0-304.9)
  physical complications of alcohol, such as:
    cerebral degeneration (331.7)
    cirrhosis of liver (571.2)
    epilepsy (345.0-345.9)
    gastritis (535.3)
    hepatitis (571.1)
    liver damage NOS (571.3)

Excludes: drunkenness NOS (305.0)

The following fifth-digit subclassification is for use with category 303:

 0 unspecified
 1 continuous
 2 episodic
 3 in remission

⑤ **303.0 Acute alcoholic intoxication**
Acute drunkenness in alcoholism

⑤ **303.9 Other and unspecified alcohol dependence**
Chronic alcoholism
Dipsomania

⑤ **304 Drug dependence**

Excludes: nondependent abuse of drugs (305.1-305.9)

The following fifth-digit subclassification is for use with category 304:

 0 unspecified
 1 continuous
 2 episodic
 3 in remission

⑤ **304.0 Opioid type dependence**
Heroin   Opium alkaloids and their derivatives
Meperidine   Synthetics with morphine-like effects
Methadone
Morphine
Opium

⑤ **304.1 Sedative, hypnotic or anxiolytic dependence**
Barbiturates
Nonbarbiturate sedatives and tranquilizers with a similar effect:
  chlordiazepoxide
  diazepam
  glutethimide
  meprobamate
  methaqualone

⑤ **304.2 Cocaine dependence**
Coca leaves and derivatives

MENTAL DISORDERS

- ⑤ 304.3 **Cannabis dependence**
    Hashish
    Hemp
    Marihuana
- ⑤ 304.4 **Amphetamine and other psychostimulant dependence**
    Methylphenidate
    Phenmetrazine
- ⑤ 304.5 **Hallucinogen dependence**
    Dimethyltryptamine [DMT]
    Lysergic acid diethylamide [LSD] and derivatives
    Mescaline
    Psilocybin
- ⑤ 304.6 **Other specified drug dependence**
    Absinthe addiction
    Glue sniffing
    Inhalant dependence
    Phencyclidine dependence
    Excludes: tobacco dependence (305.1)
- ⑤ 304.7 **Combinations of opioid type drug with any other**
- ⑤ 304.8 **Combinations of drug dependence excluding opioid type drug**
- ⑤ 304.9 **Unspecified drug dependence**
    Drug addiction NOS
    Drug dependence NOS

305 Nondependent abuse of drugs
Note: Includes cases where a person, for whom no other diagnosis is possible, has come under medical care because of the maladaptive effect of a drug on which he is not dependent and that he has taken on his own initiative to the detriment of his health or social functioning.

Excludes: alcohol dependence syndrome (303.0-303.9)
    drug dependence (304.0-304.9)
    drug withdrawal syndrome (292.0)
    poisoning by drugs or medicinal substances (960.0-979.9)

The following fifth-digit subclassification is for use with codes 305.0, 305.2-305.9:

- **0** unspecified
- **1** continuous
- **2** episodic
- **3** in remission

- ⑤ 305.0 **Alcohol abuse**
    Drunkenness NOS   "Hangover" (alcohol)
    Excessive drinking of alcohol NOS   Inebriety NOS
    Excludes: acute alcohol intoxication in alcoholism (303.0)
        alcoholic psychoses (291.0-291.9)
- 305.1 **Tobacco use disorder**
    Tobacco dependence
    Excludes: history of tobacco use (V15.82)
        smoking complicating pregnancy (649.0)
        tobacco use disorder complicating pregnancy (649.0)
- ⑤ 305.2 **Cannabis abuse**
- ⑤ 305.3 **Hallucinogen abuse**
    Acute intoxication from hallucinogens ["bad trips"]
    LSD reaction
- ⑤ 305.4 **Sedative, hypnotic or anxiolytic abuse**
- ⑤ 305.5 **Opioid abuse**
- ⑤ 305.6 **Cocaine abuse**
- ⑤ 305.7 **Amphetamine or related acting sympathomimetic abuse**
- ⑤ 305.8 **Antidepressant type abuse**

Add 4th or 5th digit	Nonspecific code	Unspecified code	Manifestation code

TABULAR LIST

⑤ **305.9** **Other, mixed, or unspecified drug abuse**
  Caffeine intoxication
  Inhalant abuse
  "Laxative habit"
  Misuse of drugs NOS
  Nonprescribed use of drugs or patent medicinals
  Phencyclidine abuse

306 **Physiological malfunction arising from mental factors**
  Includes: psychogenic:
    physical symptoms not involving tissue damage
    physiological manifestation not involving tissue damage

  Excludes: hysteria (300.11-300.19)
    physical symptoms secondary to a psychiatric disorder classified elsewhere
    psychic factors associated with physical conditions involving tissue damage classified elsewhere (316)
    specific nonpsychotic mental disorders following organic brain damage (310.0-310.9)

  306.0 **Musculoskeletal**
    Psychogenic paralysis
    Psychogenic torticollis

    Excludes: Gilles de la Tourette's syndrome (307.23)
      paralysis as hysterical or conversion reaction (300.11)
      tics (307.20-307.22)

  306.1 **Respiratory**
    Psychogenic: Psychogenic:
      air hunger   hyperventilation
      cough   yawning
      hiccough

    Excludes: psychogenic asthma (316 and 493.9)

  306.2 **Cardiovascular**
    Cardiac neurosis
    Cardiovascular neurosis
    Neurocirculatory asthenia
    Psychogenic cardiovascular disorder

    Excludes: psychogenic paroxysmal tachycardia (316 and 427.2)

  306.3 **Skin**
    Psychogenic pruritus

    Excludes: psychogenic:
      alopecia (316 and 704.00)
      dermatitis (316 and 692.9)
      eczema (316 and 691.8 or 692.9)
      urticaria (316 and 708.0-708.9)

  306.4 **Gastrointestinal**
    Aerophagy   Diarrhea, psychogenic
    Cyclical vomiting,   Nervous gastritis
      psychogenic   Psychogenic dyspepsia

    Excludes: cyclical vomiting NOS (536.2)
      globus hystericus (300.11)
      mucous colitis (316 and 564.9)
      psychogenic:
        cardiospasm (316 and 530.0)
        duodenal ulcer (316 and 532.0-532.9)
        gastric ulcer (316 and 531.0-531.9)
        peptic ulcer NOS (316 and 533.0-533.9)
        vomiting NOS (307.54)

  ⑤ **306.5** **Genitourinary**
    Excludes: enuresis, psychogenic (307.6)
      frigidity (302.72)
      impotence (302.72)
      psychogenic dyspareunia (302.76)

    306.50 **Psychogenic genitourinary malfunction, unspecified**

    306.51 **Psychogenic vaginismus**
      Functional vaginismus

    306.52 **Psychogenic dysmenorrhea**

MENTAL DISORDERS

- 306.53 Psychogenic dysuria
- **306.59** Other
- **306.6 Endocrine**
- **306.7 Organs of special sense**
  - *Excludes:* hysterical blindness or deafness (300.11)
  - psychophysical visual disturbances (368.16)
- **306.8 Other specified psychophysiological malfunction**
  - Bruxism
  - Teeth grinding
- **306.9 Unspecified psychophysiological malfunction**
  - Psychophysiologic disorder NOS
  - Psychosomatic disorder NOS

307 Special symptoms or syndromes, not elsewhere classified
Note: This category is intended for use if the psychopathology is manifested by a single specific symptom or group of symptoms which is not part of an organic illness or other mental disorder classifiable elsewhere.
Excludes: those due to mental disorders classified elsewhere
those of organic origin

- **307.0 Stuttering**
  - *Excludes:* dysphasia (784.5)
  - lisping or lalling (307.9)
  - retarded development of speech (315.31-315.39)

- **307.1 Anorexia nervosa**
  - *Excludes:* eating disturbance NOS (307.50)
  - feeding problem (783.3)
  - of nonorganic origin (307.59)
  - loss of appetite (783.0)
  - of nonorganic origin (307.59)

- ⑤ **307.2 Tics**
  - *Excludes:* nail-biting or thumb-sucking (307.9)
  - stereotypies occurring in isolation (307.3)
  - tics of organic origin (333.3)

  - **307.20 Tic disorder, unspecified**
    - Tic disorder NOS
  - **307.21 Transient tic disorder**
  - **307.22 Chronic motor or vocal tic disorder**
  - **307.23 Tourette's disorder**
    - Motor-verbal tic disorder

- **307.3 Stereotypic movement disorder**
  - Body-rocking
  - Head banging
  - Spasmus nutans
  - Stereotypies NOS
  - *Excludes:* tics (307.20-307.23)
  - of organic origin (333.3)

- ⑤ **307.4 Specific disorders of sleep of nonorganic origin**
  - *Excludes:* narcolepsy (347.00-347.11)
  - organic hypersomnia (327.10-327.19)
  - organic insomnia (327.00-327.09)
  - those of unspecified cause (780.50-780.59)

  - **307.40 Nonorganic sleep disorder, unspecified**
  - **307.41 Transient disorder of initiating or maintaining sleep**
    - Adjustment insomnia
    - Hyposomnia associated with acute or intermittent emotional reactions or conflicts
    - Insomnia associated with acute or intermittent emotional reactions or conflicts
    - Sleeplessness associated with acute or intermittent emotional reactions or conflicts

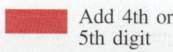 Add 4th or 5th digit
 Nonspecific code
 Unspecified code
 Manifestation code

269

TABULAR LIST

307.42 Persistent disorder of initiating or maintaining sleep
Hyposomnia, insomnia, or sleeplessness associated with:
  anxiety
  conditioned arousal
  depression (major) (minor)
  psychosis
Idiopathic insomnia
Paradoxical insomnia
Primary insomnia
Psychophysiological insomnia

307.43 Transient disorder of initiating or maintaining wakefulness
Hypersomnia associated with acute or intermittent emotional reactions or conflicts

307.44 Persistent disorder of initiating or maintaining wakefulness
Hypersomnia associated with depression (major) (minor)
Insufficient sleep syndrome
Primary hypersomnia

Excludes: sleep deprivation (V69.4)

307.45 Circadian rhythm sleep disorder of nonorganic origin

307.46 Sleep arousal disorder
Night terror disorder
Night terrors
Sleep terror disorder
Sleepwalking
Somnambulism

307.47 Other dysfunctions of sleep stages or arousal from sleep
Dyssomnia NOS
Nightmare disorder
Nightmares:
  NOS
  REM-sleep type
Parasomnia NOS
Sleep drunkenness

307.48 Repetitive intrusions of sleep
Repetitive intrusion of sleep with:
  atypical polysomnographic features
  environmental disturbances
  repeated REM-sleep interruptions

307.49 Other
"Short-sleeper"
Subjective insomnia complaint

307.5 Other and unspecified disorders of eating

Excludes: anorexia:
  nervosa (307.1)
  of unspecified cause (783.0)
overeating, of unspecified cause (783.6)
vomiting:
  NOS (787.0)
  cyclical (536.2)
  psychogenic (306.4)

307.50 Eating disorder, unspecified
Eating disorder NOS

307.51 Bulimia nervosa
Overeating of nonorganic origin

307.52 Pica
Perverted appetite of nonorganic origin

307.53 Rumination disorder
Regurgitation, of nonorganic origin, of food with reswallowing

Excludes: obsessional rumination (300.3)

307.54 Psychogenic vomiting

307.59 Other
Feeding disorder of infancy or early childhood of nonorganic origin
Infantile feeding disturbances of nonorganic origin
Loss of appetite of nonorganic origin

MENTAL DISORDERS

307.6 Enuresis
Enuresis (primary) (secondary) of nonorganic origin
Excludes: enuresis of unspecified cause (788.3)

307.7 Encopresis
Encopresis (continuous) (discontinuous) of nonorganic origin
Excludes: encopresis of unspecified cause (787.6)

307.8 Pain disorders related to psychological factors

307.80 Psychogenic pain, site unspecified

307.81 Tension headache
Excludes: headache:
NOS (784.0)
migraine (346.0-346.9)

307.89 Other
Code first to type or site of pain
Excludes: pain disorder exclusively attributed to psychological factors (307.80)
psychogenic pain (307.80)

307.9 Other and unspecified special symptoms or syndromes, not elsewhere classified
Communication disorder NOS
Hair plucking
Lalling
Lisping
Masturbation
Nail-biting
Thumb-sucking

308 Acute reaction to stress
Includes: catastrophic stress
combat fatigue
gross stress reaction (acute)
transient disorders in response to exceptional physical or mental stress which usually subside within hours or days
Excludes: adjustment reaction or disorder (309.0-309.9)
chronic stress reaction (309.1-309.9)

308.0 Predominant disturbance of emotions
Anxiety as acute reaction to exceptional [gross] stress
Emotional crisis as acute reaction to exceptional [gross] stress
Panic state as acute reaction to exceptional [gross] stress

308.1 Predominant disturbance of consciousness
Fugues as acute reaction to exceptional [gross] stress

308.2 Predominant psychomotor disturbance
Agitation states as acute reaction to exceptional [gross] stress
Stupor as acute reaction to exceptional [gross] stress

308.3 Other acute reactions to stress
Acute situational disturbance
Acute stress disorder
Excludes: prolonged posttraumatic emotional disturbance (309.81)

308.4 Mixed disorders as reaction to stress

308.9 Unspecified acute reaction to stress

309 Adjustment reaction
Includes: adjustment disorders
reaction (adjustment) to chronic stress
Excludes: acute reaction to major stress (308.0-308.9)
neurotic disorders (300.0-300.9)

309.0 Adjustment disorder with depressed mood
Grief reaction
Excludes: affective psychoses (296.0-296.9)
neurotic depression (300.4)
prolonged depressive reaction (309.1)
psychogenic depressive psychosis (298.0)

TABULAR LIST

309.1 Prolonged depressive reaction
>Excludes: *affective psychoses (296.0-296.9)*
>   *brief depressive reaction (309.0)*
>   *neurotic depression (300.4)*
>   *psychogenic depressive psychosis (298.0)*

⑤ **309.2 With predominant disturbance of other emotions**

    309.21 Separation anxiety disorder

    309.22 Emancipation disorder of adolescence and early adult life

    309.23 Specific academic or work inhibition

    309.24 Adjustment disorder with anxiety

    309.28 Adjustment disorder with mixed anxiety and depressed mood
        Adjustment reaction with anxiety and depression

    309.29 Other
        Culture shock

309.3 Adjustment disorder with disturbance of conduct
    Conduct disturbance as adjustment reaction
    Destructiveness as adjustment reaction
>Excludes: *destructiveness in child (312.9)*
>   *disturbance of conduct NOS (312.9)*
>   *dyssocial behavior without manifest psychiatric disorder (V71.01-V71.02)*
>   *personality disorder with predominantly sociopathic or asocial manifestations (301.7)*

309.4 Adjustment disorder with mixed disturbance of emotions and conduct

⑤ **309.8 Other specified adjustment reactions**

    309.81 Posttraumatic stress disorder
        Chronic posttraumatic stress disorder
        Concentration camp syndrome
        Posttraumatic stress disorder NOS
        Post-Traumatic Stress Disorder (PTSD)
>Excludes: *acute stress disorder (308.3)*
>   *posttraumatic brain syndrome:*
>   *nonpsychotic (310.2)*
>   *psychotic (293.0-293.9)*

    309.82 Adjustment reaction with physical symptoms

    309.83 Adjustment reaction with withdrawal
        Elective mutism as adjustment reaction
        Hospitalism (in children) NOS

    309.89 Other

309.9 Unspecified adjustment reaction
    Adaptation reaction NOS
    Adjustment reaction NOS

310 Specific nonpsychotic mental disorders due to brain damage
>Excludes: *neuroses, personality disorders, or other nonpsychotic conditions occurring in a form similar to that seen with functional disorders but in association with a physical condition (300.0-300.9, 301.0-301.9)*

310.0 Frontal lobe syndrome
    Lobotomy syndrome
    Postleucotomy syndrome [state]
>Excludes: *postcontusion syndrome (310.2)*

310.1 Personality change due to conditions classified elsewhere
    Cognitive or personality change of other type, of nonpsychotic severity
    Organic psychosyndrome of nonpsychotic severity
    Presbyophrenia NOS
    Senility with mental changes of nonpsychotic severity
>Excludes: *memory loss of unknown cause (780.93)*

MENTAL DISORDERS

310.2 Postconcussion syndrome
Postcontusion syndrome or encephalopathy
Posttraumatic brain syndrome, nonpsychotic
Status postcommotio cerebri

Excludes: *frontal lobe syndrome (310.0)*
postencephalitic syndrome (310.8)
any organic psychotic conditions following head injury (293.0—294.0)

310.8 Other specified nonpsychotic mental disorders following organic brain damage
Mild memory disturbance
Postencephalitic syndrome
Other focal (partial) organic psychosyndromes

310.9 Unspecified nonpsychotic mental disorder following organic brain damage

311 Depressive disorder, not elsewhere classified
Depressive disorder NOS
Depressive state NOS
Depression NOS

Excludes: *acute reaction to major stress with depressive symptoms (308.0)*
affective personality disorder (301.10-301.13)
affective psychoses (296.0-296.9)
brief depressive reaction (309.0)
depressive states associated with stressful events (309.0-309.1)
disturbance of emotions specific to childhood and adolescence, with misery and unhappiness (313.1)
mixed adjustment reaction with depressive symptoms (309.4)
neurotic depression (300.4)
prolonged depressive adjustment reaction (309.1)
psychogenic depressive psychosis (298.0)

312 Disturbance of conduct, not elsewhere classified

Excludes: *adjustment reaction with disturbance of conduct (309.3)*
drug dependence (304.0-304.9)
dyssocial behavior without manifest psychiatric disorder (V71.01-V71.02)
personality disorder with predominantly sociopathic or asocial manifestations (301.7)
sexual deviations (302.0-302.9)

The following fifth-digit subclassification is for use with categories 312.0-312.2:

- **0** unspecified
- **1** mild
- **2** moderate
- **3** severe

312.0 Undersocialized conduct disorder, aggressive type
Aggressive outburst   Unsocialized aggressive disorder
Anger reaction

312.1 Undersocialized conduct disorder, unaggressive type
Childhood truancy,   Solitary stealing
  unsocialized   Tantrums

312.2 Socialized conduct disorder
Childhood truancy, socialized
Group delinquency

Excludes: *gang activity without manifest psychiatric disorder (V71.01)*

312.3 Disorders of impulse control, not elsewhere classified

312.30 Impulse control disorder, unspecified

312.31 Pathological gambling

312.32 Kleptomania

312.33 Pyromania

312.34 Intermittent explosive disorder

312.35 Isolated explosive disorder

312.39 Other
Trichotillomania

312.4 Mixed disturbance of conduct and emotions
Neurotic delinquency

Excludes: *compulsive conduct disorder (312.3)*

 Add 4th or 5th digit
 Nonspecific code
 Unspecified code
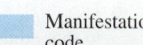 Manifestation code

TABULAR LIST

⑤ **312.8 Other specified disturbances of conduct, not elsewhere classified**

    312.81 Conduct disorder, childhood onset type

    312.82 Conduct disorder, adolescent onset type

    312.89 Other conduct disorder
        Conduct disorder of unspecified onset

312.9 Unspecified disturbance of conduct
    Delinquency (juvenile)
    Disruptive behavior disorder NOS

313 Disturbance of emotions specific to childhood and adolescence

Excludes: adjustment reaction (309.0-309.9)
        emotional disorder of neurotic type (300.0-300.9)
        masturbation, nail-biting, thumb-sucking, and other isolated symptoms (307.0-307.9)

313.0 Overanxious disorder
    Anxiety and fearfulness of childhood and adolescence
    Overanxious disorder of childhood and adolescence

Excludes: abnormal separation anxiety (309.21)
        anxiety states (300.00-300.09)
        hospitalism in children (309.83)
        phobic state (300.20-300.29)

313.1 Misery and unhappiness disorder

Excludes: depressive neurosis (300.4)

⑤ **313.2 Sensitivity, shyness, and social withdrawal disorder**

Excludes: infantile autism (299.0)
        schizoid personality (301.20-301.22)
        schizophrenia (295.0-295.9)

    313.21 Shyness disorder of childhood
        Sensitivity reaction of childhood or adolescence

    313.22 Introverted disorder of childhood
        Social withdrawal of childhood and adolescence
        Withdrawal reaction of childhood and adolescence

    313.23 Selective mutism

Excludes: elective mutism as adjustment reaction (309.83)

313.3 Relationship problems
    Sibling jealousy

Excludes: relationship problems associated with aggression, destruction, or other forms of conduct disturbance (312.0-312.9)

⑤ **313.8 Other or mixed emotional disturbances of childhood or adolescence**

    313.81 Oppositional defiant disorder

    313.82 Identity disorder
        Identity problem

    313.83 Academic underachievement disorder

    313.89 Other
        Reactive attachment disorder of infancy or early childhood

313.9 Unspecified emotional disturbance of childhood or adolescence
    Mental disorder of infancy, childhood or adolescence NOS

314 Hyperkinetic syndrome of childhood

Excludes: hyperkinesis as symptom of underlying disorder—code the underlying disorder

⑤ **314.0 Attention deficit disorder**
    Adult
    Child

    314.00 Without mention of hyperactivity
        Predominantly inattentive type

    314.01 With hyperactivity
        Combined type
        Overactivity NOS
        Predominantly hyperactive/impulsive type
        Simple disturbance of attention with overactivity

316 Psychic factors associated with diseases classified elsewhere
Psychologic factors in physical conditions classified elsewhere

Use additional code to identify the associated physical condition, as:
psychogenic:
asthma (493.9)
dermatitis (692.9)
duodenal ulcer (532.0-532.9)
eczema (691.8, 692.9)
gastric ulcer (531.0-531.9)
mucous colitis (564.9)
paroxysmal tachycardia (427.2)
ulcerative colitis (556)
urticaria (708.0-708.9)
psychosocial dwarfism (259.4)

Excludes: *physical symptoms and physiological malfunctions, not involving tissue damage, of mental origin (306.0-306.9)*

MENTAL RETARDATION (317-319)

Use additional code(s) to identify any associated psychiatric or physical condition(s)

317 Mild mental retardation
High-grade defect   Mild mental subnormality
IQ 50-70

318 Other specified mental retardation

318.0 Moderate mental retardation
IQ 35-49
Moderate mental subnormality

318.1 Severe mental retardation
IQ 20-34
Severe mental subnormality

318.2 Profound mental retardation
IQ under 20
Profound mental subnormality

319 Unspecified mental retardation
Mental deficiency NOS
Mental subnormality NOS

MENTAL DISORDERS

314.1 Hyperkinesis with developmental delay
Developmental disorder of hyperkinesis
Use additional code to identify any associated neurological disorder

314.2 Hyperkinetic conduct disorder
Hyperkinetic conduct disorder without developmental delay

Excludes: hyperkinesis with significant delays in specific skills (314.1)

314.8 Other specified manifestations of hyperkinetic syndrome

314.9 Unspecified hyperkinetic syndrome
Hyperkinetic reaction of childhood or adolescence NOS
Hyperkinetic syndrome NOS

315 Specific delays in development

Excludes: that due to a neurological disorder (320.0-389.9)

⑤ **315.0 Specific reading disorder**

315.00 Reading disorder, unspecified

315.01 Alexia

315.02 Developmental dyslexia

315.09 Other
Specific spelling difficulty

315.1 Mathematics disorder
Dyscalculia

315.2 Other specific learning difficulties
Disorder of written expression

Excludes: specific arithmetical disorder (315.1)
specific reading disorder (315.00-315.09)

⑤ **315.3 Developmental speech or language disorder**

315.31 Expressive language disorder
Developmental aphasia
Word deafness

Excludes: acquired aphasia (784.3)
elective mutism (309.83, 313.0, 313.23)

315.32 Mixed receptive-expressive language disorder
Central auditory processing disorder

Excludes: acquired auditory processing disorder (388.45)

● **315.34 Speech and language developmental delay due to hearing loss**
Use additional code to identify type of hearing loss (389.00-389.9)

315.39 Other
Developmental articulation disorder
Dyslalia
Phonological disorder

Excludes: lisping and lalling (307.9)
stammering and stuttering (307.0)

315.4 Developmental coordination disorder
Clumsiness syndrome
Dyspraxia syndrome
Specific motor development disorder

315.5 Mixed development disorder

315.8 Other specified delays in development

315.9 Unspecified delay in development
Developmental disorder NOS
Learning disorder NOS

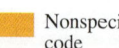 Add 4th or 5th digit
 Nonspecific code
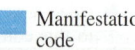 Unspecified code
Manifestation code

275

NERVOUS SYSTEM AND SENSE ORGANS

6. DISEASES OF THE NERVOUS SYSTEM AND SENSE ORGANS (320-389)

INFLAMMATORY DISEASES OF THE CENTRAL NERVOUS SYSTEM (320-326)

320 Bacterial meningitis
Includes: arachnoiditis, bacterial
leptomeningitis, bacterial
meningitis, bacterial
meningoencephalitis, bacterial
meningomyelitis, bacterial
pachymeningitis, bacterial

320.0 Hemophilus meningitis
Meningitis due to Hemophilus influenzae [H. influenzae]

320.1 Pneumococcal meningitis

320.2 Streptococcal meningitis

320.3 Staphylococcal meningitis

320.7 *Meningitis in other bacterial diseases classified elsewhere*
Code first underlying disease, as:
actinomycosis (039.8)
listeriosis (027.0)
typhoid fever (002.0)
whooping cough (033.0-033.9)

Excludes: *meningitis (in):*
epidemic (036.0)
gonococcal (098.82)
meningococcal (036.0)
salmonellosis (003.21)
syphilis:
NOS (094.2)
congenital (090.42)
meningovascular (094.2)
secondary (091.81)
tuberculous (013.0)

⑤ 320.8 Meningitis due to other specified bacteria

320.81 Anaerobic meningitis
Bacteroides (fragilis)
Gram-negative anaerobes

320.82 Meningitis due to Gram-negative bacteria, not elsewhere classified
Aerobacter aerogenes
Escherichia coli [E. coli]
Friedlander bacillus
Klebsiella pneumoniae
Proteus morganii
Pseudomonas

Excludes: *Gram-negative anaerobes (320.81)*

320.89 Meningitis due to other specified bacteria
Bacillus pyocyaneus

320.9 Meningitis due to unspecified bacterium
Meningitis: Meningitis:
  bacterial NOS   pyogenic NOS
  purulent NOS   suppurative NOS

321 Meningitis due to other organisms
Includes: arachnoiditis due to organisms other than bacteria
leptomeningitis due to organisms other than bacteria
meningitis due to organisms other than bacteria
pachymeningitis due to organisms other than bacteria

321.0 *Cryptococcal meningitis*
Code first underlying disease (117.5)

321.1 *Meningitis in other fungal diseases*
Code first underlying disease (110.0-118)

Excludes: *meningitis in:*
candidiasis (112.83)
coccidioidomycosis (114.2)
histoplasmosis (115.01, 115.11, 115.91)

 Add 4th or 5th digit   Nonspecific code   Unspecified code   Manifestation code

277

TABULAR LIST

321.2 Meningitis due to viruses not elsewhere classified
Code first underlying disease, as:
meningitis due to arbovirus (060.0-066.9)

Excludes: meningitis (due to):
abacterial (047.0-047.9)
adenovirus (049.1)
aseptic NOS (047.9)
Coxsackie (virus) (047.0)
ECHO virus (047.1)
enterovirus (047.0-047.9)
herpes simplex virus (054.72)
herpes zoster virus (053.0)
lymphocytic choriomeningitis virus (049.0)
mumps (072.1)
viral NOS (047.9)
meningo-eruptive syndrome (047.1)

321.3 Meningitis due to trypanosomiasis
Code first underlying disease (086.0-086.9)

321.4 Meningitis in sarcoidosis
Code first underlying disease (135)

321.8 Meningitis due to other nonbacterial organisms classified elsewhere
Code first underlying disease

Excludes: leptospiral meningitis (100.81)

322 Meningitis of unspecified cause
Includes: arachnoiditis with no organism specified as cause
leptomeningitis with no organism specified as cause
meningitis with no organism specified as cause
pachymeningitis with no organism specified as cause

322.0 Nonpyogenic meningitis
Meningitis with clear cerebrospinal fluid

322.1 Eosinophilic meningitis

322.2 Chronic meningitis

322.9 Meningitis, unspecified

323 Encephalitis, myelitis, and encephalomyelitis
Includes: acute disseminated encephalomyelitis
meningoencephalitis, except bacterial
meningomyelitis, except bacterial
myelitis:
ascending
transverse

Excludes: acute transverse myelitis NOS (341.20)
acute transverse myelitis in conditions classified elsewhere (341.21)
bacterial:
meningoencephalitis (320.0-320.9)
meningomyelitis (320.0-320.9)
idiopathic transverse myelitis (341.22)
idiopathic transverse myelitis (341.22)

323.0 Encephalitis, myelitis, and encephalomyelitis in viral diseases classified elsewhere
Code first underlying disease, as:
cat-scratch disease (078.3)
infectious mononucleosis (075)
ornithosis (073.7)

323.01 Encephalitis and encephalomyelitis in viral diseases classified elsewhere

Excludes: encephalitis (in):
arthropod-borne viral (062.0-064)
herpes simplex (054.3)
mumps (072.2)
other viral diseases of central nervous system (049.8-049.9)
poliomyelitis (045.0-045.9)
rubella (056.01)
slow virus infections of central nervous system (046.0-046.9)
viral NOS (049.9)
West Nile (066.41)

NERVOUS SYSTEM AND SENSE ORGANS

323.02 **Myelitis in viral diseases classified elsewhere**
Excludes: myelitis (in):
    herpes simplex (054.74)
    herpes zoster (053.14)
    poliomyelitis (045.0-045.9)
    rubella (056.01)
    other viral diseases of central nervous system (049.8-049.9)

323.1 **Encephalitis, myelitis, and encephalomyelitis in rickettsial diseases classified elsewhere**
Code first underlying disease (080-083.9)

323.2 **Encephalitis, myelitis, and encephalomyelitis in protozoal diseases classified elsewhere**
Code first underlying disease, as:
    malaria (084.0-084.9)
    trypanosomiasis (086.0-086.9)

⑤ **323.4** **Other encephalitis, myelitis, and encephalomyelitis due to infection classified elsewhere**
Code first underlying disease

323.41 **Other encephalitis and encephalomyelitis due to infection classified elsewhere**
Excludes: encephalitis (in):
    meningococcal (036.1)
    syphilis:
        NOS (094.81)
        congenital (090.41)
    toxoplasmosis (130.0)
    tuberculosis (013.6)
    meningoencephalitis due to free-living ameba [Naegleria] ((136.2)

323.42 **Other myelitis due to infection classified elsewhere**
Excludes: myelitis (in):
    syphilis (094.89)
    tuberculosis (013.6)

⑤ **323.5** **Encephalitis, myelitis, and encephalomyelitis following immunization procedures**
Use additional E code, if desired, to identify vaccine

323.51 **Encephalitis and encephalomyelitis following immunization procedures**
Encephalitis postimmunization or postvaccinal
Encephalomyelitis postimmunization or postvaccinal

323.52 **Myelitis following immunization procedures**
Myelitis postimmunization or postvaccinal

⑤ **323.6** **Postinfectious encephalitis, myelitis, and encephalomyelitis**
Code first underlying disease

323.61 **Infectious acute disseminated encephalomyelitis (ADEM)**
Acute necrotizing hemorrhagic encephalopathy
Excludes: noninfectious acute disseminated encephalomyelitis (ADEM) (323.81)

323.62 **Other postinfectious encephalitis and encephalomyelitis**
Excludes: encephalitis:
    postchickenpox (052.0)
    postmeasles (055.0)

323.63 **Postinfectious myelitis**
Excludes: postchickenpox myelitis (052.2)
    herpes simplex myelitis (054.74)
    herpes zoster myelitis (053.14)

⑤ **323.7** **Toxic encephalitis, myelitis, and encephalomyelitis**
Code first underlying cause, as:
    carbon tetrachloride (982.1)
    hydroxyquinoline derivatives (961.3)
    lead (984.0-984.9)
    mercury (985.0)
    thallium (985.8)

323.71 **Toxic encephalitis and encephalomyelitis**
323.72 **Toxic myelitis**

⑤ **323.8** **Other causes of encephalitis, myelitis, and encephalomyelitis**
323.81 **Other causes of encephalitis and encephalomyelitis**
Noninfectious acute disseminated encephalomyelitis (ADEM)

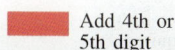 Add 4th or 5th digit   Nonspecific code   Unspecified code 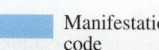 Manifestation code

323.82 Other causes of myelitis
Transverse myelitis NOS

323.9 Unspecified causes of encephalitis, myelitis, and encephalomyelitis

324 Intracranial and intraspinal abscess

324.0 Intracranial abscess
Abscess (embolic):
  cerebellar
  cerebral
Abscess (embolic) of brain [any part]:
  epidural
  extradural
  otogenic
  subdural

Excludes: tuberculous (013.3)

324.1 Intraspinal abscess
Abscess (embolic) of spinal cord [any part]:
  epidural
  extradural
  subdural

Excludes: tuberculous (013.5)

324.9 Of unspecified site
Extradural or subdural abscess NOS

325 Phlebitis and thrombophlebitis of intracranial venous sinuses
Embolism, of cavernous, lateral, or other intracranial or unspecified intracranial venous sinus
Endophlebitis, of cavernous, lateral, or other intracranial or unspecified intracranial venous sinus
Phlebitis, septic or suppurative, of cavernous, lateral, or other intracranial or unspecified intracranial venous sinus
Thrombophlebitis of cavernous, lateral, or other intracranial or unspecified intracranial venous sinus
Thrombosis of cavernous, lateral, or other intracranial or unspecified intracranial venous sinus

Excludes: that specified as:
  complicating pregnancy, childbirth, or the puerperium (671.5)
  of nonpyogenic origin (437.6)

326 Late effects of intracranial abscess or pyogenic infection
Note: This category is to be used to indicate conditions whose primary classification is to 320-325 [excluding 320.7, 321.0-321.8, 323.01-323.42, 323.61-323.72] as the cause of late effects, themselves classifiable elsewhere. The "late effects" include conditions specified as such, or as sequelae, which may occur at any time after the resolution of the causal condition.

Use additional code, if desired, to identify condition, as:
  hydrocephalus (331.4)
  paralysis (342.0-342.9, 344.0-344.9)

ORGANIC SLEEP DISORDERS (327)

327 Organic sleep disorders

327.0 Organic disorders of initiating and maintaining sleep [Organic insomnia]

Excludes: insomnia NOS (780.52)
  insomnia not due to a substance or known physiological condition (307.41-307.42)
  insomnia with sleep apnea NOS (780.51)

327.00 Organic insomnia, unspecified

327.01 Insomnia due to medical condition classified elsewhere
Code first underlying condition

Excludes: insomnia due to mental disorder (327.02)

327.02 Insomnia due to mental disorder
Code first mental disorder

Excludes: alcohol induced insomnia (291.82)
  drug induced insomnia (292.85)

327.09 Other organic insomnia

327.1 Organic disorder of excessive somnolence [Organic hypersomnia]

Excludes: hypersomnia NOS (780.54)
  hypersomnia not due to a substance or known physiological condition (307.43-307.44)
  hypersomnia with sleep apnea NOS (780.53)

327.10 Organic hypersomnia, unspecified

NERVOUS SYSTEM AND SENSE ORGANS

- 327.11 **Idiopathic hypersomnia with long sleep time**
- 327.12 **Idiopathic hypersomnia without long sleep time**
- 327.13 **Recurrent hypersomnia**
  Kleine-Levin syndrome
  Menstrual related hypersomnia
- 327.14 **Hypersomnia due to medical condition classified elsewhere**
  Code first underlying condition

  Excludes: hypersomnia due to mental disorder (327.15)

- 327.15 **Hypersomnia due to mental disorder**
  Code first mental disorder

  Excludes: alcohol induced hypersomnia (291.82)
  drug induced hypersomnia (292.85)

- 327.19 **Other organic hypersomnia**

⑤ 327.2 **Organic sleep apnea**

  Excludes: Cheyne-Stokes breathing (786.04)
  hypersomnia with sleep apnea NOS (780.53)
  insomnia with sleep apnea NOS (780.51)
  sleep apnea in newborn (770.81-770.82)
  sleep apnea NOS (780.57)

- 327.20 **Organic sleep apnea, unspecified**
- 327.21 **Primary central sleep apnea**
- 327.22 **High altitude periodic breathing**
- 327.23 **Obstructive sleep apnea (adult) (pediatric)**
- 327.24 **Idiopathic sleep related nonobstructive alveolar hypoventilation**
  Sleep related hypoxia
- 327.25 **Congenital central alveolar hypoventilation syndrome**
- 327.26 **Sleep related hypoventilation/hypoxemia in conditions classifiable elsewhere**
  Code first underlying condition
- 327.27 **Central sleep apnea in conditions classified elsewhere**
  Code first underlying condition
- 327.29 **Other organic sleep apnea**

⑤ 327.3 **Circadian rhythm sleep disorder**
  Organic disorder of sleep wake cycle
  Organic disorder of sleep wake schedule

  Excludes: alcohol induced circadian rhythm sleep disorder (291.82)
  circadian rhythm sleep disorder of nonorganic origin (307.45)
  disruption of 24 hour sleep wake cycle NOS (780.55)
  drug induced circadian rhythm sleep disorder (292.85)

- 327.30 **Circadian rhythm sleep disorder, unspecified**
- 327.31 **Circadian rhythm sleep disorder, delayed sleep phase type**
- 327.32 **Circadian rhythm sleep disorder, advanced sleep phase type**
- 327.33 **Circadian rhythm sleep disorder, irregular sleep-wake type**
- 327.34 **Circadian rhythm sleep disorder, free-running type**
- 327.35 **Circadian rhythm sleep disorder, jet lag type**
- 327.36 **Circadian rhythm sleep disorder, shift work type**
- 327.37 **Circadian rhythm sleep disorder in conditions classified elsewhere**
  Code first underlying condition
- 327.39 **Other circadian rhythm sleep disorder**

⑤ 327.4 **Organic parasomnia**

  Excludes: alcohol induced parasomnia (291.82)
  drug induced parasomnia (292.85)
  parasomnia not due to a known physiological condition (307.47)

- 327.40 **Organic parasomnia, unspecified**
- 327.41 **Confusional arousals**
- 327.42 **REM sleep behavior disorder**
- 327.43 **Recurrent isolated sleep paralysis**
- 327.44 **Parasomnia in conditions classified elsewhere**
  Code first underlying condition

 Add 4th or 5th digit   Nonspecific code   Unspecified code   Manifestation code

281

TABULAR LIST

327.49 Other organic parasomnia

⑤ **327.5 Organic sleep related movement disorders**

Excludes: restless legs syndrome (333.94)
sleep related movement disorder NOS (780.58)

327.51 Periodic limb movement disorder
Periodic limb movement sleep disorder

327.52 Sleep related leg cramps

327.53 Sleep related bruxism

327.59 Other organic sleep related movement disorders

327.8 Other organic sleep disorders

HEREDITARY AND DEGENERATIVE DISEASES OF THE CENTRAL NERVOUS SYSTEM (330-337)

Excludes: hepatolenticular degeneration (275.1)
multiple sclerosis (340)
other demyelinating diseases of central nervous system (341.0-341.9)

330 Cerebral degenerations usually manifest in childhood
Use additional code, if desired, to identify associated mental retardation

330.0 Leukodystrophy
Krabbe's disease
Leukodystrophy:
NOS
globoid cell
Leukodystrophy:
metachromatic
sudanophilic
Pelizaeus-Merzbacher disease
Sulfatide lipidosis

330.1 Cerebral lipidoses
Amaurotic (familial) idiocy
Disease:
Batten
Jansky-Bielschowsky
Disease:
Kufs'
Spielmeyer-Vogt
Tay-Sachs
Gangliosidosis

330.2 Cerebral degeneration in generalized lipidoses
Code first underlying disease, as:
Fabry's disease (272.7)
Gaucher's disease (272.7)
Neimann-Pick disease (272.7)
sphingolipidosis (272.7)

330.3 Cerebral degeneration of childhood in other diseases classified elsewhere
Code first underlying disease, as:
Hunter's disease (277.5)
mucopolysaccharidosis (277.5)

330.8 Other specified cerebral degenerations in childhood
Alpers' disease or gray-matter degeneration
Infantile necrotizing encephalomyelopathy
Leigh's disease
Subacute necrotizing encephalopathy or encephalomyelopathy

330.9 Unspecified cerebral degeneration in childhood

331 Other cerebral degenerations
Use additional code, where applicable, to identify:
with behavioral disturbance (294.11)
without behavioral disturbance (294.10)

331.0 Alzheimer's disease

⑤ **331.1 Frontotemporal dementia**

331.11 Pick's disease

331.19 Other frontotemporal dementia
Frontal dementia

331.2 Senile degeneration of brain
Excludes: senility NOS (797)

NERVOUS SYSTEM AND SENSE ORGANS

331.3 Communicating hydrocephalus
Secondary normal pressure hydrocephalus

Excludes: congenital hydrocephalus (742.3)
idiopathic normal pressure hydrocephalus (331.5)
normal pressure hydrocephalus (331.5)
spina bifida with hydrocephalus (741.0)

331.4 Obstructive hydrocephalus
Acquired hydrocephalus NOS

Excludes: congenital hydrocephalus (742.3)
idiopathic normal pressure hydrocephalus (331.5)
normal pressure hydrocephalus (331.5)
spina bifida with hydrocephalus (741.0)

● **331.5 Idiopathic normal pressure hydrocephalus (INPH)**
Normal pressure hydrocephalus NOS

Excludes: congenital hydrocephalus (742.3)
secondary normal pressure hydrocephalus (331.3)
spina bifida with hydrocephalus (741.0)

331.7 Cerebral degeneration in diseases classified elsewhere
Code first underlying disease, as:
alcoholism (303.0-303.9)
beriberi (265.0)
cerebrovascular disease (430-438)
congenital hydrocephalus (741.0, 742.3)
neoplastic disease (140.0-239.9)
myxedema (244.0-244.9)
vitamin B$_{12}$ deficiency (266.2)

Excludes: cerebral degeneration in:
Jakob-Creutzfeldt disease (046.1)
progressive multifocal leukoencephalopathy (046.3)
subacute spongiform encephalopathy (046.1)

⑤ **331.8 Other cerebral degeneration**

331.81 Reye's syndrome

331.82 Dementia with Lewy bodies
Dementia with Parkinsonism
Lewy body dementia
Lewy body disease

331.83 Mild cognitive impairment, so stated

Excludes: altered mental status (780.97)
cerebral degeneration (331.0-331.9)
change in mental status (780.97)
cognitive deficits following (late effects of) cerebral hemorrhage or infarction (438.0)
cognitive impairment due to intracranial or head injury (850-854, 959.01)
cognitive impairment due to late effect of intracranial injury (907.0)
dementia (290.0-290.43, 294.8)
mild memory disturbance (310.8)
neurologic neglect syndrome (781.8)
personality change, nonpsychotic (310.1)

331.89 Other
Cerebral ataxia

331.9 Cerebral degeneration, unspecified

332 Parkinson's disease

Excludes: dementia with Parkinsonism (331.82)

332.0 Paralysis agitans
Parkinsonism or Parkinson's disease:
NOS
idiopathic
primary

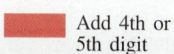 Add 4th or 5th digit
 Nonspecific code
 Unspecified code
 Manifestation code

TABULAR LIST

332.1 Secondary Parkinsonism
   Neuroleptic-induced Parkinsonism
   Parkinsonism due to drugs

Use additional E code, if desired, to identify drug, if drug-induced

Excludes: Parkinsonism (in):
   Huntington's disease (333.4)
   progressive supranuclear palsy (333.0)
   Shy-Drager syndrome (333.0)
   syphilitic (094.82)

333 Other extrapyramidal disease and abnormal movement disorders
   Includes: other forms of extrapyramidal, basal ganglia, or striatopallidal disease

Excludes: abnormal movements of head NOS (781.0)
   sleep related movement disorders (327.51-327.59)

333.0 Other degenerative diseases of the basal ganglia
   Atrophy or degeneration:
      olivopontocerebellar [Déjérine-Thomas syndrome]
      pigmentary pallidal [Hallervorden-Spatz disease]
      striatonigral
   Parkinsonian syndrome associated with:
      idiopathic orthostatic hypotension
      symptomatic orthostatic hypotension
   Progressive supranuclear ophthalmoplegia
   Shy-Drager syndrome

333.1 Essential and other specified forms of tremor
   Benign essential tremor
   Familial tremor
   Medication-induced postural tremor

Use additional E code, if desired, to identify drug, if drug-induced

Excludes: tremor NOS (781.0)

333.2 Myoclonus
   Familial essential myoclonus
   Progressive myoclonic epilepsy
   Unverricht-Lundborg disease

Use additional E code, if desired, to identify drug, if drug-induced

333.3 Tics of organic origin

Excludes: Gilles de la Tourette's syndrome (307.23)
   habit spasm (307.22)
   tic NOS (307.20)

Use additional E code, if desired, to identify drug, if drug-induced

333.4 Huntington's chorea

333.5 Other choreas
   Hemiballism(us)
   Paroxysmal choreo-athetosis

Excludes: Sydenham's or rheumatic chorea (392.0-392.9)

Use additional E code, if desired, to identify drug, if drug-induced

333.6 Genetic torsion dystonia
   Dystonia:
      deformans progressiva
      musculorum deformans
   (Schwalbe-) Ziehen-Oppenheim disease

333.7 Acquired torsion dystonia
   333.71 Athetoid cerebral palsy
      Double athetosis (syndrome)
      Vogt's disease

Excludes: infantile cerebral palsy (343.0-343.9)

NERVOUS SYSTEM AND SENSE ORGANS

333.72 Acute dystonia due to drugs
Acute dystonic reaction due to drugs
Neuroleptic induced acute dystonia

Use additional E code to identify drug

Excludes: *blepharospasm due to drugs (333.85)*
orofacial dyskinesia due to drugs (333.85)
secondary Parkinsonism (332.1)
subacute dyskinesia due to drugs (333.85)
tardive dyskinesia (333.85)

333.79 Other acquired torsion dystonia

⑤ **333.8 Fragments of torsion dystonia**
Use additional E code, if desired, to identify drug, if drug-induced

333.81 Blepharospasm

Excludes: *blepharospasm due to drugs (333.85)*

333.82 Orofacial dyskinesia

Excludes: *orofacial dyskinesia due to drugs (333.85)*

333.83 Spasmodic torticollis

Excludes: *torticollis:*
  NOS (723.5)
  hysterical (300.11)
  psychogenic (306.0)

333.84 Organic writers' cramp

Excludes: *psychogenic (300.89)*

333.85 Subacute dyskinesia due to drugs
Blepharospasm due to drugs
Orofacial dyskinesia due to drugs
Tardive dyskinesia

Use additional E code to identify drug

Excludes: *acute dystonia due to drugs (333.72)*
acute dystonic reaction due to drugs (333.72)
secondary Parkinsonism (332.1)

333.89 Other

⑤ **333.9 Other and unspecified extrapyramidal diseases and abnormal movement disorders**

333.90 Unspecified extrapyramidal disease and abnormal movement disorder
Medication-induced movement disorders NOS
Use additional E code to identify drug, if drug-induced

333.91 Stiff-man syndrome

333.92 Neuroleptic malignant syndrome
Use additional E code to identify drug

Excludes: *neuroleptic induced Parkinsonism (332.1)*

333.93 Benign shuddering attacks

333.94 Restless legs syndrome (RLS)

333.99 Other
Neuroleptic-induced acute akathisia
Use additional E code to identify drug, if drug-induced

334 Spinocerebellar disease

Excludes: *olivopontocerebellar degeneration (333.0)*
peroneal muscular atrophy (356.1)

334.0 Friedreich's ataxia

334.1 Hereditary spastic paraplegia

334.2 Primary cerebellar degeneration
Cerebellar ataxia:
  Marie's
  Sanger-Brown
Dyssynergia cerebellaris myoclonica
Primary cerebellar degeneration:
  NOS
  hereditary
  sporadic

 Add 4th or 5th digit
 Nonspecific code
 Unspecified code
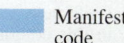 Manifestation code

TABULAR LIST

334.3 Other cerebellar ataxia
Cerebellar ataxia NOS

Use additional E code, if desired, to identify drug, if drug-induced

334.4 *Cerebellar ataxia in diseases classified elsewhere*
Code first underlying disease, as:
alcoholism (303.0-303.9)
myxedema (244.0-244.9)
neoplastic disease (140.0-239.9)

334.8 Other spinocerebellar diseases
Ataxia-telangiectasia [Louis-Bar syndrome]
Corticostriatal-spinal degeneration

334.9 Spinocerebellar disease, unspecified

335 Anterior horn cell disease

335.0 Werdnig-Hoffmann disease
Infantile spinal muscular atrophy
Progressive muscular atrophy of infancy

⑤ **335.1 Spinal muscular atrophy**

335.10 Spinal muscular atrophy, unspecified

335.11 Kugelberg-Welander disease
Spinal muscular atrophy:
familial
juvenile

335.19 Other
Adult spinal muscular atrophy

⑤ **335.2 Motor neuron disease**

335.20 Amyotrophic lateral sclerosis
Motor neuron disease (bulbar) (mixed type)

335.21 Progressive muscular atrophy
Duchenne-Aran muscular atrophy
Progressive muscular atrophy (pure)

335.22 Progressive bulbar palsy

335.23 Pseudobulbar palsy

335.24 Primary lateral sclerosis

335.29 Other

335.8 Other anterior horn cell diseases

335.9 Anterior horn cell disease, unspecified

336 Other diseases of spinal cord

336.0 Syringomyelia and syringobulbia

336.1 Vascular myelopathies
Acute infarction of spinal cord (embolic) (nonembolic)
Arterial thrombosis of spinal cord
Edema of spinal cord
Hematomyelia
Subacute necrotic myelopathy

336.2 *Subacute combined degeneration of spinal cord in diseases classified elsewhere*
Code first underlying disease, as:
pernicious anemia (281.0)
other vitamin B_{12} deficiency anemia (281.1)
vitamin B_{12} deficiency (266.2)

336.3 *Myelopathy in other diseases classified elsewhere*
Code first underlying disease, as:
myelopathy in neoplastic disease (140.0-239.9)

Excludes: myelopathy in:
intervertebral disc disorder (722.70-722.73)
spondylosis (721.1, 721.41-721.42, 721.91)

336.8 Other myelopathy
Myelopathy:
drug-induced
radiation-induced

Use additional E code, if desired, to identify cause

286 ● Code new to this edition   ▲ Revision of existing code   ④ ⑤ Fourth or fifth digit required

NERVOUS SYSTEM AND SENSE ORGANS

336.9 **Unspecified disease of spinal cord**
Cord compression NOS   Myelopathy NOS
Excludes: *myelitis (323.02, 323.1, 323.2, 323.42, 323.52, 323.63, 323.72, 323.82, 323.9)*
spinal (canal) stenosis (723.0, 724.00-724.09)

337 **Disorders of the autonomic nervous system**
Includes: disorders of peripheral autonomic, sympathetic, parasympathetic, or vegetative system
Excludes: *familial dysautonomia [Riley-Day syndrome] (742.8)*

337.0 Idiopathic peripheral autonomic neuropathy
Carotid sinus syncope or syndrome
Cervical sympathetic dystrophy or paralysis

337.1 *Peripheral autonomic neuropathy in disorders classified elsewhere*
Code first underlying disease, as:
amyloidosis (277.30-277.39)
diabetes (250.6)

⑤ **337.2 Reflex sympathetic dystrophy**

337.20 Reflex sympathetic dystrophy, unspecified

337.21 Reflex sympathetic dystrophy of the upper limb

337.22 Reflex sympathetic dystrophy of the lower limb

337.29 Reflex sympathetic dystrophy of other specified site

337.3 Autonomic dysreflexia
Use additional code to identify the cause, such as:
decubitus ulcer (707.00-707.09)
fecal impaction (560.39)
urinary tract infection (599.0)

337.9 **Unspecified disorder of autonomic nervous system**

PAIN (338)

338 **Pain, not elsewhere classified**
Use additional code to identify:
pain associated with psychological factors (307.89)
Excludes: *generalized pain (780.96)*
localized pain, unspecified type – code to pain by site
pain disorder exclusively attributed to psychological factors (307.80)

338.0 Central pain syndrome
Déjérine-Roussy syndrome
Myelopathic pain syndrome
Thalamic pain syndrome (hyperesthetic)

⑤ **338.1 Acute pain**

338.11 Acute pain due to trauma

338.12 Acute post-thoracotomy pain
Post-thoracotomy pain NOS

338.18 Other acute postoperative pain
Postoperative pain NOS

338.19 Other acute pain

Excludes: *neoplasm related acute pain (338.3)*

⑤ **338.2 Chronic pain**
Excludes: *causalgia (355.9)*
lower limb (355.71)
upper limb (354.4)
chronic pain syndrome (338.4)
myofascial pain syndrome (729.1)
neoplasm related chronic pain (338.3)
reflex sympathetic dystrophy (337.20-337.29)

338.21 Chronic pain due to trauma

338.22 Chronic post-thoracotomy pain

338.28 Other chronic postoperative pain

338.29 Other chronic pain

 Nonspecific code
 Unspecified code
 Manifestation code

TABULAR LIST

338.3 Neoplasm related pain (acute) (chronic)
Cancer associated pain
Pain due to malignancy (primary) (secondary)
Tumor associated pain

338.4 Chronic pain syndrome
Chronic pain associated with significant psychosocial dysfunction

OTHER DISORDERS OF THE CENTRAL NERVOUS SYSTEM (340-349)

340 Multiple sclerosis
Disseminated or multiple sclerosis:
NOS
brain stem
cord
generalized

341 Other demyelinating diseases of central nervous system

341.0 Neuromyelitis optica

341.1 Schilder's disease
Baló's concentric sclerosis
Encephalitis periaxialis:
concentrica [Baló's]
diffusa [Schilder's]

341.2 Acute (transverse) myelitis
Excludes: acute (transverse)myelitis (in) (due to):
following immunization procedures (323.52)
infection classified elsewhere (323.42)
postinfectious (323.63)
protozoal diseases classified elsewhere (323.2)
rickettsial diseases classified elsewhere (323.1)
toxic (323.72)
viral diseases classified elsewhere (323.02)
transverse myelitis NOS (323.82)

341.20 Acute (transverse) myelitis NOS

341.21 Acute (transverse) myelitis in conditions classified elsewhere
Code first underlying condition

341.22 Idiopathic transverse myelitis

341.8 Other demyelinating diseases of central nervous system
Central demyelination of corpus callosum
Central pontine myelinosis
Marchiafava (-Bignami) disease

341.9 Demyelinating disease of central nervous system, unspecified

342 Hemiplegia and hemiparesis
Excludes: congenital (343.1)
hemiplegia due to late effect of cerebrovascular accident (438.20-438.22)
infantile NOS (343.4)

Note: This category is to be used when hemiplegia (complete) (incomplete) is reported without further specification, or is stated to be old or long-standing but of unspecified cause. The category is also for use in multiple coding to identify these types of hemiplegia resulting from any cause.

The following fifth-digits are for use with codes 342.0-342.9

   0 affecting unspecified side
   1 affecting dominant side
   2 affecting nondominant side

342.0 Flaccid hemiplegia

342.1 Spastic hemiplegia

342.8 Other specified hemiplegia

342.9 Hemiplegia, unspecified

NERVOUS SYSTEM AND SENSE ORGANS

343 Infantile cerebral palsy
  Includes: cerebral:
      palsy NOS
      spastic infantile paralysis
    congenital spastic paralysis (cerebral)
    Little's disease
    paralysis (spastic) due to birth injury:
      intracranial
      spinal

  Excludes: athetoid cerebral palsy (333.71)
    hereditary cerebral paralysis, such as:
      hereditary spastic paraplegia (334.1)
      Vogt's disease (333.71)
    spastic paralysis specified as noncongenital or noninfantile (344.0-344.9)

  343.0 **Diplegic**
    Congenital diplegia   Congenital paraplegia

  343.1 **Hemiplegic**
    Congenital hemiplegia
    Excludes: infantile hemiplegia NOS (343.4)

  343.2 **Quadriplegic**
    Tetraplegic

  343.3 **Monoplegic**

  343.4 **Infantile hemiplegia**
    Infantile hemiplegia (postnatal) NOS

  343.8 Other specified infantile cerebral palsy

  343.9 Infantile cerebral palsy, unspecified
    Cerebral palsy NOS

344 Other paralytic syndromes
  Note: This category is to be used when the listed conditions are reported without further specification or are stated to be old or long-standing but of unspecified cause. The category is also for use in multiple coding to identify these conditions resulting from any cause.
  Includes: paralysis (complete) (incomplete), except as classifiable to 342 and 343
    Excludes: congenital or infantile cerebral palsy (343.0-343.9)
      hemiplegia (342.0-342.9)
        congenital or infantile (343.1, 343.4)

  ⑤ 344.0 **Quadriplegia and quadriparesis**
    344.00 Quadriplegia, unspecified
    344.01 C1-C4, complete
    344.02 C1-C4, incomplete
    344.03 C5-C7, complete
    344.04 C5-C7, incomplete
    344.09 Other

  344.1 **Paraplegia**
    Paralysis of both lower limbs
    Paraplegia (lower)

  344.2 **Diplegia of upper limbs**
    Diplegia (upper)
    Paralysis of both upper limbs

  ⑤ 344.3 **Monoplegia of lower limb**
    Paralysis of lower limb
    Excludes: monoplegia of lower limb due to late effect of cerebrovascular accident (438.40-438.42)
      344.30 affecting unspecified side
      344.31 affecting dominant side
      344.32 affecting nondominant side

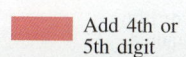 Add 4th or 5th digit   Nonspecific code   Unspecified code   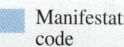 Manifestation code

289

TABULAR LIST

⑤ **344.4 Monoplegia of upper limb**
Paralysis of upper limb

Excludes: *monoplegia of upper limb due to late effect of cerebrovascular accident (438.30-438.32)*

344.40 affecting unspecified side
344.41 affecting dominant side
344.42 affecting nondominant side

344.5 Unspecified monoplegia

⑤ **344.6 Cauda equina syndrome**

344.60 Without mention of neurogenic bladder
344.61 With neurogenic bladder
Acontractile bladder
Autonomic hyperreflexia of bladder
Cord bladder
Detrusor hyperreflexia

⑤ **344.8 Other specified paralytic syndromes**

344.81 Locked-in state
344.89 Other specified paralytic syndrome

344.9 Paralysis, unspecified

345 Epilepsy and recurrent seizures
The following fifth-digit subclassification is for use with categories 345.0, 345.1, 345.4-345.9:

  0 without mention of intractable epilepsy
  1 with intractable epilepsy

Excludes: *progressive myoclonic epilepsy (333.2)*

⑤ **345.0 Generalized nonconvulsive epilepsy**
Absences:
  atonic
  typical
Minor epilepsy
Petit mal
Pykno-epilepsy
Seizures:
  akinetic
  atonic

⑤ **345.1 Generalized convulsive epilepsy**
Epileptic seizures:
  clonic
  myoclonic
  tonic
  tonic-clonic
Grand mal
Major epilepsy

Excludes: *convulsions:*
  NOS (780.39)
  infantile (780.39)
  newborn (779.0)
infantile spasms (345.6)

345.2 Petit mal status
Epileptic absence status

345.3 Grand mal status
Status epilepticus NOS

Excludes: *epilepsia partialis continua (345.7)*
  status:
    psychomotor (345.7)
    temporal lobe (345.7)

⑤ **345.4 Localization-related (focal) (partial) epilepsy and epileptic syndromes with complex partial seizures**
Epilepsy:
  limbic system
  partial:
    secondarily generalized
    with impairment of consciousness
    with memory and ideational disturbances
  psychomotor
  psychosensory
  temporal lobe
Epileptic automatism

NERVOUS SYSTEM AND SENSE ORGANS

⑤ **345.5 Localization-related (focal) (partial) epilepsy and epileptic syndromes with simple partial seizures**
Epilepsy:
 Bravais-Jacksonian NOS
 focal (motor) NOS
 Jacksonian NOS
 motor partial
 partial NOS:
  without impairment of consciousness
Epilepsy:
 sensory-induced
 somatomotor
 somatosensory
 visceral
 visual

⑤ **345.6 Infantile spasms**
Hypsarrhythmia
Lightning spasms
Salaam attacks

Excludes: salaam tic (781.0)

⑤ **345.7 Epilepsia partialis continua**
Kojevnikov's epilepsy

⑤ **345.8 Other forms of epilepsy and recurrent seizures**
Epilepsy:
 cursive [running]
 gelastic

⑤ **345.9 Epilepsy, unspecified**
Epileptic convulsions, fits, or seizures NOS
Recurrent seizures NOS
Seizure disorder NOS

Excludes: convulsion (convulsive) disorder (780.39)
 convulsive seizure or fit NOS (780.39)
 recurrent convulsions (780.39)

⑤ **346 Migraine**
The following fifth-digit subclassification is for use with category 346:

 0 without mention of intractable migraine
 1 with intractable migraine, so stated

⑤ **346.0 Classical migraine**
Migraine preceded or accompanied by transient focal neurological phenomena
Migraine with aura

⑤ **346.1 Common migraine**
Atypical migraine
Sick headache

⑤ **346.2 Variants of migraine**
Cluster headache
Histamine cephalgia
Horton's neuralgia
Migraine:
 abdominal
 basilar
Migraine:
 lower half
 retinal
Neuralgia:
 ciliary
 migrainous

⑤ **346.8 Other forms of migraine**
Migraine:
 hemiplegic
 ophthalmoplegic

⑤ **346.9 Migraine, unspecified**

347 Cataplexy and narcolepsy

⑤ **347.0 Narcolepsy**

 347.00 Without cataplexy
 Narcolepsy NOS

 347.01 With cataplexy

⑤ **347.1 Narcolepsy in conditions classified elsewhere**
Code first underlying condition

 347.10 *Without cataplexy*
 347.11 *With cataplexy*

348 Other conditions of brain

348.0 Cerebral cysts
Arachnoid cyst
Porencephalic cyst
Porencephaly, acquired
Pseudoporencephaly

Excludes: porencephaly (congenital) (742.4)

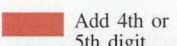 Add 4th or 5th digit
 Nonspecific code
 Unspecified code
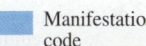 Manifestation code

TABULAR LIST

348.1 Anoxic brain damage
  Excludes: that occurring in:
        abortion (634-638 with .7, 639.8)
        ectopic or molar pregnancy (639.8)
        labor or delivery (668.2, 669.4)
        that of newborn (767.0, 768.0-768.9, 772.1-772.2)
  Use additional E code, if desired, to identify cause

348.2 Benign intracranial hypertension
    Pseudotumor cerebri
  Excludes: hypertensive encephalopathy (437.2)

⑤ **348.3 Encephalopathy, not elsewhere classified**
   348.30 Encephalopathy, unspecified
   348.31 Metabolic encephalopathy
       Septic encephalopathy
     Excludes: toxic metabolic encephalopathy (349.82)
   348.39 Other encephalopathy
  Excludes: encephalopathy:
        alcoholic (291.2)
        hepatic (572.2)
        hypertensive (437.2)
        toxic (349.82)

348.4 Compression of brain
    Compression, brain (stem)
    Herniation, brain (stem)
    Posterior fossa compression syndrome

348.5 Cerebral edema

348.8 Other conditions of brain
    Cerebral:
      calcification
      fungus

348.9 Unspecified condition of brain

349 Other and unspecified disorders of the nervous system

349.0 Reaction to spinal or lumbar puncture
    Headache following lumbar puncture

349.1 Nervous system complications from surgically implanted device

349.2 Disorders of meninges, not elsewhere classified
  Excludes: immediate postoperative complications (997.00-997.09)
          mechanical complications of nervous system device (996.2)
    Adhesions, meningeal (cerebral) (spinal)
    Cyst, spinal meninges
    Meningocele, acquired
    Pseudomeningocele, acquired

⑤ **349.8 Other specified disorders of nervous system**
   349.81 Cerebrospinal fluid rhinorrhea
     Excludes: cerebrospinal fluid otorrhea (388.61)
   349.82 Toxic encephalopathy
       Toxic metabolic encephalopathy
     Use additional E code, if desired, to identify cause
   349.89 Other

349.9 Unspecified disorders of nervous system
    Disorder of nervous system (central) NOS

NERVOUS SYSTEM AND SENSE ORGANS

DISORDERS OF THE PERIPHERAL NERVOUS SYSTEM (350-359)

Excludes: diseases of:
  acoustic [8th] nerve (388.5)
  oculomotor [3rd, 4th, 6th] nerves (378.0-378.9)
  optic [2nd] nerve (377.0-377.9)
  peripheral autonomic nerves (337.0-337.9)
  neuralgia NOS or "rheumatic" (729.2)
  neuritis NOS or "rheumatic" (729.2)
  radiculitis NOS or "rheumatic" (729.2)
  peripheral neuritis in pregnancy (646.4)

350 Trigeminal nerve disorders
Includes: disorders of 5th cranial nerve

350.1 Trigeminal neuralgia
  Tic douloureux
  Trifacial neuralgia
  Trigeminal neuralgia NOS

  Excludes: postherpetic (053.12)

350.2 Atypical face pain

350.8 Other specified trigeminal nerve disorders

350.9 Trigeminal nerve disorder, unspecified

351 Facial nerve disorders
Includes: disorders of 7th cranial nerve

  Excludes: that in newborn (767.5)

351.0 Bell's palsy
  Facial palsy

351.1 Geniculate ganglionitis
  Geniculate ganglionitis NOS

  Excludes: herpetic (053.11)

351.8 Other facial nerve disorders
  Facial myokymia
  Melkersson's syndrome

351.9 Facial nerve disorder, unspecified

352 Disorders of other cranial nerves

352.0 Disorders of olfactory [1st] nerve

352.1 Glossopharyngeal neuralgia

352.2 Other disorders of glossopharyngeal [9th] nerve

352.3 Disorders of pneumogastric [10th] nerve
  Disorders of vagal nerve

  Excludes: paralysis of vocal cords or larynx (478.30-478.34)

352.4 Disorders of accessory [11th] nerve

352.5 Disorders of hypoglossal [12th] nerve

352.6 Multiple cranial nerve palsies
  Collet-Sicard syndrome
  Polyneuritis cranialis

352.9 Unspecified disorder of cranial nerves

353 Nerve root and plexus disorders

  Excludes: conditions due to:
    intervertebral disc disorders (722.0-722.9)
    spondylosis (720.0-721.9)
    vertebrogenic disorders (723.0-724.9)

353.0 Brachial plexus lesions
  Cervical rib syndrome
  Costoclavicular syndrome
  Scalenus anticus syndrome
  Thoracic outlet syndrome

  Excludes: brachial neuritis or radiculitis NOS (723.4)
    that in newborn (767.6)

353.1 Lumbosacral plexus lesions
Code first, if applicable, associated diabetes mellitus (250.6)

353.2 Cervical root lesions, not elsewhere classified

353.3 Thoracic root lesions, not elsewhere classified

TABULAR LIST

- **353.4 Lumbosacral root lesions, not elsewhere classified**
- **353.5 Neuralgic amyotrophy**
  Parsonage-Aldren-Turner syndrome
- **353.6 Phantom limb (syndrome)**
- **353.8 Other nerve root and plexus disorders**
- **353.9 Unspecified nerve root and plexus disorder**

354 Mononeuritis of upper limb and mononeuritis multiplex

- **354.0 Carpal tunnel syndrome**
  Median nerve entrapment
  Partial thenar atrophy
- **354.1 Other lesion of median nerve**
  Median nerve neuritis
- **354.2 Lesion of ulnar nerve**
  Cubital tunnel syndrome
  Tardy ulnar nerve palsy
- **354.3 Lesion of radial nerve**
  Acute radial nerve palsy
- **354.4 Causalgia of upper limb**
  Excludes: causalgia:
    NOS (355.9)
    lower limb (355.71)
- **354.5 Mononeuritis multiplex**
  Combinations of single conditions classifiable to 354 or 355
- **354.8 Other mononeuritis of upper limb**
- **354.9 Mononeuritis of upper limb, unspecified**

355 Mononeuritis of lower limb and unspecified site

- **355.0 Lesion of sciatic nerve**
  Excludes: sciatica NOS (724.3)
- **355.1 Meralgia paresthetica**
  Lateral cutaneous femoral nerve of thigh compression or syndrome
- **355.2 Other lesion of femoral nerve**
- **355.3 Lesion of lateral popliteal nerve**
  Lesion of common peroneal nerve
- **355.4 Lesion of medial popliteal nerve**
- **355.5 Tarsal tunnel syndrome**
- **355.6 Lesion of plantar nerve**
  Morton's metatarsalgia, neuralgia, or neuroma
- ⑤ **355.7 Other mononeuritis of lower limb**
  - **355.71 Causalgia of lower limb**
    Excludes: causalgia:
      NOS (355.9)
      upper limb (354.4)
  - **355.79 Other mononeuritis of lower limb**
- **355.8 Mononeuritis of lower limb, unspecified**
- **355.9 Mononeuritis of unspecified site**
  Causalgia NOS
  Excludes: causalgia:
    lower limb (355.71)
    upper limb (354.4)

356 Hereditary and idiopathic peripheral neuropathy

- **356.0 Hereditary peripheral neuropathy**
  Déjérine-Sottas disease
- **356.1 Peroneal muscular atrophy**
  Charcot-Marie-Tooth disease
  Neuropathic muscular atrophy
- **356.2 Hereditary sensory neuropathy**

NERVOUS SYSTEM AND SENSE ORGANS

356.3 Refsum's disease
Heredopathia atactica polyneuritiformis

356.4 Idiopathic progressive polyneuropathy

356.8 Other specified idiopathic peripheral neuropathy
Supranuclear paralysis

356.9 Unspecified

357 Inflammatory and toxic neuropathy

357.0 Acute infective polyneuritis
Guillain-Barré syndrome
Postinfectious polyneuritis

357.1 *Polyneuropathy in collagen vascular disease*
Code first underlying disease, as:
disseminated lupus erythematosus (710.0)
polyarteritis nodosa (446.0)
rheumatoid arthritis (714.0)

357.2 *Polyneuropathy in diabetes*
Code first underlying disease (250.6)

357.3 *Polyneuropathy in malignant disease*
Code first underlying disease (140.0-208.9)

357.4 *Polyneuropathy in other diseases classified elsewhere*
Code first underlying disease, as:
amyloidosis (277.30-277.39)
beriberi (265.0)
chronic uremia (585.9)
deficiency of B vitamins (266.0-266.9)
diphtheria (032.0-032.9)
hypoglycemia (251.2)
pellagra (265.2)
porphyria (277.1)
sarcoidosis (135)
uremia NOS (586)

Excludes: polyneuropathy in:
herpes zoster (053.13)
mumps (072.72)

357.5 Alcoholic polyneuropathy

357.6 Polyneuropathy due to drugs
Use additional E code, if desired, to identify drug

357.7 Polyneuropathy due to other toxic agents
Use additional E code, if desired, to identify toxic agent

⑤ 357.8 Other

    357.81 Chronic inflammatory demyelinating polyneuritis

    357.82 Critical illness polyneuropathy
        Acute motor neuropathy

    357.89 Other inflammatory and toxic neuropathy

357.9 Unspecified

358 Myoneural disorders

⑤ 358.0 Myasthenia gravis

    358.00 Myasthenia gravis without (acute) exacerbation
        Myasthenia gravis NOS

    358.01 Myasthenia gravis with (acute) exacerbation
        Myasthenia gravis in crisis

358.1 *Myasthenic syndromes in diseases classified elsewhere*
Eaton-Lambert syndrome from stated cause classified elsewhere
Code first underlying disease, as:
botulism (005.1)
hypothyroidism (244.0-244.9)
malignant neoplasm (140.0-208.9)
pernicious anemia (281.0)
thyrotoxicosis (242.0-242.9)

358.2 Toxic myoneural disorders
Use additional E code, if desired, to identify toxic agent

358.8 Other specified myoneural disorders

TABULAR LIST

358.9 **Myoneural disorders, unspecified**

359 **Muscular dystrophies and other myopathies**

Excludes: idiopathic polymyositis (710.4)

359.0 **Congenital hereditary muscular dystrophy**
Benign congenital myopathy
Central core disease
Centronuclear myopathy
Myotubular myopathy
Nemaline body disease

Excludes: arthrogryposis multiplex congenita (754.89)

359.1 **Hereditary progressive muscular dystrophy**

Muscular dystrophy:
  NOS
  distal
  Duchenne
  Erb's
  fascioscapulohumeral

Muscular dystrophy:
  Gower's
  Landouzy-Déjérine
  limb-girdle
  ocular
  oculopharyngeal

⑤ **359.2** **Myotonic disorders**

Excludes: periodic paralysis (359.3)

● **359.21** **Myotonic muscular dystrophy**
Dystrophia myotonica
Myotonia atrophica
Myotonic dystrophy
Proximal myotonic myopathy (PROMM)
Steinert's disease

● **359.22** **Myotonia congenita**
Acetazolamide responsive myotonia congenita
Dominant form (Thomsen's disease)
Recessive form (Becker's disease)

● **359.23** **Myotonic chondrodystrophy**
Congenital myotonic chondrodystrophy
Schwartz-Jampel disease

● **359.24** **Drug-induced myotonia**
Use additional E code to identify drug

● **359.29** **Other specified myotonic disorder**
Myotonia fluctuans
Myotonia levior
Myotonia permanens
Paramyotonia congenita (of von Eulenburg)

▲ **359.3** **Periodic paralysis**
Familial periodic paralysis
Hyperkalemic periodic paralysis
Hypokalemic familial periodic paralysis
Hypokalemic periodic paralysis
Potassium sensitive periodic paralysis

Excludes: paramyotonia congenita (of von Eulenburg) (359.29)

359.4 **Toxic myopathy**
Use additional E code, if desired, to identify toxic agent

359.5 ***Myopathy in endocrine diseases classified elsewhere***
Code first underlying disease, as:
  Addison's disease (255.41)
  Cushing's syndrome (255.0)
  hypopituitarism (253.2)
  myxedema (244.0-244.9)
  thyrotoxicosis (242.0-242.9)

NERVOUS SYSTEM AND SENSE ORGANS

359.6 Symptomatic inflammatory myopathy in diseases classified elsewhere
Code first underlying disease, as:
amyloidosis (277.30-277.39)
disseminated lupus erythematosus (710.0)
malignant neoplasm (140.0-208.9)
polyarteritis nodosa (446.0)
rheumatoid arthritis (714.0)
sarcoidosis (135)
scleroderma (710.1)
Sjögren's disease (710.2)

359.8 Other myopathies

359.81 Critical illness myopathy
Acute necrotizing myopathy
Acute quadriplegic myopathy
Intensive care (ICU) myopathy
Myopathy of critical illness

359.89 Other myopathies

359.9 Myopathy, unspecified

DISORDERS OF THE EYE AND ADNEXA (360-379)

360 Disorders of the globe
Includes: disorders affecting multiple structures of eye

360.0 Purulent endophthalmitis
Excludes: bleb associated endophthalmitis (379.63)

360.00 Purulent endophthalmitis, unspecified

360.01 Acute endophthalmitis

360.02 Panophthalmitis

360.03 Chronic endophthalmitis

360.04 Vitreous abscess

360.1 Other endophthalmitis
Excludes: bleb associated endophthalmitis (379.63)

360.11 Sympathetic uveitis

360.12 Panuveitis

360.13 Parasitic endophthalmitis NOS

360.14 Ophthalmia nodosa

360.19 Other
Phacoanaphylactic endophthalmitis

360.2 Degenerative disorders of globe

360.20 Degenerative disorder of globe, unspecified

360.21 Progressive high (degenerative) myopia
Malignant myopia

360.23 Siderosis

360.24 Other metallosis
Chalcosis

360.29 Other
Excludes: xerophthalmia (264.7)

360.3 Hypotony of eye

360.30 Hypotony, unspecified

360.31 Primary hypotony

360.32 Ocular fistula causing hypotony

360.33 Hypotony associated with other ocular disorders

360.34 Flat anterior chamber

360.4 Degenerated conditions of globe

360.40 Degenerated globe or eye, unspecified

360.41 Blind hypotensive eye
Atrophy of globe
Phthisis bulbi

TABULAR LIST

- **360.42 Blind hypertensive eye**
  Absolute glaucoma
- **360.43 Hemophthalmos, except current injury**
  Excludes: traumatic (871.0-871.9, 921.0-921.9)
- **360.44 Leucocoria**

⑤ **360.5 Retained (old) intraocular foreign body, magnetic**
  Excludes: current penetrating injury with magnetic foreign body (871.5)
  retained (old) foreign body of orbit (376.6)
  - **360.50 Foreign body, magnetic, intraocular, unspecified**
  - **360.51 Foreign body, magnetic, in anterior chamber**
  - **360.52 Foreign body, magnetic, in iris or ciliary body**
  - **360.53 Foreign body, magnetic, in lens**
  - **360.54 Foreign body, magnetic, in vitreous**
  - **360.55 Foreign body, magnetic, in posterior wall**
  - **360.59 Foreign body, magnetic, in other or multiple sites**

⑤ **360.6 Retained (old) intraocular foreign body, nonmagnetic**
  Retained (old) foreign body:
    NOS
    nonmagnetic
  Excludes: current penetrating injury with (nonmagnetic) foreign body (871.6)
  retained (old) foreign body in orbit (376.6)
  - **360.60 Foreign body, intraocular, unspecified**
  - **360.61 Foreign body in anterior chamber**
  - **360.62 Foreign body in iris or ciliary body**
  - **360.63 Foreign body in lens**
  - **360.64 Foreign body in vitreous**
  - **360.65 Foreign body in posterior wall**
  - **360.69 Foreign body in other or multiple sites**

⑤ **360.8 Other disorders of globe**
  - **360.81 Luxation of globe**
  - **360.89 Other**

360.9 Unspecified disorder of globe

361 Retinal detachments and defects

⑤ **361.0 Retinal detachment with retinal defect**
  Rhegmatogenous retinal detachment
  Excludes: detachment of retinal pigment epithelium (362.42-362.43)
  retinal detachment (serous) (without defect) (361.2)
  - **361.00 Retinal detachment with retinal defect, unspecified**
  - **361.01 Recent detachment, partial, with single defect**
  - **361.02 Recent detachment, partial, with multiple defects**
  - **361.03 Recent detachment, partial, with giant tear**
  - **361.04 Recent detachment, partial, with retinal dialysis**
    Dialysis (juvenile) of retina (with detachment)
  - **361.05 Recent detachment, total or subtotal**
  - **361.06 Old detachment, partial**
    Delimited old retinal detachment
  - **361.07 Old detachment, total or subtotal**

⑤ **361.1 Retinoschisis and retinal cysts**
  Excludes: juvenile retinoschisis (362.73)
  microcystoid degeneration of retina (362.62)
  parasitic cyst of retina (360.13)
  - **361.10 Retinoschisis, unspecified**
  - **361.11 Flat retinoschisis**
  - **361.12 Bullous retinoschisis**
  - **361.13 Primary retinal cysts**

● Code new to this edition   ▲ Revision of existing code   ④ ⑤ Fourth or fifth digit required

NERVOUS SYSTEM AND SENSE ORGANS

    361.14 Secondary retinal cysts
    361.19 **Other**
          Pseudocyst of retina

361.2 Serous retinal detachment
    Retinal detachment without retinal defect
    Excludes: central serous retinopathy (362.41)
               retinal pigment epithelium detachment (362.42-362.43)

⑤ **361.3 Retinal defects without detachment**
    Excludes: chorioretinal scars after surgery for detachment (363.30-363.35)
               peripheral retinal degeneration without defect (362.60-362.66)

    361.30 **Retinal defect, unspecified**
          Retinal break(s) NOS

    361.31 Round hole of retina without detachment

    361.32 Horseshoe tear of retina without detachment
          Operculum of retina without mention of detachment

    361.33 Multiple defects of retina without detachment

⑤ **361.8 Other forms of retinal detachment**
    361.81 Traction detachment of retina
          Traction detachment with vitreoretinal organization

    361.89 **Other**

361.9 Unspecified retinal detachment

362 Other retinal disorders
    Excludes: chorioretinal scars (363.30-363.35)
               chorioretinitis (363.0-363.2)

⑤ **362.0 Diabetic retinopathy**
    Code first diabetes (250.5)

    362.01 *Background diabetic retinopathy*
          Diabetic retinal microaneurysms
          Diabetic retinopathy NOS

    362.02 *Proliferative diabetic retinopathy*

    362.03 Nonproliferative diabetic retinopathy NOS

    362.04 Mild nonproliferative diabetic retinopathy

    362.05 Moderate nonproliferative diabetic retinopathy

    362.06 Severe nonproliferative diabetic retinopathy

    362.07 Diabetic macular edema
          Diabetic retinal edema
    Note: Code 362.07 must be used with a code for diabetic retinopathy (362.01-362.06)

⑤ **362.1 Other background retinopathy and retinal vascular changes**

    362.10 **Background retinopathy, unspecified**

    362.11 Hypertensive retinopathy

    362.12 Exudative retinopathy
          Coats' syndrome

    362.13 Changes in vascular appearance
          Vascular sheathing of retina
    Use additional code for any associated atherosclerosis (440.8)

    362.14 Retinal microaneurysms NOS

    362.15 Retinal telangiectasia

    362.16 Retinal neovascularization NOS
          Neovascularization:
              choroidal
              subretinal

    362.17 Other intraretinal microvascular abnormalities
          Retinal varices

    362.18 Retinal vasculitis
          Eales' disease   Retinal:
          Retinal: perivasculitis
            arteritis   phlebitis
            endarteritis

 Nonspecific code Unspecified code 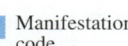 Manifestation code

TABULAR LIST

⑤ **362.2 Other proliferative retinopathy**
    362.21 Retrolental fibroplasia
    362.29 Other nondiabetic proliferative retinopathy

⑤ **362.3 Retinal vascular occlusion**
    362.30 Retinal vascular occlusion, unspecified
    362.31 Central retinal artery occlusion
    362.32 Arterial branch occlusion
    362.33 Partial arterial occlusion
        Hollenhorst plaque
        Retinal microembolism
    362.34 Transient arterial occlusion
        Amaurosis fugax
    362.35 Central retinal vein occlusion
    362.36 Venous tributary (branch) occlusion
    362.37 Venous engorgement
        Occlusion:
            incipient of retinal vein
            partial of retinal vein

⑤ **362.4 Separation of retinal layers**
    Excludes: retinal detachment (serous) (361.2)
                 rhegmatogenous (361.00-361.07)
    362.40 Retinal layer separation, unspecified
    362.41 Central serous retinopathy
    362.42 Serous detachment of retinal pigment epithelium
        Exudative detachment of retinal pigment epithelium
    362.43 Hemorrhagic detachment of retinal pigment epithelium

⑤ **362.5 Degeneration of macula and posterior pole**
    Excludes: degeneration of optic disc (377.21-377.24)
                 hereditary retinal degeneration [dystrophy] (362.70-362.77)
    362.50 Macular degeneration (senile), unspecified
    362.51 Nonexudative senile macular degeneration
        Senile macular degeneration:
            atrophic
            dry
    362.52 Exudative senile macular degeneration
        Kuhnt-Junius degeneration
        Senile macular degeneration:
            disciform
            wet
    362.53 Cystoid macular degeneration
        Cystoid macular edema
    362.54 Macular cyst, hole, or pseudohole
    362.55 Toxic maculopathy
    Use additional E code, if desired, to identify drug, if drug induced
    362.56 Macular puckering
        Preretinal fibrosis
    362.57 Drusen (degenerative)

⑤ **362.6 Peripheral retinal degenerations**
    Excludes: hereditary retinal degeneration [dystrophy] (362.70-362.77)
                 retinal degeneration with retinal defect (361.00-361.07)
    362.60 Peripheral retinal degeneration, unspecified
    362.61 Paving stone degeneration
    362.62 Microcystoid degeneration
        Blessig's cysts   Iwanoff's cysts
    362.63 Lattice degeneration
        Palisade degeneration of retina
    362.64 Senile reticular degeneration
    362.65 Secondary pigmentary degeneration
        Pseudoretinitis pigmentosa

NERVOUS SYSTEM AND SENSE ORGANS

- 362.66 Secondary vitreoretinal degenerations
- ⑤ **362.7 Hereditary retinal dystrophies**
  - 362.70 Hereditary retinal dystrophy, unspecified
  - 362.71 *Retinal dystrophy in systemic or cerebroretinal lipidoses*
    Code first underlying disease, as:
    cerebroretinal lipidoses (330.1)
    systemic lipidoses (272.7)
  - 362.72 *Retinal dystrophy in other systemic disorders and syndromes*
    Code first underlying disease, as:
    Bassen-Kornzweig syndrome (272.5)
    Refsum's disease (356.3)
  - 362.73 Vitreoretinal dystrophies
    Juvenile retinoschisis
  - 362.74 Pigmentary retinal dystrophy
    Retinal dystrophy, albipunctate
    Retinitis pigmentosa
  - 362.75 Other dystrophies primarily involving the sensory retina
    Progressive cone (-rod) dystrophy
    Stargardt's disease
  - 362.76 Dystrophies primarily involving the retinal pigment epithelium
    Fundus flavimaculatus
    Vitelliform dystrophy
  - 362.77 **Dystrophies primarily involving Bruch's membrane**
    Dystrophy:
    hyaline
    pseudoinflammatory foveal
    Hereditary drusen
- ⑤ **362.8 Other retinal disorders**
  - Excludes: chorioretinal inflammations (363.0-363.2)
    chorioretinal scars (363.30-363.35)
  - 362.81 **Retinal hemorrhage**
    Hemorrhage:
    preretinal
    retinal (deep) (superficial)
    subretinal
  - 362.82 Retinal exudates and deposits
  - 362.83 Retinal edema
    Retinal:
    cotton wool spots
    edema (localized) (macular) (peripheral)
  - 362.84 Retinal ischemia
  - 362.85 Retinal nerve fiber bundle defects
  - 362.89 Other retinal disorders
- **362.9 Unspecified retinal disorder**
- **363 Chorioretinal inflammations, scars, and other disorders of choroid**
- ⑤ **363.0 Focal chorioretinitis and focal retinochoroiditis**
  - Excludes: focal chorioretinitis or retinochoroiditis in:
    histoplasmosis (115.02, 115.12, 115.92)
    toxoplasmosis (130.2)
    congenital infection (771.2)
  - 363.00 Focal chorioretinitis, unspecified
    Focal:
    choroiditis or chorioretinitis NOS
    retinitis or retinochoroiditis NOS
  - 363.01 Focal choroiditis and chorioretinitis, juxtapapillary
  - 363.03 Focal choroiditis and chorioretinitis of other posterior pole
  - 363.04 Focal choroiditis and chorioretinitis, peripheral
  - 363.05 Focal retinitis and retinochoroiditis, juxtapapillary
    Neuroretinitis
  - 363.06 Focal retinitis and retinochoroiditis, macular or paramacular
  - 363.07 Focal retinitis and retinochoroiditis of other posterior pole

301

| Add 4th or 5th digit | Nonspecific code | Unspecified code | Manifestation code |

TABULAR LIST

    363.08   **Focal retinitis and retinochoroiditis, peripheral**

⑤ **363.1 Disseminated chorioretinitis and disseminated retinochoroiditis**
> Excludes: *disseminated choroiditis or chorioretinitis in secondary syphilis (091.51)*
> *neurosyphilitic disseminated retinitis or retinochoroiditis (094.83)*
> *retinal (peri)vasculitis (362.18)*

    363.10   **Disseminated chorioretinitis, unspecified**
        Disseminated:
          choroiditis or chorioretinitis NOS
          retinitis or retinochoroiditis NOS

    363.11   **Disseminated choroiditis and chorioretinitis, posterior pole**

    363.12   **Disseminated choroiditis and chorioretinitis, peripheral**

    363.13   **Disseminated choroiditis and chorioretinitis, generalized**
        Code first any underlying disease, as:
          tuberculosis (017.3)

    363.14   **Disseminated retinitis and retinochoroiditis, metastatic**

    363.15   **Disseminated retinitis and retinochoroiditis, pigment epitheliopathy**
        Acute posterior multifocal placoid pigment epitheliopathy

⑤ **363.2 Other and unspecified forms of chorioretinitis and retinochoroiditis**
> Excludes: *panophthalmitis (360.02)*
> *sympathetic uveitis (360.11)*
> *uveitis NOS (364.3)*

    363.20   **Chorioretinitis, unspecified**
        Choroiditis NOS
        Retinitis NOS
        Uveitis, posterior NOS

    363.21   **Pars planitis**
        Posterior cyclitis

    363.22   **Harada's disease**

⑤ **363.3 Chorioretinal scars**
    Scar (postinflammatory) (postsurgical) (posttraumatic):
      choroid
      retina

    363.30   **Chorioretinal scar, unspecified**

    363.31   **Solar retinopathy**

    363.32   **Other macular scars**

    363.33   **Other scars of posterior pole**

    363.34   **Peripheral scars**

    363.35   **Disseminated scars**

⑤ **363.4 Choroidal degenerations**

    363.40   **Choroidal degeneration, unspecified**
        Choroidal sclerosis NOS

    363.41   **Senile atrophy of choroid**

    363.42   **Diffuse secondary atrophy of choroid**

    363.43   **Angioid streaks of choroid**

⑤ **363.5 Hereditary choroidal dystrophies**
    Hereditary choroidal atrophy:
      partial [choriocapillaris]
      total [all vessels]

    363.50   **Hereditary choroidal dystrophy or atrophy, unspecified**

    363.51   **Circumpapillary dystrophy of choroid, partial**

    363.52   **Circumpapillary dystrophy of choroid, total**
        Helicoid dystrophy of choroid

    363.53   **Central dystrophy of choroid, partial**
        Dystrophy, choroidal:
          central areolar
          circinate

    363.54   **Central choroidal atrophy, total**
        Dystrophy, choroidal:
          central gyrate
          serpiginous

NERVOUS SYSTEM AND SENSE ORGANS

- 363.55 Choroideremia
- **363.56** Other diffuse or generalized dystrophy, partial
  Diffuse choroidal sclerosis
- **363.57** Other diffuse or generalized dystrophy, total
  Generalized gyrate atrophy, choroid

⑤ 363.6 Choroidal hemorrhage and rupture
- **363.61** Choroidal hemorrhage, unspecified
- 363.62 Expulsive choroidal hemorrhage
- 363.63 Choroidal rupture

⑤ 363.7 Choroidal detachment
- **363.70** Choroidal detachment, unspecified
- 363.71 Serous choroidal detachment
- 363.72 Hemorrhagic choroidal detachment

363.8 Other disorders of choroid

363.9 Unspecified disorder of choroid

364 Disorders of iris and ciliary body

⑤ 364.0 Acute and subacute iridocyclitis
  Anterior uveitis, acute, subacute
  Cyclitis, acute, subacute
  Iridocyclitis, acute, subacute
  Iritis, acute, subacute

  Excludes: gonococcal (098.41)
    herpes simplex (054.44)
    herpes zoster (053.22)

- **364.00** Acute and subacute iridocyclitis, unspecified
- 364.01 Primary iridocyclitis
- 364.02 Recurrent iridocyclitis
- 364.03 Secondary iridocyclitis, infectious
- 364.04 Secondary iridocyclitis, noninfectious
  Aqueous:
    cells
    fibrin
    flare
- 364.05 Hypopyon

⑤ 364.1 Chronic iridocyclitis

  Excludes: posterior cyclitis (363.21)

- **364.10** Chronic iridocyclitis, unspecified
- **364.11** Chronic iridocyclitis in diseases classified elsewhere
  Code first underlying disease, as:
    sarcoidosis (135)
    tuberculosis (017.3)

  Excludes: syphilitic iridocyclitis (091.52)

⑤ 364.2 Certain types of iridocyclitis

  Excludes: posterior cyclitis (363.21)
    sympathetic uveitis (360.11)

- 364.21 Fuchs' heterochromic cyclitis
- 364.22 Glaucomatocyclitic crises
- 364.23 Lens-induced iridocyclitis
- 364.24 Vogt-Koyanagi syndrome

364.3 Unspecified iridocyclitis
  Uveitis NOS

⑤ 364.4 Vascular disorders of iris and ciliary body
- 364.41 Hyphema
  Hemorrhage of iris or ciliary body
- 364.42 Rubeosis iridis
  Neovascularization of iris or ciliary body

⑤ 364.5 Degenerations of iris and ciliary body

| ■ Add 4th or 5th digit | ■ Nonspecific code | ■ Unspecified code | ■ Manifestation code |

303

TABULAR LIST

- **364.51** Essential or progressive iris atrophy
- **364.52** Iridoschisis
- **364.53** Pigmentary iris degeneration
  Acquired heterochromia of iris
  Pigment dispersion syndrome of iris
  Translucency of iris
- **364.54** Degeneration of pupillary margin
  Atrophy of sphincter of iris
  Ectropion of pigment epithelium of iris
- **364.55** Miotic cysts of pupillary margin
- **364.56** Degenerative changes of chamber angle
- **364.57** Degenerative changes of ciliary body
- **364.59** Other iris atrophy
  Iris atrophy (generalized) (sector shaped)

⑤ **364.6 Cysts of iris, ciliary body, and anterior chamber**
  Excludes: *miotic pupillary cyst (364.55)*
  parasitic cyst (360.13)

- **364.60** Idiopathic cysts
- **364.61** Implantation cysts
  Epithelial down-growth, anterior chamber
  Implantation cysts (surgical) (traumatic)
- **364.62** Exudative cysts of iris or anterior chamber
- **364.63** Primary cyst of pars plana
- **364.64** Exudative cyst of pars plana

⑤ **364.7 Adhesions and disruptions of iris and ciliary body**
  Excludes: *flat anterior chamber (360.34)*

- **364.70** Adhesions of iris, unspecified
  Synechiae (iris) NOS
- **364.71** Posterior synechiae
- **364.72** Anterior synechiae
- **364.73** Goniosynechiae
  Peripheral anterior synechiae
- **364.74** Pupillary membranes
  Iris bombé
  Pupillary:
    occlusion
    seclusion
- **364.75** Pupillary abnormalities
  Deformed pupil   Rupture of sphincter, pupil
  Ectopic pupil
- **364.76** Iridodialysis
- **364.77** Recession of chamber angle

▲ **364.8 Other disorders of iris and ciliary body**

● **364.81** Floppy iris syndrome
  Intraoperative floppy iris syndrome (IFIS)

Use additional E code to identify cause, such as:
  sympatholytics [antiadrenergics] causing adverse effect in therapeutic use (E941.3)

● **364.89** Other disorders of iris and ciliary body
  Prolapse of iris NOS
  Excludes: *prolapse of iris in recent wound (871.1)*

364.9 Unspecified disorder of iris and ciliary body

365 Glaucoma
  Excludes: *blind hypertensive eye [absolute glaucoma] (360.42)*
  congenital glaucoma (743.20-743.22)

⑤ **365.0 Borderline glaucoma [glaucoma suspect]**

- **365.00** Preglaucoma, unspecified

---

304 ● Code new to this edition   ▲ Revision of existing code   ④ ⑤ Fourth or fifth digit required

NERVOUS SYSTEM AND SENSE ORGANS

- **365.01 Open angle with borderline findings**
  Open angle with:
  borderline intraocular pressure
  cupping of optic discs
- **365.02 Anatomical narrow angle**
- **365.03 Steroid responders**
- **365.04 Ocular hypertension**

365.1 Open-angle glaucoma

- **365.10 Open-angle glaucoma, unspecified**
  Wide-angle glaucoma NOS
- **365.11 Primary open angle glaucoma**
  Chronic simple glaucoma
- **365.12 Low tension glaucoma**
- **365.13 Pigmentary glaucoma**
- **365.14 Glaucoma of childhood**
  Infantile or juvenile glaucoma
- **365.15 Residual stage of open angle glaucoma**

365.2 Primary angle-closure glaucoma

- **365.20 Primary angle-closure glaucoma, unspecified**
- **365.21 Intermittent angle-closure glaucoma**
  Angle-closure glaucoma:
  interval
  subacute
- **365.22 Acute angle-closure glaucoma**
- **365.23 Chronic angle-closure glaucoma**
- **365.24 Residual stage of angle-closure glaucoma**

365.3 Corticosteroid-induced glaucoma

- **365.31 Glaucomatous stage**
- **365.32 Residual stage**

365.4 Glaucoma associated with congenital anomalies, dystrophies, and systemic syndromes

- **365.41 *Glaucoma associated with chamber angle anomalies***
  Code first associated disorder, as:
  Axenfeld's anomaly (743.44)
  Rieger's anomaly or syndrome (743.44)
- **365.42 *Glaucoma associated with anomalies of iris***
  Code first associated disorder, as:
  aniridia (743.45)
  essential iris atrophy (364.51)
- **365.43 *Glaucoma associated with other anterior segment anomalies***
  Code first associated disorder, as:
  microcornea (743.41)
- **365.44 *Glaucoma associated with systemic syndromes***
  Code first associated disease, as:
  neurofibromatosis (237.7)
  Sturge-Weber (-Dimitri) syndrome (759.6)

365.5 Glaucoma associated with disorders of the lens

- **365.51 Phacolytic glaucoma**
  Use additional code for associated hypermature cataract (366.18)
- **365.52 Pseudoexfoliation glaucoma**
  Use additional code for associated pseudoexfoliation of capsule (366.11)
- **365.59 Glaucoma associated with other lens disorders**
  Use additional code for associated disorder, as:
  dislocation of lens (379.33-379.34)
  spherophakia (743.36)

365.6 Glaucoma associated with other ocular disorders

- **365.60 Glaucoma associated with unspecified ocular disorder**
- **365.61 Glaucoma associated with pupillary block**
  Use additional code for associated disorder, as:
  seclusion of pupil [iris bombé] (364.74)

Add 4th or 5th digit | Nonspecific code | Unspecified code | Manifestation code

TABULAR LIST

365.62 Glaucoma associated with ocular inflammations
Use additional code for associated disorder, as:
  glaucomatocyclitic crises (364.22)
  iridocyclitis (364.0-364.3)

365.63 Glaucoma associated with vascular disorders
Use additional code for associated disorder, as:
  central retinal vein occlusion (362.35)
  hyphema (364.41)

365.64 Glaucoma associated with tumors or cysts
Use additional code for associated disorder, as:
  benign neoplasm (224.0-224.9)
  epithelial down-growth (364.61)
  malignant neoplasm (190.0-190.9)

365.65 Glaucoma associated with ocular trauma
Use additional code for associated condition, as:
  contusion of globe (921.3)
  recession of chamber angle (364.77)

⑤ **365.8 Other specified forms of glaucoma**
  365.81 Hypersecretion glaucoma
  365.82 Glaucoma with increased episcleral venous pressure
  365.83 Aqueous misdirection
    Malignant glaucoma
  365.89 Other specified glaucoma

365.9 Unspecified glaucoma

366 Cataract
  Excludes: congenital cataract (743.30-743.34)

⑤ **366.0 Infantile, juvenile, and presenile cataract**
  366.00 Nonsenile cataract, unspecified
  366.01 Anterior subcapsular polar cataract
  366.02 Posterior subcapsular polar cataract
  366.03 Cortical, lamellar, or zonular cataract
  366.04 Nuclear cataract
  366.09 Other and combined forms of nonsenile cataract

⑤ **366.1 Senile cataract**
  366.10 Senile cataract, unspecified
  366.11 Pseudoexfoliation of lens capsule
  366.12 Incipient cataract
    Cataract: Water clefts
      coronary
      immature NOS
      punctate
  366.13 Anterior subcapsular polar senile cataract
  366.14 Posterior subcapsular polar senile cataract
  366.15 Cortical senile cataract
  366.16 Nuclear sclerosis
    Cataracta brunescens
    Nuclear cataract
  366.17 Total or mature cataract
  366.18 Hypermature cataract
    Morgagni cataract
  366.19 Other and combined forms of senile cataract

⑤ **366.2 Traumatic cataract**
  366.20 Traumatic cataract, unspecified
  366.21 Localized traumatic opacities
    Vossius' ring
  366.22 Total traumatic cataract
  366.23 Partially resolved traumatic cataract

306 ● Code new   ▲ Revision of   ④ ⑤ Fourth or fifth
       to this edition   existing code   digit required

NERVOUS SYSTEM AND SENSE ORGANS

- ⑤ **366.3 Cataract secondary to ocular disorders**
  - **366.30** Cataracts complicata, unspecified
  - **366.31** Glaucomatous flecks (subcapsular)
    Code first underlying glaucoma (365.0-365.9)
  - **366.32** Cataract in inflammatory disorders
    Code first underlying condition, as:
    chronic choroiditis (363.0-363.2)
  - **366.33** Cataract with neovascularization
    Code first underlying condition, as:
    chronic iridocyclitis (364.10)
  - **366.34** Cataract in degenerative disorders
    Sunflower cataract
    Code first underlying condition, as:
    chalcosis (360.24)
    degenerative myopia (360.21)
    pigmentary retinal dystrophy (362.74)
- ⑤ **366.4 Cataract associated with other disorders**
  - **366.41** Diabetic cataract
    Code first diabetes (250.5)
  - **366.42** Tetanic cataract
    Code first underlying disease, as:
    calcinosis (275.4)
    hypoparathyroidism (252.1)
  - **366.43** Myotonic cataract
    Code first underlying disorder (359.21-359.29)
  - **366.44** Cataract associated with other syndromes
    Code first underlying condition, as:
    craniofacial dysostosis (756.0)
    galactosemia (271.1)
  - 366.45 Toxic cataract
    Drug-induced cataract
    Use additional E code, if desired, to identify drug or other toxic substance
  - 366.46 Cataract associated with radiation and other physical influences
    Use additional E code, if desired, to identify cause
- ⑤ **366.5 After-cataract**
  - **366.50** After-cataract, unspecified
    Secondary cataract NOS
  - 366.51 Soemmering's ring
  - **366.52** Other after-cataract, not obscuring vision
  - 366.53 After-cataract, obscuring vision
- **366.8 Other cataract**
  Calcification of lens
- **366.9 Unspecified cataract**

367 Disorders of refraction and accommodation
- 367.0 Hypermetropia
  Far-sightedness
  Hyperopia
- 367.1 Myopia
  Near-sightedness
- ⑤ 367.2 Astigmatism
  - **367.20** Astigmatism, unspecified
  - 367.21 Regular astigmatism
  - 367.22 Irregular astigmatism
- ⑤ 367.3 Anisometropia and aniseikonia
  - 367.31 Anisometropia
  - 367.32 Aniseikonia
- 367.4 Presbyopia
- ⑤ 367.5 Disorders of accommodation
  - 367.51 Paresis of accommodation
    Cycloplegia

🟥 Add 4th or 5th digit	🟧 Nonspecific code	🟨 Unspecified code	🟦 Manifestation code

TABULAR LIST

- 367.52 Total or complete internal ophthalmoplegia
- 367.53 Spasm of accommodation
- ⑤ 367.8 **Other disorders of refraction and accommodation**
  - 367.81 Transient refractive change
  - **367.89** Other
    Drug-induced disorders of refraction and accommodation
    Toxic disorders of refraction and accommodation
- **367.9** Unspecified disorder of refraction and accommodation

368 Visual disturbances
Excludes: *electrophysiological disturbances (794.11-794.14)*

- ⑤ 368.0 **Amblyopia ex anopsia**
  - **368.00** Amblyopia, unspecified
  - 368.01 Strabismic amblyopia
    Suppression amblyopia
  - 368.02 Deprivation amblyopia
  - 368.03 Refractive amblyopia
- ⑤ 368.1 **Subjective visual disturbances**
  - **368.10** Subjective visual disturbance, unspecified
  - 368.11 Sudden visual loss
  - 368.12 Transient visual loss
    Concentric fading
    Scintillating scotoma
  - 368.13 Visual discomfort
    Asthenopia   Photophobia
    Eye strain
  - 368.14 Visual distortions of shape and size
    Macropsia   Micropsia
    Metamorphopsia
  - **368.15** Other visual distortions and entoptic phenomena
    Photopsia   Visual halos
    Refractive:
      diplopia
      polyopia
  - 368.16 Psychophysical visual disturbances
    Visual:
      agnosia
      disorientation syndrome
      hallucinations
- 368.2 **Diplopia**
  Double vision
- ⑤ 368.3 **Other disorders of binocular vision**
  - **368.30** Binocular vision disorder, unspecified
  - 368.31 Suppression of binocular vision
  - 368.32 Simultaneous visual perception without fusion
  - 368.33 Fusion with defective stereopsis
  - 368.34 Abnormal retinal correspondence
- ⑤ 368.4 **Visual field defects**
  - **368.40** Visual field defect, unspecified
  - 368.41 Scotoma involving central area
    Scotoma:
      central
      centrocecal
      paracentral
  - 368.42 Scotoma of blind spot area
    Enlarged: Paracecal scotoma
      angioscotoma
      blind spot

● Code new to this edition   ▲ Revision of existing code   ④ ⑤ Fourth or fifth digit required

NERVOUS SYSTEM AND SENSE ORGANS

- **368.43** **Sector or arcuate defects**
  Scotoma:
    arcuate
    Bjerrum
    Seidel

- **368.44** **Other localized visual field defect**
  Scotoma: Visual field defect:
    NOS   nasal step
    ring   peripheral

- **368.45** **Generalized contraction or constriction**

- **368.46** **Homonymous bilateral field defects**
  Hemianopsia (altitudinal) (homonymous)
  Quadrant anopia

- **368.47** **Heteronymous bilateral field defects**
  Hemianopsia:
    binasal
    bitemporal

- **368.5** **Color vision deficiencies**
  Color blindness

  - **368.51** **Protan defect**
    Protanomaly
    Protanopia

  - **368.52** **Deutan defect**
    Deuteranomaly
    Deuteranopia

  - **368.53** **Tritan defect**
    Tritanomaly
    Tritanopia

  - **368.54** **Achromatopsia**
    Monochromatism (cone) (rod)

  - **368.55** **Acquired color vision deficiencies**

  - **368.59** **Other color vision deficiencies**

- **368.6** **Night blindness**
  Nyctalopia

  - **368.60** **Night blindness, unspecified**

  - **368.61** **Congenital night blindness**
    Hereditary night blindness
    Oguchi's disease

  - **368.62** **Acquired night blindness**

    Excludes: that due to vitamin A deficiency (264.5)

  - **368.63** **Abnormal dark adaptation curve**
    Abnormal threshold of cones or rods
    Delayed adaptation of cones or rods

  - **368.69** **Other night blindness**

- **368.8** **Other specified visual disturbances**
  Blurred vision NOS

- **368.9** **Unspecified visual disturbance**

TABULAR LIST

369 Blindness and low vision

Note: Visual impairment refers to a functional limitation of the eye (e.g., limited visual acuity or visual field). It should be distinguished from visual disability, indicating a limitation of the abilities of the individual (e.g., limited reading skills, vocational skills), and from visual handicap, indicating a limitation of personal and socioeconomic independence (e.g., limited mobility, limited employability.)

The levels of impairment defined in the table in this section are based on the recommendations of the WHO Study Group on Prevention of Blindness (Geneva, November 6-10, 1972; WHO Technical Report Series 518), and of the International Council of Ophthalmology (1976).

Note that definitions of blindness vary in different settings.

For international reporting WHO defines blindness as profound impairment. This definition can be applied to blindness of one eye (369.1, 369.6) and to blindness of the individual (369.0).

For determination of benefits in the U.S.A., the definition of legal blindness as severe impairment is often used. This definition applies to blindness of the individual only.

Excludes: *correctable impaired vision due to refractive errors (367.0-367.9)*

⑤ **369.0 Profound impairment, both eyes**

- **369.00** Impairment level not further specified
  Blindness:
  NOS according to WHO definition
  both eyes
- **369.01** Better eye: total impairment;
  lesser eye: total impairment
- **369.02** Better eye: near-total impairment;
  lesser eye: not further specified
- **369.03** Better eye: near-total impairment;
  lesser eye: total impairment
- **369.04** Better eye: near-total impairment;
  lesser eye: near-total impairment
- **369.05** Better eye: profound impairment;
  lesser eye: not further specified
- **369.06** Better eye: profound impairment;
  lesser eye: total impairment
- **369.07** Better eye: profound impairment;
  lesser eye: near-total impairment
- **369.08** Better eye: profound impairment;
  lesser eye: profound impairment

⑤ **369.1 Moderate or severe impairment, better eye, profound impairment lesser eye**

- **369.10** Impairment level not further specified
  Blindness, one eye, low vision other eye
- **369.11** Better eye: severe impairment;
  lesser eye: blind, not further specified
- **369.12** Better eye: severe impairment;
  lesser eye: total impairment
- **369.13** Better eye: severe impairment;
  lesser eye: near-total impairment
- **369.14** Better eye: severe impairment;
  lesser eye: profound impairment
- **369.15** Better eye: moderate impairment;
  lesser eye: blind, not further specified
- **369.16** Better eye: moderate impairment;
  lesser eye: total impairment
- **369.17** Better eye: moderate impairment;
  lesser eye: near-total impairment
- **369.18** Better eye: moderate impairment;
  lesser eye: profound impairment

⑤ **369.2 Moderate or severe impairment, both eyes**

- **369.20** Impairment level not further specified
  Low vision, both eyes NOS

NERVOUS SYSTEM AND SENSE ORGANS

- **369.21** Better eye: severe impairment;
  lesser eye: not further specified
- 369.22 Better eye: severe impairment;
  lesser eye: severe impairment
- **369.23** Better eye: moderate impairment;
  lesser eye: not further specified
- 369.24 Better eye: moderate impairment;
  lesser eye: severe impairment
- 369.25 Better eye: moderate impairment;
  lesser eye: moderate impairment

369.3 Unqualified visual loss, both eyes
  Excludes: blindness NOS:
    legal [U.S.A. definition] (369.4)
    WHO definition (369.00)

369.4 Legal blindness, as defined in U.S.A.
  Blindness NOS according to U.S.A. definition
  Excludes: legal blindness with specification of impairment level (369.01-369.08, 369.11-369.14, 369.21-369.22)

⑤ 369.6 Profound impairment, one eye
- **369.60** Impairment level not further specified
  Blindness, one eye
- **369.61** One eye: total impairment; other eye: not specified
- 369.62 One eye: total impairment; other eye: near-normal vision
- 369.63 One eye: total impairment; other eye: normal vision
- **369.64** One eye: near-total impairment; other eye: not specified
- 369.65 One eye: near-total impairment; other eye: near-normal vision
- 369.66 One eye: near-total impairment; other eye: normal vision
- **369.67** One eye: profound impairment; other eye: not specified
- 369.68 One eye: profound impairment; other eye: near-normal vision
- 369.69 One eye: profound impairment; other eye: normal vision

⑤ 369.7 Moderate or severe impairment, one eye
- **369.70** Impairment level not further specified
  Low vision, one eye
- **369.71** One eye: severe impairment; other eye: not specified
- 369.72 One eye: severe impairment; other eye: near-normal vision
- 369.73 One eye: severe impairment; other eye: normal vision
- **369.74** One eye: moderate impairment; other eye: not specified
- 369.75 One eye: moderate impairment; other eye: near-normal vision
- 369.76 One eye: moderate impairment; other eye: normal vision

369.8 Unqualified visual loss, one eye

369.9 Unspecified visual loss

TABULAR LIST

Classification		LEVELS OF VISUAL IMPAIRMENT					Additional Descriptors which may be encountered
"legal"	WHO	Visual Acuity and/or Visual Field Limitation (whichever is worse)					
LEGAL BLINDNESS (USA) both eyes	(NEAR-) NORMAL VISION	**RANGE OF NORMAL VISION** 20/10 — 0.7	20/13 — 0.6	20/16 — 0.5	20/20 — 0.4	20/25 — 0.8	

(NEAR-) NORMAL VISION:
- **RANGE OF NORMAL VISION**: 20/10 (0.7), 20/13 (0.6), 20/16 (0.5), 20/20 (0.4), 20/25 (0.8)
- **NEAR-NORMAL VISION**: 20/30 (0.7), 20/40 (0.6), 20/50 (0.5), 20/60 (0.4), 20/60 (0.4)

LOW VISION:
- **MODERATE VISUAL IMPAIRMENT**: 20/70, 20/80 (0.25), 20/100 (0.20), 20/125 (0.16), 20/160 (0.12) — *Moderate low vision*
- **SEVERE VISUAL IMPAIRMENT**: 20/200 (0.10), 20/250 (0.08), 20/320 (0.06), 20/400 (0.05) — *Severe low vision, "legal blindness"*
  Visual Field: 20 degrees or less

BLINDNESS (WHO one or both eyes):
- **PROFOUND VISUAL IMPAIRMENT**: 20/500 (0.04), 20/630 (0.03), 20/800 (0.025), 20/1000 (0.02) — *Profound low vision, moderate blindness*
  Count Fingers at: less than 3 m (10ft)
  Visual Field: 10 degrees or less
- **NEAR-TOTAL VISUAL IMPAIRMENT** — *Severe blindness / Near-Total blindness*
  Visual Acuity: less than 0.02 (20/1000)
  Count Fingers at: 1 m (3 ft) or less
  Hand Movements: 5m (15ft) or less
  Light projection, light perception
  Visual Field: 5 degrees or less
- **TOTAL VISUAL IMPAIRMENT** — *Total blindness*
  No light perception (NLP)

Visual acuity refers to best achievable acuity with correction
Non-listed Snellen fractions may be classified by converting to the nearest decimal equivalent, e.g., 10/200=0.05, 6/30=0.20
CF (count fingers) without designation of distance, may be classified to profound impairment
HM (hand motion) without designation of distance, may be classified to near-total impairment.
Visual field measurements refer to the largest field diameter for a 1/100 white test object.

370 Keratitis

⑤ **370.0 Corneal ulcer**
    Excludes: that due to vitamin A deficiency (264.3)
- **370.00** Corneal ulcer, unspecified
- **370.01** Marginal corneal ulcer
- **370.02** Ring corneal ulcer
- **370.03** Central corneal ulcer
- **370.04** Hypopyon ulcer
      Serpiginous ulcer
- **370.05** Mycotic corneal ulcer
- **370.06** Perforated corneal ulcer
- **370.07** Mooren's ulcer

⑤ **370.2 Superficial keratitis without conjunctivitis**
    Excludes: dendritic [herpes simplex] keratitis (054.42)
- **370.20** Superficial keratitis, unspecified
- **370.21** Punctate keratitis
      Thygeson's superficial punctate keratitis
- **370.22** Macular keratitis
      Keratitis: areolar, nummular
      Keratitis: stellate, striate

● Code new to this edition   ▲ Revision of existing code   ④ ⑤ Fourth or fifth digit required

NERVOUS SYSTEM AND SENSE ORGANS

- **370.23** Filamentary keratitis
- **370.24** Photokeratitis
  Snow blindness
  Welders' keratitis

⑤ **370.3 Certain types of keratoconjunctivitis**

- **370.31** Phlyctenular keratoconjunctivitis
  Phlyctenulosis

  Use additional code for any associated tuberculosis (017.3)

- **370.32** Limbar and corneal involvement in vernal conjunctivitis
  Use additional code for vernal conjunctivitis (372.13)

- **370.33** Keratoconjunctivitis sicca, not specified as Sjögren's

  Excludes: Sjögren's syndrome (710.2)

- **370.34** Exposure keratoconjunctivitis
- **370.35** Neurotrophic keratoconjunctivitis

⑤ **370.4 Other and unspecified keratoconjunctivitis**

- **370.40** Keratoconjunctivitis, unspecified
  Superficial keratitis with conjunctivitis NOS

- **370.44** Keratitis or keratoconjunctivitis in exanthema
  Code first underlying condition (050.0-052.9)

  Excludes: herpes simplex (054.43)
  herpes zoster (053.21)
  measles (055.71)

- **370.49** Other

  Excludes: epidemic keratoconjunctivitis (077.1)

⑤ **370.5 Interstitial and deep keratitis**

- **370.50** Interstitial keratitis, unspecified
- **370.52** Diffuse interstitial keratitis
  Cogan's syndrome
- **370.54** Sclerosing keratitis
- **370.55** Corneal abscess
- **370.59** Other

  Excludes: disciform herpes simplex keratitis (054.43)
  syphilitic keratitis (090.3)

⑤ **370.6 Corneal neovascularization**

- **370.60** Corneal neovascularization, unspecified
- **370.61** Localized vascularization of cornea
- **370.62** Pannus (corneal)
- **370.63** Deep vascularization of cornea
- **370.64** Ghost vessels (corneal)

370.8 Other forms of keratitis

370.9 Unspecified keratitis

371 Corneal opacity and other disorders of cornea

⑤ **371.0 Corneal scars and opacities**

Excludes: that due to vitamin A deficiency (264.6)

- **371.00** Corneal opacity, unspecified
  Corneal scar NOS
- **371.01** Minor opacity of cornea
  Corneal nebula
- **371.02** Peripheral opacity of cornea
  Corneal macula not interfering with central vision
- **371.03** Central opacity of cornea
  Corneal:
    leucoma interfering with central vision
    macula interfering with central vision
- **371.04** Adherent leucoma
- **371.05** Phthisical cornea
  Code first underlying tuberculosis (017.3)

| | Add 4th or 5th digit | | Nonspecific code | | Unspecified code | | Manifestation code |

TABULAR LIST

- ⑤ **371.1 Corneal pigmentations and deposits**
  - **371.10 Corneal deposit, unspecified**
  - 371.11 **Anterior pigmentations**
    Stähli's lines
  - 371.12 **Stromal pigmentations**
    Hematocornea
  - 371.13 **Posterior pigmentations**
    Krukenberg spindle
  - 371.14 **Kayser-Fleischer ring**
  - **371.15 Other deposits associated with metabolic disorders**
  - 371.16 **Argentous deposits**

- ⑤ **371.2 Corneal edema**
  - **371.20 Corneal edema, unspecified**
  - 371.21 **Idiopathic corneal edema**
  - 371.22 **Secondary corneal edema**
  - 371.23 **Bullous keratopathy**
  - 371.24 **Corneal edema due to wearing of contact lenses**

- ⑤ **371.3 Changes of corneal membranes**
  - **371.30 Corneal membrane change, unspecified**
  - 371.31 **Folds and rupture of Bowman's membrane**
  - 371.32 **Folds in Descemet's membrane**
  - 371.33 **Rupture in Descemet's membrane**

- ⑤ **371.4 Corneal degenerations**
  - **371.40 Corneal degeneration, unspecified**
  - 371.41 **Senile corneal changes**
    Arcus senilis
    Hassall-Henle bodies
  - 371.42 **Recurrent erosion of cornea**
    Excludes: Mooren's ulcer (370.07)
  - 371.43 **Band-shaped keratopathy**
  - **371.44 Other calcerous degenerations of cornea**
  - 371.45 **Keratomalacia NOS**
    Excludes: that due to vitamin A deficiency (264.4)
  - 371.46 **Nodular degeneration of cornea**
    Salzmann's nodular dystrophy
  - 371.48 **Peripheral degenerations of cornea**
    Marginal degeneration of cornea [Terrien's]
  - **371.49 Other**
    Discrete colliquative keratopathy

- ⑤ **371.5 Hereditary corneal dystrophies**
  - **371.50 Corneal dystrophy, unspecified**
  - 371.51 **Juvenile epithelial corneal dystrophy**
  - **371.52 Other anterior corneal dystrophies**
    Corneal dystrophy:
      microscopic cystic
      ring-like
  - 371.53 **Granular corneal dystrophy**
  - 371.54 **Lattice corneal dystrophy**
  - 371.55 **Macular corneal dystrophy**
  - **371.56 Other stromal corneal dystrophies**
    Crystalline corneal dystrophy
  - 371.57 **Endothelial corneal dystrophy**
    Combined corneal dystrophy
    Cornea guttata
    Fuchs' endothelial dystrophy
  - **371.58 Other posterior corneal dystrophies**
    Polymorphous corneal dystrophy

● Code new to this edition ▲ Revision of existing code ④ ⑤ Fourth or fifth digit required

NERVOUS SYSTEM AND SENSE ORGANS

- ⑤ **371.6 Keratoconus**
  - **371.60** Keratoconus, unspecified
  - 371.61 Keratoconus, stable condition
  - 371.62 Keratoconus, acute hydrops
- ⑤ **371.7 Other corneal deformities**
  - **371.70** Corneal deformity, unspecified
  - 371.71 Corneal ectasia
  - 371.72 Descemetocele
  - 371.73 Corneal staphyloma
- ⑤ **371.8 Other corneal disorders**
  - 371.81 Corneal anesthesia and hypoesthesia
  - 371.82 Corneal disorder due to contact lens
    - Excludes: corneal edema due to contact lens (371.24)
  - **371.89** Other
- **371.9** Unspecified corneal disorder

372 Disorders of conjunctiva
  - Excludes: keratoconjunctivitis (370.3-370.4)

- ⑤ **372.0 Acute conjunctivitis**
  - **372.00** Acute conjunctivitis, unspecified
  - 372.01 Serous conjunctivitis, except viral
    - Excludes: viral conjunctivitis NOS (077.9)
  - 372.02 Acute follicular conjunctivitis
    Conjunctival folliculosis NOS
    - Excludes: conjunctivitis:
      - adenoviral (acute follicular) (077.3)
      - epidemic hemorrhagic (077.4)
      - inclusion (077.0)
      - Newcastle (077.8)
      - epidemic keratoconjunctivitis (077.1)
      - pharyngoconjunctival fever (077.2)
  - **372.03** Other mucopurulent conjunctivitis
    Catarrhal conjunctivitis
    - Excludes: blennorrhea neonatorum (gonococcal) (098.40)
      - neonatal conjunctivitis (771.6)
      - ophthalmia neonatorum NOS (771.6)
  - 372.04 Pseudomembranous conjunctivitis
    Membranous conjunctivitis
    - Excludes: diphtheritic conjunctivitis (032.81)
  - 372.05 Acute atopic conjunctivitis
- ⑤ **372.1 Chronic conjunctivitis**
  - **372.10** Chronic conjunctivitis, unspecified
  - 372.11 Simple chronic conjunctivitis
  - 372.12 Chronic follicular conjunctivitis
  - 372.13 Vernal conjunctivitis
  - **372.14** Other chronic allergic conjunctivitis
  - **372.15** *Parasitic conjunctivitis*
    Code first underlying disease, as:
    - filariasis (125.0-125.9)
    - mucocutaneous leishmaniasis (085.5)
- ⑤ **372.2 Blepharoconjunctivitis**
  - **372.20** Blepharoconjunctivitis, unspecified
  - 372.21 Angular blepharoconjunctivitis
  - 372.22 Contact blepharoconjunctivitis
- ⑤ **372.3 Other and unspecified conjunctivitis**
  - **372.30** Conjunctivitis, unspecified

| ■ Add 4th or 5th digit | ■ Nonspecific code | ■ Unspecified code | ■ Manifestation code |

315

TABULAR LIST

372.31 Rosacea conjunctivitis
Code first underlying rosacea dermatitis (695.3)

372.33 Conjunctivitis in mucocutaneous disease
Code first underlying disease, as:
erythema multiforme (695.1)
Reiter's disease (099.3)

Excludes: ocular pemphigoid (694.61)

372.39 Other

372.4 Pterygium

Excludes: pseudopterygium (372.52)

372.40 Pterygium, unspecified
372.41 Peripheral pterygium, stationary
372.42 Peripheral pterygium, progressive
372.43 Central pterygium
372.44 Double pterygium
372.45 Recurrent pterygium

372.5 Conjunctival degenerations and deposits

372.50 Conjunctival degeneration, unspecified
372.51 Pinguecula
372.52 Pseudopterygium
372.53 Conjunctival xerosis

Excludes: conjunctival xerosis due to vitamin A deficiency (264.0, 264.1, 264.7)

372.54 Conjunctival concretions
372.55 Conjunctival pigmentations
Conjunctival argyrosis
372.56 Conjunctival deposits

372.6 Conjunctival scars

372.61 Granuloma of conjunctiva
372.62 Localized adhesions and strands of conjunctiva
372.63 Symblepharon
Extensive adhesions of conjunctiva
372.64 Scarring of conjunctiva
Contraction of eye socket (after enucleation)

372.7 Conjunctival vascular disorders and cysts

372.71 Hyperemia of conjunctiva
372.72 Conjunctival hemorrhage
Hyposphagma
Subconjunctival hemorrhage
372.73 Conjunctival edema
Chemosis of conjunctiva
Subconjunctival edema
372.74 Vascular abnormalities of conjunctiva
Aneurysm(ata) of conjunctiva
372.75 Conjunctival cysts

372.8 Other disorders of conjunctiva

372.81 Conjunctivochalasis
372.89 Other disorders of conjunctiva

372.9 Unspecified disorder of conjunctiva

373 Inflammation of eyelids

373.0 Blepharitis

Excludes: blepharoconjunctivitis (372.20-372.22)

373.00 Blepharitis, unspecified
373.01 Ulcerative blepharitis
373.02 Squamous blepharitis

373.1 Hordeolum and other deep inflammation of eyelid

● Code new to this edition   ▲ Revision of existing code   ④ ⑤ Fourth or fifth digit required

NERVOUS SYSTEM AND SENSE ORGANS

  373.11 Hordeolum externum
    Hordeolum NOS
    Stye

  373.12 Hordeolum internum
    Infection of meibomian gland

  373.13 Abscess of eyelid
    Furuncle of eyelid

373.2 Chalazion
  Meibomian (gland) cyst
  [Excludes:] *infected meibomian gland (373.12)*

⑤ **373.3 Noninfectious dermatoses of eyelid**

  373.31 Eczematous dermatitis of eyelid

  373.32 Contact and allergic dermatitis of eyelid

  373.33 Xeroderma of eyelid

  373.34 Discoid lupus erythematosus of eyelid

373.4 Infective dermatitis of eyelid of types resulting in deformity
  Code first underlying disease, as:
   leprosy (030.0-030.9)
   lupus vulgaris (tuberculous) (017.0)
   yaws (102.0-102.9)

373.5 Other infective dermatitis of eyelid
  Code first underlying disease, as:
   actinomycosis (039.3)
   impetigo (684)
   mycotic dermatitis (110.0-111.9)
   vaccinia (051.0)
   postvaccination (999.0)
  [Excludes:] *herpes:*
    simplex (054.41)
    zoster (053.20)

373.6 Parasitic infestation of eyelid
  Code first underlying disease, as:
   leishmaniasis (085.0-085.9)
   loiasis (125.2)
   onchocerciasis (125.3)
   pediculosis (132.0)

373.8 Other inflammations of eyelids

373.9 Unspecified inflammation of eyelid

374 Other disorders of eyelids

 ⑤ **374.0 Entropion and trichiasis of eyelid**
   374.00 Entropion, unspecified
   374.01 Senile entropion
   374.02 Mechanical entropion
   374.03 Spastic entropion
   374.04 Cicatricial entropion
   374.05 Trichiasis without entropion

 ⑤ **374.1 Ectropion**
   374.10 Ectropion, unspecified
   374.11 Senile ectropion
   374.12 Mechanical ectropion
   374.13 Spastic ectropion
   374.14 Cicatricial ectropion

 ⑤ **374.2 Lagophthalmos**
   374.20 Lagophthalmos, unspecified
   374.21 Paralytic lagophthalmos
   374.22 Mechanical lagophthalmos
   374.23 Cicatricial lagophthalmos

 ⑤ **374.3 Ptosis of eyelid**

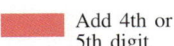 Add 4th or 5th digit   Nonspecific code   Unspecified code   Manifestation code

317

TABULAR LIST

- **374.30** Ptosis of eyelid, unspecified
- **374.31** Paralytic ptosis
- **374.32** Myogenic ptosis
- **374.33** Mechanical ptosis
- **374.34** Blepharochalasis
  Pseudoptosis

⑤ **374.4 Other disorders affecting eyelid function**

Excludes: blepharoclonus (333.81)
blepharospasm (333.81)
facial nerve palsy (351.0)
third nerve palsy or paralysis (378.51-378.52)
tic (psychogenic) (307.20-307.23)
  organic (333.3)

- **374.41** Lid retraction or lag
- **374.43** Abnormal innervation syndrome
  Jaw-blinking
  Paradoxical facial movements
- **374.44** Sensory disorders
- **374.45** Other sensorimotor disorders
  Deficient blink reflex
- **374.46** Blepharophimosis
  Ankyloblepharon

⑤ **374.5 Degenerative disorders of eyelid and periocular area**

- **374.50** Degenerative disorder of eyelid, unspecified
- **374.51** Xanthelasma
  Xanthoma (planum) (tuberosum) of eyelid
  Code first underlying condition (272.0-272.9)
- **374.52** Hyperpigmentation of eyelid
  Chloasma
  Dyspigmentation
- **374.53** Hypopigmentation of eyelid
  Vitiligo of eyelid
- **374.54** Hypertrichosis of eyelid
- **374.55** Hypotrichosis of eyelid
  Madarosis of eyelid
- **374.56** Other degenerative disorders of skin affecting eyelid

⑤ **374.8 Other disorders of eyelid**

- **374.81** Hemorrhage of eyelid

Excludes: black eye (921.0)

- **374.82** Edema of eyelid
  Hyperemia of eyelid
- **374.83** Elephantiasis of eyelid
- **374.84** Cysts of eyelids
  Sebaceous cyst of eyelid
- **374.85** Vascular anomalies of eyelid
- **374.86** Retained foreign body of eyelid
- **374.87** Dermatochalasis
- **374.89** Other disorders of eyelid

374.9 Unspecified disorder of eyelid

375 Disorders of lacrimal system

⑤ **375.0 Dacryoadenitis**

- **375.00** Dacryoadenitis, unspecified
- **375.01** Acute dacryoadenitis
- **375.02** Chronic dacryoadenitis
- **375.03** Chronic enlargement of lacrimal gland

⑤ **375.1 Other disorders of lacrimal gland**

- **375.11** Dacryops

● Code new to this edition ▲ Revision of existing code ④ ⑤ Fourth or fifth digit required

NERVOUS SYSTEM AND SENSE ORGANS

- **375.12** Other lacrimal cysts and cystic degeneration
- 375.13 Primary lacrimal atrophy
- 375.14 Secondary lacrimal atrophy
- **375.15** Tear film insufficiency, unspecified
   Dry eye syndrome
- 375.16 Dislocation of lacrimal gland
- ⑤ 375.2 Epiphora
  - **375.20** Epiphora, unspecified as to cause
  - 375.21 Epiphora due to excess lacrimation
  - 375.22 Epiphora due to insufficient drainage
- ⑤ 375.3 Acute and unspecified inflammation of lacrimal passages
  - Excludes: neonatal dacryocystitis (771.6)
  - **375.30** Dacryocystitis, unspecified
  - 375.31 Acute canaliculitis, lacrimal
  - 375.32 Acute dacryocystitis
     Acute peridacryocystitis
  - 375.33 Phlegmonous dacryocystitis
- ⑤ 375.4 Chronic inflammation of lacrimal passages
  - 375.41 Chronic canaliculitis
  - 375.42 Chronic dacryocystitis
  - 375.43 Lacrimal mucocele
- ⑤ 375.5 Stenosis and insufficiency of lacrimal passages
  - 375.51 Eversion of lacrimal punctum
  - 375.52 Stenosis of lacrimal punctum
  - 375.53 Stenosis of lacrimal canaliculi
  - 375.54 Stenosis of lacrimal sac
  - 375.55 Obstruction of nasolacrimal duct, neonatal
  - Excludes: congenital anomaly of nasolacrimal duct (743.65)
  - 375.56 Stenosis of nasolacrimal duct, acquired
  - 375.57 Dacryolith
- ⑤ 375.6 Other changes of lacrimal passages
  - 375.61 Lacrimal fistula
  - **375.69** Other
- ⑤ 375.8 Other disorders of lacrimal system
  - 375.81 Granuloma of lacrimal passages
  - **375.89** Other
- **375.9** Unspecified disorder of lacrimal system
- **376** Disorders of the orbit
  - ⑤ 376.0 Acute inflammation of orbit
    - **376.00** Acute inflammation of orbit, unspecified
    - 376.01 Orbital cellulitis
       Abscess of orbit
    - 376.02 Orbital periostitis
    - 376.03 Orbital osteomyelitis
    - 376.04 Tenonitis
  - ⑤ 376.1 Chronic inflammatory disorders of orbit
    - **376.10** Chronic inflammation of orbit, unspecified
    - 376.11 Orbital granuloma
       Pseudotumor (inflammatory) of orbit
    - 376.12 Orbital myositis
    - **376.13** Parasitic infestation of orbit
       Code first underlying disease, as:
         hydatid infestation of orbit (122.3, 122.6, 122.9)
         myiasis of orbit (134.0)

| ■ Add 4th or 5th digit | ■ Nonspecific code | ■ Unspecified code | ■ Manifestation code |

319

TABULAR LIST

- ⑤ **376.2 Endocrine exophthalmos**
  Code first underlying thyroid disorder (242.0-242.9)
  - **376.21** Thyrotoxic exophthalmos
  - **376.22** Exophthalmic ophthalmoplegia
- ⑤ **376.3 Other exophthalmic conditions**
  - **376.30** Exophthalmos, unspecified
  - 376.31 Constant exophthalmos
  - 376.32 Orbital hemorrhage
  - 376.33 Orbital edema or congestion
  - 376.34 Intermittent exophthalmos
  - 376.35 Pulsating exophthalmos
  - 376.36 Lateral displacement of globe
- ⑤ **376.4 Deformity of orbit**
  - **376.40** Deformity of orbit, unspecified
  - 376.41 Hypertelorism of orbit
  - 376.42 Exostosis of orbit
  - 376.43 Local deformities due to bone disease
  - 376.44 Orbital deformities associated with craniofacial deformities
  - 376.45 Atrophy of orbit
  - 376.46 Enlargement of orbit
  - 376.47 Deformity due to trauma or surgery
- ⑤ **376.5 Enophthalmos**
  - **376.50** Enophthalmos, unspecified as to cause
  - 376.51 Enophthalmos due to atrophy of orbital tissue
  - 376.52 Enophthalmos due to trauma or surgery
- **376.6 Retained (old) foreign body following penetrating wound of orbit**
  Retrobulbar foreign body
- ⑤ **376.8 Other orbital disorders**
  - 376.81 Orbital cysts
    Encephalocele of orbit
  - 376.82 Myopathy of extraocular muscles
  - **376.89** Other
- **376.9 Unspecified disorder of orbit**

377 Disorders of optic nerve and visual pathways
- ⑤ **377.0 Papilledema**
  - **377.00** Papilledema, unspecified
  - 377.01 Papilledema associated with increased intracranial pressure
  - 377.02 Papilledema associated with decreased ocular pressure
  - 377.03 Papilledema associated with retinal disorder
  - 377.04 Foster-Kennedy syndrome
- ⑤ **377.1 Optic atrophy**
  - **377.10** Optic atrophy, unspecified
  - 377.11 Primary optic atrophy
    Excludes: neurosyphilitic optic atrophy (094.84)
  - 377.12 Postinflammatory optic atrophy
  - 377.13 Optic atrophy associated with retinal dystrophies
  - 377.14 Glaucomatous atrophy [cupping] of optic disc
  - 377.15 Partial optic atrophy
    Temporal pallor of optic disc
  - 377.16 Hereditary optic atrophy
    Optic atrophy:
      dominant hereditary
      Leber's
- ⑤ **377.2 Other disorders of optic disc**

● Code new to this edition ▲ Revision of existing code ④ ⑤ Fourth or fifth digit required

NERVOUS SYSTEM AND SENSE ORGANS

      377.21 Drusen of optic disc
      377.22 Crater-like holes of optic disc
      377.23 Coloboma of optic disc
      377.24 Pseudopapilledema

⑤ **377.3 Optic neuritis**
    Excludes: meningococcal optic neuritis (036.81)

      377.30 Optic neuritis, unspecified
      377.31 Optic papillitis
      377.32 Retrobulbar neuritis (acute)
    Excludes: syphilitic retrobulbar neuritis (094.85)

      377.33 Nutritional optic neuropathy
      377.34 Toxic optic neuropathy
            Toxic amblyopia
      377.39 Other
    Excludes: ischemic optic neuropathy (377.41)

⑤ **377.4 Other disorders of optic nerve**
      377.41 Ischemic optic neuropathy
      377.42 Hemorrhage in optic nerve sheaths
      377.43 Optic nerve hypoplasia
      377.49 Other
            Compression of optic nerve

⑤ **377.5 Disorders of optic chiasm**
      377.51 Associated with pituitary neoplasms and disorders
      377.52 Associated with other neoplasms
      377.53 Associated with vascular disorders
      377.54 Associated with inflammatory disorders

⑤ **377.6 Disorders of other visual pathways**
      377.61 Associated with neoplasms
      377.62 Associated with vascular disorders
      377.63 Associated with inflammatory disorders

⑤ **377.7 Disorders of visual cortex**
    Excludes: visual:
          agnosia (368.16)
          hallucinations (368.16)
          halos (368.15)

      377.71 Associated with neoplasms
      377.72 Associated with vascular disorders
      377.73 Associated with inflammatory disorders
      377.75 Cortical blindness

377.9 Unspecified disorder of optic nerve and visual pathways

378 Strabismus and other disorders of binocular eye movements
    Excludes: nystagmus and other irregular eye movements (379.50-379.59)

⑤ **378.0 Esotropia**
      Convergent concomitant strabismus
    Excludes: intermittent esotropia (378.20-378.22)

      378.00 Esotropia, unspecified
      378.01 Monocular esotropia
      378.02 Monocular esotropia with A pattern
      378.03 Monocular esotropia with V pattern
      378.04 Monocular esotropia with other noncomitancies
            Monocular esotropia with X or Y pattern
      378.05 Alternating esotropia
      378.06 Alternating esotropia with A pattern

Add 4th or 5th digit	Nonspecific code	Unspecified code	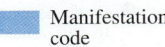 Manifestation code

TABULAR LIST

- 378.07 Alternating esotropia with V pattern
- **378.08** Alternating esotropia with other noncomitancies
  Alternating esotropia with X or Y pattern

⑤ 378.1 **Exotropia**
Divergent concomitant strabismus

Excludes: *intermittent exotropia (378.20, 378.23-378.24)*

- **378.10** Exotropia, unspecified
- 378.11 Monocular exotropia
- 378.12 Monocular exotropia with A pattern
- 378.13 Monocular exotropia with V pattern
- **378.14** Monocular exotropia with other noncomitancies
  Monocular exotropia with X or Y pattern
- 378.15 Alternating exotropia
- 378.16 Alternating exotropia with A pattern
- 378.17 Alternating exotropia with V pattern
- **378.18** Alternating exotropia with other noncomitancies
  Alternating exotropia with X or Y pattern

⑤ 378.2 **Intermittent heterotropia**

Excludes: *vertical heterotropia (intermittent) (378.31)*

- **378.20** Intermittent heterotropia, unspecified
  Intermittent:
    esotropia NOS
    exotropia NOS
- 378.21 Intermittent esotropia, monocular
- 378.22 Intermittent esotropia, alternating
- 378.23 Intermittent exotropia, monocular
- 378.24 Intermittent exotropia, alternating

⑤ 378.3 **Other and unspecified heterotropia**

- **378.30** Heterotropia, unspecified
- 378.31 Hypertropia
  Vertical heterotropia (constant) (intermittent)
- 378.32 Hypotropia
- 378.33 Cyclotropia
- 378.34 Monofixation syndrome
  Microtropia
- 378.35 Accommodative component in esotropia

⑤ 378.4 **Heterophoria**

- **378.40** Heterophoria, unspecified
- 378.41 Esophoria
- 378.42 Exophoria
- 378.43 Vertical heterophoria
- 378.44 Cyclophoria
- 378.45 Alternating hyperphoria

⑤ 378.5 **Paralytic strabismus**

- **378.50** Paralytic strabismus, unspecified
- 378.51 Third or oculomotor nerve palsy, partial
- 378.52 Third or oculomotor nerve palsy, total
- 378.53 Fourth or trochlear nerve palsy
- 378.54 Sixth or abducens nerve palsy
- 378.55 External ophthalmoplegia
- 378.56 Total ophthalmoplegia

⑤ 378.6 **Mechanical strabismus**

- **378.60** Mechanical strabismus, unspecified
- 378.61 Brown's (tendon) sheath syndrome
- **378.62** Mechanical strabismus from other musculofascial disorders

● Code new to this edition ▲ Revision of existing code ④ ⑤ Fourth or fifth digit required

NERVOUS SYSTEM AND SENSE ORGANS

- **378.63** Limited duction associated with other conditions
- ⑤ **378.7** Other specified strabismus
  - **378.71** Duane's syndrome
  - **378.72** Progressive external ophthalmoplegia
  - **378.73** Strabismus in other neuromuscular disorders
- ⑤ **378.8** Other disorders of binocular eye movements
  - Excludes: *nystagmus (379.50-379.56)*
  - **378.81** Palsy of conjugate gaze
  - **378.82** Spasm of conjugate gaze
  - **378.83** Convergence insufficiency or palsy
  - **378.84** Convergence excess or spasm
  - **378.85** Anomalies of divergence
  - **378.86** Internuclear ophthalmoplegia
  - **378.87** Other dissociated deviation of eye movements
    Skew deviation
- **378.9** Unspecified disorder of eye movements
  Ophthalmoplegia NOS
  Strabismus NOS

379 Other disorders of eye

- ⑤ **379.0** Scleritis and episcleritis
  - Excludes: *syphilitic episcleritis (095.0)*
  - **379.00** Scleritis, unspecified
    Episcleritis NOS
  - **379.01** Episcleritis periodica fugax
  - **379.02** Nodular episcleritis
  - **379.03** Anterior scleritis
  - **379.04** Scleromalacia perforans
  - **379.05** Scleritis with corneal involvement
    Scleroperikeratitis
  - **379.06** Brawny scleritis
  - **379.07** Posterior scleritis
    Sclerotenonitis
  - **379.09** Other
    Scleral abscess
- ⑤ **379.1** Other disorders of sclera
  - Excludes: *blue sclera (743.47)*
  - **379.11** Scleral ectasia
    Scleral staphyloma NOS
  - **379.12** Staphyloma posticum
  - **379.13** Equatorial staphyloma
  - **379.14** Anterior staphyloma, localized
  - **379.15** Ring staphyloma
  - **379.16** Other degenerative disorders of sclera
  - **379.19** Other
- ⑤ **379.2** Disorders of vitreous body
  - **379.21** Vitreous degeneration
    Vitreous:
      cavitation
      detachment
      liquefaction
  - **379.22** Crystalline deposits in vitreous
    Asteroid hyalitis
    Synchysis scintillans
  - **379.23** Vitreous hemorrhage
  - **379.24** Other vitreous opacities
    Vitreous floaters

■ Add 4th or 5th digit   ■ Nonspecific code   ■ Unspecified code   ■ Manifestation code

TABULAR LIST

  379.25 Vitreous membranes and strands
  379.26 Vitreous prolapse
  379.29 Other disorders of vitreous
  Excludes: *vitreous abscess (360.04)*

⑤ 379.3 **Aphakia and other disorders of lens**
  Excludes: *after-cataract (366.50-366.53)*
  379.31 Aphakia
  Excludes: *cataract extraction status (V45.61)*
  379.32 Subluxation of lens
  379.33 Anterior dislocation of lens
  379.34 Posterior dislocation of lens
  379.39 Other disorders of lens

⑤ 379.4 **Anomalies of pupillary function**
  379.40 Abnormal pupillary function, unspecified
  379.41 Anisocoria
  379.42 Miosis (persistent), not due to miotics
  379.43 Mydriasis (persistent) not due to mydriatics
  379.45 Argyll Robertson pupil, atypical
    Argyll Robertson phenomenon or pupil, nonsyphilitic
  Excludes: Argyll Robertson pupil (syphilitic) (094.89)
  379.46 Tonic pupillary reaction
    Adie's pupil or syndrome
  379.49 Other
    Hippus
    Pupillary paralysis

⑤ 379.5 **Nystagmus and other irregular eye movements**
  379.50 Nystagmus, unspecified
  379.51 Congenital nystagmus
  379.52 Latent nystagmus
  379.53 Visual deprivation nystagmus
  379.54 Nystagmus associated with disorders of the vestibular system
  379.55 Dissociated nystagmus
  379.56 Other forms of nystagmus
  379.57 Deficiencies of saccadic eye movements
    Abnormal optokinetic response
  379.58 Deficiencies of smooth pursuit movements
  379.59 Other irregularities of eye movements
    Opsoclonus

⑤ 379.6 **Inflammation (infection) of postprocedural bleb**
  Postprocedural blebitis
  379.60 Inflammation (infection) of postprocedural bleb, unspecified
  379.61 Inflammation (infection) of postprocedural bleb, stage 1
  379.62 Inflammation (infection) of postprocedural bleb, stage 2
  379.63 Inflammation (infection) of postprocedural bleb, stage 3
    Bleb associated endophthalmitis

379.8 Other specified disorders of eye and adnexa

⑤ 379.9 **Unspecified disorder of eye and adnexa**
  379.90 Disorder of eye, unspecified
  379.91 Pain in or around eye
  379.92 Swelling or mass of eye
  379.93 Redness or discharge of eye
  379.99 Other ill-defined disorders of eye
  Excludes: *blurred vision NOS (368.8)*

● Code new to this edition ▲ Revision of existing code ④ ⑤ Fourth or fifth digit required

NERVOUS SYSTEM AND SENSE ORGANS

DISEASES OF THE EAR AND MASTOID PROCESS (380-389)

380 Disorders of external ear

⑤ **380.0** Perichondritis and chondritis of pinna
Chondritis of auricle
Perichondritis of auricle

380.00 Perichondritis of pinna, unspecified
380.01 Acute perichondritis of pinna
380.02 Chronic perichondritis of pinna
380.03 Chondritis of pinna

⑤ **380.1** Infective otitis externa

380.10 Infective otitis externa, unspecified
Otitis externa (acute):
NOS
circumscribed
diffuse
hemorrhagica
infective NOS

380.11 Acute infection of pinna

Excludes: furuncular otitis externa (680.0)

380.12 Acute swimmers' ear
Beach ear
Tank ear

380.13 Other acute infections of external ear
Code first underlying disease, as:
erysipelas (035)
impetigo (684)
seborrheic dermatitis (690.10-690.18)

Excludes: herpes simplex (054.73)
herpes zoster (053.71)

380.14 Malignant otitis externa

380.15 Chronic mycotic otitis externa
Code first underlying disease, as:
aspergillosis (117.3)
otomycosis NOS (111.9)

Excludes: candidal otitis externa (112.82)

380.16 Other chronic infective otitis externa
Chronic infective otitis externa NOS

⑤ **380.2** Other otitis externa

380.21 Cholesteatoma of external ear
Keratosis obturans of external ear (canal)

Excludes: cholesteatoma NOS (385.30-385.35)
postmastoidectomy (383.32)

380.22 Other acute otitis externa
Acute otitis externa:
actinic
chemical
contact
eczematoid
reactive

380.23 Other chronic otitis externa
Chronic otitis externa NOS

⑤ **380.3** Noninfectious disorders of pinna

380.30 Disorder of pinna, unspecified
380.31 Hematoma of auricle or pinna
380.32 Acquired deformities of auricle or pinna

Excludes: cauliflower ear (738.7)

380.39 Other

Excludes: gouty tophi of ear (274.81)

380.4 Impacted cerumen
Wax in ear

325

 Add 4th or 5th digit
 Nonspecific code
 Unspecified code
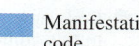 Manifestation code

TABULAR LIST

- ⑤ **380.5 Acquired stenosis of external ear canal**
  Collapse of external ear canal
  - **380.50** Acquired stenosis of external ear canal, unspecified as to cause
  - 380.51 Secondary to trauma
  - 380.52 Secondary to surgery
  - 380.53 Secondary to inflammation
- ⑤ **380.8 Other disorders of external ear**
  - 380.81 Exostosis of external ear canal
  - **380.89** Other
- **380.9 Unspecified disorder of external ear**

381 Nonsuppurative otitis media and Eustachian tube disorders

- ⑤ **381.0 Acute nonsuppurative otitis media**
  Acute tubotympanic catarrh
  Otitis media, acute or subacute:
    catarrhal
    exudative
    transudative
    with effusion

  Excludes: otitic barotrauma (993.0)

  - **381.00** Acute nonsuppurative otitis media, unspecified
  - 381.01 Acute serous otitis media
    Acute or subacute secretory otitis media
  - 381.02 Acute mucoid otitis media
    Acute or subacute seromucinous otitis media
    Blue drum syndrome
  - 381.03 Acute sanguinous otitis media
  - 381.04 Acute allergic serous otitis media
  - 381.05 Acute allergic mucoid otitis media
  - 381.06 Acute allergic sanguinous otitis media
- ⑤ **381.1 Chronic serous otitis media**
  Chronic tubotympanic catarrh
  - 381.10 Chronic serous otitis media, simple or unspecified
  - **381.19** Other
    Serosanguinous chronic otitis media
- ⑤ **381.2 Chronic mucoid otitis media**
  Glue ear

  Excludes: adhesive middle ear disease (385.10-385.19)

  - 381.20 Chronic mucoid otitis media, simple or unspecified
  - **381.29** Other
    Mucosanguinous chronic otitis media
- **381.3 Other and unspecified chronic nonsuppurative otitis media**
  Otitis media, chronic: Otitis media, chronic:
    allergic   seromucinous
    exudative   transudative
    secretory   with effusion
- **381.4 Nonsuppurative otitis media, not specified as acute or chronic**
  Otitis media: Otitis media:
    allergic   secretory
    catarrhal   seromucinous
    exudative   serous
    mucoid   transudative
                                 with effusion
- ⑤ **381.5 Eustachian salpingitis**
  - **381.50** Eustachian salpingitis, unspecified
  - 381.51 Acute Eustachian salpingitis
  - 381.52 Chronic Eustachian salpingitis
- ⑤ **381.6 Obstruction of Eustachian tube**
  Stenosis of Eustachian tube
  Stricture of Eustachian tube

● Code new to this edition ▲ Revision of existing code ④ ⑤ Fourth or fifth digit required

NERVOUS SYSTEM AND SENSE ORGANS

- **381.60** Obstruction of Eustachian tube, unspecified
- **381.61** Osseous obstruction of Eustachian tube
  Obstruction of Eustachian tube from cholesteatoma, polyp, or other osseous lesion
- **381.62** Intrinsic cartilagenous obstruction of Eustachian tube
- **381.63** Extrinsic cartilagenous obstruction of Eustachian tube
  Compression of Eustachian tube

381.7 Patulous Eustachian tube

⑤ **381.8** Other disorders of Eustachian tube
- **381.81** Dysfunction of Eustachian tube
- **381.89** Other

381.9 Unspecified Eustachian tube disorder

382 Suppurative and unspecified otitis media

⑤ **382.0** Acute suppurative otitis media
  Otitis media, acute:
    necrotizing NOS
    purulent
- **382.00** Acute suppurative otitis media without spontaneous rupture of ear drum
- **382.01** Acute suppurative otitis media with spontaneous rupture of ear drum
- **382.02** Acute suppurative otitis media in diseases classified elsewhere
  Code first underlying disease, as:
    influenza (487.8)
    scarlet fever (034.1)
  Excludes: postmeasles otitis (055.2)

382.1 Chronic tubotympanic suppurative otitis media
  Benign chronic suppurative otitis media (with anterior perforation of ear drum)
  Chronic tubotympanic disease (with anterior perforation of ear drum)

382.2 Chronic atticoantral suppurative otitis media
  Chronic atticoantral disease (with posterior or superior marginal perforation of ear drum)
  Persistent mucosal disease (with posterior or superior marginal perforation of ear drum)

382.3 Unspecified chronic suppurative otitis media
  Chronic purulent otitis media
  Excludes: tuberculous otitis media (017.4)

382.4 Unspecified suppurative otitis media
  Purulent otitis media NOS

382.9 Unspecified otitis media
  Otitis media:
    NOS
    acute NOS
    chronic NOS

383 Mastoiditis and related conditions

⑤ **383.0** Acute mastoiditis
  Abscess of mastoid
  Empyema of mastoid
- **383.00** Acute mastoiditis without complications
- **383.01** Subperiosteal abscess of mastoid
- **383.02** Acute mastoiditis with other complications
  Gradenigo's syndrome

383.1 Chronic mastoiditis
  Caries of mastoid
  Fistula of mastoid
  Excludes: tuberculous mastoiditis (015.6)

⑤ **383.2** Petrositis
  Coalescing osteitis of petrous bone
  Inflammation of petrous bone
  Osteomyelitis of petrous bone
- **383.20** Petrositis, unspecified
- **383.21** Acute petrositis
- **383.22** Chronic petrositis

TABULAR LIST

- ⑤ **383.3 Complications following mastoidectomy**
  - **383.30** Postmastoidectomy complication, unspecified
  - 383.31 Mucosal cyst of postmastoidectomy cavity
  - 383.32 Recurrent cholesteatoma of postmastoidectomy cavity
  - 383.33 Granulations of postmastoidectomy cavity
    Chronic inflammation of postmastoidectomy cavity
- ⑤ **383.8 Other disorders of mastoid**
  - 383.81 Postauricular fistula
  - **383.89** Other
- **383.9 Unspecified mastoiditis**

384 Other disorders of tympanic membrane
- ⑤ **384.0 Acute myringitis without mention of otitis media**
  - **384.00** Acute myringitis, unspecified
    Acute tympanitis NOS
  - 384.01 Bullous myringitis
    Myringitis bullosa hemorrhagica
  - **384.09** Other
- **384.1 Chronic myringitis without mention of otitis media**
  Chronic tympanitis
- ⑤ **384.2 Perforation of tympanic membrane**
  Perforation of ear drum:
    NOS
    persistent posttraumatic
    postinflammatory

  Excludes: otitis media with perforation of tympanic membrane (382.00-382.9)
  traumatic perforation [current injury] (872.61)

  - **384.20** Perforation of tympanic membrane, unspecified
  - 384.21 Central perforation of tympanic membrane
  - 384.22 Attic perforation of tympanic membrane
    Pars flaccida
  - **384.23** Other marginal perforation of tympanic membrane
  - 384.24 Multiple perforations of tympanic membrane
  - 384.25 Total perforation of tympanic membrane
- ⑤ **384.8 Other specified disorders of tympanic membrane**
  - 384.81 Atrophic flaccid tympanic membrane
    Healed perforation of ear drum
  - 384.82 Atrophic nonflaccid tympanic membrane
- **384.9 Unspecified disorder of tympanic membrane**

385 Other disorders of middle ear and mastoid
  Excludes: mastoiditis (383.0-383.9)

- ⑤ **385.0 Tympanosclerosis**
  - **385.00** Tympanosclerosis, unspecified as to involvement
  - 385.01 Tympanosclerosis involving tympanic membrane only
  - 385.02 Tympanosclerosis involving tympanic membrane and ear ossicles
  - 385.03 Tympanosclerosis involving tympanic membrane, ear ossicles, and middle ear
  - 385.09 Tympanosclerosis involving other combination of structures
- ⑤ **385.1 Adhesive middle ear disease**
  Adhesive otitis
  Otitis media:
    chronic adhesive
    fibrotic

  Excludes: glue ear (381.20-381.29)

  - **385.10** Adhesive middle ear disease, unspecified as to involvement
  - 385.11 Adhesions of drum head to incus
  - 385.12 Adhesions of drum head to stapes

328 ● Code new to this edition ▲ Revision of existing code ④ ⑤ Fourth or fifth digit required

NERVOUS SYSTEM AND SENSE ORGANS

- 385.13 Adhesions of drum head to promontorium
- **385.19** Other adhesions and combinations

⑤ 385.2 **Other acquired abnormality of ear ossicles**
- 385.21 **Impaired mobility of malleus**
  Ankylosis of malleus
- **385.22** **Impaired mobility of other ear ossicles**
  Ankylosis of ear ossicles, except malleus
- 385.23 **Discontinuity or dislocation of ear ossicles**
- 385.24 **Partial loss or necrosis of ear ossicles**

⑤ 385.3 **Cholesteatoma of middle ear and mastoid**
  Cholesterosis of (middle) ear
  Epidermosis of (middle) ear
  Keratosis of (middle) ear
  Polyp of (middle) ear

  Excludes: cholesteatoma:
    external ear canal (380.21)
    recurrent of postmastoidectomy cavity (383.32)

- **385.30** Cholesteatoma, unspecified
- 385.31 Cholesteatoma of attic
- 385.32 Cholesteatoma of middle ear
- 385.33 Cholesteatoma of middle ear and mastoid
- 385.35 Diffuse cholesteatosis

⑤ 385.8 **Other disorders of middle ear and mastoid**
- 385.82 **Cholesterin granuloma**
- 385.83 **Retained foreign body of middle ear**
- **385.89** Other

385.9 **Unspecified disorder of middle ear and mastoid**

386 **Vertiginous syndromes and other disorders of vestibular system**

  Excludes: vertigo NOS (780.4)

⑤ 386.0 **Ménière's disease**
  Endolymphatic hydrops   Ménière's syndrome or vertigo
  Lermoyez's syndrome

- **386.00** **Ménière's disease, unspecified**
  Ménière's disease (active)
- 386.01 Active Ménière's disease, cochleovestibular
- 386.02 Active Ménière's disease, cochlear
- 386.03 Active Ménière's disease, vestibular
- 386.04 Inactive Ménière's disease
  Ménière's disease in remission

⑤ 386.1 **Other and unspecified peripheral vertigo**

  Excludes: epidemic vertigo (078.81)

- **386.10** Peripheral vertigo, unspecified
- 386.11 Benign paroxysmal positional vertigo
  Benign paroxysmal positional nystagmus
- 386.12 Vestibular neuronitis
  Acute (and recurrent) peripheral vestibulopathy
- **386.19** Other
  Aural vertigo
  Otogenic vertigo

386.2 **Vertigo of central origin**
  Central positional nystagmus
  Malignant positional vertigo

⑤ 386.3 **Labyrinthitis**
- **386.30** Labyrinthitis, unspecified
- 386.31 Serous labyrinthitis
  Diffuse labyrinthitis
- 386.32 Circumscribed labyrinthitis
  Focal labyrinthitis

TABULAR LIST

- 386.33 **Suppurative labyrinthitis**
  Purulent labyrinthitis
- 386.34 **Toxic labyrinthitis**
- 386.35 **Viral labyrinthitis**

⑤ 386.4 **Labyrinthine fistula**
- 386.40 **Labyrinthine fistula, unspecified**
- 386.41 **Round window fistula**
- 386.42 **Oval window fistula**
- 386.43 **Semicircular canal fistula**
- 386.48 **Labyrinthine fistula of combined sites**

⑤ 386.5 **Labyrinthine dysfunction**
- 386.50 **Labyrinthine dysfunction, unspecified**
- 386.51 **Hyperactive labyrinth, unilateral**
- 386.52 **Hyperactive labyrinth, bilateral**
- 386.53 **Hypoactive labyrinth, unilateral**
- 386.54 **Hypoactive labyrinth, bilateral**
- 386.55 **Loss of labyrinthine reactivity, unilateral**
- 386.56 **Loss of labyrinthine reactivity, bilateral**
- 386.58 **Other forms and combinations**

386.8 Other disorders of labyrinth
386.9 Unspecified vertiginous syndromes and labyrinthine disorders

387 **Otosclerosis**
Includes: otospongiosis
- 387.0 **Otosclerosis involving oval window, nonobliterative**
- 387.1 **Otosclerosis involving oval window, obliterative**
- 387.2 **Cochlear otosclerosis**
  Otosclerosis involving:
    otic capsule
    round window

387.8 Other otosclerosis
387.9 Otosclerosis, unspecified

388 Other disorders of ear
⑤ 388.0 **Degenerative and vascular disorders of ear**
- 388.00 **Degenerative and vascular disorders, unspecified**
- 388.01 **Presbyacusis**
- 388.02 **Transient ischemic deafness**

⑤ 388.1 **Noise effects on inner ear**
- 388.10 **Noise effects on inner ear, unspecified**
- 388.11 **Acoustic trauma (explosive) to ear**
  Otitic blast injury
- 388.12 **Noise-induced hearing loss**

388.2 Sudden hearing loss, unspecified

⑤ 388.3 **Tinnitus**
- 388.30 **Tinnitus, unspecified**
- 388.31 **Subjective tinnitus**
- 388.32 **Objective tinnitus**

⑤ 388.4 **Other abnormal auditory perception**
- 388.40 **Abnormal auditory perception, unspecified**
- 388.41 **Diplacusis**
- 388.42 **Hyperacusis**
- 388.43 **Impairment of auditory discrimination**
- 388.44 **Recruitment**

● Code new to this edition   ▲ Revision of existing code   ④ ⑤ Fourth or fifth digit required

NERVOUS SYSTEM AND SENSE ORGANS

● **388.45 Acquired auditory processing disorder**
Auditory processing disorder NOS
Excludes: central auditory processing disorder (315.32)

388.5 Disorders of acoustic nerve
Acoustic neuritis
Degeneration of acoustic or eighth nerve
Disorder of acoustic or eighth nerve
Excludes: acoustic neuroma (225.1)
syphilitic acoustic neuritis (094.86)

⑤ **388.6 Otorrhea**

388.60 Otorrhea, unspecified
Discharging ear NOS

388.61 Cerebrospinal fluid otorrhea
Excludes: cerebrospinal fluid rhinorrhea (349.81)

388.69 Other
Otorrhagia

⑤ **388.7 Otalgia**

388.70 Otalgia, unspecified
Earache NOS

388.71 Otogenic pain

388.72 Referred pain

388.8 Other disorders of ear

388.9 Unspecified disorder of ear

389 Hearing loss

⑤ **389.0 Conductive hearing loss**
Conductive deafness
Excludes: mixed conductive and sensorineural hearing loss (389.20-389.22)

389.00 Conductive hearing loss, unspecified

389.01 Conductive hearing loss, external ear

389.02 Conductive hearing loss, tympanic membrane

389.03 Conductive hearing loss, middle ear

389.04 Conductive hearing loss, inner ear

● **389.05 Conductive hearing loss, unilateral**

● **389.06 Conductive hearing loss, bilateral**

389.08 Conductive hearing loss of combined types

⑤ **389.1 Sensorineural hearing loss**
Perceptive hearing loss or deafness
Excludes: abnormal auditory perception (388.40-388.44)
mixed conductive and sensorineural hearing loss (389.20-389.22)
psychogenic deafness (306.7)

389.10 Sensorineural hearing loss, unspecified

389.11 Sensory hearing loss, bilateral

389.12 Neural hearing loss, bilateral

● **389.13 Neural hearing loss, unilateral**

▲ **389.14 Central hearing loss**

389.15 Sensorineural hearing loss, unilateral

389.16 Sensorineural hearing loss, asymmetrical

● **389.17 Sensory hearing loss, unilateral**

▲ **389.18 Sensorineural hearing loss, bilateral**

⑤ **389.2 Mixed conductive and sensorineural hearing loss**
Deafness or hearing loss of type classifiable to 389.00-389.08 with type classifiable to 389.10-389.18

● **389.20 Mixed hearing loss, unspecified**

● **389.21 Mixed hearing loss, unilateral**

● **389.22 Mixed hearing loss, bilateral**

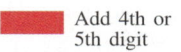 Add 4th or 5th digit
 Nonspecific code
 Unspecified code
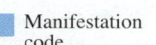 Manifestation code

331

TABULAR LIST

▲ **389.7** Deaf nonspeaking, not elsewhere classifiable
389.8 Other specified forms of hearing loss
389.9 Unspecified hearing loss
   Deafness NOS

CIRCULATORY SYSTEM

7. DISEASES OF THE CIRCULATORY SYSTEM (390-459)

ACUTE RHEUMATIC FEVER (390-392)

390 Rheumatic fever without mention of heart involvement
Arthritis, rheumatic, acute or subacute
Rheumatic fever (active) (acute)
Rheumatism, articular, acute or subacute
Excludes: that with heart involvement (391.0-391.9)

391 Rheumatic fever with heart involvement
Excludes: chronic heart diseases of rheumatic origin (393.0-398.9) unless rheumatic fever is also present or there is evidence of recrudescence or activity of the rheumatic process

391.0 Acute rheumatic pericarditis
Rheumatic:
    fever (active) (acute) with pericarditis
    pericarditis (acute)
Any condition classifiable to 390 with pericarditis
Excludes: that not specified as rheumatic (420.0-420.9)

391.1 Acute rheumatic endocarditis
Rheumatic:
    endocarditis, acute
    fever (active) (acute) with endocarditis or valvulitis
    valvulitis acute
Any condition classifiable to 390 with endocarditis or valvulitis

391.2 Acute rheumatic myocarditis
Rheumatic fever (active) (acute) with myocarditis
Any condition classifiable to 390 with myocarditis

391.8 Other acute rheumatic heart disease
Rheumatic:
    fever (active) (acute) with other or multiple types of heart involvement
    pancarditis, acute
Any condition classifiable to 390 with other or multiple types of heart involvement

391.9 Acute rheumatic heart disease, unspecified
Rheumatic:
    carditis, acute
    fever (active) (acute) with unspecified type of heart involvement
    heart disease, active or acute
Any condition classifiable to 390 with unspecified type of heart involvement

392 Rheumatic chorea
Includes: Sydenham's chorea
Excludes: chorea:
    NOS (333.5)
    Huntington's (333.4)

392.0 With heart involvement
Rheumatic chorea with heart involvement of any type classifiable to 391

392.9 Without mention of heart involvement

CHRONIC RHEUMATIC HEART DISEASE (393-398)

393 Chronic rheumatic pericarditis
Adherent pericardium, rheumatic
Chronic rheumatic:
    mediastinopericarditis
    myopericarditis
Excludes: pericarditis NOS or not specified as rheumatic (423.0-423.9)

394 Diseases of mitral valve
Excludes: that with aortic valve involvement (396.0-396.9)

394.0 Mitral stenosis
Mitral (valve):
    obstruction (rheumatic)
    stenosis NOS

333

| | Add 4th or 5th digit | | Nonspecific code | | Unspecified code | | Manifestation code |

TABULAR LIST

394.1 Rheumatic mitral insufficiency
Rheumatic mitral:
  incompetence
  regurgitation
Excludes: that not specified as rheumatic (424.0)

394.2 Mitral stenosis with insufficiency
Mitral stenosis with incompetence or regurgitation

394.9 Other and unspecified mitral valve diseases
Mitral (valve):
  disease (chronic)
  failure

395 Diseases of aortic valve
Excludes: that not specified as rheumatic (424.1)
  that with mitral valve involvement (396.0-396.9)

395.0 Rheumatic aortic stenosis
Rheumatic aortic (valve) obstruction

395.1 Rheumatic aortic insufficiency
Rheumatic aortic:
  incompetence
  regurgitation

395.2 Rheumatic aortic stenosis with insufficiency
Rheumatic aortic stenosis with incompetence or regurgitation

395.9 Other and unspecified rheumatic aortic diseases
Rheumatic aortic (valve) disease

396 Diseases of mitral and aortic valves
Includes: involvement of both mitral and aortic valves, whether specified as rheumatic or not

396.0 Mitral valve stenosis and aortic valve stenosis
Atypical aortic (valve) stenosis
Mitral and aortic (valve) obstruction (rheumatic)

396.1 Mitral valve stenosis and aortic valve insufficiency

396.2 Mitral valve insufficiency and aortic valve stenosis

396.3 Mitral valve insufficiency and aortic valve insufficiency
Mitral and aortic (valve):
  incompetence
  regurgitation

396.8 Multiple involvement of mitral and aortic valves
Stenosis and insufficiency of mitral or aortic valve with stenosis or insufficiency, or both, of the other valve

396.9 Mitral and aortic valve diseases, unspecified

397 Diseases of other endocardial structures

397.0 Diseases of tricuspid valve
Tricuspid (valve) (rheumatic):
  disease
  insufficiency
  obstruction
  regurgitation
  stenosis

397.1 Rheumatic diseases of pulmonary valve
Excludes: that not specified as rheumatic (424.3)

397.9 Rheumatic diseases of endocardium, valve unspecified
Rheumatic:
  endocarditis (chronic)
  valvulitis (chronic)
Excludes: that not specified as rheumatic (424.90-424.99)

398 Other rheumatic heart disease

398.0 Rheumatic myocarditis
Rheumatic degeneration of myocardium
Excludes: myocarditis not specified as rheumatic (429.0)

⑤ **398.9 Other and unspecified rheumatic heart diseases**

CIRCULATORY SYSTEM

398.90 Rheumatic heart disease, unspecified
Rheumatic:
  carditis
  heart disease NOS

Excludes: *carditis not specified as rheumatic (429.89)*
  heart disease NOS not specified as rheumatic (429.9)

398.91 Rheumatic heart failure (congestive)
Rheumatic left ventricular failure

398.99 Other

HYPERTENSIVE DISEASE (401-405)

Excludes: *that complicating pregnancy, childbirth, or the puerperium (642.0-642.9)*
  that involving coronary vessels (410.00-414.9)

401 Essential hypertension
Includes: high blood pressure
  hyperpiesia
  hyperpiesis
  hypertension (arterial) (essential) (primary) (systemic)
  hypertensive vascular:
    degeneration
    disease

Excludes: *elevated blood pressure without diagnosis of hypertension (796.2)*
  pulmonary hypertension (416.0-416.9)
  that involving vessels of:
    brain (430-438)
    eye (362.11)

401.0 Malignant
401.1 Benign
401.9 Unspecified

402 Hypertensive heart disease
Use additional code to specify type of heart failure (428.0-428.43), if known
Includes: hypertensive:
  cardiomegaly
  cardiopathy
  cardiovascular disease
  heart (disease) (failure)
  any condition classifiable to 429.0-429.3, 429.8, 429.9 due to hypertension

⑤ **402.0 Malignant**
  402.00 Without heart failure
  402.01 With heart failure

⑤ **402.1 Benign**
  402.10 Without heart failure
  402.11 With heart failure

⑤ **402.9 Unspecified**
  402.90 Without heart failure
  402.91 With heart failure

| ■ Add 4th or 5th digit | ■ Nonspecific code | ■ Unspecified code | ■ Manifestation code |

335

TABULAR LIST

⑤ **403 Hypertensive chronic kidney disease**
  The following fifth-digit subclassification is for use with category 403:
    0 with chronic kidney disease stage I through stage IV, or unspecified
      Use additional code to identify the stage of chronic kidney disease (585.1-585.4, 585.9)
    1 with chronic kidney disease stage V or end stage renal disease
      Use additional code to identify the stage of chronic kidney disease (585.5, 585.6)
  Includes: arteriolar nephritis
             arteriosclerosis of:
               kidney
               renal arterioles
             arteriosclerotic nephritis (chronic) (interstitial)
             hypertensive:
               nephropathy
               renal failure
               uremia (chronic)
             nephrosclerosis
             renal sclerosis with hypertension
             any condition classifiable to 585, 586, or 587 with any condition classifiable to 401
  Excludes: acute renal failure (584.5-584.9)
              renal disease stated as not due to hypertension
              renovascular hypertension (405.0-405.9 with fifth-digit 1)

⑤ 403.0 Malignant
⑤ 403.1 Benign
⑤ **403.9** Unspecified

⑤ **404 Hypertensive heart and chronic kidney disease**
  Use additional code to specify type of heart failure (428.0-428.43), if known
  The following fifth-digit subclassification is for use with category 404:
    0 without heart failure and with chronic kidney disease stage I through stage IV, or unspecified
      Use additional code to identify the stage of chronic kidney disease (585.1-585.4, 585.9)
    1 with heart failure and with chronic kidney disease stage I through stage IV, or unspecified
      Use additional code to identify the stage of chronic kidney disease (585.1-585.4, 585.9)
    2 without heart failure and with chronic kidney disease stage V or end stage renal disease
      Use additional code to identify the stage of chronic kidney disease (585.5, 585.6)
    3 with heart failure and chronic kidney disease stage V or end stage renal disease
      Use additional code to identify the stage of chronic kidney disease (585.5-585.6)
  Includes: disease:
               cardiornal
               cardiovascular renal
             any condition classifiable to 402 with any condition classifiable to 403

⑤ 404.0 Malignant
⑤ 404.1 Benign
⑤ **404.9** Unspecified

405 Secondary hypertension
  ⑤ 405.0 Malignant
       405.01 Renovascular
       405.09 Other
  ⑤ 405.1 Benign
       405.11 Renovascular
       405.19 Other
  ⑤ 405.9 Unspecified
       405.91 Renovascular
       405.99 Other

CIRCULATORY SYSTEM

ISCHEMIC HEART DISEASE (410-414)

Includes: that with mention of hypertension

Use additional code, if desired, to identify presence of hypertension (401.0-405.9)

⑤ 410 Acute myocardial infarction
ST elevation (STEMI) and non-ST elevation (NSTEMI) myocardial infarction
Includes: cardiac infarction
coronary (artery):
  embolism
  occlusion
  rupture
  thrombosis
infarction of heart, myocardium, or ventricle
rupture of heart, myocardium, or ventricle
any condition classifiable to 414.1-414.9 specified as acute or with a stated duration of 8 weeks or less

The following fifth-digit subclassification is for use with category 410:

0 episode of care unspecified
Use when the source document does not contain sufficient information for the assignment of fifth digit 1 or 2.

1 initial episode of care
Use fifth digit 1 to designate the first episode of care (regardless of facility site) for a newly diagnosed myocardial infarction. The fifth digit 1 is assigned regardless of the number of times a patient may be transferred during the initial episode of care

2 subsequent episode of care
Use fifth digit 2 to designate an episode of care following the initial episode when the patient is admitted for further observation, evaluation, or treatment for a myocardial infarction that has received initial treatment, but is still less than 8 weeks old.

⑤ 410.0 Of anterolateral wall
ST elevation myocardial infarction (STEMI) of anterolateral wall

⑤ 410.1 Of other anterior wall
ST elevation myocardial infarction (STEMI) of other anterior wall
Infarction:
anterior (wall) NOS (with contiguous portion of intraventricular septum)
anteroapical (with contiguous portion of intraventricular septum)
anteroseptal (with contiguous portion of intraventricular septum)

⑤ 410.2 Of inferolateral wall
ST elevation myocardial infarction (STEMI) of inferolateral wall

⑤ 410.3 Of inferoposterior wall
ST elevation myocardial infarction (STEMI) of inferoposterior wall

⑤ 410.4 Of other inferior wall
ST elevation myocardial infarction (STEMI) of other inferior wall
Infarction:
diaphragmatic wall NOS (with contiguous portion of intraventricular septum)
inferior (wall) NOS (with contiguous portion of intraventricular septum)

⑤ 410.5 Of other lateral wall
ST elevation myocardial infarction (STEMI) of other lateral wall
Infarction: Infarction:
  apical-lateral   high lateral
  basal-lateral   posterolateral

⑤ 410.6 True posterior wall infarction
ST elevation myocardial infarction (STEMI) of true posterior wall
Infarction:
posterobasal
strictly posterior

⑤ 410.7 Subendocardial infarction
Non-ST elevation myocardial infarction (NSTEMI)
Nontransmural infarction

⑤ 410.8 Other specified sites
ST elevation myocardial infarction (STEMI) of other specified sites
Infarction of:
atrium
papillary muscle
septum alone

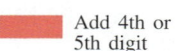 Add 4th or 5th digit
 Nonspecific code
 Unspecified code
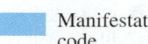 Manifestation code

TABULAR LIST

⑤ **410.9 Unspecified site**
Acute myocardial infarction NOS
Coronary occlusion NOS
Myocardial infarction NOS

411 Other acute and subacute forms of ischemic heart disease

411.0 Postmyocardial infarction syndrome
Dressler's syndrome

411.1 Intermediate coronary syndrome
Impending infarction   Preinfarction syndrome
Preinfarction angina   Unstable angina

Excludes: angina (pectoris) (413.9)
decubitus (413.0)

⑤ **411.8 Other**

411.81 Acute coronary occlusion without myocardial infarction
Acute coronary (artery):
embolism without or not resulting in myocardial infarction
obstruction without or not resulting in myocardial infarction
occlusion without or not resulting in myocardial infarction
thrombosis without or not resulting in myocardial infarction

Excludes: obstruction without infarction due to atherosclerosis (414.00-414.07)
occlusion without infarction due to atherosclerosis (414.00-414.07)

411.89 Other
Coronary insufficiency (acute)
Subendocardial ischemia

412 Old myocardial infarction
Healed myocardial infarction
Past myocardial infarction diagnosed on ECG [EKG] or other special investigation, but currently presenting no symptoms

413 Angina pectoris

413.0 Angina decubitus
Nocturnal angina

413.1 Prinzmetal angina
Variant angina pectoris

413.9 Other and unspecified angina pectoris
Angina: Anginal syndrome
  NOS   Status anginosus
  cardiac   Stenocardia
  of effort   Syncope anginosa

Excludes: preinfarction angina (411.1)

414 Other forms of chronic ischemic heart disease

Excludes: arteriosclerotic cardiovascular disease [ASCVD] (429.2)
cardiovascular:
arteriosclerosis or sclerosis (429.2)
degeneration or disease (429.2)

⑤ **414.0 Coronary atherosclerosis**
Arteriosclerotic heart disease [ASHD]
Atherosclerotic heart disease
Coronary (artery):
  arteriosclerosis
  arteritis or endarteritis
  atheroma
  sclerosis
  stricture
Use additional code, if applicable, to identify chronic total occlusion of coronary artery (414.2)

Excludes: embolism of graft (996.72)
occlusion NOS of graft (996.72)
thrombus of graft (996.72)

414.00 Of unspecified type of vessel, native or graft

414.01 Of native coronary artery

414.02 Of autologous vein bypass graft

414.03 Of nonautologous biological bypass graft

CIRCULATORY SYSTEM

414.04 Of artery bypass graft
Internal mammary artery

414.05 Of unspecified type of bypass graft
Bypass graft NOS

414.06 Of native coronary artery of transplanted heart

414.07 Of bypass graft (artery) (vein) of transplanted heart

⑤ **414.1 Aneurysm and dissection of heart**

414.10 Aneurysm of heart (wall)
Aneurysm (arteriovenous):
  mural
  ventricular

414.11 Aneurysm of coronary vessels
Aneurysm (arteriovenous) of coronary vessels

414.12 Dissection of coronary artery

414.19 Other aneurysm of heart
Arteriovenous fistula, acquired, of heart

● **414.2 Chronic total occlusion of coronary artery**
Complete occlusion of coronary artery
Total occlusion of coronary artery

Code first coronary atherosclerosis (414.00-414.07)

Excludes: acute coronary occlusion with myocardial infarction (410.00-410.92)
acute coronary occlusion without myocardial infarction (411.81)

414.8 Other specified forms of chronic ischemic heart disease
Chronic coronary insufficiency
Ischemia, myocardial (chronic)
Any condition classifiable to 410 specified as chronic, or presenting with symptoms after 8 weeks from date of infarction

Excludes: coronary insufficiency (acute) (411.89)

414.9 Chronic ischemic heart disease, unspecified
Ischemic heart disease NOS

DISEASES OF PULMONARY CIRCULATION (415-417)

415 Acute pulmonary heart disease

415.0 Acute cor pulmonale

Excludes: cor pulmonale NOS (416.9)

⑤ **415.1 Pulmonary embolism and infarction**
Pulmonary (artery) (vein):
  apoplexy
  embolism
  infarction (hemorrhagic)
  thrombosis

Excludes: that complicating:
  abortion (634-638 with .6, 639.6)
  ectopic or molar pregnancy (639.6)
  pregnancy, childbirth, or the puerperium (673.0-673.8)

415.11 Iatrogenic pulmonary embolism and infarction

● **415.12 Septic pulmonary embolism**
Septic embolism NOS

Code first underlying infection, such as:
  septicemia (038.0-038.9)

Excludes: septic arterial embolism (449)

415.19 Other

416 Chronic pulmonary heart disease

416.0 Primary pulmonary hypertension
Idiopathic pulmonary arteriosclerosis
Pulmonary hypertension (essential) (idiopathic) (primary)

416.1 Kyphoscoliotic heart disease

416.8 Other chronic pulmonary heart diseases
Pulmonary hypertension, secondary

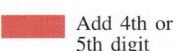 Add 4th or 5th digit
 Nonspecific code
 Unspecified code
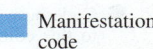 Manifestation code

416.9 Chronic pulmonary heart disease, unspecified
Chronic cardiopulmonary disease
Cor pulmonale (chronic) NOS

417 Other diseases of pulmonary circulation

417.0 Arteriovenous fistula of pulmonary vessels
Excludes: congenital arteriovenous fistula (747.3)

417.1 Aneurysm of pulmonary artery
Excludes: congenital aneurysm (747.3)

417.8 Other specified diseases of pulmonary circulation
Pulmonary:
  arteritis
  endarteritis
Rupture of pulmonary vessel
Stricture of pulmonary vessel

417.9 Unspecified disease of pulmonary circulation

OTHER FORMS OF HEART DISEASE (420-429)

420 Acute pericarditis
Includes: acute:
  mediastinopericarditis
  myopericarditis
  pericardial effusion
  pleuropericarditis
  pneumopericarditis

Excludes: acute rheumatic pericarditis (391.0)
postmyocardial infarction syndrome [Dressler's] (411.0)

420.0 Acute pericarditis in diseases classified elsewhere
Code first underlying disease, as:
  actinomycosis (039.8)
  amebiasis (006.8)
  chronic uremia (585.9)
  nocardiosis (039.8)
  tuberculosis (017.9)
  uremia NOS (586)

Excludes: pericarditis (acute) (in):
  Coxsackie (virus) (074.21)
  gonococcal (098.83)
  histoplasmosis (115.0-115.9 with fifth-digit 3)
  meningococcal infection (036.41)
  syphilitic (093.81)

⑤ **420.9 Other and unspecified acute pericarditis**

420.90 Acute pericarditis, unspecified
Pericarditis (acute):
  NOS
  infective NOS
  sicca

420.91 Acute idiopathic pericarditis
Pericarditis, acute:
  benign
  nonspecific
  viral

420.99 Other
Pericarditis (acute):   Pericarditis (acute):
  pneumococcal   streptococcal
  purulent   suppurative
  staphylococcal   Pneumopyopericardium
                           Pyopericardium

Excludes: pericarditis in diseases classified elsewhere (420.0)

CIRCULATORY SYSTEM

421 Acute and subacute endocarditis

421.0 Acute and subacute bacterial endocarditis

Endocarditis (acute) (chronic) (subacute):
  bacterial
  infective NOS
  lenta
  malignant
  purulent

Endocarditis (acute) (chronic) (subacute):
  septic
  ulcerative
  vegetative
Infective aneurysm
Subacute bacterial endocarditis [SBE]

Use additional code, if desired, to identify infectious organism [e.g., Streptococcus 041.0, Staphylococcus 041.1]

421.1 Acute and subacute infective endocarditis in diseases classified elsewhere

Code first underlying disease, as:
  blastomycosis (116.0)
  Q fever (083.0)
  typhoid (fever) (002.0)

Excludes: endocarditis (in):
  Coxsackie (virus) (074.22)
  gonococcal (098.84)
  histoplasmosis (115.0-115.9 with fifth-digit 4)
  meningococcal infection (036.42)
  monilial (112.81)

421.9 Acute endocarditis, unspecified

Endocarditis, acute or subacute
Myoendocarditis, acute or subacute
Periendocarditis, acute or subacute

Excludes: *acute rheumatic endocarditis (391.1)*

422 Acute myocarditis

Excludes: *acute rheumatic myocarditis (391.2)*

422.0 Acute myocarditis in diseases classified elsewhere

Code first underlying disease, as:
  myocarditis (acute):
    influenzal (487.8)
    tuberculous (017.9)

Excludes: *myocarditis (acute) (due to):*
  aseptic, of newborn (074.23)
  Coxsackie (virus) (074.23)
  diphtheritic (032.82)
  meningococcal infection (036.43)
  syphilitic (093.82)
  toxoplasmosis (130.3)

⑤ **422.9 Other and unspecified acute myocarditis**

422.90 Acute myocarditis, unspecified
Acute or subacute (interstitial) myocarditis

422.91 Idiopathic myocarditis
Myocarditis (acute or subacute):
  Fiedler's
  giant cell
  isolated (diffuse) (granulomatous)
  nonspecific granulomatous

422.92 Septic myocarditis
Myocarditis, acute or subacute:
  pneumococcal
  staphylococcal

Use additional code, if desired, to identify infectious organism [e.g., Staphylococcus 041.1]

Excludes: *myocarditis, acute or subacute:*
  in bacterial diseases classified elsewhere (422.0)
  streptococcal (391.2)

422.93 Toxic myocarditis

422.99 Other

341

 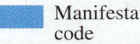

TABULAR LIST

423 Other diseases of pericardium
Excludes: that specified as rheumatic (393)

423.0 Hemopericardium

423.1 Adhesive pericarditis
Adherent pericardium
Fibrosis of pericardium
Milk spots
Pericarditis:
  adhesive
  obliterative
Soldiers' patches

423.2 Constrictive pericarditis
Concato's disease
Pick's disease of heart (and liver)

● 423.3 Cardiac tamponade
Code first the underlying cause

423.8 Other specified diseases of pericardium
Calcification of pericardium
Fistula of pericardium

423.9 Unspecified disease of pericardium

424 Other diseases of endocardium
Excludes: bacterial endocarditis (421.0-421.9)
  rheumatic endocarditis (391.1, 394.0-397.9)
  syphilitic endocarditis (093.20-093.24)

424.0 Mitral valve disorders
Mitral (valve):
  incompetence NOS of specified cause, except rheumatic
  insufficiency NOS of specified cause, except rheumatic
  regurgitation NOS of specified cause, except rheumatic

Excludes: mitral (valve):
  disease (394.9)
  failure (394.9)
  stenosis (394.0)
  the listed conditions:
    specified as rheumatic (394.1)
    unspecified as to cause but with mention of:
      diseases of aortic valve (396.0-396.9)
      mitral stenosis or obstruction (394.2)

424.1 Aortic valve disorders
Aortic (valve):
  incompetence NOS of specified cause, except rheumatic
  insufficiency NOS of specified cause, except rheumatic
  regurgitation NOS of specified cause, except rheumatic
  stenosis NOS of specified cause, except rheumatic

Excludes: hypertrophic subaortic stenosis (425.1)
  that specified as rheumatic (395.0-395.9)
  that of unspecified cause but with mention of diseases of mitral valve (396.0-396.9)

424.2 Tricuspid valve disorders, specified as nonrheumatic
Tricuspid valve:
  incompetence of specified cause, except rheumatic
  insufficiency of specified cause, except rheumatic
  regurgitation of specified cause, except rheumatic
  stenosis of specified cause, except rheumatic

Excludes: rheumatic or of unspecified cause (397.0)

424.3 Pulmonary valve disorders
Pulmonic:
  incompetence NOS
  insufficiency NOS
Pulmonic:
  regurgitation NOS
  stenosis NOS

Excludes: that specified as rheumatic (397.1)

CIRCULATORY SYSTEM

⑤ **424.9 Endocarditis, valve unspecified**

424.90 Endocarditis, valve unspecified, unspecified cause
Endocarditis (chronic):
  NOS
  nonbacterial thrombotic
Valvular:
  incompetence of unspecified valve, unspecified cause
  insufficiency of unspecified valve, unspecified cause
  regurgitation of unspecified valve, unspecified cause
  stenosis of unspecified valve, unspecified cause
Valvulitis (chronic)

424.91 *Endocarditis in diseases classified elsewhere*
Code first underlying disease, as:
  atypical verrucous endocarditis [Libman-Sacks] (710.0)
  disseminated lupus erythematosus (710.0)
  tuberculosis (017.9)

Excludes: syphilitic (093.20-093.24)

424.99 Other
Any condition classifiable to 424.90 with specified cause, except rheumatic

Excludes: endocardial fibroelastosis (425.3)
that specified as rheumatic (397.9)

425 Cardiomyopathy
Includes: myocardiopathy

425.0 Endomyocardial fibrosis

425.1 Hypertrophic obstructive cardiomyopathy
Hypertrophic subaortic stenosis (idiopathic)

425.2 Obscure cardiomyopathy of Africa
Becker's disease
Idiopathic mural endomyocardial disease

425.3 Endocardial fibroelastosis
Elastomyofibrosis

425.4 Other primary cardiomyopathies
Cardiomyopathy: Cardiomyopathy:
  NOS   idiopathic
  congestive   nonobstructive
  constrictive   obstructive
  familial   restrictive
  hypertrophic   Cardiovascular collagenosis

425.5 Alcoholic cardiomyopathy

425.7 *Nutritional and metabolic cardiomyopathy*
Code first underlying disease, as:
  amyloidosis (277.30-277.39)
  beriberi (265.0)
  cardiac glycogenosis (271.0)
  mucopolysaccharidosis (277.5)
  thyrotoxicosis (242.0-242.9)

Excludes: gouty tophi of heart (274.82)

425.8 *Cardiomyopathy in other diseases classified elsewhere*
Code first underlying disease, as:
  Friedreich's ataxia (334.0)
  myotonia atrophica (359.21)
  progressive muscular dystrophy (359.1)
  sarcoidosis (135)

Excludes: cardiomyopathy in Chagas' disease (086.0)

425.9 Secondary cardiomyopathy, unspecified

426 Conduction disorders

426.0 Atrioventricular block, complete
Third degree atrioventricular block

⑤ **426.1 Atrioventricular block, other and unspecified**

426.10 Atrioventricular block, unspecified
Atrioventricular [AV] block (incomplete) (partial)

343

  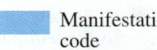

TABULAR LIST

- **426.11 First degree atrioventricular block**
  Incomplete atrioventricular block, first degree
  Prolonged P-R interval NOS

- **426.12 Mobitz (type) II atrioventricular block**
  Incomplete atrioventricular block:
    Mobitz (type) II
    second degree, Mobitz (type) II

- **426.13 Other second degree atrioventricular block**
  Incomplete atrioventricular block:
    Mobitz (type) I [Wenckebach's]
    second degree:
      NOS
      Mobitz (type) I
    with 2:1 atrioventricular response [block]
  Wenckebach's phenomenon

426.2 Left bundle branch hemiblock
Block:
  left anterior fascicular
  left posterior fascicular

426.3 Other left bundle branch block
Left bundle branch block:
  NOS
  anterior fascicular with posterior fascicular
  complete
  main stem

426.4 Right bundle branch block

⑤ **426.5 Bundle branch block, other and unspecified**

- **426.50 Bundle branch block, unspecified**
- **426.51 Right bundle branch block and left posterior fascicular block**
- **426.52 Right bundle branch block and left anterior fascicular block**
- **426.53 Other bilateral bundle branch block**
  Bifascicular block NOS
  Bilateral bundle branch block NOS
  Right bundle branch with left bundle branch block (incomplete) (main stem)
- **426.54 Trifascicular block**

426.6 Other heart block
Intraventricular block: Sinoatrial block
  NOS   Sinoauricular block
  diffuse
  myofibrillar

426.7 Anomalous atrioventricular excitation
Atrioventricular conduction:
  accelerated
  accessory
  pre-excitation
Ventricular pre-excitation
Wolff-Parkinson-White syndrome

⑤ **426.8 Other specified conduction disorders**

- **426.81 Lown-Ganong-Levine syndrome**
  Syndrome of short P-R interval, normal QRS complexes, and supraventricular tachycardias
- **426.82 Long QT syndrome**
- **426.89 Other**
  Dissociation:
    atrioventricular [AV]
    interference
    isorhythmic
  Nonparoxysmal AV nodal tachycardia

426.9 Conduction disorder, unspecified
Heart block NOS
Stokes-Adams syndrome

---

344   ● Code new to this edition   ▲ Revision of existing code   ④ ⑤ Fourth or fifth digit required

CIRCULATORY SYSTEM

427 Cardiac dysrhythmias
> *Excludes:* that complicating:
>> abortion (634-638 with .7, 639.8)
>> ectopic or molar pregnancy (639.8)
>> labor or delivery (668.1, 669.4)

- **427.0 Paroxysmal supraventricular tachycardia**
  Paroxysmal tachycardia:
  - atrial [PAT]
  - atrioventricular [AV]
  - junctional
  - nodal

- **427.1 Paroxysmal ventricular tachycardia**
  Ventricular tachycardia (paroxysmal)

- **427.2 Paroxysmal tachycardia, unspecified**
  Bouveret-Hoffmann syndrome
  Paroxysmal tachycardia:
  - NOS
  - essential

- ⑤ **427.3 Atrial fibrillation and flutter**
  - **427.31 Atrial fibrillation**
  - **427.32 Atrial flutter**

- ⑤ **427.4 Ventricular fibrillation and flutter**
  - **427.41 Ventricular fibrillation**
  - **427.42 Ventricular flutter**

- **427.5 Cardiac arrest**
  Cardiorespiratory arrest

- ⑤ **427.6 Premature beats**
  - **427.60 Premature beats, unspecified**
    - Ectopic beats
    - Extrasystoles
    - Extrasystolic arrhythmia
    - Premature contractions or systoles NOS
  - **427.61 Supraventricular premature beats**
    Atrial premature beats, contractions, or systoles
  - **427.69 Other**
    Ventricular premature beats, contractions, or systoles

- ⑤ **427.8 Other specified cardiac dysrhythmias**
  - **427.81 Sinoatrial node dysfunction**
    Sinus bradycardia: Syndrome:
      persistent   sick sinus
      severe   tachycardia-bradycardia
    > *Excludes:* sinus bradycardia NOS (427.89)
  - **427.89 Other**
    Rhythm disorder: Rhythm disorder:
      coronary sinus   nodal
      ectopic   Wandering (atrial) pacemaker
    > *Excludes:* carotid sinus syncope (337.0)
    >> neonatal bradycardia (779.81)
    >> neonatal tachycardia (779.82)
    >> reflex bradycardia (337.0)
    >> tachycardia (785.0)

- **427.9 Cardiac dysrhythmia, unspecified**
  Arrhythmia (cardiac) NOS

TABULAR LIST

428 Heart failure
Code, if applicable, heart failure due to hypertension first (402.0-402.9, with fifth-digit 1 or 404.0-404.9 with fifth digit 1 or 3)

Excludes: following cardiac surgery (429.4)
 rheumatic (398.91)
 that complicating:
  abortion (634-638 with .7, 639.8)
  ectopic or molar pregnancy (639.8)
  labor or delivery (668.1, 669.4)

428.0 Congestive heart failure, unspecified
Congestive heart disease
Right heart failure (secondary to left heart failure)

Excludes: fluid overload NOS (276.6)

428.1 Left heart failure
Acute edema of lung with heart disease NOS or heart failure
Acute pulmonary edema with heart disease NOS or heart failure
Cardiac asthma
Left ventricular failure

428.2 Systolic heart failure
Excludes: combined systolic and diastolic heart failure (428.40-428.43)

428.20 Unspecified
428.21 Acute
428.22 Chronic
428.23 Acute on chronic

428.3 Diastolic heart failure
Excludes: combined systolic and diastolic heart failure (428.40-428.43)

428.30 Unspecified
428.31 Acute
428.32 Chronic
428.33 Acute on chronic

428.4 Combined systolic and diastolic heart failure
428.40 Unspecified
428.41 Acute
428.42 Chronic
428.43 Acute on chronic

428.9 Heart failure, unspecified
Cardiac failure NOS   Myocardial failure NOS
Heart failure NOS   Weak heart

429 Ill-defined descriptions and complications of heart disease

429.0 Myocarditis, unspecified
Myocarditis:
 NOS (with mention of arteriosclerosis)
 chronic (interstitial) (with mention of arteriosclerosis)
 fibroid (with mention of arteriosclerosis)
 senile (with mention of arteriosclerosis)
Use additional code, if desired, to identify presence of arteriosclerosis

Excludes: acute or subacute (422.0-422.9)
 rheumatic (398.0)
  acute (391.2)
 that due to hypertension (402.0-402.9)

429.1 Myocardial degeneration
Degeneration of heart or myocardium:
 fatty (with mention of arteriosclerosis)
 mural (with mention of arteriosclerosis)
 muscular (with mention of arteriosclerosis)
Myocardial:
 degeneration (with mention of arteriosclerosis)
 disease (with mention of arteriosclerosis)
Use additional code, if desired, to identify presence of arteriosclerosis

Excludes: that due to hypertension (402.0-402.9)

CIRCULATORY SYSTEM

429.2 Cardiovascular disease, unspecified
  Arteriosclerotic cardiovascular disease [ASCVD]
  Cardiovascular arteriosclerosis
  Cardiovascular:
   degeneration (with mention of arteriosclerosis)
   disease (with mention of arteriosclerosis)
   sclerosis (with mention of arteriosclerosis)
Use additional code, if desired, to identify presence of arteriosclerosis
> *Excludes:* that due to hypertension (402.0-402.9)

429.3 Cardiomegaly
  Cardiac: Ventricular dilatation
   dilatation
   hypertrophy
> *Excludes:* that due to hypertension (402.0-402.9)

429.4 Functional disturbances following cardiac surgery
  Cardiac insufficiency following cardiac surgery or due to prosthesis
  Heart failure following cardiac surgery or due to prosthesis
  Postcardiotomy syndrome
  Postvalvulotomy syndrome
> *Excludes:* cardiac failure in the immediate postoperative period (997.1)

429.5 Rupture of chordae tendineae

429.6 Rupture of papillary muscle

⑤ **429.7 Certain sequelae of myocardial infarction, not elsewhere classified**
Use additional code to identify the associated myocardial infarction:
  with onset of 8 weeks or less (410.00-410.92)
  with onset of more than 8 weeks (414.8)
> *Excludes:* congenital defects of heart (745, 746)
>   coronary aneurysm (414.11)
>   disorders of papillary muscle (429.6, 429.81)
>   postmyocardial infarction syndrome (411.0)
>   rupture of chordae tendineae (429.5)

  429.71 Acquired cardiac septal defect
> *Excludes:* acute septal infarction (410.00-410.92)

  429.79 Other
    Mural thrombus (atrial) (ventricular), acquired, following myocardial infarction

⑤ **429.8 Other ill-defined heart diseases**
  429.81 Other disorders of papillary muscle
   Papillary muscle: Papillary muscle:
    atrophy   incompetence
    degeneration   incoordination
    dysfunction   scarring

  429.82 Hyperkinetic heart disease

  429.83 Takotsubo syndrome
   Broken heart syndrome
   Reversible left ventricular dysfunction following sudden emotional stress
   Stress induced cardiomyopathy
   Transient left ventricular apical ballooning syndrome

  429.89 Other
   Carditis
> *Excludes:* that due to hypertension (402.0-402.9)

429.9 Heart disease, unspecified
  Heart disease (organic) NOS
  Morbus cordis NOS
> *Excludes:* that due to hypertension (402.0-402.9)

CEREBROVASCULAR DISEASE (430-438)

  Includes: with mention of hypertension (conditions classifiable to 401-405)
Use additional code, if desired, to identify presence of hypertension
> *Excludes:* any condition classifiable to 430-434, 436, 437 occurring during pregnancy,
>   childbirth, or the puerperium, or specified as puerperal (674.0)
>   iatrogenic cerebrovascular infarction or hemorrhage (997.02)

TABULAR LIST

430 Subarachnoid hemorrhage
Meningeal hemorrhage
Ruptured:
  berry aneurysm
  (congenital) cerebral aneurysm NOS

Excludes: syphilitic ruptured cerebral aneurysm (094.87)

431 Intracerebral hemorrhage
Hemorrhage (of):
  basilar
  bulbar
  cerebellar
  cerebral
  cerebromeningeal
  cortical
  internal capsule
Hemorrhage (of):
  intrapontine
  pontine
  subcortical
  ventricular
Rupture of blood vessel in brain

432 Other and unspecified intracranial hemorrhage

432.0 Nontraumatic extradural hemorrhage
Nontraumatic epidural hemorrhage

432.1 Subdural hemorrhage
Subdural hematoma, nontraumatic

432.9 Unspecified intracranial hemorrhage
Intracranial hemorrhage NOS

433 Occlusion and stenosis of precerebral arteries
The following fifth-digit subclassification is for use with category 433:

  0 without mention of cerebral infarction
  1 with cerebral infarction

Includes: embolism of basilar, carotid, and vertebral arteries
          narrowing of basilar, carotid, and vertebral arteries
          obstruction of basilar, carotid, and vertebral arteries
          thrombosis of basilar, carotid, and vertebral arteries

Excludes: insufficiency NOS of precerebral arteries (435.0-435.9)

433.0 Basilar artery
433.1 Carotid artery
433.2 Vertebral artery
433.3 Multiple and bilateral
433.8 Other specified precerebral artery
433.9 Unspecified precerebral artery
Precerebral artery NOS

434 Occlusion of cerebral arteries
The following fifth-digit subclassification is for use with category 434:

  0 without mention of cerebral infarction
  1 with cerebral infarction

434.0 Cerebral thrombosis
Thrombosis of cerebral arteries

434.1 Cerebral embolism

434.9 Cerebral artery occlusion, unspecified

435 Transient cerebral ischemia
Includes: cerebrovascular insufficiency (acute) with transient focal neurological signs and symptoms
          insufficiency of basilar, carotid, and vertebral arteries
          spasm of cerebral arteries

Excludes: acute cerebrovascular insufficiency NOS (437.1)
            that due to any condition classifiable to 433 (433.0-433.9)

435.0 Basilar artery syndrome
435.1 Vertebral artery syndrome
435.2 Subclavian steal syndrome
435.3 Vertebrobasilar artery syndrome
435.8 Other specified transient cerebral ischemias

● Code new to this edition ▲ Revision of existing code ④ ⑤ Fourth or fifth digit required

CIRCULATORY SYSTEM

435.9 **Unspecified transient cerebral ischemia**
   Impending cerebrovascular accident
   Intermittent cerebral ischemia
   Transient ischemic attack [TIA]

436 **Acute, but ill-defined, cerebrovascular disease**
   Apoplexy, apoplectic:
      NOS
      attack
      cerebral
      seizure
   Cerebral seizure

   Excludes: any condition classifiable to categories 430-435
      cerebrovascular accident (434.91)
      CVA (ischemic) (434.91)
         embolic (434.11)
         hemorrhagic (430, 431, 432.0-432.9)
         thrombotic (434.01)
      postoperative cerebrovascular accident (997.02)
      stroke (ischemic) (434.91)
         embolic (434.11)
         hemorrhagic (430, 431, 432.0-432.9)
         thrombotic (434.01)

437 **Other and ill-defined cerebrovascular disease**

   437.0 **Cerebral atherosclerosis**
      Atheroma of cerebral arteries
      Cerebral arteriosclerosis

   437.1 **Other generalized ischemic cerebrovascular disease**
      Acute cerebrovascular insufficiency NOS
      Cerebral ischemia (chronic)

   437.2 **Hypertensive encephalopathy**

   437.3 **Cerebral aneurysm, nonruptured**
      Internal carotid artery, intracranial portion
      Internal carotid artery NOS

      Excludes: congenital cerebral aneurysm, nonruptured (747.81)
         internal carotid artery, extracranial portion (442.81)

   437.4 **Cerebral arteritis**

   437.5 **Moyamoya disease**

   437.6 **Nonpyogenic thrombosis of intracranial venous sinus**
      Excludes: pyogenic (325)

   437.7 **Transient global amnesia**

   437.8 **Other**

   437.9 **Unspecified**
      Cerebrovascular disease or lesion NOS

438 **Late effects of cerebrovascular disease**
   Note: This category is to be used to indicate conditions in 430-437 as the cause of late effects. The "late effects" include conditions specified as such, as sequelae, which may occur at any time after the onset of the causal condition.

   Excludes: personal history of:
      cerebral infarction without residual deficits (V12.54)
      PRIND (Prolonged reversible ischemic neurologic deficit) (V12.54)
      RIND (Reversible ischemic neurological deficit) (V12.54)
      transient ischemic attack (TIA) (V12.54)

   438.0 **Cognitive deficits**

   ⑤ **438.1** **Speech and language deficits**
      438.10 Speech and language deficit, unspecified
      438.11 Aphasia
      438.12 Dysphasia
      438.19 Other speech and language deficits

   ⑤ **438.2** **Hemiplegia/hemiparesis**
      438.20 Hemiplegia affecting unspecified side
      438.21 Hemiplegia affecting dominant side

349

TABULAR LIST

438.22 Hemiplegia affecting nondominant side

⑤ 438.3 **Monoplegia of upper limb**
- **438.30** Monoplegia of upper limb affecting unspecified side
- 438.31 Monoplegia of upper limb affecting dominant side
- 438.32 Monoplegia of upper limb affecting nondominant side

⑤ 438.4 **Monoplegia of lower limb**
- **438.40** Monoplegia of lower limb affecting unspecified side
- 438.41 Monoplegia of lower limb affecting dominant side
- 438.42 Monoplegia of lower limb affecting nondominant side

⑤ 438.5 **Other paralytic syndrome**

Use additional code to identify type of paralytic syndrome, such as:
  locked-in state (344.81)
  quadriplegia (344.00-344.09)

Excludes: late effects of cerebrovascular accident with:
  hemiplegia/hemiparesis (438.20-438.22)
  monoplegia of lower limb (438.40-438.42)
  monoplegia of upper limb (438.30-438.32)

- **438.50** Other paralytic syndrome affecting unspecified side
- **438.51** Other paralytic syndrome affecting dominant side
- **438.52** Other paralytic syndrome affecting nondominant side
- **438.53** Other paralytic syndrome, bilateral

438.6 **Alterations of sensations**
Use additional code to identify the altered sensation

438.7 **Disturbances of vision**
Use additional code to identify the visual disturbance

⑤ 438.8 **Other late effects of cerebrovascular disease**
- 438.81 **Apraxia**
- 438.82 **Dysphagia**
  Use additional code to identify the type of dysphagia, if known (787.20-787.29)
- 438.83 **Facial weakness**
  Facial droop
- 438.84 **Ataxia**
- 438.85 **Vertigo**
- ▲ **438.89** **Other late effects of cerebrovascular disease**
  Use additional code to identify the late effect

438.9 Unspecified late effects of cerebrovascular disease

DISEASES OF ARTERIES, ARTERIOLES, AND CAPILLARIES (440-449)

440 **Atherosclerosis**
Includes: arteriolosclerosis
  arteriosclerosis (obliterans) (senile)
  arteriosclerotic vascular disease
  atheroma
  degeneration:
    arterial
    arteriovascular
    vascular
  endarteritis deformans or obliterans
  senile arteritis
  senile endarteritis

Excludes: atheroembolism (445.01-445.89)
  atherosclerosis of bypass graft of the extremities (440.30-440.32)

440.0 **Of aorta**

440.1 **Of renal artery**

Excludes: atherosclerosis of renal arterioles (403.00-403.91)

CIRCULATORY SYSTEM

⑤ **440.2 Of native arteries of the extremities**
Use additional code, if applicable, to identify chronic total occlusion of artery of the extremities (440.4)

Excludes: *atherosclerosis of bypass graft of the extremities (440.30-440.32)*

440.20 Atherosclerosis of the extremities, unspecified

440.21 Atherosclerosis of the extremities with intermittent claudication

440.22 Atherosclerosis of the extremities with rest pain
Any condition classifiable to 440.21

440.23 Atherosclerosis of the extremities with ulceration
Any condition classifiable to 440.21 and 440.22
Use additional code for any associated ulceration (707.10-707.9)

440.24 Atherosclerosis of the extremities with gangrene
Any condition classifiable to 440.21, 440.22, and 440.23 with ischemic gangrene 785.4
Use additional code for any associated ulceration (707.10-707.9)

Excludes: *gas gangrene 040.0*

440.29 Other

⑤ **440.3 Of bypass graft of the extremities**

Excludes: *atherosclerosis of native artery of the extremity (440.21-440.24)*
embolism [occlusion NOS] [thrombus]
of graft (996.74)

440.30 Of unspecified graft

440.31 Of autologous vein bypass graft

440.32 Of nonautologous biological bypass graft

● **440.4 Chronic total occlusion of artery of the extremities**
Complete occlusion of artery of the extremities
Total occlusion of artery of the extremities
Code first atherosclerosis of arteries of the extremities (440.20-440.29, 440.30-440.32)

Excludes: *acute occlusion of artery of extremity (444.21- 444.22)*

440.8 **Of other specified arteries**

Excludes: *basilar (433.0)*
carotid (433.1)
cerebral (437.0)
coronary (414.00-414.07)
mesenteric (557.1)
precerebral (433.0-433.9)
pulmonary (416.0)
vertebral (433.2)

440.9 **Generalized and unspecified atherosclerosis**
Arteriosclerotic vascular disease NOS

Excludes: *arteriosclerotic cardiovascular disease [ASCVD] (429.2)*

441 **Aortic aneurysm and dissection**

Excludes: *syphilitic aortic aneurysm (093.0)*
traumatic aortic aneurysm (901.0, 902.0)

⑤ **441.0 Dissection of aorta**

441.00 Unspecified site

441.01 Thoracic

441.02 Abdominal

441.03 Thoracoabdominal

441.1 Thoracic aneurysm, ruptured

441.2 Thoracic aneurysm without mention of rupture

441.3 Abdominal aneurysm, ruptured

441.4 Abdominal aneurysm without mention of rupture

441.5 **Aortic aneurysm of unspecified site, ruptured**
Rupture of aorta NOS

441.6 Thoracoabdominal aneurysm, ruptured

441.7 Thoracoabdominal aneurysm, without mention of rupture

TABULAR LIST

441.9 Aortic aneurysm of unspecified site without mention of rupture
Aneurysm
Dilatation of aorta
Hyaline necrosis of aorta

442 Other aneurysm
Includes: aneurysm (ruptured) (cirsoid) (false) (varicose)
aneurysmal varix

Excludes: arteriovenous aneurysm or fistula:
acquired (447.0)
congenital (747.60-747.69)
traumatic (900.0-904.9)

442.0 Of artery of upper extremity

442.1 Of renal artery

442.2 Of iliac artery

442.3 Of artery of lower extremity
Aneurysm:
femoral artery
popliteal artery

⑤ **442.8 Of other specified artery**

442.81 Artery of neck
Aneurysm of carotid artery (common) (external) (internal, extracranial portion)

Excludes: internal carotid artery, intracranial portion (437.3)

442.82 Subclavian artery

442.83 Splenic artery

442.84 Other visceral artery
Aneurysm:
celiac artery
gastroduodenal artery
gastroepiploic artery
hepatic artery
pancreaticoduodenal artery
superior mesenteric artery

442.89 Other
Aneurysm:
mediastinal artery
spinal artery

Excludes: cerebral (nonruptured) (437.3)
congenital (747.81)
ruptured (430)
coronary (414.11)
heart (414.10)
pulmonary (417.1)

442.9 Of unspecified site

443 Other peripheral vascular disease

443.0 Raynaud's syndrome
Raynaud's:
disease
phenomenon (secondary)
Use additional code, if desired, to identify gangrene (785.4)

443.1 Thromboangiitis obliterans [Buerger's disease]
Presenile gangrene

⑤ **443.2 Other arterial dissection**

Excludes: dissection of aorta (441.00-441.03)
dissection of coronary arteries (414.12)

443.21 Dissection of carotid artery

443.22 Dissection of iliac artery

443.23 Dissection of renal artery

443.24 Dissection of vertebral artery

443.29 Dissection of other artery

CIRCULATORY SYSTEM

⑤ **443.8 Other specified peripheral vascular diseases**

443.81 Peripheral angiopathy in diseases classified elsewhere
Code first underlying disease, as:
diabetes mellitus (250.7)

443.82 Erythromelalgia

443.89 Other
Acrocyanosis
Acroparesthesia:
simple [Schultze's type]
vasomotor [Nothnagel's type]
Erythrocyanosis

Excludes: chilblains (991.5)
frostbite (991.0-991.3)
immersion foot (991.4)

443.9 Peripheral vascular disease, unspecified
Intermittent claudication NOS
Peripheral:
angiopathy NOS
vascular disease NOS
Spasm of artery

Excludes: atherosclerosis of the arteries of the extremities (440.20-440.22)
spasm of cerebral artery (435.0-435.9)

444 Arterial embolism and thrombosis
Includes: infarction:
embolic
thrombotic
occlusion

Excludes: atheroembolism (445.01-445.89)
septic arterial embolism (449)
that complicating:
abortion (634-638 with .6, 639.6)
ectopic or molar pregnancy (639.6)
pregnancy, childbirth, or the puerperium (673.0-673.8)

444.0 Of abdominal aorta
Aortic bifurcation syndrome   Leriche's syndrome
Aortoiliac obstruction   Saddle embolus

444.1 Of thoracic aorta
Embolism or thrombosis of aorta (thoracic)

⑤ **444.2 Of arteries of the extremities**

444.21 Upper extremity

444.22 Lower extremity
Arterial embolism or thrombosis:
femoral
peripheral NOS
popliteal

Excludes: iliofemoral (444.81)

⑤ **444.8 Of other specified artery**

444.81 Iliac artery

444.89 Other

Excludes: basilar (433.0)
carotid (433.1)
cerebral (434.0-434.9)
coronary (410.00-410.92)
mesenteric (557.0)
ophthalmic (362.30-362.34)
precerebral (433.0-433.9)
pulmonary (415.19)
renal (593.81)
retinal (362.30-362.34)
vertebral (433.2)

444.9 Of unspecified artery

TABULAR LIST

445 **Atheroembolism**
    Includes: Atherothrombotic microembolism
                  Cholesterol embolism

⑤ **445.0 Of extremities**
    445.01 Upper extremity
    445.02 Lower extremity

⑤ **445.8 Of other sites**
    445.81 Kidney
        Use additional code for any associated acute renal failure or chronic kidney disease (584, 585)
    445.89 Other site

446 **Polyarteritis nodosa and allied conditions**
    446.0 Polyarteritis nodosa
        Disseminated necrotizing periarteritis
        Necrotizing angiitis
        Panarteritis (nodosa)
        Periarteritis (nodosa)

    446.1 Acute febrile mucocutaneous lymph node syndrome [MLNS]
        Kawasaki disease

⑤ **446.2 Hypersensitivity angiitis**
      Excludes: *antiglomerular basement membrane disease without pulmonary hemorrhage (583.89)*
    446.20 Hypersensitivity angiitis, unspecified
    446.21 Goodpasture's syndrome
        Antiglomerular basement membrane antibody-mediated nephritis with pulmonary hemorrhage
    Use additional code, if desired, to identify renal disease (583.81)
    446.29 Other specified hypersensitivity angiitis

    446.3 Lethal midline granuloma
        Malignant granuloma of face

    446.4 Wegener's granulomatosis
        Necrotizing respiratory granulomatosis
        Wegener's syndrome

    446.5 Giant cell arteritis
        Cranial arteritis   Temporal arteritis
        Horton's disease

    446.6 Thrombotic microangiopathy
        Moschcowitz's syndrome
        Thrombotic thrombocytopenic purpura

    446.7 Takayasu's disease
        Aortic arch arteritis
        Pulseless disease

447 **Other disorders of arteries and arterioles**
    447.0 Arteriovenous fistula, acquired
        Arteriovenous aneurysm, acquired
      Excludes: *cerebrovascular (437.3)*
          coronary (414.19)
          pulmonary (417.0)
          surgically created arteriovenous shunt or fistula:
            complication (996.1, 996.61-996.62)
            status or presence (V45.1)
          traumatic (900.0-904.9)

    447.1 Stricture of artery

    447.2 Rupture of artery
        Erosion of artery
        Fistula, except arteriovenous of artery
        Ulcer of artery
      Excludes: *traumatic rupture of artery (900.0-904.9)*

    447.3 Hyperplasia of renal artery
        Fibromuscular hyperplasia of renal artery

CIRCULATORY SYSTEM

447.4 Celiac artery compression syndrome
  Celiac axis syndrome
  Marable's syndrome

447.5 Necrosis of artery

447.6 Arteritis, unspecified
  Aortitis NOS
  Endarteritis NOS

  Excludes: *arteritis, endarteritis:*
    aortic arch (446.7)
    cerebral (437.4)
    coronary (414.00-414.07)
    deformans (440.0-440.9)
    obliterans (440.0-440.9)
    pulmonary (417.8)
    senile (440.0-440.9)
  polyarteritis NOS (446.0)
  syphilitic aortitis (093.1)

447.8 Other specified disorders of arteries and arterioles
  Fibromuscular hyperplasia of arteries, except renal

447.9 Unspecified disorders of arteries and arterioles

448 Disease of capillaries

448.0 Hereditary hemorrhagic telangiectasia
  Rendu-Osler-Weber disease

448.1 Nevus, non-neoplastic
  Nevus: Nevus:
    araneus   spider
    senile   stellar

  Excludes: *neoplastic (216.0-216.9)*
    port wine (757.32)
    strawberry (757.32)

448.9 Other and unspecified capillary diseases
  Capillary:
    hemorrhage
    hyperpermeability
    thrombosis

  Excludes: *capillary fragility (hereditary) (287.8)*

● **449 Septic arterial embolism**
  Code first underlying infection, such as:
    infective endocarditis (421.0)
    lung abscess (513.0)
  Use additional code to identify the site of the embolism (433.0-433.9, 444.0-444.9)

  Excludes: *septic pulmonary embolism (415.12)*

DISEASES OF VEINS AND LYMPHATICS, AND OTHER DISEASES OF CIRCULATORY SYSTEM (451-459)

451 Phlebitis and thrombophlebitis
  Includes: endophlebitis
             inflammation, vein
             periphlebitis
             suppurative phlebitis
  Use additional E Code, if desired, to identify drug, if drug-induced

  Excludes: *that complicating:*
    abortion (634-638 with .7, 639.8)
    ectopic or molar pregnancy (639.8)
    pregnancy, childbirth, or the puerperium (671.0-671.9)
    that due to or following:
      implant or catheter device (996.61-996.62)
      infusion, perfusion, or transfusion (999.2)

  451.0 Of superficial vessels of lower extremities
    Saphenous vein (greater) (lesser)

  ⑤ **451.1 Of deep vessels of lower extremities**
    451.11 Femoral vein (deep) (superficial)

Add 4th or 5th digit	Nonspecific code	Unspecified code	Manifestation code

355

TABULAR LIST

451.19 **Other**
- Femoropopliteal vein
- Popliteal vein
- Tibial vein

451.2 **Of lower extremities, unspecified**

⑤ **451.8** **Of other sites**

Excludes: intracranial venous sinus (325)
nonpyogenic (437.6)
portal (vein) (572.1)

451.81 **Iliac vein**

451.82 **Of superficial veins of upper extremities**
- Antecubital vein
- Basilic vein
- Cephalic vein

451.83 **Of deep veins of upper extremities**
- Brachial vein
- Radial vein
- Ulnar vein

451.84 **Of upper extremities, unspecified**

451.89 **Other**
- Axillary vein
- Jugular vein
- Subclavian vein
- Thrombophlebitis of breast (Mondor's disease)

451.9 **Of unspecified site**

452 **Portal vein thrombosis**
Portal (vein) obstruction

Excludes: hepatic vein thrombosis (453.0)
phlebitis of portal vein (572.1)

453 **Other venous embolism and thrombosis**

Excludes: that complicating:
abortion (634-638 with .7, 639.8)
ectopic or molar pregnancy (639.8)
pregnancy, childbirth, or the puerperium (671.0-671.9)
that with inflammation, phlebitis, and thrombophlebitis (451.0-451.9)

453.0 **Budd-Chiari syndrome**
Hepatic vein thrombosis

453.1 **Thrombophlebitis migrans**

453.2 **Of vena cava**

453.3 **Of renal vein**

⑤ **453.4** **Venous embolism and thrombosis of deep vessels of lower extremity**

453.40 **Venous embolism and thrombosis of unspecified deep vessels of lower extremity**
- Deep vein thrombosis NOS
- DVT NOS

453.41 **Venous embolism and thrombosis of deep vessels of proximal lower extremity**
- Femoral
- Iliac
- Popliteal
- Thigh
- Upper leg NOS

453.42 **Venous embolism and thrombosis of deep vessels of distal lower extremity**
- Calf
- Lower leg NOS
- Peroneal
- Tibial

CIRCULATORY SYSTEM

453.8 Of other specified veins
> *Excludes:* cerebral (434.0-434.9)
> coronary (410.00-410.92)
> intracranial venous sinus (325)
>   nonpyogenic (437.6)
> mesenteric (557.0)
> portal (452)
> precerebral (433.0-433.9)
> pulmonary (415.19)

453.9 Of unspecified site
Embolism of vein
Thrombosis (vein)

454 Varicose veins of lower extremities
> *Excludes:* that complicating pregnancy, childbirth, or the puerperium (671.0)

454.0 With ulcer
Varicose ulcer (lower extremity, any part)
Varicose veins with ulcer of lower extremity [any part] or of unspecified site
Any condition classifiable to 454.9 with ulcer or specified as ulcerated

454.1 With inflammation
Stasis dermatitis
Varicose veins with inflammation of lower extremity [any part] or of unspecified site
Any condition classifiable to 454.9 with inflammation or specified as inflamed

454.2 With ulcer and inflammation
Varicose veins with ulcer and inflammation of lower extremity [any part] or of unspecified site
Any condition classifiable to 454.9 with ulcer and inflammation

454.8 With other complications
Edema
Pain
Swelling

454.9 Asymptomatic varicose veins
Phlebectasia of lower extremity [any part] or of unspecified site
Varicose veins NOS
Varicose veins of lower extremity [any part] or of unspecified site
Varix of lower extremity [any part] or of unspecified site

455 Hemorrhoids
Includes: hemorrhoids (anus) (rectum)
          piles
          varicose veins, anus or rectum
> *Excludes:* that complicating pregnancy, childbirth or the puerperium (671.8)

455.0 Internal hemorrhoids without mention of complication

455.1 Internal thrombosed hemorrhoids

455.2 Internal hemorrhoids with other complication
Internal hemorrhoids: Internal hemorrhoids:
   bleeding   strangulated
   prolapsed   ulcerated

455.3 External hemorrhoids without mention of complication

455.4 External thrombosed hemorrhoids

455.5 External hemorrhoids with other complication
External hemorrhoids: External hemorrhoids:
   bleeding   strangulated
   prolapsed   ulcerated

455.6 Unspecified hemorrhoids without mention of complication
Hemorrhoids NOS

455.7 Unspecified thrombosed hemorrhoids
Thrombosed hemorrhoids, unspecified whether internal or external

455.8 Unspecified hemorrhoids with other complication
Hemorrhoids, unspecified whether internal or external:
   bleeding
   prolapsed
   strangulated
   ulcerated

TABULAR LIST

455.9 Residual hemorrhoidal skin tags
Skin tags, anus or rectum

456 Varicose veins of other sites

456.0 Esophageal varices with bleeding

456.1 Esophageal varices without mention of bleeding

⑤ **456.2 Esophageal varices in diseases classified elsewhere**
Code first underlying cause, as:
cirrhosis of liver (571.0-571.9)
portal hypertension (572.3)

456.20 With bleeding

456.21 Without mention of bleeding

456.3 Sublingual varices

456.4 Scrotal varices
Varicocele

456.5 Pelvic varices
Varices of broad ligament

456.6 Vulval varices
Varices of perineum
Excludes: that complicating pregnancy, childbirth, or the puerperium (671.1)

456.8 Varices of other sites
Varicose veins of nasal septum (with ulcer)
Excludes: placental varices (656.7)
retinal varices (362.17)
varicose ulcer of unspecified site (454.0)
varicose veins of unspecified site (454.9)

457 Noninfectious disorders of lymphatic channels

457.0 Postmastectomy lymphedema syndrome
Elephantiasis due to mastectomy
Obliteration of lymphatic vessel due to mastectomy

457.1 Other lymphedema
Elephantiasis (nonfilarial) NOS
Lymphangiectasis
Lymphedema:
  acquired (chronic)
  praecox
  secondary
Obliteration, lymphatic vessel
Excludes: elephantiasis (nonfilarial):
      congenital (757.0)
      eyelid (374.83)
      vulva (624.8)

457.2 Lymphangitis
Lymphangitis:
  NOS
  chronic
  subacute
Excludes: acute lymphangitis (682.0-682.9)

457.8 Other noninfectious disorders of lymphatic channels
Chylocele (nonfilarial)   Lymph node or vessel:
Chylous: fistula
  ascites   infarction
  cyst   rupture
Excludes: chylocele:
      filarial (125.0-125.9)
      tunica vaginalis (nonfilarial) (608.84)

457.9 Unspecified noninfectious disorder of lymphatic channels

CIRCULATORY SYSTEM

458 Hypotension
Includes: hypopiesis

Excludes: cardiovascular collapse (785.50)
maternal hypotension syndrome (669.2)
shock (785.50-785.59)
Shy-Drager syndrome (333.0)

458.0 Orthostatic hypotension
Hypotension:
orthostatic (chronic)
postural

458.1 Chronic hypotension
Permanent idiopathic hypotension

458.2 Iatrogenic hypotension

458.21 Hypotension of hemodialysis
Intra-dialytic hypotension

458.29 Other iatrogenic hypotension
Postoperative hypotension

458.8 Other specified hypotension

458.9 Hypotension, unspecified
Hypotension (arterial) NOS

459 Other disorders of circulatory system

459.0 Hemorrhage, unspecified
Rupture of blood vessel NOS
Spontaneous hemorrhage NEC

Excludes: hemorrhage:
gastrointestinal NOS (578.9)
in newborn NOS (772.9)
secondary or recurrent following trauma (958.2)
traumatic rupture of blood vessel (900.0-904.9)

459.1 Postphlebitic syndrome
Chronic venous hypertension due to deep vein thrombosis

Excludes: chronic venous hyptertension without deep vein thrombosis (459.30-459.39)

459.10 Postphlebetic syndrome without complications
Asymptomatic postphlebetic syndrome
Postphlebetic syndrome NOS

459.11 Postphlebetic syndrome with ulcer

459.12 Postphlebetic syndrome with inflammation

459.13 Postphlebetic syndrome with ulcer and inflammation

459.19 Postphlebetic syndrome with other complication

459.2 Compression of vein
Stricture of vein
Vena cava syndrome (inferior) (superior)

459.3 Chronic venous hypertension (idiopathic)
Statis edema

Excludes: chronic venous hypertension due to deep vein thrombosis (459.10-459.19)
varicose veins (454.0-454.9)

459.30 Chronic venous hypertension without complications
Asymptomatic chronic venous hypertension
Chronic venous hypertension NOS

459.31 Chronic venous hypertension with ulcer

459.32 Chronic venous hypertension with inflammation

459.33 Chronic venous hypertension with ulcer and inflammation

459.39 Chronic venous hypertension with other complication

459.8 Other specified disorders of circulatory system

459.81 Venous (peripheral) insufficiency, unspecified
Chronic venous insufficiency NOS

Use additional code for any associated ulceration (707.10-707.9)

459.89 Other
  Collateral circulation (venous), any site
  Phlebosclerosis
  Venofibrosis

459.9 Unspecified circulatory system disorder

RESPIRATORY SYSTEM

8. DISEASES OF THE RESPIRATORY SYSTEM (460-519)

Use additional code, if desired, to identify infectious organism

ACUTE RESPIRATORY INFECTIONS (460-466)

Excludes: pneumonia and influenza (480.0-488)

460 Acute nasopharyngitis [common cold]
Coryza (acute)
Nasal catarrh, acute
Nasopharyngitis:
  NOS
  acute
  infective NOS
Rhinitis:
  acute
  infective

Excludes: nasopharyngitis, chronic (472.2)
  pharyngitis:
    acute or unspecified (462)
    chronic (472.1)
  rhinitis:
    allergic (477.0-477.9)
    chronic or unspecified (472.0)
  sore throat:
    acute or unspecified (462)
    chronic (472.1)

461 Acute sinusitis
Includes: abscess acute, of sinus (accessory) (nasal)
  empyema acute, of sinus (accessory) (nasal)
  infection acute, of sinus (accessory) (nasal)
  inflammation acute, of sinus (accessory) (nasal)
  suppuration acute, of sinus (accessory) (nasal)

Excludes: chronic or unspecified sinusitis (473.0-473.9)

461.0 Maxillary
  Acute antritis

461.1 Frontal

461.2 Ethmoidal

461.3 Sphenoidal

461.8 Other acute sinusitis
  Acute pansinusitis

461.9 Acute sinusitis, unspecified
  Acute sinusitis NOS

462 Acute pharyngitis
Acute sore throat NOS
Pharyngitis (acute):
  NOS
  gangrenous
  infective
  phlegmonous
  pneumococcal
Pharyngitis (acute):
  staphylococcal
  suppurative
  ulcerative
Sore throat (viral) NOS
Viral pharyngitis

Excludes: abscess:
  peritonsillar [quinsy] (475)
  pharyngeal NOS (478.29)
  retropharyngeal (478.24)
chronic pharyngitis (472.1)
infectious mononucleosis (075)
that specified as (due to):
  Coxsackie (virus) (074.0)
  gonococcus (098.6)
  herpes simplex (054.79)
  influenza (487.1)
  septic (034.0)
  streptococcal (034.0)

361

TABULAR LIST

463 Acute tonsillitis
    Tonsillitis (acute):
      NOS
      follicular
      gangrenous
      infective
      pneumococcal
    Tonsillitis (acute):
      septic
      staphylococcal
      suppurative
      ulcerative
      viral

    Excludes: *chronic tonsillitis (474.0)*
      hypertrophy of tonsils (474.1)
      peritonsillar abscess [quinsy] (475)
      sore throat:
        acute or NOS (462)
        septic (034.0)
      streptococcal tonsillitis (034.0)

464 Acute laryngitis and tracheitis

    Excludes: *that associated with influenza (487.1)*
      that due to Streptococcus (034.0)

⑤ **464.0 Acute laryngitis**
    Laryngitis (acute):
      NOS
      edematous
      Hemophilus influenza
        [H. influenzae]
    Laryngitis (acute):
      pneumococcal
      septic
      suppurative
      ulcerative

    Excludes: *chronic laryngitis (476.0-476.1)*
      influenzal laryngitis (487.1)

    464.00 Without mention of obstruction
    464.01 With obstruction

⑤ **464.1 Acute tracheitis**
    Tracheitis (acute):
      NOS
      catarrhal
      viral

    Excludes: *chronic tracheitis (491.8)*

    464.10 Without mention of obstruction
    464.11 With obstruction

⑤ **464.2 Acute laryngotracheitis**
    Laryngotracheitis (acute)
    Tracheitis (acute) with laryngitis (acute)

    Excludes: *chronic laryngotracheitis (476.1)*

    464.20 Without mention of obstruction
    464.21 With obstruction

⑤ **464.3 Acute epiglottitis**
    Viral epiglottitis

    Excludes: *epiglottitis, chronic (476.1)*

    464.30 Without mention of obstruction
    464.31 With obstruction

  464.4 Croup
    Croup syndrome

⑤ **464.5 Supraglottitis, unspecified**

    464.50 Without mention of obstruction
    464.51 With obstruction

465 Acute upper respiratory infections of multiple or unspecified sites

    Excludes: *upper respiratory infection due to:*
      influenza (487.1)
      Streptococcus (034.0)

  465.0 Acute laryngopharyngitis

  465.8 Other multiple sites
    Multiple URI

RESPIRATORY SYSTEM

465.9 Unspecified site
Acute URI NOS
Upper respiratory infection (acute)

466 Acute bronchitis and bronchiolitis
Includes: that with:
bronchospasm
obstruction

466.0 Acute bronchitis
Bronchitis, acute or subacute:
fibrinous
membranous
pneumococcal
purulent
septic
viral
with tracheitis
Croupous bronchitis
Tracheobronchitis, acute

Excludes: acute bronchitis with chronic obstructive pulmonary disease (491.22)

⑤ **466.1 Acute bronchiolitis**
Bronchiolitis (acute)
Capillary pneumonia

466.11 Acute bronchiolitis due to respiratory syncytial virus (RSV)

466.19 Acute bronchiolitis due to other infectious organisms
Use additional code to identify organism

OTHER DISEASES OF THE UPPER RESPIRATORY TRACT (470-478)

470 Deviated nasal septum
Deflected septum (nasal) (acquired)
Excludes: congenital (754.0)

471 Nasal polyps
Excludes: adenomatous polyps (212.0)

471.0 Polyp of nasal cavity
Polyp:
choanal
nasopharyngeal

471.1 Polypoid sinus degeneration
Woakes' syndrome or ethmoiditis

471.8 Other polyp of sinus
Polyp of sinus: Polyp of sinus:
accessory   maxillary
ethmoidal   sphenoidal

471.9 Unspecified nasal polyp
Nasal polyp NOS

472 Chronic pharyngitis and nasopharyngitis

472.0 Chronic rhinitis
Ozena   Rhinitis:
Rhinitis: hypertrophic
NOS   obstructive
atrophic   purulent
granulomatous   ulcerative

Excludes: allergic rhinitis (477.0-477.9)

472.1 Chronic pharyngitis
Chronic sore throat
Pharyngitis:
atrophic
granular (chronic)
hypertrophic

472.2 Chronic nasopharyngitis
Excludes: acute or unspecified nasopharyngitis (460)

TABULAR LIST

473 Chronic sinusitis
Includes: abscess (chronic) of sinus (accessory) (nasal)
empyema (chronic) of sinus (accessory) (nasal)
infection (chronic) of sinus (accessory) (nasal)
suppuration (chronic) of sinus (accessory) (nasal)

Excludes: acute sinusitis (461.0-461.9)

473.0 Maxillary
Antritis (chronic)

473.1 Frontal

473.2 Ethmoidal
Excludes: Woakes' ethmoiditis (471.1)

473.3 Sphenoidal

473.8 Other chronic sinusitis
Pansinusitis (chronic)

473.9 Unspecified sinusitis (chronic)
Sinusitis (chronic) NOS

474 Chronic disease of tonsils and adenoids

⑤ **474.0 Chronic tonsillitis and adenoiditis**
Excludes: acute or unspecified tonsillitis (463)

474.00 Chronic tonsillitis
474.01 Chronic adenoiditis
474.02 Chronic tonsillitis and adenoiditis

⑤ **474.1 Hypertrophy of tonsils and adenoids**
Enlargement of tonsils or adenoids
Hyperplasia of tonsils or adenoids
Hypertrophy of tonsils or adenoids

Excludes: that with adenoiditis (474.01)
that with adenoiditis and tonsillitis (474.02)
that with tonsillitis (474.00)

474.10 Tonsils with adenoids
474.11 Tonsils alone
474.12 Adenoids alone

474.2 Adenoid vegetations

474.8 Other chronic disease of tonsils and adenoids
Amygdalolith
Calculus, tonsil
Cicatrix of tonsil (and adenoid)
Tonsillar tag
Ulcer, tonsil

474.9 Unspecified chronic disease of tonsils and adenoids
Disease (chronic) of tonsils (and adenoids)

475 Peritonsillar abscess
Abscess of tonsil
Peritonsillar cellulitis
Quinsy

Excludes: tonsillitis:
acute or NOS (463)
chronic (474.0)

476 Chronic laryngitis and laryngotracheitis

476.0 Chronic laryngitis
Laryngitis:
catarrhal
hypertrophic
Sicca

476.1 Chronic laryngotracheitis
Laryngitis, chronic, with tracheitis (chronic)
Tracheitis, chronic, with laryngitis

Excludes: chronic tracheitis (491.8)
laryngitis and tracheitis, acute or unspecified (464.00-464.51)

RESPIRATORY SYSTEM

477 **Allergic rhinitis**
 Includes: allergic rhinitis (nonseasonal) (seasonal)
  hay fever
  spasmodic rhinorrhea

 Excludes: allergic rhinitis with asthma (bronchial) (493.0)

 477.0 Due to pollen
  Pollinosis

 477.1 Due to food

 477.2 Due to animal (cat) (dog) hair and dander

 477.8 Due to other allergen

 477.9 Cause unspecified

478 **Other diseases of upper respiratory tract**

 478.0 Hypertrophy of nasal turbinates

⑤ **478.1 Other diseases of nasal cavity and sinuses**

 Excludes: varicose ulcer of nasal septum (456.8)

  478.11 Nasal mucositis (ulcerative)
 Use additional E code to identify adverse effects of therapy, such as:
  antineoplastic and immunosuppressive drugs (E930.7, E933.1)
  radiation therapy (E879.2)

  478.19 Other disease of nasal cavity and sinuses
   Abscess of nose (septum)
   Necrosis of nose (septum)
   Ulcer of nose (septum)
   Cyst or mucocele of sinus (nasal)
   Rhinolith

⑤ **478.2 Other diseases of pharynx, not elsewhere classified**

  478.20 Unspecified disease of pharynx
  478.21 Cellulitis of pharynx or nasopharynx
  478.22 Parapharyngeal abscess
  478.24 Retropharyngeal abscess
  478.25 Edema of pharynx or nasopharynx
  478.26 Cyst of pharynx or nasopharynx
  478.29 Other
   Abscess of pharynx or nasopharynx

 Excludes: ulcerative pharyngitis (462)

⑤ **478.3 Paralysis of vocal cords or larynx**

  478.30 Paralysis, unspecified
   Laryngoplegia
   Paralysis of glottis
  478.31 Unilateral, partial
  478.32 Unilateral, complete
  478.33 Bilateral, partial
  478.34 Bilateral, complete

 478.4 Polyp of vocal cord or larynx

 Excludes: adenomatous polyps (212.1)

 478.5 Other diseases of vocal cords
  Abscess of vocal cords
  Cellulitis of vocal cords
  Granuloma of vocal cords
  Leukoplakia of vocal cords
  Chorditis (fibrinous) (nodosa) (tuberosa)
  Singers' nodes

 478.6 Edema of larynx
  Edema (of):
   glottis
   subglottic
   supraglottic

⑤ **478.7 Other diseases of larynx, not elsewhere classified**

  478.70 Unspecified disease of larynx

TABULAR LIST

- **478.71** Cellulitis and perichondritis of larynx
- **478.74** Stenosis of larynx
- **478.75** Laryngeal spasm
  Laryngismus (stridulus)
- **478.79** Other
  Abscess of larynx
  Necrosis of larynx
  Obstruction of larynx
  Pachyderma of larynx
  Ulcer of larynx
  Excludes: ulcerative laryngitis (464.00-464.01)
- **478.8** Upper respiratory tract hypersensitivity reaction, site unspecified
  Excludes: hypersensitivity reaction of lower respiratory tract, as:
    extrinsic allergic alveolitis (495.0-495.9)
    pneumoconiosis (500-505)
- **478.9** Other and unspecified diseases of upper respiratory tract
  Abscess of trachea
  Cicatrix of trachea

PNEUMONIA AND INFLUENZA (480-488)

Excludes: pneumonia:
  allergic or eosinophilic (518.3)
  aspiration:
    NOS (507.0)
    newborn (770.18)
    solids and liquids (507.0-507.8)
  congenital (770.0)
  lipoid (507.1)
  passive (514)
  rheumatic (390)

480 Viral pneumonia
- **480.0** Pneumonia due to adenovirus
- **480.1** Pneumonia due to respiratory syncytial virus
- **480.2** Pneumonia due to parainfluenza virus
- **480.3** Pneumonia due to SARS-associated coronavirus
- **480.8** Pneumonia due to other virus not elsewhere classified
  Excludes: congenital rubella pneumonitis (771.0)
    influenza with pneumonia, any form (487.0)
    pneumonia complicating viral diseases classified elsewhere (484.1-484.8)
- **480.9** Viral pneumonia, unspecified

481 Pneumococcal pneumonia [*Streptococcus pneumoniae* pneumonia]
Lobar pneumonia, organism unspecified

482 Other bacterial pneumonia
- **482.0** Pneumonia due to Klebsiella pneumoniae
- **482.1** Pneumonia due to Pseudomonas
- **482.2** Pneumonia due to Hemophilus influenzae [H. influenzae]
- ⑤ **482.3** Pneumonia due to Streptococcus
  Excludes: Streptococcus pneumoniae pneumonia (481)
  - **482.30** Streptococcus, unspecified
  - **482.31** Group A
  - **482.32** Group B
  - **482.39** Other Streptococcus
- ⑤ **482.4** Pneumonia due to Staphylococcus
  - **482.40** Pneumonia due to Staphylococcus, unspecified
  - **482.41** Pneumonia due to Staphylococcus aureus
  - **482.49** Other Staphylococcus pneumonia
- ⑤ **482.8** Pneumonia due to other specified bacteria
  Excludes: pneumonia complicating infectious disease classified elsewhere (484.1-484.8)

RESPIRATORY SYSTEM

482.81 Anaerobes
  Bacteroides (melaninogenicus)
  Gram-negative anaerobes

482.82 Escherichia coli [E. coli]

482.83 Other gram-negative bacteria
  Gram-negative pneumonia NOS
  Proteus
  Serratia marcescens

Excludes: Gram-negative anaerobes (482.81)
  Legionnaires' disease (482.84)

482.84 Legionnaires' disease

482.89 Other specified bacteria

482.9 Bacterial pneumonia unspecified

483 Pneumonia due to other specified organism

483.0 Mycoplasma pneumoniae
  Eaton's agent
  Pleuropneumonia-like organism [PPLO]

483.1 Chlamydia

483.8 Other specified organism

484 Pneumonia in infectious diseases classified elsewhere

Excludes: influenza with pneumonia, any form (487.0)

484.1 Pneumonia in cytomegalic inclusion disease
  Code first underlying disease (078.5)

484.3 Pneumonia in whooping cough
  Code first underlying disease (033.0-033.9)

484.5 Pneumonia in anthrax
  Code first underlying disease (022.1)

484.6 Pneumonia in aspergillosis
  Code first underlying disease (117.3)

484.7 Pneumonia in other systemic mycoses
  Code first underlying disease

Excludes: pneumonia in:
  candidiasis (112.4)
  coccidioidomycosis (114.0)
  histoplasmosis (115.0-115.9 with fifth-digit 5)

484.8 Pneumonia in other infectious diseases classified elsewhere
  Code first underlying disease, as:
  Q fever (083.0)
  typhoid fever (002.0)

Excludes: pneumonia in:
  actinomycosis (039.1)
  measles (055.1)
  nocardiosis (039.1)
  ornithosis (073.0)
  Pneumocystis carinii (136.3)
  salmonellosis (003.22)
  toxoplasmosis (130.4)
  tuberculosis (011.6)
  tularemia (021.2)
  varicella (052.1)

485 Bronchopneumonia, organism unspecified
  Bronchopneumonia: Pneumonia:
    hemorrhagic   lobular
    terminal   segmental
  Pleurobronchopneumonia

Excludes: bronchiolitis (acute) (466.11-466.19)
  chronic (491.8)
  lipoid pneumonia (507.1)

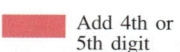 Add 4th or 5th digit   Nonspecific code   Unspecified code   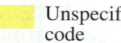 Manifestation code

367

TABULAR LIST

486 **Pneumonia, organism unspecified**
 Excludes: *hypostatic or passive pneumonia (514)*
  influenza with pneumonia, any form (487.0)
  inhalation or aspiration pneumonia due to foreign materials (507.0-507.8)
  pneumonitis due to fumes and vapors (506.0)

487 **Influenza**
 Excludes: *Hemophilus influenzae [H. influenzae]:*
   infection NOS (041.5)
   laryngitis (464.00-464.01)
   meningitis (320.0)
  influenza due to identified avian influenza virus (488)

 487.0 With pneumonia
  Influenza with pneumonia, any form
  Influenzal:
   bronchopneumonia
   pneumonia
  Use additional code to identify the type of pneumonia (480.0-480.9, 481, 482.0-482.9, 483.0-483.8, 485)

 487.1 With other respiratory manifestations
  Influenza NOS
  Influenzal:
   laryngitis
   pharyngitis
   respiratory infection (upper) (acute)

 487.8 With other manifestations
  Encephalopathy due to influenza
  Influenza with involvement of gastrointestinal tract
  Excludes: *"intestinal flu" [viral gastroenteritis] (008.8)*

● **488 Influenza due to identified avian influenza virus**
  Note: Influenza caused by influenza viruses that normally infect only birds and, less commonly, other animals
  Excludes: *influenza caused by other influenza viruses (487)*

CHRONIC OBSTRUCTIVE PULMONARY DISEASE AND ALLIED CONDITIONS (490-496)

490 **Bronchitis, not specified as acute or chronic**
  Bronchitis NOS: Tracheobronchitis NOS
   catarrhal
   with tracheitis NOS
  Excludes: *bronchitis:*
   allergic NOS (493.9)
   asthmatic NOS (493.9)
   due to fumes and vapors (506.0)

491 **Chronic bronchitis**
  Excludes: *chronic obstructive asthma (493.2)*

 491.0 Simple chronic bronchitis
  Catarrhal bronchitis, chronic
  Smokers' cough

 491.1 Mucopurulent chronic bronchitis
  Bronchitis (chronic) (recurrent):
   fetid
   mucopurulent
   purulent

 ⑤ **491.2 Obstructive chronic bronchitis**
  Bronchitis: Bronchitis with:
   emphysematous   chronic airway obstruction
   obstructive (chronic) (diffuse)   emphysema
  Excludes: *asthmatic bronchitis (acute) NOS (493.9)*
   chronic obstructive asthma (493.2)

   491.20 Without exacerbation
    Emphysema with chronic bronchitis

368 ● Code new to this edition   ▲ Revision of existing code   ④ ⑤ Fourth or fifth digit required

RESPIRATORY SYSTEM

491.21 With (acute) exacerbation
Acute exacerbation of chronic obstructive pulmonary disease [COPD]
Decompensated chronic obstructive pulmonary disease [COPD]
Decompensated chronic obstructive pulmonary disease [COPD] with exacerbation

Excludes: chronic obstructive asthma with acute exacerbation (493.22)

491.22 With acute bronchitis

491.8 Other chronic bronchitis
Chronic:
  tracheitis
  tracheobronchitis

491.9 Unspecified chronic bronchitis

492 Emphysema

492.0 Emphysematous bleb
Giant bullous emphysema
Ruptured emphysematous bleb
Tension pneumatocele
Vanishing lung

492.8 Other emphysema
Emphysema (lung or pulmonary):
  NOS
  centriacinar
  centrilobular
  obstructive
  panacinar

Emphysema (lung or pulmonary):
  panlobular
  unilateral
  vesicular
MacLeod's syndrome
Swyer-James syndrome
Unilateral hyperlucent lung

Excludes: emphysema:
  compensatory (518.2)
  due to fumes and vapors (506.4)
  interstitial (518.1)
    newborn (770.2)
  mediastinal (518.1)
  surgical (subcutaneous) (998.81)
  traumatic (958.7)
  with chronic bronchitis (491.20-491.22)

493 Asthma

Excludes: wheezing NOS (786.07)

The following fifth-digit subclassification is for use with codes 493.0-493.2, 493.9:

  0 unspecified
  1 with status asthmaticus
  2 with (acute) exacerbation

⑤ 493.0 extrinsic asthma
Asthma:
  allergic with stated cause
  atopic
  childhood
  hay
  platinum
Hay fever with asthma

Excludes: asthma:
  allergic NOS (493.9)
  detergent (507.8)
  miners' (500)
  wood (495.8)

⑤ 493.1 Intrinsic asthma
Late-onset asthma

⑤ 493.2 Chronic obstructive asthma
Asthma with chronic obstructive pulmonary disease [COPD]
Chronic asthmatic bronchitis

Excludes: chronic obstructive bronchitis (491.20-491.22)
  acute bronchitis (466.0)

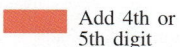 Add 4th or 5th digit   Nonspecific code   Unspecified code   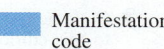 Manifestation code

TABULAR LIST

⑤ **493.8 Other forms of asthma**
    493.81 Exercise induced bronchospasm
    493.82 Cough variant asthma

⑤ **493.9 Asthma, unspecified**
    Asthma (bronchial) (allergic NOS)
    Bronchitis:
      allergic
      asthmatic

494 Bronchiectasis
    Bronchiectasis (fusiform) (postinfectious) (recurrent)
    Bronchiolectasis
    Excludes: congenital (748.61)
        tuberculous bronchiectasis (current disease) (011.5)

  494.0 Bronchiectasis without acute exacerbation
  494.1 Bronchiectasis with acute exacerbation

495 Extrinsic allergic alveolitis
    Includes: allergic alveolitis and pneumonitis due to inhaled organic dust particles of fungal, thermophilic actinomycete, or other origin

  495.0 Farmers' lung
  495.1 Bagassosis
  495.2 Bird-fanciers' lung
    Budgerigar-fanciers' disease or lung
    Pigeon-fanciers' disease or lung
  495.3 Suberosis
    Cork-handlers' disease or lung
  495.4 Malt workers' lung
    Alveolitis due to Aspergillus clavatus
  495.5 Mushroom workers' lung
  495.6 Maple bark-strippers' lung
    Alveolitis due to Cryptostroma corticale
  495.7 "Ventilation" pneumonitis
    Allergic alveolitis due to fungal, thermophilic actinomycete, and other organisms growing in ventilation [air conditioning] systems
  495.8 Other specified allergic alveolitis and pneumonitis
    Cheese-washers' lung   Pituitary snuff-takers' disease
    Coffee workers' lung   Sequoiosis or red-cedar asthma
    Fish-meal workers' lung   Wood asthma
    Furriers' lung
    Grain-handlers' disease or lung
  495.9 Unspecified allergic alveolitis and pneumonitis
    Alveolitis, allergic (extrinsic)
    Hypersensitivity pneumonitis

496 Chronic airway obstruction, not elsewhere classified
    Note: This code is not to be used with any code from categories 491-493
    Chronic:
      nonspecific lung disease
      obstructive lung disease
      obstructive pulmonary disease [COPD] NOS
    Excludes: chronic obstructive lung disease [COPD] specified (as) (with):
        allergic alveolitis (495.0-495.9)
        asthma (493.2)
        bronchiectasis (494.0-494.1)
        bronchitis (491.20-491.22)
          with emphysema (491.20-491.22)
        decompensated (491.21)
        emphysema (492.0-492.8)

RESPIRATORY SYSTEM

PNEUMOCONIOSES AND OTHER LUNG DISEASES DUE TO EXTERNAL AGENTS (500-508)

500 Coal workers' pneumoconiosis
   Anthracosilicosis
   Anthracosis
   Black lung disease
   Coal workers' lung
   Miner's asthma

501 Asbestosis

502 Pneumoconiosis due to other silica or silicates
   Pneumoconiosis due to talc
   Silicotic fibrosis (massive) of lung
   Silicosis (simple) (complicated)

503 Pneumoconiosis due to other inorganic dust
   Aluminosis (of lung)
   Bauxite fibrosis (of lung)
   Berylliosis
   Graphite fibrosis (of lung)
   Siderosis
   Stannosis

504 Pneumonopathy due to inhalation of other dust
   Byssinosis
   Cannabinosis
   Flax-dressers' disease

   Excludes: allergic alveolitis (495.0-495.9)
      asbestosis (501)
      bagassosis (495.1)
      farmers' lung (495.0)

505 Pneumoconiosis, unspecified

506 Respiratory conditions due to chemical fumes and vapors
   Use additional E code, if desired, to identify cause

   506.0 Bronchitis and pneumonitis due to fumes and vapors
      Chemical bronchitis (acute)

   506.1 Acute pulmonary edema due to fumes and vapors
      Chemical pulmonary edema (acute)

      Excludes: acute pulmonary edema NOS (518.4)
         chronic or unspecified pulmonary edema (514)

   506.2 Upper respiratory inflammation due to fumes and vapors

   506.3 Other acute and subacute respiratory conditions due to fumes and vapors

   506.4 Chronic respiratory conditions due to fumes and vapors
      Emphysema (diffuse) (chronic) due to inhalation of chemical fumes and vapors
      Obliterative bronchiolitis (chronic) (subacute) due to inhalation of chemical fumes and vapors
      Pulmonary fibrosis (chronic) due to inhalation of chemical fumes and vapors

   506.9 Unspecified respiratory conditions due to fumes and vapors
      Silo-fillers' disease

507 Pneumonitis due to solids and liquids

   Excludes: fetal aspiration pneumonitis (770.18)

   507.0 Due to inhalation of food or vomitus
      Aspiration pneumonia (due to):
         NOS
         food (regurgitated)
         gastric secretions
         milk
         saliva
         vomitus

   507.1 Due to inhalation of oils and essences
      Lipoid pneumonia (exogenous)

      Excludes: endogenous lipoid pneumonia (516.8)

   507.8 Due to other solids and liquids
      Detergent asthma

508 Respiratory conditions due to other and unspecified external agents
   Use additional E code, if desired, to identify cause

   508.0 Acute pulmonary manifestations due to radiation
      Radiation pneumonitis

   508.1 Chronic and other pulmonary manifestations due to radiation
      Fibrosis of lung following radiation

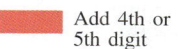 Add 4th or 5th digit
 Nonspecific code
 Unspecified code
 Manifestation code

TABULAR LIST

508.8 Respiratory conditions due to other specified external agents

508.9 Respiratory conditions due to unspecified external agent

OTHER DISEASES OF RESPIRATORY SYSTEM (510-519)

510 Empyema
Use additional code, if desired, to identify infectious organism (041.0-041.9)

Excludes: abscess of lung (513.0)

510.0 With fistula
Fistula:
 bronchocutaneous
 bronchopleural
 hepatopleural
Fistula:
 mediastinal
 pleural
 thoracic
Any condition classifiable to 510.9 with fistula

510.9 Without mention of fistula
Abscess:
 pleura
 thorax
Empyema (chest) (lung) (pleura)
Fibrinopurulent pleurisy
Pleurisy:
 purulent
 septic
 seropurulent
 suppurative
Pyopneumothorax
Pyothorax

511 Pleurisy
Excludes: malignant pleural effusion (197.2)
 pleurisy with mention of tuberculosis, current disease (012.0)

511.0 Without mention of effusion or current tuberculosis
Adhesion, lung or pleura
Calcification of pleura
Pleurisy (acute) (sterile):
 diaphragmatic
 fibrinous
 interlobar
Pleurisy:
 NOS
 pneumococcal
 staphylococcal
 streptococcal
Thickening of pleura

511.1 With effusion, with mention of a bacterial cause other than tuberculosis
Pleurisy with effusion (exudative) (serous):
 pneumococcal
 staphylococcal
 streptococcal
 other specified nontuberculous bacterial cause

511.8 Other specified forms of effusion, except tuberculous
Encysted pleurisy
Hemopneumothorax
Hemothorax
Hydropneumothorax
Hydrothorax

Excludes: traumatic (860.2-860.5, 862.29, 862.39)

511.9 Unspecified pleural effusion
Pleural effusion NOS
Pleurisy:
 exudative
 serofibrinous
Pleurisy:
 serous
 with effusion NOS

512 Pneumothorax

512.0 Spontaneous tension pneumothorax

512.1 Iatrogenic pneumothorax
Postoperative pneumothorax

512.8 Other spontaneous pneumothorax
Pneumothorax:
 NOS
 acute
 chronic

Excludes: pneumothorax:
 congenital (770.2)
 traumatic (860.0-860.1, 860.4-860.5)
 tuberculous, current disease (011.7)

RESPIRATORY SYSTEM

513 **Abscess of lung and mediastinum**

513.0 Abscess of lung
Abscess (multiple) of lung
Gangrenous or necrotic pneumonia
Pulmonary gangrene or necrosis

513.1 Abscess of mediastinum

514 Pulmonary congestion and hypostasis
Hypostatic:
  bronchopneumonia
  pneumonia
Passive pneumonia
Pulmonary congestion (chronic) (passive)
Pulmonary edema:
  NOS
  chronic

Excludes: *acute pulmonary edema:*
  NOS (518.4)
  with mention of heart disease or failure (428.1)
  hypostatic pneumonia due to or specified as a specific type of pneumonia – code to the type of pneumonia (480.0-480.9, 481, 482.0-482.49, 483.0-483.8, 485, 486, 487.0)

515 Postinflammatory pulmonary fibrosis
Cirrhosis of lung, chronic or unspecified
Fibrosis of lung (atrophic) (confluent) (massive) (perialveolar) (peribronchial), chronic or unspecified
Induration of lung, chronic or unspecified

516 **Other alveolar and parietoalveolar pneumonopathy**

516.0 Pulmonary alveolar proteinosis

516.1 Idiopathic pulmonary hemosiderosis
Essential brown induration of lung
Code first underlying disease (275.0)

516.2 Pulmonary alveolar microlithiasis

516.3 Idiopathic fibrosing alveolitis
Alveolar capillary block
Diffuse (idiopathic) (interstitial) pulmonary fibrosis
Hamman-Rich syndrome

516.8 Other specified alveolar and parietoalveolar pneumonopathies
Endogenous lipoid pneumonia
Interstitial pneumonia (desquamative) (lymphoid)

Excludes: *lipoid pneumonia, exogenous or unspecified (507.1)*

516.9 Unspecified alveolar and parietoalveolar pneumonopathy

517 **Lung involvement in conditions classified elsewhere**

Excludes: *rheumatoid lung (714.81)*

517.1 Rheumatic pneumonia
Code first underlying disease (390)

517.2 Lung involvement in systemic sclerosis
Code first underlying disease (710.1)

517.3 Acute chest syndrome
Code first sickle-cell disease in crisis (282.42, 282.62, 282.64, 282.69)

517.8 Lung involvement in other diseases classified elsewhere
Code first underlying disease, as:
  amyloidosis (277.30-277.39)
  polymyositis (710.4)
  sarcoidosis (135)
  Sjögren's disease (710.2)
  systemic lupus erythematosus (710.0)

Excludes: *syphilis (095.1)*

373

TABULAR LIST

518 Other diseases of lung

518.0 Pulmonary collapse
  Atelectasis
  Collapse of lung
  Middle lobe syndrome

  Excludes: atelectasis:
       congenital (partial) (770.5)
         primary (770.4)
       tuberculous, current disease (011.8)

518.1 Interstitial emphysema
  Mediastinal emphysema

  Excludes: surgical (subcutaneous) emphysema (998.81)
       that in fetus or newborn (770.2)
       traumatic emphysema (958.7)

518.2 Compensatory emphysema

518.3 Pulmonary eosinophilia
  Eosinophilic asthma   Tropical eosinophilia
  Löffler's syndrome
  Pneumonia:
    allergic
    eosinophilic

518.4 Acute edema of lung, unspecified
  Acute pulmonary edema NOS
  Pulmonary edema, postoperative

  Excludes: pulmonary edema:
       acute, with mention of heart disease or failure (428.1)
       chronic or unspecified (514)
       due to external agents (506.0-508.9)

518.5 Pulmonary insufficiency following trauma and surgery
  Adult respiratory distress syndrome
  Pulmonary insufficiency following:
    shock
    surgery
    trauma
  Shock lung

  Excludes: adult respiratory distress syndrome associated with other conditions (518.82)
       pneumonia:
         aspiration (507.0)
         hypostatic (514)
       respiratory failure in other conditions (518.81, 518.83-518.84)

518.6 Allergic bronchopulmonary aspergillosis

518.7 Transfusion related acute lung injury (TRALI)

⑤ **518.8 Other diseases of lung**

  518.81 Acute respiratory failure
    Respiratory failure NOS

  Excludes: acute and chronic respiratory failure (518.84)
       acute respiratory distress (518.82)
       chronic respiratory failure (518.83)
       respiratory arrest (799.1)
       respiratory failure, newborn (770.84)

  518.82 Other pulmonary insufficiency, not elsewhere classified
    Acute respiratory distress
    Acute respiratory insufficiency
    Adult respiratory distress syndrome NEC

  Excludes: adult respiratory distress syndrome associated with trauma and surgery (518.5)
       pulmonary insufficiency following trauma and surgery (518.5)
       respiratory distress:
         NOS (786.09)
         newborn (770.89)
         syndrome, newborn (769)
       shock lung (518.5)

  518.83 Chronic respiratory failure

RESPIRATORY SYSTEM

- **518.84** **Acute and chronic respiratory failure**
  Acute or chronic respiratory failure
- **518.89** **Other diseases of lung, not elsewhere classified**
  Broncholithiasis   Lung disease NOS
  Calcification of lung   Pulmolithiasis

519 Other diseases of respiratory system

- ⑤ **519.0** **Tracheostomy complications**
  - **519.00** **Tracheostomy complication, unspecified**
  - **519.01** **Infection of tracheostomy**
    Use additional code to identify type of infection, such as:
        abscess or cellulitis of neck (682.1)
        septicemia (038.0-038.9)
    Use additional code to identify organism (041.00-041.9)
  - **519.02** **Mechanical complication of tracheostomy**
    Tracheal stenosis due to tracheostomy
  - **519.09** **Other tracheostomy complications**
    Hemorrhage due to tracheostomy
    Tracheoesophageal fistula due to tracheostomy

- ⑤ **519.1** **Other diseases of trachea and bronchus, not elsewhere classified**
  - **519.11** **Acute bronchospasm**
    Bronchospasm NOS

    Excludes: acute bronchitis with bronchospasm (466.0)
              asthma (493.00-493.92)
              exercise induced bronchospasm (493.81)

  - **519.19** **Other diseases of trachea and bronchus**
    Calcification of bronchus or trachea
    Stenosis of bronchus or trachea
    Ulcer of bronchus or trachea

- **519.2** **Mediastinitis**
- **519.3** **Other diseases of mediastinum, not elsewhere classified**
  Fibrosis of mediastinum
  Hernia of mediastinum
  Retraction of mediastinum
- **519.4** **Disorders of diaphragm**
  Diaphragmitis
  Paralysis of diaphragm
  Relaxation of diaphragm

  Excludes: congenital defect of diaphragm (756.6)
            diaphragmatic hernia (551-553 with .3)
              congenital (756.6)

- **519.8** **Other diseases of respiratory system, not elsewhere classified**
- **519.9** **Unspecified disease of respiratory system**
  Respiratory disease (chronic) NOS

Add 4th or 5th digit   Nonspecific code   Unspecified code   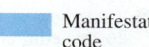 Manifestation code

TABULAR LIST

DIGESTIVE SYSTEM

9. DISEASES OF THE DIGESTIVE SYSTEM (520-579)

DISEASES OF ORAL CAVITY, SALIVARY GLANDS, AND JAWS (520-529)

520 Disorders of tooth development and eruption

520.0 Anodontia
Absence of teeth (complete) (congenital) (partial)
Hypodontia
Oligodontia

Excludes: acquired absence of teeth (525.10-525.19)

520.1 Supernumerary teeth
Distomolar
Fourth molar
Mesiodens
Paramolar
Supplemental teeth

Excludes: supernumerary roots (520.2)

520.2 Abnormalities of size and form
Concrescence of teeth
Fusion of teeth
Gemination of teeth
Dens evaginatus
Dens in dente
Dens invaginatus
Enamel pearls
Macrodontia
Microdontia
Peg-shaped [conical] teeth
Supernumerary roots
Taurodontism
Tuberculum paramolare

Excludes: that due to congenital syphilis (090.5)
tuberculum Carabelli, which is regarded as a normal variation

520.3 Mottled teeth
Dental fluorosis
Mottling of enamel
Nonfluoride enamel opacities

520.4 Disturbances of tooth formation
Aplasia and hypoplasia of cementum
Dilaceration of tooth
Enamel hypoplasia (neonatal) (postnatal) (prenatal)
Horner's teeth
Hypocalcification of teeth
Regional odontodysplasia
Turner's tooth

Excludes: Hutchinson's teeth and mulberry molars in congenital syphilis (090.5)
mottled teeth (520.3)

520.5 Hereditary disturbances in tooth structure, not elsewhere classified
Amelogenesis imperfecta
Dentinogenesis imperfecta
Odontogenesis imperfecta
Dentinal dysplasia
Shell teeth

520.6 Disturbances of tooth eruption
Teeth:
  embedded
  impacted
  natal
  neonatal
  prenatal
  primary [deciduous]:
    persistent
    shedding, premature
Tooth eruption:
  late
  obstructed
  premature

Excludes: exfoliation of teeth (attributable to disease of surrounding tissues) (525.0-525.19)

520.7 Teething syndrome

520.8 Other specified disorders of tooth development and eruption
Color changes during tooth formation
Pre-eruptive color changes

Excludes: posteruptive color changes (521.7)

520.9 Unspecified disorder of tooth development and eruption

521 Diseases of hard tissue of teeth

⑤ **521.0 Dental caries**

521.00 Dental caries, unspecified

■ Add 4th or 5th digit	■ Nonspecific code	■ Unspecified code	■ Manifestation code

377

TABULAR LIST

- **521.01 Dental caries limited to enamel**
  Initial caries
  White spot lesion
- **521.02 Dental caries extending into dentine**
- **521.03 Dental caries extending into pulp**
- **521.04 Arrested dental caries**
- **521.05 Odontoclasia**
  Infantile melanodontia
  Melanodontoclasia

  Excludes: internal and external resorption of teeth (521.40-521.49)

- **521.06 Dental caries pit and fissure**
  Primary dental caries, pit and fissure origin
- **521.07 Dental caries of smooth surface**
  Primary dental caries, smooth surface origin
- **521.08 Dental caries of root surface**
  Primary dental caries, root surface
- **521.09 Other dental caries**

⑤ **521.1 Excessive attrition (approximal wear) (occlusal wear)**
- **521.10 Excessive attrition, unspecified**
- **521.11 Excessive attrition, limited to enamel**
- **521.12 Excessive attrition, extending into dentine**
- **521.13 Excessive attrition, extending into pulp**
- **521.14 Excessive attrition, localized**
- **521.15 Excessive attrition, generalized**

⑤ **521.2 Abrasion**
  Abrasion of teeth:
    dentifrice
    habitual
    occupational
    ritual
    traditional
  Wedge defect NOS of teeth
- **521.20 Abrasion, unspecified**
- **521.21 Abrasion, limited to enamel**
- **521.22 Abrasion, extending into dentine**
- **521.23 Abrasion, extending into pulp**
- **521.24 Abrasion, localized**
- **521.25 Abrasion, generalized**

⑤ **521.3 Erosion**
  Erosion of teeth: Erosion of teeth:
    NOS   idiopathic
    due to: occupational
      medicine
      persistent vomiting
- **521.30 Erosion, unspecified**
- **521.31 Erosion, limited to enamel**
- **521.32 Erosion, extending into dentine**
- **521.33 Erosion, extending into pulp**
- **521.34 Erosion, localized**
- **521.35 Erosion, generalized**

⑤ **521.4 Pathological resorption**
- **521.40 Pathological resorption, unspecified**
- **521.41 Pathological resorption, internal**
- **521.42 Pathological resorption, external**
- **521.49 Other pathological resorption**
  Internal granuloma of pulp

521.5 Hypercementosis
  Cementation hyperplasia

● Code new to this edition ▲ Revision of existing code ④ ⑤ Fourth or fifth digit required

DIGESTIVE SYSTEM

521.6 Ankylosis of teeth

521.7 Intrinsic posteruptive color changes
Staining [discoloration] of teeth:
  NOS
  due to:
    drugs
    metals
    pulpal bleeding

Excludes: accretions [deposits] on teeth (523.6)
extrinsic color changes (523.6)
pre-eruptive color changes (520.8)

⑤ **521.8 Other specific diseases of hard tissues of teeth**

521.81 Cracked tooth

Excludes: asymptomatic craze lines in enamel – omit code
broken tooth due to trauma (873.63, 873.73)
fractured tooth due to trauma (873.63, 873.73)

521.89 Other specific diseases of hard tissues of teeth
Irradiated enamel
Sensitive dentin

521.9 Unspecified disease of hard tissues of teeth

522 Diseases of pulp and periapical tissues

522.0 Pulpitis
Pulpal: Pulpitis:
  abscess   acute
  polyp   chronic (hyperplastic) (ulcerative)
                           suppurative

522.1 Necrosis of the pulp
Pulp gangrene

522.2 Pulp degeneration
Denticles
Pulp calcifications
Pulp stones

522.3 Abnormal hard tissue formation in pulp
Secondary or irregular dentin

522.4 Acute apical periodontitis of pulpal origin

522.5 Periapical abscess without sinus
Abscess:
  dental
  dentoalveolar

Excludes: periapical abscess with sinus (522.7)

522.6 Chronic apical periodontitis
Apical or periapical granuloma
Apical periodontitis NOS

522.7 Periapical abscess with sinus
Fistula:
  alveolar process
  dental

522.8 Radicular cyst
Cyst:
  apical (periodontal)
  periapical
  radiculodental
  residual radicular

Excludes: lateral developmental or lateral periodontal cyst (526.0)

522.9 Other and unspecified diseases of pulp and periapical tissues

523 Gingival and periodontal diseases

⑤ **523.0 Acute gingivitis**

Excludes: acute necrotizing ulcerative gingivitis (101)
herpetic gingivostomatitis (054.2)

523.00 Acute gingivitis, plaque induced
Acute gingivitis NOS

523.01 Acute gingivitis, non-plaque induced

| Add 4th or 5th digit | Nonspecific code | Unspecified code | Manifestation code |

TABULAR LIST

⑤ **523.1 Chronic gingivitis**
  Gingivitis (chronic):   Gingivitis (chronic):
   desquamative   simple marginal
   hyperplastic   ulcerative
  Excludes: herpetic gingivostomatitis (054.2)

  523.10 Chronic gingivitis, plaque induced
    Chronic gingivitis NOS
    Gingivitis NOS

  523.11 Chronic gingivitis, non-plaque induced

⑤ **523.2 Gingival recession**
  Gingival recession (postinfective) (postoperative)

  523.20 Gingival recession, unspecified
  523.21 Gingival recession, minimal
  523.22 Gingival recession, moderate
  523.23 Gingival recession, severe
  523.24 Gingival recession, localized
  523.25 Gingival recession, generalized

⑤ **523.3 Aggressive and acute periodontitis**
  Acute:
   pericementitis
   pericoronitis
  Excludes: acute apical periodontitis (522.4)
      periapical abscess (522.5, 522.7)

  523.30 Aggressive periodontitis, unspecified
  523.31 Aggressive periodontitis, localized
    Periodontal abscess
  523.32 Aggressive periodontitis, generalized
  523.33 Aggressive periodontitis

⑤ **523.4 Chronic periodontitis**
  Chronic pericoronitis
  Pericementitis (chronic)
  Periodontitis:
   NOS
   complex
   simplex
  Excludes: chronic apical periodontitis (522.6)

  523.40 Chronic periodontitis, unspecified
  523.41 Chronic periodontitis, localized
  523.42 Chronic periodontitis, generalized

523.5 Periodontosis

523.6 Accretions on teeth
  Dental calculus:
   subgingival
   supragingival
  Deposits on teeth:
   betel
   materia alba
   soft
   tartar
   tobacco
  Extrinsic discoloration of teeth
  Excludes: intrinsic discoloration of teeth (521.7)

DIGESTIVE SYSTEM

523.8 **Other specified periodontal diseases**
Giant cell:
   epulis
   peripheral granuloma
Gingival:
   cysts
   enlargement NOS
   fibromatosis
Gingival polyp
Periodontal lesions due to traumatic occlusion
Peripheral giant cell granuloma

Excludes: leukoplakia of gingiva (528.6)

523.9 **Unspecified gingival and periodontal disease**

524 Dentofacial anomalies, including malocclusion

⑤ **524.0** **Major anomalies of jaw size**

Excludes: hemifacial atrophy or hypertrophy (754.0)
          unilateral condylar hyperplasia or hypoplasia of mandible (526.89)

    524.00 **Unspecified anomaly**
    524.01 **Maxillary hyperplasia**
    524.02 **Mandibular hyperplasia**
    524.03 **Maxillary hypoplasia**
    524.04 **Mandibular hypoplasia**
    524.05 **Macrogenia**
    524.06 **Microgenia**
    524.07 **Excessive tuberosity of jaw**
        Entire maxillary tuberosity
    524.09 **Other specified anomaly**

⑤ **524.1** **Anomalies of relationship of jaw to cranial base**

    524.10 **Unspecified anomaly**
        prognathism
        retrognathism
    524.11 **Maxillary asymmetry**
    524.12 **Other jaw asymmetry**
    524.19 **Other specified anomaly**

⑤ **524.2** **Anomalies of dental arch relationship**
    Anomaly of dental arch

Excludes: hemifacial atrophy or hypertrophy (754.0)
          soft tissue impingement (524.81-524.82)
          unilateral condylar hyperplasia or hypoplasia of mandible (526.89)

    524.20 **Unspecified anomaly of dental arch relationship**
    524.21 **Malocclusion, Angle's class I**
        Neutro-occlusion
    524.22 **Malocclusion, Angle's class II**
        Disto-occlusion Division I
        Disto-occlusion Division II
    524.23 **Malocclusion, Angle's class III**
        Mesio-occlusion
    524.24 **Open anterior occlusal relationship**
        Anterior open bite
    524.25 **Open posterior occlusal relationship**
        Posterior open bite
    524.26 **Excessive horizontal overlap**
        Excessive horizontal overjet
    524.27 **Reverse articulation**
        Anterior articulation
        Crossbite
        Posterior articulation
    524.28 **Anomalies of interarch distance**
        Excessive interarch distance
        Inadequate interarch distance
    524.29 **Other anomalies of dental arch relationship**
        Other anomalies of dental arch

Add 4th or 5th digit	Nonspecific code	Unspecified code	Manifestation code

TABULAR LIST

⑤ **524.3 Anomalies of tooth position of fully erupted teeth**

Excludes: impacted or embedded teeth with abnormal position of such teeth or adjacent teeth (520.6)

- **524.30** Unspecified anomaly of tooth position
  Diastema of teeth NOS
  Displacement of teeth NOS
  Transposition of teeth NOS
- 524.31 Crowding of teeth
- 524.32 Excessive spacing of teeth
- 524.33 Horizontal displacement of teeth
  Tipped teeth
  Tipping of teeth
- 524.34 Vertical displacement of teeth
  Extruded tooth
  Infraeruption of teeth
  Intruded tooth
  Supraeruption of teeth
- 524.35 Rotation of tooth/teeth
- 524.36 Insufficient interocclusal distance of teeth (ridge)
  Lack of adequate intermaxillary vertical dimension
- 524.37 Excessive interocclusal distance of teeth
  Excessive intermaxillary vertical dimension
  Loss of occlusal vertical dimension
- **524.39** Other anomalies of tooth position

524.4 Malocclusion, unspecified

⑤ **524.5 Dentofacial functional abnormalities**

- **524.50** Dentofacial functional abnormality, unspecified
- 524.51 Abnormal jaw closure
- 524.52 Limited mandibular range of motion
- 524.53 Deviation in opening and closing of the mandible
- 524.54 Insufficient anterior guidance
  Insufficient anterior occlusal guidance
- 524.55 Centric occlusion maximum intercuspation discrepancy
  Centric occlusion of teeth discrepancy
- 524.56 Non-working side interference
  Balancing side interference
- 524.57 Lack of posterior occlusal support
- **524.59** Other dentofacial functional abnormalities
  Abnormal swallowing
  Mouth breathing
  Sleep postures
  Tongue, lip, or finger habits

⑤ **524.6 Temporomandibular joint disorders**

Excludes: current temporomandibular joint:
  dislocation (830.0-830.1)
  strain (848.1)

- **524.60** Temporomandibular joint disorders, unspecified
  Temporomandibular joint-pain-dysfunction syndrome [TMJ]
- 524.61 Adhesions and ankylosis (bony or fibrous)
- 524.62 Arthralgia of temporomandibular joint
- 524.63 Articular disc disorder (reducing or non-reducing)
- 524.64 Temporomandibular joint sounds on opening and/or closing the jaw
- **524.69** Other specified temporomandibular joint disorders

⑤ **524.7 Dental alveolar anomalies**

- **524.70** Unspecified alveolar anomaly
- 524.71 Alveolar maxillary hyperplasia
- 524.72 Alveolar mandibular hyperplasia
- 524.73 Alveolar maxillary hypoplasia
- 524.74 Alveolar mandibular hypoplasia

DIGESTIVE SYSTEM

	524.75	Vertical displacement of alveolus and teeth
		Extrusion of alveolus and teeth
	524.76	Occlusal plane deviation
	524.79	Other specified alveolar anomaly
⑤ 524.8		Other specified dentofacial anomalies
	524.81	Anterior soft tissue impingement
	524.82	Posterior soft tissue impingement
	524.89	Other specified dentofacial anomalies
524.9		Unspecified dentofacial anomalies

525 Other diseases and conditions of the teeth and supporting structures

525.0 Exfoliation of teeth due to systemic causes

⑤ 525.1 Loss of teeth due to trauma, extraction, or periodontal disease
Code first class of edentulism (525.40-525.44, 525.50-525.54)

    525.10 Acquired absence of teeth, unspecified
           Tooth extraction status, NOS
    525.11 Loss of teeth due to trauma
    525.12 Loss of teeth due to periodontal disease
    525.13 Loss of teeth due to caries
    525.19 Other loss of teeth

⑤ 525.2 Atrophy of edentulous alveolar ridge

    525.20 Unspecified atrophy of edentulous alveolar ridge
           Atrophy of the mandible NOS
           Atrophy of the maxilla NOS
    525.21 Minimal atrophy of the mandible
    525.22 Moderate atrophy of the mandible
    525.23 Severe atrophy of the mandible
    525.24 Minimal atrophy of the maxilla
    525.25 Moderate atrophy of the maxilla
    525.26 Severe atrophy of the maxilla

525.3 Retained dental root

⑤ 525.4 Complete edentulism
Use additional code to identify cause of edentulism (525.10-525.19)

    525.40 Complete edentulism, unspecified
           Edentulism NOS
    525.41 Complete edentulism, class I
    525.42 Complete edentulism, class II
    525.43 Complete edentulism, class III
    525.44 Complete edentulism, class IV

⑤ 525.5 Partial edentulism
Use additional code to identify cause of edentulism (525.10-525.19)

    525.50 Partial edentulism, unspecified
    525.51 Partial edentulism, class I
    525.52 Partial edentulism, class II
    525.53 Partial edentulism, class III
    525.54 Partial edentulism, class IV

⑤ 525.6 Unsatisfactory restoration of tooth
    Defective bridge, crown, fillings
    Defective dental restoration

    Excludes: dental restoration status (V45.84)
               unsatisfactory endodontic treatment (526.61-526.69)

    525.60 Unspecified unsatisfactory restoration of tooth
           Unspecified defective dental restoration
    525.61 Open restoration margins
           Dental restoration failure of marginal integrity
           Open margin on tooth restoration

  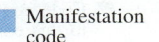

TABULAR LIST

525.62 Unrepairable overhanging of dental restorative materials
Overhanging of tooth restoration

525.63 Fractured dental restorative material without loss of material
Excludes: *cracked tooth (521.81)*
fractured tooth (873.63, 873.73)

525.64 Fractured dental restorative material with loss of material
Excludes: *cracked tooth (521.81)*
fractured tooth (873.63, 873.73)

525.65 Contour of existing restoration of tooth biologically incompatible with oral health
Dental restoration failure of periodontal anatomical integrity
Unacceptable contours of existing restoration
Unacceptable morphology of existing restoration

525.66 Allergy to existing dental restorative material
Use additional code to identify the specific type of allergy

525.67 Poor aesthetics of existing restoration
Dental restoration aesthetically inadequate or displeasing

525.69 Other unsatisfactory restoration of existing tooth

525.7 Endosseous dental implant failure

- **525.71 Osseointegration failure of dental implant**
  Hemorrhagic complications of dental implant placement
  Iatrogenic osseointegration failure of dental implant
  Osseointegration failure of dental implant due to complications of systemic disease
  Osseointegration failure of dental implant due to poor bone quality
  Pre-integration failure of dental implant NOS
  Pre-osseointegration failure of dental implant

- **525.72 Post-osseointegration biological failure of dental implant**
  Failure of dental implant due to lack of attached gingiva
  Failure of dental implant due to occlusal trauma (caused by poor prosthetic design)
  Failure of dental implant due to parafunctional habits
  Failure of dental implant due to periodontal infection (peri-implantitis)
  Failure of dental implant due to poor oral hygiene
  Iatrogenic post-osseointegration failure of dental implant
  Post-osseointegration failure of dental implant due to complications of systemic disease

- **525.73 Post-osseointegration mechanical failure of dental implant**
  Failure of dental prosthesis causing loss of dental implant
  Fracture of dental implant

  Excludes: *cracked tooth (521.81)*
  fractured dental restorative material with loss of material (525.64)
  fractured dental restorative material without loss of material (525.63)
  fractured tooth (873.63, 873.73)

- **525.79 Other endosseous dental implant failure**
  Dental implant failure NOS

525.8 Other specified disorders of the teeth and supporting structures
Enlargement of alveolar ridge NOS
Irregular alveolar process

525.9 Unspecified disorder of the teeth and supporting structures

526 Diseases of the jaws

526.0 Developmental odontogenic cysts

Cyst:
  dentigerous
  eruption
  follicular
  lateral developmental

Cyst:
  lateral periodontal
  primordial
  Keratocyst

Excludes: *radicular cyst (522.8)*

DIGESTIVE SYSTEM

- **526.1 Fissural cysts of jaw**
  Cyst:
  globulomaxillary
  incisor canal
  median anterior maxillary
  median palatal
  nasopalatine
  palatine of papilla

  Excludes: cysts of oral soft tissues (528.4)

- **526.2 Other cysts of jaws**
  Cyst of jaw: Cyst of jaw:
  NOS   hemorrhagic
  aneurysmal   traumatic

- **526.3 Central giant cell (reparative) granuloma**

  Excludes: peripheral giant cell granuloma (523.8)

- **526.4 Inflammatory conditions**
  Abscess of jaw (acute) (chronic) (suppurative)
  Osteitis of jaw (acute) (chronic) (suppurative)
  Osteomyelitis (neonatal) of jaw (acute) (chronic) (suppurative)
  Periostitis of jaw (acute) (chronic) (suppurative)
  Sequestrum of jaw bone

  Excludes: alveolar osteitis (526.5)
  osteonecrosis of jaw (733.45)

- **526.5 Alveolitis of jaw**
  Alveolar osteitis
  Dry socket

- ⑤ **526.6 Periradicular pathology associated with previous endodontic treatment**
  - **526.61** Perforation of root canal space
  - **526.62** Endodontic overfill
  - **526.63** Endodontic underfill
  - **526.69** Other periradicular pathology associated with previous endodontic treatment

- ⑤ **526.8 Other specified diseases of the jaws**
  - **526.81** Exostosis of jaw
    Torus mandibularis
    Torus palatinus
  - **526.89** Other
    Cherubism of jaw(s)
    Fibrous dysplasia of jaw(s)
    Latent bone cyst of jaw(s)
    Osteoradionecrosis of jaw(s)
    Unilateral condylar hyperplasia or hypoplasia of mandible

- **526.9 Unspecified disease of the jaws**

527 Diseases of the salivary glands

- **527.0 Atrophy**
- **527.1 Hypertrophy**
- **527.2 Sialoadenitis**
  Parotitis: Sialoangitis
  NOS   Sialodochitis
  allergic
  toxic

  Excludes: epidemic or infectious parotitis (072.0-072.9)
  uveoparotid fever (135)

- **527.3 Abscess**
- **527.4 Fistula**

  Excludes: congenital fistula of salivary glands (750.24)

- **527.5 Sialolithiasis**
  Calculus of salivary gland or duct
  Stone of salivary gland or duct
  Sialodocholithiasis

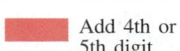 Add 4th or 5th digit Nonspecific code Unspecified code 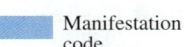 Manifestation code

TABULAR LIST

527.6 Mucocele
Mucous:
extravasation cyst of salivary gland
retention cyst of salivary gland
Ranula

527.7 Disturbance of salivary secretion
Hyposecretion   Sialorrhea
Ptyalism   Xerostomia

527.8 Other specified diseases of the salivary glands
Benign lymphoepithelial lesion of salivary gland
Sialectasia
Sialosis
Stenosis of salivary duct
Stricture of salivary duct

527.9 Unspecified disease of the salivary glands

528 Diseases of the oral soft tissues, excluding lesions specific for gingiva and tongue

⑤ **528.0 Stomatitis and mucositis (ulcerative)**
  Excludes: cellulitis and abscess of mouth (528.3)
  diphtheritic stomatitis (032.0)
  epizootic stomatitis (078.4)
  gingivitis (523.0-523.1)
  oral thrush (112.0)
  Stevens-Johnson syndrome (695.1)
  stomatitis:
    acute necrotizing ulcerative (101)
    aphthous (528.2)
    gangrenous (528.1)
    herpetic (054.2)
    Vincent's (101)

  528.00 Stomatitis and mucositis, unspecified
  Mucositis NOS
  Ulcerative mucositis NOS
  Ulcerative stomatitis NOS
  Vesicular stomatitis NOS

  528.01 Mucositis (ulcerative) due to antineoplastic therapy
  Use additional E code to identify adverse effects of therapy, such as:
  antineoplastic and immunosuppressive drugs (E930.7, E933.1)
  radiation therapy (E879.2)

  528.02 Mucositis (ulcerative) due to other drugs
  Use additional E code to identify drug

  528.09 Other stomatitis and mucositis (ulcerative)

528.1 Cancrum oris
Gangrenous stomatitis
Noma

528.2 Oral aphthae
Aphthous stomatitis   Recurrent aphthous ulcer
Canker sore   Stomatitis herpetiformis
Periadenitis mucosa necrotica recurrens
  Excludes: herpetic stomatitis (054.2)

528.3 Cellulitis and abscess
Cellulitis of mouth (floor)
Ludwig's angina
Oral fistula
  Excludes: abscess of tongue (529.0)
  cellulitis or abscess of lip (528.5)
  fistula (of):
    dental (522.7)
    lip (528.5)
  gingivitis (523.00-523.11)

386 ● Code new to this edition   ▲ Revision of existing code   ④ ⑤ Fourth or fifth digit required

DIGESTIVE SYSTEM

528.4 Cysts
 Dermoid cyst of mouth
 Epidermoid cyst of mouth
 Epstein's pearl of mouth
 Lymphoepithelial cyst of mouth
 Nasoalveolar cyst of mouth
 Nasolabial cyst of mouth

> Excludes: cyst:
> gingiva (523.8)
> tongue (529.8)

528.5 Diseases of lips
 Abscess of lip(s)   Cheilitis:
 Cellulitis of lip(s)   NOS
 Fistula of lip(s)   angular
 Hypertrophy of lip(s)   Cheilodynia
                                    Cheilosis

> Excludes: actinic cheilitis (692.79)
> congenital fistula of lip (750.25)
> leukoplakia of lips (528.6)

528.6 Leukoplakia of oral mucosa, including tongue
 Leukokeratosis of oral mucosa
 Leukoplakia of:
  gingiva
  lips
  tongue

> Excludes: carcinoma in situ (230.0, 232.0)
> leukokeratosis nicotina palati (528.79)

⑤ **528.7 Other disturbances of oral epithelium, including tongue**

> Excludes: carcinoma in situ (230.0, 232.0)
> leukokeratosis NOS (702.8)

  528.71 Minimal keratinized residual ridge mucosa
   Minimal keratinization of alveolar ridge mucosa

  528.72 Excessive keratinized residual ridge mucosa
   Excessive keratinization of alveolar ridge mucosa

  528.79 Other disturbances of oral epithelium, including tongue
   Erythroplakia of mouth or tongue
   Focal epithelial hyperplasia of mouth or tongue
   Leukoedema of mouth or tongue
   Leukokeratosis nicotina palate
   Other oral epithelium disturbances

528.8 Oral submucosal fibrosis, including of tongue

528.9 Other and unspecified diseases of the oral soft tissues
 Cheek and lip biting
 Denture sore mouth
 Denture stomatitis
 Melanoplakia
 Papillary hyperplasia of palate
 Eosinophilic granuloma of oral mucosa
 Irritative hyperplasia of oral mucosa
 Pyogenic granuloma of oral mucosa
 Ulcer (traumatic) of oral mucosa

529 Diseases and other conditions of the tongue

 529.0 Glossitis
  Abscess of tongue
  Ulceration (traumatic) of tongue

> Excludes: glossitis:
> benign migratory (529.1)
> Hunter's (529.4)
> median rhomboid (529.2)
> Moeller's (529.4)

 529.1 Geographic tongue
  Benign migratory glossitis
  Glossitis areata exfoliativa

 529.2 Median rhomboid glossitis

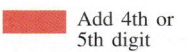 Add 4th or 5th digit
 Nonspecific code
 Unspecified code
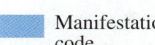 Manifestation code

387

TABULAR LIST

529.3 Hypertrophy of tongue papillae
Black hairy tongue
Coated tongue
Hypertrophy of foliate papillae
Lingua villosa nigra

529.4 Atrophy of tongue papillae
Bald tongue
Glazed tongue
Glossitis:
  Hunter's
  Moeller's
Glossodynia exfoliativa
Smooth atrophic tongue

529.5 Plicated tongue
Fissured tongue
Furrowed tongue
Scrotal tongue

Excludes: *fissure of tongue, congenital (750.13)*

529.6 Glossodynia
Glossopyrosis
Painful tongue

Excludes: *glossodynia exfoliativa (529.4)*

529.8 Other specified conditions of the tongue
Atrophy (of) tongue
Crenated (of) tongue
Enlargement (of) tongue
Hypertrophy (of) tongue
Glossocele
Glossoptosis

Excludes: *erythroplasia of tongue (528.79)*
leukoplakia of tongue (528.6)
macroglossia (congenital) (750.15)
microglossia (congenital) (750.16)
oral submucosal fibrosis (528.8)

529.9 Unspecified condition of the tongue

DISEASES OF ESOPHAGUS, STOMACH, AND DUODENUM (530-538)

530 Diseases of esophagus

Excludes: *esophageal varices (456.0-456.2)*

530.0 Achalasia and cardiospasm
Achalasia (of cardia)
Aperistalsis of esophagus
Megaesophagus

Excludes: *congenital cardiospasm (750.7)*

⑤ **530.1 Esophagitis**
Abscess of esophagus
Esophagitis:
  NOS
  chemical
  peptic
Esophagitis:
  postoperative
  regurgitant

Use additional E code, if desired, to identify cause, if induced by chemical

Excludes: *tuberculous esophagitis (017.8)*

    530.10 Esophagitis, unspecified
    530.11 **Reflux esophagitis**
    530.12 **Acute esophagitis**
    530.19 Other esophagitis

⑤ **530.2 Ulcer of esophagus**
Ulcer of esophagus
  fungal
  peptic
Ulcer of esophagus due to ingestion of:
  aspirin
  chemicals
  medicines

Use additional E code, if desired, to identify cause, if induced by chemical or drug

DIGESTIVE SYSTEM

- **530.20 Ulcer of esophagus without bleeding**
  Ulcer of esophagus NOS
- **530.21 Ulcer of esophagus with bleeding**

  Excludes: bleeding esophageal varices (456.0, 456.20)

- **530.3 Stricture and stenosis of esophagus**
  Compression of esophagus
  Obstruction of esophagus

  Excludes: congenital stricture of esophagus (750.3)

- **530.4 Perforation of esophagus**
  Rupture of esophagus

  Excludes: traumatic perforation of esophagus (862.22, 862.32, 874.4-874.5)

- **530.5 Dyskinesia of esophagus**
  Corkscrew esophagus   Esophagospasm
  Curling esophagus   Spasm of esophagus

  Excludes: cardiospasm (530.0)

- **530.6 Diverticulum of esophagus, acquired**
  Diverticulum, acquired:
    epiphrenic
    pharyngoesophageal
    pulsion
    subdiaphragmatic
    traction
    Zenker's (hypopharyngeal)
  Esophageal pouch, acquired
  Esophagocele, acquired

  Excludes: congenital diverticulum of esophagus (750.4)

- **530.7 Gastroesophageal laceration-hemorrhage syndrome**
  Mallory-Weiss syndrome

- ⑤ **530.8 Other specified disorders of esophagus**
  - **530.81 Esophageal reflux**
    Gastroesophageal reflux

    Excludes: reflux esophagitis (530.11)

  - **530.82 Esophageal hemorrhage**

    Excludes: hemorrhage due to esophageal varices (456.0-456.2)

  - **530.83 Esophageal leukoplakia**
  - **530.84 Tracheoesophageal fistula**

    Excludes: congenital tracheoesophageal fistula (750.3)

  - **530.85 Barrett's esophagus**
  - **530.86 Infection of esophagostomy**
    Use additional code to specify infection
  - **530.87 Mechanical complication of esophagostomy**
    Malfunction of esophagostomy
  - **530.89 Other**

    Excludes: Paterson-Kelly syndrome (280.8)

- **530.9 Unspecified disorder of esophagus**

- ⑤ **531 Gastric ulcer**
  Includes: ulcer (peptic):
    prepyloric
    pylorus
    stomach
  Use additional E code, if desired, to identify drug, if drug-induced

  Excludes: peptic ulcer NOS (533.0-533.9)

  The following fifth-digit subclassification is for use with category 531:
    0 without mention of obstruction
    1 with obstruction

- ⑤ **531.0 Acute with hemorrhage**
- ⑤ **531.1 Acute with perforation**
- ⑤ **531.2 Acute with hemorrhage and perforation**

389

 Add 4th or 5th digit   Nonspecific code Unspecified code 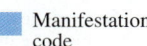 Manifestation code

TABULAR LIST

- ⑤ **531.3** Acute without mention of hemorrhage or perforation
- ⑤ **531.4** Chronic or unspecified with hemorrhage
- ⑤ **531.5** Chronic or unspecified with perforation
- ⑤ **531.6** Chronic or unspecified with hemorrhage and perforation
- ⑤ **531.7** Chronic without mention of hemorrhage or perforation
- ⑤ **531.9** Unspecified as acute or chronic, without mention of hemorrhage or perforation

⑤ **532 Duodenal ulcer**
   Includes: erosion (acute) of duodenum
   ulcer (peptic):
   duodenum
   postpyloric

Use additional E code, if desired, to identify drug, if drug-induced

Excludes: peptic ulcer NOS (533.0-533.9)

The following fifth-digit subclassification is for use with category 532:
   0   without mention of obstruction
   1   with obstruction

- ⑤ **532.0** Acute with hemorrhage
- ⑤ **532.1** Acute with perforation
- ⑤ **532.2** Acute with hemorrhage and perforation
- ⑤ **532.3** Acute without mention of hemorrhage or perforation
- ⑤ **532.4** Chronic or unspecified with hemorrhage
- ⑤ **532.5** Chronic or unspecified with perforation
- ⑤ **532.6** Chronic or unspecified with hemorrhage and perforation
- ⑤ **532.7** Chronic without mention of hemorrhage or perforation
- ⑤ **532.9** Unspecified as acute or chronic, without mention of hemorrhage or perforation

⑤ **533 Peptic ulcer, site unspecified**
   Includes: gastroduodenal ulcer NOS
   peptic ulcer NOS
   stress ulcer NOS

Use additional E code, if desired, to identify drug, if drug-induced

Excludes: peptic ulcer:
   duodenal (532.0-532.9)
   gastric (531.0-531.9)

The following fifth-digit subclassification is for use with category 533:
   0   without mention of obstruction
   1   with obstruction

- ⑤ **533.0** Acute with hemorrhage
- ⑤ **533.1** Acute with perforation
- ⑤ **533.2** Acute with hemorrhage and perforation
- ⑤ **533.3** Acute without mention of hemorrhage and perforation
- ⑤ **533.4** Chronic or unspecified with hemorrhage
- ⑤ **533.5** Chronic or unspecified with perforation
- ⑤ **533.6** Chronic or unspecified with hemorrhage and perforation
- ⑤ **533.7** Chronic without mention of hemorrhage or perforation
- ⑤ **533.9** Unspecified as acute or chronic, without mention of hemorrhage or perforation

⑤ **534 Gastrojejunal ulcer**
   Includes: ulcer (peptic) or erosion:
   anastomotic
   gastrocolic
   gastrointestinal
   gastrojejunal
   jejunal
   marginal
   stomal

Excludes: primary ulcer of small intestine (569.82)

The following fifth-digit subclassification is for use with category 534:
   0   without mention of obstruction
   1   with obstruction

DIGESTIVE SYSTEM

- ⑤ **534.0** Acute with hemorrhage
- ⑤ **534.1** Acute with perforation
- ⑤ **534.2** Acute with hemorrhage and perforation
- ⑤ **534.3** Acute without mention of hemorrhage or perforation
- ⑤ **534.4** Chronic or unspecified with hemorrhage
- ⑤ **534.5** Chronic or unspecified with perforation
- ⑤ **534.6** Chronic or unspecified with hemorrhage and perforation
- ⑤ **534.7** Chronic without mention of hemorrhage or perforation
- ⑤ **534.9** Unspecified as acute or chronic, without mention of hemorrhage or perforation

⑤ **535 Gastritis and duodenitis**

The following fifth-digit subclassification is for use with category 535

    0 without mention of hemorrhage
    1 with hemorrhage

- ⑤ **535.0 Acute gastritis**
- ⑤ **535.1 Atrophic gastritis**
  Gastritis:
    atrophic-hyperplastic
    chronic (atrophic)
- ⑤ **535.2 Gastric mucosal hypertrophy**
  Hypertrophic gastritis
- ⑤ **535.3 Alcoholic gastritis**
- ⑤ **535.4 Other specified gastritis**
  Gastritis: Gastritis:
    allergic   superficial
    bile induced   toxic
    irritant
- ⑤ **535.5 Unspecified gastritis and gastroduodenitis**
- ⑤ **535.6 Duodenitis**

536 Disorders of function of stomach

    Excludes: functional disorders of stomach specified as psychogenic (306.4)

- **536.0 Achlorhydria**
- **536.1 Acute dilatation of stomach**
  Acute distention of stomach
- **536.2 Persistent vomiting**
  Habit vomiting
  Persistent vomiting [not of pregnancy]
  Uncontrollable vomiting

    Excludes: excessive vomiting in pregnancy (643.0-643.9)
           vomiting NOS (787.0)

- **536.3 Gastroparesis**
  Gastroparalysis
  Code first underlying disease, such as:
    diabetes mellitus (250.4)
- ⑤ **536.4 Gastrostomy complications**
  - **536.40** Gastrostomy complications, unspecified
  - **536.41** Infection of gastrostomy
    Use additional code to specify type of infection, such as:
      abscess or cellulitis of abdomen (682.2)
      septicemia (038.0-038.9)
    Use additional code to identify organism (041.00-041.9)
  - **536.42** Mechanical complication of gastrostomy
  - **536.49** Other gastrostomy complications

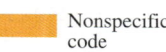 Add 4th or 5th digit   Nonspecific code   Unspecified code   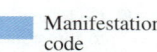 Manifestation code

391

TABULAR LIST

536.8 Dyspepsia and other specified disorders of function of stomach
Achylia gastrica
Hourglass contraction of stomach
Hyperacidity
Hyperchlorhydria
Hypochlorhydria
Indigestion
Tachygastria

Excludes: *achlorhydria (536.0)*
heartburn (787.1)

536.9 Unspecified functional disorder of stomach
Functional gastrointestinal:
  disorder
  disturbance
  irritation

537 Other disorders of stomach and duodenum

537.0 Acquired hypertrophic pyloric stenosis
Constriction of pylorus, acquired or adult
Obstruction of pylorus, acquired or adult
Stricture of pylorus, acquired or adult

Excludes: *congenital or infantile pyloric stenosis (750.5)*

537.1 Gastric diverticulum

Excludes: *congenital diverticulum of stomach (750.7)*

537.2 Chronic duodenal ileus

537.3 Other obstruction of duodenum
Cicatrix of duodenum
Stenosis of duodenum
Stricture of duodenum
Volvulus of duodenum

Excludes: *congenital obstruction of duodenum (751.1)*

537.4 Fistula of stomach or duodenum
Gastrocolic fistula
Gastrojejunocolic fistula

537.5 Gastroptosis

537.6 Hourglass stricture or stenosis of stomach
Cascade stomach

Excludes: *congenital hourglass stomach (750.7)*
hourglass contraction of stomach (536.8)

⑤ **537.8 Other specified disorders of stomach and duodenum**

537.81 Pylorospasm

Excludes: *congenital pylorospasm (750.5)*

537.82 Angiodysplasia of stomach and duodenum without mention of hemorrhage

537.83 Angiodysplasia of stomach and duodenum with hemorrhage

537.84 Dieulafoy lesion (hemorrhagic) of stomach and duodenum

537.89 Other
Gastric or duodenal:
  prolapse
  rupture
Intestinal metaplasia of gastric mucosa
Passive congestion of stomach

Excludes: *diverticula of duodenum (562.00-562.01)*
gastrointestinal hemorrhage (578.0-578.9)

537.9 Unspecified disorder of stomach and duodenum

538 Gastrointestinal mucositis (ulcerative)
Use additional E code to identify adverse effects of therapy, such as:
  antineoplastic and immunosuppressive drugs (E930.7, E933.1)
  radiation therapy (E879.2)

Excludes: *mucositis (ulcerative) of mouth and oral soft tissue (528.00-528.09)*

DIGESTIVE SYSTEM

APPENDICITIS (540-543)

540 Acute appendicitis

540.0 With generalized peritonitis
Appendicitis (acute):
  fulminating with: perforation, peritonitis (generalized), rupture
  gangrenous with: perforation, peritonitis (generalized), rupture
  obstructive with: perforation, peritonitis (generalized), rupture
Cecitis (acute) with: perforation peritonitis (generalized) rupture
Rupture of appendix

Excludes: *acute appendicitis with peritoneal abscess (540.1)*

540.1 With peritoneal abscess
Abscess of appendix
With generalized peritonitis

540.9 Without mention of peritonitis
Acute:
  appendicitis:
    fulminating without mention of perforation, peritonitis, or rupture
    gangrenous without mention of perforation, peritonitis, or rupture
    inflamed without mention of perforation, peritonitis, or rupture
    obstructive without mention of perforation, peritonitis, or rupture
    cecitis without mention of perforation, peritonitis, or rupture

541 Appendicitis, unqualified

542 Other appendicitis
Appendicitis: Appendicitis:
  chronic   relapsing
  recurrent   subacute

Excludes: *hyperplasia (lymphoid) of appendix (543.0)*

543 Other diseases of appendix

543.0 Hyperplasia of appendix (lymphoid)

543.9 Other and unspecified diseases of appendix
Appendicular or appendiceal:
  colic
  concretion
  fistula
Diverticulum of appendix
Fecalith of appendix
Intussusception of appendix
Mucocele of appendix
Stercolith of appendix

HERNIA OF ABDOMINAL CAVITY (550-553)

Includes: hernia:
  acquired
  congenital, except diaphragmatic or hiatal

⑤ 550 Inguinal hernia
Includes: bubonocele
  inguinal hernia (direct) (double) (indirect) (oblique) (sliding)
  scrotal hernia

The following fifth-digit subclassification is for use with category 550:

  0 unilateral or unspecified (not specified as recurrent)
    Unilateral NOS

  1 unilateral or unspecified, recurrent

  2 bilateral (not specified as recurrent)
    Bilateral NOS

  3 bilateral, recurrent

⑤ **550.0 Inguinal hernia, with gangrene**
Inguinal hernia with gangrene (and obstruction)

⑤ **550.1 Inguinal hernia, with obstruction, without mention of gangrene**
Inguinal hernia with mention of incarceration, irreducibility, or strangulation

⑤ **550.9 Inguinal hernia, without mention of obstruction or gangrene**
Inguinal hernia NOS

393

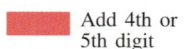 Add 4th or 5th digit
 Nonspecific code
 Unspecified code
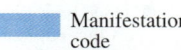 Manifestation code

TABULAR LIST

551 **Other hernia of abdominal cavity, with gangrene**
Includes: that with gangrene (and obstruction)

⑤ **551.0 Femoral hernia with gangrene**

551.00 **Unilateral or unspecified (not specified as recurrent)**
Femoral hernia NOS with gangrene

551.01 **Unilateral or unspecified, recurrent**

551.02 Bilateral (not specified as recurrent)

551.03 Bilateral, recurrent

551.1 Umbilical hernia with gangrene
Parumbilical hernia specified as gangrenous

⑤ **551.2 Ventral hernia with gangrene**

551.20 **Ventral, unspecified, with gangrene**

551.21 Incisional, with gangrene
Hernia:
postoperative specified as gangrenous
recurrent, ventral specified as gangrenous

551.29 **Other**
Epigastric hernia specified as gangrenous

551.3 Diaphragmatic hernia with gangrene
Hernia:
hiatal (esophageal) (sliding) specified as gangrenous
paraesophageal specified as gangrenous
Thoracic stomach specified as gangrenous

Excludes: congenital diaphragmatic hernia (756.6)

551.8 **Hernia of other specified sites, with gangrene**
Any condition classifiable to 553.8 if specified as gangrenous

551.9 **Hernia of unspecified site, with gangrene**
Any condition classifiable to 553.9 if specified as gangrenous

552 **Other hernia of abdominal cavity, with obstruction, but without mention of gangrene**

Excludes: that with mention of gangrene (551.0-551.9)

⑤ **552.0 Femoral hernia with obstruction**
Femoral hernia specified as incarcerated, irreducible, strangulated, or causing obstruction

552.00 **Unilateral or unspecified (not specified as recurrent)**

552.01 **Unilateral or unspecified, recurrent**

552.02 Bilateral (not specified as recurrent)

552.03 Bilateral, recurrent

552.1 Umbilical hernia with obstruction
Parumbilical hernia specified as incarcerated, irreducible, strangulated, or causing obstruction

⑤ **552.2 Ventral hernia with obstruction**
Ventral hernia specified as incarcerated, irreducible, strangulated, or causing obstruction

552.20 **Ventral, unspecified, with obstruction**

552.21 Incisional, with obstruction
Hernia:
postoperative specified as incarcerated, irreducible, strangulated, or causing obstruction
recurrent, ventral specified as incarcerated, irreducible, strangulated, or causing obstruction

552.29 **Other**
Epigastric hernia specified as incarcerated, irreducible, strangulated, or causing obstruction

552.3 Diaphragmatic hernia with obstruction
Hernia:
hiatal (esophageal) (sliding), specified as incarcerated, irreducible, strangulated, or causing obstruction
paraesophageal, specified as incarcerated, irreducible, strangulated, or causing obstruction
Thoracic stomach, specified as incarcerated, irreducible, strangulated, or causing obstruction

Excludes: congenital diaphragmatic hernia (756.6)

● Code new to this edition   ▲ Revision of existing code   ④ ⑤ Fourth or fifth digit required

DIGESTIVE SYSTEM

552.8 Hernia of other specified sites, with obstruction
Any condition classifiable to 553.8 if specified as incarcerated, irreducible, strangulated, or causing obstruction

Excludes: hernia due to adhesion with obstruction (560.81)

552.9 Hernia of unspecified site, with obstruction
Any condition classifiable to 553.9 if specified as incarcerated, irreducible, strangulated, or causing obstruction

553 Other hernia of abdominal cavity without mention of obstruction or gangrene

Excludes: the listed conditions with mention of:
  gangrene (and obstruction) (551.0-551.9)
  obstruction (552.0-552.9)

⑤ **553.0 Femoral hernia**

  553.00 Unilateral or unspecified (not specified as recurrent)
    Femoral hernia NOS

  553.01 Unilateral or unspecified, recurrent

  553.02 Bilateral (not specified as recurrent)

  553.03 Bilateral, recurrent

553.1 **Umbilical hernia**
  Parumbilical hernia

⑤ 553.2 **Ventral hernia**

  553.20 Ventral, unspecified

  553.21 **Incisional**
    Hernia:
      postoperative
      recurrent, ventral

  553.29 Other
    Hernia:
      epigastric
      spigelian

553.3 **Diaphragmatic hernia**
  Hernia:
    hiatal (esophageal) (sliding)
    paraesophageal
  Thoracic stomach

Excludes: congenital:
  diaphragmatic hernia (756.6)
  hiatal hernia (750.6)
  esophagocele (530.6)

553.8 Hernia of other specified sites
  Hernia: Hernia:
    ischiatic   retroperitoneal
    ischiorectal   sciatic
    lumbar   Other abdominal hernia of specified site
    obturator
    pudendal

Excludes: vaginal enterocele (618.6)

553.9 Hernia of unspecified site
  Enterocele   Hernia:
  Epiplocele   intestinal
  Hernia: intra-abdominal
    NOS   Rupture (nontraumatic)
    interstitial   Sarcoepiplocele

NONINFECTIOUS ENTERITIS AND COLITIS (555-558)

555 Regional enteritis
  Includes: Crohn's disease
    Granulomatous enteritis

Excludes: ulcerative colitis (556)

  555.0 **Small intestine**
    Ileitis: Regional enteritis or Crohn's disease of:
      regional   duodenum
      segmental   ileum
      terminal   jejunum

Add 4th or 5th digit | Nonspecific code | Unspecified code | Manifestation code

TABULAR LIST

555.1 Large intestine
Colitis:
  granulomatous
  regional
  transmural
Regional enteritis or Crohn's disease of:
  colon
  large bowel
  rectum

555.2 Small intestine with large intestine
Regional ileocolitis

555.9 Unspecified site
Crohn's disease NOS
Regional enteritis NOS

556 Ulcerative colitis

556.0 Ulcerative (chronic) enterocolitis

556.1 Ulcerative (chronic) ileocolitis

556.2 Ulcerative (chronic) proctitis

556.3 Ulcerative (chronic) proctosigmoiditis

556.4 Pseudopolyposis of colon

556.5 Left-sided ulcerative (chronic) colitis

556.6 Universal ulcerative (chronic) colitis
Pancolitis

556.8 Other ulcerative colitis

556.9 Ulcerative colitis, unspecified
Ulcerative enteritis NOS

557 Vascular insufficiency of intestine

Excludes: necrotizing enterocolitis of the newborn (777.5)

557.0 Acute vascular insufficiency of intestine
Acute:
  hemorrhagic enterocolitis
  ischemic colitis, enteritis, or enterocolitis
  massive necrosis of intestine
Bowel infarction
Embolism of mesenteric artery
Fulminant enterocolitis
Hemorrhagic necrosis of intestine
Infarction of appendices epiploicae
Intestinal gangrene
Intestinal infarction (acute) (agnogenic) (hemorrhagic) (nonocclusive)
Mesenteric infarction (embolic) (thrombotic)
Necrosis of intestine
Terminal hemorrhagic enteropathy
Thrombosis of mesenteric artery

557.1 Chronic vascular insufficiency of intestine
Angina, abdominal
Chronic ischemic colitis, enteritis, or enterocolitis
Ischemic stricture of intestine
Mesenteric:
  angina
  artery syndrome (superior)
  vascular insufficiency

557.9 Unspecified vascular insufficiency of intestine
Alimentary pain due to vascular insufficiency
Ischemic colitis, enteritis, or enterocolitis NOS

558 Other and unspecified noninfectious gastroenteritis and colitis

Excludes: infectious:
    colitis, enteritis, or gastroenteritis (009.0-009.1)
    diarrhea (009.2-009.3)

558.1 Gastroenteritis and colitis due to radiation
Radiation enterocolitis

558.2 Toxic gastroenteritis and colitis
Use additional E code, if desired, to identify cause

558.3 Allergic gastroenteritis and colitis
Use additional code to identify type of food allergy (V15.01-V15.05)

DIGESTIVE SYSTEM

558.9 Other and unspecified noninfectious gastroenteritis and colitis
Colitis NOS, dietetic, or noninfectious
Enteritis NOS, dietetic, or noninfectious
Gastroenteritis NOS, dietetic, or noninfectious
Ileitis NOS, dietetic, or noninfectious
Jejunitis NOS, dietetic, or noninfectious
Sigmoiditis NOS, dietetic, or noninfectious

OTHER DISEASES OF INTESTINES AND PERITONEUM (560-569)

560 Intestinal obstruction without mention of hernia

Excludes: duodenum (537.2-537.3)
  inguinal hernia with obstruction (550.1)
  intestinal obstruction complicating hernia (552.0-552.9)
  mesenteric:
    embolism (557.0)
    infarction (557.0)
    thrombosis (557.0)
  neonatal intestinal obstruction (277.01, 777.1-777.2, 777.4)

560.0 Intussusception
Intussusception (colon) (intestine) (rectum)
Invagination of intestine or colon

Excludes: intussusception of appendix (543.9)

560.1 Paralytic ileus
Adynamic ileus
Ileus (of intestine) (of bowel) (of colon)
Paralysis of intestine or colon

Excludes: gallstone ileus (560.31)

560.2 Volvulus
Knotting of intestine, bowel, or colon
Strangulation of intestine, bowel, or colon
Torsion of intestine, bowel, or colon
Twist of intestine, bowel, or colon

Ⓢ **560.3 Impaction of intestine**

560.30 Impaction of intestine, unspecified
Impaction of colon

560.31 Gallstone ileus
Obstruction of intestine by gallstone

560.39 Other
Concretion of intestine
Enterolith
Fecal impaction

Ⓢ **560.8 Other specified intestinal obstruction**

560.81 Intestinal or peritoneal adhesions with obstruction (postoperative) (postinfection)

Excludes: adhesions without obstruction (568.0)

560.89 Other
Acute pseudo-obstruction of intestine
Mural thickening causing obstruction

Excludes: ischemic stricture of intestine (557.1)

560.9 Unspecified intestinal obstruction
Enterostenosis
Obstruction of intestine or colon
Occlusion of intestine or colon
Stenosis of intestine or colon
Stricture of intestine or colon

Excludes: congenital stricture or stenosis of intestine (751.1-751.2)

562 Diverticula of intestine
Use additional code, if desired, to identify any associated:
  peritonitis (567.0-567.9)

Excludes: congenital diverticulum of colon (751.5)
  diverticulum of appendix (543.9)
  Meckel's diverticulum (751.0)

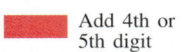 Add 4th or 5th digit
 Nonspecific code
 Unspecified code
 Manifestation code

397

TABULAR LIST

⑤ **562.0 Small intestine**

562.00 Diverticulosis of small intestine (without mention of hemorrhage)
Diverticulosis:
  duodenum without mention of diverticulitis
  ileum without mention of diverticulitis
  jejunum without mention of diverticulitis

562.01 Diverticulitis of small intestine (without mention of hemorrhage)
Diverticulitis (with diverticulosis):
  duodenum
  ileum
  jejunum
  small intestine

562.02 Diverticulosis of small intestine with hemorrhage

562.03 Diverticulitis of small intestine with hemorrhage

⑤ **562.1 Colon**

562.10 Diverticulosis of colon (without mention of hemorrhage)
Diverticulosis:
  NOS without mention of diverticulitis
  intestine (large) without mention of diverticulitis
  Diverticular disease (colon) without mention of diverticulitis

562.11 Diverticulitis of colon (without mention of hemorrhage)
Diverticulitis (with diverticulosis):
  NOS
  colon
  intestine (large)

562.12 Diverticulosis of colon with hemorrhage

562.13 Diverticulitis of colon with hemorrhage

564 Functional digestive disorders, not elsewhere classified
Excludes: *functional disorders of stomach (536.0-536.9)*
  those specified as psychogenic (306.4)

⑤ **564.0 Constipation**

564.00 Constipation, unspecified

564.01 Slow transit constipation

564.02 Outlet dysfunction constipation

564.09 Other constipation

564.1 Irritable bowel syndrome
Irritable colon   Spastic colon

564.2 Postgastric surgery syndromes
Dumping syndrome   Postgastrectomy syndrome
Jejunal syndrome   Postvagotomy syndrome
Excludes: *malnutrition following gastrointestinal surgery (579.3)*
  postgastrojejunostomy ulcer (534.0-534.9)

564.3 Vomiting following gastrointestinal surgery
Vomiting (bilious) following gastrointestinal surgery

564.4 Other postoperative functional disorders
Diarrhea following gastrointestinal surgery
Excludes: *colostomy and enterostomy complications (569.60-569.69)*

564.5 Functional diarrhea
Excludes: *diarrhea:*
  NOS (787.91)
  psychogenic (306.4)

564.6 Anal spasm
Proctalgia fugax

564.7 Megacolon, other than Hirschsprung's
Dilatation of colon
Excludes: *megacolon:*
  congenital [Hirschsprung's] (751.3)
  toxic (556)

⑤ **564.8 Other specified functional disorders of intestine**
Excludes: *malabsorption (579.0-579.9)*

DIGESTIVE SYSTEM

  564.81 Neurogenic bowel
  564.89 Other functional disorders of intestine
  Atony of colon
 564.9 Unspecified functional disorder of intestine
565 **Anal fissure and fistula**
 565.0 Anal fissure
  Excludes: anal sphincter tear (healed) (non-traumatic) (old) (569.43)
  traumatic (863.89, 863.99)
 565.1 Anal fistula
  Fistula:
   anorectal
   rectal
   rectum to skin
  Excludes: fistula of rectum to internal organs—see Alphabetic Index
  ischiorectal fistula (566)
  rectovaginal fistula (619.1)
566 **Abscess of anal and rectal regions**
 Abscess:
  ischiorectal
  perianal
  perirectal
 Cellulitis:
  anal
  perirectal
  rectal
  Ischiorectal fistula
567 **Peritonitis and retroperitoneal infections**
 Excludes: peritonitis:
  benign paroxysmal (277.31)
  pelvic, female (614.5, 614.7)
  periodic familial (277.31)
  puerperal (670)
  with or following:
   abortion (634-638 with .0, 639.0)
   appendicitis (540.0-540.1)
   ectopic or molar pregnancy (639.0)
 567.0 **Peritonitis in infectious diseases classified elsewhere**
  Code first underlying disease
  Excludes: peritonitis:
   gonococcal (098.86)
   syphilitic (095.2)
   tuberculous (014.0)
  567.1 Pneumococcal peritonitis
  ⑤ 567.2 Other suppurative peritonitis
   567.21 Peritonitis (acute) generalized
    Pelvic peritonitis, male
   567.22 Peritoneal abscess
    Abscess (of):
     abdominopelvic
     mesenteric
     omentum
     peritoneum
    Abscess (of):
     retrocecal
     subdiaphragmatic
     subhepatic
     subphrenic
   567.23 Spontaneous bacterial peritonitis
   Excludes: bacterial peritonitis NOS (567.29)
    567.29 Other suppurative peritonitis
     Subphrenic peritonitis
  ⑤ 567.3 Retroperitoneal infections
   567.31 Psoas muscle abscess
   567.38 Other retroperitoneal abscess
   567.39 Other retroperitoneal infections
  ⑤ 567.8 Other specified peritonitis
   567.81 Choleperitonitis
    Peritonitis due to bile

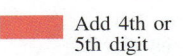 Add 4th or 5th digit
 Nonspecific code
 Unspecified code
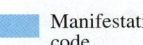 Manifestation code

399

TABULAR LIST

567.82 Sclerosing mesenteritis
Fat necrosis of peritoneum
(Idiopathic) sclerosing mesenteric fibrosis
Mesenteric lipodystrophy
Mesenteric panniculitis
Retractile mesenteritis

567.89 Other specified peritonitis
Chronic proliferative peritonitis
Mesenteric saponification
Peritonitis due to urine

567.9 Unspecified peritonitis
Peritonitis:
  NOS
  of unspecified cause

568 Other disorders of peritoneum

568.0 Peritoneal adhesions (postoperative) (postinfection)

Adhesions (of):
  abdominal (wall)
  diaphragm
  intestine
  male pelvis

Adhesions (of):
  mesenteric
  omentum
  stomach
Adhesive bands

Excludes: adhesions:
  pelvic, female (614.6)
  with obstruction:
    duodenum (537.3)
    intestine (560.81)

568.8 Other specified disorders of peritoneum

568.81 Hemoperitoneum (nontraumatic)

568.82 Peritoneal effusion (chronic)

Excludes: ascites NOS (789.51-789.59)

568.89 Other
Peritoneal:
  cyst
  granuloma

568.9 Unspecified disorder of peritoneum

569 Other disorders of intestine

569.0 Anal and rectal polyp
Anal and rectal polyp NOS

Excludes: adenomatous anal and rectal polyp (211.4)

569.1 Rectal prolapse

Procidentia:
  anus (sphincter)
  rectum (sphincter)
Proctoptosis

Prolapse:
  anal canal
  rectal mucosa

Excludes: prolapsed hemorrhoids (455.2, 455.5)

569.2 Stenosis of rectum and anus
Stricture of anus (sphincter)

569.3 Hemorrhage of rectum and anus

Excludes: gastrointestinal bleeding NOS (578.9)
  melena (578.1)

569.4 Other specified disorders of rectum and anus

569.41 Ulcer of anus and rectum
Solitary ulcer of anus (sphincter) or rectum (sphincter)
Stercoral ulcer of anus (sphincter) or rectum (sphincter)

569.42 Anal or rectal pain

● **569.43 Anal sphincter tear (healed) (old)**
Tear of anus, nontraumatic

Use additional code for any associated fecal incontinence (787.6)

Excludes: anal fissure (565.0)
  anal sphincter tear (healed) (old) complicating delivery (654.8)

---

400   ● Code new to this edition   ▲ Revision of existing code   Fourth or fifth digit required

DIGESTIVE SYSTEM

569.49 Other
Granuloma of rectum (sphincter)
Rupture of rectum (sphincter)
Hypertrophy of anal papillae
Proctitis NOS

Excludes: *fistula of rectum to:*
internal organs—see Alphabetic Index
skin (565.1)
hemorrhoids (455.0-455.9)
incontinence of sphincter ani (787.6)

569.5 Abscess of intestine

Excludes: *appendiceal abscess (540.1)*

⑤ **569.6 Colostomy and enterostomy complications**

569.60 Colostomy and enterostomy complication, unspecified

569.61 Infection of colostomy or enterostomy
Use additional code to specify type of infection, such as:
abscess or cellulitis of abdomen (682.2)
septicemia (038.0-038.9)
Use additional code to identify organism (041.00-041.9)

569.62 Mechanical complication of colostomy and enterostomy
Malfunction of colostomy and enterostomy

569.69 Other complication
Fistula
Hernia
Prolapse

⑤ **569.8 Other specified disorders of intestine**

569.81 Fistula of intestine, excluding rectum and anus
Fistula: Fistula:
  abdominal wall   enteroenteric
  enterocolic   ileorectal

Excludes: *fistula of intestine to internal organs —see Alphabetic Index*
persistent postoperative fistula (998.6)

569.82 Ulceration of intestine
Primary ulcer of intestine
Ulceration of colon

Excludes: *that with perforation (569.83)*

569.83 Perforation of intestine

569.84 Angiodysplasia of intestine (without mention of hemorrhage)

569.85 Angiodysplasia of intestine with hemorrhage

569.86 Dieulafoy lesion (hemorrhagic) of intestine

569.89 Other
Enteroptosis
Granuloma of intestine
Prolapse of intestine
Pericolitis
Perisigmoiditis
Visceroptosis

Excludes: *gangrene of intestine, mesentery, or omentum (557.0)*
hemorrhage of intestine NOS (578.9)
obstruction of intestine (560.0-560.9)

569.9 Unspecified disorder of intestine

 Nonspecific code
 Unspecified code
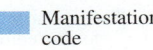 Manifestation code

401

TABULAR LIST

OTHER DISEASES OF DIGESTIVE SYSTEM (570-579)

570   Acute and subacute necrosis of liver
   Acute hepatic failure
   Acute or subacute hepatitis, not specified as infective
   Necrosis of liver (acute) (diffuse) (massive) (subacute)
   Parenchymatous degeneration of liver
   Yellow atrophy (liver) (acute) (subacute)
   Excludes: icterus gravis of newborn (773.0-773.2)
       serum hepatitis (070.2-070.3)
       that with:
           abortion (634-638 with .7, 639.8)
           ectopic or molar pregnancy (639.8)
           pregnancy, childbirth, or the puerperium (646.7)
       viral hepatitis (070.0-070.9)

571   Chronic liver disease and cirrhosis

   571.0   Alcoholic fatty liver

   571.1   Acute alcoholic hepatitis
       Acute alcoholic liver disease

   571.2   Alcoholic cirrhosis of liver
       Florid cirrhosis
       Laennec's cirrhosis (alcoholic)

   571.3   Alcoholic liver damage, unspecified

   ⑤ **571.4   Chronic hepatitis**
       Excludes: viral hepatitis (acute) (chronic) (070.0-070.9)

       571.40   Chronic hepatitis, unspecified

       571.41   Chronic persistent hepatitis

       571.49   Other
           Chronic hepatitis:
               active
               aggressive
           Recurrent hepatitis

   571.5   Cirrhosis of liver without mention of alcohol
       Cirrhosis of liver: Cirrhosis of liver:
           NOS   posthepatitic
           cryptogenic   postnecrotic
           macronodular   Healed yellow atrophy (liver)
           micronodular   Portal cirrhosis

   571.6   Biliary cirrhosis
       Chronic nonsuppurative destructive cholangitis
       Cirrhosis:
           cholangitic
           cholestatic

   571.8   Other chronic nonalcoholic liver disease
       Chronic yellow atrophy (liver)
       Fatty liver, without mention of alcohol

   571.9   Unspecified chronic liver disease without mention of alcohol

572   Liver abscess and sequelae of chronic liver disease

   572.0   Abscess of liver
       Excludes: amebic liver abscess (006.3)

   572.1   Portal pyemia
       Phlebitis of portal vein   Pylephlebitis
       Portal thrombophlebitis   Pylethrombophlebitis

   572.2   Hepatic coma
       Hepatic encephalopathy
       Hepatocerebral intoxication
       Portal-systemic encephalopathy
       Excludes: hepatic coma associated with viral hepatitis – see category 070

   572.3   Portal hypertension

   572.4   Hepatorenal syndrome
       Excludes: that following delivery (674.8)

   572.8   Other sequelae of chronic liver disease

● Code new to this edition   ▲ Revision of existing code   ④ ⑤ Fourth or fifth digit required

DIGESTIVE SYSTEM

573 **Other disorders of liver**
> *Excludes:* amyloid or lardaceous degeneration of liver (277.39)
> congenital cystic disease of liver (751.62)
> glycogen infiltration of liver (271.0)
> hepatomegaly NOS (789.1)
> portal vein obstruction (452)

573.0 **Chronic passive congestion of liver**

573.1 **Hepatitis in viral diseases classified elsewhere**
Code first underlying disease as:
Coxsackie virus disease (074.8)
cytomegalic inclusion virus disease (078.5)
infectious mononucleosis (075)
> *Excludes:* hepatitis (in):
> mumps (072.71)
> viral (070.0-070.9)
> yellow fever (060.0-060.9)

573.2 **Hepatitis in other infectious diseases classified elsewhere**
Code first underlying disease, as:
malaria (084.9)
> *Excludes:* hepatitis in:
> late syphilis (095.3)
> secondary syphilis (091.62)
> toxoplasmosis (130.5)

573.3 **Hepatitis, unspecified**
Toxic (noninfectious) hepatitis
Use additional E code, if desired, to identify cause

573.4 **Hepatic infarction**

573.8 **Other specified disorders of liver**
Hepatoptosis

573.9 **Unspecified disorder of liver**

574 **Cholelithiasis**
The following fifth-digit subclassification is for use with category 574:
  0 **without mention of obstruction**
  1 **with obstruction**

574.0 **Calculus of gallbladder with acute cholecystitis**
Biliary calculus with acute cholecystitis
Calculus of cystic duct with acute cholecystitis
Cholelithiasis with acute cholecystitis
Any condition classifiable to 574.2 with acute cholecystitis

574.1 **Calculus of gallbladder with other cholecystitis**
Biliary calculus with cholecystitis
Calculus of cystic duct with cholecystitis
Cholelithiasis with cholecystitis
Cholecystitis with cholelithiasis NOS
Any condition classifiable to 574.2 with cholecystitis (chronic)

574.2 **Calculus of gallbladder without mention of cholecystitis**
Biliary: Cholelithiasis NOS
  calculus NOS   Colic (recurrent) of gallbladder
  colic NOS   Gallstone (impacted)
Calculus of cystic duct

574.3 **Calculus of bile duct with acute cholecystitis**
Calculus of bile duct [any] with acute cholecystitis
Choledocholithiasis with acute cholecystitis
Any condition classifiable to 574.5 with acute cholecystitis

574.4 **Calculus of bile duct with other cholecystitis**
Calculus of bile duct [any] with cholecystitis (chronic)
Choledocholithiasis with cholecystitis (chronic)
Any condition classifiable to 574.5 with cholecystitis (chronic)

574.5 **Calculus of bile duct without mention of cholecystitis**
Calculus of: Choledocholithiasis
  bile duct [any]   Hepatic:
  common duct   colic (recurrent)
  hepatic duct   lithiasis

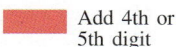 Add 4th or 5th digit   Nonspecific code   Unspecified code   Manifestation code

TABULAR LIST

- ⑤ **574.6 Calculus of gallbladder and bile duct with acute cholecystitis**
  Any condition classifiable to 574.0 and 574.3

- ⑤ **574.7 Calculus of gallbladder and bile duct with other cholecystitis**
  Any condition classifiable to 574.1 and 574.4

- ⑤ **574.8 Calculus of gallbladder and bile duct with acute and chronic cholecystitis**
  Any condition classifiable to 574.6 and 574.7

- ⑤ **574.9 Calculus of gallbladder and bile duct without cholecystitis**
  Any condition classifiable to 574.2 and 574.5

575 Other disorders of gallbladder

575.0 Acute cholecystitis
Abscess of gallbladder without mention of calculus
Angiocholecystitis without mention of calculus
Cholecystitis without mention of calculus:
  emphysematous (acute)
  gangrenous
  suppurative
Empyema of gallbladder without mention of calculus
Gangrene of gallbladder without mention of calculus

Excludes: that with:
  acute and chronic cholecystitis (575.12)
  choledocholithiasis (574.3)
  choledocholithiasis and cholelithiasis (574.6)
  cholelithiasis (574.0)

⑤ **575.1 Other cholecystitis**
Cholecystitis:
  NOS without mention of calculus
  chronic without mention of calculus

Excludes: that with:
  choledocholithiasis (574.4)
  choledocholithiasis and cholelithiasis (574.8)
  cholelithiasis (574.1)

575.10 Cholecystitis, unspecified
Cholecystitis NOS

575.11 Chronic cholecystitis

575.12 Acute and chronic cholecystits

575.2 Obstruction of gallbladder
Occlusion of cystic duct or gallbladder without mention of calculus
Stenosis of cystic duct or gallbladder without mention of calculus
Stricture of cystic duct or gallbladder without mention of calculus

Excludes: that with calculus (574.0-574.2 with fifth-digit 1)

575.3 Hydrops of gallbladder
Mucocele of gallbladder

575.4 Perforation of gallbladder
Rupture of cystic duct or gallbladder

575.5 Fistula of gallbladder
Fistula:
  cholecystoduodenal
  cholecystoenteric

575.6 Cholesterolosis of gallbladder
Strawberry gallbladder

575.8 Other specified disorders of gallbladder
Adhesions (of) cystic duct or gallbladder
Atrophy (of) cystic duct or gallbladder
Cyst (of) cystic duct or gallbladder
Hypertrophy (of) cystic duct or gallbladder
Nonfunctioning (of) cystic duct or gallbladder
Ulcer (of) cystic duct or gallbladder
Biliary dyskinesia

Excludes: nonvisualization of gallbladder (793.3)
  Hartmann's pouch of intestine (V44.3)

575.9 Unspecified disorder of gallbladder

DIGESTIVE SYSTEM

576 Other disorders of biliary tract
Excludes: that involving the:
cystic duct (575.0-575.9)
gallbladder (575.0-575.9)

576.0 Postcholecystectomy syndrome

576.1 Cholangitis
Cholangitis:
  NOS
  acute
  ascending
  chronic
  primary
Cholangitis:
  recurrent
  sclerosing
  secondary
  stenosing
  suppurative

576.2 Obstruction of bile duct
Occlusion of bile duct, except cystic duct, without mention of calculus
Stenosis of bile duct, except cystic duct, without mention of calculus
Stricture of bile duct, except cystic duct, without mention of calculus

Excludes: congenital (751.61)
that with calculus (574.3-574.5 with fifth-digit 1)

576.3 Perforation of bile duct
Rupture of bile duct, except cystic duct

576.4 Fistula of bile duct
Choledochoduodenal fistula

576.5 Spasm of sphincter of Oddi

576.8 Other specified disorders of biliary tract
Adhesions of bile duct [any]
Atrophy of bile duct [any]
Cyst of bile duct [any]
Hypertrophy of bile duct [any]
Stasis of bile duct [any]
Ulcer of bile duct [any]

Excludes: congenital choledochal cyst (751.69)

576.9 Unspecified disorder of biliary tract

577 Diseases of pancreas

577.0 Acute pancreatitis
Abscess of pancreas
Necrosis of pancreas:
  acute
  infective
Pancreatitis:
  NOS
  acute (recurrent)
  apoplectic
  hemorrhagic
  subacute
  suppurative

Excludes: mumps pancreatitis (072.3)

577.1 Chronic pancreatitis
Chronic pancreatitis:
  NOS
  infectious
  interstitial
Pancreatitis:
  painless
  recurrent
  relapsing

577.2 Cyst and pseudocyst of pancreas

577.8 Other specified diseases of pancreas
Atrophy of pancreas
Calculus of pancreas
Cirrhosis of pancreas
Fibrosis of pancreas
Pancreatic:
  infantilism
  necrosis:
    NOS
    aseptic
    fat
Pancreatolithiasis

Excludes: fibrocystic disease of pancreas (277.00-277.09)
islet cell tumor of pancreas (211.7)
pancreatic steatorrhea (579.4)

577.9 Unspecified disease of pancreas

Add 4th or 5th digit   Nonspecific code   Unspecified code   Manifestation code

TABULAR LIST

578 Gastrointestinal hemorrhage
> Excludes: that with mention of:
> angiodysplasia of stomach and duodenum (537.83)
> angiodysplasia of intestine (569.85)
> diverticulitis, intestine:
>   large (562.13)
>   small (562.03)
> diverticulosis, intestine:
>   large (562.12)
>   small (562.02)
> gastritis and duodenitis (535.0-535.6)
> ulcer:
>   duodenal (532.0-532.9)
>   gastric (531.0-531.9)
>   gastrojejunal (534.0-534.9)
>   peptic (533.0-533.9)

578.0 Hematemesis
Vomiting of blood

578.1 Blood in stool
Melena
> Excludes: occult blood (792.1)

578.9 Hemorrhage of gastrointestinal tract, unspecified
Gastric hemorrhage
Intestinal hemorrhage

579 Intestinal malabsorption

579.0 Celiac disease
Celiac: Gee (-Herter) disease
  crisis   Gluten enteropathy
  infantilism   Idiopathic steatorrhea
  rickets   Nontropical sprue

579.1 Tropical sprue
Sprue: Tropical steatorrhea
  NOS
  tropical

579.2 Blind loop syndrome
Postoperative blind loop syndrome

579.3 Other and unspecified postsurgical nonabsorption
Hypoglycemia following gastrointestinal surgery
Malnutrition following gastrointestinal surgery

579.4 Pancreatic steatorrhea

579.8 Other specified intestinal malabsorption
Enteropathy: Steatorrhea (chronic)
  exudative
  protein-losing

579.9 Unspecified intestinal malabsorption
Malabsorption syndrome NOS

GENITOURINARY SYSTEM

10. DISEASES OF THE GENITOURINARY SYSTEM (580-629)

NEPHRITIS, NEPHROTIC SYNDROME, AND NEPHROSIS (580-589)

Excludes: hypertensive chronic kidney disease (403.00-403.91, 404.00-404.93)

580 Acute glomerulonephritis
Includes: acute nephritis

580.0 With lesion of proliferative glomerulonephritis
Acute (diffuse) proliferative glomerulonephritis
Acute poststreptococcal glomerulonephritis

580.4 With lesion of rapidly progressive glomerulonephritis
Acute nephritis with lesion of necrotizing glomerulitis

⑤ **580.8 With other specified pathological lesion in kidney**

580.81 Acute glomerulonephritis in diseases classified elsewhere
Code first underlying disease, as:
infectious hepatitis (070.0-070.9)
mumps (072.79)
subacute bacterial endocarditis (421.0)
typhoid fever (002.0)

580.89 Other
Glomerulonephritis, acute, with lesion of:
exudative nephritis
interstitial (diffuse) (focal) nephritis

580.9 Acute glomerulonephritis with unspecified pathological lesion in kidney
Glomerulonephritis:
NOS specified as acute
hemorrhagic specified as acute
Nephritis specified as acute
Nephropathy specified as acute

581 Nephrotic syndrome

581.0 With lesion of proliferative glomerulonephritis

581.1 With lesion of membranous glomerulonephritis
Epimembranous nephritis
Idiopathic membranous glomerular disease
Nephrotic syndrome with lesion of:
focal glomerulosclerosis
sclerosing membranous glomerulonephritis
segmental hyalinosis

581.2 With lesion of membranoproliferative glomerulonephritis
Nephrotic syndrome with lesion (of):
endothelial glomerulonephritis
hypocomplementemic persistent glomerulonephritis
lobular glomerulonephritis
mesangiocapillary glomerulonephritis
mixed membranous and proliferative glomerulonephritis

581.3 With lesion of minimal change glomerulonephritis
Foot process disease
Lipoid nephrosis
Minimal change:
glomerular disease
glomerulitis
nephrotic syndrome

⑤ **581.8 With other specified pathological lesion in kidney**

581.81 Nephrotic syndrome in diseases classified elsewhere
Code first underlying disease, as:
amyloidosis (277.30-277.39)
diabetes mellitus (250.4)
malaria (084.9)
polyarteritis (446.0)
systemic lupus erythematosus (710.0)

Excludes: nephrosis in epidemic hemorrhagic fever (078.6)

581.89 Other
Glomerulonephritis with edema and lesion of:
exudative nephritis
interstitial (diffuse) (focal) nephritis

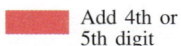 Add 4th or 5th digit
 Nonspecific code
 Unspecified code
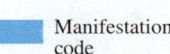 Manifestation code

407

TABULAR LIST

581.9 Nephrotic syndrome with unspecified pathological lesion in kidney
Glomerulonephritis with edema NOS
Nephritis:
  nephrotic NOS
  with edema NOS
Nephrosis NOS
Renal disease with edema NOS

582 Chronic glomerulonephritis
Includes: chronic nephritis

582.0 With lesion of proliferative glomerulonephritis
Chronic (diffuse) proliferative glomerulonephritis

582.1 With lesion of membranous glomerulonephritis
Chronic glomerulonephritis:
  membranous
  sclerosing
Focal glomerulosclerosis
Segmental hyalinosis

582.2 With lesion of membranoproliferative glomerulonephritis
Chronic glomerulonephritis:
  endothelial
  hypocomplementemic persistent
  lobular
  membranoproliferative
  mesangiocapillary
  mixed membranous and proliferative

582.4 With lesion of rapidly progressive glomerulonephritis
Chronic nephritis with lesion of necrotizing glomerulitis

⑤ 582.8 With other specified pathological lesion in kidney

582.81 Chronic glomerulonephritis in diseases classified elsewhere
Code first underlying disease, as:
  amyloidosis (277.30-277.39)
  systemic lupus erythematosus (710.0)

582.89 Other
Chronic glomerulonephritis with lesion of:
  exudative nephritis
  interstitial (diffuse) (focal) nephritis

582.9 Chronic glomerulonephritis with unspecified pathological lesion in kidney
Glomerulonephritis:
  NOS specified as chronic
  hemorrhagic specified as chronic
Nephritis specified as chronic
Nephropathy specified as chronic

583 Nephritis and nephropathy, not specified as acute or chronic
Includes: "renal disease" so stated, not specified as acute or chronic but with stated pathology or cause

583.0 With lesion of proliferative glomerulonephritis
Proliferative:
  glomerulonephritis (diffuse) NOS
  nephritis NOS
  nephropathy NOS

583.1 With lesion of membranous glomerulonephritis
Membranous: Membranous nephropathy NOS
  glomerulonephritis NOS
  nephritis NOS

583.2 With lesion of membranoproliferative glomerulonephritis
Membranoproliferative:
  glomerulonephritis NOS
  nephritis NOS
  nephropathy NOS
Nephritis NOS, with lesion of:
  hypocomplementemic persistent glomerulonephritis
  lobular glomerulonephritis
  mesangiocapillary glomerulonephritis
  mixed membranous and proliferative glomerulonephritis

GENITOURINARY SYSTEM

- **583.4 With lesion of rapidly progressive glomerulonephritis**
  Necrotizing or rapidly progressive:
    glomerulitis NOS
    glomerulonephritis NOS
    nephritis NOS
    nephropathy NOS
  Nephritis, unspecified, with lesion of necrotizing glomerulitis

- **583.6 With lesion of renal cortical necrosis**
  Nephritis NOS with (renal) cortical necrosis
  Nephropathy NOS with (renal) cortical necrosis
  Renal cortical necrosis NOS

- **583.7 With lesion of renal medullary necrosis**
  Nephritis NOS with (renal) medullary [papillary] necrosis
  Nephropathy NOS with (renal) medullary [papillary] necrosis

- ⑤ **583.8 With other specified pathological lesion in kidney**

  - **583.81 Nephritis and nephropathy, not specified as acute or chronic, in diseases classified elsewhere**
    Code first underlying disease, as:
      amyloidosis (277.30-277.39)
      diabetes mellitus (250.4)
      gonococcal infection (098.19)
      Goodpasture's syndrome (446.21)
      systemic lupus erythematosus (710.0)
      tuberculosis (016.0)

    Excludes: gouty nephropathy (274.10)
            syphilitic nephritis (095.4)

  - **583.89 Other**
    Glomerulitis with lesion of:
      exudative nephritis
      interstitial nephritis
    Glomerulonephritis with lesion of:
      exudative nephritis
      interstitial nephritis
    Nephritis with lesion of:
      exudative nephritis
      interstitial nephritis
    Nephropathy with lesion of:
      exudative nephritis
      interstitial nephritis
    Renal disease with lesion of:
      exudative nephritis
      interstitial nephritis

- **583.9 With unspecified pathological lesion in kidney**
  Glomerulitis NOS
  Glomerulonephritis NOS
  Nephritis NOS
  Nephropathy NOS

  Excludes: nephropathy complicating pregnancy, labor, or the puerperium (642.0-642.9, 646.2)
          renal disease NOS with no stated cause (593.9)

584 Acute renal failure

Excludes: following labor and delivery (669.3)
        posttraumatic (958.5)
        that complicating:
          abortion (634-638 with .3, 639.3)
          ectopic or molar pregnancy (639.3)

- **584.5 With lesion of tubular necrosis**
  Lower nephron nephrosis
  Renal failure with (acute) tubular necrosis
  Tubular necrosis:
    NOS
    acute

- **584.6 With lesion of renal cortical necrosis**

- **584.7 With lesion of renal medullary [papillary] necrosis**
  Necrotizing renal papillitis

- **584.8 With other specified pathological lesion in kidney**

- **584.9 Acute renal failure, unspecified**

409

TABULAR LIST

585 Chronic kidney disease (CKD)
Code first hypertensive chronic kidney disease, if applicable, (403.00-403.91, 404.00-404.93)
Use additional code to identify kidney transplant status, if applicable (V42.0)

    585.1 Chronic kidney disease, Stage I
    585.2 Chronic kidney disease, Stage II (mild)
    585.3 Chronic kidney disease, Stage III (moderate)
    585.4 Chronic kidney disease, Stage IV (severe)
    585.5 Chronic kidney disease, Stage V
        Excludes: *chronic kidney disease, stage V requiring chronic dialysis (585.6)*

    585.6 End stage renal disease
        Chronic kidney disease requiring chronic dialysis

    585.9 Chronic kidney disease, unspecified
        Chronic renal disease
        Chronic renal failure NOS
        Chronic renal insufficiency

586 Renal failure, unspecified
    Uremia NOS
    Excludes: *following labor and delivery (669.3)*
        posttraumatic renal failure (958.5)
        that complicating:
            abortion (634-638 with .3, 639.3)
            ectopic or molar pregnancy (639.3)
        uremia:
            extrarenal (788.9)
            prenatal (788.9)
        with any condition classifiable to 401 (403.0-403.9 with fifth-digit 1)

587 Renal sclerosis, unspecified
    Atrophy of kidney   Renal:
    Contracted kidney   cirrhosis
                                fibrosis
    Excludes: *nephrosclerosis (arteriolar) (arteriosclerotic) (403.00-403.92)*
        with hypertension (403.00-403.92)

588 Disorders resulting from impaired renal function
    588.0 Renal osteodystrophy
        Azotemic osteodystrophy   Renal:
        Phosphate-losing tubular   dwarfism
            disorders   infantilism
                                      rickets

    588.1 Nephrogenic diabetes insipidus
        Excludes: *diabetes insipidus NOS (253.5)*

    ⑤ **588.8 Other specified disorders resulting from impaired renal function**
        Excludes: *secondary hypertension (405.0-405.9)*
        588.81 Secondary hyperparathyroidism (of renal origin)
            Secondary hyperparathyroidism NOS
        588.89 Other specified disorders resulting from impaired renal function
            Hypokalemic nephropathy

    588.9 Unspecified disorder resulting from impaired renal function

589 Small kidney of unknown cause
    589.0 Unilateral small kidney
    589.1 Bilateral small kidneys
    589.9 Small kidney, unspecified

OTHER DISEASES OF URINARY SYSTEM (590-599)

590 Infections of kidney
Use additional code, if desired, to identify organism, such as Escherichia coli [E. coli] (041.4)

    ⑤ **590.0 Chronic pyelonephritis**
        Chronic pyelitis
        Chronic pyonephrosis
        Code, if applicable, any causal condition first
        590.00 Without lesion of renal medullary necrosis

GENITOURINARY SYSTEM

  590.01 With lesion of renal medullary necrosis

⑤ **590.1 Acute pyelonephritis**
  Acute pyelitis
  Acute pyonephrosis

  590.10 Without lesion of renal medullary necrosis
  590.11 With lesion of renal medullary necrosis

590.2 Renal and perinephric abscess
  Abscess: Carbuncle of kidney
   kidney
   nephritic
   perirenal

590.3 Pyeloureteritis cystica
  Infection of renal pelvis and ureter
  Ureteritis cystica

⑤ **590.8 Other pyelonephritis or pyonephrosis, not specified as acute or chronic**

  590.80 Pyelonephritis, unspecified
   Pyelitis NOS
   Pyelonephritis NOS

  590.81 Pyelitis or pyelonephritis in diseases classified elsewhere
   Code first underlying disease, as:
    tuberculosis (016.0)

590.9 Infection of kidney, unspecified
  Excludes: urinary tract infection NOS (599.0)

591 Hydronephrosis
  Hydrocalycosis   Hydroureteronephrosis
  Hydronephrosis
  Excludes: congenital hydronephrosis (753.29)
     hydroureter (593.5)

592 Calculus of kidney and ureter
  Excludes: nephrocalcinosis (275.4)

 592.0 Calculus of kidney
  Nephrolithiasis NOS Staghorn calculus
  Renal calculus or stone Stone in kidney
  Excludes: uric acid nephrolithiasis (274.11)

 592.1 Calculus of ureter
  Ureteric stone
  Ureterolithiasis

592.9 Urinary calculus, unspecified

593 Other disorders of kidney and ureter

 593.0 Nephroptosis
  Floating kidney
  Mobile kidney

 593.1 Hypertrophy of kidney

 593.2 Cyst of kidney, acquired
  Cyst (multiple) (solitary) of kidney, not congenital
  Peripelvic (lymphatic) cyst
  Excludes: calyceal or pyelogenic cyst of kidney (591)
     congenital cyst of kidney (753.1)
     polycystic (disease of) kidney (753.1)

 593.3 Stricture or kinking of ureter
  Angulation of ureter (postoperative)
  Constriction of ureter (postoperative)
  Stricture of pelviureteric junction

 593.4 Other ureteric obstruction
  Idiopathic retroperitoneal fibrosis
  Occlusion NOS of ureter
  Excludes: that due to calculus (592.1)

 593.5 Hydroureter
  Excludes: congenital hydroureter (753.22)
     hydroureteronephrosis (591)

Add 4th or 5th digit   Nonspecific code   Unspecified code   Manifestation code

TABULAR LIST

593.6 Postural proteinuria
Benign postural proteinuria
Orthostatic proteinuria

Excludes: proteinuria NOS (791.0)

⑤ **593.7 Vesicoureteral reflux**
  593.70 Unspecified or without reflux nephropathy
  593.71 With reflux nephropathy, unilateral
  593.72 With reflux nephropathy, bilateral
  593.73 With reflux nephropathy NOS

⑤ **593.8 Other specified disorders of kidney and ureter**
  593.81 Vascular disorders of kidney
  Renal (artery):   Renal infarction
    embolism
    hemorrhage
    thrombosis

  593.82 Ureteral fistula
  Intestinoureteral fistula

  Excludes: fistula between ureter and female genital tract (619.0)

  593.89 Other
  Adhesions, kidney or ureter
  Periureteritis
  Polyp of ureter
  Pyelectasia
  Ureterocele

  Excludes: tuberculosis of ureter (016.2)
  ureteritis cystica (590.3)

593.9 Unspecified disorder of kidney and ureter
Acute renal disease
Acute renal insufficiency
Renal disease NOS
Salt-losing nephritis or syndrome

Excludes: chronic renal insufficiency (585.9)
  cystic kidney disease (753.1)
  nephropathy, so stated (583.0-583.9)
  renal disease:
    arising in pregnancy or the puerperium (642.1-642.2, 642.4-642.7, 646.2)
    not specified as acute or chronic, but with stated pathology or cause (583.0-583.9)

594 Calculus of lower urinary tract

594.0 Calculus in diverticulum of bladder

594.1 Other calculus in bladder
Urinary bladder stone

Excludes: staghorn calculus (592.0)

594.2 Calculus in urethra

594.8 Other lower urinary tract calculus

594.9 Calculus of lower urinary tract, unspecified

Excludes: calculus of urinary tract NOS (592.9)

595 Cystitis

Excludes: prostatocystitis (601.3)

Use additional code, if desired, to identify organism, such as Escherichia coli [E. coli] (041.4)

595.0 Acute cystitis

Excludes: trigonitis (595.3)

595.1 Chronic interstitial cystitis
Hunner's ulcer   Submucous cystitis
Panmural fibrosis of bladder

595.2 Other chronic cystitis
Chronic cystitis NOS
Subacute cystitis

Excludes: trigonitis (595.3)

GENITOURINARY SYSTEM

595.3　Trigonitis
　　　　Follicular cystitis
　　　　Trigonitis (acute) (chronic)
　　　　Urethrotrigonitis

595.4　Cystitis in diseases classified elsewhere
　　　　Code first underlying disease, as:
　　　　　actinomycosis (039.8)
　　　　　amebiasis (006.8)
　　　　　bilharziasis (120.0-120.9)
　　　　　Echinococcus infestation (122.3, 122.6)

　　Excludes: cystitis:
　　　　　diphtheritic (032.84)
　　　　　gonococcal (098.11, 098.31)
　　　　　monilial (112.2)
　　　　　trichomonal (131.09)
　　　　　tuberculous (016.1)

⑤ **595.8　Other specified types of cystitis**

　　595.81　Cystitis cystica

　　595.82　Irradiation cystitis
　　　　Use additional E code, if desired, to identify cause

　　595.89　Other
　　　　Abscess of bladder
　　　　Cystitis:
　　　　　bullous
　　　　　emphysematous
　　　　　glandularis

595.9　Cystitis, unspecified

596　Other disorders of bladder
Use additional code, if desired, to identify urinary incontinence (625.6, 788.30-788.39)

596.0　Bladder neck obstruction
　　　　Contracture (acquired) of bladder neck or vesicourethral orifice
　　　　Obstruction (acquired) of bladder neck or vesicourethral orifice
　　　　Stenosis (acquired) of bladder neck or vesicourethral orifice

　　Excludes: congenital (753.6)

596.1　Intestinovesical fistula
　　　Fistula:　　　　　　　　　Fistula:
　　　　enterovesical　　　　　　vesicoenteric
　　　　vesicocolic　　　　　　　vesicorectal

596.2　Vesical fistula, not elsewhere classified
　　　Fistula:　　　　　　　　　Fistula:
　　　　bladder NOS　　　　　　 vesicocutaneous
　　　　urethrovesical　　　　　 vesicoperineal

　　Excludes: fistula between bladder and female genital tract (619.0)

596.3　Diverticulum of bladder
　　　　Diverticulitis of bladder
　　　　Diverticulum (acquired) (false) of bladder

　　Excludes: that with calculus in diverticulum of bladder (594.0)

596.4　Atony of bladder
　　　　High compliance bladder, of bladder
　　　　Hypotonicity of bladder
　　　　Inertia of bladder

　　Excludes: neurogenic bladder (596.54)

⑤ **596.5　Other functional disorders of bladder**

　　Excludes: cauda equina syndrome
　　　　　with neurogenic bladder (344.61)

　　596.51　Hypertonicity of bladder
　　　　Hyperactivity
　　　　Overactive bladder

　　596.52　Low bladder compliance

　　596.53　Paralysis of bladder

　　596.54　Neurogenic bladder NOS

413

　■ Add 4th or 5th digit　　■ Nonspecific code　　■ Unspecified code　　■ Manifestation code

TABULAR LIST

- **596.55** **Detrusor sphincter dyssynergia**
- **596.59** **Other functional disorder of bladder**
  Detrusor instability
- **596.6** **Rupture of bladder, nontraumatic**
- **596.7** **Hemorrhage into bladder wall**
  Hyperemia of bladder
  Excludes: acute hemorrhagic cystitis (595.0)
- **596.8** **Other specified disorders of bladder**
  Bladder: Bladder:
    calcified   hemorrhage
    contracted   hypertrophy
  Excludes: cystocele, female (618.01-618.02, 618.09, 618.2-618.4)
            hernia or prolapse of bladder, female (618.01-618.02, 618.09, 618.2-618.4)
- **596.9** **Unspecified disorder of bladder**

597 Urethritis, not sexually transmitted, and urethral syndrome
Excludes: nonspecific urethritis, so stated (099.4)

- **597.0** **Urethral abscess**
  Abscess of: Abscess:
    bulbourethral gland   periurethral
    Cowper's gland   urethral (gland)
    Littré's gland   Periurethral cellulitis
  Excludes: urethral caruncle (599.3)

- ⑤ **597.8** **Other urethritis**
  - **597.80** **Urethritis, unspecified**
  - **597.81** **Urethral syndrome NOS**
  - **597.89** **Other**
    Adenitis, Skene's   Meatitis, urethral
      glands   Ulcer, urethra (meatus)
    Cowperitis   Verumontanitis
    Excludes: trichomonal (131.02)

598 Urethral stricture
Includes: pinhole meatus
           stricture of urinary meatus
Excludes: congenital stricture of urethra and urinary meatus (753.6)
Use additional code to identify urinary incontinence (625.6, 788.30-788.39)

- ⑤ **598.0** **Urethral stricture due to infection**
  - **598.00** **Due to unspecified infection**
  - **598.01** **Due to infective diseases classified elsewhere**
    Code first underlying disease, as:
      gonococcal infection (098.2)
      schistosomiasis (120.0-120.9)
      syphilis (095.8)
- **598.1** **Traumatic urethral stricture**
  Stricture of urethra:
    late effect of injury
    postobstetric
  Excludes: postoperative following surgery on genitourinary tract (598.2)
- **598.2** **Postoperative urethral stricture**
  Postcatheterization stricture of urethra
- **598.8** **Other specified causes of urethral stricture**
- **598.9** **Urethral stricture, unspecified**

599 Other disorders of urethra and urinary tract
- **599.0** **Urinary tract infection, site not specified**
  Pyuria
  Excludes: candidiasis of urinary tract (112.2)
            urinary tract infection of newborn (771.82)
  Use additional code to identify organism, such as Escherichia coli [E. coli] (041.4)

GENITOURINARY SYSTEM

599.1 Urethral fistula
Fistula: Urinary fistula NOS
urethroperineal
urethrorectal

Excludes: fistula:
urethroscrotal (608.89)
urethrovaginal (619.0)
urethrovesicovaginal (619.0)

599.2 Urethral diverticulum

599.3 Urethral caruncle
Polyp of urethra

599.4 Urethral false passage

599.5 Prolapsed urethral mucosa
Prolapse of urethra
Urethrocele

Excludes: urethrocele, female (618.03, 618.09, 618.2-618.4)

⑤ **599.6 Urinary obstruction**

599.60 Urinary obstruction, unspecified
Obstructive uropathy NOS
Urinary (tract) obstruction NOS

599.69 Urinary obstruction, not elsewhere classified
Code, if applicable, any causal condition first, such as:
hyperplasia of prostate (600.0-600.9 with fifth-digit 1)

599.7 Hematuria
Hematuria (benign) (essential)

Excludes: hemoglobinuria (791.2)

⑤ **599.8 Other specified disorders of urethra and urinary tract**

Excludes: symptoms and other conditions classifiable to 788.0-788.9, 791.0-791.9
Use additional code, if desired, to identify urinary incontinence (625.6, 788.30-788.39)

599.81 Urethral hypermobility

599.82 Intrinsic (urethral) sphincter deficiency [ISD]

599.83 Urethral instability

599.84 Other specified disorders of urethra
Rupture of urethra (nontraumatic)
Urethral:
cyst
granuloma

599.89 Other specified disorders of urinary tract

599.9 Unspecified disorder of urethra and urinary tract

DISEASES OF MALE GENITAL ORGANS (600-608)

600 Hyperplasia of prostate
Includes: enlarged prostate

⑤ **600.0 Hypertrophy (benign) of prostate**
Benign prostatic hypertrophy
Enlargement of prostate
Smooth enlarged prostate
Soft enlarged prostate

600.00 Hypertrophy (benign) of prostate without urinary obstruction and other lower urinary tract symptoms (LUTS)
Hypertrophy (benign) of prostate NOS

TABULAR LIST

- **600.01 Hypertrophy (benign) of prostate with urinary obstruction and other lower urinary tract symptoms (LUTS)**
  Hypertrophy (benign) of prostate with urinary retention
  Use additional code to identify symptoms:
  incomplete bladder emptying (788.21)
  nocturia (788.43)
  straining on urination (788.65)
  urinary frequency (788.41)
  urinary hesitancy (788.64)
  urinary incontinence (788.30-788.39)
  urinary obstruction (599.69)
  urinary retention (788.20)
  urinary urgency (788.63)
  weak urinary stream (788.62)

⑤ **600.1 Nodular prostate**
  Hard, firm prostate
  Multinodular prostate

  Excludes: malignant neoplasm of prostate (185)

  600.10 Nodular prostate without urinary obstruction
  Nodular prostate NOS

  600.11 Nodular prostate with urinary obstruction
  Nodular prostate with urinary retention

⑤ **600.2 Benign localized hyperplasia of prostate**
  Adenofibromatous hypertrophy of prostate
  Adenoma of prostate
  Fibroadenoma of prostate
  Fibroma of prostate
  Myoma of prostate
  Polyp of prostate

  Excludes: benign neoplasms of prostate (222.2)
  hypertrophy of prostate (600.00-600.01)
  malignant neoplasm of prostate (185)

  600.20 Benign localized hyperplasia of prostate without urinary obstruction and other lower urinary tract symptoms (LUTS)
  Benign localized hyperplasia of prostate NOS

  600.21 Benign localized hyperplasia of prostate with urinary obstruction and other lower urinary tract symptoms (LUTS)
  Benign localized hyperplasia of prostate with urinary retention
  Use additional code to identify symptoms:
  incomplete bladder emptying (788.21)
  nocturia (788.43)
  straining on urination (788.65)
  urinary frequency (788.41)
  urinary hesitancy (788.64)
  urinary incontinence (788.30-788.39)
  urinary obstruction (599.69)
  urinary retention (788.20)
  urinary urgency (788.63)
  weak urinary stream (788.62)

600.3 Cyst of prostate

⑤ **600.9 Hyperplasia of prostate, unspecified**
  Median bar
  Prostatic obstruction NOS

  600.90 Hyperplasia of prostate, unspecified, without urinary obstruction and other lower urinary symptoms (LUTS)
  Hyperplasia of prostate NOS

GENITOURINARY SYSTEM

600.91 **Hyperplasia of prostate, unspecified, with urinary obstruction and other lower urinary symptoms (LUTS)**
Hyperplasia of prostate, unspecified, with urinary retention
Use additional code to identify symptoms:
- incomplete bladder emptying (788.21)
- nocturia (788.43)
- straining on urination (788.65)
- urinary frequency (788.41)
- urinary hesitancy (788.64)
- urinary incontinence (788.30-788.39)
- urinary obstruction (599.69)
- urinary retention (788.20)
- urinary urgency (788.63)
- weak urinary stream (788.62)

601 Inflammatory diseases of prostate
Use additional code, if desired, to identify organism, such as Staphylococcus (041.1), or Streptococcus (041.0).

601.0 Acute prostatitis

601.1 Chronic prostatitis

601.2 Abscess of prostate

601.3 Prostatocystitis

601.4 *Prostatitis in diseases classified elsewhere*
Code first underlying disease, as:
- actinomycosis (039.8)
- blastomycosis (116.0)
- syphilis (095.8)
- tuberculosis (016.5)

Excludes: prostatitis:
- gonococcal (098.12, 098.32)
- monilial (112.2)
- trichomonal (131.03)

601.8 Other specified inflammatory diseases of prostate
Prostatitis:
- cavitary
- diverticular
- granulomatous

601.9 Prostatitis, unspecified
Prostatitis NOS

602 Other disorders of prostate

602.0 Calculus of prostate
Prostatic stone

602.1 Congestion or hemorrhage of prostate

602.2 Atrophy of prostate

602.3 Dysplasia of prostate
Prostatic intraepithelial neoplasia I (PIN I)
Prostatic intraepithelial neoplasia II (PIN II)

Excludes: Prostatic intraepithelial neoplasia III (PIN III) (233.4)

602.8 Other specified disorders of prostate
- Fistula of prostate
- Infarction of prostate
- Stricture of prostate
- Periprostatic adhesions

602.9 Unspecified disorder of prostate

603 Hydrocele
Includes: hydrocele of spermatic cord, testis, or tunica vaginalis
Excludes: congenital (778.6)

603.0 Encysted hydrocele

603.1 Infected hydrocele
Use additional code, if desired, to identify organism

603.8 Other specified types of hydrocele

603.9 Hydrocele, unspecified

TABULAR LIST

604 Orchitis and epididymitis
Use additional code, if desired, to identify organism, such as Escherichia coli [E. coli] (041.4), Staphylococcus (041.1), or Streptococcus (041.0)

- **604.0 Orchitis, epididymitis, and epididymo-orchitis, with abscess**
  Abscess of epididymis or testis

⑤ **604.9 Other orchitis, epididymitis, and epididymo-orchitis, without mention of abscess**

- **604.90 Orchitis and epididymitis, unspecified**
- **604.91 Orchitis and epididymitis in diseases classified elsewhere**
  Code first underlying disease, as:
  diphtheria (032.89)
  filariasis (125.0-125.9)
  syphilis (095.8)

  Excludes: orchitis:
  gonococcal (098.13, 098.33)
  mumps (072.0)
  tuberculous (016.5)
  tuberculous epididymitis (016.4)

- **604.99 Other**

605 Redundant prepuce and phimosis
Adherent prepuce
Paraphimosis
Phimosis (congenital)
Tight foreskin

606 Infertility, male

- **606.0 Azoospermia**
  Absolute infertility
  Infertility due to:
  germinal (cell) aplasia
  spermatogenic arrest (complete)

- **606.1 Oligospermia**
  Infertility due to:
  germinal cell desquamation
  hypospermatogenesis
  incomplete spermatogenic arrest

- **606.8 Infertility due to extratesticular causes**
  Infertility due to:
  drug therapy
  infection
  obstruction of efferent ducts
  radiation
  systemic disease

- **606.9 Male infertility, unspecified**

607 Disorders of penis
Excludes: phimosis (605)

- **607.0 Leukoplakia of penis**
  Kraurosis of penis

  Excludes: carcinoma in situ of penis (233.5)
  erythroplasia of Queyrat (233.5)

- **607.1 Balanoposthitis**
  Balanitis
Use additional code, if desired, to identify organism

- **607.2 Other inflammatory disorders of penis**
  Abscess of corpus cavernosum or penis
  Boil of corpus cavernosum or penis
  Carbuncle of corpus cavernosum or penis
  Cellulitis of corpus cavernosum or penis
  Cavernitis (penis)
Use additional code, if desired, to identify organism
  Excludes: herpetic infection (054.13)

- **607.3 Priapism**
  Painful erection

⑤ **607.8 Other specified disorders of penis**

- **607.81 Balanitis xerotica obliterans**
  Induratio penis plastica

GENITOURINARY SYSTEM

- **607.82 Vascular disorders of penis**
  - Embolism of corpus cavernosum or penis
  - Hematoma (nontraumatic) of corpus cavernosum or penis
  - Hemorrhage of corpus cavernosum or penis
  - Thrombosis of corpus cavernosum or penis
- **607.83 Edema of penis**
- **607.84 Impotence of organic origin**
  - *Excludes:* nonorganic (302.72)
- **607.85 Peyronie's disease**
- **607.89 Other**
  - Atrophy of corpus cavernosum or penis
  - Fibrosis of corpus cavernosum or penis
  - Hypertrophy of corpus cavernosum or penis
  - Ulcer (chronic) of corpus cavernosum or penis

607.9 Unspecified disorder of penis

608 Other disorders of male genital organs

- **608.0 Seminal vesiculitis**
  - Abscess of seminal vesicle
  - Cellulitis of seminal vesicle
  - Vesiculitis (seminal)
  - Use additional code, if desired, to identify organism
  - *Excludes:* gonococcal infection (098.14, 098.34)
- **608.1 Spermatocele**
- ⑤ **608.2 Torsion of testis**
  - **608.20 Torsion of testis, unspecified**
  - **608.21 Extravaginal torsion of spermatic cord**
  - **608.22 Intravaginal torsion of spermatic cord**
    - Torsion of spermatic cord NOS
  - **608.23 Torsion of appendix testis**
  - **608.24 Torsion of appendix epididymis**
- **608.3 Atrophy of testis**
- **608.4 Other inflammatory disorders of male genital organs**
  - Abscess of scrotum, spermatic cord, testis [except abscess], tunica vaginalis, or vas deferens
  - Boil of scrotum, spermatic cord, testis [except abscess], tunica vaginalis, or vas deferens
  - Carbuncle of scrotum, spermatic cord, testis [except abscess], tunica vaginalis, or vas deferens
  - Cellulitis of scrotum, spermatic cord, testis [except abscess], tunica vaginalis, or vas deferens
  - Vasitis
  - Use additional code, if desired, to identify organism
  - *Excludes:* abscess of testis (604.0)
- ⑤ **608.8 Other specified disorders of male genital organs**
  - **608.81 Disorders of male genital organs in diseases classified elsewhere**
    - Code first underlying disease, as:
      - filariasis (125.0-125.9)
      - tuberculosis (016.5)
  - **608.82 Hematospermia**
  - **608.83 Vascular disorders**
    - Hematoma (nontraumatic) of seminal vesicle, spermatic cord, testis, scrotum, tunica vaginalis, or vas deferens
    - Hemorrhage of seminal vesicle, spermatic cord, testis, scrotum, tunica vaginalis, or vas deferens
    - Thrombosis of seminal vesicle, spermatic cord, testis, scrotum, tunica vaginalis, or vas deferens
    - Hematocele NOS, male
  - **608.84 Chylocele of tunica vaginalis**
  - **608.85 Stricture**
    - Stricture of:
      - spermatic cord
      - tunica vaginalis
      - vas deferens
  - **608.86 Edema**
  - **608.87 Retrograde ejaculation**

TABULAR LIST

608.89 Other
  Atrophy of seminal vesicle, spermatic cord, testis, scrotum, tunica vaginalis, or vas deferens
  Fibrosis of seminal vesicle, spermatic cord, testis, scrotum, tunica vaginalis, or vas deferens
  Hypertrophy of seminal vesicle, spermatic cord, testis, scrotum, tunica vaginalis, or vas deferens
  Ulcer of seminal vesicle, spermatic cord, testis, scrotum, tunica vaginalis, or vas deferens

  Excludes: atrophy of testis (608.3)

608.9 Unspecified disorder of male genital organs

DISORDERS OF BREAST (610-611)

610 Benign mammary dysplasias

  610.0 Solitary cyst of breast
    Cyst (solitary) of breast

  610.1 Diffuse cystic mastopathy
    Chronic cystic mastitis   Fibrocystic disease of breast
    Cystic breast

  610.2 Fibroadenosis of breast
    Fibroadenosis of breast: Fibroadenosis of breast:
      NOS   diffuse
      chronic   periodic
      cystic   segmental

  610.3 Fibrosclerosis of breast

  610.4 Mammary duct ectasia
    Comedomastitis   Mastitis:
    Dust ectasia   periductal
                                       plasma cell

  610.8 Other specified benign mammary dysplasias
    Mazoplasia
    Sebaceous cyst of breast

  610.9 Benign mammary dysplasia, unspecified

611 Other disorders of breast

  Excludes: that associated with lactation or the puerperium (675.0-676.9)

  611.0 Inflammatory disease of breast
    Abscess (acute) (chronic) (nonpuerperal) of:
      areola
      breast
    Mammillary fistula
    Mastitis (acute) (subacute) (nonpuerperal):
      NOS
      infective
      retromammary
      submammary

    Excludes: carbuncle of breast (680.2)
      chronic cystic mastitis (610.1)
      neonatal infective mastitis (771.5)
      thrombophlebitis of breast [Mondor's disease] (451.89)

  611.1 Hypertrophy of breast
    Gynecomastia
    Hypertrophy of breast:
      NOS
      massive pubertal

  611.2 Fissure of nipple

  611.3 Fat necrosis of breast
    Fat necrosis (segmental) of breast

  611.4 Atrophy of breast

  611.5 Galactocele

  611.6 Galactorrhea not associated with childbirth

  ⑤ **611.7** Signs and symptoms in breast

    611.71 Mastodynia
      Pain in breast

GENITOURINARY SYSTEM

611.72 Lump or mass in breast

611.79 Other
Induration of breast
Inversion of nipple
Nipple discharge
Retraction of nipple

611.8 Other specified disorders of breast
Hematoma (nontraumatic) of breast
Infarction of breast
Occlusion of breast duct
Subinvolution of breast (postlactational) (postpartum)

611.9 Unspecified breast disorder

INFLAMMATORY DISEASE OF FEMALE PELVIC ORGANS (614-616)

Use additional code, if desired, to identify organism, such as Staphylococcus (041.1), or Streptococcus (041.0)

Excludes: that associated with pregnancy, abortion, childbirth, or the puerperium (630-676.9)

614 Inflammatory disease of ovary, fallopian tube, pelvic cellular tissue, and peritoneum

Excludes: endometritis (615.0-615.9)
major infection following delivery (670)
that complicating:
abortion (634-638 with .0, 639.0)
ectopic or molar pregnancy (639.0)
pregnancy or labor (646.6)

614.0 Acute salpingitis and oophoritis
Any condition classifiable to 614.2, specified as acute or subacute

614.1 Chronic salpingitis and oophoritis
Hydrosalpinx
Salpingitis:
follicularis
isthmica nodosa
Any condition classifiable to 614.2, specified as chronic

614.2 Salpingitis and oophoritis not specified as acute, subacute, or chronic
Abscess (of):
fallopian tube
ovary
tubo-ovarian
Oophoritis
Perioophoritis
Perisalpingitis
Pyosalpinx
Salpingitis
Salpingo-oophoritisRTubo-ovarian inflammatory disease

Excludes: gonococcal infection (chronic) (098.37)
acute (098.17)
tuberculous (016.6)

614.3 Acute parametritis and pelvic cellulitis
Acute inflammatory pelvic disease
Any condition classifiable to 614.4, specified as acute

614.4 Chronic or unspecified parametritis and pelvic cellulitis
Abscess (of):
broad ligament, chronic or NOS
parametrium, chronic or NOS
pelvis, female, chronic or NOS
pouch of Douglas, chronic or NOS
Chronic inflammatory pelvic disease
Pelvic cellulitis, female

Excludes: tuberculous (016.7)

614.5 Acute or unspecified pelvic peritonitis, female

614.6 Pelvic peritoneal adhesions, female (postoperative) (postinfection)
Adhesions:
peritubal
tubo-ovarian

Use additional code, if desired, to identify any associated infertility (628.2)

614.7 Other chronic pelvic peritonitis, female
Excludes: tuberculous (016.7)

614.8 Other specified inflammatory disease of female pelvic organs and tissues

TABULAR LIST

614.9 Unspecified inflammatory disease of female pelvic organs and tissues
Pelvic infection or inflammation, female NOS
Pelvic inflammatory disease [PID]

615 Inflammatory diseases of uterus, except cervix

Excludes: following delivery (670)
  hyperplastic endometritis (621.30-621.33)
  that complicating:
    abortion (634-638 with .0, 639.0)
    ectopic or molar pregnancy (639.0)
    pregnancy or labor (646.6)

615.0 Acute
Any condition classifiable to 615.9, specified as acute or subacute

615.1 Chronic
Any condition classifiable to 615.9, specified as chronic

615.9 Unspecified inflammatory disease of uterus
Endometritis   Perimetritis
Endomyometritis   Pyometra
Metritis   Uterine abscess
Myometritis

616 Inflammatory disease of cervix, vagina, and vulva

Excludes: that complicating:
  abortion (634-638 with .0, 639.0)
  ectopic or molar pregnancy (639.0)
  pregnancy, childbirth, or the puerperium (646.6)

616.0 Cervicitis and endocervicitis
Cervicitis with or without mention of erosion or ectropion
Endocervicitis with or without mention of erosion or ectropion
Nabothian (gland) cyst or follicle

Excludes: erosion or ectropion without mention of cervicitis (622.0)

⑤ **616.1 Vaginitis and vulvovaginitis**

616.10 Vaginitis and vulvovaginitis, unspecified
Vaginitis:
  NOS
  postirradiation
Vulvitis NOS
Vulvovaginitis NOS

Use additional code, if desired, to identify organism, such as Escherichia coli [E. coli] (041.4), Staphylococcus (041.1), or Streptococcus (041.0)

Excludes: noninfective leukorrhea (623.5)
  postmenopausal or senile vaginitis (627.3)

616.11 Vaginitis and vulvovaginitis in diseases classified elsewhere
Code first underlying disease, as:
  pinworm vaginitis (127.4)

Excludes: herpetic vulvovaginitis (054.11)
  monilial vulvovaginitis (112.1)
  trichomonal vaginitis or vulvovaginitis (131.01)

616.2 Cyst of Bartholin's gland
Bartholin's duct cyst

616.3 Abscess of Bartholin's gland
Vulvovaginal gland abscess

616.4 Other abscess of vulva
Abscess of vulva
Carbuncle of vulva
Furuncle of vulva

⑤ **616.5 Ulceration of vulva**

616.50 Ulceration of vulva, unspecified
Ulcer NOS of vulva

422 ● Code new to this edition ▲ Revision of existing code ④ ⑤ Fourth or fifth digit required

GENITOURINARY SYSTEM

616.51 Ulceration of vulva in diseases classified elsewhere
Code first underlying disease, as:
Behçet's syndrome (136.1)
tuberculosis (016.7)
Excludes: vulvar ulcer (in):
gonococcal (098.0)
herpes simplex (054.12)
syphilitic (091.0)

⑤ 616.8 Other specified inflammatory diseases of cervix, vagina, and vulva
Excludes: noninflammatory disorders of:
cervix (622.0-622.9)
vagina (623.0-623.9)
vulva (624.0-624.9)

616.81 Mucositis (ulcerative) of cervix, vagina, and vulva
Use additional E code to identify adverse effects of therapy, such as:
antineoplastic and immunosuppressive drugs (E930.7, E933.1)
radiation therapy (E879.2)

616.89 Other inflammatory disease of cervix, vagina and vulva
Caruncle, vagina or labium
Ulcer, vagina

616.9 Unspecified inflammatory disease of cervix, vagina, and vulva

OTHER DISORDERS OF FEMALE GENITAL TRACT (617-629)

617 Endometriosis

617.0 Endometriosis of uterus
Adenomyosis
Endometriosis:
cervix
internal
myometrium
Excludes: stromal endometriosis (236.0)

617.1 Endometriosis of ovary
Chocolate cyst of ovary
Endometrial cystoma of ovary

617.2 Endometriosis of fallopian tube

617.3 Endometriosis of pelvic peritoneum
Endometriosis: Endometriosis:
broad ligament   parametrium
cul-de-sac (Douglas')   round ligament

617.4 Endometriosis of rectovaginal septum and vagina

617.5 Endometriosis of intestine
Endometriosis:
appendix
colon
rectum

617.6 Endometriosis in scar of skin

617.8 Endometriosis of other specified sites
Endometriosis: Endometriosis:
bladder   umbilicus
lung   vulva

617.9 Endometriosis, site unspecified

618 Genital prolapse
Use additional code, if desired, to identify urinary incontinence (625.6, 788.31, 788.33-788.39)
Excludes: that complicating pregnancy, labor, or delivery (654.4)

⑤ 618.0 Prolapse of vaginal walls without mention of uterine prolapse
Excludes: that with uterine prolapse (618.2-618.4)
enterocele (618.6)
vaginal vault prolapse following hysterectomy (618.5)

618.00 Unspecified prolapse of vaginal walls
Vaginal prolapse NOS

618.01 Cystocele, midline
Cystocele NOS

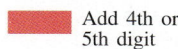 Add 4th or 5th digit
 Nonspecific code
 Unspecified code
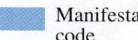 Manifestation code

423

TABULAR LIST

618.02 Cystocele, lateral
Paravaginal

618.03 Urethrocele

618.04 Rectocele
Proctocele

618.05 Perineocele

618.09 Other prolapse of vaginal walls without mention of uterine prolapse
Cystourethrocele

618.1 Uterine prolapse without mention of vaginal wall prolapse
Descensus uteri
Uterine prolapse:
  NOS
  complete
Uterine prolapse:
  first degree
  second degree
  third degree

Excludes: that with mention of cystocele, urethrocele, or rectocele (618.2-618.4)

618.2 Uterovaginal prolapse, incomplete

618.3 Uterovaginal prolapse, complete

618.4 Uterovaginal prolapse, unspecified

618.5 Prolapse of vaginal vault after hysterectomy

618.6 Vaginal enterocele, congenital or acquired
Pelvic enterocele, congenital or acquired

618.7 Old laceration of muscles of pelvic floor

618.8 Other specified genital prolapse

  618.81 Incompetence or weakening of pubocervical tissue

  618.82 Incompetence or weakening of rectovaginal tissue

  618.83 Pelvic muscle wasting
    Disuse atrophy of pelvic muscles and anal sphincter

  618.84 Cervical stump prolapse

  618.89 Other specified genital prolapse

618.9 Unspecified genital prolapse

619 Fistula involving female genital tract

Excludes: vesicorectal and intestinovesical fistula (596.1)

619.0 Urinary-genital tract fistula, female
Fistula:
  cervicovesical
  ureterovaginal
  urethrovaginal
  urethrovesicovaginal
Fistula:
  uteroureteric
  uterovesical
  vesicocervicovaginal
  vesicovaginal

619.1 Digestive-genital tract fistula, female
Fistula:
  intestinouterine
  intestinovaginal
  rectovaginal
Fistula:
  rectovulval
  sigmoidovaginal
  uterorectal

619.2 Genital tract-skin fistula, female
Fistula:
  uterus to abdominal wall
  vaginoperinea

619.8 Other specified fistulas involving female genital tract
Fistula:
  cervix
  cul-de-sac (Douglas')
Fistula:
  uterus
  vagina

619.9 Unspecified fistula involving female genital tract

620 Noninflammatory disorders of ovary, fallopian tube, and broad ligament

Excludes: hydrosalpinx (614.1)

620.0 Follicular cyst of ovary
Cyst of graafian follicle

620.1 Corpus luteum cyst or hematoma
Corpus luteum hemorrhage or rupture
Lutein cyst

GENITOURINARY SYSTEM

620.2 Other and unspecified ovarian cyst
Cyst of ovary:
NOS
corpus albicans
retention NOS
serous
theca-lutein
Simple cystoma of ovary

Excludes: cystadenoma (benign) (serous) (220)
developmental cysts (752.0)
neoplastic cysts (220)
polycystic ovaries (256.4)
Stein-Leventhal syndrome (256.4)

620.3 Acquired atrophy of ovary and fallopian tube
Senile involution of ovary

620.4 Prolapse or hernia of ovary and fallopian tube
Displacement of ovary and fallopian tube
Salpingocele

620.5 Torsion of ovary, ovarian pedicle, or fallopian tube
Torsion:
accessory tube
hydatid of Morgagni

620.6 Broad ligament laceration syndrome
Masters-Allen syndrome

620.7 Hematoma of broad ligament
Hematocele, broad ligament

620.8 Other noninflammatory disorders of ovary, fallopian tube, and broad ligament
Cyst of broad ligament or fallopian tube
Polyp of broad ligament or fallopian tube
Infarction of ovary or fallopian tube
Rupture of ovary or fallopian tube
Hematosalpinx of ovary or fallopian tube

Excludes: hematosalpinx in ectopic pregnancy (639.2)
peritubal adhesions (614.6)
torsion of ovary, ovarian pedicle, or fallopian tube (620.5)

620.9 Unspecified noninflammatory disorder of ovary, fallopian tube, and broad ligament

621 Disorders of uterus, not elsewhere classified

621.0 Polyp of corpus uteri
Polyp:
endometrium
uterus NOS

Excludes: cervical polyp NOS (622.7)

621.1 Chronic subinvolution of uterus

Excludes: puerperal (674.8)

621.2 Hypertrophy of uterus
Bulky or enlarged uterus

Excludes: puerperal (674.8)

⑤ **621.3 Endometrial hyperplasia**
Hyperplasia (adenomatous) (cystic) (glandular) of endometrium
Hyperplastic endometritis

621.30 Endometrial hyperplasia, unspecified
Endometrial hyperplasia NOS

621.31 Simple endometrial hyperplasia without atypia
621.32 Complex endometrial hyperplasia without atypia
621.33 Endometrial hyperplasia with atypia

621.4 Hematometra
Hemometra

Excludes: that in congenital anomaly (752.2-752.3)

621.5 Intrauterine synechiae
Adhesions of uterus
Band(s) of uterus

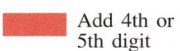 Add 4th or 5th digit   Nonspecific code   Unspecified code   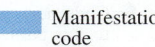 Manifestation code

425

TABULAR LIST

621.6 Malposition of uterus
Anteversion of uterus
Retroflexion of uterus
Retroversion of uterus

Excludes: malposition complicating pregnancy, labor, or delivery (654.3-654.4)
prolapse of uterus (618.1-618.4)

621.7 Chronic inversion of uterus

Excludes: current obstetrical trauma (665.2)
prolapse of uterus (618.1-618.4)

621.8 Other specified disorders of uterus, not elsewhere classified
Atrophy, acquired of uterus
Cyst of uterus
Fibrosis NOS of uterus
Old laceration (postpartum) of uterus
Ulcer of uterus

Excludes: bilharzial fibrosis (120.0-120.9)
endometriosis (617.0)
fistulas (619.0-619.8)
inflammatory diseases (615.0-615.9)

621.9 Unspecified disorder of uterus

622 Noninflammatory disorders of cervix

Excludes: abnormality of cervix complicating pregnancy, labor, or delivery (654.5-654.6)
fistula (619.0-619.8)

622.0 Erosion and ectropion of cervix
Eversion of cervix
Ulcer of cervix

Excludes: that in chronic cervicitis (616.0)

⑤ 622.1 Dysplasia of cervix (uteri)

Excludes: abnormal results from cervical cytologic examination without histologic confirmation (795.00-795.09)
carcinoma in situ of cervix (233.1)
cervical intraepithelial neoplasia III [CIN III] (233.1)

622.10 Dysplasia of cervix, unspecified
Anaplasia of cervix
Cervical atypism
Cervical dysplasia NOS

622.11 Mild dysplasia of cervix
Cervical intraepithelial neoplasia I [CIN I]

622.12 Moderate dysplasia of cervix
Cervical intraepithelial neoplasia II [CIN II]

Excludes: carcinoma in situ of cervix (233.1)
cervical intraepithelial neoplasia III [CIN III] (233.1)
severe dysplasia (233.1)

622.2 Leukoplakia of cervix (uteri)

Excludes: carcinoma in situ of cervix (233.1)

622.3 Old laceration of cervix
Adhesions of cervix
Band(s) of cervix
Cicatrix (postpartum) of cervix

Excludes: current obstetrical trauma (665.3)

622.4 Stricture and stenosis of cervix
Atresia (acquired) of cervix
Contracture of cervix
Occlusion of cervix
Pinpoint os uteri

Excludes: congenital (752.49)
that complicating labor (654.6)

622.5 Incompetence of cervix

Excludes: complicating pregnancy (654.5)
that affecting fetus or newborn (761.0)

GENITOURINARY SYSTEM

622.6 Hypertrophic elongation of cervix

622.7 Mucous polyp of cervix
Polyp NOS of cervix

Excludes: *adenomatous polyp of cervix (219.0)*

622.8 Other specified noninflammatory disorders of cervix
Atrophy (senile) of cervix
Cyst of cervix
Fibrosis of cervix
Hemorrhage of cervix

Excludes: *endometriosis (617.0)*
fistula (619.0-619.8)
inflammatory diseases (616.0)

622.9 Unspecified noninflammatory disorder of cervix

623 Noninflammatory disorders of vagina

Excludes: *abnormality of vagina complicating pregnancy, labor, or delivery (654.7)*
congenital absence of vagina (752.49)
congenital diaphragm or bands (752.49)
fistulas involving vagina (619.0-619.8)

623.0 Dysplasia of vagina
Vaginal intraepithelial neoplasia I and II [VAIN I and II]

Excludes: *carcinoma in situ of vagina (233.31)*
severe dysplasia of vagina (233.31)
vaginal intraepithelial neoplasia III [VAIN III] (233.31)

623.1 Leukoplakia of vagina

623.2 Stricture or atresia of vagina
Adhesions (postoperative) (postradiation) of vagina
Occlusion of vagina
Stenosis, vagina

Use additional E code, if desired, to identify any external cause

Excludes: *congenital atresia or stricture (752.49)*

623.3 Tight hymenal ring
Rigid hymen acquired or congenital
Tight hymenal ring acquired or congenital
Tight introitus acquired or congenital

Excludes: *imperforate hymen (752.42)*

623.4 Old vaginal laceration

Excludes: *old laceration involving muscles of pelvic floor (618.7)*

623.5 Leukorrhea, not specified as infective
Leukorrhea NOS of vagina
Vaginal discharge NOS

Excludes: *trichomonal (131.00)*

623.6 Vaginal hematoma

Excludes: *current obstetrical trauma (665.7)*

623.7 Polyp of vagina

623.8 Other specified noninflammatory disorders of vagina
Cyst of vagina
Hemorrhage of vagina

623.9 Unspecified noninflammatory disorder of vagina

624 Noninflammatory disorders of vulva and perineum

Excludes: *abnormality of vulva and perineum complicating pregnancy, labor, or delivery (654.8)*
condyloma acuminatum (078.1)
fistulas involving:
  perineum—see Alphabetic Index
  vulva (619.0-619.8)
vulval varices (456.6)
vulvar involvement in skin conditions (690-709.9)

TABULAR LIST

⑤ **624.0 Dystrophy of vulva**
  Excludes: carcinoma in situ of vulva (233.32)
        severe dysplasia of vulva (233.32)
        vulvar intraepithelial neoplasia III [VIN III] (233.32)
  ● **624.01 Vulvar intraepithelial neoplasia I [VIN I]**
        Mild dysplasia of vulva
  ● **624.02 Vulvar intraepithelial neoplasia II [VIN II]**
        Moderate dysplasia of vulva
  ● **624.09 Other dystrophy of vulva**
        Kraurosis of vulva
        Leukoplakia of vulva
 624.1 Atrophy of vulva
 624.2 Hypertrophy of clitoris
   Excludes: that in endocrine disorders (255.2, 256.1)
 624.3 Hypertrophy of labia
       Hypertrophy of vulva NOS
 624.4 Old laceration or scarring of vulva
 624.5 Hematoma of vulva
   Excludes: that complicating delivery (664.5)
 624.6 Polyp of labia and vulva
 624.8 Other specified noninflammatory disorders of vulva and perineum
       Cyst of vulva
       Edema of vulva
       Stricture of vulva
 624.9 Unspecified noninflammatory disorder of vulva and perineum

625 Pain and other symptoms associated with female genital organs
 625.0 Dyspareunia
   Excludes: psychogenic dyspareunia (302.76)
 625.1 Vaginismus
       Colpospasm
       Vulvismus
   Excludes: psychogenic vaginismus (306.51)
 625.2 Mittelschmerz
       Intermenstrual pain
       Ovulation pain
 625.3 Dysmenorrhea
       Painful menstruation
   Excludes: psychogenic dysmenorrhea (306.52)
 625.4 Premenstrual tension syndromes
       Menstrual: Premenstrual dysphoric disorder
         migraine   Premenstrual syndrome
         molimen   Premenstrual tension NOS
 625.5 Pelvic congestion syndrome
       Congestion-fibrosis syndrome
       Taylor's syndrome
 625.6 Stress incontinence, female
   Excludes: mixed incontinence (788.33)
        stress incontinence, male (788.32)
 625.8 Other specified symptoms associated with female genital organs
 625.9 Unspecified symptom associated with female genital organs

626 Disorders of menstruation and other abnormal bleeding from female genital tract
   Excludes: menopausal and premenopausal bleeding (627.0)
        pain and other symptoms associated with menstrual cycle (625.2-625.4)
        postmenopausal bleeding (627.1)
 626.0 Absence of menstruation
       Amenorrhea (primary) (secondary)

● Code new to this edition   ▲ Revision of existing code   ④ ⑤ Fourth or fifth digit required

GENITOURINARY SYSTEM

626.1 Scanty or infrequent menstruation
    Hypomenorrhea
    Oligomenorrhea

626.2 Excessive or frequent menstruation
    Heavy periods   Menorrhagia
    Menometrorrhagia   Polymenorrhea

    Excludes: *premenopausal (627.0)*
                    that in puberty (626.3)

626.3 Puberty bleeding
    Excessive bleeding associated with onset of menstrual periods
    Pubertal menorrhagia

626.4 Irregular menstrual cycle
    Irregular:
      bleeding NOS
      menstruation
      periods

626.5 Ovulation bleeding
    Regular intermenstrual bleeding

626.6 Metrorrhagia
    Bleeding unrelated to menstrual cycle
    Irregular intermenstrual bleeding

626.7 Postcoital bleeding

626.8 Other
    Dysfunctional or functional uterine hemorrhage NOS
    Menstruation:
      retained
      suppression of

626.9 Unspecified

627 Menopausal and postmenopausal disorders

    Excludes: *asymptomatic age-related (natural) postmenopausal status (V49.81)*

627.0 Premenopausal menorrhagia
    Excessive bleeding associated with onset of menopause
    Menorrhagia:
      climacteric
      menopausal
      preclimacteric

627.1 Postmenopausal bleeding

627.2 Symptomatic menopausal or female climacteric states
    Symptoms, such as flushing, sleeplessness, headache, lack of concentration, associated with the menopause

627.3 Postmenopausal atrophic vaginitis
    Senile (atrophic) vaginitis

627.4 Symptomatic states associated with artificial menopause
    Postartificial menopause syndromes
    Any condition classifiable to 627.1, 627.2, or 627.3 which follows induced menopause

627.8 Other specified menopausal and postmenopausal disorders
    Excludes: *premature menopause NOS (256.31)*

627.9 Unspecified menopausal and postmenopausal disorder

628 Infertility, female
    Includes: primary and secondary sterility

628.0 Associated with anovulation
    Anovulatory cycle
Use additional code for any associated Stein-Leventhal syndrome (256.4)

628.1 Of pituitary-hypothalamic origin
    Code first underlying cause, as:
      adiposogenital dystrophy (253.8)
      anterior pituitary disorder (253.0-253.4)

TABULAR LIST

628.2 Of tubal origin
Infertility associated with congenital anomaly of tube
Tubal:
  block
  occlusion
  stenosis

Use additional code for any associated peritubal adhesions (614.6)

628.3 Of uterine origin
Infertility associated with congenital anomaly of uterus
Nonimplantation

Use additional code for any associated tuberculous endometritis (016.7)

628.4 Of cervical or vaginal origin
Infertility associated with:
  anomaly of cervical mucus
  congenital structural anomaly
  dysmucorrhea

628.8 Of other specified origin

628.9 Of unspecified origin

629 Other disorders of female genital organs

629.0 Hematocele, female, not elsewhere classified

Excludes: hematocele or hematoma:
  broad ligament (620.7)
  fallopian tube (620.8)
  that associated with ectopic pregnancy (633.00-633.91)
  uterus (621.4)
  vagina (623.6)
  vulva (624.5)

629.1 Hydrocele, canal of Nuck
Cyst of canal of Nuck (acquired)

Excludes: *congenital (752.41)*

⑤ **629.2 Female genital mutilation status**
Female circumcision status
Female genital cutting

629.20 Female genital mutilation status, unspecified
Female genital cutting status, unspecified
Female genital mutilation status NOS
Female genital mutilation status, type 4

629.21 Female genital mutilation Type I status
Clitorectomy status
Female genital cutting Type I status

629.22 Female genital mutilation Type II status
Clitorectomy with excision of labia minor status
Female genital cutting Type II status

629.23 Female genital mutilation Type III status
Female genital cutting Type III status
Infibulation status

629.29 Other female genital mutilation status
Female genital cutting Type IV status
Female genital mutilation Type IV status
Other female genital cutting status

⑤ **629.8 Other specified disorders of female genital organs**

629.81 Habitual aborter without current pregnancy

Excludes: *habitual aborter with current pregnancy (646.3)*

629.89 Other specified disorders of female genital organs

629.9 Unspecified disorder of female genital organs

PREGNANCY, CHILDBIRTH, PUERPERIUM

11. COMPLICATIONS OF PREGNANCY, CHILDBIRTH, AND THE PUERPERIUM (630–677)

ECTOPIC AND MOLAR PREGNANCY (630–633)

Use additional code from category 639 to identify any complications

630 Hydatidiform mole
Trophoblastic disease NOS
Vesicular mole
Excludes: *chorioadenoma (destruens) (236.1)*
chorionepithelioma (181)
malignant hydatidiform mole (236.1)

631 Other abnormal product of conception
Blighted ovum
Mole:
  NOS
  carneous
Mole:
  fleshy
  stone

632 Missed abortion
Early fetal death before completion of 22 weeks' gestation with retention of dead fetus
Retained products of conception, not following spontaneous or induced abortion or delivery
Excludes: *failed induced abortion (638.0-638.9)*
fetal death (intrauterine) (late) (656.4)
missed delivery (656.4)
that with abnormal product of conception (630, 631)

633 Ectopic pregnancy
Includes: ruptured ectopic pregnancy

⑤ **633.0 Abdominal pregnancy**
Intraperitoneal pregnancy

    633.00 Abdominal pregnancy without intrauterine pregnancy

    633.01 Abdominal pregnancy with intrauterine pregnancy

⑤ **633.1 Tubal pregnancy**
Fallopian pregnancy
Rupture of (fallopian) tube due to pregnancy
Tubal abortion

    633.10 Tubal pregnancy without intrauterine pregnancy

    633.11 Tubal pregnancy with intrauterine pregnancy

⑤ **633.2 Ovarian pregnancy**

    633.20 Ovarian pregnancy without intrauterine pregnancy

    633.21 Ovarian pregnancy with intrauterine pregnancy

⑤ **633.8 Other ectopic pregnancy**
Pregnancy:
  cervical
  combined
  cornual
Pregnancy:
  intraligamentous
  mesometric
  mural

    633.80 Other ectopic pregnancy without intrauterine pregnancy

    633.81 Other ectopic pregnancy with intrauterine pregnancy

⑤ **633.9 Unspecified ectopic pregnancy**

    633.90 Unspecified ectopic pregnancy without intrauterine pregnancy

    633.91 Unspecified ectopic pregnancy with intrauterine pregnancy

---

▮ Add 4th or 5th digit   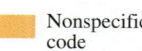 Nonspecific code   ▮ Unspecified code   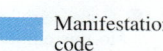 Manifestation code

TABULAR LIST

OTHER PREGNANCY WITH ABORTIVE OUTCOME (634-639)

Note: Use the following fifth-digit subclassification with categories 634-637:

0 Unspecified
1 Incomplete
2 Complete

The following fourth-digit subdivisions are for use with categories 634-638:

.0 Complicated by genital tract and pelvic infection
Endometritis
Salpingo-oophoritis
Sepsis NOS
Septicemia NOS
Any condition classifiable to 639.0, with condition classifiable to 634-638

Excludes: urinary tract infection (634-638 with .7)

.1 Complicated by delayed or excessive hemorrhage
Afibrinogenemia
Defibrination syndrome
Intravascular hemolysis
Any condition classifiable to 639.1, with condition classifiable to 634-638

.2 Complicated by damage to pelvic organs and tissues
Laceration, perforation, or tear of:
  bladder
  uterus
Any condition classifiable to 639.2, with condition classifiable to 634-638

.3 Complicated by renal failure
Oliguria
Uremia
Any condition classifiable to 639.3, with condition classifiable to 634-638

.4 Complicated by metabolic disorder
Electrolyte imbalance with conditions classifiable to 634-638

.5 Complicated by shock
Circulatory collapse
Shock (postoperative) (septic)
Any condition classifiable to 639.5, with condition classifiable to 634-638

.6 Complicated by embolism
Embolism:
  NOS
  amniotic fluid
  pulmonary
Any condition classifiable to 639.6, with condition classifiable to 634-638

.7 With other specified complications
Cardiac arrest or failure
Urinary tract infection
Any condition classifiable to 639.8, with condition classifiable to 634-638

.8 With unspecified complication

.9 Without mention of complication

634 Abortion
Includes: miscarriage
           spontaneous abortion

- 634.0 **Complicated by genital tract and pelvic infection**
- 634.1 **Complicated by delayed or excessive hemorrhage**
- 634.2 **Complicated by damage to pelvic organs or tissues**
- 634.3 **Complicated by renal failure**
- 634.4 **Complicated by metabolic disorder**
- 634.5 **Complicated by shock**
- 634.6 **Complicated by embolism**
- **634.7** **With other specified complications**
- **634.8** **With unspecified complication**
- 634.9 **Without mention of complication**

PREGNANCY, CHILDBIRTH, PUERPERIUM

⑤ 635 **Legally induced abortion**
  Includes: abortion or termination of pregnancy:
     elective
     legal
     therapeutic
  Excludes: menstrual extraction or regulation (V25.3)

  ⑤ 635.0 **Complicated by genital tract and pelvic infection**
  ⑤ 635.1 **Complicated by delayed or excessive hemorrhage**
  ⑤ 635.2 **Complicated by damage to pelvic organs or tissues**
  ⑤ 635.3 **Complicated by renal failure**
  ⑤ 635.4 **Complicated by metabolic disorder**
  ⑤ 635.5 **Complicated by shock**
  ⑤ 635.6 **Complicated by embolism**
  ⑤ 635.7 **With other specified complications**
  ⑤ 635.8 **With unspecified complication**
  ⑤ 635.9 **Without mention of complication**

⑤ 636 **Illegally induced abortion**
  Includes: abortion:
     criminal
     illegal
     self-induced

  ⑤ 636.0 **Complicated by genital tract and pelvic infection**
  ⑤ 636.1 **Complicated by delayed or excessive hemorrhage**
  ⑤ 636.2 **Complicated by damage to pelvic organs or tissues**
  ⑤ 636.3 **Complicated by renal failure**
  ⑤ 636.4 **Complicated by metabolic disorder**
  ⑤ 636.5 **Complicated by shock**
  ⑤ 636.6 **Complicated by embolism**
  ⑤ 636.7 **With other specified complications**
  ⑤ 636.8 **With unspecified complication**
  ⑤ 636.9 **Without mention of complication**

⑤ 637 **Unspecified abortion**
  Includes: abortion NOS
     retained products of conception following abortion, not classifiable elsewhere

  ⑤ 637.0 **Complicated by genital tract and pelvic infection**
  ⑤ 637.1 **Complicated by delayed or excessive hemorrhage**
  ⑤ 637.2 **Complicated by damage to pelvic organs or tissues**
  ⑤ 637.3 **Complicated by renal failure**
  ⑤ 637.4 **Complicated by metabolic disorder**
  ⑤ 637.5 **Complicated by shock**
  ⑤ 637.6 **Complicated by embolism**
  ⑤ 637.7 **With other specified complications**
  ⑤ 637.8 **With unspecified complication**
  ⑤ 637.9 **Without mention of complication**

638 **Failed attempted abortion**
  Includes: failure of attempted induction of (legal) abortion
  Excludes: incomplete abortion (634.0-637.9)

  638.0 **Complicated by genital tract and pelvic infection**
  638.1 **Complicated by delayed or excessive hemorrhage**
  638.2 **Complicated by damage to pelvic organs or tissues**
  638.3 **Complicated by renal failure**
  638.4 **Complicated by metabolic disorder**
  638.5 **Complicated by shock**
  638.6 **Complicated by embolism**
  638.7 **With other specified complications**

TABULAR LIST

638.8 With unspecified complication

638.9 Without mention of complication

639 **Complications following abortion and ectopic and molar pregnancies**

Note: This category is provided for use when it is required to classify separately the complications classifiable to the fourth-digit level in categories 634-638; for example:
- a) when the complication itself was responsible for an episode of medical care, the abortion, ectopic or molar pregnancy itself having been dealt with at a previous episode
- b) when these conditions are immediate complications of ectopic or molar pregnancies classifiable to 630-633 where they cannot be identified at fourth-digit level.

639.0 Genital tract and pelvic infection
Endometritis following conditions classifiable to 630-638
Parametritis following conditions classifiable to 630-638
Pelvic peritonitis following conditions classifiable to 630-638
Salpingitis following conditions classifiable to 630-638
Salpingo-oophoritis following conditions classifiable to 630-638
Sepsis NOS following conditions classifiable to 630-638
Septicemia NOS following conditions classifiable to 630-638

Excludes: *urinary tract infection (639.8)*

639.1 Delayed or excessive hemorrhage
Afibrinogenemia following conditions classifiable to 630-638
Defibrination syndrome following conditions classifiable to 630-638
Intravascular hemolysis following conditions classifiable to 630-638

639.2 Damage to pelvic organs and tissues
Laceration, perforation, or tear of:
  bladder following conditions classifiable to 630-638
  bowel following conditions classifiable to 630-638
  broad ligament following conditions classifiable to 630-638
  cervix following conditions classifiable to 630-638
  periurethral tissue following conditions classifiable to 630-638
  uterus following conditions classifiable to 630-638
  vagina following conditions classifiable to 630-638

639.3 Renal failure
Oliguria following conditions classifiable to 630-638
Renal:
  failure (acute) following conditions classifiable to 630-638
  shutdown following conditions classifiable to 630-638
  tubular necrosis following conditions classifiable to 630-638
Uremia following conditions classifiable to 630-638

639.4 Metabolic disorders
Electrolyte imbalance following conditions classifiable to 630-638

639.5 Shock
Circulatory collapse following conditions classifiable to 630-638
Shock (postoperative) (septic) following conditions classifiable to 630-638

639.6 Embolism
Embolism:
  NOS following conditions classifiable to 630-638
  air following conditions classifiable to 630-638
  amniotic fluid following conditions classifiable to 630-638
  blood-clot following conditions classifiable to 630-638
  fat following conditions classifiable to 630-638
  pulmonary following conditions classifiable to 630-638
  pyemic following conditions classifiable to 630-638
  septic following conditions classifiable to 630-638
  soap following conditions classifiable to 630-638

639.8 **Other specified complications following abortion or ectopic and molar pregnancy**
Acute yellow atrophy or necrosis of liver following conditions classifiable to 630-638
Cardiac arrest or failure following conditions classifiable to 630-638
Cerebral anoxia following conditions classifiable to 630-638
Urinary tract infection following conditions classifiable to 630-638

639.9 **Unspecified complication following abortion or ectopic and molar pregnancy**
Complication(s) not further specified following conditions classifiable to 630-638

PREGNANCY, CHILDBIRTH, PUERPERIUM

COMPLICATIONS MAINLY RELATED TO PREGNANCY (640-649)

Includes: the listed conditions even if they arose or were present during labor, delivery, or the puerperium

The following fifth-digit subclassification is for use with categories 640-649 to denote the current episode of care:

0 unspecified as to episode of care or not applicable

1 delivered, with or without mention of antepartum condition
   Antepartum condition with delivery
   Delivery NOS (with mention of antepartum complication during current episode of care)
   Intrapartum obstetric condition (with mention of antepartum complication during current episode of care)
   Pregnancy, delivered (with mention of antepartum complication during current episode of care)

2 delivered, with mention of postpartum complication
   Delivery with mention of puerperal complication during current episode of care

3 antepartum condition or complication
   Antepartum obstetric condition, not delivered during the current episode of care

4 postpartum condition or complication
   Postpartum or puerperal obstetric condition or complication following delivery that occurred:
      during previous episode of care
      outside hospital, with subsequent admission for observation or care

⑤ 640 Hemorrhage in early pregnancy
Includes: hemorrhage before completion of 22 weeks' gestation

⑤ 640.0 Threatened abortion
[0,1,3]

⑤ 640.8 Other specified hemorrhage in early pregnancy
[0,1,3]

⑤ 640.9 Unspecified hemorrhage in early pregnancy
[0,1,3]

⑤ 641 Antepartum hemorrhage, abruptio placentae, and placenta previa

⑤ 641.0 Placenta previa without hemorrhage
[0,1,3]
Low implantation of placenta without hemorrhage
Placenta previa noted:
   during pregnancy without hemorrhage
   before labor (and delivered by cesarean delivery) without hemorrhage

⑤ 641.1 Hemorrhage from placenta previa
[0,1,3]
Low-lying placenta NOS or with hemorrhage (intrapartum)
Placenta previa:
   incomplete NOS or with hemorrhage (intrapartum)
   marginal NOS or with hemorrhage (intrapartum)
   partial NOS or with hemorrhage (intrapartum)
   total NOS or with hemorrhage (intrapartum)

Excludes: *hemorrhage from vasa previa (663.5)*

⑤ 641.2 Premature separation of placenta
[0,1,3]
Ablatio placentae
Abruptio placentae
Accidental antepartum hemorrhage
Couvelaire uterus
Detachment of placenta (premature)
Premature separation of normally implanted placenta

⑤ 641.3 Antepartum hemorrhage associated with coagulation defects
[0,1,3]
Antepartum or intrapartum hemorrhage associated with:
   afibrinogenemia
   hyperfibrinolysis
   hypofibrinogenemia

Excludes: *coagulation defects not associated with antepartum hemorrhage (649.3)*

⑤ 641.8 Other antepartum hemorrhage
[0,1,3]
Antepartum or intrapartum hemorrhage associated with:
   trauma
   uterine leiomyoma

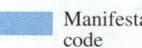

TABULAR LIST

⑤ **641.9 Unspecified antepartum hemorrhage**
[0,1,3]   Hemorrhage:
                antepartum NOS
                intrapartum NOS
                of pregnancy NOS

⑤ **642 Hypertension complicating pregnancy, childbirth, and the puerperium**

  ⑤ **642.0 Benign essential hypertension complicating pregnancy, childbirth, and the puerperium**
  [0-4]   Hypertension:
                benign essential specified as complicating, or as a reason for obstetric care during
                    pregnancy, childbirth, or the puerperium
                chronic NOS specified as complicating, or as a reason for obstetric care during
                    pregnancy, childbirth, or the puerperium
                essential specified as complicating, or as a reason for obstetric care during
                    pregnancy, childbirth, or the puerperium
                pre-existing NOS specified as complicating, or as a reason for obstetric care during
                    pregnancy, childbirth, or the puerperium

  ⑤ **642.1 Hypertension secondary to renal disease, complicating pregnancy, childbirth, and the puerperium**
  [0-4]   Hypertension secondary to renal disease, specified as complicating, or as a reason for
                obstetric care during pregnancy, childbirth, or the puerperium

  ⑤ **642.2 Other pre-existing hypertension complicating pregnancy, childbirth, and the puerperium**
  [0-4]   Hypertensive:
                chronic kidney disease specified as complicating, or as a reason for obstetric care
                    during pregnancy, childbirth, or the puerperium
                heart and chronic kidney disease specified as complicating, or as a reason for obstetric
                    care during pregnancy, childbirth, or the puerperium
                heart disease specified as complicating, or as a reason for obstetric care during
                    pregnancy, childbirth, or the puerperium
                Malignant hypertension specified as complicating, or as a reason for obstetric care
                    during pregnancy, childbirth, or the puerperium

  ⑤ **642.3 Transient hypertension of pregnancy**
  [0-4]   Gestational hypertension
            Transient hypertension, so described, in pregnancy, childbirth, or the puerperium

  ⑤ **642.4 Mild or unspecified pre-eclampsia**
  [0-4]   Hypertension in pregnancy, childbirth, or the puerperium, not specified as pre-existing,
                with either albuminuria or edema, or both; mild or unspecified
            Pre-eclampsia: Toxemia (pre-eclamptic):
                NOS   NOS
                mild   mild
            Excludes: albuminuria in pregnancy, without mention of hypertension (646.2)
                      edema in pregnancy, without mention of hypertension (646.1)

  ⑤ **642.5 Severe pre-eclampsia**
  [0-4]   Hypertension in pregnancy, childbirth, or the puerperium, not specified as pre-existing,
                with either albuminuria or edema, or both; specified as severe
            Pre-eclampsia, severe
            Toxemia (pre-eclamptic), severe

  ⑤ **642.6 Eclampsia**
  [0-4]   Toxemia:
                eclamptic
                with convulsions

  ⑤ **642.7 Pre-eclampsia or eclampsia superimposed on pre-existing hypertension**
  [0-4]   Conditions classifiable to 642.4-642.6, with conditions classifiable to 642.0-642.2

  ⑤ **642.9 Unspecified hypertension complicating pregnancy, childbirth, or the puerperium**
  [0-4]   Hypertension NOS, without mention of albuminuria or edema, complicating pregnancy,
                childbirth, or the puerperium

⑤ **643 Excessive vomiting in pregnancy**
        Includes: hyperemesis arising during pregnancy
                   vomiting:
                       persistent arising during pregnancy
                       vicious arising during pregnancy
                   hyperemesis gravidarum

  ⑤ **643.0 Mild hyperemesis gravidarum**
  [0,1,3]   Hyperemesis gravidarum, mild or unspecified, starting before the end of the 22nd week
                of gestation

---

436   ● Code new   ▲ Revision of   ④ ⑤ Fourth or fifth
            to this edition   existing code   digit required

PREGNANCY, CHILDBIRTH, PUERPERIUM

⑤ **643.1 Hyperemesis gravidarum with metabolic disturbance**
[0,1,3]   Hyperemesis gravidarum, starting before the end of the 22nd week of gestation, with metabolic disturbance, such as:
    carbohydrate depletion
    dehydration
    electrolyte imbalance

⑤ **643.2 Late vomiting of pregnancy**
[0,1,3]   Excessive vomiting starting after 22 completed weeks of gestation

⑤ **643.8 Other vomiting complicating pregnancy**
[0,1,3]   Vomiting due to organic disease or other cause, specified as complicating pregnancy, or as a reason for obstetric care during pregnancy
Use additional code, if desired, to specify cause

⑤ **643.9 Unspecified vomiting of pregnancy**
[0,1,3]   Vomiting as a reason for care during pregnancy, length of gestation unspecified

⑤ **644 Early or threatened labor**

⑤ **644.0 Threatened premature labor**
[0,3]   Premature labor after 22 weeks, but before 37 completed weeks of gestation without delivery
    Excludes: that occurring before 22 completed weeks of gestation (640.0)

⑤ **644.1 Other threatened labor**
[0,3]   False labor:
    NOS without delivery
    after 37 completed weeks of gestation without delivery
Threatened labor NOS without delivery

⑤ **644.2 Early onset of delivery**
[0,1]   Onset (spontaneous) of delivery before 37 completed weeks of gestation
Premature labor with onset of delivery before 37 completed weeks of gestation

⑤ **645 Late pregnancy**

⑤ **645.1 Post term pregnancy**
[0,1,3]   Pregnancy over 40 completed weeks to 42 completed weeks gestation

⑤ **645.2 Prolonged pregnancy**
[0,1,3]   Pregnancy which has advanced beyond 42 completed weeks gestation

⑤ **646 Other complications of pregnancy, not elsewhere classified**
Use additional code(s) to further specify complication

⑤ **646.0 Papyraceous fetus**
[0,1,3]

⑤ **646.1 Edema or excessive weight gain in pregnancy, without mention of hypertension**
[0-4]   Gestational edema
    Maternal obesity syndrome
    Excludes: that with mention of hypertension (642.0-642.9)

⑤ **646.2 Unspecified renal disease in pregnancy, without mention of hypertension**
[0-4]   Albuminuria in pregnancy or the puerperium, without mention of hypertension
Nephropathy NOS in pregnancy or the puerperium, without mention of hypertension
Renal disease NOS in pregnancy or the puerperium, without mention of hypertension
Uremia in pregnancy or the puerperium, without mention of hypertension
Gestational proteinuria in pregnancy or the puerperium, without mention of hypertension
    Excludes: that with mention of hypertension (642.0-642.9)

⑤ **646.3 Habitual aborter**
[0,1,3]
    Excludes: with current abortion (634.0-634.9)
        without current pregnancy (629.81)

⑤ **646.4 Peripheral neuritis in pregnancy**
[0-4]

⑤ **646.5 Asymptomatic bacteriuria in pregnancy**
[0-4]

⑤ **646.6 Infections of genitourinary tract in pregnancy**
[0-4]   Conditions classifiable to 590, 595, 597, 599.0, 616 complicating pregnancy, childbirth, or the puerperium
Conditions classifiable to (614.0-614.5, 617.7-614.9, 615) complicating pregnancy or labor
    Excludes: major puerperal infection (670)

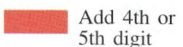 Add 4th or 5th digit
 Nonspecific code
Unspecified code
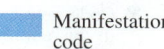 Manifestation code

437

TABULAR LIST

⑤ **646.7 Liver disorders in pregnancy**
[0,1,3]   Acute yellow atrophy of liver (obstetric) (true) of pregnancy
Icterus gravis of pregnancy
Necrosis of liver of pregnancy

> Excludes: hepatorenal syndrome following delivery (674.8)
> viral hepatitis (647.6)

⑤ **646.8 Other specified complications of pregnancy**
[0-4]   Fatigue during pregnancy
Herpes gestationis
Insufficient weight gain of pregnancy

⑤ **646.9 Unspecified complication of pregnancy**
[0,1,3]

⑤ **647 Infectious and parasitic conditions in the mother classifiable elsewhere, but complicating pregnancy, childbirth, or the puerperium**
Includes: the listed conditions when complicating the pregnant state, aggravated by the pregnancy, or when a main reason for obstetric care

> Excludes: those conditions in the mother known or suspected to have affected the fetus (655.0-655.9)

Use additional code(s) to further specify complication

⑤ **647.0 Syphilis**
[0-4]   Conditions classifiable to 090-097

⑤ **647.1 Gonorrhea**
[0-4]   Conditions classifiable to 098

⑤ **647.2 Other venereal diseases**
[0-4]   Conditions classifiable to 099

⑤ **647.3 Tuberculosis**
[0-4]   Conditions classifiable to 010-018

⑤ **647.4 Malaria**
[0-4]   Conditions classifiable to 084

⑤ **647.5 Rubella**
[0-4]   Conditions classifiable to 056

⑤ **647.6 Other viral diseases**
[0-4]   Conditions classifiable to 042 and 050-079, except 056

⑤ **647.8 Other specified infectious and parasitic diseases**
[0-4]

⑤ **647.9 Unspecified infection or infestation**
[0-4]

⑤ **648 Other current conditions in the mother classifiable elsewhere, but complicating pregnancy, childbirth, or the puerperium**
Includes: the listed conditions when complicating the pregnant state, aggravated by the pregnancy, or when a main reason for obstetric care

> Excludes: those conditions in the mother known or suspected to have affected the fetus (655.0-655.9)

Use additional code(s) to identify the condition

⑤ **648.0 Diabetes mellitus**
[0-4]   Conditions classifiable to 250

> Excludes: gestational diabetes (648.8)

⑤ **648.1 Thyroid dysfunction**
[0-4]   Conditions classifiable to 240-246

⑤ **648.2 Anemia**
[0-4]   Conditions classifiable to 280-285

⑤ **648.3 Drug dependence**
[0-4]   Conditions classifiable to 304

⑤ **648.4 Mental disorders**
[0-4]   Conditions classifiable to 290-303, 305.0, 305.2-305.9, 306-316, 317-319

⑤ **648.5 Congenital cardiovascular disorders**
[0-4]   Conditions classifiable to 745-747

PREGNANCY, CHILDBIRTH, PUERPERIUM

- ⑤ **648.6 Other cardiovascular diseases**
  [0-4]   Conditions classifiable to 390-398, 410-429

  Excludes: *cerebrovascular disorders in the puerperium (674.0)*
  peripartum cardiomyopathy (674.5)
  venous complications (671.0-671.9)

- ⑤ **648.7 Bone and joint disorders of back, pelvis, and lower limbs**
  [0-4]   Conditions classifiable to 720-724, and those classifiable to 711-719 or 725-738, specified as affecting the lower limbs

- ⑤ **648.8 Abnormal glucose tolerance**
  [0-4]   Conditions classifiable to 790.21-790.29
  Gestational diabetes
  Use additional code, if applicable, for associated long-term (current) insulin use (V58.67)

- ⑤ **648.9 Other current conditions classifiable elsewhere**
  [0-4]   Conditions classifiable to 440-459
  Nutritional deficiencies [conditions classifiable to 260-269]

649 Other conditions or status of the mother complicating pregnancy, childbirth, or the puerperium

The following fifth-digit subclassification is for use with categories 640-649 to denote the current episode of care:

  0 unspecified as to episode of care or not applicable

  1 delivered, with or without mention of antepartum condition
   Antepartum condition with delivery
   Delivery NOS (with mention of antepartum complication during current episode of care)
   Intrapartum obstetric condition (with mention of antepartum complication during current episode of care)
   Pregnancy, delivered (with mention of antepartum complication during current episode of care)

  2 delivered, with mention of postpartum complication
   Delivery with mention of puerperal complication during current episode of care

  3 antepartum condition or complication
   Antepartum obstetric condition, not delivered during the current episode of care

  4 postpartum condition or complication
   Postpartum or puerperal obstetric condition or complication following delivery that occurred:
    during previous episode of care
    outside hospital, with subsequent admission for observation or care

- ⑤ **649.0 Tobacco use disorder complicating pregnancy, childbirth, or the puerperium**
  [0-4]   Smoking complicating pregnancy, childbirth, or the puerperium

- ⑤ **649.1 Obesity complicating pregnancy, childbirth, or the puerperium**
  [0-4]
  Use additional code to identify the obesity (278.00, 278.01)

- ⑤ **649.2 Bariatric surgery status complicating pregnancy, childbirth, or the puerperium**
  [0-4]   Gastric banding status complicating pregnancy, childbirth, or the puerperium
  Gastric bypass status for obesity complicating pregnancy, childbirth, or the puerperium
  Obesity surgery status complicating pregnancy, childbirth, or the puerperium

- ⑤ **649.3 Coagulation defects complicating pregnancy, childbirth, or the puerperium**
  [0-4]   Conditions classifiable to 286
  Use additional code to identify the specific coagulation defect (286.0-286.9)

  Excludes: *coagulation defects causing antepartum hemorrhage (641.3)*
  postpartum coagulation defects (666.3)

- ⑤ **649.4 Epilepsy complicating pregnancy, childbirth, or the puerperium**
  [0-4]   Conditions classifiable to 345
  Use additional code to identify the specific type of epilepsy (345.00-345.91)

  Excludes: *eclampsia (642.6)*

- ⑤ **649.5 Spotting complicating pregnancy**
  [0,1,3]

  Excludes: *antepartum hemorrhage (641.0-641.9)*
  hemorrhage in early pregnancy (640.0-640.9)

- ⑤ **649.6 Uterine size date discrepancy**
  [0-4]

439

TABULAR LIST

NORMAL DELIVERY, AND OTHER INDICATIONS FOR CARE IN PREGNANCY, LABOR, AND DELIVERY (650-659)

650 Normal delivery
    Delivery requiring minimal or no assistance, with or without episiotomy, without fetal manipulation [e.g., rotation version] or instrumentation [forceps] of spontaneous, cephalic, vaginal, full-term, single, live born infant. This code is for use as a single diagnosis code and is not to be used with any other code in the range 630-676.

  Excludes: breech delivery (assisted) (spontaneous) NOS (652.2)
                delivery by vacuum extractor, forceps, cesarean section, or breech extraction, without specified complication (669.5-669.7)

    Use additional code to indicate outcome of delivery (V27.0)

The following fifth-digit subclassification is for use with categories 651-659 to denote the current episode of care:

  0 unspecified as to episode of care or not applicable
  1 delivered, with or without mention of antepartum condition
  2 delivered, with mention of postpartum complication
  3 antepartum condition or complication
  4 postpartum condition or complication

⑤ **651 Multiple gestation**

  ⑤ **651.0 Twin pregnancy**
      [0,1,3]

  ⑤ **651.1 Triplet pregnancy**
      [0,1,3]

  ⑤ **651.2 Quadruplet pregnancy**
      [0,1,3]

  ⑤ **651.3 Twin pregnancy with fetal loss and retention of one fetus**
      [0,1,3]

  ⑤ **651.4 Triplet pregnancy with fetal loss and retention of one or more fetus(es)**
      [0,1,3]

  ⑤ **651.5 Quadruplet pregnancy with fetal loss and retention of one or more fetus(es)**
      [0,1,3]

  ⑤ **651.6 Other multiple pregnancy with fetal loss and retention of one or more fetus(es)**
      [0,1,3]

  ⑤ **651.7 Multiple gestation following (elective) fetal reduction**
      [0,1,3]   Fetal reduction of multiple fetuses reduced to single fetus

      651.70 Multiple gestation following (elective) fetal reduction, unspecified as to episode of care or not applicable

      651.71 Multiple gestation following (elective) fetal reduction, delivered, with or without mention of antepartum condition

      651.73 Multiple gestation following (elective) fetal reduction, antepartum condition or complication

  ⑤ **651.8 Other specified multiple gestation**
      [0,1,3]

  ⑤ **651.9 Unspecified multiple gestation**
      [0,1,3]

⑤ **652 Malposition and malpresentation of fetus**
    Code first any associated obstructed labor (660.0)

  ⑤ **652.0 Unstable lie**
      [0,1,3]

  ⑤ **652.1 Breech or other malpresentation successfully converted to cephalic presentation**
      [0,1,3]   Cephalic version NOS

  ⑤ **652.2 Breech presentation without mention of version**
      [0,1,3]   Breech delivery (assisted) (spontaneous) NOS
                Buttocks presentation
                Complete breech
                Frank breech

      Excludes: footling presentation (652.8)
                incomplete breech (652.8)

● Code new to this edition   ▲ Revision of existing code   ④ ⑤ Fourth or fifth digit required

PREGNANCY, CHILDBIRTH, PUERPERIUM

- ⑤ **652.3 Transverse or oblique presentation**
  [0,1,3]   Oblique lie   Transverse lie
  Excludes: transverse arrest of fetal head (660.3)

- ⑤ **652.4 Face or brow presentation**
  [0,1,3]   Mentum presentation

- ⑤ **652.5 High head at term**
  [0,1,3]   Failure of head to enter pelvic brim

- ⑤ **652.6 Multiple gestation with malpresentation of one fetus or more**
  [0,1,3]

- ⑤ **652.7 Prolapsed arm**
  [0,1,3]

- ⑤ **652.8 Other specified malposition or malpresentation**
  [0,1,3]   Compound presentation

- ⑤ **652.9 Unspecified malposition or malpresentation**
  [0,1,3]

⑤ **653 Disproportion**
Code first any associated obstructed labor (660.1)

- ⑤ **653.0 Major abnormality of bony pelvis, not further specified**
  [0,1,3]   Pelvic deformity NOS

- ⑤ **653.1 Generally contracted pelvis**
  [0,1,3]   Contracted pelvis NOS

- ⑤ **653.2 Inlet contraction of pelvis**
  [0,1,3]   Inlet contraction (pelvis)

- ⑤ **653.3 Outlet contraction of pelvis**
  [0,1,3]   Outlet contraction (pelvis)

- ⑤ **653.4 Fetopelvic disproportion**
  [0,1,3]   Cephalopelvic disproportion NOS
            Disproportion of mixed maternal and fetal origin, with normally formed fetus

- ⑤ **653.5 Unusually large fetus causing disproportion**
  [0,1,3]   Disproportion of fetal origin with normally formed fetus
            Fetal disproportion NOS
  Excludes: that when the reason for medical care was concern for the fetus (656.6)

- ⑤ **653.6 Hydrocephalic fetus causing disproportion**
  [0,1,3]
  Excludes: that when the reason for medical care was concern for the fetus (655.0)

- ⑤ **653.7 Other fetal abnormality causing disproportion**
  [0,1,3]   Conjoined twins   Fetal:
            Fetal: myelomeningocele
              ascites   sacral teratoma
              hydrops   tumor

- ⑤ **653.8 Disproportion of other origin**
  [0,1,3]
  Excludes: shoulder (girdle) dystocia (660.4)

- ⑤ **653.9 Unspecified disproportion**
  [0,1,3]

⑤ **654 Abnormality of organs and soft tissues of pelvis**
Includes: the listed conditions during pregnancy, childbirth, or the puerperium
Code first any associated obstructed labor (660.2)
Excludes: trauma to perineum and vulva complicating current delivery (664.0-664.9)

- ⑤ **654.0 Congenital abnormalities of uterus**
  [0-4]   Double uterus   Uterus bicornis

- ⑤ **654.1 Tumors of body of uterus**
  [0-4]   Uterine fibroids

- ⑤ **654.2 Previous cesarean delivery NOS**
  [0,1,3] Uterine scar from previous cesarean delivery

- ⑤ **654.3 Retroverted and incarcerated gravid uterus**
  [0-4]

 Add 4th or 5th digit   Nonspecific code   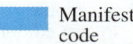 Unspecified code   Manifestation code

441

TABULAR LIST

- ⑤ **654.4** **Other abnormalities in shape or position of gravid uterus and of neighboring structures**
  - [0-4]
    - Cystocele
    - Pelvic floor repair
    - Pendulous abdomen
    - Prolapse of gravid uterus
    - Rectocele
    - Rigid pelvic floor

- ⑤ **654.5** **Cervical incompetence**
  - [0-4] Presence of Shirodkar suture with or without mention of cervical incompetence

- ⑤ **654.6** **Other congenital or acquired abnormality of cervix**
  - [0-4]
    - Cicatricial cervix
    - Polyp of cervix
    - Previous surgery to cervix
    - Rigid cervix (uteri)
    - Stenosis or stricture of cervix
    - Tumor of cervix

- ⑤ **654.7** **Congenital or acquired abnormality of vagina**
  - [0-4]
    - Previous surgery to vagina
    - Septate vagina
    - Stenosis of vagina (acquired) (congenital)
    - Stricture of vagina
    - Tumor of vagina

- ⑤ **654.8** **Congenital or acquired abnormality of vulva**
  - [0-4]
    - Anal sphincter tear (healed) (old) complicating delivery
    - Fibrosis of perineum
    - Persistent hymen
    - Previous surgery to perineum or vulva
    - Rigid perineum
    - Tumor of vulva

  Excludes: anal sphincter tear (healed) (old) not associated with delivery (569.43)
  varicose veins of vulva (671.1)

- ⑤ **654.9** **Other and unspecified**
  - [0-4] Uterine scar NEC

- ⑤ **655** **Known or suspected fetal abnormality affecting management of mother**
  Includes: the listed conditions in the fetus as a reason for observation or obstetrical care of the mother, or for termination of pregnancy

- ⑤ **655.0** **Central nervous system malformation in fetus**
  - [0,1,3] Fetal or suspected fetal:
    - anencephaly
    - hydrocephalus
    - spina bifida (with myelomeningocele)

- ⑤ **655.1** **Chromosomal abnormality in fetus**
  - [0,1,3]

- ⑤ **655.2** **Hereditary disease in family possibly affecting fetus**
  - [0,1,3]

- ⑤ **655.3** **Suspected damage to fetus from viral disease in the mother**
  - [0,1,3] Suspected damage to fetus from maternal rubella

- ⑤ **655.4** **Suspected damage to fetus from other disease in the mother**
  - [0,1,3] Suspected damage to fetus from maternal:
    - alcohol addiction
    - listeriosis
    - toxoplasmosis

- ⑤ **655.5** **Suspected damage to fetus from drugs**
  - [0,1,3]

- ⑤ **655.6** **Suspected damage to fetus from radiation**
  - [0,1,3]

- ⑤ **655.7** **Decreased fetal movements**
  - [0,1,3]

- ⑤ **655.8** **Other known or suspected fetal abnormality, not elsewhere classified**
  - [0,1,3] Suspected damage to fetus from:
    - environmental toxins
    - intrauterine contraceptive device

- ⑤ **655.9** **Unspecified**
  - [0,1,3]

● Code new to this edition   ▲ Revision of existing code   ④ ⑤ Fourth or fifth digit required

PREGNANCY, CHILDBIRTH, PUERPERIUM

656 Other fetal and placental problems affecting management of mother

656.0 Fetal-maternal hemorrhage
[0,1,3] Leakage (microscopic) of fetal blood into maternal circulation

656.1 Rhesus isoimmunization
[0,1,3] Anti-D [Rh] antibodies
Rh incompatibility

656.2 Isoimmunization from other and unspecified blood-group incompatibility
[0,1,3] ABO isoimmunization

656.3 Fetal distress
[0,1,3] Fetal metabolic acidemia

Excludes: *abnormal fetal acid-base balance (656.8)*
abnormality in fetal heart rate or rhythm (659.7)
fetal bradycardia (659.7)
fetal tachycardia (659.7)
meconium in liquor (656.8)

656.4 Intrauterine death
[0,1,3] Fetal death:
NOS
after completion of 22 weeks' gestation
late
Missed delivery

Excludes: *missed abortion (632)*

656.5 Poor fetal growth
[0,1,3] "Light-for-dates"   "Small-for-dates"
"Placental insufficiency"

656.6 Excessive fetal growth
[0,1,3] "Large-for-dates"

656.7 Other placental conditions
[0,1,3] Abnormal placenta   Placental infarct

Excludes: *placental polyp (674.4)*
placentitis (658.4)

656.8 Other specified fetal and placental problems
[0,1,3] Abnormal acid-base balance
Intrauterine acidosis
Lithopedian
Meconium in liquor

656.9 Unspecified fetal and placental problem
[0,1,3]

657 Polyhydramnios
[0,1,3] Hydramnios
Use 0 as fourth-digit for this category

658 Other problems associated with amniotic cavity and membranes

Excludes: *amniotic fluid embolism (673.1)*

658.0 Oligohydramnios
[0,1,3] Oligohydramnios without mention of rupture of membranes

658.1 Premature rupture of membranes
[0,1,3] Rupture of amniotic sac less than 24 hours prior to the onset of labor

658.2 Delayed delivery after spontaneous or unspecified rupture of membranes
[0,1,3] Prolonged rupture of membranes NOS
Rupture of amniotic sac 24 hours or more prior to the onset of labor

658.3 Delayed delivery after artificial rupture of membranes
[0,1,3]

658.4 Infection of amniotic cavity
[0,1,3] Amnionitis
Chorioamnionitis
Membranitis
Placentitis

658.8 Other
[0,1,3] Amnion nodosum
Amniotic cyst

TABULAR LIST

⑤ **658.9** Unspecified
[0,1,3]

⑤ **659** Other indications for care or intervention related to labor and delivery, not elsewhere classified

⑤ 659.0 **Failed mechanical induction**
[0,1,3]   Failure of induction of labor by surgical or other instrumental methods

⑤ 659.1 **Failed medical or unspecified induction**
[0,1,3]   Failed induction NOS
    Failure of induction of labor by medical methods, such as oxytocic drugs

⑤ **659.2** Maternal pyrexia during labor, unspecified
[0,1,3]

⑤ 659.3 **Generalized infection during labor**
[0,1,3]   Septicemia during labor

⑤ 659.4 **Grand multiparity**
[0,1,3]

Excludes: *supervision only, in pregnancy (V23.3)*
without current pregnancy (V61.5)

⑤ 659.5 **Elderly primigravida**
[0,1,3]   First pregnancy in a woman who will be 35 years of age or older at expected date of delivery

Excludes: *supervision only, in pregnancy (V23.81)*

⑤ 659.6 **Elderly multigravida**
[0,1,3]   Second or more pregnancy in a woman who will be 35 years of age or older at expected date of delivery

Excludes: *elderly primigravida 659.5*
supervision only, in pregnancy (V23.82)

⑤ 659.7 **Abnormality in fetal heart rate or rhythm**
[0,1,3]   Depressed fetal heart tones
    Fetal:
      bradycardia
      tachycardia
    Fetal heart rate decelerations
    Non-reassuring fetal heart rate or rhythm

⑤ **659.8** Other specified indications for care or intervention related to labor and delivery
[0,1,3]   Pregnancy in female less than 16 years old at expected date of delivery
    Very young maternal age

⑤ **659.9** Unspecified indication for care or intervention related to labor and delivery
[0,1,3]

PREGNANCY, CHILDBIRTH, PUERPERIUM

COMPLICATIONS OCCURRING MAINLY IN THE COURSE OF LABOR AND DELIVERY (660-669)

The following fifth-digit subclassification is for use with categories 660-669 to denote the current episode of care:

   0 unspecified as to episode of care or not applicable
   1 delivered, with or without mention of antepartum condition
   2 delivered, with mention of postpartum complication
   3 antepartum condition or complication
   4 postpartum condition or complication

660 Obstructed labor

660.0 Obstruction caused by malposition of fetus at onset of labor
[0,1,3]   Any condition classifiable to 652, causing obstruction during labor
Use additional code from 652.0-652.9, if desired, to identify condition

660.1 Obstruction by bony pelvis
[0,1,3]   Any condition classifiable to 653, causing obstruction during labor
Use additional code from 653.0-653.9, if desired, to identify condition

660.2 Obstruction by abnormal pelvic soft tissues
[0,1,3]   Prolapse of anterior lip of cervix
    Any condition classifiable to 654, causing obstruction during labor
Use additional code from 654.0-654.9, if desired, to identify condition

660.3 Deep transverse arrest and persistent occipitoposterior position
[0,1,3]

660.4 Shoulder (girdle) dystocia
[0,1,3]   Impacted shoulders

660.5 Locked twins
[0,1,3]

660.6 Failed trial of labor, unspecified
[0,1,3]   Failed trial of labor, without mention of condition or suspected condition

660.7 Failed forceps or vacuum extractor, unspecified
[0,1,3]   Application of ventouse or forceps, without mention of condition

660.8 Other causes of obstructed labor
[0,1,3]   Use additional code to identify condition

660.9 Unspecified obstructed labor
[0,1,3]   Dystocia:
      NOS
      fetal NOS
      maternal NOS

661 Abnormality of forces of labor

661.0 Primary uterine inertia
[0,1,3]   Failure of cervical dilation
    Hypotonic uterine dysfunction, primary
    Prolonged latent phase of labor

661.1 Secondary uterine inertia
[0,1,3]   Arrested active phase of labor
    Hypotonic uterine dysfunction, secondary

661.2 Other and unspecified uterine inertia
[0,1,3]   Atony of uterus without hemorrhage
    Desultory labor   Poor contractions
    Irregular labor   Slow slope active phase of labor
    Excludes: atony of uterus with hemorrhage (666.1)
                  postpartum atony of uterus without hemorrhage (669.8)

661.3 Precipitate labor
[0,1,3]

  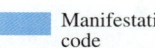

445

TABULAR LIST

- ⑤ **661.4 Hypertonic, incoordinate, or prolonged uterine contractions**
  [0,1,3]
  Cervical spasm
  Contraction ring (dystocia)
  Dyscoordinate labor
  Hourglass contraction of uterus
  Hypertonic uterine dysfunction
  Incoordinate uterine action
  Retraction ring (Bandl's) (pathological)
  Tetanic contractions
  Uterine dystocia NOS
  Uterine spasm

- ⑤ **661.9 Unspecified abnormality of labor**
  [0,1,3]

- ⑤ **662 Long labor**
  - ⑤ **662.0 Prolonged first stage**
    [0,1,3]
  - ⑤ **662.1 Prolonged labor, unspecified**
    [0,1,3]
  - ⑤ **662.2 Prolonged second stage**
    [0,1,3]
  - ⑤ **662.3 Delayed delivery of second twin, triplet, etc.**
    [0,1,3]

- ⑤ **663 Umbilical cord complications**
  - ⑤ **663.0 Prolapse of cord**
    [0,1,3]
    Presentation of cord
  - ⑤ **663.1 Cord around neck, with compression**
    [0,1,3]
    Cord tightly around neck
  - ⑤ **663.2 Other and unspecified cord entanglement, with compression**
    [0,1,3]
    Entanglement of cords of twins in mono-amniotic sac
    Knot in cord (with compression)
  - ⑤ **663.3 Other and unspecified cord entanglement, without mention of compression**
    [0,1,3]
  - ⑤ **663.4 Short cord**
    [0,1,3]
  - ⑤ **663.5 Vasa previa**
    [0,1,3]
  - ⑤ **663.6 Vascular lesions of cord**
    [0,1,3]
    Bruising of cord
    Hematoma of cord
    Thrombosis of vessels of cord
  - ⑤ **663.8 Other umbilical cord complications**
    [0,1,3]
    Velamentous insertion of umbilical cord
  - ⑤ **663.9 Unspecified umbilical cord complication**
    [0,1,3]

- ⑤ **664 Trauma to perineum and vulva during delivery**
  Includes: damage from instruments
  that from extension of episiotomy
  - ⑤ **664.0 First-degree perineal laceration**
    [0,1,4]
    Perineal laceration, rupture, or tear involving:
    fourchette
    hymen
    labia
    skin
    vagina
    vulva
  - ⑤ **664.1 Second-degree perineal laceration**
    [0,1,4]
    Perineal laceration, rupture, or tear (following episiotomy) involving:
    pelvic floor
    perineal muscles
    vaginal muscles

    Excludes: that involving anal sphincter (664.2)

446 ● Code new to this edition ▲ Revision of existing code ④ ⑤ Fourth or fifth digit required

PREGNANCY, CHILDBIRTH, PUERPERIUM

⑤ **664.2 Third-degree perineal laceration**
[0,1,4]   Perineal laceration, rupture, or tear (following episiotomy) involving:
  anal sphincter
  rectovaginal septum
  sphincter NOS

> Excludes: anal sphincter tear during delivery not associated with third-degree perineal laceration (664.6)
> that with anal or rectal mucosal laceration (664.3)

⑤ **664.3 Fourth-degree perineal laceration**
[0,1,4]   Perineal laceration, rupture, or tear as classifiable to 664.2 and involving also:
  anal mucosa
  rectal mucosa

⑤ **664.4 Unspecified perineal laceration**
[0,1,4]   Central laceration

● **664.6 Anal sphincter tear complicating delivery, not associated with third-degree perineal laceration**
[0,1,4]

> Excludes: third-degree perineal laceration (664.2)

⑤ **664.5 Vulval and perineal hematoma**
[0,1,4]

⑤ **664.8 Other specified trauma to perineum and vulva**
[0,1,4]

⑤ **664.9 Unspecified trauma to perineum and vulva**
[0,1,4]

⑤ **665 Other obstetrical trauma**
  Includes: damage from instruments

⑤ **665.0 Rupture of uterus before onset of labor**
[0,1,3]

⑤ **665.1 Rupture of uterus during labor**
[0,1]   Rupture of uterus NOS

⑤ **665.2 Inversion of uterus**
[0,2,4]

⑤ **665.3 Laceration of cervix**
[0,1,4]

⑤ **665.4 High vaginal laceration**
[0,1,4]   Laceration of vaginal wall or sulcus without mention of perineal laceration

⑤ **665.5 Other injury to pelvic organs**
[0,1,4]   Injury to:
  bladder
  urethra

⑤ **665.6 Damage to pelvic joints and ligaments**
[0,1,4]   Avulsion of inner symphyseal cartilage
  Damage to coccyx
  Separation of symphysis (pubis)

⑤ **665.7 Pelvic hematoma**
[0,1,2,4]   Hematoma of vagina

⑤ **665.8 Other specified obstetrical trauma**
[0-4]

⑤ **665.9 Unspecified obstetrical trauma**
[0-4]

⑤ **666 Postpartum hemorrhage**

⑤ **666.0 Third-stage hemorrhage**
[0,2,4]   Hemorrhage associated with retained, trapped, or adherent placenta
  Retained placenta NOS

⑤ **666.1 Other immediate postpartum hemorrhage**
[0,2,4]   Atony of uterus with hemorrhage
  Hemorrhage within the first 24 hours following delivery of placenta
  Postpartum atony of uterus with hemorrhage
  Postpartum hemorrhage (atonic) NOS

> Excludes: atony of uterus without hemorrhage (661.2)
> postpartum atony of uterus without hemorrhage (669.8)

TABULAR LIST

- ⑤ **666.2 Delayed and secondary postpartum hemorrhage**
  [0,2,4] Hemorrhage:
  after the first 24 hours following delivery
  associated with retained portions of placenta or membranes
  Postpartum hemorrhage specified as delayed or secondary
  Retained products of conception NOS, following delivery

- ⑤ **666.3 Postpartum coagulation defects**
  [0,2,4] Postpartum afibrinogenemia
  Postpartum fibrinolysis

⑤ **667 Retained placenta or membranes, without hemorrhage**

- ⑤ **667.0 Retained placenta without hemorrhage**
  [0,2,4] Placenta accreta without hemorrhage
  Retained placenta: without hemorrhage
    NOS without hemorrhage
    total without hemorrhage

- ⑤ **667.1 Retained portions of placenta or membranes, without hemorrhage**
  [0,2,4] Retained products of conception following delivery, without hemorrhage

⑤ **668 Complications of the administration of anesthetic or other sedation in labor and delivery**
Includes: complications arising from the administration of a general or local anesthetic, analgesic, or other sedation in labor and delivery

Excludes: reaction to spinal or lumbar puncture (349.0)
spinal headache (349.0)

Use additional code(s) to further specify complication

- ⑤ **668.0 Pulmonary complications**
  [0-4] Inhalation [aspiration] of stomach contents or secretions following anesthesia or other sedation in labor or delivery
  Mendelson's syndrome following anesthesia or other sedation in labor or delivery
  Pressure collapse of lung following anesthesia or other sedation in labor or delivery

- ⑤ **668.1 Cardiac complications**
  [0-4] Cardiac arrest or failure following anesthesia or other sedation in labor and delivery

- ⑤ **668.2 Central nervous system complications**
  [0-4] Cerebral anoxia following anesthesia or other sedation in labor and delivery

- ⑤ **668.8 Other complications of anesthesia or other sedation in labor and delivery**
  [0-4]

- ⑤ **668.9 Unspecified complication of anesthesia and other sedation**
  [0-4]

⑤ **669 Other complications of labor and delivery, not elsewhere classified**

- ⑤ **669.0 Maternal distress**
  [0-4] Metabolic disturbance in labor and delivery

- ⑤ **669.1 Shock during or following labor and delivery**
  [0-4] Obstetric shock

- ⑤ **669.2 Maternal hypotension syndrome**
  [0-4]

- ⑤ **669.3 Acute renal failure following labor and delivery**
  [0,2,4]

- ⑤ **669.4 Other complications of obstetrical surgery and procedures**
  [0-4] Cardiac:
  arrest following cesarean or other obstetrical surgery or procedure, including delivery NOS
  failure following cesarean or other obstetrical surgery or procedure, including delivery NOS
  Cerebral anoxia following cesarean or other obstetrical surgery or procedure, including delivery NOS

  Excludes: complications of obstetrical surgical wounds (674.1-674.3)

- ⑤ **669.5 Forceps or vacuum extractor delivery without mention of indication**
  [0,1] Delivery by ventouse, without mention of indication

- ⑤ **669.6 Breech extraction, without mention of indication**
  [0,1]

  Excludes: breech delivery NOS (652.2)

- ⑤ **669.7 Cesarean delivery, without mention of indication**
  [0,1]

| ● Code new to this edition | ▲ Revision of existing code | ④ ⑤ Fourth or fifth digit required |

PREGNANCY, CHILDBIRTH, PUERPERIUM

⑤ **669.8** Other complications of labor and delivery
[0-4]

⑤ **669.9** Unspecified complication of labor and delivery
[0-4]

COMPLICATIONS OF THE PUERPERIUM (670-677)

Note: Categories 671 and 673-676 include the listed conditions even if they occur during pregnancy or childbirth.

The following fifth-digit subclassification is for use with categories 670-676 to denote the current episode of care:

0 unspecified as to episode of care or not applicable
1 delivered, with or without mention of antepartum condition
2 delivered, with mention of postpartum complication
3 antepartum condition or complication
4 postpartum condition or complication

⑤ **670** Major puerperal infection
[0,2,4]

Puerperal:
    endometritis
    fever (septic)
    pelvic:
        cellulitis
    sepsis

Puerperal:
    peritonitis
    pyemia
    salpingitis
    septicemia

Use 0 as fourth-digit for this category

| Excludes: | infection following abortion (639.0)
    minor genital tract infection following delivery (646.6)
    puerperal pyrexia NOS (672)
    puerperal fever NOS (672)
    puerperal pyrexia of unknown origin (672)
    urinary tract infection following delivery (646.6)

⑤ **671** Venous complications in pregnancy and the puerperium

⑤ **671.0** Varicose veins of legs
[0-4]   Varicose veins NOS

⑤ **671.1** Varicose veins of vulva and perineum
[0-4]

⑤ **671.2** Superficial thrombophlebitis
[0-4]   Thrombophlebitis (superficial)

⑤ **671.3** Deep phlebothrombosis, antepartum
[0,1,3]   Deep-vein thrombosis, antepartum

⑤ **671.4** Deep phlebothrombosis, postpartum
[0,2,4]   Deep-vein thrombosis, postpartum
    Pelvic thrombophlebitis, postpartum
    Phlegmasia alba dolens (puerperal)

⑤ **671.5** Other phlebitis and thrombosis
[0-4]   Cerebral venous thrombosis
    Thrombosis of intracranial venous sinus

⑤ **671.8** Other venous complications
[0-4]   Hemorrhoids

⑤ **671.9** Unspecified venous complication
[0-4]   Phlebitis NOS
    Thrombosis NOS

⑤ **672** Pyrexia of unknown origin during the puerperium
[0,2,4]   Puerperal fever NOS
    Postpartum fever NOS

Use 0 as fourth-digit for this category

⑤ **673** Obstetrical pulmonary embolism
Includes: pulmonary emboli in pregnancy, childbirth, or the puerperium, or specified as puerperal

| Excludes: | embolism following abortion (639.6)

 Add 4th or 5th digit
 Unspecified code
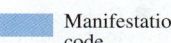 Manifestation code

449

TABULAR LIST

⑤ **673.0 Obstetrical air embolism**
  [0-4]

⑤ **673.1 Amniotic fluid embolism**
  [0-4]

⑤ **673.2 Obstetrical blood-clot embolism**
  [0-4]   Puerperal pulmonary embolism NOS

⑤ **673.3 Obstetrical pyemic and septic embolism**
  [0-4]

⑤ **673.8 Other pulmonary embolism**
  [0-4]   Fat embolism

⑤ **674 Other and unspecified complications of the puerperium, not elsewhere classified**

⑤ **674.0 Cerebrovascular disorders in the puerperium**
  [0-4]   Any condition classifiable to 430-434, 436-437 occurring during pregnancy, childbirth, or the puerperium, or specified as puerperal
      Excludes: intracranial venous sinus thrombosis (671.5)

⑤ **674.1 Disruption of cesarean wound**
  [0,2,4] Dehiscence or disruption of uterine wound
      Excludes: uterine rupture before onset of labor (665.0)
              uterine rupture during labor (665.1)

⑤ **674.2 Disruption of perineal wound**
  [0,2,4] Breakdown of perineum
      Disruption of wound of:
        episiotomy
        perineal laceration
      Secondary perineal tear

⑤ **674.3 Other complications of obstetrical surgical wounds**
  [0,2,4] Hematoma of cesarean section or perineal wound
      Hemorrhage of cesarean section or perineal wound
      Infection of cesarean section or perineal wound
      Excludes: damage from instruments in delivery (664.0-665.9)

⑤ **674.4 Placental polyp**
  [0,2,4]

⑤ **674.5 Peripartum cardiomyopathy**
  [0-4]   Postpartum cardiomyopathy

⑤ **674.8 Other**
  [0,2,4] Hepatorenal syndrome, following delivery
      Postpartum:
        subinvolution of uterus
        uterine hypertrophy

⑤ **674.9 Unspecified**
  [0,2,4] Sudden death of unknown cause during the puerperium

⑤ **675 Infections of the breast and nipple associated with childbirth**
  Includes: the listed conditions during pregnancy, childbirth, or the puerperium

⑤ **675.0 Infections of nipple**
  [0-4]   Abscess of nipple

⑤ **675.1 Abscess of breast**
  [0-4]   Abscess:
        mammary
        subareolar
        submammary
      Mastitis:
        purulent
        retromammary
        submammary

⑤ **675.2 Nonpurulent mastitis**
  [0-4]   Lymphangitis of breast
      Mastitis:
        NOS
        interstitial
        parenchymatous

⑤ **675.8 Other specified infections of the breast and nipple**
  [0-4]

450 ● Code new to this edition   ▲ Revision of existing code   ④ ⑤ Fourth or fifth digit required

PREGNANCY, CHILDBIRTH, PUERPERIUM

⑤ **675.9** Unspecified infection of the breast and nipple
[0-4]

⑤ **676** Other disorders of the breast associated with childbirth and disorders of lactation
Includes: the listed conditions during pregnancy, the puerperium, or lactation

⑤ 676.0 Retracted nipple
[0-4]

⑤ 676.1 Cracked nipple
[0-4]   Fissure of nipple

⑤ 676.2 Engorgement of breasts
[0-4]

⑤ **676.3** Other and unspecified disorder of breast
[0-4]

⑤ 676.4 Failure of lactation
[0-4]   Agalactia

⑤ 676.5 Suppressed lactation
[0-4]

⑤ 676.6 Galactorrhea
[0-4]
Excludes: *galactorrhea not associated with childbirth (611.6)*

⑤ **676.8** Other disorders of lactation
[0-4]   Galactocele

⑤ **676.9** Unspecified disorder of lactation
[0-4]

677 Late effect of complication of pregnancy, childbirth, and the puerperium
Note: This category is to be used to indicate conditions in 632-648.9 and 651-676.9 as the cause of the late effect, themselves classifiable elsewhere. The "late effects" include conditions specified as such, or as sequelae, which may occur at any time after the puerperium.
Code first any sequelae

TABULAR LIST

INFECTIOUS AND PARASITIC DISEASES

12. DISEASES OF THE SKIN AND SUBCUTANEOUS TISSUE (680-709)

INFECTIONS OF SKIN AND SUBCUTANEOUS TISSUE (680-686)

Excludes: certain infections of skin classified under "Infectious and Parasitic Diseases," such as:
   erysipelas (035)
   erysipeloid of Rosenbach (027.1)
   herpes:
      simplex (054.0-054.9)
      zoster (053.0-053.9)
   molluscum contagiosum (078.0)
   viral warts (078.1)

680 Carbuncle and furuncle
Includes: boil
furunculosis

680.0 Face
Ear [any part]
Face [any part, except eye]
Nose (septum)
Temple (region)

Excludes: eyelid (373.13)
lacrimal apparatus (375.31)
orbit (376.01)

680.1 Neck

680.2 Trunk
Abdominal wall
Back [any part, except buttocks]
Breast
Chest wall
Flank
Groin
Pectoral region
Perineum
Umbilicus

Excludes: buttocks (680.5)
external genital organs:
   female (616.4)
   male (607.2, 608.4)

680.3 Upper arm and forearm
Arm [any part, except hand]
Axilla
Shoulder

680.4 Hand
Finger [any]
Thumb
Wrist

680.5 Buttock
Anus
Gluteal region

680.6 Leg, except foot
Ankle
Hip
Knee
Thigh

680.7 Foot
Heel
Toe

680.8 Other specified sites
Head [any part, except face]
Scalp

Excludes: external genital organs:
   female (616.4)
   male (607.2, 608.4)

680.9 Unspecified site
Boil NOS
Carbuncle NOS
Furuncle NOS

681 Cellulitis and abscess of finger and toe
Includes: that with lymphangitis
Use additional code, if desired, to identify organism, such as Staphylococcus (041.1)

⑤ **681.0 Finger**
681.00 Cellulitis and abscess, unspecified

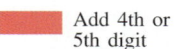

453

Add 4th or 5th digit   Nonspecific code   Unspecified code   Manifestation code

TABULAR LIST

681.01 Felon
Pulp abscess
Whitlow

Excludes: herpetic whitlow (054.6)

681.02 Onychia and paronychia of finger
Panaritium of finger
Perionychia of finger

⑤ **681.1 Toe**

681.10 Cellulitis and abscess, unspecified

681.11 Onychia and paronychia of toe
Panaritium of toe
Perionychia of toe

681.9 Cellulitis and abscess of unspecified digit
Infection of nail NOS

682 Other cellulitis and abscess
Includes: abscess (acute) (with lymphangitis) except of finger or toe
cellulitis (diffuse) (with lymphangitis) except of finger or toe
lymphangitis, acute (with lymphangitis) except of finger or toe

Use additional code, if desired, to identify organism, such as Staphylococcus (041.1)

Excludes: lymphangitis (chronic) (subacute) (457.2)

682.0 Face
Cheek, external
Chin
Forehead
Nose, external
Submandibular
Temple (region)

Excludes: ear [any part] (380.10-380.16)
eyelid (373.13)
lacrimal apparatus (375.31)
lip (528.5)
mouth (528.3)
nose (internal) (478.1)
orbit (376.01)

682.1 Neck

682.2 Trunk
Abdominal wall
Back [any part, except buttock]
Chest wall
Flank
Groin
Pectoral region
Perineum
Umbilicus, except newborn

Excludes: anal and rectal regions (566)
breast:
NOS (611.0)
puerperal (675.1)
external genital organs:
female (616.3-616.4)
male (604.0, 607.2, 608.4)
umbilicus, newborn (771.4)

682.3 Upper arm and forearm
Arm [any part, except hand]
Axilla
Shoulder

Excludes: hand (682.4)

682.4 Hand, except fingers and thumb
Wrist

Excludes: finger and thumb (681.00-681.02)

682.5 Buttock
Gluteal region

Excludes: anal and rectal regions (566)

682.6 Leg, except foot
Ankle
Hip
Knee
Thigh

SKIN AND SUBCUTANEOUS TISSUE

682.7 Foot, except toes
Heel

Excludes: toe (681.10-681.11)

682.8 Other specified sites
Head [except face]
Scalp

Excludes: face (682.0)

682.9 Unspecified site
Abscess NOS
Cellulitis NOS
Lymphangitis, acute NOS

Excludes: lymphangitis NOS (457.2)

683 Acute lymphadenitis
Abscess (acute), lymph gland or node, except mesenteric
Adenitis, acute, lymph gland or node, except mesenteric
Lymphadenitis, acute, lymph gland or node, except mesenteric

Use additional code, if desired, to identify organism, such as Staphylococcus (041.1)

Excludes: enlarged glands NOS (785.6)
    lymphadenitis:
      chronic or subacute, except mesenteric (289.1)
      mesenteric (acute) (chronic) (subacute) (289.2)
      unspecified (289.3)

684 Impetigo
Impetiginization of other dermatoses
Impetigo (contagiosa) [any site] [any organism]:
  bullous
  circinate
  neonatorum
  simplex
Pemphigus neonatorum

Excludes: impetigo herpetiformis (694.3)

685 Pilonidal cyst
Includes:
    fistula, coccygeal or pilonidal
    sinus, coccygeal or pilonidal

685.0 With abscess

685.1 Without mention of abscess

686 Other local infections of skin and subcutaneous tissue
Use additional code, if desired, to identify any infectious organism (041.0-041.8)

⑤ **686.0 Pyoderma**
Dermatitis:
  purulent
  septic
  suppurative

  686.00 Pyoderma, unspecified

  686.01 Pyoderma gangrenosum

  686.09 Other pyoderma

686.1 Pyogenic granuloma
Granuloma:
  septic
  suppurative
  telangiectaticum

Excludes: pyogenic granuloma of oral mucosa (528.9)

686.8 Other specified local infections of skin and subcutaneous tissue
Bacterid (pustular)
Dermatitis vegetans
Ecthyma
Perlèche

Excludes: dermatitis infectiosa eczematoides (690.8)
    panniculitis (729.30-729.39)

686.9 Unspecified local infection of skin and subcutaneous tissue
Fistula of skin NOS
Skin infection NOS

Excludes: fistula to skin from internal organs—see Alphabetic Index

TABULAR LIST

OTHER INFLAMMATORY CONDITIONS OF SKIN AND SUBCUTANEOUS TISSUE (690-698)

Excludes: panniculitis (729.30-729.39)

690 Erythematosquamous dermatosis

Excludes: eczematous dermatitis of eyelid (373.31)
parakeratosis variegata (696.2)
psoriasis (696.0-696.1)
seborrheic keratosis (702.11-702.19)

⑤ **690.1 Seborrheic dermatitis**

690.10 Seborrheic dermatitis, unspecified
Seborrheic dermatitis NOS

690.11 Seborrhea capitis
Cradle cap

690.12 Seborrheic infantile dermatitis

690.18 Other seborrheic dermatitis

690.8 Other erythematosquamous dermatosis

691 Atopic dermatitis and related conditions

691.0 Diaper or napkin rash
Ammonia dermatitis
Diaper or napkin:
  dermatitis
  erythema
  rash
Psoriasiform napkin eruption

691.8 Other atopic dermatitis and related conditions
Atopic dermatitis   Neurodermatitis:
Besnier's prurigo   atopic
Eczema: diffuse (of Brocq)
  atopic
  flexural
  intrinsic (allergic)

692 Contact dermatitis and other eczema
Includes:
  dermatitis: eczema (acute) (chronic):
    NOS   NOS
    contact   allergic
    occupational   erythematous
    venenata   occupational

Excludes: allergy NOS (995.3)
contact dermatitis of eyelids (373.32)
dermatitis due to substances taken internally (693.0-693.9)
eczema of external ear (380.22)
perioral dermatitis (695.3)
urticarial reactions (708.0-708.9, 995.1)

692.0 Due to detergents

692.1 Due to oils and greases

692.2 Due to solvents
Dermatitis due to solvents of:
  chlorocompound group
  cyclohexane group
  ester group
  glycol group
  hydrocarbon group
  ketone group

SKIN AND SUBCUTANEOUS TISSUE

692.3 Due to drugs and medicines in contact with skin
Dermatitis (allergic) (contact) due to:
arnica
fungicides
iodine
keratolytics
mercurials
neomycin
pediculocides
phenols
scabicides
any drug applied to skin
Dermatitis medicamentosa due to drug applied to skin
Use additional E code, if desired, to identify drug

Excludes: allergy NOS due to drugs (995.27)
dermatitis due to ingested drugs (693.0)
dermatitis medicamentosa NOS (693.0)

692.4 Due to other chemical products
Dermatitis due to:
acids
adhesive plaster
alkalis
caustics
dichromate

Dermatitis due to:
insecticide
nylon
plastic
rubber

692.5 Due to food in contact with skin
Dermatitis, contact, due to:
cereals
fish
flour

Dermatitis, contact, due to:
fruit
meat
milk

Excludes: dermatitis due to:
dyes (692.89)
ingested foods (693.1)
preservatives (692.89)

692.6 Due to plants [except food]
Dermatitis due to:
lacquer tree [Rhus verniciflua]
poison ivy [Rhus toxicodendron]
poison oak [Rhus diversiloba]
poison sumac [Rhus venenata]
poison vine [Rhus radicans]
primrose [Primula]
ragweed [Senecio jacobae]
other plants in contact with the skin

Excludes: allergy NOS due to pollen (477.0)
nettle rash (708.8)

⑤ **692.7 Due to solar radiation**

Excludes: sunburn due to other ultraviolet radiation exposure (692.82)

692.70 Unspecified dermatitis due to sun

692.71 Sunburn
First degree sunburn
Sunburn NOS

692.72 Acute dermatitis due to solar radiation
Berloque dermatitis
Photoallergic response
Phototoxic response
Polymorphus light eruption
Acute solar skin damage NOS

Excludes: sunburn (692.71, 692.76-692.77)
Use additional E code, if desired, to identify drug, if drug induced

692.73 Actinic reticuloid and actinic granuloma

692.74 Other chronic dermatitis due to solar radiation
Solar elastosis
Chronic solar skin damage NOS

Excludes: actinic [solar] keratosis (702.0)

457

Add 4th or 5th digit | Nonspecific code | Unspecified code | Manifestation code

TABULAR LIST

- **692.75** Disseminated superficial actinic porokeratosis (DSAP)
- **692.76** Sunburn of second degree
- **692.77** Sunburn of third degree
- **692.79** Other dermatitis due to solar radiation
  Hydroa aestivale
  Photodermatitis due to sun
  Photosensitiveness due to sun
  Solar skin damage NOS

⑤ **692.8 Due to other specified agents**
- **692.81** Dermatitis due to cosmetics
- **692.82** Dermatitis due to other radiation
  Infrared rays
  Light, except from sun
  Radiation NOS
  Ultraviolet rays, except from sun
  X-rays
  Tanning bed

  Excludes: that due to solar radiation (692.70-692.79)

- **692.83** Dermatitis due to metals
  Jewelry
- **692.84** Due to animal (cat) (dog) dander
  Due to animal (cat) (dog) hair
- **692.89** Other
  Dermatitis due to:
    cold weather
    dyes
    hot weather
    preservatives

  Excludes: allergy (NOS) (rhinitis) due to animal hair or dander (477.2)
  allergy to dust (477.8)
  sunburn (692.71, 692.76-692.77)

692.9 Unspecified cause
  Dermatitis: Eczema NOS
    NOS
    contact NOS
    venenata NOS

693 Dermatitis due to substances taken internally

  Excludes: adverse effect NOS of drugs and medicines (995.20)
  allergy NOS (995.3)
  contact dermatitis (692.0-692.9)
  urticarial reactions (708.0-708.9, 995.1)

- **693.0 Due to drugs and medicines**
  Dermatitis medicamentosa NOS

  Use additional E code, if desired, to identify drug

  Excludes: that due to drugs in contact with skin (692.3)

- **693.1 Due to food**
- **693.8 Due to other specified substances taken internally**
- **693.9 Due to unspecified substance taken internally**

  Excludes: dermatitis NOS (692.9)

694 Bullous dermatoses

- **694.0 Dermatitis herpetiformis**
  Dermatosis herpetiformis
  Duhring's disease
  Hydroa herpetiformis

  Excludes: herpes gestationis (646.8)
  dermatitis herpetiformis:
    juvenile (694.2)
    senile (694.5)

- **694.1 Subcorneal pustular dermatosis**
  Sneddon-Wilkinson disease or syndrome

SKIN AND SUBCUTANEOUS TISSUE

694.2 Juvenile dermatitis herpetiformis
Juvenile pemphigoid

694.3 Impetigo herpetiformis

694.4 Pemphigus
Pemphigus:
  NOS
  erythematosus
  foliaceus
Pemphigus:
  malignant
  vegetans
  vulgaris

Excludes: pemphigus neonatorum (684)

694.5 Pemphigoid
Benign pemphigus NOS
Bullous pemphigoid
Herpes circinatus bullosus
Senile dermatitis herpetiformis

⑤ **694.6 Benign mucous membrane pemphigoid**
Cicatricial pemphigoid
Mucosynechial atrophic bullous dermatitis

694.60 Without mention of ocular involvement

694.61 With ocular involvement
Ocular pemphigus

694.8 Other specified bullous dermatoses
Excludes: herpes gestationis (646.8)

694.9 Unspecified bullous dermatoses

695 Erythematous conditions

695.0 Toxic erythema
Erythema venenatum

695.1 Erythema multiforme
Erythema iris
Herpes iris
Lyell's syndrome
Scalded skin syndrome
Stevens-Johnson syndrome
Toxic epidermal necrolysis

695.2 Erythema nodosum
Excludes: tuberculous erythema nodosum (017.1)

695.3 Rosacea
Acne:
  erythematosa
  rosacea
Perioral dermatitis
Rhinophyma

695.4 Lupus erythematosus
Lupus:
  erythematodes (discoid)
  erythematosus (discoid), not disseminated

Excludes: lupus (vulgaris) NOS (017.0)
systemic [disseminated] lupus erythematosus (710.0)

⑤ **695.8 Other specified erythematous conditions**

695.81 Ritter's disease
Dermatitis exfoliativa neonatorum

695.89 Other
Erythema intertrigo
Intertrigo
Pityriasis rubra (Hebra)

Excludes: mycotic intertrigo (111.0-111.9)

695.9 Unspecified erythematous condition
Erythema NOS
Erythroderma (secondary)

696 Psoriasis and similar disorders

696.0 Psoriatic arthropathy

696.1 Other psoriasis
Acrodermatitis continua
Dermatitis repens
Psoriasis:
  NOS
  any type, except arthropathic

Excludes: psoriatic arthropathy (696.0)

459

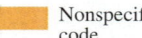 Add 4th or 5th digit
 Nonspecific code
 Unspecified code
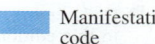 Manifestation code

TABULAR LIST

696.2 Parapsoriasis
Parakeratosis variegata
Parapsoriasis lichenoides chronica
Pityriasis lichenoides et varioliformis

696.3 Pityriasis rosea
Pityriasis circinata (et maculata)

696.4 Pityriasis rubra pilaris
Devergie's disease
Lichen ruber acuminatus
Excludes: *pityriasis rubra (Hebra) (695.89)*

696.5 Other and unspecified pityriasis
Pityriasis:
  NOS
  alba
  streptogenes
Excludes: *pityriasis simplex (690.18)*
          pityriasis versicolor (111.0)

696.8 Other

697 Lichen
Excludes: *lichen:*
  obtusus corneus (698.3)
  pilaris (congenital) (757.39)
  ruber acuminatus (696.4)
  sclerosus et atrophicus (701.0)
  scrofulosus (017.0)
  simplex chronicus (698.3)
  spinulosus (congenital) (757.39)
  urticatus (698.2)

697.0 Lichen planus
Lichen:
  planopilaris
  ruber planus

697.1 Lichen nitidus
Pinkus' disease

697.8 Other lichen, not elsewhere classified
Lichen:
  ruber moniliforme
  striata

697.9 Lichen, unspecified

698 Pruritus and related conditions
Excludes: *pruritus specified as psychogenic (306.3)*

698.0 Pruritus ani
Perianal itch

698.1 Pruritus of genital organs

698.2 Prurigo
Lichen urticatus
Prurigo:
  NOS
  Hebra's
  mitis
  simplex
Urticaria papulosa (Hebra)
Excludes: *prurigo nodularis (698.3)*

698.3 Lichenification and lichen simplex chronicus
Hyde's disease
Neurodermatitis (circumscripta) (local)
Prurigo nodularis
Excludes: *neurodermatitis, diffuse (of Brocq) (691.8)*

698.4 Dermatitis factitia [artefacta]
Dermatitis ficta
Neurotic excoriation
Use additional code, if desired, to identify any associated mental disorder

SKIN AND SUBCUTANEOUS TISSUE

698.8 **Other specified pruritic conditions**
Pruritus:
 hiemalis
 senilis
Winter itch

698.9 **Unspecified pruritic disorder**
Itch NOS
Pruritus NOS

OTHER DISEASES OF SKIN AND SUBCUTANEOUS TISSUE (700-709)

Excludes: conditions confined to eyelids (373.0-374.9)
 congenital conditions of skin, hair, and nails (757.0-757.9)

700 **Corns and callosities**
Callus
Clavus

701 **Other hypertrophic and atrophic conditions of skin**
Excludes: dermatomyositis (710.3)
 hereditary edema of legs (757.0)
 scleroderma (generalized) (710.1)

701.0 **Circumscribed scleroderma**
Addison's keloid
Dermatosclerosis, localized
Lichen sclerosus et atrophicus
Morphea
Scleroderma, circumscribed or localized

701.1 **Keratoderma, acquired**
Acquired:
 ichthyosis
 keratoderma palmaris et plantaris
Elastosis perforans serpiginosa
Hyperkeratosis:
 NOS
 follicularis in cutem penetrans
 palmoplantaris climacterica
Keratoderma:
 climactericum
 tylodes, progressive
Keratosis (blennorrhagica)

Excludes: Darier's disease [keratosis follicularis] (congenital) (757.39)
 keratosis:
 arsenical (692.4)
 gonococcal (098.81)

701.2 **Acquired acanthosis nigricans**
Keratosis nigricans

701.3 **Striae atrophicae**
Atrophic spots of skin
Atrophoderma maculatum
Atrophy blanche (of Milian)
Degenerative colloid atrophy
Senile degenerative atrophy
Striae distensae

701.4 **Keloid scar**
Cheloid
Hypertrophic scar
Keloid

701.5 **Other abnormal granulation tissue**
Excessive granulation

701.8 **Other specified hypertrophic and atrophic conditions of skin**
Acrodermatitis atrophicans chronica
Atrophia cutis senilis
Atrophoderma neuriticum
Confluent and reticulate papillomatosis
Cutis laxa senilis
Elastosis senilis
Folliculitis ulerythematosa reticulata
Gougerot-Carteaud syndrome or disease

TABULAR LIST

701.9 Unspecified hypertrophic and atrophic conditions of skin
Atrophoderma

702 Other dermatoses
Excludes: carcinoma in situ (232.0-232.9)

702.0 Actinic keratosis

⑤ **702.1 Seborrheic keratosis**

702.11 Inflamed seborrheic keratosis

702.19 Other seborrheic keratosis
Seborrheic keratosis NOS

702.8 Other specified dermatoses

703 Diseases of nail
Excludes: congenital anomalies (757.5)
onychia and paronychia (681.02, 681.11)

703.0 Ingrowing nail
Ingrowing nail with infection
Unguis incarnatus

Excludes: infection, nail NOS (681.9)

703.8 Other specified diseases of nail
Dystrophia unguium   Onychauxis
Hypertrophy of nail   Onychogryposis
Koilonychia   Onycholysis
Leukonychia (punctata) (striata)

703.9 Unspecified disease of nail

704 Diseases of hair and hair follicles
Excludes: congenital anomalies (757.4)

⑤ **704.0 Alopecia**
Excludes: madarosis (374.55)
syphilitic alopecia (091.82)

704.00 Alopecia, unspecified
Baldness
Loss of hair

704.01 Alopecia areata
Ophiasis

704.02 Telogen effluvim

704.09 Other
Folliculitis decalvans
Hypotrichosis:
  NOS
  postinfectional NOS
Pseudopelade

704.1 Hirsutism
Hypertrichosis:
  NOS
  lanuginosa, acquired
Polytrichia

Excludes: hypertrichosis of eyelid (374.54)

704.2 Abnormalities of the hair
Atrophic hair   Trichiasis:
Clastothrix   NOS
Fragilitas crinium   cicatrical
                      Trichorrhexis (nodosa)

Excludes: trichiasis of eyelid (374.05)

704.3 Variations in hair color
Canities (premature)   Poliosis:
Grayness, hair (premature)   NOS
Heterochromia of hair   circumscripta, acquired

● Code new to this edition ▲ Revision of existing code ④ ⑤ Fourth or fifth digit required

SKIN AND SUBCUTANEOUS TISSUE

704.8 **Other specified diseases of hair and hair follicles**
Folliculitis:
  NOS
  abscedens et suffodiens
  pustular
Perifolliculitis:
  NOS
  capitis abscedens et suffodiens
  scalp
Sycosis:
  NOS
  barbae [not parasitic]
  lupoid
  vulgaris

704.9 **Unspecified disease of hair and hair follicles**

705 **Disorders of sweat glands**

705.0 **Anhidrosis**
Hypohidrosis
Oligohidrosis

705.1 **Prickly heat**
Heat rash
Miliaria rubra (tropicalis)
Sudamina

⑤ **705.2** **Focal hyperhidrosis**
Excludes: generalized (secondary) hyperhidrosis (780.8)

705.21 **Primary focal hyperhidrosis**
Focal hyperhidrosis NOS
Hyperhidrosis NOS
Hyperhidrosis of:
  axilla
  face
  palms
  soles

705.22 **Secondary focal hyperhidrosis**
Frey's syndrome

⑤ **705.8** **Other specified disorders of sweat glands**

705.81 **Dyshidrosis**
Cheiropompholyx
Pompholyx

705.82 **Fox-Fordyce disease**

705.83 **Hidradenitis**
Hidradenitis suppurativa

705.89 **Other**
Bromhidrosis   Granulosis rubra nasi
Chromhidrosis   Urhidrosis

Excludes: generalized hyperhidrosis (780.8)
          hidrocystoma (216.0-216.9)

705.9 **Unspecified disorder of sweat glands**
Disorder of sweat glands NOS

706 **Diseases of sebaceous glands**

706.0 **Acne varioliformis**
Acne:
  frontalis
  necrotica

706.1 **Other acne**
Acne: Blackhead
  NOS   Comedo
  conglobata
  cystic
  pustular
  vulgaris

Excludes: acne rosacea (695.3)

706.2 **Sebaceous cyst**
Atheroma, skin
Keratin cyst
Wen

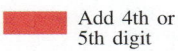 Add 4th or 5th digit   Nonspecific code   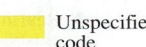 Unspecified code   Manifestation code

463

TABULAR LIST

706.3 Seborrhea

Excludes: seborrhea:
capitis (690.11)
sicca (690.18)
seborrheic dermatitis (690.11)
seborrheic keratosis (702.11-702.19)

706.8 Other specified diseases of sebaceous glands
Asteatosis (cutis)
Xerosis cutis

706.9 Unspecified disease of sebaceous glands

707 Chronic ulcer of skin
Includes: non-infected sinus of skin
non-healing ulcer

Excludes: specific infections classified under "Infectious and Parasitic Diseases" (001.0-136.9)
varicose ulcer (454.0, 454.2)

707.0 Decubitus ulcer
Bed sore   Plaster ulcer
Decubitus ulcer [any site]   Pressure ulcer

- **707.00** Unspecified site
- **707.01** Elbow
- **707.02** Upper back
  Shoulder blades
- **707.03** Lower back
  Sacrum
- **707.04** Hip
- **707.05** Buttock
- **707.06** Ankle
- **707.07** Heel
- **707.09** Other site
  Head

707.1 Ulcer of lower limbs, except decubitus
Ulcer, chronic, of lower limb:
neurogenic of lower limb
trophic of lower limb

Code, if applicable, any causal condition first:
atherosclerosis of the extremities with ulceration (440.23)
chronic venous hypertension with ulcer (459.31)
chronic venous hypertension with ulcer and inflammation (459.33)
diabetes mellitus (250.80-250.83)
postphlebetic syndrome with ulcer (459.11)
postphlebetic syndrome with ulcer and inflammation (459.13)

- **707.10** Ulcer of lower limb, unspecified
- **707.11** Ulcer of thigh
- **707.12** Ulcer of calf
- **707.13** Ulcer of ankle
- **707.14** Ulcer of heel and midfoot
  Plantar surface of midfoot
- **707.15** Ulcer of other part of foot
  Toes
- **707.19** Ulcer of other part of lower limb

707.8 Chronic ulcer of other specified sites
Ulcer, chronic, of other specified sites:
neurogenic of other specified sites
trophic of other specified sites

707.9 Chronic ulcer of unspecified site
Chronic ulcer NOS   Tropical ulcer NOS
Trophic ulcer NOS   Ulcer of skin NOS

SKIN AND SUBCUTANEOUS TISSUE

708 Urticaria

Excludes: edema:
 angioneurotic (995.1)
 Quincke's (995.1)
 hereditary angioedema (277.6)
 urticaria:
  giant (995.1)
  papulosa (Hebra) (698.2)
  pigmentosa (juvenile) (congenital) (757.33)

708.0 Allergic urticaria

708.1 Idiopathic urticaria

708.2 Urticaria due to cold and heat
 Thermal urticaria

708.3 Dermatographic urticaria
 Dermatographia
 Factitial urticaria

708.4 Vibratory urticaria

708.5 Cholinergic urticaria

708.8 Other specified urticaria
 Nettle rash
 Urticaria:
  chronic
  recurrent periodic

708.9 Urticaria, unspecified
 Hives NOS

709 Other disorders of skin and subcutaneous tissue

⑤ **709.0 Dyschromia**

Excludes: albinism (270.2)
 pigmented nevus (216.0-216.9)
 that of eyelid (374.52-374.53)

 709.00 Dyschromia, unspecified

 709.01 Vitiligo

 709.09 Other

709.1 Vascular disorders of skin
 Angioma serpiginosum
 Purpura (primary) annularis telangiectodes

709.2 Scar conditions and fibrosis of skin
 Adherent scar (skin)
 Cicatrix
 Disfigurement (due to scar)
 Fibrosis, skin NOS
 Scar NOS

Excludes: keloid scar (701.4)

709.3 Degenerative skin disorders
 Calcinosis: Degeneration, skin
  circumscripta   Deposits, skin
  cutis   Senile dermatosis NOS
 Colloid milium   Subcutaneous calcification

709.4 Foreign body granuloma of skin and subcutaneous tissue

Excludes: residual foreign body without granuloma of skin and subcutaneous tissue (729.6)
 that of muscle (728.82)

709.8 Other specified disorders of skin
 Epithelial hyperplasia
 Menstrual dermatosis
 Vesicular eruption

709.9 Unspecified disorder of skin and subcutaneous tissue
 Dermatosis NOS

465

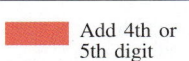 Add 4th or 5th digit
 Nonspecific code
 Unspecified code
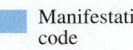 Manifestation code

TABULAR LIST

MUSCULOSKELETAL SYSTEM AND CONNECTIVE TISSUE

13. DISEASES OF THE MUSCULOSKELETAL SYSTEM AND CONNECTIVE TISSUE (710-739)

The following fifth-digit subclassification is for use with categories 711-712, 715-716, 718-719, and 730:

0 site unspecified

1 shoulder region
Acromioclavicular joint(s)
Glenohumeral joint(s)
Sternoclavicular joint(s)
Clavicle
Scapula

2 upper arm
Elbow joint   Humerus

3 forearm
Radius   Wrist joint
Ulna

4 hand
Carpus   Phalanges [fingers]
Metacarpus

5 pelvic region and thigh
Buttock   Hip (joint)
Femur

6 lower leg
Fibula   Patella
Knee joint   Tibia

7 ankle and foot
Ankle joint   Phalanges, foot
Digits [toes]   Tarsus
Metatarsus   Other joints in foot

8 other specified sites
Head   Skull
Neck   Trunk
Ribs   Vertebral column

9 multiple sites

ARTHROPATHIES AND RELATED DISORDERS (710-719)

Excludes: *disorders of spine (720.0-724.9)*

710 Diffuse diseases of connective tissue
Includes: all collagen diseases whose effects are not mainly confined to a single system

Excludes: *those affecting mainly the cardiovascular system, i.e., polyarteritis nodosa and allied conditions (446.0-446.7)*

710.0 Systemic lupus erythematosus
Disseminated lupus erythematosus
Libman-Sacks disease

Use additional code, if desired, to identify manifestation, as:
endocarditis (424.91)
nephritis (583.81)
chronic (582.81)
nephrotic syndrome (581.81)

Excludes: *lupus erythematosus (discoid) NOS (695.4)*

710.1 Systemic sclerosis
Acrosclerosis
CRST syndrome
Progressive systemic sclerosis
Scleroderma

Use additional code, if desired, to identify manifestation, as:
lung involvement (517.2)
myopathy (359.6)

Excludes: *circumscribed scleroderma (701.0)*

710.2 Sicca syndrome
Keratoconjunctivitis sicca
Sjögren's disease

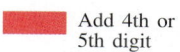 Add 4th or 5th digit
 Nonspecific code
 Unspecified code
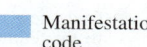 Manifestation code

TABULAR LIST

710.3 Dermatomyositis
Poikilodermatomyositis
Polymyositis with skin involvement

710.4 Polymyositis

710.5 Eosinophilia myalgia syndrome
Toxic oil syndrome

Use additional E code, if desired, to identify drug, if drug induced

710.8 Other specified diffuse diseases of connective tissue
Multifocal fibrosclerosis (idiopathic) NEC
Systemic fibrosclerosing syndrome

710.9 Unspecified diffuse connective tissue disease
Collagen disease NOS

711 Arthropathy associated with infections
Includes: arthritis associated with conditions classifiable below
arthropathy associated with conditions classifiable below
polyarthritis associated with conditions classifiable below
polyarthropathy associated with conditions classifiable below

Excludes: rheumatic fever (390)

The following fifth-digit subclassification is for use with category 711; valid digits are in [brackets] under each code. For definitions, see the beginning of this chapter:

0   site unspecified
1   shoulder region
2   upper arm
3   forearm
4   hand
5   pelvic region and thigh
6   lower leg
7   ankle and foot
8   other specified sites
9   multiple sites

711.0 Pyogenic arthritis
[0-9]   Arthritis or polyarthritis (due to):
coliform [Escherichia coli]
Hemophilus influenzae [H. influenzae]
pneumococcal
Pseudomonas
staphylococcal
streptococcal
Pyarthrosis

Use additional code, if desired, to identify infectious organism (041.0-041.8)

711.1 Arthropathy associated with Reiter's disease and nonspecific urethritis
[0-9]   Code first underlying disease, as:
nonspecific urethritis (099.4)
Reiter's disease (099.3)

711.2 Arthropathy in Behçet's syndrome
[0-9]   Code first underlying disease (136.1)

711.3 Postdysenteric arthropathy
[0-9]   Code first underlying disease, as:
dysentery (009.0)
enteritis, infectious (008.0-009.3)
paratyphoid fever (002.1-002.9)
typhoid fever (002.0)

Excludes: salmonella arthritis (003.23)

711.4 Arthropathy associated with other bacterial diseases
[0-9]   Code first underlying disease, as:
diseases classifiable to 010-040, 090-099, except as in 711.1, 711.3, and 713.5
leprosy (030.0-030.9)
tuberculosis (015.0-015.9)

Excludes: gonococcal arthritis (098.50)
meningococcal arthritis (036.82)

MUSCULOSKELETAL SYSTEM AND CONNECTIVE TISSUE

⑤ **711.5** *Arthropathy associated with other viral diseases*
[0-9]   Code first underlying disease, as:
         diseases classifiable to 045-049, 050-079, 480, 487
         O'nyong nyong (066.3)
   Excludes: that due to rubella (056.71)

⑤ **711.6** *Arthropathy associated with mycoses*
[0-9]   Code first underlying disease (110.0-118)

⑤ **711.7** *Arthropathy associated with helminthiasis*
[0-9]   Code first underlying disease, as:
         filariasis (125.0-125.9)

⑤ **711.8** *Arthropathy associated with other infectious and parasitic diseases*
[0-9]   Code first underlying disease, as:
         diseases classifiable to 080-088, 100-104, 130-136
   Excludes: arthropathy associated with sarcoidosis (713.7)

⑤ **711.9** Unspecified infective arthritis
[0-9]   Infective arthritis or polyarthritis (acute) (chronic) (subacute) NOS

⑤ **712** Crystal arthropathies
   Includes: crystal-induced arthritis and synovitis
   Excludes: gouty arthropathy (274.0)

The following fifth-digit subclassification is for use with category 712; valid digits are in [brackets] under each code. See beginning of this chapter for definitions:

0 site unspecified
1 shoulder region
2 upper arm
3 forearm
4 hand
5 pelvic region and thigh
6 lower leg
7 ankle and foot
8 other specified sites
9 multiple sites

⑤ **712.1** *Chondrocalcinosis due to dicalcium phosphate crystals*
[0-9]   Chondrocalcinosis due to dicalcium phosphate crystals (with other crystals)
         Code first underlying disease (275.4)

⑤ **712.2** *Chondrocalcinosis due to pyrophosphate crystals*
[0-9]   Code first underlying disease (275.4)

⑤ **712.3** *Chondrocalcinosis, unspecified*
[0-9]   Code first underlying disease (275.4)

⑤ **712.8** Other specified crystal arthropathies
[0-9]

⑤ **712.9** Unspecified crystal arthropathy
[0-9]

713 Arthropathy associated with other disorders classified elsewhere
   Includes: arthritis associated with conditions classifiable below
             arthropathy associated with conditions classifiable below
             polyarthritis associated with conditions classifiable below
             polyarthropathy associated with conditions classifiable below

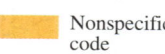 Add 4th or 5th digit
 Nonspecific code
Unspecified code
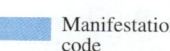 Manifestation code

469

TABULAR LIST

713.0 Arthropathy associated with other endocrine and metabolic disorders
Code first underlying disease, as:
acromegaly (253.0)
hemochromatosis (275.0)
hyperparathyroidism (252.00-252.08)
hypogammaglobulinemia (279.00-279.09)
hypothyroidism (243-244.9)
lipoid metabolism disorder (272.0-272.9)
ochronosis (270.2)

Excludes: arthropathy associated with:
amyloidosis (713.7)
crystal deposition disorders, except gout (712.1-712.9)
diabetic neuropathy (713.5)
gouty arthropathy (274.0)

713.1 Arthropathy associated with gastrointestinal conditions other than infections
Code first underlying disease, as:
regional enteritis (555.0-555.9)
ulcerative colitis (556)

713.2 Arthropathy associated with hematological disorders
Code first underlying disease, as:
hemoglobinopathy (282.4-282.7)
hemophilia (286.0-286.2)
leukemia (204.0-208.9)
malignant reticulosis (202.3)
multiple myelomatosis (203.0)

Excludes: arthropathy associated with Henoch-Schönlein purpura (713.6)

713.3 Arthropathy associated with dermatological disorders
Code first underlying disease, as:
erythema multiforme (695.1)
erythema nodosum (695.2)

Excludes: psoriatic arthropathy (696.0)

713.4 Arthropathy associated with respiratory disorders
Code first underlying disease, as:
diseases classifiable to 490-519

Excludes: arthropathy associated with respiratory infections (711.0, 711.4-711.8)

713.5 Arthropathy associated with neurological disorders
Charcot's arthropathy associated with diseases classifiable elsewhere
Neuropathic arthritis associated with diseases classifiable elsewhere
Code first underlying disease, as:
neuropathic joint disease [Charcot's joints]:
NOS (094.0)
diabetic (250.6)
syringomyelic (336.0)
tabetic [syphilitic] (094.0)

713.6 Arthropathy associated with hypersensitivity reaction
Code first underlying disease, as:
Henoch (-Schönlein) purpura (287.0)
serum sickness (999.5)

Excludes: allergic arthritis NOS (716.2)

713.7 Other general diseases with articular involvement
Code first underlying disease, as:
amyloidosis (277.30-277.39)
familial Mediterranean fever (277.31)
sarcoidosis (135)

713.8 Arthropathy associated with other conditions classifiable elsewhere
Code first underlying disease, as:
conditions classifiable elsewhere except as in 711.1-711.8, 712, and 713.0-713.7

714 Rheumatoid arthritis and other inflammatory polyarthropathies

Excludes: rheumatic fever (390)
rheumatoid arthritis of spine NOS (720.0)

● Code new to this edition
▲ Revision of existing code
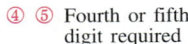 Fourth or fifth digit required

MUSCULOSKELETAL SYSTEM AND CONNECTIVE TISSUE

714.0 Rheumatoid arthritis
Arthritis or polyarthritis:
  atrophic
  rheumatic (chronic)

Use additional code, if desired, to identify manifestation, as:
  myopathy (359.6)
  polyneuropathy (357.1)

Excludes: juvenile rheumatoid arthritis NOS (714.30)

714.1 Felty's syndrome
Rheumatoid arthritis with splenoadenomegaly and leukopenia

714.2 Other rheumatoid arthritis with visceral or systemic involvement
Rheumatoid carditis

⑤ **714.3 Juvenile chronic polyarthritis**

    714.30 Polyarticular juvenile rheumatoid arthritis, chronic or unspecified
        Juvenile rheumatoid arthritis NOS
        Still's disease

    714.31 Polyarticular juvenile rheumatoid arthritis, acute

    714.32 Pauciarticular juvenile rheumatoid arthritis

    714.33 Monoarticular juvenile rheumatoid arthritis

714.4 Chronic postrheumatic arthropathy
Chronic rheumatoid nodular fibrositis
Jaccoud's syndrome

⑤ **714.8 Other specified inflammatory polyarthropathies**

    714.81 Rheumatoid lung
        Caplan's syndrome
        Diffuse interstitial rheumatoid disease of lung
        Fibrosing alveolitis, rheumatoid

    714.89 Other

714.9 Unspecified inflammatory polyarthropathy
Inflammatory polyarthropathy or polyarthritis NOS

Excludes: polyarthropathy NOS (716.5)

⑤ **715 Osteoarthrosis and allied disorders**
Note: Localized, in the subcategories below, includes bilateral involvement of the same site.
Includes: arthritis or polyarthritis:
  degenerative
  hypertrophic
  degenerative joint disease
  osteoarthritis

Excludes: Marie-Strümpell spondylitis (720.0)
  osteoarthrosis [osteoarthritis] of spine (721.0-721.9)

The following fifth-digit subclassification is for use with category 715; valid digits are in [brackets] under each code. See beginning of this chapter for definitions:

  0 site unspecified
  1 shoulder region
  2 upper arm
  3 forearm
  4 hand
  5 pelvic region and thigh
  6 lower leg
  7 ankle and foot
  8 other specified sites
  9 multiple sites

⑤ **715.0 Osteoarthrosis, generalized**
[0,4,9] Degenerative joint disease, involving multiple joints
       Primary generalized hypertrophic osteoarthrosis

⑤ **715.1 Osteoarthrosis, localized, primary**
[0-8] Localized osteoarthropathy, idiopathic

⑤ **715.2 Osteoarthrosis, localized, secondary**
[0-8] Coxae malum senilis

Add 4th or 5th digit	Nonspecific code	Unspecified code	Manifestation code

471

TABULAR LIST

- ⑤ **715.3** Osteoarthrosis, localized, not specified whether primary or secondary
  [0-8] Otto's pelvis
- ⑤ **715.8** Osteoarthrosis involving, or with mention of more than one site, but not specified as generalized
  [0,9]
- ⑤ **715.9** Osteoarthrosis, unspecified whether generalized or localized
  [0-8]

⑤ **716 Other and unspecified arthropathies**

Excludes: cricoarytenoid arthropathy (478.79)

The following fifth-digit subclassification is for use with category 716; valid digits are in [brackets] under each code. See beginning of this chapter for definitions:

- **0** site unspecified
- 1 shoulder region
- 2 upper arm
- 3 forearm
- 4 hand
- 5 pelvic region and thigh
- 6 lower leg
- 7 ankle and foot
- **8** other specified sites
- **9** multiple sites

- ⑤ **716.0** Kaschin-Beck disease
  [0-9] Endemic polyarthritis
- ⑤ **716.1** Traumatic arthropathy
  [0-9]
- ⑤ **716.2** Allergic arthritis
  [0-9]

  Excludes: arthritis associated with Henoch-Schönlein purpura or serum sickness (713.6)

- ⑤ **716.3** Climacteric arthritis
  [0-9] Menopausal arthritis
- ⑤ **716.4** Transient arthropathy
  [0-9]

  Excludes: palindromic rheumatism (719.3)

- ⑤ **716.5** Unspecified polyarthropathy or polyarthritis
  [0-9]
- ⑤ **716.6** Unspecified monoarthritis
  [0-8] Coxitis
- ⑤ **716.8** Other specified arthropathy
  [0-9]
- ⑤ **716.9** Arthropathy, unspecified
  [0-9] Arthritis (acute) (chronic) (subacute)
  Arthropathy (acute) (chronic) (subacute)
  Articular rheumatism (chronic)
  Inflammation of joint NOS

717 Internal derangement of knee

Includes: degeneration of articular cartilage or meniscus of knee
rupture, old, of articular cartilage or meniscus of knee
tear, old, of articular cartilage or meniscus of knee

Excludes: acute derangement of knee (836.0-836.6)
ankylosis (718.5)
contracture (718.4)
current injury (836.0-836.6)
deformity (736.4-736.6)
recurrent dislocation (718.3)

- **717.0** Old bucket handle tear of medial meniscus
  Old bucket handle tear of unspecified cartilage
- **717.1** Derangement of anterior horn of medial meniscus
- **717.2** Derangement of posterior horn of medial meniscus
- **717.3** Other and unspecified derangement of medial meniscus
  Degeneration of internal semilunar cartilage

● Code new to this edition ▲ Revision of existing code ④ ⑤ Fourth or fifth digit required

MUSCULOSKELETAL SYSTEM AND CONNECTIVE TISSUE

⑤ **717.4 Derangement of lateral meniscus**
   717.40 Derangement of lateral meniscus, unspecified
   717.41 Bucket handle tear of lateral meniscus
   717.42 Derangement of anterior horn of lateral meniscus
   717.43 Derangement of posterior horn of lateral meniscus
   717.49 Other

717.5 Derangement of meniscus, not elsewhere classified
   Congenital discoid meniscus
   Cyst of semilunar cartilage
   Derangement of semilunar cartilage NOS

717.6 Loose body in knee
   Joint mice, knee
   Rice bodies, knee (joint)

717.7 Chondromalacia of patella
   Chondromalacia patellae
   Degeneration [softening] of articular cartilage of patella

⑤ **717.8 Other internal derangement of knee**
   717.81 Old disruption of lateral collateral ligament
   717.82 Old disruption of medial collateral ligament
   717.83 Old disruption of anterior cruciate ligament
   717.84 Old disruption of posterior cruciate ligament
   717.85 Old disruption of other ligaments of knee
      Capsular ligament of knee
   717.89 Other
      Old disruption of ligaments of knee NOS

717.9 Unspecified internal derangement of knee
   Derangement NOS of knee

⑤ **718 Other derangement of joint**
   Excludes: current injury (830.0-848.9)
              jaw (524.60-524.69)

The following fifth-digit subclassification is for use with category 718; valid digits are in [brackets] under each code. See beginning of this chapter for definitions:

   0 site unspecified
   1 shoulder region
   2 upper arm
   3 forearm
   4 hand
   5 pelvic region and thigh
   6 lower leg
   7 ankle and foot
   8 other specified sites
   9 multiple sites

⑤ **718.0 Articular cartilage disorder**
   [0-5, 7-9] Meniscus:
      disorder
      rupture, old
      tear, old
      Old rupture of ligament(s) of joint NOS

   Excludes: articular cartilage disorder:
      in ochronosis (270.2)
      knee (717.0-717.9)
      chondrocalcinosis (275.4)
      metastatic calcification (275.4)

⑤ **718.1 Loose body in joint**
   [0-5, 7-9] Joint mice
   Excludes: knee (717.6)

⑤ **718.2 Pathological dislocation**
   [0-9] Dislocation or displacement of joint, not recurrent and not current injury
      Spontaneous dislocation (joint)

473

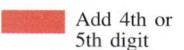 Add 4th or 5th digit
 Nonspecific code
 Unspecified code
 Manifestation code

TABULAR LIST

⑤ **718.3 Recurrent dislocation of joint**
[0-9]

⑤ **718.4 Contracture of joint**
[0-9]

⑤ **718.5 Ankylosis of joint**
[0-9]   Ankylosis of joint (fibrous) (osseous)
Excludes: spine (724.9)
stiffness of joint without mention of ankylosis (719.5)

⑤ **718.6 Unspecified intrapelvic protrusion of acetabulum**
[0, 5]   Protrusio acetabuli, unspecified

⑤ **718.7 Developmental dislocation of joint**
[0-9]
Excludes: congenital dislocation of joint (754.0-755.8)
traumatic dislocation of joint (830-839)

⑤ **718.8 Other joint derangement, not elsewhere classified**
[0-9]   Flail joint (paralytic)   Instability of joint
Excludes: deformities classifiable to 736 (736.0-736.9)

⑤ **718.9 Unspecified derangement of joint**
[0-5, 7-9]
Excludes: knee (717.9)

719 Other and unspecified disorders of joint
Excludes: jaw (524.60-524.69)
The following fifth-digit subclassification is for use with codes 719.0-719.6, 719.8-719.9; valid digits are in [brackets] under each code. See list at beginning of chapter for definitions:

0 site unspecified
1 shoulder region
2 upper arm
3 forearm
4 hand
5 pelvic region and thigh
6 lower leg
7 ankle and foot
8 other specified sites
9 multiple sites

⑤ **719.0 Effusion of joint**
[0-9]   Hydrarthrosis
Swelling of joint, with or without pain
Excludes: intermittent hydrarthrosis (719.3)

⑤ **719.1 Hemarthrosis**
[0-9]
Excludes: current injury (840.0-848.9)

⑤ **719.2 Villonodular synovitis**
[0-9]

⑤ **719.3 Palindromic rheumatism**
[0-9]   Hench-Rosenberg syndrome
Intermittent hydrarthrosis

⑤ **719.4 Pain in joint**
[0-9]   Arthralgia

⑤ **719.5 Stiffness of joint, not elsewhere classified**
[0-9]

⑤ **719.6 Other symptoms referable to joint**
[0-9]   Joint crepitus   Snapping hip

719.7 Difficulty in walking
Excludes: abnormality of gait (781.2)

MUSCULOSKELETAL SYSTEM AND CONNECTIVE TISSUE

⑤ **719.8 Other specified disorders of joint**
[0-9]   Calcification of joint   Fistula of joint
          Excludes: temporomandibular joint-pain-dysfunction syndrome [Costen's syndrome] (524.60)

⑤ **719.9 Unspecified disorder of joint**
[0-9]

DORSOPATHIES (720-724)

Excludes: curvature of spine (737.0-737.9)
            osteochondrosis of spine (juvenile) (732.0)
                adult (732.8)

720 Ankylosing spondylitis and other inflammatory spondylopathies

720.0 Ankylosing spondylitis
Rheumatoid arthritis of spine NOS
Spondylitis:
  Marie-Strümpell
  rheumatoid

720.1 Spinal enthesopathy
Disorder of peripheral ligamentous or muscular attachments of spine
Romanus lesion

720.2 Sacroiliitis, not elsewhere classified
Inflammation of sacroiliac joint NOS

⑤ **720.8 Other inflammatory spondylopathies**

720.81 Inflammatory spondylopathies in diseases classified elsewhere
Code first underlying disease, as:
  tuberculosis (015.0)

720.89 Other

720.9 Unspecified inflammatory spondylopathy
Spondylitis NOS

721 Spondylosis and allied disorders

721.0 Cervical spondylosis without myelopathy
Cervical or cervicodorsal:
  arthritis
  osteoarthritis
  spondylarthritis

721.1 Cervical spondylosis with myelopathy
Anterior spinal artery compression syndrome
Spondylogenic compression of cervical spinal cord
Vertebral artery compression syndrome

721.2 Thoracic spondylosis without myelopathy
Thoracic:
  arthritis
  osteoarthritis
  spondylarthritis

721.3 Lumbosacral spondylosis without myelopathy
Lumbar or lumbosacral:
  arthritis
  osteoarthritis
  spondylarthritis

⑤ **721.4 Thoracic or lumbar spondylosis with myelopathy**

721.41 Thoracic region
Spondylogenic compression of thoracic spinal cord

721.42 Lumbar region
Spondylogenic compression of lumbar spinal cord

721.5 Kissing spine
Baastrup's syndrome

721.6 Ankylosing vertebral hyperostosis

721.7 Traumatic spondylopathy
Kümmell's disease or spondylitis

721.8 Other allied disorders of spine

⑤ **721.9 Spondylosis of unspecified site**

■ Add 4th or 5th digit	■ Nonspecific code	■ Unspecified code	■ Manifestation code

TABULAR LIST

721.90 **Without mention of myelopathy**
  Spinal:
    arthritis (deformans) (degenerative) (hypertrophic)
    osteoarthritis NOS
  Spondylarthrosis NOS

721.91 **With myelopathy**
  Spondylogenic compression of spinal cord NOS

722 Intervertebral disc disorders

722.0 **Displacement of cervical intervertebral disc without myelopathy**
  Neuritis (brachial) or radiculitis due to displacement or rupture of cervical intervertebral disc
  Any condition classifiable to 722.2 of the cervical or cervicothoracic intervertebral disc

722.1 **Displacement of thoracic or lumbar intervertebral disc without myelopathy**

  722.10 **Lumbar intervertebral disc without myelopathy**
    Lumbago or sciatica due to displacement of intervertebral disc
    Neuritis or radiculitis due to displacement or rupture of lumbar intervertebral disc
    Any condition classifiable to 722.2 of the lumbar or lumbosacral intervertebral disc

  722.11 **Thoracic intervertebral disc without myelopathy**
    Any condition classifiable to 722.2 of thoracic intervertebral disc

722.2 **Displacement of intervertebral disc, site unspecified, without myelopathy**
  Discogenic syndrome NOS
  Herniation of nucleus pulposus NOS
  Intervertebral disc NOS:
    extrusion
    prolapse
    protrusion
    rupture
  Neuritis or radiculitis due to displacement or rupture of intervertebral disc

722.3 **Schmorl's nodes**

  722.30 **Unspecified region**
  722.31 **Thoracic region**
  722.32 **Lumbar region**
  722.39 **Other**

722.4 **Degeneration of cervical intervertebral disc**
  Degeneration of cervicothoracic intervertebral disc

722.5 **Degeneration of thoracic or lumbar intervertebral disc**

  722.51 **Thoracic or thoracolumbar intervertebral disc**
  722.52 **Lumbar or lumbosacral intervertebral disc**

722.6 **Degeneration of intervertebral disc, site unspecified**
  Degenerative disc disease NOS
  Narrowing of intervertebral disc or space NOS

722.7 **Intervertebral disc disorder with myelopathy**

  722.70 **Unspecified region**
  722.71 **Cervical region**
  722.72 **Thoracic region**
  722.73 **Lumbar region**

722.8 **Postlaminectomy syndrome**

  722.80 **Unspecified region**
  722.81 **Cervical region**
  722.82 **Thoracic region**
  722.83 **Lumbar region**

722.9 **Other and unspecified disc disorder**
  Calcification of intervertebral cartilage or disc
  Discitis

  722.90 **Unspecified region**
  722.91 **Cervical region**
  722.92 **Thoracic region**
  722.93 **Lumbar region**

MUSCULOSKELETAL SYSTEM AND CONNECTIVE TISSUE

723 **Other disorders of cervical region**
Excludes: conditions due to:
intervertebral disc disorders (722.0-722.9)
spondylosis (721.0-721.9)

723.0 Spinal stenosis in cervical region

723.1 Cervicalgia
Pain in neck

723.2 Cervicocranial syndrome
Barré-Liéou syndrome
Posterior cervical sympathetic syndrome

723.3 Cervicobrachial syndrome (diffuse)

723.4 Brachial neuritis or radiculitis NOS
Cervical radiculitis
Radicular syndrome of upper limbs

723.5 Torticollis, unspecified
Contracture of neck
Excludes: congenital (754.1)
due to birth injury (767.8)
hysterical (300.11)
ocular torticollis (781.93)
psychogenic (306.0)
spasmodic (333.83)
traumatic, current (847.0)

723.6 Panniculitis specified as affecting neck

723.7 Ossification of posterior longitudinal ligament in cervical region

723.8 Other syndromes affecting cervical region
Cervical syndrome NEC
Klippel's disease
Occipital neuralgia

723.9 Unspecified musculoskeletal disorders and symptoms referable to neck
Cervical (region) disorder NOS

724 **Other and unspecified disorders of back**
Excludes: collapsed vertebra (code to cause, e.g., osteoporosis, 733.00-733.09)
conditions due to:
intervertebral disc disorders (722.0-722.9)
spondylosis (721.0-721.9)

⑤ **724.0 Spinal stenosis, other than cervical**
  724.00 Spinal stenosis, unspecified region
  724.01 Thoracic region
  724.02 Lumbar region
  724.09 Other

724.1 Pain in thoracic spine

724.2 Lumbago
Low back pain
Low back syndrome
Lumbalgia

724.3 Sciatica
Neuralgia or neuritis of sciatic nerve
Excludes: specified lesion of sciatic nerve (355.0)

724.4 Thoracic or lumbosacral neuritis or radiculitis, unspecified
Radicular syndrome of lower limbs

724.5 Backache, unspecified
Vertebrogenic (pain) syndrome NOS

724.6 Disorders of sacrum
Ankylosis, lumbosacral or sacroiliac (joint)
Instability, lumbosacral or sacroiliac (joint)

⑤ **724.7 Disorders of coccyx**
  724.70 Unspecified disorder of coccyx
  724.71 Hypermobility of coccyx

477

 Add 4th or 5th digit
 Nonspecific code
 Unspecified code
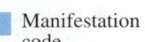 Manifestation code

TABULAR LIST

724.79 **Other**
Coccygodynia

724.8 **Other symptoms referable to back**
Ossification of posterior longitudinal ligament NOS
Panniculitis specified as sacral or affecting back

724.9 **Other unspecified back disorders**
Ankylosis of spine NOS
Compression of spinal nerve root NEC
Spinal disorder NOS

Excludes: sacroiliitis (720.2)

RHEUMATISM, EXCLUDING THE BACK (725-729)

Includes: disorders of muscles and tendons and their attachments, and of other soft tissues

725 Polymyalgia rheumatica

726 Peripheral enthesopathies and allied syndromes
Note: Enthesopathies are disorders of peripheral ligamentous or muscular attachments.

Excludes: spinal enthesopathy (720.1)

726.0 Adhesive capsulitis of shoulder

⑤ **726.1 Rotator cuff syndrome of shoulder and allied disorders**

726.10 **Disorders of bursae and tendons in shoulder region, unspecified**
Rotator cuff syndrome NOS
Supraspinatus syndrome NOS

726.11 Calcifying tendinitis of shoulder

726.12 Bicipital tenosynovitis

726.19 **Other specified disorders**

Excludes: complete rupture of rotator cuff, nontraumatic (727.61)

726.2 **Other affections of shoulder region, not elsewhere classified**
Periarthritis of shoulder
Scapulohumeral fibrositis

⑤ **726.3 Enthesopathy of elbow region**

726.30 **Enthesopathy of elbow, unspecified**

726.31 Medial epicondylitis

726.32 Lateral epicondylitis
Epicondylitis NOS
Golfers' elbow
Tennis elbow

726.33 Olecranon bursitis
Bursitis of elbow

726.39 **Other**

726.4 Enthesopathy of wrist and carpus
Bursitis of hand or wrist
Periarthritis of wrist

726.5 Enthesopathy of hip region
Bursitis of hip   Psoas tendinitis
Gluteal tendinitis   Trochanteric tendinitis
Iliac crest spur

⑤ **726.6 Enthesopathy of knee**

726.60 **Enthesopathy of knee, unspecified**
Bursitis of knee NOS

726.61 Pes anserinus tendinitis or bursitis

726.62 Tibial collateral ligament bursitis
Pellegrini-Stieda syndrome

726.63 Fibular collateral ligament bursitis

726.64 Patellar tendinitis

726.65 Prepatellar bursitis

726.69 **Other**
Bursitis:
  infrapatellar
  subpatellar

MUSCULOSKELETAL SYSTEM AND CONNECTIVE TISSUE

⑤ **726.7 Enthesopathy of ankle and tarsus**

726.70 Enthesopathy of ankle and tarsus, unspecified
Metatarsalgia NOS

Excludes: Morton's metatarsalgia (355.6)

726.71 Achilles bursitis or tendinitis

726.72 Tibialis tendinitis
Tibialis (anterior) (posterior) tendinitis

726.73 Calcaneal spur

726.79 Other
Peroneal tendinitis

726.8 Other peripheral enthesopathies

⑤ **726.9 Unspecified enthesopathy**

726.90 Enthesopathy of unspecified site
Capsulitis NOS
Periarthritis NOS
Tendinitis NOS

726.91 Exostosis of unspecified site
Bone spur NOS

727 Other disorders of synovium, tendon, and bursa

⑤ **727.0 Synovitis and tenosynovitis**

727.00 Synovitis and tenosynovitis, unspecified
Synovitis NOS
Tenosynovitis NOS

727.01 Synovitis and tenosynovitis in diseases classified elsewhere
Code first underlying disease, as:
tuberculosis (015.0-015.9)

Excludes: crystal-induced (275.4)
gonococcal (098.51)
gouty (274.0)
syphilitic (095.7)

727.02 Giant cell tumor of tendon sheath

727.03 Trigger finger (acquired)

727.04 Radial styloid tenosynovitis
de Quervain's disease

727.05 Other tenosynovitis of hand and wrist

727.06 Tenosynovitis of foot and ankle

727.09 Other

727.1 Bunion

727.2 Specific bursitides often of occupational origin
Beat:
elbow
hand
knee
Chronic crepitant synovitis of wrist
Miners':
elbow
knee

727.3 Other bursitis
Bursitis NOS

Excludes: bursitis:
gonococcal (098.52)
subacromial (726.19)
subcoracoid (726.19)
subdeltoid (726.19)
syphilitic (095.7)
"frozen shoulder" (726.0)

⑤ **727.4 Ganglion and cyst of synovium, tendon, and bursa**

727.40 Synovial cyst, unspecified

Excludes: that of popliteal space (727.51)

727.41 Ganglion of joint

479

TABULAR LIST

- **727.42** Ganglion of tendon sheath
- **727.43** Ganglion, unspecified
- **727.49** Other
  - Cyst of bursa

⑤ **727.5 Rupture of synovium**
- **727.50** Rupture of synovium, unspecified
- **727.51** Synovial cyst of popliteal space
  - Baker's cyst (knee)
- **727.59** Other

⑤ **727.6 Rupture of tendon, nontraumatic**
- **727.60** Nontraumatic rupture of unspecified tendon
- **727.61** Complete rupture of rotator cuff
- **727.62** Tendons of biceps (long head)
- **727.63** Extensor tendons of hand and wrist
- **727.64** Flexor tendons of hand and wrist
- **727.65** Quadriceps tendon
- **727.66** Patellar tendon
- **727.67** Achilles tendon
- **727.68** Other tendons of foot and ankle
- **727.69** Other

⑤ **727.8 Other disorders of synovium, tendon, and bursa**
- **727.81** Contracture of tendon (sheath)
  - Short Achilles tendon (acquired)
- **727.82** Calcium deposits in tendon and bursa
  - Calcification of tendon NOS
  - Calcific tendinitis NOS

  Excludes: peripheral ligamentous or muscular attachments (726.0-726.9)

- **727.83** Plica syndrome
  - Plica knee
- **727.89** Other
  - Abscess of bursa or tendon

  Excludes: xanthomatosis localized to tendons (272.7)

- **727.9** Unspecified disorder of synovium, tendon, and bursa

728 Disorders of muscle, ligament, and fascia

Excludes: enthesopathies (726.0-726.9)
muscular dystrophies (359.0-359.1)
myoneural disorders (358.00-358.9)
myopathies (359.2-359.9)
old disruption of ligaments of knee (717.81-717.89)

728.0 Infective myositis
Myositis:
  purulent
  suppurative

Excludes: myositis:
  epidemic (074.1)
  interstitial (728.81)
  syphilitic (095.6)
  tropical (040.81)

⑤ **728.1 Muscular calcification and ossification**
- **728.10** Calcification and ossification, unspecified
  - Massive calcification (paraplegic)
- **728.11** Progressive myositis ossificans
- **728.12** Traumatic myositis ossificans
  - Myositis ossificans (circumscripta)
- **728.13** Postoperative heterotopic calcification
- **728.19** Other
  - Polymyositis ossificans

480 ● Code new to this edition   ▲ Revision of existing code   ④ ⑤ Fourth or fifth digit required

MUSCULOSKELETAL SYSTEM AND CONNECTIVE TISSUE

728.2 Muscular wasting and disuse atrophy, not elsewhere classified
Amyotrophia NOS
Myofibrosis

Excludes: neuralgic amyotrophy (353.5)
pelvic muscle wasting and disuse atrophy (618.83)
progressive muscular atrophy (335.0-335.9)

728.3 Other specific muscle disorders
Arthrogryposis
Immobility syndrome (paraplegic)

Excludes: arthrogryposis multiplex congenita (754.89)
stiff-man syndrome (333.91)

728.4 Laxity of ligament

728.5 Hypermobility syndrome

728.6 Contracture of palmar fascia
Dupuytren's contracture

⑤ **728.7 Other fibromatoses**

728.71 Plantar fascial fibromatosis
Contracture of plantar fascia
Plantar fasciitis (traumatic)

728.79 Other
Garrod's or knuckle pads
Nodular fasciitis
Pseudosarcomatous fibromatosis (proliferative) (subcutaneous)

⑤ **728.8 Other disorders of muscle, ligament, and fascia**

728.81 Interstitial myositis

728.82 Foreign body granuloma of muscle
Talc granuloma of muscle

728.83 Rupture of muscle, nontraumatic

728.84 Diastasis of muscle
Diastasis recti (abdomen)

Excludes: diastasis recti complicating pregnancy, labor, and delivery (665.8)

728.85 Spasm of muscle

728.86 Necrotizing fasciitis
Use additional code to identify:
infectious organism (041.00 - 041.89)
gangrene (785.4), if applicable

728.87 Muscle weakness (generalized)

Excludes: generalized weakness (780.79)

728.88 Rhabdomyolysis

728.89 Other
Eosinophilic fasciitis
Use additional E code, if desired, to identify drug, if drug induced

728.9 Unspecified disorder of muscle, ligament, and fascia

729 Other disorders of soft tissues

Excludes: acroparesthesia (443.89)
carpal tunnel syndrome (354.0)
disorders of the back (720.0-724.9)
entrapment syndromes (354.0-355.9)
palindromic rheumatism (719.3)
periarthritis (726.0-726.9)
psychogenic rheumatism (306.0)

729.0 Rheumatism, unspecified and fibrositis

729.1 Myalgia and myositis, unspecified
Fibromyositis NOS

481

TABULAR LIST

729.2 Neuralgia, neuritis, and radiculitis, unspecified

Excludes: brachial radiculitis (723.4)
cervical radiculitis (723.4)
lumbosacral radiculitis (724.4)
mononeuritis (354.0-355.9)
radiculitis due to intervertebral disc involvement (722.0-722.2, 722.7)
sciatica (724.3)

⑤ **729.3 Panniculitis, unspecified**

    729.30 Panniculitis, unspecified site
        Weber-Christian disease

    729.31 Hypertrophy of fat pad, knee
        Hypertrophy of infrapatellar fat pad

    729.39 Other site

Excludes: panniculitis specified as (affecting):
back (724.8)
neck (723.6)
sacral (724.8)

729.4 Fasciitis, unspecified

Excludes: necrotizing fasciitis (728.86)
nodular fasciitis (728.79)

729.5 Pain in limb

729.6 Residual foreign body in soft tissue

Excludes: foreign body granuloma:
muscle (728.82)
skin and subcutaneous tissue (709.4)

⑤ **729.7 Nontraumatic compartment syndrome**

Excludes: compartment syndrome NOS (958.90)
traumatic compartment syndrome (958.90-958.99)

    729.71 Nontraumatic compartment syndrome of upper extremity
        Nontraumatic compartment syndrome of shoulder, arm, forearm, wrist, hand and fingers

    729.72 Nontraumatic compartment syndrome of lower extremity
        Nontraumatic compartment syndrome of hip, buttock, thigh, leg, foot and toes

    729.73 Nontraumatic compartment syndrome of abdomen

    729.79 Nontraumatic compartment syndrome of other sites

⑤ **729.8 Other musculoskeletal symptoms referable to limbs**

    729.81 Swelling of limb

    729.82 Cramp

    729.89 Other

Excludes: abnormality of gait (781.2)
tetany (781.7)
transient paralysis of limb (781.4)

729.9 Other and unspecified disorders of soft tissue
    Polyalgia

MUSCULOSKELETAL SYSTEM AND CONNECTIVE TISSUE

OSTEOPATHIES, CHONDROPATHIES, AND ACQUIRED MUSCULOSKELETAL DEFORMITIES (730-739)

⑤ **730 Osteomyelitis, periostitis, and other infections involving bone**

Excludes: jaw (526.4-526.5)
petrous bone (383.2)

Use additional code, if desired, to identify organism, such as Staphylococcus (041.1)

The following fifth-digit subclassification is for use with category 730; valid digits are in [brackets] under each code. See beginning of this chapter for definitions:

0 site unspecified
1 shoulder region
2 upper arm
3 forearm
4 hand
5 pelvic region and thigh
6 lower leg
7 ankle and foot
8 other specified sites
9 multiple sites

⑤ **730.0 Acute osteomyelitis**
[0-9]
Abscess of any bone except accessory sinus, jaw, or mastoid
Acute or subacute osteomyelitis, with or without mention of periostitis
Use additional code to identify major osseous defect, if applicable (731.3)

⑤ **730.1 Chronic osteomyelitis**
[0-9]
Brodie's abscess
Chronic or old osteomyelitis, with or without mention of periostitis
Sequestrum of bone
Sclerosing osteomyelitis of Garré
Use additional code to identify major osseous defect, if applicable (731.3)

Excludes: aseptic necrosis of bone (733.40-733.49)

⑤ **730.2 Unspecified osteomyelitis**
[0-9]
Osteitis or osteomyelitis NOS, with or without mention of periostitis
Use additional code to identify major osseous defect, if applicable (731.3)

⑤ **730.3 Periostitis without mention of osteomyelitis**
[0-9]
Abscess of periosteum without mention of osteomyelitis
Periostosis without mention of osteomyelitis

Excludes: that in secondary syphilis (091.61)

⑤ **730.7 Osteopathy resulting from poliomyelitis**
[0-9]
Code first underlying disease (045.0-045.9)

⑤ **730.8 Other infections involving bone in diseases classified elsewhere**
[0-9]
Code first underlying disease, as:
tuberculosis (015.0-015.9)
typhoid fever (002.0)

Excludes: syphilis of bone NOS (095.5)

⑤ **730.9 Unspecified infection of bone**
[0-9]

731 Osteitis deformans and osteopathies associated with other disorders classified elsewhere

731.0 Osteitis deformans without mention of bone tumor
Paget's disease of bone

731.1 Osteitis deformans in diseases classified elsewhere
Code first underlying disease, as:
malignant neoplasm of bone (170.0-170.9)

731.2 Hypertrophic pulmonary osteoarthropathy
Bamberger-Marie disease

 Add 4th or 5th digit
 Nonspecific code
Unspecified code
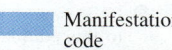 Manifestation code

731.3 Major osseous defects
  Code first underlying disease, if known, such as:
    aseptic necrosis (733.40-733.49)
    malignant neoplasm of bone (170.0-170.9)
    osteomyelitis (730.00-730.29)
    osteoporosis (733.00-733.09)
    peri-prosthetic osteolysis (996.45)

731.8 Other bone involvement in diseases classified elsewhere
  Code first underlying disease, as:
    diabetes mellitus (250.8)
  Use additional code to specify bone condition, such as:
    acute osteomyelitis (730.00-730.09)

732 Osteochondropathies

732.0 Juvenile osteochondrosis of spine
  Juvenile osteochondrosis (of):
    marginal or vertebral epiphysis (of Scheuermann)
    spine NOS
  Vertebral epiphysitis

  Excludes: adolescent postural kyphosis (737.0)

732.1 Juvenile osteochondrosis of hip and pelvis
  Coxa plana
  Ischiopubic synchondrosis (of van Neck)
  Osteochondrosis (juvenile) of:
    acetabulum
    head of femur (of Legg-Calvé-Perthes)
    iliac crest (of Buchanan)
    symphysis pubis (of Pierson)
  Pseudocoxalgia

732.2 Nontraumatic slipped upper femoral epiphysis
  Slipped upper femoral epiphysis NOS

732.3 Juvenile osteochondrosis of upper extremity
  Osteochondrosis (juvenile) of:
    capitulum of humerus (of Panner)
    carpal lunate (of Kienbock)
    hand NOS
    head of humerus (of Haas)
    heads of metacarpals (of Mauclaire)
    lower ulna (of Burns)
    radial head (of Brailsford)
    upper extremity NOS

732.4 Juvenile osteochondrosis of lower extremity, excluding foot
  Osteochondrosis (juvenile) of:
    lower extremity NOS
    primary patellar center (of Köhler)
    proximal tibia (of Blount)
    secondary patellar center (of Sinding-Larsen)
    tibial tubercle (of Osgood-Schlatter)
  Tibia vara

732.5 Juvenile osteochondrosis of foot
  Calcaneal apophysitis
  Epiphysitis, os calcis
  Osteochondrosis (juvenile) of:
    astragalus (of Diaz)
    calcaneum (of Sever)
    foot NOS
    metatarsal
      second (of Freiberg)
      fifth (of Iselin)
    os tibiale externum (Haglund)
    tarsal navicular (of Köhler)

732.6 Other juvenile osteochondrosis
  Apophysitis specified as juvenile, of other site, or site NOS
  Epiphysitis specified as juvenile, of other site, or site NOS
  Osteochondritis specified as juvenile, of other site, or site NOS
  Osteochondrosis specified as juvenile, of other site, or site NOS

732.7 Osteochondritis dissecans

MUSCULOSKELETAL SYSTEM AND CONNECTIVE TISSUE

732.8 Other specified forms of osteochondropathy
Adult osteochondrosis of spine

732.9 Unspecified osteochondropathy
Apophysitis
  NOS
  not specified as adult or juvenile, of unspecified site
Epiphysitis
  NOS
  not specified as adult or juvenile, of unspecified site
Osteochondritis
  NOS
  not specified as adult or juvenile, of unspecified site
Osteochondrosis
  NOS
  not specified as adult or juvenile, of unspecified site

733 Other disorders of bone and cartilage

Excludes: bone spur (726.91)
cartilage of, or loose body in, joint (717.0-717.9, 718.0-718.9)
giant cell granuloma of jaw (526.3)
osteitis fibrosa cystica generalisata (252.01)
osteomalacia (268.2)
polyostotic fibrous dysplasia of bone (756.54)
prognathism, retrognathism (524.1)
xanthomatosis localized to bone (272.7)

⑤ **733.0 Osteoporosis**
Use additional code to identify major osseous defect, if applicable (731.3)

    733.00 Osteoporosis, unspecified
      Wedging of vertebra NOS

    733.01 **Senile osteoporosis**
      Postmenopausal osteoporosis

    733.02 **Idiopathic osteoporosis**

    733.03 **Disuse osteoporosis**

    733.09 Other
      Drug-induced osteoporosis
    Use additional E code, if desired, to identify drug

⑤ **733.1 Pathologic fracture**
Spontaneous fracture
Excludes: traumatic fracture (800-829)
stress fracture (733.93-733.95)

    733.10 Pathologic fracture, unspecified site

    733.11 **Pathologic fracture of humerus**

    733.12 **Pathologic fracture of distal radius and ulna**
      Wrist NOS

    733.13 **Pathologic fracture of vertebrae**
      Collapse of vertebra NOS

    733.14 **Pathologic fracture of neck of femur**
      Femur NOS
      Hip NOS

    733.15 **Pathologic fracture of other specified part of femur**

    733.16 **Pathologic fracture of tibia or fibula**
      Ankle NOS

    733.19 Pathologic fracture of other specified site

⑤ **733.2 Cyst of bone**

    733.20 Cyst of bone (localized), unspecified

    733.21 **Solitary bone cyst**
      Unicameral bone cyst

    733.22 **Aneurysmal bone cyst**

    733.29 Other
      Fibrous dysplasia (monostotic)

Excludes: cyst of jaw (526.0-526.2, 526.89)
osteitis fibrosa cystica (252.01)
polyostotic fibrous dysplasia of bone (756.54)

TABULAR LIST

733.3 Hyperostosis of skull
  Hyperostosis interna frontalis
  Leontiasis ossium

⑤ **733.4 Aseptic necrosis of bone**
Use additional code to identify major osseous defect, if applicable (731.3)
Excludes: osteochondropathies (732.0-732.9)

    733.40 Aseptic necrosis of bone, site unspecified

    733.41 Head of humerus

    733.42 Head and neck of femur
        Femur NOS
    Excludes: Legg-Calvé-Perthes disease (732.1)

    733.43 Medial femoral condyle

    733.44 Talus

    ● **733.45 Jaw**
    Use additional E code to identify drug, if drug-induced
    Excludes: osteoradionecrosis of jaw (526.89)

    733.49 Other

733.5 Osteitis condensans
  Piriform sclerosis of ilium

733.6 Tietze's disease
  Costochondral junction syndrome
  Costochondritis

733.7 Algoneurodystrophy
  Disuse atrophy of bone
  Sudeck's atrophy

⑤ **733.8 Malunion and nonunion of fracture**

    733.81 Malunion of fracture

    733.82 Nonunion of fracture
        Pseudoarthrosis (bone)

⑤ **733.9 Other and unspecified disorders of bone and cartilage**

    733.90 Disorder of bone and cartilage, unspecified

    733.91 Arrest of bone development or growth
        Epiphyseal arrest

    733.92 Chondromalacia
        Chondromalacia:
          NOS
          localized, except patella
          systemic
          tibial plateau
    Excludes: chondromalacia of patella (717.7)

    733.93 Stress fracture of tibia or fibula
        Stress reaction of tibia or fibula

    733.94 Stress fracture of the metatarsals
        Stress reaction of metatarsals

    733.95 Stress fracture of other bone
        Stress reaction of other bone

    733.99 Other
        Diaphysitis
        Hypertrophy of bone
        Relapsing polychondritis

734 Flat foot
  Pes planus (acquired)
  Talipes planus (acquired)
  Excludes: congenital (754.61)
      rigid flat foot (754.61)
      spastic (everted) flat foot (754.61)

735 Acquired deformities of toe
  Excludes: congenital (754.60-754.69, 755.65-755.66)

  735.0 Hallux valgus (acquired)

MUSCULOSKELETAL SYSTEM AND CONNECTIVE TISSUE

- 735.1 **Hallux varus (acquired)**
- 735.2 **Hallux rigidus**
- 735.3 **Hallux malleus**
- 735.4 **Other hammer toe (acquired)**
- 735.5 **Claw toe (acquired)**
- 735.8 **Other acquired deformities of toe**
- 735.9 **Unspecified acquired deformity of toe**

736 Other acquired deformities of limbs
Excludes: congenital (754.3-755.9)

⑤ 736.0 **Acquired deformities of forearm, excluding fingers**
- 736.00 **Unspecified deformity**
  Deformity of elbow, forearm, hand, or wrist (acquired) NOS
- 736.01 **Cubitus valgus (acquired)**
- 736.02 **Cubitus varus (acquired)**
- 736.03 **Valgus deformity of wrist (acquired)**
- 736.04 **Varus deformity of wrist (acquired)**
- 736.05 **Wrist drop (acquired)**
- 736.06 **Claw hand (acquired)**
- 736.07 **Club hand, acquired**
- 736.09 **Other**

736.1 **Mallet finger**

⑤ 736.2 **Other acquired deformities of finger**
- 736.20 **Unspecified deformity**
  Deformity of finger (acquired) NOS
- 736.21 **Boutonniere deformity**
- 736.22 **Swan-neck deformity**
- 736.29 **Other**

Excludes: trigger finger (727.03)

⑤ 736.3 **Acquired deformities of hip**
- 736.30 **Unspecified deformity**
  Deformity of hip (acquired) NOS
- 736.31 **Coxa valga (acquired)**
- 736.32 **Coxa vara (acquired)**
- 736.39 **Other**

⑤ 736.4 **Genu valgum or varum (acquired)**
- 736.41 **Genu valgum (acquired)**
- 736.42 **Genu varum (acquired)**

736.5 **Genu recurvatum (acquired)**

736.6 **Other acquired deformities of knee**
Deformity of knee (acquired) NOS

⑤ 736.7 **Other acquired deformities of ankle and foot**
Excludes: deformities of toe (acquired) (735.0-735.9)
  pes planus (acquired) (734)
- 736.70 **Unspecified deformity of ankle and foot, acquired**
- 736.71 **Acquired equinovarus deformity**
  Clubfoot, acquired

Excludes: clubfoot not specified as acquired (754.5-754.7)
- 736.72 **Equinus deformity of foot, acquired**
- 736.73 **Cavus deformity of foot**

Excludes: that with claw foot (736.74)
- 736.74 **Claw foot, acquired**
- 736.75 **Cavovarus deformity of foot, acquired**
- 736.76 **Other calcaneus deformity**

487

 Nonspecific code
 Unspecified code
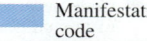 Manifestation code

Add 4th or 5th digit

TABULAR LIST

736.79 Other
Acquired:
pes not elsewhere classified
talipes not elsewhere classified

⑤ **736.8 Acquired deformities of other parts of limbs**

736.81 Unequal leg length (acquired)

736.89 Other
Deformity (acquired):
arm or leg, not elsewhere classified
shoulder

736.9 Acquired deformity of limb, site unspecified

737 Curvature of spine
Excludes: congenital (754.2)

737.0 Adolescent postural kyphosis
Excludes: osteochondrosis of spine (juvenile) (732.0)
adult (732.8)

⑤ **737.1 Kyphosis (acquired)**

737.10 Kyphosis (acquired) (postural)

737.11 Kyphosis due to radiation

737.12 Kyphosis, postlaminectomy

737.19 Other
Excludes: that associated with conditions classifiable elsewhere (737.41)

⑤ **737.2 Lordosis (acquired)**

737.20 Lordosis (acquired) (postural)

737.21 Lordosis, postlaminectomy

737.22 Other postsurgical lordosis

737.29 Other
Excludes: that associated with conditions classifiable elsewhere (737.42)

⑤ **737.3 Kyphoscoliosis and scoliosis**

737.30 Scoliosis [and kyphoscoliosis], idiopathic

737.31 Resolving infantile idiopathic scoliosis

737.32 Progressive infantile idiopathic scoliosis

737.33 Scoliosis due to radiation

737.34 Thoracogenic scoliosis

737.39 Other
Excludes: that associated with conditions classifiable elsewhere (737.43)
that in kyphoscoliotic heart disease (416.1)

⑤ **737.4 Curvature of spine associated with other conditions**
Code first associated condition, as:
Charcot-Marie-Tooth disease (356.1)
mucopolysaccharidosis (277.5)
neurofibromatosis (237.7)
osteitis deformans (731.0)
osteitis fibrosa cystica (252.01)
osteoporosis (733.00-733.09)
poliomyelitis (138)
tuberculosis [Pott's curvature] (015.0)

737.40 Curvature of spine, unspecified

737.41 Kyphosis

737.42 Lordosis

737.43 Scoliosis

737.8 Other curvatures of spine

737.9 Unspecified curvature of spine
Curvature of spine (acquired) (idiopathic) NOS
Hunchback, acquired
Excludes: deformity of spine NOS (738.5)

MUSCULOSKELETAL SYSTEM AND CONNECTIVE TISSUE

738 Other acquired deformity
  Excludes: congenital (754.0-756.9, 758.0-759.9)
  dentofacial anomalies (524.0-524.9)

  738.0 Acquired deformity of nose
    Deformity of nose (acquired)
    Overdevelopment of nasal bones
   Excludes: deflected or deviated nasal septum (470)

  ⑤ **738.1 Other acquired deformity of head**
    738.10 Unspecified deformity
    738.11 Zygomatic hyperplasia
    738.12 Zygomatic hypoplasia
    738.19 Other specified deformity

  738.2 Acquired deformity of neck

  738.3 Acquired deformity of chest and rib
    Deformity: Pectus:
      chest (acquired)   carinatum, acquired
      rib (acquired)   excavatum, acquired

  738.4 Acquired spondylolisthesis
    Degenerative spondylolisthesis
    Spondylolysis, acquired
   Excludes: congenital (756.12)

  738.5 Other acquired deformity of back or spine
    Deformity of spine NOS
   Excludes: curvature of spine (737.0-737.9)

  738.6 Acquired deformity of pelvis
    Pelvic obliquity
   Excludes: intrapelvic protrusion of acetabulum (718.6)
     that in relation to labor and delivery (653.0-653.4, 653.8-653.9)

  738.7 Cauliflower ear

  738.8 Acquired deformity of other specified site
    Deformity of clavicle

  738.9 Acquired deformity of unspecified site

739 Nonallopathic lesions, not elsewhere classified
  Includes: segmental dysfunction
    somatic dysfunction

  739.0 Head region
    Occipitocervical region

  739.1 Cervical region
    Cervicothoracic region

  739.2 Thoracic region
    Thoracolumbar region

  739.3 Lumbar region
    Lumbosacral region

  739.4 Sacral region
    Sacrococcygeal region
    Sacroiliac region

  739.5 Pelvic region
    Hip region
    Pubic region

  739.6 Lower extremities

  739.7 Upper extremities
    Acromioclavicular region
    Sternoclavicular region

  739.8 Rib cage
    Costochondral region   Sternochondral region
    Costovertebral region

  739.9 Abdomen and other

TABULAR LIST

CONGENITAL ANOMALIES

14. CONGENITAL ANOMALIES (740-759)

740 Anencephalus and similar anomalies

740.0 Anencephalus
Acrania
Amyelencephalus
Hemianencephaly
Hemicephaly

740.1 Craniorachischisis

740.2 Iniencephaly

⑤ 741 Spina bifida

Excludes: spina bifida occulta (756.17)

The following fifth-digit subclassification is for use with category 741:

0 unspecified region
1 cervical region
2 dorsal [thoracic] region
3 lumbar region

⑤ 741.0 With hydrocephalus
Arnold-Chiari syndrome, type II
Any condition classifiable to 741.9 with any condition classifiable to 742.3
Chiari malformation, type II

⑤ 741.9 Without mention of hydrocephalus
Hydromeningocele (spinal)
Hydromyelocele
Meningocele (spinal)
Meningomyelocele
Myelocele
Myelocystocele
Rachischisis
Spina bifida (aperta)
Syringomyelocele

742 Other congenital anomalies of nervous system

Excludes: congenital central alveolar hypoventilation syndrome (327.25)

742.0 Encephalocele
Encephalocystocele
Encephalomyelocele
Hydroencephalocele
Hydromeningocele, cranial
Meningocele, cerebral
Meningoencephalocele

742.1 Microcephalus
Hydromicrocephaly
Micrencephaly

742.2 Reduction deformities of brain
Absence of part of brain
Agenesis of part of brain
Agyria
Aplasia of part of brain
Arhinencephaly
Hypoplasia of part of brain
Holoprosencephaly
Microgyria

742.3 Congenital hydrocephalus
Aqueduct of Sylvius:
  anomaly
  obstruction, congenital
  stenosis
Atresia of foramina of Magendie and Luschka
Hydrocephalus in newborn

Excludes: hydrocephalus:
  acquired (331.3-331.4)
  due to congenital toxoplasmosis (771.2)
  with any condition classifiable to 741.9 (741.0)

742.4 Other specified anomalies of brain
Congenital cerebral cyst
Macroencephaly
Macrogyria
Megalencephaly
Multiple anomalies of brain NOS
Porencephaly
Ulegyria

⑤ 742.5 Other specified anomalies of spinal cord

742.51 Diastematomyelia

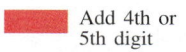 Add 4th or 5th digit
 Nonspecific code
 Unspecified code
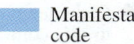 Manifestation code

491

TABULAR LIST

742.53 Hydromyelia
Hydrorhachis

742.59 Other
Amyelia
Atelomyelia
Congenital anomaly of spinal meninges
Defective development of cauda equina
Hypoplasia of spinal cord
Myelatelia
Myelodysplasia

742.8 Other specified anomalies of nervous system
Agenesis of nerve
Displacement of brachial
  plexus
Familial dysautonomia
Jaw-winking syndrome
Marcus-Gunn syndrome
Riley-Day syndrome

Excludes: neurofibromatosis (237.7)

742.9 Unspecified anomaly of brain, spinal cord, and nervous system
Anomaly of brain, nervous system, and spinal cord
Congenital:
  disease of brain, nervous system, and spinal cord
  lesion of brain, nervous system, and spinal cord
Deformity of brain, nervous system, and spinal cord

743 Congenital anomalies of eye

743.0 Anophthalmos

743.00 Clinical anophthalmos, unspecified
Agenesis of eye
Congenital absence of eye
Anophthalmos NOS

743.03 Cystic eyeball, congenital

743.06 Cryptophthalmos

743.1 Microphthalmos
Dysplasia of eye
Hypoplasia of eye
Rudimentary eye

743.10 Microphthalmos, unspecified

743.11 Simple microphthalmos

743.12 Microphthalmos associated with other anomalies of eye and adnexa

743.2 Buphthalmos
Glaucoma:
  congenital
  newborn
Hydrophthalmos

Excludes: glaucoma of childhood (365.14)
         traumatic glaucoma due to birth injury (767.8)

743.20 Buphthalmos, unspecified

743.21 Simple buphthalmos

743.22 Buphthalmos associated with other ocular anomalies
Keratoglobus, congenital associated with buphthalmos
Megalocornea associated with buphthalmos

743.3 Congenital cataract and lens anomalies

Excludes: infantile cataract (366.00-366.09)

743.30 Congenital cataract, unspecified

743.31 Capsular and subcapsular cataract

743.32 Cortical and zonular cataract

743.33 Nuclear cataract

743.34 Total and subtotal cataract, congenital

743.35 Congenital aphakia
Congenital absence of lens

743.36 Anomalies of lens shape
Microphakia
Spherophakia

743.37 Congenital ectopic lens

CONGENITAL ANOMALIES

- **743.39** Other
- ⑤ **743.4** Coloboma and other anomalies of anterior segment
  - **743.41** Anomalies of corneal size and shape
    - Microcornea
    - *Excludes:* *that associated with buphthalmos (743.22)*
  - **743.42** Corneal opacities, interfering with vision, congenital
  - **743.43** Other corneal opacities, congenital
  - **743.44** Specified anomalies of anterior chamber, chamber angle, and related structures
    - Anomaly:
      - Axenfeld's
      - Peters'
      - Rieger's
  - **743.45** Aniridia
  - **743.46** Other specified anomalies of iris and ciliary body
    - Anisocoria, congenital
    - Atresia of pupil
    - Coloboma of iris
    - Corectopia
  - **743.47** Specified anomalies of sclera
  - **743.48** Multiple and combined anomalies of anterior segment
  - **743.49** Other
- ⑤ **743.5** Congenital anomalies of posterior segment
  - **743.51** Vitreous anomalies
    - Congenital vitreous opacity
  - **743.52** Fundus coloboma
  - **743.53** Chorioretinal degeneration, congenital
  - **743.54** Congenital folds and cysts of posterior segment
  - **743.55** Congenital macular changes
  - **743.56** Other retinal changes, congenital
  - **743.57** Specified anomalies of optic disc
    - Coloboma of optic disc (congenital)
  - **743.58** Vascular anomalies
    - Congenital retinal aneurysm
  - **743.59** Other
- ⑤ **743.6** Congenital anomalies of eyelids, lacrimal system, and orbit
  - **743.61** Congenital ptosis
  - **743.62** Congenital deformities of eyelids
    - Ablepharon
    - Absence of eyelid
    - Accessory eyelid
    - Congenital:
      - ectropion
      - entropion
  - **743.63** Other specified congenital anomalies of eyelid
    - Absence, agenesis, of cilia
  - **743.64** Specified congenital anomalies of lacrimal gland
  - **743.65** Specified congenital anomalies of lacrimal passages
    - Absence, agenesis of:
      - lacrimal apparatus
      - punctum lacrimale
    - Accessory lacrimal canal
  - **743.66** Specified congenital anomalies of orbit
  - **743.69** Other
    - Accessory eye muscles
- **743.8** Other specified anomalies of eye
  - *Excludes:* *congenital nystagmus (379.51)*
    - *ocular albinism (270.2)*
    - *optic nerve hypoplasia (377.43)*
    - *retinitis pigmentosa (362.74)*

743.9 Unspecified anomaly of eye
Congenital:
anomaly NOS of eye [any part]
deformity NOS of eye [any part]

744 Congenital anomalies of ear, face, and neck

Excludes: anomaly of:
cervical spine (754.2, 756.10-756.19)
larynx (748.2-748.3)
nose (748.0-748.1)
parathyroid gland (759.2)
thyroid gland (759.2)
cleft lip (749.10-749.25)

⑤ **744.0 Anomalies of ear causing impairment of hearing**

Excludes: congenital deafness without mention of cause (389.0-389.9)

744.00 Unspecified anomaly of ear with impairment of hearing

744.01 Absence of external ear
Absence of:
auditory canal (external)
auricle (ear) (with stenosis or atresia of auditory canal)

744.02 Other anomalies of external ear with impairment of hearing
Atresia or stricture of auditory canal (external)

744.03 Anomaly of middle ear, except ossicles
Atresia or stricture of osseous meatus (ear)

744.04 Anomalies of ear ossicles
Fusion of ear ossicles

744.05 Anomalies of inner ear
Congenital anomaly of:
membranous labyrinth
organ of Corti

744.09 Other
Absence of ear, congenital

744.1 Accessory auricle
Accessory tragus   Supernumerary:
Polyotia   ear
Preauricular appendage   lobule

⑤ **744.2 Other specified anomalies of ear**

Excludes: that with impairment of hearing (744.00-744.09)

744.21 Absence of ear lobe, congenital

744.22 Macrotia

744.23 Microtia

744.24 Specified anomalies of Eustachian tube
Absence of Eustachian tube

744.29 Other
Bat ear   Prominence of auricle
Darwin's tubercle   Ridge ear
Pointed ear

Excludes: preauricular sinus (744.46)

744.3 Unspecified anomaly of ear
Congenital:
anomaly NOS of ear, not elsewhere classified
deformity NOS of ear, not elsewhere classified

⑤ **744.4 Branchial cleft cyst or fistula; preauricular sinus**

744.41 Branchial cleft sinus or fistula
Branchial:
sinus (external) (internal)
vestige

744.42 Branchial cleft cyst

744.43 Cervical auricle

744.46 Preauricular sinus or fistula

744.47 Preauricular cyst

CONGENITAL ANOMALIES

744.49 Other
   Fistula (of):
      auricle, congenital
      cervicoaural

744.5 Webbing of neck
   Pterygium colli

⑤ **744.8 Other specified anomalies of face and neck**

   744.81 Macrocheilia
      Hypertrophy of lip, congenital

   744.82 Microcheilia

   744.83 Macrostomia

   744.84 Microstomia

   744.89 Other

   Excludes: *congenital fistula of lip (750.25)*
              musculoskeletal anomalies (754.0-754.1, 756.0)

744.9 Unspecified anomalies of face and neck
   Congenital:
      anomaly NOS of face [any part] or neck [any part]
      deformity NOS of face [any part] or neck [any part]

745 Bulbus cordis anomalies and anomalies of cardiac septal closure

   745.0 Common truncus
      Absent septum between aorta and pulmonary artery
      Communication (abnormal) between aorta and pulmonary artery
      Aortic septal defect
      Common aortopulmonary trunk
      Persistent truncus arteriosus

   ⑤ **745.1 Transposition of great vessels**

      745.10 Complete transposition of great vessels
         Transposition of great vessels:
            NOS
            classical

      745.11 Double outlet right ventricle
         Dextratransposition of aorta
         Incomplete transposition of great vessels
         Origin of both great vessels from right ventricle
         Taussig-Bing syndrome or defect

      745.12 Corrected transposition of great vessels

      745.19 Other

   745.2 Tetralogy of Fallot
      Fallot's pentalogy
      Ventricular septal defect with pulmonary stenosis or atresia, dextraposition of aorta, and
         hypertrophy of right ventricle

      Excludes: *Fallot's triad (746.09)*

   745.3 Common ventricle
      Cor triloculare biatriatum
      Single ventricle

   745.4 Ventricular septal defect
      Eisenmenger's defect or complex
      Gerbode defect
      Interventricular septal defect
      Left ventricular-right atrial communication
      Roger's disease

      Excludes: *common atrioventricular canal type (745.69)*
                 single ventricle (745.3)

   745.5 Ostium secundum type atrial septal defect
      Defect: Patent or persistent:
         atrium secundum   foramen ovale
         fossa ovalis   ostium secundum
      Lutembacher's syndrome

   ⑤ **745.6 Endocardial cushion defects**

      745.60 Endocardial cushion defect, unspecified type

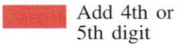 Add 4th or 5th digit
 Nonspecific code
 Unspecified code
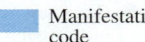 Manifestation code

495

TABULAR LIST

745.61 Ostium primum defect
Persistent ostium primum

745.69 Other
Absence of atrial septum
Atrioventricular canal type ventricular septal defect
Common atrioventricular canal
Common atrium

745.7 Cor biloculare
Absence of atrial and ventricular septa

745.8 Other

745.9 Unspecified defect of septal closure
Septal defect NOS

746 Other congenital anomalies of heart
Excludes: endocardial fibroelastosis (425.3)

746.0 Anomalies of pulmonary valve
Excludes: infundibular or subvalvular pulmonic stenosis (746.83)
tetralogy of Fallot (745.2)

746.00 Pulmonary valve anomaly, unspecified

746.01 Atresia, congenital
Congenital absence of pulmonary valve

746.02 Stenosis, congenital

746.09 Other
Congenital insufficiency of pulmonary valve
Fallot's triad or trilogy

746.1 Tricuspid atresia and stenosis, congenital
Absence of tricuspid valve

746.2 Ebstein's anomaly

746.3 Congenital stenosis of aortic valve
Congenital aortic stenosis
Excludes: congenital:
subaortic stenosis (746.81)
supravalvular aortic stenosis (747.22)

746.4 Congenital insufficiency of aortic valve
Bicuspid aortic valve
Congenital aortic insufficiency

746.5 Congenital mitral stenosis
Fused commissure of mitral valve
Parachute deformity of mitral valve
Supernumerary cusps of mitral valve

746.6 Congenital mitral insufficiency

746.7 Hypoplastic left heart syndrome
Atresia, or marked hypoplasia, of aortic orifice or valve, with hypoplasia of ascending aorta and defective development of left ventricle (with mitral valve atresia)

746.8 Other specified anomalies of heart

746.81 Subaortic stenosis

746.82 Cor triatriatum

746.83 Infundibular pulmonic stenosis
Subvalvular pulmonic stenosis

746.84 Obstructive anomalies of heart, not elsewhere classified
Uhl's disease

746.85 Coronary artery anomaly
Anomalous origin or communication of coronary artery
Arteriovenous malformation of coronary artery
Coronary artery:
absence
arising from aorta or pulmonary trunk
single

746.86 Congenital heart block
Complete or incomplete atrioventricular [AV] block

CONGENITAL ANOMALIES

746.87 Malposition of heart and cardiac apex
Abdominal heart   Levocardia (isolated)
Dextrocardia   Mesocardia
Ectopia cordis

Excludes: *dextrocardia with complete transposition of viscera (759.3)*

746.89 Other
Atresia of cardiac vein
Hypoplasia of cardiac vein
Congenital:
  cardiomegaly
  diverticulum, left ventricle
  pericardial defect

746.9 Unspecified anomaly of heart
Congenital:
  anomaly of heart NOS
  heart disease NOS

747 Other congenital anomalies of circulatory system

747.0 Patent ductus arteriosus
Patent ductus Botalli
Persistent ductus arteriosus

747.1 Coarctation of aorta

747.10 Coarctation of aorta (preductal) (postductal)
Hypoplasia of aortic arch

747.11 Interruption of aortic arch

747.2 Other anomalies of aorta

747.20 Anomaly of aorta, unspecified

747.21 Anomalies of aortic arch
Anomalous origin, right subclavian artery
Dextraposition of aorta
Double aortic arch
Kommerell's diverticulum
Overriding aorta
Persistent:
  convolutions, aortic arch
  right aortic arch
Vascular ring

Excludes: *hypoplasia of aortic arch (747.10)*

747.22 Atresia and stenosis of aorta
Absence of aorta
Aplasia of aorta
Hypoplasia of aorta
Stricture of aorta
Supra (valvular)-aortic stenosis

Excludes: *congenital aortic (valvular) stenosis or stricture, so stated (746.3)*
hypoplasia of aorta in hypoplastic left heart syndrome (746.7)

747.29 Other
Aneurysm of sinus of Valsalva
Congenital:
  aneurysm of aorta
  dilation of aorta

747.3 Anomalies of pulmonary artery
Agenesis of pulmonary artery
Anomaly of pulmonary artery
Atresia of pulmonary artery
Coarctation of pulmonary artery
Hypoplasia of pulmonary artery
Stenosis of pulmonary artery
Pulmonary arteriovenous aneurysm

747.4 Anomalies of great veins

747.40 Anomaly of great veins, unspecified
Anomaly NOS of:
  pulmonary veins
  vena cava

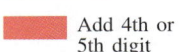 Add 4th or 5th digit   Nonspecific code   Unspecified code   Manifestation code

TABULAR LIST

- **747.41 Total anomalous pulmonary venous connection**
  Total anomalous pulmonary venous return [TAPVR]:
  - subdiaphragmatic
  - supradiaphragmatic

- **747.42 Partial anomalous pulmonary venous connection**
  Partial anomalous pulmonary venous return

- **747.49 Other anomalies of great veins**
  Absence of vena cava (inferior) (superior)
  Congenital stenosis of vena cava (inferior) (superior)
  Persistent:
  - left posterior cardinal vein
  - left superior vena cava
  Scimitar syndrome
  Transposition of pulmonary veins NOS

747.5 Absence or hypoplasia of umbilical artery
  Single umbilical artery

⑤ **747.6 Other anomalies of peripheral vascular system**
  Absence of artery or vein, not elsewhere classified
  Anomaly of artery or vein, not elsewhere classified
  Atresia of artery or vein, not elsewhere classified
  Arteriovenous aneurysm (peripheral)
  Arteriovenous malformation of the peripheral vascular system
  Congenital:
  - aneurysm (peripheral)
  - phlebectasia
  - stricture, artery
  - varix
  Multiple renal arteries

  Excludes: anomalies of:
  - cerebral vessels (747.81)
  - pulmonary artery (747.3)
  - congenital retinal aneurysm (743.58)
  - hemangioma (228.00-228.09)
  - lymphangioma (228.1)

- **747.60 Anomaly of the peripheral vascular system, unspecified site**
- **747.61 Gastrointestinal vessel anomaly**
- **747.62 Renal vessel anomaly**
- **747.63 Upper limb vessel anomaly**
- **747.64 Lower limb vessel anomaly**
- **747.69 Anomalies of other specified sites of peripheral vascular system**

⑤ **747.8 Other specified anomalies of circulatory system**

- **747.81 Anomalies of cerebrovascular system**
  Arteriovenous malformation of brain
  Cerebral arteriovenous aneurysm, congenital
  Congenital anomalies of cerebral vessels

  Excludes: ruptured cerebral (arteriovenous) aneurysm (430)

- **747.82 Spinal vessel anomaly**
  Arteriovenous malformation of spinal vessel

- **747.83 Persistent fetal circulation**
  Persistent pulmonary hypertension
  Primary pulmonary hypertension of newborn

- **747.89 Other**
  Aneurysm, congenital, specified site not elsewhere classified

  Excludes: congenital aneurysm:
  - coronary (746.85)
  - peripheral (747.6)
  - pulmonary (747.3)
  - retinal (743.58)

747.9 Unspecified anomaly of circulatory system

748 Congenital anomalies of respiratory system

  Excludes: congenital central alveolar hypoventilation syndrome (327.25)
  congenital defect of diaphragm (756.6)

CONGENITAL ANOMALIES

748.0 Choanal atresia
Atresia of nares (anterior) (posterior)
Congenital stenosis of nares (anterior) (posterior)

748.1 Other anomalies of nose
Absent nose
Accessory nose
Cleft nose
Deformity of wall of nasal sinus

Congenital:
deformity of nose
notching of tip of nose
perforation of wall of nasal sinus

Excludes: congenital deviation of nasal septum (754.0)

748.2 Web of larynx
Web of larynx:
NOS
glottic
subglottic

748.3 Other anomalies of larynx, trachea, and bronchus
Absence or agenesis of:
bronchus
larynx
trachea
Anomaly (of):
cricoid cartilage
epiglottis
thyroid cartilage
tracheal cartilage
Atresia (of):
epiglottis
glottis
larynx
trachea
Cleft thyroid, cartilage, congenital

Congenital:
dilation, trachea
stenosis:
larynx
trachea
tracheocele
Diverticulum:
bronchus
trachea
Fissure of epiglottis
Laryngocele
Posterior cleft of cricoid cartilage (congenital)
Rudimentary tracheal bronchus
Stridor, laryngeal, congenital

748.4 Congenital cystic lung
Disease, lung:
cystic, congenital
polycystic, congenital

Honeycomb lung, congenital

Excludes: acquired or unspecified cystic lung (518.89)

748.5 Agenesis, hypoplasia, and dysplasia of lung
Absence of lung (fissures) (lobe)
Aplasia of lung
Hypoplasia of lung (lobe)
Sequestration of lung

⑤ **748.6 Other anomalies of lung**

748.60 Anomaly of lung, unspecified

748.61 Congenital bronchiectasis

748.69 Other
Accessory lung (lobe)
Azygos lobe (fissure), lung

748.8 Other specified anomalies of respiratory system
Abnormal communication between pericardial and pleural sacs
Anomaly, pleural folds
Atresia of nasopharynx
Congenital cyst of mediastinum

748.9 Unspecified anomaly of respiratory system
Anomaly of respiratory system NOS

749 Cleft palate and cleft lip

⑤ **749.0 Cleft palate**

749.00 Cleft palate, unspecified

749.01 Unilateral, complete

749.02 Unilateral, incomplete
Cleft uvula

749.03 Bilateral, complete

749.04 Bilateral, incomplete

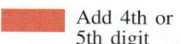 Add 4th or 5th digit
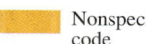 Nonspecific code
Unspecified code
Manifestation code

499

TABULAR LIST

- ⑤ **749.1 Cleft lip**
  Cheiloschisis
  Congenital fissure of lip
  Harelip
  Labium leporinum
  - **749.10** Cleft lip, unspecified
  - 749.11 Unilateral, complete
  - 749.12 Unilateral, incomplete
  - 749.13 Bilateral, complete
  - 749.14 Bilateral, incomplete

- ⑤ **749.2 Cleft palate with cleft lip**
  Cheilopalatoschisis
  - **749.20** Cleft palate with cleft lip, unspecified
  - 749.21 Unilateral, complete
  - 749.22 Unilateral, incomplete
  - 749.23 Bilateral, complete
  - 749.24 Bilateral, incomplete
  - **749.25** Other combinations

750 Other congenital anomalies of upper alimentary tract
Excludes: dentofacial anomalies (524.0-524.9)

- **750.0 Tongue tie**
  Ankyloglossia

- ⑤ **750.1 Other anomalies of tongue**
  - **750.10** Anomaly of tongue, unspecified
  - 750.11 Aglossia
  - 750.12 Congenital adhesions of tongue
  - 750.13 Fissure of tongue
    Bifid tongue
    Double tongue
  - 750.15 Macroglossia
    Congenital hypertrophy of tongue
  - 750.16 Microglossia
    Hypoplasia of tongue
  - **750.19** Other

- ⑤ **750.2 Other specified anomalies of mouth and pharynx**
  - 750.21 Absence of salivary gland
  - 750.22 Accessory salivary gland
  - 750.23 Atresia, salivary duct
    Imperforate salivary duct
  - 750.24 Congenital fistula of salivary gland
  - 750.25 Congenital fistula of lip
    Congenital (mucus) lip pits
  - **750.26** Other specified anomalies of mouth
    Absence of uvula
  - 750.27 Diverticulum of pharynx
    Pharyngeal pouch
  - **750.29** Other specified anomalies of pharynx
    Imperforate pharynx

- **750.3 Tracheoesophageal fistula, esophageal atresia and stenosis**
  Absent esophagus
  Atresia of esophagus
  Congenital:
    esophageal ring
    stenosis of esophagus
    stricture of esophagus
  Congenital fistula:
    esophagobronchial
    esophagotracheal
  Imperforate esophagus
  Webbed esophagus

CONGENITAL ANOMALIES

750.4 Other specified anomalies of esophagus
　　Dilatation, congenital (of) esophagus
　　Displacement, congenital (of) esophagus
　　Diverticulum (of) esophagus
　　Duplication (of) esophagus
　　Giant esophagus
　　Esophageal pouch
　Excludes: congenital hiatus hernia (750.6)

750.5 Congenital hypertrophic pyloric stenosis
　　Congenital or infantile:
　　　constriction of pylorus
　　　hypertrophy of pylorus
　　　spasm of pylorus
　　　stenosis of pylorus
　　　stricture of pylorus

750.6 Congenital hiatus hernia
　　Displacement of cardia through esophageal hiatus
　Excludes: congenital diaphragmatic hernia (756.6)

750.7 Other specified anomalies of stomach
　　Congenital:　　　　　　　Duplication of stomach
　　　cardiospasm　　　　　　Megalogastria
　　　hourglass stomach　　　Microgastria
　　Displacement of stomach　Transposition of stomach
　　Diverticulum of stomach,
　　　congenital

750.8 Other specified anomalies of upper alimentary tract

750.9 Unspecified anomaly of upper alimentary tract
　　Congenital:
　　　anomaly NOS of upper alimentary tract [any part, except tongue]
　　　deformity NOS of upper alimentary tract [any part, except tongue]

751 Other congenital anomalies of digestive system

751.0 Meckel's diverticulum
　　Meckel's diverticulum (displaced) (hypertrophic)
　　Persistent:
　　　omphalomesenteric duct
　　　vitelline duct

751.1 Atresia and stenosis of small intestine
　　Atresia of:
　　　duodenum
　　　ileum
　　　intestine NOS
　　Congenital:
　　　absence of small intestine or intestine NOS
　　　obstruction of small intestine or intestine NOS
　　　stenosis of small intestine or intestine NOS
　　　stricture of small intestine or intestine NOS
　　Imperforate jejunum

751.2 Atresia and stenosis of large intestine, rectum, and anal canal
　　Absence:　　　　　　　　Congenital or infantile:
　　　anus (congenital)　　　　obstruction of large intestine
　　　appendix, congenital　　　occlusion of anus
　　　large intestine, congenital　stricture of anus
　　　rectum　　　　　　　　Imperforate:
　　Atresia of:　　　　　　　　anus
　　　anus　　　　　　　　　　rectum
　　　colon　　　　　　　　Stricture of rectum, congenital
　　　rectum

751.3 Hirschsprung's disease and other congenital functional disorders of colon
　　Aganglionosis　　　　　Congenital megacolon
　　Congenital dilation of colon　Macrocolon

751.4 Anomalies of intestinal fixation
　　Congenital adhesions:　　Rotation of cecum or colon:
　　　omental, anomalous　　　failure of
　　　peritoneal　　　　　　　incomplete
　　Jackson's membrane　　　insufficient
　　Malrotation of colon　　　Universal mesentery

TABULAR LIST

751.5 Other anomalies of intestine
Congenital diverticulum, colon
Dolichocolon
Duplication of:
    anus
    appendix
    cecum
    intestine
Ectopic anus
Megaloappendix
Megaloduodenum
Microcolon
Persistent cloaca
Transposition of:
    appendix
    colon
    intestine

⑤ **751.6 Anomalies of gallbladder, bile ducts, and liver**

751.60 Unspecified anomaly of gallbladder, bile ducts, and liver

751.61 Biliary atresia
Congenital:
    absence of bile duct (common) or passage
    hypoplasia of bile duct (common) or passage
    obstruction of bile duct (common) or passage
    stricture of bile duct (common) or passage

751.62 Congenital cystic disease of liver
Congenital polycystic disease of liver
Fibrocystic disease of liver

751.69 Other anomalies of gallbladder, bile ducts, and liver
Absence of:
    gallbladder, congenital
    liver (lobe)
Accessory:
    hepatic ducts
    liver
Congenital:
    choledochal cyst
    hepatomegaly
Duplication of:
    biliary duct
    cystic duct
    gallbladder
    liver
Floating:
    gallbladder
    liver
Intrahepatic gallbladder

751.7 Anomalies of pancreas
Absence of pancreas
Accessory pancreas
Agenesis of pancreas
Annular pancreas
Ectopic pancreatic tissue
Hypoplasia of pancreas
Pancreatic heterotopia

Excludes: diabetes mellitus:
        congenital (250.0-250.9)
        neonatal (775.1)
    fibrocystic disease of pancreas (277.00-277.09)

751.8 Other specified anomalies of digestive system
Absence (complete) (partial) of alimentary tract NOS
Duplication of digestive organs NOS
Malposition, congenital of digestive organs NOS

Excludes: congenital diaphragmatic hernia (756.6)
    congenital hiatus hernia (750.6)

751.9 Unspecified anomaly of digestive system
Congenital:
    anomaly NOS of digestive system NOS
    deformity NOS of digestive system NOS

752 Congenital anomalies of genital organs

Excludes: syndromes associated with anomalies in the number and form of chromosomes (758.0-758.9)
    testicular feminization syndrome (259.5)

752.0 Anomalies of ovaries
Absence, congenital (of) ovary
Accessory ovary
Ectopic ovary
Streak of ovary

⑤ **752.1 Anomalies of fallopian tubes and broad ligaments**

752.10 Unspecified anomaly of fallopian tubes and broad ligaments

CONGENITAL ANOMALIES

- **752.11 Embryonic cyst of fallopian tubes and broad ligaments**
  Cyst:
    epoophoron
    fimbrial
    parovarian
- **752.19 Other**
  Absence of fallopian tube or broad ligament
  Accessory fallopian tube or broad ligament
  Atresia of fallopian tube or broad ligament

752.2 Doubling of uterus
  Didelphic uterus
  Doubling of uterus [any degree] (associated with doubling of cervix and vagina)

752.3 Other anomalies of uterus
  Absence, congenital, of uterus
  Agenesis of uterus
  Aplasia of uterus
  Bicornuate uterus
  Uterus unicornis
  Uterus with only one functioning horn

⑤ **752.4 Anomalies of cervix, vagina, and external female genitalia**
- **752.40 Unspecified anomaly of cervix, vagina, and external female genitalia**
- **752.41 Embryonic cyst of cervix, vagina, and external female genitalia**
  Cyst of: Cyst of:
    canal of Nuck, congenital   vagina, embryonal
    Gartner's duct   vulva, congenital
- **752.42 Imperforate hymen**
- **752.49 Other anomalies of cervix, vagina, and external female genitalia**
  Absence of cervix, clitoris, vagina, or vulva
  Agenesis of cervix, clitoris, vagina, or vulva
  Congenital stenosis or stricture of:
    cervical canal
    vagina

  Excludes: double vagina associated with total duplication (752.2)

⑤ **752.5 Undescended and retractile testicle**
- **752.51 Undescended testis**
  Cryptorchism
  Ectopic testis
- **752.52 Retractile testis**

⑤ **752.6 Hypospadias and epispadias and other penile anomalies**
- **752.61 Hypospadias**
- **752.62 Epispadias**
  Anaspadias
- **752.63 Congenital chordee**
- **752.64 Micropenis**
- **752.65 Hidden penis**
- **752.69 Other penile anomalies**

752.7 Indeterminate sex and pseudohermaphroditism
  Gynandrism   Pseudohermaphroditism (male) (female)
  Hermaphroditism   Pure gonadal dysgenesis
  Ovotestis

  Excludes: pseudohermaphroditism:
    female, with adrenocortical disorder (255.2)
    male, with gonadal disorder (257.8)
    with specified chromosomal anomaly (758.0-758.9)
    testicular feminization syndrome (259.5)

⑤ **752.8 Other specified anomalies of genital organs**
  Excludes: congenital hydrocele (778.6)
    penile anomalies (752.61-752.69)
    phimosis or paraphimosis (605)

- **752.81 Scrotal transposition**

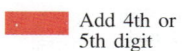 Add 4th or 5th digit   Nonspecific code   Unspecified code   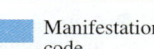 Manifestation code

503

TABULAR LIST

752.89 **Other specified anomalies of genital organs**
Absence of:
  prostate
  spermatic cord
  vas deferens
Anorchism
Aplasia (congenital) of:
  prostate
  round ligament
  testicle
Atresia of:
  ejaculatory duct
  vas deferens
Fusion of testes
Hypoplasia of testes
Monorchism
Polyorchism

752.9 **Unspecified anomaly of genital organs**
Congenital:
  anomaly NOS of genital organ, NEC
  deformity NOS of genital organ, NEC

753 Congenital anomalies of urinary system

753.0 **Renal agenesis and dysgenesis**
Atrophy of kidney: Congenital absence of kidney(s)
  congenital   Hypoplasia of kidney(s)
  infantile

⑤ **753.1** **Cystic kidney disease**
Excludes: acquired cyst of kidney (593.2)

  753.10 Cystic kidney disease, unspecified
  753.11 Congenital single renal cyst
  753.12 Polycystic kidney, unspecified type
  753.13 Polycystic kidney, autosomal dominant
  753.14 Polycystic kidney, autosomal recessive
  753.15 Renal dysplasia
  753.16 Medullary cystic kidney
    Nephronopthisis
  753.17 Medullary sponge kidney
  753.19 Other specified cystic kidney disease
    Multicystic kidney

⑤ **753.2** **Obstructive defects of renal pelvis and ureter**

  753.20 Unspecified obstructive defect of renal pelvis and ureter
  753.21 Congenital obstruction of ureteropelvic junction
  753.22 Congenital obstruction of ureterovesical junction
    Adynamic ureter
    Congenital hydroureter
  753.23 Congenital ureterocele
  753.29 Other

753.3 **Other specified anomalies of kidney**
Accessory kidney   Fusion of kidneys
Congenital: Giant kidney
  calculus of kidney   Horseshoe kidney
  displaced kidney   Hyperplasia of kidney
Discoid kidney   Lobulation of kidney
Double kidney with double   Malrotation of kidney
  pelvis   Trifid kidney (pelvis)
Ectopic kidney

753.4 **Other specified anomalies of ureter**
Absent ureter   Double ureter
Accessory ureter   Ectopic ureter
Deviation of ureter   Implantation, anomalous of ureter
Displaced ureteric orifice

753.5 **Exstrophy of urinary bladder**
Ectopia vesicae   Extroversion of bladder

504 ● Code new to this edition   ▲ Revision of existing code   ④ ⑤ Fourth or fifth digit required

CONGENITAL ANOMALIES

753.6 Atresia and stenosis of urethra and bladder neck
  Congenital obstruction: Imperforate urinary meatus
    bladder neck   Impervious urethra
    urethra   Urethral valve formation
  Congenital stricture of:
    urethra (valvular)
    urinary meatus
    vesicourethral orifice

753.7 Anomalies of urachus
  Cyst (of) urachus   Persistent umbilical sinus
  Fistula (of) urachus
  Patent (of) urachus

753.8 Other specified anomalies of bladder and urethra
  Absence, congenital of: Congenital urethrorectal fistula
    bladder   Congenital prolapse of:
    urethra   bladder (mucosa)
  Accessory: urethra
    bladder   Double:
    urethra   urethra
  Congenital: urinary meatus
    diverticulum of bladder
    hernia of bladder

753.9 Unspecified anomaly of urinary system
  Congenital:
    anomaly NOS of urinary system [any part, except urachus]
    deformity NOS of urinary system [any part, except urachus]

754 Certain congenital musculoskeletal deformities
  Includes: nonteratogenic deformities which are considered to be due to intrauterine malposition and pressure

754.0 Of skull, face, and jaw
  Asymmetry of face   Dolichocephaly
  Compression facies   Plagiocephaly
  Depressions in skull   Potter's facies
  Deviation of nasal   Squashed or bent nose, congenital
    septum, congenital

  Excludes: dentofacial anomalies (524.0-524.9)
             syphilitic saddle nose (090.5)

754.1 Of sternocleidomastoid muscle
  Congenital sternomastoid torticollis
  Congenital wryneck
  Contracture of sternocleidomastoid (muscle)
  Sternomastoid tumor

754.2 Of spine
  Congenital postural:
    lordosis
    scoliosis

754.3 Congenital dislocation of hip

  754.30 Congenital dislocation of hip, unilateral
    Congenital dislocation of hip NOS

  754.31 Congenital dislocation of hip, bilateral

  754.32 Congenital subluxation of hip, unilateral
    Congenital flexion deformity, hip or thigh
    Predislocation status of hip at birth
    Preluxation of hip, congenital

  754.33 Congenital subluxation of hip, bilateral

  754.35 Congenital dislocation of one hip with subluxation of other hip

754.4 Congenital genu recurvatum and bowing of long bones of leg

  754.40 Genu recurvatum

  754.41 Congenital dislocation of knee (with genu recurvatum)

  754.42 Congenital bowing of femur

  754.43 Congenital bowing of tibia and fibula

  754.44 Congenital bowing of unspecified long bones of leg

TABULAR LIST

- ⑤ **754.5 Varus deformities of feet**
  - *Excludes:* acquired (736.71, 736.75, 736.79)
  - **754.50 Talipes varus**
    Congenital varus deformity of foot, unspecified
    Pes varus
  - **754.51 Talipes equinovarus**
    Equinovarus (congenital)
  - **754.52 Metatarsus primus varus**
  - **754.53 Metatarsus varus**
  - **754.59 Other**
    Talipes calcaneovarus

- ⑤ **754.6 Valgus deformities of feet**
  - *Excludes:* valgus deformity of foot (acquired) (736.79)
  - **754.60 Talipes valgus**
    Congenital valgus deformity of foot, unspecified
  - **754.61 Congenital pes planus**
    Congenital rocker bottom flat foot
    Flat foot, congenital
    - *Excludes:* pes planus (acquired) (734)
  - **754.62 Talipes calcaneovalgus**
  - **754.69 Other**
    Talipes:
       equinovalgus
       planovalgus

- ⑤ **754.7 Other deformities of feet**
  - *Excludes:* acquired (736.70-736.79)
  - **754.70 Talipes, unspecified**
    Congenital deformity of foot NOS
  - **754.71 Talipes cavus**
    Cavus foot (congenital)
  - **754.79 Other**
    Asymmetric talipes
    Talipes:
       calcaneus
       equinus

- ⑤ **754.8 Other specified nonteratogenic anomalies**
  - **754.81 Pectus excavatum**
    Congenital funnel chest
  - **754.82 Pectus carinatum**
    Congenital pigeon chest [breast]
  - **754.89 Other**
    Club hand (congenital)
    Congenital:
       deformity of chest wall
       dislocation of elbow
    Generalized flexion contractures of lower limb joints, congenital
    Spade-like hand (congenital)

- **755 Other congenital anomalies of limbs**
  - *Excludes:* those deformities classifiable to 754.0-754.8
  - ⑤ **755.0 Polydactyly**
    - **755.00 Polydactyly, unspecified digits**
      Supernumerary digits
    - **755.01 Of fingers**
      Accessory fingers
    - **755.02 Of toes**
      Accessory toes
  - ⑤ **755.1 Syndactyly**
    Symphalangy
    Webbing of digits
    - **755.10 Of multiple and unspecified sites**

CONGENITAL ANOMALIES

      755.11   Of fingers without fusion of bone
      755.12   Of fingers with fusion of bone
      755.13   Of toes without fusion of bone
      755.14   Of toes with fusion of bone

⑤ **755.2 Reduction deformities of upper limb**

      755.20   **Unspecified reduction deformity of upper limb**
                    Ectromelia NOS of upper limb
                    Hemimelia NOS of upper limb
                    Shortening of arm, congenital

      755.21   **Transverse deficiency of upper limb**
                    Amelia of upper limb
                    Congenital absence of:
                      fingers, all (complete or partial)
                      forearm, including hand and fingers
                      upper limb, complete
                    Congenital amputation of upper limb
                    Transverse hemimelia of upper limb

      755.22   **Longitudinal deficiency of upper limb, not elsewhere classified**
                    Phocomelia NOS of upper limb
                    Rudimentary arm

      755.23   **Longitudinal deficiency, combined, involving humerus, radius, and ulna (complete or incomplete)**
                    Congenital absence of arm and forearm (complete or incomplete) with or without metacarpal deficiency and/or phalangeal deficiency, incomplete
                    Phocomelia, complete, of upper limb

      755.24   **Longitudinal deficiency, humeral, complete or partial (with or without distal deficiencies, incomplete)**
                    Congenital absence of humerus (with or without absence of some [but not all] distal elements)
                    Proximal phocomelia of upper limb

      755.25   **Longitudinal deficiency, radioulnar, complete or partial (with or without distal deficiencies, incomplete)**
                    Congenital absence of radius and ulna (with or without absence of some [but not all] distal elements)
                    Distal phocomelia of upper limb

      755.26   **Longitudinal deficiency, radial, complete or partial (with or without distal deficiencies, incomplete)**
                    Agenesis of radius
                    Congenital absence of radius (with or without absence of some [but not all] distal elements)

      755.27   **Longitudinal deficiency, ulnar, complete or partial (with or without distal deficiencies, incomplete)**
                    Agenesis of ulna
                    Congenital absence of ulna (with or without absence of some [but not all] distal elements)

      755.28   **Longitudinal deficiency, carpals or metacarpals, complete or partial (with or without incomplete phalangeal deficiency)**

      755.29   **Longitudinal deficiency, phalanges, complete or partial**
                    Absence of finger, congenital
                    Aphalangia of upper limb, terminal, complete or partial

          Excludes: terminal deficiency of all five digits (755.21)
                    transverse deficiency of phalanges (755.21)

⑤ **755.3 Reduction deformities of lower limb**

      755.30   **Unspecified reduction deformity of lower limb**
                    Ectromelia NOS of lower limb
                    Hemimelia NOS of lower limb
                    Shortening of leg, congenital

      755.31   **Transverse deficiency of lower limb**
                    Amelia of lower limb
                    Congenital absence of:
                      foot
                      leg, including foot and toes
                      lower limb, complete
                      toes, all, complete
                    Transverse hemimelia of lower limb

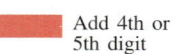 Add 4th or 5th digit
 Nonspecific code
 Unspecified code
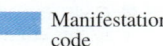 Manifestation code

TABULAR LIST

- **755.32 Longitudinal deficiency of lower limb, not elsewhere classified**
  Phocomelia NOS of lower limb
- **755.33 Longitudinal deficiency, combined, involving femur, tibia, and fibula (complete or incomplete)**
  Congenital absence of thigh and (lower) leg (complete or incomplete) with or without metacarpal deficiency and/or phalangeal deficiency, incomplete
  Phocomelia, complete, of lower limb
- **755.34 Longitudinal deficiency, femoral, complete or partial (with or without distal deficiencies, incomplete)**
  Congenital absence of femur (with or without absence of some [but not all] distal elements)
  Proximal phocomelia of lower limb
- **755.35 Longitudinal deficiency, tibiofibular, complete or partial (with or without distal deficiencies, incomplete)**
  Congenital absence of tibia and fibula (with or without absence of some [but not all] distal elements)
  Distal phocomelia of lower limb
- **755.36 Longitudinal deficiency, tibia, complete or partial (with or without distal deficiencies, incomplete)**
  Agenesis of tibia
  Congenital absence of tibia (with or without absence of some [but not all] distal elements)
- **755.37 Longitudinal deficiency, fibular, complete or partial (with or without distal deficiencies, incomplete)**
  Agenesis of fibula
  Congenital absence of fibula (with or without absence of some [but not all] distal elements)
- **755.38 Longitudinal deficiency, tarsals or metatarsals, complete or partial (with or without incomplete phalangeal deficiency)**
- **755.39 Longitudinal deficiency, phalanges, complete or partial**
  Absence of toe, congenital
  Aphalangia of lower limb, terminal, complete or partial

  Excludes: *terminal deficiency of all five digits (755.31)*
  transverse deficiency of phalanges (755.31)

- **755.4 Reduction deformities, unspecified limb**
  Absence, congenital (complete or partial) of limb NOS
  Amelia of unspecified limb
  Ectromelia of unspecified limb
  Hemimelia of unspecified limb
  Phocomelia of unspecified limb

⑤ **755.5 Other anomalies of upper limb, including shoulder girdle**
- **755.50 Unspecified anomaly of upper limb**
- **755.51 Congenital deformity of clavicle**
- **755.52 Congenital elevation of scapula**
  Sprengel's deformity
- **755.53 Radioulnar synostosis**
- **755.54 Madelung's deformity**
- **755.55 Acrocephalosyndactyly**
  Apert's syndrome
- **755.56 Accessory carpal bones**
- **755.57 Macrodactylia (fingers)**
- **755.58 Cleft hand, congenital**
  Lobster-claw hand
- **755.59 Other**
  Cleidocranial dysostosis
  Cubitus:
    valgus, congenital
    varus, congenital

  Excludes: *club hand (congenital) (754.89)*
  congenital dislocation of elbow (754.89)

⑤ **755.6 Other anomalies of lower limb, including pelvic girdle**
- **755.60 Unspecified anomaly of lower limb**
- **755.61 Coxa valga, congenital**

CONGENITAL ANOMALIES

- **755.62** Coxa vara, congenital
- **755.63** **Other congenital deformity of hip (joint)**
  Congenital anteversion of femur (neck)

  Excludes: congenital dislocation of hip (754.30-754.35)

- **755.64** **Congenital deformity of knee (joint)**
  Congenital:
    absence of patella
    genu valgum [knock-knee]
    genu varum [bowleg]
  Rudimentary patella

- **755.65** **Macrodactylia of toes**
- **755.66** **Other anomalies of toes**
  Congenital:
    hallux valgus
    hallux varus
    hammer toe

- **755.67** **Anomalies of foot, not elsewhere classified**
  Astragaloscaphoid synostosis
  Calcaneonavicular bar
  Coalition of calcaneus
  Talonavicular synostosis
  Tarsal coalitions

- **755.69** **Other**
  Congenital:
    angulation of tibia
    deformity (of):
      ankle (joint)
      sacroiliac (joint)
    fusion of sacroiliac joint

- **755.8** **Other specified anomalies of unspecified limb**
- **755.9** **Unspecified anomaly of unspecified limb**
  Congenital:
    anomaly NOS of unspecified limb
    deformity NOS of unspecified limb

  Excludes: reduction deformity of unspecified limb (755.4)

756 Other congenital musculoskeletal anomalies

Excludes: those deformities classifiable to 754.0-754.8

- **756.0** **Anomalies of skull and face bones**
  Absence of skull bones
  Acrocephaly
  Congenital deformity of
    forehead
  Craniosynostosis
  Crouzon's disease
  Hypertelorism
  Imperfect fusion of skull
  Oxycephaly
  Platybasia
  Premature closure of cranial sutures
  Tower skull
  Trigonocephaly

  Excludes: acrocephalosyndactyly [Apert's syndrome] (755.55)
    dentofacial anomalies (524.0-524.9)
    skull defects associated with brain anomalies, such as:
      anencephalus (740.0)
      encephalocele (742.0)
      hydrocephalus (742.3)
      microcephalus (742.1)

- ⑤ **756.1** **Anomalies of spine**
  - **756.10** **Anomaly of spine, unspecified**
  - **756.11** **Spondylolysis, lumbosacral region**
    Prespondylolisthesis (lumbosacral)
  - **756.12** **Spondylolisthesis**
  - **756.13** **Absence of vertebra, congenital**
  - **756.14** **Hemivertebra**
  - **756.15** **Fusion of spine [vertebra], congenital**
  - **756.16** **Klippel-Feil syndrome**

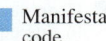

509

TABULAR LIST

756.17 Spina bifida occulta

Excludes: *spina bifida (aperta) (741.0-741.9)*

756.19 Other
Platyspondylia
Supernumerary vertebra

756.2 Cervical rib
Supernumerary rib in the cervical region

756.3 Other anomalies of ribs and sternum
Congenital absence of:
  rib
  sternum
Congenital:
  fissure of sternum
  fusion of ribs
Sternum bifidum

Excludes: *nonteratogenic deformity of chest wall (754.81-754.89)*

756.4 Chondrodystrophy
Achondroplasia
Chondrodystrophia (fetalis)
Dyschondroplasia
Enchondromatosis
Ollier's disease

Excludes: *congenital myotonic chondrodystrophy (359.23)*
lipochondrodystrophy [Hurler's syndrome] (277.5)
Morquio's disease (277.5)

⑤ **756.5 Osteodystrophies**

756.50 Osteodystrophy, unspecified

756.51 Osteogenesis imperfecta
Fragilitas ossium
Osteopsathyrosis

756.52 Osteopetrosis

756.53 Osteopoikilosis

756.54 Polyostotic fibrous dysplasia of bone

756.55 Chondroectodermal dysplasia
Ellis-van Creveld syndrome

756.56 Multiple epiphyseal dysplasia

756.59 Other
Albright (-McCune)-Sternberg syndrome

756.6 Anomalies of diaphragm
Absence of diaphragm
Congenital hernia:
  diaphragmatic
  foramen of Morgagni
Eventration of diaphragm

Excludes: *congenital hiatus hernia (750.6)*

⑤ **756.7 Anomalies of abdominal wall**

756.70 Anomaly of abdominal wall, unspecified

756.71 Prune belly syndrome
Eagle-Barrett syndrome
Prolapse of bladder mucosa

756.79 Other congenital anomalies of abdominal wall
Exomphalos
Gastroschisis
Omphalocele

Excludes: *umbilical hernia (551-553 with .1)*

⑤ **756.8 Other specified anomalies of muscle, tendon, fascia, and connective tissue**

756.81 Absence of muscle and tendon
Absence of muscle (pectoral)

756.82 Accessory muscle

756.83 Ehlers-Danlos syndrome

CONGENITAL ANOMALIES

756.89 **Other**
Amyotrophia congenita
Congenital shortening of tendon

756.9 **Other and unspecified anomalies of musculoskeletal system**
Congenital:
anomaly NOS of musculoskeletal system, not elsewhere classified
deformity NOS of musculoskeletal system, not elsewhere classified

757 **Congenital anomalies of the integument**
Includes: anomalies of skin, subcutaneous tissue, hair, nails, and breast

Excludes: hemangioma (228.00-228.09)
pigmented nevus (216.0-216.9)

757.0 **Hereditary edema of legs**
Congenital lymphedema   Milroy's disease
Hereditary trophedema

757.1 **Ichthyosis congenita**
Congenital ichthyosis
Harlequin fetus
Ichthyosiform erythroderma

757.2 **Dermatoglyphic anomalies**
Abnormal palmar creases

⑤ **757.3** **Other specified anomalies of skin**

757.31 **Congenital ectodermal dysplasia**

757.32 **Vascular hamartomas**
Birthmarks
Port-wine stain
Strawberry nevus

757.33 **Congenital pigmentary anomalies of skin**
Congenital poikiloderma
Urticaria pigmentosa
Xeroderma pigmentosum

Excludes: albinism (270.2)

757.39 **Other**
Accessory skin tags, congenital
Congenital scar
Epidermolysis bullosa
Keratoderma (congenital)

Excludes: pilonidal cyst (685.0-685.1)

757.4 **Specified anomalies of hair**
Congenital: Congenital:
  alopecia   hypertrichosis
  atrichosis   monilethrix
  beaded hair   Persistent lanugo

757.5 **Specified anomalies of nails**
Anonychia   Congenital:
Congenital: leukonychia
  clubnail   onychauxis
  koilonychia   pachyonychia

757.6 **Specified anomalies of breast**
Absent breast or nipple
Accessory breast or nipple
Supernumerary breast or nipple
Hypoplasia of breast

Excludes: absence of pectoral muscle (756.81)

757.8 **Other specified anomalies of the integument**

757.9 **Unspecified anomaly of the integument**
Congenital:
anomaly NOS of integument
deformity NOS of integument

758 **Chromosomal anomalies**
Includes: syndromes associated with anomalies in the number and form of chromosomes
Use additional codes for conditions associated with the chromosomal anomalies

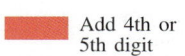 Add 4th or 5th digit
 Nonspecific code
 Unspecified code
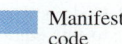 Manifestation code

TABULAR LIST

758.0 Down's syndrome
Mongolism
Translocation Down's syndrome
Trisomy:
21 or 22
G

758.1 Patau's syndrome
Trisomy:
13
D₁

758.2 Edwards' syndrome
Trisomy:
18
E₃

⑤ **758.3 Autosomal deletion syndromes**

758.31 Cri-du-chat syndrome
Deletion 5p

758.32 Velo-cardio-facial syndrome
Deletion 22q11.2

758.33 Other microdeletions
Miller-Dieker syndrome
Smith-Magenis syndrome

758.39 Other autosomal deletions

758.4 Balanced autosomal translocation in normal individual

758.5 Other conditions due to autosomal anomalies
Accessory autosomes NEC

758.6 Gonadal dysgenesis
Ovarian dysgenesis
Turner's syndrome
XO syndrome

Excludes: pure gonadal dysgenesis (752.7)

758.7 Klinefelter's syndrome
XXY syndrome

⑤ **758.8 Other conditions due to chromosome anomalies**

758.81 Other conditions due to sex chromosome anomalies

758.89 Other

758.9 Conditions due to anomaly of unspecified chromosome

759 Other and unspecified congenital anomalies

759.0 Anomalies of spleen
Aberrant spleen
Absent spleen
Accessory spleen
Congenital splenomegaly
Ectopic spleen
Lobulation of spleen

759.1 Anomalies of adrenal gland
Aberrant adrenal gland
Absent adrenal gland
Accessory adrenal gland

Excludes: adrenogenital disorders (255.2)
congenital disorders of steroid metabolism (255.2)

759.2 Anomalies of other endocrine glands
Absent parathyroid gland
Accessory thyroid gland
Persistent thyroglossal or thyrolingual duct
Thyroglossal (duct) cyst

Excludes: congenital:
goiter (246.1)
hypothyroidism (243)

759.3 Situs inversus
Situs inversus or transversus:
abdominalis
thoracis
Transposition of viscera:
abdominal
thoracic

Excludes: dextrocardia without mention of complete transposition (746.87)

CONGENITAL ANOMALIES

759.4 Conjoined twins
Craniopagus
Dicephalus
Pygopagus
Thoracopagus
Xiphopagus

759.5 Tuberous sclerosis
Bourneville's disease
Epiloia

759.6 Other hamartoses, not elsewhere classified
Syndrome:
  Peutz-Jeghers
  Sturge-Weber (-Dimitri)
  von Hippel-Lindau

Excludes: *neurofibromatosis (237.7)*

759.7 Multiple congenital anomalies, so described
Congenital:
  anomaly, multiple NOS
  deformity, multiple NOS

759.8 Other specified anomalies
  759.81 Prader-Willi syndrome
  759.82 Marfan syndrome
  759.83 Fragile X syndrome
  759.89 Other
    Congenital malformation syndromes affecting multiple systems, not elsewhere classified
    Laurence-Moon-Biedl syndrome

759.9 Congenital anomaly, unspecified

TABULAR LIST

CONDITIONS IN THE PERINATAL PERIOD

15. CERTAIN CONDITIONS ORIGINATING IN THE PERINATAL PERIOD (760-779)

Includes: conditions which have their origin in the perinatal period, before birth through the first 28 days after birth, even though death or morbidity occurs later

Use additional code(s) to further specify condition

MATERNAL CAUSES OF PERINATAL MORBIDITY AND MORTALITY (760-763)

760 Fetus or newborn affected by maternal conditions which may be unrelated to present pregnancy
Includes: the listed maternal conditions only when specified as a cause of mortality or morbidity of the fetus or newborn

Excludes: maternal endocrine and metabolic disorders affecting fetus or newborn (775.0-775.9)

760.0 Maternal hypertensive disorders
Fetus or newborn affected by maternal conditions classifiable to 642

760.1 Maternal renal and urinary tract diseases
Fetus or newborn affected by maternal conditions classifiable to 580-599

760.2 Maternal infections
Fetus or newborn affected by maternal infectious disease classifiable to 001-136 and 487, but fetus or newborn not manifesting that disease

Excludes: congenital infectious diseases (771.0-771.8)
maternal genital tract and other localized infections (760.8)

760.3 Other chronic maternal circulatory and respiratory diseases
Fetus or newborn affected by chronic maternal conditions classifiable to 390-459, 490-519, 745-748

760.4 Maternal nutritional disorders
Fetus or newborn affected by:
 maternal disorders classifiable to 260-269
 maternal malnutrition NOS

Excludes: fetal malnutrition (764.10-764.29)

760.5 Maternal injury
Fetus or newborn affected by maternal conditions classifiable to 800-995

760.6 Surgical operation on mother
Excludes: cesarean section for present delivery (763.4)
damage to placenta from amniocentesis, cesarean section, or surgical induction (762.1)
previous surgery to uterus or pelvic organs (763.89)

⑤ **760.7 Noxious influences affecting fetus or newborn via placenta or breast milk**
Fetus or newborn affected by noxious substance transmitted via placenta or breast milk

Excludes: anesthetic and analgesic drugs administered during labor and delivery (763.5)
drug withdrawal syndrome in newborn (779.5)

760.70 Unspecified noxious substance
Fetus or newborn affected by:
 Drug NEC

760.71 Alcohol
Fetal alcohol syndrome

760.72 Narcotics

760.73 Hallucinogenic agents

760.74 Anti-infectives
Antibiotics
Antifungals

760.75 Cocaine

760.76 Diethylstilbestrol (DES)

760.77 Anticonvulsants
Carbamazepine
Phenobarbital
Phenytoin
Valproic acid

760.78 Antimetabolic agents
Methotrexate
Retinoic acid
Statins

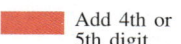 Add 4th or 5th digit   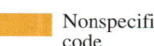 Nonspecific code   Unspecified code   Manifestation code

515

TABULAR LIST

760.79 **Other**
Fetus or newborn affected by:
immune sera transmitted via placenta or breast milk
medicinal agents NEC transmitted via placenta or breast milk
toxic substance NEC transmitted via placenta or breast milk

760.8 **Other specified maternal conditions affecting fetus or newborn**
Maternal genital tract and other localized infection affecting fetus or newborn, but fetus or newborn not manifesting that disease

Excludes: maternal urinary tract infection affecting fetus or newborn (760.1)

760.9 **Unspecified maternal condition affecting fetus or newborn**

761 **Fetus or newborn affected by maternal complications of pregnancy**
Includes: the listed maternal conditions only when specified as a cause of mortality or morbidity of the fetus or newborn

761.0 **Incompetent cervix**

761.1 **Premature rupture of membranes**

761.2 **Oligohydramnios**

Excludes: that due to premature rupture of membranes (761.1)

761.3 **Polyhydramnios**
Hydramnios (acute) (chronic)

761.4 **Ectopic pregnancy**
Pregnancy:
abdominal
intraperitoneal
tubal

761.5 **Multiple pregnancy**
Triplet (pregnancy)
Twin (pregnancy)

761.6 **Maternal death**

761.7 **Malpresentation before labor**
Breech presentation before labor
External version before labor
Oblique lie before labor
Transverse lie before labor
Unstable lie before labor

761.8 **Other specified maternal complications of pregnancy affecting fetus or newborn**
Spontaneous abortion, fetus

761.9 **Unspecified maternal complication of pregnancy affecting fetus or newborn**

762 **Fetus or newborn affected by complications of placenta, cord, and membranes**
Includes: the listed maternal conditions only when specified as a cause of mortality or morbidity in the fetus or newborn

762.0 **Placenta previa**

762.1 **Other forms of placental separation and hemorrhage**
Abruptio placentae
Antepartum hemorrhage
Damage to placenta from amniocentesis, cesarean section, or surgical induction
Maternal blood loss
Premature separation of placenta
Rupture of marginal sinus

762.2 **Other and unspecified morphological and functional abnormalities of placenta**
Placental:
dysfunction
infarction
insufficiency

762.3 **Placental transfusion syndromes**
Placental and cord abnormality resulting in twin-to-twin or other transplacental transfusion

Use additional code, if desired, to indicate resultant condition in fetus or newborn:
fetal blood loss (772.0)
polycythemia neonatorum (776.4)

762.4 **Prolapsed cord**
Cord presentation

CONDITIONS IN THE PERINATAL PERIOD

762.5 **Other compression of umbilical cord**
  Cord around neck   Knot in cord
  Entanglement of cord   Torsion of cord

762.6 **Other and unspecified conditions of umbilical cord**
  Short umbilical cord
  Thrombosis of umbilical cord
  Varices of umbilical cord
  Velamentous insertion of umbilical cord
  Vasa previa

  Excludes: infection of umbilical cord (771.4)
           single umbilical artery (747.5)

762.7 **Chorioamnionitis**
  Amnionitis
  Membranitis
  Placentitis

762.8 **Other specified abnormalities of chorion and amnion**

762.9 **Unspecified abnormality of chorion and amnion**

763 **Fetus or newborn affected by other complications of labor and delivery**
  Includes: the listed conditions only when specified as a cause of mortality or morbidity in the fetus or newborn

763.0 **Breech delivery and extraction**

763.1 **Other malpresentation, malposition, and disproportion during labor and delivery**
  Fetus or newborn affected by:
    abnormality of bony pelvis
    contracted pelvis
    persistent occipitoposterior position
    shoulder presentation
    transverse lie
    conditions classifiable to 652, 653, and 660

763.2 **Forceps delivery**
  Fetus or newborn affected by forceps extraction

763.3 **Delivery by vacuum extractor**

763.4 **Cesarean delivery**
  Excludes: placental separation or hemorrhage from cesarean section (762.1)

763.5 **Maternal anesthesia and analgesia**
  Reactions and intoxications from maternal opiates and tranquilizers during labor and delivery
  Excludes: drug withdrawal syndrome in newborn (779.5)

763.6 **Precipitate delivery**
  Rapid second stage

763.7 **Abnormal uterine contractions**
  Fetus or newborn affected by:
    contraction ring
    hypertonic labor
    hypotonic uterine dysfunction
    uterine inertia or dysfunction
    conditions classifiable to 661, except 661.3

⑤ 763.8 **Other specified complications of labor and delivery affecting fetus or newborn**
  763.81 **Abnormality in fetal heart rate or rhythm before the onset of labor**
  763.82 **Abnormality in fetal heart rate or rhythm during labor**
  763.83 **Abnormality in fetal heart rate or rhythm, unspecified as to time of onset**
  763.84 **Meconium passage during delivery**
    Excludes: meconium aspiration (770.11, 770.12)
             meconium staining (779.84)

TABULAR LIST

763.89 **Other specified complications of labor and delivery affecting fetus or newborn**
Fetus or newborn affected by:
abnormality of maternal soft tissues
destructive operation on live fetus to facilitate delivery
induction of labor (medical)
previous surgery to uterus or pelvic organs
other conditions classifiable to 650-669
other procedures used in labor and delivery

763.9 Unspecified complication of labor and delivery affecting fetus or newborn

OTHER CONDITIONS ORIGINATING IN THE PERINATAL PERIOD (764-779)

The following fifth-digit subclassification is for use with categories 764 and codes 765.0 and 765.1 to denote birthweight:

0 unspecified [weight]
1 less than 500 grams
2 500-749 grams
3 750-999 grams
4 1,000- 1,249 grams
5 1,250-1,499 grams
6 1,500-1,749 grams
7 1,750-1,999 grams
8 2,000-2,499 grams
9 2,500 grams and over

764 Slow fetal growth and fetal malnutrition

⑤ 764.0 **"Light-for-dates" without mention of fetal malnutrition**
Infants underweight for gestational age
"Small-for-dates"

⑤ 764.1 **"Light-for-dates" with signs of fetal malnutrition**
Infants "light-for-dates" classifiable to 764.0, who in addition show signs of fetal malnutrition, such as dry peeling skin and loss of subcutaneous tissue

⑤ 764.2 **Fetal malnutrition without mention of "light-for-dates"**
Infants, not underweight for gestational age, showing signs of fetal malnutrition, such as dry peeling skin and loss of subcutaneous tissue
Intrauterine malnutrition

⑤ **764.9** **Fetal growth retardation, unspecified**
Intrauterine growth retardation

765 Disorders relating to short gestation and low birthweight
Includes: the listed conditions, without further specification, as causes of mortality, morbidity, or additional care, in fetus or newborn

⑤ 765.0 **Extreme immaturity**
Note: Usually implies a birthweight of less than 1000 grams
Use additional code for weeks of gestation (765.20-765.29)

⑤ 765.1 **Other preterm infants**
Prematurity NOS
Prematurity or small size, not classifiable to 765.0 or as "light-for-dates" in 764
Note: Usually implies a birthweight of 1000-2499 grams
Use additional code for weeks of gestation (765.20-765.29)

⑤ 765.2 **Weeks of gestation**

765.20 **Unspecified weeks of gestation**
765.21 Less than 24 completed weeks of gestation
765.22 24 completed weeks of gestation
765.23 25-26 completed weeks of gestation
765.24 27-28 completed weeks of gestation
765.25 29-30 completed weeks of gestation
765.26 31-32 completed weeks of gestation
765.27 33-34 completed weeks of gestation
765.28 35-36 completed weeks of gestation
765.29 37 or more completed weeks of gestation

CONDITIONS IN THE PERINATAL PERIOD

766 Disorders relating to long gestation and high birthweight
Includes: the listed conditions, without further specification, as causes of mortality, morbidity, or additional care, in fetus or newborn

766.0 Exceptionally large baby
Note: Usually implies a birthweight of 4500 grams or more.

766.1 Other "heavy-for-dates" infants
Other fetus or infant "heavy-" or "large-for-dates" regardless of period of gestation

⑤ **766.2 Late infant, not "heavy-for-dates"**

766.21 Post-term infant
Infant with gestation period over 40 completed weeks to 42 completed weeks

766.22 Prolonged gestation of infant
Infant with gestation period over 42 completed weeks
Postmaturity NOS

767 Birth trauma

767.0 Subdural and cerebral hemorrhage
Subdural and cerebral hemorrhage, whether described as due to birth trauma or to intrapartum anoxia or hypoxia
Subdural hematoma (localized)
Tentorial tear
Use additional code, if desired, to identify cause
Excludes: intraventricular hemorrhage (772.10-772.14)
subarachnoid hemorrhage (772.2)

⑤ **767.1 Injuries to scalp**

767.11 Epicranial subaponeurotic hemorrhage (massive)
Subgaleal hemorrhage

767.19 Other injuries to scalp
Caput succedaneum
Cephalhematoma
Chignon (from vacuum extraction)

767.2 Fracture of clavicle

767.3 Other injuries to skeleton
Fracture of:
long bones
skull
Excludes: congenital dislocation of hip (754.30-754.35)
fracture of spine, congenital (767.4)

767.4 Injury to spine and spinal cord
Dislocation of spine or spinal cord due to birth trauma
Fracture of spine or spinal cord due to birth trauma
Laceration of spine or spinal cord due to birth trauma
Rupture of spine or spinal cord due to birth trauma

767.5 Facial nerve injury
Facial palsy

767.6 Injury to brachial plexus
Palsy or paralysis:
brachial
Erb (-Duchenne)
Klumpke (-Déjérine)

767.7 Other cranial and peripheral nerve injuries
Phrenic nerve paralysis

767.8 Other specified birth trauma
Eye damage
Hematoma of:
liver (subcapsular)
testes
vulva
Rupture of:
liver
spleen
Scalpel wound
Traumatic glaucoma
Excludes: hemorrhage classifiable to 772.0-772.9

767.9 Birth trauma, unspecified
Birth injury NOS

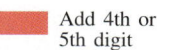 Add 4th or 5th digit
 Nonspecific code
Unspecified code
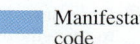 Manifestation code

519

TABULAR LIST

768 Intrauterine hypoxia and birth asphyxia
Use only when associated with newborn morbidity classifiable elsewhere

> Excludes: acidemia NOS of newborn (775.81)
> acidosis NOS of newborn (775.81)
> cerebral ischemia NOS (779.2)
> hypoxia NOS of newborn (770.88)
> mixed metabolic and respiratory acidosis of newborn (775.81)
> respiratory arrest of newborn (770.87)

768.0 Fetal death from asphyxia or anoxia before onset of labor or at unspecified time

768.1 Fetal death from asphyxia or anoxia during labor

768.2 Fetal distress before onset of labor, in liveborn infant
Fetal metabolic acidemia before onset of labor, in liveborn infant

768.3 Fetal distress first noted during labor and delivery, in liveborn infant
Fetal metabolic acidemia first noted during labor and delivery, in liveborn infant

768.4 Fetal distress, unspecified as to time of onset, in liveborn infant
Fetal metabolic acidemia unspecified as to time of onset, in liveborn infant

768.5 Severe birth asphyxia
Birth asphyxia with neurologic involvement

> Excludes: hypoxic-ischemic encephalopathy (HIE) (768.7)

768.6 Mild or moderate birth asphyxia
Other specified birth asphyxia (without mention of neurologic involvement)

> Excludes: hypoxic-ischemic encephalopathy (HIE) (768.7)

768.7 Hypoxic-ischemic encephalopathy (HIE)

768.9 Unspecified birth asphyxia in liveborn infant
Anoxia NOS, in liveborn infant
Asphyxia NOS, in liveborn infant

769 Respiratory distress syndrome
Cardiorespiratory distress syndrome of newborn
Hyaline membrane disease (pulmonary)
Idiopathic respiratory distress syndrome [IRDS or RDS] of newborn
Pulmonary hypoperfusion syndrome

> Excludes: transient tachypnea of newborn (770.6)

770 Other respiratory conditions of fetus and newborn

770.0 Congenital pneumonia
Infective pneumonia acquired prenatally

> Excludes: pneumonia from infection acquired after birth (480.0-486)

⑤ **770.1 Fetal and newborn aspiration**

> Excludes: aspiration of postnatal stomach contents (770.85, 770.86)
> meconium passage during delivery (763.84)
> meconium staining (779.84)

770.10 Fetal and newborn aspiration, unspecified

770.11 Meconium aspiration without respiratory symptoms
Meconium aspiration NOS

770.12 Meconium aspiration with respiratory symptoms
Meconium aspiration pneumonia
Meconium aspiration pneumonitis
Meconium aspiration syndrome NOS
Use additional code to identify any secondary pulmonary hypertension (416.8), if applicable

770.13 Aspiration of clear amniotic fluid without respiratory symptoms
Aspiration of clear amniotic fluid NOS

770.14 Aspiration of clear amniotic fluid with respiratory symptoms
Aspiration of clear amniotic fluid with pneumonia
Aspiration of clear amniotic fluid with pneumonitis
Use additional code to identify any secondary pulmonary hypertension (416.8), if applicable

770.15 Aspiration of blood without respiratory symptoms
Aspiration of blood NOS

CONDITIONS IN THE PERINATAL PERIOD

- 770.16 **Aspiration of blood with respiratory symptoms**
  Aspiration of blood with pneumonia
  Aspiration of blood with pneumonitis
  Use additional code to identify any secondary pulmonary hypertension (416.8), if applicable

- 770.17 **Other fetal and newborn aspiration without respiratory symptoms**

- 770.18 **Other fetal and newborn aspiration with respiratory symptoms**
  Other aspiration pneumonia
  Other aspiration pneumonitis
  Use additional code to identify any secondary pulmonary hypertension (416.8), if applicable

770.2 **Interstitial emphysema and related conditions**
  Pneumomediastinum originating in the perinatal period
  Pneumopericardium originating in the perinatal period
  Pneumothorax originating in the perinatal period

770.3 **Pulmonary hemorrhage**
  Hemorrhage:
    alveolar (lung) originating in the perinatal period
    intra-alveolar (lung) originating in the perinatal period
    massive pulmonary originating in the perinatal period

770.4 **Primary atelectasis**
  Pulmonary immaturity NOS

770.5 **Other and unspecified atelectasis**
  Atelectasis:
    NOS, originating in the perinatal period
    partial, originating in the perinatal period
    secondary, originating in the perinatal period
  Pulmonary collapse, originating in the perinatal period

770.6 **Transitory tachypnea of newborn**
  Idiopathic tachypnea of newborn
  Wet lung syndrome
  Excludes: respiratory distress syndrome (769)

770.7 **Chronic respiratory disease arising in the perinatal period**
  Bronchopulmonary dysplasia
  Interstitial pulmonary fibrosis of prematurity
  Wilson-Mikity syndrome

⑤ 770.8 **Other respiratory problems after birth**
  Excludes: mixed metabolic and respiratory acidosis of newborn (775.81)

- 770.81 **Primary apnea of newborn**
  Apneic spells of newborn NOS
  Essential apnea of newborn
  Sleep apnea of newborn

- 770.82 **Other apnea of newborn**
  Obstructure apnea of newborn

- 770.83 **Cyanotic attacks of newborn**

- 770.84 **Respiratory failure of newborn**
  Excludes: respiratory distress syndrome (769)

- 770.85 **Aspiration of postnatal stomach contents without respiratory symptoms**
  Aspiration of postnatal stomach contents NOS

- 770.86 **Aspiration of postnatal stomach contents with respiratory symptoms**
  Aspiration of postnatal stomach contents with pneumonia
  Aspiration of postnatal stomach contents with pneumonitis
  Use additional code to identify any secondary pulmonary hypertension (416.8), if applicable

- 770.87 **Respiratory arrest of newborn**

- 770.88 **Hypoxemia of newborn**
  Hypoxia NOS of newborn

- 770.89 **Other respiratory problems after birth**

770.9 **Unspecified respiratory condition of fetus and newborn**

TABULAR LIST

771 Infections specific to the perinatal period
   Includes: infections acquired before or during birth via the umbilicus or during the first 28 days after birth

   Excludes: *congenital pneumonia (770.0)*
   congenital syphilis (090.0-090.9)
   infant botulism (040.41)
   maternal infectious disease as a cause of mortality or morbidity in fetus or newborn, but fetus or newborn not manifesting the disease (760.2)
   ophthalmia neonatorum due to gonococcus (098.40)
   other infections not specifically classified to this category

   771.0 Congenital rubella
   Congenital rubella pneumonitis

   771.1 Congenital cytomegalovirus infection
   Congenital cytomegalic inclusion disease

   771.2 Other congenital infections
   Congenital:
      herpes simplex
      listeriosis
      malaria
   Congenital:
      toxoplasmosis
      tuberculosis

   771.3 Tetanus neonatorum
   Tetanus omphalitis

   Excludes: *hypocalcemic tetany (775.4)*

   771.4 Omphalitis of the newborn
   Infection:
      navel cord
      umbilical stump

   Excludes: *tetanus omphalitis (771.3)*

   771.5 Neonatal infective mastitis

   Excludes: *noninfective neonatal mastitis (778.7)*

   771.6 Neonatal conjunctivitis and dacryocystitis
   Ophthalmia neonatorum NOS

   Excludes: *ophthalmia neonatorum due to gonococcus (098.40)*

   771.7 Neonatal Candida infection
   Neonatal moniliasis
   Thrush in newborn

   ⑤ **771.8 Other infection specific to the perinatal period**
   Use additional code to identify organism (041.00-041.9)

   771.81 Septicemia [sepsis] of newborn

   771.82 Urinary tract infection of newborn

   771.83 Bacteremia of newborn

   771.89 Other infections specific to the perinatal period
   Intra-amniotic infection of fetus NOS
   Infection of newborn NOS

772 Fetal and neonatal hemorrhage

   Excludes: *hematological disorders of fetus and newborn (776.0-776.9)*

   772.0 Fetal blood loss
   Fetal blood loss from:
      cut end of co-twin's cord
      placenta
      ruptured cord
      vasa previa
   Fetal exsanguination
   Fetal hemorrhage into:
      co-twin
      mother's circulation

   ⑤ **772.1 Intraventricular hemorrhage**
   Intraventricular hemorrhage from any perinatal cause

   772.10 Unspecified grade

   772.11 Grade I
   Bleeding into germinal matrix

   772.12 Grade II
   Bleeding into ventricle

   772.13 Grade III
   Bleeding with enlargement of ventricle

522 ● Code new to this edition   ▲ Revision of existing code   ④ ⑤ Fourth or fifth digit required

CONDITIONS IN THE PERINATAL PERIOD

- **772.14 Grade IV**
  Bleeding into cerebral cortex
- **772.2 Subarachnoid hemorrhage**
  Subarachnoid hemorrhage from any perinatal cause
  Excludes: subdural and cerebral hemorrhage (767.0)
- **772.3 Umbilical hemorrhage after birth**
  Slipped umbilical ligature
- **772.4 Gastrointestinal hemorrhage**
  Excludes: swallowed maternal blood (777.3)
- **772.5 Adrenal hemorrhage**
- **772.6 Cutaneous hemorrhage**
  Bruising in fetus or newborn
  Ecchymoses in fetus or newborn
  Petechiae in fetus or newborn
  Superficial hematoma in fetus or newborn
- **772.8 Other specified hemorrhage of fetus or newborn**
  Excludes: hemorrhagic disease of newborn (776.0)
  pulmonary hemorrhage (770.3)
- **772.9 Unspecified hemorrhage of newborn**

773 Hemolytic disease of fetus or newborn, due to isoimmunization

- **773.0 Hemolytic disease due to Rh isoimmunization**
  Anemia due to RH:
    antibodies
    isoimmunization
    maternal/fetal incompatibility
  Erythroblastosis (fetalis) due to RH:
    antibodies
    isoimmunization
    maternal/fetal incompatibility
  Hemolytic disease (fetus) (newborn) due to RH:
    antibodies
    isoimmunization
    maternal/fetal incompatibility
  Jaundice due to RH:
    antibodies
    isoimmunization
    maternal/fetal incompatibility
  Rh hemolytic disease
  Rh isoimmunization
- **773.1 Hemolytic disease due to ABO isoimmunization**
  ABO hemolytic disease
  ABO isoimmunization
  Anemia due to ABO: antibodies, isoimmunization, or maternal/fetal incompatibility
  Erythroblastosis (fetalis) due to ABO:
    antibodies
    isoimmunization
    maternal/fetal incompatibility
  Hemolytic disease (fetus) (newborn) due to ABO:
    antibodies
    isoimmunization
    maternal/fetal incompatibility
  Jaundice due to ABO:
    antibodies
    isoimmunization
    maternal/fetal incompatibility
- **773.2 Hemolytic disease due to other and unspecified isoimmunization**
  Erythroblastosis (fetalis) (neonatorum) NOS
  Hemolytic disease (fetus) (newborn) NOS
  Jaundice or anemia due to other and unspecified blood-group incompatibility
- **773.3 Hydrops fetalis due to isoimmunization**
  Use additional code, if desired, to identify type of isoimmunization (773.0-773.2)
- **773.4 Kernicterus due to isoimmunization**
  Use additional code, if desired, to identify type of isoimmunization (773.0-773.2)
- **773.5 Late anemia due to isoimmunization**

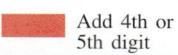

523

TABULAR LIST

774 Other perinatal jaundice

774.0 Perinatal jaundice from hereditary hemolytic anemias
Code first underlying disease (282.0-282.9)

774.1 Perinatal jaundice from other excessive hemolysis
Fetal or neonatal jaundice from:
  bruising
  drugs or toxins transmitted from mother
  infection
  polycythemia
  swallowed maternal blood
Use additional code, if desired, to identify cause
Excludes: jaundice due to isoimmunization (773.0-773.2)

774.2 Neonatal jaundice associated with preterm delivery
Hyperbilirubinemia of prematurity
Jaundice due to delayed conjugation associated with preterm delivery

⑤ **774.3 Neonatal jaundice due to delayed conjugation from other causes**

774.30 Neonatal jaundice due to delayed conjugation, cause unspecified

774.31 Neonatal jaundice due to delayed conjugation in diseases classified elsewhere
Code first underlying diseases, as:
  congenital hypothyroidism (243)
  Crigler-Najjar syndrome (277.4)
  Gilbert's syndrome (277.4)

774.39 Other
Jaundice due to delayed conjugation from causes, such as:
  breast milk inhibitors
  delayed development of conjugating system

774.4 Perinatal jaundice due to hepatocellular damage
Fetal or neonatal hepatitis
Giant cell hepatitis
Inspissated bile syndrome

774.5 Perinatal jaundice from other causes
Code first underlying cause, as:
  congenital obstruction of bile duct (751.61)
  galactosemia (271.1)
  mucoviscidosis (277.00-277.09)

774.6 Unspecified fetal and neonatal jaundice
Icterus neonatorum
Neonatal hyperbilirubinemia (transient)
Physiologic jaundice NOS in newborn
Excludes: that in preterm infants (774.2)

774.7 Kernicterus not due to isoimmunization
Bilirubin encephalopathy
Kernicterus of newborn NOS
Excludes: kernicterus due to isoimmunization (773.4)

775 Endocrine and metabolic disturbances specific to the fetus and newborn
Includes: transitory endocrine and metabolic disturbances caused by the infant's response to maternal endocrine and metabolic factors, its removal from them, or its adjustment to extrauterine existence

775.0 Syndrome of "infant of a diabetic mother"
Maternal diabetes mellitus affecting fetus or newborn (with hypoglycemia)

775.1 Neonatal diabetes mellitus
Diabetes mellitus syndrome in newborn infant

775.2 Neonatal myasthenia gravis

775.3 Neonatal thyrotoxicosis
Neonatal hyperthyroidism (transient)

775.4 Hypocalcemia and hypomagnesemia of newborn
Cow's milk hypocalcemia
Hypocalcemic tetany, neonatal
Neonatal hypoparathyroidism
Phosphate-loading hypocalcemia

775.5 Other transitory neonatal electrolyte disturbances
Dehydration, neonatal

● Code new to this edition   ▲ Revision of existing code   ④ ⑤ Fourth or fifth digit required

CONDITIONS IN THE PERINATAL PERIOD

775.6 Neonatal hypoglycemia
Excludes: infant of mother with diabetes mellitus (775.0)

775.7 Late metabolic acidosis of newborn

⑤ **775.8 Other neonatal endocrine and metabolic disturbances**

775.81 Other acidosis of newborn
Acidemia NOS of newborn
Acidosis of newborn NOS
Mixed metabolic and respiratory acidosis of newborn

775.89 Other neonatal endocrine and metabolic disturbances
Amino-acid metabolic disorders described as transitory

775.9 Unspecified endocrine and metabolic disturbances specific to the fetus and newborn

776 Hematological disorders of fetus and newborn
Includes: disorders specific to the fetus or newborn

776.0 Hemorrhagic disease of newborn
Hemorrhagic diathesis of newborn
Vitamin K deficiency of newborn
Excludes: fetal or neonatal hemorrhage (772.0-772.9)

776.1 Transient neonatal thrombocytopenia
Neonatal thrombocytopenia due to:
  exchange transfusion
  idiopathic maternal thrombocytopenia
  isoimmunization

776.2 Disseminated intravascular coagulation in newborn

776.3 Other transient neonatal disorders of coagulation
Transient coagulation defect, newborn

776.4 Polycythemia neonatorum
Plethora of newborn
Polycythemia due to:
  donor twin transfusion
  maternal-fetal transfusion

776.5 Congenital anemia
Anemia following fetal blood loss
Excludes: anemia due to isoimmunization (773.0-773.2, 773.5)
  hereditary hemolytic anemias (282.0-282.9)

776.6 Anemia of prematurity

776.7 Transient neonatal neutropenia
Isoimmune neutropenia
Maternal transfer neutropenia
Excludes: congenital neutropenia (nontransient) (288.01)

776.8 Other specified transient hematological disorders

776.9 Unspecified hematological disorder specific to fetus or newborn

777 Perinatal disorders of digestive system
Includes: disorders specific to the fetus and newborn
Excludes: intestinal obstruction classifiable to 560.0-560.9

777.1 Meconium obstruction
Congenital fecaliths
Delayed passage of meconium
Meconium ileus NOS
Meconium plug syndrome
Excludes: meconium ileus in cystic fibrosis (277.01)

777.2 Intestinal obstruction due to inspissated milk

777.3 Hematemesis and melena due to swallowed maternal blood
Swallowed blood syndrome in newborn
Excludes: that not due to swallowed maternal blood (772.4)

777.4 Transitory ileus of newborn
Excludes: Hirschsprung's disease (751.3)

777.5 Necrotizing enterocolitis in fetus or newborn
Pseudomembranous enterocolitis in newborn

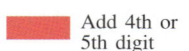 Add 4th or 5th digit   Nonspecific code   Unspecified code 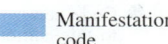 Manifestation code

525

TABULAR LIST

- **777.6 Perinatal intestinal perforation**
  Meconium peritonitis
- **777.8 Other specified perinatal disorders of digestive system**
- **777.9 Unspecified perinatal disorder of digestive system**

778 Conditions involving the integument and temperature regulation of fetus and newborn

- **778.0 Hydrops fetalis not due to isoimmunization**
  Idiopathic hydrops
  Excludes: hydrops fetalis due to isoimmunization (773.3)
- **778.1 Sclerema neonatorum**
  Subcutaneous fat necrosis
- **778.2 Cold injury syndrome of newborn**
- **778.3 Other hypothermia of newborn**
- **778.4 Other disturbances of temperature regulation of newborn**
  Dehydration fever in newborn
  Environmentally-induced pyrexia
  Hyperthermia in newborn
  Transitory fever of newborn
- **778.5 Other and unspecified edema of newborn**
  Edema neonatorum
- **778.6 Congenital hydrocele**
  Congenital hydrocele of tunica vaginalis
- **778.7 Breast engorgement in newborn**
  Noninfective mastitis of newborn
  Excludes: infective mastitis of newborn (771.5)
- **778.8 Other specified conditions involving the integument of fetus and newborn**
  Urticaria neonatorum
  Excludes: impetigo neonatorum (684)
  pemphigus neonatorum (684)
- **778.9 Unspecified condition involving the integument and temperature regulation of fetus and newborn**

779 Other and ill-defined conditions originating in the perinatal period

- **779.0 Convulsions in newborn**
  Fits in newborn
  Seizures in newborn
- **779.1 Other and unspecified cerebral irritability in newborn**
- **779.2 Cerebral depression, coma, and other abnormal cerebral signs**
  Cerebral ischemia NOS of newborn
  CNS dysfunction in newborn NOS
  Excludes: cerebral ischemia due to birth trauma (767.0)
  intrauterine cerebral ischemia (768.2-768.9)
  intraventricular hemorrhage (772.10-772.14)
- **779.3 Feeding problems in newborn**
  Regurgitation of food in newborn
  Slow feeding in newborn
  Vomiting in newborn
- **779.4 Drug reactions and intoxications specific to newborn**
  Gray syndrome from chloramphenicol administration in newborn
  Excludes: fetal alcohol syndrome (760.71)
  reactions and intoxications from maternal opiates and tranquilizers (763.5)
- **779.5 Drug withdrawal syndrome in newborn**
  Drug withdrawal syndrome in infant of dependent mother
  Excludes: fetal alcohol syndrome (760.71)
- **779.6 Termination of pregnancy (fetus)**
  Fetus death due to:
    induced abortion
    termination of pregnancy
  Excludes: spontaneous abortion (fetus) (761.8)
- **779.7 Periventricular leukomalacia**
- ⑤ **779.8 Other specified conditions originating in the perinatal period**

● Code new to this edition   ▲ Revision of existing code   Fourth or fifth digit required

CONDITIONS IN THE PERINATAL PERIOD

779.81 Neonatal bradycardia
Excludes: *abnormality in fetal heart rate or rhythm complicating labor and delivery (763.81-763.83)*
bradycardia due to birth asphyxia (768.5-768.9)

779.82 Neonatal tachycardia
Excludes: *abnormality in fetal heart rate or rhythm complicating labor and delivery (763.81-763.83)*

779.83 Delayed separation of umbilical cord

779.84 Meconium staining
Excludes: *meconium aspiration (770.11, 770.12)*
meconium passage during delivery (763.84)

779.85 Cardiac arrest of newborn

779.89 Other specified conditions originating in the perinatal period
Use additional code to specify condition

779.9 Unspecified condition originating in the perinatal period
Congenital debility NOS
Stillbirth NEC

TABULAR LIST

SYMPTOMS, SIGNS, AND ILL-DEFINED CONDITIONS

16. SYMPTOMS, SIGNS, AND ILL-DEFINED CONDITIONS (780-799)

This section includes symptoms, signs, abnormal results of laboratory or other investigative procedures, and ill-defined conditions regarding which no diagnosis classifiable elsewhere is recorded.

Signs and symptoms that point rather definitely to a given diagnosis are assigned to some category in the preceding part of the classification. In general, categories 780-796 include the more ill-defined conditions and symptoms that point with perhaps equal suspicion to two or more diseases or to two or more systems of the body, and without the necessary study of the case to make a final diagnosis. Practically all categories in this group could be designated as "not otherwise specified," or as "unknown etiology," or as "transient." The Alphabetic Index should be consulted to determine which symptoms and signs are to be allocated here and which to more specific sections of the classification; the residual subcategories numbered .9 are provided for other relevant symptoms which cannot be allocated elsewhere in the classification.

The conditions and signs or symptoms included in categories 780-796 consist of: (a) cases for which no more specific diagnosis can be made even after all facts bearing on the case have been investigated; (b) signs or symptoms existing at the time of initial encounter that proved to be transient and whose causes could not be determined; (c) provisional diagnoses in a patient who failed to return for further investigation or care; (d) cases referred elsewhere for investigation or treatment before the diagnosis was made; (e) cases in which a more precise diagnosis was not available for any other reason; (f) certain symptoms which represent important problems in medical care and which it might be desired to classify in addition to a known cause.

SYMPTOMS (780-789)

780   General symptoms

⑤ **780.0   Alteration of consciousness**

Excludes: coma:
    diabetic (250.2-250.3)
    hepatic (572.2)
    originating in the perinatal period (779.2)

    780.01   Coma

    780.02   Transient alteration of awareness

    780.03   Persistent vegetative state

    780.09   Other
        Drowsiness   Somnolence
        Semicoma   Stupor
        Unconsciousness

780.1   Hallucinations
    Hallucinations: Hallucinations:
        NOS   olfactory
        auditory   tactile
        gustatory

Excludes: those associated with mental disorders, as functional psychoses (295.0-298.9)
    organic brain syndromes (290.0-294.9, 310.0-310.9)
    visual hallucinations (368.16)

780.2   Syncope and collapse
    Blackout   (Near) (Pre) syncope
    Fainting   Vasovagal attack

Excludes: carotid sinus syncope (337.0)
    heat syncope (992.1)
    neurocirculatory asthenia (306.2)
    orthostatic hypotension (458.0)
    shock NOS (785.50)

⑤ **780.3   Convulsions**

Excludes: convulsions:
    epileptic (345.10-345.91)
    in newborn (779.0)

    780.31   Febrile convulsions (simple), unspecified
        Febrile seizure NOS

    780.32   Complex febrile convulsions
        Febrile seizure:
           atypical
           complex
           complicated

Excludes: status epilepticus (345.3)

 Add 4th or 5th digit   Nonspecific code   Unspecified code   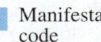 Manifestation code

TABULAR LIST

780.39 **Other convulsions**
    Convulsive disorder NOS
    Fit NOS
    Recurrent convulsions NOS
    Seizure NOS

780.4 Dizziness and giddiness
    Light-headedness
    Vertigo NOS
    Excludes: *Ménière's disease and other specified vertiginous syndromes (386.0-386.9)*

⑤ **780.5 Sleep disturbances**
    Excludes: *circadian rhythm sleep disorders (327.30-327.39)*
        organic hypersomnia (327.10-327.19)
        organic insomnia (327.00-327.09)
        organic sleep apnea (327.20-327.29)
        organic sleep related movement disorders (327.51-327.59)
        parasomnias (327.40-327.49)
        that of nonorganic origin (307.40-307.49)

780.50 **Sleep disturbance, unspecified**

780.51 **Insomnia with sleep apnea, unspecified**

780.52 **Insomnia, unspecified**

780.53 **Hypersomnia with sleep apnea, unspecified**

780.54 **Hypersomnia, unspecified**

780.55 **Disruption of 24 hour sleep wake cycle, unspecified**

780.56 **Dysfunctions associated with sleep stages or arousal from sleep**

780.57 **Unspecified sleep apnea**

780.58 **Sleep related movement disorder, unspecified**
    Excludes: *restless legs syndrome (333.94)*

780.59 **Other**

780.6 Fever
    Chills with fever   Hyperpyrexia NOS
    Fever NOS   Pyrexia NOS
    Fever of unknown origin   Pyrexia of unknown origin
      (FUO)
  Code first underlying condition when associated fever is present,
    such as with:
        leukemia (codes from categories 204-208)
        neutropenia (288.00-288.09)
        sickle-cell disease (282.60-282.69)
    Excludes: *pyrexia of unknown origin (during):*
            in newborn (778.4)
            labor (659.2)
            the puerperium (672)

⑤ **780.7 Malaise and fatigue**
    Excludes: *debility, unspecified (799.3)*
        fatigue (during):
          combat (308.0-308.9)
          heat (992.6)
          pregnancy (646.8)
        neurasthenia (300.5)
        senile asthenia (797.5)

780.71 **Chronic fatigue syndrome**

780.79 **Other malaise and fatigue**
    Asthenia NOS
    Lethargy
    Postviral (asthenic) syndrome
    Tiredness

780.8 Generalized hyperhidrosis
    Diaphoresis
    Excessive sweating
    Secondary hyperhidrosis
    Excludes: *focal (localized) (primary) (secondary) hyperhidrosis (705.21-705.22)*
         Frey's syndrome (705.22)

SYMPTOMS, SIGNS, AND ILL-DEFINED CONDITIONS

⑤ **780.9 Other general symptoms**
Excludes: *hypothermia:*
NOS (accidental) (991.6)
due to anesthesia (995.89)
of newborn (778.2-778.3)
memory disturbance as part of a pattern of mental disorder

780.91 Fussy infant (baby)

780.92 Excessive crying of infant (baby)
Excludes: *excessive crying of child, adolescent or adult (780.95)*

780.93 Memory loss
Amnesia (retrograde)
Memory loss NOS
Excludes: *mild memory disturbance due to organic brain damage (310.1)*
transient global amnesia (437.7)

780.94 Early satiety

780.95 Excessive crying of child, adolescent, or adult
Excludes: *excessive crying of infant (baby) (780.92)*

780.96 Generalized pain
Pain NOS

780.97 Altered mental status
Change in mental status
Excludes: *altered level of consciousness (780.01-780.09)*
altered mental status due to known condition — code to condition
delirium NOS (780.09)

780.99 Other general symptoms
Chill(s) NOS
Hypothermia, not associated with low environmental temperature

781 Symptoms involving nervous and musculoskeletal systems
Excludes: *depression NOS (311)*
disorders specifically relating to:
back (724.0-724.9)
hearing (388.0-389.9)
joint (718.0-719.9)
limb (729.0-729.9)
neck (723.0-723.9)
vision (368.0-369.9)
pain in limb (729.5)

781.0 Abnormal involuntary movements
Abnormal head movements
Fasciculation
Spasms NOS
Tremor NOS
Excludes: *abnormal reflex (796.1)*
chorea NOS (333.5)
infantile spasms (345.60-345.61)
spastic paralysis (342.1, 343.0-344.9)
specified movement disorders classifiable to 333 (333.0-333.9)
that of nonorganic origin (307.2-307.3)

781.1 Disturbances of sensation of smell and taste
Anosmia   Parosmia
Parageusia

781.2 Abnormality of gait
Gait: Gait:
  ataxic   spastic
  paralytic   staggering
Excludes: *ataxia:*
NOS (781.3)
locomotor (progressive) (094.0)
difficulty in walking (719.7)

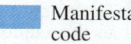

TABULAR LIST

781.3 Lack of coordination
　　Ataxia NOS
　　Muscular incoordination
Excludes: ataxic gait (781.2)
　　　　cerebellar ataxia (334.0-334.9)
　　　　difficulty in walking (719.7)
　　　　vertigo NOS (780.4)

781.4 Transient paralysis of limb
　　Monoplegia, transient NOS
Excludes: paralysis (342.0-344.9)

781.5 Clubbing of fingers

781.6 Meningismus
　　Dupré's syndrome
　　Meningism

781.7 Tetany
　　Carpopedal spasm
Excludes: tetanus neonatorum (771.3)
　　　tetany:
　　　　hysterical (300.11)
　　　　newborn (hypocalcemic) (775.4)
　　　　parathyroid (252.1)
　　　　psychogenic (306.0)

781.8 Neurologic neglect syndrome
　　Asomatognosia　　　　Left-sided neglect
　　Hemi-akinesia　　　　Sensory extinction
　　Hemi-inattention　　　Sensory neglect
　　Hemispatial neglect　　Visuospatial neglect

⑤ **781.9 Other symptoms involving nervous and musculoskeletal systems**

　　781.91 Loss of height
Excludes: osteoporosis (733.00-733.09)

　　781.92 Abnormal posture

　　781.93 Ocular torticollis

　　781.94 Facial weakness
　　　　Facial droop
Excludes: facial weakness due to late effect of cerebrovascular accident (438.83)

　　781.99 Other symptoms involving nervous and musculoskeletal systems

782 Symptoms involving skin and other integumentary tissue
Excludes: symptoms relating to breast (611.71-611.79)

782.0 Disturbance of skin sensation
　　Anesthesia of skin　　　Hypoesthesia
　　Burning or prickling　　Numbness
　　　sensation　　　　　　Paresthesia
　　Hyperesthesia　　　　　Tingling

782.1 Rash and other nonspecific skin eruption
　　Exanthem
Excludes: vesicular eruption (709.8)

782.2 Localized superficial swelling, mass, or lump
　　Subcutaneous nodules
Excludes: localized adiposity (278.1)

782.3 Edema
　　Anasarca　　　　　Localized edema NOS
　　Dropsy
Excludes: ascites (789.51-789.59)
　　　edema of:
　　　　newborn NOS (778.5)
　　　　pregnancy (642.0-642.9, 646.1)
　　　fluid retention (276.6)
　　　hydrops fetalis (773.3, 778.0)
　　　hydrothorax (511.8)
　　　nutritional edema (260, 262)

SYMPTOMS, SIGNS, AND ILL-DEFINED CONDITIONS

782.4 Jaundice, unspecified, not of newborn
  Cholemia NOS
  Icterus NOS
  Excludes: jaundice in newborn (774.0-774.7)
      due to isoimmunization (773.0-773.2, 773.4)

782.5 Cyanosis
  Excludes: newborn (770.83)

⑤ **782.6 Pallor and flushing**
  782.61 Pallor
  782.62 Flushing
      Excessive blushing

782.7 Spontaneous ecchymoses
  Petechiae
  Excludes: ecchymosis in fetus or newborn (772.6)
      purpura (287.0-287.9)

782.8 Changes in skin texture
  Induration of skin
  Thickening of skin

782.9 Other symptoms involving skin and integumentary tissues

783 Symptoms concerning nutrition, metabolism, and development

783.0 Anorexia
  Loss of appetite
  Excludes: anorexia nervosa (307.1)
      loss of appetite of nonorganic origin (307.59)

783.1 Abnormal weight gain
  Excludes: excessive weight gain in pregnancy (646.1)
      obesity (278.00)
      morbid (278.01)

⑤ **783.2 Abnormal loss of weight and underweight**
  Use additional code to identify Body Mass Index (BMI), if known (V85.0-V85.54)
  783.21 Loss of weight
  783.22 Underweight

783.3 Feeding difficulties and mismanagement
  Feeding problem (elderly) (infant)
  Excludes: feeding disturbance or problems:
      in newborn (779.3)
      of nonorganic origin (307.50-307.59)

⑤ **783.4 Lack of expected normal physiological development in childhood**
  Excludes: delay in sexual development and puberty (259.0)
      gonadal dysgenesis (758.6)
      pituitary dwarfism (253.3)
      slow fetal growth and fetal malnutrition (764.00-764.99)
      specific delays in mental development (315.0-315.9)

  783.40 Lack of normal physiological development, unspecified
      Inadequate development
      Lack of development

  783.41 Failure to thrive
      Failure to gain weight

  783.42 Delayed milestones
      Late talker
      Late walker

  783.43 Short stature
      Growth failure
      Growth retardation
      Lack of growth
      Physical retardation

783.5 Polydipsia
  Excessive thirst

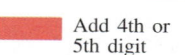 Add 4th or 5th digit
 Nonspecific code
 Unspecified code
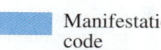 Manifestation code

TABULAR LIST

783.6 Polyphagia
Excessive eating
Hyperalimentation NOS
Excludes: disorders of eating of nonorganic origin (307.50-307.59)

783.7 Adult failure to thrive

783.9 Other symptoms concerning nutrition, metabolism, and development
Hypometabolism
Excludes: abnormal basal metabolic rate (794.7)
dehydration (276.51)
other disorders of fluid, electrolyte, and acid-base balance (276.0-276.9)

784 Symptoms involving head and neck
Excludes: encephalopathy NOS (348.30)
specific symptoms involving neck classifiable to 723 (723.0-723.9)

784.0 Headache
Facial pain
Pain in head NOS
Excludes: atypical face pain (350.2)
migraine (346.0-346.9)
tension headache (307.81)

784.1 Throat pain
Excludes: dysphagia (787.20-787.29)
neck pain (723.1)
sore throat (462)
chronic (472.1)

784.2 Swelling, mass, or lump in head and neck
Space-occupying lesion, intracranial NOS

784.3 Aphasia
Excludes: aphasia due to late effects of cerebrovascular disease (438.11)
developmental aphasia (315.31)

⑤ **784.4 Voice disturbance**

    784.40 Voice disturbance, unspecified

    784.41 Aphonia
        Loss of voice

    784.49 Other
        Change in voice   Hypernasality
        Dysphonia   Hyponasality
        Hoarseness

784.5 Other speech disturbance
Dysarthria   Slurred speech
Dysphasia
Excludes: stammering and stuttering (307.0)
that of nonorganic origin (307.0, 307.9)

⑤ **784.6 Other symbolic dysfunction**
Excludes: developmental learning delays (315.0-315.9)

    784.60 Symbolic dysfunction, unspecified

    784.61 Alexia and dyslexia
        Alexia (with agraphia)

    784.69 Other
        Acalculia   Agraphia NOS
        Agnosia   Apraxia

784.7 Epistaxis
Hemorrhage from nose
Nosebleed

784.8 Hemorrhage from throat
Excludes: hemoptysis (786.3)

⑤ **784.9 Other symptoms involving head and neck**

    784.91 Postnasal drip

SYMPTOMS, SIGNS, AND ILL-DEFINED CONDITIONS

784.99 Other symptoms involving head and neck
Choking sensation
Feeling of foreign body in throat
Halitosis
Mouth breathing
Sneezing

Excludes: *foreign body in throat (933.0)*

785 Symptoms involving cardiovascular system

Excludes: *heart failure NOS (428.9)*

785.0 Tachycardia, unspecified
Rapid heart beat

Excludes: *neonatal tachycardia (779.82)*
paroxysmal tachycardia (427.0-427.2)

785.1 Palpitations
Awareness of heart beat

Excludes: *specified dysrhythmias (427.0-427.9)*

785.2 Undiagnosed cardiac murmurs
Heart murmur NOS

785.3 Other abnormal heart sounds
Cardiac dullness, increased or decreased
Friction fremitus, cardiac
Precordial friction

785.4 Gangrene
Gangrene NOS
Gangrene spreading cutaneous
Gangrenous cellulitis
Phagedena

Code first any associated underlying condition, as:
diabetes (250.7)
Raynaud's syndrome (443.0)

Excludes: *gangrene of certain sites—see Alphabetic Index*
gangrene with atherosclerosis of the extremities (440.24)
gas gangrene (040.0)

⑤ 785.5 Shock without mention of trauma

785.50 Shock, unspecified
Failure of peripheral circulation

785.51 Cardiogenic shock

785.52 Septic shock
endotoxic
gram-negative

Code first systemic inflammatory response syndrome due to infectious process with organ dysfunction (995.92)

785.59 Other
Shock:
hypovolemic

Excludes: *shock (due to):*
anesthetic (995.4)
anaphylactic (995.0)
due to serum (999.4)
electric (994.8)
following abortion (639.5)
lightning (994.0)
obstetrical (669.1)
postoperative (998.0)
traumatic (958.4)

785.6 Enlargement of lymph nodes
Lymphadenopathy
"Swollen glands"

Excludes: *lymphadenitis (chronic) (289.1-289.3)*
acute (683)

785.9 Other symptoms involving cardiovascular system
Bruit (arterial)
Weak pulse

TABULAR LIST

786 Symptoms involving respiratory system and other chest symptoms

⑤ **786.0 Dyspnea and respiratory abnormalities**

786.00 Respiratory abnormality, unspecified

786.01 Hyperventilation

Excludes: hyperventilation, psychogenic (306.1)

786.02 Orthopnea

786.03 Apnea

Excludes: apnea of newborn (770.81, 770.82)
sleep apnea (780.51, 780.53, 780.57)

786.04 Cheyne-Stokes respiration

786.05 Shortness of breath

786.06 Tachypnea

Excludes: transitory tachypnea of newborn (770.6)

786.07 Wheezing

Excludes: asthma (493.00-493.92)

786.09 Other
Respiratory:
   distress
   insufficiency

Excludes: respiratory distress:
   following trauma and surgery (518.5)
   newborn (770.89)
   syndrome (newborn) (769)
      adult (518.5)
   respiratory failure (518.81, 518.83-518.84)
   newborn (770.84)

786.1 Stridor

Excludes: congenital laryngeal stridor (748.3)

786.2 Cough

Excludes: cough:
   psychogenic (306.1)
   smokers' (491.0)
   with hemorrhage (786.3)

786.3 Hemoptysis
Cough with hemorrhage
Pulmonary hemorrhage NOS

Excludes: pulmonary hemorrhage of newborn (770.3)

786.4 Abnormal sputum
Abnormal:
   amount (of) sputum
   color (of) sputum
   odor (of) sputum
Excessive sputum

⑤ **786.5 Chest pain**

786.50 Chest pain, unspecified

786.51 Precordial pain

786.52 Painful respiration
Pain:
   anterior chest wall
   pleuritic
Pleurodynia

Excludes: epidemic pleurodynia (074.1)

786.59 Other
Discomfort in chest
Pressure in chest
Tightness in chest

Excludes: pain in breast (611.71)

SYMPTOMS, SIGNS, AND ILL-DEFINED CONDITIONS

786.6 Swelling, mass, or lump in chest
Excludes: lump in breast (611.72)

786.7 Abnormal chest sounds
Abnormal percussion, chest
Friction sounds, chest
Rales
Tympany, chest
Excludes: wheezing (786.07)

786.8 Hiccough
Excludes: psychogenic hiccough (306.1)

786.9 Other symptoms involving respiratory system and chest
Breath-holding spell

787 Symptoms involving digestive system
Excludes: constipation (564.00-564.09)
pylorospasm (537.81)
congenital (750.5)

787.0 Nausea and vomiting
Emesis
Excludes: hematemesis NOS (578.0)
vomiting:
bilious, following gastrointestinal surgery (564.3)
cyclical (536.2)
psychogenic (306.4)
excessive, in pregnancy (643.0-643.9)
habit (536.2)
of newborn (779.3)
psychogenic NOS (307.54)

  787.01 Nausea with vomiting
  787.02 Nausea alone
  787.03 Vomiting alone

787.1 Heartburn
Pyrosis
Waterbrash
Excludes: dyspepsia or indigestion (536.8)

787.2 Dysphagia
Code first, if applicable, dysphagia due to late effect of cerebrovascular accident (438.82)

- **787.20 Dysphagia, unspecified**
  Difficulty in swallowing NOS
- **787.21 Dysphagia, oral phase**
- **787.22 Dysphagia, oropharyngeal phase**
- **787.23 Dysphagia, pharyngeal phase**
- **787.24 Dysphagia, pharyngoesophageal phase**
- **787.29 Other dysphagia**
  Cervical dysphagia
  Neurogenic dysphagia

787.3 Flatulence, eructation, and gas pain
Abdominal distention (gaseous)
Bloating
Tympanites (abdominal) (intestinal)
Excludes: aerophagy (306.4)

787.4 Visible peristalsis
Hyperperistalsis

787.5 Abnormal bowel sounds
Absent bowel sounds
Hyperactive bowel sounds

787.6 Incontinence of feces
Encopresis NOS
Incontinence of sphincter ani
Excludes: that of nonorganic origin (307.7)

537

 Add 4th or 5th digit
 Nonspecific code
Unspecified code
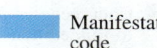 Manifestation code

TABULAR LIST

787.7 Abnormal feces
Bulky stools

Excludes: abnormal stool content (792.1)
melena:
NOS (578.1)
newborn (772.4, 777.3)

⑤ **787.9 Other symptoms involving digestive system**

Excludes: gastrointestinal hemorrhage (578.0-578.9)
intestinal obstruction (560.0-560.9)
specific functional digestive disorders:
esophagus (530.0-530.9)
stomach and duodenum (536.0-536.9)
those not elsewhere classified (564.00-564.9)

787.91 Diarrhea
Diarrhea NOS

787.99 Other
Change in bowel habits
Tenesmus (rectal)

788 Symptoms involving urinary system

Excludes: hematuria (599.7)
nonspecific findings on examination of the urine (791.0-791.9)
small kidney of unknown cause (589.0-589.9)
uremia NOS (586)
urinary obstruction (599.60, 599.69)

788.0 Renal colic
Colic (recurrent) of:
kidney
ureter

788.1 Dysuria
Painful urination
Strangury

⑤ **788.2 Retention of urine**
Code, if applicable, any causal condition first, such as:
hyperplasia of prostate (600.0-600.9 with fifth-digit 1)

788.20 Retention of urine, unspecified

788.21 Incomplete bladder emptying

788.29 Other specified retention of urine

⑤ **788.3 Urinary incontinence**

Excludes: that of nonorganic origin (307.6)
Code, if applicable, any causal condition first, such as:
congenital ureterocele (753.23)
genital prolapse (618.00-618.9)
hyperplasia of prostate (600.0-600.9 with fifth-digit 1)

788.30 Urinary incontinence, unspecified
Enuresis NOS

788.31 Urge incontinence

788.32 Stress incontinence, male

Excludes: stress incontinence (female) (625.6)

788.33 Mixed incontinence (male) (female)
Urge and stress

788.34 Incontinence without sensory awareness

788.35 Post-void dribbling

788.36 Nocturnal enuresis

788.37 Continuous leakage

788.38 Overflow incontinence

788.39 Other urinary incontinence

⑤ **788.4 Frequency of urination and polyuria**
Code, if applicable, any causal condition first, such as:
hyperplasia of prostate (600.0-600.9 with fifth-digit 1)

SYMPTOMS, SIGNS, AND ILL-DEFINED CONDITIONS

- **788.41 Urinary frequency**
  Frequency of micturition
- **788.42 Polyuria**
- **788.43 Nocturia**

788.5 Oliguria and anuria
Deficient secretion of urine
Suppression of urinary secretion

Excludes: that complicating:
  abortion (634-638 with .3, 639.3)
  ectopic or molar pregnancy (639.3)
  pregnancy, childbirth, or the puerperium (642.0-642.9, 646.2)

⑤ **788.6 Other abnormality of urination**
Code, if applicable, any causal condition first, such as:
  hyperplasia of prostate (600.0-600.9 with fifth-digit 1)

- **788.61 Splitting of urinary stream**
  Intermittent urinary stream
- **788.62 Slowing of urinary stream**
  Weak stream
- **788.63 Urgency of urination**

Excludes: urge incontinence (788.31, 788.33)

- **788.64 Urinary hesitancy**
- **788.65 Straining on urination**
- **788.69 Other**

788.7 Urethral discharge
Penile discharge
Urethrorrhea

788.8 Extravasation of urine

788.9 Other symptoms involving urinary system
Extrarenal uremia
Vesical:
  pain
  tenesmus

789 Other symptoms involving abdomen and pelvis
The following fifth-digit subclassification is to be used for codes 789.0, 789.3, 789.4, 789.6

- **0 unspecified site**
- **1 right upper quadrant**
- **2 left upper quadrant**
- **3 right lower quadrant**
- **4 left lower quadrant**
- **5 periumbilic**
- **6 epigastric**
- **7 generalized**
- **9 other specified site**
  multiple sites

Excludes: symptoms referable to genital organs:
  female (625.0-625.9)
  male (607.0-608.9)
  psychogenic (302.70-302.79)

⑤ **789.0 Abdominal pain**
Colic:
  NOS
  infantile
Cramps, abdominal

Excludes: renal colic (788.0)

789.1 Hepatomegaly
Enlargement of liver

789.2 Splenomegaly
Enlargement of spleen

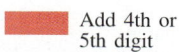 Add 4th or 5th digit Nonspecific code Unspecified code 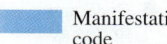 Manifestation code

TABULAR LIST

⑤ **789.3 Abdominal or pelvic swelling, mass, or lump**
Diffuse or generalized swelling or mass:
  abdominal NOS
  umbilical

Excludes: *abdominal distention (gaseous) (787.3)*
  ascites (789.51-789.59)

⑤ **789.4 Abdominal rigidity**

⑤ **789.5 Ascites**
Fluid in peritoneal cavity

● **789.51 Malignant ascites**
Code first malignancy, such as:
  malignant neoplasm of ovary (183.0)
  secondary malignant neoplasm of retroperitoneum and peritoneum (197.6)

● **789.59 Other ascites**

⑤ **789.6 Abdominal tenderness**
Rebound tenderness

789.9 Other symptoms involving abdomen and pelvis
Umbilical:
  bleeding
  discharge

NONSPECIFIC ABNORMAL FINDINGS (790-796)

790 Nonspecific findings on examination of blood

Excludes: *abnormalities of:*
  platelets (287.0-287.9)
  thrombocytes (287.0-287.9)
  white blood cells (288.00-288.9)

⑤ **790.0 Abnormality of red blood cells**

Excludes: *anemia:*
  congenital (776.5)
  newborn, due to isoimmunization (773.0-773.2, 773.5)
  of premature infant (776.6)
  other specified types (280.0-285.9)
  hemoglobin disorders (282.5-282.7)
  polycythemia:
    familial (289.6)
    neonatorum (776.4)
    secondary (289.0)
    vera (238.4)

790.01 Precipitous drop in hematocrit
Drop in hematocrit

790.09 Other abnormality of red blood cells
Abnormal red cell morphology NOS
Abnormal red cell volume NOS
Anisocytosis
Poikilocytosis

790.1 Elevated sedimentation rate

⑤ **790.2 Abnormal glucose**

Excludes: *diabetes mellitus (250.00-250.93)*
  dysmetabolic syndrome X (277.7)
  gestational diabetes (648.8)
  glycosuria (791.5)
  hypoglycemia (251.2)
  that complicating pregnancy, childbirth, or the puerperium (648.8)

790.21 Impaired fasting glucose
Elevated fasting glucose

790.22 Impaired glucose tolerance test (oral)
Elevated glucose tolerance test

790.29 Other abnormal glucose
Abnormal glucose NOS
Abnormal non-fasting glucose
Hyperglycemia NOS
Pre-diabetes NOS

SYMPTOMS, SIGNS, AND ILL-DEFINED CONDITIONS

- **790.3 Excessive blood level of alcohol**
  Elevated blood-alcohol
- **790.4 Nonspecific elevation of levels of transaminase or lactic acid dehydrogenase [LDH]**
- **790.5 Other nonspecific abnormal serum enzyme levels**
  Abnormal serum level of:
   acid phosphatase
   alkaline phosphatase
  Abnormal serum level of:
   amylase
   lipase

  Excludes: deficiency of circulating enzymes (277.6)

- **790.6 Other abnormal blood chemistry**
  Abnormal blood level of:
   cobalt
   copper
   iron
   lead
  Abnormal blood level of:
   lithium
   magnesium
   mineral
   zinc

  Excludes: abnormality of electrolyte or acid-base balance (276.0-276.9)
   hypoglycemia NOS (251.2)
   lead poisoning (984.0-984.9)
   specific finding indicating abnormality of:
    amino-acid transport and metabolism (270.0-270.9)
    carbohydrate transport and metabolism (271.0-271.9)
    lipid metabolism (272.0-272.9)
   uremia NOS (586)

- **790.7 Bacteremia**

  Excludes: bacteremia of newborn (771.83)
   septicemia (038)

  Use additional code, if desired, to identify organism (041)

- **790.8 Viremia, unspecified**
- ⑤ 790.9 **Other nonspecific findings on examination of blood**
    - **790.91 Abnormal arterial blood gases**
    - **790.92 Abnormal coagulation profile**
      Abnormal or prolonged:
       bleeding time
       coagulation time
       partial thromboplastin time [PTT]
       prothrombin time [PT]

      Excludes: coagulation (hemorrhagic) disorders (286.0-286.9)

    - **790.93 Elevated prostate specific antigen (PSA)**
    - **790.94 Euthyroid sick syndrome**
    - **790.95 Elevated C-reactive protein (CRP)**
    - **790.99 Other**

791 Nonspecific findings on examination of urine

Excludes: hematuria NOS (599.7)
 specific findings indicating abnormality of:
  amino-acid transport and metabolism (270.0-270.9)
  carbohydrate transport and metabolism (271.0-271.9)

- **791.0 Proteinuria**
  Albuminuria
  Bence-Jones proteinuria

  Excludes: postural proteinuria (593.6)
   that arising during pregnancy or the puerperium (642.0-642.9, 646.2)

- **791.1 Chyluria**

  Excludes: filarial (125.0-125.9)

- **791.2 Hemoglobinuria**
- **791.3 Myoglobinuria**
- **791.4 Biliuria**
- **791.5 Glycosuria**

  Excludes: renal glycosuria (271.4)

- **791.6 Acetonuria**
  Ketonuria

TABULAR LIST

791.7 Other cells and casts in urine

791.9 Other nonspecific findings on examination of urine
- Crystalluria
- Elevated urine levels of:
  - 17-ketosteroids
  - catecholamines
  - indolacetic acid
  - vanillylmandelic acid [VMA]
- Melanuria

792 Nonspecific abnormal findings in other body substances

Excludes: that in chromosomal analysis (795.2)

792.0 Cerebrospinal fluid

792.1 Stool contents
- Abnormal stool color
- Fat in stool
- Mucus in stool
- Occult blood
- Pus in stool

Excludes: blood in stool [melena] (578.1)
newborn (772.4, 777.3)

792.2 Semen
- Abnormal spermatozoa

Excludes: azoospermia (606.0)
oligospermia (606.1)

792.3 Amniotic fluid

792.4 Saliva

Excludes: that in chromosomal analysis (795.2)

792.5 Cloudy (hemodialysis) (peritoneal) dialysis effluent

792.9 Other nonspecific abnormal findings in body substances
- Peritoneal fluid
- Pleural fluid
- Synovial fluid
- Vaginal fluids

793 Nonspecific abnormal findings on radiological and other examinations of body structure

Includes: nonspecific abnormal findings of:
- thermography
- ultrasound examination [echogram]
- x-ray examination

Excludes: abnormal results of function studies and radioisotope scans (794.0-794.9)

793.0 Skull and head

Excludes: nonspecific abnormal echoencephalogram (794.01)

793.1 Lung field
- Coin lesion of lung
- Shadow, lung

793.2 Other intrathoracic organ
- Abnormal:
  - echocardiogram
  - heart shadow
  - ultrasound cardiogram
- Mediastinal shift

793.3 Biliary tract
- Nonvisualization of gallbladder

793.4 Gastrointestinal tract

793.5 Genitourinary organs
- Filling defect:
  - bladder
  - kidney
  - ureter

793.6 Abdominal area, including retroperitoneum

793.7 Musculoskeletal system

⑤ **793.8** Breast

793.80 Abnormal mammogram, unspecified

SYMPTOMS, SIGNS, AND ILL-DEFINED CONDITIONS

793.81 Mammographic microcalcification
Excludes: mammographic calcification (793.89)
mammographic calculus (793.89)

793.89 Other abnormal findings on radiological examination of breast
Mammographic calcification
Mammographic calculus

793.9 Other
Excludes: abnormal finding by radioisotope localization of placenta (794.9)

793.91 Image test inconclusive due to excess body fat
Use additional code to identify Body Mass Index (BMI), if known (V85.0-V85.54)

793.99 Other nonspecific abnormal findings on radiological and other examinations of body structure
Abnormal:
placental finding by x-ray or ultrasound method
radiological findings in skin and subcutaneous tissue

794 Nonspecific abnormal results of function studies
Includes: radioisotope:
scans
uptake studies
scintiphotography

794.0 Brain and central nervous system

794.00 Abnormal function study, unspecified

794.01 Abnormal echoencephalogram

794.02 Abnormal electroencephalogram [EEG]

794.09 Other
Abnormal brain scan

794.1 Peripheral nervous system and special senses

794.10 Abnormal response to nerve stimulation, unspecified

794.11 Abnormal retinal function studies
Abnormal electroretinogram [ERG]

794.12 Abnormal electro-oculogram [EOG]

794.13 Abnormal visually evoked potential

794.14 Abnormal oculomotor studies

794.15 Abnormal auditory function studies

794.16 Abnormal vestibular function studies

794.17 Abnormal electromyogram [EMG]
Excludes: that of eye (794.14)

794.19 Other

794.2 Pulmonary
Abnormal lung scan
Reduced:
ventilatory capacity
vital capacity

794.3 Cardiovascular

794.30 Abnormal function study, unspecified

794.31 Abnormal electrocardiogram [ECG] [EKG]
Excludes: long QT syndrome (426.82)

794.39 Other
Abnormal:
ballistocardiogram
phonocardiogram
vectorcardiogram

794.4 Kidney
Abnormal renal function test

794.5 Thyroid
Abnormal thyroid:
scan
uptake

TABULAR LIST

794.6 Other endocrine function study

794.7 **Basal metabolism**
Abnormal basal metabolic rate [BMR]

794.8 **Liver**
Abnormal liver scan

794.9 **Other**
Bladder
Pancreas
Placenta
Spleen

795 Other and nonspecific abnormal cytological, histological, immunological and DNA test findings

> Excludes: nonspecific abnormalities of red blood cells (790.01-790.09)

⑤ **795.0** **Abnormal Papanicolaou smear of cervix and cervical HPV**
Abnormal thin preparation smear of cervix
Abnormal cervical cytology

> Excludes: carcinoma in-situ of cervix (233.1)
> cervical intraepithelial neoplasia I [CIN I] (622.11)
> cervical intraepithelial neoplasia II [CIN II] (622.12)
> cervical intraepithelial neoplasia III [CIN III] (233.1)
> dysplasia (histologically confirmed) of cervix (uteri) NOS (622.10)
> mild dysplasia (histologically confirmed) (622.11)
> moderate dysplasia (histologically confirmed) (622.12)
> severe dysplasia (histologically confirmed) (233.1)

795.00 **Abnormal glandular Papanicolaou smear of cervix**
Atypical endocervical cells NOS
Atypical endometrial cells NOS
Atypical glandular cells NOS

795.01 Papanicolaou smear of cervix with atypical squamous cells of undetermined significance (ASC-US)

795.02 Papanicolaou smear of cervix with atypical squamous cells cannot exclude high grade squamous intraepithelial lesion (ASC-H)

795.03 Papanicolaou smear of cervix with low grade squamous intraepithelial lesion (LGSIL)

795.04 Papanicolaou smear of cervix with high grade squamous intraepithelial lesion (HGSIL)

795.05 Cervical high risk human papillomavirus (HPV) DNA test positive

795.06 Papanicolaou smear of cervix with cytologic evidence of malignancy

795.08 **Unsatisfactory smear**
Inadequate sample

795.09 **Other abnormal Papanicolaou smear of cervix and cervical HPV**
Cervical low risk human papillomavirus (HPV) DNA test positive
Papanicolaou smear of cervix with low risk human papillomavirus (HPV) DNA test positive

Use additional code for associated human papillomavirus (HPV) (079.4)

> Excludes: encounter for Papanicolaou cervical smear to confirm findings of recent normal smear following initial abnormal smear (V72.32)

795.1 Nonspecific abnormal Papanicolaou smear of other site

795.2 **Nonspecific abnormal findings on chromosomal analysis**
Abnormal karyotype

⑤ **795.3** **Nonspecific positive culture findings**
Positive culture findings in:
nose
sputum
throat
wound

> Excludes: that of:
> blood (790.7-790.8)
> urine (791.9)

795.31 **Nonspecific positive findings for anthrax**
Positive findings by nasal swab

795.39 Other nonspecific positive culture findings

SYMPTOMS, SIGNS, AND ILL-DEFINED CONDITIONS

795.4 Other nonspecific abnormal histological findings

795.5 Nonspecific reaction to tuberculin skin test without active tuberculosis
Abnormal result of Mantoux test
PPD positive
Tuberculin (skin test):
   positive
   reactor

795.6 False positive serological test for syphilis
False positive Wassermann reaction

⑤ **795.7 Other nonspecific immunological findings**

Excludes: abnormal tumor markers (795.81-795.89)
   elevated prostate specific antigen [PSA] (790.93)
   elevated tumor associated antigens (795.81-795.89)
   isoimmunization, in pregnancy (656.1-656.2)
      affecting fetus or newborn (773.0-773.2)

795.71 Nonspecific serologic evidence of human immunodeficiency virus [HIV]
Inconclusive human immunodeficiency virus [HIV] test (adult) (infant)

Note: This code is ONLY to be used when a test finding is reported as nonspecific. Asymptomatic positive findings are coded to V08. If any HIV infection symptom or condition is present, see code 042. Negative findings are not coded.

Excludes: acquired immunodeficiency syndrome [AIDS] (042)
   asymptomatic human immunodeficiency virus, [HIV] infection status (V08)
   HIV infection, symptomatic (042)
   human immunodeficiency virus [HIV] disease (042)
   positive (status) NOS (V08)

795.79 Other and unspecified nonspecific immunological findings
Raised antibody titer
Raised level of immunoglobulins

⑤ **795.8 Abnormal tumor markers**
Elevated tumor associated antigens [TAA]
Elevated tumor specific antigens [TSA]

Excludes: elevated prostate specific antigen [PSA] (790.93)

795.81 Elevated carcinoembryonic antigen (CEA)

795.82 Elevated cancer antigen 125 (CA 125)

795.89 Other abnormal tumor markers

796 Other nonspecific abnormal findings

796.0 Nonspecific abnormal toxicological findings
Abnormal levels of heavy metals or drugs in blood, urine, or other tissue

Excludes: excessive blood level of alcohol (790.3)

796.1 Abnormal reflex

796.2 Elevated blood pressure reading without diagnosis of hypertension
Note: This category is to be used to record an episode of elevated blood pressure in a patient in whom no formal diagnosis of hypertension has been made, or as an incidental finding.

796.3 Nonspecific low blood pressure reading

796.4 Other abnormal clinical findings

796.5 Abnormal finding on antenatal screening

796.6 Abnormal findings on neonatal screening

Excludes: nonspecific serologic evidence of human immunodeficiency virus [HIV] (795.71)

796.9 Other

ILL-DEFINED AND UNKNOWN CAUSES OF MORBIDITY AND MORTALITY (797-799)

797 Senility without mention of psychosis
Old age
Senescence
Senile asthenia
Senile debility
Senile exhaustion

Excludes: senile psychoses (290.0-290.9)

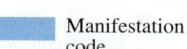

TABULAR LIST

798 Sudden death, cause unknown

    798.0 Sudden infant death syndrome
        Cot death
        Crib death
        Sudden death of nonspecific cause in infancy

    798.1 Instantaneous death

    798.2 Death occurring in less than 24 hours from onset of symptoms, not otherwise explained
        Death known not to be violent or instantaneous, for which no cause could be discovered
        Died without sign of disease

    798.9 Unattended death
        Death in circumstances where the body of the deceased was found and no cause could be discovered
        Found dead

799 Other ill-defined and unknown causes of morbidity and mortality

    799.0 Asphyxia and hypoxemia
        Excludes: asphyxia and hypoxemia (due to)
                hypercapnia (786.09)

        799.01 Asphyxia

        799.02 Hypoxemia

    799.1 Respiratory arrest
        Cardiorespiratory failure
        Excludes: cardiac arrest (427.5)
                failure of peripheral circulation (785.50)
                respiratory distress:
                  NOS (786.09)
                  acute (518.82)
                  following trauma and surgery (518.5)
                  newborn (770.89)
                  syndrome (newborn) (769)
                    adult (following trauma and surgery) (518.5)
                    other (518.82)
                respiratory failure (518.81, 518.83-518.84)
                  newborn (770.84)
                respiratory insufficiency (786.09)
                  acute (518.82)

    799.2 Nervousness
        "Nerves"

    799.3 Debility, unspecified
        Excludes: asthenia (780.79)
                nervous debility (300.5)
                neurasthenia (300.5)
                senile asthenia (797)

    799.4 Cachexia
        Wasting disease
    Code first underlying condition, if known

    799.8 Other ill-defined conditions

        799.81 Decreased libido
            Decreased sexual desire
        Excludes: psychosexual dysfunction with inhibited sexual desire (302.71)

        799.89 Other ill-defined conditions

    799.9 Other unknown and unspecified cause
        Undiagnosed disease, not specified as to site or system involved
        Unknown cause of morbidity or mortality

INJURY AND POISONING

17. INJURY AND POISONING (800-999)
Use E code(s) to identify the cause and intent of the injury or poisoning (E800-E999)
Note:
1. The principle of multiple coding of injuries should be followed wherever possible. Combination categories for multiple injuries are provided for use when there is insufficient detail as to the nature of the individual conditions, or for primary tabulation purposes when it is more convenient to record a single code; otherwise, the component injuries should be coded separately.

    Where multiple sites of injury are specified in the titles, the word "with" indicates involvement of both sites, and the word "and" indicates involvement of either or both sites. The word "finger" includes thumb.
2. Categories for "late effect" of injuries are to be found at 905-909.

FRACTURES (800-829)

Excludes: malunion (733.81)
nonunion (733.82)
pathologic or spontaneous fracture (733.10-733.19)
stress fractures (733.93-733.95)

The terms "condyle," "coronoid process," "ramus," and "symphysis" indicate the portion of the bone fractured, not the name of the bone involved.
The descriptions "closed" and "open" used in the fourth-digit subdivisions include the following terms:

closed (with or without delayed healing):
- comminuted
- depressed
- elevated
- fissured
- fracture NOS
- greenstick
- impacted
- linear
- simple
- slipped epiphysis
- spiral

open (with or without delayed healing):
- compound
- infected
- missile
- puncture
- with foreign body

A fracture not indicated as closed or open should be classified as closed.

FRACTURE OF SKULL (800-804)

The following fifth-digit subclassification is for use with the appropriate codes in categories 800, 801, 803, and 804:

0 unspecified state of consciousness

1 with no loss of consciousness

2 with brief [less than one hour] loss of consciousness

3 with moderate [1-24 hours] loss of consciousness and return to pre-existing conscious level

4 with prolonged [more than 24 hours] loss of consciousness and return to pre-existing conscious level

5 with prolonged [more than 24 hours] loss of consciousness, without return to pre-existing conscious level
    Use fifth-digit 5 to designate when a patient is unconscious and dies before regaining consciousness, regardless of the duration of the loss of consciousness

6 with loss of consciousness of unspecified duration

9 with concussion, unspecified

800 Fracture of vault of skull
Includes: frontal bone
parietal bone

- **800.0** Closed without mention of intracranial injury
- **800.1** Closed with cerebral laceration and contusion
- **800.2** Closed with subarachnoid, subdural, and extradural hemorrhage
- **800.3** Closed with other and unspecified intracranial hemorrhage
- **800.4** Closed with intracranial injury of other and unspecified nature
- **800.5** Open without mention of intracranial injury
- **800.6** Open with cerebral laceration and contusion
- **800.7** Open with subarachnoid, subdural, and extradural hemorrhage

TABULAR LIST

⑤ **800.8** Open with other and unspecified intracranial hemorrhage

⑤ **800.9** Open with intracranial injury of other and unspecified nature

⑤ **801** Fracture of base of skull
Includes:
    fossa: sinus:
      anterior   ethmoid
      middle   frontal
      posterior   sphenoid bone
    occiput bone   temporal bone
    orbital roof

⑤ **801.0** Closed without mention of intracranial injury

⑤ **801.1** Closed with cerebral laceration and contusion

⑤ **801.2** Closed with subarachnoid, subdural, and extradural hemorrhage

⑤ **801.3** Closed with other and unspecified intracranial hemorrhage

⑤ **801.4** Closed with intracranial injury of other and unspecified nature

⑤ **801.5** Open without mention of intracranial injury

⑤ **801.6** Open with cerebral laceration and contusion

⑤ **801.7** Open with subarachnoid, subdural, and extradural hemorrhage

⑤ **801.8** Open with other and unspecified intracranial hemorrhage

⑤ **801.9** Open with intracranial injury of other and unspecified nature

802 Fracture of face bones

  802.0 Nasal bones, closed

  802.1 Nasal bones, open

  ⑤ **802.2** Mandible, closed
    Inferior maxilla
    Lower jaw (bone)

    802.20 Unspecified site
    802.21 Condylar process
    802.22 Subcondylar
    802.23 Coronoid process
    802.24 Ramus, unspecified
    802.25 Angle of jaw
    802.26 Symphysis of body
    802.27 Alveolar border of body
    802.28 Body, other and unspecified
    802.29 Multiple sites

  ⑤ **802.3** Mandible, open

    802.30 Unspecified site
    802.31 Condylar process
    802.32 Subcondylar
    802.33 Coronoid process
    802.34 Ramus, unspecified
    802.35 Angle of jaw
    802.36 Symphysis of body
    802.37 Alveolar border of body
    802.38 Body, other and unspecified
    802.39 Multiple sites

  802.4 Malar and maxillary bones, closed
    Superior maxilla   Zygoma
    Upper jaw (bone)   Zygomatic arch

  802.5 Malar and maxillary bones, open

  802.6 Orbital floor (blow-out), closed

  802.7 Orbital floor (blow-out), open

INJURY AND POISONING

802.8 Other facial bones, closed
  Alveolus
  Orbit:
    NOS
    part other than roof or floor
  Palate
  Excludes: orbital:
    floor (802.6)
    roof (801.0-801.9)

802.9 Other facial bones, open

⑤ **803** Other and unqualified skull fractures
  Includes: skull NOS
    skull multiple NOS

⑤ **803.0** Closed without mention of intracranial injury
⑤ **803.1** Closed with cerebral laceration and contusion
⑤ **803.2** Closed with subarachnoid, subdural, and extradural hemorrhage
⑤ **803.3** Closed with other and unspecified intracranial hemorrhage
⑤ **803.4** Closed with intracranial injury of other and unspecified nature
⑤ **803.5** Open without mention of intracranial injury
⑤ **803.6** Open with cerebral laceration and contusion
⑤ **803.7** Open with subarachnoid, subdural, and extradural hemorrhage
⑤ **803.8** Open with other and unspecified intracranial hemorrhage
⑤ **803.9** Open with intracranial injury of other and unspecified nature

⑤ **804** Multiple fractures involving skull or face with other bones

⑤ **804.0** Closed without mention of intracranial injury
⑤ **804.1** Closed with cerebral laceration and contusion
⑤ **804.2** Closed with subarachnoid, subdural, and extradural hemorrhage
⑤ **804.3** Closed with other and unspecified intracranial hemorrhage
⑤ **804.4** Closed with intracranial injury of other and unspecified nature
⑤ **804.5** Open without mention of intracranial injury
⑤ **804.6** Open with cerebral laceration and contusion
⑤ **804.7** Open with subarachnoid, subdural, and extradural hemorrhage
⑤ **804.8** Open with other and unspecified intracranial hemorrhage
⑤ **804.9** Open with intracranial injury of other and unspecified nature

FRACTURE OF NECK AND TRUNK (805-809)

805 Fracture of vertebral column without mention of spinal cord injury
  Includes: neural arch
    spine
    spinous process
    transverse process
    vertebra

  The following fifth-digit subclassification is for use with codes 805.0-805.1:

  0 cervical vertebra, unspecified level
  1 first cervical vertebra
  2 second cervical vertebra
  3 third cervical vertebra
  4 fourth cervical vertebra
  5 fifth cervical vertebra
  6 sixth cervical vertebra
  7 seventh cervical vertebra
  8 multiple cervical vertebrae

⑤ **805.0** Cervical, closed
  Atlas
  Axis

⑤ **805.1** Cervical, open

805.2 Dorsal [thoracic], closed

Add 4th or 5th digit | Nonspecific code | Unspecified code | Medicare secondary payer (MSP) alert

TABULAR LIST

- **805.3** Dorsal [thoracic], open
- **805.4** Lumbar, closed
- **805.5** Lumbar, open
- **805.6** Sacrum and coccyx, closed
- **805.7** Sacrum and coccyx, open
- **805.8** Unspecified, closed
- **805.9** Unspecified, open

806 **Fracture of vertebral column with spinal cord injury**
Includes: any condition classifiable to 805 with:
  complete or incomplete transverse lesion (of cord)
  hematomyelia
  injury to:
    cauda equina
    nerve
  paralysis
  paraplegia
  quadriplegia
  spinal concussion

⑤ **806.0 Cervical, closed**

- **806.00** C_1-C_4 level with unspecified spinal cord injury
  Cervical region NOS with spinal cord injury NOS
- **806.01** C_1-C_4 level with complete lesion of cord
- **806.02** C_1-C_4 level with anterior cord syndrome
- **806.03** C_1-C_4 level with central cord syndrome
- **806.04** C_1-C_4 level with other specified spinal cord injury
  C_1-C_4 level with:
    incomplete spinal cord lesion NOS
    posterior cord syndrome
- **806.05** C_5-C_7 level with unspecified spinal cord injury
- **806.06** C_5-C_7 level with complete lesion of cord
- **806.07** C_5-C_7 level with anterior cord syndrome
- **806.08** C_5-C_7 level with central cord syndrome
- **806.09** C_5-C_7 level with other specified spinal cord injury
  C_5-C_7 level with:
    incomplete spinal cord lesion NOS
    posterior cord syndrome

⑤ **806.1 Cervical, open**

- **806.10** C_1-C_4 level with unspecified spinal cord injury
- **806.11** C_1-C_4 level with complete lesion of cord
- **806.12** C_1-C_4 level with anterior cord syndrome
- **806.13** C_1-C_4 level with central cord syndrome
- **806.14** C_1-C_4 level with other specified spinal cord injury
  C_1-C_4 level with:
    incomplete spinal cord lesion NOS
    posterior cord syndrome
- **806.15** C_5-C_7 level with unspecified spinal cord injury
- **806.16** C_5-C_7 level with complete lesion of cord
- **806.17** C_5-C_7 level with anterior cord syndrome
- **806.18** C_5-C_7 level with central cord syndrome
- **806.19** C_5-C_7 level with other specified spinal cord injury
  C_5-C_7 level with:
    incomplete spinal cord lesion NOS
    posterior cord syndrome

⑤ **806.2 Dorsal [thoracic], closed**

- **806.20** T_1-T_6 level with unspecified spinal cord injury
  Thoracic region NOS with spinal cord injury NOS
- **806.21** T_1-T_6 level with complete lesion of cord
- **806.22** T_1-T_6 level with anterior cord syndrome
- **806.23** T_1-T_6 level with central cord syndrome

INJURY AND POISONING

- **806.24** T$_1$-T$_6$ level with other specified spinal cord injury
  T$_1$-T$_6$ level with:
  incomplete spinal cord lesion NOS
  posterior cord syndrome
- **806.25** T$_7$-T$_{12}$ level with unspecified spinal cord injury
- **806.26** T$_7$-T$_{12}$ level with complete lesion of cord
- **806.27** T$_7$-T$_{12}$ level with anterior cord syndrome
- **806.28** T$_7$-T$_{12}$ level with central cord syndrome
- **806.29** T$_7$-T$_{12}$ level with other specified spinal cord injury
  T$_7$-T$_{12}$ level with:
  incomplete spinal cord lesion NOS
  posterior cord syndrome

⑤ **806.3 Dorsal [thoracic], open**
- **806.30** T$_1$-T$_6$ level with unspecified spinal cord injury
- **806.31** T$_1$-T$_6$ level with complete lesion of cord
- **806.32** T$_1$-T$_6$ level with anterior cord syndrome
- **806.33** T$_1$-T$_6$ level with central cord syndrome
- **806.34** T$_1$-T$_6$ level with other specified spinal cord injury
  T$_1$-T$_6$ level with:
  incomplete spinal cord lesion NOS
  posterior cord syndrome
- **806.35** T$_7$-T$_{12}$ level with unspecified spinal cord injury
- **806.36** T$_7$-T$_{12}$ level with complete lesion of cord
- **806.37** T$_7$-T$_{12}$ level with anterior cord syndrome
- **806.38** T$_7$-T$_{12}$ level with central cord syndrome
- **806.39** T$_7$-T$_{12}$ level with other specified spinal cord injury
  T$_7$-T$_{12}$ level with:
  incomplete spinal cord lesion NOS
  posterior cord syndrome

806.4 Lumbar, closed

806.5 Lumbar, open

⑤ **806.6 Sacrum and coccyx, closed**
- **806.60** With unspecified spinal cord injury
- **806.61** With complete cauda equina lesion
- **806.62** With other cauda equina injury
- **806.69** With other spinal cord injury

⑤ **806.7 Sacrum and coccyx, open**
- **806.70** With unspecified spinal cord injury
- **806.71** With complete cauda equina lesion
- **806.72** With other cauda equina injury
- **806.79** With other spinal cord injury

806.8 Unspecified, closed

806.9 Unspecified, open

807 Fracture of rib(s), sternum, larynx, and trachea
The following fifth-digit subclassification is for use with codes 807.0-807.1:
- 0 rib(s), unspecified
- 1 one rib
- 2 two ribs
- 3 three ribs
- 4 four ribs
- 5 five ribs
- 6 six ribs
- 7 seven ribs
- 8 eight or more ribs
- 9 multiple ribs, unspecified

Add 4th or 5th digit | Nonspecific code | Unspecified code | Medicare secondary payer (MSP) alert

TABULAR LIST

⑤ **807.0** **Rib(s), closed**
⑤ **807.1** **Rib(s), open**
   807.2 **Sternum, closed**
   807.3 **Sternum, open**
   807.4 **Flail chest**
   807.5 **Larynx and trachea, closed**
       Hyoid bone   Trachea
       Thyroid cartilage
   807.6 **Larynx and trachea, open**

808 **Fracture of pelvis**
   808.0 **Acetabulum, closed**
   808.1 **Acetabulum, open**
   808.2 **Pubis, closed**
   808.3 **Pubis, open**
⑤ **808.4** **Other specified part, closed**
      808.41 **Ilium**
      808.42 **Ischium**
      808.43 **Multiple pelvic fractures with disruption of pelvic circle**
      808.49 **Other**
          Innominate bone
          Pelvic rim
⑤ **808.5** **Other specified part, open**
      808.51 **Ilium**
      808.52 **Ischium**
      808.53 **Multiple pelvic fractures with disruption of pelvic circle**
      808.59 **Other**
   808.8 **Unspecified, closed**
   808.9 **Unspecified, open**

809 **Ill-defined fractures of bones of trunk**
   Includes: bones of trunk with other bones except those of skull and face
                  multiple bones of trunk

   Excludes: multiple fractures of:
          pelvic bones alone (808.0-808.9)
          ribs alone (807.0-807.1, 807.4)
          ribs or sternum with limb bones (819.0-819.1, 828.0-828.1)
          skull or face with other bones (804.0-804.9)

   809.0 **Fracture of bones of trunk, closed**
   809.1 **Fracture of bones of trunk, open**

FRACTURE OF UPPER LIMB (810-819)

⑤ **810** **Fracture of clavicle**
   Includes: collar bone
                  interligamentous part of clavicle
   The following fifth-digit subclassification is for use with category 810:

      0 **unspecified part**
          Clavicle NOS
      1 **sternal end of clavicle**
      2 **shaft of clavicle**
      3 **acromial end of clavicle**

⑤ **810.0** **Closed**
⑤ **810.1** **Open**

INJURY AND POISONING

⑤ **811** Fracture of scapula
    Includes: shoulder blade
The following fifth-digit subclassification is for use with category 811:
    0 unspecified part
    1 acromial process
        Acromion (process)
    2 coracoid process
    3 glenoid cavity and neck of scapula
    9 other
        Scapula body

⑤ **811.0** Closed
⑤ **811.1** Open

812 Fracture of humerus
  ⑤ **812.0** Upper end, closed
      812.00 Upper end, unspecified part
          Proximal end
          Shoulder
      812.01 Surgical neck
          Neck of humerus NOS
      812.02 Anatomical neck
      812.03 Greater tuberosity
      812.09 Other
          Head
          Upper epiphysis
  ⑤ **812.1** Upper end, open
      812.10 Upper end, unspecified part
      812.11 Surgical neck
      812.12 Anatomical neck
      812.13 Greater tuberosity
      812.19 Other
  ⑤ **812.2** Shaft or unspecified part, closed
      812.20 Unspecified part of humerus
          Humerus NOS
          Upper arm NOS
      812.21 Shaft of humerus
  ⑤ **812.3** Shaft or unspecified part, open
      812.30 Unspecified part of humerus
      812.31 Shaft of humerus
  ⑤ **812.4** Lower end, closed
      Distal end of humerus
      Elbow
      812.40 Lower end, unspecified part
      812.41 Supracondylar fracture of humerus
      812.42 Lateral condyle
          External condyle
      812.43 Medial condyle
          Internal epicondyle
      812.44 Condyle(s), unspecified
          Articular process NOS
          Lower epiphysis NOS
      812.49 Other
          Multiple fractures of lower end
          Trochlea
  ⑤ **812.5** Lower end, open
      812.50 Lower end, unspecified part
      812.51 Supracondylar fracture of humerus
      812.52 Lateral condyle
      812.53 Medial condyle

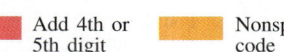 Add 4th or 5th digit   Nonspecific code   Unspecified code   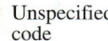 Medicare secondary payer (MSP) alert

553

TABULAR LIST

812.54 Condyle(s), unspecified
812.59 Other

813 Fracture of radius and ulna

⑤ 813.0 Upper end, closed
  Proximal end
  813.00 Upper end of forearm, unspecified
  813.01 Olecranon process of ulna
  813.02 Coronoid process of ulna
  813.03 Monteggia's fracture
  813.04 Other and unspecified fractures of proximal end of ulna (alone)
    Multiple fractures of ulna, upper end
  813.05 Head of radius
  813.06 Neck of radius
  813.07 Other and unspecified fractures of proximal end of radius (alone)
    Multiple fractures of radius, upper end
  813.08 Radius with ulna, upper end [any part]

⑤ 813.1 Upper end, open
  813.10 Upper end of forearm, unspecified
  813.11 Olecranon process of ulna
  813.12 Coronoid process of ulna
  813.13 Monteggia's fracture
  813.14 Other and unspecified fractures of proximal end of ulna (alone)
  813.15 Head of radius
  813.16 Neck of radius
  813.17 Other and unspecified fractures of proximal end of radius (alone)
  813.18 Radius with ulna, upper end [any part]

⑤ 813.2 Shaft, closed
  813.20 Shaft, unspecified
  813.21 Radius (alone)
  813.22 Ulna (alone)
  813.23 Radius with ulna

⑤ 813.3 Shaft, open
  813.30 Shaft, unspecified
  813.31 Radius (alone)
  813.32 Ulna (alone)
  813.33 Radius with ulna

⑤ 813.4 Lower end, closed
  Distal end
  813.40 Lower end of forearm, unspecified
  813.41 Colles' fracture
    Smith's fracture
  813.42 Other fractures of distal end of radius (alone)
    Dupuytren's fracture, radius
    Radius, lower end
  813.43 Distal end of ulna (alone)
    Ulna: Ulna:
      head   lower epiphysis
      lower end   styloid process
  813.44 Radius with ulna, lower end
  813.45 Torus fracture of radius

⑤ 813.5 Lower end, open
  813.50 Lower end of forearm, unspecified
  813.51 Colles' fracture
  813.52 Other fractures of distal end of radius (alone)
  813.53 Distal end of ulna (alone)

● Code new to this edition   ▲ Revision of existing code   ④ ⑤ Fourth or fifth digit required

INJURY AND POISONING

- 813.54 Radius with ulna, lower end
- ⑤ 813.8 Unspecified part, closed
  - 813.80 Forearm, unspecified
  - 813.81 Radius (alone)
  - 813.82 Ulna (alone)
  - 813.83 Radius with ulna
- ⑤ 813.9 Unspecified part, open
  - 813.90 Forearm, unspecified
  - 813.91 Radius (alone)
  - 813.92 Ulna (alone)
  - 813.93 Radius with ulna

⑤ **814 Fracture of carpal bone(s)**

The following fifth-digit subclassification is for use with category 814:

- **0** carpal bone, unspecified
  Wrist NOS
- **1** navicular [scaphoid] of wrist
- **2** lunate [semilunar] bone of wrist
- **3** triquetral [cuneiform] bone of wrist
- **4** pisiform
- **5** trapezium bone [larger multangular]
- **6** trapezoid bone [smaller multangular]
- **7** capitate bone [os magnum]
- **8** hamate [unciform] bone
- **9** other

- ⑤ 814.0 Closed
- ⑤ 814.1 Open

⑤ **815 Fracture of metacarpal bone(s)**
Includes: hand [except finger]
          metacarpus

The following fifth-digit subclassification is for use with category 815:

- **0** metacarpal bone(s), site unspecified
- **1** base of thumb [first] metacarpal
  Bennett's fracture
- **2** base of other metacarpal bone(s)
- **3** shaft of metacarpal bone(s)
- **4** neck of metacarpal bone(s)
- **9** multiple sites of metacarpus

- ⑤ 815.0 Closed
- ⑤ 815.1 Open

⑤ **816 Fracture of one or more phalanges of hand**
Includes: finger(s)
          thumb

The following fifth-digit subclassification is for use with category 816:

- **0** phalanx or phalanges, unspecified
- **1** middle or proximal phalanx or phalanges
- **2** distal phalanx or phalanges
- **3** multiple sites

- ⑤ 816.0 Closed
- ⑤ 816.1 Open

817 Multiple fractures of hand bones
Includes: metacarpal bone(s) with phalanx or phalanges of same hand

- 817.0 Closed
- 817.1 Open

TABULAR LIST

818 **Ill-defined fractures of upper limb**
　　Includes:　arm NOS
　　　　　　　multiple bones of same upper limb
　　Excludes:　multiple fractures of:
　　　　　　　　metacarpal bone(s) with phalanx or phalanges (817.0-817.1)
　　　　　　　　phalanges of hand alone (816.0-816.1)
　　　　　　　　radius with ulna (813.0-813.9)

　818.0　Closed
　818.1　Open

819 **Multiple fractures involving both upper limbs, and upper limb with rib(s) and sternum**
　　Includes:　arm(s) with rib(s) or sternum
　　　　　　　both arms [any bones]

　819.0　Closed
　819.1　Open

FRACTURE OF LOWER LIMB (820-829)

820 **Fracture of neck of femur**
　⑤　820.0　Transcervical fracture, closed
　　　　　820.00　Intracapsular section, unspecified
　　　　　820.01　Epiphysis (separation) (upper)
　　　　　　　　　Transepiphyseal
　　　　　820.02　Midcervical section
　　　　　　　　　Transcervical NOS
　　　　　820.03　Base of neck
　　　　　　　　　Cervicotrochanteric section
　　　　　820.09　Other
　　　　　　　　　Head of femur
　　　　　　　　　Subcapital

　⑤　820.1　Transcervical fracture, open
　　　　　820.10　Intracapsular section, unspecified
　　　　　820.11　Epiphysis (separation) (upper)
　　　　　820.12　Midcervical section
　　　　　820.13　Base of neck
　　　　　820.19　Other

　⑤　820.2　Pertrochanteric fracture, closed
　　　　　820.20　Trochanteric section, unspecified
　　　　　　　　　Trochanter:
　　　　　　　　　　NOS
　　　　　　　　　　greater
　　　　　　　　　　lesser
　　　　　820.21　Intertrochanteric section
　　　　　820.22　Subtrochanteric section

　⑤　820.3　Pertrochanteric fracture, open
　　　　　820.30　Trochanteric section, unspecified
　　　　　820.31　Intertrochanteric section
　　　　　820.32　Subtrochanteric section

　　820.8　Unspecified part of neck of femur, closed
　　　　　Hip NOS
　　　　　Neck of femur NOS
　　820.9　Unspecified part of neck of femur, open

821 **Fracture of other and unspecified parts of femur**
　⑤　821.0　Shaft or unspecified part, closed
　　　　　821.00　Unspecified part of femur
　　　　　　　　　Thigh
　　　　　　　　　Upper leg
　　　　　Excludes:　hip NOS (820.8)
　　　　　821.01　Shaft

　⑤　821.1　Shaft or unspecified part, open

556　　● Code new　　　▲ Revision of　　　④ ⑤ Fourth or fifth
　　　　to this edition　　　existing code　　　digit required

INJURY AND POISONING

- **821.10** Unspecified part of femur
- **821.11** Shaft
- ⑤ **821.2** Lower end, closed
  Distal end
  - **821.20** Lower end, unspecified part
  - **821.21** Condyle, femoral
  - **821.22** Epiphysis, lower (separation)
  - **821.23** Supracondylar fracture of femur
  - **821.29** Other
    Multiple fractures of lower end
- ⑤ **821.3** Lower end, open
  - **821.30** Lower end, unspecified part
  - **821.31** Condyle, femoral
  - **821.32** Epiphysis, lower (separation)
  - **821.33** Supracondylar fracture of femur
  - **821.39** Other

822 Fracture of patella
- **822.0** Closed
- **822.1** Open

⑤ **823** Fracture of tibia and fibula

> Excludes: *Dupuytren's fracture (824.4-824.5)*
>   *ankle (824.4-824.5)*
>   *radius (813.42, 813.52)*
> *Pott's fracture (824.4-824.5)*
> *that involving ankle (824.0-824.9)*

The following fifth-digit subclassification is for use with category 823:
- **0** tibia alone
- **1** fibula alone
- **2** fibula with tibia

- ⑤ **823.0** Upper end, closed
  Head   Tibia:
  Proximal end   condyles
                             tuberosity
- ⑤ **823.1** Upper end, open
- ⑤ **823.2** Shaft, closed
- ⑤ **823.3** Shaft, open
- ⑤ **823.4** Torus fracture
- ⑤ **823.8** Unspecified part, closed
  Lower leg NOS
- ⑤ **823.9** Unspecified part, open

824 Fracture of ankle
- **824.0** Medial malleolus, closed
  Tibia involving:
    ankle
    malleolus
- **824.1** Medial malleolus, open
- **824.2** Lateral malleolus, closed
  Fibula involving:
    ankle
    malleolus
- **824.3** Lateral malleolus, open
- **824.4** Bimalleolar, closed
  Dupuytren's fracture, fibula
  Pott's fracture
- **824.5** Bimalleolar, open
- **824.6** Trimalleolar, closed
  Lateral and medial malleolus with anterior or posterior lip of tibia

TABULAR LIST

- 824.7 Trimalleolar, open
- **824.8** Unspecified, closed
  Ankle NOS
- **824.9** Unspecified, open

825 Fracture of one or more tarsal and metatarsal bones
- 825.0 Fracture of calcaneus, closed
  Heel bone
  Os calcis
- 825.1 Fracture of calcaneus, open
- ⑤ 825.2 Fracture of other tarsal and metatarsal bones, closed
  - **825.20** Unspecified bone(s) of foot [except toes]
    Instep
  - 825.21 Astragalus
    Talus
  - 825.22 Navicular [scaphoid], foot
  - 825.23 Cuboid
  - 825.24 Cuneiform, foot
  - 825.25 Metatarsal bone(s)
  - **825.29** Other
    Tarsal with metatarsal bone(s) only

  Excludes: calcaneus (825.0)

- ⑤ 825.3 Fracture of other tarsal and metatarsal bones, open
  - **825.30** Unspecified bone(s) of foot [except toes]
  - 825.31 Astragalus
  - 825.32 Navicular [scaphoid], foot
  - 825.33 Cuboid
  - 825.34 Cuneiform, foot
  - 825.35 Metatarsal bone(s)
  - **825.39** Other

826 Fracture of one or more phalanges of foot
  Includes: toe(s)
- 826.0 Closed
- 826.1 Open

827 Other, multiple, and ill-defined fractures of lower limb
  Includes: leg NOS
    multiple bones of same lower limb

  Excludes: multiple fractures of:
    ankle bones alone (824.4-824.9)
    phalanges of foot alone (826.0-826.1)
    tarsal with metatarsal bones (825.29, 825.39)
    tibia with fibula (823.0-823.9 with fifth-digit 2)

- **827.0** Closed
- **827.1** Open

828 Multiple fractures involving both lower limbs, lower with upper limb, and lower limb(s) with rib(s) and sternum
  Includes: arm(s) with leg(s) [any bones]
    both legs [any bones]
    leg(s) with rib(s) or sternum

- **828.0** Closed
- **828.1** Open

829 Fracture of unspecified bones
- **829.0** Unspecified bone, closed
- **829.1** Unspecified bone, open

INJURY AND POISONING

DISLOCATION (830-839)

Includes: displacement
subluxation

Excludes: congenital dislocation (754.0-755.8)
pathological dislocation (718.2)
recurrent dislocation (718.3)

The descriptions "closed" and "open", used in the fourth-digit subdivisions, include the following terms:

closed:
  complete
  dislocation NOS
  partial
  simple
  uncomplicated

open:
  compound
  infected
  with foreign body

A dislocation not indicated as closed or open should be classified as closed.

830 Dislocation of jaw
Includes: jaw (cartilage) (meniscus)
mandible
maxilla (inferior)
temporomandibular (joint)

  830.0 Closed dislocation
  830.1 Open dislocation

831 Dislocation of shoulder

Excludes: sternoclavicular joint (839.61, 839.71)
sternum (839.61, 839.71)

The following fifth-digit subclassification is for use with category 831:

0 shoulder, unspecified
  Humerus NOS

1 anterior dislocation of humerus

2 posterior dislocation of humerus

3 inferior dislocation of humerus

4 acromioclavicular (joint)
  Clavicle

9 other
  Scapula

  831.0 Closed dislocation
  831.1 Open dislocation

832 Dislocation of elbow
The following fifth-digit subclassification is for use with category 832:

0 elbow unspecified

1 anterior dislocation of elbow

2 posterior dislocation of elbow

3 medial dislocation of elbow

4 lateral dislocation of elbow

9 other

  832.0 Closed dislocation
  832.1 Open dislocation

833 Dislocation of wrist
The following fifth-digit subclassification is for use with category 833:

0 wrist, unspecified part
  Carpal (bone)   Radius, distal end

1 radioulnar (joint), distal

2 radiocarpal (joint)

3 midcarpal (joint)

4 carpometacarpal (joint)

5 metacarpal (bone), proximal end

9 other
  Ulna, distal end

| | Add 4th or 5th digit | | Nonspecific code | | Unspecified code | | Medicare secondary payer (MSP) alert |

TABULAR LIST

- ⑤ **833.0** Closed dislocation
- ⑤ **833.1** Open dislocation
- ⑤ **834** **Dislocation of finger**
    Includes: finger(s)
    phalanx of hand
    thumb

  The following fifth-digit subclassification is for use with category 834:

  - **0** finger, unspecified part
  - **1** metacarpophalangeal (joint)
      Metacarpal (bone), distal end
  - **2** interphalangeal (joint), hand

- ⑤ **834.0** Closed dislocation
- ⑤ **834.1** Open dislocation
- ⑤ **835** **Dislocation of hip**

  The following fifth-digit subclassification is for use with category 835:

  - **0** dislocation of hip, unspecified
  - **1** posterior dislocation
  - **2** obturator dislocation
  - **3** other anterior dislocation

- ⑤ **835.0** Closed dislocation
- ⑤ **835.1** Open dislocation
- **836** **Dislocation of knee**

    Excludes: dislocation of knee:
        old or pathological (718.2)
        recurrent (718.3)
      internal derangement of knee joint (717.0-717.5, 717.8-717.9)
      old tear of cartilage or meniscus of knee (717.0-717.5, 717.8-717.9)

  - **836.0** **Tear of medial cartilage or meniscus of knee, current**
      Bucket handle tear:
        NOS current injury
        medial meniscus current injury
  - **836.1** **Tear of lateral cartilage or meniscus of knee, current**
  - **836.2** **Other tear of cartilage or meniscus of knee, current**
      Tear of:
        cartilage (semilunar) current injury, not specified as medial or lateral
        meniscus current injury, not specified as medial or lateral
  - **836.3** **Dislocation of patella, closed**
  - **836.4** **Dislocation of patella, open**
  - ⑤ **836.5** **Other dislocation of knee, closed**
    - **836.50** Dislocation of knee, unspecified
    - **836.51** Anterior dislocation of tibia, proximal end
        Posterior dislocation of femur, distal end
    - **836.52** Posterior dislocation of tibia, proximal end
        Anterior dislocation of femur, distal end
    - **836.53** Medial dislocation of tibia, proximal end
    - **836.54** Lateral dislocation of tibia, proximal end
    - **836.59** Other
  - ⑤ **836.6** **Other dislocation of knee, open**
    - **836.60** Dislocation of knee, unspecified
    - **836.61** Anterior dislocation of tibia, proximal end
    - **836.62** Posterior dislocation of tibia, proximal end
    - **836.63** Medial dislocation of tibia, proximal end
    - **836.64** Lateral dislocation of tibia, proximal end
    - **836.69** Other

560 ● Code new to this edition ▲ Revision of existing code ④ ⑤ Fourth or fifth digit required

INJURY AND POISONING

837 Dislocation of ankle
  Includes: astragalus
  fibula, distal end
  navicular, foot
  scaphoid, foot
  tibia, distal end
  837.0 Closed dislocation
  837.1 Open dislocation

838 Dislocation of foot
  The following fifth-digit subclassification is for use with category 838:
  0 foot, unspecified
  1 tarsal (bone), joint unspecified
  2 midtarsal (joint)
  3 tarsometatarsal (joint)
  4 metatarsal (bone), joint unspecified
  5 metatarsophalangeal (joint)
  6 interphalangeal (joint), foot
  9 other
  Phalanx of foot
  Toe(s)

  838.0 Closed dislocation
  838.1 Open dislocation

839 Other, multiple, and ill-defined dislocations
  839.0 Cervical vertebra, closed
  Cervical spine
  Neck
  839.00 Cervical vertebra, unspecified
  839.01 First cervical vertebra
  839.02 Second cervical vertebra
  839.03 Third cervical vertebra
  839.04 Fourth cervical vertebra
  839.05 Fifth cervical vertebra
  839.06 Sixth cervical vertebra
  839.07 Seventh cervical vertebra
  839.08 Multiple cervical vertebrae

  839.1 Cervical vertebra, open
  839.10 Cervical vertebra, unspecified
  839.11 First cervical vertebra
  839.12 Second cervical vertebra
  839.13 Third cervical vertebra
  839.14 Fourth cervical vertebra
  839.15 Fifth cervical vertebra
  839.16 Sixth cervical vertebra
  839.17 Seventh cervical vertebra
  839.18 Multiple cervical vertebrae

  839.2 Thoracic and lumbar vertebra, closed
  839.20 Lumbar vertebra
  839.21 Thoracic vertebra
  Dorsal [thoracic] vertebra

  839.3 Thoracic and lumbar vertebra, open
  839.30 Lumbar vertebra
  839.31 Thoracic vertebra

  839.4 Other vertebra, closed
  839.40 Vertebra, unspecified site
  Spine NOS

TABULAR LIST

- 839.41 **Coccyx**
- 839.42 **Sacrum**
  - Sacroiliac (joint)
- **839.49** **Other**

⑤ 839.5 **Other vertebra, open**
- **839.50** **Vertebra, unspecified site**
- 839.51 **Coccyx**
- 839.52 **Sacrum**
- **839.59** **Other**

⑤ 839.6 **Other location, closed**
- 839.61 **Sternum**
  - Sternoclavicular joint
- **839.69** **Other**
  - Pelvis

⑤ 839.7 **Other location, open**
- **839.71** **Sternum**
- **839.79** **Other**

839.8 **Multiple and ill-defined, closed**
  - Arm
  - Back
  - Hand
  - Multiple locations, except fingers or toes alone
  - Other ill-defined locations
  - Unspecified location

839.9 **Multiple and ill-defined, open**

SPRAINS AND STRAINS OF JOINTS AND ADJACENT MUSCLES (840-848)

Includes: avulsion of: joint capsule, ligament, muscle, tendon
  hemarthrosis of: joint capsule, ligament, muscle, tendon
  laceration of: joint capsule, ligament, muscle, tendon
  rupture of: joint capsule, ligament, muscle, tendon
  sprain of: joint capsule, ligament, muscle, tendon
  strain of: joint capsule, ligament, muscle, tendon
  tear of: joint capsule, ligament, muscle, tendon

Excludes: laceration of tendon in open wounds (880-884 and 890-894 with .2)

840 **Sprains and strains of shoulder and upper arm**
- 840.0 **Acromioclavicular (joint) (ligament)**
- 840.1 **Coracoclavicular (ligament)**
- 840.2 **Coracohumeral (ligament)**
- 840.3 **Infraspinatus (muscle) (tendon)**
- 840.4 **Rotator cuff (capsule)**

  Excludes: complete rupture of rotator cuff, nontraumatic (727.61)

- 840.5 **Subscapularis (muscle)**
- 840.6 **Supraspinatus (muscle) (tendon)**
- 840.7 **Superior glenoid labrum lesion**
  - SLAP lesion
- **840.8** **Other specified sites of shoulder and upper arm**
- **840.9** **Unspecified site of shoulder and upper arm**
  - Arm NOS
  - Shoulder NOS

841 **Sprains and strains of elbow and forearm**
- 841.0 **Radial collateral ligament**
- 841.1 **Ulnar collateral ligament**
- 841.2 **Radiohumeral (joint)**
- 841.3 **Ulnohumeral (joint)**
- **841.8** **Other specified sites of elbow and forearm**
- **841.9** **Unspecified site of elbow and forearm**
  - Elbow NOS

INJURY AND POISONING

842 Sprains and strains of wrist and hand
⑤ 842.0 Wrist
842.00 Unspecified site
842.01 Carpal (joint)
842.02 Radiocarpal (joint) (ligament)
842.09 Other
Radioulnar joint, distal
⑤ 842.1 Hand
842.10 Unspecified site
842.11 Carpometacarpal (joint)
842.12 Metacarpophalangeal (joint)
842.13 Interphalangeal (joint)
842.19 Other
Midcarpal (joint)

843 Sprains and strains of hip and thigh
843.0 Iliofemoral (ligament)
843.1 Ischiocapsular (ligament)
843.8 Other specified sites of hip and thigh
843.9 Unspecified site of hip and thigh
Hip NOS
Thigh NOS

844 Sprains and strains of knee and leg
844.0 Lateral collateral ligament of knee
844.1 Medial collateral ligament of knee
844.2 Cruciate ligament of knee
844.3 Tibiofibular (joint) (ligament), superior
844.8 Other specified sites of knee and leg
844.9 Unspecified site of knee and leg
Knee NOS
Leg NOS

845 Sprains and strains of ankle and foot
⑤ 845.0 Ankle
845.00 Unspecified site
845.01 Deltoid (ligament), ankle
Internal collateral (ligament), ankle
845.02 Calcaneofibular (ligament)
845.03 Tibiofibular (ligament), distal
845.09 Other
Achilles tendon
⑤ 845.1 Foot
845.10 Unspecified site
845.11 Tarsometatarsal (joint) (ligament)
845.12 Metatarsophalangeal (joint)
845.13 Interphalangeal (joint), toe
845.19 Other

846 Sprains and strains of sacroiliac region
846.0 Lumbosacral (joint) (ligament)
846.1 Sacroiliac ligament
846.2 Sacrospinatus (ligament)
846.3 Sacrotuberous (ligament)
846.8 Other specified sites of sacroiliac region
846.9 Unspecified site of sacroiliac region

847 Sprains and strains of other and unspecified parts of back
Excludes: lumbosacral (846.0)

TABULAR LIST

847.0 Neck
　　Anterior longitudinal (ligament), cervical
　　Atlanto-axial (joints)
　　Atlanto-occipital (joints)
　　Whiplash injury
　　Excludes: neck injury NOS (959.0)
　　　　　　thyroid region (848.2)

847.1 Thoracic

847.2 Lumbar

847.3 Sacrum
　　Sacrococcygeal (ligament)

847.4 Coccyx

847.9 Unspecified site of back
　　Back NOS

848 Other and ill-defined sprains and strains

848.0 Septal cartilage of nose

848.1 Jaw
　　Temporomandibular (joint) (ligament)

848.2 Thyroid region
　　Cricoarytenoid (joint) (ligament)
　　Cricothyroid (joint) (ligament)
　　Thyroid cartilage

848.3 Ribs
　　Chondrocostal (joint) without mention of injury to sternum
　　Costal cartilage without mention of injury to sternum

⑤ **848.4 Sternum**

　　848.40   Unspecified site

　　848.41   Sternoclavicular (joint) (ligament)

　　848.42   Chondrosternal (joint)

　　848.49   Other
　　　　Xiphoid cartilage

848.5 Pelvis
　　Symphysis pubis
　　Excludes: that in childbirth (665.6)

848.8 Other specified sites of sprains and strains

848.9 Unspecified site of sprain and strain

INTRACRANIAL INJURY, EXCLUDING THOSE WITH SKULL FRACTURE (850-854)

Excludes: intracranial injury with skull fracture (800-801 and 803-804, except .0 and .5)
　　　　open wound of head without intracranial injury (870.0-873.9)
　　　　skull fracture alone (800-801 and 803-804 with .0, .5)

The description "with open intracranial wound," used in the fourth-digit subdivisions, includes those specified as open or with mention of infection or foreign body.

The following fifth-digit subclassification is for use with categories 851-854:

0 unspecified state of consciousness

1 with no loss of consciousness

2 with brief [less than one hour] loss of consciousness

3 with moderate [1-24 hours] loss of consciousness

4 with prolonged [more than 24 hours] loss of consciousness and return to pre-existing conscious level

5 with prolonged [more than 24 hours] loss of consciousness, without return to pre-existing conscious level
　　Use fifth-digit 5 to designate when a patient is unconscious and dies before regaining consciousness, regardless of the duration of the loss of consciousness

6 with loss of consciousness of unspecified duration

9 with concussion, unspecified

564　　● Code new to this edition　　▲ Revision of existing code　　④ ⑤ Fourth or fifth digit required

INJURY AND POISONING

850 Concussion
Includes: commotio cerebri

Excludes: concussion with:
cerebral laceration or contusion (851.0-851.9)
cerebral hemorrhage (852-853)
head injury NOS (959.01)

- **850.0 With no loss of consciousness**
  Concussion with mental confusion or disorientation, without loss of consciousness
- **850.1 With brief loss of consciousness**
  Loss of consciousness for less than one hour
  - **850.11 With loss of consciousness of 30 minutes or less**
  - **850.12 With loss of consciousness from 31 to 59 minutes**
- **850.2 With moderate loss of consciousness**
  Loss of consciousness for 1-24 hours
- **850.3 With prolonged loss of consciousness and return to pre-existing conscious level**
  Loss of consciousness for more than 24 hours with complete recovery
- **850.4 With prolonged loss of consciousness, without return to pre-existing conscious level**
- **850.5 With loss of consciousness of unspecified duration**
- **850.9 Concussion, unspecified**

851 Cerebral laceration and contusion

- **851.0 Cortex (cerebral) contusion without mention of open intracranial wound**
- **851.1 Cortex (cerebral) contusion with open intracranial wound**
- **851.2 Cortex (cerebral) laceration without mention of open intracranial wound**
- **851.3 Cortex (cerebral) laceration with open intracranial wound**
- **851.4 Cerebellar or brain stem contusion without mention of open intracranial wound**
- **851.5 Cerebellar or brain stem contusion with open intracranial wound**
- **851.6 Cerebellar or brain stem laceration without mention of open intracranial wound**
- **851.7 Cerebellar or brain stem laceration with open intracranial wound**
- **851.8 Other and unspecified cerebral laceration and contusion, without mention of open intracranial wound**
  Brain (membrane) NOS
- **851.9 Other and unspecified cerebral laceration and contusion, with open intracranial wound**

852 Subarachnoid, subdural, and extradural hemorrhage, following injury

Excludes: Cerebral contusion or laceration (with hemorrhage) (851.0-851.9)

- **852.0 Subarachnoid hemorrhage following injury without mention of open intracranial wound**
  Middle meningeal hemorrhage following injury
- **852.1 Subarachnoid hemorrhage following injury with open intracranial wound**
- **852.2 Subdural hemorrhage following injury without mention of open intracranial wound**
- **852.3 Subdural hemorrhage following injury with open intracranial wound**
- **852.4 Extradural hemorrhage following injury without mention of open intracranial wound**
  Epidural hematoma following injury
- **852.5 Extradural hemorrhage following injury with open intracranial wound**

853 Other and unspecified intracranial hemorrhage following injury

- **853.0 Without mention of open intracranial wound**
  Cerebral compression due to injury
  Intracranial hematoma following injury
  Traumatic cerebral hemorrhage
- **853.1 With open intracranial wound**

854 Intracranial injury of other and unspecified nature
Includes: brain injury NOS
cavernous sinus
intracranial injury

Excludes: any condition classifiable to 850-853
head injury NOS (959.01)

TABULAR LIST

⑤ **854.0** Without mention of open intracranial wound

⑤ **854.1** With open intracranial wound

INTERNAL INJURY OF THORAX, ABDOMEN, AND PELVIS (860-869)

Includes:
- blast injuries of internal organs
- blunt trauma of internal organs
- bruise of internal organs
- concussion injuries (except cerebral) of internal organs
- crushing of internal organs
- hematoma of internal organs
- laceration of internal organs
- puncture of internal organs
- tear of internal organs
- traumatic rupture of internal organs

Excludes: concussion NOS (850.0-850.9)
flail chest (807.4)
foreign body entering through orifice (930.0-939.9)
injury to blood vessels (901.0-902.9)

The description "with open wound," used in the fourth-digit subdivisions, includes those with mention of infection or foreign body.

860 Traumatic pneumothorax and hemothorax

860.0 Pneumothorax without mention of open wound into thorax

860.1 Pneumothorax with open wound into thorax

860.2 Hemothorax without mention of open wound into thorax

860.3 Hemothorax with open wound into thorax

860.4 Pneumohemothorax without mention of open wound into thorax

860.5 Pneumohemothorax with open wound into thorax

861 Injury to heart and lung

Excludes: injury to blood vessels of thorax (901.0-901.9)

⑤ **861.0** Heart, without mention of open wound into thorax

  861.00 Unspecified injury

  861.01 Contusion
  Cardiac contusion
  Myocardial contusion

  861.02 Laceration without penetration of heart chambers

  861.03 Laceration with penetration of heart chambers

⑤ **861.1** Heart, with open wound into thorax

  861.10 Unspecified injury

  861.11 Contusion

  861.12 Laceration without penetration of heart chambers

  861.13 Laceration with penetration of heart chambers

⑤ **861.2** Lung, without mention of open wound into thorax

  861.20 Unspecified injury

  861.21 Contusion

  861.22 Laceration

⑤ **861.3** Lung, with open wound into thorax

  861.30 Unspecified injury

  861.31 Contusion

  861.32 Laceration

862 Injury to other and unspecified intrathoracic organs

Excludes: injury to blood vessels of thorax (901.0-901.9)

862.0 Diaphragm, without mention of open wound into cavity

862.1 Diaphragm, with open wound into cavity

⑤ **862.2** Other specified intrathoracic organs, without mention of open wound into cavity

  862.21 Bronchus

  862.22 Esophagus

INJURY AND POISONING

- **862.29** Other
  - Pleura
  - Thymus gland
- ⑤ **862.3** Other specified intrathoracic organs, with open wound into cavity
  - **862.31** Bronchus
  - **862.32** Esophagus
  - **862.39** Other
- **862.8** Multiple and unspecified intrathoracic organs, without mention of open wound into cavity
  - Crushed chest
  - Multiple intrathoracic organs
- **862.9** Multiple and unspecified intrathoracic organs, with open wound into cavity

863 Injury to gastrointestinal tract

> *Excludes:* anal sphincter laceration during delivery (664.2)
> bile duct (868.0-868.1 with fifth-digit 2)
> gallbladder (868.0-868.1 with fifth-digit 2)

- **863.0** Stomach, without mention of open wound into cavity
- **863.1** Stomach, with open wound into cavity
- ⑤ **863.2** Small intestine, without mention of open wound into cavity
  - **863.20** Small intestine, unspecified site
  - **863.21** Duodenum
  - **863.29** Other
- ⑤ **863.3** Small intestine, with open wound into cavity
  - **863.30** Small intestine, unspecified site
  - **863.31** Duodenum
  - **863.39** Other
- ⑤ **863.4** Colon or rectum, without mention of open wound into cavity
  - **863.40** Colon, unspecified site
  - **863.41** Ascending [right] colon
  - **863.42** Transverse colon
  - **863.43** Descending [left] colon
  - **863.44** Sigmoid colon
  - **863.45** Rectum
  - **863.46** Multiple sites in colon and rectum
  - **863.49** Other
- ⑤ **863.5** Colon or rectum, with open wound into cavity
  - **863.50** Colon, unspecified site
  - **863.51** Ascending [right] colon
  - **863.52** Transverse colon
  - **863.53** Descending [left] colon
  - **863.54** Sigmoid colon
  - **863.55** Rectum
  - **863.56** Multiple sites in colon and rectum
  - **863.59** Other
- ⑤ **863.8** Other and unspecified gastrointestinal sites, without mention of open wound into cavity
  - **863.80** Gastrointestinal tract, unspecified site
  - **863.81** Pancreas, head
  - **863.82** Pancreas, body
  - **863.83** Pancreas, tail
  - **863.84** Pancreas, multiple and unspecified sites
  - **863.85** Appendix
  - **863.89** Other
    - Intestine NOS

| | Add 4th or 5th digit | | Nonspecific code | | Unspecified code | | Medicare secondary payer (MSP) alert |

TABULAR LIST

⑤ **863.9 Other and unspecified gastrointestinal sites, with open wound into cavity**
- **863.90** Gastrointestinal tract, unspecified site
- **863.91** Pancreas, head
- **863.92** Pancreas, body
- **863.93** Pancreas, tail
- **863.94** Pancreas, multiple and unspecified sites
- **863.95** Appendix
- **863.99** Other

⑤ **864 Injury to liver**

The following fifth-digit subclassification is for use with category 864:

- **0** unspecified injury
- **1** hematoma and contusion
- **2** laceration, minor
  Laceration involving capsule only, or without significant involvement of hepatic parenchyma [i.e., less than 1 cm deep]
- **3** laceration, moderate
  Laceration involving parenchyma but without major disruption of parenchyma [i.e., less than 10 cm long and less than 3 cm deep]
- **4** laceration, major
  Laceration with significant disruption of hepatic parenchyma [i.e., 10 cm long and 3 cm deep]
  Multiple moderate lacerations, with or without hematoma
  Stellate lacerations of liver
- **5** laceration, unspecified
- **9** other

⑤ **864.0 Without mention of open wound into cavity**
⑤ **864.1 With open wound into cavity**

⑤ **865 Injury to spleen**

The following fifth-digit subclassification is for use with category 865:

- **0** unspecified injury
- **1** hematoma without rupture of capsule
- **2** capsular tears, without major disruption of parenchyma
- **3** laceration extending into parenchyma
- **4** massive parenchymal disruption
- **9** other

⑤ **865.0 Without mention of open wound into cavity**
⑤ **865.1 With open wound into cavity**

⑤ **866 Injury to kidney**

The following fifth-digit subclassification is for use with category 866:

- **0** unspecified injury
- **1** hematoma without rupture of capsule
- **2** laceration
- **3** complete disruption of kidney parenchyma

⑤ **866.0 Without mention of open wound into cavity**
⑤ **866.1 With open wound into cavity**

867 Injury to pelvic organs

Excludes: *injury during delivery (664.0-665.9)*

- **867.0** Bladder and urethra, without mention of open wound into cavity
- **867.1** Bladder and urethra, with open wound into cavity
- **867.2** Ureter, without mention of open wound into cavity
- **867.3** Ureter, with open wound into cavity
- **867.4** Uterus, without mention of open wound into cavity
- **867.5** Uterus, with open wound into cavity

● Code new to this edition ▲ Revision of existing code ④ ⑤ Fourth or fifth digit required

INJURY AND POISONING

867.6 Other specified pelvic organs, without mention of open wound into cavity
  Fallopian tube   Seminal vesicle
  Ovary   Vas deferens
  Prostate

867.7 Other specified pelvic organs, with open wound into cavity

867.8 Unspecified pelvic organs, without mention of open wound into cavity

867.9 Unspecified pelvic organ, with open wound into cavity

⑤ **868** Injury to other intra-abdominal organs
The following fifth-digit subclassification is for use with category 868:

  0 unspecified intra-abdominal organ
  1 adrenal gland
  2 bile duct and gallbladder
  3 peritoneum
  4 retroperitoneum
  9 other and multiple intra-abdominal organs

⑤ **868.0** Without mention of open wound into cavity
⑤ **868.1** With open wound into cavity

869 Internal injury to unspecified or ill-defined organs
  Includes: internal injury NOS
            multiple internal injury NOS

869.0 Without mention of open wound into cavity
869.1 With open wound into cavity

OPEN WOUND (870-897)

Includes: animal bite
          avulsion
          cut
          laceration
          puncture wound
          traumatic amputation

Excludes: *burn (940.0-949.5)*
            crushing (925-929.9)
            puncture of internal organs (860.0-869.1)
            superficial injury (910.0-919.9)
            that incidental to:
              dislocation (830.0-839.9)
              fracture (800.0-829.1)
              internal injury (860.0-869.1)
              intracranial injury (851.0-854.1)

Note: The description "complicated" used in the fourth-digit subdivisions includes those with mention of delayed healing, delayed treatment, foreign body, or infection.
Use additional code to identify infection.

OPEN WOUND OF HEAD, NECK, AND TRUNK (870-879)

870 Open wound of ocular adnexa
  870.0 Laceration of skin of eyelid and periocular area
  870.1 Laceration of eyelid, full-thickness, not involving lacrimal passages
  870.2 Laceration of eyelid involving lacrimal passages
  870.3 Penetrating wound of orbit, without mention of foreign body
  870.4 Penetrating wound of orbit with foreign body
    Excludes: *retained (old) foreign body in orbit (376.6)*
  870.8 Other specified open wounds of ocular adnexa
  870.9 Unspecified open wound of ocular adnexa

871 Open wound of eyeball
  Excludes: *2nd cranial nerve [optic] injury (950.0-950.9)*
              3rd cranial nerve [oculomotor] injury (951.0)
  871.0 Ocular laceration without prolapse of intraocular tissue
  871.1 Ocular laceration with prolapse or exposure of intraocular tissue
  871.2 Rupture of eye with partial loss of intraocular tissue

Add 4th or 5th digit | Nonspecific code | Unspecified code | Medicare secondary payer (MSP) alert

569

TABULAR LIST

- 871.3 **Avulsion of eye**
  Traumatic enucleation
- **871.4** **Unspecified laceration of eye**
- 871.5 **Penetration of eyeball with magnetic foreign body**
  Excludes: retained (old) magnetic foreign body in globe (360.50-360.59)
- 871.6 **Penetration of eyeball with (nonmagnetic) foreign body**
  Excludes: retained (old) (nonmagnetic) foreign body in globe (360.60-360.69)
- **871.7** **Unspecified ocular penetration**
- **871.9** **Unspecified open wound of eyeball**

872 **Open wound of ear**
- ⑤ 872.0 **External ear, without mention of complication**
  - **872.00** **External ear, unspecified site**
  - 872.01 **Auricle, ear**
    Pinna
  - 872.02 **Auditory canal**
- ⑤ 872.1 **External ear, complicated**
  - **872.10** **External ear, unspecified site**
  - 872.11 **Auricle, ear**
  - 872.12 **Auditory canal**
- ⑤ 872.6 **Other specified parts of ear, without mention of complication**
  - 872.61 **Ear drum**
    Drumhead
    Tympanic membrane
  - 872.62 **Ossicles**
  - 872.63 **Eustachian tube**
  - 872.64 **Cochlea**
  - **872.69** **Other and multiple sites**
- ⑤ 872.7 **Other specified parts of ear, complicated**
  - 872.71 **Ear drum**
  - 872.72 **Ossicles**
  - 872.73 **Eustachian tube**
  - 872.74 **Cochlea**
  - **872.79** **Other and multiple sites**
- **872.8** **Ear, part unspecified, without mention of complication**
  Ear NOS
- **872.9** **Ear, part unspecified, complicated**

873 **Other open wound of head**
- 873.0 **Scalp, without mention of complication**
- 873.1 **Scalp, complicated**
- ⑤ 873.2 **Nose, without mention of complication**
  - **873.20** **Nose, unspecified site**
  - 873.21 **Nasal septum**
  - 873.22 **Nasal cavity**
  - 873.23 **Nasal sinus**
  - **873.29** **Multiple sites**
- ⑤ 873.3 **Nose, complicated**
  - **873.30** **Nose, unspecified site**
  - 873.31 **Nasal septum**
  - 873.32 **Nasal cavity**
  - 873.33 **Nasal sinus**
  - **873.39** **Multiple sites**
- ⑤ 873.4 **Face, without mention of complication**
  - **873.40** **Face, unspecified site**

● Code new to this edition ▲ Revision of existing code ④ ⑤ Fourth or fifth digit required

INJURY AND POISONING

- 873.41 Cheek
- 873.42 Forehead
    Eyebrow
- 873.43 Lip
- 873.44 Jaw
- 873.49 Other and multiple sites

⑤ 873.5 **Face, complicated**
- 873.50 Face, unspecified site
- 873.51 Cheek
- 873.52 Forehead
- 873.53 Lip
- 873.54 Jaw
- 873.59 Other and multiple sites

⑤ 873.6 **Internal structures of mouth, without mention of complication**
- 873.60 Mouth, unspecified site
- 873.61 Buccal mucosa
- 873.62 Gum (alveolar process)
- 873.63 Tooth (broken) (fractured) (due to trauma)
    Excludes: *cracked tooth (521.81)*
- 873.64 Tongue and floor of mouth
- 873.65 Palate
- 873.69 Other and multiple sites

⑤ 873.7 **Internal structures of mouth, complicated**
- 873.70 Mouth, unspecified site
- 873.71 Buccal mucosa
- 873.72 Gum (alveolar process)
- 873.73 Tooth (broken) (fractured) (due to trauma)
    Excludes: *cracked tooth (521.81)*
- 873.74 Tongue and floor of mouth
- 873.75 Palate
- 873.79 Other and multiple sites

- 873.8 Other and unspecified open wound of head without mention of complication
    Head NOS
- 873.9 Other and unspecified open wound of head, complicated

874 Open wound of neck

⑤ 874.0 **Larynx and trachea, without mention of complication**
- 874.00 Larynx with trachea
- 874.01 Larynx
- 874.02 Trachea

⑤ 874.1 **Larynx and trachea, complicated**
- 874.10 Larynx with trachea
- 874.11 Larynx
- 874.12 Trachea

- 874.2 Thyroid gland, without mention of complication
- 874.3 Thyroid gland, complicated
- 874.4 Pharynx, without mention of complication
    Cervical esophagus
- 874.5 Pharynx, complicated
- 874.8 Other and unspecified parts, without mention of complication
    Nape of neck   Throat NOS
    Supraclavicular region
- 874.9 Other and unspecified parts, complicated

Add 4th or 5th digit | Nonspecific code | Unspecified code | Medicare secondary payer (MSP) alert

571

TABULAR LIST

875 Open wound of chest (wall)
> Excludes: open wound into thoracic cavity (860.0-862.9)
> traumatic pneumothorax and hemothorax (860.1, 860.3, 860.5)

- 875.0 Without mention of complication
- 875.1 Complicated

876 Open wound of back
Includes: loin
lumbar region
> Excludes: open wound into thoracic cavity (860.0-862.9)
> traumatic pneumothorax and hemothorax (860.1, 860.3, 860.5)

- 876.0 Without mention of complication
- 876.1 Complicated

877 Open wound of buttock
Includes: sacroiliac region

- 877.0 Without mention of complication
- 877.1 Complicated

878 Open wound of genital organs (external), including traumatic amputation
> Excludes: injury during delivery (664.0-665.9)
> internal genital organs (867.0-867.9)

- 878.0 Penis, without mention of complication
- 878.1 Penis, complicated
- 878.2 Scrotum and testes, without mention of complication
- 878.3 Scrotum and testes, complicated
- 878.4 Vulva, without mention of complication
  Labium (majus) (minus)
- 878.5 Vulva, complicated
- 878.6 Vagina, without mention of complication
- 878.7 Vagina, complicated
- 878.8 Other and unspecified parts, without mention of complication
- 878.9 Other and unspecified parts, complicated

879 Open wound of other and unspecified sites, except limbs

- 879.0 Breast, without mention of complication
- 879.1 Breast, complicated
- 879.2 Abdominal wall, anterior, without mention of complication
  Abdominal wall NOS   Pubic region
  Epigastric region   Umbilical region
  Hypogastric region
- 879.3 Abdominal wall, anterior, complicated
- 879.4 Abdominal wall, lateral, without mention of complication
  Flank   Iliac (region)
  Groin   Inguinal region
  Hypochondrium
- 879.5 Abdominal wall, lateral, complicated
- 879.6 Other and unspecified parts of trunk, without mention of complication
  Pelvic region   Trunk NOS
  Perineum
- 879.7 Other and unspecified parts of trunk, complicated
- 879.8 Open wound(s) (multiple) of unspecified site(s) without mention of complication
  Multiple open wounds NOS
  Open wound NOS
- 879.9 Open wound(s) (multiple) of unspecified site(s), complicated

INJURY AND POISONING

OPEN WOUND OF UPPER LIMB (880-887)

⑤ **880** Open wound of shoulder and upper arm
The following fifth-digit subclassification is for use with category 880:
    0 shoulder region
    1 scapular region
    2 axillary region
    3 upper arm
    9 multiple sites

⑤ 880.0 Without mention of complication
⑤ 880.1 Complicated
⑤ 880.2 With tendon involvement

⑤ **881** Open wound of elbow, forearm, and wrist
The following fifth-digit subclassification is for use with category 881:
    0 forearm
    1 elbow
    2 wrist

⑤ 881.0 Without mention of complication
⑤ 881.1 Complicated
⑤ 881.2 With tendon involvement

882 Open wound of hand except finger(s) alone
  882.0 Without mention of complication
  882.1 Complicated
  882.2 With tendon involvement

883 Open wound of finger(s)
Includes: fingernail
            thumb (nail)

  883.0 Without mention of complication
  883.1 Complicated
  883.2 With tendon involvement

884 Multiple and unspecified open wound of upper limb
Includes: arm NOS
            multiple sites of one upper limb
            upper limb NOS

  884.0 Without mention of complication
  884.1 Complicated
  884.2 With tendon involvement

885 Traumatic amputation of thumb (complete) (partial)
Includes: thumb(s) (with finger(s) of either hand)

  885.0 Without mention of complication
  885.1 Complicated

886 Traumatic amputation of other finger(s) (complete) (partial)
Includes: finger(s) of one or both hands, without mention of thumb(s)

  886.0 Without mention of complication
  886.1 Complicated

887 Traumatic amputation of arm and hand (complete) (partial)
  887.0 Unilateral, below elbow, without mention of complication
  887.1 Unilateral, below elbow, complicated
  887.2 Unilateral, at or above elbow, without mention of complication
  887.3 Unilateral, at or above elbow, complicated
  887.4 Unilateral, level not specified, without mention of complication
  887.5 Unilateral, level not specified, complicated
  887.6 Bilateral [any level], without mention of complication
          One hand and other arm
  887.7 Bilateral [any level], complicated

OPEN WOUND OF LOWER LIMB (890-897)

890 Open wound of hip and thigh
    890.0 Without mention of complication
    890.1 Complicated
    890.2 With tendon involvement

891 Open wound of knee, leg [except thigh], and ankle
    Includes: leg NOS
             multiple sites of leg, except thigh
    Excludes: that of thigh (890.0-890.2)
             with multiple sites of lower limb (894.0-894.2)
    891.0 Without mention of complication
    891.1 Complicated
    891.2 With tendon involvement

892 Open wound of foot except toe(s) alone
    Includes: heel
    892.0 Without mention of complication
    892.1 Complicated
    892.2 With tendon involvement

893 Open wound of toe(s)
    Includes: toenail
    893.0 Without mention of complication
    893.1 Complicated
    893.2 With tendon involvement

894 Multiple and unspecified open wound of lower limb
    Includes: lower limb NOS
             multiple sites of one lower limb, with thigh
    894.0 Without mention of complication
    894.1 Complicated
    894.2 With tendon involvement

895 Traumatic amputation of toe(s) (complete) (partial)
    Includes: toe(s) of one or both feet
    895.0 Without mention of complication
    895.1 Complicated

896 Traumatic amputation of foot (complete) (partial)
    896.0 Unilateral, without mention of complication
    896.1 Unilateral, complicated
    896.2 Bilateral, without mention of complication
    Excludes: one foot and other leg (897.6-897.7)
    896.3 Bilateral, complicated

897 Traumatic amputation of leg(s) (complete) (partial)
    897.0 Unilateral, below knee, without mention of complication
    897.1 Unilateral, below knee, complicated
    897.2 Unilateral, at or above knee, without mention of complication
    897.3 Unilateral, at or above knee, complicated
    897.4 Unilateral, level not specified, without mention of complication
    897.5 Unilateral, level not specified, complicated
    897.6 Bilateral [any level], without mention of complication
            One foot and other leg
    897.7 Bilateral [any level], complicated

INJURY AND POISONING

INJURY TO BLOOD VESSELS (900-904)

Includes: arterial hematoma of blood vessel, secondary to other injuries e.g., fracture or open wound
avulsion of blood vessel, secondary to other injuries e.g., fracture or open wound
cut of blood vessel, secondary to other injuries e.g., fracture or open wound
laceration of blood vessel, secondary to other injuries e.g., fracture or open wound
rupture of blood vessel, secondary to other injuries e.g., fracture or open wound
traumatic aneurysm or fistula (arteriovenous) of blood vessel, secondary to other injuries e.g., fracture or open wound

Excludes: *accidental puncture or laceration during medical procedure (998.2)*
intracranial hemorrhage following injury (851.0-854.1)

900 Injury to blood vessels of head and neck
  ⑤ 900.0 **Carotid artery**
      900.00 Carotid artery, unspecified
      900.01 Common carotid artery
      900.02 External carotid artery
      900.03 Internal carotid artery
  900.1 **Internal jugular vein**
  ⑤ 900.8 **Other specified blood vessels of head and neck**
      900.81 External jugular vein
            Jugular vein NOS
      900.82 Multiple blood vessels of head and neck
      900.89 Other
  900.9 **Unspecified blood vessel of head and neck**

901 Injury to blood vessels of thorax
      Excludes: *traumatic hemothorax (860.2-860.5)*
  901.0 **Thoracic aorta**
  901.1 **Innominate and subclavian arteries**
  901.2 **Superior vena cava**
  901.3 **Innominate and subclavian veins**
  ⑤ 901.4 **Pulmonary blood vessels**
      901.40 Pulmonary vessel(s), unspecified
      901.41 Pulmonary artery
      901.42 Pulmonary vein
  ⑤ 901.8 **Other specified blood vessels of thorax**
      901.81 Intercostal artery or vein
      901.82 Internal mammary artery or vein
      901.83 Multiple blood vessels of thorax
      901.89 Other
            Azygos vein
            Hemiazygos vein
  901.9 **Unspecified blood vessel of thorax**

902 Injury to blood vessels of abdomen and pelvis
  902.0 **Abdominal aorta**
  ⑤ 902.1 **Inferior vena cava**
      902.10 Inferior vena cava, unspecified
      902.11 Hepatic veins
      902.19 Other
  ⑤ 902.2 **Celiac and mesenteric arteries**
      902.20 Celiac and mesenteric arteries, unspecified
      902.21 Gastric artery
      902.22 Hepatic artery
      902.23 Splenic artery
      902.24 Other specified branches of celiac axis
      902.25 Superior mesenteric artery (trunk)

■	Add 4th or 5th digit	■	Nonspecific code	■	Unspecified code	■ Medicare secondary payer (MSP) alert

TABULAR LIST

- 902.26 **Primary branches of superior mesenteric artery**
  Ileo-colic artery
- 902.27 **Inferior mesenteric artery**
- 902.29 **Other**

⑤ 902.3 **Portal and splenic veins**
- 902.31 **Superior mesenteric vein and primary subdivisions**
  Ileo-colic vein
- 902.32 **Inferior mesenteric vein**
- 902.33 **Portal vein**
- 902.34 **Splenic vein**
- 902.39 **Other**
  Cystic vein
  Gastric vein

⑤ 902.4 **Renal blood vessels**
- 902.40 **Renal vessel(s), unspecified**
- 902.41 **Renal artery**
- 902.42 **Renal vein**
- 902.49 **Other**
  Suprarenal arteries

⑤ 902.5 **Iliac blood vessels**
- 902.50 **Iliac vessel(s), unspecified**
- 902.51 **Hypogastric artery**
- 902.52 **Hypogastric vein**
- 902.53 **Iliac artery**
- 902.54 **Iliac vein**
- 902.55 **Uterine artery**
- 902.56 **Uterine vein**
- 902.59 **Other**

⑤ 902.8 **Other specified blood vessels of abdomen and pelvis**
- 902.81 **Ovarian artery**
- 902.82 **Ovarian vein**
- 902.87 **Multiple blood vessels of abdomen and pelvis**
- 902.89 **Other**

902.9 **Unspecified blood vessel of abdomen and pelvis**

903 Injury to blood vessels of upper extremity
⑤ 903.0 **Axillary blood vessels**
- 903.00 **Axillary vessel(s), unspecified**
- 903.01 **Axillary artery**
- 903.02 **Axillary vein**

903.1 **Brachial blood vessels**
903.2 **Radial blood vessels**
903.3 **Ulnar blood vessels**
903.4 **Palmar artery**
903.5 **Digital blood vessels**
903.8 **Other specified blood vessels of upper extremity**
  Multiple blood vessels of upper extremity
903.9 **Unspecified blood vessel of upper extremity**

904 Injury to blood vessels of lower extremity and unspecified sites
904.0 **Common femoral artery**
  Femoral artery above profunda origin
904.1 **Superficial femoral artery**
904.2 **Femoral veins**
904.3 **Saphenous veins**
  Saphenous vein (greater) (lesser)
⑤ 904.4 **Popliteal blood vessels**

● Code new to this edition ▲ Revision of existing code ④ ⑤ Fourth or fifth digit required

INJURY AND POISONING

- **904.40** Popliteal vessel(s), unspecified
- 904.41 Popliteal artery
- 904.42 Popliteal vein

⑤ 904.5 **Tibial blood vessels**
- **904.50** Tibial vessel(s), unspecified
- 904.51 Anterior tibial artery
- 904.52 Anterior tibial vein
- 904.53 Posterior tibial artery
- 904.54 Posterior tibial vein

904.6 Deep plantar blood vessels

904.7 Other specified blood vessels of lower extremity
Multiple blood vessels of lower extremity

904.8 Unspecified blood vessel of lower extremity

904.9 Unspecified site
Injury to blood vessel NOS

LATE EFFECTS OF INJURIES, POISONINGS, TOXIC EFFECTS, AND OTHER EXTERNAL CAUSES (905-909)

Note: These categories are to be used to indicate conditions classifiable to 800-999 as the cause of late effects, which are themselves classified elsewhere. The "late effects" include those specified as such, or as sequelae, which may occur at any time after the acute injury.

905 Late effects of musculoskeletal and connective tissue injuries

905.0 Late effect of fracture of skull and face bones
Late effect of injury classifiable to 800-804

905.1 Late effect of fracture of spine and trunk without mention of spinal cord lesion
Late effect of injury classifiable to 805, 807-809

905.2 Late effect of fracture of upper extremities
Late effect of injury classifiable to 810-819

905.3 Late effect of fracture of neck of femur
Late effect of injury classifiable to 820

905.4 Late effect of fracture of lower extremities
Late effect of injury classifiable to 821-827

905.5 Late effect of fracture of multiple and unspecified bones
Late effect of injury classifiable to 828-829

905.6 Late effect of dislocation
Late effect of injury classifiable to 830-839

905.7 Late effect of sprain and strain without mention of tendon injury
Late effect of injury classifiable to 840-848, except tendon injury

905.8 Late effect of tendon injury
Late effect of tendon injury due to:
open wound [injury classifiable to 880-884 with .2, 890-894 with .2]
sprain and strain [injury classifiable to 840-848]

905.9 Late effect of traumatic amputation
Late effect of injury classifiable to 885-887, 895-897

Excludes: late amputation stump complication (997.60-997.69)

906 Late effects of injuries to skin and subcutaneous tissues

906.0 Late effect of open wound of head, neck, and trunk
Late effect of injury classifiable to 870-879

906.1 Late effect of open wound of extremities without mention of tendon injury
Late effect of injury classifiable to 880-884, 890-894 except .2

906.2 Late effect of superficial injury
Late effect of injury classifiable to 910-919

906.3 Late effect of contusion
Late effect of injury classifiable to 920-924

906.4 Late effect of crushing
Late effect of injury classifiable to 925-929

906.5 Late effect of burn of eye, face, head, and neck
Late effect of injury classifiable to 940-941

TABULAR LIST

- **906.6** **Late effect of burn of wrist and hand**
  Late effect of injury classifiable to 944
- **906.7** **Late effect of burn of other extremities**
  Late effect of injury classifiable to 943 or 945
- **906.8** **Late effect of burns of other specified sites**
  Late effect of injury classifiable to 942, 946-947
- **906.9** **Late effect of burn of unspecified site**
  Late effect of injury classifiable to 948-949

907 Late effects of injuries to the nervous system

- **907.0** **Late effect of intracranial injury without mention of skull fracture**
  Late effect of injury classifiable to 850-854
- **907.1** **Late effect of injury to cranial nerve**
  Late effect of injury classifiable to 950-951
- **907.2** **Late effect of spinal cord injury**
  Late effect of injury classifiable to 806, 952
- **907.3** **Late effect of injury to nerve root(s), spinal plexus(es), and other nerves of trunk**
  Late effect of injury classifiable to 953-954
- **907.4** **Late effect of injury to peripheral nerve of shoulder girdle and upper limb**
  Late effect of injury classifiable to 955
- **907.5** **Late effect of injury to peripheral nerve of pelvic girdle and lower limb**
  Late effect of injury classifiable to 956
- **907.9** **Late effect of injury to other and unspecified nerve**
  Late effect of injury classifiable to 957

908 Late effects of other and unspecified injuries

- **908.0** **Late effect of internal injury to chest**
  Late effect of injury classifiable to 860-862
- **908.1** **Late effect of internal injury to intra-abdominal organs**
  Late effect of injury classifiable to 863-866, 868
- **908.2** **Late effect of internal injury to other internal organs**
  Late effect of injury classifiable to 867 or 869
- **908.3** **Late effect of injury to blood vessel of head, neck, and extremities**
  Late effect of injury classifiable to 900, 903-904
- **908.4** **Late effect of injury to blood vessel of thorax, abdomen, and pelvis**
  Late effect of injury classifiable to 901-902
- **908.5** **Late effect of foreign body in orifice**
  Late effect of injury classifiable to 930-939
- **908.6** **Late effect of certain complications of trauma**
  Late effect of complications classifiable to 958
- **908.9** **Late effect of unspecified injury**
  Late effect of injury classifiable to 959

909 Late effects of other and unspecified external causes

- **909.0** **Late effect of poisoning due to drug, medicinal or biological substance**
  Late effect of conditions classifiable to 960-979

  Excludes: late effect of adverse effect of drug, medicinal or biological substance (909.5)

- **909.1** **Late effect of toxic effects of nonmedical substances**
  Late effect of conditions classifiable to 980-989
- **909.2** **Late effect of radiation**
  Late effect of conditions classifiable to 990
- **909.3** **Late effect of complications of surgical and medical care**
  Late effect of conditions classifiable to 996-999
- **909.4** **Late effect of certain other external causes**
  Late effect of conditions classifiable to 991-994
- **909.5** **Late effect of adverse effect of drug, medicinal or biological substance**

  Excludes: late effect of poisoning due to drug, medicinal or biological substance (909.0)

- **909.9** **Late effect of other and unspecified external causes**

INJURY AND POISONING

SUPERFICIAL INJURY (910-919)

Excludes: burn (blisters) (940.0-949.5)
contusion (920-924.9)
foreign body:
    granuloma (728.82)
    inadvertently left in operative wound (998.4)
    residual, in soft tissue (729.6)
insect bite, venomous (989.5)
open wound with incidental foreign body (870.0-897.7)

910 Superficial injury of face, neck, and scalp except eye
Includes: cheek
ear
gum
lip
nose
throat

Excludes: eye and adnexa (918.0-918.9)

- 910.0 Abrasion or friction burn without mention of infection
- 910.1 Abrasion or friction burn, infected
- 910.2 Blister without mention of infection
- 910.3 Blister, infected
- 910.4 Insect bite, nonvenomous, without mention of infection
- 910.5 Insect bite, nonvenomous, infected
- 910.6 Superficial foreign body (splinter) without major open wound and without mention of infection
- 910.7 Superficial foreign body (splinter) without major open wound, infected
- 910.8 Other and unspecified superficial injury of face, neck, and scalp without mention of infection
- 910.9 Other and unspecified superficial injury of face, neck, and scalp, infected

911 Superficial injury of trunk
Includes:
abdominal wall   interscapular region
anus   labium (majus) (minus)
back   penis
breast   perineum
buttock   scrotum
chest wall   testis
flank   vagina
groin   vulva

Excludes: hip (916.0-916.9)
scapular region (912.0-912.9)

- 911.0 Abrasion or friction burn without mention of infection
- 911.1 Abrasion or friction burn, infected
- 911.2 Blister without mention of infection
- 911.3 Blister, infected
- 911.4 Insect bite, nonvenomous, without mention of infection
- 911.5 Insect bite, nonvenomous, infected
- 911.6 Superficial foreign body (splinter) without major open wound and without mention of infection
- 911.7 Superficial foreign body (splinter) without major open wound, infected
- 911.8 Other and unspecified superficial injury of trunk without mention of infection
- 911.9 Other and unspecified superficial injury of trunk, infected

912 Superficial injury of shoulder and upper arm
Includes: axilla   scapular region

- 912.0 Abrasion or friction burn without mention of infection
- 912.1 Abrasion or friction burn, infected
- 912.2 Blister without mention of infection
- 912.3 Blister, infected
- 912.4 Insect bite, nonvenomous, without mention of infection

TABULAR LIST

- 912.5 Insect bite, nonvenomous, infected
- 912.6 Superficial foreign body (splinter) without major open wound and without mention of infection
- 912.7 Superficial foreign body (splinter) without major open wound, infected
- 912.8 Other and unspecified superficial injury of shoulder and upper arm without mention of infection
- 912.9 Other and unspecified superficial injury of shoulder and upper arm, infected

913 Superficial injury of elbow, forearm, and wrist
- 913.0 Abrasion or friction burn without mention of infection
- 913.1 Abrasion or friction burn, infected
- 913.2 Blister without mention of infection
- 913.3 Blister, infected
- 913.4 Insect bite, nonvenomous, without mention of infection
- 913.5 Insect bite, nonvenomous, infected
- 913.6 Superficial foreign body (splinter) without major open wound and without mention of infection
- 913.7 Superficial foreign body (splinter) without major open wound, infected
- 913.8 Other and unspecified superficial injury of elbow, forearm, and wrist without mention of infection
- 913.9 Other and unspecified superficial injury of elbow, forearm, and wrist, infected

914 Superficial injury of hand(s) except finger(s) alone
- 914.0 Abrasion or friction burn without mention of infection
- 914.1 Abrasion or friction burn, infected
- 914.2 Blister without mention of infection
- 914.3 Blister, infected
- 914.4 Insect bite, nonvenomous, without mention of infection
- 914.5 Insect bite, nonvenomous, infected
- 914.6 Superficial foreign body (splinter) without major open wound and without mention of infection
- 914.7 Superficial foreign body (splinter) without major open wound, infected
- 914.8 Other and unspecified superficial injury of hand without mention of infection
- 914.9 Other and unspecified superficial injury of hand, infected

915 Superficial injury of finger(s)
  Includes: fingernail   thumb (nail)
- 915.0 Abrasion or friction burn without mention of infection
- 915.1 Abrasion or friction burn, infected
- 915.2 Blister without mention of infection
- 915.3 Blister, infected
- 915.4 Insect bite, nonvenomous, without mention of infection
- 915.5 Insect bite, nonvenomous, infected
- 915.6 Superficial foreign body (splinter) without major open wound and without mention of infection
- 915.7 Superficial foreign body (splinter) without major open wound, infected
- 915.8 Other and unspecified superficial injury of fingers without mention of infection
- 915.9 Other and unspecified superficial injury of fingers, infected

916 Superficial injury of hip, thigh, leg, and ankle
- 916.0 Abrasion or friction burn without mention of infection
- 916.1 Abrasion or friction burn, infected
- 916.2 Blister without mention of infection
- 916.3 Blister, infected
- 916.4 Insect bite, nonvenomous, without mention of infection
- 916.5 Insect bite, nonvenomous, infected
- 916.6 Superficial foreign body (splinter) without major open wound and without mention of infection

INJURY AND POISONING

- **916.7** Superficial foreign body (splinter) without major open wound, infected
- **916.8** Other and unspecified superficial injury of hip, thigh, leg, and ankle without mention of infection
- **916.9** Other and unspecified superficial injury of hip, thigh, leg, and ankle, infected

917 **Superficial injury of foot and toe(s)**
Includes: heel   toenail

- **917.0** Abrasion or friction burn without mention of infection
- **917.1** Abrasion or friction burn, infected
- **917.2** Blister without mention of infection
- **917.3** Blister, infected
- **917.4** Insect bite, nonvenomous, without mention of infection
- **917.5** Insect bite, nonvenomous, infected
- **917.6** Superficial foreign body (splinter) without major open wound and without mention of infection
- **917.7** Superficial foreign body (splinter) without major open wound, infected
- **917.8** Other and unspecified superficial injury of foot and toes without mention of infection
- **917.9** Other and unspecified superficial injury of foot and toes, infected

918 **Superficial injury of eye and adnexa**
Excludes: burn (940.0-940.9)
foreign body on external eye (930.0-930.9)

- **918.0** Eyelids and periocular area
  Abrasion   Superficial foreign body (splinter)
  Insect bite
- **918.1** Cornea
  Corneal abrasion
  Superficial laceration
  Excludes: corneal injury due to contact lens (371.82)
- **918.2** Conjunctiva
- **918.9** Other and unspecified superficial injuries of eye
  Eye (ball) NOS

919 **Superficial injury of other, multiple, and unspecified sites**
Excludes: multiple sites classifiable to the same three-digit category (910.0-918.9)

- **919.0** Abrasion or friction burn without mention of infection
- **919.1** Abrasion or friction burn, infected
- **919.2** Blister without mention of infection
- **919.3** Blister, infected
- **919.4** Insect bite, nonvenomous, without mention of infection
- **919.5** Insect bite, nonvenomous, infected
- **919.6** Superficial foreign body (splinter) without major open wound and without mention of infection
- **919.7** Superficial foreign body (splinter) without major open wound, infected
- **919.8** Other and unspecified superficial injury without mention of infection
- **919.9** Other and unspecified superficial injury, infected

TABULAR LIST

CONTUSION WITH INTACT SKIN SURFACE (920-924)

Includes: bruise without fracture or open wound
hematoma without fracture or open wound

Excludes: concussion (850.0-850.9)
hemarthrosis (840.0-848.9)
internal organs (860.0-869.1)
that incidental to:
 crushing injury (925-929.9)
 dislocation (830.0-839.9)
 fracture (800.0-829.1)
 internal injury (860.0-869.1)
 intracranial injury (850.0-854.1)
 nerve injury (950.0-957.9)
 open wound (870.0-897.7)

920 Contusion of face, scalp, and neck except eye(s)
- Cheek
- Ear (auricle)
- Gum
- Lip
- Mandibular joint area
- Nose
- Throat

921 Contusion of eye and adnexa
- **921.0** Black eye, not otherwise specified
- **921.1** Contusion of eyelids and periocular area
- **921.2** Contusion of orbital tissues
- **921.3** Contusion of eyeball
- **921.9** Unspecified contusion of eye
  - Injury of eye NOS

922 Contusion of trunk
- **922.0** Breast
- **922.1** Chest wall
- **922.2** Abdominal wall
  - Flank
  - Groin
- ⑤ **922.3** Back
  - Excludes: scapular region (923.01)
  - **922.31** Back
    - Excludes: interscapular region (922.33)
  - **922.32** Buttock
  - **922.33** Interscapular region
- **922.4** Genital organs
  - Labium (majus) (minus)
  - Penis
  - Perineum
  - Scrotum
  - Testis
  - Vagina
  - Vulva
- **922.8** Multiple sites of trunk
- **922.9** Unspecified part
  - Trunk NOS

923 Contusion of upper limb
- ⑤ **923.0** Shoulder and upper arm
  - **923.00** Shoulder region
  - **923.01** Scapular region
  - **923.02** Axillary region
  - **923.03** Upper arm
  - **923.09** Multiple sites
- ⑤ **923.1** Elbow and forearm
  - **923.10** Forearm
  - **923.11** Elbow
- ⑤ **923.2** Wrist and hand(s), except finger(s) alone
  - **923.20** Hand(s)

● Code new to this edition ▲ Revision of existing code ④ ⑤ Fourth or fifth digit required

INJURY AND POISONING

      923.21   Wrist
  923.3 **Finger**
      Fingernail
      Thumb (nail)
  923.8 **Multiple sites of upper limb**
  923.9 **Unspecified part of upper limb**
      Arm NOS

924 **Contusion of lower limb and of other and unspecified sites**
  ⑤ **924.0** **Hip and thigh**
      924.00   Thigh
      924.01   Hip
  ⑤ **924.1** **Knee and lower leg**
      924.10   Lower leg
      924.11   Knee
  ⑤ **924.2** **Ankle and foot, excluding toe(s)**
      924.20   Foot
                Heel
      924.21   Ankle
  924.3 **Toe**
      Toenail
  924.4 **Multiple sites of lower limb**
  924.5 **Unspecified part of lower limb**
      Leg NOS
  924.8 **Multiple sites, not elsewhere classified**
  924.9 **Unspecified site**

CRUSHING INJURY (925-929)

  Use additional code to identify any associated injuries, such as:
      fractures (800-829)
      internal injuries (860.0-869.1)
      intracranial injury (850.0-854.1)

925 **Crushing injury of face, scalp, and neck**
      Cheek   Pharynx
      Ear   Throat
      Larynx
  925.1 **Crushing injury of face and scalp**
      Cheek   Ear
  925.2 **Crushing injury of neck**
      Larynx   Throat
      Pharynx

926 **Crushing injury of trunk**
  926.0 **External genitalia**
      Labium (majus) (minus)   Testis
      Penis   Vulva
      Scrotum
  ⑤ **926.1** **Other specified sites**
      926.11   Back
      926.12   Buttock
      926.19   Other
                Breast
  926.8 **Multiple sites of trunk**
  926.9 **Unspecified site**
      Trunk NOS

927 **Crushing injury of upper limb**
  ⑤ **927.0** **Shoulder and upper arm**
      927.00   Shoulder region
      927.01   Scapular region
      927.02   Axillary region

Add 4th or 5th digit   Nonspecific code   Unspecified code   Medicare secondary payer (MSP) alert

TABULAR LIST

       927.03   Upper arm
       927.09   Multiple sites

⑤ 927.1 Elbow and forearm
       927.10   Forearm
       927.11   Elbow

⑤ 927.2 Wrist and hand(s), except finger(s) alone
       927.20   Hand(s)
       927.21   Wrist

   927.3 Finger(s)

927.8 Multiple sites of upper limb

927.9 Unspecified site
       Arm NOS

928 Crushing injury of lower limb

⑤ 928.0 Hip and thigh
       928.00   Thigh
       928.01   Hip

⑤ 928.1 Knee and lower leg
       928.10   Lower leg
       928.11   Knee

⑤ 928.2 Ankle and foot, excluding toe(s) alone
       928.20   Foot
                 Heel
       928.21   Ankle

   928.3 Toe(s)

928.8 Multiple sites of lower limb

928.9 Unspecified site
       Leg NOS

929 Crushing injury of multiple and unspecified sites

929.0 Multiple sites, not elsewhere classified

929.9 Unspecified site

EFFECTS OF FOREIGN BODY ENTERING THROUGH ORIFICE (930-939)

Excludes: foreign body:
    granuloma (728.82)
    inadvertently left in operative wound (998.4, 998.7)
    in open wound (800-839, 851-897)
    residual, in soft tissues (729.6)
    superficial without major open wound (910-919 with .6 or .7)

930 Foreign body on external eye

Excludes: foreign body in penetrating wound of:
    eyeball (871.5-871.6)
      retained (old) (360.5-360.6)
    ocular adnexa (870.4)
      retained (old) (376.6)

   930.0 Corneal foreign body

   930.1 Foreign body in conjunctival sac

   930.2 Foreign body in lacrimal punctum

930.8 Other and combined sites

930.9 Unspecified site
       External eye NOS

931 Foreign body in ear
    Auditory canal
    Auricle

932 Foreign body in nose
    Nasal sinus
    Nostril

933 Foreign body in pharynx and larynx

INJURY AND POISONING

- **933.0 Pharynx**
  Nasopharynx
  Throat NOS
- **933.1 Larynx**
  Asphyxia due to foreign body
  Choking due to:
     food (regurgitated)
     phlegm

934 Foreign body in trachea, bronchus, and lung
- **934.0** Trachea
- **934.1** Main bronchus
- **934.8** Other specified parts
  Bronchioles
  Lung
- **934.9** Respiratory tree, unspecified
  Inhalation of liquid or vomitus, lower respiratory tract NOS

935 Foreign body in mouth, esophagus, and stomach
- **935.0** Mouth
- **935.1** Esophagus
- **935.2** Stomach

936 Foreign body in intestine and colon

937 Foreign body in anus and rectum
Rectosigmoid (junction)

938 Foreign body in digestive system, unspecified
Alimentary tract NOS
Swallowed foreign body

939 Foreign body in genitourinary tract
- **939.0** Bladder and urethra
- **939.1** Uterus, any part
  Excludes: intrauterine contraceptive device:
     complications from (996.32, 996.65)
     presence of (V45.51)
- **939.2** Vulva and vagina
- **939.3** Penis
- **939.9** Unspecified site

BURNS (940-949)

Includes: burns from:
   electrical heating appliance
   electricity
   flame
   hot object
   lightning
   radiation
   chemical burns (external) (internal)
   scalds

Excludes: friction burns (910-919 with .0, .1)
   sunburn (692.71, 692.76-692.77)

940 Burn confined to eye and adnexa
- **940.0** Chemical burn of eyelids and periocular area
- **940.1** Other burns of eyelids and periocular area
- **940.2** Alkaline chemical burn of cornea and conjunctival sac
- **940.3** Acid chemical burn of cornea and conjunctival sac
- **940.4** Other burn of cornea and conjunctival sac
- **940.5** Burn with resulting rupture and destruction of eyeball
- **940.9** Unspecified burn of eye and adnexa

TABULAR LIST

⑤ **941** **Burn of face, head, and neck**
Excludes: mouth (947.0)
The following fifth-digit subclassification is for use with category 941:
- **0** face and head, unspecified site
- 1 ear [any part]
- 2 eye (with other parts of face, head, and neck)
- 3 lip(s)
- 4 chin
- 5 nose (septum)
- 6 scalp [any part]
  Temple (region)
- 7 forehead and cheek
- 8 neck
- **9** multiple sites [except with eye] of face, head, and neck

⑤ **941.0** Unspecified degree
⑤ 941.1 Erythema [first degree]
⑤ 941.2 Blisters, epidermal loss [second degree]
⑤ 941.3 Full-thickness skin loss [third degree NOS]
⑤ 941.4 Deep necrosis of underlying tissues [deep third degree] without mention of loss of a body part
⑤ 941.5 Deep necrosis of underlying tissues [deep third degree] with loss of a body part

⑤ **942** **Burn of trunk**
Excludes: scapular region (943.0-943.5 with fifth-digit 6)
The following fifth-digit subclassification is for use with category 942:
- **0** trunk, unspecified site
- 1 breast
- 2 chest wall, excluding breast and nipple
- 3 abdominal wall
  Flank   Groin
- 4 back [any part]
  Buttock   Interscapular region
- 5 genitalia
  Labium (majus) (minus)   Scrotum
  Penis   Testis
  Perineum   Vulva
- **9** other and multiple sites of trunk

⑤ **942.0** Unspecified degree
⑤ 942.1 Erythema [first degree]
⑤ 942.2 Blisters, epidermal loss [second degree]
⑤ 942.3 Full-thickness skin loss [third degree NOS]
⑤ 942.4 Deep necrosis of underlying tissues [deep third degree] without mention of loss of a body part
⑤ 942.5 Deep necrosis of underlying tissues [deep third degree] with loss of a body part

⑤ **943** **Burn of upper limb, except wrist and hand**
The following fifth-digit subclassification is for use with category 943:
- **0** upper limb, unspecified site
- 1 forearm
- 2 elbow
- 3 upper arm
- 4 axilla
- 5 shoulder
- 6 scapular region
- **9** multiple sites of upper limb, except wrist and hand

⑤ **943.0** Unspecified degree
⑤ 943.1 Erythema [first degree]

● Code new to this edition   ▲ Revision of existing code   ④ ⑤ Fourth or fifth digit required

INJURY AND POISONING

⑤ 943.2 Blisters, epidermal loss [second degree]
⑤ 943.3 Full-thickness skin loss [third degree NOS]
⑤ 943.4 Deep necrosis of underlying tissues [deep third degree] without mention of loss of a body part
⑤ 943.5 Deep necrosis of underlying tissues [deep third degree] with loss of a body part

⑤ **944** Burn of wrist(s) and hand(s)
The following fifth-digit subclassification is for use with category 944:
- **0** hand, unspecified site
- 1 single digit [finger (nail)] other than thumb
- 2 thumb (nail)
- 3 two or more digits, not including thumb
- 4 two or more digits including thumb
- 5 palm
- 6 back of hand
- 7 wrist
- **8** multiple sites of wrist(s) and hand(s)

⑤ **944.0** Unspecified degree
⑤ 944.1 Erythema [first degree]
⑤ 944.2 Blisters, epidermal loss [second degree]
⑤ 944.3 Full-thickness skin loss [third degree NOS]
⑤ 944.4 Deep necrosis of underlying tissues [deep third degree] without mention of loss of a body part
⑤ 944.5 Deep necrosis of underlying tissues [deep third degree] with loss of a body part

⑤ **945** Burn of lower limb(s)
The following fifth-digit subclassification is for use with category 945:
- **0** lower limb [leg], unspecified site
- 1 toe(s) (nail)
- 2 foot
- 3 ankle
- 4 lower leg
- 5 knee
- 6 thigh [any part]
- **9** multiple sites of lower limb(s)

⑤ **945.0** Unspecified degree
⑤ 945.1 Erythema [first degree]
⑤ 945.2 Blisters, epidermal loss [second degree]
⑤ 945.3 Full-thickness skin loss [third degree NOS]
⑤ 945.4 Deep necrosis of underlying tissues [deep third degree] without mention of loss of a body part
⑤ 945.5 Deep necrosis of underlying tissues [deep third degree] with loss of a body part

946 Burns of multiple specified sites
Includes: burns of sites classifiable to more than one three-digit category in 940-945
Excludes: multiple burns NOS (949.0-949.5)

946.0 Unspecified degree
946.1 Erythema [first degree]
946.2 Blisters, epidermal loss [second degree]
946.3 Full-thickness skin loss [third degree NOS]
946.4 Deep necrosis of underlying tissues [deep third degree] without mention of loss of a body part
946.5 Deep necrosis of underlying tissues [deep third degree] with loss of a body part

947 Burn of internal organs
Includes: burns from chemical agents (ingested)

947.0 Mouth and pharynx
Gum
Tongue

TABULAR LIST

- **947.1** Larynx, trachea, and lung
- **947.2** Esophagus
- **947.3** Gastrointestinal tract
  - Colon
  - Rectum
  - Small intestine
  - Stomach
- **947.4** Vagina and uterus
- **947.8** Other specified sites
- **947.9** Unspecified site

⑤ **948** **Burns classified according to extent of body surface involved**

> *Excludes:* sunburn (692.71, 692.76-692.77)

Note: This category is to be used when the site of the burn is unspecified, or with categories 940-947 when the site is specified.

The following fifth-digit subclassification is for use with category 948 to indicate the percent of *body surface* with *third degree burn*; valid digits are in [brackets] under each code:

- **0** less than 10 percent or unspecified
- **1** 10-19%
- **2** 20-29%
- **3** 30-39%
- **4** 40-49%
- **5** 50-59%
- **6** 60-69%
- **7** 70-79%
- **8** 80-89%
- **9** 90% or more of body surface

⑤ **948.0** Burn [any degree] involving less than 10 percent of body surface
[0]

⑤ **948.1** 10-19 percent of body surface
[0-1]

⑤ **948.2** 20-29 percent of body surface
[0-2]

⑤ **948.3** 30-39 percent of body surface
[0-3]

⑤ **948.4** 40-49 percent of body surface
[0-4]

⑤ **948.5** 50-59 percent of body surface
[0-5]

⑤ **948.6** 60-69 percent of body surface
[0-6]

⑤ **948.7** 70-79 percent of body surface
[0-7]

⑤ **948.8** 80-89 percent of body surface
[0-8]

⑤ **948.9** 90 percent or more of body surface
[0-9]

949 **Burn, unspecified**
Includes: burn NOS
multiple burns NOS

> *Excludes:* burn of unspecified site but with statement of the extent of body surface involved (948.0-948.9)

- **949.0** Unspecified degree
- **949.1** Erythema [first degree]
- **949.2** Blisters, epidermal loss [second degree]
- **949.3** Full-thickness skin loss [third degree NOS]
- **949.4** Deep necrosis of underlying tissues [deep third degree] without mention of loss of a body part
- **949.5** Deep necrosis of underlying tissues [deep third degree] with loss of a body part

INJURY AND POISONING

INJURY TO NERVES AND SPINAL CORD (950-957)

Includes:
- division of nerve (with open wound)
- lesion in continuity (with open wound)
- traumatic neuroma (with open wound)
- traumatic transient paralysis (with open wound)

Excludes: accidental puncture or laceration during medical procedure (998.2)

950 Injury to optic nerve and pathways

- **950.0 Optic nerve injury**
  Second cranial nerve
- **950.1 Injury to optic chiasm**
- **950.2 Injury to optic pathways**
- **950.3 Injury to visual cortex**
- **950.9 Unspecified**
  Traumatic blindness NOS

951 Injury to other cranial nerve(s)

- **951.0 Injury to oculomotor nerve**
  Third cranial nerve
- **951.1 Injury to trochlear nerve**
  Fourth cranial nerve
- **951.2 Injury to trigeminal nerve**
  Fifth cranial nerve
- **951.3 Injury to abducens nerve**
  Sixth cranial nerve
- **951.4 Injury to facial nerve**
  Seventh cranial nerve
- **951.5 Injury to acoustic nerve**
  Auditory nerve   Traumatic deafness NOS
  Eighth cranial nerve
- **951.6 Injury to accessory nerve**
  Eleventh cranial nerve
- **951.7 Injury to hypoglossal nerve**
  Twelfth cranial nerve
- **951.8 Injury to other specified cranial nerves**
  Glossopharyngeal [9th cranial] nerve
  Olfactory [1st cranial] nerve
  Pneumogastric [10th cranial] nerve
  Traumatic anosmia NOS
  Vagus [10th cranial] nerve
- **951.9 Injury to unspecified cranial nerve**

952 Spinal cord injury without evidence of spinal bone injury

⑤ **952.0 Cervical**

- **952.00** C_1-C_4 level with unspecified spinal cord injury
  Spinal cord injury, cervical region NOS
- **952.01** C_1-C_4 level with complete lesion of spinal cord
- **952.02** C_1-C_4 level with anterior cord syndrome
- **952.03** C_1-C_4 level with central cord syndrome
- **952.04** C_1-C_4 level with other specified spinal cord injury
  Incomplete spinal cord lesion at C_1-C_4 level:
    NOS
    with posterior cord syndrome
- **952.05** C_5-C_7 level with unspecified spinal cord injury
- **952.06** C_5-C_7 level with complete lesion of spinal cord
- **952.07** C_5-C_7 level with anterior cord syndrome
- **952.08** C_5-C_7 level with central cord syndrome
- **952.09** C_5-C_7 level with other specified spinal cord injury
  Incomplete spinal cord lesion at C_5-C_7 level:
    NOS
    with posterior cord syndrome

⑤ **952.1 Dorsal [thoracic]**

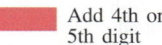

Add 4th or 5th digit | Nonspecific code | Unspecified code | Medicare secondary payer (MSP) alert

TABULAR LIST

- **952.10** **T$_1$-T$_6$ level with unspecified spinal cord injury**
  Spinal cord injury, thoracic region NOS
- 952.11 T$_1$-T$_6$ level with complete lesion of spinal cord
- 952.12 T$_1$-T$_6$ level with anterior cord syndrome
- 952.13 T$_1$-T$_6$ level with central cord syndrome
- **952.14** **T$_1$-T$_6$ level with other specified spinal cord injury**
  Incomplete spinal cord lesion at T$_1$-T$_6$ level:
    NOS
    with posterior cord syndrome
- **952.15** **T$_7$-T$_{12}$ level with unspecified spinal cord injury**
- 952.16 T$_7$-T$_{12}$ level with complete lesion of spinal cord
- 952.17 T$_7$-T$_{12}$ level with anterior cord syndrome
- 952.18 T$_7$-T$_{12}$ level with central cord syndrome
- **952.19** **T$_7$-T$_{12}$ level with other specified spinal cord injury**
  Incomplete spinal cord lesion at T$_7$-T$_{12}$ level:
    NOS
    with posterior cord syndrome
- 952.2 Lumbar
- 952.3 Sacral
- 952.4 Cauda equina
- **952.8** **Multiple sites of spinal cord**
- **952.9** **Unspecified site of spinal cord**

953 Injury to nerve roots and spinal plexus
- 953.0 Cervical root
- 953.1 Dorsal root
- 953.2 Lumbar root
- 953.3 Sacral root
- 953.4 Brachial plexus
- 953.5 Lumbosacral plexus
- **953.8** **Multiple sites**
- **953.9** **Unspecified site**

954 Injury to other nerve(s) of trunk, excluding shoulder and pelvic girdles
- 954.0 Cervical sympathetic
- **954.1** **Other sympathetic**
  Celiac ganglion or plexus   Splanchnic nerve(s)
  Inferior mesenteric plexus   Stellate ganglion
- **954.8** **Other specified nerve(s) of trunk**
- **954.9** **Unspecified nerve of trunk**

955 Injury to peripheral nerve(s) of shoulder girdle and upper limb
- 955.0 Axillary nerve
- 955.1 Median nerve
- 955.2 Ulnar nerve
- 955.3 Radial nerve
- 955.4 Musculocutaneous nerve
- 955.5 Cutaneous sensory nerve, upper limb
- 955.6 Digital nerve
- **955.7** **Other specified nerve(s) of shoulder girdle and upper limb**
- **955.8** **Multiple nerves of shoulder girdle and upper limb**
- **955.9** **Unspecified nerve of shoulder girdle and upper limb**

956 Injury to peripheral nerve(s) of pelvic girdle and lower limb
- 956.0 Sciatic nerve
- 956.1 Femoral nerve
- 956.2 Posterior tibial nerve
- 956.3 Peroneal nerve
- 956.4 Cutaneous sensory nerve, lower limb

INJURY AND POISONING

- **956.5** Other specified nerve(s) of pelvic girdle and lower limb
- **956.8** Multiple nerves of pelvic girdle and lower limb
- **956.9** Unspecified nerve of pelvic girdle and lower limb

957 Injury to other and unspecified nerves
- **957.0** Superficial nerves of head and neck
- **957.1** Other specified nerve(s)
- **957.8** Multiple nerves in several parts
  Multiple nerve injury NOS
- **957.9** Unspecified site
  Nerve injury NOS

CERTAIN TRAUMATIC COMPLICATIONS AND UNSPECIFIED INJURIES (958-959)

958 Certain early complications of trauma
Excludes: *adult respiratory distress syndrome (518.5)*
   flail chest (807.4)
   shock lung (518.5)
   that occurring during or following medical procedures (996.0-999.9)

- **958.0** Air embolism
  Pneumathemia
  Excludes: *that complicating:*
     abortion (634-638 with .6, 639.6)
     ectopic or molar pregnancy (639.6)
     pregnancy, childbirth, or the puerperium (673.0)

- **958.1** Fat embolism
  Excludes: *that complicating:*
     abortion (634-638 with .6, 639.6)
     pregnancy, childbirth, or the puerperium (673.8)

- **958.2** Secondary and recurrent hemorrhage
- **958.3** Posttraumatic wound infection, not elsewhere classified
  Excludes: *infected open wounds—code to complicated open wound of site*

- **958.4** Traumatic shock
  Shock (immediate) (delayed) following injury
  Excludes: *shock:*
     anaphylactic (995.0)
        due to serum (999.4)
     anesthetic (995.4)
     electric (994.8)
     following abortion (639.5)
     lightning (994.0)
     nontraumatic NOS (785.50)
     obstetric (669.1)
     postoperative (998.0)

- **958.5** Traumatic anuria
  Crush syndrome
  Renal failure following crushing
  Excludes: *that due to a medical procedure (997.5)*

- **958.6** Volkmann's ischemic contracture
  Posttraumatic muscle contracture

- **958.7** Traumatic subcutaneous emphysema
  Excludes: *subcutaneous emphysema resulting from a procedure (998.81)*

- **958.8** Other early complications of trauma
- ⑤ **958.9** Traumatic compartment syndrome
  Excludes: *nontraumatic compartment syndrome (729.71-729.79)*

  - **958.90** Compartment syndrome, unspecified
  - **958.91** Traumatic compartment syndrome of upper extremity
    Traumatic compartment syndrome of shoulder, arm, forearm, wrist, hand, and fingers
  - **958.92** Traumatic compartment syndrome of lower extremity
    Traumatic compartment syndrome of hip, buttock, thigh, leg, foot, and toes

TABULAR LIST

    958.93   Traumatic compartment syndrome of abdomen
    958.99   Traumatic compartment syndrome of other sites

959 Injury, other and unspecified
    Includes: injury NOS

    Excludes: *injury NOS of:*
        blood vessels (900.0-904.9)
        eye (921.0-921.9)
        internal organs (860.0-869.1)
        intracranial sites (854.0-854.1)
        nerves (950.0-951.9, 953.0-957.9)
        spinal cord (952.0-952.9)

⑤ **959.0 Head, face and neck**
    Cheek   Mouth
    Ear   Nose
    Eyebrow   Throat
    Lip

    959.01 Head injury, unspecified
    Excludes: *concussion (850.1-850.9)*
            with head injury NOS (850.1-850.9)
            head injury NOS with loss of consciousness (850.1-850.5)
            specified intracranial injuries (850.0-854.1)

    959.09   Injury of face and neck

⑤ **959.1 Trunk**
    Excludes: *scapular region (959.2)*

    959.11   Other injury of chest wall
    959.12   Other injury of abdomen
    959.13   Fracture of corpus cavernosum penis
    959.14   Other injury of external genitals
    959.19   Other injury of other sites of trunk
                 Injury of trunk NOS

959.2 Shoulder and upper arm
    Axilla
    Scapular region

959.3 Elbow, forearm, and wrist

959.4 Hand, except finger

959.5 Finger
    Fingernail
    Thumb (nail)

959.6 Hip and thigh
    Upper leg

959.7 Knee, leg, ankle, and foot

959.8 Other specified sites, including multiple
    Excludes: *multiple sites classifiable to the same four-digit category (959.0-959.7)*

959.9 Unspecified site

INJURY AND POISONING

POISONING BY DRUGS, MEDICINAL AND BIOLOGICAL SUBSTANCES (960-979)

Includes: overdose of these substances
wrong substances given or taken in error

Excludes: adverse effects ["hypersensitivity," "reaction," etc.] of correct substance properly administered. Such cases are to be classified according to the nature of the adverse effect, such as:
adverse effect NOS (995.20)
allergic lymphadenitis (289.3)
aspirin gastritis (535.4)
blood disorders (280.0-289.9)
dermatitis:
  contact (692.0-692.9)
  due to ingestion (693.0-693.9)
nephropathy (583.9)
[The drug giving rise to the adverse effect may be identified by use of categories E930-E949]
drug dependence (304.0-304.9)
drug reaction and poisoning affecting the newborn (760.0-779.9)
nondependent abuse of drugs (305.0-305.9)
pathological drug intoxication (292.2)

Use additional code to specify the effects of the poisoning

960 Poisoning by antibiotics

Excludes: antibiotics:
ear, nose, and throat (976.6)
eye (976.5)
local (976.0)

960.0 Penicillins
Ampicillin
Carbenicillin
Cloxacillin
Penicillin G

960.1 Antifungal antibiotics
Amphotericin B
Griseofulvin
Nystatin
Trichomycin

Excludes: preparations intended for topical use (976.0-976.9)

960.2 Chloramphenicol group
Chloramphenicol
Thiamphenicol

960.3 Erythromycin and other macrolides
Oleandomycin
Spiramycin

960.4 Tetracycline group
Doxycycline
Minocycline
Oxytetracycline

960.5 Cephalosporin group
Cephalexin
Cephaloglycin
Cephaloridine
Cephalothin

960.6 Antimycobacterial antibiotics
Cycloserine
Kanamycin
Rifampin
Streptomycin

960.7 Antineoplastic antibiotics
Actinomycin such as:
  Cactinomycin
  Dactinomycin
Bleomycin
Daunorubicin
Mitomycin

960.8 Other specified antibiotics

960.9 Unspecified antibiotic

961 Poisoning by other anti-infectives

Excludes: anti-infectives:
ear, nose, and throat (976.6)
eye (976.5)
local (976.0)

961.0 Sulfonamides
Sulfadiazine
Sulfafurazole
Sulfamethoxazole

961.1 Arsenical anti-infectives

593

TABULAR LIST

961.2 Heavy metal anti-infectives
Compounds of:
  antimony
  bismuth
Compounds of:
  lead
  mercury

Excludes: mercurial diuretics (974.0)

961.3 Quinoline and hydroxyquinoline derivatives
  Chiniofon
  Diiodohydroxyquin

Excludes: antimalarial drugs (961.4)

961.4 Antimalarials and drugs acting on other blood protozoa
  Chloroquine
  Cycloguanil
  Primaquine
  Proguanil [chloroguanide]
  Pyrimethamine
  Quinine

961.5 Other antiprotozoal drugs
  Emetine

961.6 Anthelmintics
  Hexylresorcinol
  Piperazine
  Thiabendazole

961.7 Antiviral drugs
  Methisazone

Excludes: amantadine (966.4)
  cytarabine (963.1)
  idoxuridine (976.5)

961.8 Other antimycobacterial drugs
  Ethambutol
  Ethionamide
  Isoniazid
  Para-aminosalicylic acid derivatives
  Sulfones

961.9 Other and unspecified anti-infectives
  Flucytosine
  Nitrofuran derivatives

962 Poisoning by hormones and synthetic substitutes

Excludes: oxytocic hormones (975.0)

962.0 Adrenal cortical steroids
  Cortisone derivatives
  Desoxycorticosterone derivatives
  Fluorinated corticosteroids

962.1 Androgens and anabolic congeners
  Methandriol
  Nandrolone
  Oxymetholone
  Testosterone

962.2 Ovarian hormones and synthetic substitutes
  Contraceptives, oral
  Estrogens
  Estrogens and progestogens, combined
  Progestogens

962.3 Insulins and antidiabetic agents
  Acetohexamide
  Biguanide derivatives, oral
  Chlorpropamide
  Glucagon
  Insulin
  Phenformin
  Sulfonylurea derivatives, oral
  Tolbutamide

962.4 Anterior pituitary hormones
  Corticotropin
  Gonadotropin
  Somatotropin [growth hormone]

962.5 Posterior pituitary hormones
  Vasopressin

Excludes: oxytocic hormones (975.0)

962.6 Parathyroid and parathyroid derivatives

962.7 Thyroid and thyroid derivatives
  Dextrothyroxin
  Levothyroxine sodium
  Liothyronine
  Thyroglobulin

INJURY AND POISONING

962.8 Antithyroid agents
    Iodides   Thiourea
    Thiouracil

962.9 Other and unspecified hormones and synthetic substitutes

963 Poisoning by primarily systemic agents

963.0 Antiallergic and antiemetic drugs
    Antihistamines   Diphenylpyraline
    Chlorpheniramine   Thonzylamine
    Diphenhydramine   Tripelennamine
      Excludes: phenothiazine-based tranquilizers (969.1)

963.1 Antineoplastic and immunosuppressive drugs
    Azathioprine   Cytarabine
    Busulfan   Fluorouracil
    Chlorambucil   Mercaptopurine
    Cyclophosphamide   thio-TEPA
      Excludes: antineoplastic antibiotics (960.7)

963.2 Acidifying agents

963.3 Alkalizing agents

963.4 Enzymes, not elsewhere classified
    Penicillinase

963.5 Vitamins, not elsewhere classified
    Vitamin A
    Vitamin D
      Excludes: nicotinic acid (972.2)
                    vitamin K (964.3)

963.8 Other specified systemic agents
    Heavy metal antagonists

963.9 Unspecified systemic agent

964 Poisoning by agents primarily affecting blood constituents

964.0 Iron and its compounds
    Ferric salts
    Ferrous sulfate and other ferrous salts

964.1 Liver preparations and other antianemic agents
    Folic acid

964.2 Anticoagulants
    Coumarin   Phenindione
    Heparin   Warfarin sodium

964.3 Vitamin K [phytonadione]

964.4 Fibrinolysis-affecting drugs
    Aminocaproic acid   Streptokinase
    Streptodornase   Urokinase

964.5 Anticoagulant antagonists and other coagulants
    Hexadimethrine
    Protamine sulfate

964.6 Gamma globulin

964.7 Natural blood and blood products
    Blood plasma   Packed red cells
    Human fibrinogen   Whole blood
      Excludes: transfusion reactions (999.4-999.8)

964.8 Other specified agents affecting blood constituents
    Macromolecular blood substitutes
    Plasma expanders

964.9 Unspecified agent affecting blood constituents

965 Poisoning by analgesics, antipyretics, and antirheumatics

      Excludes: drug dependence (304.0-304.9)
                  nondependent abuse (305.0-305.9)

⑤ **965.0 Opiates and related narcotics**
        965.00 Opium (alkaloids), unspecified

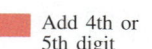

TABULAR LIST

  965.01 Heroin
    Diacetylmorphine
  965.02 Methadone
  965.09 Other
    Codeine [methylmorphine]
    Meperidine [pethidine]
    Morphine

965.1 Salicylates
  Acetylsalicylic acid [aspirin]
  Salicylic acid salts

965.4 Aromatic analgesics, not elsewhere classified
  Acetanilid
  Paracetamol [acetaminophen]
  Phenacetin [acetophenetidin]

965.5 Pyrazole derivatives
  Aminophenazone [aminopyrine]
  Phenylbutazone

⑤ **965.6 Antirheumatics [antiphlogistics]**
  Excludes: *salicylates (965.1)*
      steroids (962.0-962.9)

  965.61 Propionic acid derivatives
    Fenoprofen Ketoprofen
    Flurbiprofen Naproxen
    Ibuprofen   Oxaprozin

  965.69 Other antirheumatics
    Gold salts
    Indomethacin

965.7 Other non-narcotic analgesics
  Pyrabital

965.8 Other specified analgesics and antipyretics
  Pentazocine

965.9 Unspecified analgesic and antipyretic

966 Poisoning by anticonvulsants and anti-Parkinsonism drugs

  966.0 Oxazolidine derivatives
    Paramethadione
    Trimethadione

  966.1 Hydantoin derivatives
    Phenytoin

  966.2 Succinimides
    Ethosuximide
    Phensuximide

  966.3 Other and unspecified anticonvulsants
    Primidone
    Excludes: *barbiturates (967.0)*
        sulfonamides (961.0)

  966.4 Anti-Parkinsonism drugs
    Amantadine
    Ethopropazine [profenamine]
    Levodopa [L-dopa]

967 Poisoning by sedatives and hypnotics
  Excludes: *drug dependence (304.0-304.9)*
      nondependent abuse (305.0-305.9)

  967.0 Barbiturates
    Amobarbital [amylobarbitone]
    Barbital [barbitone]
    Butabarbital [butabarbitone]
    Pentobarbital [pentobarbitone]
    Phenobarbital [phenobarbitone]
    Secobarbital [quinalbarbitone]
    Excludes: *thiobarbiturate anesthetics (968.3)*

  967.1 Chloral hydrate group
  967.2 Paraldehyde

---

596 ● Code new ▲ Revision of ④ ⑤ Fourth or fifth
    to this edition   existing code   digit required

INJURY AND POISONING

- **967.3 Bromine compounds**
  - Bromide
  - Carbromal (derivatives)
- **967.4 Methaqualone compounds**
- **967.5 Glutethimide group**
- **967.6 Mixed sedatives, not elsewhere classified**
- **967.8 Other sedatives and hypnotics**
- **967.9 Unspecified sedative or hypnotic**
  - Sleeping:
    - drug NOS
    - pill NOS
    - tablet NOS

968 Poisoning by other central nervous system depressants and anesthetics
  Excludes: drug dependence (304.0-304.9)
  nondependent abuse (305.0-305.9)

- **968.0 Central nervous system muscle-tone depressants**
  - Chlorphenesin (carbamate)   Methocarbamol
  - Mephenesin
- **968.1 Halothane**
- **968.2 Other gaseous anesthetics**
  - Ether
  - Halogenated hydrocarbon derivatives, except halothane
  - Nitrous oxide
- **968.3 Intravenous anesthetics**
  Excludes: Methohexital [methohexitone]
  Thiobarbiturates, such as thiopental sodium
- **968.4 Other and unspecified general anesthetics**
- **968.5 Surface [topical] and infiltration anesthetics**
  - Cocaine   Procaine
  - Lidocaine [lignocaine]   Tetracaine
- **968.6 Peripheral nerve and plexus-blocking anesthetics**
- **968.7 Spinal anesthetics**
- **968.9 Other and unspecified local anesthetics**

969 Poisoning by psychotropic agents
  Excludes: drug dependence (304.0-304.9)
  nondependent abuse (305.0-305.9)

- **969.0 Antidepressants**
  - Amitriptyline   Monoamine oxidase [MAO] inhibitors
  - Imipramine
- **969.1 Phenothiazine-based tranquilizers**
  - Chlorpromazine   Prochlorperazine
  - Fluphenazine   Promazine
- **969.2 Butyrophenone-based tranquilizers**
  - Haloperidol   Trifluperidol
  - Spiperone
- **969.3 Other antipsychotics, neuroleptics, and major tranquilizers**
- **969.4 Benzodiazepine-based tranquilizers**
  - Chlordiazepoxide   Lorazepam
  - Diazepam   Medazepam
  - Flurazepam   Nitrazepam
- **969.5 Other tranquilizers**
  - Hydroxyzine
  - Meprobamate
- **969.6 Psychodysleptics [hallucinogens]**
  - Cannabis (derivatives)   Mescaline
  - Lysergide [LSD]   Psilocin
  - Marihuana (derivatives)   Psilocybin

597

TABULAR LIST

969.7 Psychostimulants
　　Amphetamine
　　Caffeine
　Excludes: central appetite depressants (977.0)

969.8 Other specified psychotropic agents

969.9 Unspecified psychotropic agent

970 Poisoning by central nervous system stimulants

970.0 Analeptics
　　Lobeline
　　Nikethamide

970.1 Opiate antagonists
　　Levallorphan　　　　Naloxone
　　Nalorphine

970.8 Other specified central nervous system stimulants

970.9 Unspecified central nervous system stimulant

971 Poisoning by drugs primarily affecting the autonomic nervous system

971.0 Parasympathomimetics [cholinergics]
　　Acetylcholine　　　　Pilocarpine
　　Anticholinesterase:
　　　organophosphorus
　　　reversible

971.1 Parasympatholytics [anticholinergics and antimuscarinics] and spasmolytics
　　Atropine　　　　　　Hyoscine [scopalamine]
　　Homatropine　　　　Quaternary ammonium derivatives
　Excludes: papaverine (972.5)

971.2 Sympathomimetics [adrenergics]
　　Epinephrine [adrenalin]
　　Levarterenol [noradrenalin]

971.3 Sympatholytics [antiadrenergics]
　　Phenoxybenzamine
　　Tolazoline hydrochloride

971.9 Unspecified drug primarily affecting autonomic nervous system

972 Poisoning by agents primarily affecting the cardiovascular system

972.0 Cardiac rhythm regulators
　　Practolol　　　　　　Propranolol
　　Procainamide　　　　Quinidine
　Excludes: lidocaine (968.5)

972.1 Cardiotonic glycosides and drugs of similar action
　　Digitalis glycosides　　Strophanthins
　　Digoxin

972.2 Antilipemic and antiarteriosclerotic drugs
　　Clofibrate
　　Nicotinic acid derivatives

972.3 Ganglion-blocking agents
　　Pentamethonium bromide

972.4 Coronary vasodilators
　　Dipyridamole　　　　Nitrites
　　Nitrates [nitroglycerin]

972.5 Other vasodilators
　　Cyclandelate　　　　Papaverine
　　Diazoxide
　Excludes: nicotinic acid (972.2)

972.6 Other antihypertensive agents
　　Clonidine　　　　　　Rauwolfia alkaloids
　　Guanethidine　　　　Reserpine

972.7 Antivaricose drugs, including sclerosing agents
　　Sodium morrhuate
　　Zinc salts

598　　● Code new to this edition　　▲ Revision of existing code　　④ ⑤ Fourth or fifth digit required

INJURY AND POISONING

- **972.8 Capillary-active drugs**
  - Adrenochrome derivatives
  - Metaraminol
- **972.9 Other and unspecified agents primarily affecting the cardiovascular system**

973 Poisoning by agents primarily affecting the gastrointestinal system

- **973.0 Antacids and antigastric secretion drugs**
  - Aluminum hydroxide
  - Magnesium trisilicate
- **973.1 Irritant cathartics**
  - Bisacodyl
  - Castor oil
  - Phenolphthalein
- **973.2 Emollient cathartics**
  - Dioctyl sulfosuccinates
- **973.3 Other cathartics, including intestinal atonia drugs**
  - Magnesium sulfate
- **973.4 Digestants**
  - Pancreatin
  - Papain
  - Pepsin
- **973.5 Antidiarrheal drugs**
  - Kaolin
  - Pectin

  Excludes: anti-infectives (960.0-961.9)
- **973.6 Emetics**
- **973.8 Other specified agents primarily affecting the gastrointestinal system**
- **973.9 Unspecified agent primarily affecting the gastrointestinal system**

974 Poisoning by water, mineral, and uric acid metabolism drugs

- **974.0 Mercurial diuretics**
  - Chlormerodrin
  - Mercaptomerin
  - Mersalyl
- **974.1 Purine derivative diuretics**
  - Theobromine
  - Theophylline

  Excludes: aminophylline [theophylline ethylenediamine] (975.7)
  caffeine (969.7)
- **974.2 Carbonic acid anhydrase inhibitors**
  - Acetazolamide
- **974.3 Saluretics**
  - Benzothiadiazides
  - Chlorothiazide group
- **974.4 Other diuretics**
  - Ethacrynic acid
  - Furosemide
- **974.5 Electrolytic, caloric, and water-balance agents**
- **974.6 Other mineral salts, not elsewhere classified**
- **974.7 Uric acid metabolism drugs**
  - Allopurinol
  - Colchicine
  - Probenecid

975 Poisoning by agents primarily acting on the smooth and skeletal muscles and respiratory system

- **975.0 Oxytocic agents**
  - Ergot alkaloids
  - Oxytocin
  - Prostaglandins
- **975.1 Smooth muscle relaxants**
  - Adiphenine
  - Metaproterenol [orciprenaline]

  Excludes: papaverine (972.5)
- **975.2 Skeletal muscle relaxants**
- **975.3 Other and unspecified drugs acting on muscles**

599

TABULAR LIST

- **975.4** **Antitussives**
  - Dextromethorphan
  - Pipazethate
- **975.5** **Expectorants**
  - Acetylcysteine
  - Guaifenesin
  - Terpin hydrate
- **975.6** **Anti-common cold drugs**
- **975.7** **Antiasthmatics**
  - Aminophylline [theophylline ethylenediamine]
- **975.8** **Other and unspecified respiratory drugs**

976 Poisoning by agents primarily affecting skin and mucous membrane, ophthalmological, otorhinolaryngological, and dental drugs

- **976.0** **Local anti-infectives and anti-inflammatory drugs**
- **976.1** **Antipruritics**
- **976.2** **Local astringents and local detergents**
- **976.3** **Emollients, demulcents, and protectants**
- **976.4** **Keratolytics, keratoplastics, other hair treatment drugs and preparations**
- **976.5** **Eye anti-infectives and other eye drugs**
  - Idoxuridine
- **976.6** **Anti-infectives and other drugs and preparations for ear, nose, and throat**
- **976.7** **Dental drugs topically applied**
  - Excludes: anti-infectives (976.0)
  - local anesthetics (968.5)
- **976.8** **Other agents primarily affecting skin and mucous membrane**
  - Spermicides [vaginal contraceptives]
- **976.9** **Unspecified agent primarily affecting skin and mucous membrane**

977 Poisoning by other and unspecified drugs and medicinal substances

- **977.0** **Dietetics**
  - Central appetite depressants
- **977.1** **Lipotropic drugs**
- **977.2** **Antidotes and chelating agents, not elsewhere classified**
- **977.3** **Alcohol deterrents**
- **977.4** **Pharmaceutical excipients**
  - Pharmaceutical adjuncts
- **977.8** **Other specified drugs and medicinal substances**
  - Contrast media used for diagnostic x-ray procedures
  - Diagnostic agents and kits
- **977.9** **Unspecified drug or medicinal substance**

978 Poisoning by bacterial vaccines

- **978.0** **BCG**
- **978.1** **Typhoid and paratyphoid**
- **978.2** **Cholera**
- **978.3** **Plague**
- **978.4** **Tetanus**
- **978.5** **Diphtheria**
- **978.6** **Pertussis vaccine, including combinations with a pertussis component**
- **978.8** **Other and unspecified bacterial vaccines**
- **978.9** **Mixed bacterial vaccines, except combinations with a pertussis component**

979 Poisoning by other vaccines and biological substances

Excludes: gamma globulin (964.6)

- **979.0** **Smallpox vaccine**
- **979.1** **Rabies vaccine**
- **979.2** **Typhus vaccine**
- **979.3** **Yellow fever vaccine**
- **979.4** **Measles vaccine**

INJURY AND POISONING

979.5 Poliomyelitis vaccine

979.6 Other and unspecified viral and rickettsial vaccines
Mumps vaccine

979.7 Mixed viral-rickettsial and bacterial vaccines, except combinations with a pertussis component

Excludes: combinations with a pertussis component (978.6)

979.9 Other and unspecified vaccines and biological substances

TOXIC EFFECTS OF SUBSTANCES CHIEFLY NONMEDICINAL AS TO SOURCE (980-989)

Excludes: burns from chemical agents (ingested) (947.0-947.9)
localized toxic effects indexed elsewhere (001.0-799.9)
respiratory conditions due to external agents (506.0-508.9)

Use additional code to specify the nature of the toxic effect

980 Toxic effect of alcohol

980.0 Ethyl alcohol
Denatured alcohol
Ethanol
Grain alcohol

Use additional code to identify any associated:
acute alcohol intoxication (305.0)
in alcoholism (303.0)
drunkenness (simple) (305.0)
pathological (291.4)

980.1 Methyl alcohol
Methanol   Wood alcohol

980.2 Isopropyl alcohol
Dimethyl carbinol   Rubbing alcohol
Isopropanol

980.3 Fusel oil
Alcohol:
  amyl
  butyl
  propyl

980.8 Other specified alcohols

980.9 Unspecified alcohol

981 Toxic effect of petroleum products
Benzine   Petroleum:
Gasoline   ether
Kerosene   naphtha
Paraffin wax   spirit

982 Toxic effect of solvents other than petroleum-based

982.0 Benzene and homologues

982.1 Carbon tetrachloride

982.2 Carbon disulfide
Carbon bisulfide

982.3 Other chlorinated hydrocarbon solvents
Tetrachloroethylene
Trichloroethylene

Excludes: chlorinated hydrocarbon preparations other than solvents (989.2)

982.4 Nitroglycol

982.8 Other nonpetroleum-based solvents
Acetone

983 Toxic effect of corrosive aromatics, acids, and caustic alkalis

983.0 Corrosive aromatics
Carbolic acid or phenol
Cresol

983.1 Acids
Acid:
  hydrochloric
  nitric
  sulfuric

Add 4th or 5th digit | Nonspecific code | Unspecified code | Medicare secondary payer (MSP) alert

601

TABULAR LIST

983.2 Caustic alkalis
Lye
Potassium hydroxide
Sodium hydroxide

983.9 Caustic, unspecified

984 Toxic effect of lead and its compounds (including fumes)
Includes: that from all sources except medicinal substances

984.0 Inorganic lead compounds
Lead dioxide
Lead salts

984.1 Organic lead compounds
Lead acetate
Tetraethyl lead

984.8 Other lead compounds

984.9 Unspecified lead compound

985 Toxic effect of other metals
Includes: that from all sources except medicinal substances

985.0 Mercury and its compounds
Minamata disease

985.1 Arsenic and its compounds

985.2 Manganese and its compounds

985.3 Beryllium and its compounds

985.4 Antimony and its compounds

985.5 Cadmium and its compounds

985.6 Chromium

985.8 Other specified metals
Brass fumes
Copper salts
Iron compounds
Nickel compounds

985.9 Unspecified metal

986 Toxic effect of carbon monoxide
Carbon monoxide from any source

987 Toxic effect of other gases, fumes, or vapors

987.0 Liquefied petroleum gases
Butane
Propane

987.1 Other hydrocarbon gas

987.2 Nitrogen oxides
Nitrogen dioxide
Nitrous fumes

987.3 Sulfur dioxide

987.4 Freon
Dichloromonofluoromethane

987.5 Lacrimogenic gas
Bromobenzyl cyanide
Chloroacetophenone
Ethyliodoacetate

987.6 Chlorine gas

987.7 Hydrocyanic acid gas

987.8 Other specified gases, fumes, or vapors
Phosgene
Polyester fumes

987.9 Unspecified gas, fume, or vapor

988 Toxic effect of noxious substances eaten as food
Excludes: allergic reaction to food, such as:
gastroenteritis (558.3)
rash (692.5, 693.1)
food poisoning (bacterial) (005.0-005.9)
toxic effects of food contaminants, such as:
aflatoxin and other mycotoxin (989.7)
mercury (985.0)

988.0 Fish and shellfish

INJURY AND POISONING

- **988.1** Mushrooms
- **988.2** Berries and other plants
- **988.8** Other specified noxious substances eaten as food
- **988.9** Unspecified noxious substance eaten as food

989 Toxic effect of other substances, chiefly nonmedicinal as to source

- **989.0** Hydrocyanic acid and cyanides
  - Potassium cyanide
  - Sodium cyanide

  Excludes: gas and fumes (987.7)

- **989.1** Strychnine and salts
- **989.2** Chlorinated hydrocarbons
  - Aldrin
  - Chlordane
  - DDT
  - Dieldrin

  Excludes: chlorinated hydrocarbon solvents (982.0-982.3)

- **989.3** Organophosphate and carbamate
  - Carbaryl
  - Dichlorvos
  - Malathion
  - Parathion
  - Phorate
  - Phosdrin

- **989.4** Other pesticides, not elsewhere classified
  - Mixtures of insecticides

- **989.5** Venom
  - Bites of venomous snakes, lizards, and spiders
  - Tick paralysis

- **989.6** Soaps and detergents
- **989.7** Aflatoxin and other mycotoxin [food contaminants]
- ⑤ **989.8** Other substances, chiefly nonmedicinal as to source
  - **989.81** Asbestos

    Excludes: asbestosis (501)
    exposure to asbestos (V15.84)

  - **989.82** Latex
  - **989.83** Silicone

    Excludes: silicone used in medical devices, implants and grafts (996.00-996.79)

  - **989.84** Tobacco
  - **989.89** Other

- **989.9** Unspecified substance, chiefly nonmedicinal as to source

OTHER AND UNSPECIFIED EFFECTS OF EXTERNAL CAUSES (990-995)

990 Effects of radiation, unspecified
  - Complication of phototherapy
  - Complication of radiation therapy
  - Radiation sickness

  Excludes: specified adverse effects of radiation
  Such conditions are to be classified according to the nature of the adverse effect, as:
  burns (940.0-949.5)
  dermatitis (692.7-692.8)
  leukemia (204.0-208.9)
  pneumonia (508.0)
  sunburn (692.71, 692.76-692.77)
  [The type of radiation giving rise to the adverse effect may be identified by use of the E codes.]

991 Effects of reduced temperature
- **991.0** Frostbite of face
- **991.1** Frostbite of hand
- **991.2** Frostbite of foot
- **991.3** Frostbite of other and unspecified sites
- **991.4** Immersion foot
  - Trench foot

TABULAR LIST

991.5 Chilblains
   Erythema pernio
   Perniosis

991.6 Hypothermia
   Hypothermia (accidental)
   Excludes: hypothermia following anesthesia (995.89)
   hypothermia not associated with low environmental temperature (780.99)

991.8 Other specified effects of reduced temperature

991.9 Unspecified effect of reduced temperature
   Effects of freezing or excessive cold NOS

992 Effects of heat and light
   Excludes: burns (940.0-949.5)
   diseases of sweat glands due to heat (705.0-705.9)
   malignant hyperpyrexia following anesthesia (995.86)
   sunburn (692.71, 692.76-692.77)

992.0 Heat stroke and sunstroke
   Heat apoplexy
   Heat pyrexia
   Ictus solaris
   Siriasis
   Thermoplegia

992.1 Heat syncope
   Heat collapse

992.2 Heat cramps

992.3 Heat exhaustion, anhydrotic
   Heat prostration due to water depletion
   Excludes: that associated with salt depletion (992.4)

992.4 Heat exhaustion due to salt depletion
   Heat prostration due to salt (and water) depletion

992.5 Heat exhaustion, unspecified
   Heat prostration NOS

992.6 Heat fatigue, transient

992.7 Heat edema

992.8 Other specified heat effects

992.9 Unspecified

993 Effects of air pressure

993.0 Barotrauma, otitic
   Aero-otitis media
   Effects of high altitude on ears

993.1 Barotrauma, sinus
   Aerosinusitis
   Effects of high altitude on sinuses

993.2 Other and unspecified effects of high altitude
   Alpine sickness
   Andes disease
   Anoxia due to high altitude
   Hypobaropathy
   Mountain sickness

993.3 Caisson disease
   Bends
   Compressed-air disease
   Decompression sickness
   Divers' palsy or paralysis

993.4 Effects of air pressure caused by explosion

993.8 Other specified effects of air pressure

993.9 Unspecified effect of air pressure

994 Effects of other external causes
   Excludes: certain adverse effects not elsewhere classified (995.0-995.8)

994.0 Effects of lightning
   Shock from lightning
   Struck by lightning NOS
   Excludes: burns (940.0-949.5)

994.1 Drowning and nonfatal submersion
   Bathing cramp
   Immersion

INJURY AND POISONING

994.2 Effects of hunger
Deprivation of food
Starvation

994.3 Effects of thirst
Deprivation of water

994.4 Exhaustion due to exposure

994.5 Exhaustion due to excessive exertion
Overexertion

994.6 Motion sickness
Air sickness
Seasickness
Travel sickness

994.7 Asphyxiation and strangulation
Suffocation (by):
  bedclothes
  cave-in
  constriction
  mechanical
Suffocation (by):
  plastic bag
  pressure
  strangulation

Excludes: asphyxia from:
  carbon monoxide (986)
  inhalation of food or foreign body (932-934.9)
  other gases, fumes, and vapors (987.0-987.9)

994.8 Electrocution and nonfatal effects of electric current
Shock from electric current

Excludes: electric burns (940.0-949.5)

994.9 Other effects of external causes
Effects of:
  abnormal gravitational [G] forces or states
  weightlessness

995 Certain adverse effects not elsewhere classified

Excludes: complications of surgical and medical care (996.0-999.9)

995.0 Other anaphylactic shock
Allergic shock NOS or due to adverse effect of correct medicinal substance properly administered
Anaphylactic reaction NOS or due to adverse effect of correct medicinal substance properly administered
Anaphylaxis NOS or due to adverse effect of correct medicinal substance properly administered

Excludes: anaphylactic reaction to serum (999.4)
  anaphylactic shock due to adverse food reaction (995.60-995.69)

Use additional E code, if desired, to identify external cause, such as:
  adverse effects of correct medicinal substance properly administered (E930-E949)

995.1 Angioneurotic edema
Giant urticaria

Excludes: Urticaria:
  due to serum (999.5)
  other specified (698.2, 708.0-708.9, 757.33)

995.2 Other and unspecified adverse effect of drug, medicinal and biological substance
Adverse effect to correct medicinal substance properly administered
Allergic reaction to correct medicinal substance properly administered
Hypersensitivity to correct medicinal substance properly administered
Idiosyncrasy due to correct medicinal substance properly administered
Drug:
  hypersensitivity NOS
  reaction NOS

Excludes: pathological drug intoxication (292.2)

  995.20 Unspecified adverse effect of unspecified drug, medicinal and biological substance

  995.21 Arthus phenomenon
    Arthus reaction

  995.22 Unspecified adverse effect of anesthesia

  995.23 Unspecified adverse effect of insulin

TABULAR LIST

995.27 **Other drug allergy**
  Drug allergy NOS
  Drug hypersensitivity NOS

995.29 **Unspecified adverse effect of other drug, medicinal and biological substance**

995.3 **Allergy, unspecified**
  Allergic reaction NOS   Idiosyncrasy NOS
  Hypersensitivity NOS

  Excludes: *allergic reaction NOS to correct medicinal substance properly administered (995.27)*
  allergy to existing dental restorative materials (525.66)
  specific types of allergic reaction, such as:
    allergic diarrhea (558.3)
    dermatitis (691.0-693.9)
    hay fever (477.0-477.9)

995.4 **Shock due to anesthesia**
  Shock due to anesthesia in which the correct substance was properly administered

  Excludes: *complications of anesthesia in labor or delivery (668.0-668.9)*
  overdose or wrong substance given (968.0-969.9)
  postoperative shock NOS (998.0)
  specified adverse effects of anesthesia classified elsewhere, such as:
    anoxic brain damage (348.1)
    hepatitis (070.0-070.9), etc.
  unspecified adverse effect of anesthesia (995.22)

⑤ **995.5** **Child maltreatment syndrome**
  Use additional code(s), if applicable, to identify any associated injuries
  Use additional E code to identify:
    nature of abuse (E960-E968)
    perpetrator (E967.0-E967.9)

  995.50 **Child abuse, unspecified**

  995.51 **Child emotional/psychological abuse**

  995.52 **Child neglect (nutritional)**

  995.53 **Child sexual abuse**

  995.54 **Child physical abuse**
    Battered baby or child syndrome

  Excludes: *Shaken infant syndrome (995.55)*

  995.55 **Shaken infant syndrome**
  Use additional code(s) to identify any associated injuries

  995.59 **Other child abuse and neglect**
    Multiple forms of abuse

⑤ **995.6** **Anaphylactic shock due to adverse food reaction**
  Anaphylactic shock due to nonpoisonous foods

  995.60 **Due to unspecified food**

  995.61 **Due to peanuts**

  995.62 **Due to crustaceans**

  995.63 **Due to fruits and vegetables**

  995.64 **Due to tree nuts and seeds**

  995.65 **Due to fish**

  995.66 **Due to food additives**

  995.67 **Due to milk products**

  995.68 **Due to eggs**

  995.69 **Due to other specified food**

INJURY AND POISONING

995.7 Other adverse food reactions, not elsewhere classified
Use additional code to identify the type of reaction, such as:
    hives (708.0)
    wheezing (786.07)

Excludes: anaphylactic shock due to adverse food reaction (995.60-995.69)
    asthma (493.0, 493.9)
    dermatitis due to food (693.1)
      in contact with the skin (692.5)
    gastroenteritis and colitis due to food (558.3)
    rhinitis due to food (477.1)

⑤ **995.8 Other specified adverse effects, not elsewhere classified**

995.80 Adult maltreatment, unspecified
    Abused person NOS
Use additional code to identify:
    any associated injury
    perpetrator (E967.0-E967.9)

995.81 Adult physical abuse
    Battered:
      person syndrome NEC
      man
      spouse
      woman
Use additional code to identify:
    any associated injury
    nature of abuse (E960-E968)
    perpetrator (E967.0-E967.9)

995.82 Adult emotional/psychological abuse
Use additional E code to identify perpetrator (E967.0-E967.9)

995.83 Adult sexual abuse
Use additional code to identify:
    any associated injury
    perpetrator (E967.0-E967.9)

995.84 Adult neglect (nutritional)
Use additional code to identify:
    intent of neglect (E904.0, E968.4)
    perpetrator (E967.0-967.9)

995.85 Other adult abuse and neglect
    Multiple forms of abuse and neglect
Use additional code to identify:
    any associated injury
    intent of neglect (E904.0, E968.4)
    nature of abuse (E960-E968)
    perpetrator (E967.0-E967.9)

995.86 Malignant hyperthermia
    Malignant hyperpyrexia due to anesthesia

995.89 Other
    Hypothermia due to anesthesia

⑤ **995.9 Systemic inflammatory response syndrome (SIRS)**

995.90 Systemic inflammatory response syndrome, unspecified
    SIRS NOS

995.91 Sepsis
    Systemic inflammatory response syndrome due to infectious process without acute organ dysfunction
Code first underlying infection
Excludes: sepsis with acute organ dysfunction (995.92)
    sepsis with multiple organ dysfunction (995.92)
    severe sepsis (995.92)

TABULAR LIST

995.92 Severe sepsis
Sepsis with acute organ dysfunction
Sepsis with multiple organ dysfunction (MOD)
Systemic inflammatory response syndrome due to infectious process with acute organ dysfunction

Code first underlying infection

Use additional code to specify acute organ dysfunction, such as:
acute renal failure (584.5-584.9)
acute respiratory failure (518.81)
critical illness myopathy (359.81)
critical illness polyneuropathy (357.82)
disseminated intravascular coagulopathy (DIC) syndrome (286.6)
encephalopathy (348.31)
hepatic failure (570)
septic shock (785.52)

995.93 Systemic inflammatory response syndrome due to noninfectious process without acute organ dysfunction

Code first underlying conditions, such as:
acute pancreatitis (577.0)
trauma

| Excludes: | systemic inflammatory response syndrome due to noninfectious process with acute organ dysfunction (995.94) |

995.94 Systemic inflammatory response syndrome due to noninfectious process with acute organ dysfunction

Code first underlying condition, such as:
acute pancreatitis (577.0)
trauma

Use additional code to specify acute organ dysfunction, such as:
acute renal failure (584.5-584.9)
acute respiratory failure (518.81)
critical illness myopathy (359.81)
critical illness polyneuropathy (357.82)
disseminated intravascular coagulopathy (DIC) syndrome (286.6)
encephalopathy (348.31)
hepatic failure (570)

| Excludes: | severe sepsis (995.92) |

COMPLICATIONS OF SURGICAL AND MEDICAL CARE, NOT ELSEWHERE CLASSIFIED (996-999)

| Excludes: | adverse effects of medicinal agents (001.0-799.9, 995.0-995.8)
burns from local applications and irradiation (940.0-949.5)
complications of:
  conditions for which the procedure was performed
  surgical procedures during abortion, labor, and delivery (630-676.9)
poisoning and toxic effects of drugs and chemicals (960.0-989.9)
postoperative conditions in which no complications are present, such as:
  artificial opening status (V44.0-V44.9)
  closure of external stoma (V55.0-V55.9)
  fitting of prosthetic device (V52.0-V52.9)
specified complications classified elsewhere
  anesthetic shock (995.4)
  electrolyte imbalance (276.0-276.9)
  postlaminectomy syndrome (772.80-722.83)
  postmastectomy lymphedema syndrome (457.0)
  postoperative psychosis (293.0-293.9)
  any other condition classified elsewhere in the Alphabetic Index when described as due to a procedure |

INJURY AND POISONING

996 Complications peculiar to certain specified procedures
Includes: complications, not elsewhere classified, in the use of artificial substitutes [e.g., Dacron, metal, Silastic, Teflon] or natural sources [e.g., bone] involving:
  anastomosis (internal)
  graft (bypass) (patch)
  implant
  internal device:
    catheter
    electronic
    fixation
    prosthetic
  reimplant
  transplant

Excludes: accidental puncture or laceration during procedure (998.2)
  complications of internal anastomosis of:
    gastrointestinal tract (997.4)
    urinary tract (997.5)
  endosseous dental implant failures (525.71-525.79)
  intraoperative floppy iris syndrome (IFIS) (364.81)
  mechanical complication of respirator (V46.14)
  other specified complications classified elsewhere, such as:
    hemolytic anemia (283.1)
    functional cardiac disturbances (429.4)
    serum hepatitis (070.2-070.3)

⑤ 996.0 Mechanical complication of cardiac device, implant, and graft
Breakdown (mechanical)   Obstruction, mechanical
Displacement   Perforation
Leakage   Protrusion

  996.00 Unspecified device, implant, and graft
  996.01 Due to cardiac pacemaker (electrode)
  996.02 Due to heart valve prosthesis
  996.03 Due to coronary bypass graft
    Excludes: atherosclerosis of graft (414.02, 414.03)
      embolism [occlusion NOS] [thrombus] of graft (996.72)
  996.04 Due to automatic implantable cardiac defibrillator
  996.09 Other

996.1 Mechanical complication of other vascular device, implant, and graft
Mechanical complications involving:
  aortic (bifurcation) graft (replacement)
  arteriovenous:
    dialysis catheter
    fistula surgically created
    shunt surgicall created
  balloon (counterpulsation) device, intra-aortic
  carotid artery bypass graft
  femoral-popliteal bypass graft
  umbrella device, vena cava

Excludes: atherosclerosis of biological graft (440.30-440.32)
  embolism [occlusion NOS] [thrombus] of (biological) (synthetic) graft (996.74)
  peritoneal dialysis catheter (996.56)

996.2 Mechanical complication of nervous system device, implant, and graft
Mechanical complications involving:
  dorsal column stimulator
  electrodes implanted in brain [brain "pacemaker"]
  peripheral nerve graft
  ventricular (communicating) shunt

⑤ 996.3 Mechanical complication of genitourinary device, implant, and graft
  996.30 Unspecified device, implant, and graft
  996.31 Due to urethral [indwelling] catheter
  996.32 Due to intrauterine contraceptive device

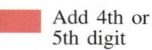 Add 4th or 5th digit   Nonspecific code   Unspecified code   Medicare secondary payer (MSP) alert

609

TABULAR LIST

996.39 Other
Cystostomy catheter
Prosthetic reconstruction of vas deferens
Repair (graft) of ureter without mention of resection

Excludes: *complications due to:*
external stoma of urinary tract (997.5)
internal anastomosis of urinary tract (997.5)

⑤ **996.4 Mechanical complication of internal orthopedic device, implant, and graft**
Use additional code to identify prosthetic joint with mechanical complication (V43.60-V43.69)

996.40 Unspecified mechanical complication of internal orthopedic device, implant, and graft

996.41 Mechanical loosening of prosthetic joint
Aseptic loosening

996.42 Dislocation of prosthetic joint
Instability of prosthetic joint
Subluxation of prosthetic joint

996.43 Prosthetic joint implant failure
Breakage (fracture) of prosthetic joint

996.44 Peri-prosthetic fracture around prosthetic joint

996.45 Peri-prosthetic osteolysis
Use additional code to identify major osseous defect, if applicable (731.3)

996.46 Articular bearing surface wear of prosthetic joint

996.47 Other mechanical complication of prosthetic joint implant
Mechanical complication of prosthetic joint NOS

996.49 Other mechanical complication of other internal orthopedic device, implant, and graft

Excludes: *mechanical complication of prosthetic joint implant (996.41-996.47)*

⑤ **996.5 Mechanical complication of other specified prosthetic device, implant, and graft**
Mechanical complications involving:
    prosthetic implant in:
        bile duct
        breast
        chin
        orbit of eye
    nonabsorbable surgical material NOS
    other graft, implant, and internal device, not elsewhere classified

996.51 Due to corneal graft

996.52 Due to graft of other tissue, not elsewhere classified
Skin graft failure or rejection

Excludes: *failure of artificial skin graft (996.55)*
failure of decellularized allodermis (996.55)
sloughing of temporary skin allografts or xenografts (pigskin)—omit code

996.53 Due to ocular lens prosthesis

Excludes: *contact lenses—code to condition*

996.54 Due to breast prosthesis
Breast capsule (prosthesis)
Mammary implant

996.55 Due to artificial skin graft and decellularized allodermis
Dislodgement   Displacement
Failure   Non-adherence
Poor incorporation   Shearing

996.56 Due to peritoneal dialysis catheter

Excludes: *mechanical complication of arteriovenous dialysis catheter (996.1)*

996.57 Due to insulin pump

996.59 Due to other implant and internal device, not elsewhere classified
Nonabsorbable surgical material NOS
Prosthetic implant in:
    bile duct
    chin
    orbit of eye

INJURY AND POISONING

⑤ **996.6 Infection and inflammatory reaction due to internal prosthetic device, implant, and graft**
    Infection (causing obstruction) due to (presence of) any device, implant and graft classifiable to 996.0-996.5
    Inflammation due to (presence of) any device, implant and graft classifiable to 996.0-996.5
Use additional code to identify specified infections

    996.60 Due to unspecified device, implant, and graft

    996.61 Due to cardiac device, implant, and graft
        Cardiac pacemaker or defibrillator:
            electrode(s), lead(s)
            pulse generator
            subcutaneous pocket
        Coronary artery bypass graft
        Heart valve prosthesis

    996.62 Due to other vascular device, implant, and graft
        Arterial graft
        Arteriovenous fistula or shunt
        Infusion pump
        Vascular catheter (arterial) (dialysis) (peripheral venous)
    Excludes: *infection due to:*
        central venous catheter (999.31)
        Hickman catheter (999.31)
        peripherally inserted central catheter (PICC) (999.31)
        triple lumen catheter (999.31)

    996.63 Due to nervous system device, implant, and graft
        Electrodes implanted in brain
        Peripheral nerve graft
        Spinal canal catheter
        Ventricular (communicating) shunt (catheter)

    996.64 Due to indwelling urinary catheter
Use additional code to identify specified infections, such as:
    Cystitis (595.0-595.9)
    Sepsis (038.0-038.9)

    996.65 Due to other genitourinary device, implant, and graft
        Intrauterine contraceptive device

    996.66 Due to internal joint prosthesis
Use additional code to identify infected prosthetic joint (V43.60-V43.69)

    996.67 Due to other internal orthopedic device, implant, and graft
        Bone growth stimulator (electrode)
        Internal fixation device (pin) (rod) (screw)

    996.68 Due to peritoneal dialysis catheter
        Exit-site infection or inflammation

    996.69 Due to other internal prosthetic device, implant, and graft
        Breast prosthesis
        Ocular lens prosthesis
        Prosthetic orbital implant

⑤ **996.7 Other complications of internal (biological) (synthetic) prosthetic device, implant, and graft**
    Complication NOS due to (presence of) any device, implant, and graft classifiable to 996.0-996.5
        occlusion NOS
    Embolism due to (presence of) any device, implant, and graft classifiable to 996.0-996.5
    Fibrosis due to (presence of) any device, implant, and graft classifiable to 996.0-996.5
    Hemorrhage due to (presence of) any device, implant, and graft classifiable to 996.0-996.5
    Pain due to (presence of) any device, implant, and graft classifiable to 996.0-996.5
    Stenosis due to (presence of) any device, implant, and graft classifiable to 996.0-996.5
    Thrombus due to (presence of) any device, implant, and graft classifiable to 996.0-996.5
Use additional code to identify complication, such as:
    pain due to presence of device, implant or graft (338.18-338.19,338.28-338.29)
Excludes: *transplant rejection (996.8)*

    996.70 Due to unspecified device, implant, and graft

    996.71 Due to heart valve prosthesis

TABULAR LIST

996.72 **Due to other cardiac device, implant, and graft**
　　　Cardiac pacemaker or defibrillator:
　　　　electrode(s), lead(s)
　　　　subcutaneous pocket
　　　Coronary artery bypass (graft)

Excludes: occlusion due to atherosclerosis (414.02-414.06)

996.73 **Due to renal dialysis device, implant, and graft**

996.74 **Due to other vascular device, implant, and graft**

Excludes: occlusion of biological graft due to atherosclerosis (440.30-440.32)

996.75 **Due to nervous system device, implant, and graft**

996.76 **Due to genitourinary device, implant, and graft**

996.77 **Due to internal joint prosthesis**
　　　Use additional code to identify prosthetic joint (V43.60 - V43.69)

996.78 **Due to other internal orthopedic device, implant, and graft**

996.79 **Due to other internal prosthetic device, implant, and graft**

⑤ **996.8** **Complications of transplanted organ**
　　Use additional code, if desired, to identify nature of complication, such as:
　　　　Cytomegalovirus (CMV) infection (078.5)
　　　　Transplant failure or rejection

996.80 **Transplanted organ, unspecified**

996.81 **Kidney**

996.82 **Liver**

996.83 **Heart**

996.84 **Lung**

996.85 **Bone Marrow**
　　　Graft-versus-host disease (acute) (chronic)

996.86 **Pancreas**

996.87 **Intestine**

996.89 **Other specified transplanted organ**

⑤ **996.9** **Complications of reattached extremity or body part**

996.90 **Unspecified extremity**

996.91 **Forearm**

996.92 **Hand**

996.93 **Finger(s)**

996.94 **Upper extremity, other and unspecified**

996.95 **Foot and toe(s)**

996.96 **Lower extremity, other and unspecified**

996.99 **Other specified body part**

997 **Complications affecting specified body systems, not elsewhere classified**
Use additional code to identify complication

Excludes: the listed conditions when specified as:
　　　causing shock (998.0)
　　　complications of:
　　　　anesthesia:
　　　　　adverse effect (001.0-799.9, 995.0-995.8)
　　　　　in labor or delivery (668.0-668.9)
　　　　　poisoning (968.0-969.9)
　　　　implanted device or graft (996.0-996.9)
　　　　obstetrical procedures (669.0-669.4)
　　　　reattached extremity (996.90-996.96)
　　　　transplanted organ (996.80-996.89)

⑤ **997.0** **Nervous system complications**

997.00 **Nervous system complication, unspecified**

997.01 **Central nervous system complication**
　　　Anoxic brain damage
　　　Cerebral hypoxia

Excludes: cerebrovascular hemorrhage or infarction (997.02)

612　　● Code new　　▲ Revision of　　④ ⑤ Fourth or fifth
　　　to this edition　　existing code　　digit required

INJURY AND POISONING

997.02 Iatrogenic cerebrovascular infarction or hemorrhage
Postoperative stroke

997.09 Other nervous system complications

997.1 Cardiac complications
Cardiac arrest during or resulting from a procedure
Cardiac insufficiency during or resulting from a procedure
Cardiorespiratory failure during or resulting from a procedure
Heart failure during or resulting from a procedure

Excludes: the listed conditions as long-term effects of cardiac surgery or due to the presence of cardiac prosthetic device (429.4)

997.2 Peripheral vascular complications
Phlebitis or thrombophlebitis during or resulting from a procedure

Excludes: the listed conditions due to:
    implant or catheter device (996.62)
    infusion, perfusion, or transfusion (999.2)
    complications affecting blood vessels (997.71-997.79)

997.3 Respiratory complications
Mendelson's syndrome resulting from a procedure
Pneumonia (aspiration) resulting from a procedure

Excludes: iatrogenic [postoperative] pneumothorax (512.1)
    iatrogenic pulmonary embolism (415.11)
    Mendelson's syndrome in labor and delivery (668.0)
    specified complications classified elsewhere, such as:
      adult respiratory distress syndrome (518.5)
      pulmonary edema, postoperative (518.4)
      respiratory insufficiency, acute, postoperative (518.5)
      shock lung (518.5)
      tracheostomy complications (519.00-519.09)
      transfusion related acute lung injury (TRALI) (518.7)

997.4 Digestive system complications
Complications of intestinal (internal) anastomosis and bypass, not elsewhere classified, except that involving urinary tract
Hepatic failure specified as due to a procedure
Hepatorenal syndrome specified as due to a procedure
Intestinal obstruction NOS specified as due to a procedure

Excludes: specified gastrointestinal complications classified elsewhere, such as:
    blind loop syndrome (579.2)
    colostomy or enterostomy complications (569.60-569.69)
    gastrostomy complications (536.40-536.49)
    gastrojejunal ulcer (534.0-534.9)
    infection of esophagostomy (530.86)
    infection of external stoma (569.61)
    mechanical complication of esophagostomy (530.87)
    pelvic peritoneal adhesions, female (614.6)
    peritoneal adhesions (568.0)
    peritoneal adhesions with obstruction (560.81)
    postcholecystectomy syndrome (576.0)
    postgastric surgery syndromes (564.2)
    vomiting following gastrointestinal surgery (564.3)

997.5 Urinary complications
Complications of:
  external stoma of urinary tract
  internal anastomosis and bypass of urinary tract, including that involving intestinal tract
Oliguria or anuria specified as due to procedure
Renal:
  failure (acute) specified as due to procedure
  insufficiency (acute) specified as due to procedure
Tubular necrosis (acute) specified as due to procedure

Excludes: specified complications classified elsewhere, such as:
    postoperative stricture of:
      ureter (593.3)
      urethra (598.2)

TABULAR LIST

⑤ **997.6 Amputation stump complication**
> *Excludes:* admission for treatment for a current traumatic amputation; code to complicated traumatic amputation
> phantom limb (syndrome) (353.6)

997.60 Unspecified complication
997.61 Neuroma of amputation stump
997.62 Infection (chronic)
Use additional code to identify the organism
997.69 Other

⑤ **997.7 Vascular complications of other vessels**
> *Excludes:* peripheral vascular complications (997.2)

997.71 Vascular complications of mesenteric artery
997.72 Vascular complications of renal artery
997.79 Vascular complications of other vessels

⑤ **997.9 Complications affecting other specified body systems, not elsewhere classified**
> *Excludes:* specified complications classified elsewhere, such as:
> broad ligament laceration syndrome (620.6)
> postartificial menopause syndrome (627.4)
> postoperative stricture of vagina (623.2)

997.91 Hypertension
> *Excludes:* essential hypertension (401.0-401.9)

997.99 Other
Vitreous touch syndrome

998 Other complications of procedures, NEC

998.0 Postoperative shock
Collapse NOS during or resulting from a surgical procedure
Shock (endotoxic) (hypovolemic) (septic) during or resulting from a surgical procedure
> *Excludes:* shock:
> anaphylactic due to serum (999.4)
> anesthetic (995.4)
> electric (994.8)
> following abortion (639.5)
> obstetric (669.1)
> traumatic (958.4)

⑤ **998.1 Hemorrhage or hematoma or seroma complicating a procedure**
> *Excludes:* hemorrhage due to implanted device or graft (996.70-996.79)
> hemorrhage, hematoma or seroma complicating cesarean section or puerperal perineal wound (674.3)

998.11 Hemorrhage complicating a procedure
998.12 Hematoma complicating a procedure
998.13 Seroma complicating a procedure

998.2 Accidental puncture or laceration during a procedure
Accidental perforation by catheter or other instrument during a procedure on:
blood vessel
nerve
organ
> *Excludes:* iatrogenic [postoperative] pneumothorax (512.1)
> puncture or laceration caused by implanted device intentionally left in operation wound (996.0-996.5)
> specified complications classified elsewhere, such as:
> broad ligament laceration syndrome (620.6)
> trauma from instruments during delivery (664.0-665.9)

⑤ **998.3 Disruption of operation wound**
Dehiscence of operation wound
Rupture of operation wound
> *Excludes:* disruption of:
> cesarean wound (674.1)
> perineal wound, puerperal (674.2)

998.31 Disruption of internal operation wound

INJURY AND POISONING

998.32 Disruption of external operation wound
Disruption of operation wound NOS

998.4 **Foreign body accidentally left during a procedure**
Adhesions due to foreign body accidentally left in operative wound or body cavity during a procedure
Obstruction due to foreign body accidentally left in operative wound or body cavity during a procedure
Perforation due to foreign body accidentally left in operative wound or body cavity during a procedure

Excludes: *obstruction or perforation caused by implanted device intentionally left in body (996.0-996.5)*

⑤ **998.5** **Postoperative infection**

Excludes: *bleb associated endophthalmitis (379.63)*
infection due to:
  implanted device (996.60-996.69)
  infusion, perfusion, or transfusion (999.31-999.39)
postoperative obstetrical wound infection (674.3)

998.51 Infected postoperative seroma
Use additional code to identify organism

998.59 Other postoperative infection
Abscess: postoperative
  intra-abdominal postoperative
  stitch postoperative
  subphrenic postoperative
  wound postoperative
Septicemia postoperative

Use additional code to identify infection

998.6 Persistent postoperative fistula

998.7 **Acute reaction to foreign substance accidentally left during a procedure**
Peritonitis:
  aseptic
  chemical

⑤ **998.8** **Other specified complications of procedures, not elsewhere classified**

998.81 Emphysema (subcutaneous) (surgical) resulting from a procedure
998.82 Cataract fragments in eye following cataract surgery
998.83 Non-healing surgical wound
998.89 Other specified complications

998.9 **Unspecified complication of procedure, not elsewhere classified**
Postoperative complication NOS

Excludes: *complication NOS of obstetrical surgery or procedure (669.4)*

615

Add 4th or 5th digit   Nonspecific code   Unspecified code   Medicare secondary payer (MSP) alert

TABULAR LIST

999 Complications of medical care, not elsewhere classified
Use additional code, where applicable, to identify specific complication
Includes: complications, not elsewhere classified, of:
dialysis (hemodialysis) (peritoneal) (renal)
extracorporeal circulation
hyperalimentation therapy
immunization
infusion
inhalation therapy
injection
inoculation
perfusion
transfusion
vaccination
ventilation therapy

Excludes: specified complications classified elsewhere such as:
complications of implanted device (996.0-996.9)
contact dermatitis due to drugs (692.3)
dementia dialysis (294.8)
  transient (293.9)
dialysis disequilibrium syndrome (276.0-276.9)
poisoning and toxic effects of drugs and chemicals (960.0-989.9)
postvaccinal encephalitis (323.51)
water and electrolyte imbalance (276.0-276.9)

999.0 Generalized vaccinia

999.1 Air embolism
Air embolism to any site following infusion, perfusion, or transfusion

Excludes: embolism specified as:
complicating:
  abortion (634-638 with .6, 639.6)
  ectopic or molar pregnancy (639.6)
  pregnancy, childbirth, or the puerperium (673.0)
due to implanted device (996.7)
traumatic (958.0)

999.2 Other vascular complications
Phlebitis following infusion, perfusion, or transfusion
Thromboembolism following infusion, perfusion, or transfusion
Thrombophlebitis following infusion, perfusion, or transfusion

Excludes: the listed conditions when specified as:
due to implanted device (996.61-996.62, 996.72-996.74)
postoperative NOS (997.2, 997.71-997.79)

⑤ **999.3 Other infection**
Infection following infusion, injection, transfusion, or vaccination
Sepsis following infusion, injection, transfusion, or vaccination
Septicemia following infusion, injection, transfusion, or vaccination
Use additional code to identify the specified infection, such as:
septicemia (038.0-038.9)

Excludes: the listed conditions when specified as:
due to implanted device (996.60-996.69)
postoperative NOS (998.51-998.59)

● **999.31 Infection due to central venous catheter**
Catheter-related bloodstream infection (CRBSI)
Infection due to:
  Hickman catheter
  Peripherally inserted central catheter (PICC)
  Triple lumen catheter

Excludes: infection due to:
arterial catheter (996.62)
catheter NOS (996.69)
peripheral venous catheter (996.62)
urinary catheter (996.64)

● **999.39 Infection following other infusion, injection, transfusion, or vaccination**

---

616 ● Code new to this edition ▲ Revision of existing code ④ ⑤ Fourth or fifth digit required

INJURY AND POISONING

999.4 Anaphylactic shock due to serum
  Excludes: shock:
    allergic NOS (995.0)
    anaphylactic:
      NOS (995.0)
      due to drugs and chemicals (995.0)

999.5 Other serum reaction
  Intoxication by serum   Serum sickness
  Protein sickness   Urticaria due to serum
  Serum rash

  Excludes: serum hepatitis (070.2-070.3)

999.6 ABO incompatibility reaction
  Incompatible blood transfusion
  Reaction to blood group incompatibility in infusion or transfusion

999.7 Rh incompatibility reaction
  Reactions due to Rh factor in infusion or transfusion

999.8 Other transfusion reaction
  Septic shock due to transfusion
  Transfusion reaction NOS

  Excludes: postoperative shock (998.0)
    transfusion related acute lung injury (TRALI) (518.7)

999.9 Other and unspecified complications of medical care, not elsewhere classified
  Complications, not elsewhere classified, of:
    electroshock therapy
    inhalation therapy
    ultrasound therapy
    ventilation therapy
  Unspecified misadventure of medical care

  Excludes: unspecified complication of:
    phototherapy (990)
    radiation therapy (990)

TABULAR LIST

● Code new to this edition   ▲ Revision of existing code   ④ ⑤ Fourth or fifth digit required

V CODES

SUPPLEMENTARY CLASSIFICATION OF FACTORS INFLUENCING HEALTH STATUS AND CONTACT WITH HEALTH SERVICES (V01-V86)

This classification is provided to deal with occasions when circumstances other than a disease or injury classifiable to categories 001-999 (the main part of ICD) are recorded as "diagnoses" or "problems." This can arise mainly in three ways:

a) When a person who is not currently sick encounters the health services for some specific purpose, such as to act as a donor of an organ or tissue, to receive prophylactic vaccination, or to discuss a problem which is in itself not a disease or injury. This will be a fairly rare occurrence among hospital inpatients, but will be relatively more common among hospital outpatients and patients of family practitioners, health clinics, etc.

b) When a person with a known disease or injury, whether it is current or resolving, encounters the health care system for a specific treatment of that disease or injury (e.g., dialysis for renal disease; chemotherapy for malignancy; cast change).

c) When some circumstance or problem is present which influences the person's health status but is not in itself a current illness or injury. Such factors may be elicited during population surveys, when the person may or may not be currently sick, or be recorded as an additional factor to be borne in mind when the person is receiving care for some current illness or injury classifiable to categories 001-999.

In the latter circumstances the V code should be used only as a supplementary code and should not be the one selected for use in primary, single cause tabulations. Examples of these circumstances are a personal history of certain diseases, or a person with an artificial heart valve in situ.

PERSONS WITH POTENTIAL HEALTH HAZARDS RELATED TO COMMUNICABLE DISEASES (V01-V06)

Excludes: family history of infectious and parasitic diseases (V18.8)
personal history of infectious and parasitic diseases (V12.0)

V01 Contact with or exposure to communicable diseases

V01.0 Cholera
Conditions classifiable to 001

V01.1 Tuberculosis
Conditions classifiable to 010-018

V01.2 Poliomyelitis
Conditions classifiable to 045

V01.3 Smallpox
Conditions classifiable to 050

V01.4 Rubella
Conditions classifiable to 056

V01.5 Rabies
Conditions classifiable to 071

V01.6 Venereal diseases
Conditions classifiable to 090-099

⑤ V01.7 Other viral diseases
Conditions classifiable to 042-078 and V08, except as above

V01.71 Varicella

V01.79 Other viral diseases

⑤ V01.8 Other communicable diseases
Conditions classifiable to 001-136, except as above

V01.81 Anthrax

V01.82 Exposure to SARS-associated coronavirus

V01.83 Escherichia coli (E. coli)

V01.84 Meningococcus

V01.89 Other communicable diseases

V01.9 Unspecified communicable disease

V02 Carrier or suspected carrier of infectious diseases

V02.0 Cholera

V02.1 Typhoid

V02.2 Amebiasis

V02.3 Other gastrointestinal pathogens

V02.4 Diphtheria

619

TABULAR LIST

⑤ **V02.5 Other specified bacterial diseases**
    V02.51 Group B streptococcus
    V02.52 Other streptococcus
    V02.59 Other specified bacterial diseases
        Meningococcal
        Staphylococcal

⑤ **V02.6 Viral hepatitis**
    Hepatitis Australian-antigen [HAA] [SH] carrier
    Serum hepatitis carrier
    V02.60 Viral hepatitis carrier, unspecified
    V02.61 Hepatitis B carrier
    V02.62 Hepatitis C carrier
    V02.69 Other viral hepatitis carrier

V02.7 Gonorrhea
V02.8 Other venereal diseases
V02.9 Other specified infectious organism

V03 Need for prophylactic vaccination and inoculation against bacterial diseases
    Excludes: vaccination not carried out (V64.00-V64.09)
              vaccines against combinations of diseases (V06.0-V06.9)

V03.0 Cholera alone
V03.1 Typhoid-paratyphoid alone [TAB]
V03.2 Tuberculosis [BCG]
V03.3 Plague
V03.4 Tularemia
V03.5 Diphtheria alone
V03.6 Pertussis alone
V03.7 Tetanus toxoid alone

⑤ **V03.8 Other specified vaccinations against single bacterial diseases**
    V03.81 Hemophilus influenza, type B [Hib]
    V03.82 Streptococcus pneumoniae [pneumococcus]
    V03.89 Other specified vaccination

V03.9 Unspecified single bacterial disease

V04 Need for prophylactic vaccination and inoculation against certain viral diseases
    Excludes: vaccines against combinations of diseases (V06.0-V06.9)

V04.0 Poliomyelitis
V04.1 Smallpox
V04.2 Measles alone
V04.3 Rubella alone
V04.4 Yellow fever
V04.5 Rabies
V04.6 Mumps alone
V04.7 Common cold

⑤ **V04.8 Other viral diseases**
    V04.81 Influenza
    V04.82 Respiratory syncytial virus (RSV)
    V04.89 Other viral diseases

V05 Need for other prophylactic vaccination and inoculation against single diseases
    Excludes: vaccines against combinations of diseases (V06.0-V06.9)

V05.0 Arthropod-borne viral encephalitis
V05.1 Other arthropod-borne viral diseases
V05.2 Leishmaniasis
V05.3 Viral hepatitis

V CODES

V05.4 Varicella
Chickenpox

V05.8 Other specified disease

V05.9 Unspecified single disease

V06 Need for prophylactic vaccination and inoculation against combinations of diseases
Note: Use additional single vaccination codes from categories V03-V05 to identify any vaccinations not included in a combination code.

V06.0 Cholera with typhoid-paratyphoid [cholera + TAB]

V06.1 Diphtheria-tetanus-pertussis, combined [DTP] [DTaP]

V06.2 Diphtheria-tetanus-pertussis with typhoid-paratyphoid [DTP + TAB]

V06.3 Diphtheria-tetanus-pertussis with poliomyelitis [DTP + polio]

V06.4 Measles-mumps-rubella [MMR]

V06.5 Tetanus-diphtheria [Td] [DT]

V06.6 Streptococcus pneumoniae [pneumococcus] and influenza

V06.8 Other combinations
Excludes: multiple single vaccination codes (V03.0-V05.9)

V06.9 Unspecified combined vaccine

PERSONS WITH NEED FOR ISOLATION, OTHER POTENTIAL HEALTH HAZARDS AND PROPHYLACTIC MEASURES (V07-V09)

V07 Need for isolation and other prophylactic measures
Excludes: prophylactic organ removal (V50.41-V50.49)

V07.0 Isolation
Admission to protect the individual from his surroundings or for isolation of individual after contact with infectious diseases

V07.1 Desensitization to allergens

V07.2 Prophylactic immunotherapy
Administration of:
antivenin
immune sera [gamma globulin]
RhoGAM
tetanus antitoxin

⑤ **V07.3 Other prophylactic chemotherapy**

V07.31 Prophylactic fluoride administration

V07.39 Other prophylactic chemotherapy
Excludes: maintenance chemotherapy following disease (V58.11)

V07.4 Hormone replacement therapy (postmenopausal)

V07.8 Other specified prophylactic measure

V07.9 Unspecified prophylactic measure

V08 Asymptomatic human immunodeficiency virus [HIV] infection status
HIV positive NOS

Note: This code is ONLY to be used when NO HIV infection symptoms or conditions are present. If any HIV infection symptoms or conditions are present, see code 042.

Excludes: AIDS (042)
human immunodeficiency virus [HIV] disease (042)
exposure to HIV (V01.79)
nonspecific serologic evidence of HIV (795.71)
symptomatic human immunodeficiency virus [HIV] infection (042)

V09 Infection with drug-resistant microorganisms
Note: This category is intended for use as an additional code for infectious conditions classified elsewhere to indicate the presence of drug-resistance of the infectious organism.

V09.0 Infection with microorganisms resistant to penicillins
Methicillin-resistant staphylococcus aureus (MRSA)

V09.1 Infection with microorganisms resistant to cephalosporins and other B-lactam antibiotics

V09.2 Infection with microorganisms resistant to macrolides

V09.3 Infection with microorganisms resistant to tetracyclines

V09.4 Infection with microorganisms resistant to aminoglycosides

TABULAR LIST

⑤ **V09.5 Infection with microorganisms resistant to quinolones and fluoroquinolones**

V09.50 Without mention of resistance to multiple quinolones and fluoroquinolones

V09.51 With resistance to multiple quinolones and fluoroquinolones

V09.6 Infection with microorganisms resistant to sulfonamides

⑤ **V09.7 Infection with microorganisms resistant to other specified antimycobacterial agents**

Excludes: Amikacin (V09.4)
Kanamycin (V09.4)
Streptomycin [SM] (V09.4)

V09.70 Without mention of resistance to multiple antimycobacterial agents

V09.71 With resistance to multiple antimycobacterial agents

⑤ **V09.8 Infection with microorganisms resistant to other specified drugs**
Vancomycin (glycopeptide) intermediate staphylococcus aureus (VISA/GISA)
Vancomycin (glycopeptide) resistant enterococcus (VRE)
Vancomycin (glycopeptide) resistant staphylococcus aureus (VRSA/GRSA)

V09.80 Without mention of resistance to multiple drugs

V09.81 With resistance to multiple drugs

⑤ **V09.9 Infection with drug-resistant microorganisms, unspecified**
Drug resistance NOS

V09.90 Without mention of multiple drug resistance

V09.91 With multiple drug resistance
Multiple drug resistance NOS

PERSONS WITH POTENTIAL HEALTH HAZARDS RELATED TO PERSONAL AND FAMILY HISTORY (V10-V19)

Excludes: obstetric patients where the possibility that the fetus might be affected is the reason for observation or management during pregnancy (655.0-655.9)

V10 Personal history of malignant neoplasm

⑤ **V10.0 Gastrointestinal tract**
History of conditions classifiable to 140-159

V10.00 Gastrointestinal tract, unspecified

V10.01 Tongue

V10.02 Other and unspecified oral cavity and pharynx

V10.03 Esophagus

V10.04 Stomach

V10.05 Large intestine

V10.06 Rectum, rectosigmoid junction, and anus

V10.07 Liver

V10.09 Other

⑤ **V10.1 Trachea, bronchus, and lung**
History of conditions classifiable to 162

V10.11 Bronchus and lung

V10.12 Trachea

⑤ **V10.2 Other respiratory and intrathoracic organs**
History of conditions classifiable to 160, 161, 163-165

V10.20 Respiratory organ, unspecified

V10.21 Larynx

V10.22 Nasal cavities, middle ear, and accessory sinuses

V10.29 Other

V10.3 Breast
History of conditions classifiable to 174 and 175

⑤ **V10.4 Genital organs**
History of conditions classifiable to 179-187

V10.40 Female genital organ, unspecified

V10.41 Cervix uteri

V10.42 Other parts of uterus

V10.43 Ovary

● Code new to this edition ▲ Revision of existing code ④ ⑤ Fourth or fifth digit required

V CODES

- **V10.44** Other female genital organs
- **V10.45** Male genital organ, unspecified
- V10.46 Prostate
- V10.47 Testis
- V10.48 Epididymis
- **V10.49** Other male genital organs

⑤ V10.5 **Urinary organs**
History of conditions classifiable to 188 and 189

- **V10.50** Urinary organ, unspecified
- V10.51 Bladder
- V10.52 Kidney

Excludes: renal pelvis (V10.53)

- V10.53 Renal pelvis
- **V10.59** Other

⑤ V10.6 **Leukemia**
Conditions classifiable to 204-208

Excludes: leukemia in remission (204-208)

- **V10.60** Leukemia, unspecified
- V10.61 Lymphoid leukemia
- V10.62 Myeloid leukemia
- V10.63 Monocytic leukemia
- **V10.69** Other

⑤ V10.7 **Other lymphatic and hematopoietic neoplasms**
Conditions classifiable to 200-203

Excludes: listed conditions in 200-203 in remission

- V10.71 Lymphosarcoma and reticulosarcoma
- V10.72 Hodgkin's disease
- **V10.79** Other

⑤ V10.8 **Personal history of malignant neoplasm of other sites**
History of conditions classifiable to 170-173, 190-195

- V10.81 Bone
- V10.82 Malignant melanoma of skin
- **V10.83** Other malignant neoplasm of skin
- V10.84 Eye
- V10.85 Brain
- **V10.86** Other parts of nervous system

Excludes: peripheral, sympathetic, and parasympathetic nerves (V10.89)

- V10.87 Thyroid
- **V10.88** Other endocrine glands and related structures
- **V10.89** Other

V10.9 Unspecified personal history of malignant neoplasm

V11 Personal history of mental disorder

V11.0 Schizophrenia

Excludes: that in remission (295.0-295.9 with fifth-digit 5)

V11.1 Affective disorders
Personal history of manic-depressive psychosis

Excludes: that in remission (296.0-296.6 with fifth-digit 5, 6)

V11.2 Neurosis

V11.3 Alcoholism

V11.8 Other mental disorders

V11.9 Unspecified mental disorder

Add 4th or 5th digit   Nonspecific code   Unspecific code   Secondary Dx Only   Primary Dx Only

TABULAR LIST

V12 Personal history of certain other diseases
- ⑤ **V12.0** Infectious and parasitic diseases
  - *Excludes:* personal history of infectious diseases specific to a body system
    - **V12.00** Unspecified infectious and parasitic disease
    - V12.01 Tuberculosis
    - V12.02 Poliomyelitis
    - V12.03 Malaria
    - **V12.09** Other
- **V12.1** Nutritional deficiency
- **V12.2** Endocrine, metabolic, and immunity disorders
  - *Excludes:* history of allergy (V14.0-V14.9, V15.01-V15.09)
- **V12.3** Diseases of blood and blood-forming organs
- ⑤ **V12.4** Disorders of nervous system and sense organs
    - **V12.40** Unspecified disorder of nervous system and sense organs
    - V12.41 Benign neoplasm of the brain
    - V12.42 Infections of the central nervous system
      Encephalitis
      Meningitis
    - **V12.49** Other disorders of nervous system and sense organs
- ⑤ **V12.5** Diseases of circulatory system
  - *Excludes:* old myocardial infarction (412)
    postmyocardial infarction syndrome (411.0)
    - **V12.50** Unspecified circulatory disease
    - V12.51 Venous thrombosis and embolism
      Pulmonary embolism
    - V12.52 Thrombophlebitis
    - ● V12.53 Sudden cardiac arrest
      Sudden cardiac death successfully resuscitated
    - ● V12.54 Transient ischemic attack (TIA), and cerebral infarction without residual deficits
      Prolonged reversible ischemic neurological deficit (PRIND)
      Reversible ischemic neurologic deficit (RIND)
      Stroke NOS without residual deficits
  - *Excludes:* late effects of cerebrovascular disease (438.0-438.9)
    - **V12.59** Other
      Note: Assign code V12.59 (and not a code from category 438) as an additional code for history of cerebrovascular disease when no neurologic deficits are present.
- ⑤ **V12.6** Diseases of respiratory system
  - *Excludes:* tuberculosis (V12.01)
    - **V12.60** Unspecified disease of respiratory system
    - V12.61 Pneumonia (recurrent)
    - **V12.69** Other diseases of respiratory system
- ⑤ **V12.7** Diseases of digestive system
    - **V12.70** Unspecified digestive disease
    - V12.71 Peptic ulcer disease
    - V12.72 Colonic polyps
    - **V12.79** Other

V13 Personal history of other diseases
- ⑤ **V13.0** Disorders of urinary system
    - **V13.00** Unspecified urinary disorder
    - V13.01 Urinary calculi
    - V13.02 Urinary (tract) infection
    - V13.03 Nephrotic syndrome
    - **V13.09** Other

● Code new to this edition   ▲ Revision of existing code   ④ ⑤ Fourth or fifth digit required

V CODES

V13.1 Trophoblastic disease
Excludes: supervision during a current pregnancy (V23.1)

⑤ **V13.2 Other genital system and obstetric disorders**
Excludes: supervision during a current pregnancy of a woman with poor obstetric history (V23.0-V23.9)
habitual aborter (646.3)
without current pregnancy (629.81)

V13.21 Personal history of pre-term labor
Excludes: current pregnancy with history of pre-term labor (V23.41)

● **V13.22 Personal history of cervical dysplasia**
Personal history of conditions classifiable to 622.10-622.12
Excludes: personal history of malignant neoplasm of cervix uteri (V10.41)

V13.29 Other genital system and obstetric disorders

V13.3 Diseases of skin and subcutaneous tissue
V13.4 Arthritis
V13.5 Other musculoskeletal disorders
⑤ **V13.6 Congenital malformations**
 V13.61 Hypospadias
 V13.69 Other congenital malformations
V13.7 Perinatal problems
Excludes: low birth weight status (V21.30-V21.35)

V13.8 Other specified diseases
V13.9 Unspecified disease

V14 Personal history of allergy to medicinal agents
V14.0 Penicillin
V14.1 Other antibiotic agent
V14.2 Sulfonamides
V14.3 Other anti-infective agent
V14.4 Anesthetic agent
V14.5 Narcotic agent
V14.6 Analgesic agent
V14.7 Serum or vaccine
V14.8 Other specified medicinal agents
V14.9 Unspecified medicinal agent

V15 Other personal history presenting hazards to health
⑤ **V15.0 Allergy, other than to medicinal agents**
Excludes: allergy to food substance used as base for medicinal agent (V14.0-V14.9)

 V15.01 Allergy to peanuts
 V15.02 Allergy to milk products
Excludes: lactose intolerance (271.3)

 V15.03 Allergy to eggs
 V15.04 Allergy to seafood
 Seafood (octopus) (squid) ink
 Shellfish

 V15.05 Allergy to other foods
 Food additives
 Nuts other than peanuts

 V15.06 Allergy to insects
 Bugs
 Insect bites and stings
 Spiders

 V15.07 Allergy to latex
 Latex sensitivity

 V15.08 Allergy to radiographic dye
 Contrast media used for diagnostic x-ray procedures

625

| Add 4th or 5th digit | Nonspecific code | Unspecific code | Secondary Dx Only | Primary Dx Only |

TABULAR LIST

V15.09 Other allergy, other than to medicinal agents

V15.1 Surgery to heart and great vessels
Excludes: replacement by transplant or other means (V42.1-V42.2, V43.2-V43.4)

V15.2 Surgery to other major organs
Excludes: replacement by transplant or other means (V42.0-V43.8)

V15.3 Irradiation
Previous exposure to therapeutic or other ionizing radiation

⑤ **V15.4** Psychological trauma
Excludes: history of condition classifiable to 290-316 (V11.0-V11.9)

    V15.41 History of physical abuse
        Rape

    V15.42 History of emotional abuse
        Neglect

    V15.49 Other

V15.5 Injury

V15.6 Poisoning

V15.7 Contraception
Excludes: current contraceptive management (V25.0-V25.4)
         presence of intrauterine contraceptive device as incidental finding (V45.5)

⑤ **V15.8** Other specified personal history presenting hazards to health

    V15.81 Noncompliance with medical treatment

    V15.82 History of tobacco use
Excludes: tobacco dependence (305.1)

    V15.84 Exposure to asbestos

    V15.85 Exposure to potentially hazardous body fluids

    V15.86 Exposure to lead

    V15.87 History of extracorporeal membrane oxygenation [ECMO]

    V15.88 History of fall
        At risk for falling

    V15.89 Other

V15.9 Unspecified personal history presenting hazards to health

V16 Family history of malignant neoplasm

    V16.0 Gastrointestinal tract
        Family history of condition classifiable to 140-159

    V16.1 Trachea, bronchus, and lung
        Family history of condition classifiable to 162

    V16.2 Other respiratory and intrathoracic organs
        Family history of condition classifiable to 160-161, 163-165

    V16.3 Breast
        Family history of condition classifiable to 174

⑤   V16.4 Genital organs
        Family history of condition classifiable to 179-187

    V16.40 Genital organ, unspecified

    V16.41 Ovary

    V16.42 Prostate

    V16.43 Testis

    V16.49 Other

⑤   V16.5 Urinary organs
        Family history of condition classifiable to 188-189

    V16.51 Kidney

●   V16.52 Bladder

    V16.59 Other

    V16.6 Leukemia
        Family history of condition classifiable to 204-208

V CODES

V16.7 **Other lymphatic and hematopoietic neoplasms**
Family history of condition classifiable to 200-203

V16.8 **Other specified malignant neoplasm**
Family history of other condition classifiable to 140-199

V16.9 **Unspecified malignant neoplasm**

V17 **Family history of certain chronic disabling diseases**

V17.0 **Psychiatric condition**
Excludes: family history of mental retardation (V18.4)

V17.1 **Stroke (cerebrovascular)**

V17.2 **Other neurological diseases**
Epilepsy
Huntington's chorea

V17.3 **Ischemic heart disease**

⑤ **V17.4** **Other cardiovascular diseases**
● **V17.41** **Family history of sudden cardiac death (SCD)**
Excludes: family history of ischemic heart disease (V17.3)
family history of myocardial infarction (V17.3)

● **V17.49** **Family history of other cardiovascular diseases**
Family history of cardiovascular disease NOS

V17.5 **Asthma**

V17.6 **Other chronic respiratory conditions**

V17.7 **Arthritis**

⑤ **V17.8** **Other musculoskeletal diseases**
V17.81 **Osteoporosis**
V17.89 **Other musculoskeletal diseases**

V18 **Family history of certain other specific conditions**

V18.0 **Diabetes mellitus**

⑤ **V18.1** **Other endocrine and metabolic diseases**
● **V18.11** **Multiple endocrine neoplasia [MEN] syndrome**
● **V18.19** **Other endocrine and metabolic diseases**

V18.2 **Anemia**

V18.3 **Other blood disorders**

V18.4 **Mental retardation**

⑤ **V18.5** **Digestive disorders**
V18.51 **Colonic polyps**
Excludes: family history of malignant neoplasm of gastrointestinal tract (V16.0)
V18.59 **Other digestive disorders**

⑤ **V18.6** **Kidney diseases**
V18.61 **Polycystic kidney**
V18.69 **Other kidney diseases**

V18.7 **Other genitourinary diseases**

V18.8 **Infectious and parasitic diseases**

V18.9 **Genetic disease carrier**

V19 **Family history of other conditions**

V19.0 **Blindness or visual loss**

V19.1 **Other eye disorders**

V19.2 **Deafness or hearing loss**

V19.3 **Other ear disorders**

V19.4 **Skin conditions**

V19.5 **Congenital anomalies**

V19.6 **Allergic disorders**

V19.7 **Consanguinity**

V19.8 **Other condition**

TABULAR LIST

PERSONS ENCOUNTERING HEALTH SERVICES IN CIRCUMSTANCES RELATED TO REPRODUCTION AND DEVELOPMENT (V20-V29)

V20 Health supervision of infant or child

- **V20.0 Foundling**
- **V20.1 Other healthy infant or child receiving care**
  Medical or nursing care supervision of healthy infant in cases of:
    maternal illness, physical or psychiatric
    socioeconomic adverse condition at home
    too many children at home preventing or interfering with normal care
- **V20.2 Routine infant or child health check**
  Developmental testing of infant or child
  Immunizations appropriate for age
  Initial and subsequent routine newborn check
  Routine vision and hearing testing

  Excludes: special screening for developmental handicaps (V79.3)
  Use additional code(s) to identify:
    Special screening examination(s) performed (V73.0-V82.9)

V21 Constitutional states in development

- **V21.0 Period of rapid growth in childhood**
- **V21.1 Puberty**
- **V21.2 Other adolescence**
- **V21.3 Low birth weight status**

  Excludes: history of perinatal problems (V13.7)

    - **V21.30 Low birth weight status, unspecified**
    - **V21.31 Low birth weight status, less than 500 grams**
    - **V21.32 Low birth weight status, 500-999 grams**
    - **V21.33 Low birth weight status, 1000-1499 grams**
    - **V21.34 Low birth weight status, 1500-1999 grams**
    - **V21.35 Low birth weight status, 2000-2500 grams**

- **V21.8 Other specified constitutional states in development**
- **V21.9 Unspecified constitutional state in development**

V22 Normal pregnancy

  Excludes: pregnancy examination or test, pregnancy unconfirmed (V72.40)

- **V22.0 Supervision of normal first pregnancy**
- **V22.1 Supervision of other normal pregnancy**
- **V22.2 Pregnant state, incidental**
  Pregnant state NOS

V23 Supervision of high-risk pregnancy

- **V23.0 Pregnancy with history of infertility**
- **V23.1 Pregnancy with history of trophoblastic disease**
  Pregnancy with history of:
    hydatidiform mole
    vesicular mole

  Excludes: that without current pregnancy (V13.1)

- **V23.2 Pregnancy with history of abortion**
  Pregnancy with history of conditions classifiable to 634-638

  Excludes: habitual aborter:
      care during pregnancy (646.3)
      that without current pregnancy (629.81)

- **V23.3 Grand multiparity**

  Excludes: care in relation to labor and delivery (659.4)
      that without current pregnancy (V61.5)

- **V23.4 Pregnancy with other poor obstetric history**
  Pregnancy with history of other conditions classifiable to 630-676

    - **V23.41 Pregnancy with history of pre-term labor**
    - **V23.49 Pregnancy with other poor obstetric history**

V CODES

V23.5 Pregnancy with other poor reproductive history
Pregnancy with history of stillbirth or neonatal death

V23.7 Insufficient prenatal care
History of little or no prenatal care

⑤ **V23.8 Other high-risk pregnancy**

  V23.81 Elderly primigravida
  First pregnancy in a woman who will be 35 years of age or older at expected date of delivery

  Excludes: elderly primigravida complicating pregnancy (659.5)

  V23.82 Elderly multigravida
  Second or more pregnancy in a woman who will be 35 years of age or older at expected date of delivery

  Excludes: elderly multigravida complicating pregnancy (659.6)

  V23.83 Young primigravida
  First pregnancy in a female less than 16 years old at expected date of delivery

  Excludes: young primigravida complicating pregnancy (659.8)

  V23.84 Young multigravida
  Second or more pregnancy in a female less than 16 years old at expected date of delivery

  Excludes: young multigravida complicating pregnancy (659.8)

  V23.89 Other high-risk pregnancy

V23.9 Unspecified high-risk pregnancy

V24 Postpartum care and examination

  V24.0 Immediately after delivery
  Care and observation in uncomplicated cases

  V24.1 Lactating mother
  Supervision of lactation

  V24.2 Routine postpartum follow-up

V25 Encounter for contraceptive management

  ⑤ **V25.0 General counseling and advice**

   V25.01 Prescription of oral contraceptives

   V25.02 Initiation of other contraceptive measures
   Fitting of diaphragm
   Prescription of foams, creams, or other agents

   V25.03 Encounter for emergency contraceptive counseling and prescription
   Encounter for postcoital contraceptive counseling and prescription

   ● **V25.04 Counseling and instruction in natural family planning to avoid pregnancy**

   V25.09 Other
   Family planning advice

  V25.1 Insertion of intrauterine contraceptive device

  V25.2 Sterilization
  Admission for interruption of fallopian tubes or vas deferens

  V25.3 Menstrual extraction
  Menstrual regulation

  ⑤ **V25.4 Surveillance of previously prescribed contraceptive methods**
  Checking, reinsertion, or removal of contraceptive device
  Repeat prescription for contraceptive method
  Routine examination in connection with contraceptive maintenance

  Excludes: presence of intrauterine contraceptive device as incidental finding (V45.5)

   V25.40 Contraceptive surveillance, unspecified

   V25.41 Contraceptive pill

   V25.42 Intrauterine contraceptive device
   Checking, reinsertion, or removal of intrauterine device

   V25.43 Implantable subdermal contraceptive

   V25.49 Other contraceptive method

  V25.5 Insertion of implantable subdermal contraceptive

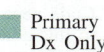

TABULAR LIST

V25.8 **Other specified contraceptive management**
Postvasectomy sperm count
Excludes: *sperm count following sterilization reversal (V26.22)*
sperm count for fertility testing (V26.21)

V25.9 **Unspecified contraceptive management**

V26 Procreative management

V26.0 **Tuboplasty or vasoplasty after previous sterilization**

V26.1 **Artificial insemination**

⑤ **V26.2** **Investigation and testing**
Excludes: *postvasectomy sperm count (V25.8)*

V26.21 **Fertility testing**
Fallopian insufflation
Sperm count for fertility testing
Excludes: *genetic counseling and testing (V26.31-V26.39)*

V26.22 **Aftercare following sterilization reversal**
Fallopian insufflation following sterilization reversal
Sperm count following sterilization reversal

V26.29 **Other investigation and testing**

⑤ **V26.3** **Genetic counseling and testing**
Excludes: *fertility testing (V26.21)*
nonprocreative genetic screening (V82.71, V82.79)

V26.31 **Testing of female for genetic disease carrier status**

V26.32 **Other genetic testing of female**
Use additional code to identify habitual aborter (629.81, 646.3)

V26.33 **Genetic counseling**

V26.34 **Testing of male for genetic disease carrier status**

V26.35 **Encounter for testing of male partner of habitual aborter**

V26.39 **Other genetic testing of male**

⑤ **V26.4** **General counseling and advice**
● **V26.41** **Procreative counseling and advice using natural family planning**
● **V26.49** **Other procreative management counseling and advice**

⑤ **V26.5** **Sterilization status**

V26.51 **Tubal ligation status**
Excludes: *infertility not due to previous tubal ligation (628.0-628.9)*

V26.52 **Vasectomy status**

⑤ **V26.8** **Other specified procreative management**
● **V26.81** **Encounter for assisted reproductive fertility procedure cycle**
Patient undergoing in vitro fertilization cycle
Use additional code to identify the type of infertility
Excludes: *pre-cycle diagnosis and testing – code to reason for encounter*

● **V26.89** **Other specified procreative management**

V26.9 **Unspecified procreative management**

V27 Outcome of delivery
Note: This category is intended for the coding of the outcome of delivery on the mother's record.

V27.0 **Single liveborn**

V27.1 **Single stillborn**

V27.2 **Twins, both liveborn**

V27.3 **Twins, one liveborn and one stillborn**

V27.4 **Twins, both stillborn**

V27.5 **Other multiple birth, all liveborn**

V27.6 **Other multiple birth, some liveborn**

V27.7 **Other multiple birth, all stillborn**

● Code new to this edition   ▲ Revision of existing code   ④ ⑤ Fourth or fifth digit required

V CODES

V27.9 Unspecified outcome of delivery
    Single birth, outcome to infant unspecified
    Multiple birth, outcome to infant unspecified

V28 Encounter for antenatal screening of mother
    Excludes: abnormal findings on screening—code to findings
        routine prenatal care (V22.0-V23.9)

    V28.0 Screening for chromosomal anomalies by amniocentesis
    V28.1 Screening for raised alpha-fetoprotein levels in amniotic fluid
    V28.2 Other screening based on amniocentesis
    V28.3 Screening for malformation using ultrasonics
    V28.4 Screening for fetal growth retardation using ultrasonics
    V28.5 Screening for isoimmunization
    V28.6 Screening for Streptococcus B
    V28.8 Other specified antenatal screening
    V28.9 Unspecified antenatal screening

V29 Observation and evaluation of newborns for suspected condition not found
    Note: This category is to be used for newborns, within the neonatal period, (the first 28 days of life) who are suspected of having an abnormal condition resulting from exposure from the mother or the birth process, but without signs or symptoms, and, which after examination and observation, is found not to exist.

    V29.0 Observation for suspected infectious condition
    V29.1 Observation for suspected neurological condition
    V29.2 Observation for suspected respiratory condition
    V29.3 Observation for suspected genetic or metabolic condition
    V29.8 Observation for other specified suspected condition
    V29.9 Observation for unspecified suspected condition

LIVEBORN INFANTS ACCORDING TO TYPE OF BIRTH (V30-V39)

    Note: These categories are intended for the coding of liveborn infants who are consuming health care [e.g., crib or bassinet occupancy].

    The following fourth-digit subdivisions are for use with categories V30-V39:
        ⑤ .0 **Born in hospital**
           .1 **Born before admission to hospital**
           .2 **Born outside hospital and not hospitalized**

    The following two fifth-digits are for use with the fourth-digit .0, Born in hospital:
        0 delivered without mention of cesarean delivery
        1 delivered by cesarean delivery

④ **V30** Single liveborn
④ **V31** Twin, mate liveborn
④ **V32** Twin, mate stillborn
④ **V33** Twin, unspecified
④ **V34** Other multiple, mates all liveborn
④ **V35** Other multiple, mates all stillborn
④ **V36** Other multiple, mates live- and stillborn
④ **V37** Other multiple, unspecified
④ **V39** Unspecified

PERSONS WITH A CONDITION INFLUENCING THEIR HEALTH STATUS (V40-V49)

    Note: These categories are intended for use when these conditions are recorded as "diagnoses" or "problems."

V40 Mental and behavioral problems
    V40.0 Problems with learning
    V40.1 Problems with communication [including speech]
    V40.2 Other mental problems
    V40.3 Other behavioral problems
    V40.9 Unspecified mental or behavioral problem

Add 4th or 5th digit   Nonspecific code   Unspecific code   Secondary Dx Only   Primary Dx Only

TABULAR LIST

V41 **Problems with special senses and other special functions**
- **V41.0** Problems with sight
- **V41.1** Other eye problems
- **V41.2** Problems with hearing
- **V41.3** Other ear problems
- **V41.4** Problems with voice production
- **V41.5** Problems with smell and taste
- **V41.6** Problems with swallowing and mastication
- **V41.7** Problems with sexual function

  Excludes: marital problems (V61.10)
  psychosexual disorders (302.0-302.9)
- **V41.8** Other problems with special functions
- **V41.9** Unspecified problem with special function

V42 **Organ or tissue replaced by transplant**
Includes: homologous or heterologous (animal) (human) transplant organ status
- **V42.0** Kidney
- **V42.1** Heart
- **V42.2** Heart valve
- **V42.3** Skin
- **V42.4** Bone
- **V42.5** Cornea
- **V42.6** Lung
- **V42.7** Liver
- ⑤ V42.8 Other specified organ or tissue
  - **V42.81** Bone marrow
  - **V42.82** Peripheral stem cells
  - **V42.83** Pancreas
  - **V42.84** Intestines
  - **V42.89** Other
- **V42.9** Unspecified organ or tissue

V43 **Organ or tissue replaced by other means**
Includes: organ or tissue assisted by other means
replacement of organ by:
artificial device
mechanical device
prosthesis

Excludes: cardiac pacemaker in situ (V45.01)
fitting and adjustment of prosthetic device (V52.0-V52.9)
renal dialysis status (V45.1)

- **V43.0** Eye globe
- **V43.1** Lens
  Pseudophakos
- ⑤ V43.2 Heart
  - **V43.21** Heart assist device
  - V43.22 Fully implantable artificial heart
- **V43.3** Heart valve
- **V43.4** Blood vessel
- **V43.5** Bladder
- ⑤ V43.6 Joint
  - **V43.60** Unspecified joint
  - **V43.61** Shoulder
  - **V43.62** Elbow
  - **V43.63** Wrist
  - **V43.64** Hip
  - **V43.65** Knee

V CODES

        V43.66 Ankle
        V43.69 Other
    V43.7 Limb
 ⑤ V43.8 Other organ or tissue
        V43.81 Larynx
        V43.82 Breast
        V43.83 Artificial skin
        V43.89 Other

V44 Artificial opening status
    Excludes: artificial openings requiring attention or management (V55.0-V55.9)
    V44.0 Tracheostomy
    V44.1 Gastrostomy
    V44.2 Ileostomy
    V44.3 Colostomy
    V44.4 Other artificial opening of gastrointestinal tract
 ⑤ V44.5 Cystostomy
        V44.50 Cystostomy, unspecified
        V44.51 Cutaneous-vesicostomy
        V44.52 Appendico-vesicostomy
        V44.59 Other cystostomy
    V44.6 Other artificial opening of urinary tract
        Nephrostomy
        Ureterostomy
        Urethrostomy
    V44.7 Artificial vagina
    V44.8 Other artificial opening status
    V44.9 Unspecified artificial opening status

V45 Other postprocedural states
    Excludes: aftercare management (V51-V58.9)
               malfunction or other complication—code to condition
 ⑤ V45.0 Cardiac device in situ
      Excludes: artificial heart (V43.22)
                heart assist device (V43.21)
        V45.06 Unspecified cardiac device
        V45.01 Cardiac pacemaker
        V45.02 Automatic implantable cardiac defibrillator
        V45.09 Other specified cardiac device
            Carotid sinus pacemaker in situ
    V45.1 Renal dialysis status
        Hemodialysis status
        Peritoneal dialysis status
        Patient requiring intermittent renal dialysis
        Presence of arterial-venous shunt (for dialysis)
    Excludes: admission for dialysis treatment, or session (V56.0)
    V45.2 Presence of cerebrospinal fluid drainage device
        Cerebral ventricle (communicating) shunt, valve, or device in situ
    Excludes: malfunction (996.2)
    V45.3 Intestinal bypass or anastomosis status
    Excludes: bariatric surgery status (V45.86)
             gastric bypass status (V45.86)
             obesity surgery status (V45.86)
    V45.4 Arthrodesis status

633

| Add 4th or 5th digit | Nonspecific code | Unspecific code | Secondary Dx Only | Primary Dx Only |

TABULAR LIST

- ⑤ **V45.5 Presence of contraceptive device**
  Excludes: *checking, reinsertion, or removal of device (V25.42)*
  complication from device (996.32)
  insertion of device (V25.1)
  - **V45.51** Intrauterine contraceptive device
  - **V45.52** Subdermal contraceptive implant
  - **V45.59** Other

- ⑤ **V45.6 States following surgery of eye and adnexa**
  Cataract extraction state following eye surgery
  Filtering bleb state following eye surgery
  Surgical eyelid adhesion state following eye surgery
  Excludes: *aphakia (379.31)*
  artificial eye globe (V43.0)
  - **V45.61** Cataract extraction status
    Use additional code for associated artificial lens status (V43.1)
  - **V45.69** Other states following surgery of eye and adnexa

- ⑤ **V45.7 Acquired absence of organ**
  - **V45.71** Acquired absence of breast
  - **V45.72** Acquired absence of intestine (large) (small)
  - **V45.73** Acquired absence of kidney
  - **V45.74** Other parts of urinary tract
    Bladder
  - **V45.75** Stomach
  - **V45.76** Lung
  - **V45.77** Genital organs
    Excludes: *female genital mutilation status (629.20-629.29)*
  - **V45.78** Eye
  - **V45.79** Other acquired absence of organ

- ⑤ **V45.8 Other postprocedural status**
  - **V45.81** Aortocoronary bypass status
  - **V45.82** Percutaneous transluminal coronary angioplasty status
  - **V45.83** Breast implant removal status
  - **V45.84** Dental restoration status
    Dental crowns status
    Dental fillings status
  - **V45.85** Insulin pump status
  - **V45.86** Bariatric surgery status
    Gastric banding status
    Gastric bypass status for obesity
    Obesity surgery status
    Excludes: *bariatric surgery status complicating pregnancy, childbirth or the puerperium (649.2)*
    intestinal bypass or anastomosis status (V45.3)
  - **V45.89** Other
    Presence of neuropacemaker or other electronic device
  Excludes: *artificial heart valve in situ (V43.3)*
  vascular prosthesis in situ (V43.4)

- **V46 Other dependence on machines**
  - **V46.0** Aspirator
  - ⑤ **V46.1 Respirator [Ventilator]**
    Iron lung
    - **V46.11** Dependence on respirator, status
    - **V46.12** Encounter for respirator dependence during power failure
    - **V46.13** Encounter for weaning from respirator [ventilator]
    - **V46.14** Mechanical complication of respirator [ventilator]
      Mechanical failure of respirator [ventilator]

V CODES

V46.2 Supplemental oxygen
  Long-term oxygen therapy

V46.8 Other enabling machines
  Hyperbaric chamber
  Possum [Patient-Operated-Selector-Mechanism]
  Excludes: cardiac pacemaker (V45.0)
           kidney dialysis machine (V45.1)

V46.9 Unspecified machine dependence

V47 Other problems with internal organs

V47.0 Deficiencies of internal organs

V47.1 Mechanical and motor problems with internal organs

V47.2 Other cardiorespiratory problems
  Cardiovascular exercise intolerance with pain (with):
    at rest
    less than ordinary activity
    ordinary activity

V47.3 Other digestive problems

V47.4 Other urinary problems

V47.5 Other genital problems

V47.9 Unspecified

V48 Problems with head, neck, and trunk

V48.0 Deficiencies of head
  Excludes: deficiencies of ears, eyelids, and nose (V48.8)

V48.1 Deficiencies of neck and trunk

V48.2 Mechanical and motor problems with head

V48.3 Mechanical and motor problems with neck and trunk

V48.4 Sensory problem with head

V48.5 Sensory problem with neck and trunk

V48.6 Disfigurements of head

V48.7 Disfigurements of neck and trunk

V48.8 Other problems with head, neck, and trunk

V48.9 Unspecified problem with head, neck, or trunk

V49 Other conditions influencing health status

V49.0 Deficiencies of limbs

V49.1 Mechanical problems with limbs

V49.2 Motor problems with limbs

V49.3 Sensory problems with limbs

V49.4 Disfigurements of limbs

V49.5 Other problems of limbs

⑤ **V49.6** Upper limb amputation status
  V49.60 Unspecified level
  V49.61 Thumb
  V49.62 Other finger(s)
  V49.63 Hand
  V49.64 Wrist
    Disarticulation of wrist
  V49.65 Below elbow
  V49.66 Above elbow
    Disarticulation of elbow
  V49.67 Shoulder
    Disarticulation of shoulder

⑤ **V49.7** Lower limb amputation status
  V49.70 Unspecified level
  V49.71 Great toe
  V49.72 Other toe(s)

635

Add 4th or 5th digit | Nonspecific code | Unspecific code | Secondary Dx Only | Primary Dx Only

TABULAR LIST

  V49.73 **Foot**

  V49.74 **Ankle**
    Disarticulation of ankle

  V49.75 **Below knee**

  V49.76 **Above knee**
    Disarticulation of knee

  V49.77 **Hip**
    Disarticulation of hip

⑤ V49.8 **Other specified conditions influencing health status**

  V49.81 **Asymptomatic postmenopausal status (age-related) (natural)**

    Excludes: menopausal and premenopausal disorders (627.0-627.9)
      postsurgical menopause (256.2)
      premature menopause (256.31)
      symptomatic menopause (627.0-627.9)

  V49.82 **Dental sealant status**

  V49.83 **Awaiting organ transplant status**

  V49.84 **Bed confinement status**

 ● V49.85 **Dual sensory impairment**
    Blindness with deafness
    Combined visual hearing impairment

 Code first:
  hearing impairment (389.00-389.9)
  visual impairment (369.00-369.9)

  V49.89 **Other specified conditions influencing health status**

 V49.9 **Unspecified**

PERSONS ENCOUNTERING HEALTH SERVICES FOR SPECIFIC PROCEDURES AND AFTERCARE (V50-V59)

 Note: Categories V51-V58 are intended for use to indicate a reason for care in patients who may have already been treated for some disease or injury not now present, but who are receiving care to consolidate the treatment, to deal with residual states, or to prevent recurrence.

 Excludes: follow-up examination for medical surveillance following treatment (V67.0-V67.9)

V50 **Elective surgery for purposes other than remedying health states**

 V50.0 **Hair transplant**

 V50.1 **Other plastic surgery for unacceptable cosmetic appearance**
  Breast augmentation or reduction
  Face-lift

  Excludes: plastic surgery following healed injury or operation (V51)

 V50.2 **Routine or ritual circumcision**
  Circumcision in the absence of significant medical indication

 V50.3 **Ear piercing**

⑤ V50.4 **Prophylactic organ removal**
  Excludes: organ donations (V59.0-V59.9)
    therapeutic organ removal—code to condition

  V50.41 **Breast**

  V50.42 **Ovary**

  V50.49 **Other**

 V50.8 **Other**

 V50.9 **Unspecified**

V51 **Aftercare involving the use of plastic surgery**
 Plastic surgery following healed injury or operation

 Excludes: cosmetic plastic surgery (V50.1)
   plastic surgery as treatment for current injury—code to condition
   repair of scarred tissue—code to scar

V52 **Fitting and adjustment of prosthetic device and implant**
 Includes: removal of device

 Excludes: malfunction or complication of prosthetic device (996.0-996.7)
   status only, without need for care (V43.0-V43.8)

V CODES

- **V52.0** Artificial arm (complete) (partial)
- **V52.1** Artificial leg (complete) (partial)
- **V52.2** Artificial eye
- **V52.3** Dental prosthetic device
- **V52.4** Breast prosthesis and implant
  - *Excludes:* admission for implant insertion (V50.1)
- **V52.8** Other specified prosthetic device
- **V52.9** Unspecified prosthetic device

V53 Fitting and adjustment of other device
  - Includes: removal of device
  - replacement of device
  - *Excludes:* status only, without need for care (V45.0-V45.8)

- ⑤ **V53.0** Devices related to nervous system and special senses
  - **V53.01** Fitting and adjustment of cerebral ventricular (communicating) shunt
  - **V53.02** Neuropacemaker (brain) (peripheral nerve) (spinal cord)
  - **V53.09** Fitting and adjustment of other devices related to nervous system and special senses
    - Auditory substitution device
    - Visual substitution device
- **V53.1** Spectacles and contact lenses
- **V53.2** Hearing aid
- ⑤ **V53.3** Cardiac device
  - Reprogramming
  - **V53.31** Cardiac pacemaker
    - *Excludes:* mechanical complication of cardiac pacemaker (996.01)
  - **V53.32** Automatic implantable cardiac defibrillator
  - **V53.39** Other cardiac device
- **V53.4** Orthodontic devices
- **V53.5** Other intestinal appliance
  - *Excludes:* colostomy (V55.3)
    - ileostomy (V55.2)
    - other artificial opening of digestive tract (V55.4)
- **V53.6** Urinary devices
  - Urinary catheter
  - *Excludes:* cystostomy (V55.5)
    - nephrostomy (V55.6)
    - ureterostomy (V55.6)
    - urethrostomy (V55.6)
- **V53.7** Orthopedic devices
  - Orthopedic:
    - brace
    - cast
  - Orthopedic:
    - corset
    - shoes
  - *Excludes:* other orthopedic aftercare (V54)
- **V53.8** Wheelchair
- ⑤ **V53.9** Other and unspecified device
  - **V53.90** Unspecified device
  - **V53.91** Fitting and adjustment of insulin pump
    - Insulin pump titration
  - **V53.99** Other device

V54 Other orthopedic aftercare
  - *Excludes:* fitting and adjustment of orthopedic devices (V53.7)
    - malfunction of internal orthopedic device (996.40-996.49)
    - other complication of nonmechanical nature (996.60-996.79)
- ⑤ **V54.0** Aftercare involving internal fixation device
  - *Excludes:* malfunction of internal orthopedic device (996.40-996.49)
    - removal of external fixation device (V54.89)

637

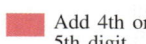 Add 4th or 5th digit
 Nonspecific code
 Unspecific code
 Secondary Dx Only
 Primary Dx Only

TABULAR LIST

    V54.01 Encounter for removal of internal fixation device
    V54.02 Encounter for lengthening/adjustment of growth rod
    V54.09 Other aftercare involving internal fixation device

⑤ V54.1 Aftercare for healing traumatic fracture
    Excludes: *aftercare for amputation stump (V54.89)*

    V54.10 Aftercare for healing traumatic fracture of arm, unspecified
    V54.11 Aftercare for healing traumatic fracture of upper arm
    V54.12 Aftercare for healing traumatic fracture of lower arm
    V54.13 Aftercare for healing traumatic fracture of hip
    V54.14 Aftercare for healing traumatic fracture of leg, unspecified
    V54.15 Aftercare for healing traumatic fracture of upper leg
    Excludes: *aftercare for healing traumatic fracture of hip (V54.13)*

    V54.16 Aftercare for healing traumatic fracture of lower leg
    V54.17 Aftercare for healing traumatic fracture of vertebrae
    V54.19 Aftercare for healing traumatic fracture of other bone

⑤ V54.2 Aftercare for healing pathologic fracture
    V54.20 Aftercare for healing pathologic fracture of arm, unspecified
    V54.21 Aftercare for healing pathologic fracture of upper arm
    V54.22 Aftercare for healing pathologic fracture of lower arm
    V54.23 Aftercare for healing pathologic fracture of hip
    V54.24 Aftercare for healing pathologic fracture of leg, unspecified
    V54.25 Aftercare for healing pathologic fracture of upper leg
    Excludes: *aftercare for healing pathologic fracture of hip (V54.23)*

    V54.26 Aftercare for healing pathologic fracture of lower leg
    V54.27 Aftercare for healing pathologic fracture of vertebrae
    V54.29 Aftercare for healing pathologic fracture of other bone

⑤ V54.8 Other orthopedic aftercare
    V54.81 Aftercare following joint replacement
        Use additional code to identify joint replacement site (V43.60-V43.69)
    V54.89 Other orthopedic aftercare
        Aftercare for healing fracture NOS

V54.9 Unspecified orthopedic aftercare

V55 Attention to artificial openings
    Includes: adjustment or repositioning of catheter
              closure
              passage of sounds or bougies
               reforming
               removal or replacement of catheter
               toilet or cleansing
    Excludes: *complications of external stoma (519.00-519.09, 569.60-569.69, 997.4, 997.5)*
                  status only, without need for care (V44.0-V44.9)

V55.0 Tracheostomy
V55.1 Gastrostomy
V55.2 Ileostomy
V55.3 Colostomy
V55.4 Other artificial opening of digestive tract
V55.5 Cystostomy
V55.6 Other artificial opening of urinary tract
    Nephrostomy   Urethrostomy
    Ureterostomy
V55.7 Artificial vagina
V55.8 Other specified artificial opening
V55.9 Unspecified artificial opening

V CODES

V56 Encounter for dialysis and dialysis catheter care
Use additional code to identify the associated condition
Excludes: dialysis preparation—code to condition

V56.0 Extracorporeal dialysis
Dialysis (renal) NOS
Excludes: dialysis status (V45.1)

V56.1 Fitting and adjustment of extracorporeal dialysis catheter
Removal or replacement of catheter
Toilet or cleansing
Use additional code for any concurrent extracorporeal dialysis (V56.0)

V56.2 Fitting and adjustment of peritoneal dialysis catheter
Use additional code for any concurrent peritoneal dialysis (V56.8)

V56.3 Encounter for adequacy testing for dialysis

  V56.31 Encounter for adequacy testing for hemodialysis

  V56.32 Encounter for adequacy testing for peritoneal dialysis
  Peritoneal equilibration test

V56.8 Other dialysis
Peritoneal dialysis

V57 Care involving use of rehabilitation procedures
Use additional code to identify underlying condition

V57.0 Breathing exercises

V57.1 Other physical therapy
Therapeutic and remedial exercises, except breathing

V57.2 Occupational therapy and vocational rehabilitation

  V57.21 Encounter for occupational therapy

  V57.22 Encounter for vocational therapy

V57.3 Speech therapy

V57.4 Orthoptic training

V57.8 Other specified rehabilitation procedure

  V57.81 Orthotic training
  Gait training in the use of artificial limbs

  V57.89 Other
  Multiple training or therapy

V57.9 Unspecified rehabilitation procedure

V58 Encounter for other and unspecified procedures and aftercare
Excludes: convalescence and palliative care (V66)

V58.0 Radiotherapy
Encounter or admission for radiotherapy
Excludes: encounter for radioactive implant—code to condition
radioactive iodine therapy—code to condition

V58.1 Encounter for antineoplastic chemotherapy and immunotherapy
Encounter or admission for chemotherapy
Excludes: chemotherapy and immunotherapy for nonneoplastic conditions—code to condition
prophylactic chemotherapy against disease which has never been present (V03.0-V07.9)

  V58.11 Encounter for antineoplastic chemotherapy

  V58.12 Encounter for antineoplastic immunotherapy

V58.2 Blood transfusion, without reported diagnosis

V58.3 Attention to dressings and sutures
Change or removal of wound packing
Excludes: attention to drains (V58.49)
planned postoperative wound closure (V58.41)

  V58.30 Encounter for change or removal of nonsurgical wound dressing
  Encounter for change or removal of wound dressing NOS

  V58.31 Encounter for change or removal of surgical wound dressing

  V58.32 Encounter for removal of sutures
  Encounter for removal of staples

639

| Add 4th or 5th digit | Nonspecific code | Unspecific code | Secondary Dx Only | Primary Dx Only |

TABULAR LIST

⑤ **V58.4 Other aftercare following surgery**
Note: Codes from this subcategory should be used in conjunction with other aftercare codes to fully identify the reason for the aftercare encounter

Excludes: *aftercare following sterilization reversal surgery (V26.22)*
attention to artificial openings (V55.0-V55.9)
orthopedic aftercare (V54.0-V54.9)

V58.41 Encounter for planned postoperative wound closure
Excludes: *disruption of operative wound (998.3)*
encounter for dressings and suture aftercare (V58.30-V58.32)

V58.42 Aftercare following surgery for neoplasm
Conditions classifiable to 140-239

V58.43 Aftercare following surgery for injury and trauma
Conditions classifiable to 800-999

Excludes: *aftercare for healing traumatic fracture (V54.10-V54.19)*

V58.44 Aftercare following organ transplant
Use additional code to identify the organ transplanted (V42.0-V42.9)

V58.49 Other specified aftercare following surgery
Change or removal of drains

V58.5 Orthodontics
Excludes: *fitting and adjustment of orthodontic device (V53.4)*

⑤ **V58.6 Long-term (current) drug use**
Excludes: *drug abuse (305.00-305.93)*
drug dependence (304.00-304.93)
hormone replacement therapy (postmenopausal) (V07.4)

V58.61 Long-term (current) use of anticoagulants
Excludes: *long-term (current) use of aspirin (V58.66)*

V58.62 Long-term (current) use of antibiotics

V58.63 Long-term (current) use of antiplatelets/antithrombotics
Excludes: *long-term (current) use of aspirin (V58.66)*

V58.64 Long-term (current) use of non-steroidal anti-inflammatories (NSAID)
Excludes: *long-term (current) use of aspirin (V58.66)*

V58.65 Long-term (current) use of steroids
V58.66 Long-term (current) use of aspirin
V58.67 Long-term (current) use of insulin
V58.69 Long-term (current) use of other medications
Other high-risk medications

⑤ **V58.7 Aftercare following surgery to specified body systems, not elsewhere classified**
Note: Codes from this subcategory should be used in conjunction with other aftercare codes to fully identify the reason for the aftercare encounter

Excludes: *aftercare following organ transplant (V58.44)*
aftercare following surgery for neoplasm (V58.42)

V58.71 Aftercare following surgery of the sense organs, NEC
Conditions classifiable to 360-379, 380-389

V58.72 Aftercare following surgery of the nervous system, NEC
Conditions classifiable to 320-359

Excludes: *aftercare following surgery of the sense organs, NEC (V58.71)*

V58.73 Aftercare following surgery of the circulatory system, NEC
Conditions classifiable to 390-459

V58.74 Aftercare following surgery of the respiratory system, NEC
Conditions classifiable to 460-519

V58.75 Aftercare following surgery of the teeth, oral cavity and digestive system, NEC
Conditions classifiable to 520-579

V58.76 Aftercare following surgery of the genitourinary system, NEC
Conditions classifiable to 580-629

Excludes: *aftercare following sterilization reversal (V26.22)*

V CODES

V58.77 Aftercare following surgery of the skin and subcutaneous tissue, NEC
Conditions classifiable to 680-709

V58.78 Aftercare following surgery of the musculoskeletal system, NEC
Conditions classifiable to 710-739

Excludes: orthopedic aftercare (V54.01-V54.9)

V58.8 Other specified procedures and aftercare

V58.81 Fitting and adjustment of vascular catheter
Removal or replacement of catheter
Toilet or cleansing

Excludes: complication of renal dialysis catheter (996.73)
complication of vascular catheter (996.74)
dialysis preparation — code to condition
encounter for dialysis (V56.0-V56.8)
fitting and adjustment of dialysis catheter (V56.1)

V58.82 Fitting and adjustment of non-vascular catheter NEC
Removal or replacement of catheter
Toilet or cleansing

Excludes: fitting and adjustment of peritoneal dialysis catheter (V56.2)
fitting and adjustment of urinary catheter (V53.6)

V58.83 Encounter for therapeutic drug monitoring
Use additional code for any associated long-term (current) drug use (V58.61-V58.69)

Excludes: blood-drug testing for medicolegal reasons (V70.4)

V58.89 Other specified aftercare

V58.9 Unspecified aftercare

V59 Donors

Excludes: examination of potential donor (V70.8)
self-donation of organ or tissue—code to condition

V59.0 Blood

V59.01 Whole blood

V59.02 Stem cells

V59.09 Other

V59.1 Skin

V59.2 Bone

V59.3 Bone marrow

V59.4 Kidney

V59.5 Cornea

V59.6 Liver

V59.7 Egg (oocyte) (ovum)

V59.70 Egg (oocyte) (ovum) donor, unspecified

V59.71 Egg (oocyte) (ovum) donor, under age 35, anonymous recipient
Egg donor, under age 35 NOS

V59.72 Egg (oocyte) (ovum) donor, under age 35, designated recipient

V59.73 Egg (oocyte) (ovum) donor, age 35 and over, anonymous recipient
Egg donor, age 35 and over NOS

V59.74 Egg (oocyte) (ovum) donor, age 35 and over, designated recipient

V59.8 Other specified organ or tissue

V59.9 Unspecified organ or tissue

PERSONS ENCOUNTERING HEALTH SERVICES IN OTHER CIRCUMSTANCES (V60-V69)

V60 Housing, household, and economic circumstances

V60.0 Lack of housing
Hobos
Social migrants
Tramps
Transients
Vagabonds

V60.1 Inadequate housing
Lack of heating
Restriction of space
Technical defects in home preventing adequate care

641

Add 4th or 5th digit | Nonspecific code | Unspecific code | Secondary Dx Only | Primary Dx Only

TABULAR LIST

V60.2 **Inadequate material resources**
Economic problem
Poverty NOS

V60.3 **Person living alone**

V60.4 **No other household member able to render care**
Person requiring care (has) (is):
family member too handicapped, ill, or otherwise unsuited to render care
partner temporarily away from home
temporarily away from usual place of abode

Excludes: *holiday relief care (V60.5)*

V60.5 **Holiday relief care**
Provision of health care facilities to a person normally cared for at home, to enable relatives to take a vacation

V60.6 **Person living in residential institution**
Boarding school resident

V60.8 **Other specified housing or economic circumstances**

V60.9 **Unspecified housing or economic circumstance**

V61 **Other family circumstances**
Includes: when these circumstances or fear of them, affecting the person directly involved or others, are mentioned as the reason, justified or not, for seeking or receiving medical advice or care

V61.0 **Family disruption**
Divorce
Estrangement

⑤ **V61.1** **Counseling for marital and partner problems**

Excludes: *problems related to:*
psychosexual disorders (302.0-302.9)
sexual function (V41.7)

V61.10 **Counseling for marital and partner problems, unspecified**
Marital conflict
Marital relationship problem
Partner conflict
Partner relationship problem

V61.11 **Counseling for victim of spousal and partner abuse**

Excludes: *encounter for treatment of current injuries due to abuse (995.80-995.85)*

V61.12 **Counseling for perpetrator of spousal and partner abuse**

⑤ **V61.2** **Parent-child problems**

V61.20 **Counseling for parent-child problem, unspecified**
Concern about behavior of child
Parent-child conflict
Parent-child relationship problem

V61.21 **Counseling for victim of child abuse**
Child battering
Child neglect

Excludes: *current injuries due to abuse (995.50-995.59)*

V61.22 **Counseling for perpetrator of parental child abuse**

Excludes: *counseling for non-parental abuser (V62.83)*

V61.29 **Other**
Problem concerning adopted or foster child

V61.3 **Problems with aged parents or in-laws**

⑤ **V61.4** **Health problems within family**

V61.41 **Alcoholism in family**

V61.49 **Other**
Care of sick or handicapped person in family or household
Presence of sick or handicapped person in family or household

V61.5 **Multiparity**

V61.6 **Illegitimacy or illegitimate pregnancy**

V61.7 **Other unwanted pregnancy**

V CODES

V61.8 **Other specified family circumstances**
　　Problems with family members NEC
　　Sibling relationship problem

V61.9 **Unspecified family circumstance**

V62 **Other psychosocial circumstances**
　Includes: those circumstances or fear of them, affecting the person directly involved or others, mentioned as the reason, justified or not, for seeking or receiving medical advice or care
　Excludes: previous psychological trauma (V15.41-V15.49)

V62.0 **Unemployment**
　Excludes: circumstances when main problem is economic inadequacy or poverty (V60.2)

V62.1 **Adverse effects of work environment**

V62.2 **Other occupational circumstances or maladjustment**
　　Career choice problem
　　Dissatisfaction with employment
　　Occupational problem

V62.3 **Educational circumstances**
　　Academic problem
　　Dissatisfaction with school environment
　　Educational handicap

V62.4 **Social maladjustment**
　　Acculturation problem　　　Social:
　　Cultural deprivation　　　　　isolation
　　Political, religious, or sex　　persecution
　　　discrimination

V62.5 **Legal circumstances**
　　Imprisonment　　　　Litigation
　　Legal investigation　　Prosecution

V62.6 **Refusal of treatment for reasons of religion or conscience**

⑤ **V62.8** **Other psychological or physical stress, not elsewhere classified**

　　V62.81 **Interpersonal problems, not elsewhere classified**
　　　　Relational problem NOS

　　V62.82 **Bereavement, uncomplicated**
　　Excludes: bereavement as adjustment reaction (309.0)

　　V62.83 **Counseling for perpetrator of physical/sexual abuse**
　　Excludes: counseling for perpetrator of parental child abuse (V61.22)
　　　　　　counseling for perpetrator of spousal and partner abuse (V61.12)

　　V62.84 **Suicidal ideation**
　　Excludes: suicidal tendencies (300.9)

　　V62.89 **Other**
　　　　Borderline intellectual functioning
　　　　Life circumstance problems
　　　　Phase of life problems
　　　　Religious or spiritual problem

V62.9 **Unspecified psychosocial circumstance**

V63 **Unavailability of other medical facilities for care**

　V63.0 **Residence remote from hospital or other health care facility**

　V63.1 **Medical services in home not available**
　　Excludes: no other household member able to render care (V60.4)

　V63.2 **Person awaiting admission to adequate facility elsewhere**

　V63.8 **Other specified reasons for unavailability of medical facilities**
　　　Person on waiting list undergoing social agency investigation

　V63.9 **Unspecified reason for unavailability of medical facilities**

V64 **Persons encountering health services for specific procedures, not carried out**

　⑤ **V64.0** **Vaccination not carried out**

　　　V64.00 Vaccination not carried out, unspecified reason

　　　V64.01 Vaccination not carried out because of acute illness

　　　V64.02 Vaccination not carried out because of chronic illness or condition

643

TABULAR LIST

V64.03 Vaccination not carried out because of immune compromised state
V64.04 Vaccination not carried out because of allergy to vaccine or component
V64.05 Vaccination not carried out because of caregiver refusal
  Guardian refusal
  Parent refusal
V64.06 Vaccination not carried out because of patient refusal
V64.07 Vaccination not carried out for religious reasons
V64.08 Vaccination not carried out because patient had disease being vaccinated against
V64.09 Vaccination not carried out for other reason

V64.1 Surgical or other procedure not carried out because of contraindication
V64.2 Surgical or other procedure not carried out because of patient's decision
V64.3 Procedure not carried out for other reasons
⑤ **V64.4** Closed surgical procedure converted to open procedure

V64.41 Laparoscopic surgical procedure converted to open procedure
V64.42 Thoracoscopic surgical procedure converted to open procedure
V64.43 Arthroscopic surgical procedure converted to open procedure

V65 Other persons seeking consultation

V65.0 Healthy person accompanying sick person
  Boarder

⑤ **V65.1** Person consulting on behalf of another person
  Advice or treatment for nonattending third party

  Excludes: concern (normal) about sick person in family (V61.41-V61.49)

  V65.11 Pediatric pre-birth visit for expectant mother
  V65.19 Other person consulting on behalf of another person

V65.2 Person feigning illness
  Malingerer
  Peregrinating patient

V65.3 Dietary surveillance and counseling
  Dietary surveillance and counseling (in):
    NOS
    colitis
    diabetes mellitus
    food allergies or intolerance
    gastritis
    hypercholesterolemia
    hypoglycemia
    obesity
  Use additional code to identify Body Mass Index (BMI), if known (V85.0-V85.54)

⑤ **V65.4** Other counseling, not elsewhere classified
  Health:
    advice
    education
    instruction

  Excludes: counseling (for):
    contraception (V25.40-V25.49)
    genetic (V26.31-V26.39)
    on behalf of third party (V65.11, V65.19)
    procreative management (V26.41-V26.49)

  V65.40 Counseling NOS
  V65.41 Exercise counseling
  V65.42 Counseling on substance use and abuse
  V65.43 Counseling on injury prevention
  V65.44 Human immunodeficiency virus [HIV] counseling
  V65.45 Counseling on other sexually transmitted diseases
  V65.46 Encounter for insulin pump training
  V65.49 Other specified counseling

● Code new to this edition ▲ Revision of existing code ④ ⑤ Fourth or fifth digit required

V CODES

V65.5 Person with feared complaint in whom no diagnosis was made
Feared condition not demonstrated
Problem was normal state
"Worried well"

V65.8 Other reasons for seeking consultation
Excludes: specified symptoms

V65.9 Unspecified reason for consultation

V66 Convalescence and palliative care

V66.0 Following surgery

V66.1 Following radiotherapy

V66.2 Following chemotherapy

V66.3 Following psychotherapy and other treatment for mental disorder

V66.4 Following treatment of fracture

V66.5 Following other treatment

V66.6 Following combined treatment

V66.7 Encounter for palliative care
End-of-life care
Hospice care
Terminal care

Code first underlying disease

V66.9 Unspecified convalescence

V67 Follow-up examination
Includes: surveillance only following completed treatment
Excludes: surveillance of contraception (V25.40-V25.49)

V67.0 Following surgery

V67.00 Following surgery, unspecified

V67.01 Follow-up vaginal pap smear
Vaginal pap smear, status-post hysterectomy for malignant condition
Use additional code to identify:
acquired absence of uterus (V45.77)
personal history of malignant neoplasm (V10.40-V10.44)

Excludes: vaginal pap smear status-post hysterectomy for non-malignant condition (V76.47)

V67.09 Following other surgery

Excludes: sperm count following sterilization reversal (V26.22)
sperm count for fertility testing (V26.21)

V67.1 Following radiotherapy

V67.2 Following chemotherapy
Cancer chemotherapy follow-up

V67.3 Following psychotherapy and other treatment for mental disorder

V67.4 Following treatment of healed fracture
Excludes: current (healing) fracture aftercare (V54.0-V54.9)

V67.5 Following other treatment

V67.51 Following completed treatment with high-risk medication, NEC
Excludes: long-term (current) drug use (V58.61-V58.69)

V67.59 Other

V67.6 Following combined treatment

V67.9 Unspecified follow-up examination

V68 Encounters for administrative purposes

V68.0 Issue of medical certificates
Excludes: encounter for general medical examination (V70.0-V70.9)

● **V68.01 Disability examination**
Use additional code(s) to identify:
specific examination(s), screening and testing performed (V72.0-V82.9)

● **V68.09 Other issue of medical certificates**

TABULAR LIST

V68.1 Issue of repeat prescriptions
Issue of repeat prescription for:
  appliance
  glasses
  medications
Excludes: repeat prescription for contraceptives (V25.41-V25.49)

V68.2 Request for expert evidence

V68.8 Other specified administrative purpose

  V68.81 Referral of patient without examination or treatment

  V68.89 Other

V68.9 Unspecified administrative purpose

V69 Problems related to lifestyle

V69.0 Lack of physical exercise

V69.1 Inappropriate diet and eating habits
Excludes: anorexia nervosa (307.1)
  bulimia (783.6)
  malnutrition and other nutritional deficiencies (260-269.9)
  other and unspecified eating disorders (307.50-307.59)

V69.2 High-risk sexual behavior

V69.3 Gambling and betting
Excludes: pathological gambling (312.31)

V69.4 Lack of adequate sleep
Sleep deprivation
Excludes: insomnia (780.52)

V69.5 Behavioral insomnia of childhood

V69.8 Other problems related to lifestyle
Self-damaging behavior

V69.9 Problem related to lifestyle, unspecified

PERSONS WITHOUT REPORTED DIAGNOSIS ENCOUNTERED DURING EXAMINATION AND INVESTIGATION OF INDIVIDUALS AND POPULATIONS (V70-V82)

Note: Nonspecific abnormal findings disclosed at the time of these examinations are classifiable to categories 790-796.

V70 General medical examination
Use additional code(s) to identify any special screening examination(s) performed (V73.0-V82.9)

V70.0 Routine general medical examination at a health care facility
Health checkup
Excludes: health checkup of infant or child (V20.2)
  pre-procedural general physical examination (V72.83)

V70.1 General psychiatric examination, requested by the authority

V70.2 General psychiatric examination, other and unspecified

V70.3 Other medical examination for administrative purposes
General medical examination for:
  admission to old age home   marriage
  adoption   prison
  camp   school admission
  driving license   sports competition
  immigration and naturalization
  insurance certification
Excludes: attendance for issue of medical certificates (V68.0)
  pre-employment screening (V70.5)

V CODES

V70.4 Examination for medicolegal reasons
  Blood-alcohol tests
  Blood-drug tests
  Paternity testing

  Excludes: examination and observation following:
      accidents (V71.3, V71.4)
      assault (V71.6)
      rape (V71.5)

V70.5 Health examination of defined subpopulations
  Armed forces personnel   Preschool children
  Inhabitants of institutions   Prisoners
  Occupational health   Prostitutes
    examinations   Refugees
  Pre-employment screening School children
                            Students

V70.6 Health examination in population surveys
  Excludes: special screening (V73.0-V82.9)

V70.7 Examination of participant in clinical trial
  Examination of participant or control in clinical research

V70.8 Other specified general medical examinations
  Examination of potential donor of organ or tissue

V70.9 Unspecified general medical examination

V71 Observation and evaluation for suspected conditions not found
  Note: This category is to be used when persons without a diagnosis are suspected of having an abnormal condition, without signs or symptoms, which requires study, but after examination and observation, is found not to exist. This category is also for use for administrative and legal observation status.

⑤ **V71.0 Observation for suspected mental condition**

  V71.01 Adult antisocial behavior
    Dyssocial behavior or gang activity in adult without manifest psychiatric disorder

  V71.02 Childhood or adolescent antisocial behavior
    Dyssocial behavior or gang activity in child or adolescent without manifest psychiatric disorder

  V71.09 Other suspected mental condition

V71.1 Observation for suspected malignant neoplasm

V71.2 Observation for suspected tuberculosis

V71.3 Observation following accident at work

V71.4 Observation following other accident
  Examination of individual involved in motor vehicle traffic accident

V71.5 Observation following alleged rape or seduction
  Examination of victim or culprit

V71.6 Observation following other inflicted injury
  Examination of victim or culprit

V71.7 Observation for suspected cardiovascular disease

⑤ **V71.8 Observation and evaluation for other specified suspected conditions**

  V71.81 Abuse and neglect
    Excludes: adult abuse and neglect (995.80-995.85)
        child abuse and neglect (995.50-995.59)

  V71.82 Observation and evaluation for suspected exposure to anthrax

  V71.83 Observation and evaluation for suspected exposure to other biological agent

  V71.89 Other specified suspected conditions

V71.9 Observation for unspecified suspected condition

V72 Special investigations and examinations
  Includes: routine examination of specific system

  Excludes: general medical examination (V70.0-V70.4)
      general screening examination of defined population groups (V70.5, V70.6, V70.7)
      routine examination of infant or child (V20.2)

  Use additional code(s) to identify any special screening examination(s) performed (V73.0-V82.9)

647

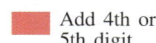 Add 4th or 5th digit
 Nonspecific code
 Unspecific code
 Secondary Dx Only
 Primary Dx Only

TABULAR LIST

V72.0 Examination of eyes and vision

⑤ **V72.1 Examination of ears and hearing**

    V72.11 Encounter for hearing examination following failed hearing screening

    ● **V72.12 Encounter for hearing conservation and treatment**

    V72.19 Other examination of ears and hearing

V72.2 Dental examination

⑤ **V72.3 Gynecological examination**

    Excludes: cervical Papanicolaou smear without general gynecological examination (V76.2)
             routine examination in contraceptive management (V25.40-V25.49)

    V72.31 Routine gynecological examination
        General gynecological examination with or without Papanicolaou cervical smear
        Pelvic examination (annual) (periodic)

    Use additional code to identify routine:
        human papillomavirus (HPV) screening (V73.81)
        routine vaginal Papanicolaou smear (V76.47)

    V72.32 Encounter for Papanicolaou cervical smear to confirm findings of recent normal smear following initial abnormal smear

⑤ **V72.4 Pregnancy examination or test**

    V72.40 Pregnancy examination or test, pregnancy unconfirmed
        Possible pregnancy, not (yet) confirmed

    V72.41 Pregnancy examination or test, negative result

    V72.42 Pregnancy examination or test, positive result

V72.5 Radiological examination, not elsewhere classified
    Routine chest x-ray

    Excludes: examination for suspected tuberculosis (V71.2)

V72.6 Laboratory examination

    Excludes: that for suspected disorder (V71.0-V71.9)

V72.7 Diagnostic skin and sensitization tests
    Allergy tests
    Skin tests for hypersensitivity

    Excludes: diagnostic skin tests for bacterial diseases (V74.0-V74.9)

⑤ **V72.8 Other specified examinations**

    V72.81 Pre-operative cardiovascular examination
        Pre-procedural cardiovascular examination

    V72.82 Pre-operative respiratory examination
        Pre-procedural respiratory examination

    V72.83 Other specified pre-operative examination
        Other pre-procedural examination
        Pre-procedural general physical examination

    Excludes: routine general medical examination (V70.0)

    V72.84 Pre-operative examination, unspecified
        Pre-procedural examination, unspecified

    V72.85 Other specified examination

    V72.86 Encounter for blood typing

V72.9 Unspecified examination

V73 Special screening examination for viral and chlamydial diseases

    V73.0 Poliomyelitis

    V73.1 Smallpox

    V73.2 Measles

    V73.3 Rubella

    V73.4 Yellow fever

    V73.5 Other arthropod-borne viral diseases
        Dengue fever   Viral encephalitis:
        Hemorrhagic fever   mosquito-borne
                                      tick-borne

V CODES

V73.6 **Trachoma**

⑤ V73.8 **Other specified viral and chlamydial diseases**
- ● V73.81 Human papillomavirus (HPV)
- V73.88 Other specified chlamydial diseases
- V73.89 Other specified viral diseases

⑤ V73.9 **Unspecified viral and chlamydial disease**
- V73.98 Unspecified chlamydial disease
- V73.99 Unspecified viral disease

V74 Special screening examination for bacterial and spirochetal diseases
Includes: diagnostic skin tests for these diseases

V74.0 **Cholera**

V74.1 **Pulmonary tuberculosis**

V74.2 **Leprosy [Hansen's disease]**

V74.3 **Diphtheria**

V74.4 **Bacterial conjunctivitis**

V74.5 **Venereal disease**
Screening for bacterial and spirochetal sexually transmitted diseases
Screening for sexually transmitted diseases NOS

Excludes: special screening for nonbacterial sexually transmitted diseases (V73.81-V73.89, V75.4, V75.8)

V74.6 **Yaws**

V74.8 **Other specified bacterial and spirochetal diseases**
- Brucellosis
- Leptospirosis
- Plague
- Tetanus
- Whooping cough

V74.9 **Unspecified bacterial and spirochetal disease**

V75 Special screening examination for other infectious diseases

V75.0 **Rickettsial diseases**

V75.1 **Malaria**

V75.2 **Leishmaniasis**

V75.3 **Trypanosomiasis**
Chagas' disease
Sleeping sickness

V75.4 **Mycotic infections**

V75.5 **Schistosomiasis**

V75.6 **Filariasis**

V75.7 **Intestinal helminthiasis**

V75.8 **Other specified parasitic infections**

V75.9 **Unspecified infectious disease**

V76 Special screening for malignant neoplasms

V76.0 **Respiratory organs**

⑤ V76.1 **Breast**
- V76.10 Breast screening, unspecified
- V76.11 Screening mammogram for high-risk patient
- V76.12 Other screening mammogram
- V76.19 Other screening breast examination

V76.2 **Cervix**
Routine cervical Papanicolaou smear

Excludes: special screening for human papillomavirus (V73.81)
that as part of a general gynecological examination (V72.31)

V76.3 **Bladder**

⑤ V76.4 **Other sites**
- V76.41 Rectum
- V76.42 Oral cavity
- V76.43 Skin

649

| Add 4th or 5th digit | Nonspecific code | Unspecific code | Secondary Dx Only | Primary Dx Only |

TABULAR LIST

- V76.44 **Prostate**
- V76.45 **Testis**
- V76.46 **Ovary**
- V76.47 **Vagina**
  Vaginal pap smear status-post hysterectomy for non-malignant condition
  Use additional code to identify acquired absence of uterus (V45.77)
  Excludes: *vaginal pap smear status-post hysterectomy for malignant condition (V67.01)*
- **V76.49** Other sites
- ⑤ V76.5 **Intestine**
  - **V76.50** Intestine, unspecified
  - V76.51 **Colon**
    Excludes: *rectum (V76.41)*
  - V76.52 **Small intestine**
- ⑤ V76.8 **Other neoplasm**
  - V76.81 **Nervous system**
  - **V76.89** Other neoplasm
- **V76.9** Unspecified

V77 Special screening for endocrine, nutritional, metabolic, and immunity disorders
- V77.0 **Thyroid disorders**
- V77.1 **Diabetes mellitus**
- V77.2 **Malnutrition**
- V77.3 **Phenylketonuria [PKU]**
- V77.4 **Galactosemia**
- V77.5 **Gout**
- V77.6 **Cystic fibrosis**
  Screening for mucoviscidosis
- **V77.7** Other inborn errors of metabolism
- V77.8 **Obesity**
- ⑤ V77.9 **Other and unspecified endocrine, nutritional, metabolic, and immunity disorders**
  - V77.91 **Screening for lipoid disorders**
    Screening cholesterol level
    Screening for hypercholesterolemia
    Screening for hyperlipidemia
  - **V77.99** Other and unspecified endocrine, nutritional, metabolic, and immunity disorders

V78 Special screening for disorders of blood and blood-forming organs
- V78.0 **Iron deficiency anemia**
- **V78.1** Other and unspecified deficiency anemia
- V78.2 **Sickle-cell disease or trait**
- **V78.3** Other hemoglobinopathies
- **V78.8** Other disorders of blood and blood-forming organs
- **V78.9** Unspecified disorder of blood and blood-forming organs

V79 Special screening for mental disorders and developmental handicaps
- V79.0 **Depression**
- V79.1 **Alcoholism**
- V79.2 **Mental retardation**
- V79.3 **Developmental handicaps in early childhood**
- **V79.8** Other specified mental disorders and developmental handicaps
- **V79.9** Unspecified mental disorder and developmental handicap

V80 Special screening for neurological, eye, and ear diseases
- V80.0 **Neurological conditions**
- V80.1 **Glaucoma**

V CODES

V80.2 Other eye conditions
  Screening for:
    cataract
    congenital anomaly of eye
    senile macular lesions
  Excludes: general vision examination (V72.0)

V80.3 Ear diseases
  Excludes: general hearing examination (V72.11-V72.19)

V81 Special screening for cardiovascular, respiratory, and genitourinary diseases
  V81.0 Ischemic heart disease
  V81.1 Hypertension
  V81.2 Other and unspecified cardiovascular conditions
  V81.3 Chronic bronchitis and emphysema
  V81.4 Other and unspecified respiratory conditions
    Excludes: screening for:
      lung neoplasm (V76.0)
      pulmonary tuberculosis (V74.1)
  V81.5 Nephropathy
    Screening for asymptomatic bacteriuria
  V81.6 Other and unspecified genitourinary conditions

V82 Special screening for other conditions
  V82.0 Skin conditions
  V82.1 Rheumatoid arthritis
  V82.2 Other rheumatic disorders
  V82.3 Congenital dislocation of hip
  V82.4 Maternal postnatal screening for chromosomal anomalies
    Excludes: antenatal screening by amniocentesis (V28.0)
  V82.5 Chemical poisoning and other contamination
    Screening for:
      heavy metal poisoning
      ingestion of radioactive substance
      poisoning from contaminated water supply
      radiation exposure
  V82.6 Multiphasic screening
  ⑤ **V82.7 Genetic screening**
    Excludes: genetic testing for procreative management (V26.31-V26.39)
      V82.71 Screening for genetic disease carrier status
      V82.79 Other genetic screening
  ⑤ **V82.8 Other specified conditions**
      V82.81 Osteoporosis
        Use additional code to identify:
          hormone replacement therapy (postmenopausal) status (V07.4)
          postmenopausal (natural) status (V49.81)
      V82.89 Other specified conditions
  V82.9 Unspecified condition

GENETICS (V83-V84)

V83 Genetic carrier status
  ⑤ **V83.0 Hemophilia A carrier**
      V83.01 Asymptomatic hemophilia A carrier
      V83.02 Symptomatic hemophilia A carrier
  ⑤ **V83.8 Other genetic carrier status**
      V83.81 Cystic fibrosis gene carrier
      V83.89 Other genetic carrier status

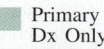

TABULAR LIST

V84 Genetic susceptibility to disease
Includes: Confirmed abnormal gene
Use additional code, if applicable, for any associated family history of the disease (V16-V19)

⑤ **V84.0 Genetic susceptibility to malignant neoplasm**
Code first, if applicable, any current malignant neoplasms (140.0-195.8, 200.0-208.9, 230.0-234.9)
Use additional code, if applicable, for any personal history of malignant neoplasm (V10.0-V10.9)

- **V84.01** Genetic susceptibility to malignant neoplasm of breast
- **V84.02** Genetic susceptibility to malignant neoplasm of ovary
- **V84.03** Genetic susceptibility to malignant neoplasm of prostate
- **V84.04** Genetic susceptibility to malignant neoplasm of endometrium
- **V84.09** Genetic susceptibility to other malignant neoplasm

⑤ **V84.8 Genetic susceptibility to other disease**
- ● **V84.81** Genetic susceptibility to multiple endocrine neoplasia [MEN]
- ● **V84.89** Genetic susceptibility to other disease

BODY MASS INDEX (V85)

V85 Body Mass Index [BMI]
Kilograms per meters squared
Note: BMI adult codes are for use for persons over 20 years old

- **V85.0** Body Mass Index less than 19, adult
- **V85.1** Body Mass Index between 19-24, adult

⑤ **V85.2** Body Mass Index between 25-29, adult
- **V85.21** Body Mass Index 25.0-25.9, adult
- **V85.22** Body Mass Index 26.0-26.9, adult
- **V85.23** Body Mass Index 27.0-27.9, adult
- **V85.24** Body Mass Index 28.0-28.9, adult
- **V85.25** Body Mass Index 29.0-29.9, adult

⑤ **V85.3** Body Mass Index between 30-39, adult
- **V85.30** Body Mass Index 30.0-30.9, adult
- **V85.31** Body Mass Index 31.0-31.9, adult
- **V85.32** Body Mass Index 32.0-32.9, adult
- **V85.33** Body Mass Index 33.0-33.9, adult
- **V85.34** Body Mass Index 34.0-34.9, adult
- **V85.35** Body Mass Index 35.0-35.9, adult
- **V85.36** Body Mass Index 36.0-36.9, adult
- **V85.37** Body Mass Index 37.0-37.9, adult
- **V85.38** Body Mass Index 38.0-38.9, adult
- **V85.39** Body Mass Index 39.0-39.9, adult

- **V85.4** Body Mass Index 40 and over, adult

⑤ **85.5** Body Mass Index, pediatric
Note: BMI pediatric codes are for use for persons age 2-20 years old. These percentiles are based on the growth charts published by the Centers for Disease Control and Prevention (CDC)

- **V85.51** Body Mass Index, pediatric, less than 5th percentile for age
- **V85.52** Body Mass Index, pediatric, 5th percentile to less than 85th percentile for age
- **V85.53** Body Mass Index, pediatric, 85th percentile to less than 95th percentile for age
- **V85.54** Body Mass Index, pediatric, greater than or equal to 95th percentile for age

ESTROGEN RECEPTOR STATUS (V86)

V86 Estrogen receptor status
Code first malignant neoplasm of breast (174.0-174.9, 175.0-175.9)

- **V86.0** Estrogen receptor positive status (ER+)
- **V86.1** Estrogen receptor negative status (ER−)

● Code new to this edition ▲ Revision of existing code ④ ⑤ Fourth or fifth digit required

E CODES

SUPPLEMENTARY CLASSIFICATION OF EXTERNAL CAUSES OF INJURY AND POISONING (E800-E999)

This section is provided to permit the classification of environmental events, circumstances, and conditions as the cause of injury, poisoning, and other adverse effects. Where a code from this section is applicable, it is intended that it shall be used in addition to a code from one of the main chapters of *ICD-9-CM*, indicating the nature of the condition. Certain other conditions which may be stated to be due to external causes are classified in Chapters 1 to 16 of *ICD-9-CM*. For these, the "E" code classification should be used for more detailed analysis.

Machinery accidents [other than those connected with transport] are classifiable to category E919, in which the fourth-digit allows a broad classification of the type of machinery involved. If a more detailed classification of type of machinery is required, it is suggested that the "Classification of Industrial Accidents according to Agency," prepared by the International Labor Office, be used in addition. This is reproduced in Appendix D, for optional use.

Categories for "late effects" of accidents and other external causes are to be found at E929, E959, E969, E977, E989, and E999.

Definitions and examples related to transport accidents

    (a) A **transport accident** (E800-E848) is any accident involving a device designed primarily for, or being used at the time primarily for, conveying persons or goods from one place to another.
        Includes: accidents involving:
                aircraft and spacecraft (E840-E845)
                watercraft (E830-E838)
                motor vehicle (E810-E825)
                railway (E800-E807)
                other road vehicles (E826-E829)

        In classifying accidents which involve more than one kind of transport, the above order of precedence of transport accidents should be used.

        Accidents involving agriculture and construction machines, such as tractors, cranes, and bulldozers, are regarded as transport accidents only when these vehicles are under their own power on a highway [otherwise the vehicles are regarded as machinery]. Vehicles which can travel on land or water, such as hovercraft and other amphibious vehicles, are regarded as watercraft when on the water, as motor vehicles when on the highway, and as off-road motor vehicles when on land, but off the highway.

        Excludes: accidents:
            in sports which involve the use of transport but where the transport vehicle itself was not involved in the accident
            involving vehicles which are part of industrial equipment used entirely on industrial premises
            occurring during transportation but unrelated to the hazards associated with the means of transportation [e.g., injuries received in a fight on board ship; transport vehicle involved in a cataclysm such as an earthquake]
            to persons engaged in the maintenance or repair of transport equipment or vehicle not in motion, unless injured by another vehicle in motion

    (b) A **railway accident** is a transport accident involving a railway train or other railway vehicle operated on rails, whether in motion or not.
        Excludes: accidents:
            in repair shops
            in roundhouse or on turntable
            on railway premises but not involving a train or other railway vehicle

    (c) A **railway train** or **railway vehicle** is any device with or without cars coupled to it, designed for traffic on a railway.
        Includes: interurban:
                electric car (operated chiefly on its own right-of-way, not open to other traffic)
                streetcar (operated chiefly on its own right-of-way, not open to other traffic)
                railway train, any power [diesel] [electric] [steam]
                funicular
                monorail or two-rail
                subterranean or elevated
                other vehicle designed to run on a railway track

        Excludes: interurban electric cars [streetcars] specified to be operating on a right-of-way that forms part of the public street or highway [definition (n)]

    (d) A **railway** or **railroad** is a right-of-way designed for traffic on rails, which is used by carriages or wagons transporting passengers or freight, and by other rolling stock, and which is not open to other public vehicular traffic.

653

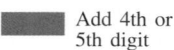 Add 4th or 5th digit   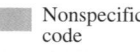 Nonspecific code   Unspecified code   Manifestation code

TABULAR LIST

(e) A **motor vehicle accident** is a transport accident involving a motor vehicle. It is defined as a motor vehicle traffic accident or as a motor vehicle nontraffic accident according to whether the accident occurs on a public highway or elsewhere.

  Excludes: injury or damage due to cataclysm
  injury or damage while a motor vehicle, not under its own power, is being loaded on, or unloaded from, another conveyance

(f) A **motor vehicle traffic accident** is any motor vehicle accident occurring on a public highway [i.e., originating, terminating, or involving a vehicle partially on the highway]. A motor vehicle accident is assumed to have occurred on the highway unless another place is specified, except in the case of accidents involving only off-road motor vehicles which are classified as nontraffic accidents unless the contrary is stated.

(g) A **motor vehicle nontraffic accident** is any motor vehicle accident which occurs entirely in any place other than a public highway.

(h) A **public highway [trafficway]** or **street** is the entire width between property lines [or other boundary lines] of every way or place, of which any part is open to the use of the public for purposes of vehicular traffic as a matter of right or custom. A roadway is that part of the public highway designed, improved, and ordinarily used, for vehicular travel.
  Includes: approaches (public) to:
       docks
       public building
       station

  Excludes: driveway (private)
       parking lot
       ramp
       roads in:
       airfield
       farm
       industrial premises
       mine
       private grounds
       quarry

(i) A **motor vehicle** is any mechanically or electrically powered device, not operated on rails, upon which any person or property may be transported or drawn upon a highway. Any object such as a trailer, coaster, sled, or wagon being towed by a motor vehicle is considered a part of the motor vehicle.
  Includes: automobile [any type]
       bus
       construction machinery, farm and industrial machinery, steam roller, tractor, army tank, highway grader, or similar vehicle on wheels or treads, while in transport under own power
       fire engine (motorized)
       motorcycle
       motorized bicycle [moped] or scooter
       trolley bus not operating on rails
       truck
       van

  Excludes: devices used solely to move persons or materials within the confines of a building and its premises, such as:
       building elevator
       coal car in mine
       electric baggage or mail truck used solely within a railroad station
       electric truck used solely within an industrial plant
       moving overhead crane

(j) A **motorcycle** is a two-wheeled motor vehicle having one or two riding saddles and sometimes having a third wheel for the support of a sidecar. The sidecar is considered part of the motorcycle.
  Includes: motorized:
       bicycle [moped]
       scooter
       tricycle

(k) An **off-road motor vehicle** is a motor vehicle of special design, to enable it to negotiate rough or soft terrain or snow. Examples of special design are high construction, special wheels and tires, driven by treads, or support on a cushion of air.
  Includes: all terrain vehicle [ATV]
       army tank
       hovercraft, on land or swamp
       snowmobile

E CODES

(l) A **driver** of a motor vehicle is the occupant of the motor vehicle operating it or intending to operate it. A **motorcyclist** is the driver of a motorcycle. Other authorized occupants of a motor vehicle are **passengers**.

(m) An **other road vehicle** is any device, except a motor vehicle, in, on, or by which any person or property may be transported on a highway.
  Includes: animal carrying a person or goods
  animal-drawn vehicle
  animal harnessed to conveyance
  bicycle [pedal cycle]
  streetcar
  tricycle (pedal)
  Excludes: pedestrian conveyance [definition (q)]

(n) A **streetcar** is a device designed and used primarily for transporting persons within a municipality, running on rails, usually subject to normal traffic control signals, and operated principally on a right-of-way that forms part of the traffic way. A trailer being towed by a streetcar is considered a part of the streetcar.
  Includes: interurban or intraurban electric or streetcar, when specified to be operating on a street or public highway
  tram (car)
  trolley (car)

(o) A **pedal cycle** is any road transport vehicle operated solely by pedals.
  Includes: bicycle
  pedal cycle
  tricycle
  Excludes: motorized bicycle [definition (i)]

(p) A **pedal cyclist** is any person riding on a pedal cycle or in a sidecar attached to such a vehicle.

(q) A **pedestrian conveyance** is any human powered device by which a pedestrian may move other than by walking or by which a walking person may move another pedestrian.
  Includes:

baby carriage	roller skates
coaster wagon	scooter
ice skates	skateboard
perambulator	skis
pushcart	sled
pushchair	wheelchair

(r) A **pedestrian** is any person involved in an accident who was not at the time of the accident riding in or on a motor vehicle, railroad train, streetcar, animal-drawn or other vehicle, or on a bicycle or animal.
  Includes: person:
  changing tire of vehicle
  in or operating a pedestrian conveyance
  making adjustment to motor of vehicle
  on foot

(s) A **watercraft** is any device for transporting passengers or goods on the water.

(t) A **small boat** is any watercraft propelled by paddle, oars, or small motor, with a passenger capacity of less than ten.
  Includes:

boat NOS	rowboat
canoe	rowing shell
coble	scull
dinghy	skiff
punt	small motorboat
raft	

  Excludes: barge
  lifeboat (used after abandoning ship)
  raft (anchored) being used as diving platform
  yacht

(u) An **aircraft** is any device for transporting passengers or goods in the air.
  Includes: airplane [any type]
  balloon
  bomber
  dirigible
  glider (hang)
  military aircraft
  parachute

(v) A **commercial transport aircraft** is any device for collective passenger or freight transportation by air, whether run on commercial lines for profit or by government authorities, with the exception of military craft.

TABULAR LIST

RAILWAY ACCIDENTS (E800-E807)

Note: For definitions of railway accident and related terms see definitions (a) to (d).

Excludes: accidents involving railway train and:
- aircraft (E840.0-E845.9)
- motor vehicle (E810.0-E825.9)
- watercraft (E830.0-E838.9)

The following fourth-digit subdivisions are for use with categories E800-E807 to identify the injured person:

.0 Railway employee
Any person who by virtue of his employment in connection with a railway, whether by the railway company or not, is at increased risk of involvement in a railway accident, such as:
- catering staff of train
- driver
- guard
- porter
- postal staff on train
- railway fireman
- shunter
- sleeping car attendant

.1 Passenger on railway
Any authorized person traveling on a train, except a railway employee.

Excludes: intending passenger waiting at station (.8)
unauthorized rider on railway vehicle (.8)

.2 Pedestrian
See definition (r)

.3 Pedal cyclist
See definition (p)

.8 Other specified person
Intending passenger or bystander waiting at station
Unauthorized rider on railway vehicle

.9 Unspecified person

E800 Railway accident involving collision with rolling stock
Includes: collision between railway trains or railway vehicles, any kind
collision NOS on railway
derailment with antecedent collision with rolling stock or NOS

E801 Railway accident involving collision with other object
Includes: collision of railway train with:
- buffers
- fallen tree on railway
- gates
- platform
- rock on railway
- streetcar
- other nonmotor vehicle
- other object

Excludes: collision with:
aircraft (E840.0-E842.9)
motor vehicle (E810.0-E810.9, E820.0-E822.9)

E802 Railway accident involving derailment without antecedent collision

E803 Railway accident involving explosion, fire, or burning

Excludes: explosion or fire, with antecedent derailment (E802.0-E802.9)
explosion or fire, with mention of antecedent collision (E800.0-E801.9)

E804 Fall in, on, or from railway train
Includes: fall while alighting from or boarding railway train

Excludes: fall related to collision, derailment, or explosion of railway train (E800.0-E803.9)

E805 Hit by rolling stock
Includes: crushed by railway train or part
injured by railway train or part
killed by railway train or part
knocked down by railway train or part
run over by railway train or part

Excludes: pedestrian hit by object set in motion by railway train (E806.0-E806.9)

● Code new to this edition ▲ Revision of existing code ④ ⑤ Fourth or fifth digit required

E CODES

④ **E806** Other specified railway accident
    Includes: hit by object falling in railway train
              injured by door or window on railway train
              nonmotor road vehicle or pedestrian hit by object set in motion by railway train
              railway train hit by falling:
                earth NOS
                rock
                tree
                other object

    Excludes: *railway accident due to cataclysm (E908-E909)*

④ **E807** Railway accident of unspecified nature
    Includes:
                 found dead on railway right-of-way NOS
                injured on railway right-of-way NOS
                railway accident NOS

MOTOR VEHICLE TRAFFIC ACCIDENTS (E810-E819)

    Note: For definitions of motor vehicle traffic accident, and related terms, see definitions (e) to (k).

    Excludes: *accidents involving motor vehicle and aircraft (E840.0-E845.9)*

    The following fourth-digit subdivisions are for use with categories E810-E819 to identify the injured person:

    .0 Driver of motor vehicle other than motorcycle
        See definition (l)

    .1 Passenger in motor vehicle other than motorcycle
        See definition (l)

    .2 Motorcyclist
        See definition (l)

    .3 Passenger on motorcycle
        See definition (l)

    .4 Occupant of streetcar

    .5 Rider of animal; occupant of animal-drawn vehicle

    .6 Pedal cyclist
        See definition (p)

    .7 Pedestrian
        See definition (r)

    .8 Other specified person
        Occupant of vehicle other than above
        Person in railway train involved in accident
        Unauthorized rider of motor vehicle

    .9 Unspecified person

④ **E810** Motor vehicle traffic accident involving collision with train

    Excludes: *motor vehicle collision with object set in motion by railway train (E815.0-E815.9)*
                  railway train hit by object set in motion by motor vehicle (E818.0-E818.9)

④ **E811** Motor vehicle traffic accident involving re-entrant collision with another motor vehicle
    Includes: collision between motor vehicle which accidentally leaves the roadway then re-enters the same roadway, or the opposite roadway on a divided highway, and another motor vehicle

    Excludes: *collision on the same roadway when none of the motor vehicles involved have left and re-entered the roadway (E812.0-E812.9)*

④ **E812** Other motor vehicle traffic accident involving collision with motor vehicle
    Includes: collision with another motor vehicle parked, stopped, stalled, disabled, or abandoned on the highway
              motor vehicle collision NOS

    Excludes: *collision with object set in motion by another motor vehicle (E815.0-E815.9)*
                  re-entrant collision with another motor vehicle (E811.0-E811.9)

TABULAR LIST

④ **E813** **Motor vehicle traffic accident involving collision with other vehicle**
Includes: collision between motor vehicle, any kind, and:
other road (nonmotor transport) vehicle, such as:
animal carrying a person
animal-drawn vehicle
pedal cycle
streetcar

Excludes: collision with:
object set in motion by nonmotor road vehicle (E815.0-E815.9)
pedestrian (E814.0-E814.9)
nonmotor road vehicle hit by object set in motion by motor vehicle (E818.0-E818.9)

④ **E814** **Motor vehicle traffic accident involving collision with pedestrian**
Includes: collision between motor vehicle, any kind, and pedestrian
pedestrian dragged, hit, or run over by motor vehicle, any kind

Excludes: pedestrian hit by object set in motion by motor vehicle (E818.0-E818.9)

④ **E815** **Other motor vehicle traffic accident involving collision on the highway**
Includes: collision (due to loss of control) (on highway) between motor vehicle, any kind, and:
abutment (bridge) (overpass)
animal (herded) (unattended)
fallen stone, traffic sign, tree, utility pole
guard rail or boundary fence
interhighway divider
landslide (not moving)
object set in motion by railway train or road vehicle (motor) (nonmotor)
object thrown in front of motor vehicle
safety island
temporary traffic sign or marker
wall of cut made for road
other object, fixed, movable, or moving

Excludes: collision with:
any object off the highway (resulting from loss of control) (E816.0-E816.9)
any object which normally would have been off the highway and is not stated to have been on it (E816.0-E816.9)
motor vehicle parked, stopped, stalled, disabled, or abandoned on highway (E812.0-E812.9)
moving landslide (E909)
motor vehicle hit by object:
set in motion by railway train or road vehicle (motor) (nonmotor) (E818.0-E818.9)
thrown into or on vehicle (E818.0-E818.9)

E CODES

④ **E816** **Motor vehicle traffic accident due to loss of control, without collision on the highway**
    Includes: motor vehicle:
        failing to make curve and:
            colliding with object off the highway
            overturning
            stopping abruptly off the highway
        going out of control (due to):
            blowout and:
                colliding with object off the highway
                overturning
                stopping abruptly off the highway
            burst tire and:
                colliding with object off the highway
                overturning
                stopping abruptly off the highway
            driver falling asleep and:
                colliding with object off the highway
                overturning
                stopping abruptly off the highway
            driver inattention and:
                colliding with object off the highway
                overturning
                stopping abruptly off the highway
            excessive speed and:
                colliding with object off the highway
                overturning
                stopping abruptly off the highway
            failure of mechanical part and:
                colliding with object off the highway
                overturning
                stopping abruptly off the highway
    Excludes: collision on highway following loss of control (E810.0-E815.9)
              loss of control of motor vehicle following collision on the highway
                  (E810.0-E815.9)

④ **E817** **Noncollision motor vehicle traffic accident while boarding or alighting**
    Includes: fall down stairs of motor bus while boarding or alighting
              fall from car in street while boarding or alighting
              injured by moving part of the vehicle while boarding or alighting
              trapped by door of motor bus while boarding or alighting

④ **E818** **Other noncollision motor vehicle traffic accident**
    Includes: accidental poisoning from exhaust gas generated by motor vehicle while in motion
              breakage of any part of motor vehicle while in motion
              explosion of any part of motor vehicle while in motion
              fall, jump, or being accidentally pushed from motor vehicle while in motion
              fire starting in motor vehicle while in motion
              hit by object thrown into or on motor vehicle while in motion
              injured by being thrown against some part of, or object in motor vehicle while in motion
              injury from moving part of motor vehicle while in motion
              object falling in or on motor vehicle while in motion
              object thrown on motor vehicle while in motion
              collision of railway train or road vehicle except motor vehicle, with object set in motion by motor vehicle
              motor vehicle hit by object set in motion by railway train or road vehicle (motor) (nonmotor)
              pedestrian, railway train, or road vehicle (motor) (nonmotor) hit by object set in motion by motor vehicle
    Excludes: collision between motor vehicle and:
              object set in motion by railway train or road vehicle (motor) (nonmotor)
                  (E815.0-E815.9)
              object thrown towards the motor vehicle (E815.0-E815.9)
              person overcome by carbon monoxide generated by stationary motor vehicle off the roadway with motor running (E868.2)

④ **E819** **Motor vehicle traffic accident of unspecified nature**
    Includes: motor vehicle traffic accident NOS
              traffic accident NOS

TABULAR LIST

MOTOR VEHICLE NONTRAFFIC ACCIDENTS (E820-E825)

Note: For definitions of motor vehicle nontraffic accident and related terms see definitions (a) to (k).

Includes: accidents involving motor vehicles being used in recreational or sporting activities off the highway
collision and noncollision motor vehicle accidents occurring entirely off the highway

Excludes: accidents involving motor vehicle and:
aircraft (E840.0-E845.9)
watercraft (E830.0-E838.9)
accidents, not on the public highway, involving agricultural and construction machinery but not involving another motor vehicle (E919.0, E919.2, E919.7)

The following fourth-digit subdivisions are for use with categories E820-E825 to identify the injured person:

.0 Driver of motor vehicle other than motorcycle
See definition (l)

.1 Passenger in motor vehicle other than motorcycle
See definition (l)

.2 Motorcyclist
See definition (l)

.3 Passenger on motorcycle
See definition (l)

.4 Occupant of streetcar

.5 Rider of animal; occupant of animal-drawn vehicle

.6 Pedal cyclist
See definition (p)

.7 Pedestrian
See definition (r)

.8 Other specified person
Occupant of vehicle other than above
Person on railway train involved in accident
Unauthorized rider of motor vehicle

.9 Unspecified person

④ **E820 Nontraffic accident involving motor-driven snow vehicle**
Includes: breakage of part of motor-driven snow vehicle (not on public highway)
fall from motor-driven snow vehicle (not on public highway)
hit by motor-driven snow vehicle (not on public highway)
overturning of motor-driven snow vehicle (not on public highway)
run over or dragged by motor-driven snow vehicle (not on public highway)
collision of motor-driven snow vehicle with:
animal (being ridden) (-drawn vehicle)
another off-road motor vehicle
other motor vehicle, not on public highway
railway train
other object, fixed or movable
injury caused by rough landing of motor-driven snow vehicle (after leaving ground on rough terrain)

Excludes: accident on the public highway involving motor driven snow vehicle (E810.0-E819.9)

● Code new to this edition ▲ Revision of existing code ④ ⑤ Fourth or fifth digit required

E CODES

④ **E821** **Nontraffic accident involving other off-road motor vehicle**
   Includes: breakage of part of off-road motor vehicle, except snow vehicle (not on public highway)
   fall from off-road motor vehicle, except snow vehicle (not on public highway)
   hit by off-road motor vehicle, except snow vehicle (not on public highway)
   overturning of off-road motor vehicle, except snow vehicle (not on public highway)
   run over or dragged by off-road motor vehicle, except snow vehicle (not on public highway)
   thrown against some part of or object in off-road motor vehicle, except snow vehicle (not on public highway)
   collision with:
     animal (being ridden) (-drawn vehicle)
     another off-road motor vehicle, except snow vehicle
     other motor vehicle, not on public highway
     other object, fixed or movable
   Excludes: accident on public highway involving off-road motor vehicle (E810.0-E819.9)
   collision between motor driven snow vehicle and other off-road motor vehicle (E820.0-E820.9)
   hovercraft accident on water (E830.0-E838.9)

④ **E822** **Other motor vehicle nontraffic accident involving collision with moving object**
   Includes: collision, not on public highway, between motor vehicle, except off-road motor vehicle and:
     animal
     nonmotor vehicle
     other motor vehicle, except off-road motor vehicle
     pedestrian
     railway train
     other moving object
   Excludes: collision with:
     motor-driven snow vehicle (E820.0-E820.9)
     other off-road motor vehicle (E821.0-E821.9)

④ **E823** **Other motor vehicle nontraffic accident involving collision with stationary object**
   Includes: collision, not on public highway, between motor vehicle, except off-road motor vehicle, and any object, fixed or movable, but not in motion

④ **E824** **Other motor vehicle nontraffic accident while boarding and alighting**
   Includes: fall while boarding or alighting from motor vehicle, except off-road motor vehicle, not on public highway
   injury from moving part of motor vehicle while boarding or alighting from motor vehicle, except off-road motor vehicle, not on public highway
   trapped by door of motor vehicle while boarding or alighting from motor vehicle, except off-road motor vehicle, not on public highway

④ **E825** **Other motor vehicle nontraffic accident of other and unspecified nature**
   Includes: accidental poisoning from carbon monoxide generated by motor vehicle while in motion, not on public highway
   breakage of any part of motor vehicle while in motion, not on public highway
   explosion of any part of motor vehicle while in motion, not on public highway
   fall, jump, or being accidentally pushed from motor vehicle while in motion, not on public highway
   fire starting in motor vehicle while in motion, not on public highway
   hit by object thrown into, towards, or on motor vehicle while in motion, not on public highway
   injured by being thrown against some part of, or object in motor vehicle while in motion, not on public highway
   injury from moving part of motor vehicle while in motion, not on public highway
   object falling in or on motor vehicle while in motion, not on public highway
   motor vehicle nontraffic accident NOS
   Excludes: fall from or in stationary motor vehicle (E884.9, E885.9)
   overcome by carbon monoxide or exhaust gas generated by stationary motor vehicle off the roadway with motor running (E868.2)
   struck by falling object from or in stationary motor vehicle (E916)

TABULAR LIST

OTHER ROAD VEHICLE ACCIDENTS (E826-E829)

Note: Other road vehicle accidents are transport accidents involving road vehicles other than motor vehicles. For definitions of other road vehicle and related terms see definitions (m) to (o).

Includes: accidents involving other road vehicles being used in recreational or sporting activities

Excludes: collision of other road vehicle [any] with:
- aircraft (E840.0-E845.9)
- motor vehicle (E813.0-E813.9, E820.0-E822.9)
- railway train (E801.0-E801.9)

The following fourth-digit subdivisions are for use with categories E826-E829 to identify the injured person:

.0 **Pedestrian**
   See definition (r)

.1 **Pedal cyclist**
   See definition (p)

.2 **Rider of animal**

.3 **Occupant of animal-drawn vehicle**

.4 **Occupant of streetcar**

.8 **Other specified person**

.9 **Unspecified person**

④ **E826 Pedal cycle accident**
[0-9]

Includes: breakage of any part of pedal cycle
collision between pedal cycle and:
- animal (being ridden) (herded) (unattended)
- another pedal cycle
- nonmotor road vehicle, any
- pedestrian
- other object, fixed, movable, or moving, not set in motion by motor vehicle, railway train, or aircraft

entanglement in wheel of pedal cycle
fall from pedal cycle
hit by object falling or thrown on the pedal cycle
pedal cycle accident NOS
pedal cycle overturned

④ **E827 Animal-drawn vehicle accident**
[0,2-4,8,9]

Includes: breakage of any part of vehicle
collision between animal-drawn vehicle and:
- animal (being ridden) (herded) (unattended)
- nonmotor road vehicle, except pedal cycle
- pedestrian, pedestrian conveyance, or pedestrian vehicle
- other object, fixed, movable, or moving, not set in motion by motor vehicle, railway train, or aircraft

fall from animal-drawn vehicle
knocked down by animal-drawn vehicle
overturning of animal-drawn vehicle
run over by animal-drawn vehicle
thrown from animal-drawn vehicle

Excludes: collision of animal-drawn vehicle with pedal cycle (E826.0-E826.9)

E CODES

④ **E828** **Accident involving animal being ridden**
[0,2,4,8,9]

    Includes: collision between animal being ridden and:
        another animal
        nonmotor road vehicle, except pedal cycle, and animal-drawn vehicle
        pedestrian, pedestrian conveyance, or pedestrian vehicle
        other object, fixed, movable, or moving, not set in motion by motor vehicle, railway train, or aircraft
    fall from animal being ridden
    knocked down by animal being ridden
    thrown from animal being ridden
    trampled by animal being ridden
    ridden animal stumbled and fell

    Excludes: *collision of animal being ridden with:*
        animal-drawn vehicle (E827.0-E827.9)
        pedal cycle (E826.0-E826.9)

④ **E829** **Other road vehicle accidents**
[0,4,8,9]

    Includes: accident while boarding or alighting from:
        streetcar
        nonmotor road vehicle not classifiable to E826-E828
    blow from object in:
        streetcar
        nonmotor road vehicle not classifiable to E826-E828
    breakage of any part of:
        streetcar
        nonmotor road vehicle not classifiable to E826-E828
    caught in door of:
        streetcar
        nonmotor road vehicle not classifiable to E826-E828
    derailment of:
        streetcar
        nonmotor road vehicle not classifiable to E826-E828
    fall in, on, or from:
        streetcar
        nonmotor road vehicle not classifiable to E826-E828
    fire in:
        streetcar
        nonmotor road vehicle not classifiable to E826-E828
    collision between streetcar or nonmotor road vehicle, except as in E826-E828, and:
        animal (not being ridden)
        another nonmotor road vehicle not classifiable to E826-E828
        pedestrian
        other object, fixed, movable, or moving, not set in motion by motor vehicle, railway train, or aircraft
    nonmotor road vehicle accident NOS
    streetcar accident NOS

    Excludes: *collision with:*
        animal being ridden (E828.0-E828.9)
        animal-drawn vehicle (E827.0-E827.9)
        pedal cycle (E826.0-E826.9)

TABULAR LIST

WATER TRANSPORT ACCIDENTS (E830-E838)

Note: For definitions of water transport accident and related terms see definitions (a), (s), and (t).

Includes: watercraft accidents in the course of recreational activities

Excludes: accidents involving both aircraft, including objects set in motion by aircraft, and watercraft (E840.0-E845.9)

The following fourth-digit subdivisions are for use with categories E830-E838 to identify the injured person:

.0 Occupant of small boat, unpowered

.1 Occupant of small boat, powered
See definition (t)

Excludes: water skier (.4)

.2 Occupant of other watercraft—crew
Persons:
engaged in operation of watercraft
providing passenger services [cabin attendants, ship's physician, catering personnel]
working on ship during voyage in other capacity [musician in band, operators of shops and beauty parlors]

.3 Occupant of other watercraft—other than crew
Passenger
Occupant of lifeboat, other than crew, after abandoning ship

.4 Water skier

.5 Swimmer

.6 Dockers, stevedores
Longshoreman employed on the dock in loading and unloading ships

.8 Other specified person
Immigration and custom officials on board ship
Person:
accompanying passenger or member of crew
visiting boat
Pilot (guiding ship into port)

.9 Unspecified person

E830 Accident to watercraft causing submersion
Includes: submersion and drowning due to:
boat overturning
boat submerging
falling or jumping from burning ship
falling or jumping from crushed watercraft
ship sinking
other accident to watercraft

E831 Accident to watercraft causing other injury
Includes: any injury, except submersion and drowning, as a result of an accident to watercraft
burned while ship on fire
crushed between ships in collision
crushed by lifeboat after abandoning ship
fall due to collision or other accident to watercraft
hit by falling object due to accident to watercraft
injured in watercraft accident involving collision
struck by boat or part thereof after fall or jump from damaged boat

Excludes: burns from localized fire or explosion on board ship (E837.0-E837.9)

E832 Other accidental submersion or drowning in water transport accident
Includes: submersion or drowning as a result of an accident other than accident to the watercraft, such as:
fall:
from gangplank
from ship
overboard
thrown overboard by motion of ship
washed overboard

Excludes: submersion or drowning of swimmer or diver who voluntarily jumps from boat not involved in an accident (E910.0-E910.9)

E833 Fall on stairs or ladders in water transport

Excludes: fall due to accident to watercraft (E831.0-E831.9)

E CODES

④ **E834** **Other fall from one level to another in water transport**
Excludes: fall due to accident to watercraft (E831.0-E831.9)

④ **E835** **Other and unspecified fall in water transport**
Excludes: fall due to accident to watercraft (E831.0-E831.9)

④ **E836** **Machinery accident in water transport**
Includes: injuries in water transport caused by:
deck machinery
engine room machinery
galley machinery
laundry machinery
loading machinery

④ **E837** **Explosion, fire, or burning in watercraft**
Includes: explosion of boiler on steamship
localized fire on ship

Excludes: burning ship (due to collision or explosion) resulting in:
submersion or drowning (E830.0-E830.9)
other injury (E831.0-E831.9)

④ **E838** **Other and unspecified water transport accident**
Includes: accidental poisoning by gases or fumes on ship
atomic power plant malfunction in watercraft
crushed between ship and stationary object [wharf]
crushed between ships without accident to watercraft
crushed by falling object on ship or while loading or unloading
hit by boat while water skiing
struck by boat or part thereof (after fall from boat)
watercraft accident NOS

665

TABULAR LIST

AIR AND SPACE TRANSPORT ACCIDENTS (E840-E845)

Note: For definition of aircraft and related terms see definitions (u) and (v).

The following fourth-digit subdivisions are for use with categories E840-E845 to identify the injured person:

.0 Occupant of spacecraft

.1 Occupant of military aircraft, any
Crew in military aircraft [air force] [army] [national guard] [navy]
Passenger (civilian) (military) in military aircraft [air force] [army] [national guard] [navy]
Troops in military aircraft [air force] [army] [national guard] [navy]

Excludes: occupants of aircraft operated under jurisdiction of police departments (.5)
parachutist (.7)

.2 Crew of commercial aircraft (powered) in surface to surface transport

.3 Other occupant of commercial aircraft (powered) in surface to surface transport
Flight personnel:
  not part of crew
  on familiarization flight
Passenger on aircraft (powered) NOS

.4 Occupant of commercial aircraft (powered) in surface to air transport
Occupant [crew] [passenger] of aircraft (powered) engaged in activities, such as:
  aerial spraying (crops) (fire retardants)
  air drops of emergency supplies
  air drops of parachutists, except from military craft
  crop dusting
  lowering of construction material [bridge or telephone pole]
  sky writing

.5 Occupant of other powered aircraft
Occupant [crew] [passenger] of aircraft [powered] engaged in activities, such as:
  aerobatic flying
  aircraft racing
  rescue operation
  storm surveillance
  traffic surveillance
Occupant of private plane NOS

.6 Occupant of unpowered aircraft, except parachutist
Occupant of aircraft classifiable to E842

.7 Parachutist (military) (other)
Person making voluntary descent

Excludes: person making descent after accident to aircraft (.1-.6)

.8 Ground crew, airline employee
Persons employed at airfields (civil) (military) or launching pads, not occupants of aircraft

.9 Other person

④ **E840 Accident to powered aircraft at takeoff or landing**
Includes: collision of aircraft with any object, fixed, movable, or moving while taking off or landing
crash while taking off or landing
explosion on aircraft while taking off or landing
fire on aircraft while taking off or landing
forced landing

④ **E841 Accident to powered aircraft, other and unspecified**
Includes: aircraft accident NOS
aircraft crash or wreck NOS
any accident to powered aircraft while in transit or when not specified whether in transit, taking off, or landing
collision of aircraft with another aircraft, bird, or any object, while in transit
explosion on aircraft while in transit
fire on aircraft while in transit

E CODES

④ **E842** **Accident to unpowered aircraft**
[6-9]
    Includes: any accident, except collision with powered aircraft, to:
        balloon
        glider
        hang glider
        kite carrying a person
        hit by object falling from unpowered aircraft

④ **E843** **Fall in, on, or from aircraft**
[0-9]
    Includes: accident in boarding or alighting from aircraft, any kind
        fall in, on, or from aircraft [any kind], while in transit, taking off, or landing,
            except when as a result of an accident to aircraft

④ **E844** **Other specified air transport accidents**
[0-9]
    Includes: hit by:
        aircraft without accident to aircraft
        object falling from aircraft without accident to aircraft
      injury by or from:
        machinery on aircraft without accident to aircraft
        rotating propeller without accident to aircraft
        voluntary parachute descent without accident to aircraft
      poisoning by carbon monoxide from aircraft while in transit without accident to
        aircraft
      sucked into jet without accident to aircraft
      any accident involving other transport vehicle (motor) (nonmotor) due to being hit
        by object set in motion by aircraft (powered)
    Excludes: air sickness (E903)
      effects of:
        high altitude (E902.0-E902.1)
        pressure change (E902.0-E902.1)
      injury in parachute descent due to accident to aircraft (840.0-E842.9)

④ **E845** **Accident involving spacecraft**
[0,8,9]
    Includes: launching pad accident
    Excludes: effects of weightlessness in spacecraft (E928.0)

VEHICLE ACCIDENTS NOT ELSEWHERE CLASSIFIABLE (E846-E848)

E846 Accidents involving powered vehicles used solely within the buildings and premises of industrial or commercial establishment
    Accident to, on, or involving:
      battery powered airport passenger vehicle
      battery powered trucks (baggage) (mail)
      coal car in mine
      logging car
      self propelled truck, industrial
      station baggage truck (powered)
      tram, truck, or tub (powered) in mine or quarry
    Breakage of any part of vehicle
    Collision with:
      pedestrian
      other vehicle or object within premises
    Explosion of powered vehicle, industrial or commercial
    Fall from powered vehicle, industrial or commercial
    Overturning of powered vehicle, industrial or commercial
    Struck by powered vehicle, industrial or commercial
    Excludes: accidental poisoning by exhaust gas from vehicle not elsewhere classifiable
        (E868.2)
      injury by crane, lift (fork), or elevator (E919.2)

TABULAR LIST

E847 **Accidents involving cable cars not running on rails**
Accident to, on, or involving:
- cable car, not on rails
- ski chair-lift
- ski-lift with gondola
- téléférique

Breakage of cable
Caught or dragged by cable car, not on rails
Fall or jump from cable car, not on rails
Object thrown from or in cable car, not on rails

E848 **Accidents involving other vehicles, not elsewhere classifiable**
Accident to, on, or involving:
- ice yacht
- land yacht
- nonmotor, nonroad vehicle NOS

E849 **Place of occurrence**
The following category is for use to denote the place where the injury or poisoning occurred.

E849.0 **Home**
- Apartment
- Boarding house
- Farm house
- Home premises
- House (residential)
- Noninstitutional place of residence
- Private:
  - driveway
  - garage
  - garden
  - home
  - walk
- Swimming pool in private house or garden
- Yard of home

Excludes: home under construction but not yet occupied (E849.3)
institutional place of residence (E849.7)

E849.1 **Farm**
Farm:
- buildings
- land under cultivation

Excludes: farm house and home premises of farm (E849.0)

E849.2 **Mine and quarry**
- Gravel pit
- Sand pit
- Tunnel under construction

E849.3 **Industrial place and premises**
- Building under construction
- Dockyard
- Dry dock
- Factory
  - building
  - premises
- Garage (place of work)
- Industrial yard
- Loading platform (factory) (store)
- Plant, industrial
- Railway yard
- Shop (place of work)
- Warehouse
- Workhouse

E849.4 **Place for recreation and sport**
- Amusement park
- Baseball field
- Basketball court
- Beach resort
- Cricket ground
- Fives court
- Football field
- Golf course
- Gymnasium
- Hockey field
- Holiday camp
- Ice palace
- Lake resort
- Mountain resort
- Playground, including school playground
- Public park
- Racecourse
- Resort NOS
- Riding school
- Rifle range
- Seashore resort
- Skating rink
- Sports ground
- Sports palace
- Stadium
- Swimming pool, public
- Tennis court
- Vacation resort

Excludes: that in private house or garden (E849.0)

E849.5 **Street and highway**

668 ● Code new to this edition   ▲ Revision of existing code   ④ ⑤ Fourth or fifth digit required

E CODES

E849.6 Public building
Building (including adjacent grounds) used by the general public or by a particular group of the public, such as:

- airport
- bank
- café
- casino
- church
- cinema
- clubhouse
- courthouse
- dance hall
- garage building (for car storage)
- hotel
- market (grocery or other commodity)
- movie house
- music hall
- nightclub
- office
- office building
- opera house
- post office
- public hall
- radio broadcasting station
- restaurant
- school (state) (public) (private)
- shop, commercial
- station (bus) (railway)
- store
- theater

Excludes: home garage (E849.0)
industrial building or workplace (E849.3)

E849.7 Residential institution
- Children's home
- Dormitory
- Hospital
- Jail
- Old people's home
- Orphanage
- Prison
- Reform school

E849.8 Other specified places
- Beach NOS
- Canal
- Caravan site NOS
- Derelict house
- Desert
- Dock
- Forest
- Harbor
- Hill
- Lake NOS
- Mountain
- Parking lot
- Parking place
- Pond or pool (natural)
- Prairie
- Public place NOS
- Railway line
- Reservoir
- River
- Sea
- Seashore NOS
- Stream
- Swamp
- Trailer court
- Woods

E849.9 Unspecified place

ACCIDENTAL POISONING BY DRUGS, MEDICINAL SUBSTANCES, AND BIOLOGICALS (E850-E858)

Includes: accidental overdose of drug, wrong drug given or taken in error, and drug taken inadvertently
accidents in the use of drugs and biologicals in medical and surgical procedures

Excludes: administration with suicidal or homicidal intent or intent to harm, or in circumstances classifiable to E980-E989 (E950.0-E950.5, E962.0, E980.0-E980.5)
correct drug properly administered in therapeutic or prophylactic dosage, as the cause of adverse effect (E930.0-E949.9)

See Alphabetic Index for more complete list of specific drugs to be classified under the fourth-digit subdivisions. The American Hospital Formulary numbers can be used to classify new drugs listed by the American Hospital Formulary Service (AHFS). See appendix C.

E850 Accidental poisoning by analgesics, antipyretics, and antirheumatics

E850.0 Heroin
Diacetylmorphine

E850.1 Methadone

E850.2 Other opiates and related narcotics
- Codeine [methylmorphine]
- Meperidine [pethidine]
- Morphine
- Opium (alkaloids)

E850.3 Salicylates
- Acetylsalicylic acid [aspirin]
- Amino derivatives of salicylic acid
- Salicylic acid salts

TABULAR LIST

- **E850.4 Aromatic analgesics, not elsewhere classified**
  Acetanilid
  Paracetamol [acetaminophen]
  Phenacetin [acetophenetidin]
- **E850.5 Pyrazole derivatives**
  Aminophenazone [amidopyrine]
  Phenylbutazone
- **E850.6 Antirheumatics [antiphlogistics]**
  Gold salts   Indomethacin
  Excludes: salicylates (E850.3)
            steroids (E858.0)
- **E850.7 Other non-narcotic analgesics**
  Pyrabital
- **E850.8 Other specified analgesics and antipyretics**
  Pentazocine
- **E850.9 Unspecified analgesic or antipyretic**

E851 Accidental poisoning by barbiturates
  Amobarbital [amylobarbitone]
  Barbital [barbitone]
  Butabarbital [butabarbitone]
  Pentobarbital [pentobarbitone]
  Phenobarbital [phenobarbitone]
  Secobarbital [quinalbarbitone]
  Excludes: thiobarbiturates (E855.1)

E852 Accidental poisoning by other sedatives and hypnotics
- **E852.0 Chloral hydrate group**
- **E852.1 Paraldehyde**
- **E852.2 Bromine compounds**
  Bromides   Carbromal (derivatives)
- **E852.3 Methaqualone compounds**
- **E852.4 Glutethimide group**
- **E852.5 Mixed sedatives, not elsewhere classified**
- **E852.8 Other specified sedatives and hypnotics**
- **E852.9 Unspecified sedative or hypnotic**
  Sleeping:
    drug NOS
    pill NOS
    tablet NOS

E853 Accidental poisoning by tranquilizers
- **E853.0 Phenothiazine-based tranquilizers**
  Chlorpromazine   Prochlorperazine
  Fluphenazine   Promazine
- **E853.1 Butyrophenone-based tranquilizers**
  Haloperidol   Trifluperidol
  Spiperone
- **E853.2 Benzodiazepine-based tranquilizers**
  Chlordiazepoxide   Lorazepam
  Diazepam   Medazepam
  Flurazepam   Nitrazepam
- **E853.8 Other specified tranquilizers**
  Hydroxyzine   Meprobamate
- **E853.9 Unspecified tranquilizer**

E854 Accidental poisoning by other psychotropic agents
- **E854.0 Antidepressants**
  Amitriptyline   Monoamine oxidase [MAO] inhibitors
  Imipramine
- **E854.1 Psychodysleptics [hallucinogens]**
  Cannabis derivatives   Mescaline
  Lysergide [LSD]   Psilocin
  Marihuana (derivatives) Psilocybin

E CODES

E854.2 Psychostimulants
  Amphetamine   Caffeine
  Excludes: central appetite depressants (E858.8)

E854.3 Central nervous system stimulants
  Analeptics   Opiate antagonists

E854.8 Other psychotropic agents

E855 Accidental poisoning by other drugs acting on central and autonomic nervous system

  E855.0 Anticonvulsant and anti-Parkinsonism drugs
    Amantadine
    Hydantoin derivatives
    Levodopa [L-dopa]
    Oxazolidine derivatives [paramethadione] [trimethadione]
    Succinimides

  E855.1 Other central nervous system depressants
    Ether   Intravenous anesthetics
    Gaseous anesthetics   Thiobarbiturates, such as thiopental sodium
    Halogenated hydrocarbon
      derivatives

  E855.2 Local anesthetics
    Cocaine   Procaine
    Lidocaine [lignocaine]   Tetracaine

  E855.3 Parasympathomimetics [cholinergics]
    Acetylcholine   Pilocarpine
    Anticholinesterase:
      organophosphorus
      reversible

  E855.4 Parasympatholytics [anticholinergics and antimuscarinics] and spasmolytics
    Atropine   Hyoscine [scopolamine]
    Homatropine   Quaternary ammonium derivatives

  E855.5 Sympathomimetics [adrenergics]
    Epinephrine [adrenalin]
    Levarterenol [noradrenalin]

  E855.6 Sympatholytics [antiadrenergics]
    Phenoxybenzamine   Tolazoline hydrochloride

  E855.8 Other specified drugs acting on central and autonomic nervous systems

  E855.9 Unspecified drug acting on central and autonomic nervous systems

E856 Accidental poisoning by antibiotics

E857 Accidental poisoning by other anti-infectives

E858 Accidental poisoning by other drugs

  E858.0 Hormones and synthetic substitutes

  E858.1 Primarily systemic agents

  E858.2 Agents primarily affecting blood constituents

  E858.3 Agents primarily affecting cardiovascular system

  E858.4 Agents primarily affecting gastrointestinal system

  E858.5 Water, mineral, and uric acid metabolism drugs

  E858.6 Agents primarily acting on the smooth and skeletal muscles and respiratory system

  E858.7 Agents primarily affecting skin and mucous membrane, ophthalmological, otorhinolaryngological, and dental drugs

  E858.8 Other specified drugs
    Central appetite depressants

  E858.9 Unspecified drug

ACCIDENTAL POISONING BY OTHER SOLID AND LIQUID SUBSTANCES, GASES, AND VAPORS (E860-E869)

  Note: Categories in this section are intended primarily to indicate the external cause of poisoning states classifiable to 980-989. They may also be used to indicate external causes of localized effects classifiable to 001-799.

E860 Accidental poisoning by alcohol, not elsewhere classified

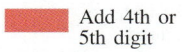 Add 4th or 5th digit   Nonspecific code   Unspecified code   Manifestation code

671

TABULAR LIST

E860.0   **Alcoholic beverages**
    Alcohol in preparations intended for consumption

E860.1   **Other and unspecified ethyl alcohol and its products**
    Denatured alcohol   Grain alcohol NOS
    Ethanol NOS   Methylated spirit

E860.2   **Methyl alcohol**
    Methanol   Wood alcohol

E860.3   **Isopropyl alcohol**
    Dimethyl carbinol   Secondary propyl alcohol
    Isopropanol
    Rubbing alcohol substitute

E860.4   **Fusel oil**
    Alcohol:
      amyl
      butyl
      propyl

E860.8   **Other specified alcohols**

E860.9   **Unspecified alcohol**

E861   **Accidental poisoning by cleansing and polishing agents, disinfectants, paints, and varnishes**

E861.0   **Synthetic detergents and shampoos**

E861.1   **Soap products**

E861.2   **Polishes**

E861.3   **Other cleansing and polishing agents**
    Scouring powders

E861.4   **Disinfectants**
    Household and other disinfectants not ordinarily used on the person
    Excludes: carbolic acid or phenol (E864.0)

E861.5   **Lead paints**

E861.6   **Other paints and varnishes**
    Lacquers   Paints, other than lead
    Oil colors   White washes

E861.9   **Unspecified**

E862   **Accidental poisoning by petroleum products, other solvents and their vapors, not elsewhere classified**

E862.0   **Petroleum solvents**
    Petroleum:
      ether
      benzine
      naphtha

E862.1   **Petroleum fuels and cleaners**
    Antiknock additives to petroleum fuels
    Gas oils
    Gasoline or petrol
    Kerosene
    Excludes: kerosene insecticides (E863.4)

E862.2   **Lubricating oils**

E862.3   **Petroleum solids**
    Paraffin wax

E862.4   **Other specified solvents**
    Benzene

E862.9   **Unspecified solvent**

E863   **Accidental poisoning by agricultural and horticultural chemical and pharmaceutical preparations other than plant foods and fertilizers**
    Excludes: plant foods and fertilizers (E866.5)

E863.0   **Insecticides of organochlorine compounds**
    Benzene hexachloride   Dieldrin
    Chlordane   Endrine
    DDT   Toxaphene

E CODES

E863.1 **Insecticides of organophosphorus compounds**
    Demeton
    Diazinon
    Dichlorvos
    Malathion
    Methyl parathion
    Parathion
    Phenylsulphthion
    Phorate
    Phosdrin

E863.2 **Carbamates**
    Aldicarb
    Carbaryl
    Propoxur

E863.3 **Mixtures of insecticides**

E863.4 **Other and unspecified insecticides**
    Kerosene insecticides

E863.5 **Herbicides**
    2, 4-Dichlorophenoxyacetic acid [2, 4-D]
    2, 4, 5-Trichlorophenoxyacetic acid [2, 4, 5-T]
    Chlorates
    Diquat
    Mixtures of plant food and fertilizers with herbicides
    Paraquat

E863.6 **Fungicides**
    Organic mercurials (used in seed dressing)
    Pentachlorophenols

E863.7 **Rodenticides**
    Fluoroacetates
    Squill and derivatives
    Thallium
    Warfarin
    Zinc phosphide

E863.8 **Fumigants**
    Cyanides
    Methyl bromide
    Phosphine

E863.9 **Other and unspecified**

E864 **Accidental poisoning by corrosives and caustics, not elsewhere classified**
    Excludes: those as components of disinfectants (E861.4)

E864.0 **Corrosive aromatics**
    Carbolic acid or phenol

E864.1 **Acids**
    Acid:
      hydrochloric
      nitric
      sulfuric

E864.2 **Caustic alkalis**
    Lye

E864.3 **Other specified corrosives and caustics**

E864.4 **Unspecified corrosives and caustics**

E865 **Accidental poisoning from poisonous foodstuffs and poisonous plants**
    Includes: any meat, fish, or shellfish
               plants, berries, and fungi eaten as, or in mistake for, food, or by a child
    Excludes: anaphylactic shock due to adverse food reaction (995.6)
              food poisoning (bacterial) (005.0-005.9)
              poisoning and toxic reactions to venomous plants (E905.6-E905.7)

E865.0 Meat
E865.1 Shellfish
E865.2 Other fish
E865.3 Berries and seeds
E865.4 Other specified plants
E865.5 Mushrooms and other fungi
E865.8 Other specified foods
E865.9 Unspecified foodstuff or poisonous plant

TABULAR LIST

E866 Accidental poisoning by other and unspecified solid and liquid substances

> Excludes: these substances as a component of:
> medicines (E850.0-E858.9)
> paints (E861.5-E861.6)
> pesticides (E863.0-E863.9)
> petroleum fuels (E862.1)

- E866.0 Lead and its compounds and fumes
- E866.1 Mercury and its compounds and fumes
- E866.2 Antimony and its compounds and fumes
- E866.3 Arsenic and its compounds and fumes
- **E866.4** Other metals and their compounds and fumes
    - Beryllium (compounds)
    - Brass fumes
    - Cadmium (compounds)
    - Copper salts
    - Iron (compounds)
    - Manganese (compounds)
    - Nickel (compounds)
    - Thallium (compounds)
- E866.5 Plant foods and fertilizers
    > Excludes: mixtures with herbicides (E863.5)
- E866.6 Glues and adhesives
- E866.7 Cosmetics
- **E866.8** Other specified solid or liquid substances
- **E866.9** Unspecified solid or liquid substance

E867 Accidental poisoning by gas distributed by pipeline
Carbon monoxide from incomplete combustion of piped gas
Coal gas NOS
Liquefied petroleum gas distributed through pipes (pure or mixed with air)
Piped gas (natural) (manufactured)

E868 Accidental poisoning by other utility gas and other carbon monoxide

- E868.0 Liquefied petroleum gas distributed in mobile containers
    - Butane or carbon monoxide from incomplete combustion of this gas
    - Liquefied hydrocarbon gas NOS or carbon monoxide from incomplete combustion of this gas
    - Propane or carbon monoxide from incomplete combustion of this gas
- **E868.1** Other and unspecified utility gas
    - Acetylene or or carbon monoxide from incomplete combustion of these gases
    - Gas NOS used for lighting, heating, cooking, or carbon monoxide from incomplete combustion of these gases
    - Water gas or carbon monoxide from incomplete combustion of these gases
- E868.2 Motor vehicle exhaust gas
    - Exhaust gas from:
        - farm tractor, not in transit
        - gas engine
        - motor pump
        - motor vehicle, not in transit
        - any type of combustion engine not in watercraft
    > Excludes: poisoning by carbon monoxide from:
    > aircraft while in transit (E844.0-E844.9)
    > motor vehicle while in transit (E818.0-E818.9)
    > watercraft whether or not in transit (E838.0-E838.9)
- **E868.3** Carbon monoxide from incomplete combustion of other domestic fuels
    - Carbon monoxide from incomplete combustion of:
        - coal in domestic stove or fireplace
        - coke in domestic stove or fireplace
        - kerosene in domestic stove or fireplace
        - wood in domestic stove or fireplace
    > Excludes: carbon monoxide from smoke and fumes due to conflagration (E890.0-E893.9)
- E868.8 Carbon monoxide from other sources
    - Carbon monoxide from:
        - blast furnace gas
        - incomplete combustion of fuels in industrial use
        - kiln vapor
- **E868.9** Unspecified carbon monoxide

E CODES

E869 Accidental poisoning by other gases and vapors
> *Excludes:* effects of gases used as anesthetics (E855.1, E938.2)
> fumes from heavy metals (E866.0-E866.4)
> smoke and fumes due to conflagration or explosion (E890.0-E899)

- E869.0 **Nitrogen oxides**
- E869.1 **Sulfur dioxide**
- E869.2 **Freon**
- E869.3 **Lacrimogenic gas [tear gas]**
  - Bromobenzyl cyanide
  - Chloroacetophenone
  - Ethyliodoacetate
- E869.4 **Second-hand tobacco smoke**
- **E869.8** **Other specified gases and vapors**
  - Chlorine
  - Hydrocyanic acid gas
- **E869.9** **Unspecified gases and vapors**

MISADVENTURES TO PATIENTS DURING SURGICAL AND MEDICAL CARE (E870-E876)

> *Excludes:* accidental overdose of drug and wrong drug given in error (E850.0-E858.9)
> surgical and medical procedures as the cause of abnormal reaction by the patient, without mention of misadventure at the time of procedure (E878.0-E879.9)

E870 Accidental cut, puncture, perforation, or hemorrhage during medical care
- E870.0 **Surgical operation**
- E870.1 **Infusion or transfusion**
- **E870.2** **Kidney dialysis or other perfusion**
- E870.3 **Injection or vaccination**
- E870.4 **Endoscopic examination**
- E870.5 **Aspiration of fluid or tissue, puncture, and catheterization**
  - Abdominal paracentesis
  - Aspirating needle biopsy
  - Blood sampling
  - Lumbar puncture
  - Thoracentesis
  > *Excludes:* heart catheterization (E870.6)
- E870.6 **Heart catheterization**
- E870.7 **Administration of enema**
- **E870.8** **Other specified medical care**
- **E870.9** **Unspecified medical care**

E871 Foreign object left in body during procedure
- E871.0 **Surgical operation**
- E871.1 **Infusion or transfusion**
- E871.2 **Kidney dialysis or other perfusion**
- E871.3 **Injection or vaccination**
- E871.4 **Endoscopic examination**
- E871.5 **Aspiration of fluid or tissue, puncture, and catheterization**
  - Abdominal paracentesis
  - Aspiration needle biopsy
  - Blood sampling
  - Lumbar puncture
  - Thoracentesis
  > *Excludes:* heart catheterization (E871.6)
- E871.6 **Heart catheterization**
- E871.7 **Removal of catheter or packing**
- **E871.8** **Other specified procedures**
- **E871.9** **Unspecified procedure**

E872 Failure of sterile precautions during procedure
- E872.0 **Surgical operation**
- E872.1 **Infusion or transfusion**
- E872.2 **Kidney dialysis and other perfusion**
- E872.3 **Injection or vaccination**
- E872.4 **Endoscopic examination**

TABULAR LIST

E872.5 Aspiration of fluid or tissue, puncture, and catheterization
    Abdominal paracentesis   Lumbar puncture
    Aspirating needle biopsy   Thoracentesis
    Blood sampling

    Excludes: heart catheterization (E872.6)

E872.6 Heart catheterization
E872.8 Other specified procedures
E872.9 Unspecified procedure

E873 Failure in dosage
    Excludes: accidental overdose of drug, medicinal or biological substance (E850.0-E858.9)

E873.0 Excessive amount of blood or other fluid during transfusion or infusion
E873.1 Incorrect dilution of fluid during infusion
E873.2 Overdose of radiation in therapy
E873.3 Inadvertent exposure of patient to radiation during medical care
E873.4 Failure in dosage in electroshock or insulin-shock therapy
E873.5 Inappropriate [too hot or too cold] temperature in local application and packing
E873.6 Nonadministration of necessary drug or medicinal substance
E873.8 Other specified failure in dosage
E873.9 Unspecified failure in dosage

E874 Mechanical failure of instrument or apparatus during procedure

E874.0 Surgical operation
E874.1 Infusion and transfusion
    Air in system
E874.2 Kidney dialysis and other perfusion
E874.3 Endoscopic examination
E874.4 Aspiration of fluid or tissue, puncture, and catheterization
    Abdominal paracentesis   Lumbar puncture
    Aspirating needle biopsy   Thoracentesis
    Blood sampling

    Excludes: heart catheterization (E874.5)

E874.5 Heart catheterization
E874.8 Other specified procedures
E874.9 Unspecified procedure

E875 Contaminated or infected blood, other fluid, drug, or biological substance
    Includes: presence of:
            bacterial pyrogens
            endotoxin-producing bacteria
            serum hepatitis-producing agent

E875.0 Contaminated substance transfused or infused
E875.1 Contaminated substance injected or used for vaccination
E875.2 Contaminated drug or biological substance administered by other means
E875.8 Other
E875.9 Unspecified

E876 Other and unspecified misadventures during medical care

E876.0 Mismatched blood in transfusion
E876.1 Wrong fluid in infusion
E876.2 Failure in suture and ligature during surgical operation
E876.3 Endotracheal tube wrongly placed during anesthetic procedure
E876.4 Failure to introduce or to remove other tube or instrument
    Excludes: foreign object left in body during procedure (E871.0-E871.9)
E876.5 Performance of inappropriate operation
E876.8 Other specified misadventures during medical care
    Performance of inappropriate treatment NEC
E876.9 Unspecified misadventure during medical care

---

676   ● Code new to this edition   ▲ Revision of existing code   ④ ⑤ Fourth or fifth digit required

E CODES

SURGICAL AND MEDICAL PROCEDURES AS THE CAUSE OF ABNORMAL REACTION OF PATIENT OR LATER COMPLICATION, WITHOUT MENTION OF MISADVENTURE AT THE TIME OF PROCEDURE (E878-E879)

Includes: procedures as the cause of abnormal reaction, such as:
  displacement or malfunction of prosthetic device
  hepatorenal failure, postoperative
  malfunction of external stoma
  postoperative intestinal obstruction
  rejection of transplanted organ

Excludes: anesthetic management properly carried out as the cause of adverse effect (E937.0-E938.9)
  infusion and transfusion, without mention of misadventure in the technique of procedure (E930.0-E949.9)

E878 Surgical operation and other surgical procedures as the cause of abnormal reaction of patient, or of later complication, without mention of misadventure at the time of operation

E878.0 **Surgical operation with transplant of whole organ**
  Transplantation of:
    heart
    kidney
    liver

E878.1 **Surgical operation with implant of artificial internal device**
  Cardiac pacemaker   Heart valve prosthesis
  Electrodes implanted in brain   Internal orthopedic device

E878.2 **Surgical operation with anastomosis, bypass, or graft, with natural or artificial tissues used as implant**
  Anastomosis: Graft of blood vessel, tendon, or skin
    arteriovenous
    gastrojejunal

  Excludes: external stoma (E878.3)

E878.3 **Surgical operation with formation of external stoma**
  Colostomy   Gastrostomy
  Cystostomy   Ureterostomy
  Duodenostomy

E878.4 Other restorative surgery

E878.5 Amputation of limb(s)

E878.6 Removal of other organ (partial) (total)

E878.8 Other specified surgical operations and procedures

E878.9 Unspecified surgical operations and procedures

E879 Other procedures, without mention of misadventure at the time of procedure, as the cause of abnormal reaction of patient, or of later complication

E879.0 **Cardiac catheterization**

E879.1 **Kidney dialysis**

E879.2 **Radiological procedure and radiotherapy**

  Excludes: radio-opaque dyes for diagnostic x-ray procedures (E947.8)

E879.3 **Shock therapy**
  Electroshock therapy   Insulin-shock therapy

E879.4 **Aspiration of fluid**
  Lumbar puncture   Thoracentesis

E879.5 **Insertion of gastric or duodenal sound**

E879.6 **Urinary catheterization**

E879.7 **Blood sampling**

E879.8 Other specified procedures
  Blood transfusion

E879.9 Unspecified procedure

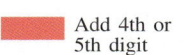 Add 4th or 5th digit   Nonspecific code   Unspecified code   Manifestation code

677

ACCIDENTAL FALLS (E880-E888)

> Excludes: falls (in or from):
> burning building (E890.8, E891.8)
> into fire (E890.0-E899)
> into water (with submersion or drowning) (E910.0-E910.9)
> machinery (in operation) (E919.0-E919.9)
> on edged, pointed, or sharp object (E920.0-E920.9)
> transport vehicle (E800.0-E845.9)
> vehicle not elsewhere classifiable (E846-E848)

E880 Fall on or from stairs or steps

    E880.0 Escalator

    E880.1 Fall on or from sidewalk curb

> Excludes: fall from moving sidewalk (E885.9)

    E880.9 Other stairs or steps

E881 Fall on or from ladders or scaffolding

    E881.0 Fall from ladder

    E881.1 Fall from scaffolding

E882 Fall from or out of building or other structure

Fall from:
- balcony
- bridge
- building
- flagpole
- tower

Fall from:
- turret
- viaduct
- wall
- window

Fall through roof

> Excludes: collapse of a building or structure (E916)
> fall or jump from burning building (E890.8, E891.8)

E883 Fall into hole or other opening in surface

Includes:

fall into:
- cavity
- dock
- hole
- pit
- quarry

fall into:
- shaft
- swimming pool
- tank
- well

> Excludes: fall into water NOS (E910.9)
> that resulting in drowning or submersion without mention of injury (E910.0-E910.9)

    E883.0 Accident from diving or jumping into water [swimming pool]

Strike or hit:
- against bottom when jumping or diving into water
- wall or board of swimming pool
- water surface

> Excludes: diving with insufficient air supply (E913.2)
> effects of air pressure from diving (E902.2)

    E883.1 Accidental fall into well

    E883.2 Accidental fall into storm drain or manhole

    E883.9 Fall into other hole or other opening in surface

E884 Other fall from one level to another

    E884.0 Fall from playground equipment

> Excludes: recreational machinery (E919.8)

    E884.1 Fall from cliff

    E884.2 Fall from chair

    E884.3 Fall from wheelchair

    E884.4 Fall from bed

    E884.5 Fall from other furniture

    E884.6 Fall from commode

Toilet

E CODES

E884.9 **Other fall from one level to another**
Fall from:
  embankment
  haystack
Fall from:
  stationary vehicle
  tree

E885 **Fall on same level from slipping, tripping, or stumbling**

E885.0 **Fall from (nonmotorized) scooter**

E885.1 **Fall from roller skates**
In-line skates

E885.2 **Fall from skateboard**

E885.3 **Fall from skis**

E885.4 **Fall from snowboard**

E885.9 **Fall from other slipping, tripping or stumbling**
Fall on moving sidewalk

E886 **Fall on same level from collision, pushing, or shoving, by or with other person**

Excludes: crushed or pushed by a crowd or human stampede (E917.1, E917.6)

E886.0 **In sports**
Tackles in sports

Excludes: kicked, stepped on, struck by object, in sports (E917.0, E917.5)

E886.9 **Other and unspecified**
Fall from collision of pedestrian (conveyance) with another pedestrian (conveyance)

E887 **Fracture, cause unspecified**

E888 **Other and unspecified fall**
Accidental fall NOS
Fall on same level NOS

E888.0 **Fall resulting in striking against sharp object**
Use additional external cause code to identify object (E920)

E888.1 **Fall resulting in striking against other object**

E888.8 **Other fall**

E888.9 **Unspecified fall**
Fall NOS

ACCIDENTS CAUSED BY FIRE AND FLAMES (E890-E899)

Includes: asphyxia or poisoning due to conflagration or ignition
burning by fire
secondary fires resulting from explosion

Excludes: arson (E968.0)
fire in or on:
  machinery (in operation) (E919.0-E919.9)
  transport vehicle other than stationary vehicle (E800.0-E845.9)
  vehicle not elsewhere classifiable (E846-E848)

E890 **Conflagration in private dwelling**
Includes: conflagration in:
  apartment
  boarding house
  camping place
  caravan
  farmhouse
  house
  lodging house
  mobile home
  private garage
  rooming house
  tenement
conflagration originating from sources classifiable to E893-E898 in the above buildings

E890.0 **Explosion caused by conflagration**

E890.1 **Fumes from combustion of polyvinylchloride [PVC] and similar material in conflagration**

E890.2 **Other smoke and fumes from conflagration**
Carbon monoxide from conflagration in private building
Fumes NOS from conflagration in private building
Smoke NOS from conflagration in private building

Add 4th or 5th digit | Nonspecific code | Unspecified code | Manifestation code

TABULAR LIST

E890.3 **Burning caused by conflagration**

E890.8 **Other accident resulting from conflagration**
Collapse of burning private building
Fall from burning private building
Hit by object falling from burning private building
Jump from burning private building

E890.9 **Unspecified accident resulting from conflagration in private dwelling**

E891 **Conflagration in other and unspecified building or structure**

Conflagration in:	Conflagration in:
barn	farm outbuildings
church	hospital
convalescent and other residential home	hotel
	school
dormitory of educational institution	store
	theater
factory	

Conflagration originating from sources classifiable to E893-E898, in the above buildings

E891.0 **Explosion caused by conflagration**

E891.1 **Fumes from combustion of polyvinylchloride [PVC] and similar material in conflagration**

E891.2 **Other smoke and fumes from conflagration**
Carbon monoxide from conflagration in building or structure
Fumes NOS from conflagration in building or structure
Smoke NOS from conflagration in building or structure

E891.3 **Burning caused by conflagration**

E891.8 **Other accident resulting from conflagration**
Collapse of burning building or structure
Fall from burning building or structure
Hit by object falling from burning building or structure
Jump from burning building or structure

E891.9 **Unspecified accident resulting from conflagration of other and unspecified building or structure**

E892 **Conflagration not in building or structure**
Fire (uncontrolled) (in) (of):
forest
grass
hay
lumber
mine
prairie
transport vehicle [any], except while in transit
tunnel

E893 **Accident caused by ignition of clothing**
Excludes: ignition of clothing:
from highly inflammable material (E894)
with conflagration (E890.0-E892)

E893.0 **From controlled fire in private dwelling**
Ignition of clothing from:
normal fire (charcoal) (coal) (electric) (gas) (wood) in:
brazier in private dwelling (as listed in E890)
fireplace in private dwelling (as listed in E890)
furnace in private dwelling (as listed in E890)
stove in private dwelling (as listed in E890)

E893.1 **From controlled fire in other building or structure**
Ignition of clothing from:
normal fire (charcoal) (coal) (electric) (gas) (wood) in:
brazier in other building or structure (as listed in E891)
fireplace in other building or structure (as listed in E891)
furnace in other building or structure (as listed in E891)
stove in other building or structure (as listed in E891)

● Code new to this edition   ▲ Revision of existing code   ④ ⑤ Fourth or fifth digit required

E CODES

E893.2 From controlled fire not in building or structure
Ignition of clothing from:
   bonfire (controlled)
   brazier fire (controlled), not in building or structure
   trash fire (controlled)

Excludes: conflagration not in building (E892)
   trash fire out of control (E892)

E893.8 From other specified sources
Ignition of clothing from: Ignition of clothing from:
   blowlamp   cigarette
   blowtorch   lighter
   burning bedspread   matches
   candle   pipe
   cigar   welding torch

E893.9 Unspecified source
Ignition of clothing (from controlled fire NOS) (in building NOS) NOS

E894 Ignition of highly inflammable material
Ignition of:
   benzine (with ignition of clothing)
   gasoline (with ignition of clothing)
   fat (with ignition of clothing)
   kerosene (with ignition of clothing)
   paraffin (with ignition of clothing)
   petrol (with ignition of clothing)

Excludes: ignition of highly inflammable material with:
   conflagration (E890.0-E892)
   explosion (E923.0-E923.9)

E895 Accident caused by controlled fire in private dwelling
Burning by (flame of) normal fire (charcoal) (coal) (electric) (gas) (wood) in:
   brazier in private dwelling (as listed in E890)
   fireplace in private dwelling (as listed in E890)
   furnace in private dwelling (as listed in E890)
   stove in private dwelling (as listed in E890)

Excludes: burning by hot objects not producing fire or flames (E924.0-E924.9)
   ignition of clothing from these sources (E893.0)
   poisoning by carbon monoxide from incomplete combustion of fuel (E867-E868.9)
   that with conflagration (E890.0-E890.9)

E896 Accident caused by controlled fire in other and unspecified building or structure
Burning by (flame of) normal fire (charcoal) (coal) (electric) (gas) (wood) in:
   brazier in other building or structure (as listed in E891)
   fireplace in other building or structure (as listed in E891)
   furnace in other building or structure (as listed in E891)
   stove in other building or structure (as listed in E891)

Excludes: burning by hot objects not producing fire or flames (E924.0-E924.9)
   ignition of clothing from these sources (E893.1)
   poisoning by carbon monoxide from incomplete combustion of fuel (E867-E868.9)
   that with conflagration (E891.0-E891.9)

E897 Accident caused by controlled fire not in building or structure
Burns from flame of:
   bonfire (controlled)
   brazier fire (controlled), not in building or structure
   trash fire (controlled)

Excludes: ignition of clothing from these sources (E893.2)
   trash fire out of control (E892)
   that with conflagration (E892)

E898 Accident caused by other specified fire and flames
Excludes: conflagration (E890.0-E892)
   that with ignition of:
      clothing (E893.0-E893.9)
      highly inflammable material (E894)

E898.0 Burning bedclothes
Bed set on fire NOS

681

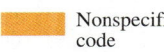 Add 4th or 5th digit   Nonspecific code   Unspecified code   Manifestation code

TABULAR LIST

E898.1 **Other**
    Burning by:
      blowlamp
      blowtorch
      candle
      cigar
      cigarette
      fire in room NOS

    Burning by:
      lamp
      lighter
      matches
      pipe
      welding torch

E899 **Accident caused by unspecified fire**
    Burning NOS

ACCIDENTS DUE TO NATURAL AND ENVIRONMENTAL FACTORS (E900-E909)

E900 **Excessive heat**

  E900.0 **Due to weather conditions**
    Excessive heat as the external cause of:
      ictus solaris
      siriasis
      sunstroke

  E900.1 **Of man-made origin**
    Heat (in):
      boiler room
      drying room
      factory
      furnace room

    Heat (in):
      generated in transport vehicle
      kitchen

  E900.9 **Of unspecified origin**

E901 **Excessive cold**

  E901.0 **Due to weather conditions**
    Excessive cold as the cause of:
      chilblains NOS
      immersion foot

  E901.1 **Of man-made origin**
    Contact with or inhalation of:
      dry ice
      liquid air
      liquid hydrogen
      liquid nitrogen
    Prolonged exposure in:
      deep freeze unit
      refrigerator

  E901.8 **Other specified origin**

  E901.9 **Of unspecified origin**

E902 **High and low air pressure and changes in air pressure**

  E902.0 **Residence or prolonged visit at high altitude**
    Residence or prolonged visit at high altitude as the cause of:
      Acosta syndrome
      Alpine sickness
      altitude sickness
      Andes disease
      anoxia, hypoxia
      barotitis, barodontalgia, barosinusitis, otitic barotrauma
      hypobarism, hypobaropathy
      mountain sickness
      range disease

  E902.1 **In aircraft**
    Sudden change in air pressure in aircraft during ascent or descent as the cause of:
      aeroneurosis
      aviators' disease

E CODES

E902.2 Due to diving
High air pressure from rapid descent in water as the cause of:
  caisson disease
  divers' disease
  divers' palsy or paralysis
Reduction in atmospheric pressure while surfacing from deep water diving as the cause of:
  caisson disease
  divers' disease
  divers' palsy or paralysis

E902.8 Due to other specified causes
Reduction in atmospheric pressure while surfacing from underground

E902.9 Unspecified cause

E903 Travel and motion

E904 Hunger, thirst, exposure, and neglect
Excludes: any condition resulting from homicidal intent (E968.0-E968.9)
  hunger, thirst, and exposure resulting from accidents connected with transport (E800.0-E848)

E904.0 Abandonment or neglect of infants and helpless persons
Exposure to weather conditions resulting from abandonment or neglect
Hunger or thirst resulting from abandonment or neglect
Desertion of newborn
Inattention at or after birth
Lack of care (helpless person) (infant)
Excludes: criminal [purposeful] neglect (E968.4)

E904.1 Lack of food
Lack of food as the cause of:
  inanition
  insufficient nourishment
  starvation
Excludes: hunger resulting from abandonment or neglect (E904.0)

E904.2 Lack of water
Lack of water as the cause of:
  dehydration
  inanition
Excludes: dehydration due to acute fluid loss (276.51)

E904.3 Exposure (to weather conditions), not elsewhere classifiable
Exposure NOS   Struck by hailstones
Humidity
Excludes: struck by lightning (E907)

E904.9 Privation, unqualified
Destitution

E905 Venomous animals and plants as the cause of poisoning and toxic reactions
Includes: chemical released by animal
  insects
  release of venom through fangs, hairs, spines, tentacles, and other venom apparatus
Excludes: eating of poisonous animals or plants (E865.0-E865.9)

E905.0 Venomous snakes and lizards
Cobra   Mamba
Copperhead snake   Rattlesnake
Coral snake   Sea snake
Fer de lance   Snake (venomous)
Gila monster   Viper
Krait   Water moccasin
Excludes: bites of snakes and lizards known to be nonvenomous (E906.2)

E905.1 Venomous spiders
Black widow spider   Tarantula (venomous)
Brown spider

E905.2 Scorpion

E905.3 Hornets, wasps, and bees
Yellow jacket

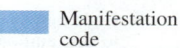

683

TABULAR LIST

E905.4 Centipede and venomous millipede (tropical)

E905.5 Other venomous arthropods
  Sting of:
    ant
    caterpillar

E905.6 Venomous marine animals and plants
  Puncture by sea urchin spine
  Sting of:
    coral
    jelly fish
  Sting of:
    nematocysts
    sea anemone
    sea cucumber
    other marine animal or plant

  Excludes: bites and other injuries caused by nonvenomous marine animal (E906.2-E906.8)
    bite of sea snake (venomous) (E905.0)

E905.7 Poisoning and toxic reactions caused by other plants
  Injection of poisons or toxins into or through skin by plant thorns, spines, or other mechanisms

  Excludes: puncture wound NOS by plant thorns or spines (E920.8)

E905.8 Other specified

E905.9 Unspecified
  Sting NOS   Venomous bite NOS

E906 Other injury caused by animals

  Excludes: poisoning and toxic reactions caused by venomous animals and insects (E905.0-E905.9)
    road vehicle accident involving animals (E827.0-E828.9)
    tripping or falling over an animal (E885.9)

E906.0 Dog bite

E906.1 Rat bite

E906.2 Bite of nonvenomous snakes and lizards

E906.3 Bite of other animal except arthropod
  Cats   Rodents, except rats
  Moray eel   Shark

E906.4 Bite of nonvenomous arthropod
  Insect bite NOS

E906.5 Bite by unspecified animal
  Animal bite NOS

E906.8 Other specified injury caused by animal
  Butted by animal
  Fallen on by horse or other animal, not being ridden
  Gored by animal
  Implantation of quills of porcupine
  Pecked by bird
  Run over by animal, not being ridden
  Stepped on by animal, not being ridden

  Excludes: injury by animal being ridden (E828.0-E828.9)

E906.9 Unspecified injury caused by animal

E907 Lightning

  Excludes: injury from:
    fall of tree or other object caused by lightning (E916)
    fire caused by lightning (E890.0-E892)

E908 Cataclysmic storms, and floods resulting from storms

  Excludes: collapse of dam or man-made structure causing flood (E909.3)

E908.0 Hurricane
  Storm surge
  "Tidal wave" caused by storm action
  Typhoon

E908.1 Tornado
  Cyclone
  Twisters

E CODES

E908.2 Floods
    Torrential rainfall
    Flash flood

> *Excludes:* collapse of dam or man-made structure causing flood (909.3)

E908.3 Blizzard (snow) (ice)

E908.4 Dust storm

E908.8 Other cataclysmic storms

E908.9 Unspecified cataclysmic storms, and floods resulting from storms
    Storm NOS

E909 Cataclysmic earth surface movements and eruptions

> *Excludes:* "tidal wave" caused by storm action (E908.0)
> transport accident involving collision with avalanche or landslide not in motion (E800.0-E848)

E909.0 Earthquakes

E909.1 Volcanic eruptions
    Burns from lava
    Ash inhalation

E909.2 Avalanche, landslide, or mudslide

E909.3 Collapse of dam or man-made structure

E909.4 Tidal wave caused by earthquake
    Tidal wave NOS
    Tsunami

> *Excludes:* tidal wave caused by tropical storm (E908.0)

E909.8 Other cataclysmic earth surface movements and eruptions

E909.9 Unspecified cataclysmic earth surface movements and eruptions

ACCIDENTS CAUSED BY SUBMERSION, SUFFOCATION, AND FOREIGN BODIES (E910-E915)

E910 Accidental drowning and submersion
    Includes: immersion
                 swimmers' cramp

> *Excludes:* diving accident (NOS) (resulting in injury except drowning) (E883.0)
>   diving with insufficient air supply (E913.2)
>   drowning and submersion due to:
>   cataclysm (E908-E909)
>   machinery accident (E919.0-E919.9)
>   transport accident (E800.0-E845.9)
>   effect of high and low air pressure (E902.2)
>   injury from striking against objects while in running water (E917.2)

E910.0 While water-skiing
    Fall from water skis with submersion or drowning

> *Excludes:* accident to water-skier involving a watercraft and resulting in submersion or other injury (E830.4, E831.4)

E910.1 While engaged in other sport or recreational activity with diving equipment
    Scuba diving NOS
    Skin diving NOS
    Underwater spear fishing NOS

E910.2 While engaged in other sport or recreational activity without diving equipment
    Fishing or hunting, except from boat or with diving equipment
    Ice skating
    Playing in water
    Surfboarding
    Swimming NOS
    Voluntarily jumping from boat, not involved in accident, for swim NOS
    Wading in water

> *Excludes:* jumping into water to rescue another person (E910.3)

E910.3 While swimming or diving for purposes other than recreation or sport
    Marine salvage (with diving equipment)
    Pearl diving (with diving equipment)
    Placement of fishing nets (with diving equipment)
    Rescue (attempt) of another person (with diving equipment)
    Underwater construction or repairs (with diving equipment)

TABULAR LIST

E910.4 **In bathtub**

E910.8 **Other accidental drowning or submersion**
Drowning in:
quenching tank
swimming pool

E910.9 **Unspecified accidental drowning or submersion**
Accidental fall into water NOS
Drowning NOS

E911 **Inhalation and ingestion of food causing obstruction of respiratory tract or suffocation**
Aspiration and inhalation of food [any] (into respiratory tract) NOS
Asphyxia by food [including bone, seed in food, regurgitated food]
Choked on food [including bone, seed in food, regurgitated food]
Suffocation by food [including bone, seed in food, regurgitated food]
Compression of trachea by food lodged in esophagus
Interruption of respiration by food lodged in esophagus
Obstruction of respiration by food lodged in esophagus
Obstruction of pharynx by food (bolus)

Excludes: injury, except asphyxia and obstruction of respiratory passage, caused by food (E915)
obstruction of esophagus by food without mention of asphyxia or obstruction of respiratory passage (E915)

E912 **Inhalation and ingestion of other object causing obstruction of respiratory tract or suffocation**
Aspiration and inhalation of foreign body except food (into respiratory tract) NOS
Foreign object [bean] [marble] in nose
Obstruction of pharynx by foreign body
Compression by foreign body in esophagus
Interruption of respiration by foreign body in esophagus
Obstruction of respiration by foreign body in esophagus

Excludes: injury, except asphyxia and obstruction of respiratory passage, caused by foreign body (E915)
obstruction of esophagus by foreign body without mention of asphyxia or obstruction in respiratory passage (E915)

E913 **Accidental mechanical suffocation**

Excludes: mechanical suffocation from or by:
accidental inhalation or ingestion of:
food (E911)
foreign object (E912)
cataclysm (E908-E909)
explosion (E921.0-E921.9, E923.0-E923.9)
machinery accident (E919.0-E919.9)

E913.0 **In bed or cradle**

Excludes: suffocation by plastic bag (E913.1)

E913.1 **By plastic bag**

E913.2 **Due to lack of air (in closed place)**
Accidentally closed up in refrigerator or other airtight enclosed space
Diving with insufficient air supply

Excludes: suffocation by plastic bag (E913.1)

E913.3 **By falling earth or other substance**
Cave-in NOS

Excludes: cave-in caused by cataclysmic earth surface movements and eruptions (E909)
struck by cave-in without asphyxiation or suffocation (E916)

E913.8 **Other specified means**
Accidental hanging, except in bed or cradle

E913.9 **Unspecified means**
Asphyxia, mechanical NOS
Strangulation NOS
Suffocation NOS

E914 **Foreign body accidentally entering eye and adnexa**

Excludes: corrosive liquid (E924.1)

E915 **Foreign body accidentally entering other orifice**

Excludes: aspiration and inhalation of foreign body, any, (into respiratory tract) NOS (E911-E912)

E CODES

OTHER ACCIDENTS (E916-E928)

E916 Struck accidentally by falling object
    Collapse of building, except on fire   Object falling from:
    Falling: machine, not in operation
       rock   stationary vehicle
       snowslide NOS
       stone
       tree
    Code first: collapse of building on fire (E890.0-E891.9)
                falling object in:
                     cataclysm (E908-E909)
                     machinery accidents (E919.0-E919.9)
                     transport accidents (E800.0-E845.9)
                     vehicle accidents not elsewhere classifiable (E846-E848)
                object set in motion by:
                     explosion (E921.0-E921.9, E923.0-E923.9)
                     firearm (E922.0-E922.9)
                projected object (E917.0-E917.9)

E917 Striking against or struck accidentally by objects or persons
    Includes: bumping into or against:
                  object (moving) (projected) (stationary)
                  pedestrian conveyance
                  person
            colliding with:
                object (moving) (projected) (stationary)
                pedestrian conveyance
                person
            kicking against:
                object (moving) (projected) (stationary)
                pedestrian conveyance
                person
            stepping on:
                object (moving) (projected) (stationary)
                pedestrian conveyance
                person
            struck by:
                object (moving) (projected) (stationary)
                pedestrian conveyance
                person
    Excludes: fall from collision with another person, except when caused by a crowd
                (E886.0-E886.9)
            fall from stumbling over object (E885.9)
            fall resulting in striking against object (E888.0, E888.1)
            injury caused by:
                assault (E960.0-E960.1, E967.0-E967.9)
                cutting or piercing instrument (E920.0-E920.9)
                explosion (E921.0-E921.9, E923.0-E923.9)
                firearm (E922.0-E922.9)
                machinery (E919.0-E919.9)
                transport vehicle (E800.0-E845.9)
                vehicle not elsewhere classifiable (E846-E848)

    E917.0 In sports without subsequent fall
            Kicked or stepped on during game (football) (rugby)
            Struck by hit or thrown ball
            Struck by hockey stick or puck

    E917.1 Caused by a crowd, by collective fear or panic without subsequent fall
            Crushed by crown or human stampede
            Pushed by crown or human stampede
            Stepped on by crown or human stampede

    E917.2 In running water without subsequent fall
        Excludes: drowning or submersion (E910.0-E910.9)
                that in sports (E917.0, E917.5)

    E917.3 Furniture without subsequent fall
        Excludes: fall from furniture (E884.2, E884.4-E884.5)

    E917.4 Other stationary object without subsequent fall
            Bath tub
            Fence
            Lamp-post

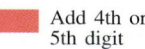 Add 4th or 5th digit   Nonspecific code   Unspecified code   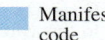 Manifestation code

TABULAR LIST

E917.5 **Object in sports with subsequent fall**
Knocked down while boxing

E917.6 **Caused by a crowd, by collective fear or panic with subsequent fall**

E917.7 **Furniture with subsequent fall**
Excludes: fall from furniture (E884.2, E884.4-E884.5)

E917.8 **Other stationary object with subsequent fall**
Bath tub
Fence
Lamp-post

E917.9 **Other striking against with or without subsequent fall**

E918 **Caught accidentally in or between objects**
Caught, crushed, jammed, or pinched in or between moving or stationary objects, such as:
escalator
folding object
hand tools, appliances, or implements
sliding door and door frame
under packing crate
washing machine wringer

Excludes: injury caused by:
    cutting or piercing instrument (E920.0-E920.9)
    machinery (E919.0-E919.9)
    transport vehicle (E800.0-E845.9)
    vehicle not elsewhere classifiable (E846-E848)
struck accidentally by:
    falling object (E916)
    object (moving) (projected) (E917.0-E917.9)

E919 **Accidents caused by machinery**
Includes:
burned by machinery (accident)
caught in (moving parts of) machinery (accident)
collapse of machinery (accident)
crushed by machinery (accident)
cut or pierced by machinery (accident)
drowning or submersion caused by machinery (accident)
explosion of, on, in machinery (accident)
fall from or into moving part of machinery (accident)
fire starting in or on machinery (accident)
mechanical suffocation caused by machinery (accident)
object falling from, on, in motion by machinery (accident)
overturning of machinery (accident)
pinned under machinery (accident)
run over by machinery (accident)
struck by machinery (accident)
thrown from machinery (accident)
caught between machinery and other object
machinery accident NOS

Excludes: accidents involving machinery, not in operation (E884.9, E916-E918)
injury caused by:
    electric current in connection with machinery (E925.0-E925.9)
    escalator (E880.0, E918)
    explosion of pressure vessel in connection with machinery (E921.0-E921.9)
    moving sidewalk (E885.9)
    powered hand tools, appliances, and implements (E916-E918, E920.0-E921.9, E923.0-E926.9)
    transport vehicle accidents involving machinery (E800.0-E848.9)
    poisoning by carbon monoxide generated by machine (E868.8)

E919.0 **Agriculture machines**
Animal-powered agricultural machine
Combine
Derrick, hay
Farm machinery NOS
Farm tractor
Harvester
Hay mower or rake
Reaper
Thresher

Excludes: that in transport under own power on the highway (E810.0-E819.9)
that being towed by another vehicle on the highway (E810.0-E819.9, E827.0-E827.9, E829.0-E829.9)
that involved in accident classifiable to E820-E829 (E820.0-E829.9)

E CODES

E919.1 Mining and earth-drilling machinery
  Bore or drill (land)   Shaft lift
  (seabed)   Under-cutter
  Shaft hoist

  Excludes: coal car, tram, truck, and tub in mine (E846)

E919.2 Lifting machines and appliances
  Chain hoist except in agricultural or mining operations
  Crane except in agricultural or mining operations
  Derrick except in agricultural or mining operations
  Elevator (building) (grain) except in agricultural or mining operations
  Forklift truck except in agricultural or mining operations
  Lift except in agricultural or mining operations
  Pulley block except in agricultural or mining operations
  Winch except in agricultural or mining operations

  Excludes: that being towed by another vehicle on the highway (E810.0-E819.9, E827.0-E827.9, E829.0-E829.9)
           that in transport under own power on the highway (E810.0-E819.9)
           that involved in accident classifiable to E820-E829 (E820.0-E829.9)

E919.3 Metalworking machines
  Abrasive wheel   Metal:
  Forging machine   drilling machine
  Lathe   milling machine
  Mechanical shears   power press
                                 rolling-mill
                                 sawing machine

E919.4 Woodworking and forming machines
  Band saw   Powered saw
  Bench saw   Radial saw
  Circular saw   Sander
  Molding machine
  Overhead plane

  Excludes: hand saw (E920.1)

E919.5 Prime movers, except electrical motors
  Gas turbine   Steam engine
  Internal combustion engine   Water driven turbine

  Excludes: that being towed by other vehicle on the highway (E810.0-E819.9, E827.0-E827.9, E829.0-E829.9)
           that in transport under own power on the highway (E810.0-E819.9)

E919.6 Transmission machinery
  Transmission: Transmission:
    belt   pinion
    cable   pulley
    chain   shaft
    gear

E919.7 Earth moving, scraping, and other excavating machines
  Bulldozer   Steam shovel
  Road scraper

  Excludes: that being towed by other vehicle on the highway (E810.0-E819.9, E827.0-E827.9, E829.0-E829.9)
           that in transport under own power on the highway (E810.0-E819.9)

E919.8 Other specified machinery
  Machines for manufacture of: Printing machine
    clothing   Recreational machinery
    foodstuffs and beverages   Spinning, weaving, and textile machines
    paper

E919.9 Unspecified machinery

E920 Accidents caused by cutting and piercing instruments or objects
  Includes: accidental injury (by) object:
               edged
               pointed
               sharp

E920.0 Powered lawn mower

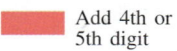 Add 4th or 5th digit
 Nonspecific code
 Unspecified code
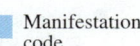 Manifestation code

689

TABULAR LIST

E920.1 **Other powered hand tools**
Any powered hand tool [compressed air] [electric] [explosive cartridge] [hydraulic power], such as:
- drill
- hand saw
- hedge clipper
- rivet gun
- snow blower
- staple gun

Excludes: band saw (E919.4)
bench saw (E919.4)

E920.2 **Powered household appliances and implements**
- Blender
- Electric:
  - beater or mixer
  - can opener
  - fan
- Electric:
  - knife
  - sewing machine
- Garbage disposal appliance

E920.3 **Knives, swords, and daggers**

E920.4 **Other hand tools and implements**
- Axe
- Can opener NOS
- Chisel
- Fork
- Hand saw
- Hoe
- Ice pick
- Needle (sewing)
- Paper cutter
- Pitchfork
- Rake
- Scissors
- Screwdriver
- Sewing machine, not powered
- Shovel

E920.5 **Hypodermic needle**
- Contaminated needle
- Needle stick

E920.8 **Other specified cutting and piercing instruments or objects**
- Arrow
- Broken glass
- Dart
- Edge of stiff paper
- Lathe turnings
- Nail
- Plant thorn
- Splinter
- Tin can lid

Excludes: animal spines or quills (E906.8)
flying glass due to explosion (E921.0-E923.9)

E920.9 **Unspecified cutting and piercing instrument or object**

E921 **Accident caused by explosion of pressure vessel**
Includes: accidental explosion of pressure vessels, whether or not part of machinery

Excludes: explosion of pressure vessel on transport vehicle (E800.0-E845.9)

E921.0 **Boilers**

E921.1 **Gas cylinders**
- Air tank
- Pressure gas tank

E921.8 **Other specified pressure vessels**
- Aerosol can
- Automobile tire
- Pressure cooker

E921.9 **Unspecified pressure vessel**

E922 **Accident caused by firearm and air gun missile**

E922.0 **Handgun**
- Pistol
- Revolver

Excludes: Verey pistol (E922.8)

E922.1 **Shotgun (automatic)**

E922.2 **Hunting rifle**

E922.3 **Military firearms**
- Army rifle
- Machine gun

E922.4 **Air gun**
- BB gun
- Pellet gun

E922.5 **Paintball gun**

E922.8 **Other specified firearm missile**
- Verey pistol [flare]

E922.9 **Unspecified firearm missile**
- Gunshot wound NOS
- Shot NOS

E CODES

E923 **Accident caused by explosive material**
    Includes: flash burns and other injuries resulting from explosion of explosive material
                       ignition of highly explosive material with explosion

    Excludes: explosion:
                 in or on machinery (E919.0-E919.9)
                 on any transport vehicle, except stationary motor vehicle (E800.0-E848)
                 with conflagration (E890.0, E891.0, E892)
                 secondary fires resulting from explosion (E890.0-E899)

    E923.0   **Fireworks**

    E923.1   **Blasting materials**
            Blasting cap   Explosive [any] used in blasting operations
            Detonator
            Dynamite

    E923.2   **Explosive gases**
            Acetylene   Fire damp
            Butane   Gasoline fumes
            Coal gas   Methane
            Explosion in mine NOS   Propane

    E923.8   **Other explosive materials**
            Bomb   Torpedo
            Explosive missile   Explosion in munitions:
            Grenade   dump
            Mine   factory
            Shell

    E923.9   **Unspecified explosive material**
            Explosion NOS

E924 **Accident caused by hot substance or object, caustic or corrosive material, and steam**

    Excludes: burning NOS (E899)
                 chemical burn resulting from swallowing a corrosive substance (E860.0-E864.4)
                 fire caused by these substances and objects (E890.0-E894)
                 radiation burns (E926.0-E926.9)
                 therapeutic misadventures (E870.0-E876.9)

    E924.0   **Hot liquids and vapors, including steam**
            Burning or scalding by:
                boiling water
                hot or boiling liquids not primarily caustic or corrosive
                liquid metal
                steam
                other hot vapor

        Excludes: hot (boiling) tap water (E924.2)

    E924.1   **Caustic and corrosive substances**
            Burning by:
                acid [any kind]
                ammonia
                caustic oven cleaner or other substance
                corrosive substance
                lye
                vitriol

    E924.2   **Hot (boiling) tap water**

    E924.8   **Other**
            Burning by:
                heat from electric heating appliance
                hot object NOS
                light bulb
                steam pipe

    E924.9   **Unspecified**

TABULAR LIST

E925 **Accident caused by electric current**
Includes: electric current from exposed wire, faulty appliance, high voltage cable, live rail, or open electric socket as the cause of:
burn
cardiac fibrillation
convulsion
electric shock
electrocution
puncture wound
respiratory paralysis

Excludes: burn by heat from electrical appliance (E924.8)
lightning (E907)

E925.0 **Domestic wiring and appliances**

E925.1 **Electric power generating plants, distribution stations, transmission lines**
Broken power line

E925.2 **Industrial wiring, appliances, and electrical machinery**
Conductors
Control apparatus
Electrical equipment and machinery
Transformers

E925.8 **Other electric current**
Wiring and appliances in or on:
farm [not farmhouse]
outdoors
public building
residential institutions
schools

E925.9 **Unspecified electric current**
Burns or other injury from electric current NOS
Electric shock NOS
Electrocution NOS

E926 **Exposure to radiation**

Excludes: abnormal reaction to or complication of treatment without mention of misadventure (E879.2)
atomic power plant malfunction in water transport (E838.0-E838.9)
misadventure to patient in surgical and medical procedures (E873.2-E873.3)
use of radiation in war operations (E996-E997.9)

E926.0 **Radiofrequency radiation**
Overexposure to:
microwave radiation from:
high-powered radio and television transmitters
industrial radiofrequency induction heaters
radar installations
radar radiation from:
high-powered radio and television transmitters
industrial radiofrequency induction heaters
radar installations
radiofrequency from:
high-powered radio and television transmitters
industrial radiofrequency induction heaters
radar installations
radiofrequency radiation [any] from:
high-powered radio and television transmitters
industrial radiofrequency induction heaters
radar installations

E926.1 **Infra-red heaters and lamps**
Exposure to infra-red radiation from heaters and lamps as the cause of:
blistering
burning
charring
inflammatory change

Excludes: physical contact with heater or lamp (E924.8)

E CODES

E926.2 Visible and ultraviolet light sources
Arc lamps
Black light sources
Electrical welding arc
Oxygas welding torch
Sun rays
Tanning bed

Excludes: excessive heat from these sources (E900.1-E900.9)

E926.3 X-rays and other electromagnetic ionizing radiation
Gamma rays
X-rays (hard) (soft)

E926.4 Lasers

E926.5 Radioactive isotopes
Radiobiologicals
Radiopharmaceuticals

E926.8 Other specified radiation
Artificially accelerated beams of ionized particles generated by:
  betatrons
  synchrotrons

E926.9 Unspecified radiation
Radiation NOS

E927 Overexertion and strenuous movements
Excessive physical exercise
Overexertion (from):
  lifting
  pulling
  pushing
Strenuous movements in:
  recreational activities
  other activities

E928 Other and unspecified environmental and accidental causes

E928.0 Prolonged stay in weightless environment
Weightlessness in spacecraft (simulator)

E928.1 Exposure to noise
Noise (pollution)
Sound waves
Supersonic waves

E928.2 Vibration

E928.3 Human bite

E928.4 External constriction caused by hair

E928.5 External constriction caused by other object

● **E928.6 Environmental exposure to harmful algae and toxins**
Algae bloom NOS
Blue-green algae bloom
Brown tide
Cyanobacteria bloom
Florida red tide
Harmful algae bloom
Pfisteria piscicida
Red tide

E928.8 Other

E928.9 Unspecified accident
Accident NOS stated as accidentally inflicted
Blow NOS stated as accidentally inflicted
Casualty (not due to war), stated as accidentally inflicted, but not otherwise specified
Decapitation, stated as accidentally inflicted, but not otherwise specified
Injury [any part of body, or unspecified], stated as accidentally inflicted, but not otherwise specified
Killed, stated as accidentally inflicted, but not otherwise specified
Knocked down, stated as accidentally inflicted, but not otherwise specified
Mangled, stated as accidentally inflicted, but not otherwise specified
Wound, stated as accidentally inflicted, but not otherwise specified

Excludes: fracture, cause unspecified (E887)
injuries undetermined whether accidentally or purposely inflicted (E980.0-E989)

TABULAR LIST

LATE EFFECTS OF ACCIDENTAL INJURY (E929)

Note: This category is to be used to indicate accidental injury as the cause of death or disability from late effects, which are themselves classifiable elsewhere. The "late effects" include conditions reported as such or as sequelae which may occur at any time after the acute injury.

E929 Late effects of accidental injury

Excludes: late effects of:
surgical and medical procedures (E870.0-E879.9)
therapeutic use of drugs and medicines (E930.0-E949.9)

E929.0 Late effects of motor vehicle accident
Late effects of accidents classifiable to E810-E825

E929.1 Late effects of other transport accident
Late effects of accidents classifiable to E800-E807, E826-E838, E840-E848

E929.2 Late effects of accidental poisoning
Late effects of accidents classifiable to E850-E858, E860-E869

E929.3 Late effects of accidental fall
Late effects of accidents classifiable to E880-E888

E929.4 Late effects of accident caused by fire
Late effects of accidents classifiable to E890-E899

E929.5 Late effects of accident due to natural and environmental factors
Late effects of accidents classifiable to E900-E909

E929.8 Late effects of other accidents
Late effects of accidents classifiable to E910-E928.8

E929.9 Late effects of unspecified accident
Late effects of accidents classifiable to E928.9

DRUGS, MEDICINAL AND BIOLOGICAL SUBSTANCES CAUSING ADVERSE EFFECTS IN THERAPEUTIC USE (E930-E949)

Includes: correct drug properly administered in therapeutic or prophylactic dosage, as the cause of any adverse effect including allergic or hypersensitivity reactions

Excludes: accidental overdose of drug and wrong drug given or taken in error (E850.0-E858.9)
accidents in the technique of administration of drug or biological substance, such as accidental puncture during injection, or contamination of drug (E870.0-E876.9)
administration with suicidal or homicidal intent or intent to harm, or in circumstances classifiable to E980-E989 (E950.0-E950.5, E962.0, E980.0-E980.5)

See Alphabetic Index for more complete list of specific drugs to be classified under the fourth-digit subdivisions. The American Hospital Formulary numbers can be used to classify new drugs listed by the American Hospital Formulary Service (AHFS). See appendix C.

E930 Antibiotics

Excludes: that used as eye, ear, nose, and throat [ENT], and local anti-infectives (E946.0-E946.9)

E930.0 **Penicillins**
Natural
Synthetic
Semisynthetic, such as:
ampicillin
cloxacillin
nafcillin
oxacillin

E930.1 **Antifungal antibiotics**
Amphotericin B
Griseofulvin
Hachimycin [trichomycin]
Nystatin

E930.2 **Chloramphenicol group**
Chloramphenicol
Thiamphenicol

E930.3 **Erythromycin and other macrolides**
Oleandomycin
Spiramycin

E CODES

E930.4 **Tetracycline group**
- Doxycycline
- Minocycline
- Oxytetracycline

E930.5 **Cephalosporin group**
- Cephalexin
- Cephaloglycin
- Cephaloridine
- Cephalothin

E930.6 **Antimycobacterial antibiotics**
- Cycloserine
- Kanamycin
- Rifampin
- Streptomycin

E930.7 **Antineoplastic antibiotics**
- Actinomycins, such as:
  - Cactinomycin
  - Dactinomycin
- Bleomycin
- Daunorubicin
- Mitomycin

Excludes: other antineoplastic drugs (E933.1)

E930.8 **Other specified antibiotics**

E930.9 **Unspecified antibiotic**

E931 Other anti-infectives

Excludes: ENT, and local anti-infectives (E946.0-E946.9)

E931.0 **Sulfonamides**
- Sulfadiazine
- Sulfafurazole
- Sulfamethoxazole

E931.1 **Arsenical anti-infectives**

E931.2 **Heavy metal anti-infectives**
- Compounds of:
  - antimony
  - bismuth
  - lead
  - mercury

Excludes: mercurial diuretics (E944.0)

E931.3 **Quinoline and hydroxyquinoline derivatives**
- Chiniofon
- Diiodohydroxyquin

Excludes: antimalarial drugs (E931.4)

E931.4 **Antimalarials and drugs acting on other blood protozoa**
- Chloroquine phosphate
- Cycloguanil
- Primaquine
- Proguanil [chloroguanide]
- Pyrimethamine
- Quinine (sulphate)

E931.5 **Other antiprotozoal drugs**
- Emetine

E931.6 **Anthelmintics**
- Hexylresorcinol
- Male fern oleoresin
- Piperazine
- Thiabendazole

E931.7 **Antiviral drugs**
- Methisazone

Excludes: amantadine (E936.4)
cytarabine (E933.1)
idoxuridine (E946.5)

E931.8 **Other antimycobacterial drugs**
- Ethambutol
- Ethionamide
- Isoniazid
- Para-aminosalicylic acid derivatives
- Sulfones

E931.9 **Other and unspecified anti-infectives**
- Flucytosine
- Nitrofuran derivatives

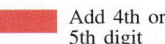 Add 4th or 5th digit
 Nonspecific code
 Unspecified code
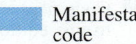 Manifestation code

TABULAR LIST

E932 **Hormones and synthetic substitutes**

- **E932.0** **Adrenal cortical steroids**
  - Cortisone derivatives
  - Desoxycorticosterone derivatives
  - Fluorinated corticosteroids

- **E932.1** **Androgens and anabolic congeners**
  - Nandrolone phenpropionate
  - Oxymetholone
  - Testosterone and preparations

- **E932.2** **Ovarian hormones and synthetic substitutes**
  - Contraceptives, oral
  - Estrogens
  - Estrogens and progestogens combined
  - Progestogens

- **E932.3** **Insulins and antidiabetic agents**
  - Acetohexamide
  - Biguanide derivatives, oral
  - Chlorpropamide
  - Glucagon
  - Insulin
  - Phenformin
  - Sulfonylurea derivatives, oral
  - Tolbutamide

  Excludes: adverse effect of insulin administered for shock therapy (E879.3)

- **E932.4** **Anterior pituitary hormones**
  - Corticotropin
  - Gonadotropin
  - Somatotropin [growth hormone]

- **E932.5** **Posterior pituitary hormones**
  - Vasopressin

  Excludes: oxytocic agents (E945.0)

- **E932.6** **Parathyroid and parathyroid derivatives**

- **E932.7** **Thyroid and thyroid derivatives**
  - Dextrothyroxine
  - Levothyroxine sodium
  - Liothyronine
  - Thyroglobulin

- **E932.8** **Antithyroid agents**
  - Iodides
  - Thiouracil
  - Thiourea

- **E932.9** **Other and unspecified hormones and synthetic substitutes**

E933 **Primarily systemic agents**

- **E933.0** **Antiallergic and antiemetic drugs**
  - Antihistamines
  - Chlorpheniramine
  - Diphenhydramine
  - Diphenylpyraline
  - Thonzylamine
  - Tripelennamine

  Excludes: phenothiazine-based tranquilizers (E939.1)

- **E933.1** **Antineoplastic and immunosuppressive drugs**
  - Azathioprine
  - Busulfan
  - Chlorambucil
  - Cyclophosphamide
  - Cytarabine
  - Fluorouracil
  - Mechlorethamine hydrochloride
  - Mercaptopurine
  - Triethylenethiophosphoramide [thio-TEPA]

  Excludes: antineoplastic antibiotics (E930.7)

- **E933.2** **Acidifying agents**

- **E933.3** **Alkalizing agents**

- **E933.4** **Enzymes, not elsewhere classified**
  - Penicillinase

- **E933.5** **Vitamins, not elsewhere classified**
  - Vitamin A
  - Vitamin D

  Excludes: nicotinic acid (E942.2)
  vitamin K (E934.3)

- ● **E933.6** **Oral bisphosphonates**

- ● **E933.7** **Intravenous bisphosphonates**

- **E933.8** **Other systemic agents, not elsewhere classified**
  - Heavy metal antagonists

E CODES

- **E933.9** Unspecified systemic agent

E934 Agents primarily affecting blood constituents

- **E934.0** Iron and its compounds
  - Ferric salts
  - Ferrous sulphate and other ferrous salts

- **E934.1** Liver preparations and other antianemic agents
  - Folic acid

- **E934.2** Anticoagulants
  - Coumarin
  - Heparin
  - Phenindione
  - Prothrombin synthesis inhibitor
  - Warfarin sodium

- **E934.3** Vitamin K [phytonadione]

- **E934.4** Fibrinolysis-affecting drugs
  - Aminocaproic acid
  - Streptodornase
  - Streptokinase
  - Urokinase

- **E934.5** Anticoagulant antagonists and other coagulants
  - Hexadimethrine bromide
  - Protamine sulfate

- **E934.6** Gamma globulin

- **E934.7** Natural blood and blood products
  - Blood plasma
  - Human fibrinogen
  - Packed red cells
  - Whole blood

- **E934.8** Other agents affecting blood constituents
  - Macromolecular blood substitutes

- **E934.9** Unspecified agent affecting blood constituents

E935 Analgesics, antipyretics, and antirheumatics

- **E935.0** Heroin
  - Diacetylmorphine

- **E935.1** Methadone

- **E935.2** Other opiates and related narcotics
  - Codeine [methylmorphine]
  - Morphine
  - Opium (alkaloids)
  - Meperidine [pethidine]

- **E935.3** Salicylates
  - Acetylsalicylic acid [aspirin]
  - Amino derivatives of salicylic acid
  - Salicylic acid salts

- **E935.4** Aromatic analgesics, not elsewhere classified
  - Acetanilid
  - Paracetamol [acetaminophen]
  - Phenacetin [acetophenetidin]

- **E935.5** Pyrazole derivatives
  - Aminophenazone [aminopyrine]
  - Phenylbutazone

- **E935.6** Antirheumatics [antiphlogistics]
  - Gold salts
  - Indomethacin
  - *Excludes:* salicylates (E935.3)
    steroids (E932.0)

- **E935.7** Other non-narcotic analgesics
  - Pyrabital

- **E935.8** Other specified analgesics and antipyretics
  - Pentazocine

- **E935.9** Unspecified analgesic and antipyretic

E936 Anticonvulsants and anti-Parkinsonism drugs

- **E936.0** Oxazolidine derivatives
  - Paramethadione
  - Trimethadione

- **E936.1** Hydantoin derivatives
  - Phenytoin

- **E936.2** Succinimides
  - Ethosuximide
  - Phensuximide

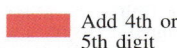 Add 4th or 5th digit
 Nonspecific code
 Unspecified code
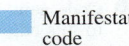 Manifestation code

697

TABULAR LIST

E936.3 **Other and unspecified anticonvulsants**
 Beclamide
 Primidone

E936.4 **Anti-Parkinsonism drugs**
 Amantadine
 Ethopropazine [profenamine]
 Levodopa [L-dopa]

E937 **Sedatives and hypnotics**

E937.0 **Barbiturates**
 Amobarbital [amylobarbitone]
 Barbital [barbitone]
 Butabarbital [butabarbitone]
 Pentobarbital [pentobarbitone]
 Phenobarbital [phenobarbitone]
 Secobarbital [quinalbarbitone]
 Excludes: thiobarbiturates (E938.3)

E937.1 **Chloral hydrate group**

E937.2 **Paraldehyde**

E937.3 **Bromine compounds**
 Bromide
 Carbromal (derivatives)

E937.4 **Methaqualone compounds**

E937.5 **Glutethimide group**

E937.6 **Mixed sedatives, not elsewhere classified**

E937.8 **Other sedatives and hypnotics**

E937.9 **Unspecified**
 Sleeping:
  drug NOS
  pill NOS
  tablet NOS

E938 **Other central nervous system depressants and anesthetics**

E938.0 **Central nervous system muscle-tone depressants**
 Chlorphenesin (carbamate) Methocarbamol
 Mephenesin

E938.1 **Halothane**

E938.2 **Other gaseous anesthetics**
 Ether
 Halogenated hydrocarbon derivatives, except halothane
 Nitrous oxide

E938.3 **Intravenous anesthetics**
 Ketamine Thiobarbiturates, such as thiopental sodium
 Methohexital
 [methohexitone]

E938.4 **Other and unspecified general anesthetics**

E938.5 **Surface and infiltration anesthetics**
 Cocaine Procaine
 Lidocaine [lignocaine] Tetracaine

E938.6 **Peripheral nerve- and plexus-blocking anesthetics**

E938.7 **Spinal anesthetics**

E938.9 **Other and unspecified local anesthetics**

E939 **Psychotropic agents**

E939.0 **Antidepressants**
 Amitriptyline Monoamine oxidase [MAO] inhibitors
 Imipramine

E939.1 **Phenothiazine-based tranquilizers**
 Chlorpromazine Prochlorperazine
 Fluphenazine Promazine
 Phenothiazine

E939.2 **Butyrophenone-based tranquilizers**
 Haloperidol Trifluperidol
 Spiperone

E CODES

E939.3 **Other antipsychotics, neuroleptics, and major tranquilizers**

E939.4 **Benzodiazepine-based tranquilizers**
    Chlordiazepoxide   Lorazepam
    Diazepam   Medazepam
    Flurazepam   Nitrazepam

E939.5 **Other tranquilizers**
    Hydroxyzine   Meprobamate

E939.6 **Psychodysleptics [hallucinogens]**
    Cannabis (derivatives)   Mescaline
    Lysergide [LSD]   Psilocin
    Marihuana (derivatives)   Psilocybin

E939.7 **Psychostimulants**
    Amphetamine   Caffeine
    Excludes: central appetite depressants (E947.0)

E939.8 **Other psychotropic agents**

E939.9 **Unspecified psychotropic agent**

E940 **Central nervous system stimulants**

  E940.0 **Analeptics**
    Lobeline
    Nikethamide

  E940.1 **Opiate antagonists**
    Levallorphan
    Nalorphine
    Naloxone

  E940.8 **Other specified central nervous system stimulants**

  E940.9 **Unspecified central nervous system stimulant**

E941 **Drugs primarily affecting the autonomic nervous system**

  E941.0 **Parasympathomimetics [cholinergics]**
    Acetylcholine   Pilocarpine
    Anticholinesterase:
      organophosphorus
      reversible

  E941.1 **Parasympatholytics [anticholinergics and antimuscarinics] and spasmolytics**
    Atropine   Hyoscine [scopolamine]
    Homatropine   Quaternary ammonium derivatives
    Excludes: papaverine (E942.5)

  E941.2 **Sympathomimetics [adrenergics]**
    Epinephrine [adrenalin]
    Levarterenol [noradrenalin]

  E941.3 **Sympatholytics [antiadrenergics]**
    Phenoxybenzamine
    Tolazoline hydrochloride

  E941.9 **Unspecified drug primarily affecting the autonomic nervous system**

E942 **Agents primarily affecting the cardiovascular system**

  E942.0 **Cardiac rhythm regulators**
    Practolol   Propranolol
    Procainamide   Quinidine

  E942.1 **Cardiotonic glycosides and drugs of similar action**
    Digitalis glycosides   Strophantins
    Digoxin

  E942.2 **Antilipemic and antiarteriosclerotic drugs**
    Cholestyramine   Nicotinic acid derivatives
    Clofibrate   Sitosterols
    Excludes: dextrothyroxine (E932.7)

  E942.3 **Ganglion-blocking agents**
    Pentamethonium bromide

  E942.4 **Coronary vasodilators**
    Dipyridamole   Nitrites
    Nitrates [nitroglycerin]   Prenylamine

TABULAR LIST

E942.5 **Other vasodilators**
    Cyclandelate   Hydralazine
    Diazoxide   Papaverine

E942.6 **Other antihypertensive agents**
    Clonidine   Rauwolfia alkaloids
    Guanethidine   Reserpine

E942.7 **Antivaricose drugs, including sclerosing agents**
    Monoethanolamine   Zinc salts

E942.8 **Capillary-active drugs**
    Adrenochrome derivatives   Metaraminol
    Bioflavonoids

E942.9 **Other and unspecified agents primarily affecting the cardiovascular system**

E943 **Agents primarily affecting gastrointestinal system**

E943.0 **Antacids and antigastric secretion drugs**
    Aluminum hydroxide   Magnesium trisilicate

E943.1 **Irritant cathartics**
    Bisacodyl   Phenolphthalein
    Castor oil

E943.2 **Emollient cathartics**
    Sodium dioctyl sulfosuccinate

E943.3 **Other cathartics, including intestinal atonia drugs**
    Magnesium sulfate

E943.4 **Digestants**
    Pancreatin   Pepsin
    Papain

E943.5 **Antidiarrheal drugs**
    Bismuth subcarbonate   Pectin
    Kaolin
    Excludes: anti-infectives (E930.0-E931.9)

E943.6 **Emetics**

E943.8 **Other specified agents primarily affecting the gastrointestinal system**

E943.9 **Unspecified agent primarily affecting the gastrointestinal system**

E944 **Water, mineral, and uric acid metabolism drugs**

E944.0 **Mercurial diuretics**
    Chlormerodrin   Mercurophylline
    Mercaptomerin   Mersalyl

E944.1 **Purine derivative diuretics**
    Theobromine   Theophylline
    Excludes: aminophylline [theophylline ethylenediamine] (E945.7)

E944.2 **Carbonic acid anhydrase inhibitors**
    Acetazolamide

E944.3 **Saluretics**
    Benzothiadiazides
    Chlorothiazide group

E944.4 **Other diuretics**
    Ethacrynic acid
    Furosemide

E944.5 **Electrolytic, caloric, and water-balance agents**

E944.6 **Other mineral salts, not elsewhere classified**

E944.7 **Uric acid metabolism drugs**
    Cinchophen and congeners   Phenoquin
    Colchicine   Probenecid

E945 **Agents primarily acting on the smooth and skeletal muscles and respiratory system**

E945.0 **Oxytocic agents**
    Ergot alkaloids
    Prostaglandins

E945.1 **Smooth muscle relaxants**
    Adiphenine
    Metaproterenol [orciprenaline]
    Excludes: papaverine (E942.5)

E CODES

E945.2 Skeletal muscle relaxants
    Alcuronium chloride
    Suxamethonium chloride

E945.3 Other and unspecified drugs acting on muscles

E945.4 Antitussives
    Dextromethorphan
    Pipazethate hydrochloride

E945.5 Expectorants
    Acetylcysteine   Ipecacuanha
    Cocillana   Terpin hydrate
    Guaifenesin [glyceryl guaiacolate]

E945.6 Anti-common cold drugs

E945.7 Antiasthmatics
    Aminophylline [theophylline ethylenediamine]

E945.8 Other and unspecified respiratory drugs

E946 Agents primarily affecting skin and mucous membrane, ophthalmological, otorhinolaryngological, and dental drugs

E946.0 Local anti-infectives and anti-inflammatory drugs

E946.1 Antipruritics

E946.2 Local astringents and local detergents

E946.3 Emollients, demulcents, and protectants

E946.4 Keratolytics, keratoplastics, other hair treatment drugs and preparations

E946.5 Eye anti-infectives and other eye drugs
    Idoxuridine

E946.6 Anti-infectives and other drugs and preparations for ear, nose, and throat

E946.7 Dental drugs topically applied

E946.8 Other agents primarily affecting skin and mucous membrane
    Spermicides

E946.9 Unspecified agent primarily affecting skin and mucous membrane

E947 Other and unspecified drugs and medicinal substances

E947.0 Dietetics

E947.1 Lipotropic drugs

E947.2 Antidotes and chelating agents, not elsewhere classified

E947.3 Alcohol deterrents

E947.4 Pharmaceutical excipients

E947.8 Other drugs and medicinal substances
    Contrast media used for diagnostic x-ray procedures
    Diagnostic agents and kits

E947.9 Unspecified drug or medicinal substance

E948 Bacterial vaccines

E948.0 BCG vaccine

E948.1 Typhoid and paratyphoid

E948.2 Cholera

E948.3 Plague

E948.4 Tetanus

E948.5 Diphtheria

E948.6 Pertussis vaccine, including combinations with a pertussis component

E948.8 Other and unspecified bacterial vaccines

E948.9 Mixed bacterial vaccines, except combinations with a pertussis component

E949 Other vaccines and biological substances
    Excludes: gamma globulin (E934.6)

E949.0 Smallpox vaccine

E949.1 Rabies vaccine

E949.2 Typhus vaccine

E949.3 Yellow fever vaccine

E949.4 Measles vaccine

Add 4th or 5th digit   Nonspecific code   Unspecified code   Manifestation code

TABULAR LIST

E949.5 Poliomyelitis vaccine
E949.6 Other and unspecified viral and rickettsial vaccines
    Mumps vaccine
E949.7 Mixed viral-rickettsial and bacterial vaccines, except combinations with a pertussis component
    Excludes: combinations with a pertussis component (E948.6)
E949.9 Other and unspecified vaccines and biological substances

SUICIDE AND SELF-INFLICTED INJURY (E950-E959)

    Includes: injuries in suicide and attempted suicide
              self-inflicted injuries specified as intentional

E950 Suicide and self-inflicted poisoning by solid or liquid substances
    E950.0 Analgesics, antipyretics, and antirheumatics
    E950.1 Barbiturates
    E950.2 Other sedatives and hypnotics
    E950.3 Tranquilizers and other psychotropic agents
    E950.4 Other specified drugs and medicinal substances
    E950.5 Unspecified drug or medicinal substances
    E950.6 Agricultural and horticultural chemical and pharmaceutical preparations other than plant foods and fertilizers
    E950.7 Corrosive and caustic substances
            Suicide and self-inflicted poisoning by substances classifiable to E864
    E950.8 Arsenic and its compounds
    E950.9 Other and unspecified solid and liquid substances
E951 Suicide and self-inflicted poisoning by gases in domestic use
    E951.0 Gas distributed by pipeline
    E951.1 Liquefied petroleum gas distributed in mobile containers
    E951.8 Other utility gas
E952 Suicide and self-inflicted poisoning by other gases and vapors
    E952.0 Motor vehicle exhaust gas
    E952.1 Other carbon monoxide
    E952.8 Other specified gases and vapors
    E952.9 Unspecified gases and vapors
E953 Suicide and self-inflicted injury by hanging, strangulation, and suffocation
    E953.0 Hanging
    E953.1 Suffocation by plastic bag
    E953.8 Other specified means
    E953.9 Unspecified means
E954 Suicide and self-inflicted injury by submersion [drowning]
E955 Suicide and self-inflicted injury by firearms, air guns and explosives
    E955.0 Handgun
    E955.1 Shotgun
    E955.2 Hunting rifle
    E955.3 Military firearms
    E955.4 Other and unspecified firearm
            Gunshot NOS
            Shot NOS
    E955.5 Explosives
    E955.6 Air gun
            BB gun
            Pellet gun
    E955.7 Paintball gun
    E955.9 Unspecified
E956 Suicide and self-inflicted injury by cutting and piercing instrument
E957 Suicide and self-inflicted injuries by jumping from high place

E CODES

- **E957.0** Residential premises
- **E957.1** Other man-made structures
- **E957.2** Natural sites
- **E957.9** Unspecified

E958 Suicide and self-inflicted injury by other and unspecified means
- **E958.0** Jumping or lying before moving object
- **E958.1** Burns, fire
- **E958.2** Scald
- **E958.3** Extremes of cold
- **E958.4** Electrocution
- **E958.5** Crashing of motor vehicle
- **E958.6** Crashing of aircraft
- **E958.7** Caustic substances, except poisoning
  - *Excludes:* poisoning by caustic substance (E950.7)
- **E958.8** Other specified means
- **E958.9** Unspecified means

E959 Late effects of self-inflicted injury
Note: This category is to be used to indicate circumstances classifiable to E950-E958 as the cause of death or disability from late effects, which are themselves classifiable elsewhere. The "late effects" include conditions reported as such or as sequelae which may occur at any time after the attempted suicide or self-inflicted injury.

HOMICIDE AND INJURY PURPOSELY INFLICTED BY OTHER PERSONS (E960-E969)

Includes: injuries inflicted by another person with intent to injure or kill, by any means

Excludes: injuries due to:
  legal intervention (E970-E978)
  operations of war (E990-E999)
  terrorism (E979)

E960 Fight, brawl, rape
- **E960.0** Unarmed fight or brawl
  Beatings NOS
  Brawl or fight with hands, fists, feet
  Injured or killed in fight NOS
  - *Excludes:* homicidal:
    injury by weapons (E965.0-E966, E969)
    strangulation (E963)
    submersion (E964)
- **E960.1** Rape

E961 Assault by corrosive or caustic substance, except poisoning
Injury or death purposely caused by corrosive or caustic substance, such as:
  acid [any]
  corrosive substance
  vitriol
- *Excludes:* burns from hot liquid (E968.3)
  chemical burns from swallowing a corrosive substance (E962.0-E962.9)

E962 Assault by poisoning
- **E962.0** Drugs and medicinal substances
  Homicidal poisoning by any drug or medicinal substance
- **E962.1** Other solid and liquid substances
- **E962.2** Other gases and vapors
- **E962.9** Unspecified poisoning

E963 Assault by hanging and strangulation
Homicidal (attempt):
  garrotting or ligature
  hanging
  strangulation
  suffocation

E964 Assault by submersion [drowning]

E965 Assault by firearms and explosives

703

TABULAR LIST

E965.0 Handgun
  Pistol
  Revolver

E965.1 Shotgun

E965.2 Hunting rifle

E965.3 Military firearms

E965.4 Other and unspecified firearm

E965.5 Antipersonnel bomb

E965.6 Gasoline bomb

E965.7 Letter bomb

E965.8 Other specified explosive
  Bomb NOS (placed in) car
  Bomb NOS (placed in) house
  Dynamite

E965.9 Unspecified explosive

E966 Assault by cutting and piercing instrument
  Assassination (attempt), homicide (attempt) by any instrument classifiable under E920
  Homicidal cut, any part of the body
  Homicidal puncture, any part of the body
  Homicidal stab, any part of the body
  Stabbed, any part of the body

E967 Perpetrator of child and adult abuse
  Note: selection of the correct perpetrator code is based on the relationship between the perpetrator and the victim

E967.0 By father, stepfather or boyfriend
  Male partner of child's parent or guardian

E967.1 By other specified person

E967.2 By mother, stepmother or girlfriend
  Female partner of child's parent or guardian

E967.3 By spouse or partner
  Abuse of spouse or partner by ex-spouse or ex-partner

E967.4 By child

E967.5 By sibling

E967.6 By grandparent

E967.7 By other relative

E967.8 By non-related caregiver

E967.9 By unspecified person

E968 Assault by other and unspecified means

E968.0 Fire
  Arson
  Homicidal burns NOS
  Excludes: burns from hot liquid (E968.3)

E968.1 Pushing from a high place

E968.2 Striking by blunt or thrown object

E968.3 Hot liquid
  Homicidal burns by scalding

E968.4 Criminal neglect
  Abandonment of child, infant, or other helpless person with intent to injure or kill

E968.5 Transport vehicle
  Being struck by other vehicle or run down with intent to injure
  Pushed in front of, thrown from, or dragged by moving vehicle with intent to injure

E968.6 Air gun
  BB gun
  Pellet gun

E968.7 Human bite

E968.8 Other specified means

E CODES

E968.9   **Unspecified means**
        Assassination (attempt) NOS   Manslaughter (nonaccidental)
        Homicidal (attempt):   Murder (attempt) NOS
           injury NOS   Violence, non-accidental
           wound NOS

E969   **Late effects of injury purposely inflicted by other person**
      Note: This category is to be used to indicate circumstances classifiable to E960-E968 as the cause of death or disability from late effects, which are themselves classifiable elsewhere. The "late effects" include conditions reported as such, or as sequelae which may occur at any time after the acute injury.

LEGAL INTERVENTION (E970-E978)

      Includes: injuries inflicted by the police or other law-enforcing agents, including military on duty, in the course of arresting or attempting to arrest lawbreakers, suppressing disturbances, maintaining order, and other legal action
                     legal execution
      Excludes: injuries caused by civil insurrections (E990.0-E999)

E970   **Injury due to legal intervention by firearms**
      Gunshot wound
      Injury by:
          machine gun
          revolver
          rifle pellet or rubber bullet
          shot NOS

E971   **Injury due to legal intervention by explosives**
      Injury by:
          dynamite
          explosive shell
          grenade
          mortar bomb

E972   **Injury due to legal intervention by gas**
      Asphyxiation by gas
      Injury by tear gas
      Poisoning by gas

E973   **Injury due to legal intervention by blunt object**
      Hit, struck by:
          baton (nightstick)
          blunt object
          stave

E974   **Injury due to legal intervention by cutting and piercing instrument**
      Cut
      Incised wound
      Injured by bayonet
      Stab wound

E975   **Injury due to legal intervention by other specified means**
      Blow
      Manhandling

E976   **Injury due to legal intervention by unspecified means**

E977   **Late effects of injuries due to legal intervention**
      Note: This category is to be used to indicate circumstances classifiable to E970-E976 as the cause of death or disability from late effects, which are themselves classifiable elsewhere. The "late effects" include conditions reported as such, or as sequelae which may occur at any time after the acute injury due to legal intervention.

E978   **Legal execution**
      All executions performed at the behest of the judiciary or ruling authority [whether permanent or temporary] as:
          asphyxiation by gas   hanging
          beheading, decapitation   poisoning
             (by guillotine)   shooting
          capital punishment   other specified means
          electrocution

       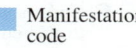

705

TERRORISM (E979)

E979 **Terrorism**
Injuries resulting from the unlawful use of force or violence against persons or property to intimidate or coerce a Government, the civilian population, or any segment thereof, in furtherance of political or social objective

E979.0 **Terrorism involving explosion of marine weapons**
Depth-charge
Marine mine
Mine NOS, at sea or in harbor
Sea-based artillery shell
Torpedo
Underwater blast

E979.1 **Terrorism involving destruction of aircraft**
Aircraft used as a weapon
Aircraft:
  burned
  exploded
  shot down
Crushed by falling aircraft

E979.2 **Terrorism involving other explosions and fragments**
Antipersonnel bomb (fragments)
Blast NOS
Explosion (of):
  artillery shell
  breech-block
  cannon block
  mortar bomb
  munitions being used in terrorism
  NOS
Fragments from:
  artillery shell
  bomb
  grenade
  guided missile
  land-mine
  rocket
  shell
  shrapnel
Mine NOS

E979.3 **Terrorism involving fires, conflagration and hot substances**
Burning building or structure:
  collapse of
  fall from
  hit by falling object in
  jump from
Conflagration NOS
Fire (causing):
  asphyxia
  burns
  NOS
  other injury
Melting of fittings and furniture in burning
Petrol bomb
Smouldering building or structure

E979.4 **Terrorism involving firearms**
Bullet:
  carbine
  machine gun
  pistol
  rifle
  rubber (rifle)
Pellets (shotgun)

E979.5 **Terrorism involving nuclear weapons**
Blast effects
Exposure to ionizing radiation from nuclear weapon
Fireball effects
Heat from nuclear weapon
Other direct and secondary effects of nuclear weapons

E CODES

- **E979.6** Terrorism involving biological weapons
  - Anthrax
  - Cholera
  - Smallpox
- **E979.7** Terrorism involving chemical weapons
  - Gases, fumes, chemicals
  - Hydrogen cyanide
  - Phosgene
  - Sarin
- **E979.8** Terrorism involving other means
  - Drowning and submersion
  - Lasers
  - Piercing or stabbing instruments
  - Terrorism NOS
- **E979.9** Terrorism, secondary effects
  Note: This code is for use to identify conditions occuring subsequent to a terrorist attack not those that are due to the intial terrorist act
  Excludes: late effect of terroist attack (E999.1)

INJURY UNDETERMINED WHETHER ACCIDENTALLY OR PURPOSELY INFLICTED (E980-E989)

Note: Categories E980-E989 are for use when it is unspecified or it cannot be determined whether the injuries are accidental (unintentional), suicide (attempted), or assault.

- **E980** Poisoning by solid or liquid substances, undetermined whether accidentally or purposely inflicted
  - E980.0 Analgesics, antipyretics, and antirheumatics
  - E980.1 Barbiturates
  - **E980.2** Other sedatives and hypnotics
  - **E980.3** Tranquilizers and other psychotropic agents
  - **E980.4** Other specified drugs and medicinal substances
  - **E980.5** Unspecified drug or medicinal substance
  - E980.6 Corrosive and caustic substances
    Poisoning, undetermined whether accidental or purposeful, by substances classifiable to E864
  - E980.7 Agricultural and horticultural chemical and pharmaceutical preparations other than plant foods and fertilizers
  - E980.8 Arsenic and its compounds
  - **E980.9** Other and unspecified solid and liquid substances
- **E981** Poisoning by gases in domestic use, undetermined whether accidentally or purposely inflicted
  - E981.0 Gas distributed by pipeline
  - E981.1 Liquefied petroleum gas distributed in mobile containers
  - **E981.8** Other utility gas
- **E982** Poisoning by other gases, undetermined whether accidentally or purposely inflicted
  - E982.0 Motor vehicle exhaust gas
  - **E982.1** Other carbon monoxide
  - **E982.8** Other specified gases and vapors
  - **E982.9** Unspecified gases and vapors
- **E983** Hanging, strangulation, or suffocation, undetermined whether accidentally or purposely inflicted
  - E983.0 Hanging
  - E983.1 Suffocation by plastic bag
  - **E983.8** Other specified means
  - **E983.9** Unspecified means
- E984 Submersion [drowning], undetermined whether accidentally or purposely inflicted
- **E985** Injury by firearms, air guns and explosives, undetermined whether accidentally or purposely inflicted
  - E985.0 Handgun
  - E985.1 Shotgun

707

TABULAR LIST

- **E985.2** Hunting rifle
- **E985.3** Military firearms
- **E985.4** Other and unspecified firearm
- **E985.5** Explosives
- **E985.6** Air gun
  - BB gun
  - Pellet gun
- **E985.7** Paintball gun

E986 Injury by cutting and piercing instruments, undetermined whether accidentally or purposely inflicted

E987 Falling from high place, undetermined whether accidentally or purposely inflicted
- **E987.0** Residential premises
- **E987.1** Other man-made structures
- **E987.2** Natural sites
- **E987.9** Unspecified site

E988 Injury by other and unspecified means, undetermined whether accidentally or purposely inflicted
- **E988.0** Jumping or lying before moving object
- **E988.1** Burns, fire
- **E988.2** Scald
- **E988.3** Extremes of cold
- **E988.4** Electrocution
- **E988.5** Crashing of motor vehicle
- **E988.6** Crashing of aircraft
- **E988.7** Caustic substances, except poisoning
- **E988.8** Other specified means
- **E988.9** Unspecified means

E989 Late effects of injury, undetermined whether accidentally or purposely inflicted

> Note: This category is to be used to indicate circumstances classifiable to E980-E988 as the cause of death or disability from late effects, which are themselves classifiable elsewhere. The "late effects" include conditions reported as such or as sequelae which may occur at any time after the acute injury, undetermined whether accidentally or purposely inflicted.

INJURY RESULTING FROM OPERATIONS OF WAR (E990-E999)

Includes: injuries to military personnel and civilians caused by war and civil insurrections and occurring during the time of war and insurrection

Excludes: *accidents during training of military personnel, manufacture of war material and transport, unless attributable to enemy action*

E990 Injury due to war operations by fires and conflagrations
Includes: asphyxia, burns, or other injury originating from fire caused by a fire-producing device or indirectly by any conventional weapon
- **E990.0** From gasoline bomb
- **E990.9** From other and unspecified source

E991 Injury due to war operations by bullets and fragments
- **E991.0** Rubber bullets (rifle)
- **E991.1** Pellets (rifle)
- **E991.2** Other bullets
  - Bullet [any, except rubber bullets and pellets]
    - carbine
    - machine gun
    - pistol
    - rifle
    - shotgun
- **E991.3** Antipersonnel bomb (fragments)

E CODES

E991.9 **Other and unspecified fragments**
  Fragments from:
    artillery shell
    bombs, except antipersonnel
    grenade
    guided missile
  Fragments from:
    land mine
    rockets
    shell
    Shrapnel

E992 **Injury due to war operations by explosion of marine weapons**
  Depth charge
  Marine mines
  Mine NOS, at sea or in harbor
  Sea-based artillery shell
  Torpedo
  Underwater blast

E993 **Injury due to war operations by other explosion**
  Accidental explosion of munitions being used in war
  Accidental explosion of own weapons
  Air blast NOS
  Blast NOS
  Explosion NOS
  Explosion of:
    artillery shell
    breech block
    cannon block
    mortar bomb
  Injury by weapon burst

E994 **Injury due to war operations by destruction of aircraft**
  Airplane:
    burned
    exploded
    shot down
  Crushed by falling airplane

E995 **Injury due to war operations by other and unspecified forms of conventional warfare**
  Battle wounds
  Bayonet injury
  Drowned in war operations

E996 **Injury due to war operations by nuclear weapons**
  Blast effects
  Exposure to ionizing radiation from nuclear weapons
  Fireball effects
  Heat
  Other direct and secondary effects of nuclear weapons

E997 **Injury due to war operations by other forms of unconventional warfare**

  E997.0 Lasers

  E997.1 Biological warfare

  E997.2 Gases, fumes, and chemicals

  E997.8 Other specified forms of unconventional warfare

  E997.9 Unspecified form of unconventional warfare

E998 **Injury due to war operations but occurring after cessation of hostilities**
  Injuries due to operations of war but occurring after cessation of hostilities by any means classifiable under E990-E997
  Injuries by explosion of bombs or mines placed in the course of operations of war, if the explosion occurred after cessation of hostilities

E999 **Late effect of injury due to war operations and terrorism**
  Note: This category is to be used to indicate circumstances classifiable to E979, E990-E998 as the cause of death or disability from late effects, which are themselves classifiable elsewhere. The "late effects" include conditions reported as such or as sequelae which may occur at any time after the acute injury, resulting from operations of war or terrorism.

  E999.0 Late effect of injury due to war operations

  E999.1 Late effect of injury due to terrorism

TABULAR LIST

APPENDIX A: MORPHOLOGY OF NEOPLASMS

The World Health Organization has published an adaptation of the International Classification of Diseases for oncology (ICD-O). It contains a coded nomenclature for the morphology of neoplasms, which is reproduced here for those who wish to use it in conjunction with Chapter 2 of the *International Classification of Diseases, 9th Revision, Clinical Modification*.

The morphology code numbers consist of five digits; the first four identify the histological type of the neoplasm and the fifth indicates its behavior. The one-digit behavior code is as follows:

/0 Benign

/1 Uncertain whether benign or malignant
    Borderline malignancy

/2 Carcinoma in situ
    Intraepithelial
    Noninfiltrating
    Noninvasive

/3 Malignant, primary site

/6 Malignant, metastatic site
    Secondary site

/9 Malignant, uncertain whether primary or metastatic site

In the nomenclature below, the morphology code numbers include the behavior code appropriate to the histological type of neoplasm, but this behavior code should be changed if other reported information makes this necessary. For example, "chordoma (M9370/3)" is assumed to be malignant; the term "benign chordoma" should be coded M9370/0. Similarly, "superficial spreading adenocarcinoma (M8143/3)" described as "noninvasive" should be coded M8143/2 and "melanoma (M8720/3)" described as "secondary" should be coded M8720/6.

The following table shows the correspondence between the morphology code and the different sections of Chapter 2:

Morphology code Histology/Behavior			ICD-9-CM Chapter 2
Any	0	210-229	Benign neoplasms
M8000-M8004	1	239	Neoplasms of unspecified nature
M8010+	1	235-238	Neoplasms of uncertain behavior
Any	2	230-234	Carcinoma in situ
Any	3	140-195 200-208	Malignant neoplasms, stated or presumed to be primary
Any	6	196-198	Malignant neoplasms, stated or presumed to be secondary

The ICD-O behavior digit /9 is inapplicable in an ICD context, since all malignant neoplasms are presumed to be primary (/3) or secondary (/6) according to other information on the medical record.

Only the first-listed term of the full ICD-O morphology nomenclature appears against each code number in the list below. The ICD-9-CM Alphabetical Index (Volume 2), however, includes all the ICD-O synonyms as well as a number of other morphological names still likely to be encountered on medical records but omitted from ICD-O as outdated or otherwise undesirable.

A coding difficulty sometimes arises where a morphological diagnosis contains two qualifying adjectives that have different code numbers. An example is "transitional cell epidermoid carcinoma." "Transitional cell carcinoma NOS" is M8120/3 and "epidermoid carcinoma NOS" is M8070/3. In such circumstances, the higher number (M8120/3 in this example) should be used, as it is usually more specific.

APPENDIX A

CODED NOMENCLATURE FOR MORPHOLOGY OF NEOPLASMS

M800   **Neoplasms NOS**
M8000/0   *Neoplasm, benign*
M8000/1   *Neoplasm, uncertain whether benign or malignant*
M8000/3   *Neoplasm, malignant*
M8000/6   *Neoplasm, metastatic*
M8000/9   *Neoplasm, malignant, uncertain whether primary or metastatic*
M8001/0   *Tumor cells, benign*
M8001/1   *Tumor cells, uncertain whether benign or malignant*
M8001/3   *Tumor cells, malignant*
M8002/3   *Malignant tumor, small cell type*
M8003/3   *Malignant tumor, giant cell type*
M8004/3   *Malignant tumor, fusiform cell type*

M801-M804   **Epithelial neoplasms NOS**
M8010/0   *Epithelial tumor, benign*
M8010/2   *Carcinoma in situ NOS*
M8010/3   *Carcinoma NOS*
M8010/6   *Carcinoma, metastatic NOS*
M8010/9   *Carcinomatosis*
M8011/0   *Epithelioma, benign*
M8011/3   *Epithelioma, malignant*
M8012/3   *Large cell carcinoma NOS*
M8020/3   *Carcinoma, undifferentiated type NOS*
M8021/3   *Carcinoma, anaplastic type NOS*
M8022/3   *Pleomorphic carcinoma*
M8030/3   *Giant cell and spindle cell carcinoma*
M8031/3   *Giant cell carcinoma*
M8032/3   *Spindle cell carcinoma*
M8033/3   *Pseudosarcomatous carcinoma*
M8034/3   *Polygonal cell carcinoma*
M8035/3   *Spheroidal cell carcinoma*
M8040/1   *Tumorlet*
M8041/3   *Small cell carcinoma NOS*
M8042/3   *Oat cell carcinoma*
M8043/3   *Small cell carcinoma, fusiform cell type*

M805-M808   **Papillary and squamous cell neoplasms**
M8050/0   *Papilloma NOS (except Papilloma of urinary bladder M8120/1)*
M8050/2   *Papillary carcinoma in situ*
M8050/3   *Papillary carcinoma NOS*
M8051/0   *Verrucous papilloma*
M8051/3   *Verrucous carcinoma NOS*
M8052/0   *Squamous cell papilloma*
M8052/3   *Papillary squamous cell carcinoma*
M8053/0   *Inverted papilloma*
M8060/0   *Papillomatosis NOS*
M8070/2   *Squamous cell carcinoma in situ NOS*
M8070/3   *Squamous cell carcinoma NOS*
M8070/6   *Squamous cell carcinoma, metastatic NOS*
M8071/3   *Squamous cell carcinoma, keratinizing type NOS*
M8072/3   *Squamous cell carcinoma, large cell, nonkeratinizing type*
M8073/3   *Squamous cell carcinoma, small cell, nonkeratinizing type*
M8074/3   *Squamous cell carcinoma, spindle cell type*
M8075/3   *Adenoid squamous cell carcinoma*
M8076/2   *Squamous cell carcinoma in situ with questionable stromal invasion*
M8076/3   *Squamous cell carcinoma, microinvasive*
M8080/2   *Queyrat's erythroplasia*
M8081/2   *Bowen's disease*
M8082/3   *Lymphoepithelial carcinoma*

M809-M811   **Basal cell neoplasms**
M8090/1   *Basal cell tumor*
M8090/3   *Basal cell carcinoma NOS*
M8091/3   *Multicentric basal cell carcinoma*
M8092/3   *Basal cell carcinoma, morphea type*
M8093/3   *Basal cell carcinoma, fibroepithelial type*
M8094/3   *Basosquamous carcinoma*
M8095/3   *Metatypical carcinoma*
M8096/0   *Intraepidermal epithelioma of Jadassohn*
M8100/0   *Trichoepithelioma*
M8101/0   *Trichofolliculoma*

MORPHOLOGY OF NEOPLASMS

M8102/0   *Tricholemmoma*
M8110/0   *Pilomatrixoma*

M812-M813 Transitional cell papillomas and carcinomas
M8120/0   *Transitional cell papilloma NOS*
M8120/1   *Urothelial papilloma*
M8120/2   *Transitional cell carcinoma in situ*
M8120/3   *Transitional cell carcinoma NOS*
M8121/0   *Schneiderian papilloma*
M8121/1   *Transitional cell papilloma, inverted type*
M8121/3   *Schneiderian carcinoma*
M8122/3   *Transitional cell carcinoma, spindle cell type*
M8123/3   *Basaloid carcinoma*
M8124/3   *Cloacogenic carcinoma*
M8130/3   *Papillary transitional cell carcinoma*

M814-M838 Adenomas and adenocarcinomas
M8140/0   *Adenoma NOS*
M8140/1   *Bronchial adenoma NOS*
M8140/2   *Adenocarcinoma in situ*
M8140/3   *Adenocarcinoma NOS*
M8140/6   *Adenocarcinoma, metastatic NOS*
M8141/3   *Scirrhous adenocarcinoma*
M8142/3   *Linitis plastica*
M8143/3   *Superficial spreading adenocarcinoma*
M8144/3   *Adenocarcinoma, intestinal type*
M8145/3   *Carcinoma, diffuse type*
M8146/0   *Monomorphic adenoma*
M8147/0   *Basal cell adenoma*
M8150/0   *Islet cell adenoma*
M8150/3   *Islet cell carcinoma*
M8151/0   *Insulinoma NOS*
M8151/3   *Insulinoma, malignant*
M8152/0   *Glucagonoma NOS*
M8152/3   *Glucagonoma, malignant*
M8153/1   *Gastrinoma NOS*
M8153/3   *Gastrinoma, malignant*
M8154/3   *Mixed islet cell and exocrine adenocarcinoma*
M8160/0   *Bile duct adenoma*
M8160/3   *Cholangiocarcinoma*
M8161/0   *Bile duct cystadenoma*
M8161/3   *Bile duct cystadenocarcinoma*
M8170/0   *Liver cell adenoma*
M8170/3   *Hepatocellular carcinoma NOS*
M8180/0   *Hepatocholangioma, benign*
M8180/3   *Combined hepatocellular carcinoma and cholangiocarcinoma*
M8190/0   *Trabecular adenoma*
M8190/3   *Trabecular adenocarcinoma*
M8191/0   *Embryonal adenoma*
M8200/0   *Eccrine dermal cylindroma*
M8200/3   *Adenoid cystic carcinoma*
M8201/3   *Cribriform carcinoma*
M8210/0   *Adenomatous polyp NOS*
M8210/3   *Adenocarcinoma in adenomatous polyp*
M8211/0   *Tubular adenoma NOS*
M8211/3   *Tubular adenocarcinoma*
M8220/0   *Adenomatous polyposis coli*
M8220/3   *Adenocarcinoma in adenomatous polyposis coli*
M8221/0   *Multiple adenomatous polyps*
M8230/3   *Solid carcinoma NOS*
M8231/3   *Carcinoma simplex*
M8240/1   *Carcinoid tumor NOS*
M8240/3   *Carcinoid tumor, malignant*
M8241/1   *Carcinoid tumor, argentaffin NOS*
M8241/3   *Carcinoid tumor, argentaffin, malignant*
M8242/1   *Carcinoid tumor, nonargentaffin NOS*
M8242/3   *Carcinoid tumor, nonargentaffin, malignant*
M8243/3   *Mucocarcinoid tumor, malignant*
M8244/3   *Composite carcinoid*
M8250/1   *Pulmonary adenomatosis*
M8250/3   *Bronchiolo-alveolar adenocarcinoma*
M8251/0   *Alveolar adenoma*

APPENDIX A

M8251/3	*Alveolar adenocarcinoma*
M8260/0	*Papillary adenoma NOS*
M8260/3	*Papillary adenocarcinoma NOS*
M8261/1	*Villous adenoma NOS*
M8261/3	*Adenocarcinoma in villous adenoma*
M8262/3	*Villous adenocarcinoma*
M8263/0	*Tubulovillous adenoma*
M8270/0	*Chromophobe adenoma*
M8270/3	*Chromophobe carcinoma*
M8280/0	*Acidophil adenoma*
M8280/3	*Acidophil carcinoma*
M8281/0	*Mixed acidophil-basophil adenoma*
M8281/3	*Mixed acidophil-basophil carcinoma*
M8290/0	*Oxyphilic adenoma*
M8290/3	*Oxyphilic adenocarcinoma*
M8300/0	*Basophil adenoma*
M8300/3	*Basophil carcinoma*
M8310/0	*Clear cell adenoma*
M8310/3	*Clear cell adenocarcinoma NOS*
M8311/1	*Hypernephroid tumor*
M8312/3	*Renal cell carcinoma*
M8313/0	*Clear cell adenofibroma*
M8320/3	*Granular cell carcinoma*
M8321/0	*Chief cell adenoma*
M8322/0	*Water-clear cell adenoma*
M8322/3	*Water-clear cell adenocarcinoma*
M8323/0	*Mixed cell adenoma*
M8323/3	*Mixed cell adenocarcinoma*
M8324/0	*Lipoadenoma*
M8330/0	*Follicular adenoma*
M8330/3	*Follicular adenocarcinoma NOS*
M8331/3	*Follicular adenocarcinoma, well differentiated type*
M8332/3	*Follicular adenocarcinoma, trabecular type*
M8333/0	*Microfollicular adenoma*
M8334/0	*Macrofollicular adenoma*
M8340/3	*Papillary and follicular adenocarcinoma*
M8350/3	*Nonencapsulated sclerosing carcinoma*
M8360/1	*Multiple endocrine adenomas*
M8361/1	*Juxtaglomerular tumor*
M8370/0	*Adrenal cortical adenoma NOS*
M8370/3	*Adrenal cortical carcinoma*
M8371/0	*Adrenal cortical adenoma, compact cell type*
M8372/0	*Adrenal cortical adenoma, heavily pigmented variant*
M8373/0	*Adrenal cortical adenoma, clear cell type*
M8374/0	*Adrenal cortical adenoma, glomerulosa cell type*
M8375/0	*Adrenal cortical adenoma, mixed cell type*
M8380/0	*Endometrioid adenoma NOS*
M8380/1	*Endometrioid adenoma, borderline malignancy*
M8380/3	*Endometrioid carcinoma*
M8381/0	*Endometrioid adenofibroma NOS*
M8381/1	*Endometrioid adenofibroma, borderline malignancy*
M8381/3	*Endometrioid adenofibroma, malignant*
M839-M842	**Adnexal and skin appendage neoplasms**
M8390/0	*Skin appendage adenoma*
M8390/3	*Skin appendage carcinoma*
M8400/0	*Sweat gland adenoma*
M8400/1	*Sweat gland tumor NOS*
M8400/3	*Sweat gland adenocarcinoma*
M8401/0	*Apocrine adenoma*
M8401/3	*Apocrine adenocarcinoma*
M8402/0	*Eccrine acrospiroma*
M8403/0	*Eccrine spiradenoma*
M8404/0	*Hidrocystoma*
M8405/0	*Papillary hydradenoma*
M8406/0	*Papillary syringadenoma*
M8407/0	*Syringoma NOS*
M8410/0	*Sebaceous adenoma*
M8410/3	*Sebaceous adenocarcinoma*
M8420/0	*Ceruminous adenoma*
M8420/3	*Ceruminous adenocarcinoma*

MORPHOLOGY OF NEOPLASMS

M843	**Mucoepidermoid neoplasms**
M8430/1	*Mucoepidermoid tumor*
M8430/3	*Mucoepidermoid carcinoma*
M844-M849	**Cystic, mucinous, and serous neoplasms**
M8440/0	*Cystadenoma NOS*
M8440/3	*Cystadenocarcinoma NOS*
M8441/0	*Serous cystadenoma NOS*
M8441/1	*Serous cystadenoma, borderline malignancy*
M8441/3	*Serous cystadenocarcinoma NOS*
M8450/0	*Papillary cystadenoma NOS*
M8450/1	*Papillary cystadenoma, borderline malignancy*
M8450/3	*Papillary cystadenocarcinoma NOS*
M8460/0	*Papillary serous cystadenoma NOS*
M8460/1	*Papillary serous cystadenoma, borderline malignancy*
M8460/3	*Papillary serous cystadenocarcinoma*
M8461/0	*Serous surface papilloma NOS*
M8461/1	*Serous surface papilloma, borderline malignancy*
M8461/3	*Serous surface papillary carcinoma*
M8470/0	*Mucinous cystadenoma NOS*
M8470/1	*Mucinous cystadenoma, borderline malignancy*
M8470/3	*Mucinous cystadenocarcinoma NOS*
M8471/0	*Papillary mucinous cystadenoma NOS*
M8471/1	*Papillary mucinous cystadenoma, borderline malignancy*
M8471/3	*Papillary mucinous cystadenocarcinoma*
M8480/0	*Mucinous adenoma*
M8480/3	*Mucinous adenocarcinoma*
M8480/6	*Pseudomyxoma peritonei*
M8481/3	*Mucin-producing adenocarcinoma*
M8490/3	*Signet ring cell carcinoma*
M8490/6	*Metastatic signet ring cell carcinoma*
M850-M854	**Ductal, lobular, and medullary neoplasms**
M8500/2	*Intraductal carcinoma, noninfiltrating NOS*
M8500/3	*Infiltrating duct carcinoma*
M8501/2	*Comedocarcinoma, noninfiltrating*
M8501/3	*Comedocarcinoma NOS*
M8502/3	*Juvenile carcinoma of the breast*
M8503/0	*Intraductal papilloma*
M8503/2	*Noninfiltrating intraductal papillary adenocarcinoma*
M8504/0	*Intracystic papillary adenoma*
M8504/2	*Noninfiltrating intracystic carcinoma*
M8505/0	*Intraductal papillomatosis NOS*
M8506/0	*Subareolar duct papillomatosis*
M8510/3	*Medullary carcinoma NOS*
M8511/3	*Medullary carcinoma with amyloid stroma*
M8512/3	*Medullary carcinoma with lymphoid stroma*
M8520/2	*Lobular carcinoma in situ*
M8520/3	*Lobular carcinoma NOS*
M8521/3	*Infiltrating ductular carcinoma*
M8530/3	*Inflammatory carcinoma*
M8540/3	*Paget's disease, mammary*
M8541/3	*Paget's disease and infiltrating duct carcinoma of breast*
M8542/3	*Paget's disease, extramammary (except Paget's disease of bone)*
M855	**Acinar cell neoplasms**
M8550/0	*Acinar cell adenoma*
M8550/1	*Acinar cell tumor*
M8550/3	*Acinar cell carcinoma*
M856-M858	**Complex epithelial neoplasms**
M8560/3	*Adenosquamous carcinoma*
M8561/0	*Adenolymphoma*
M8570/3	*Adenocarcinoma with squamous metaplasia*
M8571/3	*Adenocarcinoma with cartilaginous and osseous metaplasia*
M8572/3	*Adenocarcinoma with spindle cell metaplasia*
M8573/3	*Adenocarcinoma with apocrine metaplasia*
M8580/0	*Thymoma, benign*
M8580/3	*Thymoma, malignant*
M859-M867	**Specialized gonadal neoplasms**
M8590/1	*Sex cord-stromal tumor*
M8600/0	*Thecoma NOS*
M8600/3	*Theca cell carcinoma*

APPENDIX A

M8610/0	Luteoma NOS
M8620/1	Granulosa cell tumor NOS
M8620/3	Granulosa cell tumor, malignant
M8621/1	Granulosa cell-theca cell tumor
M8630/0	Androblastoma, benign
M8630/1	Androblastoma NOS
M8630/3	Androblastoma, malignant
M8631/0	Sertoli-Leydig cell tumor
M8632/1	Gynandroblastoma
M8640/0	Tubular androblastoma NOS
M8640/3	Sertoli cell carcinoma
M8641/0	Tubular androblastoma with lipid storage
M8650/0	Leydig cell tumor, benign
M8650/1	Leydig cell tumor NOS
M8650/3	Leydig cell tumor, malignant
M8660/0	Hilar cell tumor
M8670/0	Lipid cell tumor of ovary
M8671/0	Adrenal rest tumor

M868-M871 Paragangliomas and glomus tumors

M8680/1	Paraganglioma NOS
M8680/3	Paraganglioma, malignant
M8681/1	Sympathetic paraganglioma
M8682/1	Parasympathetic paraganglioma
M8690/1	Glomus jugulare tumor
M8691/1	Aortic body tumor
M8692/1	Carotid body tumor
M8693/1	Extra-adrenal paraganglioma NOS
M8693/3	Extra-adrenal paraganglioma, malignant
M8700/0	Pheochromocytoma NOS
M8700/3	Pheochromocytoma, malignant
M8710/3	Glomangiosarcoma
M8711/0	Glomus tumor
M8712/0	Glomangioma

M872-M879 Nevi and melanomas

M8720/0	Pigmented nevus NOS
M8720/3	Malignant melanoma NOS
M8721/3	Nodular melanoma
M8722/0	Balloon cell nevus
M8722/3	Balloon cell melanoma
M8723/0	Halo nevus
M8724/0	Fibrous papule of the nose
M8725/0	Neuronevus
M8726/0	Magnocellular nevus
M8730/0	Nonpigmented nevus
M8730/3	Amelanotic melanoma
M8740/0	Junctional nevus
M8740/3	Malignant melanoma in junctional nevus
M8741/2	Precancerous melanosis NOS
M8741/3	Malignant melanoma in precancerous melanosis
M8742/2	Hutchinson's melanotic freckle
M8742/3	Malignant melanoma in Hutchinson's melanotic freckle
M8743/3	Superficial spreading melanoma
M8750/0	Intradermal nevus
M8760/0	Compound nevus
M8761/1	Giant pigmented nevus
M8761/3	Malignant melanoma in giant pigmented nevus
M8770/0	Epithelioid and spindle cell nevus
M8771/3	Epithelioid cell melanoma
M8772/3	Spindle cell melanoma NOS
M8773/3	Spindle cell melanoma, type A
M8774/3	Spindle cell melanoma, type B
M8775/3	Mixed epithelioid and spindle cell melanoma
M8780/0	Blue nevus NOS
M8780/3	Blue nevus, malignant
M8790/0	Cellular blue nevus

M880 Soft tissue tumors and sarcomas NOS

M8800/0	Soft tissue tumor, benign
M8800/3	Sarcoma NOS
M8800/9	Sarcomatosis NOS
M8801/3	Spindle cell sarcoma

MORPHOLOGY OF NEOPLASMS

M8802/3	Giant cell sarcoma (except of bone M9250/3)
M8803/3	Small cell sarcoma
M8804/3	Epithelioid cell sarcoma

M881-M883 Fibromatous neoplasms

M8810/0	Fibroma NOS
M8810/3	Fibrosarcoma NOS
M8811/0	Fibromyxoma
M8811/3	Fibromyxosarcoma
M8812/0	Periosteal fibroma
M8812/3	Periosteal fibrosarcoma
M8813/0	Fascial fibroma
M8813/3	Fascial fibrosarcoma
M8814/3	Infantile fibrosarcoma
M8820/0	Elastofibroma
M8821/1	Aggressive fibromatosis
M8822/1	Abdominal fibromatosis
M8823/1	Desmoplastic fibroma
M8830/0	Fibrous histiocytoma NOS
M8830/1	Atypical fibrous histiocytoma
M8830/3	Fibrous histiocytoma, malignant
M8831/0	Fibroxanthoma NOS
M8831/1	Atypical fibroxanthoma
M8831/3	Fibroxanthoma, malignant
M8832/0	Dermatofibroma NOS
M8832/1	Dermatofibroma protuberans
M8832/3	Dermatofibrosarcoma NOS

M884 Myxomatous neoplasms

M8840/0	Myxoma NOS
M8840/3	Myxosarcoma

M885-M888 Lipomatous neoplasms

M8850/0	Lipoma NOS
M8850/3	Liposarcoma NOS
M8851/0	Fibrolipoma
M8851/3	Liposarcoma, well differentiated type
M8852/0	Fibromyxolipoma
M8852/3	Myxoid liposarcoma
M8853/3	Round cell liposarcoma
M8854/3	Pleomorphic liposarcoma
M8855/3	Mixed type liposarcoma
M8856/0	Intramuscular lipoma
M8857/0	Spindle cell lipoma
M8860/0	Angiomyolipoma
M8860/3	Angiomyoliposarcoma
M8861/0	Angiolipoma NOS
M8861/1	Angiolipoma, infiltrating
M8870/0	Myelolipoma
M8880/0	Hibernoma
M8881/0	Lipoblastomatosis

M889-M892 Myomatous neoplasms

M8890/0	Leiomyoma NOS
M8890/1	Intravascular leiomyomatosis
M8890/3	Leiomyosarcoma NOS
M8891/1	Epithelioid leiomyoma
M8891/3	Epithelioid leiomyosarcoma
M8892/1	Cellular leiomyoma
M8893/0	Bizarre leiomyoma
M8894/0	Angiomyoma
M8894/3	Angiomyosarcoma
M8895/0	Myoma
M8895/3	Myosarcoma
M8900/0	Rhabdomyoma NOS
M8900/3	Rhabdomyosarcoma NOS
M8901/3	Pleomorphic rhabdomyosarcoma
M8902/3	Mixed type rhabdomyosarcoma
M8903/0	Fetal rhabdomyoma
M8904/0	Adult rhabdomyoma
M8910/3	Embryonal rhabdomyosarcoma
M8920/3	Alveolar rhabdomyosarcoma

APPENDIX A

M893-M899 Complex mixed and stromal neoplasms
M8930/3   *Endometrial stromal sarcoma*
M8931/1   *Endolymphatic stromal myosis*
M8932/0   *Adenomyoma*
M8940/0   *Pleomorphic adenoma*
M8940/3   *Mixed tumor, malignant NOS*
M8950/3   *Mullerian mixed tumor*
M8951/3   *Mesodermal mixed tumor*
M8960/1   *Mesoblastic nephroma*
M8960/3   *Nephroblastoma NOS*
M8961/3   *Epithelial nephroblastoma*
M8962/3   *Mesenchymal nephroblastoma*
M8970/3   *Hepatoblastoma*
M8980/3   *Carcinosarcoma NOS*
M8981/3   *Carcinosarcoma, embryonal type*
M8982/0   *Myoepithelioma*
M8990/0   *Mesenchymoma, benign*
M8990/1   *Mesenchymoma, NOS*
M8990/3   *Mesenchymoma, malignant*
M8991/3   *Embryonal sarcoma*

M900-M903 Fibroepithelial neoplasms
M9000/0   *Brenner tumor NOS*
M9000/1   *Brenner tumor, borderline malignancy*
M9000/3   *Brenner tumor, malignant*
M9010/0   *Fibroadenoma NOS*
M9011/0   *Intracanalicular fibroadenoma NOS*
M9012/0   *Pericanalicular fibroadenoma*
M9013/0   *Adenofibroma NOS*
M9014/0   *Serous adenofibroma*
M9015/0   *Mucinous adenofibroma*
M9020/0   *Cellular intracanalicular fibroadenoma*
M9020/1   *Cystosarcoma phyllodes NOS*
M9020/3   *Cystosarcoma phyllodes, malignant*
M9030/0   *Juvenile fibroadenoma*

M904 Synovial neoplasms
M9040/0   *Synovioma, benign*
M9040/3   *Synovial sarcoma NOS*
M9041/3   *Synovial sarcoma, spindle cell type*
M9042/3   *Synovial sarcoma, epithelioid cell type*
M9043/3   *Synovial sarcoma, biphasic type*
M9044/3   *Clear cell sarcoma of tendons and aponeuroses*

M905 Mesothelial neoplasms
M9050/0   *Mesothelioma, benign*
M9050/3   *Mesothelioma, malignant*
M9051/0   *Fibrous mesothelioma, benign*
M9051/3   *Fibrous mesothelioma, malignant*
M9052/0   *Epithelioid mesothelioma, benign*
M9052/3   *Epithelioid mesothelioma, malignant*
M9053/0   *Mesothelioma, biphasic type, benign*
M9053/3   *Mesothelioma, biphasic type, malignant*
M9054/0   *Adenomatoid tumor NOS*

M906-M909 Germ cell neoplasms
M9060/3   *Dysgerminoma*
M9061/3   *Seminoma NOS*
M9062/3   *Seminoma, anaplastic type*
M9063/3   *Spermatocytic seminoma*
M9064/3   *Germinoma*
M9070/3   *Embryonal carcinoma NOS*
M9071/3   *Endodermal sinus tumor*
M9072/3   *Polyembryoma*
M9073/1   *Gonadoblastoma*
M9080/0   *Teratoma, benign*
M9080/1   *Teratoma NOS*
M9080/3   *Teratoma, malignant NOS*
M9081/3   *Teratocarcinoma*
M9082/3   *Malignant teratoma, undifferentiated type*
M9083/3   *Malignant teratoma, intermediate type*
M9084/0   *Dermoid cyst*
M9084/3   *Dermoid cyst with malignant transformation*

MORPHOLOGY OF NEOPLASMS

M9090/0	*Struma ovarii NOS*
M9090/3	*Struma ovarii, malignant*
M9091/1	*Strumal carcinoid*

M910 Trophoblastic neoplasms
M9100/0	*Hydatidiform mole NOS*
M9100/1	*Invasive hydatidiform mole*
M9100/3	*Choriocarcinoma*
M9101/3	*Choriocarcinoma combined with teratoma*
M9102/3	*Malignant teratoma, trophoblastic*

M911 Mesonephromas
M9110/0	*Mesonephroma, benign*
M9110/1	*Mesonephric tumor*
M9110/3	*Mesonephroma, malignant*
M9111/1	*Endosalpingioma*

M912-M916 Blood vessel tumors
M9120/0	*Hemangioma NOS*
M9120/3	*Hemangiosarcoma*
M9121/0	*Cavernous hemangioma*
M9122/0	*Venous hemangioma*
M9123/0	*Racemose hemangioma*
M9124/3	*Kupffer cell sarcoma*
M9130/0	*Hemangioendothelioma, benign*
M9130/1	*Hemangioendothelioma NOS*
M9130/3	*Hemangioendothelioma, malignant*
M9131/0	*Capillary hemangioma*
M9132/0	*Intramuscular hemangioma*
M9140/3	*Kaposi's sarcoma*
M9141/0	*Angiokeratoma*
M9142/0	*Verrucous keratotic hemangioma*
M9150/0	*Hemangiopericytoma, benign*
M9150/1	*Hemangiopericytoma NOS*
M9150/3	*Hemangiopericytoma, malignant*
M9160/0	*Angiofibroma NOS*
M9161/1	*Hemangioblastoma*

M917 Lymphatic vessel tumors
M9170/0	*Lymphangioma NOS*
M9170/3	*Lymphangiosarcoma*
M9171/0	*Capillary lymphangioma*
M9172/0	*Cavernous lymphangioma*
M9173/0	*Cystic lymphangioma*
M9174/0	*Lymphangiomyoma*
M9174/1	*Lymphangiomyomatosis*
M9175/0	*Hemolymphangioma*

M918-M920 Osteomas and osteosarcomas
M9180/0	*Osteoma NOS*
M9180/3	*Osteosarcoma NOS*
M9181/3	*Chondroblastic osteosarcoma*
M9182/3	*Fibroblastic osteosarcoma*
M9183/3	*Telangiectatic osteosarcoma*
M9184/3	*Osteosarcoma in Paget's disease of bone*
M9190/3	*Juxtacortical osteosarcoma*
M9191/0	*Osteoid osteoma NOS*
M9200/0	*Osteoblastoma*

M921-M924 Chondromatous neoplasms
M9210/0	*Osteochondroma*
M9210/1	*Osteochondromatosis NOS*
M9220/0	*Chondroma NOS*
M9220/1	*Chondromatosis NOS*
M9220/3	*Chondrosarcoma NOS*
M9221/0	*Juxtacortical chondroma*
M9221/3	*Juxtacortical chondrosarcoma*
M9230/0	*Chondroblastoma NOS*
M9230/3	*Chondroblastoma, malignant*
M9240/3	*Mesenchymal chondrosarcoma*
M9241/0	*Chondromyxoid fibroma*

M925 Giant cell tumors
M9250/1	*Giant cell tumor of bone NOS*
M9250/3	*Giant cell tumor of bone, malignant*

APPENDIX A

M9251/1	Giant cell tumor of soft parts NOS
M9251/3	Malignant giant cell tumor of soft parts
M926	**Miscellaneous bone tumors**
M9260/3	Ewing's sarcoma
M9261/3	Adamantinoma of long bones
M9262/0	Ossifying fibroma
M927-M934	**Odontogenic tumors**
M9270/0	Odontogenic tumor, benign
M9270/1	Odontogenic tumor NOS
M9270/3	Odontogenic tumor, malignant
M9271/0	Dentinoma
M9272/0	Cementoma NOS
M9273/0	Cementoblastoma, benign
M9274/0	Cementifying fibroma
M9275/0	Gigantiform cementoma
M9280/0	Odontoma NOS
M9281/0	Compound odontoma
M9282/0	Complex odontoma
M9290/0	Ameloblastic fibro-odontoma
M9290/3	Ameloblastic odontosarcoma
M9300/0	Adenomatoid odontogenic tumor
M9301/0	Calcifying odontogenic cyst
M9310/0	Ameloblastoma NOS
M9310/3	Ameloblastoma, malignant
M9311/0	Odontoameloblastoma
M9312/0	Squamous odontogenic tumor
M9320/0	Odontogenic myxoma
M9321/0	Odontogenic fibroma NOS
M9330/0	Ameloblastic fibroma
M9330/3	Ameloblastic fibrosarcoma
M9340/0	Calcifying epithelial odontogenic tumor
M935-M937	**Miscellaneous tumors**
M9350/1	Craniopharyngioma
M9360/1	Pinealoma
M9361/1	Pineocytoma
M9362/3	Pineoblastoma
M9363/0	Melanotic neuroectodermal tumor
M9370/3	Chordoma
M938-M948	**Gliomas**
M9380/3	Glioma, malignant
M9381/3	Gliomatosis cerebri
M9382/3	Mixed glioma
M9383/1	Subependymal glioma
M9384/1	Subependymal giant cell astrocytoma
M9390/0	Choroid plexus papilloma NOS
M9390/3	Choroid plexus papilloma, malignant
M9391/3	Ependymoma NOS
M9392/3	Ependymoma, anaplastic type
M9393/1	Papillary ependymoma
M9394/1	Myxopapillary ependymoma
M9400/3	Astrocytoma NOS
M9401/3	Astrocytoma, anaplastic type
M9410/3	Protoplasmic astrocytoma
M9411/3	Gemistocytic astrocytoma
M9420/3	Fibrillary astrocytoma
M9421/3	Pilocytic astrocytoma
M9422/3	Spongioblastoma NOS
M9423/3	Spongioblastoma polare
M9430/3	Astroblastoma
M9440/3	Glioblastoma NOS
M9441/3	Giant cell glioblastoma
M9442/3	Glioblastoma with sarcomatous component
M9443/3	Primitive polar spongioblastoma
M9450/3	Oligodendroglioma NOS
M9451/3	Oligodendroglioma, anaplastic type
M9460/3	Oligodendroblastoma
M9470/3	Medulloblastoma NOS
M9471/3	Desmoplastic medulloblastoma
M9472/3	Medullomyoblastoma

MORPHOLOGY OF NEOPLASMS

M9480/3	Cerebellar sarcoma NOS
M9481/3	Monstrocellular sarcoma

M949-M952 Neuroepitheliomatous neoplasms

M9490/0	Ganglioneuroma
M9490/3	Ganglioneuroblastoma
M9491/0	Ganglioneuromatosis
M9500/3	Neuroblastoma NOS
M9501/3	Medulloepithelioma NOS
M9502/3	Teratoid medulloepithelioma
M9503/3	Neuroepithelioma NOS
M9504/3	Spongioneuroblastoma
M9505/1	Ganglioglioma
M9506/0	Neurocytoma
M9507/0	Pacinian tumor
M9510/3	Retinoblastoma NOS
M9511/3	Retinoblastoma, differentiated type
M9512/3	Retinoblastoma, undifferentiated type
M9520/3	Olfactory neurogenic tumor
M9521/3	Esthesioneurocytoma
M9522/3	Esthesioneuroblastoma
M9523/3	Esthesioneuroepithelioma

M953 Meningiomas

M9530/0	Meningioma NOS
M9530/1	Meningiomatosis NOS
M9530/3	Meningioma, malignant
M9531/0	Meningotheliomatous meningioma
M9532/0	Fibrous meningioma
M9533/0	Psammomatous meningioma
M9534/0	Angiomatous meningioma
M9535/0	Hemangioblastic meningioma
M9536/0	Hemangiopericytic meningioma
M9537/0	Transitional meningioma
M9538/1	Papillary meningioma
M9539/3	Meningeal sarcomatosis

M954-M957 Nerve sheath tumor

M9540/0	Neurofibroma NOS
M9540/1	Neurofibromatosis NOS
M9540/3	Neurofibrosarcoma
M9541/0	Melanotic neurofibroma
M9550/0	Plexiform neurofibroma
M9560/0	Neurilemmoma NOS
M9560/1	Neurinomatosis
M9560/3	Neurilemmoma, malignant
M9570/0	Neuroma NOS

M958 Granular cell tumors and alveolar soft part sarcoma

M9580/0	Granular cell tumor NOS
M9580/3	Granular cell tumor, malignant
M9581/3	Alveolar soft part sarcoma

M959-M963 Lymphomas, NOS or diffuse

M9590/0	Lymphomatous tumor, benign
M9590/3	Malignant lymphoma NOS
M9591/3	Malignant lymphoma, non Hodgkin's type
M9600/3	Malignant lymphoma, undifferentiated cell type NOS
M9601/3	Malignant lymphoma, stem cell type
M9602/3	Malignant lymphoma, convoluted cell type NOS
M9610/3	Lymphosarcoma NOS
M9611/3	Malignant lymphoma, lymphoplasmacytoid type
M9612/3	Malignant lymphoma, immunoblastic type
M9613/3	Malignant lymphoma, mixed lymphocytic-histiocytic NOS
M9614/3	Malignant lymphoma, centroblastic-centrocytic, diffuse
M9615/3	Malignant lymphoma, follicular center cell NOS
M9620/3	Malignant lymphoma, lymphocytic, well differentiated NOS
M9621/3	Malignant lymphoma, lymphocytic, intermediate differentiation NOS
M9622/3	Malignant lymphoma, centrocytic
M9623/3	Malignant lymphoma, follicular center cell, cleaved NOS
M9630/3	Malignant lymphoma, lymphocytic, poorly differentiated NOS
M9631/3	Prolymphocytic lymphosarcoma
M9632/3	Malignant lymphoma, centroblastic type NOS
M9633/3	Malignant lymphoma, follicular center cell, noncleaved NOS

APPENDIX A

M964	**Reticulosarcomas**
M9640/3	*Reticulosarcoma NOS*
M9641/3	*Reticulosarcoma, pleomorphic cell type*
M9642/3	*Reticulosarcoma, nodular*
M965-M966	**Hodgkin's disease**
M9650/3	*Hodgkin's disease NOS*
M9651/3	*Hodgkin's disease, lymphocytic predominance*
M9652/3	*Hodgkin's disease, mixed cellularity*
M9653/3	*Hodgkin's disease, lymphocytic depletion NOS*
M9654/3	*Hodgkin's disease, lymphocytic depletion, diffuse fibrosis*
M9655/3	*Hodgkin's disease, lymphocytic depletion, reticular type*
M9656/3	*Hodgkin's disease, nodular sclerosis NOS*
M9657/3	*Hodgkin's disease, nodular sclerosis, cellular phase*
M9660/3	*Hodgkin's paragranuloma*
M9661/3	*Hodgkin's granuloma*
M9662/3	*Hodgkin's sarcoma*
M969	**Lymphomas, nodular or follicular**
M9690/3	*Malignant lymphoma, nodular NOS*
M9691/3	*Malignant lymphoma, mixed lymphocytic-histiocytic, nodular*
M9692/3	*Malignant lymphoma, centroblastic-centrocytic, follicular*
M9693/3	*Malignant lymphoma, lymphocytic, well differentiated, nodular*
M9694/3	*Malignant lymphoma, lymphocytic, intermediate differentiation, nodular*
M9695/3	*Malignant lymphoma, follicular center cell, cleaved, follicular*
M9696/3	*Malignant lymphoma, lymphocytic, poorly differentiated, nodular*
M9697/3	*Malignant lymphoma, centroblastic type, follicular*
M9698/3	*Malignant lymphoma, follicular center cell, noncleaved, follicular*
M970	**Mycosis fungoides**
M9700/3	*Mycosis fungoides*
M9701/3	*Sezary's disease*
M971-M972	**Miscellaneous reticuloendothelial neoplasms**
M9710/3	*Microglioma*
M9720/3	*Malignant histiocytosis*
M9721/3	*Histiocytic medullary reticulosis*
M9722/3	*Letterer-Siwe's disease*
M973	**Plasma cell tumors**
M9730/3	*Plasma cell myeloma*
M9731/0	*Plasma cell tumor, benign*
M9731/1	*Plasmacytoma NOS*
M9731/3	*Plasma cell tumor, malignant*
M974	**Mast cell tumors**
M9740/1	*Mastocytoma NOS*
M9740/3	*Mast cell sarcoma*
M9741/3	*Malignant mastocytosis*
M975	**Burkitt's tumor**
M9750/3	*Burkitt's tumor*
M980-M994	**Leukemias**
M980	**Leukemias NOS**
M9800/3	*Leukemia NOS*
M9801/3	*Acute leukemia NOS*
M9802/3	*Subacute leukemia NOS*
M9803/3	*Chronic leukemia NOS*
M9804/3	*Aleukemic leukemia NOS*
M981	**Compound leukemias**
M9810/3	*Compound leukemia*
M982	**Lymphoid leukemias**
M9820/3	*Lymphoid leukemia NOS*
M9821/3	*Acute lymphoid leukemia*
M9822/3	*Subacute lymphoid leukemia*
M9823/3	*Chronic lymphoid leukemia*
M9824/3	*Aleukemic lymphoid leukemia*
M9825/3	*Prolymphocytic leukemia*
M983	**Plasma cell leukemias**
M9830/3	*Plasma cell leukemia*
M984	**Erythroleukemias**
M9840/3	*Erythroleukemia*
M9841/3	*Acute erythremia*

MORPHOLOGY OF NEOPLASMS

M9842/3	*Chronic erythremia*
M985	**Lymphosarcoma cell leukemias**
M9850/3	*Lymphosarcoma cell leukemia*
M986	**Myeloid leukemias**
M9860/3	*Myeloid leukemia NOS*
M9861/3	*Acute myeloid leukemia*
M9862/3	*Subacute myeloid leukemia*
M9863/3	*Chronic myeloid leukemia*
M9864/3	*Aleukemic myeloid leukemia*
M9865/3	*Neutrophilic leukemia*
M9866/3	*Acute promyelocytic leukemia*
M987	**Basophilic leukemias**
M9870/3	*Basophilic leukemia*
M988	**Eosinophilic leukemias**
M9880/3	*Eosinophilic leukemia*
M989	**Monocytic leukemias**
M9890/3	*Monocytic leukemia NOS*
M9891/3	*Acute monocytic leukemia*
M9892/3	*Subacute monocytic leukemia*
M9893/3	*Chronic monocytic leukemia*
M9894/3	*Aleukemic monocytic leukemia*
M990-M994	**Miscellaneous leukemias**
M9900/3	*Mast cell leukemia*
M9910/3	*Megakaryocytic leukemia*
M9920/3	*Megakaryocytic myelosis*
M9930/3	*Myeloid sarcoma*
M9940/3	*Hairy cell leukemia*
M995-M997	**Miscellaneous myeloproliferative and lymphoproliferative disorders**
M9950/1	*Polycythemia vera*
M9951/1	*Acute panmyelosis*
M9960/1	*Chronic myeloproliferative disease*
M9961/1	*Myelosclerosis with myeloid metaplasia*
M9962/1	*Idiopathic thrombocythemia*
M9970/1	*Chronic lymphoproliferative disease*

APPENDIX A

APPENDIX B:
GLOSSARY OF MENTAL DISORDERS

Note: *Appendix B Glossary of Mental Disorders* has been removed from the official ICD-9-CM CD-Rom effective with the FY2005 update.

APPENDIX B

APPENDIX C:
CLASSIFICATION OF DRUGS BY AMERICAN HOSPITAL FORMULARY SERVICE LIST NUMBER AND THEIR ICD-9-CM EQUIVALENTS

The coding of adverse effects of drugs is keyed to the continually revised Hospital Formulary of the American Hospital Formulary Service (AHFS) published under the direction of the American Society of Hospital Pharmacists.

AHFS*LIST	ICD-9-CM Diagnosis Code

The following section gives the ICD-9-CM diagnosis code for each AHFS list.

4:00	**ANTIHISTAMINE DRUGS**	963.0
8:00	**ANTI-INFECTIVE AGENTS**	
8:04	Amebacides	961.5
	hydroxyquinoline derivatives	961.3
	arsenical anti-infectives	961.1
8:08	Anthelmintics	961.6
	quinoline derivatives	961.3
8:12.04	Antifungal Antibiotics	960.1
	nonantibiotics	961.9
8:12.06	Cephalosporins	960.5
8:12.08	Chloramphenicol	960.2
8:12.12	The Erythromycins	960.3
8:12.16	The Penicillins	960.0
8:12.20	The Streptomycins	960.6
8:12.24	The Tetracyclines	960.4
8:12.28	Other Antibiotics	960.8
	antimycobacterial antibiotics	960.6
	macrolides	960.3
8:16	Antituberculars	961.8
	antibiotics	960.6
8:18	Antivirals	961.7
8:20	Plasmodicides (antimalarials)	961.4
8:24	Sulfonamides	961.0
8:26	The Sulfones	961.8
8:28	Treponemicides	961.2
8:32	Trichomonacides	961.5
	hydroxyquinoline derivatives	961.3
	nitrofuran derivatives	961.9
8:36	Urinary Germicides	961.9
	quinoline derivatives	961.3
8:40	Other Anti-Infectives	961.9
10:00	**ANTINEOPLASTIC AGENTS**	963.1
	antibiotics	960.7
	progestogens	962.2
12:00	**AUTONOMIC DRUGS**	
12:04	Parasympathomimetic (Cholinergic) Agents	971.0
12:08	Parasympatholytic (Cholinergic Blocking) Agents	971.1
12:12	Sympathomimetic (Adrenergic) Agents	971.2
12:16	Sympatholytic (Adrenergic Blocking) Agents	971.3

APPENDIX C

AHFS*LIST	ICD-9-CM Diagnosis Code

12:20	Skeletal Muscle Relaxants	975.2
	central nervous system muscle-tone depressants	968.0
16:00	**BLOOD DERIVATIVES**	964.7
20:00	**BLOOD FORMATION AND COAGULATION**	
20:04	Antianemia Drugs	964.1
20:04.04	Iron Preparations	964.0
20:04.08	Liver and Stomach Preparations	964.1
20:12.04	Anticoagulants	964.2
20:12.08	Antiheparin agents	964.5
20:12.12	Coagulants	964.5
20:12.16	Hemostatics	964.5
	capillary-active drugs	972.8
	fibrinolysis-affecting agents	964.4
	natural products	964.7
24:00	**CARDIOVASCULAR DRUGS**	
24:04	Cardiac Drugs	972.9
	cardiotonic agents	972.1
	rhythm regulators	972.0
24:06	Antilipemic Agents	972.2
	thyroid derivatives	962.7
24:08	Hypotensive Agents	972.6
	adrenergic blocking agents	971.3
	ganglion-blocking agents	972.3
	vasodilators	972.5
24:12	Vasodilating Agents	972.5
	coronary	972.4
	nicotinic acid derivatives	972.2
24:16	Sclerosing Agents	972.7
28:00	**CENTRAL NERVOUS SYSTEM DRUGS**	
28:04	General Anesthetics	968.4
	gaseous anesthetics	968.2
	halothane	968.1
	intravenous anesthetics	968.3
28:08	Analgesics and Antipyretics	965.9
	antirheumatics	965.6
	aromatic analgesics	965.4
	non-narcotics NEC	965.7
	opium alkaloids	965.00
	heroin	965.01
	methadone	965.02
	specified type NEC	965.09
	pyrazole derivatives	965.5
	salicylates	965.1
	specified type NEC	965.8
28:10	Narcotic Antagonists	970.1
28:12	Anticonvulsants	966.3
	barbiturates	967.0
	benzodiazepine-based tranquilizers	969.4
	bromides	967.3
	hydantoin derivatives	966.1
	oxazolidine derivative	966.0
	succinimides	966.2
28:16.04	Antidepressants	969.0

*American Hospital Formulary Service

CLASSIFICATION OF DRUGS BY AHFS LIST

AHFS*LIST		ICD-9-CM Diagnosis Code
28:16.08	Tranquilizers	969.5
	benzodiazepine-based	969.4
	butyrophenone-based	969.2
	major NEC	969.3
	phenothiazine-based	969.1
28:16.12	Other Psychotherapeutic Agents	969.8
28:20	Respiratory and Cerebral Stimulants	970.9
	analeptics	970.0
	anorexigenic agents	977.0
	psychostimulants	969.7
	specified type NEC	970.8
28:24	Sedatives and Hypnotics	967.9
	barbiturates	967.0
	benzodiazepine-based tranquilizers	969.4
	chloral hydrate group	967.1
	glutethamide group	967.5
	intravenous anesthetics	968.3
	methaqualone	967.4
	paraldehyde	967.2
	phenothiazine-based tranquilizers	969.1
	specified type NEC	967.8
	thiobarbiturates	968.3
	tranquilizer NEC	969.5
36:00	**DIAGNOSTIC AGENTS**	977.8
40:00	**ELECTROLYTE, CALORIC, AND WATER BALANCE AGENTS NEC**	974.5
40:04	Acidifying Agents	963.2
40:08	Alkalinizing Agents	963.3
40:10	Ammonia Detoxicants	974.5
40:12	Replacement Solutions NEC	974.5
	plasma volume expanders	964.8
40:16	Sodium-Removing Resins	974.5
40:18	Potassium-Removing Resins	974.5
40:20	Caloric Agents	974.5
40:24	Salt and Sugar Substitutes	974.5
40:28	Diuretics NEC	974.4
	carbonic acid anhydrase inhibitors	974.2
	mercurials	974.0
	purine derivatives	974.1
	saluretics	974.3
40:36	Irrigating Solutions	974.5
40:40	Uricosuric Agents	974.7
44:00	**ENZYMES NEC**	963.4
	fibrinolysis-affecting agents	964.4
	gastric agents	973.4
48:00	**EXPECTORANTS AND COUGH PREPARATIONS**	
	antihistamine agents	963.0
	antitussives	975.4
	codeine derivatives	965.09
	expectorants	975.5
	narcotic agents NEC	965.09

APPENDIX C

	AHFS*LIST	ICD-9-CM Diagnosis Code
52:00	**EYE, EAR, NOSE, AND THROAT PREPARATIONS**	
52:04	Anti-Infectives	
	ENT	976.6
	ophthalmic	976.5
52:04.04	Antibiotics	
	ENT	976.6
	ophthalmic	976.5
52:04.06	Antivirals	
	ENT	976.6
	ophthalmic	976.5
52:04.08	Sulfonamides	
	ENT	976.6
	ophthalmic	976.5
52:04.12	Miscellaneous Anti-Infectives	
	ENT	976.6
	ophthalmic	976.5
52:08	Anti-Inflammatory Agents	
	ENT	976.6
	ophthalmic	976.5
52:10	Carbonic Anhydrase Inhibitors	974.2
52:12	Contact Lens Solutions	976.5
52:16	Local Anesthetics	968.5
52:20	Miotics	971.0
52:24	Mydriatics	
	adrenergics	971.2
	anticholinergics	971.1
	antimuscarinics	971.1
	parasympatholytics	971.1
	spasmolytics	971.1
	sympathomimetics	971.2
52:28	Mouth Washes and Gargles	976.6
52:32	Vasoconstrictors	971.2
52:36	Unclassified Agents	
	ENT	976.6
	ophthalmic	976.5
56:00	**GASTROINTESTINAL DRUGS**	
56:04	Antacids and Absorbants	973.0
56:08	Anti-Diarrhea Agents	973.5
56:10	Antiflatulents	973.8
56:12	Cathartics NEC	973.3
	emollients	973.2
	irritants	973.1
56:16	Digestants	973.4
56:20	Emetics and Antiemetics	
	antiemetics	963.0
	emetics	973.6
56:24	Lipotropic Agents	977.1
60:00	**GOLD COMPOUNDS**	965.6
64:00	**HEAVY METAL ANTAGONISTS**	963.8
68:00	**HORMONES AND SYNTHETIC SUBSTITUTES**	
68:04	Adrenals	962.0
68:08	Androgens	962.1

*American Hospital Formulary Service

CLASSIFICATION OF DRUGS BY AHFS LIST

	AHFS*LIST	ICD-9-CM Diagnosis Code
68:12	Contraceptives	962.2
68:16	Estrogens	962.2
68:18	Gonadotropins	962.4
68:20	Insulins and Antidiabetic Agents	962.3
68:20.08	Insulins	962.3
68:24	Parathyroid	962.6
68:28	Pituitary	
	anterior	962.4
	posterior	962.5
68:32	Progestogens	962.2
68:34	Other Corpus Luteum Hormones	962.2
68:36	Thyroid and Antithyroid	
	antithyroid	962.8
	thyroid	962.7
72:00	**LOCAL ANESTHETICS NEC**	968.9
	topical (surface) agents	968.5
	infiltrating agents (intradermal) (subcutaneous) (submucosal)	968.5
	nerve blocking agents (peripheral) (plexus)(regional)	968.6
	spinal	968.7
76:00	**OXYTOCICS**	975.0
78:00	**RADIOACTIVE AGENTS**	990
80:00	**SERUMS, TOXOIDS, AND VACCINES**	
80:04	Serums	979.9
	immune globulin (gamma) (human)	964.6
80:08	Toxoids NEC	978.8
	diphtheria	978.5
	and tetanus	978.9
	with pertussis component	978.6
	tetanus	978.4
	and diphtheria	978.9
	with pertussis component	978.6
80:12	Vaccines NEC	979.9
	bacterial NEC	978.8
	with	
	other bacterial component	978.9
	pertussis component	978.6
	viral and rickettsial component	979.7
	rickettsial NEC	979.6
	with	
	bacterial component	979.7
	pertussis component	978.6
	viral component	979.7
	viral NEC	979.6
	with	
	bacterial component	979.7
	pertussis component	978.6
	rickettsial component	979.7
84:00	**SKIN AND MUCOUS MEMBRANE PREPARATIONS**	
84:04	Anti-Infectives	976.0
84:04.04	Antibiotics	976.0
84:04.08	Fungicides	976.0
84:04.12	Scabicides and Pediculicides	976.0
84:04.16	Miscellaneous Local Anti-Infectives	976.0

APPENDIX C

	AHFS*LIST	ICD-9-CM Diagnosis Code
84:06	Anti-Inflammatory Agents	976.0
84:08	Antipruritics and Local Anesthetics	
	antipruritics	976.1
	local anesthetics	968.5
84:12	Astringents	976.2
84:16	Cell Stimulants and Proliferants	976.8
84:20	Detergents	976.2
84:24	Emollients, Demulcents, and Protectants	976.3
84:28	Keratolytic Agents	976.4
84:32	Keratoplastic Agents	976.4
84:36	Miscellaneous Agents	976.8
86:00	**SPASMOLYTIC AGENTS**	975.1
	antiasthmatics	975.7
	papaverine	972.5
	theophyllin	974.1
88:00	**VITAMINS**	
88:04	Vitamin A	963.5
88:08	Vitamin B Complex	963.5
	hematopoietic vitamin	964.1
	nicotinic acid derivatives	972.2
88:12	Vitamin C	963.5
88:16	Vitamin D	963.5
88:20	Vitamin E	963.5
88:24	Vitamin K Activity	964.3
88:28	Multivitamin Preparations	963.5
92:00	**UNCLASSIFIED THERAPEUTIC AGENTS**	

*American Hospital Formulary Service

APPENDIX D:
CLASSIFICATION OF INDUSTRIAL ACCIDENTS ACCORDING TO AGENCY

Annex B to the Resolution concerning Statistics of Employment Injuries adopted by the Tenth International Conference of Labor Statisticians on 12 October 1962

1 MACHINES

    11 Prime-Movers, except Electrical Motors
        111 Steam engines
        112 Internal combustion engines
        119 Others

    12 Transmission Machinery
        121 Transmission shafts
        122 Transmission belts, cables, pulleys, pinions, chains, gears
        129 Others

    13 Metalworking Machines
        131 Power presses
        132 Lathes
        133 Milling machines
        134 Abrasive wheels
        135 Mechanical shears
        136 Forging machines
        137 Rolling-mills
        139 Others

    14 Wood and Assimilated Machines
        141 Circular saws
        142 Other saws
        143 Molding machines
        144 Overhand planes
        149 Others

    15 Agricultural Machines
        151 Reapers (including combine reapers)
        152 Threshers
        159 Others

    16 Mining Machinery
        161 Under-cutters
        169 Others

    19 Other Machines Not Elsewhere Classified
        191 Earth-moving machines, excavating and scraping machines, except means of transport
        192 Spinning, weaving and other textile machines
        193 Machines for the manufacture of foodstuffs and beverages
        194 Machines for the manufacture of paper
        195 Printing machines
        199 Others

2 MEANS OF TRANSPORT AND LIFTING EQUIPMENT

    21 Lifting Machines and Appliances
        211 Cranes
        212 Lifts and elevators
        213 Winches
        214 Pulley blocks
        219 Others

    22 Means of Rail Transport
        221 Inter-urban railways
        222 Rail transport in mines, tunnels, quarries, industrial establishments, docks, etc.
        229 Others

    23 Other Wheeled Means of Transport, Excluding Rail Transport
        231 Tractors
        232 Lorries

APPENDIX D

2 MEANS OF TRANSPORT AND LIFTING EQUIPMENT continued
- 233 Trucks
- 234 Motor vehicles, not elsewhere classified
- 235 Animal-drawn vehicles
- 236 Hand-drawn vehicles
- 239 Others

24 Means of Air Transport

25 Means of Water Transport
- 251 Motorized means of water transport
- 252 Non-motorized means of water transport

26 Other Means of Transport
- 261 Cable-cars
- 262 Mechanical conveyors, except cable-cars
- 269 Others

3 OTHER EQUIPMENT

31 Pressure Vessels
- 311 Boilers
- 312 Pressurized containers
- 313 Pressurized piping and accessories
- 314 Gas cylinders
- 315 Caissons, diving equipment
- 319 Others

32 Furnaces, Ovens, Kilns
- 321 Blast furnaces
- 322 Refining furnaces
- 323 Other furnaces
- 324 Kilns
- 325 Ovens

33 Refrigerating Plants

34 Electrical Installations, Including Electric Motors, but Excluding Electric Hand Tools
- 341 Rotating machines
- 342 Conductors
- 343 Transformers
- 344 Control apparatus
- 349 Others

35 Electric Hand Tools

36 Tools, Implements, and Appliances, Except Electric Hand Tools
- 361 Power-driven hand tools, except electric hand tools
- 362 Hand tools, not power-driven
- 369 Others

37 Ladders, Mobile Ramps

38 Scaffolding

39 Other Equipment, Not Elsewhere Classified

4 MATERIALS, SUBSTANCES AND RADIATIONS

41 Explosives

42 Dusts, Gases, Liquids and Chemicals, Excluding Explosives
- 421 Dusts
- 422 Gases, vapors, fumes
- 423 Liquids, not elsewhere classified
- 424 Chemicals, not elsewhere classified

43 Flying Fragments

44 Radiations
- 441 Ionizing radiations
- 449 Others

49 Other Materials and Substances Not Elsewhere Classified

INDUSTRIAL ACCIDENTS ACCORDING TO AGENCY

5 WORKING ENVIRONMENT

    51 Outdoor
- 511 Weather
- 512 Traffic and working surfaces
- 513 Water
- 519 Others

    52 Indoor
- 521 Floors
- 522 Confined quarters
- 523 Stairs
- 524 Other traffic and working surfaces
- 525 Floor openings and wall openings
- 526 Environmental factors (lighting, ventilation, temperature, noise, etc.)
- 529 Others

    53 Underground
- 531 Roofs and faces of mine roads and tunnels, etc.
- 532 Floors of mine roads and tunnels, etc.
- 533 Working-faces of mines, tunnels, etc.
- 534 Mine shafts
- 535 Fire
- 536 Water
- 539 Others

6 OTHER AGENCIES, NOT ELSEWHERE CLASSIFIED

    61 Animals
- 611 Live animals
- 612 Animals products

    69 Other Agencies, Not Elsewhere Classified

7 AGENCIES NOT CLASSIFIED FOR LACK OF SUFFICIENT DATA

APPENDIX D

APPENDIX E:
LIST OF THREE-DIGIT CATEGORIES

1. INFECTIOUS AND PARASITIC DISEASES

Intestinal infectious diseases (001-009)
- 001 Cholera
- 002 Typhoid and paratyphoid fevers
- 003 Other salmonella infections
- 004 Shigellosis
- 005 Other food poisoning (bacterial)
- 006 Amebiasis
- 007 Other protozoal intestinal diseases
- 008 Intestinal infections due to other organisms
- 009 Ill-defined intestinal infections

Tuberculosis (010-018)
- 010 Primary tuberculous infection
- 011 Pulmonary tuberculosis
- 012 Other respiratory tuberculosis
- 013 Tuberculosis of meninges and central nervous system
- 014 Tuberculosis of intestines, peritoneum, and mesenteric glands
- 015 Tuberculosis of bones and joints
- 016 Tuberculosis of genitourinary system
- 017 Tuberculosis of other organs
- 018 Miliary tuberculosis

Zoonotic bacterial diseases (020-027)
- 020 Plague
- 021 Tularemia
- 022 Anthrax
- 023 Brucellosis
- 024 Glanders
- 025 Melioidosis
- 026 Rat-bite fever
- 027 Other zoonotic bacterial diseases

Other bacterial diseases (030-041)
- 030 Leprosy
- 031 Diseases due to other mycobacteria
- 032 Diphtheria
- 033 Whooping cough
- 034 Streptococcal sore throat and scarlet fever
- 035 Erysipelas
- 036 Meningococcal infection
- 037 Tetanus
- 038 Septicemia
- 039 Actinomycotic infections
- 040 Other bacterial diseases
- 041 Bacterial infection in conditions classified elsewhere and of unspecified site

Human immunodeficiency virus (HIV) infection (042)
- 042 Human immunodeficiency virus [HIV] disease

Poliomyelitis and other non-arthropod-borne viral diseases of central nervous system (045-049)
- 045 Acute poliomyelitis
- 046 Slow virus infection of central nervous system
- 047 Meningitis due to enterovirus
- 048 Other enterovirus diseases of central nervous system
- 049 Other non-arthropod-borne viral diseases of central nervous system

Viral diseases accompanied by exanthem (050-057)
- 050 Smallpox
- 051 Cowpox and paravaccinia
- 052 Chickenpox
- 053 Herpes zoster
- 054 Herpes simplex
- 055 Measles
- 056 Rubella

APPENDIX E

1. INFECTIOUS AND PARASITIC DISEASES continued

    057   Other viral exanthemata

Other Human Herpesviruses (058)
    058   Other human herpesviruses

Arthropod-borne viral diseases (060-066)
    060   Yellow fever
    061   Dengue
    062   Mosquito-borne viral encephalitis
    063   Tick-borne viral encephalitis
    064   Viral encephalitis transmitted by other and unspecified arthropods
    065   Arthropod-borne hemorrhagic fever
    066   Other arthropod-borne viral diseases

Other diseases due to viruses and Chlamydiae (070-079)
    070   Viral hepatitis
    071   Rabies
    072   Mumps
    073   Ornithosis
    074   Specific diseases due to Coxsackie virus
    075   Infectious mononucleosis
    076   Trachoma
    077   Other diseases of conjunctiva due to viruses and Chlamydiae
    078   Other diseases due to viruses and Chlamydiae
    079   Viral and Chlamydial infection in conditions classified elsewhere and of unspecified site

Rickettsioses and other arthropod-borne diseases (080-088)
    080   Louse-borne [epidemic] typhus
    081   Other typhus
    082   Tick-borne rickettsioses
    083   Other rickettsioses
    084   Malaria
    085   Leishmaniasis
    086   Trypanosomiasis
    087   Relapsing fever
    088   Other arthropod-borne diseases

Syphilis and other venereal diseases (090-099)
    090   Congenital syphilis
    091   Early syphilis, symptomatic
    092   Early syphilis, latent
    093   Cardiovascular syphilis
    094   Neurosyphilis
    095   Other forms of late syphilis, with symptoms
    096   Late syphilis, latent
    097   Other and unspecified syphilis
    098   Gonococcal infections
    099   Other venereal diseases

Other spirochetal diseases (100-104)
    100   Leptospirosis
    101   Vincent's angina
    102   Yaws
    103   Pinta
    104   Other spirochetal infection

Mycoses (110-118)
    110   Dermatophytosis
    111   Dermatomycosis, other and unspecified
    112   Candidiasis
    114   Coccidioidomycosis
    115   Histoplasmosis
    116   Blastomycotic infection
    117   Other mycoses
    118   Opportunistic mycoses

Helminthiases (120-129)
    120   Schistosomiasis [bilharziasis]
    121   Other trematode infections

THREE DIGIT CATEGORIES

1. INFECTIOUS AND PARASITIC DISEASES *continued*

- 122 Echinococcosis
- 123 Other cestode infection
- 124 Trichinosis
- 125 Filarial infection and dracontiasis
- 126 Ancylostomiasis and necatoriasis
- 127 Other intestinal helminthiases
- 128 Other and unspecified helminthiases
- 129 Intestinal parasitism, unspecified

Other infectious and parasitic diseases (130-136)
- 130 Toxoplasmosis
- 131 Trichomoniasis
- 132 Pediculosis and phthirus infestation
- 133 Acariasis
- 134 Other infestation
- 135 Sarcoidosis
- 136 Other and unspecified infectious and parasitic diseases

Late effects of infectious and parasitic diseases (137-139)
- 137 Late effects of tuberculosis
- 138 Late effects of acute poliomyelitis
- 139 Late effects of other infectious and parasitic diseases

2. NEOPLASMS

Malignant neoplasm of lip, oral cavity, and pharynx (140-149)
- 140 Malignant neoplasm of lip
- 141 Malignant neoplasm of tongue
- 142 Malignant neoplasm of major salivary glands
- 143 Malignant neoplasm of gum
- 144 Malignant neoplasm of floor of mouth
- 145 Malignant neoplasm of other and unspecified parts of mouth
- 146 Malignant neoplasm of oropharynx
- 147 Malignant neoplasm of nasopharynx
- 148 Malignant neoplasm of hypopharynx
- 149 Malignant neoplasm of other and ill-defined sites within the lip, oral cavity, and pharynx

Malignant neoplasm of digestive organs and peritoneum (150-159)
- 150 Malignant neoplasm of esophagus
- 151 Malignant neoplasm of stomach
- 152 Malignant neoplasm of small intestine, including duodenum
- 153 Malignant neoplasm of colon
- 154 Malignant neoplasm of rectum, rectosigmoid junction, and anus
- 155 Malignant neoplasm of liver and intrahepatic bile ducts
- 156 Malignant neoplasm of gallbladder and extrahepatic bile ducts
- 157 Malignant neoplasm of pancreas
- 158 Malignant neoplasm of retroperitoneum and peritoneum
- 159 Malignant neoplasm of other and ill-defined sites within the digestive organs and peritoneum

Malignant neoplasm of respiratory and intrathoracic organs (160-165)
- 160 Malignant neoplasm of nasal cavities, middle ear, and accessory sinuses
- 161 Malignant neoplasm of larynx
- 162 Malignant neoplasm of trachea, bronchus, and lung
- 163 Malignant neoplasm of pleura
- 164 Malignant neoplasm of thymus, heart, and mediastinum
- 165 Malignant neoplasm of other and ill-defined sites within the respiratory system and intrathoracic organs

Malignant neoplasm of bone, connective tissue, skin, and breast (170-176)
- 170 Malignant neoplasm of bone and articular cartilage
- 171 Malignant neoplasm of connective and other soft tissue
- 172 Malignant melanoma of skin
- 173 Other malignant neoplasm of skin
- 174 Malignant neoplasm of female breast
- 175 Malignant neoplasm of male breast
- 176 Kaposi's sarcoma

APPENDIX E

2. NEOPLASMS continued

Malignant neoplasm of genitourinary organs (179-189)
- 179 Malignant neoplasm of uterus, part unspecified
- 180 Malignant neoplasm of cervix uteri
- 181 Malignant neoplasm of placenta
- 182 Malignant neoplasm of body of uterus
- 183 Malignant neoplasm of ovary and other uterine adnexa
- 184 Malignant neoplasm of other and unspecified female genital organs
- 185 Malignant neoplasm of prostate
- 186 Malignant neoplasm of testis
- 187 Malignant neoplasm of penis and other male genital organs
- 188 Malignant neoplasm of bladder
- 189 Malignant neoplasm of kidney and other and unspecified urinary organs

Malignant neoplasm of other and unspecified sites (190-199)
- 190 Malignant neoplasm of eye
- 191 Malignant neoplasm of brain
- 192 Malignant neoplasm of other and unspecified parts of nervous system
- 193 Malignant neoplasm of thyroid gland
- 194 Malignant neoplasm of other endocrine glands and related structures
- 195 Malignant neoplasm of other and ill-defined sites
- 196 Secondary and unspecified malignant neoplasm of lymph nodes
- 197 Secondary malignant neoplasm of respiratory and digestive systems
- 198 Secondary malignant neoplasm of other specified sites
- 199 Malignant neoplasm without specification of site

Malignant neoplasm of lymphatic and hematopoietic tissue (200-208)
- 200 Lymphosarcoma and reticulosarcoma and other specified malignant tumors of lymphatic tissue
- 201 Hodgkin's disease
- 202 Other malignant neoplasm of lymphoid and histiocytic tissue
- 203 Multiple myeloma and immunoproliferative neoplasms
- 204 Lymphoid leukemia
- 205 Myeloid leukemia
- 206 Monocytic leukemia
- 207 Other specified leukemia
- 208 Leukemia of unspecified cell type

Benign neoplasms (210-229)
- 210 Benign neoplasm of lip, oral cavity, and pharynx
- 211 Benign neoplasm of other parts of digestive system
- 212 Benign neoplasm of respiratory and intrathoracic organs
- 213 Benign neoplasm of bone and articular cartilage
- 214 Lipoma
- 215 Other benign neoplasm of connective and other soft tissue
- 216 Benign neoplasm of skin
- 217 Benign neoplasm of breast
- 218 Uterine leiomyoma
- 219 Other benign neoplasm of uterus
- 220 Benign neoplasm of ovary
- 221 Benign neoplasm of other female genital organs
- 222 Benign neoplasm of male genital organs
- 223 Benign neoplasm of kidney and other urinary organs
- 224 Benign neoplasm of eye
- 225 Benign neoplasm of brain and other parts of nervous system
- 226 Benign neoplasm of thyroid gland
- 227 Benign neoplasm of other endocrine glands and related structures
- 228 Hemangioma and lymphangioma, any site
- 229 Benign neoplasm of other and unspecified sites

Carcinoma in situ (230-234)
- 230 Carcinoma in situ of digestive organs
- 231 Carcinoma in situ of respiratory system
- 232 Carcinoma in situ of skin
- 233 Carcinoma in situ of breast and genitourinary system
- 234 Carcinoma in situ of other and unspecified sites

Neoplasms of uncertain behavior (235-238)
- 235 Neoplasm of uncertain behavior of digestive and respiratory systems

THREE DIGIT CATEGORIES

2. **NEOPLASMS** continued
        236   Neoplasm of uncertain behavior of genitourinary organs
        237   Neoplasm of uncertain behavior of endocrine glands and nervous system
        238   Neoplasm of uncertain behavior of other and unspecified sites and tissues

Neoplasm of unspecified nature (239)
        239   Neoplasm of unspecified nature

3. **ENDOCRINE, NUTRITIONAL AND METABOLIC DISEASES, AND IMMUNITY DISORDERS**

Disorders of thyroid gland (240-246)
        240   Simple and unspecified goiter
        241   Nontoxic nodular goiter
        242   Thyrotoxicosis with or without goiter
        243   Congenital hypothyroidism
        244   Acquired hypothyroidism
        245   Thyroiditis
        246   Other disorders of thyroid

Diseases of other endocrine glands (250-259)
        250   Diabetes mellitus
        251   Other disorders of pancreatic internal secretion
        252   Disorders of parathyroid gland
        253   Disorders of the pituitary gland and its hypothalamic control
        254   Diseases of thymus gland
        255   Disorders of adrenal glands
        256   Ovarian dysfunction
        257   Testicular dysfunction
        258   Polyglandular dysfunction and related disorders
        259   Other endocrine disorders

Nutritional deficiencies (260-269)
        260   Kwashiorkor
        261   Nutritional marasmus
        262   Other severe protein-calorie malnutrition
        263   Other and unspecified protein-calorie malnutrition
        264   Vitamin A deficiency
        265   Thiamine and niacin deficiency states
        266   Deficiency of B-complex components
        267   Ascorbic acid deficiency
        268   Vitamin D deficiency
        269   Other nutritional deficiencies

Other metabolic and immunity disorders (270-279)
        270   Disorders of amino-acid transport and metabolism
        271   Disorders of carbohydrate transport and metabolism
        272   Disorders of lipoid metabolism
        273   Disorders of plasma protein metabolism
        274   Gout
        275   Disorders of mineral metabolism
        276   Disorders of fluid, electrolyte, and acid-base balance
        277   Other and unspecified disorders of metabolism
        278   Overweight, obesity and other hyperalimentation
        279   Disorders involving the immune mechanism

4. **DISEASES OF THE BLOOD AND BLOOD-FORMING ORGANS**

Diseases of blood and blood-forming organs (280-289)
        280   Iron deficiency anemias
        281   Other deficiency anemias
        282   Hereditary hemolytic anemias
        283   Acquired hemolytic anemias
        284   Aplastic anemia and other bone marrow failure syndromes
        285   Other and unspecified anemias
        286   Coagulation defects
        287   Purpura and other hemorrhagic conditions
        288   Diseases of white blood cells
        289   Other diseases of blood and blood-forming organs

APPENDIX E

5. MENTAL DISORDERS
Organic psychotic conditions (290-294)
- 290 Dementias
- 291 Alcohol-induced mental disorders
- 292 Drug-induced mental disorders
- 293 Transient mental disorders due to conditions classified elsewhere
- 294 Persistent mental disorders due to conditions classified elsewhere

Other psychoses (295-299)
- 295 Schizophrenic disorders
- 296 Episodic mood disorders
- 297 Delusional disorders
- 298 Other nonorganic psychoses
- 299 Pervasive developmental disorders

Neurotic disorders, personality disorders, and other nonpsychotic mental disorders (300-316)
- 300 Anxiety, dissociative and somatoform disorders
- 301 Personality disorders
- 302 Sexual and gender identity disorders
- 303 Alcohol dependence syndrome
- 304 Drug dependence
- 305 Nondependent abuse of drugs
- 306 Physiological malfunction arising from mental factors
- 307 Special symptoms or syndromes, not elsewhere classified
- 308 Acute reaction to stress
- 309 Adjustment reaction
- 310 Specific nonpsychotic mental disorders due to brain damage
- 311 Depressive disorder, not elsewhere classified
- 312 Disturbance of conduct, not elsewhere classified
- 313 Disturbance of emotions specific to childhood and adolescence
- 314 Hyperkinetic syndrome of childhood
- 315 Specific delays in development
- 316 Psychic factors associated with diseases classified elsewhere

Mental retardation (317-319)
- 317 Mild mental retardation
- 318 Other specified mental retardation
- 319 Unspecified mental retardation

6. DISEASES OF THE NERVOUS SYSTEM AND SENSE ORGANS
Inflammatory diseases of the central nervous system (320-326)
- 320 Bacterial meningitis
- 321 Meningitis due to other organisms
- 322 Meningitis of unspecified cause
- 323 Encephalitis, myelitis, and encephalomyelitis
- 324 Intracranial and intraspinal abscess
- 325 Phlebitis and thrombophlebitis of intracranial venous sinuses
- 326 Late effects of intracranial abscess or pyogenic infection

Organic sleep disorders (327)
- 327 Organic sleep disorders

Hereditary and degenerative diseases of the central nervous system (330-337)
- 330 Cerebral degenerations usually manifest in childhood
- 331 Other cerebral degenerations
- 332 Parkinson's disease
- 333 Other extrapyramidal disease and abnormal movement disorders
- 334 Spinocerebellar disease
- 335 Anterior horn cell disease
- 336 Other diseases of spinal cord
- 337 Disorders of the autonomic nervous system

Pain (338)
- 338 Pain, not elsewhere classified

Other disorders of the central nervous system (340-349)
- 340 Multiple sclerosis
- 341 Other demyelinating diseases of central nervous system
- 342 Hemiplegia and hemiparesis

THREE DIGIT CATEGORIES

6. DISEASES OF THE NERVOUS SYSTEM AND SENSE ORGANS *continued*

- 343 Infantile cerebral palsy
- 344 Other paralytic syndromes
- 345 Epilepsy and recurrent seizures
- 346 Migraine
- 347 Cataplexy and narcolepsy
- 348 Other conditions of brain
- 349 Other and unspecified disorders of the nervous system

Disorders of the peripheral nervous system (350-359)
- 350 Trigeminal nerve disorders
- 351 Facial nerve disorders
- 352 Disorders of other cranial nerves
- 353 Nerve root and plexus disorders
- 354 Mononeuritis of upper limb and mononeuritis multiplex
- 355 Mononeuritis of lower limb and unspecified site
- 356 Hereditary and idiopathic peripheral neuropathy
- 357 Inflammatory and toxic neuropathy
- 358 Myoneural disorders
- 359 Muscular dystrophies and other myopathies

Disorders of the eye and adnexa (360-379)
- 360 Disorders of the globe
- 361 Retinal detachments and defects
- 362 Other retinal disorders
- 363 Chorioretinal inflammations, scars and other disorders of choroid
- 364 Disorders of iris and ciliary body
- 365 Glaucoma
- 366 Cataract
- 367 Disorders of refraction and accommodation
- 368 Visual disturbances
- 369 Blindness and low vision
- 370 Keratitis
- 371 Corneal opacity and other disorders of cornea
- 372 Disorders of conjunctiva
- 373 Inflammation of eyelids
- 374 Other disorders of eyelids
- 375 Disorders of lacrimal system
- 376 Disorders of the orbit
- 377 Disorders of optic nerve and visual pathways
- 378 Strabismus and other disorders of binocular eye movements
- 379 Other disorders of eye

Diseases of the ear and mastoid process (380-389)
- 380 Disorders of external ear
- 381 Nonsuppurative otitis media and Eustachian tube disorders
- 382 Suppurative and unspecified otitis media
- 383 Mastoiditis and related conditions
- 384 Other disorders of tympanic membrane
- 385 Other disorders of middle ear and mastoid
- 386 Vertiginous syndromes and other disorders of vestibular system
- 387 Otosclerosis
- 388 Other disorders of ear
- 389 Hearing loss

7. DISEASES OF THE CIRCULATORY SYSTEM

Acute rheumatic fever (390-392)
- 390 Rheumatic fever without mention of heart involvement
- 391 Rheumatic fever with heart involvement
- 392 Rheumatic chorea

Chronic rheumatic heart disease (393-398)
- 393 Chronic rheumatic pericarditis
- 394 Diseases of mitral valve
- 395 Diseases of aortic valve
- 396 Diseases of mitral and aortic valves
- 397 Diseases of other endocardial structures

7. DISEASES OF THE CIRCULATORY SYSTEM *continued*

    398   Other rheumatic heart disease

Hypertensive disease (401-405)
- 401   Essential hypertension
- 402   Hypertensive heart disease
- 403   Hypertensive chronic kidney disease
- 404   Hypertensive heart and chronic kidney disease
- 405   Secondary hypertension

Ischemic heart disease (410-414)
- 410   Acute myocardial infarction
- 411   Other acute and subacute form of ischemic heart disease
- 412   Old myocardial infarction
- 413   Angina pectoris
- 414   Other forms of chronic ischemic heart disease

Diseases of pulmonary circulation (415-417)
- 415   Acute pulmonary heart disease
- 416   Chronic pulmonary heart disease
- 417   Other diseases of pulmonary circulation

Other forms of heart disease (420-429)
- 420   Acute pericarditis
- 421   Acute and subacute endocarditis
- 422   Acute myocarditis
- 423   Other diseases of pericardium
- 424   Other diseases of endocardium
- 425   Cardiomyopathy
- 426   Conduction disorders
- 427   Cardiac dysrhythmias
- 428   Heart failure
- 429   Ill-defined descriptions and complications of heart disease

Cerebrovascular disease (430-438)
- 430   Subarachnoid hemorrhage
- 431   Intracerebral hemorrhage
- 432   Other and unspecified intracranial hemorrhage
- 433   Occlusion and stenosis of precerebral arteries
- 434   Occlusion of cerebral arteries
- 435   Transient cerebral ischemia
- 436   Acute but ill-defined cerebrovascular disease
- 437   Other and ill-defined cerebrovascular disease
- 438   Late effects of cerebrovascular disease

Diseases of arteries, arterioles, and capillaries (440-449)
- 440   Atherosclerosis
- 441   Aortic aneurysm and dissection
- 442   Other aneurysm
- 443   Other peripheral vascular disease
- 444   Arterial embolism and thrombosis
- 445   Atheroembolism
- 446   Polyarteritis nodosa and allied conditions
- 447   Other disorders of arteries and arterioles
- 448   Diseases of capillaries
- 449   Septic arterial embolism

Diseases of veins and lymphatics, and other diseases of circulatory system (451-459)
- 451   Phlebitis and thrombophlebitis
- 452   Portal vein thrombosis
- 453   Other venous embolism and thrombosis
- 454   Varicose veins of lower extremities
- 455   Hemorrhoids
- 456   Varicose veins of other sites
- 457   Noninfective disorders of lymphatic channels
- 458   Hypotension
- 459   Other disorders of circulatory system

THREE DIGIT CATEGORIES

8. DISEASES OF THE RESPIRATORY SYSTEM

Acute respiratory infections (460-466)
- 460 Acute nasopharyngitis [common cold]
- 461 Acute sinusitis
- 462 Acute pharyngitis
- 463 Acute tonsillitis
- 464 Acute laryngitis and tracheitis
- 465 Acute upper respiratory infections of multiple or unspecified sites
- 466 Acute bronchitis and bronchiolitis

Other diseases of upper respiratory tract (470-478)
- 470 Deviated nasal septum
- 471 Nasal polyps
- 472 Chronic pharyngitis and nasopharyngitis
- 473 Chronic sinusitis
- 474 Chronic disease of tonsils and adenoids
- 475 Peritonsillar abscess
- 476 Chronic laryngitis and laryngotracheitis
- 477 Allergic rhinitis
- 478 Other diseases of upper respiratory tract

Pneumonia and influenza (480-488)
- 480 Viral pneumonia
- 481 Pneumococcal pneumonia [*Streptococcus pneumoniae* pneumonia]
- 482 Other bacterial pneumonia
- 483 Pneumonia due to other specified organism
- 484 Pneumonia in infectious diseases classified elsewhere
- 485 Bronchopneumonia, organism unspecified
- 486 Pneumonia, organism unspecified
- 487 Influenza
- 488 Influenza due to identified avian influenza virus

Chronic obstructive pulmonary disease and allied conditions (490-496)
- 490 Bronchitis, not specified as acute or chronic
- 491 Chronic bronchitis
- 492 Emphysema
- 493 Asthma
- 494 Bronchiectasis
- 495 Extrinsic allergic alveolitis
- 496 Chronic airway obstruction, not elsewhere classified

Pneumoconioses and other lung diseases due to external agents (500-508)
- 500 Coal workers' pneumoconiosis
- 501 Asbestosis
- 502 Pneumoconiosis due to other silica or silicates
- 503 Pneumoconiosis due to other inorganic dust
- 504 Pneumopathy due to inhalation of other dust
- 505 Pneumoconiosis, unspecified
- 506 Respiratory conditions due to chemical fumes and vapors
- 507 Pneumonitis due to solids and liquids
- 508 Respiratory conditions due to other and unspecified external agents

Other diseases of respiratory system (510-519)
- 510 Empyema
- 511 Pleurisy
- 512 Pneumothorax
- 513 Abscess of lung and mediastinum
- 514 Pulmonary congestion and hypostasis
- 515 Postinflammatory pulmonary fibrosis
- 516 Other alveolar and parietoalveolar pneumopathy
- 517 Lung involvement in conditions classified elsewhere
- 518 Other diseases of lung
- 519 Other diseases of respiratory system

9. DISEASES OF THE DIGESTIVE SYSTEM

Diseases of oral cavity, salivary glands, and jaws (520-529)
- 520 Disorders of tooth development and eruption
- 521 Diseases of hard tissues of teeth
- 522 Diseases of pulp and periapical tissues

APPENDIX E

9. DISEASES OF THE DIGESTIVE SYSTEM *continued*

    523   Gingival and periodontal diseases
    524   Dentofacial anomalies, including malocclusion
    525   Other diseases and conditions of the teeth and supporting structures
    526   Diseases of the jaws
    527   Diseases of the salivary glands
    528   Diseases of the oral soft tissues, excluding lesions specific for gingiva and tongue
    529   Diseases and other conditions of the tongue

Diseases of esophagus, stomach, and duodenum (530-538)
    530   Diseases of esophagus
    531   Gastric ulcer
    532   Duodenal ulcer
    533   Peptic ulcer, site unspecified
    534   Gastrojejunal ulcer
    535   Gastritis and duodenitis
    536   Disorders of function of stomach
    537   Other disorders of stomach and duodenum
    538   Gastrointestinal mucositis (ulcerative)

Appendicitis (540-543)
    540   Acute appendicitis
    541   Appendicitis, unqualified
    542   Other appendicitis
    543   Other diseases of appendix

Hernia of abdominal cavity (550-553)
    550   Inguinal hernia
    551   Other hernia of abdominal cavity, with gangrene
    552   Other hernia of abdominal cavity, with obstruction, but without mention of gangrene
    553   Other hernia of abdominal cavity without mention of obstruction or gangrene

Noninfectious enteritis and colitis (555-558)
    555   Regional enteritis
    556   Ulcerative colitis
    557   Vascular insufficiency of intestine
    558   Other and unspecified noninfectious gastroenteritis and colitis

Other diseases of intestines and peritoneum (560-569)
    560   Intestinal obstruction without mention of hernia
    562   Diverticula of intestine
    564   Functional digestive disorders, not elsewhere classified
    565   Anal fissure and fistula
    566   Abscess of anal and rectal regions
    567   Peritonitis and retroperitoneal infections
    568   Other disorders of peritoneum
    569   Other disorders of intestine

Other diseases of digestive system (570-579)
    570   Acute and subacute necrosis of liver
    571   Chronic liver disease and cirrhosis
    572   Liver abscess and sequelae of chronic liver disease
    573   Other disorders of liver
    574   Cholelithiasis
    575   Other disorders of gallbladder
    576   Other disorders of biliary tract
    577   Diseases of pancreas
    578   Gastrointestinal hemorrhage
    579   Intestinal malabsorption

10. DISEASES OF THE GENITOURINARY SYSTEM

Nephritis, nephrotic syndrome, and nephrosis (580-589)
    580   Acute glomerulonephritis
    581   Nephrotic syndrome
    582   Chronic glomerulonephritis
    583   Nephritis and nephropathy, not specified as acute or chronic
    584   Acute renal failure
    585   Chronic kidney disease (CKD)

THREE DIGIT CATEGORIES

10. DISEASES OF THE GENITOURINARY SYSTEM continued
- 586 Renal failure, unspecified
- 587 Renal sclerosis, unspecified
- 588 Disorders resulting from impaired renal function
- 589 Small kidney of unknown cause

Other diseases of urinary system (590-599)
- 590 Infections of kidney
- 591 Hydronephrosis
- 592 Calculus of kidney and ureter
- 593 Other disorders of kidney and ureter
- 594 Calculus of lower urinary tract
- 595 Cystitis
- 596 Other disorders of bladder
- 597 Urethritis, not sexually transmitted, and urethral syndrome
- 598 Urethral stricture
- 599 Other disorders of urethra and urinary tract

Diseases of male genital organs (600-608)
- 600 Hyperplasia of prostate
- 601 Inflammatory diseases of prostate
- 602 Other disorders of prostate
- 603 Hydrocele
- 604 Orchitis and epididymitis
- 605 Redundant prepuce and phimosis
- 606 Infertility, male
- 607 Disorders of penis
- 608 Other disorders of male genital organs

Disorders of breast (610-611)
- 610 Benign mammary dysplasias
- 611 Other disorders of breast

Inflammatory disease of female pelvic organs (614-616)
- 614 Inflammatory disease of ovary, fallopian tube, pelvic cellular tissue, and peritoneum
- 615 Inflammatory diseases of uterus, except cervix
- 616 Inflammatory disease of cervix, vagina, and vulva

Other disorders of female genital tract (617-629)
- 617 Endometriosis
- 618 Genital prolapse
- 619 Fistula involving female genital tract
- 620 Noninflammatory disorders of ovary, fallopian tube, and broad ligament
- 621 Disorders of uterus, not elsewhere classified
- 622 Noninflammatory disorders of cervix
- 623 Noninflammatory disorders of vagina
- 624 Noninflammatory disorders of vulva and perineum
- 625 Pain and other symptoms associated with female genital organs
- 626 Disorders of menstruation and other abnormal bleeding from female genital tract
- 627 Menopausal and postmenopausal disorders
- 628 Infertility, female
- 629 Other disorders of female genital organs

11. COMPLICATIONS OF PREGNANCY, CHILDBIRTH AND THE PUERPERIUM

Ectopic and molar pregnancy (630-633)
- 630 Hydatidiform mole
- 631 Other abnormal product of conception
- 632 Missed abortion
- 633 Ectopic pregnancy

Other pregnancy with abortive outcome (634-639)
- 634 Abortion
- 635 Legally induced abortion
- 636 Illegally induced abortion
- 637 Unspecified abortion
- 638 Failed attempted abortion
- 639 Complications following abortion and ectopic and molar pregnancies

APPENDIX E

11. COMPLICATIONS OF PREGNANCY, CHILDBIRTH AND THE PUERPERIUM continued

Complications mainly related to pregnancy (640-649)
- 640 Hemorrhage in early pregnancy
- 641 Antepartum hemorrhage, abruptio placentae, and placenta previa
- 642 Hypertension complicating pregnancy, childbirth, and the puerperium
- 643 Excessive vomiting in pregnancy
- 644 Early or threatened labor
- 645 Late pregnancy
- 646 Other complications of pregnancy, not elsewhere classified
- 647 Infectious and parasitic conditions in the mother classifiable elsewhere but complicating pregnancy, childbirth, and the puerperium
- 648 Other current conditions in the mother classifiable elsewhere but complicating pregnancy, childbirth, and the puerperium
- 649 Other conditions or status of the mother complicating pregnancy, childbirth or the puerperium

Normal delivery, and other indications for care in pregnancy, labor, and delivery (650-659)
- 650 Normal delivery
- 651 Multiple gestation
- 652 Malposition and malpresentation of fetus
- 653 Disproportion
- 654 Abnormality of organs and soft tissues of pelvis
- 655 Known or suspected fetal abnormality affecting management of mother
- 656 Other fetal and placental problems affecting management of mother
- 657 Polyhydramnios
- 658 Other problems associated with amniotic cavity and membranes
- 659 Other indications for care or intervention related to labor and delivery and not elsewhere classified

Complications occurring mainly in the course of labor and delivery (660-669)
- 660 Obstructed labor
- 661 Abnormality of forces of labor
- 662 Long labor
- 663 Umbilical cord complications
- 664 Trauma to perineum and vulva during delivery
- 665 Other obstetrical trauma
- 666 Postpartum hemorrhage
- 667 Retained placenta or membranes, without hemorrhage
- 668 Complications of the administration of anesthetic or other sedation in labor and delivery
- 669 Other complications of labor and delivery, not elsewhere classified

Complications of the puerperium (670-677)
- 670 Major puerperal infection
- 671 Venous complications in pregnancy and the puerperium
- 672 Pyrexia of unknown origin during the puerperium
- 673 Obstetrical pulmonary embolism
- 674 Other and unspecified complications of the puerperium, not elsewhere classified
- 675 Infections of the breast and nipple associated with childbirth
- 676 Other disorders of the breast associated with childbirth, and disorders of lactation
- 677 Late effect of complication of pregnancy, childbirth, and the puerperium

12. DISEASES OF THE SKIN AND SUBCUTANEOUS TISSUE

Infections of skin and subcutaneous tissue (680-686)
- 680 Carbuncle and furuncle
- 681 Cellulitis and abscess of finger and toe
- 682 Other cellulitis and abscess
- 683 Acute lymphadenitis
- 684 Impetigo
- 685 Pilonidal cyst
- 686 Other local infections of skin and subcutaneous tissue

Other inflammatory conditions of skin and subcutaneous tissue (690-698)
- 690 Erythematosquamous dermatosis
- 691 Atopic dermatitis and related conditions
- 692 Contact dermatitis and other eczema
- 693 Dermatitis due to substances taken internally
- 694 Bullous dermatoses

THREE DIGIT CATEGORIES

12. DISEASES OF THE SKIN AND SUBCUTANEOUS TISSUE *continued*
- 695 Erythematous conditions
- 696 Psoriasis and similar disorders
- 697 Lichen
- 698 Pruritus and related conditions

Other diseases of skin and subcutaneous tissue (700-709)
- 700 Corns and callosities
- 701 Other hypertrophic and atrophic conditions of skin
- 702 Other dermatoses
- 703 Diseases of nail
- 704 Diseases of hair and hair follicles
- 705 Disorders of sweat glands
- 706 Diseases of sebaceous glands
- 707 Chronic ulcer of skin
- 708 Urticaria
- 709 Other disorders of skin and subcutaneous tissue

13. DISEASES OF THE MUSCULOSKELETAL SYSTEM AND CONNECTIVE TISSUE

Arthropathies and related disorders (710-719)
- 710 Diffuse diseases of connective tissue
- 711 Arthropathy associated with infections
- 712 Crystal arthropathies
- 713 Arthropathy associated with other disorders classified elsewhere
- 714 Rheumatoid arthritis and other inflammatory polyarthropathies
- 715 Osteoarthrosis and allied disorders
- 716 Other and unspecified arthropathies
- 717 Internal derangement of knee
- 718 Other derangement of joint
- 719 Other and unspecified disorder of joint

Dorsopathies (720-724)
- 720 Ankylosing spondylitis and other inflammatory spondylopathies
- 721 Spondylosis and allied disorders
- 722 Intervertebral disc disorders
- 723 Other disorders of cervical region
- 724 Other and unspecified disorders of back

Rheumatism, excluding the back (725-729)
- 725 Polymyalgia rheumatica
- 726 Peripheral enthesopathies and allied syndromes
- 727 Other disorders of synovium, tendon, and bursa
- 728 Disorders of muscle, ligament, and fascia
- 729 Other disorders of soft tissues

Osteopathies, chondropathies, and acquired musculoskeletal deformities (730-739)
- 730 Osteomyelitis, periostitis, and other infections involving bone
- 731 Osteitis deformans and osteopathies associated with other disorders classified elsewhere
- 732 Osteochondropathies
- 733 Other disorders of bone and cartilage
- 734 Flat foot
- 735 Acquired deformities of toe
- 736 Other acquired deformities of limbs
- 737 Curvature of spine
- 738 Other acquired deformity
- 739 Nonallopathic lesions, not elsewhere classified

14. CONGENITAL ANOMALIES
- 740 Anencephalus and similar anomalies
- 741 Spina bifida
- 742 Other congenital anomalies of nervous system
- 743 Congenital anomalies of eye
- 744 Congenital anomalies of ear, face, and neck
- 745 Bulbus cordis anomalies and anomalies of cardiac septal closure
- 746 Other congenital anomalies of heart
- 747 Other congenital anomalies of circulatory system

APPENDIX E

14. CONGENITAL ANOMALIES continued
- 748 Congenital anomalies of respiratory system
- 749 Cleft palate and cleft lip
- 750 Other congenital anomalies of upper alimentary tract
- 751 Other congenital anomalies of digestive system
- 752 Congenital anomalies of genital organs
- 753 Congenital anomalies of urinary system
- 754 Certain congenital musculoskeletal deformities
- 755 Other congenital anomalies of limbs
- 756 Other congenital musculoskeletal anomalies
- 757 Congenital anomalies of the integument
- 758 Chromosomal anomalies
- 759 Other and unspecified congenital anomalies

15. CERTAIN CONDITIONS ORIGINATING IN THE PERINATAL PERIOD

Maternal causes of perinatal morbidity and mortality (760-763)
- 760 Fetus or newborn affected by maternal conditions which may be unrelated to present pregnancy
- 761 Fetus or newborn affected by maternal complications of pregnancy
- 762 Fetus or newborn affected by complications of placenta, cord, and membranes
- 763 Fetus or newborn affected by other complications of labor and delivery

Other conditions originating in the perinatal period (764-779)
- 764 Slow fetal growth and fetal malnutrition
- 765 Disorders relating to short gestation and low birthweight
- 766 Disorders relating to long gestation and high birthweight
- 767 Birth trauma
- 768 Intrauterine hypoxia and birth asphyxia
- 769 Respiratory distress syndrome
- 770 Other respiratory conditions of fetus and newborn
- 771 Infections specific to the perinatal period
- 772 Fetal and neonatal hemorrhage
- 773 Hemolytic disease of fetus or newborn, due to isoimmunization
- 774 Other perinatal jaundice
- 775 Endocrine and metabolic disturbances specific to the fetus and newborn
- 776 Hematological disorders of fetus and newborn
- 777 Perinatal disorders of digestive system
- 778 Conditions involving the integument and temperature regulation of fetus and newborn
- 779 Other and ill-defined conditions originating in the perinatal period

16. SYMPTOMS, SIGNS, AND ILL-DEFINED CONDITIONS

Symptoms (780-789)
- 780 General symptoms
- 781 Symptoms involving nervous and musculoskeletal systems
- 782 Symptoms involving skin and other integumentary tissue
- 783 Symptoms concerning nutrition, metabolism, and development
- 784 Symptoms involving head and neck
- 785 Symptoms involving cardiovascular system
- 786 Symptoms involving respiratory system and other chest symptoms
- 787 Symptoms involving digestive system
- 788 Symptoms involving urinary system
- 789 Other symptoms involving abdomen and pelvis

Nonspecific abnormal findings (790-796)
- 790 Nonspecific findings on examination of blood
- 791 Nonspecific findings on examination of urine
- 792 Nonspecific abnormal findings in other body substances
- 793 Nonspecific abnormal findings on radiological and other examination of body structure
- 794 Nonspecific abnormal results of function studies
- 795 Other and nonspecific abnormal cytological, histological, immunological and DNA test findings
- 796 Other nonspecific abnormal findings

Ill-defined and unknown causes of morbidity and mortality (797-799)
- 797 Senility without mention of psychosis
- 798 Sudden death, cause unknown
- 799 Other ill-defined and unknown causes of morbidity and mortality

THREE DIGIT CATEGORIES

17. INJURY AND POISONING

Fracture of skull (800-804)
- 800 Fracture of vault of skull
- 801 Fracture of base of skull
- 802 Fracture of face bones
- 803 Other and unqualified skull fractures
- 804 Multiple fractures involving skull or face with other bones

Fracture of neck and trunk (805-809)
- 805 Fracture of vertebral column without mention of spinal cord injury
- 806 Fracture of vertebral column with spinal cord injury
- 807 Fracture of rib(s), sternum, larynx, and trachea
- 808 Fracture of pelvis
- 809 Ill-defined fractures of bones of trunk

Fracture of upper limb (810-819)
- 810 Fracture of clavicle
- 811 Fracture of scapula
- 812 Fracture of humerus
- 813 Fracture of radius and ulna
- 814 Fracture of carpal bone(s)
- 815 Fracture of metacarpal bone(s)
- 816 Fracture of one or more phalanges of hand
- 817 Multiple fractures of hand bones
- 818 Ill-defined fractures of upper limb
- 819 Multiple fractures involving both upper limbs, and upper limb with rib(s) and sternum

Fracture of lower limb (820-829)
- 820 Fracture of neck of femur
- 821 Fracture of other and unspecified parts of femur
- 822 Fracture of patella
- 823 Fracture of tibia and fibula
- 824 Fracture of ankle
- 825 Fracture of one or more tarsal and metatarsal bones
- 826 Fracture of one or more phalanges of foot
- 827 Other, multiple, and ill-defined fractures of lower limb
- 828 Multiple fractures involving both lower limbs, lower with upper limb, and lower limb(s) with rib(s) and sternum
- 829 Fracture of unspecified bones

Dislocation (830-839)
- 830 Dislocation of jaw
- 831 Dislocation of shoulder
- 832 Dislocation of elbow
- 833 Dislocation of wrist
- 834 Dislocation of finger
- 835 Dislocation of hip
- 836 Dislocation of knee
- 837 Dislocation of ankle
- 838 Dislocation of foot
- 839 Other, multiple, and ill-defined dislocations

Sprains and strains of joints and adjacent muscles (840-848)
- 840 Sprains and strains of shoulder and upper arm
- 841 Sprains and strains of elbow and forearm
- 842 Sprains and strains of wrist and hand
- 843 Sprains and strains of hip and thigh
- 844 Sprains and strains of knee and leg
- 845 Sprains and strains of ankle and foot
- 846 Sprains and strains of sacroiliac region
- 847 Sprains and strains of other and unspecified parts of back
- 848 Other and ill-defined sprains and strains

Intracranial injury, excluding those with skull fracture (850-854)
- 850 Concussion
- 851 Cerebral laceration and contusion
- 852 Subarachnoid, subdural, and extradural hemorrhage, following injury
- 853 Other and unspecified intracranial hemorrhage following injury
- 854 Intracranial injury of other and unspecified nature

APPENDIX E

17. INJURY AND POISONING *continued*

Internal injury of thorax, abdomen, and pelvis (860-869)
- 860 Traumatic pneumothorax and hemothorax
- 861 Injury to heart and lung
- 862 Injury to other and unspecified intrathoracic organs
- 863 Injury to gastrointestinal tract
- 864 Injury to liver
- 865 Injury to spleen
- 866 Injury to kidney
- 867 Injury to pelvic organs
- 868 Injury to other intra-abdominal organs
- 869 Internal injury to unspecified or ill-defined organs

Open wound of head, neck, and trunk (870-879)
- 870 Open wound of ocular adnexa
- 871 Open wound of eyeball
- 872 Open wound of ear
- 873 Other open wound of head
- 874 Open wound of neck
- 875 Open wound of chest (wall)
- 876 Open wound of back
- 877 Open wound of buttock
- 878 Open wound of genital organs (external), including traumatic amputation
- 879 Open wound of other and unspecified sites, except limbs

Open wound of upper limb (880-887)
- 880 Open wound of shoulder and upper arm
- 881 Open wound of elbow, forearm, and wrist
- 882 Open wound of hand except finger(s) alone
- 883 Open wound of finger(s)
- 884 Multiple and unspecified open wound of upper limb
- 885 Traumatic amputation of thumb (complete) (partial)
- 886 Traumatic amputation of other finger(s) (complete) (partial)
- 887 Traumatic amputation of arm and hand (complete) (partial)

Open wound of lower limb (890-897)
- 890 Open wound of hip and thigh
- 891 Open wound of knee, leg [except thigh], and ankle
- 892 Open wound of foot except toe(s) alone
- 893 Open wound of toe(s)
- 894 Multiple and unspecified open wound of lower limb
- 895 Traumatic amputation of toe(s) (complete) (partial)
- 896 Traumatic amputation of foot (complete) (partial)
- 897 Traumatic amputation of leg(s) (complete) (partial)

Injury to blood vessels (900-904)
- 900 Injury to blood vessels of head and neck
- 901 Injury to blood vessels of thorax
- 902 Injury to blood vessels of abdomen and pelvis
- 903 Injury to blood vessels of upper extremity
- 904 Injury to blood vessels of lower extremity and unspecified sites

Late effects of injuries, poisonings, toxic effects, and other external causes (905-909)
- 905 Late effects of musculoskeletal and connective tissue injuries
- 906 Late effects of injuries to skin and subcutaneous tissues
- 907 Late effects of injuries to the nervous system
- 908 Late effects of other and unspecified injuries
- 909 Late effects of other and unspecified external causes

Superficial injury (910-919)
- 910 Superficial injury of face, neck, and scalp except eye
- 911 Superficial injury of trunk
- 912 Superficial injury of shoulder and upper arm
- 913 Superficial injury of elbow, forearm, and wrist
- 914 Superficial injury of hand(s) except finger(s) alone
- 915 Superficial injury of finger(s)
- 916 Superficial injury of hip, thigh, leg, and ankle
- 917 Superficial injury of foot and toe(s)

THREE DIGIT CATEGORIES

17. INJURY AND POISONING *continued*
- 918 Superficial injury of eye and adnexa
- 919 Superficial injury of other, multiple, and unspecified sites

Contusion with intact skin surface (920-924)
- 920 Contusion of face, scalp, and neck except eye(s)
- 921 Contusion of eye and adnexa
- 922 Contusion of trunk
- 923 Contusion of upper limb
- 924 Contusion of lower limb and of other and unspecified sites

Crushing injury (925-929)
- 925 Crushing injury of face, scalp, and neck
- 926 Crushing injury of trunk
- 927 Crushing injury of upper limb
- 928 Crushing injury of lower limb
- 929 Crushing injury of multiple and unspecified sites

Effects of foreign body entering through orifice (930-939)
- 930 Foreign body on external eye
- 931 Foreign body in ear
- 932 Foreign body in nose
- 933 Foreign body in pharynx and larynx
- 934 Foreign body in trachea, bronchus, and lung
- 935 Foreign body in mouth, esophagus, and stomach
- 936 Foreign body in intestine and colon
- 937 Foreign body in anus and rectum
- 938 Foreign body in digestive system, unspecified
- 939 Foreign body in genitourinary tract

Burns (940-949)
- 940 Burn confined to eye and adnexa
- 941 Burn of face, head, and neck
- 942 Burn of trunk
- 943 Burn of upper limb, except wrist and hand
- 944 Burn of wrist(s) and hand(s)
- 945 Burn of lower limb(s)
- 946 Burns of multiple specified sites
- 947 Burn of internal organs
- 948 Burns classified according to extent of body surface involved
- 949 Burn, unspecified

Injury to nerves and spinal cord (950-957)
- 950 Injury to optic nerve and pathways
- 951 Injury to other cranial nerve(s)
- 952 Spinal cord injury without evidence of spinal bone injury
- 953 Injury to nerve roots and spinal plexus
- 954 Injury to other nerve(s) of trunk excluding shoulder and pelvic girdles
- 955 Injury to peripheral nerve(s) of shoulder girdle and upper limb
- 956 Injury to peripheral nerve(s) of pelvic girdle and lower limb
- 957 Injury to other and unspecified nerves

Certain traumatic complications and unspecified injuries (958-959)
- 958 Certain early complications of trauma
- 959 Injury, other and unspecified

Poisoning by drugs, medicinal and biological substances (960-979)
- 960 Poisoning by antibiotics
- 961 Poisoning by other anti-infectives
- 962 Poisoning by hormones and synthetic substitutes
- 963 Poisoning by primarily systemic agents
- 964 Poisoning by agents primarily affecting blood constituents
- 965 Poisoning by analgesics, antipyretics, and antirheumatics
- 966 Poisoning by anticonvulsants and anti-Parkinsonism drugs
- 967 Poisoning by sedatives and hypnotics
- 968 Poisoning by other central nervous system depressants and anesthetics
- 969 Poisoning by psychotropic agents
- 970 Poisoning by central nervous system stimulants
- 971 Poisoning by drugs primarily affecting the autonomic nervous system

APPENDIX E

17. INJURY AND POISONING *continued*

- 972 Poisoning by agents primarily affecting the cardiovascular system
- 973 Poisoning by agents primarily affecting the gastrointestinal system
- 974 Poisoning by water, mineral, and uric acid metabolism drugs
- 975 Poisoning by agents primarily acting on the smooth and skeletal muscles and respiratory system
- 976 Poisoning by agents primarily affecting skin and mucous membrane, ophthalmological, otorhinolaryngological, and dental drugs
- 977 Poisoning by other and unspecified drugs and medicinals
- 978 Poisoning by bacterial vaccines
- 979 Poisoning by other vaccines and biological substances

Toxic effects of substances chiefly nonmedicinal as to source (980-989)
- 980 Toxic effect of alcohol
- 981 Toxic effect of petroleum products
- 982 Toxic effect of solvents other than petroleum-based
- 983 Toxic effect of corrosive aromatics, acids, and caustic alkalis
- 984 Toxic effect of lead and its compounds (including fumes)
- 985 Toxic effect of other metals
- 986 Toxic effect of carbon monoxide
- 987 Toxic effect of other gases, fumes, or vapors
- 988 Toxic effect of noxious substances eaten as food
- 989 Toxic effect of other substances, chiefly nonmedicinal as to source

Other and unspecified effects of external causes (990-995)
- 990 Effects of radiation, unspecified
- 991 Effects of reduced temperature
- 992 Effects of heat and light
- 993 Effects of air pressure
- 994 Effects of other external causes
- 995 Certain adverse effects, not elsewhere classified

Complications of surgical and medical care, not elsewhere classified (996-999)
- 996 Complications peculiar to certain specified procedures
- 997 Complications affecting specified body systems, not elsewhere classified
- 998 Other complications of procedures, not elsewhere classified
- 999 Complications of medical care, not elsewhere classified

SUPPLEMENTARY CLASSIFICATION OF FACTORS INFLUENCING HEALTH STATUS AND CONTACT WITH HEALTH SERVICES

Persons with potential health hazards related to communicable diseases (V01-V06)
- V01 Contact with or exposure to communicable diseases
- V02 Carrier or suspected carrier of infectious diseases
- V03 Need for prophylactic vaccination and inoculation against bacterial diseases
- V04 Need for prophylactic vaccination and inoculation against certain viral diseases
- V05 Need for other prophylactic vaccination and inoculation against single diseases
- V06 Need for prophylactic vaccination and inoculation against combinations of diseases

Persons with need for isolation, other potential health hazards and prophylactic measures (V07-V09)
- V07 Need for isolation and other prophylactic measures
- V08 Asymptomatic human immunodeficiency virus (HIV) infection status
- V09 Infection with drug-resistant microorganisms

Persons with potential health hazards related to personal and family history (V10-V19)
- V10 Personal history of malignant neoplasm
- V11 Personal history of mental disorder
- V12 Personal history of certain other diseases
- V13 Personal history of other diseases
- V14 Personal history of allergy to medicinal agents
- V15 Other personal history presenting hazards to health
- V16 Family history of malignant neoplasm
- V17 Family history of certain chronic disabling diseases
- V18 Family history of certain other specific conditions
- V19 Family history of other conditions

Persons encountering health services in circumstances related to reproduction and development (V20-V29)
- V20 Health supervision of infant or child
- V21 Constitutional states in development

THREE DIGIT CATEGORIES

SUPPLEMENTARY CLASSIFICATION...HEALTH STATUS/HEALTH SERVICES *continued*

- V22 Normal pregnancy
- V23 Supervision of high-risk pregnancy
- V24 Postpartum care and examination
- V25 Encounter for contraceptive management
- V26 Procreative management
- V27 Outcome of delivery
- V28 Encounter for antenatal screening of mother
- V29 Observation and evaluation of newborns and infants for suspected condition not found

Liveborn infants according to type of birth (V30-V39)

- V30 Single liveborn
- V31 Twin, mate liveborn
- V32 Twin, mate stillborn
- V33 Twin, unspecified
- V34 Other multiple, mates all liveborn
- V35 Other multiple, mates all stillborn
- V36 Other multiple, mates live- and stillborn
- V37 Other multiple, unspecified
- V39 Unspecified

Persons with a condition influencing their health status (V40-V49)

- V40 Mental and behavioral problems
- V41 Problems with special senses and other special functions
- V42 Organ or tissue replaced by transplant
- V43 Organ or tissue replaced by other means
- V44 Artificial opening status
- V45 Other postprocedural states
- V46 Other dependence on machines
- V47 Other problems with internal organs
- V48 Problems with head, neck, and trunk
- V49 Other conditions influencing health status

Persons encountering health services for specific procedures and aftercare (V50-V59)

- V50 Elective surgery for purposes other than remedying health states
- V51 Aftercare involving the use of plastic surgery
- V52 Fitting and adjustment of prosthetic device and implant
- V53 Fitting and adjustment of other device
- V54 Other orthopedic aftercare
- V55 Attention to artificial openings
- V56 Encounter for dialysis and dialysis catheter care
- V57 Care involving use of rehabilitation procedures
- V58 Encounter for other and unspecified procedures and aftercare
- V59 Donors

Persons encountering health services in other circumstances (V60-V69)

- V60 Housing, household, and economic circumstances
- V61 Other family circumstances
- V62 Other psychosocial circumstances
- V63 Unavailability of other medical facilities for care
- V64 Persons encountering health services for specific procedures, not carried out
- V65 Other persons seeking consultation
- V66 Convalescence and palliative care
- V67 Follow-up examination
- V68 Encounters for administrative purposes
- V69 Problems related to lifestyle

Persons without reported diagnosis encountered during examination and investigation of individuals and populations (V70-V86)

- V70 General medical examination
- V71 Observation and evaluation for suspected conditions not found
- V72 Special investigations and examinations
- V73 Special screening examination for viral and chlamydial diseases
- V74 Special screening examination for bacterial and spirochetal diseases
- V75 Special screening examination for other infectious diseases
- V76 Special screening for malignant neoplasms
- V77 Special screening for endocrine, nutritional, metabolic, and immunity disorders
- V78 Special screening for disorders of blood and blood-forming organs

APPENDIX E

SUPPLEMENTARY CLASSIFICATION...HEALTH STATUS/HEALTH SERVICES *continued*

- V79 Special screening for mental disorders and developmental handicaps
- V80 Special screening for neurological, eye, and ear diseases
- V81 Special screening for cardiovascular, respiratory, and genitourinary diseases
- V82 Special screening for other conditions
- V83 Genetic carrier status
- V84 Genetic susceptibility to disease
- V85 Body mass index
- V86 Estrogen receptor status

SUPPLEMENTARY CLASSIFICATION OF EXTERNAL CAUSES OF INJURY AND POISONING

Railway accidents (E800-E807)
- E800 Railway accident involving collision with rolling stock
- E801 Railway accident involving collision with other object
- E802 Railway accident involving derailment without antecedent collision
- E803 Railway accident involving explosion, fire, or burning
- E804 Fall in, on, or from railway train
- E805 Hit by rolling stock
- E806 Other specified railway accident
- E807 Railway accident of unspecified nature

Motor vehicle traffic accidents (E810-E819)
- E810 Motor vehicle traffic accident involving collision with train
- E811 Motor vehicle traffic accident involving re-entrant collision with another motor vehicle
- E812 Other motor vehicle traffic accident involving collision with another motor vehicle
- E813 Motor vehicle traffic accident involving collision with other vehicle
- E814 Motor vehicle traffic accident involving collision with pedestrian
- E815 Other motor vehicle traffic accident involving collision on the highway
- E816 Motor vehicle traffic accident due to loss of control, without collision on the highway
- E817 Noncollision motor vehicle traffic accident while boarding or alighting
- E818 Other noncollision motor vehicle traffic accident
- E819 Motor vehicle traffic accident of unspecified nature

Motor vehicle nontraffic accidents (E820-E825)
- E820 Nontraffic accident involving motor-driven snow vehicle
- E821 Nontraffic accident involving other off-road motor vehicle
- E822 Other motor vehicle nontraffic accident involving collision with moving object
- E823 Other motor vehicle nontraffic accident involving collision with stationary object
- E824 Other motor vehicle nontraffic accident while boarding and alighting
- E825 Other motor vehicle nontraffic accident of other and unspecified nature

Other road vehicle accidents (E826-E829)
- E826 Pedal cycle accident
- E827 Animal-drawn vehicle accident
- E828 Accident involving animal being ridden
- E829 Other road vehicle accidents

Water transport accidents (E830-E838)
- E830 Accident to watercraft causing submersion
- E831 Accident to watercraft causing other injury
- E832 Other accidental submersion or drowning in water transport accident
- E833 Fall on stairs or ladders in water transport
- E834 Other fall from one level to another in water transport
- E835 Other and unspecified fall in water transport
- E836 Machinery accident in water transport
- E837 Explosion, fire, or burning in watercraft
- E838 Other and unspecified water transport accident

Air and space transport accidents (E840-E845)
- E840 Accident to powered aircraft at takeoff or landing
- E841 Accident to powered aircraft, other and unspecified
- E842 Accident to unpowered aircraft
- E843 Fall in, on, or from aircraft
- E844 Other specified air transport accidents
- E845 Accident involving spacecraft

THREE DIGIT CATEGORIES

SUPPLEMENTARY CLASSIFICATION...INJURY AND POISONING *continued*

Vehicle accidents, not elsewhere classifiable (E846-E849)
- E846 Accidents involving powered vehicles used solely within the buildings and premises of an industrial or commercial establishment
- E847 Accidents involving cable cars not running on rails
- E848 Accidents involving other vehicles, not elsewhere classifiable
- E849 Place of occurrence

Accidental poisoning by drugs, medicinal substances, and biologicals (E850-E858)
- E850 Accidental poisoning by analgesics, antipyretics, and antirheumatics
- E851 Accidental poisoning by barbiturates
- E852 Accidental poisoning by other sedatives and hypnotics
- E853 Accidental poisoning by tranquilizers
- E854 Accidental poisoning by other psychotropic agents
- E855 Accidental poisoning by other drugs acting on central and autonomic nervous systems
- E856 Accidental poisoning by antibiotics
- E857 Accidental poisoning by other anti-infectives
- E858 Accidental poisoning by other drugs

Accidental poisoning by other solid and liquid substances, gases, and vapors (E860-E869)
- E860 Accidental poisoning by alcohol, not elsewhere classified
- E861 Accidental poisoning by cleansing and polishing agents, disinfectants, paints, and varnishes
- E862 Accidental poisoning by petroleum products, other solvents and their vapors, not elsewhere classified
- E863 Accidental poisoning by agricultural and horticultural chemical and pharmaceutical preparations other than plant foods and fertilizers
- E864 Accidental poisoning by corrosives and caustics, not elsewhere classified
- E865 Accidental poisoning from poisonous foodstuffs and poisonous plants
- E866 Accidental poisoning by other and unspecified solid and liquid substances
- E867 Accidental poisoning by gas distributed by pipeline
- E868 Accidental poisoning by other utility gas and other carbon monoxide
- E869 Accidental poisoning by other gases and vapors

Misadventures to patients during surgical and medical care (E870-E876)
- E870 Accidental cut, puncture, perforation, or hemorrhage during medical care
- E871 Foreign object left in body during procedure
- E872 Failure of sterile precautions during procedure
- E873 Failure in dosage
- E874 Mechanical failure of instrument or apparatus during procedure
- E875 Contaminated or infected blood, other fluid, drug, or biological substance
- E876 Other and unspecified misadventures during medical care

Surgical and medical procedures as the cause of abnormal reaction of patient or later complication, without mention of misadventure at the time of procedure (E878-E879)
- E878 Surgical operation and other surgical procedures as the cause of abnormal reaction of patient, or of later complication, without mention of misadventure at the time of operation
- E879 Other procedures, without mention of misadventure at the time of procedure, as the cause of abnormal reaction of patient, or of later complication

Accidental falls (E880-E888)
- E880 Fall on or from stairs or steps
- E881 Fall on or from ladders or scaffolding
- E882 Fall from or out of building or other structure
- E883 Fall into hole or other opening in surface
- E884 Other fall from one level to another
- E885 Fall on same level from slipping, tripping, or stumbling
- E886 Fall on same level from collision, pushing or shoving, by or with other person
- E887 Fracture, cause unspecified
- E888 Other and unspecified fall

Accidents caused by fire and flames (E890-E899)
- E890 Conflagration in private dwelling
- E891 Conflagration in other and unspecified building or structure
- E892 Conflagration not in building or structure
- E893 Accident caused by ignition of clothing
- E894 Ignition of highly inflammable material
- E895 Accident caused by controlled fire in private dwelling
- E896 Accident caused by controlled fire in other and unspecified building or structure

APPENDIX E

SUPPLEMENTARY CLASSIFICATION...INJURY AND POISONING continued

    E897 Accident caused by controlled fire not in building or structure
    E898 Accident caused by other specified fire and flames
    E899 Accident caused by unspecified fire

Accidents due to natural and environmental factors (E900-E909)
    E900 Excessive heat
    E901 Excessive cold
    E902 High and low air pressure and changes in air pressure
    E903 Travel and motion
    E904 Hunger, thirst, exposure, and neglect
    E905 Venomous animals and plants as the cause of poisoning and toxic reactions
    E906 Other injury caused by animals
    E907 Lightning
    E908 Cataclysmic storms, and floods resulting from storms
    E909 Cataclysmic earth surface movements and eruptions

Accidents caused by submersion, suffocation, and foreign bodies (E910-E915)
    E910 Accidental drowning and submersion
    E911 Inhalation and ingestion of food causing obstruction of respiratory tract or suffocation
    E912 Inhalation and ingestion of other object causing obstruction of respiratory tract or suffocation
    E913 Accidental mechanical suffocation
    E914 Foreign body accidentally entering eye and adnexa
    E915 Foreign body accidentally entering other orifice

Other accidents (E916-E928)
    E916 Struck accidentally by falling object
    E917 Striking against or struck accidentally by objects or persons
    E918 Caught accidentally in or between objects
    E919 Accidents caused by machinery
    E920 Accidents caused by cutting and piercing instruments or objects
    E921 Accident caused by explosion of pressure vessel
    E922 Accident caused by firearm and air gun missile
    E923 Accident caused by explosive material
    E924 Accident caused by hot substance or object, caustic or corrosive material, and steam
    E925 Accident caused by electric current
    E926 Exposure to radiation
    E927 Overexertion and strenuous movements
    E928 Other and unspecified environmental and accidental causes

Late effects of accidental injury (E929)
    E929 Late effects of accidental injury

Drugs, medicinal and biological substances causing adverse effects in therapeutic use (E930-E949)
    E930 Antibiotics
    E931 Other anti-infectives
    E932 Hormones and synthetic substitutes
    E933 Primarily systemic agents
    E934 Agents primarily affecting blood constituents
    E935 Analgesics, antipyretics, and antirheumatics
    E936 Anticonvulsants and anti-Parkinsonism drugs
    E937 Sedatives and hypnotics
    E938 Other central nervous system depressants and anesthetics
    E939 Psychotropic agents
    E940 Central nervous system stimulants
    E941 Drugs primarily affecting the autonomic nervous system
    E942 Agents primarily affecting the cardiovascular system
    E943 Agents primarily affecting gastrointestinal system
    E944 Water, mineral, and uric acid metabolism drugs
    E945 Agents primarily acting on the smooth and skeletal muscles and respiratory system
    E946 Agents primarily affecting skin and mucous membrane, ophthalmological, otorhinolaryngological, and dental drugs
    E947 Other and unspecified drugs and medicinal substances
    E948 Bacterial vaccines
    E949 Other vaccines and biological substances

THREE DIGIT CATEGORIES

SUPPLEMENTARY CLASSIFICATION...INJURY AND POISONING continued

Suicide and self-inflicted injury (E950-E959)
- E950 Suicide and self-inflicted poisoning by solid or liquid substances
- E951 Suicide and self-inflicted poisoning by gases in domestic use
- E952 Suicide and self-inflicted poisoning by other gases and vapors
- E953 Suicide and self-inflicted injury by hanging, strangulation, and suffocation
- E954 Suicide and self-inflicted injury by submersion [drowning]
- E955 Suicide and self-inflicted injury by firearms, air guns and explosives
- E956 Suicide and self-inflicted injury by cutting and piercing instruments
- E957 Suicide and self-inflicted injuries by jumping from high place
- E958 Suicide and self-inflicted injury by other and unspecified means
- E959 Late effects of self-inflicted injury

Homicide and injury purposely inflicted by other persons (E960-E969)
- E960 Fight, brawl, and rape
- E961 Assault by corrosive or caustic substance, except poisoning
- E962 Assault by poisoning
- E963 Assault by hanging and strangulation
- E964 Assault by submersion [drowning]
- E965 Assault by firearms and explosives
- E966 Assault by cutting and piercing instrument
- E967 Perpetrator of child and adult abuse
- E968 Assault by other and unspecified means
- E969 Late effects of injury purposely inflicted by other person

Legal intervention (E970-E978)
- E970 Injury due to legal intervention by firearms
- E971 Injury due to legal intervention by explosives
- E972 Injury due to legal intervention by gas
- E973 Injury due to legal intervention by blunt object
- E974 Injury due to legal intervention by cutting and piercing instruments
- E975 Injury due to legal intervention by other specified means
- E976 Injury due to legal intervention by unspecified means
- E977 Late effects of injuries due to legal intervention
- E978 Legal execution
- E979 Terrorism

Injury undetermined whether accidentally or purposely inflicted (E980-E989)
- E980 Poisoning by solid or liquid substances, undetermined whether accidentally or purposely inflicted
- E981 Poisoning by gases in domestic use, undetermined whether accidentally or purposely inflicted
- E982 Poisoning by other gases, undetermined whether accidentally or purposely inflicted
- E983 Hanging, strangulation, or suffocation, undetermined whether accidentally or purposely inflicted
- E984 Submersion [drowning], undetermined whether accidentally or purposely inflicted
- E985 Injury by firearms, air guns and explosives, undetermined whether accidentally or purposely inflicted
- E986 Injury by cutting and piercing instruments, undetermined whether accidentally or purposely inflicted
- E987 Falling from high place, undetermined whether accidentally or purposely inflicted
- E988 Injury by other and unspecified means, undetermined whether accidentally or purposely inflicted
- E989 Late effects of injury, undetermined whether accidentally or purposely inflicted

Injury resulting from operations of war (E990-E999)
- E990 Injury due to war operations by fires and conflagrations
- E991 Injury due to war operations by bullets and fragments
- E992 Injury due to war operations by explosion of marine weapons
- E993 Injury due to war operations by other explosion
- E994 Injury due to war operations by destruction of aircraft
- E995 Injury due to war operations by other and unspecified forms of conventional warfare
- E996 Injury due to war operations by nuclear weapons
- E997 Injury due to war operations by other forms of unconventional warfare
- E998 Injury due to war operations but occurring after cessation of hostilities
- E999 Late effects of injury due to war operations and terrorism

APPENDIX E

DISEASES: ALPHABETIC INDEX

VOLUME 2

INDEX TO DISEASES

A

AAT (alpha-1 antitrypsin) deficiency 273.4
AAV (disease) (illness) (infection)—*see* Human immunodeficiency virus (disease) (illness) (infection)
Abactio —*see* Abortion, induced
Abactus venter —*see* Abortion, induced
Abarognosis 781.99
Abasia (-astasia) 307.9
   atactica 781.3
   choreic 781.3
   hysterical 300.11
   paroxysmal trepidant 781.3
   spastic 781.3
   trembling 781.3
   trepidans 781.3
Abderhalden-Kaufmann-Lignac syndrome (cystinosis) 270.0
Abdomen, abdominal —*see also* condition
   accordion 306.4
   acute 789.0
   angina 557.1
   burst 868.00
   convulsive equivalent (*see also* Epilepsy) 345.5
   heart 746.87
   muscle deficiency syndrome 756.79
   obstipum 756.79
Abdominalgia 789.0
   periodic 277.31
Abduction contracture, hip or other joint —*see* Contraction, joint
Abercrombie's syndrome (amyloid degeneration) 277.39
Aberrant (congenital)—*see also* Malposition, congenital
   adrenal gland 759.1
   blood vessel NEC 747.60
      arteriovenous NEC 747.60
      cerebrovascular 747.81
      gastrointestinal 747.61
      lower limb 747.64
      renal 747.62
      spinal 747.82
      upper limb 747.63
   breast 757.6
   endocrine gland NEC 759.2
   gastrointestinal vessel (peripheral) 747.61
   hepatic duct 751.69
   lower limb vessel (peripheral) 747.64
   pancreas 751.7
   parathyroid gland 759.2
   peripheral vascular vessel NEC 747.60
   pituitary gland (pharyngeal) 759.2
   renal blood vessel 747.62
   sebaceous glands, mucous membrane, mouth 750.26
   spinal vessel 747.82
   spleen 759.0
   testis (descent) 752.51
   thymus gland 759.2
   thyroid gland 759.2
   upper limb vessel (peripheral) 747.63
Aberratio
   lactis 757.6
   testis 752.51
Aberration —*see also* Anomaly
   chromosome—*see* Anomaly, chromosome(s)
   distantial 368.9

Aberration—*continued*
   mental (*see also* Disorder, mental, nonpsychotic) 300.9
Abetalipoproteinemia 272.5
Abionarce 780.79
Abiotrophy 799.89
Ablatio
   placentae—*see* Placenta, ablatio
   retinae (*see also* Detachment, retina) 361.9
Ablation
   pituitary (gland) (with hypofunction) 253.7
   placenta—*see* Placenta, ablatio
   uterus 621.8
Ablepharia, ablepharon, ablephary 743.62
Ablepsia —*see* Blindness
Ablepsy —*see* Blindness
Ablutomania 300.3
Abnormal, abnormality, abnormalities —*see also* Anomaly
   acid-base balance 276.4
      fetus or newborn—*see* Distress, fetal
   adaptation curve, dark 368.63
   alveolar ridge 525.9
   amnion 658.9
      affecting fetus or newborn 762.9
   anatomical relationship NEC 759.9
   apertures, congenital, diaphragm 756.6
   auditory perception NEC 388.40
   autosomes NEC 758.5
      13 758.1
      18 758.2
      21 or 22 758.0
      D_1 758.1
      E_3 758.2
      G 758.0
   ballistocardiogram 794.39
   basal metabolic rate (BMR) 794.7
   biosynthesis, testicular androgen 257.2
   blood level (of)
      cobalt 790.6
      copper 790.6
      iron 790.6
      lead 790.6
      lithium 790.6
      magnesium 790.6
      mineral 790.6
      zinc 790.6
   blood pressure
      elevated (without diagnosis of hypertension) 796.2
      low (*see also* Hypotension) 458.9
      reading (incidental) (isolated) (nonspecific) 796.3
   blood sugar 790.29
   bowel sounds 787.5
   breathing behavior—*see* Respiration
   caloric test 794.19
   cervix (acquired) NEC 622.9
      congenital 752.40
      in pregnancy or childbirth 654.6
         causing obstructed labor 660.2
            affecting fetus or newborn 763.1
   chemistry, blood NEC 790.6
   chest sounds 786.7
   chorion 658.9
      affecting fetus or newborn 762.9
   chromosomal NEC 758.89
      analysis, nonspecific result 795.2

INDEX TO DISEASES

Abnormal, abnormality—*continued*
  autosomes (*see also* Abnormal, autosomes NEC) 758.5
  fetal, (suspected) affecting management of pregnancy 655.1
  sex 758.81
clinical findings NEC 796.4
communication—*see* Fistula
configuration of pupils 379.49
coronary
  artery 746.85
  vein 746.9
cortisol-binding globulin 255.8
course, Eustachian tube 744.24
dentofacial NEC 524.9
  functional 524.50
  specified type NEC 524.89
development, developmental NEC 759.9
  bone 756.9
  central nervous system 742.9
direction, teeth 524.30
Dynia (*see also* Defect, coagulation) 286.9
Ebstein 746.2
echocardiogram 793.2
echoencephalogram 794.01
echogram NEC—*see* Findings, abnormal, structure
electrocardiogram (ECG) (EKG) 794.31
electroencephalogram (EEG) 794.02
electromyogram (EMG) 794.17
  ocular 794.14
electro-oculogram (EOG) 794.12
electroretinogram (ERG) 794.11
erythrocytes 289.9
  congenital, with perinatal jaundice 282.9 [774.0]
Eustachian valve 746.9
excitability under minor stress 301.9
fat distribution 782.9
feces 787.7
fetal heart rate—*see* Distress, fetal
fetus NEC
  affecting management of pregnancy—*see* Pregnancy, management affected by, fetal
  causing disproportion 653.7
    affecting fetus or newborn 763.1
    causing obstructed labor 660.1
      affecting fetus or newborn 763.1
findings without manifest disease—*see* Findings, abnormal
fluid
  amniotic 792.3
  cerebrospinal 792.0
  peritoneal 792.9
  pleural 792.9
  synovial 792.9
  vaginal 792.9
forces of labor NEC 661.9
  affecting fetus or newborn 763.7
form, teeth 520.2
function studies
  auditory 794.15
  bladder 794.9
  brain 794.00
  cardiovascular 794.30
  endocrine NEC 794.6
  kidney 794.4
  liver 794.8
  nervous system
    central 794.00
    peripheral 794.19

Abnormal, abnormality—*continued*
  oculomotor 794.14
  pancreas 794.9
  placenta 794.9
  pulmonary 794.2
  retina 794.11
  special senses 794.19
  spleen 794.9
  thyroid 794.5
  vestibular 794.16
gait 781.2
  hysterical 300.11
gastrin secretion 251.5
globulin
  cortisol-binding 255.8
  thyroid-binding 246.8
glucagon secretion 251.4
glucose 790.29
  in pregnancy, childbirth, or puerperium 648.8
    fetus or newborn 775.0
  non-fasting 790.29
gravitational (G) forces or states 994.9
hair NEC 704.2
hard tissue formation in pulp 522.3
head movement 781.0
heart
  rate
    fetus, affecting liveborn infant
      before the onset of labor 763.81
      during labor 763.82
      unspecified as to time of onset 763.83
    intrauterine
      before the onset of labor 763.81
      during labor 763.82
      unspecified as to time of onset 763.83
    newborn
      before the onset of labor 763.81
      during labor 763.82
      unspecified as to time of onset 763.83
  shadow 793.2
  sounds NEC 785.3
hemoglobin (*see also* Disease, hemoglobin) 282.7
  trait—*see* Trait, hemoglobin, abnormal
hemorrhage, uterus—*see* Hemorrhage, uterus
histology NEC 795.4
increase in
  appetite 783.6
  development 783.9
involuntary movement 781.0
jaw closure 524.51
karyotype 795.2
knee jerk 796.1
labor NEC 661.9
  affecting fetus or newborn 763.7
laboratory findings—*see* Findings, abnormal
length, organ or site, congenital—*see* Distortion
loss of height 781.91
loss of weight 783.21
lung shadow 793.1
mammogram 793.80
  calcification 793.89
  calculus 793.89
  microcalcification 793.81
Mantoux test 795.5
membranes (fetal)
  affecting fetus or newborn 762.9
  complicating pregnancy 658.8
menstruation—*see* Menstruation
metabolism (*see also* condition) 783.9

INDEX TO DISEASES — **Abnormal, abnormality**

Abnormal, abnormality —*continued*
  movement 781.0
    disorder, NEC 333.90
      sleep related, unspecified 780.58
      specified, NEC 333.99
    head 781.0
    involuntary 781.0
    specified type NEC 333.99
  muscle contraction, localized 728.85
  myoglobin (Aberdeen) (Annapolis) 289.9
  narrowness, eyelid 743.62
  optokinetic response 379.57
  organs or tissues of pelvis NEC
    in pregnancy or childbirth 654.9
      affecting fetus or newborn 763.89
      causing obstructed labor 660.2
        affecting fetus or newborn 763.1
  origin—*see* Malposition, congenital
  palmar creases 757.2
  Papanicolaou (smear)
    cervix 795.00
      with
        atypical squamous cell
          cannot exclude high grade squamous
            intraepithelial lesion (ASC-H)
            795.02
          of undetermined significance (ASC-US)
            795.01
        cytologic evidence of malignancy 795.06
        favor benign (ASCUS favor benign)
          795.01
        favor dysplasia (ASCUS favor dysplasia)
          795.02
        high grade squamous intraepithelial lesion
          (HGSIL) 795.04
        low grade squamous intraepithelial lesion
          (LGSIL) 795.03
      nonspecific finding NEC 795.09
    other site 795.1
  parturition
    affecting fetus or newborn 763.9
    mother—*see* Delivery, complicated
  pelvis (bony)—*see* Deformity, pelvis
  percussion, chest 786.7
  periods (grossly) (*see also* Menstruation) 626.9
  phonocardiogram 794.39
  placenta—*see* Placenta, abnormal
  plantar reflex 796.1
  plasma protein—*see* Deficiency, plasma, protein
  pleural folds 748.8
  position—*see also* Malposition
    gravid uterus 654.4
      causing obstructed labor 660.2
        affecting fetus or newborn 763.1
  posture NEC 781.92
  presentation (fetus)—*see* Presentation, fetus,
    abnormal
  product of conception NEC 631
  puberty—*see* Puberty
  pulmonary
    artery 747.3
    function, newborn 770.89
    test results 794.2
    ventilation, newborn 770.89
      hyperventilation 786.01
  pulsations in neck 785.1
  pupil reflexes 379.40
  quality of milk 676.8
  radiological examination 793.99
    abdomen NEC 793.6
    biliary tract 793.3

Abnormal, abnormality —*continued*
  breast 793.89
    mammogram NOS 793.80
    mammographic
      calcification 793.89
      calculus 793.89
      microcalcification 793.81
  gastrointestinal tract 793.4
  genitourinary organs 793.5
  head 793.0
  image test inconclusive due to excess body fat
    793.91
  intrathoracic organ NEC 793.2
  lung (field) 793.1
  musculoskeletal system 793.7
  retroperitoneum 793.6
  skin and subcutaneous tissue 793.99
  skull 793.0
  red blood cells 790.09
    morphology 790.09
    volume 790.09
  reflex NEC 796.1
  renal function test 794.4
  respiration signs—*see* Respiration
  response to nerve stimulation 794.10
  retinal correspondence 368.34
  rhythm, heart—*see also* Arrhythmia fetus—*see*
    Distress, fetal
  saliva 792.4
  scan
    brain 794.09
    kidney 794.4
    liver 794.8
    lung 794.2
    thyroid 794.5
  secretion
    gastrin 251.5
    glucagon 251.4
  semen 792.2
  serum level (of)
    acid phosphatase 790.5
    alkaline phosphatase 790.5
    amylase 790.5
    enzymes NEC 790.5
    lipase 790.5
  shape
    cornea 743.41
    gallbladder 751.69
    gravid uterus 654.4
      affecting fetus or newborn 763.89
      causing obstructed labor 660.2
        affecting fetus or newborn 763.1
    head (*see also* Anomaly, skull) 756.0
    organ or site, congenital NEC—*see* Distortion
  sinus venosus 747.40
  size
    fetus, complicating delivery 653.5
      causing obstructed labor 660.1
    gallbladder 751.69
    head (*see also* Anomaly, skull) 756.0
    organ or site, congenital NEC—*see* Distortion
    teeth 520.2
  skin and appendages, congenital NEC 757.9
  soft parts of pelvis—*see* Abnormal, organs or
    tissues of pelvis
  spermatozoa 792.2
  sputum (amount) (color) (excessive) (odor)
    (purulent) 786.4
  stool NEC 787.7
    bloody 578.1
      occult 792.1

Abnormal, abnormality   **INDEX TO DISEASES**

Abnormal, abnormality —*continued*
    bulky 787.7
    color (dark) (light) 792.1
    content (fat) (mucus) (pus) 792.1
    occult blood 792.1
  synchondrosis 756.9
  test results without manifest disease—*see* Findings, abnormal
  thebesian valve 746.9
  thermography—*see* Findings, abnormal, structure
  threshold, cones or rods (eye) 368.63
  thyroid-binding globulin 246.8
  thyroid product 246.8
  toxicology (findings) NEC 796.0
  tracheal cartilage (congenital) 748.3
  transport protein 273.8
  ultrasound results—*see* Findings, abnormal, structure
  umbilical cord
    affecting fetus or newborn 762.6
    complicating delivery 663.9
    specified NEC 663.8
  union
    cricoid cartilage and thyroid cartilage 748.3
    larynx and trachea 748.3
    thyroid cartilage and hyoid bone 748.3
  urination NEC 788.69
    psychogenic 306.53
    stream
      intermittent 788.61
      slowing 788.62
      splitting 788.61
      weak 788.62
    urgency 788.63
  urine (constituents) NEC 791.9
  uterine hemorrhage (*see also* Hemorrhage, uterus) 626.9
    climacteric 627.0
    postmenopausal 627.1
  vagina (acquired) (congenital)
    in pregnancy or childbirth 654.7
      affecting fetus or newborn 763.89
      causing obstructed labor 660.2
        affecting fetus or newborn 763.1
  vascular sounds 785.9
  vectorcardiogram 794.39
  visually evoked potential (VEP) 794.13
  vulva (acquired) (congenital)
    in pregnancy or childbirth 654.8
      affecting fetus or newborn 763.89
      causing obstructed labor 660.2
        affecting fetus or newborn 763.1
  weight
    gain 783.1
      of pregnancy 646.1
        with hypertension—*see* Toxemia, of pregnancy
    loss 783.21
  x-ray examination—*see* Abnormal, radiological examination
Abnormally formed uterus —*see* Anomaly, uterus
Abnormity (any organ or part)—*see* Anomaly
ABO
  hemolytic disease 773.1
  incompatibility reaction 999.6
Abocclusion 524.20
Abolition, language 784.69

Aborter, habitual or recurrent NEC
  without current pregnancy 629.81
  current abortion (*see also* Abortion, spontaneous) 634.9
    affecting fetus or newborn 761.8
  observation in current pregnancy 646.3
Abortion (complete) (incomplete) (inevitable) (with retained products of conception) 637.9

> Note—Use the following fifth-digit subclassification with categories 634-637:
>
> 0 unspecified
> 1 incomplete
> 2 complete

  with
    complication(s) (any) following previous abortion—*see* category 639
    damage to pelvic organ (laceration) (rupture) (tear) 637.2
    embolism (air) (amniotic fluid) (blood clot) (pulmonary) (pyemic) (septic) (soap) 637.6
    genital tract and pelvic infection 637.0
    hemorrhage, delayed or excessive 637.1
    metabolic disorder 637.4
    renal failure (acute) 637.3
    sepsis (genital tract) (pelvic organ) 637.0
    urinary tract 637.7
    shock (postoperative) (septic) 637.5
    specified complication NEC 637.7
    toxemia 637.3
    unspecified complication(s) 637.8
    urinary tract infection 637.7
  accidental—*see* Abortion, spontaneous
  artificial—*see* Abortion, induced
  attempted (failed)—*see* Abortion, failed
  criminal—*see* Abortion, illegal
  early—*see* Abortion, spontaneous
  elective—*see* Abortion, legal
  failed (legal) 638.9
    with
      damage to pelvic organ (laceration) (rupture) (tear) 638.2
      embolism (air) (amniotic fluid) (blood clot) (pulmonary) (pyemic) (septic) (soap) 638.6
      genital tract and pelvic infection 638.0
      hemorrhage, delayed or excessive 638.1
      metabolic disorder 638.4
      renal failure (acute) 638.3
      sepsis (genital tract) (pelvic organ) 638.0
      urinary tract 638.7
      shock (postoperative) (septic) 638.5
      specified complication NEC 638.7
      toxemia 638.3
      unspecified complication(s) 638.8
      urinary tract infection 638.7
  fetal indication—*see* Abortion, legal
  fetus 779.6
  following threatened abortion—*see* Abortion, by type
  habitual or recurrent (care during pregnancy) 646.3
    with current abortion (*see also* Abortion, spontaneous) 634.9
      affecting fetus or newborn 761.8
    without current pregnancy 629.81
  homicidal—*see* Abortion, illegal

INDEX TO DISEASES

Abortion—*continued*
  illegal 636.9
    with
      damage to pelvic organ (laceration) (rupture) (tear) 636.2
      embolism (air) (amniotic fluid) (blood clot) (pulmonary) (pyemic) (septic) (soap) 636.6
      genital tract and pelvic infection 636.0
      hemorrhage, delayed or excessive 636.1
      metabolic disorder 636.4
      renal failure 636.3
      sepsis (genital tract) (pelvic organ) 636.0
        urinary tract 636.7
      shock (postoperative) (septic) 636.5
      specified complication NEC 636.7
      toxemia 636.3
      unspecified complication(s) 636.8
      urinary tract infection 636.7
    fetus 779.6
  induced 637.9
    illegal—*see* Abortion, illegal
    legal indications—*see* Abortion, legal
    medical indications—*see* Abortion, legal
    therapeutic—*see* Abortion, legal
  late—*see* Abortion, spontaneous
  legal (legal indication) (medical indication) (under medical supervision) 635.9
    with
      damage to pelvic organ (laceration) (rupture) (tear) 635.2
      embolism (air) (amniotic fluid) (blood clot) (pulmonary) (pyemic) (septic) (soap) 635.6
      genital tract and pelvic infection 635.0
      hemorrhage, delayed or excessive 635.1
      metabolic disorder 635.4
      renal failure (acute) 635.3
      sepsis (genital tract) (pelvic organ) 635.0
        urinary tract 635.7
      shock (postoperative) (septic) 635.5
      specified complication NEC 635.7
      toxemia 635.3
      unspecified complication(s) 635.8
      urinary tract infection 635.7
    fetus 779.6
  medical indication—*see* Abortion, legal
  mental hygiene problem—*see* Abortion, legal
  missed 632
  operative—*see* Abortion, legal
  psychiatric indication—*see* Abortion, legal
  recurrent—*see* Abortion, spontaneous
  self-induced—*see* Abortion, illegal
  septic—*see* Abortion, by type, with sepsis
  spontaneous 634.9
    with
      damage to pelvic organ (laceration) (rupture) (tear) 634.2
      embolism (air) (amniotic fluid) (blood clot) (pulmonary) (pyemic) (septic) (soap) 634.6
      genital tract and pelvic infection 634.0
      hemorrhage, delayed or excessive 634.1
      metabolic disorder 634.4
      renal failure 634.3
      sepsis (genital tract) (pelvic organ) 634.0
        urinary tract 634.7
      shock (postoperative) (septic) 634.5
      specified complication NEC 634.7
      toxemia 634.3
      unspecified complication(s) 634.8
      urinary tract infection 634.7

Abortion—*continued*
  fetus 761.8
  threatened 640.0
    affecting fetus or newborn 762.1
  surgical—*see* Abortion, legal
  therapeutic—*see* Abortion, legal
  threatened 640.0
    affecting fetus or newborn 762.1
  tubal—*see* Pregnancy, tubal
  voluntary—*see* Abortion, legal
Abortus fever 023.9
Aboulomania 301.6
Abrachia 755.20
Abrachiatism 755.20
Abrachiocephalia 759.89
Abrachiocephalus 759.89
Abrami's disease (acquired hemolytic jaundice) 283.9
Abramov-Fiedler myocarditis (acute isolated myocarditis) 422.91
Abrasion —*see also* Injury, superficial, by site
  cornea 918.1
  dental 521.20
    extending into
      dentine 521.22
      pulp 521.23
    generalized 521.25
    limited to enamel 521.21
    localized 521.24
  teeth, tooth (dentifrice) (habitual) (hard tissues) (occupational) (ritual) (traditional) (wedge defect) (*see also* Abrasion, dental) 521.20
Abrikossov's tumor (M9580/0)—*see also* Neoplasm, connective tissue, benign
  malignant (M9580/3)—*see* Neoplasm, connective tissue, malignant
Abrism 988.8
Abruption, placenta —*see* Placenta, abruptio
Abruptio placentae —*see* Placenta, abruptio
Abscess (acute) (chronic) (infectional) (lymphangitic) (metastatic) (multiple) (pyogenic) (septic) (with lymphangitis) (*see also* Cellulitis) 682.9
  abdomen, abdominal
    cavity 567.22
    wall 682.2
  abdominopelvic 567.22
  accessory sinus (chronic) (*see also* Sinusitis) 473.9
  adrenal (capsule) (gland) 255.8
  alveolar 522.5
    with sinus 522.7
  amebic 006.3
    bladder 006.8
    brain (with liver or lung abscess) 006.5
    liver (without mention of brain or lung abscess) 006.3
      with
        brain abscess (and lung abscess) 006.5
        lung abscess 006.4
    lung (with liver abscess) 006.4
      with brain abscess 006.5
    seminal vesicle 006.8
    specified site NEC 006.8
    spleen 006.8
  anaerobic 040.0
  ankle 682.6
  anorectal 566
  antecubital space 682.3
  antrum (chronic) (Highmore) (*see also* Sinusitis, maxillary) 473.0

Abscess—*continued*
  anus 566
  apical (tooth) 522.5
    with sinus (alveolar) 522.7
  appendix 540.1
  areola (acute) (chronic) (nonpuerperal) 611.0
    puerperal, postpartum 675.1
  arm (any part, above wrist) 682.3
  artery (wall) 447.2
  atheromatous 447.2
  auditory canal (external) 380.10
  auricle (ear) (staphylococcal) (streptococcal) 380.10
  axilla, axillary (region) 682.3
    lymph gland or node 683
  back (any part) 682.2
  Bartholin's gland 616.3
    with
      abortion—*see* Abortion, by type, with sepsis
      ectopic pregnancy (*see also* categories 633.0-633.9) 639.0
      molar pregnancy (*see also* categories 630-632) 639.0
    complicating pregnancy or puerperium 646.6
    following
      abortion 639.0
      ectopic or molar pregnancy 639.0
  bartholinian 616.3
  Bezold's 383.01
  bile, biliary, duct or tract (*see also* Cholecystitis) 576.8
  bilharziasis 120.1
  bladder (wall) 595.89
    amebic 006.8
  bone (subperiosteal) (*see also* Osteomyelitis) 730.0
    accessory sinus (chronic) (*see also* Sinusitis) 473.9
    acute 730.0
    chronic or old 730.1
    jaw (lower) (upper) 526.4
    mastoid—*see* Mastoiditis, acute
    petrous (*see also* Petrositis) 383.20
    spinal (tuberculous) (*see also* Tuberculosis) 015.0 *[730.88]*
    nontuberculous 730.08
  bowel 569.5
  brain (any part) 324.0
    amebic (with liver or lung abscess) 006.5
    cystic 324.0
    late effect—*see* category 326
    otogenic 324.0
    tuberculous (*see also* Tuberculosis) 013.3
  breast (acute) (chronic) (nonpuerperal) 611.0
    newborn 771.5
    puerperal, postpartum 675.1
    tuberculous (*see also* Tuberculosis) 017.9
  broad ligament (chronic) (*see also* Disease, pelvis, inflammatory) 614.4
    acute 614.3
  Brodie's (chronic) (localized) (*see also* Osteomyelitis) 730.1
  bronchus 519.19
  buccal cavity 528.3
  bulbourethral gland 597.0
  bursa 727.89
    pharyngeal 478.29
  buttock 682.5
  canaliculus, breast 611.0
  canthus 372.20
  cartilage 733.99

Abscess—*continued*
  cecum 569.5
    with appendicitis 540.1
  cerebellum, cerebellar 324.0
    late effect—*see* category 326
  cerebral (embolic) 324.0
    late effect—*see* category 326
  cervical (neck region) 682.1
    lymph gland or node 683
    stump (*see also* Cervicitis) 616.0
  cervix (stump) (uteri) (*see also* Cervicitis) 616.0
  cheek, external 682.0
    inner 528.3
  chest 510.9
    with fistula 510.0
    wall 682.2
  chin 682.0
  choroid 363.00
  ciliary body 364.3
  circumtonsillar 475
  cold (tuberculous)—*see also* Tuberculosis, abscess
    articular—*see* Tuberculosis, joint
  colon (wall) 569.5
  colostomy or enterostomy 569.6
  conjunctiva 372.00
  connective tissue NEC 682.9
  cornea 370.55
    with ulcer 370.00
  corpus
    cavernosum 607.2
    luteum (*see also* Salpingo-oophoritis) 614.2
  Cowper's gland 597.0
  cranium 324.0
  cul-de-sac (Douglas') (posterior) (*see also* Disease, pelvis, inflammatory) 614.4
    acute 614.3
  dental 522.5
    with sinus (alveolar) 522.7
  dentoalveolar 522.5
    with sinus (alveolar) 522.7
  diaphragm, diaphragmatic 567.22
  digit NEC 681.9
  Douglas' cul-de-sac or pouch (*see also* Disease, pelvis, inflammatory) 614.4
    acute 614.3
  Dubois' 090.5
  ductless gland 259.8
  ear
    acute 382.00
    external 380.10
    inner 386.30
    middle—*see* Otitis media
  elbow 682.3
  endamebic—*see* Abscess, amebic
  entamebic—*see* Abscess, amebic
  enterostomy 569.6
  epididymis 604.0
  epidural 324.9
    brain 324.0
    late effect—*see* category 326
    spinal cord 324.1
  epiglottis 478.79
  epiploon, epiploic 567.22
  erysipelatous (*see also* Erysipelas) 035
  esophagostomy 530.86
  esophagus 530.19
  ethmoid (bone) (chronic) (sinus) (*see also* Sinusitis, ethmoidal) 473.2
  external auditory canal 380.10

INDEX TO DISEASES

Abscess—*continued*
  extradural 324.9
    brain 324.0
      late effect—*see* category 326
    spinal cord 324.1
  extraperitoneal—*see* Abscess, peritoneum
  eye 360.00
  eyelid 373.13
  face (any part, except eye) 682.0
  fallopian tube (*see also* Salpingo-oophoritis) 614.2
  fascia 728.89
  fauces 478.29
  fecal 569.5
  femoral (region) 682.6
  filaria, filarial (*see also* Infestation, filarial) 125.9
  finger (any) (intrathecal) (periosteal) (subcutaneous) (subcuticular) 681.00
  fistulous NEC 682.9
  flank 682.2
  foot (except toe) 682.7
  forearm 682.3
  forehead 682.0
  frontal (sinus) (chronic) (*see also* Sinusitis, frontal) 473.1
  gallbladder (*see also* Cholecystitis, acute) 575.0
  gastric 535.0
  genital organ or tract NEC
    female 616.9
      with
        abortion—*see* Abortion, by type, with sepsis
        ectopic pregnancy (*see also* categories 633.0-633.9) 639.0
        molar pregnancy (*see also* categories 630-632) 639.0
      following
        abortion 639.0
        ectopic or molar pregnancy 639.0
      puerperal, postpartum, childbirth 670
    male 608.4
  genitourinary system, tuberculous (*see also* Tuberculosis) 016.9
  gingival 523.30
  gland, glandular (lymph) (acute) NEC 683
  glottis 478.79
  gluteal (region) 682.5
  gonorrheal NEC (*see also* Gonococcus) 098.0
  groin 682.2
  gum 523.30
  hand (except finger or thumb) 682.4
  head (except face) 682.8
  heart 429.89
  heel 682.7
  helminthic (*see also* Infestation, by specific parasite) 128.9
  hepatic 572.0
    amebic (*see also* Abscess, liver, amebic) 006.3
    duct 576.8
  hip 682.6
    tuberculous (active) (*see also* Tuberculosis) 015.1
  ileocecal 540.1
  ileostomy (bud) 569.6
  iliac (region) 682.2
    fossa 540.1
  iliopsoas 567.31
    tuberculous (see also Tuberculosis) 015.0 *[730.88]*
  infraclavicular (fossa) 682.3

Abscess—*continued*
  inguinal (region) 682.2
    lymph gland or node 683
  intersphincteric (anus) 566
  intestine, intestinal 569.5
    rectal 566
  intra-abdominal (*see also* Abscess, peritoneum) 567.22
    postoperative 998.59
  intracranial 324.0
    late effect—*see* category 326
  intramammary—*see* Abscess, breast
  intramastoid (*see also* Mastoiditis, acute) 383.00
  intraorbital 376.01
  intraperitoneal 567.22
  intraspinal 324.1
    late effect—*see* category 326
  intratonsillar 475
  iris 364.3
  ischiorectal 566
  jaw (bone) (lower) (upper) 526.4
    skin 682.0
  joint (*see also* Arthritis, pyogenic) 711.0
    vertebral (tuberculous) (*see also* Tuberculosis) 015.0 *[730.88]*
    nontuberculous 724.8
  kidney 590.2
    with
      abortion—*see* Abortion, by type, with urinary tract infection
      calculus 592.0
      ectopic pregnancy (*see also* categories 633.0-633.9) 639.8
      molar pregnancy (*see also* categories 630-632) 639.8
    complicating pregnancy or puerperium 646.6
      affecting fetus or newborn 760.1
    following
      abortion 639.8
      ectopic or molar pregnancy 639.8
  knee 682.6
    joint 711.06
    tuberculous (active) (*see also* Tuberculosis) 015.2
  labium (majus) (minus) 616.4
    complicating pregnancy, childbirth, or puerperium 646.6
  lacrimal (passages) (sac) (*see also* Dacryocystitis) 375.30
    caruncle 375.30
    gland (*see also* Dacryoadenitis) 375.00
  lacunar 597.0
  larynx 478.79
  lateral (alveolar) 522.5
    with sinus 522.7
  leg, except foot 682.6
  lens 360.00
  lid 373.13
  lingual 529.0
    tonsil 475
  lip 528.5
  Littre's gland 597.0
  liver 572.0
    amebic 006.3
      with
        brain abscess (and lung abscess) 006.5
        lung abscess 006.4
      due to Entamoeba histolytica 006.3
      dysenteric (*see also* Abscess, liver, amebic) 006.3
    pyogenic 572.0

Abscess—*continued*
  tropical (*see also* Abscess, liver, amebic) 006.3
  loin (region) 682.2
  lumbar (tuberculous) (*see also* Tuberculosis) 015.0 *[730.88]*
    nontuberculous 682.2
  lung (miliary) (putrid) 513.0
    amebic (with liver abscess) 006.4
      with brain abscess 006.5
  lymph, lymphatic, gland or node (acute) 683
    any site, except mesenteric 683
    mesentery 289.2
  lymphangitic, acute—*see* Cellulitis
  malar 526.4
  mammary gland—*see* Abscess, breast
  marginal (anus) 566
  mastoid (process) (*see also* Mastoiditis, acute) 383.00
    subperiosteal 383.01
  maxilla, maxillary 526.4
    molar (tooth) 522.5
      with sinus 522.7
    premolar 522.5
    sinus (chronic) (*see also* Sinusitis, maxillary) 473.0
  mediastinum 513.1
  meibomian gland 373.12
  meninges (*see also* Meningitis) 320.9
  mesentery, mesenteric 567.22
  mesosalpinx (*see also* Salpingo-oophoritis) 614.2
  milk 675.1
  Monro's (psoriasis) 696.1
  mons pubis 682.2
  mouth (floor) 528.3
  multiple sites NEC 682.9
  mural 682.2
  muscle 728.89
    psoas 567.31
  myocardium 422.92
  nabothian (follicle) (*see also* Cervicitis) 616.0
  nail (chronic) (with lymphangitis) 681.9
    finger 681.02
    toe 681.11
  nasal (fossa) (septum) 478.19
    sinus (chronic) (*see also* Sinusitis) 473.9
  nasopharyngeal 478.29
  nates 682.5
  navel 682.2
    newborn NEC 771.4
  neck (region) 682.1
    lymph gland or node 683
  nephritic (*see also* Abscess, kidney) 590.2
  nipple 611.0
    puerperal, postpartum 675.0
  nose (septum) 478.19
    external 682.0
  omentum 567.22
  operative wound 998.59
  orbit, orbital 376.01
  ossifluent—*see* Abscess, bone
  ovary, ovarian (corpus luteum) (*see also* Salpingo-oophoritis) 614.2
  oviduct (*see also* Salpingo-oophoritis) 614.2
  palate (soft) 528.3
    hard 526.4
  palmar (space) 682.4
  pancreas (duct) 577.0
  paradontal 523.30
  parafrenal 607.2

Abscess—*continued*
  parametric, parametrium (chronic) (*see also* Disease, pelvis, inflammatory) 614.4
    acute 614.3
  paranephric 590.2
  parapancreatic 577.0
  parapharyngeal 478.22
  pararectal 566
  parasinus (*see also* Sinusitis) 473.9
  parauterine (*see also* Disease, pelvis, inflammatory) 614.4
    acute 614.3
  paravaginal (*see also* Vaginitis) 616.10
  parietal region 682.8
  parodontal 523.30
  parotid (duct) (gland) 527.3
    region 528.3
  parumbilical 682.2
    newborn 771.4
  pectoral (region) 682.2
  pelvirectal 567.22
  pelvis, pelvic
    female (chronic) (*see also* Disease, pelvis, inflammatory) 614.4
      acute 614.3
    male, peritoneal (cellular tissue)—*see* Abscess, peritoneum
    tuberculous (*see also* Tuberculosis) 016.9
  penis 607.2
    gonococcal (acute) 098.0
      chronic or duration of 2 months or over 098.2
  perianal 566
  periapical 522.5
    with sinus (alveolar) 522.7
  periappendiceal 540.1
  pericardial 420.99
  pericecal 540.1
  pericemental 523.30
  pericholecystic (*see also* Cholecystitis, acute) 575.0
  pericoronal 523.30
  peridental 523.30
  perigastric 535.0
  perimetric (*see also* Disease, pelvis, inflammatory) 614.4
    acute 614.3
  perinephric, perinephritic (*see also* Abscess, kidney) 590.2
  perineum, perineal (superficial) 682.2
    deep (with urethral involvement) 597.0
    urethra 597.0
  periodontal (parietal) 523.31
    apical 522.5
  periosteum, periosteal (*see also* Periostitis) 730.3
    with osteomyelitis (*see also* Osteomyelitis) 730.2
    acute or subacute 730.0
    chronic or old 730.1
  peripleuritic 510.9
    with fistula 510.0
  periproctic 566
  periprostatic 601.2
  perirectal (staphylococcal) 566
  perirenal (tissue) (*see also* Abscess, kidney) 590.2
  perisinuous (nose) (*see also* Sinusitis) 473.9
  peritoneum, peritoneal (perforated) (ruptured) 567.22

INDEX TO DISEASES   **Abscess**

Abscess—*continued*
  with
    abortion—*see* Abortion, by type, with sepsis
    appendicitis 540.1
    ectopic pregnancy (*see also* categories
      633.0-633.9) 639.0
    molar pregnancy (*see also* categories
      630-632) 639.0
  following
    abortion 639.0
    ectopic or molar pregnancy 639.0
  pelvic, female (*see also* Disease, pelvis,
    inflammatory) 614.4
    acute 614.3
  postoperative 998.59
  puerperal, postpartum, childbirth 670
  tuberculous (*see also* Tuberculosis) 014.0
  peritonsillar 475
  perityphlic 540.1
  periureteral 593.89
  periurethral 597.0
    gonococcal (acute) 098.0
      chronic or duration of 2 months or over
        098.2
  periuterine (*see also* Disease, pelvis,
    inflammatory) 614.4
    acute 614.3
  perivesical 595.89
  pernicious NEC 682.9
  petrous bone—*see* Petrositis
  phagedenic NEC 682.9
    chancroid 099.0
  pharynx, pharyngeal (lateral) 478.29
  phlegmonous NEC 682.9
  pilonidal 685.0
  pituitary (gland) 253.8
  pleura 510.9
    with fistula 510.0
  popliteal 682.6
  postanal 566
  postcecal 540.1
  postlaryngeal 478.79
  postnasal 478.19
  postpharyngeal 478.24
  posttonsillar 475
  posttyphoid 002.0
  Pott's (*see also* Tuberculosis) 015.0 *[730.88]*
  pouch of Douglas (chronic) (*see also* Disease,
    pelvis, inflammatory) 614.4
  premammary—*see* Abscess, breast
  prepatellar 682.6
  prostate (*see also* Prostatitis) 601.2
    gonococcal (acute) 098.12
      chronic or duration of 2 months or over 098.32
  psoas 567.31
    tuberculous (*see also* Tuberculosis) 015.0
      [730.88]
  pterygopalatine fossa 682.8
  pubis 682.2
  puerperal—Puerperal, abscess, by site
  pulmonary—*see* Abscess, lung
  pulp, pulpal (dental) 522.0
    finger 681.01
    toe 681.10
  pyemic—*see* Septicemia
  pyloric valve 535.0
  rectovaginal septum 569.5
  rectovesical 595.89
  rectum 566
  regional NEC 682.9
  renal (*see also* Abscess, kidney) 590.2

Abscess—*continued*
  retina 363.00
  retrobulbar 376.01
  retrocecal 567.22
  retrolaryngeal 478.79
  retromammary—*see* Abscess, breast
  retroperineal 682.2
  retroperitoneal 567.38
    postprocedural 998.59
  retropharyngeal 478.24
    tuberculous (*see also* Tuberculosis) 012.8
  retrorectal 566
  retrouterine (*see also* Disease, pelvis,
    inflammatory) 614.4
    acute 614.3
  retrovesical 595.89
  root, tooth 522.5
    with sinus (alveolar) 522.7
  round ligament (*see also* Disease, pelvis,
    inflammatory) 614.4
    acute 614.3
  rupture (spontaneous) NEC 682.9
  sacrum (tuberculous) (*see also* Tuberculosis)
    015.0 *[730.88]*
    nontuberculous 730.08
  salivary duct or gland 527.3
  scalp (any part) 682.8
  scapular 730.01
  sclera 379.09
  scrofulous (*see also* Tuberculosis) 017.2
  scrotum 608.4
  seminal vesicle 608.0
    amebic 006.8
  septal, dental 522.5
    with sinus (alveolar) 522.7
  septum (nasal) 478.19
  serous (*see also* Periostitis) 730.3
  shoulder 682.3
  side 682.2
  sigmoid 569.5
  sinus (accessory) (chronic) (nasal) (*see also*
    Sinusitis) 473.9
    intracranial venous (any) 324.0
      late effect—*see* category 326
  Skene's duct or gland 597.0
  skin NEC 682.9
    tuberculous (primary) (*see also* Tuberculosis)
      017.0
  sloughing NEC 682.9
  specified site NEC 682.8
    amebic 006.8
  spermatic cord 608.4
  sphenoidal (sinus) (*see also* Sinusitis,
    sphenoidal) 473.3
  spinal
    cord (any part) (staphylococcal) 324.1
      tuberculous (*see also* Tuberculosis) 013.5
    epidural 324.1
  spine (column) (tuberculous) (*see also*
    Tuberculosis) 015.0 *[730.88]*
    nontuberculous 730.08
  spleen 289.59
    amebic 006.8
  staphylococcal NEC 682.9
  stitch 998.59
  stomach (wall) 535.0
  strumous (tuberculous) (*see also* Tuberculosis)
    017.2
  subarachnoid 324.9
    brain 324.0
    cerebral 324.0

Abscess — INDEX TO DISEASES

Abscess—*continued*
  late effect—*see* category 326
    spinal cord 324.1
  subareolar—*see also* Abscess, breast
    puerperal, postpartum 675.1
  subcecal 540.1
  subcutaneous NEC 682.9
  subdiaphragmatic 567.22
  subdorsal 682.2
  subdural 324.9
    brain 324.0
    late effect—*see* category 326
    spinal cord 324.1
  subgaleal 682.8
  subhepatic 567.22
  sublingual 528.3
    gland 527.3
  submammary—*see* Abscess, breast
  submandibular (region) (space) (triangle) 682.0
    gland 527.3
  submaxillary (region) 682.0
    gland 527.3
  submental (pyogenic) 682.0
    gland 527.3
  subpectoral 682.2
  subperiosteal—*see* Abscess, bone
  subperitoneal 567.22
  subphrenic—*see also* Abscess, peritoneum 567.22
    postoperative 998.59
  subscapular 682.2
  subungual 681.9
  suburethral 597.0
  sudoriparous 705.89
  suppurative NEC 682.9
  supraclavicular (fossa) 682.3
  suprahepatic 567.22
  suprapelvic (*see also* Disease, pelvis, inflammatory) 614.4
    acute 614.3
  suprapubic 682.2
  suprarenal (capsule) (gland) 255.8
  sweat gland 705.89
  syphilitic 095.8
  teeth, tooth (root) 522.5
    with sinus (alveolar) 522.7
    supporting structures NEC 523.30
  temple 682.0
  temporal region 682.0
  temporosphenoidal 324.0
    late effect—*see* category 326
  tendon (sheath) 727.89
  testicle—*see* Orchitis
  thecal 728.89
  thigh (acquired) 682.6
  thorax 510.9
    with fistula 510.0
  throat 478.29
  thumb (intrathecal) (periosteal) (subcutaneous) (subcuticular) 681.00
  thymus (gland) 254.1
  thyroid (gland) 245.0
  toe (any) (intrathecal) (periosteal) (subcutaneous) (subcuticular) 681.10
  tongue (staphylococcal) 529.0
  tonsil(s) (lingual) 475
  tonsillopharyngeal 475
  tooth, teeth (root) 522.5
    with sinus (alveolar) 522.7
    supporting structure NEC 523.30
  trachea 478.9

Abscess—*continued*
  trunk 682.2
  tubal (*see also* Salpingo-oophoritis) 614.2
  tuberculous—*see* Tuberculosis, abscess
  tubo-ovarian (*see also* Salpingo-oophoritis) 614.2
  tunica vaginalis 608.4
  umbilicus NEC 682.2
    newborn 771.4
  upper arm 682.3
  upper respiratory 478.9
  urachus 682.2
  urethra (gland) 597.0
  urinary 597.0
  uterus, uterine (wall) (*see also* Endometritis) 615.9
    ligament (*see also* Disease, pelvis, inflammatory) 614.4
      acute 614.3
    neck (*see also* Cervicitis) 616.0
  uvula 528.3
  vagina (wall) (*see also* Vaginitis) 616.10
  vaginorectal (*see also* Vaginitis) 616.10
  vas deferens 608.4
  vermiform appendix 540.1
  vertebra (column) (tuberculous) (*see also* Tuberculosis) 015.0 *[730.88]*
    nontuberculous 730.0
  vesical 595.89
  vesicouterine pouch (*see also* Disease, pelvis, inflammatory) 614.4
  vitreous (humor) (pneumococcal) 360.04
  vocal cord 478.5
  von Bezold's 383.01
  vulva 616.4
    complicating pregnancy, childbirth, or puerperium 646.6
  vulvovaginal gland (*see also* Vaginitis) 616.3
  web-space 682.4
  wrist 682.4
Absence (organ or part) (complete or partial)
  acoustic nerve 742.8
  adrenal (gland) (congenital) 759.1
    acquired V45.79
  albumin (blood) 273.8
  alimentary tract (complete) (congenital) (partial) 751.8
    lower 751.5
    upper 750.8
  alpha-fucosidase 271.8
  alveolar process (acquired) 525.8
    congenital 750.26
  anus, anal (canal) (congenital) 751.2
  aorta (congenital) 747.22
  aortic valve (congenital) 746.89
  appendix, congenital 751.2
  arm (acquired) V49.60
    above elbow V49.66
    below elbow V49.65
    congenital (*see also* Deformity, reduction, upper limb) 755.20
      lower—*see* Absence, forearm, congenital
      upper (complete) (partial) (with absence of distal elements, incomplete) 755.24
        with
          complete absence of distal elements 755.21
          forearm (incomplete) 755.23
  artery (congenital) (peripheral) NEC (*see also* Anomaly, peripheral vascular system) 747.60

INDEX TO DISEASES   **Absence**

Absence—*continued*
  brain 747.81
  cerebral 747.81
  coronary 746.85
  pulmonary 747.3
  umbilical 747.5
  atrial septum 745.69
  auditory canal (congenital) (external) 744.01
  auricle (ear) (with stenosis or atresia of auditory canal), congenital 744.01
  bile, biliary duct (common) or passage (congenital) 751.61
    bladder (acquired) V45.74
    congenital 753.8
  bone (congenital) NEC 756.9
    marrow 284.9
      acquired (secondary) 284.89
      congenital 284.09
      hereditary 284.09
      idiopathic 284.9
    skull 756.0
  bowel sounds 787.5
  brain 740.0
    specified part 742.2
  breast(s) (acquired) V45.71
    congenital 757.6
  broad ligament (congenital) 752.19
  bronchus (congenital) 748.3
  calvarium, calvaria (skull) 756.0
  canaliculus lacrimalis, congenital 743.65
  carpal(s) (congenital) (complete) (partial) (with absence of distal elements, incomplete) (*see also* Deformity, reduction, upper limb) 755.28
    with complete absence of distal elements 755.21
  cartilage 756.9
  caudal spine 756.13
  cecum (acquired) (postoperative) (posttraumatic) V45.72
    congenital 751.2
  cementum 520.4
  cerebellum (congenital) (vermis) 742.2
  cervix (acquired) (uteri) V45.77
    congenital 752.49
  chin, congenital 744.89
  cilia (congenital) 743.63
    acquired 374.89
  circulatory system, part NEC 747.89
  clavicle 755.51
  clitoris (congenital) 752.49
  coccyx, congenital 756.13
  cold sense (*see also* Disturbance, sensation) 782.0
  colon (acquired) (postoperative) V45.72
    congenital 751.2
  congenital
    lumen—*see* Atresia
    organ or site NEC—*see* Agenesis
    septum—*see* Imperfect, closure
  corpus callosum (congenital) 742.2
  cricoid cartilage 748.3
  diaphragm (congenital) (with hernia) 756.6
    with obstruction 756.6
  digestive organ(s) or tract, congenital (complete) (partial) 751.8
    acquired V45.79
    lower 751.5
    upper 750.8
  ductus arteriosus 747.89

Absence—*continued*
  duodenum (acquired) (postoperative) V45.72
    congenital 751.1
  ear, congenital 744.09
    acquired V45.79
    auricle 744.01
    external 744.01
    inner 744.05
    lobe, lobule 744.21
    middle, except ossicles 744.03
      ossicles 744.04
    ossicles 744.04
  ejaculatory duct (congenital) 752.89
  endocrine gland NEC (congenital) 759.2
  epididymis (congenital) 752.89
    acquired V45.77
  epiglottis, congenital 748.3
  epileptic (atonic) (typical) (*see also* Epilepsy) 345.0
  erythrocyte 284.9
  erythropoiesis 284.9
    congenital 284.01
  esophagus (congenital) 750.3
  Eustachian tube (congenital) 744.24
  extremity (acquired)
    congenital (*see also* Deformity, reduction) 755.4
    lower V49.70
    upper V49.60
  extrinsic muscle, eye 743.69
  eye (acquired) V45.78
    adnexa (congenital) 743.69
    congenital 743.00
    muscle (congenital) 743.69
  eyelid (fold), congenital 743.62
    acquired 374.89
  face
    bones NEC 756.0
    specified part NEC 744.89
  fallopian tube(s) (acquired) V45.77
    congenital 752.19
  femur, congenital (complete) (partial) (with absence of distal elements, incomplete) (*see also* Deformity, reduction, lower limb) 755.34
    with
      complete absence of distal elements 755.31
      tibia and fibula (incomplete) 755.33
  fibrin 790.92
    fibrinogen (congenital) 286.3
    acquired 286.6
  fibula, congenital (complete) (partial) (with absence of distal elements, incomplete) (*see also* Deformity, reduction, lower limb) 755.37
    with
      complete absence of distal elements 755.31
      tibia 755.35
        with
          complete absence of distal elements 755.31
      femur (incomplete) 755.33
        with complete absence of distal elements 755.31
  finger (acquired) V49.62
    congenital (complete) (partial) (*see also* Deformity, reduction, upper limb) 755.29
      meaning all fingers (complete) (partial) 755.21
      transverse 755.21
  fissures of lungs (congenital) 748.5

Absence — *continued*
  foot (acquired) V49.73
    congenital (complete) 755.31
  forearm (acquired) V49.65
    congenital (complete) (partial) (with absence
      of distal elements, incomplete) (*see also*
      Deformity, reduction, upper limb) 755.25
    with
      complete absence of distal elements (hand
        and fingers) 755.21
      humerus (incomplete) 755.23
  fovea centralis 743.55
  fucosidase 271.8
    gallbladder (acquired) V45.79
      congenital 751.69
  gamma globulin (blood) 279.00
  genital organs
    acquired V45.77
    congenital
      female 752.89
        external 752.49
        internal NEC 752.89
      male 752.89
        penis 752.69
  genitourinary organs, congenital NEC 752.89
  glottis 748.3
  gonadal, congenital NEC 758.6
  hair (congenital) 757.4
    acquired—*see* Alopecia
  hand (acquired) V49.63
    congenital (complete) (*see also* Deformity,
      reduction, upper limb) 755.21
  heart (congenital) 759.89
    acquired—*see* Status, organ replacement
  heat sense (*see also* Disturbance, sensation)
    782.0
  humerus, congenital (complete) (partial) (with
    absence of distal elements, incomplete) (*see
    also* Deformity, reduction, upper limb)
    755.24
    with
      complete absence of distal elements 755.21
      radius and ulna (incomplete) 755.23
  hymen (congenital) 752.49
  ileum (acquired) (postoperative) (posttraumatic)
    V45.72
    congenital 751.1
  immunoglobulin, isolated NEC 279.03
    IgA 279.01
    IgG 279.03
    IgM 279.02
  incus (acquired) 385.24
    congenital 744.04
  internal ear (congenital) 744.05
  intestine (acquired) (small) V45.72
    congenital 751.1
      large 751.2
    large V45.72
      congenital 751.2
  iris (congenital) 743.45
  jaw—*see* Absence, mandible
  jejunum (acquired) V45.72
    congenital 751.1
  joint, congenital NEC 755.8
  kidney(s) (acquired) V45.73
    congenital 753.0
  labium (congenital) (majus) (minus) 752.49
  labyrinth, membranous 744.05
  lacrimal apparatus (congenital) 743.65
  larynx (congenital) 748.3

Absence — *continued*
  leg (acquired) V49.70
    above knee V49.76
    below knee V49.75
    congenital (partial) (unilateral) (*see also*
      Deformity, reduction, lower limb) 755.31
    lower (complete) (partial) (with absence of
      distal elements, incomplete) 755.35
    with
      complete absence of distal elements
        (foot and toes) 755.31
      thigh (incomplete) 755.33
        with complete absence of distal
          elements 755.31
    upper—*see* Absence, femur
  lens (congenital) 743.35
    acquired 379.31
  ligament, broad (congenital) 752.19
  limb (acquired)
    congenital (complete) (partial) (*see also*
      Deformity, reduction) 755.4
    lower 755.30
      complete 755.31
      incomplete 755.32
      longitudinal—*see* Deficiency, lower limb,
        longitudinal
      transverse 755.31
    upper 755.20
      complete 755.21
      incomplete 755.22
      longitudinal—*see* Deficiency, upper limb,
        longitudinal
      transverse 755.21
    lower NEC V49.70
    upper NEC V49.60
  lip 750.26
  liver (congenital) (lobe) 751.69
  lumbar (congenital) (vertebra) 756.13
    isthmus 756.11
    pars articularis 756.11
  lumen—*see* Atresia
  lung (bilateral) (congenital) (fissure) (lobe)
    (unilateral) 748.5
    acquired (any part) V45.76
  mandible (congenital) 524.09
  maxilla (congenital) 524.09
  menstruation 626.0
  metacarpal(s), congenital (complete) (partial)
    (with absence of distal elements,
    incomplete) (*see also* Deformity, reduction,
    upper limb) 755.28
    with all fingers, complete 755.21
  metatarsal(s), congenital (complete) (partial)
    (with absence of distal elements,
    incomplete) (*see also* Deformity, reduction,
    lower limb) 755.38
    with complete absence of distal elements
      755.31
  muscle (congenital) (pectoral) 756.81
    ocular 743.69
  musculoskeletal system (congenital) NEC 756.9
  nail(s) (congenital) 757.5
  neck, part 744.89
  nerve 742.8
  nervous system, part NEC 742.8
  neutrophil 288.00
  nipple (congenital) 757.6
  nose (congenital) 748.1
    acquired 738.0
  nuclear 742.8
  ocular muscle (congenital) 743.69

INDEX TO DISEASES   Absence

Absence—*continued*
  organ
    of Corti (congenital) 744.05
    or site
      acquired V45.79
      congenital NEC 759.89
  osseous meatus (ear) 744.03
  ovary (acquired) V45.77
    congenital 752.0
  oviduct (acquired) V45.77
    congenital 752.19
  pancreas (congenital) 751.7
    acquired (postoperative) (posttraumatic) V45.79
  parathyroid gland (congenital) 759.2
  parotid gland(s) (congenital) 750.21
  patella, congenital 755.64
  pelvic girdle (congenital) 755.69
  penis (congenital) 752.69
    acquired V45.77
  pericardium (congenital) 746.89
  perineal body (congenital) 756.81
  phalange(s), congenital 755.4
    lower limb (complete) (intercalary) (partial) (terminal) (*see also* Deformity, reduction, lower limb) 755.39
      meaning all toes (complete) (partial) 755.31
      transverse 755.31
    upper limb (complete) (intercalary) (partial) (terminal) (*see also* Deformity, reduction, upper limb) 755.29
      meaning all digits (complete) (partial) 755.21
      transverse 755.21
  pituitary gland (congenital) 759.2
  postoperative—*see* Absence, by site, acquired
  prostate (congenital) 752.89
    acquired V45.77
  pulmonary
    artery 747.3
    trunk 747.3
    valve (congenital) 746.01
    vein 747.49
  punctum lacrimale (congenital) 743.65
  radius, congenital (complete) (partial) (with absence of distal elements, incomplete) 755.26
    with
      complete absence of distal elements 755.21
      ulna 755.25
        with
          complete absence of distal elements 755.21
          humerus (incomplete) 755.23
  ray, congenital 755.4
    lower limb (complete) (partial) (*see also* Deformity, reduction, lower limb) 755.38
      meaning all rays 755.31
      transverse 755.31
    upper limb (complete) (partial) (*see also* Deformity, reduction, upper limb) 755.28
      meaning all rays 755.21
      transverse 755.21
  rectum (congenital) 751.2
    acquired V45.79
  red cell 284.9
    acquired (secondary) 284.81
    congenital 284.01
    hereditary 284.01
    idiopathic 284.9
  respiratory organ (congenital) NEC 748.9

Absence—*continued*
  rib (acquired) 738.3
    congenital 756.3
  roof of orbit (congenital) 742.0
  round ligament (congenital) 752.89
  sacrum, congenital 756.13
  salivary gland(s) (congenital) 750.21
  scapula 755.59
  scrotum, congenital 752.89
  seminal tract or duct (congenital) 752.89
    acquired V45.77
  septum (congenital)—*see also* Imperfect, closure, septum
    atrial 745.69
    and ventricular 745.7
    between aorta and pulmonary artery 745.0
    ventricular 745.3
      and atrial 745.7
  sex chromosomes 758.81
  shoulder girdle, congenital (complete) (partial) 755.59
  skin (congenital) 757.39
  skull bone 756.0
    with
      anencephalus 740.0
      encephalocele 742.0
      hydrocephalus 742.3
        with spina bifida (*see also* Spina bifida) 741.0
      microcephalus 742.1
  spermatic cord (congenital) 752.89
  spinal cord 742.59
  spine, congenital 756.13
  spleen (congenital) 759.0
    acquired V45.79
  sternum, congenital 756.3
  stomach (acquired) (partial) (postoperative) V45.75
    congenital 750.7
    with postgastric surgery syndrome 564.2
  submaxillary gland(s) (congenital) 750.21
  superior vena cava (congenital) 747.49
  tarsal(s), congenital (complete) (partial) (with absence of distal elements, incomplete) (*see also* Deformity, reduction, lower limb) 755.38
  teeth, tooth (congenital) 520.0
    with abnormal spacing 524.30
    acquired 525.10
      due to
        caries 525.13
        extraction 525.10
        periodontal disease 525.12
        trauma 525.11
      with malocclusion 524.30
  tendon (congenital) 756.81
  testis (congenital) 752.89
    acquired V45.77
  thigh (acquired) 736.89
  thumb (acquired) V49.61
    congenital 755.29
  thymus gland (congenital) 759.2
  thyroid (gland) (surgical) 246.8
    with hypothyroidism 244.0
    cartilage, congenital 748.3
    congenital 243
  tibia, congenital (complete) (partial) (with absence of distal elements, incomplete) (*see also* Deformity, reduction, lower limb) 755.36

Absence INDEX TO DISEASES

Absence—*continued*
  with
    complete absence of distal elements 755.31
    fibula 755.35
      with
        complete absence of distal elements 755.31
        femur (incomplete) 755.33
          with complete absence of distal elements 755.31
  toe (acquired) V49.72
    congenital (complete) (partial) 755.39
      meaning all toes 755.31
      transverse 755.31
    great V49.71
  tongue (congenital) 750.11
  tooth, teeth, (congenital) 520.0
    with abnormal spacing 524.30
    acquired 525.10
      due to
        caries 525.13
        extraction 525.10
        periodontal disease 525.12
        trauma 525.11
      with malocclusion 524.30
  trachea (cartilage) (congenital) (rings) 748.3
  transverse aortic arch (congenital) 747.21
  tricuspid valve 746.1
  ulna, congenital (complete) (partial) (with absence of distal elements, incomplete) (*see also* Deformity, reduction, upper limb) 755.27
    with
      complete absence of distal elements 755.21
      radius 755.25
        with
          complete absence of distal elements 755.21
          humerus (incomplete) 755.23
  umbilical artery (congenital) 747.5
  ureter (congenital) 753.4
    acquired V45.74
  urethra, congenital 753.8
    acquired V45.74
  urinary system, part NEC, congenital 753.8
    acquired V45.74
  uterus (acquired)V45.77
    congenital 752.3
  uvula (congenital) 750.26
  vagina, congenital 752.49
    acquired V45.77
  vas deferens (congenital) 752.89
    acquired V45.77
  vein (congenital) (peripheral) NEC (*see also* Anomaly, peripheral vascular system) 747.60
    brain 747.81
    great 747.49
    portal 747.49
    pulmonary 747.49
  vena cava (congenital) (inferior) (superior) 747.49
  ventral horn cell 742.59
  ventricular septum 745.3
  vermis of cerebellum 742.2
  vertebra, congenital 756.13
  vulva, congenital 752.49
Absentia epileptica (*see also* Epilepsy) 345.0
Absinthemia (*see also* Dependence) 304.6
Absinthism (*see also* Dependence) 304.6
Absorbent system disease 459.89

Absorption
  alcohol, through placenta or breast milk 760.71
  antibiotics, through placenta or breast milk 760.74
  anticonvulsants, through placenta or breast milk 760.77
  antifungals, through placenta or breast milk 760.74
  anti-infective, through placenta or breast milk 760.74
  antimetabolics, through placenta or breast milk 760.78
  chemical NEC 989.9
    specified chemical or substance—*see* Table of drugs and chemicals
    through placenta or breast milk (fetus or newborn) 760.70
      alcohol 760.71
      anticonvulsants 760.77
      antifungals 760.74
      anti-infective agents 760.74
      antimetabolics 760.78
      cocaine 760.75
      "crack" 760.75
      diethylstilbestrol *[DES]* 760.76
      hallucinogenic agents 760.73
      medicinal agents NEC 760.79
      narcotics 760.72
      obstetric anesthetic or analgesic drug 763.5
      specified agent NEC 760.79
      suspected, affecting management of pregnancy 655.5
  cocaine, through placenta or breast milk 760.75
  drug NEC (*see also* Reaction, drug)
    through placenta or breast milk (fetus or newborn) 760.70
      alcohol 760.71
      anticonvulsants 760.77
      antifungals 760.74
      anti-infective agents 760.74
      antimetabolics 760.78
      cocaine 760.75
      "crack" 760.75
      diethylstilbestrol (DES) 760.76
      hallucinogenic agents 760.73
      medicinal agents NEC 760.79
      narcotics 760.72
      obstetric anesthetic or analgesic drug 763.5
      specified agent NEC 760.79
      suspected, affecting management of pregnancy 655.5
  fat, disturbance 579.8
  hallucinogenic agents, through placenta or breast milk 760.73
  immune sera, through placenta or breast milk 760.79
  lactose defect 271.3
  medicinal agents NEC, through placenta or breast milk 760.79
  narcotics, through placenta or breast milk 760.72
  noxious substance,—*see* Absorption, chemical
  protein, disturbance 579.8
  pus or septic, general—*see* Septicemia
  quinine, through placenta or breast milk 760.74
  toxic substance—*see* Absorption, chemical
  uremic—*see* Uremia
Abstinence symptoms or syndrome
  alcohol 291.81
  drug 292.0
Abt-Letterer-Siwe syndrome (acute histiocytosis X) (M9722/3) 202.5

INDEX TO DISEASES

Abulia 799.89
Abulomania 301.6
Abuse
  adult 995.80
    emotional 995.82
    multiple forms 995.85
    neglect (nutritional) 995.84
    physical 995.81
    psychological 995.82
    sexual 995.83
  alcohol (*see also* Alcoholism) 305.0
    dependent 303.9
    non-dependent 305.0
  child 995.50
    counseling
      perpetrator
        non-parent V62.83
        parent V61.22
      victim V61.21
    emotional 995.51
    multiple forms 995.59
    neglect (nutritional) 995.52
    physical 995.54
      shaken infant syndrome 995.55
    psychological 995.51
    sexual 995.53
  drugs, nondependent 305.9

> Note—Use the following fifth-digit subclassification with the following codes: 305.0, 305.2-305.9:
>
> 0 *unspecifidd*
> 1 *continuous*
> 2 *episodic*
> 3 *in remission*

    amphetamine type 305.7
    antidepressants 305.8
    anxiolytic 305.4
    barbiturates 305.4
    caffeine 305.9
    cannabis 305.2
    cocaine type 305.6
    hallucinogens 305.3
    hashish 305.2
    hypnotic 305.4
    inhalant 305.9
    LSD 305.3
    marijuana 305.2
    mixed 305.9
    morphine type 305.5
    opioid type 305.5
    phencyclidine (PCP) 305.9
    sedative 305.4
    specified NEC 305.9
    tranquilizers 305.4
  spouse 995.80
  tobacco 305.1
Acalcerosis 275.40
Acalcicosis 275.40
Acalculia 784.69
  developmental 315.1
Acanthocheilonemiasis 125.4
Acanthocytosis 272.5
Acanthokeratodermia 701.1
Acantholysis 701.8
  bullosa 757.39
Acanthoma (benign) (M8070/0)—*see also* Neoplasm, by site, benign
  malignant (M8070/3)—*see* Neoplasm, by site, malignant

Acanthosis (acquired) (nigricans) 701.2
  adult 701.2
  benign (congenital) 757.39
  congenital 757.39
  glycogenic
    esophagus 530.8
  juvenile 701.2
  tongue 529.8
Acanthrocytosis 272.5
Acapnia 276.3
Acarbia 276.2
Acardia 759.89
Acardiacus amorphus 759.89
Acardiotrophia 429.1
Acardius 759.89
Acariasis 133.9
  sarcoptic 133.0
Acaridiasis 133.9
Acarinosis 133.9
Acariosis 133.9
Acarodermatitis 133.9
  urticarioides 133.9
Acarophobia 300.29
Acatalasemia 277.89
Acatalasia 277.89
Acatamathesia 784.69
Acataphasia 784.5
Acathisia 781.0
  due to drugs 333.99
Acceleration, accelerated
  atrioventricular conduction 426.7
  idioventricular rhythm 427.89
Accessory (congenital)
  adrenal gland 759.1
  anus 751.5
  appendix 751.5
  atrioventricular conduction 426.7
  auditory ossicles 744.04
  auricle (ear) 744.1
  autosome(s) NEC 758.5
    21 or 22 758.0
  biliary duct or passage 751.69
  bladder 753.8
  blood vessels (peripheral) (congenital) NEC (*see also* Anomaly, peripheral vascular system) 747.60
    cerebral 747.81
    coronary 746.85
  bone NEC 756.9
    foot 755.67
  breast tissue, axilla 757.6
  carpal bones 755.56
  cecum 751.5
  cervix 752.49
  chromosome(s) NEC 758.5
    13-15 758.1
    16-18 758.2
    21 or 22 758.0
    autosome(s) NEC 758.5
    D_1 758.1
    E_3 758.2
    G 758.0
    sex 758.81
  coronary artery 746.85
  cusp(s), heart valve NEC 746.89
    pulmonary 746.09
  cystic duct 751.69
  digits 755.00
  ear (auricle) (lobe) 744.1
  endocrine gland NEC 759.2

Accessory—*continued*
  external os 752.49
  eyelid 743.62
  eye muscle 743.69
  face bone(s) 756.0
  fallopian tube (fimbria) (ostium) 752.19
  fingers 755.01
  foreskin 605
  frontonasal process 756.0
  gallbladder 751.69
  genital organ(s)
    female 752.89
      external 752.49
      internal NEC 752.89
    male NEC 752.89
      penis 752.69
  genitourinary organs NEC 752.89
  heart 746.89
    valve NEC 746.89
      pulmonary 746.09
  hepatic ducts 751.69
  hymen 752.49
  intestine (large) (small) 751.5
  kidney 753.3
  lacrimal canal 743.65
  leaflet, heart valve NEC 746.89
    pulmonary 746.09
  ligament, broad 752.19
  liver (duct) 751.69
  lobule (ear) 744.1
  lung (lobe) 748.69
  muscle 756.82
  navicular of carpus 755.56
  nervous system, part NEC 742.8
  nipple 757.6
  nose 748.1
  organ or site NEC—*see* Anomaly, specified type NEC
  ovary 752.0
  oviduct 752.19
  pancreas 751.7
  parathyroid gland 759.2
  parotid gland (and duct) 750.22
  pituitary gland 759.2
  placental lobe—*see* Placenta, abnormal
  preauricular appendage 744.1
  prepuce 605
  renal arteries (multiple) 747.62
  rib 756.3
    cervical 756.2
  roots (teeth) 520.2
  salivary gland 750.22
  sesamoids 755.8
  sinus—*see* condition
  skin tags 757.39
  spleen 759.0
  sternum 756.3
  submaxillary gland 750.22
  tarsal bones 755.67
  teeth, tooth 520.1
    causing crowding 524.31
  tendon 756.89
  thumb 755.01
  thymus gland 759.2
  thyroid gland 759.2
  toes 755.02
  tongue 750.13
  tragus 744.1
  ureter 753.4
  urethra 753.8
  urinary organ or tract NEC 753.8
  uterus 752.2

Accessory—*continued*
  vagina 752.49
  valve, heart NEC 746.89
    pulmonary 746.09
  vertebra 756.19
  vocal cords 748.3
  vulva 752.49
Accident, accidental —*see also* condition
  birth NEC 767.9
  cardiovascular (*see also* Disease, cardiovascular) 429.2
  cerebral (*see also* Disease, cerebrovascular, acute) 434.91
  cerebrovascular (current) (CVA) (*see also* Disease, cerebrovascular, acute) 434.91
    aborted 434.91
    embolic 434.11
    healed or old V12.54
    hemorrhagic—*see* Hemorrhage, brain
    impending 435.9
    ischemic 434.91
    late effect—*see* Late effect(s) (of) cerebrovascular disease
    postoperative 997.02
    thrombotic 434.01
  coronary (*see also* Infarct, myocardium) 410.9
  craniovascular (*see also* Disease, cerebrovascular, acute) 436
  during pregnancy, to mother
    affecting fetus or newborn 760.5
  heart, cardiac (*see also* Infarct, myocardium) 410.9
  intrauterine 779.89
  vascular—*see* Disease, cerebrovascular, acute
Accommodation
  disorder of 367.51
    drug-induced 367.89
    toxic 367.89
  insufficiency of 367.4
  paralysis of 367.51
    hysterical 300.11
  spasm of 367.53
Accouchement —*see* Delivery
Accreta placenta (without hemorrhage) 667.0
  with hemorrhage 666.0
Accretio cordis (nonrheumatic) 423.1
Accretions on teeth 523.6
Accumulation secretion, prostate 602.8
Acephalia, acephalism, acephaly 740.0
Acephalic monster 740.0
Acephalobrachia monster 759.89
Acephalocardia 759.89
Acephalocardius 759.89
Acephalochiria 759.89
Acephalochirus monster 759.89
Acephalogaster 759.89
Acephalostomus monster 759.89
Acephalothorax 759.89
Acephalus 740.0
Acetonemia 790.6
  diabetic 250.1
Acetonglycosuria 982.8
Acetonuria 791.6
Achalasia 530.0
  cardia 530.0
  digestive organs congenital NEC 751.8
  esophagus 530.0
  pelvirectal 751.3
  psychogenic 306.4
  pylorus 750.5
  sphincteral NEC 564.89

INDEX TO DISEASES

Achard-Thiers syndrome (adrenogenital) 255.2
Ache (s)—*see* Pain
Acheilia 750.26
Acheiria 755.21
Achillobursitis 726.71
Achillodynia 726.71
Achlorhydria, achlorhydric 536.0
   anemia 280.9
   diarrhea 536.0
   neurogenic 536.0
   postvagotomy 564.2
   psychogenic 306.4
   secondary to vagotomy 564.2
Achloroblepsia 368.52
Achloropsia 368.52
Acholia 575.8
Acholuric jaundice (familial) (splenomegalic)
   (*see also* Spherocytosis) 282.0
   acquired 283.9
Achondroplasia 756.4
Achrestic anemia 281.8
Achroacytosis, lacrimal gland 375.00
   tuberculous (*see also* Tuberculosis) 017.3
Achroma, cutis 709.00
Achromate (congenital) 368.54
Achromatopia 368.54
Achromatopsia (congenital) 368.54
Achromia
   congenital 270.2
   parasitica 111.0
   unguium 703.8
Achylia
   gastrica 536.8
     neurogenic 536.3
     psychogenic 306.4
   pancreatica 577.1
Achylosis 536.8
Acid
   burn—*see also* Burn, by site
     from swallowing acid—*see* Burn, internal
       organs
   deficiency
     amide nicotinic 265.2
     amino 270.9
     ascorbic 267
     folic 266.2
     nicotinic (amide) 265.2
     pantothenic 266.2
   intoxication 276.2
   peptic disease 536.8
   stomach 536.8
     psychogenic 306.4
Acidemia 276.2
   arginosuccinic 270.6
   fetal
     affecting management of pregnancy 656.3
     before onset of labor, in liveborn infant 768.2
     during labor and delivery, in liveborn infant
       768.3
     intrauterine—*see* Distress, fetal 656.3
     unspecified as to time of onset, in liveborn
       infant 768.4
   newborn 775.81
   pipecolic 270.7
Acidity, gastric (high) (low) 536.8
   psychogenic 306.4
Acidocytopenia 288.59
Acidocytosis 288.3
Acidopenia 288.59

Acomia

Acidosis 276.2
   diabetic 250.1
   fetal, affecting management of pregnancy 656.8
   fetal, affecting newborn 775.81
   kidney tubular 588.89
   lactic 276.2
   metabolic NEC 276.2
     with respiratory acidosis 276.4
       of newborn 775.81
     late, of newborn 775.7
   newborn 775.81
   renal
     hyperchloremic 588.89
     tubular (distal) (proximal) 588.89
   respiratory 276.2
     complicated by
       metabolic acidosis 276.4
         of newborn 775.81
       metabolic alkalosis 276.4
Aciduria 791.9
   arginosuccinic 270.6
   beta-aminoisobutyric (BAIB) 277.2
   glutaric
     type I 270.7
     type II (type IIA, IIB, IIC) 277.85
     type III 277.86
   glycolic 271.8
   methylmalonic 270.3
     with glycinemia 270.7
   organic 270.9
   orotic (congenital) (hereditary) (pyrimidine
     deficiency) 281.4
Acladiosis 111.8
   skin 111.8
Aclasis
   diaphyseal 756.4
   tarsoepiphyseal 756.59
Acleistocardia 745.5
Aclusion 524.4
Acmesthesia 782.0
Acne (pustular) (vulgaris) 706.1
   agminata (*see also* Tuberculosis) 017.0
   artificialis 706.1
   atrophica 706.0
   cachecticorum (Hebra) 706.1
   conglobata 706.1
   conjunctiva 706.1
   cystic 706.1
   decalvans 704.09
   erythematosa 695.3
   eyelid 706.1
   frontalis 706.0
   indurata 706.1
   keloid 706.1
   lupoid 706.0
   necrotic, necrotica 706.0
     miliaris 704.8
   neonatal 706.1
   nodular 706.1
   occupational 706.1
   papulosa 706.1
   rodens 706.0
   rosacea 695.3
   scorbutica 267
   scrofulosorum (Bazin) (*see also* Tuberculosis)
     017.0
   summer 692.72
   tropical 706.1
   varioliformis 706.0
Acneiform drug eruptions 692.3
Acnitis (primary) (*see also* Tuberculosis) 017.0
Acomia 704.00

Acontractile bladder   INDEX TO DISEASES

Acontractile bladder 344.61
Aconuresis (*see also* Incontinence) 788.30
Acosta's disease 993.2
Acousma 780.1
Acoustic —*see* condition
Acousticophobia 300.29
Acquired —*see* condition
Acquired immunodeficiency syndrome —*see* Human immunodeficiency virus (disease) (illness) (infection)
Acragnosis 781.99
Acrania (monster) 740.0
Acroagnosis 781.99
Acroasphyxia, chronic 443.89
Acrobrachycephaly 756.0
Acrobystiolith 608.89
Acrobystitis 607.2
Acrocephalopolysyndactyly 755.55
Acrocephalosyndactyly 755.55
Acrocephaly 756.0
Acrochondrohyperplasia 759.82
Acrocyanosis 443.89
   newborn 770.83
Acrodermatitis 686.8
   atrophicans (chronica) 701.8
   continua (Hallopeau) 696.1
   enteropathica 686.8
   Hallopeau's 696.1
   perstans 696.1
   pustulosa continua 696.1
   recalcitrant pustular 696.1
Acrodynia 985.0
Acrodysplasia 755.55
Acrohyperhidrosis (*see also* Hyperhidrosis) 780.8
Acrokeratosis verruciformis 757.39
Acromastitis 611.0
Acromegaly, acromegalia (skin) 253.0
Acromelalgia 443.82
Acromicria, acromikria 756.59
Acronyx 703.0
Acropachy, thyroid (*see also* Thyrotoxicosis) 242.9
Acropachyderma 757.39
Acroparesthesia 443.89
   simple (Schultz's type) 443.89
   vasomotor (Nothnagel's type) 443.89
Acropathy thyroid (*see also* Thyrotoxicosis) 242.9
Acrophobia 300.29
Acroposthitis 607.2
Acroscleriasis (*see also* Scleroderma) 710.1
Acroscleroderma (*see also* Scleroderma) 710.1
Acrosclerosis (*see also* Scleroderma) 710.1
Acrosphacelus 785.4
Acrosphenosyndactylia 755.55
Acrospiroma, eccrine (M8402/0)—*see* Neoplasm, skin, benign
Acrostealgia 732.9
Acrosyndactyly (*see also* Syndactylism) 755.10
Acrotrophodynia 991.4
Actinic —*see also* condition
   cheilitis (due to sun) 692.72
      chronic NEC 692.74
      due to radiation, except from sun 692.82
   conjunctivitis 370.24
   dermatitis (due to sun) (*see also* Dermatitis, actinic) 692.70
   due to

Actinic—*continued*
      roentgen rays or radioactive substance 692.82
      ultraviolet radiation, except from sun 692.82
      sun NEC 692.70
   elastosis solare 692.74
   granuloma 692.73
   keratitis 370.24
   ophthalmia 370.24
   reticuloid 692.73
Actinobacillosis, general 027.8
Actinobacillus
   lignieresii 027.8
   mallei 024
   muris 026.1
Actinocutitis NEC (*see also* Dermatitis, actinic) 692.70
Actinodermatitis NEC (*see also* Dermatitis, actinic) 692.70
Actinomyces
   israelii (infection)—*see* Actinomycosis
   muris-ratti (infection) 026.1
Actinomycosis actinomycotic 039.9
   with
      pneumonia 039.1
   abdominal 039.2
   cervicofacial 039.3
   cutaneous 039.0
   pulmonary 039.1
   specified site NEC 039.8
   thoracic 039.1
Actinoneuritis 357.89
Action, heart
   disorder 427.9
      postoperative 997.1
   irregular 427.9
      postoperative 997.1
      psychogenic 306.2
Active —*see* condition
Activity decrease, functional 780.99
Acute —*see also* condition
   abdomen NEC 789.0
   gallbladder (*see also* Cholecystitis, acute) 575.0
Acyanoblepsia 368.53
Acyanopsia 368.53
Acystia 753.8
Acystinervia —*see* Neurogenic, bladder
Acystineuria —*see* Neurogenic, bladder
Adactylia, adactyly (congenital) 755.4
   lower limb (complete) (intercalary) (partial) (terminal) (*see also* Deformity, reduction, lower limb) 755.39
      meaning all digits (complete) (partial) 755.31
      transverse (complete) (partial) 755.31
   upper limb (complete) (intercalary) (partial) (terminal) (*see also* Deformity, reduction, upper limb) 755.29
      meaning all digits (complete) (partial) 755.21
      transverse (complete) (partial) 755.21
Adair-Dighton syndrome (brittle bones and blue sclera, deafness) 756.51
Adamantinoblastoma (M9310/0)—*see* Ameloblastoma
Adamantinoma (M9310/0)—*see* Ameloblastoma
Adamantoblastoma (M9310/0)—*see* Ameloblastoma
Adams-Stokes (-Morgagni) disease or syndrome (syncope with heart block) 426.9
Adaptation reaction (*see also* Reaction, adjustment) 309.9

INDEX TO DISEASES

Addiction —*see also* Dependence
  absinthe 304.6
  alcoholic (ethyl) (methyl) (wood) 303.9
    complicating pregnancy, childbirth, or
      puerperium 648.4
      affecting fetus or newborn 760.71
    suspected damage to fetus affecting
      management of pregnancy 655.4
  drug (*see also* Dependence) 304.9
  ethyl alcohol 303.9
  heroin 304.0
  hospital 301.51
  methyl alcohol 303.9
  methylated spirit 303.9
  morphine (-like substances) 304.0
  nicotine 305.1
  opium 304.0
  tobacco 305.1
  wine 303.9
Addison's
  anemia (pernicious) 281.0
  disease (bronze) (primary adrenal insufficiency)
    255.41
    tuberculous (*see also* Tuberculosis) 017.6
  keloid (morphea) 701.0
  melanoderma (adrenal cortical hypofunction)
    255.41
Addison-Biermer anemia (pernicious) 281.0
Addison-Gull disease —*see* Xanthoma
Addisonian crisis or melanosis (acute
  adrenocortical insufficiency) 255.41
Additional —*see also* Accessory
  chromosome(s) 758.5
    13-15 758.1
    16-18 758.2
    21 758.0
    autosome(s) NEC 758.5
    sex 758.81
Adduction contracture, hip or other joint —*see*
  Contraction, joint
ADEM (acute disseminated encephalomyelitis)
  (postinfectious) 136.9 *[323.61]*
  infectious 136.9 *[323.61]*
  noninfectious 323.81
Adenasthenia gastrica 536.0
Aden fever 061
Adenitis (*see also* Lymphadenitis) 289.3
  acute, unspecified site 683
    epidemic infectious 075
  axillary 289.3
    acute 683
    chronic or subacute 289.1
  Bartholin's gland 616.89
  bulbourethral gland (*see also* Urethritis) 597.89
  cervical 289.3
    acute 683
    chronic or subacute 289.1
  chancroid (Ducrey's bacillus) 099.0
  chronic (any lymph node, except mesenteric)
    289.1
    mesenteric 289.2
  Cowper's gland (*see also* Urethritis) 597.89
  epidemic, acute 075
  gangrenous 683
  gonorrheal NEC 098.89
  groin 289.3
    acute 683
    chronic or subacute 289.1
  infectious 075
  inguinal (region) 289.3
    acute 683

Adenocarcinoma

Adenitis—*continued*
  chronic or subacute 289.1
  lymph gland or node, except mesenteric 289.3
    acute 683
    chronic or subacute 289.1
  mesenteric (acute) (chronic) (nonspecific)
    (subacute) 289.2
  mesenteric (acute) (chronic) (nonspecific)
    (subacute) 289.2
    due to Pasteurella multocida (P. septica) 027.2
  parotid gland (suppurative) 527.2
  phlegmonous 683
  salivary duct or gland (any) (recurring)
    (suppurative) 527.2
  scrofulous (*see also* Tuberculosis) 017.2
  septic 289.3
  Skene's duct or gland (*see also* Urethritis)
    597.89
  strumous, tuberculous (*see also* Tuberculosis)
    017.2
  subacute, unspecified site 289.1
  sublingual gland (suppurative) 527.2
  submandibular gland (suppurative) 527.2
  submaxillary gland (suppurative) 527.2
  suppurative 683
  tuberculous—*see* Tuberculosis, lymph gland
  urethral gland (*see also* Urethritis) 597.89
  venereal NEC 099.8
  Wharton's duct (suppurative) 527.2
Adenoacanthoma (M8570/3)—*see* Neoplasm, by
  site, malignant
Adenoameloblastoma (M9300/0) 213.1
  upper jaw (bone) 213.0
Adenocarcinoma (M8140/3)—*see also*
  Neoplasm, by site, malignant

> Note—The list of adjectival modifiers below is
> not exhaustive. A description of
> adenocarcinoma that does not appear in this list
> should be coded in the same manner as
> carcinoma with that description. Thus, "mixed
> acidophil-basophil adenocarcinoma," should be
> coded in the same manner as "mixed
> acidophil-basophil carcinoma," which appears
> in the list under "Carcinoma."
>
> Except where otherwise indicated, the
> morphological varieties of adenocarcinoma in
> the list below should be coded by site as for
> "Neoplasm, malignant."

  with
    apocrine metaplasia (M8573/3)
    cartilaginous (and osseous) metaplasia
      (M8571/3)
    osseous (and cartilaginous) metaplasia
      (M8571/3)
    spindle cell metaplasia (M8572/3)
    squamous metaplasia (M8570/3)
  acidophil (M8280/3)
    specified site—*see* Neoplasm, by site,
      malignant
    unspecified site 194.3
  acinar (M8550/3)
  acinic cell (M8550/3)
  adrenal cortical (M8370/3) 194.0
  alveolar (M8251/3)
  and
    epidermoid carcinoma, mixed (M8560/3)
    squamous cell carcinoma, mixed (M8560/3)
  apocrine (M8401/3)
    breast—*see* Neoplasm, breast, malignant

Adenocarcinoma—*continued*
  specified site NEC—*see* Neoplasm, skin, malignant
  unspecified site 173.9
  basophil (M8300/3)
    specified site—*see* Neoplasm, by site, malignant
    unspecified site 194.3
  bile duct type (M8160/3)
    sliver 155.1
    specified site NEC—*see* Neoplasm, by site, malignant
    unspecified site 155.1
  bronchiolar (M8250/3)—*see* Neoplasm, lung, malignant
  ceruminous (M8420/3) 173.2
  chromophobe (M8270/3)
    specified site—*see* Neoplasm, by site, malignant
    unspecified site 194.3
  clear cell (mesonephroid type) (M8310/3)
  colloid (M8480/3)
  cylindroid type (M8200/3)
  diffuse type (M8145/3)
    pecified site—*see* Neoplasm, by site, malignant
    unspecified site 151.9
  duct (infiltrating) (M8500/3)
    with Paget's disease (M8541/3)—*see* Neoplasm, breast, malignant
    specified site—*see* Neoplasm, by site, malignant
    unspecified site 174.9
  embryonal (M9070/3)
  endometrioid (M8380/3)—*see* Neoplasm, by site, malignant
  eosinophil (M8280/3)
    specified site—*see* Neoplasm, by site, malignant
    unspecified site 194.3
  follicular (M8330/3)
    and papillary (M8340/3) 193
    moderately differentiated type (M8332/3) 193
    pure follicle type (M8331/3) 193
    specified site—*see* Neoplasm, by site, malignant
    trabecular type (M8332/3) 193
    unspecified type 193
    well differentiated type (M8331/3) 193
  gelatinous (M8480/3)
  granular cell (M8320/3)
  Hürthle cell (M8290/3) 193
  in
    adenomatous
      polyp (M8210/3)
      polyposis coli (M8220/3) 153.9
    polypoid adenoma (M8210/3)
    tubular adenoma (M8210/3)
    villous adenoma (M8261/3)
  infiltrating duct (M8500/3)
    with Paget's disease (M8541/3)—*see* Neoplasm, breast, malignant
    specified site—*see* Neoplasm, by site, malignant
    unspecified site 174.9
  inflammatory (M8530/3)
    specified site—*see* Neoplasm, by site, malignant
    unspecified site 174.9
  in situ (M8140/2)—*see* Neoplasm, by site, in situ

Adenocarcinoma—*continued*
  intestinal type (M8144/3)
    specified site—*see* Neoplasm, by site, malignant
    unspecified site 151.9
  intraductal (noninfiltrating) (M8500/2)
    papillary (M8503/2)
      specified site—*see* Neoplasm, by site, in situ
      unspecified site 233.0
    specified site—*see* Neoplasm, by site, in situ
    unspecified site 233.0
  islet cell (M8150/3)
    and exocrine, mixed (M8154/3)
      specified site—*see* Neoplasm, by site, malignant
      unspecified site 157.9
    pancreas 157.4
    specified site NEC—*see* Neoplasm, by site, malignant
    unspecified site 157.4
  lobular (M8520/3)
    specified site—*see* Neoplasm, by site, malignant
    unspecified site 174.9
  medullary (M8510/3)
  mesonephric (M9110/3)
  mixed cell (M8323/3)
  mucinous (M8480/3)
  mucin-producing (M8481/3)
  mucoid (M8480/3)—*see also* Neoplasm, by site, malignant
    cell (M8300/3)
      specified site—*see* Neoplasm, by site, malignant
      unspecified site 194.3
  nonencapsulated sclerosing (M8350/3) 193
  oncocytic (M8290/3)
  oxyphilic (M8290/3)
  papillary (M8260/3)
    and follicular (M8340/3) 193
    intraductal (noninfiltrating) (M8503/2)
      specified site—*see* Neoplasm, by site, in situ
      unspecified site 233.0
    serous (M8460/3)
      specified site—*see* Neoplasm, by site, malignant
      unspecified site 183.0
  papillocystic (M8450/3)
    specified site—*see* Neoplasm, by site, malignant
    unspecified site 183.0
  pseudomucinous (M8470/3)
    specified site—*see* Neoplasm, by site, malignant
    unspecified site 183.0
  renal cell (M8312/3) 189.0
  sebaceous (M8410/3)
  serous (M8441/3)—*see also* Neoplasm, by site, malignant
    papillary
      specified site—*see* Neoplasm, by site, malignant
      unspecified site 183.0
  signet ring cell (M8490/3)
  superficial spreading (M8143/3)
  sweat gland (M8400/3)—*see* Neoplasm, skin, malignant
  trabecular (M8190/3)
  tubular (M8211/3)
  villous (M8262/3)
  water-clear cell (M8322/3) 194.1

Adenofibroma (M9013/0)
  clear cell (M8313/0)—*see* Neoplasm, by site, benign
  endometrioid (M8381/0) 220
    borderline malignancy (M8381/1) 236.2
    malignant (M8381/3) 183.0
  mucinous (M9015/0)
    specified site—*see* Neoplasm, by site, benign
    unspecified site 220
  prostate 600.20
    with
      other lower urinary tract symptoms (LUTS) 600.21
      urinary
        obstruction 600.21
        retention 600.21
  serous (M9014/0)
    specified site—*see* Neoplasm, by site, benign
    unspecified site 220
  specified site—*see* Neoplasm, by site, benign
  unspecified site 220

Adenofibrosis
  breast 610.2
  endometrioid 617.0

Adenoiditis 474.01
  acute 463
  chronic 474.01
    with chronic tonsillitis 474.02

Adenoids (congenital) (of nasal fossa) 474.9
  hypertrophy 474.12
  vegetations 474.2

Adenolipomatosis (symmetrical) 272.8

Adenolymphoma (M8561/0)
  specified site—*see* Neoplasm, by site, benign
  unspecified 210.2

Adenoma (sessile) (M8140/0)—*see also* Neoplasm, by site, benign

> Note—Except where otherwise indicated, the morphological varieties of adenoma in the list below should be coded by site as for "Neoplasm, benign."

  acidophil (M8280/0)
    specified site—*see* Neoplasm, by site, benign
    unspecified site 227.3
  acinar (cell) (M8550/0)
  acinic cell (M8550/0)
  adrenal (cortex) (cortical) (functioning) (M8370/0) 227.0
    clear cell type (M8373/0) 227.0
    compact cell type (M8371/0) 227.0
    glomerulosa cell type (M8374/0) 227.0
    heavily pigmented variant (M8372/0) 227.0
    mixed cell type (M8375/0) 227.0
  alpha cell (M8152/0)
    pancreas 211.7
    specified site NEC—*see* Neoplasm, by site, benign
    unspecified site 211.7
  alveolar (M8251/0)
  apocrine (M8401/0)
    breast 217
    specified site NEC—*see* Neoplasm, skin, benign
    unspecified site 216.9
  basal cell (M8147/0)
  basophil (M8300/0)
    specified site—*see* Neoplasm, by site, benign
    unspecified site 227.3
  beta cell (M8151/0)
    pancreas 211.7

Adenoma—*continued*
    specified site NEC—*see* Neoplasm, by site, benign
    unspecified site 211.7
  bile duct (M8160/0) 211.5
  black (M8372/0) 227.0
  bronchial (M8140/1) 235.7
    carcinoid type (M8240/3)—*see* Neoplasm, lung, malignant
    cylindroid type (M8200/3)—*see* Neoplasm, lung, malignant
  ceruminous (M8420/0) 216.2
  chief cell (M8321/0) 227.1
    chromophobe (M8270/0)
    (specified site—*see* Neoplasm, by site, benign
    unspecified site 227.3
  clear cell (M8310/0)
  colloid (M8334/0)
    specified site—*see* Neoplasm, by site, benign
    unspecified site 226
  cylindroid type, bronchus (M8200/3)—*see* Neoplasm, lung, malignant
  duct (M8503/0)
  embryonal (M8191/0)
  endocrine, multiple (M8360/1)
    single specified site—*see* Neoplasm, by site, uncertain behavior
    two or more specified sites 237.4
    unspecified site 237.4
  endometrioid (M8380/0)—*see also* Neoplasm, by site, benign
    borderline malignancy (M8380/1)—*see* Neoplasm, by site, uncertain behavior
  eosinophil (M8280/0)
    specified site—*see* Neoplasm, by site, benign
    unspecified site 227.3
  fetal (M8333/0)
    specified site—*see* Neoplasm, by site, benign
    unspecified site 226
  follicular (M8330/0)
    specified site—*see* Neoplasm, by site, benign
    unspecified site 226
  hepatocellular (M8170/0) 211.5
  Hürthle cell (M8290/0) 226
  intracystic papillary (M8504/0)
  islet cell (functioning) (M8150/0)
    pancreas 211.7
    specified site NEC—*see* Neoplasm, by site, benign
    unspecified site 211.7
  liver cell (M8170/0) 211.5
  macrofollicular (M8334/0)
    specified site NEC—*see* Neoplasm, by site, benign
    unspecified site 226
  malignant, malignum (M8140/3)—*see* Neoplasm, by site, malignant
  mesonephric (M9110/0)
  microfollicular (M8333/0)
    specified site—*see* Neoplasm, by site, benign
    unspecified site 226
  mixed cell (M8323/0)
  monomorphic (M8146/0)
  mucinous (M8480/0)
  mucoid cell (M8300/0)
    specified site—*see* Neoplasm, by site, benign
    unspecified site 227.3
  multiple endocrine (M8360/1)
    single specified site—*see* Neoplasm, by site, uncertain behavior
    two or more specified sites 237.4

Adenoma—*continued*
   unspecified site 237.4
   nipple (M8506/0) 217
   oncocytic (M8290/0)
   oxyphilic (M8290/0)
   papillary (M8260/0)—*see also* Neoplasm, by site, benign
     intracystic (M8504/0)
   papillotubular (M8263/0)
   Pick's tubular (M8640/0)
     specified site—*see* Neoplasm, by site, benign
     unspecified site
       female 220
       male 222.0
   pleomorphic (M8940/0)
   polypoid (M8210/0)
   prostate (benign) 600.20
     with
       other lower urinary tract symptoms (LUTS) 600.21
       urinary
         obstruction 600.21
         retention 600.21
   rete cell 222.0
   sebaceous, sebaceum (gland) (senile) (M8410/0)—*see also* Neoplasm, skin, benign
     disseminata 759.5
   Sertoli cell (M8640/0)
     specified site—*see* Neoplasm, by site, benign
     unspecified site
       female 220
       male 222.0
   skin appendage (M8390/0)—*see* Neoplasm, skin, benign
   sudoriferous gland (M8400/0)—*see* Neoplasm, skin, benign
   sweat gland or duct (M8400/0)—*see* Neoplasm, skin, benign
   testicular (M8640/0)
     specified site—*see* Neoplasm, by site, benign
     unspecified site
       female 220
       male 222.0
   thyroid 226
   trabecular (M8190/0)
   tubular (M8211/0)—*see also* Neoplasm, by site, benign
     papillary (M8460/3)
     Pick's (M8640/0)
       specified site—*see* Neoplasm, by site, benign
       unspecified site
         female 220
         male 222.0
   tubulovillous (M8263/0)
   villoglandular (M8263/0)
   villous (M8261/1)—*see* Neoplasm, by site, uncertain behavior
   water-clear cell (M8322/0) 227.1
   wolffian duct (M9110/0)
Adenomatosis (M8220/0)
   endocrine (multiple) (M8360/1)
     single specified site—*see* Neoplasm, by site, uncertain behavior
     two or more specified sites 237.4
     unspecified site 237.4
   erosive of nipple (M8506/0) 217
   pluriendocrine—*see* Adenomatosis, endocrine

Adenomatosis—*continued*
   pulmonary (M8250/1) 235.7
     malignant (M8250/3)—*see* Neoplasm, lung, malignant
   specified site—*see* Neoplasm, by site, benign
   unspecified site 211.3
Adenomatous
   cyst, thyroid (gland)—*see* Goiter, nodular
   goiter (nontoxic) (*see also* Goiter, nodular) 241.9
     toxic or with hyperthyroidism 242.3
Adenomyoma (M8932/0)—*see also* Neoplasm, by site, benign
   prostate 600.20
     with
       other lower urinary tract symptoms (LUTS) 600.21
       urinary
         obstruction 600.21
         retention 600.21
Adenomyometritis 617.0
Adenomyosis (uterus) (internal) 617.0
Adenopathy (lymph gland) 785.6
   inguinal 785.6
   mediastinal 785.6
   mesentery 785.6
   syphilitic (secondary) 091.4
   tracheobronchial 785.6
   tuberculous (*see also* Tuberculosis) 012.1
     primary, progressive 010.8
   tuberculous (*see also* Tuberculosis, lymph gland) 017.2
     tracheobronchial 012.1
       primary, progressive 010.8
Adenopharyngitis 462
Adenophlegmon 683
Adenosalpingitis 614.1
Adenosarcoma (M8960/3) 189.0
Adenosclerosis 289.3
Adenosis
   breast (sclerosing) 610.2
   vagina, congenital 752.49
Adentia (complete) (partial) (*see also* Absence, teeth) 520.0
Adherent
   labium (minus) 624.4
   pericardium (nonrheumatic) 423.1
     rheumatic 393
   placenta 667.0
     with hemorrhage 666.0
   prepuce 605
   scar (skin) NEC 709.2
   tendon in scar 709.2
Adhesion(s), adhesive (postinfectional)(postoperative)
   abdominal (wall) (*see also* Adhesions, peritoneum) 568.0
   amnion to fetus 658.8
     affecting fetus or newborn 762.8
   appendix 543.9
   arachnoiditis—*see* Meningitis
   auditory tube (Eustachian) 381.89
   bands—*see also* Adhesions, peritoneum
     cervix 622.3
     uterus 621.5
   bile duct (any) 576.8
   bladder (sphincter) 596.8
   bowel (*see also* Adhesions, peritoneum) 568.0
   cardiac 423.1
     rheumatic 398.99
   cecum (*see also* Adhesions, peritoneum) 568.0

Adhesion(s)—*continued*
  cervicovaginal 622.3
    congenital 752.49
    postpartal 674.8
    old 622.3
  cervix 622.3
  clitoris 624.4
  colon (*see also* Adhesions, peritoneum) 568.0
  common duct 576.8
  congenital—*see also* Anomaly, specified type NEC
    fingers (*see also* Syndactylism, fingers) 755.11
    labium (majus) (minus) 752.49
    omental, anomalous 751.4
    ovary 752.0
    peritoneal 751.4
    toes (*see also* Syndactylism, toes) 755.13
    tongue (to gum or roof of mouth) 750.12
  conjunctiva (acquired) (localized) 372.62
    congenital 743.63
    extensive 372.63
  cornea—*see* Opacity, cornea
  cystic duct 575.8
  diaphragm (*see also* Adhesions, peritoneum) 568.0
  due to foreign body—*see* Foreign body
  duodenum (*see also* Adhesions, peritoneum) 568.0
    with obstruction 537.3
  ear, middle—*see* Adhesions, middle ear
  epididymis 608.89
  epidural—*see* Adhesions, meninges
  epiglottis 478.79
  Eustachian tube 381.89
  eyelid 374.46
    postoperative 997.99
    surgically created V45.69
  gallbladder (*see also* Disease, gallbladder) 575.8
  globe 360.89
  heart 423.1
    rheumatic 398.99
  ileocecal (coil) (*see also* Adhesions, peritoneum) 568.0
  ileum (*see also* Adhesions, peritoneum) 568.0
  intestine (postoperative) (*see also* Adhesions, peritoneum) 568.0
    with obstruction 560.81
      with hernia—*see also* Hernia, by site, with obstruction
        gangrenous—*see* Hernia, by site, with gangrene
  intra-abdominal (*see also* Adhesions, peritoneum) 568.0
  iris 364.70
    to corneal graft 996.79
  joint (*see also* Ankylosis) 718.5
  kidney 593.89
  labium (majus) (minus), congenital 752.49
  liver 572.8
  lung 511.0
  mediastinum 519.3
  meninges 349.2
    cerebral (any) 349.2
      congenital 742.4
    congenital 742.8
    spinal (any) 349.2
      congenital 742.59
    tuberculous (cerebral) (spinal) (*see also* Tuberculosis, meninges) 013.0

Adhesion(s)—*continued*
  mesenteric (*see also* Adhesions, peritoneum) 568.0
  middle ear (fibrous) 385.10
    drum head 385.19
      to
        incus 385.11
        promontorium 385.13
        stapes 385.12
    specified NEC 385.19
  nasal (septum) (to turbinates) 478.19
  nerve NEC 355.9
    spinal 355.9
      root 724.9
        cervical NEC 723.4
        lumbar NEC 724.4
        lumbosacral 724.4
        thoracic 724.4
  ocular muscle 378.60
  omentum (*see also* Adhesions, peritoneum) 568.0
  organ or site, congenital NEC—*see* Anomaly, specified type NEC
  ovary 614.6
    congenital (to cecum, kidney, or omentum) 752.0
  parauterine 614.6
  parovarian 614.6
  pelvic (peritoneal)
    female 614.6
    male (*see also* Adhesions, peritoneum) 568.0
    postpartal (old) 614.6
    tuberculous (*see also* Tuberculosis) 016.9
  penis to scrotum (congenital) 752.69
  periappendiceal (*see also* Adhesions, peritoneum) 568.0
  pericardium (nonrheumatic) 423.1
    rheumatic 393
    tuberculous (*see also* Tuberculosis) 017.9 [420.0]
  pericholecystic 575.8
  perigastric (*see also* Adhesions, peritoneum) 568.0
  periovarian 614.6
  periprostatic 602.8
  perirectal (*see also* Adhesions, peritoneum) 568.0
  perirenal 593.89
  peritoneum, peritoneal (fibrous) (postoperative) 568.0
    with obstruction (intestinal) 560.81
      with hernia—*see also* Hernia, by site, with obstruction
        gangrenous—*see* Hernia, by site, with gangrene
    duodenum 537.3
    congenital 751.4
    female, (postoperative) (postinfective) 614.6
    pelvic, female 614.6
    pelvic, male 568.0
    postpartal, pelvic 614.6
    to uterus 614.6
  peritubal 614.6
  periureteral 593.89
  periuterine 621.5
  perivesical 596.7
  perivesicular (seminal vesicle) 608.89
  pleura, pleuritic 511.0
    tuberculous (*see also* Tuberculosis, pleura) 012.0
  pleuropericardial 511.0

Adhesion(s) — continued
- postoperative (gastrointestinal tract) (*See also* Adhesions, peritoneum) 568.0
  - eyelid 997.99
    - surgically created V45.69
  - urethra 598.2
- postpartal, old 624.4
- preputial, prepuce 605
- pulmonary 511.0
- pylorus (*see also* Adhesions, peritoneum) 568.0
- Rosenmüller's fossa 478.29
- sciatic nerve 355.0
- seminal vesicle 608.89
- shoulder (joint) 726.0
- sigmoid flexure (*see also* Adhesions, peritoneum) 568.0
- spermatic cord (acquired) 608.89
  - congenital 752.89
- spinal canal 349.2
  - nerve 355.9
    - root 724.9
      - cervical NEC 723.4
      - lumbar NEC 724.4
      - lumbosacral 724.4
      - thoracic 724.4
- stomach (*see also* Adhesions, peritoneum) 568.0
- subscapular 726.2
- tendonitis 726.90
  - shoulder 726.0
- testicle 608.89
- tongue (congenital) (to gum or roof of mouth) 750.12
  - acquired 529.8
- trachea 519.19
- tubo-ovarian 614.6
- tunica vaginalis 608.89
- ureter 593.89
- uterus 621.5
  - to abdominal wall 614.6
    - in pregnancy or childbirth 654.4
      - affecting fetus or newborn 763.89
- vagina (chronic) (postoperative) (postradiation) 623.2
- vaginitis (congenital) 752.49
- vesical 596.8
- vitreous 379.29

Adie (-Holmes) syndrome (tonic pupillary reaction) 379.46
Adiponecrosis neonatorum 778.1
Adiposa dolorosa 272.8
Adiposalgia 272.8
Adiposis 278.0
- cerebralis 253.8
- dolorosa 272.8
- tuberosa simplex 272.8

Adiposity 278.02
- heart (*see also* Degeneration, myocardial) 429.1
- localized 278.1

Adiposogenital dystrophy 253.8
Adjustment
- prosthesis or other device—*see* Fitting of
- reaction—*see* Reaction, adjustment

Administration, prophylactic
- antibiotics V07.39
- antitoxin, any V07.2
- antivenin V07.2
- chemotherapeutic agent NEC V07.39
- chemotherapy NEC V07.39
- diphtheria antitoxin V07.2
- fluoride V07.31
- gamma globulin V07.2

Administration, prophylactic — continued
- immune sera (gamma globulin) V07.2
- passive immunization agent V07.2
- RhoGAM V07.2

Admission (encounter)
- as organ donor—*see* Donor
- by mistake V68.9
- for
  - adequacy testing (for)
    - hemodialysis V56.31
    - peritoneal dialysis V56.32
  - adjustment (of)
    - artificial
      - arm (complete) (partial) V52.0
      - eye V52.2
      - leg (complete) (partial) V52.1
    - brain neuropacemaker V53.02
    - breast
      - implant V52.4
      - prosthesis V52.4
    - cardiac device V53.39
      - defibrillator, automatic implantable V53.32
      - pacemaker V53.31
        - carotid sinus V53.39
    - catheter
      - non-vascular V58.82
      - vascular V58.81
    - cerebral ventricle (communicating) shunt V53.01
    - colostomy belt V53.5
    - contact lenses V53.1
    - cystostomy device V53.6
    - dental prosthesis V52.3
    - device, unspecified type V53.90
      - abdominal V53.5
      - cardiac V53.39
        - defibrillator, automatic implantable V53.32
        - pacemaker V53.31
          - carotid sinus V53.39
      - cerebral ventricle (communicating) shunt V53.01
      - insulin pump V53.91
      - intrauterine contraceptive V25.1
      - nervous system V53.09
      - orthodontic V53.4
      - other device V53.99
      - prosthetic V52.9
        - breast V52.4
        - dental V52.3
        - eye V52.2
        - specified type NEC V52.8
      - special senses V53.09
      - substitution
        - auditory V53.09
        - nervous system V53.09
        - visual V53.09
      - urinary V53.6
    - dialysis catheter
      - extracorporeal V56.1
      - peritoneal V56.2
    - diaphragm (contraceptive) V25.02
    - growth rod V54.02
    - hearing aid V53.2
    - ileostomy device V53.5
    - intestinal appliance or device NEC V53.5
    - intrauterine contraceptive device V25.1
    - neuropacemaker (brain) (peripheral nerve) (spinal cord) V53.02
    - orthodontic device V53.4

INDEX TO DISEASES

Admission

Admission—*continued*
  for —*continued*
    orthopedic (device) V53.7
      brace V53.7
      cast V53.7
      shoes V53.7
    pacemaker
      brain V53.02
      cardiac V53.31
      carotid sinus V53.39
      peripheral nerve V53.02
      spinal cord V53.02
    prosthesis V52.9
      arm (complete) (partial) V52.0
      breast V52.4
      dental V52.3
      eye V52.2
      leg (complete) (partial) V52.1
      specified type NEC V52.8
    spectacles V53.1
    wheelchair V53.8
  adoption referral or proceedings V68.89
  aftercare (*see also* Aftercare) V58.9
    cardiac pacemaker V53.31
    chemotherapy V58.11
    dialysis
      extracorporeal (renal) V56.0
      peritoneal V56.8
      renal V56.0
    fracture (*see also* Aftercare, fracture) V54.9
    medical NEC V58.89
    organ transplant V58.44
    orthopedic V54.9
      specified type NEC V54.89
    pacemaker device
      brain V53.02
      cardiac V53.31
      carotid sinus V53.39
      nervous system V53.02
      spinal cord V53.02
    postoperative NEC V58.49
      wound closure, planned V58.41
    postpartum
      immediately after delivery V24.0
      routine follow-up V24.2
    postradiation V58.0
    radiation therapy V58.0
    removal of
      non-vascular catheter V58.82
      vascular catheter V58.81
    specified NEC V58.89
      removal of vascular catheter V58.81
    surgical NEC V58.49
      wound closure, planned V58.41
  antineoplastic
    chemotherapy V58.11
    immunotherapy V58.12
  assisted reproductive fertility procedure cycle V26.81
  artificial insemination V26.1
  attention to artificial opening (of) V55.9
    artificial vagina V55.7
    colostomy V55.3
    cystostomy V55.5
    enterostomy V55.4
    gastrostomy V55.1
    ileostomy V55.2
    jejunostomy V55.4
    nephrostomy V55.6
    specified site NEC V55.8
      intestinal tract V55.4

Admission—*continued*
  for —*continued*
      urinary tract V55.6
    tracheostomy V55.0
    ureterostomy V55.6
    urethrostomy V55.6
  battery replacement
    cardiac pacemaker V53.31
  blood typing V72.86
    Rh typing V72.86
  boarding V65.0
  breast
    augmentation or reduction V50.1
    removal, prophylactic V50.41
  change of
    cardiac pacemaker (battery) V53.31
    carotid sinus pacemaker V53.39
    catheter in artificial opening—*see* Attention to, artificial, opening
    drains V58.49
    dressing
      wound V58.30
        nonsurgical V58.30
        surgical V58.31
    fixation device
      external V54.89
      internal V54.01
    Kirschner wire V54.89
    neuropacemaker device (brain) (peripheral nerve) (spinal cord) V53.02
    nonsurgical wound dressing V58.30
    pacemaker device
      brain V53.02
      cardiac V53.31
      carotid sinus V53.39
      nervous system V53.02
    plaster cast V54.89
    splint, external V54.89
    Steinmann pin V54.89
    surgical wound dressing V58.31
    traction device V54.89
    wound packing V58.30
      nonsurgical V58.30
      surgical V58.31
  checkup only V70.0
  chemotherapy, antineoplastic V58.11
  circumcision, ritual or routine (in absence of medical indication) V50.2
  clinical research investigation (control) (normal comparison) (participant) V70.7
  closure of artificial opening—*see* Attention to, artificial, opening
  contraceptive
    counseling V25.09
      emergency V25.03
      postcoital V25.03
    management V25.9
      specified type NEC V25.8
  convalescence following V66.9
    chemotherapy V66.2
    psychotherapy V66.3
    radiotherapy V66.1
    surgery V66.0
    treatment (for) V66.5
      combined V66.6
      fracture V66.4
      mental disorder NEC V66.3
      specified condition NEC V66.5
  cosmetic surgery NEC V50.1
    following healed injury or operation V51

Admission

Admission—*continued*
for —*continued*
counseling (*see also* Counseling) V65.40
without complaint or sickness V65.49
contraceptive management V25.09
emergency V25.03
postcoital V25.03
dietary V65.3
exercise V65.41
for
nonattending third party V65.19
pediatric pre-birth visit for expectant mother V65.11
victim of abuse
child V61.21
partner or spouse V61.11
genetic V26.33
gonorrhea V65.45
HIV V65.44
human immunodeficiency virus V65.44
injury prevention V65.43
insulin pump training V65.46
natural family planning
procreative V26.41
to avoid pregnancy V25.04
procreative management V26.49
using natural family planning V26.41
sexually transmitted disease NEC V65.45
HIV V65.44
specified reason NEC V65.49
substance use and abuse V65.42
syphilis V65.45
victim of abuse
child V61.21
partner or spouse V61.11
desensitization to allergens V07.1
dialysis V56.0
catheter
fitting and adjustment
extracorporeal V56.1
peritoneal V56.2
removal or replacement
extracorporeal V56.1
peritoneal V56.2
extracorporeal (renal) V56.0
peritoneal V56.8
renal V56.0
dietary surveillance and counseling V65.3
drug monitoring, therapeutic V58.83
ear piercing V50.3
elective surgery V50.9
breast
augmentation or reduction V50.1
removal, prophylactic V50.41
circumcision, ritual or routine (in absence of medical indication) V50.2
cosmetic NEC V50.1
following healed injury or operation V51
ear piercing V50.3
face-lift V50.1
hair transplant V50.0
plastic
cosmetic NEC V50.1
following healed injury or operation V51
prophylactic organ removal V50.49
breast V50.41
ovary V50.42
repair of scarred tissue (following healed injury or operation) V51
specified type NEC V50.8
end-of-life care V66.7

INDEX TO DISEASES

Admission—*continued*
for —*continued*
examination (*see also* Examination) V70.9
administrative purpose NEC V70.3
adoption V70.3
allergy V72.7
at health care facility V70.0
athletic team V70.3
camp V70.3
cardiovascular, preoperative V72.81
clinical research investigation (control) (participant) V70.7
dental V72.2
developmental testing (child) (infant) V20.2
donor (potential) V70.8
driver's license V70.3
ear V72.19
employment V70.5
eye V72.0
follow-up (routine)—*see* Examination, follow-up
for admission to
old age home V70.3
school V70.3
general V70.9
specified reason NEC V70.8
gynecological V72.31
health supervision (child) (infant) V20.2
hearing V72.19
following failed hearing screening V72.11
immigration V70.3
infant, routine V20.2
insurance certification V70.3
laboratory V72.6
marriage license V70.3
medical (general) (*see also* Examination, medical) V70.9
medicolegal reasons V70.4
naturalization V70.3
pelvic (annual) (periodic) V72.31
postpartum checkup V24.2
pregnancy (possible) (unconfirmed) V72.40
negative result V72.41
positive result V72.42
preoperative V72.84
cardiovascular V72.81
respiratory V72.82
specified NEC V72.83
preprocedural V72.84
cardiovascular V72.81
general physical V72.83
respiratory V72.82
specified NEC V72.83
prison V70.3
psychiatric (general) V70.2
requested by authority V70.1
radiological NEC V72.5
respiratory, preoperative V72.82
school V70.3
screening—*see* Screening
skin hypersensitivity V72.7
specified type NEC V72.85
sport competition V70.3
vision V72.0
well baby and child care V20.2
exercise therapy V57.1
face-lift, cosmetic reason V50.1
fitting (of)
artificial
arm (complete) (partial) V52.0
eye V52.2

788

INDEX TO DISEASES

Admission

Admission—*continued*
  for —*continued*
    leg (complete) (partial) V52.1
    biliary drainage tube V58.82
    brain neuropacemaker V53.02
    breast V52.4
      implant V50.1
      prosthesis V52.4
    cardiac pacemaker V53.31
    catheter
      non-vascular V58.82
      vascular V58.81
    cerebral ventricle (communicating) shunt V53.01
    chest tube V58.82
    colostomy belt V53.5
    contact lenses V53.1
    cystostomy device V53.6
    dental prosthesis V52.3
    device, unspecified type V53.90
      abdominal V53.5
      cerebral ventricle (communicating) shunt V53.01
      insulin pump V53.91
      intrauterine contraceptive V25.1
      nervous system V53.09
      orthodontic V53.4
      other device V53.99
      prosthetic V52.9
        breast V52.4
        dental V52.3
        eye V52.2
      special senses V53.09
      substitution
        auditory V53.09
        nervous system V53.09
        visual V53.09
    diaphragm (contraceptive) V25.02
    fistula (sinus tract) drainage tube V58.82
    growth rod V54.02
    hearing aid V53.2
    ileostomy device V53.5
    intestinal appliance or device NEC V53.5
    intrauterine contraceptive device V25.1
    neuropacemaker (brain) (peripheral nerve) (spinal cord) V53.02
    orthodontic device V53.4
    orthopedic (device) V53.7
      brace V53.7
      cast V53.7
      shoes V53.7
    pacemaker
      brain V53.02
      cardiac V53.31
      carotid sinus V53.39
      spinal cord V53.02
    pleural drainage tube V58.82
    prosthesis V52.9
      arm (complete) (partial) V52.0
      breast V52.4
      dental V52.3
      eye V52.2
      leg (complete) (partial) V52.1
      specified type NEC V52.8
    spectacles V53.1
    wheelchair V53.8
    follow-up examination (routine) (following) V67.9
      cancer chemotherapy V67.2
      chemotherapy V67.2
      high-risk medication NEC V67.51

Admission—*continued*
  for —*continued*
      injury NEC V67.59
      psychiatric V67.3
      psychotherapy V67.3
      radiotherapy V67.1
      specified surgery NEC V67.09
        surgery V67.00
      treatment (for) V67.9
        combined V67.6
        fracture V67.4
        involving high-risk medication NEC V67.51
        mental disorder V67.3
        specified NEC V67.59
      vaginal pap smear V67.01
    hair transplant, for cosmetic reason V50.0
    health advice, education, or instruction V65.4
    hearing conservation and treatment V72.12
    hormone replacement therapy (postmenopausal) V07.4
    hospice care V66.7
    immunotherapy, antineoplastic V58.12
    in vitro fertilization cycle V26.81
    insertion (of)
      subdermal implantable contraceptive V25.5
    insulin pump titration V53.91
    insulin pump training V65.46
    intrauterine device
      insertion V25.1
      management V25.42
    investigation to determine further disposition V63.8
    isolation V07.0
    issue of
      disability examination certificate V68.01
      medical certificate NEC V68.09
      repeat prescription NEC V68.1
        contraceptive device NEC V25.49
    kidney dialysis V56.0
    lengthening of growth rod V54.02
    mental health evaluation V70.2
      requested by authority V70.1
    natural family planning counseling and advice
      procreative V26.41
      to avoid pregnancy V25.04
    nonmedical reason NEC V68.89
    nursing care evaluation V63.8
    observation (without need for further medical care) (*see also* Observation) V71.9
      accident V71.4
      alleged rape or seduction V71.5
      criminal assault V71.6
      following accident V71.4
        at work V71.3
      foreign body ingestion V71.89
      growth and development variations, childhood V21.0
      inflicted injury NEC V71.6
      ingestion of deleterious agent or foreign body V71.89
      injury V71.6
      malignant neoplasm V71.1
      mental disorder V71.09
      newborn—*see* Observation, suspected condition, newborn
      rape V71.5
      specified NEC V71.89

Admission—*continued*
  for —*continued*
    suspected disorder V71.9
      abuse V71.81
      accident V71.4
        at work V71.3
      benign neoplasm V71.89
      cardiovascular V71.7
      exposure
        anthrax V71.82
        biological agent NEC V71.83
        SARS V71.83
      heart V71.7
      inflicted injury NEC V71.6
      malignant neoplasm V71.1
      mental NEC V71.09
      neglect V71.81
      specified condition NEC V71.89
      tuberculosis V71.2
    tuberculosis V71.2
    occupational therapy V57.21
    organ transplant, donor—*see* Donor
    ovary, ovarian removal, prophylactic V50.42
    palliative care V66.7
    Papanicolaou smear
      cervix V76.2
        for suspected malignant neoplasm V76.2
        no disease found V71.1
        routine, as part of gynecological examination V72.31
        to confirm findings of recent normal smear following initial abnormal smear V72.32
      vaginal V76.47
        following hysterectomy for malignant condition V67.01
    passage of sounds or bougie in artificial opening—*see* Attention to, artificial, opening
    paternity testing V70.4
    peritoneal dialysis V56.8
    physical therapy NEC V57.1
    plastic surgery
      cosmetic NEC V50.1
      following healed injury or operation V51
    postmenopausal hormone replacement therapy V07.4
    postpartum observation
      immediately after delivery V24.0
      routine follow-up V24.2
    poststerilization (for restoration) V26.0
    procreative management V26.9
      assisted reproductive fertility procedure cycle V26.81
      in vitro fertilization cycle V26.81
      specified type NEC V26.89
    prophylactic
      administration of
        antibiotics V07.39
        antitoxin, any V07.2
        antivenin V07.2
        chemotherapeutic agent NEC V07.39
        chemotherapy NEC V07.39
        diphtheria antitoxin V07.2
        fluoride V07.31
        gamma globulin V07.2
        immune sera (gamma globulin) V07.2
        RhoGAM V07.2
        tetanus antitoxin V07.2
      breathing exercises V57.0
      chemotherapy NEC V07.39
        fluoride V07.31

Admission—*continued*
  for —*continued*
    measure V07.9
      specified type NEC V07.8
    organ removal V50.49
      breast V50.41
      ovary V50.42
    psychiatric examination (general) V70.2
      requested by authority V70.1
    radiation management V58.0
    radiotherapy V58.0
    reforming of artificial opening—*see* Attention to, artificial, opening
    rehabilitation V57.9
      multiple types V57.89
      occupational V57.21
      orthoptic V57.4
      orthotic V57.81
      physical NEC V57.1
      specified type NEC V57.89
      speech V57.3
      vocational V57.22
    removal of
      cardiac pacemaker V53.31
      cast (plaster) V54.89
      catheter from artificial opening—*see* Attention to, artificial, opening
      cerebral ventricle (communicating) shunt V53.01
      cystostomy catheter V55.5
      device
        cerebral ventricle (communicating) shunt V53.01
        fixation
          external V54.89
          internal V54.01
        intrauterine contraceptive V25.42
        traction, external V54.89
      drains V58.49
      dressing
        wound V58.30
          nonsurgical V58.30
          surgical V58.31
      fixation device
        external V54.89
        internal V54.01
      intrauterine contraceptive device V25.42
      Kirschner wire V54.89
      neuropacemaker (brain) (peripheral nerve) (spinal cord) V53.02
      nonsurgical wound dressing V58.30
      orthopedic fixation device
        external V54.89
        internal V54.01
      pacemaker device
        brain V53.02
        cardiac V53.31
        carotid sinus V53.39
        nervous system V53.02
      plaster cast V54.89
      plate (fracture) V54.01
      rod V54.01
      screw (fracture) V54.01
      splint, traction V54.89
      staples V58.32
      Steinmann pin V54.89
      subdermal implantable contraceptive V25.43
      surgical wound dressing V58.31
      sutures V58.32
      traction device, external V54.89
      ureteral stent V53.6

INDEX TO DISEASES   **Admission**

Admission—*continued*
  for —*continued*
    wound packing V58.30
      nonsurgical V58.30
      surgical V58.31
    repair of scarred tissue (following healed injury or operation) V51
    reprogramming of cardiac pacemaker V53.31
    respirator (ventilator) dependence
      during
        mechanical failure V46.14
        power failure V46.12
      for weaning V46.13
    restoration of organ continuity (poststerilization) (tuboplasty) (vasoplasty) V26.0
    Rh typing V72.86
    sensitivity test—*see also* Test, skin
      allergy NEC V72.7
      bacterial disease NEC V74.9
      Dick V74.8
      Kveim V82.89
      Mantoux V74.1
      mycotic infection NEC V75.4
      parasitic disease NEC V75.8
      Schick V74.3
      Schultz-Charlton V74.8
    social service (agency) referral or evaluation V63.8
    speech therapy V57.3
    sterilization V25.2
    suspected disorder (ruled out) (without need for further care)—*see* Observation
    terminal care V66.7
    tests only—*see* Test
    therapeutic drug monitoring V58.83
    therapy
      blood transfusion, without reported diagnosis V58.2
      breathing exercises V57.0
      chemotherapy, antineoplastic V58.11
        prophylactic NEC V07.39
          fluoride V07.31
      dialysis (intermittent) (treatment)
        extracorporeal V56.0
        peritoneal V56.8
        renal V56.0
        specified type NEC V56.8
      exercise (remedial) NEC V57.1
        breathing V57.0
      immunotherapy, antineoplastic V58.12
      long-term (current) drug use NEC V58.69
        antibiotics V58.62
        anticoagulants V58.61
        anti-inflammatories, non-steroidal (NSAID) V58.64
        antiplatelets V58.63
        antithrombotics V58.63
        aspirin V58.66
        high-risk medications NEC V58.69
        insulin V58.67
        steroids V58.65
      occupational V57.21
      orthoptic V57.4
      physical NEC V57.1
      radiation V58.0
      speech V57.3
      vocational V57.22

Admission—*continued*
  for —*continued*
    toilet or cleaning
      of artificial opening — *see* Attention to, artificial, opening
      of non-vascular catheter V58.82
      of vascular catheter V58.81
    tubal ligation V25.2
    tuboplasty for previous sterilization V26.0
    vaccination, prophylactic (against)
      arthropod-borne virus, viral NEC V05.1
        disease NEC V05.1
        encephalitis V05.0
      Bacille Calmette Guérin (BCG) V03.2
      BCG V03.2
      chickenpox V05.4
      cholera alone V03.0
        with typhoid-paratyphoid (cholera + TAB) V06.0
      common cold V04.7
      dengue V05.1
      diphtheria alone V03.5
      diphtheria-tetanus-pertussis (DTP) (DTaP) V06.1
        with
          poliomyelitis (DTP + polio) V06.3
          typhoid-paratyphoid (DTP + TAB) V06.2
      diphtheria-tetanus [Td] [DT] without pertussis V06.5
      disease (single) NEC V05.9
        bacterial NEC V03.9
          specified type NEC V03.89
        combinations NEC V06.9
          specified type NEC V06.8
        specified type NEC V05.8
        viral NEC V04.89
      encephalitis, viral, arthropod-borne V05.0
      Hemophilus influenzae, type B [Hib] V03.81
      hepatitis, viral V05.3
      human papillomavirus (HPV) V04.89
      immune sera (gamma globulin) V07.2
      influenza V04.81
        with
          Streptococcus pneumoniae [pneumococcus] V06.6
      Leishmaniasis V05.2
      measles alone V04.2
      measles-mumps-rubella (MMR) V06.4
      mumps alone V04.6
        with measles and rubella (MMR) V06.4
      not done because of contraindication V64.09
      pertussis alone V03.6
      plague V03.3
      pneumonia V03.82
      poliomyelitis V04.0
        with diphtheria-tetanus-pertussis (DTP + polio) V06.3
      rabies V04.5
      respiratory syncytial virus (RSV) V04.82
      rubella alone V04.3
        with measles and mumps (MMR) V06.4
      smallpox V04.1
      specified type NEC V05.8
        Streptococcus pneumoniae [pneumococcus] V03.82
        with
          influenza V06.6

Admission—continued
for —continued
- tetanus toxoid alone V03.7
  - with diphtheria [Td] [DT] V06.5
    - and pertussis (DTP) (DTaP) V06.1
- tuberculosis (BCG) V03.2
- tularemia V03.4
- typhoid alone V03.1
  - with diphtheria-tetanus-pertussis (TAB + DTP) V06.2
- typhoid-paratyphoid alone (TAB) V03.1
- typhus V05.8
- varicella V05.4
- viral encephalitis, arthropod-borne V05.0
- viral hepatitis V05.3
- yellow fever V04.4
- vasectomy V25.2
- vasoplasty for previous sterilization V26.0
- vision examination V72.0
- vocational therapy V57.22
- waiting period for admission to other facility V63.2
  - undergoing social agency investigation V63.8
- well baby and child care V20.2
- x-ray of chest
  - for suspected tuberculosis V71.2
  - routine V72.5

Adnexitis (suppurative) (*see also* Salpingo-oophoritis) 614.2
Adolescence NEC V21.2
Adoption
- agency referral V68.89
- examination V70.3
- held for V68.89

Adrenal gland —*see* condition
Adrenalism 255.9
- tuberculous (*see also* Tuberculosis) 017.6

Adrenalitis, adrenitis 255.8
- meningococcal hemorrhagic 036.3

Adrenarche, precocious 259.1
Adrenocortical syndrome 255.2
Adrenogenital syndrome (acquired) (congenital) 255.2
- iatrogenic, fetus or newborn 760.79

Adrenoleukodystrophy 277.86
- neonatal 277.86
- x-linked 277.86

Adrenomyeloneuropathy 277.86
Adventitious bursa —*see* Bursitis
Adynamia (episodica) (hereditary) (periodic) 359.3
Adynamic
- ileus or intestine (*see also* ileus) 560.1
- ureter 753.22

Aeration lung imperfect, newborn 770.5
Aerobullosis 993.3
Aerocele —*see* Embolism, air
Aerodermectasia
- subcutaneous (traumatic) 958.7
  - surgical 998.81
- surgical 998.81

Aerodontalgia 993.2
Aeroembolism 993.3
Aerogenes capsulatus infection (*see also* Gangrene, gas) 040.0
Aero-otitis media 993.0
Aerophagy, aerophagia 306.4
- psychogenic 306.4

Aerosinusitis 993.1
Aerotitis 993.0

Affection, affections —*see also* Disease
- sacroiliac (joint), old 724.6
- shoulder region NEC 726.2

Afibrinogenemia 286.3
- acquired 286.6
- congenital 286.3
- postpartum 666.3

African
- sleeping sickness 086.5
- tick fever 087.1
- trypanosomiasis 086.5
  - Gambian 086.3
  - Rhodesian 086.4

Aftercare V58.9
- amputation stump V54.89
- artificial openings—*see* Attention to, artificial, opening
- blood transfusion without reported diagnosis V58.2
- breathing exercise V57.0
- cardiac device V53.39
  - defibrillator, automatic implantable V53.32
  - pacemaker V53.31
    - carotid sinus V53.39
- carotid sinus pacemaker V53.39
- cerebral ventricle (communicating) shunt V53.01
- chemotherapy session (adjunctive) (maintenance) V58.11
- defibrillator, automatic implantable cardiac V53.32
- exercise (remedial) (therapeutic) V57.1
  - breathing V57.0
- extracorporeal dialysis (intermittent) (treatment) V56.0
- following surgery NEC V58.49
  - wound closure, planned V58.41
  - for
    - injury V58.43
    - neoplasm V58.42
    - organ transplant V58.44
    - trauma V58.43
  - joint replacement V54.81
  - of
    - circulatory system V58.73
    - digestive system V58.75
    - genital organs V58.76
    - genitourinary system V58.76
    - musculoskeletal system V58.78
    - nervous system V58.72
    - oral cavity V58.75
    - respiratory system V58.74
    - sense organs V58.71
    - skin V58.77
    - subcutaneous tissue V58.77
    - teeth V58.75
    - urinary system V58.76
  - spinal —*see* Aftercare, following surgery, of, specified body system
- fracture V54.9
  - healing V54.89
    - pathologic
      - ankle V54.29
      - arm V54.20
        - lower V54.22
        - upper V54.21
      - finger V54.29
      - foot V54.29
      - hand V54.29
      - hip V54.23
      - leg V54.24
        - lower V54.26

Aftercare—*continued*
    upper V54.25
    pelvis V54.29
    specified site NEC V54.29
    toe(s) V54.29
    vertebrae V54.27
    wrist V54.29
  traumatic
    ankle V54.19
    arm V54.10
      lower V54.12
      upper V54.11
    finger V54.19
    foot V54.19
    hand V54.19
    hip V54.13
    leg V54.14
      lower V54.16
      upper V54.15
    pelvis V54.19
    specified site NEC V54.19
    toe(s) V54.19
    vertebrae V54.17
    wrist V54.19
  removal of
    external fixation device V54.89
    internal fixation device V54.01
  specified care NEC V54.89
  gait training V57.1
    for use of artificial limb(s) V57.81
  internal fixation device V54.09
  involving
    dialysis (intermittent) (treatment)
      extracorporeal V56.0
      peritoneal V56.8
      renal V56.0
    gait training V57.1
      for use of artificial limb(s) V57.81
    growth rod
      adjustment V54.02
      lengthening V54.02
    internal fixation device V54.09
    orthoptic training V57.4
    orthotic training V57.81
    radiotherapy session V58.0
    removal of
      drains V58.49
      dressings
        wound V58.30
          nonsurgical V58.30
          surgical V58.31
      fixation device
        external V54.89
        internal V54.01
      fracture plate V54.01
      nonsurgical wound dressing V58.30
      pins V54.01
      plaster cast V54.89
      rods V54.01
      screws V54.01
      staples V58.32
      surgical wound dressings V58.31
      sutures V58.32
      traction device, external V54.89
      wound packing V58.30
        nonsurgical V58.30
        surgical V58.31
    neuropacemaker (brain) (peripheral nerve)
      (spinal cord) V53.02
    occupational therapy V57.21
    orthodontic V58.5

Aftercare—*continued*
  orthopedic V54.9
    change of external fixation or traction device
      V54.8
    following joint replacement V54.81
    internal fixation device V54.09
    removal of fixation device
      external V54.89
      internal V54.01
    specified care NEC V54.89
  orthoptic training V57.4
  orthotic training V57.81
  pacemaker
    brain V53.02
    cardiac V53.31
    carotid sinus V53.39
    peripheral nerve V53.02
    spinal cord V53.02
  peritoneal dialysis (intermittent) (treatment)
    V56.8
  physical therapy NEC V57.1
    breathing exercises V57.0
  radiotherapy session V58.0
  rehabilitation procedure V57.9
    breathing exercises V57.0
    multiple types V57.89
    occupational V57.21
    orthoptic V57.4
    orthotic V57.81
    physical therapy NEC V57.1
    remedial exercises V57.1
    specified type NEC V57.89
    speech V57.3
    therapeutic exercises V57.1
    vocational V57.22
  renal dialysis (intermittent) (treatment) V56.0
  specified type NEC V58.89
    removal of non-vascular catheter V58.82
    removal of vascular catheter V58.81
  speech therapy V57.3
  stump, amputation V54.89
  vocational rehabilitation V57.22
After-cataract 366.50
  obscuring vision 366.53
  specified type, not obscuring vision 366.52
Agalactia 676.4
Agammaglobulinemia 279.00
  with lymphopenia 279.2
  acquired (primary) (secondary) 279.06
  Bruton's X-linked 279.04
  infantile sex-linked (Bruton's) (congenital)
    279.04
  Swiss-type 279.2
Aganglionosis (bowel) (colon) 751.3
Age (old) (*see also* Senile) 797
Agenesis—*see also* Absence, by site, congenital
  acoustic nerve 742.8
  adrenal (gland) 759.1
  alimentary tract (complete) (partial) NEC 751.8
    lower 751.2
    upper 750.8
  anus, anal (canal) 751.2
  aorta 747.22
  appendix 751.2
  arm (complete) (partial) (*see also* Deformity,
    reduction, upper limb) 755.20
  artery (peripheral) NEC (*see also* Anomaly,
    peripheral vascular system) 747.60
    brain 747.81
    coronary 746.85
    pulmonary 747.3
    umbilical 747.5

Agenesis—*continued*
auditory (canal) (external) 744.01
auricle (ear) 744.01
bile, biliary duct or passage 751.61
bone NEC 756.9
brain 740.0
    specified part 742.2
breast 757.6
bronchus 748.3
canaliculus lacrimalis 743.65
carpus NEC (*see also* Deformity, reduction, upper limb) 755.28
cartilage 756.9
cecum 751.2
cerebellum 742.2
cervix 752.49
chin 744.89
cilia 743.63
circulatory system, part NEC 747.89
clavicle 755.51
clitoris 752.49
coccyx 756.13
colon 751.2
corpus callosum 742.2
cricoid cartilage 748.3
diaphragm (with hernia) 756.6
digestive organ(s) or tract (complete) (partial) NEC 751.8
    lower 751.2
    upper 750.8
ductus arteriosus 747.89
duodenum 751.1
ear NEC 744.09
    auricle 744.01
    lobe 744.21
ejaculatory duct 752.89
endocrine (gland) NEC 759.2
epiglottis 748.3
esophagus 750.3
Eustachian tube 744.24
extrinsic muscle, eye 743.69
eye 743.00
    adnexa 743.69
eyelid (fold) 743.62
face
    bones NEC 756.0
    specified part NEC 744.89
fallopian tube 752.19
femur NEC (*see also* Absence, femur, congenital) 755.34
fibula NEC (*see also* Absence, fibula, congenital) 755.37
finger NEC (*see also* Absence, finger, congenital) 755.29
foot (complete) (*see also* Deformity, reduction, lower limb) 755.31
gallbladder 751.69
gastric 750.8
genitalia, genital (organ)
    female 752.89
        external 752.49
        internal NEC 752.89
    male 752.89
        penis 752.69
glottis 748.3
gonadal 758.6
hair 757.4
hand (complete) (*see also* Deformity, reduction, upper limb) 755.21
heart 746.89
    valve NEC 746.89
        aortic 746.89

Agenesis—*continued*
    mitral 746.89
    pulmonary 746.01
hepatic 751.69
humerus NEC (*see also* Absence, humerus, congenital) 755.24
hymen 752.49
ileum 751.1
incus 744.04
intestine (small) 751.1
    large 751.2
iris (dilator fibers) 743.45
jaw 524.09
jejunum 751.1
kidney(s) (partial) (unilateral) 753.0
labium (majus) (minus) 752.49
labyrinth, membranous 744.05
lacrimal apparatus (congenital) 743.65
larynx 748.3
leg NEC (*see also* Deformity, reduction, lower limb) 755.30
lens 743.35
limb (complete) (partial) (*see also* Deformity, reduction) 755.4
    lower NEC 755.30
    upper 755.20
lip 750.26
liver 751.69
lung (bilateral) (fissures) (lobe) (unilateral) 748.5
mandible 524.09
maxilla 524.09
metacarpus NEC 755.28
metatarsus NEC 755.38
muscle (any) 756.81
musculoskeletal system NEC 756.9
nail(s) 757.5
neck, part 744.89
nerve 742.8
nervous system, part NEC 742.8
nipple 757.6
nose 748.1
nuclear 742.8
organ
    of Corti 744.05
    or site not listed—*see* Anomaly, specified type NEC
osseous meatus (ear) 744.03
ovary 752.0
oviduct 752.19
pancreas 751.7
parathyroid (gland) 759.2
patella 755.64
pelvic girdle (complete) (partial) 755.69
penis 752.69
pericardium 746.89
perineal body 756.81
pituitary (gland) 759.2
prostate 752.89
pulmonary
    artery 747.3
    trunk 747.3
    vein 747.49
punctum lacrimale 743.65
radioulnar NEC (*see also* Absence, forearm, congenital) 755.25
radius NEC (*see also* Absence, radius, congenital) 755.26
rectum 751.2
renal 753.0
respiratory organ NEC 748.9
rib 756.3

Agenesis—continued
  roof of orbit 742.0
  round ligament 752.89
  sacrum 756.13
  salivary gland 750.21
  scapula 755.59
  scrotum 752.89
  seminal duct or tract 752.89
  septum
    atrial 745.69
    between aorta and pulmonary artery 745.0
    ventricular 745.3
  shoulder girdle (complete) (partial) 755.59
  skull (bone) 756.0
    with
      anencephalus 740.0
      encephalocele 742.0
      hydrocephalus 742.3
        with spina bifida (*see also* Spina bifida) 741.0
      microcephalus 742.1
  spermatic cord 752.89
  spinal cord 742.59
  spine 756.13
    lumbar 756.13
      isthmus 756.11
      pars articularis 756.11
  spleen 759.0
  sternum 756.3
  stomach 750.7
  tarsus NEC 755.38
  tendon 756.81
  testicular 752.89
  testis 752.89
  thymus (gland) 759.2
  thyroid (gland) 243
    cartilage 748.3
  tibia NEC (*see also* Absence, tibia, congenital) 755.36
  tibiofibular NEC 755.35
  toe (complete) (partial) (*see also* Absence, toe, congenital) 755.39
  tongue 750.11
  trachea (cartilage) 748.3
  ulna NEC (*see also* Absence, ulna, congenital) 755.27
  ureter 753.4
  urethra 753.8
  urinary tract NEC 753.8
  uterus 752.3
  uvula 750.26
  vagina 752.49
  vas deferens 752.89
  vein(s) (peripheral) NEC (*see also* Anomaly, peripheral vascular system) 747.60
    brain 747.81
    great 747.49
    portal 747.49
    pulmonary 747.49
  vena cava (inferior) (superior) 747.49
  vermis of cerebellum 742.2
  vertebra 756.13
    lumbar 756.13
      isthmus 756.11
      pars articularis 756.11
  vulva 752.49
Ageusia (*see also* Disturbance, sensation) 781.1
Aggressiveness 301.3
Aggressive outburst (*see also* Disturbance, conduct) 312.0
  in children or adolescents 313.9
Aging skin 701.8

Agitated —*see* condition
Agitation 307.9
  catatonic (*see also* Schizophrenia) 295.2
Aglossia (congenital) 750.11
Aglycogenosis 271.0
Agnail (finger) (with lymphangitis) 681.02
Agnosia (body image) (tactile) 784.69
  verbal 784.69
    auditory 784.69
      secondary to organic lesion 784.69
    developmental 315.8
    secondary to organic lesion 784.69
  visual 784.69
    developmental 315.8
    secondary to organic lesion 784.69
  visual 368.16
    developmental 315.31
Agoraphobia 300.22
  with panic disorder 300.21
Agrammatism 784.69
Agranulocytopenia (see also Agranulocytosis) 288.09
Agranulocytosis (angina) 288.09
  chronic 288.09
  cyclical 288.02
  genetic 288.01
  infantile 288.01
  periodic 288.02
  pernicious 288.09
Agraphia (absolute) 784.69
  with alexia 784.61
  developmental 315.39
Agrypnia (*see also* Insomnia) 780.52
Ague (*see also* Malaria) 084.6
  brass-founders' 985.8
  dumb 084.6
  tertian 084.1
Agyria 742.2
Ahumada-del Castillo syndrome (nonpuerperal galactorrhea and amenorrhea) 253.1
AIDS 042
AIDS-associated retrovirus (disease) (illness) 042
  infection—*see* Human immunodeficiency virus, infection
AIDS-associated virus (disease) (illness) 042
  infection—*see* Human immunodeficiency virus, infection
AIDS-like disease (illness) (syndrome) 042
AIDS-related complex 042
AIDS-related conditions 042
AIDS-related virus (disease) (illness) 042
  infection—*see* Human immunodeficiency virus, infection
AIDS virus (disease) (illness) 042
  infection—*see* Human immunodeficiency virus, infection
Ailment, heart —*see* Disease, heart
Ailurophobia 300.29
Ainhum (disease) 136.0
Air
  anterior mediastinum 518.1
  compressed, disease 993.3
  embolism (any site) (artery) (cerebral) 958.0
    with
      abortion—*see* Abortion, by type, with embolism
      ectopic pregnancy (*see also* categories 633.0-633.9) 639.6
      molar pregnancy (*see also* categories 630-632) 639.6

Air —*continued*
　due to implanted device—*see* Complications, due to (presence of) any device, implant, or graft classified to 996.0-996.5 NEC
　following
　　abortion 639.6
　　ectopic or molar pregnancy 639.6
　　infusion, perfusion, or transfusion 999.1
　　in pregnancy, childbirth, or puerperium 673.0
　　traumatic 958.0
　hunger 786.09
　　psychogenic 306.1
　leak (lung) (pulmonary) (thorax) 512.8
　　iatrogenic 512.1
　　postoperative 512.1
　rarefied, effects of—*see* Effect, adverse, high altitude
　sickness 994.6
Airplane sickness 994.6
Akathisia, acathisia 781.0
　due to drugs 333.99
　neuroleptic-induced acute 333.99
Akinesia algeria 352.6
Akiyami 100.89
Akureyri disease (epidemic neuromyasthenia) 049.8
Alacrima (congenital) 743.65
Alactasia (hereditary) 271.3
Alagille syndrome 759.89
Alalia 784.3
　developmental 315.31
　　receptive-expressive 315.32
　secondary to organic lesion 784.3
Alaninemia 270.8
Alastrim 050.1
Albarrán's disease (colibacilluria) 791.9
Albers-Schönberg's disease (marble bones) 756.52
Albert's disease 726.71
Albinism, albino (choroid) (cutaneous) (eye) (generalized) (isolated) (ocular) (oculocutaneous) (partial) 270.2
Albinismus 270.2
Albright (-Martin) (-Bantam) **disease** (pseudohypoparathyroidism) 275.49
Albright (-McCune) (-Sternberg) **syndrome** (osteitis fibrosa disseminata) 756.59
Albuminous —*see* condition
Albuminuria, albuminuric (acute) (chronic) (subacute) 791.0
　Bence-Jones 791.0
　cardiac 785.9
　complicating pregnancy, childbirth, or puerperium 646.2
　　with hypertension—*see* Toxemia, of pregnancy
　　affecting fetus or newborn 760.1
　cyclic 593.6
　gestational 646.2
　gravidarum 646.2
　　with hypertension—*see* Toxemia, of pregnancy
　　affecting fetus or newborn 760.1
　heart 785.9
　idiopathic 593.6
　orthostatic 593.6
　postural 593.6
　pre-eclamptic (mild) 642.4
　　affecting fetus or newborn 760.0
　　severe 642.5
　　　affecting fetus or newborn 760.0
　recurrent physiologic 593.6
　scarlatinal 034.1

Albumosuria 791.0
　Bence-Jones 791.0
　myelopathic (M9730/3) 203.0
Alcaptonuria 270.2
Alcohol, alcoholic
　abstinance 291.81
　acute intoxication 305.0
　　with dependence 303.0
　addiction (*see also* Alcoholism) 303.9
　　maternal
　　　with suspected fetal damage affecting management of pregnancy 655.4
　　　affecting fetus or newborn 760.71
　amnestic disorder, persisting 291.1
　anxiety 291.89
　brain syndrome, chronic 291.2
　cardiopathy 425.5
　chronic (*see also* Alcoholism) 303.9
　cirrhosis (liver) 571.2
　delirium 291.0
　　acute 291.0
　　chronic 291.1
　　tremens 291.0
　　withdrawal 291.0
　dementia NEC 291.2
　deterioration 291.2
　drunkenness (simple) 305.0
　hallucinosis (acute) 291.3
　induced
　　circadian rhythm sleep disorder 291.82
　　hypersomnia 291.82
　　insomnia 291.82
　　mental disorder 291.9
　　　anxiety 291.89
　　　mood 291.89
　　　sexual 291.89
　　　sleep 291.82
　　　specified type 291.89
　　parasomnia 291.82
　　persisting
　　　amnestic disorder 291.1
　　　dementia 291.2
　　psychotic disorder
　　　with
　　　　delusions 291.5
　　　　hallucinations 291.3
　　sleep disorder 291.82
　insanity 291.9
　intoxication (acute) 305.0
　　with dependence 303.0
　　pathological 291.4
　jealousy 291.5
　Korsakoff's, Korsakov's, Korsakow's 291.1
　liver NEC 571.3
　　acute 571.1
　　chronic 571.2
　mania (acute) (chronic) 291.9
　mood 291.89
　paranoia 291.5
　paranoid (type) psychosis 291.5
　pellagra 265.2
　poisoning, accidental (acute) NEC 980.9
　　specified type of alcohol—*see* Table of drugs and chemicals
　psychosis (*see also* Psychosis, alcoholic) 291.9
　　Korsakoff's, Korsakov's, Korsakow's 291.1
　　polyneuritic 291.1
　　　with
　　　　delusions 291.5
　　　　hallucinations 291.3
　related disorder 291.9

INDEX TO DISEASES

Allergy, allergic

Alcohol, alcoholic—*continued*
  withdrawal symptoms, syndrome NEC 291.81
    delirium 291.0
    hallucinosis 291.3
Alcoholism 303.9

> *Note—Use the following fifth-digit subclassification with category 303:*
>
> 0 *unspecifhed*
> 1 *continuous*
> 2 *episodic*
> 3 *in remission*

  with psychosis (*see also* Psychosis, alcoholic) 291.9
  acute 303.0
  chronic 303.9
    with psychosis 291.9
  complicating pregnancy, childbirth, or puerperium 648.4
    affecting fetus or newborn 760.71
  history V11.3
  Korsakoff's, Korsakov's, Korsakow's 291.1
  suspected damage to fetus affecting management of pregnancy 655.4
Alder's anomaly or syndrome (leukocyte granulation anomaly) 288.2
Alder-Reilly anomaly (leukocyte granulation) 288.2
Aldosteronism (primary) 255.10
  congenital 255.10
  familial type I 255.11
  glucocorticoid-remediable 255.11
  secondary 255.14
Aldosteronoma (M8370/1) 237.2
Aldrich (-Wiskott) syndrome (eczema-thrombocytopenia) 279.12
Aleppo boil 085.1
Aleukemic —*see* condition
Aleukia
  congenital 288.09
  hemorrhagica 284.9
    acquired (secondary) 284.89
    congenital 284.09
    idiopathic 284.9
  splenica 289.4
Alexia (congenital) (developmental) 315.01
  secondary to organic lesion 784.61
Algoneurodystrophy 733.7
Algophobia 300.29
Alibert's disease (mycosis fungoides) (M9700/3) 202.1
Alibert-Bazin disease (M9700/3) 202.1
Alice in Wonderland syndrome 293.89
Alienation, mental (*see also* Psychosis) 298.9
Alkalemia 276.3
Alkalosis 276.3
  metabolic 276.3
    with respiratory acidosis 276.4
  respiratory 276.3
Alkaptonuria 270.2
Allen-Masters syndrome 620.6
Allergic bronchopulmonary aspergillosis 518.6
Allergy, allergic (reaction) 995.3
  air-borne substance (*see also* Fever, hay) 477.9
    specified allergen NEC 477.8
  alveolitis (extrinsic) 495.9
    due to
      Aspergillus clavatus 495.4
      cryptostroma corticale 495.6

Allergy, allergic—*continued*
      organisms (fungal, thermophilic actinomycete, other) growing in ventilation (air conditioning systems) 495.7
    specified type NEC 495.8
  anaphylactic shock 999.4
    due to
      food—*see* Anaphylactic shock, due to, food
  angioneurotic edema 995.1
  animal (cat) (dog) (epidermal) 477.8
    dander 477.2
    hair 477.2
  arthritis (*see also* Arthritis, allergic) 716.2
  asthma—*see* Asthma
  bee sting (anaphylactic shock) 989.5
  biological—*see* Allergy, drug
  bronchial asthma—*see* Asthma
  conjunctivitis (eczematous) 372.14
  dander, animal (cat) (dog) 477.2
  dandruff 477.8
  dermatitis (venenata)—*see* Dermatitis
  diathesis V15.09
  drug, medicinal substance, and biological (any) (correct medicinal substance properly administered) (external) (internal) 995.27
    wrong substance given or taken NEC 977.9
    specified drug or substance—*see* Table of drugs and chemicals
  dust (house) (stock) 477.8
  eczema—*see* Eczema
  endophthalmitis 360.19
  epidermal (animal) 477.8
  existing dental restorative material 525.66
  feathers 477.8
  food (any) (ingested) 693.1
    atopic 691.8
    in contact with skin 692.5
  gastritis 535.4
  gastroenteritis 558.3
  gastrointestinal 558.3
  grain 477.0
  grass (pollen) 477.0
    asthma (*see also* Asthma) 493.0
    hay fever 477.0
  hair, animal (cat) (dog) 477.2
  hay fever (grass) (pollen) (ragweed) (tree) (*see also* Fever, hay) 477.9
  history (of) V15.09
    to
      eggs V15.03
      food additives V15.05
      insect bite V15.06
      latex V15.07
      milk products V15.02
      nuts V15.05
        peanuts V15.01
      radiographic dye V15.08
      seafood V15.04
      specified food NEC V15.05
      spider bite V15.06
  horse serum—*see* Allergy, serum
  inhalant 477.9
    dust 477.8
    pollen 477.0
    specified allergen other than pollen 477.8
  kapok 477.8
  medicine—*see* Allergy, drug
  migraine 346.2
  milk protein 558.3
  pannus 370.62

Allergy, allergic—*continued*
  pneumonia 518.3
  pollen (any) (hay fever) 477.0
    asthma (*see also* Asthma) 493.0
  primrose 477.0
  primula 477.0
  purpura 287.0
  ragweed (pollen) (Senecio jacobae) 477.0
    asthma (*see also* Asthma) 493.0
    hay fever 477.0
  respiratory (*see also* Allergy, inhalant) 477.9
    due to
      drug—*see* Allergy, drug
      food—*see* Allergy, food
  rhinitis (*see also* Fever, hay) 477.9
    due to food 477.1
  rose 477.0
  Senecio jacobae 477.0
  serum (prophylactic) (therapeutic) 999.5
    anaphylactic shock 999.4
  shock (anaphylactic)
    due to
      adverse effect of correct medicinal substance properly administered 995.0
      food—*see* Anaphylactic shock, due to, food
    from serum or immunization 999.5
      anaphylactic 999.4
  sinusitis (*see also* Fever, hay) 477.9
  skin reaction 692.9
    specified substance—*see* Dermatitis, due to
  tree (any) (hay fever) (pollen) 477.0
    asthma (*see also* Asthma) 493.0
  upper respiratory (*see also* Fever, hay) 477.9
  urethritis 597.89
  urticaria 708.0
  vaccine—*see* Allergy, serum
Allescheriosis 117.6
Alligator skin disease (ichthyosis congenita) 757.1
  acquired 701.1
Allocheiria, allochiria (*see also* Disturbance, sensation) 782.0
Almeida's disease (Brazilian blastomycosis) 116.1
Alopecia (atrophicans) (pregnancy) (premature) (senile) 704.00
  adnata 757.4
  areata 704.01
  celsi 704.01
  cicatrisata 704.09
  circumscripta 704.01
  congenital, congenitalis 757.4
  disseminata 704.01
  effluvium (telogen) 704.02
  febrile 704.09
  generalisata 704.09
  hereditaria 704.09
  marginalis 704.01
  mucinosa 704.09
  postinfectional 704.09
  seborrheica 704.09
  specific 091.82
  syphilitic (secondary) 091.82
  telogen effluvium 704.02
  totalis 704.09
  toxica 704.09
  universalis 704.09
  x-ray 704.09
Alper's disease 330.8
Alpha-lipoproteinemia 272.4
Alpha thalassemia 282.49

Alphos 696.1
Alpine sickness 993.2
Alport's syndrome (hereditary hematuria-nephropathy-deafness) 759.89
Alteration (of), altered
  awareness 780.09
    transient 780.02
  consciousness 780.09
    persistent vegetative state 780.03
    transient 780.02
  mental status 780.97
    amnesia (retrograde) 780.93
    memory loss 780.93
Alternaria (infection) 118
Alternating —*see* condition
Altitude, high (effects)—*see* Effect, adverse, high altitude
Aluminosis (of lung) 503
Alvarez syndrome (transient cerebral ischemia) 435.9
Alveolar capillary block syndrome 516.3
Alveolitis
  allergic (extrinsic) 495.9
    due to organisms (fungal, thermophilic actinomycete, other) growing in ventilation (air conditioning systems) 495.7
    specified type NEC 495.8
  due to
    Aspergillus clavatus 495.4
    Cryptostroma corticale 495.6
  fibrosing (chronic) (cryptogenic) (lung) 516.3
    idiopathic 516.3
    rheumatoid 714.81
  jaw 526.5
  sicca dolorosa 526.5
Alveolus, alveolar —*see* condition
Alymphocytosis (pure) 279.2
Alymphoplasia, thymic 279.2
Alzheimer's
  dementia (senile)
    with behavioral disturbance 331.0 *[294.11]*
    without behavioral disturbance 331.0 *[294.10]*
  disease or sclerosis 331.0
    with dementia—*see* Alzheimer's, dementia
Amastia (*see also* Absence, breast) 611.8
Amaurosis (acquired) (congenital) (*see also* Blindness) 369.00
  fugax 362.34
  hysterical 300.11
  Leber's (congenital) 362.76
  tobacco 377.34
  uremic—*see* Uremia
Amaurotic familial idiocy (infantile) (juvenile) (late) 330.1
Ambisexual 752.7
Amblyopia (acquired) (congenital) (partial) 368.00
  color 368.59
    acquired 368.55
  deprivation 368.02
  ex anopsia 368.00
  hysterical 300.11
  nocturnal 368.60
    vitamin A deficiency 264.5
  refractive 368.03
  strabismic 368.01
  suppression 368.01
  tobacco 377.34
  toxic NEC 377.34
  uremic—*see* Uremia

Ameba, amebic (histolytica)–*see also* Amebiasis
  abscess 006.3
    bladder 006.8
    brain (with liver and lung abscess) 006.5
    liver 006.3
      with
        brain abscess (and lung abscess) 006.5
        lung abscess 006.4
    lung (with liver abscess) 006.4
      with brain abscess 006.5
    seminal vesicle 006.8
    spleen 006.8
  carrier (suspected of) V02.2
  meningoencephalitis
    due to Naegleria (gruberi) 136.2
    primary 136.2
Amebiasis NEC 006.9
  with
    brain abscess (with liver or lung abscess) 006.5
    liver abscess (without mention of brain or lung abscess) 006.3
    lung abscess (with liver abscess) 006.4
      with brain abscess 006.5
  acute 006.0
  bladder 006.8
  chronic 006.1
  cutaneous 006.6
  cutis 006.6
  due to organism other than Entamoeba histolytica 007.8
  hepatic (*see also* Abscess, liver, amebic) 006.3
  nondysenteric 006.2
  seminal vesicle 006.8
  specified
    organism NEC 007.8
    site NEC 006.8
Ameboma 006.8
Amelia 755.4
  lower limb 755.31
  upper limb 755.21
Ameloblastoma (M9310/0) 213.1
  jaw (bone) (lower) 213.1
    upper 213.0
  long bones (M9261/3)—*see* Neoplasm, bone, malignant
  malignant (M9310/3) 170.1
    jaw (bone) (lower) 170.1
      upper 170.0
  mandible 213.1
  tibial (M9261/3) 170.7
Amelogenesis imperfecta 520.5
  nonhereditaria (segmentalis) 520.4
Amenorrhea (primary) (secondary) 626.0
  due to ovarian dysfunction 256.8
  hyperhormonal 256.8
Amentia (*see also* Retardation, mental) 319
  Meynert's (nonalcoholic) 294.0
    alcoholic 291.1
  nevoid 759.6
American
  leishmaniasis 085.5
  mountain tick fever 066.1
  trypanosomiasis—*see* Trypanosomiasis, American
Ametropia (*see also* Disorder, accommodation) 367.9
Amianthosis 501
Amimia 784.69
Amino acid
  deficiency 270.9
    anemia 281.4
  metabolic disorder (*see also* Disorder, amino acid) 270.9

Aminoaciduria 270.9
  imidazole 270.5
Amnesia (retrograde) 780.93
  auditory 784.69
    developmental 315.31
    secondary to organic lesion 784.69
  dissociative 300.12
  hysterical or dissociative type 300.12
  psychogenic 300.12
  transient global 437.7
Amnestic (confabulatory) syndrome 294.0
  alcohol-induced persisting 291.1
  drug-induced persisting 292.83
  posttraumatic 294.0
Amniocentesis screening (for) V28.2
  alphafetoprotein level, raised V28.1
  chromosomal anomalies V28.0
Amnion, amniotic —*see also* condition
  nodosum 658.8
Amnionitis (complicating pregnancy) 658.4
  affecting fetus or newborn 762.7
Amoral trends 301.7
Amotio retinae (*see also* Detachment, retina) 361.9
Ampulla
  lower esophagus 530.89
  phrenic 530.89
Amputation
  any part of fetus, to facilitate delivery 763.89
  cervix (supravaginal) (uteri) 622.8
    in pregnancy or childbirth 654.6
      affecting fetus or newborn 763.89
  clitoris—*see* Wound, open, clitoris
  congenital
    lower limb 755.31
    upper limb 755.21
  neuroma (traumatic)—*see also* Injury, nerve, by site
  surgical complications (late) 997.61
  penis—*see* Amputation, traumatic, penis
  status (without complication)—*see* Absence, by site, acquired
  stump (surgical)(posttraumatic)
    abnormal, painful, or with complication (late) 997.60
    healed or old NEC —*see also* Absence, by site, acquired
      lower V49.70
      upper V49.60
  traumatic (complete) (partial)

> Note—"Complicated" includes traumatic amputation with delayed healing, delayed treatment, foreign body, or infection.

    arm 887.4
      at or above elbow 887.2
        complicated 887.3
      below elbow 887.0
        complicated 887.1
      both (bilateral) (any level(s)) 887.6
        complicated 887.7
      complicated 887.5
    finger(s) (one or both hands) 886.0
      with thumb(s) 885.0
        complicated 885.1
      complicated 886.1
    foot (except toe(s) only) 896.0
      and other leg 897.6
        complicated 897.7
      both (bilateral) 896.2
        complicated 896.3
      complicated 896.1

Amputation

Amputation—*continued*
    toe(s) only (one or both feet) 895.0
        complicated 895.1
    genital organ(s) (external) NEC 878.8
        complicated 878.9
    hand (except finger(s) only) 887.0
        and other arm 887.6
            complicated 887.7
        both (bilateral) 887.6
            complicated 887.7
        complicated 887.1
        finger(s) (one or both hands) 886.0
            with thumb(s) 885.0
                complicated 885.1
            complicated 886.1
        thumb(s) (with fingers of either hand) 885.0
            complicated 885.1
    head 874.9
    late effect—*see* Late, effects (of), amputation
    leg 897.4
        and other foot 897.6
            complicated 897.7
        at or above knee 897.2
            complicated 897.3
        below knee 897.0
            complicated 897.1
        both (bilateral) 897.6
            complicated 897.7
        complicated 897.5
    lower limb(s) except toe(s)—*see* Amputation, traumatic, leg
    nose—*see* Wound, open, nose
    penis 878.0
        complicated 878.1
    sites other than limbs—*see* Wound, open, by site
    thumb(s) (with finger(s) of either hand) 885.0
        complicated 885.1
    toe(s) (one or both feet) 895.0
        complicated 895.1
    upper limb(s)—*see* Amputation, traumatic, arm

Amputee (bilateral) (old) —*see also* Absence, by site, acquired V49.70

Amusia 784.69
    developmental 315.39
    secondary to organic lesion 784.69

Amyelencephalus 740.0

Amyelia 742.59

Amygdalitis— *see* Tonsillitis

Amygdalolith 474.8

Amyloid disease or degeneration 277.30
    heart 277.39 *[425.7]*

Amyloidosis (familial) (general) (generalized) (genetic) (primary) 277.39
    with lung involvement 277.39 *[517.8]*
    cardiac, hereditary 277.39
    heart 277.39 *[425.7]*
    nephropathic 277.39 *[583.81]*
    neuropathic (Portuguese) (Swiss) 277.39 *[357.4]*
    pulmonary 277.39 *[517.8]*
    secondary 277.39
    systemic, inherited 277.39

Amylopectinosis (brancher enzyme deficiency) 271.0

Amylophagia 307.52

Amyoplasia, congenita 756.89

Amyotonia 728.2
    congenita 358.8

INDEX TO DISEASES

Amyotrophia, amyotrophy, amyotrophic 728.2
    congenita 756.89
    diabetic 250.6 *[353.1]*
    lateral sclerosis (syndrome) 335.20
    neuralgic 353.5
    sclerosis (lateral) 335.20
    spinal progressive 335.21

Anacidity
    gastric 536.0
    psychogenic 306.4

Anaerosis of newborn 770.88

Analbuminemia 273.8

Analgesia (*see also* Anesthesia) 782.0

Analphalipoproteinemia 272.5

Anaphylactic shock or reaction (correct substance properly administered) 995.0
    due to
        food 995.60
            additives 995.66
            crustaceans 995.62
            eggs 995.68
            fish 995.65
            fruits 995.63
            milk products 995.67
            nuts (tree) 995.64
            peanuts 995.61
            *see*ds 995.64
            specified NEC 995.69
            tree nuts 995.64
            vegetables 995.63
        immunization 999.4
        overdose or wrong substance given or taken 977.9
            specified drug—*see* Table of drugs and chemicals
    following sting(s) 989.5
    purpura 287.0
    serum 999.4

Anaphylactoid shock or reaction —*see* Anaphylactic shock

Anaphylaxis —*see* Anaphylactic shock

Anaplasia, cervix 622.10

Anarthria 784.5

Anarthritic rheumatoid disease 446.5

Anasarca 782.3
    cardiac (*see also* Failure, heart) 428.0
    fetus or newborn 778.0
    lung 514
    nutritional 262
    pulmonary 514
    renal (*see also* Nephrosis) 581.9

Anaspadias 752.62

Anastomosis
    aneurysmal—*see* Aneurysm
    arteriovenous, congenital NEC (*see also* Anomaly, arteriovenous) 747.60
        ruptured, of brain (*see also* Hemorrhage, subarachnoid) 430
    intestinal 569.89
        complicated NEC 997.4
            involving urinary tract 997.5
    retinal and choroidal vessels 743.58
        acquired 362.17

Anatomical narrow angle (glaucoma) 365.02

Ancylostoma (infection) (infestation) 126.9
    americanus 126.1
    braziliense 126.2
    caninum 126.8
    ceylanicum 126.3
    duodenale 126.0
    Necator americanus 126.1

INDEX TO DISEASES — Anemia

Ancylostomiasis (intestinal) 126.9
  Ancylostoma
    americanus 126.1
    caninum 126.8
    ceylanicum 126.3
    duodenale 126.0
  braziliense 126.2
  Necator americanus 126.1
Anders' disease or syndrome (adiposis tuberosa simplex) 272.8
Andersen's glycogen storage disease 271.0
Anderson's disease 272.7
Andes disease 993.2
Andrews' disease (bacterid) 686.8
Androblastoma (M8630/1)
  benign (M8630/0)
    specified site—see Neoplasm, by site, benign
    unspecified site
      female 220
      male 222.0
  malignant (M8630/3)
    specified site—see Neoplasm, by site, malignant
    unspecified site
      female 183.0
      male 186.9
  specified site—see Neoplasm, by site, uncertain behavior
  tubular (M8640/0)
    with lipid storage (M8641/0)
      specified site—see Neoplasm, by site, benign
      unspecified site
        female 220
        male 222.0
    specified site—see Neoplasm, by site, benign
    unspecified site
      female 220
      male 222.0
    unspecified site
      female 236.2
      male 236.4
Android pelvis 755.69
  with disproportion (fetopelvic) 653.3
    affecting fetus or newborn 763.1
    causing obstructed labor 660.1
      affecting fetus or newborn 763.1
Anectasis, pulmonary (newborn or fetus) 770.5
Anemia 285.9
  in
    chronic illness NEC 285.29
    chronic kidney disease 285.21
    end-stage renal disease 285.21
    neoplastic disease 285.22
  with
    disorder of
      anaerobic glycolysis 282.3
      pentose phosphate pathway 282.2
    koilonychia 280.9
    6-phosphogluconic dehydrogenase deficiency 282.2
  achlorhydric 280.9
  achrestic 281.8
  Addison's (pernicious) 281.0
  Addison-Biermer (pernicious) 281.0
  agranulocytic 288.09
  amino acid deficiency 281.4
  aplastic 284.9
    acquired (secondary) 284.81
    congenital 284.01
    constitutional 284.01

Anemia—continued
  due to
    chronic systemic disease 284.89
    drugs 284.89
    infection 284.89
    radiation 284.89
  idiopathic 284.9
  myxedema 244.9
  of or complicating pregnancy 648.2
  red cell (acquired) (adult) (with thymoma) 284.81
    congenital 284.01
    pure 284.01
  specified type NEC 284.89
  toxic (paralytic) 284.89
  aregenerative 284.9
    congenital 284.01
  asiderotic 280.9
  atypical (primary) 285.9
  autohemolysis of Selwyn and Dacie (type I) 282.2
  autoimmune hemolytic 283.0
  Baghdad Spring 282.2
  Balantidium coli 007.0
  Biermer's (pernicious) 281.0
  blood loss (chronic) 280.0
    acute 285.1
  bothriocephalus 123.4
  brickmakers' (see also Ancylostomiasis) 126.9
  cerebral 437.8
  childhood 282.9
  chlorotic 280.9
  chronica congenita aregenerativa 284.01
  chronic simple 281.9
  combined system disease NEC 281.0 [336.2]
    due to dietary deficiency 281.1 [336.2]
  complicating pregnancy or childbirth 648.2
  congenital (following fetal blood loss) 776.5
    aplastic 284.01
    due to isoimmunization NEC 773.2
    Heinz-body 282.7
    hereditary hemolytic NEC 282.9
    nonspherocytic
      Type I 282.2
      Type II 282.3
    pernicious 281.0
    spherocytic (see also Spherocytosis) 282.0
  Cooley's (erythroblastic) 282.49
  crescent—see Disease, sickle-cell
  cytogenic 281.0
  Dacie's (nonspherocytic)
    Type I 282.2
    Type II 282.3
  Davidson's (refractory) 284.9
  deficiency 281.9
    2, 3 diphosphoglycurate mutase 282.3
    2, 3 PG 282.3
    6-PGD 282.2
    6-phosphoguronic dehydrogenase 282.2
    amino acid 281.4
    combined B$_{12}$ and folate 281.3
    enzyme, drug-induced (hemolytic) 282.2
    erythrocytic glutathione 282.2
    folate 281.2
      dietary 281.2
      drug-induced 281.2
    folic acid 281.2
      dietary 281.2
      drug-induced 281.2
    G-6-PD 282.2
    GGS-R 282.2

801

Anemia—*continued*
- glucose-6-phosphate dehydrogenase (G-6-PD) 282.2
- glucose-phosphate isomerase 282.3
- glutathione peroxidase 282.2
- glutathione reductase 282.2
- glyceraldehyde phosphate dehydrogenase 282.3
- GPI 282.3
- G SH 282.2
- hexokinase 282.3
- iron (Fe) 280.9
    - specified NEC 280.8
- nutritional 281.9
    - with
        - poor iron absorption 280.9
        - specified deficiency NEC 281.8
    - due to inadequate dietary iron intake 280.1
    - specified type NEC 281.8
- of or complicating pregnancy 648.2
- pentose phosphate pathway 282.2
- PFK 282.3
- phosphofructo-aldolase 282.3
- phosphofructokinase 282.3
- phosphoglycerate kinase 282.3
- PK 282.3
- protein 281.4
- pyruvate kinase (PK) 282.3
    - TPI 282.3
    - triosephosphate isomerase 282.3
    - vitamin B_{12} NEC 281.1
        - dietary 281.1
        - pernicious 281.0
- Diamond-Blackfan (congenital hypoplastic) 284.01
- dibothriocephalus 123.4
- dimorphic 281.9
- diphasic 281.8
- diphtheritic 032.89
- Diphyllobothrium 123.4
- drepanocytic (*see also* Disease, sickle-cell) 282.60
- due to
    - blood loss (chronic) 280.0
        - acute 285.1
    - defect of Embden-Meyerhof pathway glycolysis 282.3
    - disorder of glutathione metabolism 282.2
    - fetal blood loss 776.5
    - fish tapeworm (D. latum) infestation 123.4
    - glutathione metabolism disorder 282.2
    - hemorrhage (chronic) 280.0
        - acute 285.1
    - hexose monophosphate (HMP) shunt deficiency 282.2
    - impaired absorption 280.9
    - loss of blood (chronic) 280.0
        - acute 285.1
    - myxedema 244.9
    - Necator americanus 126.1
    - prematurity 776.6
    - selective vitamin B_{12} malabsorption with proteinuria 281.1
- Dyke-Young type (secondary) (symptomatic) 283.9
- dyserythropoietic (congenital) (types I, II, III) 285.8
- dyshemopoietic (congenital) 285.8
- Egypt (*see also* Ancylostomiasis) 126.9
- elliptocytosis (*see also* Elliptocytosis) 282.1
- enzyme deficiency, drug-induced 282.2

Anemia—*continued*
- epidemic (*see also* Ancylostomiasis) 126.9
- EPO resistant 285.21
- erythroblastic
    - familial 282.49
    - fetus or newborn (*see also* Disease, hemolytic) 773.2
        - late 773.5
- erythrocytic glutathione deficiency 282.2
- erythropoietin-resistant (EPO resistant anemia) 285.21
- essential 285.9
- Faber's (achlorhydric anemia) 280.9
- factitious (self-induced blood letting) 280.0
- familial erythroblastic (microcytic) 282.49
- Fanconi's (congenital pancytopenia) 284.09
- favism 282.2
- fetal, following blood loss 776.5
- fetus or newborn
    - due to
        - ABO
            - antibodies 773.1
            - incompatibility, maternal/fetal 773.1
            - isoimmunization 773.1
        - Rh
            - antibodies 773.0
            - incompatibility, maternal/fetal 773.0
            - isoimmunization 773.0
    - following fetal blood loss 776.5
- fish tapeworm (D. latum) infestation 123.4
- folate (folic acid) deficiency 281.2
    - dietary 281.2
    - drug-induced 281.2
- folate malabsorption, congenital 281.2
- folic acid deficiency 281.2
    - dietary 281.2
    - drug-induced 281.2
- G-6-PD 282.2
- general 285.9
- glucose-6-phosphate dehydrogenase deficiency 282.2
- glutathione-reductase deficiency 282.2
- goat's milk 281.2
- granulocytic 288.09
- Heinz-body, congenital 282.7
- hemoglobin deficiency 285.9
- hemolytic 283.9
    - acquired 283.9
        - with hemoglobinuria NEC 283.2
        - autoimmune (cold type) (idiopathic) (primary) (secondary) (symptomatic) (warm type) 283.0
            - due to
                - cold reactive antibodies 283.0
                - drug exposure 283.0
                - warm reactive antibodies 283.0
        - fragmentation 283.19
        - idiopathic (chronic) 283.9
        - infectious 283.19
            - autoimmune 283.0
        - non-autoimmune NEC 283.10
        - toxic 283.19
        - traumatic cardiac 283.19
    - acute 283.9
        - due to enzyme deficiency NEC 282.3
        - fetus or newborn (*see also* Disease, hemolytic) 773.2
            - late 773.5
        - Lederer's (acquired infectious hemolytic anemia) 283.19
    - autoimmune (acquired) 283.0

INDEX TO DISEASES — Anemia

Anemia—*continued*
  chronic 282.9
    idiopathic 283.9
  cold type (secondary) (symptomatic) 283.0
  congenital (spherocytic) (*see also* Spherocytosis) 282.0
    nonspherocytic—*see* Anemia, hemolytic, nonspherocytic, congenital
  drug-induced 283.0
    enzyme deficiency 282.2
  due to
    cardiac conditions 283.19
    drugs 283.0
    enzyme deficiency NEC 282.3
      drug-induced 282.2
    presence of shunt or other internal prosthetic device 283.19
    thrombotic thrombocytopenic purpura 446.6
  elliptocytotic (*see also* Elliptocytosis) 282.1
  familial 282.9
  hereditary 282.9
    due to enzyme deficiency NEC 282.3
    specified NEC 282.8
  idiopathic (chronic) 283.9
  infectious (acquired) 283.19
  mechanical 283.19
  microangiopathic 283.19
  non-autoimmune NEC 283.10
  nonspherocytic
    congenital or hereditary NEC 282.3
      glucose-6-phosphate dehydrogenase deficiency 282.2
      pyruvate kinase (PK) deficiency 282.3
      type I 282.2
      type II 282.3
      type I 282.2
      type II 282.3
  of or complicating pregnancy 648.2
  resulting from presence of shunt or other internal prosthetic device 283.19
  secondary 283.19
    autoimmune 283.0
  sickle-cell—*see* Disease, sickle-cell
  Stransky-Regala type (Hb-E) (*see also* Disease, hemoglobin) 282.7
  symptomatic 283.19
    autoimmune 283.0
  toxic (acquired) 283.19
  uremic (adult) (child) 283.11
  warm type (secondary) (symptomatic) 283.0
  hemorrhagic (chronic) 280.0
    acute 285.1
  HEMPAS 285.8
  hereditary erythroblast multinuclearity- positive acidified serum test 285.8
  Herrick's (hemoglobin S disease) 282.61
  hexokinase deficiency 282.3
  high A_2 282.49
  hookworm (*see also* Ancylostomiasis) 126.9
  hypochromic (idiopathic) (microcytic) (normoblastic) 280.9
    with iron loading 285.0
    due to blood loss (chronic) 280.0
      acute 285.1
    familial sex linked 285.0
    pyridoxine-responsive 285.0
  hypoplasia, red blood cells 284.81
    congenital or familial 284.01
  hypoplastic (idiopathic) 284.9
    congenital 284.01
    familial 284.01

Anemia—*continued*
  of childhood 284.09
  idiopathic 285.9
    hemolytic, chronic 283.9
  infantile 285.9
  infective, infectional 285.9
  intertropical (*see also* Ancylostomiasis) 126.9
  iron (Fe) deficiency 280.9
    due to blood loss (chronic) 280.0
      acute 285.1
    of or complicating pregnancy 648.2
    specified NEC 280.8
  Jaksch's (pseudoleukemia infantum) 285.8
  Joseph-Diamond-Blackfan (congenital hypoplastic) 284.01
  labyrinth 386.50
  Lederer's (acquired infectious hemolytic anemia) 283.19
  leptocytosis (hereditary) 282.49
  leukoerythroblastic 284.2
  macrocytic 281.9
    nutritional 281.2
    of or complicating pregnancy 648.2
    tropical 281.2
  malabsorption (familial), selective B_{12} with proteinuria 281.1
  malarial (*see also* Malaria) 084.6
  malignant (progressive) 281.0
  malnutrition 281.9
  marsh (*see also* Malaria) 084.6
  Mediterranean (with hemoglobinopathy) 282.49
  megaloblastic 281.9
    combined B_{12} and folate deficiency 281.3
    nutritional (of infancy) 281.2
    of infancy 281.2
    of or complicating pregnancy 648.2
    refractory 281.3
    specified NEC 281.3
  megalocytic 281.9
  microangiopathic hemolytic 283.19
  microcytic (hypochromic) 280.9
    due to blood loss (chronic) 280.0
      acute 285.1
    familial 282.49
    hypochromic 280.9
  microdrepanocytosis 282.49
  miners' (*see also* Ancylostomiasis) 126.9
  myelopathic 285.8
  myelophthisic (normocytic) 284.2
  newborn (*see also* Disease, hemolytic) 773.2
    due to isoimmunization (*see also* Disease, hemolytic) 773.2
    late, due to isoimmunization 773.5
    posthemorrhagic 776.5
  nonregenerative 284.9
  nonspherocytic hemolytic—*see* Anemia, hemolytic, nonspherocytic
  normocytic (infectional) (not due to blood loss) 285.9
    due to blood loss (chronic) 280.0
      acute 285.1
    myelophthisic 284.2
  nutritional (deficiency) 281.9
    with
      poor iron absorption 280.9
      specified deficiency NEC 281.8
    due to inadequate dietary iron intake 280.1
    megaloblastic (of infancy) 281.2
  of childhood 282.9
  of chronic
    disease NEC 285.29

Anemia — *continued*
  illness NEC 285.29
  of or complicating pregnancy 648.2
    affecting fetus or newborn 760.8
  of prematurity 776.6
  orotic aciduric (congenital) (hereditary) 281.4
  osteosclerotic 289.89
  ovalocytosis (hereditary) (*see also* Elliptocytosis) 282.1
  paludal (*see also* Malaria) 084.6
  pentose phosphate pathway deficiency 282.2
  pernicious (combined system disease) (congenital) (dorsolateral spinal degeneration) (juvenile) (myelopathy) (neuropathy) (posterior sclerosis) (primary) (progressive) (spleen) 281.0
    of or complicating pregnancy 648.2
  pleochromic 285.9
    of sprue 281.8
  portal 285.8
  posthemorrhagic (chronic) 280.0
    acute 285.1
    newborn 776.5
  postoperative
    due to (acute) blood loss 285.1
      chronic blood loss 280.0
    other 285.9
  postpartum 648.2
  pressure 285.9
  primary 285.9
  profound 285.9
  progressive 285.9
    malignant 281.0
    pernicious 281.0
  protein-deficiency 281.4
  pseudoleukemica infantum 285.8
  puerperal 648.2
  pure red cell 284.81
    congenital 284.01
  pyridoxine-responsive (hypochromic) 285.0
  pyruvate kinase (PK) deficiency 282.3
  refractoria sideroblastica 238.72
  refractory (primary) 238.72
    with
      excess
        blasts-1 (RAEB-1) 238.73
        blasts-2 (RAEB-2) 238.73
      hemochromatosis 238.72
      ringed sideroblasts (RARS) 238.72
    megaloblastic 281.3
    sideroblastic 238.72
    sideropenic 280.9
  Rietti-Greppi-Micheli (thalassemia minor) 282.49
  scorbutic 281.8
  secondary (to) 285.9
    blood loss (chronic) 280.0
      acute 285.1
    hemorrhage 280.0
      acute 285.1
    inadequate dietary iron intake 280.1
  semiplastic 284.9
  septic 285.9
  sickle-cell (*see also* Disease, sickle-cell) 282.60
  sideroachrestic 285.0
  sideroblastic (acquired) (any type) (congenital) (drug-induced) (due to disease) (hereditary) (primary) (secondary) (sex-linked hypochromic) (vitamin B$_6$ responsive) 285.0
    refractory 238.72

Anemia — *continued*
  sideropenic (refractory) 280.9
    due to blood loss (chronic) 280.0
      acute 285.1
  simple chronic 281.9
  specified type NEC 285.8
  spherocytic (hereditary) (*see also* Spherocytosis) 282.0
  splenic 285.8
    familial (Gaucher's) 272.7
  splenomegalic 285.8
  stomatocytosis 282.8
  syphilitic 095.8
  target cell (oval) 282.49
  thalassemia 282.49
  thrombocytopenic (*see also* Thrombocytopenia) 287.5
  toxic 284.89
  triosephosphate isomerase deficiency 282.3
  tropical, macrocytic 281.2
  tuberculous (*see also* Tuberculosis) 017.9
  vegan's 281.1
  vitamin
    B$_6$-responsive 285.0
    B$_{12}$ deficiency (dietary) 281.1
      pernicious 281.0
  von Jaksch's (pseudoleukemia infantum) 285.8
  Witts' (achlorhydric anemia) 280.9
  Zuelzer (-Ogden) (nutritional megaloblastic anemia) 281.2
Anencephalus, anencephaly 740.0
  fetal, affecting management of pregnancy 655.0
Anergasia (*see also* Psychosis, organic) 294.9
  senile 290.0
Anesthesia, anesthetic 782.0
  complication or reaction NEC 995.22
    due to
      correct substance properly administered 995.22
      overdose or wrong substance given 968.4
        specified anesthetic—*see* Table of drugs and chemicals
  cornea 371.81
  death from
    correct substance properly administered 995.4
    during delivery 668.9
    overdose or wrong substance given 968.4
      specified anesthetic—*see* Table of drugs and chemicals
  eye 371.81
  functional 300.11
  hyperesthetic, thalamic 338.0
  hysterical 300.11
  local skin lesion 782.0
  olfactory 781.1
  sexual (psychogenic) 302.72
  shock
    due to
      correct substance properly administered 995.4
      overdose or wrong substance given 968.4
        specified anesthetic—*see* Table of drugs and chemicals
  skin 782.0
  tactile 782.0
  testicular 608.9
  thermal 782.0
Anetoderma (maculosum) 701.3
Aneuploidy NEC 758.5
Aneurin deficiency 265.1

INDEX TO DISEASES

Aneurysm

Aneurysm (anastomotic) (artery) (cirsoid) (diffuse) (false) (fusiform) (multiple) (ruptured) (saccular) (varicose) 442.9
  abdominal (aorta) 441.4
    ruptured 441.3
    syphilitic 093.0
  aorta, aortic (nonsyphilitic) 441.9
    abdominal 441.4
      dissecting 441.02
      ruptured 441.3
      syphilitic 093.0
    arch 441.2
      ruptured 441.1
    arteriosclerotic NEC 441.9
      ruptured 441.5
    ascending 441.2
      ruptured 441.1
    congenital 747.29
    descending 441.9
      abdominal 441.4
        ruptured 441.3
      ruptured 441.5
      thoracic 441.2
        ruptured 441.1
    dissecting 441.00
      abdominal 441.02
      thoracic 441.01
      thoracoabdominal 441.03
    due to coarctation (aorta) 747.10
    ruptured 441.5
    sinus, right 747.29
    syphilitic 093.0
    thoracoabdominal 441.7
      ruptured 441.6
    thorax, thoracic (arch) (nonsyphilitic) 441.2
      dissecting 441.01
      ruptured 441.1
      syphilitic 093.0
    transverse 441.2
      ruptured 441.1
    valve (heart) (*see also* Endocarditis, aortic) 424.1
  arteriosclerotic NEC 442.9
    cerebral 437.3
      ruptured (*see also* Hemorrhage, subarachnoid) 430
  arteriovenous (congenital) (peripheral) NEC (*see also* Anomaly, arteriovenous) 747.60
    acquired NEC 447.0
      brain 437.3
        ruptured (*see also* Hemorrhage, subarachnoid) 430
      coronary 414.11
      pulmonary 417.0
    brain (cerebral) 747.81
      ruptured (*see also* Hemorrhage, subarachnoid) 430
    coronary 746.85
    pulmonary 747.3
    retina 743.58
    specified site NEC 747.89
      acquired 447.0
    traumatic (*see also* Injury, blood vessel, by site) 904.9
  basal—*see* Aneurysm, brain
  berry (congenital) (ruptured) (*see also* Hemorrhage, subarachnoid) 430
  brain 437.3
    arteriosclerotic 437.3
      ruptured (*see also* Hemorrhage, subarachnoid) 430

Aneurysm—*continued*
  arteriovenous 747.81
    acquired 437.3
      ruptured (*see also* Hemorrhage, subarachnoid) 430
    ruptured (*see also* Hemorrhage, subarachnoid) 430
  berry (congenital) (ruptured) (*see also* Hemorrhage, subarachnoid) 430
  congenital 747.81
    ruptured (*see also* Hemorrhage, subarachnoid) 430
  meninges 437.3
    ruptured (*see also* Hemorrhage, subarachnoid) 430
  miliary (congenital) (ruptured) (*see also* Hemorrhage, subarachnoid) 430
  mycotic 421.0
    ruptured (*see also* Hemorrhage, subarachnoid) 430
  nonruptured 437.3
  ruptured (*see also* Hemorrhage, subarachnoid) 430
  syphilitic 094.87
  syphilitic (hemorrhage) 094.87
  traumatic—*see* Injury, intracranial
  cardiac (false) (*see also* Aneurysm, heart) 414.10
  carotid artery (common) (external) 442.81
    internal (intracranial portion) 437.3
      extracranial portion 442.81
      ruptured into brain (*see also* Hemorrhage, subarachnoid) 430
    syphilitic 093.89
      intracranial 094.87
  cavernous sinus (*see also* Aneurysm, brain) 437.3
    arteriovenous 747.81
      ruptured (*see also* Hemorrhage, subarachnoid) 430
    congenital 747.81
      ruptured (*see also* Hemorrhage, subarachnoid) 430
  celiac 442.84
  central nervous system, syphilitic 094.89
  cerebral—*see* Aneurysm, brain
  chest—*see* Aneurysm, thorax
  circle of Willis (*see also* Aneurysm, brain) 437.3
    congenital 747.81
      ruptured (*see also* Hemorrhage, subarachnoid) 430
    ruptured (*see also* Hemorrhage, subarachnoid) 430
  common iliac artery 442.2
  congenital (peripheral) NEC 747.60
    brain 747.81
      ruptured (*see also* Hemorrhage, subarachnoid) 430
    cerebral—*see* Aneurysm, brain, congenital
    coronary 746.85
    gastrointestinal 747.61
    lower limb 747.64
    pulmonary 747.3
    renal 747.62
    retina 743.58
    specified site NEC 747.89
    spinal 747.82
    upper limb 747.63
  conjunctiva 372.74
  conus arteriosus (*see also* Aneurysm, heart) 414.10

Aneurysm INDEX TO DISEASES

Aneurysm—*continued*
  coronary (arteriosclerotic) (artery) (vein) (*see also* Aneurysm, heart) 414.11
    arteriovenous 746.85
    congenital 746.85
    syphilitic 093.89
  cylindrical 441.9
    ruptured 441.5
    syphilitic 093.9
  dissecting 442.9
    aorta 441.00
      abdominal 441.02
      thoracic 441.01
      thoracoabdominal 441.03
    syphilitic 093.9
  ductus arteriosus 747.0
  embolic—*see* Embolism, artery
  endocardial, infective (any valve) 421.0
  femoral 442.3
  gastroduodenal 442.84
  gastroepiploic 442.84
  heart (chronic or with a stated duration of over 8 weeks) (infectional) (wall) 414.10
    acute or with a stated duration of 8 weeks or less (*see also* Infarct, myocardium) 410.9
    congenital 746.89
    valve—*see* Endocarditis
  hepatic 442.84
  iliac (common) 442.2
  infective (any valve) 421.0
  innominate (nonsyphilitic) 442.89
    syphilitic 093.89
  interauricular septum (*see also* Aneurysm, heart) 414.10
  interventricular septum (*see also* Aneurysm, heart) 414.10
  intracranial—*see* Aneurysm, brain
  intrathoracic (nonsyphilitic) 441.2
    ruptured 441.1
    syphilitic 093.0
  jugular vein 453.8
  lower extremity 442.3
  lung (pulmonary artery) 417.1
  malignant 093.9
  mediastinal (nonsyphilitic) 442.89
    syphilitic 093.89
  miliary (congenital) (ruptured) (*see also* Hemorrhage, subarachnoid) 430
  mitral (heart) (valve) 424.0
  mural (arteriovenous) (heart) (*see also* Aneurysm, heart) 414.10
  mycotic, any site 421.0
    ruptured, brain (*see also* Hemorrhage, subarachnoid) 430
    without endocarditis —*see* Aneurysm, by site
  myocardium (*see also* Aneurysm, heart) 414.10
  neck 442.81
  pancreaticoduodenal 442.84
  patent ductus arteriosus 747.0
  peripheral NEC 442.89
    congenital NEC (*see also* Aneurysm, congenital) 747.60
  popliteal 442.3
  pulmonary 417.1
    arteriovenous 747.3
      acquired 417.0
    syphilitic 093.89
    valve (heart) (*see also* Endocarditis, pulmonary) 424.3
  racemose 442.9
    congenital (peripheral) NEC 747.60

Aneurysm—*continued*
  radial 442.0
  Rasmussen's (*see also* Tuberculosis) 011.2
  renal 442.1
  retinal (acquired) 362.17
    congenital 743.58
    diabetic 250.5 *[362.01]*
  sinus, aortic (of Valsalva) 747.29
  specified site NEC 442.89
  spinal (cord) 442.89
    congenital 747.82
    syphilitic (hemorrhage) 094.89
  spleen, splenic 442.83
  subclavian 442.82
    syphilitic 093.89
  superior mesenteric 442.84
  syphilitic 093.9
    aorta 093.0
    central nervous system 094.89
    congenital 090.5
    spine, spinal 094.89
  thoracoabdominal 441.7
    ruptured 441.6
  thorax, thoracic (arch) (nonsyphilitic) 441.2
    dissecting 441.01
    ruptured 441.1
    syphilitic 093.0
  traumatic (complication) (early)—*see* Injury, blood vessel, by site
  tricuspid (heart) (valve)—*see* Endocarditis, tricuspid
  ulnar 442.0
  upper extremity 442.0
  valve, valvular—*see* Endocarditis
  venous 456.8
    congenital NEC (*see also* Aneurysm, congenital) 747.60
  ventricle (arteriovenous) (*see also* Aneurysm, heart) 414.10
  visceral artery NEC 442.84
Angiectasis 459.89
Angiectopia 459.9
Angiitis 447.6
  allergic granulomatous 446.4
  hypersensitivity 446.20
    Goodpasture's syndrome 446.21
    specified NEC 446.29
  necrotizing 446.0
  Wegener's (necrotizing respiratory granulomatosis) 446.4
Angina (attack) (cardiac) (chest) (effort) (heart) (pectoris) (syndrome) (vasomotor) 413.9
  abdominal 557.1
  accelerated 411.1
  agranulocytic 288.03
  aphthous 074.0
  catarrhal 462
  crescendo 411.1
  croupous 464.4
  cruris 443.9
    due to atherosclerosis NEC (*see also* Arteriosclerosis, extremities) 440.20
  decubitus 413.0
  diphtheritic (membranous) 032.0
  erysipelatous 034.0
  erythematous 462
  exudative, chronic 476.0
  faucium 478.29
  gangrenous 462
    diphtheritic 032.0
  infectious 462

Angina—*continued*
  initial 411.1
  intestinal 557.1
  ludovici 528.3
  Ludwig's 528.3
  malignant 462
    diphtheritic 032.0
  membranous 464.4
    diphtheritic 032.0
  mesenteric 557.1
  monocytic 075
  nocturnal 413.0
  phlegmonous 475
    diphtheritic 032.0
  preinfarctional 411.1
  Prinzmetal's 413.1
  progressive 411.1
  pseudomembranous 101
  psychogenic 306.2
  pultaceous, diphtheritic 032.0
  scarlatinal 034.1
  septic 034.0
  simple 462
  stable NEC 413.9
  staphylococcal 462
  streptococcal 034.0
  stridulous, diphtheritic 032.3
  syphilitic 093.9
    congenital 090.5
  tonsil 475
  trachealis 464.4
  unstable 411.1
  variant 413.1
  Vincent's 101
Angioblastoma (M9161/1)—*see* Neoplasm, connective tissue, uncertain behavior
Angiocholecystitis (*see also* Cholecystitis, acute) 575.0
Angiocholitis (*see also* Cholecystitis, acute) 576.1
Angiodysgensis spinalis 336.1
Angiodysplasia (intestinalis) (intestine) 569.84
  with hemorrhage 569.85
  duodenum 537.82
    with hemorrhage 537.83
  stomach 537.82
    with hemorrhage 537.83
Angioedema (allergic) (any site) (with urticaria) 995.1
  hereditary 277.6
Angioendothelioma (M9130/1)—*see also* Neoplasm, by site, uncertain behavior
  benign (M9130/0) (*see also* Hemangioma, by site) 228.00
  bone (M9260/3)—*see* Neoplasm, bone, malignant
  Ewing's (M9260/3)—*see* Neoplasm, bone, malignant
  nervous system (M9130/0) 228.09
Angiofibroma (M9160/0)—*see also* Neoplasm, by site, benign
  juvenile (M9160/0) 210.7
    specified site—*see* Neoplasm, by site, benign
    unspecified site 210.7
Angiohemophilia (A) (B) 286.4
Angioid streaks (choroid) (retina) 363.43
Angiokeratoma (M9141/0)—*see also* Neoplasm, skin, benign
  corporis diffusum 272.7
Angiokeratosis
  diffuse 272.7

Angioleiomyoma (M8894/0)—*see* Neoplasm, connective tissue, benign
Angioleucitis 683
Angiolipoma (M8861/0) (*see also* Lipoma, by site) 214.9
  infiltrating (M8861/1)—*see* Neoplasm, connective tissue, uncertain behavior
Angioma (M9120/0) (*see also* Hemangioma, by site) 228.00
  capillary 448.1
  hemorrhagicum hereditaria 448.0
  malignant (M9120/3)—*see* Neoplasm, connective tissue, malignant
  pigmentosum et atrophicum 757.33
  placenta—*see* Placenta, abnormal
  plexiform (M9131/0)—*see* Hemangioma, by site
  senile 448.1
  serpiginosum 709.1
  spider 448.1
  stellate 448.1
Angiomatosis 757.32
  bacillary 083.8
  corporis diffusum universale 272.7
  cutaneocerebral 759.6
  encephalocutaneous 759.6
  encephalofacial 759.6
  encephalotrigeminal 759.6
  hemorrhagic familial 448.0
  hereditary familial 448.0
  heredofamilial 448.0
  meningo-oculofacial 759.6
  multiple sites 228.09
  neuro-oculocutaneous 759.6
  retina (Hippel's disease) 759.6
  retinocerebellosa 759.6
  retinocerebral 759.6
  systemic 228.09
Angiomyolipoma (M8860/0)
  specified site—*see* Neoplasm, connective tissue, benign
  unspecified site 223.0
Angiomyoliposarcoma (M8860/3)—*see* Neoplasm, connective tissue, malignant
Angiomyoma (M8894/0)—*see* Neoplasm, connective tissue, benign
Angiomyosarcoma (M8894/3)—*see* Neoplasm, connective tissue, malignant
Angioneurosis 306.2
Angioneurotic edema (allergic) (any site) (with urticaria) 995.1
  hereditary 277.6
Angiopathia, angiopathy 459.9
  diabetic (peripheral) 250.7 *[443.81]*
  peripheral 443.9
    diabetic 250.7 *[443.81]*
    specified type NEC 443.89
  retinae syphilitica 093.89
  retinalis (juvenilis) 362.18
    background 362.10
    diabetic 250.5 *[362.01]*
    proliferative 362.29
    tuberculous (*see also* Tuberculosis) 017.3 *[362.18]*
Angiosarcoma (M9120/3)—*see* Neoplasm, connective tissue, malignant
Angiosclerosis —*see* Arteriosclerosis
Angioscotoma, enlarged 368.42
Angiospasm 443.9
  brachial plexus 353.0
  cerebral 435.9

Angiospasm—*continued*
  cervical plexus 353.2
  nerve
    arm 354.9
      axillary 353.0
      median 354.1
      ulnar 354.2
    autonomic (*see also* Neuropathy, peripheral, autonomic) 337.9
    axillary 353.0
    leg 355.8
      plantar 355.6
    lower extremity—*see* Angiospasm, nerve, leg
    median 354.1
    peripheral NEC 355.9
    spinal NEC 355.9
    sympathetic (*see also* Neuropathy, peripheral, autonomic) 337.9
    ulnar 354.2
    upper extremity—*see* Angiospasm, nerve, arm
  peripheral NEC 443.9
  traumatic 443.9
    foot 443.9
    leg 443.9
    vessel 443.9
Angiospastic disease or edema 443.9
Angle's
  class I 524.21
  class II 524.22
  class III 524.23
Anguillulosis 127.2
Angulation
  cecum (*see also* Obstruction, intestine) 560.9
  coccyx (acquired) 738.6
    congenital 756.19
  femur (acquired) 736.39
    congenital 755.69
  intestine (large) (small) (*see also* Obstruction, intestine) 560.9
  sacrum (acquired) 738.5
    congenital 756.19
  sigmoid (flexure) (*see also* Obstruction, intestine) 560.9
  spine (*see also* Curvature, spine) 737.9
  tibia (acquired) 736.89
    congenital 755.69
  ureter 593.3
  wrist (acquired) 736.09
    congenital 755.59
Angulus infectiosus 686.8
Anhedonia 780.99
Anhidrosis (lid) (neurogenic) (thermogenic) 705.0
Anhydration 276.51
  with
    hypernatremia 276.0
    hyponatremia 276.1
Anhydremia 276.52
  with
    hypernatremia 276.0
    hyponatremia 276.1
Anidrosis 705.0
Aniridia (congenital) 743.45
Anisakiasis (infection) (infestation) 127.1
Anisakis larva infestation 127.1
Aniseikonia 367.32
Anisocoria (pupil) 379.41
  congenital 743.46
Anisocytosis 790.09
Anisometropia (congenital) 367.31
Ankle —*see* condition

Ankyloblepharon (acquired) (eyelid) 374.46
  filiforme (adnatum) (congenital) 743.62
  total 743.62
Ankylodactly (*see also* Syndactylism) 755.10
Ankyloglossia 750.0
Ankylosis (fibrous) (osseous) 718.50
  ankle 718.57
  any joint, produced by surgical fusion V45.4
  cricoarytenoid (cartilage) (joint) (larynx) 478.79
  dental 521.6
  ear ossicle NEC 385.22
    malleus 385.21
  elbow 718.52
  finger 718.54
  hip 718.55
  incostapedial joint (infectional) 385.22
  joint, produced by surgical fusion NEC V45.4
  knee 718.56
  lumbosacral (joint) 724.6
  malleus 385.21
  multiple sites 718.59
  postoperative (status) V45.4
  sacroiliac (joint) 724.6
  shoulder 718.51
  specified site NEC 718.58
  spine NEC 724.9
  surgical V45.4
  teeth, tooth (hard tissues) 521.6
  temporomandibular joint 524.61
  wrist 718.53
Ankylostoma —*see* Ancylostoma
Ankylostomiasis (intestinal)—*see* Ancylostomiasis
Ankylurethria (*see also* Stricture, urethra) 598.9
Annular —*see also* condition
  detachment, cervix 622.8
  organ or site, congenital NEC—*see* Distortion
  pancreas (congenital) 751.7
Anodontia (complete) (partial) (vera) 520.0
  with abnormal spacing 524.30
  acquired 525.10
    causing malocclusion 524.30
    due to
      caries 525.13
      extraction 525.10
      periodontal disease 525.12
      trauma 525.11
Anomaly, anomalous (congenital) (unspecified type) 759.9
  abdomen 759.9
  abdominal wall 756.70
  acoustic nerve 742.9
  adrenal (gland) 759.1
  Alder (-Reilly) (leukocyte granulation) 288.2
  alimentary tract 751.9
    lower 751.5
    specified type NEC 751.8
    upper (any part, except tongue) 750.9
      tongue 750.10
        specified type NEC 750.19
  alveolar 524.70
    ridge (process) 525.8
    specified NEC 524.79
  ankle (joint) 755.69
  anus, anal (canal) 751.5
  aorta, aortic 747.20
    arch 747.21
    coarctation (postductal) (preductal) 747.10
    cusp or valve NEC 746.9
    septum 745.0
    specified type NEC 747.29

Anomaly, anomalous—*continued*
  aorticopulmonary septum 745.0
  apertures, diaphragm 756.6
  appendix 751.5
  aqueduct of Sylvius 742.3
    with spina bifida (*see also* Spina bifida) 741.0
  arm 755.50
    reduction (*see also* Deformity, reduction, upper limb) 755.20
  arteriovenous (congenital) (peripheral) NEC 747.60
    brain 747.81
    cerebral 747.81
    coronary 746.85
    gastrointestinal 747.61
      acquired—*see* Angiodysplasia
    lower limb 747.64
    renal 747.62
    specified site NEC 747.69
    spinal 747.82
    upper limb 747.63
  artery (*see also* Anomaly, peripheral vascular system) NEC 747.60
    brain 747.81
    cerebral 747.81
    coronary 746.85
    eye 743.9
    pulmonary 747.3
    renal 747.62
    retina 743.9
    umbilical 747.5
  arytenoepiglottic folds 748.3
  atrial
    bands 746.9
    folds 746.9
    septa 745.5
  atrioventricular
    canal 745.69
    common 745.69
    conduction 426.7
    excitation 426.7
    septum 745.4
  atrium—*see* Anomaly, atrial
  auditory canal 744.3
    specified type NEC 744.29
      with hearing impairment 744.02
  auricle
    ear 744.3
      causing impairment of hearing 744.02
    heart 746.9
      septum 745.5
  autosomes, autosomal NEC 758.5
  Axenfeld's 743.44
  back 759.9
  band
    atrial 746.9
    heart 746.9
    ventricular 746.9
  Bartholin's duct 750.9
  biliary duct or passage 751.60
    atresia 751.61
  bladder (neck) (sphincter) (trigone) 753.9
    specified type NEC 753.8
  blood vessel 747.9
    artery—*see* Anomaly, artery
    peripheral vascular—*see* Anomaly, peripheral vascular system
    vein—*see* Anomaly, vein
  bone NEC 756.9
    ankle 755.69
    arm 755.50

Anomaly, anomalous—*continued*
  chest 756.3
  cranium 756.0
  face 756.0
  finger 755.50
  foot 755.67
  forearm 755.50
  frontal 756.0
  head 756.0
  hip 755.63
  leg 755.60
  lumbosacral 756.10
  nose 748.1
  pelvic girdle 755.60
  rachitic 756.4
  rib 756.3
  shoulder girdle 755.50
  skull 756.0
    with
      anencephalus 740.0
      encephalocele 742.0
      hydrocephalus 742.3
        with spina bifida (*see also* Spina bifida) 741.0
      microcephalus 742.1
  toe 755.66
  brain 742.9
    multiple 742.4
    reduction 742.2
    specified type NEC 742.4
    vessel 747.81
  branchial cleft NEC 744.49
    cyst 744.42
    fistula 744.41
    persistent 744.41
    sinus (external) (internal) 744.41
  breast 757.9
  broad ligament 752.10
    specified type NEC 752.19
  bronchus 748.3
  bulbar septum 745.0
  bulbus cordis 745.9
    persistent (in left ventricle) 745.8
  bursa 756.9
  canal of Nuck 752.9
  canthus 743.9
  capillary NEC (*see also* Anomaly, peripheral vascular system) 747.60
  cardiac 746.9
    septal closure 745.9
      acquired 429.71
    valve NEC 746.9
      pulmonary 746.00
      specified type NEC 746.89
  cardiovascular system 746.9
    complicating pregnancy, childbirth, or puerperium 648.5
  carpus 755.50
  cartilage, trachea 748.3
  cartilaginous 756.9
  caruncle, lacrimal, lachrymal 743.9
  cascade stomach 750.7
  cauda equina 742.59
  cecum 751.5
  cerebral—*see also* Anomaly, brain
    vessels 747.81
  cerebrovascular system 747.81
  cervix (uterus) 752.40
    with doubling of vagina and uterus 752.2
    in pregnancy or childbirth 654.6
      affecting fetus or newborn 763.89

Anomaly, anomalous—continued
    causing obstructed labor 660.2
        affecting fetus or newborn 763.1
  Chédiak-Higashi (-Steinbrinck) (congenital gigantism of peroxidase granules) 288.2
  cheek 744.9
  chest (wall) 756.3
  chin 744.9
    specified type NEC 744.89
  chordae tendineae 746.9
  choroid 743.9
    plexus 742.9
  chromosomes, chromosomal 758.9
    13 (13-15) 758.1
    18 (16-18) 758.2
    21 or 22 758.0
    autosomes NEC (*see also* Abnormality, autosomes) 758.5
      deletion 758.39
    Christchurch 758.39
    D$_1$ 758.1
    E$_3$ 758.2
    G 758.0
    mitochondrial 758.9
    mosaics 758.89
    sex 758.81
      complement, XO 758.6
      complement, XXX 758.81
      complement, XYY 758.81
      gonadal dysgenesis 758.6
      Klinefelter's 758.7
      Turner's 758.6
    trisomy 21 758.0
  cilia 743.9
  circulatory system 747.9
    specified type NEC 747.89
  clavicle 755.51
  clitoris 752.40
  coccyx 756.10
  colon 751.5
  common duct 751.60
  communication
    coronary artery 746.85
    left ventricle with right atrium 745.4
  concha (ear) 744.3
  connection
    renal vessels with kidney 747.62
    total pulmonary venous 747.41
  connective tissue 756.9
    specified type NEC 756.89
  cornea 743.9
    shape 743.41
    size 743.41
    specified type NEC 743.49
  coronary
    artery 746.85
    vein 746.89
  cranium—*see* Anomaly, skull
  cricoid cartilage 748.3
  cushion, endocardial 745.60
    specified type NEC 745.69
  cystic duct 751.60
  dental arch 524.20
    specified NEC 524.29
  dental arch relationship 524.20
    angle's class I 524.21
    angle's class II 524.22
    angle's class III 524.23
    articulation
      anterior 524.27
      posterior 524.27

Anomaly, anomalous—continued
    reverse 524.27
    disto-occlusion 524.22
      division I 524.22
      division II 524.22
    excessive horizontal overlap 524.26
    interarch distance (excessive) (inadequate) 524.28
    mesio-occlusion 524.23
    neutro-occlusion 524.21
    open
      anterior occlusal relationship 524.24
      posterior occlusal relationship 524.25
    specified NEC 524.29
  dentition 520.6
  dentofacial NEC 524.9
    functional 524.50
    specified type NEC 524.89
  dermatoglyphic 757.2
  Descemet's membrane 743.9
    specified type NEC 743.49
  development
    cervix 752.40
    vagina 752.40
    vulva 752.40
  diaphragm, diaphragmatic (apertures) NEC 756.6
  digestive organ(s) or system 751.9
    lower 751.5
    specified type NEC 751.8
    upper 750.9
  distribution, coronary artery 746.85
  ductus
    arteriosus 747.0
    Botalli 747.0
  duodenum 751.5
  dura 742.9
    brain 742.4
    spinal cord 742.59
  ear 744.3
    causing impairment of hearing 744.00
      specified type NEC 744.09
    external 744.3
      causing impairment of hearing 744.02
      specified type NEC 744.29
    inner (causing impairment of hearing) 744.05
    middle, except ossicles (causing impairment of hearing) 744.03
      ossicles 744.04
    ossicles 744.04
    prominent auricle 744.29
    specified type NEC 744.29
      with hearing impairment 744.09
  Ebstein's (heart) 746.2
    tricuspid valve 746.2
  ectodermal 757.9
  Eisenmenger's (ventricular septal defect) 745.4
  ejaculatory duct 752.9
    specified type NEC 752.89
  elbow (joint) 755.50
  endocardial cushion 745.60
    specified type NEC 745.69
  endocrine gland NEC 759.2
  epididymis 752.9
  epiglottis 748.3
  esophagus 750.9
    specified type NEC 750.4
  Eustachian tube 744.3
    specified type NEC 744.24
  eye (any part) 743.9
    adnexa 743.9

Anomaly, anomalous—*continued*
   specified type NEC 743.69
  anophthalmos 743.00
  anterior
    chamber and related structures 743.9
     angle 743.9
      specified type NEC 743.44
     specified type NEC 743.44
    segment 743.9
     combined 743.48
     multiple 743.48
     specified type NEC 743.49
  cataract (*see also* Cataract) 743.30
  glaucoma (*see also* Buphthalmia) 743.20
  lid 743.9
    specified type NEC 743.63
  microphthalmos (*see also* Microphthalmos) 743.10
  posterior segment 743.9
    specified type NEC 743.59
    vascular 743.58
    vitreous 743.9
     specified type NEC 743.51
  ptosis (eyelid) 743.61
  retina 743.9
    specified type NEC 743.59
  sclera 743.9
    specified type NEC 743.47
  specified type NEC 743.8
  eyebrow 744.89
  eyelid 743.9
    specified type NEC 743.63
  face (any part) 744.9
    bone(s) 756.0
    specified type NEC 744.89
  fallopian tube 752.10
    specified type NEC 752.19
  fascia 756.9
    specified type NEC 756.89
  femur 755.60
  fibula 755.60
  finger 755.50
    supernumerary 755.01
    webbed (*see also* Syndactylism, fingers) 755.11
  fixation, intestine 751.4
  flexion (joint) 755.9
    hip or thigh (*see also* Dislocation, hip, congenital) 754.30
  folds, heart 746.9
  foot 755.67
  foramen
    Botalli 745.5
    ovale 745.5
  forearm 755.50
  forehead (*see also* Anomaly, skull) 756.0
  form, teeth 520.2
  fovea centralis 743.9
  frontal bone (*see also* Anomaly, skull) 756.0
  gallbladder 751.60
  Gartner's duct 752.41
  gastrointestinal tract 751.9
    specified type NEC 751.8
    vessel 747.61
  genitalia, genital organ(s) or system
    female 752.9
     external 752.40
      specified type NEC 752.49
     internal NEC 752.9
    male (external and internal) 752.9
     epispadias 752.62
     hidden penis 752.65
     hydrocele, congenital 778.6

Anomaly, anomalous—*continued*
     hypospadias 752.61
     micropenis 752.64
     testis, undescended 752.51
      retractile 752.52
     specified type NEC 752.89
    genitourinary NEC 752.9
  Gerbode 745.4
  globe (eye) 743.9
  glottis 748.3
  granulation or granulocyte, genetic 288.2
    constitutional 288.2
    leukocyte 288.2
  gum 750.9
  gyri 742.9
  hair 757.9
    specified type NEC 757.4
  hand 755.50
  hard tissue formation in pulp 522.3
  head (*see also* Anomaly, skull) 756.0
  heart 746.9
    auricle 746.9
    bands 746.9
    fibroelastosis cordis 425.3
    folds 746.9
    malposition 746.87
    maternal, affecting fetus or newborn 760.3
    obstructive NEC 746.84
    patent ductus arteriosus (Botalli) 747.0
    septum 745.9
     acquired 429.71
     aortic 745.0
     aorticopulmonary 745.0
     atrial 745.5
     auricular 745.5
     between aorta and pulmonary artery 745.0
     endocardial cushion type 745.60
      specified type NEC 745.69
     interatrial 745.5
     interventricular 745.4
      with pulmonary stenosis or atresia, dextraposition of aorta, and hypertrophy of right ventricle 745.2
      acquired 429.71
     specified type NEC 745.8
     ventricular 745.4
      with pulmonary stenosis or atresia, dextraposition of aorta, and hypertrophy of right ventricle 745.2
      acquired 429.71
    specified type NEC 746.89
    tetralogy of Fallot 745.2
    valve NEC 746.9
     aortic 746.9
      atresia 746.89
      bicuspid valve 746.4
      insufficiency 746.4
      specified type NEC 746.89
      stenosis 746.3
       subaortic 746.81
       supravalvular 747.22
     mitral 746.9
      atresia 746.89
      insufficiency 746.6
      specified type NEC 746.89
      stenosis 746.5
     pulmonary 746.00
      atresia 746.01
      insufficiency 746.09
      stenosis 746.02
       infundibular 746.83

Anomaly, anomalous—*continued*
    subvalvular 746.83
    tricuspid 746.9
      atresia 746.1
      stenosis 746.1
    ventricle 746.9
  heel 755.67
  Hegglin's 288.2
  hemianencephaly 740.0
  hemicephaly 740.0
  hemicrania 740.0
  hepatic duct 751.60
  hip (joint) 755.63
  hourglass
    bladder 753.8
    gallbladder 751.69
    stomach 750.7
  humerus 755.50
  hymen 752.40
  hypersegmentation of neutrophils, hereditary 288.2
  hypophyseal 759.2
  ileocecal (coil) (valve) 751.5
  ileum (intestine) 751.5
  ilium 755.60
  integument 757.9
    specified type NEC 757.8
  interarch distance (excessive) (inadequate) 524.28
  intervertebral cartilage or disc 756.10
  intestine (large) (small) 751.5
    fixational type 751.4
  iris 743.9
    specified type NEC 743.46
  ischium 755.60
  jaw NEC 524.9
    closure 524.51
    size NEC 524.00
    specified type NEC 524.89
  jaw-cranial base relationship 524.10
    specified NEC 524.19
  jejunum 751.5
  joint 755.9
    hip
      dislocation (*see also* Dislocation, hip, congenital) 754.30
      predislocation (*see also* Subluxation, congenital, hip) 754.32
      preluxation (*see also* Subluxation, congenital, hip) 754.32
      subluxation (*see also* Subluxation, congenital, hip) 754.32
    lumbosacral 756.10
      spondylolisthesis 756.12
      spondylosis 756.11
    multiple arthrogryposis 754.89
    sacroiliac 755.69
  Jordan's 288.2
  kidney(s) (calyx) (pelvis) 753.9
    vessel 747.62
  Klippel-Feil (brevicollis) 756.16
  knee (joint) 755.64
  labium (majus) (minus) 752.40
  labyrinth, membranous (causing impairment of hearing) 744.05
  lacrimal
    apparatus, duct or passage 743.9
      specified type NEC 743.65
    gland 743.9
      specified type NEC 743.64
  Langdon Down (mongolism) 758.0

Anomaly, anomalous—*continued*
  larynx, laryngeal (muscle) 748.3
    web, webbed 748.2
  leg (lower) (upper) 755.60
    reduction NEC (*see also* Deformity, reduction, lower limb) 755.30
  lens 743.9
    shape 743.36
    specified type NEC 743.39
  leukocytes, genetic 288.2
    granulation (constitutional) 288.2
  lid (fold) 743.9
  ligament 756.9
    broad 752.10
    round 752.9
  limb, except reduction deformity 755.9
    lower 755.60
      reduction deformity (*see also* Deformity, reduction, lower limb) 755.30
      specified type NEC 755.69
    upper 755.50
      reduction deformity (*see also* Deformity, reduction, upper limb) 755.20
      specified type NEC 755.59
  lip 750.9
    harelip (*see also* Cleft, lip) 749.10
    specified type NEC 750.26
  liver (duct) 751.60
    atresia 751.69
  lower extremity 755.60
    vessel 747.64
  lumbosacral (joint) (region) 756.10
  lung (fissure) (lobe) NEC 748.60
    agenesis 748.5
    specified type NEC 748.69
  lymphatic system 759.9
  Madelung's (radius) 755.54
  mandible 524.9
    size NEC 524.00
  maxilla 524.9
    size NEC 524.00
  May (-Hegglin) 288.2
  meatus urinarius 753.9
    specified type NEC 753.8
  meningeal bands or folds, constriction of 742.8
  meninges 742.9
    brain 742.4
    spinal 742.59
  meningocele (*see also* Spina bifida) 741.9
  mesentery 751.9
  metacarpus 755.50
  metatarsus 755.67
  middle ear, except ossicles (causing impairment of hearing) 744.03
    ossicles 744.04
  mitral (leaflets) (valve) 746.9
    atresia 746.89
    insufficiency 746.6
    specified type NEC 746.89
    stenosis 746.5
  mouth 750.9
    specified type NEC 750.26
  multiple NEC 759.7
    specified type NEC 759.89
  muscle 756.9
    eye 743.9
      specified type NEC 743.69
    specified type NEC 756.89
  musculoskeletal system, except limbs 756.9
    specified type NEC 756.9

INDEX TO DISEASES

Anomaly, anomalous—*continued*
  nail 757.9
    specified type NEC 757.5
  narrowness, eyelid 743.62
  nasal sinus or septum 748.1
  neck (any part) 744.9
    specified type NEC 744.89
  nerve 742.9
    acoustic 742.9
      specified type NEC 742.8
    optic 742.9
      specified type NEC 742.8
    specified type NEC 742.8
  nervous system NEC 742.9
    brain 742.9
      specified type NEC 742.4
    specified type NEC 742.8
  neurological 742.9
  nipple 757.6
  nonteratogenic NEC 754.89
  nose, nasal (bone) (cartilage) (septum) (sinus) 748.1
  ocular muscle 743.9
  omphalomesenteric duct 751.0
  opening, pulmonary veins 747.49
  optic
    disc 743.9
      specified type NEC 743.57
    nerve 742.9
  opticociliary vessels 743.9
  orbit (eye) 743.9
    specified type NEC 743.66
  organ
    of Corti (causing impairment of hearing) 744.05
    or site 759.9
      specified type NEC 759.89
  origin
    both great arteries from same ventricle 745.11
    coronary artery 746.85
    innominate artery 747.69
    left coronary artery from pulmonary artery 746.85
    pulmonary artery 747.3
    renal vessels 747.62
    subclavian artery (left) (right) 747.21
  osseous meatus (ear) 744.03
  ovary 752.0
  oviduct 752.10
  palate (hard) (soft) 750.9
    cleft (*see also* Cleft, palate) 749.00
  pancreas (duct) 751.7
  papillary muscles 746.9
  parathyroid gland 759.2
  paraurethral ducts 753.9
  parotid (gland) 750.9
  patella 755.64
  Pelger-Huët (hereditary hyposegmentation) 288.2
  pelvic girdle 755.60
    specified type NEC 755.69
  pelvis (bony) 755.60
    complicating delivery 653.0
    rachitic 268.1
      fetal 756.4
  penis (glans) 752.69
  pericardium 746.89
  peripheral vascular system NEC 747.60
    gastrointestinal 747.61
    lower limb 747.64
    renal 747.62

Anomaly, anomalous—*continued*
    specified site NEC 747.69
    spinal 747.82
    upper limb 747.63
  Peter's 743.44
  pharynx 750.9
    branchial cleft 744.41
    specified type NEC 750.29
  Pierre Robin 756.0
  pigmentation NEC 709.00
    congenital 757.33
  pituitary (gland) 759.2
  pleural folds 748.8
  portal vein 747.40
  position tooth, teeth 524.30
    crowding 524.31
    displacement 524.30
      horizontal 524.33
      vertical 524.34
    distance
      interocclusal
        excessive 524.37
        insufficient 524.36
    excessive spacing 524.32
    rotation 524.35
    specified NEC 524.39
  preauricular sinus 744.46
  prepuce 752.9
  prostate 752.9
  pulmonary 748.60
    artery 747.3
    circulation 747.3
    specified type NEC 748.69
    valve 746.00
      atresia 746.01
      insufficiency 746.09
      specified type NEC 746.09
      stenosis 746.02
        infundibular 746.83
        subvalvular 746.83
    vein 747.40
    venous
      connection 747.49
        partial 747.42
        total 747.41
      return 747.49
        partial 747.42
        total (TAPVR) (complete) (subdiaphragmatic) (supradiaphragmatic) 747.41
  pupil 743.9
  pylorus 750.9
    hypertrophy 750.5
    stenosis 750.5
  rachitic, fetal 756.4
  radius 755.50
  rectovaginal (septum) 752.40
  rectum 751.5
  refraction 367.9
  renal 753.9
    vessel 747.62
  respiratory system 748.9
    specified type NEC 748.8
  rib 756.3
    cervical 756.2
  Rieger's 743.44
  rings, trachea 748.3
  rotation—*see also* Malrotation
    hip or thigh (*see also* Subluxation, congenital, hip) 754.32
  round ligament 752.9

Anomaly, anomalous—*continued*
  sacroiliac (joint) 755.69
  sacrum 756.10
  saddle
    back 754.2
    nose 754.0
      syphilitic 090.5
  salivary gland or duct 750.9
    specified type NEC 750.26
  scapula 755.50
  sclera 743.9
    specified type NEC 743.47
  scrotum 752.9
  sebaceous gland 757.9
  seminal duct or tract 752.9
  sense organs 742.9
    specified type NEC 742.8
  septum
    heart—*see* Anomaly, heart, septum
    nasal 748.1
  sex chromosomes NEC (*see also* Anomaly, chromosomes) 758.81
    shoulder (girdle) (joint) 755.50
    specified type NEC 755.59
  sigmoid (flexure) 751.5
  sinus of Valsalva 747.29
  site NEC 759.9
  skeleton generalized NEC 756.50
  skin (appendage) 757.9
    specified type NEC 757.39
  skull (bone) 756.0
    with
      anencephalus 740.0
      encephalocele 742.0
      hydrocephalus 742.3
        with spina bifida (*see also* Spina bifida) 741.0
      microcephalus 742.1
  specified type NEC
    adrenal (gland) 759.1
    alimentary tract (complete) (partial) 751.8
      lower 751.5
      upper 750.8
    ankle 755.69
    anus, anal (canal) 751.5
    aorta, aortic 747.29
      arch 747.21
    appendix 751.5
    arm 755.59
    artery (peripheral) NEC (*see also* Anomaly, peripheral vascular system) 747.60
      brain 747.81
      coronary 746.85
      eye 743.58
      pulmonary 747.3
      retinal 743.58
      umbilical 747.5
    auditory canal 744.29
      causing impairment of hearing 744.02
    bile duct or passage 751.69
    bladder 753.8
      neck 753.8
    bone(s) 756.9
      arm 755.59
      face 756.0
      leg 755.69
      pelvic girdle 755.69
      shoulder girdle 755.59
      skull 756.0
        with
          anencephalus 740.0

Anomaly, anomalous—*continued*
        encephalocele 742.0
        hydrocephalus 742.3
          with spina bifida (*see also* Spina bifida) 741.0
        microcephalus 742.1
  brain 742.4
  breast 757.6
  broad ligament 752.19
  bronchus 748.3
  canal of Nuck 752.89
  cardiac septal closure 745.8
  carpus 755.59
  cartilaginous 756.9
  cecum 751.5
  cervix 752.49
  chest (wall) 756.3
  chin 744.89
  ciliary body 743.46
  circulatory system 747.89
  clavicle 755.51
  clitoris 752.49
  coccyx 756.19
  colon 751.5
  common duct 751.69
  connective tissue 756.89
  cricoid cartilage 748.3
  cystic duct 751.69
  diaphragm 756.6
  digestive organ(s) or tract 751.8
    lower 751.5
    upper 750.8
  duodenum 751.5
  ear 744.29
    auricle 744.29
      causing impairment of hearing 744.02
    causing impairment of hearing 744.09
    inner (causing impairment of hearing) 744.05
    middle, except ossicles 744.03
      ossicles 744.04
  ejaculatory duct 752.89
  endocrine 759.2
  epiglottis 748.3
  esophagus 750.4
  Eustachian tube 744.24
  eye 743.8
    lid 743.63
    muscle 743.69
  face 744.89
    bone(s) 756.0
  fallopian tube 752.19
  fascia 756.89
  femur 755.69
  fibula 755.69
  finger 755.59
  foot 755.67
  fovea centralis 743.55
  gallbladder 751.69
  Gartner's duct 752.89
  gastrointestinal tract 751.8
  genitalia, genital organ(s)
    female 752.89
      external 752.49
      internal NEC 752.89
    male 752.89
      penis 752.69
      scrotal transposition 752.81
  genitourinary tract NEC 752.89
  glottis 748.3
  hair 757.4

INDEX TO DISEASES

Anomaly, anomalous

Anomaly, anomalous—*continued*
  hand 755.59
  heart 746.89
    valve NEC 746.89
      pulmonary 746.09
  hepatic duct 751.69
  hydatid of Morgagni 752.89
  hymen 752.49
  integument 757.8
  intestine (large) (small) 751.5
    fixational type 751.4
  iris 743.46
  jejunum 751.5
  joint 755.8
  kidney 753.3
  knee 755.64
  labium (majus) (minus) 752.49
  labyrinth, membranous 744.05
  larynx 748.3
  leg 755.69
  lens 743.39
  limb, except reduction deformity 755.8
    lower 755.69
      reduction deformity (*see also* Deformity, reduction, lower limb) 755.30
    upper 755.59
      reduction deformity (*see also* Deformity, reduction, upper limb) 755.20
  lip 750.26
  liver 751.69
  lung (fissure) (lobe) 748.69
  meatus urinarius 753.8
  metacarpus 755.59
  mouth 750.26
  muscle 756.89
    eye 743.69
  musculoskeletal system, except limbs 756.9
  nail 757.5
  neck 744.89
  nerve 742.8
    acoustic 742.8
    optic 742.8
  nervous system 742.8
  nipple 757.6
  nose 748.1
  organ NEC 759.89
    of Corti 744.05
  osseous meatus (ear) 744.03
  ovary 752.0
  oviduct 752.19
  pancreas 751.7
  parathyroid 759.2
  patella 755.64
  pelvic girdle 755.69
  penis 752.69
  pericardium 746.89
  peripheral vascular system NEC (*see also* Anomaly, peripheral vascular system) 747.60
  pharynx 750.29
  pituitary 759.2
  prostate 752.89
  radius 755.59
  rectum 751.5
  respiratory system 748.8
  rib 756.3
  round ligament 752.89
  sacrum 756.19
  salivary duct or gland 750.26
  scapula 755.59
  sclera 743.47

Anomaly, anomalous—*continued*
  scrotum 752.89
    transposition 752.81
  seminal duct or tract 752.89
  shoulder girdle 755.59
  site NEC 759.89
  skin 757.39
  skull (bone(s)) 756.0
    with
      anencephalus 740.0
      encephalocele 742.0
      hydrocephalus 742.3
        with spina bifida (*see also* Spina bifida) 741.0
      microcephalus 742.1
  specified organ or site NEC 759.89
  spermatic cord 752.89
  spinal cord 742.59
  spine 756.19
  spleen 759.0
  sternum 756.3
  stomach 750.7
  tarsus 755.67
  tendon 756.89
  testis 752.89
  thorax (wall) 756.3
  thymus 759.2
  thyroid (gland) 759.2
    cartilage 748.3
  tibia 755.69
  toe 755.66
  tongue 750.19
  trachea (cartilage) 748.3
  ulna 755.59
  urachus 753.7
  ureter 753.4
    obstructive 753.29
  urethra 753.8
    obstructive 753.6
  urinary tract 753.8
  uterus 752.3
  uvula 750.26
  vagina 752.49
  vascular NEC (*see also* Anomaly, peripheral vascular system) 747.60
    brain 747.81
  vas deferens 752.89
  vein(s) (peripheral) NEC (*see also* Anomaly, peripheral vascular system) 747.60
    brain 747.81
    great 747.49
    portal 747.49
    pulmonary 747.49
  vena cava (inferior) (superior) 747.49
  vertebra 756.19
  vulva 752.49
spermatic cord 752.9
spine, spinal 756.10
  column 756.10
  cord 742.9
    meningocele (*see also* Spina bifida) 741.9
    specified type NEC 742.59
    spina bifida (*see also* Spina bifida) 741.9
    vessel 747.82
  meninges 742.59
  nerve root 742.9
spleen 759.0
Sprengel's 755.52
sternum 756.3
stomach 750.9
  specified type NEC 750.7

815

Anomaly, anomalous—*continued*
  submaxillary gland 750.9
  superior vena cava 747.40
  talipes—*see* Talipes
  tarsus 755.67
    with complete absence of distal elements 755.31
  teeth, tooth NEC 520.9
    position 524.30
      crowding 524.31
      displacement 524.30
        horizontal 524.33
        vertical 524.34
      distance
        interocclusal
          excessive 524.37
          insufficient 524.36
      excessive spacing 524.32
      rotation 524.35
      specified NEC 524.39
    spacing 524.30
  tendon 756.9
    specified type NEC 756.89
  termination
    coronary artery 746.85
  testis 752.9
  thebesian valve 746.9
  thigh 755.60
    flexion (*see also* Subluxation, congenital, hip) 754.32
  thorax (wall) 756.3
  throat 750.9
  thumb 755.50
    supernumerary 755.01
  thymus gland 759.2
  thyroid (gland) 759.2
    cartilage 748.3
  tibia 755.60
    saber 090.5
  toe 755.66
    supernumerary 755.02
    webbed (*see also* Syndactylism, toes) 755.13
  tongue 750.10
    specified type NEC 750.19
  trachea, tracheal 748.3
    cartilage 748.3
    rings 748.3
  tragus 744.3
  transverse aortic arch 747.21
  trichromata 368.59
  trichromatopsia 368.59
  tricuspid (leaflet) (valve) 746.9
    atresia 746.1
    Ebstein's 746.2
    specified type NEC 746.89
    stenosis 746.1
  trunk 759.9
  Uhl's (hypoplasia of myocardium, right ventricle) 746.84
  ulna 755.50
  umbilicus 759.9
    artery 747.5
  union, trachea with larynx 748.3
  unspecified site 759.9
  upper extremity 755.50
    vessel 747.63
  urachus 753.7
    specified type NEC 753.7

Anomaly, anomalous—*continued*
  ureter 753.9
    obstructive 753.20
    specified type NEC 753.4
    obstructive 753.29
  urethra (valve) 753.9
    obstructive 753.6
    specified type NEC 753.8
  urinary tract or system (any part, except urachus) 753.9
    specified type NEC 753.8
    urachus 753.7
  uterus 752.3
    with only one functioning horn 752.3
    in pregnancy or childbirth 654.0
      affecting fetus or newborn 763.89
      causing obstructed labor 660.2
        affecting fetus or newborn 763.1
  uvula 750.9
  vagina 752.40
  valleculae 748.3
  valve (heart) NEC 746.9
    formation, ureter 753.29
    pulmonary 746.00
    specified type NEC 746.89
  vascular NEC (*see also* Anomaly, peripheral vascular system) 747.60
    ring 747.21
  vas deferens 752.9
  vein(s) (peripheral) NEC (*see also* Anomaly, peripheral vascular system) 747.60
    brain 747.81
    cerebral 747.81
    coronary 746.89
    great 747.40
      specified type NEC 747.49
    portal 747.40
    pulmonary 747.40
    retina 743.9
  vena cava (inferior) (superior) 747.40
  venous return (pulmonary) 747.49
    partial 747.42
    total 747.41
  ventricle, ventricular (heart) 746.9
    bands 746.9
    folds 746.9
    septa 745.4
  vertebra 756.10
  vesicourethral orifice 753.9
  vessels NEC (*see also* Anomaly, peripheral vascular system) 747.60
    optic papilla 743.9
  vitelline duct 751.0
  vitreous humor 743.9
    specified type NEC 743.51
  vulva 752.40
  wrist (joint) 755.50
Anomia 784.69
Anonychia 757.5
  acquired 703.8
Anophthalmos, anophthalmus (clinical) (congenital) (globe) 743.00
  acquired V45.78
Anopsia (altitudinal) (quadrant) 368.46
Anorchia 752.89
Anorchism, anorchidism 752.89
Anorexia 783.0
  hysterical 300.11
  nervosa 307.1

INDEX TO DISEASES   Anuria

Anosmia (*see also* Disturbance, sensation) 781.1
  hysterical 300.11
  postinfectional 478.9
  psychogenic 306.7
  traumatic 951.8
Anosognosia 780.99
Anosphrasia 781.1
Anosteoplasia 756.50
Anotia 744.09
Anovulatory cycle 628.0
Anoxemia 799.02
  newborn 770.88
Anoxia 799.02
  altitude 993.2
  cerebral 348.1
    with
      abortion—*see* Abortion, by type,
        with specified complication NEC
      ectopic pregnancy (*see also* categories
        633.0-633.9) 639.8
      molar pregnancy (*see also* categories
        630-632) 639.8
    complicating
      delivery (cesarean) (instrumental) 669.4
      ectopic or molar pregnancy 639.8
      obstetric anesthesia or sedation 668.2
      during or resulting from a procedure 997.01
    following
      abortion 639.8
      ectopic or molar pregnancy 639.8
    newborn (*see also* Distress, fetal, liveborn
      infant) 770.88
  due to drowning 994.1
  fetal, affecting newborn 770.88
  heart—*see* Insufficiency, coronary
  high altitude 993.2
  intrauterine
    fetal death (before onset of labor) 768.0
      during labor 768.1
    liveborn infant—*see* Distress, fetal, liveborn
      infant
  myocardial—*see* Insufficiency, coronary
  newborn 768.9
    mild or moderate 768.6
    severe 768.5
  pathological 799.02
Anteflexion —*see* Anteversion
Antenatal
  care, normal pregnancy V22.1
    first V22.0
  screening of mother (for) V28.9
    based on amniocentesis NEC V28.2
      chromosomal anomalies V28.0
      raised alphafetoprotein levels V28.1
    chromosomal anomalies V28.0
    fetal growth retardation using ultrasonics
      V28.4
    isoimmunization V28.5
    malformations using ultrasonics V28.3
    raised alphafetoprotein levels in amniotic fluid
      V28.1
    specified condition NEC V28.8
    Streptococcus B V28.6
Antepartum —*see* condition
Anterior —*see also* condition
  spinal artery compression syndrome 721.1
Antero-occlusion 524.24

Anteversion
  cervix (—*see* Anteversion, uterus)
  femur (neck), congenital 755.63
  uterus, uterine (cervix) (postinfectional)
    (postpartal, old) 621.6
    congenital 752.3
    in pregnancy or childbirth 654.4
      affecting fetus or newborn 763.89
      causing obstructed labor 660.2
        affecting fetus or newborn 763.1
Anthracosilicosis (occupational) 500
Anthracosis (lung) (occupational) 500
  lingua 529.3
Anthrax 022.9
  with pneumonia 022.1 *[484.5]*
  colitis 022.2
  cutaneous 022.0
  gastrointestinal 022.2
  intestinal 022.2
  pulmonary 022.1
  respiratory 022.1
  septicemia 022.3
  specified manifestation NEC 022.8
Anthropoid pelvis 755.69
  with disproportion (fetopelvic) 653.2
    affecting fetus or newborn 763.1
    causing obstructed labor 660.1
      affecting fetus or newborn 763.1
Anthropophobia 300.29
Antibioma, breast 611.0
Antibodies
  maternal (blood group) (*see also*
    Incompatibility) 656.2
  anti-D, cord blood 656.1
  fetus or newborn 773.0
Antibody deficiency syndrome
  agammaglobulinemic 279.00
  congenital 279.04
  hypogammaglobulinemic 279.00
Anticoagulant, circulating (*see also* Circulating
  anticoagulants) 286.5
Antimongolism syndrome 758.39
Antimonial cholera 985.4
Antisocial personality 301.7
Antithrombinemia (*see also* Circulating
  anticoagulants) 286.5
Antithromboplastinemia (*see also* Circulating
  anticoagulants) 286.5
Antithromboplastinogenemia (*see also*
  Circulating anticoagulants) 286.5
Antitoxin complication or reaction —*see*
  Complications, vaccination
Anton (-Babinski) syndrome
  (hemiasomatognosia) 307.9
Antritis (chronic) 473.0
  maxilla 473.0
    acute 461.0
  stomach 535.4
Antrum, antral —*see* condition
Anuria 788.5
  with
    abortion—*see* Abortion, by type, with renal
      failure
    ectopic pregnancy (*see also* categories
      633.0-633.9) 639.3
    molar pregnancy (*see also* categories 630-632)
      639.3
  calculus (impacted) (recurrent) 592.9
    kidney 592.0
    ureter 592.1
  congenital 753.3

Anuria—*continued*
  due to a procedure 997.5
  following
    abortion 639.3
    ectopic or molar pregnancy 639.3
  newborn 753.3
  postrenal 593.4
  puerperal, postpartum, childbirth 669.3
  specified as due to a procedure 997.5
  sulfonamide
    correct substance properly administered 788.5
    overdose or wrong substance given or taken 961.0
  traumatic (following crushing) 958.5
Anus, anal —*see* condition
Anusitis 569.49
Anxiety (neurosis) (reaction) (state) 300.00
  alcohol-induced 291.89
  depression 300.4
  drug-induced 292.89
  due to or associated with physical condition 293.84
  generalized 300.02
  hysteria 300.20
  in
    acute stress reaction 308.0
    transient adjustment reaction 309.24
  panic type 300.01
  separation, abnormal 309.21
  syndrome (organic) (transient) 293.84
Aorta, aortic —*see* condition
Aortectasia 441.9
Aortitis (nonsyphilitic) 447.6
  arteriosclerotic 440.0
  calcific 447.6
  Döhle-Heller 093.1
  luetic 093.1
  rheumatic (*see also* Endocarditis, acute, rheumatic) 391.1
  rheumatoid—*see* Arthritis, rheumatoid
  specific 093.1
  syphilitic 093.1
    congenital 090.5
Apathetic thyroid storm (*see also* Thyrotoxicosis) 242.9
Apepsia 536.8
  achlorhydric 536.0
  psychogenic 306.4
Aperistalsis, esophagus 530.0
Apert's syndrome (acrocephalosyndactyly) 755.55
Apert-Gallais syndrome (adrenogenital) 255.2
Apertognathia 524.20
Aphagia 787.20
  psychogenic 307.1
Aphakia (acquired) (bilateral) (postoperative) (unilateral) 379.31
  congenital 743.35
Aphalangia (congenital) 755.4
  lower limb (complete) (intercalary) (partial) (terminal) 755.39
    meaning all digits (complete) (partial) 755.31
    transverse 755.31
  upper limb (complete) (intercalary) (partial) (terminal) 755.29
    meaning all digits (complete) (partial) 755.21
    transverse 755.21

Aphasia (amnestic) (ataxic) (auditory) (Broca's) (choreatic) (classic) (expressive) (global) (ideational) (ideokinetic) (ideomotor) (jargon) (motor) (nominal) (receptive) (semantic) (sensory) (syntactic) (verbal) (visual) (Wernicke's) 784.3
  developmental 315.31
  syphilis, tertiary 094.89
  uremic—*see* Uremia
Aphemia 784.3
  uremic—*see* Uremia
Aphonia 784.41
  clericorum 784.49
  hysterical 300.11
  organic 784.41
  psychogenic 306.1
Aphthae, aphthous —*see also* condition
  Bednar's 528.2
  cachectic 529.0
  epizootic 078.4
  fever 078.4
  oral 528.2
  stomatitis 528.2
  thrush 112.0
  ulcer (oral) (recurrent) 528.2
    genital organ(s) NEC
      female 616.50
      male 608.89
    larynx 478.79
Apical —*see* condition
Apical ballooning syndrome 429.83
Aplasia —*see also* Agenesis
  alveolar process (acquired) 525.8
    congenital 750.26
  aorta (congenital) 747.22
  aortic valve (congenital) 746.89
  axialis extracorticalis (congenital) 330.0
  bone marrow (myeloid) 284.9
    acquired (secondary) 284.89
    congenital 284.01
    idiopathic 284.9
  brain 740.0
    specified part 742.2
  breast 757.6
  bronchus 748.3
  cementum 520.4
  cerebellar 742.2
  congenital (pure) red cell 284.01
  corpus callosum 742.2
  erythrocyte 284.81
    congenital 284.01
  extracortical axial 330.0
  eye (congenital) 743.00
  fovea centralis (congenital) 743.55
  germinal (cell) 606.0
  iris 743.45
  labyrinth, membranous 744.05
  limb (congenital) 755.4
    lower NEC 755.30
    upper NEC 755.20
  lung (bilateral) (congenital) (unilateral) 748.5
  nervous system NEC 742.8
  nuclear 742.8
  ovary 752.0
  Pelizaeus-Merzbacher 330.0
  prostate (congenital) 752.89

INDEX TO DISEASES

Aplasia—*continued*
  red cell (with thymoma) (adult) 284.81
    acquired (secondary) 284.81
    congenital 284.01
    hereditary 284.01
    of infants 284.01
    primary 284.01
    pure 284.01
  round ligament (congenital) 752.89
  salivary gland 750.21
  skin (congenital) 757.39
  spinal cord 742.59
  spleen 759.0
  testis (congenital) 752.89
  thymic, with immunodeficiency 279.2
  thyroid 243
  uterus 752.3
  ventral horn cell 742.59
Apleuria 756.3
Apnea, apneic (spells) 786.03
  newborn, neonatorum 770.81
    essential 770.81
    obstructive 770.82
    primary 770.81
    sleep 770.81
    specified NEC 770.82
  psychogenic 306.1
  sleep, unspecified 780.57
    with
      hypersomnia, unspecified 780.53
      hyposomnia, unspecified 780.51
      insomnia, unspecified 780.51
      sleep disturbance 780.57
    central, in conditions classified elsewhere 327.27
    obstructive (adult) (pediatric) 327.23
    organic 327.20
      other 327.29
    primary central 327.21
Apneumatosis newborn 770.4
Apodia 755.31
Apophysitis (bone) (*see also* Osteochondrosis) 732.9
  calcaneus 732.5
  juvenile 732.6
Apoplectiform convulsions (*see also* Disease, cerebrovascular, acute) 436
Apoplexia, apoplexy, apoplectic (*see also* Disease, cerebrovascular, acute) 436
  abdominal 569.89
  adrenal 036.3
  attack 436
  basilar (*see also* Disease, cerebrovascular, acute) 436
  brain (*see also* Disease, cerebrovascular, acute) 436
  bulbar (*see also* Disease, cerebrovascular, acute) 436
  capillary (*see also* Disease, cerebrovascular, acute) 436
  cardiac (*see also* Infarct, myocardium) 410.9
  cerebral (*see also* Disease, cerebrovascular, acute) 436
  chorea (*see also* Disease, cerebrovascular, acute) 436
  congestive (*see also* Disease, cerebrovascular, acute) 436
    newborn 767.4
  embolic (*see also* Embolism, brain) 434.1
  fetus 767.0
  fit (*see also* Disease, cerebrovascular, acute) 436

Appendicitis

Apoplexia, apoplexy, apoplectic—*continued*
  healed or old V12.54
  heart (auricle) (ventricle) (*see also* Infarct, myocardium) 410.9
  heat 992.0
  hemiplegia (*see also* Disease, cerebrovascular, acute) 436
  hemorrhagic (stroke) (*see also* Hemorrhage, brain) 432.9
  ingravescent (*see also* Disease, cerebrovascular, acute) 436
  late effect—*see* Late effect(s) (of) cerebrovascular disease
  lung—*see* Embolism, pulmonary
  meninges, hemorrhagic (*see also* Hemorrhage, subarachnoid) 430
  neonatorum 767.0
  newborn 767.0
  pancreatitis 577.0
  placenta 641.2
  progressive (*see also* Disease, cerebrovascular, acute) 436
  pulmonary (artery) (vein)—*see* Embolism, pulmonary
  sanguineous (*see also* Disease, cerebrovascular, acute) 436
  seizure (*see also* Disease, cerebrovascular, acute) 436
  serous (*see also* Disease, cerebrovascular, acute) 436
  spleen 289.59
  stroke (*see also* Disease, cerebrovascular, acute) 436
  thrombotic (*see also* Thrombosis, brain) 434.0
  uremic—*see* Uremia
  uteroplacental 641.2
Appendage
  fallopian tube (cyst of Morgagni) 752.11
  intestine (epiploic) 751.5
  preauricular 744.1
  testicular (organ of Morgagni) 752.89
Appendicitis 541
  with
    perforation, peritonitis (generalized), or rupture 540.0
      with peritoneal abscess 540.1
    peritoneal abscess 540.1
  acute (catarrhal) (fulminating) (gangrenous) (inflammatory) (obstructive) (retrocecal) (suppurative) 540.9
    with
      perforation, peritonitis, or rupture 540.0
        with peritoneal abscess 540.1
      peritoneal abscess 540.1
  amebic 006.8
  chronic (recurrent) 542
  exacerbation—*see* Appendicitis, acute
  fulminating—*see* Appendicitis, acute
  gangrenous—*see* Appendicitis, acute
  healed (obliterative) 542
  interval 542
  neurogenic 542
  obstructive 542
  pneumococcal 541
  recurrent 542
  relapsing 542
  retrocecal 541
  subacute (adhesive) 542
  subsiding 542
  suppurative—*see* Appendicitis, acute
  tuberculous (*see also* Tuberculosis) 014.8

Appendiclausis 543.9
Appendicolithiasis 543.9
Appendicopathia oxyurica 127.4
Appendix, appendicular —*see also* condition
   Morgagni (male) 752.89
      fallopian tube 752.11
Appetite
   depraved 307.52
   excessive 783.6
      psychogenic 307.51
   lack or loss (*see also* Anorexia) 783.0
      nonorganic origin 307.59
   perverted 307.52
      hysterical 300.11
Apprehension, apprehensiveness (abnormal) (state) 300.00
   specified type NEC 300.09
Approximal wear 521.10
Apraxia (classic) (ideational) (ideokinetic) (ideomotor) (motor) 784.69
   oculomotor, congenital 379.51
   verbal 784.69
Aptyalism 527.7
Aqueous misdirection 365.83
Arabicum elephantiasis (*see also* Infestation, filarial) 125.9
Arachnidism 989.5
Arachnitis —*see* Meningitis
Arachnodactyly 759.82
Arachnoidism 989.5
Arachnoiditis (acute) (adhesive) (basic) (brain) (cerebrospinal) (chiasmal) (chronic) (spinal) (*see also* Meningitis) 322.9
   meningococcal (chronic) 036.0
   syphilitic 094.2
   tuberculous (*see also* Tuberculosis, meninges) 013.0
Araneism 989.5
Arboencephalitis, Australian 062.4
Arborization block (heart) 426.6
Arbor virus, arbovirus (infection) NEC 066.9
ARC 042
Arches —*see* condition
Arcuatus uterus 752.3
Arcus (cornea)
   juvenilis 743.43
      interfering with vision 743.42
   senilis 371.41
Arc-welders' lung 503
Arc-welders' syndrome (photokeratitis) 370.24
Areflexia 796.1
Areola —*see* condition
Argentaffinoma (M8241/1)—*see also* Neoplasm, by site, uncertain behavior
   benign (M8241/0)—*see* Neoplasm, by site, benign
   malignant (M8241/3)—*see* Neoplasm, by site, malignant
   syndrome 259.2
Argentinian hemorrhagic fever 078.7
Arginosuccinicaciduria 270.6
Argonz-Del Castillo syndrome (nonpuerperal galactorrhea and amenorrhea) 253.1
Argyll-Robertson phenomenon pupil, or syndrome (syphilitic) 094.89
   atypical 379.45
   nonluetic 379.45
   nonsyphilitic 379.45
   reversed 379.45

Argyria, argyriasis NEC 985.8
   conjunctiva 372.55
   cornea 371.16
   from drug or medicinal agent
      correct substance properly administered 709.09
      overdose or wrong substance given or taken 961.2
Arhinencephaly 742.2
Arias-Stella phenomenon 621.30
Ariboflavinosis 266.0
Arizona enteritis 008.1
Arm —*see* condition
Armenian disease 277.31
Arnold-Chiari obstruction or syndrome (*see also* Spina bifida) 741.0
   type I 348.4
   type II (*see also* Spina bifida) 741.0
   type III 742.0
   type IV 742.2
Arousals
   confusional 327.41
Arrest, arrested
   active phase of labor 661.1
      affecting fetus or newborn 763.7
   any plane in pelvis
      complicating delivery 660.1
         affecting fetus or newborn 763.1
   bone marrow (*see also* Anemia, aplastic) 284.9
   cardiac 427.5
      with
         abortion—*see* Abortion, by type, with specified complication NEC
         ectopic pregnancy (*see also* categories 633.0-633.9) 639.8
         molar pregnancy (*see also* categories 630-632) 639.8
      complicating
         anesthesia
            correct substance properly administered 427.5
            obstetric 668.1
            overdose or wrong substance given 968.4
               specified anesthetic—*see* Table of drugs and chemicals
         delivery (cesarean) (instrumental) 669.4
         ectopic or molar pregnancy 639.8
         surgery (nontherapeutic) (therapeutic) 997.1
      fetus or newborn 779.85
      following
         abortion 639.8
         ectopic or molar pregnancy 639.8
      personal history, successfully rescucitated V12.53
      postoperative (immediate) 997.1
         long-term effect of cardiac surgery 429.4
   cardiorespiratory (*see also* Arrest, cardiac) 427.5
   deep transverse 660.3
      affecting fetus or newborn 763.1
   development or growth
      bone 733.91
      child 783.40
      fetus 764.9
         affecting management of pregnancy 656.5
      tracheal rings 748.3
   epiphyseal 733.91
   granulopoiesis 288.09
   heart—*see* Arrest, cardiac
   respiratory 799.1
      newborn 770.87
   sinus 426.6
   transverse (deep) 660.3
      affecting fetus or newborn 763.1

INDEX TO DISEASES

Arteriosclerosis, arteriosclerotic

Arrhenoblastoma (M8630.1)
  benign (M8630/0)
    specified site—*see* Neoplasm, by site, benign
    unspecified site
      female 220
      male 222.0
  malignant (M8630/3)
    specified site— *see* Neoplasm, by site, malignant
    unspecified site
      female 183.0
      male 186.9
  specified site—*see* Neoplasm, by site, uncertain behavior
  unspecified site
    female 236.2
    male 236.4
Arrhinencephaly 742.2
  due to
    trisomy 13 (13-15) 758.1
    trisomy 18 (16-18) 758.2
Arrhythmia (auricle) (cardiac) (cordis) (gallop rhythm) (juvenile) (nodal) (reflex) (sinus) (supraventricular) (transitory) (ventricle) 427.9
  bigeminal rhythm 427.89
  block 426.9
  bradycardia 427.89
  contractions, premature 427.60
  coronary sinus 427.89
  ectopic 427.89
  extrasystolic 427.60
  postoperative 997.1
  psychogenic 306.2
  vagal 780.2
Arrillaga-Ayerza syndrome (pulmonary artery sclerosis with pulmonary hypertension) 416.0
Arsenical
  dermatitis 692.4
  keratosis 692.4
  pigmentation 985.1
    from drug or medicinal agent
      correct substance properly administered 709.09
      overdose or wrong substance given or taken 961.1
Arsenism 985.1
  from drug or medicinal agent
    correct substance properly administered 692.4
    overdose or wrong substance given or taken 961.1
Arterial —*see* condition
Arteriectasis 447.8
Arteriofibrosis —*see* Arteriosclerosis
Arteriolar sclerosis —*see* Arteriosclerosis
Arteriolith —*see* Arteriosclerosis
Arteriolitis 447.6
  necrotizing, kidney 447.5
  renal—*see* Hypertension, kidney
Arteriolosclerosis —*see* Arteriosclerosis
Arterionephrosclerosis (*see also* Hypertension, kidney) 403.90
Arteriopathy 447.9
Arteriosclerosis, arteriosclerotic (artery) (deformans) (diffuse) (disease) (endarteritis) (general) (obliterans) (obliterative) (occlusive) (senile) (with calcification) 440.9
  with
    gangrene 440.24
    psychosis (*see also* Psychosis, arteriosclerotic) 290.40
    ulceration 440.23

Arteriosclerosis, arteriosclerotic—*continued*
  aorta 440.0
  arteries of extremities NEC — *see* Arteriosclerosis, extremities
  basilar (artery) (*see also* Occlusion, artery, basilar) 433.0
  brain 437.0
  bypass graft
    coronary artery 414.05
      autologous artery (gastroepiploic) (internal mammary) 414.04
      autologous vein 414.02
      nonautologous biological 414.03
      of transplanted heart 414.07
    extremity 440.30
      autologous vein 440.31
      nonautologous biological 440.32
  cardiac — *see* Arteriosclerosis, coronary
  cardiopathy — *see* Arteriosclerosis, coronary
  cardiorenal (*see also* Hypertension, cardiorenal) 404.90
  cardiovascular (*see also* Disease, cardiovascular) 429.2
  carotid (artery) (common) (internal) (*see also* Occlusion, artery, carotid) 433.1
  central nervous system 437.0
  cerebral 437.0
    late effect—*see* Late effect(s) (of) cerebrovascular disease
  cerebrospinal 437.0
  cerebrovascular 437.0
  coronary (artery) 414.00
    graft—*see* Arteriosclerosis, bypass graft
    native artery 414.01
    of transplanted heart 414.06
  of transplanted heart 414.06
  extremities (native artery) 440.20
    bypass graft 440.30
      autologous vein 440.31
      nonautologous biological 440.32
    claudication (intermittent) 440.21
    and
      gangrene 440.24
      rest pain 440.22
        and
          gangrene 440.24
          ulceration 440.23
            and gangrene 440.24
      ulceration 440.23
        and gangrene 440.24
    gangrene 440.24
    rest pain 440.22
      and
        gangrene 440.24
        ulceration 440.23
          and gangrene 440.24
    specified site NEC 440.29
    ulceration 440.23
      and gangrene 440.24
  heart (disease) — *see also* Arteriosclerosis, coronary
    valve 424.99
      aortic 424.1
      mitral 424.0
      pulmonary 424.3
      tricuspid 424.2
  kidney (*see also* Hypertension, kidney) 403.90
  labyrinth, labyrinthine 388.00
  medial NEC 440.20
  mesentery (artery) 557.1
  Mönckeberg's 440.20

Arteriosclerosis, arteriosclerotic—*continued*
    myocarditis 429.0
    nephrosclerosis (*see also* Hypertension, kidney) 403.90
    peripheral (of extremities) *see* Arteriosclerosis, extremities
    precerebral 433.9
        specified artery NEC 433.8
    pulmonary (idiopathic) 416.0
    renal (*see also* Hypertension, kidney) 403.90
        arterioles (*see also* Hypertension, kidney) 403.90
        artery 440.1
    retinal (vascular) 440.8 *[362.13]*
    specified artery NEC 440.8
        with gangrene 440.8 *[785.4]*
    spinal (cord) 437.0
    vertebral (artery) (*see also* Occlusion, artery, vertebral) 433.2
Arteriospasm 443.9
Arteriovenous —*see* condition
Arteritis 447.6
    allergic (*see also* Angiitis, hypersensitivity) 446.20
    aorta (nonsyphilitic) 447.6
        syphilitic 093.1
    aortic arch 446.7
    brachiocephalica 446.7
    brain 437.4
        syphilitic 094.89
    branchial 446.7
    cerebral 437.4
        late effect—*see* Late effect(s) (of) cerebrovascular disease
        syphilitic 094.89
    coronary (artery) —*see also* Arteriosclerosis, coronary
        rheumatic 391.9
            chronic 398.99
        syphilitic 093.89
    cranial (left) (right) 446.5
    deformans—*see* Arteriosclerosis
    giant cell 446.5
    necrosing or necrotizing 446.0
    nodosa 446.0
    obliterans—*see also* Arteriosclerosis
        subclaviocarotica 446.7
    pulmonary 417.8
    retina 362.18
    rheumatic—*see* Fever, rheumatic
    senile—*see* Arteriosclerosis
    suppurative 447.2
    syphilitic (general) 093.89
        brain 094.89
        coronary 093.89
        spinal 094.89
    temporal 446.5
    young female, syndrome 446.7
Artery, arterial —*see* condition
Arthralgia (*see also* Pain, joint) 719.4
    allergic (*see also* Pain, joint) 719.4
    in caisson disease 993.3
    psychogenic 307.89
    rubella 056.71
    Salmonella 003.23
    temporomandibular joint 524.62

Arthritis, arthritic (acute) (chronic) (subacute) 716.9

> Note—Use the following fifth-digit subclassification with categories 711-712, 715-716:
>
> 0 site unspecified
> 1 shoulder region
> 2 upper arm
> 3 forearm
> 4 hand
> 5 pelvic region and thigh
> 6 lower leg
> 7 ankle and foot
> 8 other specified sites
> 9 multiple sites

allergic 716.2
ankylosing (crippling) (spine) 720.0
    sites other than spine 716.9
atrophic 714.0
    spine 720.9
back (*see also* Arthritis, spine) 721.90
Bechterew's (ankylosing spondylitis) 720.0
blennorrhagic 098.50
cervical, cervicodorsal (*see also* Spondylosis, cervical) 721.0
Charcot's 094.0 *[713.5]*
    diabetic 250.6 *[713.5]*
    syringomyelic 336.0 *[713.5]*
    tabetic 094.0 *[713.5]*
chylous (*see also* Filariasis) 125.9 *[711.7]*
climacteric NEC 716.3
coccyx 721.8
cricoarytenoid 478.79
crystal (-induced)—*see* Arthritis, due to crystals
deformans (*see also* Osteoarthrosis) 715.9
    spine 721.90
        with myelopathy 721.91
degenerative (*see also* Osteoarthrosis) 715.9
    idiopathic 715.09
    polyarticular 715.09
    spine 721.90
        with myelopathy 721.91
dermatoarthritis, lipoid 272.8 *[713.0]*
due to or associated with
    acromegaly 253.0 *[713.0]*
    actinomycosis 039.8 *[711.4]*
    amyloidosis 277.39 *[713.7]*
    bacterial disease NEC 040.89 *[711.4]*
    Behçet's syndrome 136.1 *[711.2]*
    blastomycosis 116.0 *[711.6]*
    brucellosis (*see also* Brucellosis) 023.9 *[711.4]*
    caisson disease 993.3
    coccidioidomycosis 114.3 *[711.6]*
    coliform (Escherichia coli) 711.0
    colitis, ulcerative (*see also* Colitis, ulcerative) 556.9 *[713.1]*
    cowpox 051.0 *[711.5]*
    crystals (*see also* Gout)
        dicalcium phosphate 275.49 *[712.1]*
        pyrophosphate 275.49 *[712.2]*
        specified NEC 275.49 *[712.8]*
    dermatoarthritis, lipoid 272.8 *[713.0]*
    dermatological disorder NEC 709.9 *[713.3]*
    diabetes 250.6 *[713.5]*
    diphtheria 032.89 *[711.4]*
    dracontiasis 125.7 *[711.7]*
    dysentery 009.0 *[711.3]*
    endocrine disorder NEC 259.9 *[713.0]*

INDEX TO DISEASES

Arthritis, arthritic

Arthritis, arthritic—*continued*
- enteritis NEC 009.1 *[711.3]*
  - infectious (*see also* Enteritis, infectious) 009.0 *[711.3]*
    - specified organism NEC 008.8 *[711.3]*
  - regional (*see also* Enteritis, regional) 555.9 *[713.1]*
    - specified organism NEC 008.8 *[711.3]*
- epiphyseal slip, nontraumatic (old) 716.8
- erysipelas 035 *[711.4]*
- erythema
  - epidemic 026.1
  - multiforme 695.1 *[713.3]*
  - nodosum 695.2 *[713.3]*
- Escherichia coli 711.0
- filariasis NEC 125.9 *[711.7]*
- gastrointestinal condition NEC 569.9 *[713.1]*
- glanders 024 *[711.4]*
- Gonococcus 098.50
- gout 274.0
- H. influenzae 711.0
- helminthiasis NEC 128.9 *[711.7]*
- hematological disorder NEC 289.9 *[713.2]*
- hemochromatosis 275.0 *[713.0]*
- hemoglobinopathy NEC (*see also* Disease, hemoglobin) 282.7 *[713.2]*
- hemophilia (*see also* Hemophilia) 286.0 *[713.2]*
- Hemophilus influenzae (H. influenzae) 711.0
- Henoch (-Schönlein) purpura 287.0 *[713.6]*
- histoplasmosis NEC (*see also* Histoplasmosis) 115.99 *[711.6]*
- human parvovirus 079.83 *[711.5]*
- hyperparathyroidism 252.00 *[713.0]*
- hypersensitivity reaction NEC 995.3 *[713.6]*
- hypogammaglobulinemia (*see also* Hypogammaglobulinemia) 279.00 *[713.0]*
- hypothyroidism NEC 244.9 *[713.0]*
- infection (*see also* Arthritis, infectious) 711.9
- infectious disease NEC 136.9 *[711.8]*
- leprosy (*see also* Leprosy) 030.9 *[711.4]*
- leukemia NEC (M9800/3) 208.9 *[713.2]*
- lipoid dermatoarthritis 272.8 *[713.0]*
- Lyme disease 088.81 *[711.8]*
- meaning Osteoarthritis—*see* Osteoarthrosis
- Mediterranean fever, familial 277.31 *[713.7]*
- meningococcal infection 036.82
- metabolic disorder NEC 277.9 *[713.0]*
- multiple myelomatosis (M9730/3) 203.0 *[713.2]*
- mumps 072.79 *[711.5]*
- mycobacteria 031.8 *[711.4]*
- mycosis NEC 117.9 *[711.6]*
- neurological disorder NEC 349.9 *[713.5]*
- ochronosis 270.2 *[713.0]*
- O'Nyong Nyong 066.3 *[711.5]*
- parasitic disease NEC 136.9 *[711.8]*
- paratyphoid fever (*see also* Fever, paratyphoid) 002.9 *[711.3]*
- parvovirus B19 079.83 *[711.5]*
- Pneumococcus 711.0
- poliomyelitis (*see also* Poliomyelitis) 045.9 *[711.5]*
- Pseudomonas 711.0
- psoriasis 696.0
- pyogenic organism (E. coli) (H. influenzae) (Pseudomonas) (Streptococcus) 711.0
- rat-bite fever 026.1 *[711.4]*
- regional enteritis (*see also* Enteritis, regional) 555.9 *[713.1]*
- Reiter's disease 099.3 *[711.1]*

Arthritis, arthritic—*continued*
- respiratory disorder NEC 519.9 *[713.4]*
- reticulosis, malignant (M9720/3) 202.3 *[713.2]*
- rubella 056.71
- salmonellosis 003.23
- sarcoidosis 135 *[713.7]*
- serum sickness 999.5 *[713.6]*
- Staphylococcus 711.0
- Streptococcus 711.0
- syphilis (*see also* Syphilis) 094.0 *[711.4]*
- syringomyelia 336.0 *[713.5]*
- thalassemia 282.49 *[713.2]*
- tuberculosis (*see also* Tuberculosis, arthritis) 015.9 *[711.4]*
- typhoid fever 002.0 *[711.3]*
- ulcerative colitis (*see also* Colitis, ulcerative) 556.9 *[713.1]*
- urethritis
  - nongonococcal (*see also* Urethritis, nongonococcal) 099.40 *[711.1]*
  - nonspecific (*see also* Urethritis, nongonococcal) 099.40 *[711.1]*
  - Reiter's 099.3 *[711.1]*
- viral disease NEC 079.99 *[711.5]*
- erythema epidemic 026.1
- gonococcal 098.50
- gouty (acute) 274.0
- hypertrophic (*see also* Osteoarthrosis) 715.9
  - spine 721.90
    - with myelopathy 721.91
- idiopathic, blennorrheal 099.3
- in caisson disease 993.3 *[713.8]*
- infectious or infective (acute) (chronic) (subacute) NEC 711.9
- nonpyogenic 711.9
  - spine 720.9
- inflammatory NEC 714.9
- juvenile rheumatoid (chronic) (polyarticular) 714.30
  - acute 714.31
  - monoarticular 714.33
  - pauciarticular 714.32
- lumbar (*see also* Spondylosis, lumbar) 721.3
- meningococcal 036.82
- menopausal NEC 716.3
- migratory—*see* Fever, rheumatic
- neuropathic (Charcot's) 094.0 *[713.5]*
  - diabetic 250.6 *[713.5]*
  - nonsyphilitic NEC 349.9 *[713.5]*
  - syringomyelic 336.0 *[713.5]*
  - tabetic 094.0 *[713.5]*
- nodosa (*see also* Osteoarthrosis) 715.9
  - spine 721.90
    - with myelopathy 721.91
- nonpyogenic NEC 716.9
  - spine 721.90
    - with myelopathy 721.91
- ochronotic 270.2 *[713.0]*
- palindromic (*see also* Rheumatism, palindromic) 719.3
- pneumococcal 711.0
- postdysenteric 009.0 *[711.3]*
- postrheumatic, chronic (Jaccoud's) 714.4
- primary progressive 714.0
  - spine 720.9
- proliferative 714.0
  - spine 720.0
- psoriatic 696.0
- purulent 711.0
- pyogenic or pyemic 711.0

823

Arthritis, arthritic — *continued*
  rheumatic 714.0
    acute or subacute—*see* Fever, rheumatic
    chronic 714.0
    spine 720.9
  rheumatoid (nodular) 714.0
    with
      splenoadenomegaly and leukopenia 714.1
      visceral or systemic involvement 714.2
    aortitis 714.89
    carditis 714.2
    heart disease 714.2
    juvenile (chronic) (polyarticular) 714.30
      acute 714.31
      monoarticular 714.33
      pauciarticular 714.32
    spine 720.0
  rubella 056.71
  sacral, sacroiliac, sacrococcygeal (*see also*
    Spondylosis, sacral) 721.3
  scorbutic 267
  senile or senescent (*see also* Osteoarthrosis)
    715.9
    spine 721.90
      with myelopathy 721.91
  septic 711.0
  serum (nontherapeutic) (therapeutic) 999.5
    [713.6]
  specified form NEC 716.8
  spine 721.90
    with myelopathy 721.91
    atrophic 720.9
    degenerative 721.90
      with myelopathy 721.91
    hypertrophic (with deformity) 721.90
      with myelopathy 721.91
    infectious or infective NEC 720.9
    Marie-Strümpell 720.0
    nonpyogenic 721.90
      with myelopathy 721.91
    pyogenic 720.9
    rheumatoid 720.0
    traumatic (old) 721.7
    tuberculous (*see also* Tuberculosis) 015.0
      [720.81]
  staphylococcal 711.0
  streptococcal 711.0
  suppurative 711.0
  syphilitic 094.0 *[713.5]*
    congenital 090.49 *[713.5]*
  syphilitica deformans (Charcot) 094.0 *[713.5]*
  temporomandibular joint 524.69
  thoracic (*see also* Spondylosis, thoracic) 721.2
  toxic of menopause 716.3
  transient 716.4
  traumatic (chronic) (old) (post) 716.1
    current injury—*see* nature of injury
  tuberculous (*see also* Tuberculosis, arthritis)
    015.9 *[711.4]*
  urethritica 099.3 *[711.1]*
  urica, uratic 274.0
  venereal 099.3 *[711.1]*
  vertebral (*see also* Arthritis, spine) 721.90
  villous 716.8
  von Bechterew's 720.0
Arthrocele (*see also* Effusion, joint) 719.0
Arthrochondritis —*see* Arthritis
Arthrodesis status V45.4
Arthrodynia (*see also* Pain, joint) 719.4
  psychogenic 307.89

Arthrodysplasia 755.9
Arthrofibrosis, joint (*see also* Ankylosis) 718.5
Arthrogryposis 728.3
  multiplex, congenita 754.89
Arthrokatadysis 715.35
Arthrolithiasis 274.0
Arthro-onychodysplasia 756.89
Arthro-osteo-onychodysplasia 756.89
Arthropathy (*see also* Arthritis) 716.9

> Note—Use the following fifth-digit
> subclassification with categories 711-712, 716:
>
> 0 site unspecified
> 1 shoulder region
> 2 upper arm
> 3 forearm
> 4 hand
> 5 pelvic region and thigh
> 6 lower leg
> 7 ankle and foot
> 8 other specified sites
> 9 multiple sites

  Behçet's 136.1 *[711.2]*
  Charcot's 094.0 *[713.5]*
    diabetic 250.6 *[713.5]*
    syringomyelic 336.0 *[713.5]*
    tabetic 094.0 *[713.5]*
  crystal (-induced)—*see* Arthritis, due to crystals
  gouty 274.0
  neurogenic, neuropathic (Charcot's) (tabetic)
    094.0 *[713.5]*
    diabetic 250.6 *[713.5]*
    nonsyphilitic NEC 349.9 *[713.5]*
    syringomyelic 336.0 *[713.5]*
  postdysenteric NEC 009.0 *[711.3]*
  postrheumatic, chronic (Jaccoud's) 714.4
  psoriatic 696.0
  pulmonary 731.2
  specified NEC 716.8
  syringomyelia 336.0 *[713.5]*
  tabes dorsalis 094.0 *[713.5]*
  tabetic 094.0 *[713.5]*
  transient 716.4
  traumatic 716.1
  uric acid 274.0
Arthrophyte (*see also* Loose, body, joint) 718.1
Arthrophytis 719.80
  ankle 719.87
  elbow 719.82
  foot 719.87
  hand 719.84
  hip 719.85
  knee 719.86
  multiple sites 719.89
  pelvic region 719.85
  shoulder (region) 719.81
  specified site NEC 719.88
  wrist 719.83
Arthropyosis (*see also* Arthritis, pyogenic) 711.0
Arthroscopic surgical procedure converted to
  open procedure V64.43
Arthrosis (deformans) (degenerative) (*see also*
  Osteoarthrosis) 715.9
  Charcot's 094.0 *[713.5]*
  polyarticular 715.09
  spine (*see also* Spondylosis) 721.90

INDEX TO DISEASES

Arthus' phenomenon 995.21
  due to
    correct substance properly administered 995.21
    overdose or wrong substance given or taken 977.9
    specified drug—*see* Table of drugs and chemicals
  serum 999.5
Articular —*see also* condition
  disc disorder (reducing or non-reducing) 524.63
  spondylolisthesis 756.12
Articulation
  anterior 524.27
  posterior 524.27
  reverse 524.27
Artificial
  device (prosthetic)—*see* Fitting, device
  insemination V26.1
  menopause (states) (symptoms) (syndrome) 627.4
  opening status (functioning) (without complication) V44.9
    anus (colostomy) V44.3
    colostomy V44.3
    cystostomy V44.50
      appendico-vesicostomy V44.52
      cutaneous-vesicostomy V44.51
      specified type NEC V44.59
    enterostomy V44.4
    gastrostomy V44.1
    ileostomy V44.2
    intestinal tract NEC V44.4
    jejunostomy V44.4
    nephrostomy V44.6
    specified site NEC V44.8
    tracheostomy V44.0
    ureterostomy V44.6
    urethrostomy V44.6
    urinary tract NEC V44.6
    vagina V44.7
  vagina status V44.7
ARV (disease) (illness) (infection)—*see* Human immunodeficiency virus (disease) (illness) (infection)
Arytenoid —*see* condition
Asbestosis (occupational) 501
Asboe-Hansen's disease (incontinentia pigmenti) 757.33
Ascariasis (intestinal) (lung) 127.0
Ascaridiasis 127.0
Ascaridosis 127.0
Ascaris 127.0
  lumbricoides (infestation) 127.0
  pneumonia 127.0
Ascending —*see* condition
ASC-H (atypical squamous cells cannot exclude high grade squamous intraepithelial lesion) 795.02
Aschoff's bodies (*see also* Myocarditis, rheumatic) 398.0
Ascites 789.59
  abdominal NEC 789.59
  cancerous (M8000/6) 789.51
  cardiac 428.0
  chylous (nonfilarial) 457.8
    filarial (*see also* Infestation, filarial) 125.9
  congenital 778.0
  due to S. japonicum 120.2
  fetal, causing fetopelvic disproportion 653.7
  heart 428.0

Asphyxia, asphyxiation

Ascites—*continued*
  joint (*see also* Effusion, joint) 719.0
  malignant (M8000/6) 789.51
  pseudochylous 789.59
  syphilitic 095.2
  tuberculous (*see also* Tuberculosis) 014.0
Ascorbic acid (vitamin C) deficiency (scurvy) 267
ASC-US (atypical squamous cells of undetermined significance) 795.01
ASCVD (arteriosclerotic cardiovascular disease) 429.2
Aseptic —*see* condition
Asherman's syndrome 621.5
Asialia 527.7
Asiatic cholera (*see also* Cholera) 001.9
Asocial personality or trends 301.7
Asomatognosia 781.8
Aspergillosis 117.3
  with pneumonia 117.3 [484.6]
  allergic bronchopulmonary 518.6
  nonsyphilitic NEC 117.3
Aspergillus (flavus) (fumigatus) (infection) (terreus) 117.3
Aspermatogenesis 606.0
Aspermia (testis) 606.0
Asphyxia, asphyxiation (by) 799.01
  antenatal—*see* Distress, fetal
  bedclothes 994.7
  birth (*see also* Asphyxia, newborn) 768.9
  bunny bag 994.7
  carbon monoxide 986
  caul (*see also* Asphyxia, newborn) 768.9
  cave-in 994.7
    crushing—*see* Injury, internal, intrathoracic organs
  constriction 994.7
  crushing—*see* Injury, internal, intrathoracic organs
  drowning 994.1
  fetal, affecting newborn 768.9
  food or foreign body (in larynx) 933.1
    bronchioles 934.8
    bronchus (main) 934.1
    lung 934.8
    nasopharynx 933.0
    nose, nasal passages 932
    pharynx 933.0
    respiratory tract 934.9
      specified part NEC 934.8
    throat 933.0
    trachea 934.0
  gas, fumes, or vapor NEC 987.9
    specified—*see* Table of drugs and chemicals
  gravitational changes 994.7
  hanging 994.7
  inhalation—*see* Inhalation
  intrauterine
    fetal death (before onset of labor) 768.0
    during labor 768.1
    liveborn infant—*see* Distress, fetal, liveborn infant
  local 443.0
  mechanical 994.7
    during birth (*see also* Distress, fetal) 768.9
  mucus 933.1
    bronchus (main) 934.1
    larynx 933.1
    lung 934.8
    nasal passages 932
    newborn 770.18

825

Asphyxia, asphyxiation—*continued*
  pharynx 933.0
  respiratory tract 934.9
    specified part NEC 934.8
  throat 933.0
  trachea 934.0
  vaginal (fetus or newborn) 770.18
  newborn 768.9
    blue 768.6
    livida 768.6
    mild or moderate 768.6
    pallida 768.5
    severe 768.5
    white 768.5
    with neurologic involvement 768.5
  pathological 799.01
  plastic bag 994.7
  postnatal (*see also* Asphyxia, newborn) 768.9
    mechanical 994.7
  pressure 994.7
  reticularis 782.61
  strangulation 994.7
  submersion 994.1
  traumatic NEC—*see* Injury, internal, intrathoracic organs
  vomiting, vomitus—*see* Asphyxia, food or foreign body
Aspiration
  acid pulmonary (syndrome) 997.3
    obstetric 668.0
  amniotic fluid 770.13
    with respiratory symptoms 770.14
  bronchitis 507.0
  clear amniotic fluid 770.13
    with
      pneumonia 770.14
      pneumonitis 770.14
      respiratory symptoms 770.14
  contents of birth canal 770.17
    with respiratory symptoms 770.18
  fetal 770.10
    blood 770.15
      with
        pneumonia 770.16
        pneumonitis 770.16
    pneumonitis 770.18
  food, foreign body, or gasoline (with asphyxiation)—*see* Asphyxia, food or foreign body
  meconium 770.11
    with
      pneumonia 770.12
      pneumonitis 770.12
      respiratory symptoms 770.12
    below vocal cords 770.11
      with respiratory symptoms 770.12
  mucus 933.1
    into
      bronchus (main) 934.1
      lung 934.8
      respiratory tract 934.9
        specified part NEC 934.8
      trachea 934.0
    newborn 770.17
    vaginal (fetus or newborn) 770.17

Aspiration—*continued*
  newborn 770.10
    with respiratory symptoms 770.18
    blood 770.15
      with
        pneumonia 770.16
        pneumonitis 770.16
        respiratory symptoms 770.16
    pneumonia 507.0
      fetus or newborn 770.18
      meconium 770.12
    pneumonitis 507.0
      fetus or newborn 770.18
      meconium 770.12
      obstetric 668.0
    postnatal stomach contents 770.85
      with
        pneumonia 770.86
        pneumonitis 770.86
        respiratory symptoms 770.86
    syndrome of newborn (massive) 770.18
      meconium 770.12
    vernix caseosa 770.17
Asplenia 759.0
  with mesocardia 746.87
Assam fever 085.0
Assimilation, pelvis
  with disproportion 653.2
    affecting fetus or newborn 763.1
    causing obstructed labor 660.1
      affecting fetus or newborn 763.1
Assmann's focus (*see also* Tuberculosis) 011.0
Astasia (-abasia) 307.9
  hysterical 300.11
Asteatosis 706.8
  cutis 706.8
Astereognosis 780.99
Asterixis 781.3
  in liver disease 572.8
Asteroid hyalitis 379.22
Asthenia, asthenic 780.79
  cardiac (*see also* Failure, heart) 428.9
    psychogenic 306.2
  cardiovascular (*see also* Failure, heart) 428.9
    psychogenic 306.2
  heart (*see also* Failure, heart) 428.9
    psychogenic 306.2
  hysterical 300.11
  myocardial (*see also* Failure, heart) 428.9
    psychogenic 306.2
  nervous 300.5
  neurocirculatory 306.2
  neurotic 300.5
  psychogenic 300.5
  psychoneurotic 300.5
  psychophysiologic 300.5
  reaction, psychoneurotic 300.5
  senile 797
  Stiller's 780.79
  tropical anhidrotic 705.1
Asthenopia 368.13
  accommodative 367.4
  hysterical (muscular) 300.11
  psychogenic 306.7
Asthenospermia 792.2

INDEX TO DISEASES

Asthma, asthmatic (bronchial) (catarrh) (spasmodic) 493.9

> Note—The following fifth digit subclassification is for use with codes 493.0-493.2, 493.9:
>
> 0 unspecified
> 1 with status asthmaticus
> 2 with (acute) exacerbation

with
   chronic obstructive pulmonary disease (COPD) 493.2
   hay fever 493.0
   rhinitis, allergic 493.0
allergic 493.9
   stated cause (external allergen) 493.0
atopic 493.0
cardiac (*see also* Failure, ventricular, left) 428.1
cardiobronchial (*see also* Failure, ventricular, left) 428.1
cardiorenal (*see also* Hypertension, cardiorenal) 404.90
childhood 493.0
colliers' 500
cough variant 493.82
croup 493.9
detergent 507.8
due to
   detergent 507.8
   inhalation of fumes 506.3
   internal immunological process 493.0
endogenous (intrinsic) 493.1
eosinophilic 518.3
exercise induced bronchospasm 493.81
exogenous (cosmetics) (dander or dust) (drugs) (dust) (feathers) (food) (hay) (platinum) (pollen) 493.0
extrinsic 493.0
grinders' 502
hay 493.0
heart (*see also* Failure, ventricular, left) 428.1
IgE 493.0
infective 493.1
intrinsic 493.1
Kopp's 254.8
late-onset 493.1
meat-wrappers' 506.9
Millar's (laryngismus stridulus) 478.75
millstone makers' 502
miners' 500
Monday morning 504
New Orleans (epidemic) 493.0
platinum 493.0
pneumoconiotic (occupational) NEC 505
potters' 502
psychogenic 316 *[493.9]*
pulmonary eosinophilic 518.3
red cedar 495.8
Rostan's (*see also* Failure, ventricular, left) 428.1
sandblasters' 502
sequoiosis 495.8
stonemasons' 502
thymic 254.8
tuberculous (*see also* Tuberculosis, pulmonary) 011.9
Wichmann's (laryngismus stridulus) 478.75
wood 495.8
Astigmatism (compound) (congenital) 367.20
   irregular 367.22
   regular 367.21

Ataxia, ataxy, ataxic

Astroblastoma (M9430/3)
   nose 748.1
   specified site—*see* Neoplasm, by site, malignant
   unspecified site 191.9
Astrocytoma (cystic) (M9400/3)
   anaplastic type (M9401/3)
     specified site—*see* Neoplasm, by site, malignant
     unspecified site 191.9
   fibrillary (M9420/3)
     specified site—*see* Neoplasm, by site, malignant
     unspecified site 191.9
   fibrous (M9420/3)
     specified site—*see* Neoplasm, by site, malignant
     unspecified site 191.9
   gemistocytic (M9411/3)
     specified site—*see* Neoplasm, by site, malignant
     unspecified site 191.9
   juvenile (M9421/3)
     specified site—*see* Neoplasm, by site, malignant
     unspecified site 191.9
   nose 748.1
   pilocytic (M9421/3)
     specified site—*see* Neoplasm, by site, malignant
     unspecified site 191.9
   piloid (M9421/3)
     specified site—*see* Neoplasm, by site, malignant
     unspecified site 191.9
   protoplasmic (M9410/3)
     specified site—*see* Neoplasm, by site, malignant
     unspecified site 191.9
   specified site—*see* Neoplasm, by site, malignant
   subependymal (M9383/1) 237.5
     giant cell (M9384/1) 237.5
   unspecified site 191.9
Astroglioma (M9400/3)
   nose 748.1
   specified site—*see* Neoplasm, by site, malignant
   unspecified site 191.9
Asymbolia 784.60
Asymmetrical breathing 786.09
Asymmetry —*see also* Distortion
   chest 786.9
   face 754.0
   jaw NEC 524.12
     maxillary 524.11
   pelvis with disproportion 653.0
     affecting fetus or newborn 763.1
     causing obstructed labor 660.1
       affecting fetus or newborn 763.1
Asynergia 781.3
Asynergy 781.3
   ventricular 429.89
Asystole (heart) (*see also* Arrest, cardiac) 427.5
At risk for falling V15.88
Ataxia, ataxy, ataxic 781.3
   acute 781.3
   brain 331.89
   cerebellar 334.3
     hereditary (Marie's) 334.2
     in
       alcoholism 303.9 *[334.4]*
       myxedema (*see also* Myxedema) 244.9 *[334.4]*

Ataxia, ataxy, ataxic—*continued*
  neoplastic disease NEC 239.9 *[334.4]*
  cerebral 331.89
  family, familial 334.2
    cerebral (Marie's) 334.2
    spinal (Friedreich's) 334.0
    Friedreich's (heredofamilial) (spinal) 334.0
  frontal lobe 781.3
  gait 781.2
    hysterical 300.11
  general 781.3
  hereditary NEC 334.2
    cerebellar 334.2
    spastic 334.1
    spinal 334.0
  heredofamilial (Marie's) 334.2
  hysterical 300.11
  locomotor (progressive) 094.0
    diabetic 250.6 *[337.1]*
  Marie's (cerebellar) (heredofamilial) 334.2
  nonorganic origin 307.9
  partial 094.0
  postchickenpox 052.7
  progressive locomotor 094.0
  psychogenic 307.9
  Sanger-Brown's 334.2
  spastic 094.0
    hereditary 334.1
    syphilitic 094.0
  spinal
    hereditary 334.0
    progressive locomotor 094.0
  telangiectasia 334.8
Ataxia-telangiectasia 334.8
Atelectasis (absorption collapse) (complete) (compression) (massive) (partial) (postinfective) (pressure collapse) (pulmonary) (relaxation) 518.0
  newborn (congenital) (partial) 770.5
    primary 770.4
  primary 770.4
  tuberculous (*see also* Tuberculosis, pulmonary) 011.9
Ateleiosis, ateliosis 253.3
Atelia —*see* Distortion
Ateliosis 253.3
Atelocardia 746.9
Atelomyelia 742.59
Athelia 757.6
Atheroembolism
  extremity
    lower 445.02
    upper 445.01
  kidney 445.81
  specified site NEC 445.89
Atheroma, atheromatous (*see also* Arteriosclerosis) 440.9
  aorta, aortic 440.0
  valve (*see also* Endocarditis, aortic) 424.1
  artery—*see* Arteriosclerosis
  basilar, (artery) (*see also* Occlusion, artery, basilar) 433.0
  carotid (artery) (common) (internal) (*see also* Occlusion, artery, carotid) 433.1
  cerebral (arteries) 437.0
  coronary (artery)—*see* Arteriosclerosis, coronary
  degeneration—*see* Arteriosclerosis
  heart, cardiac —*see* Arteriosclerosis, coronary
  mitral (valve) 424.0
  myocardium, myocardial —*see* Arteriosclerosis, coronary

Atheroma, atheromatous—*continued*
  pulmonary valve (heart) (*see also* Endocarditis, pulmonary) 424.3
  skin 706.2
  tricuspid (heart) (valve) 424.2
  valve, valvular—*see* Endocarditis
  vertebral (artery) (*see also* Occlusion, artery, vertebral) 433.2
Atheromatosis —*see also* Arteriosclerosis
  arterial, congenital 272.8
Atherosclerosis —*see* Arteriosclerosis
Athetosis (acquired) 781.0
  bilateral 333.79
  congenital (bilateral) 333.6
  double 333.71
  unilateral 781.0
Athlete's
  foot 110.4
  heart 429.3
Athletic team examination V70.3
Athrepsia 261
Athyrea (acquired) (*see also* Hypothyroidism) 244.9
  congenital 243
Athyreosis (congenital) 243
  acquired—*see* Hypothyroidism
Athyroidism (acquired) (*see also* Hypothyroidism) 244.9
  congenital 243
Atmospheric pyrexia 992.0
Atonia, atony, atonic
  abdominal wall 728.2
  bladder (sphincter) 596.4
    neurogenic NEC 596.54
      with cauda equina syndrome 344.61
  capillary 448.9
  cecum 564.89
    psychogenic 306.4
  colon 564.89
    psychogenic 306.4
    congenital 779.89
  dyspepsia 536.3
    psychogenic 306.4
  intestine 564.89
    psychogenic 306.4
  stomach 536.3
    neurotic or psychogenic 306.4
    psychogenic 306.4
  uterus 661.2
    affecting fetus or newborn 763.7
    with hemorrhage (postpartum) 666.1
    without hemorrhage
      intrapartum 661.2
      postpartum 669.8
  vesical 596.4
Atopy NEC V15.09
Atransferrinemia, congenital 273.8
Atresia, atretic (congenital) 759.89
  alimentary organ or tract NEC 751.8
    lower 751.2
    upper 750.8
  ani, anus, anal (canal) 751.2
  aorta 747.22
    with hypoplasia of ascending aorta and defective development of left ventricle (with mitral valve atresia) 746.7
    arch 747.11
    ring 747.21
  aortic (orifice) (valve) 746.89
    arch 747.11
  aqueduct of Sylvius 742.3
    with spina bifida (*see also* Spina bifida) 741.0

Atresia, atretic—*continued*
  artery NEC (*see also* Atresia, blood vessel) 747.60
    cerebral 747.81
    coronary 746.85
    eye 743.58
    pulmonary 747.3
    umbilical 747.5
  auditory canal (external) 744.02
  bile, biliary duct (common) or passage 751.61
    acquired (*see also* Obstruction, biliary) 576.2
  bladder (neck) 753.6
  blood vessel (peripheral) NEC 747.60
    cerebral 747.81
    gastrointestinal 747.61
    lower limb 747.64
    pulmonary artery 747.3
    renal 747.62
    spinal 747.82
    upper limb 747.63
  bronchus 748.3
  canal, ear 744.02
  cardiac
    valve 746.89
      aortic 746.89
      mitral 746.89
      pulmonary 746.01
      tricuspid 746.1
  cecum 751.2
  cervix (acquired) 622.4
    congenital 752.49
    in pregnancy or childbirth 654.6
      affecting fetus or newborn 763.89
      causing obstructed labor 660.2
        affecting fetus or newborn 763.1
  choana 748.0
  colon 751.2
  cystic duct 751.61
    acquired 575.8
      with obstruction (*see also* Obstruction, gallbladder) 575.2
  digestive organs NEC 751.8
  duodenum 751.1
  ear canal 744.02
  ejaculatory duct 752.89
  epiglottis 748.3
  esophagus 750.3
  Eustachian tube 744.24
  fallopian tube (acquired) 628.2
    congenital 752.19
  follicular cyst 620.0
  foramen of
    Luschka 742.3
      with spina bifida (*see also* Spina bifida) 741.0
    Magendie 742.3
      with spina bifida (*see also* Spina bifida) 741.0
  gallbladder 751.69
  genital organ
    external
      female 752.49
      male NEC 752.89
        penis 752.69
    internal
      female 752.89
      male 752.89
  glottis 748.3
  gullet 750.3
  heart
    valve NEC 746.89
      aortic 746.89

Atresia, atretic—*continued*
      mitral 746.89
      pulmonary 746.01
      tricuspid 746.1
  hymen 752.42
    acquired 623.3
    postinfective 623.3
  ileum 751.1
  intestine (small) 751.1
    large 751.2
  iris, filtration angle (*see also* Buphthalmia) 743.20
  jejunum 751.1
  kidney 753.3
  lacrimal, apparatus 743.65
    acquired—*see* Stenosis, lacrimal
  larynx 748.3
  ligament, broad 752.19
  lung 748.5
  meatus urinarius 753.6
  mitral valve 746.89
    with atresia or hypoplasia of aortic orifice or valve, with hypoplasia of ascending aorta and defective development of left ventricle 746.7
  nares (anterior) (posterior) 748.0
  nasolacrimal duct 743.65
  nasopharynx 748.8
  nose, nostril 748.0
    acquired 738.0
  organ or site NEC—*see* Anomaly, specified type NEC
  osseous meatus (ear) 744.03
  oviduct (acquired) 628.2
    congenital 752.19
  parotid duct 750.23
    acquired 527.8
  pulmonary (artery) 747.3
    valve 746.01
    vein 747.49
  pulmonic 746.01
  pupil 743.46
  rectum 751.2
  salivary duct or gland 750.23
    acquired 527.8
  sublingual duct 750.23
    acquired 527.8
  submaxillary duct or gland 750.23
    acquired 527.8
  trachea 748.3
  tricuspid valve 746.1
  ureter 753.29
  ureteropelvic junction 753.21
  ureterovesical orifice 753.22
  urethra (valvular) 753.6
  urinary tract NEC 753.29
  uterus 752.3
    acquired 621.8
  vagina (acquired) 623.2
    congenital 752.49
    postgonococcal (old) 098.2
    postinfectional 623.2
    senile 623.2
  vascular NEC (*see also* Atresia, blood vessel) 747.60
    cerebral 747.81
  vas deferens 752.89
  vein NEC (*see also* Atresia, blood vessel) 747.60
    cardiac 746.89
    great 747.49

Atresia, atretic—*continued*
    portal 747.49
    pulmonary 747.49
    vena cava (inferior) (superior) 747.49
    vesicourethral orifice 753.6
    vulva 752.49
        acquired 624.8
Atrichia, atrichosis 704.00
    congenital (universal) 757.4
Atrioventricularis commune 745.69
Atrophia —*see also* Atrophy
    alba 709.09
    cutis 701.8
        idiopathica progressiva 701.8
        senilis 701.8
    dermatological, diffuse (idiopathic) 701.8
    flava hepatis (acuta) (subacuta) (*see also* Necrosis, liver) 570
    gyrata of choroid and retina (central) 363.54
        generalized 363.57
    senilis 797
        dermatological 701.8
    unguium 703.8
        congenita 757.5
Atrophoderma, atrophodermia 701.9
    diffusum (idiopathic) 701.8
    maculatum 701.3
    et striatum 701.3
        due to syphilis 095.8
    syphilitic 091.3
    neuriticum 701.8
    pigmentosum 757.33
    reticulatum symmetricum faciei 701.8
    senile 701.8
    symmetrical 701.8
    vermiculata 701.8
Atrophy, atrophic
    adrenal (autoimmune) (capsule) (cortex) (gland) 255.41
        with hypofunction 255.41
    alveolar process or ridge (edentulous) 525.20
        mandible 525.20
            minimal 525.21
            moderate 525.22
            severe 525.23
        maxilla 525.20
            minimal 525.24
            moderate 525.25
            severe 525.26
    appendix 543.9
    Aran-Duchenne muscular 335.21
    arm 728.2
    arteriosclerotic—*see* Arteriosclerosis
    arthritis 714.0
        spine 720.9
    bile duct (any) 576.8
    bladder 596.8
    blanche (of Milian) 701.3
    bone (senile) 733.99
        due to
            disuse 733.7
            infection 733.99
            tabes dorsalis (neurogenic) 094.0
        posttraumatic 733.99
    brain (cortex) (progressive) 331.9
        with dementia 290.10
            Alzheimer's 331.0
                with dementia—*see* Alzheimer's dementia
        circumscribed (Pick's) 331.11
            with dementia

Atrophy, atrophic—*continued*
        with behavioral disturbance 331.11
            [294.11]
        without behavioral disturbance 331.11
            [294.10]
    congenital 742.4
    hereditary 331.9
    senile 331.2
    breast 611.4
        puerperal, postpartum 676.3
    buccal cavity 528.9
    cardiac (brown) (senile) (*see also* Degeneration, myocardial) 429.1
    cartilage (infectional) (joint) 733.99
    cast, plaster of Paris 728.2
    cerebellar—*see* Atrophy, brain
    cerebral—*see* Atrophy, brain
    cervix (endometrium) (mucosa) (myometrium) (senile) (uteri) 622.8
        menopausal 627.8
    Charcot-Marie-Tooth 356.1
    choroid 363.40
        diffuse secondary 363.42
        hereditary (*see also* Dystrophy, choroid) 363.50
        gyrate
            central 363.54
            diffuse 363.57
            generalized 363.57
        senile 363.41
    ciliary body 364.57
    colloid, degenerative 701.3
    conjunctiva (senile) 372.89
    corpus cavernosum 607.89
    cortical (*see also* Atrophy, brain) 331.9
    Cruveilhier's 335.21
    cystic duct 576.8
    dacryosialadenopathy 710.2
    degenerative
        colloid 701.3
        senile 701.3
    Déjérine-Thomas 333.0
    diffuse idiopathic, dermatological 701.8
    disuse
        bone 733.7
        muscle 728.2
        pelvic muscles and anal sphincter 618.83
    Duchenne-Aran 335.21
    ear 388.9
    edentulous alveolar ridge 525.20
        mandible 525.20
            minimal 525.21
            moderate 525.22
            severe 525.23
        maxilla 525.20
            minimal 525.24
            moderate 525.25
            severe 525.26
    emphysema, lung 492.8
    endometrium (senile) 621.8
        cervix 622.8
    enteric 569.89
    epididymis 608.3
    eyeball, cause unknown 360.41
    eyelid (senile) 374.50
    facial (skin) 701.9
    facioscapulohumeral (Landouzy-Déjérine) 359.1
    fallopian tube (senile), acquired 620.3
    fatty, thymus (gland) 254.8
    gallbladder 575.8
    gastric 537.89

Atrophy, atrophic—*continued*
  gastritis (chronic) 535.1
  gastrointestinal 569.89
  genital organ, male 608.89
  glandular 289.3
  globe (phthisis bulbi) 360.41
  gum (*see also* Recession, gingival) 523.20
  hair 704.2
  heart (brown) (senile) (*see also* Degeneration, myocardial) 429.1
  hemifacial 754.0
    Romberg 349.89
  hydronephrosis 591
  infantile 261
    paralysis, acute (*see also* Poliomyelitis, with paralysis) 045.1
  intestine 569.89
  iris (generalized) (postinfectional) (sector shaped) 364.59
    essential 364.51
    progressive 364.51
    sphincter 364.54
  kidney (senile) (*see also* Sclerosis, renal) 587
    with hypertension (*see also* Hypertension, kidney) 403.90
    congenital 753.0
    hydronephrotic 591
    infantile 753.0
  lacrimal apparatus (primary) 375.13
    secondary 375.14
  Landouzy-Déjérine 359.1
  laryngitis, infection 476.0
  larynx 478.79
  Leber's optic 377.16
  lip 528.5
  liver (acute) (subacute) (*see also* Necrosis, liver) 570
    chronic (yellow) 571.8
    yellow (congenital) 570
      with
        abortion—*see* Abortion, by type, with specified complication NEC
        ectopic pregnancy (*see also* categories 633.0-633.9) 639.8
        molar pregnancy (*see also* categories 630-632) 639.8
      chronic 571.8
      complicating pregnancy 646.7
      following
        abortion 639.8
        ectopic or molar pregnancy 639.8
      from injection, inoculation or transfusion (onset within 8 months after administration)—*see* Hepatitis, viral
      healed 571.5
      obstetric 646.7
      postabortal 639.8
      postimmunization—*see* Hepatitis, viral
      posttransfusion—*see* Hepatitis, viral
      puerperal, postpartum 674.8
  lung (senile) 518.89
    congenital 748.69
  macular (dermatological) 701.3
    syphilitic, skin 091.3
      striated 095.8
  muscle, muscular 728.2
    disuse 728.2
    Duchenne-Aran 335.21
    extremity (lower) (upper) 728.2
    familial spinal 335.11
    general 728.2

Atrophy, atrophic—*continued*
    idiopathic 728.2
    infantile spinal 335.0
    myelopathic (progressive) 335.10
    myotonic 359.21
    neuritic 356.1
    neuropathic (peroneal) (progressive) 356.1
    peroneal 356.1
    primary (idiopathic) 728.2
    progressive (familial) (hereditary) (pure) 335.21
      adult (spinal) 335.19
      infantile (spinal) 335.0
      juvenile (spinal) 335.11
    spinal 335.10
      adult 335.19
      hereditary or familial 335.11
      infantile 335.0
    pseudohypertrophic 359.1
      spinal (progressive) 335.10
      adult 335.19
      Aran-Duchenne 335.21
      familial 335.11
      hereditary 335.11
      infantile 335.0
      juvenile 335.11
    syphilitic 095.6
  myocardium (*see also* Degeneration, myocardial) 429.1
  myometrium (senile) 621.8
    cervix 622.8
  myotatic 728.2
  myotonia 359.21
  nail 703.8
    congenital 757.5
  nasopharynx 472.2
  nerve—*see also* Disorder, nerve
    abducens 378.54
    accessory 352.4
    acoustic or auditory 388.5
    cranial 352.9
      first (olfactory) 352.0
      second (optic) (*see also* Atrophy, optic nerve) 377.10
      third (oculomotor) (partial) 378.51
        total 378.52
      fourth (trochlear) 378.53
      fifth (trigeminal) 350.8
      sixth (abducens) 378.54
      seventh (facial) 351.8
      eighth (auditory) 388.5
      ninth (glossopharyngeal) 352.2
      tenth (pneumogastric) (vagus) 352.3
      eleventh (accessory) 352.4
      twelfth (hypoglossal) 352.5
    facial 351.8
    glossopharyngeal 352.2
    hypoglossal 352.5
    oculomotor (partial) 378.51
      total 378.52
    olfactory 352.0
    peripheral 355.9
    pneumogastric 352.3
    trigeminal 350.8
    trochlear 378.53
    vagus (pneumogastric) 352.3
  nervous system, congenital 742.8
  neuritic (*see also* Disorder, nerve) 355.9
  neurogenic NEC 355.9
    bone
      tabetic 094.0

Atrophy, atrophic—*continued*
  nutritional 261
  old age 797
  olivopontocerebellar 333.0
  optic nerve (ascending) (descending)
    (infectional) (nonfamilial) (papillomacular
    bundle) (postretinal) (secondary NEC)
    (simple) 377.10
    associated with retinal dystrophy 377.13
    dominant hereditary 377.16
    glaucomatous 377.14
    hereditary (dominant) (Leber's) 377.16
    Leber's (hereditary) 377.16
    partial 377.15
    postinflammatory 377.12
    primary 377.11
    syphilitic 094.84
      congenital 090.49
      tabes dorsalis 094.0
  orbit 376.45
  ovary (senile), acquired 620.3
  oviduct (senile), acquired 620.3
  palsy, diffuse 335.20
  pancreas (duct) (senile) 577.8
  papillary muscle 429.81
  paralysis 355.9
  parotid gland 527.0
  patches skin 701.3
    senile 701.8
  penis 607.89
  pharyngitis 472.1
  pharynx 478.29
  pluriglandular 258.8
  polyarthritis 714.0
  prostate 602.2
  pseudohypertrophic 359.1
  renal (*see also* Sclerosis, renal) 587
  reticulata 701.8
  retina (*see also* Degeneration, retina) 362.60
    hereditary (*see also* Dystrophy, retina) 362.70
  rhinitis 472.0
  salivary duct or gland 527.0
  scar NEC 709.2
  sclerosis, lobar (of brain) 331.0
    with dementia
      with behavioral disturbance 331.0 *[294.11]*
      without behavioral disturbance 331.0
        [294.10]
  scrotum 608.89
  seminal vesicle 608.89
  senile 797
    degenerative, of skin 701.3
  skin (patches) (senile) 701.8
  spermatic cord 608.89
  spinal (cord) 336.8
    acute 336.8
    muscular (chronic) 335.10
      adult 335.19
      familial 335.11
      juvenile 335.10
    paralysis 335.10
      acute (*see also* Poliomyelitis, with paralysis)
        045.1
  spine (column) 733.99
  spleen (senile) 289.59
  spots (skin) 701.3
    senile 701.8
  stomach 537.89
  striate and macular 701.3
    syphilitic 095.8

Atrophy, atrophic—*continued*
  subcutaneous 701.9
    due to injection 999.9
  sublingual gland 527.0
  submaxillary gland 527.0
  Sudeck's 733.7
  suprarenal (autoimmune) (capsule) (gland)
    255.41
    with hypofunction 255.41
  tarso-orbital fascia, congenital 743.66
  testis 608.3
  thenar, partial 354.0
  throat 478.29
  thymus (fat) 254.8
  thyroid (gland) 246.8
    with
      cretinism 243
      myxedema 244.9
    congenital 243
  tongue (senile) 529.8
    papillae 529.4
    smooth 529.4
  trachea 519.19
  tunica vaginalis 608.89
  turbinate 733.99
  tympanic membrane (nonflaccid) 384.82
    flaccid 384.81
  ulcer (*see also* Ulcer, skin) 707.9
  upper respiratory tract 478.9
  uterus, uterine (acquired) (senile) 621.8
    cervix 622.8
    due to radiation (intended effect) 621.8
  vagina (senile) 627.3
  vascular 459.89
  vas deferens 608.89
  vertebra (senile) 733.99
  vulva (primary) (senile) 624.1
  Werdnig-Hoffmann 335.0
  yellow (acute) (congenital) (liver) (subacute)
    (*see also* Necrosis, liver) 570
    chronic 571.8
    resulting from administration of blood,
      plasma, serum, or other biological
      substance (within 8 months of
      administration)—*see* Hepatitis, viral

Attack
  akinetic (*see also* Epilepsy) 345.0
  angina—*see* Angina
  apoplectic (*see also* Disease, cerebrovascular,
    acute) 436
  benign shuddering 333.93
  bilious—*see* Vomiting
  cataleptic 300.11
  cerebral (*see also* Disease, cerebrovascular,
    acute) 436
  coronary (*see also* Infarct, myocardium) 410.9
  cyanotic, newborn 770.83
  epileptic (*see also* Epilepsy) 345.9
  epileptiform 780.39
  heart (*see also* Infarct, myocardium) 410.9
  hemiplegia (*see also* Disease, cerebrovascular,
    acute) 436
  hysterical 300.11
  jacksonian (*see also* Epilepsy) 345.5
  myocardium, myocardial (*see also* Infarct,
    myocardium) 410.9
  myoclonic (*see also* Epilepsy) 345.1
  panic 300.01
  paralysis (*see also* Disease, cerebrovascular,
    acute) 436
  paroxysmal 780.39

Attack—*continued*
  psychomotor (*see also* Epilepsy) 345.4
  salaam (*see also* Epilepsy) 345.6
  schizophreniform (*see also* Schizophrenia) 295.4
  sensory and motor 780.39
  syncope 780.2
  toxic, cerebral 780.39
  transient ischemic (TIA) 435.9
  unconsciousness 780.2
    hysterical 300.11
  vasomotor 780.2
  vasovagal (idiopathic) (paroxysmal) 780.2
Attention to
  artificial
    opening (of) V55.9
      digestive tract NEC V55.4
      specified site NEC V55.8
      urinary tract NEC V55.6
    vagina V55.7
  colostomy V55.3
  cystostomy V55.5
  dressing
    wound V58.30
      nonsurgical V58.30
      surgical V58.31
  gastrostomy V55.1
  ileostomy V55.2
  jejunostomy V55.4
  nephrostomy V55.6
  surgical dressings V58.31
  sutures V58.32
  tracheostomy V55.0
  ureterostomy V55.6
  urethrostomy V55.6
Attrition
  gum (*see also* Recession, gingival) 523.20
  teeth (hard tissues) 521.10
    excessive 521.10
      extending into
        dentine 521.12
        pulp 521.13
      generalized 521.15
      limited to enamel 521.11
      localized 521.14
Atypical —*see also* condition
  cells
    endocervical 795.00
    endometrial 795.00
    glandular 795.00
  distribution, vessel (congenital) (peripheral) NEC 747.60
  endometrium 621.9
  kidney 593.89
Atypism, cervix 622.10
Audible tinnitus (*see also* Tinnitus) 388.30
Auditory —*see* condition
Audry's syndrome (acropachyderma) 757.39
Aujeszky's disease 078.89
Aura, jacksonian (*see also* Epilepsy) 345.5
Aurantiasis, cutis 278.3
Auricle, auricular —*see* condition
Auriculotemporal syndrome 350.8
Australian
  Q fever 083.0
  X disease 062.4
Autism, autistic (child) (infantile) 299.0
Autodigestion 799.89
Autoerythrocyte sensitization 287.2
Autographism 708.3

Autoimmune
  cold sensitivity 283.0
  disease NEC 279.4
  hemolytic anemia 283.0
  thyroiditis 245.2
Autoinfection, septic —*see* Septicemia
Autointoxication 799.89
Automatism 348.8
  epileptic (*see also* Epilepsy) 345.4
  paroxysmal, idiopathic (*see also* Epilepsy) 345.4
Autonomic, autonomous
  bladder 596.54
    neurogenic 596.54
      with cauda equine 344.61
  dysreflexia 337.3
  faciocephalalgia (*see also* Neuropathy, peripheral, autonomic) 337.9
  hysterical seizure 300.11
  imbalance (*see also* Neuropathy, peripheral, autonomic) 337.9
Autophony 388.40
Autosensitivity, erythrocyte 287.2
Autotopagnosia 780.99
Autotoxemia 799.89
Autumn —*see* condition
Avellis' syndrome 344.89
Aviators
  disease or sickness (*see also* Effect, adverse, high altitude) 993.2
  ear 993.0
  effort syndrome 306.2
Avitaminosis (multiple NEC) (*see also* Deficiency, vitamin) 269.2
  A 264.9
  B 266.9
    with
      beriberi 265.0
      pellagra 265.2
  B_1 265.1
  B_2 266.0
  B_6 266.1
  B_{12} 266.2
  C (with scurvy) 267
  D 268.9
    with
      osteomalacia 268.2
      rickets 268.0
  E 269.1
  G 266.0
  H 269.1
  K 269.0
  multiple 269.2
  nicotinic acid 265.2
  P 269.1
Avulsion (traumatic) 879.8
  blood vessel—*see* Injury, blood vessel, by site
  cartilage—*see also* Dislocation, by site
    knee, current (*see also* Tear, meniscus) 836.2
    symphyseal (inner), complicating delivery 665.6
  complicated 879.9
  diaphragm—*see* Injury, internal, diaphragm
  ear—*see* Wound, open, ear
  epiphysis of bone—*see* Fracture, by site
  external site other than limb—*see* Wound, open, by site
  eye 871.3
  fingernail—*see* Wound, open, finger
  fracture—*see* Fracture, by site
  genital organs, external—*see* Wound, open, genital organs

Avulsion—*continued*
  head (intracranial) NEC—*see also* Injury,
     intracranial, with open intracranial wound
    complete 874.9
    external site NEC 873.8
     complicated 873.9
  internal organ or site—*see* Injury, internal, by site
  joint—*see also* Dislocation, by site
    capsule—*see* Sprain, by site
  ligament—*see* Sprain, by site
  limb—*see also* Amputation, traumatic, by site
    skin and subcutaneous tissue—*see* Wound,
     open, by site
  muscle—*see* Sprain, by site
  nerve (root)—*see* Injury, nerve, by site
  scalp—*see* Wound, open, scalp
  skin and subcutaneous tissue—*see* Wound,
    open, by site
  symphyseal cartilage (inner), complicating
    delivery 665.6
  tendon—*see also* Sprain, by site
    with open wound—*see* Wound, open, by site
  toenail—*see* Wound, open, toe(s)
  tooth 873.63
    complicated 873.73
Awaiting organ transplant status V49.83
Awareness of heart beat 785.1
Axe grinders' disease 502
Axenfeld's anomaly or syndrome 743.44
Axilla, axillary —*see also* condition
  breast 757.6
Axonotmesis —*see* Injury, nerve, by site
Ayala's disease 756.89
Ayerza's disease or syndrome (pulmonary
    artery sclerosis with pulmonary hypertension)
    416.0
Azoospermia 606.0
Azorean disease (of the nervous system) 334.8
Azotemia 790.6
  meaning uremia (*see also* Uremia) 586
Aztec ear 744.29
Azygos lobe, lung (fissure) 748.69

INDEX TO DISEASES

B

Baader's syndrome (erythema multiforme exudativum) 695.1
Baastrup's syndrome 721.5
Babesiasis 088.82
Babesiosis 088.82
Babington's disease (familial hemorrhagic telangiectasia) 448.0
Babinski's syndrome (cardiovascular syphilis) 093.89
Babinski-Fröhlich syndrome (adiposogenital dystrophy) 253.8
Babinski-Nageotte syndrome 344.89
Bacillary —*see* condition
Bacilluria 791.9
  asymptomatic, in pregnancy or puerperium 646.5
  tuberculous (*see also* Tuberculosis) 016.9
Bacillus —*see also* Infection, bacillus
  abortus infection 023.1
  anthracis infection 022.9
  coli
    infection 041.4
      generalized 038.42
      intestinal 008.00
      pyemia 038.42
      septicemia 038.42
  Flexner's 004.1
  fusiformis infestation 101
  mallei infection 024
  Shiga's 004.0
  suipestifer infection (*see also* Infection, Salmonella) 003.9
Back —*see* condition
Backache (postural) 724.5
  psychogenic 307.89
  sacroiliac 724.6
Backflow (pyelovenous) (*see also* Disease, renal) 593.9
Backknee (*see also* Genu, recurvatum) 736.5
Bacteremia (*see also* Infection, bacillus) 790.7
  newborn 771.83
Bacteria
  in blood (*see also* Bacteremia) 790.7
  in urine (*see also* Bacteriuria) 599.0
Bacterial —*see* condition
Bactericholia (*see also* Cholecystitis, acute) 575.0
Bacterid, bacteride (Andrews' pustular) 686.8
Bacteriuria, bacteruria 791.9
  with
    urinary tract infection 599.0
  asymptomatic 791.9
    in pregnancy or puerperium 646.5
      affecting fetus or newborn 760.1
Bad
  breath 784.99
  heart—*see* Disease, heart
  trip (*see also* Abuse, drugs, nondependent) 305.3
Baehr-Schiffrin disease (thrombotic thrombocytopenic purpura) 446.6
Baelz's disease (cheilitis glandularis apostematosa) 528.5
Baerensprung's disease (eczema marginatum) 110.3
Bagassosis (occupational) 495.1
Baghdad boil 085.1

Bagratuni's syndrome (temporal arteritis) 446.5
Baker's
  cyst (knee) 727.51
    tuberculous (*see also* Tuberculosis) 015.2
  itch 692.89
Bakwin-Krida syndrome (craniometaphyseal dysplasia) 756.89
Balanitis (circinata) (gangraenosa) (infectious) (vulgaris) 607.1
  amebic 006.8
  candidal 112.2
  chlamydial 099.53
  due to Ducrey's bacillus 099.0
  erosiva circinata et gangraenosa 607.1
  gangrenous 607.1
  gonococcal (acute) 098.0
    chronic or duration of 2 months or over 098.2
  nongonococcal 607.1
  phagedenic 607.1
  venereal NEC 099.8
  xerotica obliterans 607.81
Balanoposthitis 607.1
  chlamydial 099.53
  gonococcal (acute) 098.0
    chronic or duration of 2 months or over 098.2
  ulcerative NEC 099.8
Balanorrhagia —*see* Balanitis
Balantidiasis 007.0
Balantidiosis 007.0
Balbuties, balbutio 307.0
Bald
  patches on scalp 704.00
  tongue 529.4
Baldness (*see also* Alopecia) 704.00
Balfour's disease (chloroma) 205.3
Balint's syndrome (psychic paralysis of visual fixation) 368.16
Balkan grippe 083.0
Ball
  food 938
  hair 938
Ballantyne (-Runge) **syndrome** (postmaturity) 766.22
Balloon disease (*see also* Effect, adverse, high altitude) 993.2
Ballooning posterior leaflet syndrome 424.0
Baló's disease or concentric sclerosis 341.1
Bamberger's disease (hypertrophic pulmonary osteoarthropathy) 731.2
Bamberger-Marie disease (hypertrophic pulmonary osteoarthropathy) 731.2
Bamboo spine 720.0
Bancroft's filariasis 125.0
Band(s)
  adhesive (*see also* Adhesions, peritoneum) 568.0
  amniotic 658.8
    affecting fetus or newborn 762.8
  anomalous or congenital—*see also* Anomaly, specified type NEC
    atrial 746.9
    heart 746.9
    intestine 751.4
    omentum 751.4
    ventricular 746.9
  cervix 622.3
  gallbladder (congenital) 751.69

835

Band(s)—*continued*
 intestinal (adhesive) (*see also* Adhesions, peritoneum) 568.0
   congenital 751.4
   obstructive (*see also* Obstruction, intestine) 560.81
   periappendiceal (congenital) 751.4
   peritoneal (adhesive) (*see also* Adhesions, peritoneum) 568.0
     with intestinal obstruction 560.81
     congenital 751.4
   uterus 621.5
   vagina 623.2
Bandemia (without diagnosis of specific infection) 288.66
Bandl's ring (contraction)
 complicating delivery 661.4
 affecting fetus or newborn 763.7
Bang's disease (Brucella abortus) 023.1
Bangkok hemorrhagic fever 065.4
Bannister's disease 995.1
Bantam-Albright-Martin disease (pseudohypoparathyroidism) 275.49
Banti's disease or syndrome (with cirrhosis) (with portal hypertension)—*see* Cirrhosis, liver
Bar
 calcaneocuboid 755.67
 calcaneonavicular 755.67
 cubonavicular 755.67
 prostate 600.90
   with
     other lower urinary tract symptoms (LUTS) 600.91
     urinary
       obstruction 600.91
       retention 600.91
 talocalcaneal 755.67
Baragnosis 780.99
Barasheh, barashek 266.2
Barcoo disease or rot (*see also* Ulcer, skin) 707.9
Bard-Pic syndrome (carcinoma, head of pancreas) 157.0
Bärensprung's disease (eczema marginatum) 110.3
Baritosis 503
Barium lung disease 503
Barlow's syndrome (meaning mitral valve prolapse) 424.0
Barlow (-Möller) disease or syndrome (meaning infantile scurvy) 267
Barodontalgia 993.2
Baron Münchausen syndrome 301.51
Barosinusitis 993.1
Barotitis 993.0
Barotrauma 993.2
 odontalgia 993.2
 otitic 993.0
 sinus 993.1
Barraquer's disease or syndrome (progressive lipodystrophy) 272.6
Barré-Guillain syndrome 357.0
Barré-Liéou syndrome (posterior cervical sympathetic) 723.2
Barrel chest 738.3
Barrett's esophagus 530.85
Barrett's syndrome or ulcer (chronic peptic ulcer of esophagus) 530.85
Bársony-Polgár syndrome (corkscrew esophagus) 530.5
Bársony-Teschendorf syndrome (corkscrew esophagus) 530.5

Barth syndrome 759.89
Bartholin's
 adenitis (*see also* Bartholinitis) 616.89
 gland—*see* condition
Bartholinitis (suppurating) 616.89
 gonococcal (acute) 098.0
 chronic or duration of 2 months or over 098.2
Bartonellosis 088.0
Bartter's syndrome (secondary hyperaldosteronism with juxtaglomerular hyperplasia) 255.13
Basal—*see* condition
Basan's (hidrotic) ectodermal dysplasia 757.31
Baseball finger 842.13
Basedow's disease or syndrome (exophthalmic goiter) 242.0
Basic —*see* condition
Basilar —*see* condition
Bason's (hidrotic) ectodermal dysplasia 757.31
Basopenia 288.59
Basophilia 288.65
Basophilism (corticoadrenal) (Cushing's) (pituitary) (thymic) 255.0
Bassen-Kornzweig syndrome (abetalipoproteinemia) 272.5
Bat ear 744.29
Bateman's
 disease 078.0
 purpura (senile) 287.2
Bathing cramp 994.1
Bathophobia 300.23
Batten's disease, retina 330.1 *[362.71]*
Batten-Mayou disease 330.1 *[362.71]*
Batten-Steinert syndrome 359.21
Battered
 adult (syndrome) 995.81
 baby or child (syndrome) 995.54
 spouse (syndrome) 995.81
Battey mycobacterium infection 031.0
Battledore placenta —*see* Placenta, abnormal
Battle exhaustion (*see also* Reaction, stress, acute) 308.9
Baumgarten-Cruveilhier (cirrhosis) disease, or syndrome 571.5
Bauxite
 fibrosis (of lung) 503
 workers' disease 503
Bayle's disease (dementia paralytica) 094.1
Bazin's disease (primary) (*see also* Tuberculosis) 017.1
Beach ear 380.12
Beaded hair (congenital) 757.4
Beals syndrome 759.82
Beard's disease (neurasthenia) 300.5
Bearn-Kunkel (-Slater) syndrome (lupoid hepatitis) 571.49
Beat
 elbow 727.2
 hand 727.2
 knee 727.2
Beats
 ectopic 427.60
 escaped, heart 427.60
   postoperative 997.1
 premature (nodal) 427.60
   atrial 427.61
   auricular 427.61
   postoperative 997.1
   specified type NEC 427.69
   supraventricular 427.61
   ventricular 427.69

INDEX TO DISEASES

Beau's
 disease or syndrome (*see also* Degeneration, myocardial) 429.1
 lines (transverse furrows on fingernails) 703.8
Bechterew's disease (ankylosing spondylitis) 720.0
Bechterew-Strümpell-Marie syndrome (ankylosing spondylitis) 720.0
Beck's syndrome (anterior spinal artery occlusion) 433.8
Becker's
 disease
  idiopathic mural endomyocardial disease 425.2
  myotonia congenita, recessive form 359.22
 dystrophy 359.22
Beckwith (-Wiedemann) syndrome 759.89
Bed confinement status V49.84
Bedclothes, asphyxiation or suffocation by 994.7
Bednar's aphthae 528.2
Bedsore 707.00
 with gangrene 707.00 *[785.4]*
Bedwetting (*see also* Enuresis) 788.36
Beer-drinkers' heart (disease) 425.5
Bee sting (with allergic or anaphylactic shock) 989.5
Begbie's disease (exophthalmic goiter) 242.0
Behavior disorder, disturbance —*see also* Disturbance, conduct
 antisocial, without manifest psychiatric disorder
  adolescent V71.02
  adult V71.01
  child V71.02
 dyssocial, without manifest psychiatric disorder
  adolescent V71.02
  adult V71.01
  child V71.02
 high-risk—*see* Problem
Behçet's syndrome 136.1
Behr's disease 362.50
Beigel's disease or morbus (white piedra) 111.2
Bejel 104.0
Bekhterev's disease (ankylosing spondylitis) 720.0
Bekhterev-Strümpell-Marie syndrome (ankylosing spondylitis) 720.0
Belching (*see also* Eructation) 787.3
Bell's
 disease (*see also* Psychosis, affective) 296.0
 mania (*see also* Psychosis, affective) 296.0
 palsy, paralysis 351.0
  infant 767.5
  newborn 767.5
  syphilitic 094.89
 spasm 351.0
Bence-Jones albuminuria, albuminosuria, or proteinuria 791.0
Bends 993.3
Benedikt's syndrome (paralysis) 344.89
Benign —*see also* condition
 cellular changes, cervix 795.09
 prostate
  hyperplasia 600.20
   with urinary retention 600.21
  neoplasm 222.2
  with
   other lower urinary tract symptoms (LUTS) 600.21
   urinary
    obstruction 600.21
    retention 600.21

Bennett's
 disease (leukemia) 208.9
 fracture (closed) 815.01
  open 815.11
Benson's disease 379.22
Bent
 back (hysterical) 300.11
 nose 738.0
  congenital 754.0
Bereavement V62.82
 as adjustment reaction 309.0
Berger's paresthesia (lower limb) 782.0
Bergeron's disease (hysteroepilepsy) 300.11
Beriberi (acute) (atrophic) (chronic) (dry) (subacute) (wet) 265.0
 with polyneuropathy 265.0 *[357.4]*
 heart (disease) 265.0 *[425.7]*
 leprosy 030.1
 neuritis 265.0 *[357.4]*
Berlin's disease or edema (traumatic) 921.3
Berloque dermatitis 692.72
Bernard-Horner syndrome (*see also* Neuropathy, peripheral, autonomic) 337.9
Bernard-Sergent syndrome (acute adrenocortical insufficiency) 255.41
Bernard-Soulier disease or thrombopathy 287.1
Bernhardt's disease or paresthesia 355.1
Bernhardt-Roth disease or syndrome (paresthesia) 355.1
Bernheim's syndrome (*see also* Failure, heart) 428.0
Bertielliasis 123.8
Bertolotti's syndrome (sacralization of fifth lumbar vertebra) 756.15
Berylliosis (acute) (chronic) (lung) (occupational) 503
Besnier's
 lupus pernio 135
 prurigo (atopic dermatitis) (infantile eczema) 691.8
Besnier-Boeck disease or sarcoid 135
Besnier-Boeck-Schaumann disease (sarcoidosis) 135
Best's disease 362.76
Bestiality 302.1
Beta-adrenergic hyperdynamic circulatory state 429.82
Beta-aminoisobutyric aciduria 277.2
Beta-mercaptolactate-cysteine disulfiduria 270.0
Beta thalassemia (major) (minor) (mixed) 282.49
Beurmann's disease (sporotrichosis) 117.1
Bezoar 938
 intestine 936
 stomach 935.2
Bezold's abscess (*see also* Mastoiditis) 383.01
Bianchi's syndrome (aphasia-apraxia-alexia) 784.69
Bicornuate or bicornis uterus 752.3
 in pregnancy or childbirth 654.0
  with obstructed labor 660.2
   affecting fetus or newborn 763.1
  affecting fetus or newborn 763.89
Bicuspid aortic valve 746.4
Biedl-Bardet syndrome 759.89
Bielschowsky's disease 330.1
Bielschowsky-Jansky
 amaurotic familial idiocy 330.1
 disease 330.1
Biemond's syndrome (obesity, polydactyly, and mental retardation) 759.89

Biermer's anemia or disease (pernicious anemia) 281.0
Biett's disease 695.4
Bifid (congenital)—*see also* Imperfect, closure
  apex, heart 746.89
  clitoris 752.49
  epiglottis 748.3
  kidney 753.3
  nose 748.1
  patella 755.64
  scrotum 752.89
  toe 755.66
  tongue 750.13
  ureter 753.4
  uterus 752.3
  uvula 749.02
    with cleft lip (*see also* Cleft, palate, with cleft lip) 749.20
Biforis uterus (suprasimplex) 752.3
Bifurcation (congenital)—*see also* Imperfect, closure
  gallbladder 751.69
  kidney pelvis 753.3
  renal pelvis 753.3
  rib 756.3
  tongue 750.13
  trachea 748.3
  ureter 753.4
  urethra 753.8
  uvula 749.02
    with cleft lip (*see also* Cleft, palate, with cleft lip) 749.20
  vertebra 756.19
Bigeminal pulse 427.89
Bigeminy 427.89
Big spleen syndrome 289.4
Bilateral —*see* condition
Bile duct —*see* condition
Bile pigments in urine 791.4
Bilharziasis (*see also* Schistosomiasis) 120.9
  chyluria 120.0
  cutaneous 120.3
  galacturia 120.0
  hematochyluria 120.0
  intestinal 120.1
  lipemia 120.9
  lipuria 120.0
  Oriental 120.2
  piarhemia 120.9
  pulmonary 120.2
  tropical hematuria 120.0
  vesical 120.0
Biliary —*see* condition
Bilious (attack)—*see also* Vomiting
  fever, hemoglobinuric 084.8
Bilirubinuria 791.4
Biliuria 791.4
Billroth's disease
  meningocele (*see also* Spina bifida) 741.9
Bilobate placenta —*see* Placenta, abnormal
Bilocular
  heart 745.7
  stomach 536.8
Bing-Horton syndrome (histamine cephalgia) 346.2
Binswanger's disease or dementia 290.12
Biörck (-Thorson) syndrome (malignant carcinoid) 259.2

Biparta, bipartite —*see also* Imperfect, closure
  carpal scaphoid 755.59
  patella 755.64
  placenta—*see* Placenta, abnormal
  vagina 752.49
Bird
  face 756.0
  fanciers' lung or disease 495.2
Bird's disease (oxaluria) 271.8
Birth
  abnormal fetus or newborn 763.9
  accident, fetus or newborn—*see* Birth, injury
  complications in mother—*see* Delivery, complicated
  compression during NEC 767.9
  defect—*see* Anomaly
  delayed, fetus 763.9
  difficult NEC, affecting fetus or newborn 763.9
  dry, affecting fetus or newborn 761.1
  forced, NEC, affecting fetus or newborn 763.89
  forceps, affecting fetus or newborn 763.2
  hematoma of sternomastoid 767.8
  immature 765.1
    extremely 765.0
  inattention, after or at 995.52
  induced, affecting fetus or newborn 763.89
  infant—*see* Newborn
  injury NEC 767.9
    adrenal gland 767.8
    basal ganglia 767.0
    brachial plexus (paralysis) 767.6
    brain (compression) (pressure) 767.0
    cerebellum 767.0
    cerebral hemorrhage 767.0
    conjunctiva 767.8
    eye 767.8
    fracture
      bone, any except clavicle or spine 767.3
      clavicle 767.2
      femur 767.3
      humerus 767.3
      long bone 767.3
      radius and ulna 767.3
      skeleton NEC 767.3
      skull 767.3
      spine 767.4
      tibia and fibula 767.3
    hematoma 767.8
      liver (subcapsular) 767.8
      mastoid 767.8
      skull 767.19
      sternomastoid 767.8
      testes 767.8
      vulva 767.8
    intracranial (edema) 767.0
    laceration
      brain 767.0
      by scalpel 767.8
      peripheral nerve 767.7
    liver 767.8
    meninges
      brain 767.0
      spinal cord 767.4
    nerves (cranial, peripheral) 767.7
      brachial plexus 767.6
      facial 767.5
    paralysis 767.7
      brachial plexus 767.6
      Erb (-Duchenne) 767.6
      facial nerve 767.5
      Klumpke (-Déjérine) 767.6

INDEX TO DISEASES — Bleeding

Birth—*continued*
    radial nerve 767.6
    spinal (cord) (hemorrhage) (laceration)
        (rupture) 767.4
    rupture
        intracranial 767.0
        liver 767.8
        spinal cord 767.4
        spleen 767.8
        viscera 767.8
    scalp 767.19
    scalpel wound 767.8
    skeleton NEC 767.3
    specified NEC 767.8
    spinal cord 767.4
    spleen 767.8
    subdural hemorrhage 767.0
    tentorial, tear 767.0
    testes 767.8
    vulva 767.8
  instrumental, NEC, affecting fetus or newborn 763.2
  lack of care, after or at 995.52
  multiple
    affected by maternal complications of pregnancy 761.5
    healthy liveborn—*see* Newborn, multiple
  neglect, after or at 995.52
  newborn—*see* Newborn
  palsy or paralysis NEC 767.7
  precipitate, fetus or newborn 763.6
  premature (infant) 765.1
  prolonged, affecting fetus or newborn 763.9
  retarded, fetus or newborn 763.9
  shock, newborn 779.89
  strangulation or suffocation
    due to aspiration of clear amniotic fluid 770.13
      with respiratory symptoms 770.14
    mechanical 767.8
  trauma NEC 767.9
  triplet
    affected by maternal complications of pregnancy 761.5
    healthy liveborn—*see* Newborn, multiple
  twin
    affected by maternal complications of pregnancy 761.5
    healthy liveborn—*see* Newborn, twin
  ventouse, affecting fetus or newborn 763.3
Birthmark 757.32
Bisalbuminemia 273.8
Biskra button 085.1
Bite(s)
  with intact skin surface—*see* Contusion
  animal—*see* Wound, open, by site
    intact skin surface—*see* Contusion
  centipede 989.5
  chigger 133.8
  fire ant 989.5
  flea—*see* Injury, superficial, by site
  human (open wound)—*see also* Wound, open, by site
    intact skin surface—*see* Contusion
  insect
    nonvenomous—*see* Injury, superficial, by site
    venomous 989.5
  mad dog (death from) 071
  open
    anterior 524.24
    posterior 524.25
  poisonous 989.5

Bite(s)—*continued*
  red bug 133.8
  reptile 989.5
    nonvenomous—*see* Wound, open, by site
  snake 989.5
    nonvenomous—*see* Wound, open, by site
  spider (venomous) 989.5
    nonvenomous—*see* Injury, superficial, by site
  venomous 989.5
Biting
  cheek or lip 528.9
  nail 307.9
Black
  death 020.9
  eye NEC 921.0
  hairy tongue 529.3
  heel 924.20
  lung disease 500
  palm 923.20
Blackfan-Diamond anemia or syndrome (congenital hypoplastic anemia) 284.01
Blackhead 706.1
Blackout 780.2
Blackwater fever 084.8
Bladder —*see* Condition
Blast
  blindness 921.3
  concussion—*see* Blast, injury
  injury 869.0
    with open wound into cavity 869.1
    abdomen or thorax—*see* Injury, internal, by site
    brain (*see also* Concussion, brain) 850.9
      with skull fracture—*see* Fracture, skull
    ear (acoustic nerve trauma) 951.5
      with perforation, tympanic membrane—*see* Wound, open, ear, drum
    lung (*see also* Injury, internal, lung) 861.20
    otitic (explosive) 388.11
Blastomycosis, blastomycotic (chronic) (cutaneous) (disseminated) (lung) (pulmonary) (systemic) 116.0
  Brazilian 116.1
  European 117.5
  keloidal 116.2
  North American 116.0
  primary pulmonary 116.0
  South American 116.1
Bleb(s) 709.8
  emphysematous (bullous) (diffuse) (lung) (ruptured) (solitary) 492.0
  filtering, eye (postglaucoma) (status) V45.69
    with complication 997.99
    postcataract extraction (complication) 997.99
  lung (ruptured) 492.0
    congenital 770.5
  subpleural (emphysematous) 492.0
Bleeder (familial) (hereditary) (*see also* Defect, coagulation) 286.9
  nonfamilial 286.9
Bleeding (*see also* Hemorrhage) 459.0
  anal 569.3
  anovulatory 628.0
  atonic, following delivery 666.1
  capillary 448.9
  due to subinvolution 621.1
    puerperal 666.2
  ear 388.69
  excessive, associated with menopausal onset 627.0
  familial (*see also* Defect, coagulation) 286.9

Bleeding—*continued*
  following intercourse 626.7
  gastrointestinal 578.9
  gums 523.8
  hemorrhoids—*see* Hemorrhoids, bleeding
  intermenstrual
    irregular 626.6
    regular 626.5
  intraoperative 998.11
  irregular NEC 626.4
  menopausal 627.0
  mouth 528.9
  nipple 611.79
  nose 784.7
  ovulation 626.5
  postclimacteric 627.1
  postcoital 626.7
  postmenopausal 627.1
    following induced menopause 627.4
  postoperative 998.11
  preclimacteric 627.0
  puberty 626.3
    excessive, with onset of menstrual periods 626.3
  rectum, rectal 569.3
  tendencies (*see also* Defect, coagulation) 286.9
  throat 784.8
  umbilical stump 772.3
  umbilicus 789.9
  unrelated to menstrual cycle 626.6
  uterus, uterine 626.9
    climacteric 627.0
    dysfunctional 626.8
    functional 626.8
    unrelated to menstrual cycle 626.6
  vagina, vaginal 623.8
    functional 626.8
  vicarious 625.8
Blennorrhagia, blennorrhagic —*see* Blennorrhea
Blennorrhea (acute) 098.0
  adultorum 098.40
  alveolaris 523.40
  chronic or duration of 2 months or over 098.2
  gonococcal (neonatorum) 098.40
  inclusion (neonatal) (newborn) 771.6
  neonatorum 098.40
Blepharelosis (*see also* Entropion) 374.00
Blepharitis (eyelid) 373.00
  angularis 373.01
  ciliaris 373.00
    with ulcer 373.01
  marginal 373.00
    with ulcer 373.01
  scrofulous (*see also* Tuberculosis) 017.3 [373.00]
  squamous 373.02
  ulcerative 373.01
Blepharochalasis 374.34
  congenital 743.62
Blepharoclonus 333.81
Blepharoconjunctivitis (*see also* Conjunctivitis) 372.20
  angular 372.21
  contact 372.22
Blepharophimosis (eyelid) 374.46
  congenital 743.62
Blepharoplegia 374.89
Blepharoptosis 374.30
  congenital 743.61
Blepharopyorrhea 098.49

Blepharospasm 333.81
  due to drugs 333.85
Blessig's cyst 362.62
Blighted ovum 631
Blind
  bronchus (congenital) 748.3
  eye—*see also* Blindness
    hypertensive 360.42
    hypotensive 360.41
  loop syndrome (postoperative) 579.2
  sac, fallopian tube (congenital) 752.19
  spot, enlarged 368.42
  tract or tube (congenital) NEC—*see* Atresia
Blindness (acquired) (congenital) (both eyes) 369.00
  with deafness V49.85
  blast 921.3
    with nerve injury—*see* Injury, nerve, optic
  Bright's—*see* Uremia
  color (congenital) 368.59
    acquired 368.55
    blue 368.53
    green 368.52
    red 368.51
    total 368.54
  concussion 950.9
  cortical 377.75
  day 368.10
    acquired 368.10
    congenital 368.10
    hereditary 368.10
    specified type NEC 368.10
  due to
    injury NEC 950.9
    refractive error—*see* Error, refractive
  eclipse (total) 363.31
  emotional 300.11
  hysterical 300.11
  legal (both eyes) (USA definition) 369.4
    with impairment of better (less impaired) eye
      near-total 369.02
        with
          lesser eye impairment 369.02
            near-total 369.04
            total 369.03
      profound 369.05
        with
          lesser eye impairment 369.05
            near-total 369.07
            profound 369.08
            total 369.06
      severe 369.21
        with
          lesser eye impairment 369.21
            blind 369.11
            near-total 369.13
            profound 369.14
            severe 369.22
            total 369.12
      total
        with lesser eye impairment total 369.01
  mind 784.69
  moderate
    both eyes 369.25
      with impairment of lesser eye (specified as)
        blind, not further specified 369.15
        low vision, not further specified 369.23
        near-total 369.17
        profound 369.18
        severe 369.24
        total 369.16

Blindness—*continued*
  one eye 369.74
    with vision of other eye (specified as)
      near-normal 369.75
      normal 369.76
  near-total
    both eyes 369.04
      with impairment of lesser eye (specified as)
        blind, not further specified 369.02
        total 369.03
    one eye 369.64
      with vision of other eye (specified as)
        near-normal 369.65
        normal 369.66
  night 368.60
    acquired 368.62
    congenital (Japanese) 368.61
    hereditary 368.61
    specified type NEC 368.69
    vitamin A deficiency 264.5
  nocturnal—*see* Blindness, night
  one eye 369.60
    with low vision of other eye 369.10
  profound
    both eyes 369.08
      with impairment of lesser eye (specified as)
        blind, not further specified 369.05
        near-total 369.07
        total 369.06
    one eye 369.67
      with vision of other eye (specified as)
        near-normal 369.68
        normal 369.69
  psychic 784.69
  severe
    both eyes 369.22
      with impairment of lesser eye (specified as)
        blind, not further specified 369.11
        low vision, not further specified 369.21
        near-total 369.13
        profound 369.14
        total 369.12
    one eye 369.71
      with vision of other eye (specified as)
        near-normal 369.72
        normal 369.73
  snow 370.24
  sun 363.31
  temporary 368.12
  total
    both eyes 369.01
    one eye 369.61
      with vision of other eye (specified as)
        near-normal 369.62
        normal 369.63
  transient 368.12
  traumatic NEC 950.9
  word (developmental) 315.01
    acquired 784.61
    secondary to organic lesion 784.61
Blister —*see also* Injury, superficial, by site
  beetle dermatitis 692.89
  due to burn—*see* Burn, by site, second degree
  fever 054.9
  multiple, skin, nontraumatic 709.8
Bloating 787.3
Bloch-Siemens syndrome (incontinentia pigmenti) 757.33
Bloch-Stauffer dyshormonal dermatosis 757.33
Bloch-Sulzberger disease or syndrome
  (incontinentia pigmenti) (melanoblastosis) 757.33

Block
  alveolar capillary 516.3
  arborization (heart) 426.6
  arrhythmic 426.9
  atrioventricular (AV) (incomplete) (partial) 426.10
    with
      2:1 atrioventricular response block 426.13
      atrioventricular dissociation 426.0
      first degree (incomplete) 426.11
      second degree (Mobitz type I) 426.13
        Mobitz (type) II 426.12
      third degree 426.0
    complete 426.0
      congenital 746.86
    congenital 746.86
    Mobitz (incomplete)
      type I (Wenckebach's) 426.13
      type II 426.12
    partial 426.13
  auriculoventricular (*see also* Block, atrioventricular) 426.10
    complete 426.0
      congenital 746.86
    congenital 746.86
  bifascicular (cardiac) 426.53
  bundle branch (complete) (false) (incomplete) 426.50
    bilateral 426.53
    left (complete) (main stem) 426.3
      with right bundle branch block 426.53
      anterior fascicular 426.2
        with
          posterior fascicular block 426.3
          right bundle branch block 426.52
      hemiblock 426.2
      incomplete 426.2
        with right bundle branch block 426.53
      posterior fascicular 426.2
        with
          anterior fascicular block 426.3
          right bundle branch block 426.51
    right 426.4
      with
        left bundle branch block (incomplete) (main stem) 426.53
        left fascicular block 426.53
          anterior 426.52
          posterior 426.51
    Wilson's type 426.4
  cardiac 426.9
  conduction 426.9
    complete 426.0
  Eustachian tube (*see also* Obstruction, Eustachian tube) 381.60
  fascicular (left anterior) (left posterior) 426.2
  foramen Magendie (acquired) 331.3
    congenital 742.3
      with spina bifida (*see also* Spina bifida) 741.0
  heart 426.9
    first degree (atrioventricular) 426.11
    second degree (atrioventricular) 426.13
    third degree (atrioventricular) 426.0
    bundle branch (complete) (false) (incomplete) 426.50
      bilateral 426.53
      left (*see also* Block, bundle branch, left) 426.3
      right (*see also* Block, bundle branch, right) 426.4

Block

Block—*continued*
   complete (atrioventricular) 426.0
      congenital 746.86
   incomplete 426.13
   intra-atrial 426.6
   intraventricular NEC 426.6
   sinoatrial 426.6
   specified type NEC 426.6
  hepatic vein 453.0
  intraventricular (diffuse) (myofibrillar) 426.6
    bundle branch (complete) (false) (incomplete) 426.50
      bilateral 426.53
      left (*see also* Block, bundle branch, left) 426.3
      right (*see also* Block, bundle branch, right) 426.4
  kidney (*see also* Disease, renal) 593.9
    postcystoscopic 997.5
  myocardial (*see also* Block, heart) 426.9
  nodal 426.10
  optic nerve 377.49
  organ or site (congenital) NEC—*see* Atresia
  parietal 426.6
  peri-infarction 426.6
  portal (vein) 452
  sinoatrial 426.6
  sinoauricular 426.6
  spinal cord 336.9
  trifascicular 426.54
  tubal 628.2
  vein NEC 453.9
Blocq's disease or syndrome (astasia-abasia) 307.9
Blood
  constituents, abnormal NEC 790.6
  disease 289.9
    specified NEC 289.89
  donor V59.01
    other blood components V59.09
    stem cells V59.02
    whole blood V59.01
  dyscrasia 289.9
    with
      abortion—*see* Abortion, by type, with hemorrhage, delayed or excessive
      ectopic pregnancy (*see also* categories 633.0-633.9) 639.1
      molar pregnancy (*see also* categories 630-632) 639.1
      fetus or newborn NEC 776.9
    following
      abortion 639.1
      ectopic or molar pregnancy 639.1
    puerperal, postpartum 666.3
  flukes NEC (*see also* Infestation, Schistosoma) 120.9
  in
    feces (*see also* Melena) 578.1
      occult 792.1
    urine (*see also* Hematuria) 599.7
  mole 631
  occult 792.1
  poisoning (*see also* Septicemia) 038.9
  pressure
    decreased, due to shock following injury 958.4
    fluctuating 796.4
    high (*see also* Hypertension) 401.9
      incidental reading (isolated) (nonspecific), without diagnosis of hypertension 796.2
    low (*see also* Hypotension) 458.9

INDEX TO DISEASES

Blood—*continued*
    incidental reading (isolated) (nonspecific), without diagnosis of hypotension 796.3
  spitting (*see also* Hemoptysis) 786.3
  staining cornea 371.12
  transfusion
    without reported diagnosis V58.2
    donor V59.01
      stem cells V59.02
    reaction or complication—*see* Complications, transfusion
  tumor—*see* Hematoma
  vessel rupture—*see* Hemorrhage
  vomiting (*see also* Hematemesis) 578.0
Blood-forming organ disease 289.9
Bloodgood's disease 610.1
Bloodshot eye 379.93
Bloom (-Machacek) (-Torre) syndrome 757.39
Blotch, palpebral 372.55
Blount's disease (tibia vara) 732.4
Blount-Barber syndrome (tibia vara) 732.4
Blue
  baby 746.9
  bloater 491.20
    with acute bronchitis 491.22
    with exacerbation (acute) 491.21
  diaper syndrome 270.0
  disease 746.9
  dome cyst 610.0
  drum syndrome 381.02
  sclera 743.47
    with fragility of bone and deafness 756.51
  toe syndrome 445.02
Blueness (cyanosis) 782.5
Blurred vision 368.8
Blushing (abnormal) (excessive) 782.62
BMI (body mass index)
  adult
    25.0-25.9 V85.21
    26.0-26.9 V85.22
    27.0-27.9 V85.23
    28.0-28.9 V85.24
    29.0-29.9 V85.25
    30.0-30.9 V85.30
    31.0-31.9 V85.31
    32.0-32.9 V85.32
    33.0-33.9 V85.33
    34.0-34.9 V85.34
    35.0-35.9 V85.35
    36.0-36.9 V85.36
    37.0-37.9 V85.37
    38.0-38.9 V85.38
    39.0-39.9 V85.39
    40 and over V85.4
    between 19-24 V85.1
    less than 19 V85.0
  pediatric
    5th percentile to less than 85th percentile for age V85.52
    85th percentile to less than 95th percentile for age V85.53
    greater than or equal to 95th percentile for age V85.54
    less than 5th percentile for age V85.51
Boarder, hospital V65.0
  infant V65.0
Bockhart's impetigo (superficial folliculitis) 704.8
Bodechtel-Guttmann disease (subacute sclerosing panencephalitis) 046.2
Boder-Sedgwick syndrome (ataxia-telangiectasia) 334.8

Body, bodies
  Aschoff (*see also* Myocarditis, rheumatic) 398.0
  asteroid, vitreous 379.22
  choroid, colloid (degenerative) 362.57
    hereditary 362.77
  cytoid (retina) 362.82
  drusen (retina) (*see also* Drusen) 362.57
    optic disc 377.21
  fibrin, pleura 511.0
  foreign—*see* Foreign body
  Hassall-Henle 371.41
  loose
    joint (*see also* Loose, body, joint) 718.1
      knee 717.6
    knee 717.6
    sheath, tendon 727.82
  Mallory's 034.1
  mass index (BMI)
    adult
      25.0-25.9 V85.21
      26.0-26.9 V85.22
      27.0-27.9 V85.23
      28.0-28.9 V85.24
      29.0-29.9 V85.25
      30.0-30.9 V85.30
      31.0-31.9 V85.31
      32.0-32.9 V85.32
      33.0-33.9 V85.33
      34.0-34.9 V85.34
      35.0-35.9 V85.35
      36.0-36.9 V85.36
      37.0-37.9 V85.37
      38.0-38.9 V85.38
      39.0-39.9 V85.39
      40 and over V85.4
      between 19-24 V85.1
      less than 19 V85.0
    pediatric
      5th percentile to less than 85th percentile for age V85.52
      85th percentile to less than 95th percentile for age V85.53
      greater than or equal to 95th percentile for age V85.54
      less than 5th percentile for age V85.51
  Mooser 081.0
  Negri 071
  rice (joint) (*see also* Loose, body, joint) 718.1
    knee 717.6
  rocking 307.3
Boeck's
  disease (sarcoidosis) 135
  lupoid (miliary) 135
  sarcoid 135
Boerhaave's syndrome (spontaneous esophageal rupture) 530.4
Boggy
  cervix 622.8
  uterus 621.8
Boil (*see also* Carbuncle) 680.9
  abdominal wall 680.2
  Aleppo 085.1
  ankle 680.6
  anus 680.5
  arm (any part, above wrist) 680.3
  auditory canal, external 680.0
  axilla 680.3
  back (any part) 680.2
  Baghdad 085.1
  breast 680.2
  buttock 680.5

Boil —*continued*
  chest wall 680.2
  corpus cavernosum 607.2
  Delhi 085.1
  ear (any part) 680.0
  eyelid 373.13
  face (any part, except eye) 680.0
  finger (any) 680.4
  flank 680.2
  foot (any part) 680.7
  forearm 680.3
  Gafsa 085.1
  genital organ, male 608.4
  gluteal (region) 680.5
  groin 680.2
  hand (any part) 680.4
  head (any part, except face) 680.8
  heel 680.7
  hip 680.6
  knee 680.6
  labia 616.4
  lacrimal (*see also* Dacryocystitis) 375.30
    gland (*see also* Dacryoadenitis) 375.00
    passages (duct) (sac) (*see also* Dacryocystitis) 375.30
  leg, any part except foot 680.6
  multiple sites 680.9
  Natal 085.1
  neck 680.1
  nose (external) (septum) 680.0
  orbit, orbital 376.01
  partes posteriores 680.5
  pectoral region 680.2
  penis 607.2
  perineum 680.2
  pinna 680.0
  scalp (any part) 680.8
  scrotum 608.4
  seminal vesicle 608.0
  shoulder 680.3
  skin NEC 680.9
  specified site NEC 680.8
  spermatic cord 608.4
  temple (region) 680.0
  testis 608.4
  thigh 680.6
  thumb 680.4
  toe (any) 680.7
  tropical 085.1
  trunk 680.2
  tunica vaginalis 608.4
  umbilicus 680.2
  upper arm 680.3
  vas deferens 608.4
  vulva 616.4
  wrist 680.4
Bold hives (*see also* Urticaria) 708.9
Bolivian hemorrhagic fever 078.7
Bombé, iris 364.74
Bomford-Rhoads anemia (refractory) 238.72
Bone —*see* condition
Bonnevie-Ullrich syndrome 758.6
Bonnier's syndrome 386.19
Bonvale Dam fever 780.79
Bony block of joint 718.80
  ankle 718.87
  elbow 718.82
  foot 718.87
  hand 718.84
  hip 718.85
  knee 718.86

Bony block of joint—*continued*
　multiple sites 718.89
　pelvic region 718.85
　shoulder (region) 718.81
　specified site NEC 718.88
　wrist 718.83
Borderline
　intellectual functioning V62.89
　pelvis 653.1
　　with obstruction during labor 660.1
　　　affecting fetus or newborn 763.1
　　psychosis (*see also* Schizophrenia) 295.5
　　　of childhood (*see also* Psychosis, childhood) 299.8
　　schizophrenia (*see also* Schizophrenia) 295.5
Borna disease 062.9
Bornholm disease (epidemic pleurodynia) 074.1
Borrelia vincentii (mouth) (pharynx) (tonsils) 101
Bostock's catarrh (*see also* Fever, hay) 477.9
Boston exanthem 048
Botalli, ductus (patent) (persistent) 747.0
Bothriocephalus latus infestation 123.4
Botulism 005.1
　food poisoning 005.1
　infant 040.41
　non-foodborne 040.42
　wound 040.42
Bouba (*see also* Yaws) 102.9
Bouffée délirante 298.3
Bouillaud's disease or syndrome (rheumatic heart disease) 391.9
Bourneville's disease (tuberous sclerosis) 759.5
Boutonneuse fever 082.1
Boutonniere
　deformity (finger) 736.21
　hand (intrinsic) 736.21
Bouveret (-Hoffmann) disease or syndrome (paroxysmal tachycardia) 427.2
Bovine heart —*see* Hypertrophy, cardiac
Bowel —*see* condition
Bowen's
　dermatosis (precancerous) (M8081/2)—*see* Neoplasm, skin, in situ
　disease (M8081/2)—*see* Neoplasm, skin, in situ
　epithelioma (M8081/2)—*see* Neoplasm, skin, in situ
　type
　　epidermoid carcinoma in situ (M8081/2)—*see* Neoplasm, skin, in situ
　　intraepidermal squamous cell carcinoma (M8081/2)–*see* Neoplasm, skin, in situ
Bowing
　femur 736.89
　　congenital 754.42
　fibula 736.89
　　congenital 754.43
　forearm 736.09
　　away from midline (cubitus valgus) 736.01
　　toward midline (cubitus varus) 736.02
　leg(s), long bones, congenital 754.44
　radius 736.09
　　away from midline (cubitus valgus) 736.01
　　toward midline (cubitus varus) 736.02
　tibia 736.89
　　congenital 754.43
Bowleg (s) 736.42
　congenital 754.44
　rachitic 268.1
Boyd's dysentery 004.2
Brachial —*see* condition

Brachman-de Lange syndrome (Amsterdam dwarf, mental retardation, and brachycephaly) 759.89
Brachycardia 427.89
Brachycephaly 756.0
Brachymorphism and ectopia lentis 759.89
Bradley's disease (epidemic vomiting) 078.82
Bradycardia 427.89
　chronic (sinus) 427.81
　newborn 779.81
　nodal 427.89
　postoperative 997.1
　reflex 337.0
　sinoatrial 427.89
　　with paroxysmal tachyarrhythmia or tachycardia 427.81
　　chronic 427.81
　sinus 427.89
　　with paroxysmal tachyarrhythmia or tachycardia 427.81
　　chronic 427.81
　　persistent 427.81
　　severe 427.81
　tachycardia syndrome 427.81
　vagal 427.89
Bradypnea 786.09
Brailsford's disease 732.3
　radial head 732.3
　tarsal scaphoid 732.5
Brailsford-Morquio disease or syndrome (mucopolysaccharidosis IV) 277.5
Brain —*see also* condition
　death 348.8
　syndrome (acute) (chronic) (nonpsychotic) (organic) (with neurotic reaction) (with behavioral reaction) (*see also* Syndrome, brain) 310.9
　　with
　　　presenile brain disease 290.10
　　　psychosis, psychotic reaction (*see also* Psychosis, organic) 294.9
　　congenital (*see also* Retardation, mental) 319
Branched-chain amino-acid disease 270.3
Branchial —*see* condition
Brandt's syndrome (acrodermatitis enteropathica) 686.8
Brash (water) 787.1
Brass-founders' ague 985.8
Bravais-Jacksonian epilepsy (*see also* Epilepsy) 345.5
Braxton Hicks contractions 644.1
Braziers' disease 985.8
Brazilian
　blastomycosis 116.1
　leishmaniasis 085.5
BRBPR (bright red blood per rectum) 569.3
Break
　cardiorenal—*see* Hypertension, cardiorenal
　retina (*see also* Defect, retina) 361.30
Breakbone fever 061
Breakdown
　device, implant, or graft—*see* Complications, mechanical
　nervous (*see also* Disorder, mental, nonpsychotic) 300.9
　perineum 674.2
Breast —*see* condition
Breast feeding difficulties 676.8

Breath
 foul 784.99
 holder, child 312.81
 holding spells 786.9
 shortness 786.05
Breathing
 asymmetrical 786.09
 bronchial 786.09
 exercises V57.0
 labored 786.09
 mouth 784.99
  causing malocclusion 524.59
 periodic 786.09
  high altitude 327.22
 tic 307.20
Breathlessness 786.09
Breda's disease (*see also* Yaws) 102.9
Breech
 delivery, affecting fetus or newborn 763.0
 extraction, affecting fetus or newborn 763.0
 presentation (buttocks) (complete) (frank) 652.2
  with successful version 652.1
   before labor, affecting fetus or newborn 761.7
   during labor, affecting fetus or newborn 763.0
Breisky's disease (kraurosis vulvae) 624.09
Brennemann's syndrome (acute mesenteric lymphadenitis) 289.2
Brenner's
 tumor (benign) (M9000/0) 220
  borderline malignancy (M9000/1) 236.2
  malignant (M9000/3) 183.0
  proliferating (M9000/1) 236.2
Bretonneau's disease (diphtheritic malignant angina) 032.0
Breus' mole 631
Brevicollis 756.16
Bricklayers' itch 692.89
Brickmakers' anemia 126.9
Bridge
 myocardial 746.85
Bright's
 blindness—*see* Uremia
 disease (*see also* Nephritis) 583.9
  arteriosclerotic (*see also* Hypertension, kidney) 403.90
Bright red blood per rectum (BRBPR) 569.3
Brill's disease (recrudescent typhus) 081.1
 flea-borne 081.0
 louse-borne 081.1
Brill-Symmers disease (follicular lymphoma) (M9690/3) 202.0
Brill-Zinsser disease (recrudescent typhus) 081.1
Brinton's disease (linitis plastica) (M8142/3) 151.9
Brion-Kayser disease (*see also* Fever, paratyphoid) 002.9
Briquet's disorder or syndrome 300.81
Brissaud's
 infantilism (infantile myxedema) 244.9
 motor-verbal tic 307.23
Brissaud-Meige syndrome (infantile myxedema) 244.9
Brittle
 bones (congenital) 756.51
 nails 703.8
  congenital 757.5
Broad —*see also* condition
 beta disease 272.2
 ligament laceration syndrome 620.6
Brock's syndrome (atelectasis due to enlarged lymph nodes) 518.0

Brocq's disease 691.8
 atopic (diffuse) neurodermatitis 691.8
 lichen simplex chronicus 698.3
 parakeratosis psoriasiformis 696.2
 parapsoriasis 696.2
Brocq-Duhring disease (dermatitis herpetiformis) 694.0
Brodie's
 abscess (localized) (chronic) (*see also* Osteomyelitis) 730.1
 disease (joint) (*see also* Osteomyelitis) 730.1
Broken
 arches 734
  congenital 755.67
 back—*see* Fracture, vertebra, by site
 bone—*see* Fracture, by site
 compensation—*see* Disease, heart
 heart syndrome 429.83
 implant or internal device—*see* listing under Complications, mechanical
 neck—*see* Fracture, vertebra, cervical
 nose 802.0
  open 802.1
 tooth, teeth 873.63
  complicated 873.73
Bromhidrosis 705.89
Bromidism, bromism
 acute 967.3
  correct substance properly administered 349.82
  overdose or wrong substance given or taken 967.3
 chronic (*see also* Dependence) 304.1
Bromidrosiphobia 300.23
Bromidrosis 705.89
Bronchi, bronchial —*see* condition
Bronchiectasis (cylindrical) (diffuse) (fusiform) (localized) (moniliform) (postinfectious) (recurrent) (saccular) 494.0
 with acute exacerbation 494.1
 congenital 748.61
 tuberculosis (*see also* Tuberculosis) 011.5
Bronchiolectasis —*see* Bronchiectasis
Bronchiolitis (acute) (infectious) (subacute) 466.19
 with
  bronchospasm or obstruction 466.19
  influenza, flu, or grippe 487.1
 catarrhal (acute) (subacute) 466.19
 chemical 506.0
  chronic 506.4
 chronic (obliterative) 491.8
 due to external agent—*see* Bronchitis, acute, due to
 fibrosa obliterans 491.8
 influenzal 487.1
 obliterans 491.8
  status post lung transplant 996.84
  with organizing pneumonia (B.O.O.P.) 516.8
 obliterative (chronic) (diffuse) (subacute) 491.8
  due to fumes or vapors 506.4
 respiratory syncytial virus 466.11
 vesicular—*see* Pneumonia, broncho-
Bronchitis (diffuse) (hypostatic) (infectious) (inflammatory) (simple) 490
 with
  emphysema—*see* Emphysema
  influenza, flu, or grippe 487.1
  obstruction airway, chronic 491.20
   with
    acute bronchitis 491.22

Bronchitis—*continued*
    exacerbation (acute) 491.21
  tracheitis 490
    acute or subacute 466.0
      with bronchospasm or obstruction 466.0
    chronic 491.8
acute or subacute 466.0
  with
    bronchospasm 466.0
    obstruction 466.0
    tracheitis 466.0
  chemical (due to fumes or vapors) 506.0
  due to
    fumes or vapors 506.0
    radiation 508.8
allergic (acute) (*see also* Asthma) 493.9
arachidic 934.1
aspiration 507.0
  due to fumes or vapors 506.0
asthmatic (acute) 493.90
  with
    acute exacerbation 493.92
    status asthmaticus 493.91
  chronic 493.2
capillary 466.19
  with bronchospasm or obstruction 466.19
  chronic 491.8
caseous (*see also* Tuberculosis) 011.3
Castellani's 104.8
catarrhal 490
  acute—*see* Bronchitis, acute
  chronic 491.0
chemical (acute) (subacute) 506.0
  chronic 506.4
  due to fumes or vapors (acute) (subacute) 506.0
    chronic 506.4
chronic 491.9
  with
    tracheitis (chronic) 491.8
  asthmatic 493.2
  catarrhal 491.0
  chemical (due to fumes and vapors) 506.4
  due to
    fumes or vapors (chemical) (inhalation) 506.4
    radiation 508.8
    tobacco smoking 491.0
  mucopurulent 491.1
  obstructive 491.20
    with
      acute bronchitis 491.22
      exacerbation (acute) 491.21
  purulent 491.1
  simple 491.0
  specified type NEC 491.8
croupous 466.0
  with bronchospasm or obstruction 466.0
  due to fumes or vapors 506.0
emphysematous 491.20
  with
    acute bronchitis 491.22
    exacerbation (acute) 491.21
exudative 466.0
fetid (chronic) (recurrent) 491.1
fibrinous, acute or subacute 466.0
  with bronchospasm or obstruction 466.0
grippal 487.1
influenzal 487.1
membranous, acute or subacute 466.0
  with bronchospasm or obstruction 466.0

Bronchitis—*continued*
  moulders' 502
  mucopurulent (chronic) (recurrent) 491.1
    acute or subacute 466.0
  non-obstructive 491.0
  obliterans 491.8
  obstructive (chronic) 491.20
    with
      acute bronchitis 491.22
      exacerbation (acute) 491.21
  pituitous 491.1
  plastic (inflammatory) 466.0
  pneumococcal, acute or subacute 466.0
    with bronchospasm or obstruction 466.0
  pseudomembranous 466.0
  purulent (chronic) (recurrent) 491.1
    acute or subacute 466.0
      with bronchospasm or obstruction 466.0
  putrid 491.1
  scrofulous (*see also* Tuberculosis) 011.3
  senile 491.9
  septic, acute or subacute 466.0
    with bronchospasm or obstruction 466.0
  smokers' 491.0
  spirochetal 104.8
  suffocative, acute or subacute 466.0
  summer (*see also* Asthma) 493.9
  suppurative (chronic) 491.1
    acute or subacute 466.0
  tuberculous (*see also* Tuberculosis) 011.3
  ulcerative 491.8
  Vincent's 101
  Vincent's 101
  viral, acute or subacute 466.0
    with bronchospasm or obstruction 466.0
Bronchoalveolitis 485
Bronchoaspergillosis 117.3
Bronchocele
  meaning
    dilatation of bronchus 519.19
    goiter 240.9
Bronchogenic carcinoma 162.9
Bronchohemisporosis 117.9
Broncholithiasis 518.89
  tuberculous (*see also* Tuberculosis) 011.3
Bronchomalacia 748.3
Bronchomoniliasis 112.89
Bronchomycosis 112.89
Bronchonocardiosis 039.1
Bronchopleuropneumonia —*see* Pneumonia, broncho-
Bronchopneumonia —*see* Pneumonia, broncho-
Bronchopneumonitis —*see* Pneumonia, broncho-
Bronchopulmonary —*see* condition
Bronchopulmonitis —*see* Pneumonia, broncho-
Bronchorrhagia 786.3
  newborn 770.3
  tuberculous (*see also* Tuberculosis) 011.3
Bronchorrhea (chronic) (purulent) 491.0
  acute 466.0
Bronchospasm 519.11
  with
    asthma—*see* Asthma
    bronchiolitis, acute 466.19
      due to respiratory syncytial virus 466.11
    bronchitis—*see* Bronchitis
    chronic obstructive pulmonary disease (COPD) 496
    emphysema—*see* Emphysema

Bronchospasm—*continued*
due to external agent—*see* Condition, respiratory, acute, due to
acute 519.11
due to external agent—*see* Condition, respiratory, acute, due to
exercise induced 493.81
Bronchospirochetosis 104.8
Bronchostenosis 519.19
Bronchus —*see* condition
Bronze, bronzed
diabetes 275.0
disease (Addison's) (skin) 255.41
tuberculous (*see also* Tuberculosis) 017.6
Brooke's disease or tumor (M8100/0)—*see* Neoplasm, skin, benign
Brow presentation complicating delivery 652.4
Brown's tendon sheath syndrome 378.61
Brown enamel of teeth (hereditary) 520.5
Brown-Séquard's paralysis (syndrome) 344.89
Brucella, brucellosis (infection) 023.9
abortus 023.1
canis 023.3
dermatitis, skin 023.9
melitensis 023.0
mixed 023.8
suis 023.2
Bruck's disease 733.99
Bruck-de Lange disease or syndrome (Amsterdam dwarf, mental retardation, and brachycephaly) 759.89
Brugada syndrome 746.89
Brug's filariasis 125.1
Brugsch's syndrome (acropachyderma) 757.39
Bruhl's disease (splenic anemia with fever) 285.8
Bruise (skin surface intact)—*see also* Contusion
with
fracture—*see* Fracture, by site
open wound—*see* Wound, open, by site
internal organ (abdomen, chest, or pelvis)—*see* Injury, internal, by site
umbilical cord 663.6
affecting fetus or newborn 762.6
Bruit 785.9
arterial (abdominal) (carotid) 785.9
supraclavicular 785.9
Brushburn —*see* Injury, superficial, by site
Bruton's X-linked agammaglobulinemia 279.04
Bruxism 306.8
sleep related 327.53
Bubbly lung syndrome 770.7
Bubo 289.3
blennorrhagic 098.89
chancroidal 099.0
climatic 099.1
due to Hemophilus ducreyi 099.0
gonococcal 098.89
indolent NEC 099.8
inguinal NEC 099.8
chancroidal 099.0
climatic 099.1
due to H. ducreyi 099.0
scrofulous (*see also* Tuberculosis) 017.2
soft chancre 099.0
suppurating 683
syphilitic 091.0
congenital 090.0
tropical 099.1
venereal NEC 099.8
virulent 099.0

Bubonic plague 020.0
Bubonocele —*see* Hernia, inguinal
Buccal —*see* condition
Buchanan's disease (juvenile osteochondrosis of iliac crest) 732.1
Buchem's syndrome (hyperostosis corticalis) 733.3
Buchman's disease (osteochondrosis, juvenile) 732.1
Bucket handle fracture (semilunar cartilage) (*see also* Tear, meniscus) 836.2
Budd-Chiari syndrome (hepatic vein thrombosis) 453.0
Budgerigar-fanciers' disease or lung 495.2
Büdinger-Ludloff-Läwen disease 717.89
Buerger's disease (thromboangiitis obliterans) 443.1
Bulbar —*see* condition
Bulbus cordis 745.9
persistent (in left ventricle) 745.8
Bulging fontanels (congenital) 756.0
Bulimia 783.6
nervosa 307.51
nonorganic origin 307.51
Bulky uterus 621.2
Bulla(e) 709.8
lung (emphysematous) (solitary) 492.0
Bullet wound —*see also* Wound, open, by site
fracture—*see* Fracture, by site, open
internal organ (abdomen, chest, or pelvis)—*see* Injury, internal, by site, with open wound
intracranial—*see* Laceration, brain, with open wound
Bullis fever 082.8
Bullying (*see also* Disturbance, conduct) 312.0
Bundle
branch block (complete) (false) (incomplete) 426.50
bilateral 426.53
left (*see also* Block, bundle branch, left) 426.3
hemiblock 426.2
right (*see also* Block, bundle branch, right) 426.4
of His—*see* condition
of Kent syndrome (anomalous atrioventricular excitation) 426.7
Bungpagga 040.81
Bunion 727.1
Bunionette 727.1
Bunyamwera fever 066.3
Buphthalmia, buphthalmos (congenital) 743.20
associated with
keratoglobus, congenital 743.22
megalocornea 743.22
ocular anomalies NEC 743.22
isolated 743.21
simple 743.21
Bürger-Grütz disease or syndrome (essential familial hyperlipemia) 272.3
Buried roots 525.3
Burke's syndrome 577.8
Burkitt's
tumor (M9750/3) 200.2
type malignant, lymphoma, lymphoblastic, or undifferentiated (M9750/3) 200.2

Burn (acid) (cathode ray) (caustic) (chemical) (electric heating appliance) (electricity) (fire) (flame) (hot liquid or object) (irradiation) (lime) (radiation) (steam) (thermal) (x-ray) 949.0

> *Note—Use the following fifth-digit subclassification with category 948 to indicate the percent of body surface with third degree burn:*
>
> 0 *less than 10% or unspecified*
> 1 *10-19%*
> 2 *20-29%*
> 3 *30-39%*
> 4 *40-49%*
> 5 *50-59%*
> 6 *60-69%*
> 7 *70-79%*
> 8 *80-89%*
> 9 *90% or more of body surface*

with
    blisters—*see* Burn, by site, second degree
    erythema—*see* Burn, by site, first degree
    skin loss (epidermal)—*see also* Burn, by site, second degree
        full thickness—*see also* Burn, by site, third degree
            with necrosis of underlying tissues—*see* Burn, by site, third degree, deep
    first degree—*see* Burn, by site, first degree
    second degree—*see* Burn, by site, second degree
    third degree—*see also* Burn, by site, third degree
        deep—*see* Burn, by site, third degree, deep
abdomen, abdominal (muscle) (wall) 942.03
    with
        trunk—*see* Burn, trunk, multiple sites
    first degree 942.13
    second degree 942.23
    third degree 942.33
        deep 942.43
            with loss of body part 942.53
ankle 945.03
    with
        lower limb(s)–*see* Burn, leg, multiple sites
    first degree 945.13
    second degree 945.23
    third degree 945.33
        deep 945.43
            with loss of body part 945.53
anus—*see* Burn, trunk, specified site NEC
arm(s) 943.00
    first degree 943.10
    second degree 943.20
    third degree 943.30
        deep 943.40
            with loss of body part 943.50
    lower—*see* Burn, forearm(s)
    multiple sites, except hand(s) or wrist(s) 943.09
        first degree 943.19
        second degree 943.29
        third degree 943.39
            deep 943.49
                with loss of body part 943.59
    upper 943.03
        first degree 943.13
        second degree 943.23
        third degree 943.33
            deep 943.43
                with loss of body part 943.53
auditory canal (external)—*see* Burn, ear

Burn—*continued*
    auricle (ear)—*see* Burn, ear
    axilla 943.04
        with
            upper limb(s) except hand(s) or wrist(s)—*see* Burn, arm(s), multiple sites
        first degree 943.14
        second degree 943.24
        third degree 943.34
            deep 943.44
                with loss of body part 943.54
    back 942.04
        with
            trunk—*see* Burn, trunk, multiple sites
        first degree 942.14
        second degree 942.24
        third degree 942.34
            deep 942.44
                with loss of body part 942.54
    biceps
        brachii—*see* Burn, arm(s), upper
        femoris—*see* Burn, thigh
    breast(s) 942.01
        with
            trunk—*see* Burn, trunk, multiple sites
        first degree 942.11
        second degree 942.21
        third degree 942.31
            deep 942.41
                with loss of body part 942.51
    brow—*see* Burn, forehead
    buttock(s)—*see* Burn, back
    canthus (eye) 940.1
        chemical 940.0
    cervix (uteri) 947.4
    cheek (cutaneous) 941.07
        with
            face or head—*see* Burn, head, multiple sites
        first degree 941.17
        second degree 941.27
        third degree 941.37
            deep 941.47
                with loss of body part 941.57
    chest wall (anterior) 942.02
        with
            trunk—*see* Burn, trunk, multiple sites
        first degree 942.12
        second degree 942.22
        third degree 942.32
            deep 942.42
                with loss of body part 942.52
    chin 941.04
        with
            face or head—*see* Burn, head, multiple sites
        first degree 941.14
        second degree 941.24
        third degree 941.34
            deep 941.44
                with loss of body part 941.54
    clitoris—*see* Burn, genitourinary organs, external
    colon 947.3
    conjunctiva (and cornea) 940.4
        chemical
            acid 940.3
            alkaline 940.2
    cornea (and conjunctiva) 940.4
        chemical
            acid 940.3
            alkaline 940.2
    costal region—*see* Burn, chest wall

INDEX TO DISEASES   Burn

Burn—*continued*
  due to ingested chemical agent—*see* Burn,
      internal organs
  ear (auricle) (canal) (drum) (external) 941.01
    with
      face or head—*see* Burn, head, multiple sites
    first degree 941.11
    second degree 941.21
    third degree 941.31
      deep 941.41
        with loss of a body part 941.51
  elbow 943.02
    with
      hand(s) and wrist(s)—*see* Burn, multiple
          specified sites
      upper limb(s) except hand(s) or
          wrist(s)—*see also* Burn, arm(s), multiple
          sites
    first degree 943.12
    second degree 943.22
    third degree 943.32
      deep 943.42
        with loss of body part 943.52
  electricity, electric current—*see* Burn, by site
  entire body—*see* Burn, multiple, specified sites
  epididymis—*see* Burn, genitourinary organs,
      external
  epigastric region—*see* Burn, abdomen
  epiglottis 947.1
  esophagus 947.2
  extent (percent of body surface)
    less than 10 percent 948.0
    10-19 percent 948.1
    20-29 percent 948.2
    30-39 percent 948.3
    40-49 percent 948.4
    50-59 percent 948.5
    60-69 percent 948.6
    70-79 percent 948.7
    80-89 percent 948.8
    90 percent or more 948.9
  extremity
    lower—*see* Burn, leg
    upper—*see* Burn, arm(s)
  eye(s) (and adnexa) (only) 940.9
    with
      face, head, or neck 941.02
      first degree 941.12
      second degree 941.22
      third degree 941.32
        deep 941.42
          with loss of body part 941.52
      other sites (classifiable to more than one
          category in 940-945)—*see* Burn,
          multiple, specified sites
      resulting rupture and destruction of eyeball
          940.5
    specified part—*see* Burn, by site
  eyeball—*see also* Burn, eye
    with resulting rupture and destruction of
        eyeball 940.5
  eyelid(s) 940.1
    chemical 940.0
  face—*see* Burn, head
  finger (nail) (subungual) 944.01
    with
      hand(s)—*see* Burn, hand(s), multiple sites
      other sites—*see* Burn, multiple, specified
          sites
      thumb 944.04
        first degree 944.14

Burn—*continued*
    second degree 944.24
    third degree 944.34
      deep 944.44
        with loss of body part 944.54
    first degree 944.11
    second degree 944.21
    third degree 944.31
      deep 944.41
        with loss of body part 944.51
    multiple (digits) 944.03
      with thumb—*see* Burn, finger, with thumb
      first degree 944.13
      second degree 944.23
      third degree 944.33
        deep 944.43
          with loss of body part 944.53
  flank—*see* Burn, abdomen
  foot 945.02
    with
      lower limb(s)—*see* Burn, leg, multiple sites
    first degree 945.12
    second degree 945.22
    third degree 945.32
      deep 945.42
        with loss of body part 945.52
  forearm(s) 943.01
    with
      upper limb(s) except hand(s) or
          wrist(s)—*see* Burn, arm(s), multiple sites
    first degree 943.11
    second degree 943.21
    third degree 943.31
      deep 943.41
        with loss of body part 943.51
  forehead 941.07
    with
      face or head—*see* Burn, head, multiple sites
    first degree 941.17
    second degree 941.27
    third degree 941.37
      deep 941.47
        with loss of body part 941.57
  fourth degree—*see* Burn, by site, third degree,
      deep
  friction—*see* Injury, superficial, by site
  from swallowing caustic or corrosive substance
      NEC—*see* Burn, internal organs
  full thickness—*see* Burn, by site, third degree
  gastrointestinal tract 947.3
  genitourinary organs
    external 942.05
      with
        trunk—*see* Burn, trunk, multiple sites
      first degree 942.15
      second degree 942.25
      third degree 942.35
        deep 942.45
          with loss of body part 942.55
    internal 947.8
  globe (eye)—*see* Burn, eyeball
  groin—*see* Burn, abdomen
  gum 947.0
  hand(s) (phalanges) (and wrist) 944.00
    first degree 944.10
    second degree 944.20
    third degree 944.30
      deep 944.40
        with loss of body part 944.50
    back (dorsal surface) 944.06
      first degree 944.16

849

Burn—*continued*
    second degree 944.26
    third degree 944.36
      deep 944.46
        with loss of body part 944.56
    multiple sites 944.08
      first degree 944.18
      second degree 944.28
      third degree 944.38
        deep 944.48
          with loss of body part 944.58
  head (and face) 941.00
    eye(s) only 940.9
    specified part—*see* Burn, by site
    first degree 941.10
    second degree 941.20
    third degree 941.30
      deep 941.40
        with loss of body part 941.50
    multiple sites 941.09
      with eyes—*see* Burn, eyes, with face, head, or neck
      first degree 941.19
      second degree 941.29
      third degree 941.39
        deep 941.49
          with loss of body part 941.59
  heel—*see* Burn, foot
  hip—*see* Burn, trunk, specified site NEC
  iliac region—*see* Burn, trunk, specified site NEC
  infected 958.3
  inhalation (*see also* Burn, internal organs) 947.9
  internal organs 947.9
    from caustic or corrosive substance (swallowing) NEC 947.9
    specified NEC (*see also* Burn, by site) 947.8
  interscapular region—*see* Burn, back
  intestine (large) (small) 947.3
  iris—*see* Burn, eyeball
  knee 945.05
    with
      lower limb(s)—*see* Burn, leg, multiple sites
    first degree 945.15
    second degree 945.25
    third degree 945.35
      deep 945.45
        with loss of body part 945.55
  labium (majus) (minus)—*see* Burn, genitourinary organs, external
  lacrimal apparatus, duct, gland, or sac 940.1
    chemical 940.0
  larynx 947.1
  late effect—*see* Late, effects (of), burn
  leg 945.00
    first degree 945.10
    second degree 945.20
    third degree 945.30
      deep 945.40
        with loss of body part 945.50
    lower 945.04
      with other part(s) of lower limb(s)—*see* Burn, leg, multiple sites
      first degree 945.14
      second degree 945.24
      third degree 945.34
        deep 945.44
          with loss of body part 945.54
    multiple sites 945.09
      first degree 945.19
      second degree 945.29

Burn—*continued*
      third degree 945.39
        deep 945.49
          with loss of body part 945.59
    upper—*see* Burn, thigh
  lightning—*see* Burn, by site
  limb(s)
    lower (including foot or toe(s))—*see* Burn, leg
    upper (except wrist and hand)—*see* Burn, arm(s)
  lip(s) 941.03
    with
      face or head—*see* Burn, head, multiple sites
    first degree 941.13
    second degree 941.23
    third degree 941.33
      deep 941.43
        with loss of body part 941.53
  lumbar region—*see* Burn, back
  lung 947.1
  malar region—*see* Burn, cheek
  mastoid region—*see* Burn, scalp
  membrane, tympanic—*see* Burn, ear
  midthoracic region—*see* Burn, chest wall
  mouth 947.0
  multiple (*see also* Burn, unspecified) 949.0
    specified sites (classifiable to more than one category in 940-945) 946.0
      first degree 946.1
      second degree 946.2
      third degree 946.3
        deep 946.4
          with loss of body part 946.5
  muscle, abdominal—*see* Burn, abdomen
  nasal (septum)—*see* Burn, nose
  neck 941.08
    with
      face or head—*see* Burn, head, multiple sites
    first degree 941.18
    second degree 941.28
    third degree 941.38
      deep 941.48
        with loss of body part 941.58
  nose (septum) 941.05
    with
      face or head—*see* Burn, head, multiple sites
    first degree 941.15
    second degree 941.25
    third degree 941.35
      deep 941.45
        with loss of body part 941.55
  occipital region—*see* Burn, scalp
  orbit region 940.1
    chemical 940.0
  oronasopharynx 947.0
  palate 947.0
  palm(s) 944.05
    with
      hand(s) and wrist(s)—*see* Burn, hand(s), multiple sites
    first degree 944.15
    second degree 944.25
    third degree 944.35
      deep 944.45
        with loss of a body part 944.55
  parietal region—*see* Burn, scalp
  penis–*see* Burn, genitourinary organs, external
  perineum—*see* Burn, genitourinary organs, external
  periocular area 940.1
    chemical 940.0

INDEX TO DISEASES — Burn

Burn—*continued*
 pharynx 947.0
 pleura 947.1
 popliteal space—*see* Burn, knee
 prepuce—*see* Burn, genitourinary organs, external
 pubic region—*see* Burn, genitourinary organs, external
 pudenda—*see* Burn, genitourinary organs, external
 rectum 947.3
 sac, lacrimal 940.1
  chemical 940.0
 sacral region—*see* Burn, back
 salivary (ducts) (glands) 947.0
 scalp 941.06
  with
   face or neck—*see* Burn, head, multiple sites
  first degree 941.16
  second degree 941.26
  third degree 941.36
   deep 941.46
    with loss of body part 941.56
 scapular region 943.06
  with
   upper limb(s), except hand(s) or wrist(s)—*see* Burn, arm(s), multiple sites
  first degree 943.16
  second degree 943.26
  third degree 943.36
   deep 943.46
    with loss of body part 943.56
 sclera—*see* Burn, eyeball
 scrotum—*see* Burn, genitourinary organs, external
 septum, nasal—*see* Burn, nose
 shoulder(s) 943.05
  with
   hand(s) and wrist(s)—*see* Burn, multiple, specified sites
   upper limb(s), except hand(s) or wrist(s)—*see* Burn, arm(s), multiple sites
  first degree 943.15
  second degree 943.25
  third degree 943.35
   deep 943.45
    with loss of body part 943.55
 skin NEC (*see also* Burn, unspecified) 949.0
 skull—*see* Burn, head
 small intestine 947.3
 sternal region—*see* Burn, chest wall
 stomach 947.3
 subconjunctival—*see* Burn, conjunctiva
 subcutaneous—*see* Burn, by site, third degree
 submaxillary region—*see* Burn, head
 submental region—*see* Burn, chin
 sun—*see* Sunburn
 supraclavicular fossa—*see* Burn, neck
 supraorbital—*see* Burn, forehead
 temple—*see* Burn, scalp
 temporal region—*see* Burn, scalp
 testicle—*see* Burn, genitourinary organs, external
 testis—*see* Burn, genitourinary organs, external
 thigh 945.06
  with
   lower limb(s)–*see* Burn, leg, multiple sites
  first degree 945.16
  second degree 945.26

Burn—*continued*
  third degree 945.36
   deep 945.46
    with loss of body part 945.56
 thorax (external)—*see* Burn, chest wall
 throat 947.0
 thumb(s) (nail) (subungual) 944.02
  with
   finger(s)—*see* Burn, finger, with other sites, thumb
   hand(s) and wrist(s)—*see* Burn, hand(s), multiple sites
  first degree 944.12
  second degree 944.22
  third degree 944.32
   deep 944.42
    with loss of body part 944.52
 toe (nail) (subungual) 945.01
  with
   lower limb(s)—*see* Burn, leg, multiple sites
  first degree 945.11
  second degree 945.21
  third degree 945.31
   deep 945.41
    with loss of body part 945.51
 tongue 947.0
 tonsil 947.0
 trachea 947.1
 trunk 942.00
  first degree 942.10
  second degree 942.20
  third degree 942.30
   deep 942.40
    with loss of body part 942.50
  multiple sites 942.09
   first degree 942.19
   second degree 942.29
   third degree 942.39
    deep 942.49
     with loss of body part 942.59
  specified site NEC 942.09
   first degree 942.19
   second degree 942.29
   third degree 942.39
    deep 942.49
     with loss of body part 942.59
 tunica vaginalis—*see* Burn, genitourinary organs, external
 tympanic membrane—*see* Burn, ear
 tympanum—*see* Burn, ear
 ultraviolet 692.82
 unspecified site (multiple) 949.0
  with extent of body surface involved specified
   less than 10 percent 948.0
   10-19 percent 948.1
   20-29 percent 948.2
   30-39 percent 948.3
   40-49 percent 948.4
   50-59 percent 948.5
   60-69 percent 948.6
   70-79 percent 948.7
   80-89 percent 948.8
   90 percent or more 948.9
  first degree 949.1
  second degree 949.2
  third degree 949.3
   deep 949.4
    with loss of body part 949.5
 uterus 947.4
 uvula 947.0

Burn—*continued*
vagina 947.4
vulva—*see* Burn, genitourinary organs, external
wrist(s) 944.07
  with
    hand(s)—*see* Burn, hand(s), multiple sites
  first degree 944.17
  second degree 944.27
  third degree 944.37
    deep 944.47
      with loss of body part 944.57
Burnett's syndrome (milk-alkali) 275.42
Burnier's syndrome (hypophyseal dwarfism) 253.3
Burning
  feet syndrome 266.2
  sensation (*see also* Disturbance, sensation) 782.0
  tongue 529.6
Burns' disease (osteochondrosis, lower ulna) 732.3
Bursa —*see also* condition
  pharynx 478.29
Bursitis NEC 727.3
  Achilles tendon 726.71
  adhesive 726.90
    shoulder 726.0
  ankle 726.79
  buttock 726.5
  calcaneal 726.79
  collateral ligament
    fibular 726.63
    tibial 726.62
  Duplay's 726.2
  elbow 726.33
  finger 726.8
  foot 726.79
  gonococcal 098.52
  hand 726.4
  hip 726.5
  infrapatellar 726.69
  ischiogluteal 726.5
  knee 726.60
  occupational NEC 727.2
  olecranon 726.33
  pes anserinus 726.61
  pharyngeal 478.29
  popliteal 727.51
  prepatellar 726.65
  radiohumeral 727.3
  scapulohumeral 726.19
    adhesive 726.0
  shoulder 726.10
    adhesive 726.0
  subacromial 726.19
    adhesive 726.0
  subcoracoid 726.19
  subdeltoid 726.19
    adhesive 726.0
  subpatellar 726.69
  syphilitic 095.7
  Thornwaldt's, Tornwaldt's (pharyngeal) 478.29
  toe 726.79
  trochanteric area 726.5
  wrist 726.4
Burst stitches or sutures (complication of surgery) (external) 998.32
  internal 998.31
Buruli ulcer 031.1
Bury's disease (erythema elevatum diutinum) 695.89

Buschke's disease or scleredema (adultorum) 710.1
Busquet's disease (osteoperiostitis) (*see also* Osteomyelitis) 730.1
Busse-Buschke disease (cryptococcosis) 117.5
Buttock —*see* condition
Button
  Biskra 085.1
  Delhi 085.1
  oriental 085.1
Buttonhole hand (intrinsic) 736.21
Bwamba fever (encephalitis) 066.3
Byssinosis (occupational) 504
Bywaters' syndrome 958.5

C

Cacergasia 300.9
Cachexia 799.4
  cancerous —*see also* Neoplasm, by site, malignant 799.4
  cardiac—*see* Disease, heart
  dehydration 276.51
    with
      hypernatremia 276.0
      hyponatremia 276.1
    due to malnutrition 799.4
  exophthalmic 242.0
  heart—*see* Disease, heart
  hypophyseal 253.2
  hypopituitary 253.2
  lead 984.9
    specified type of lead—*see* Table of drugs and chemicals
  malaria 084.9
  malignant —*see also* Neoplasm, by site, malignant 799.4
  marsh 084.9
  nervous 300.5
  old age 797
  pachydermic—*see* Hypothyroidism
  paludal 084.9
  pituitary (postpartum) 253.2
  renal (*see also* Disease, renal) 593.9
  saturnine 984.9
    specified type of lead—*see* Table of drugs and chemicals
  senile 797
  Simmonds' (pituitary cachexia) 253.2
  splenica 289.59
  strumipriva (*see also* Hypothyroidism) 244.9
  tuberculous NEC (*see also* Tuberculosis) 011.9
café au lait spots 709.09
Caffey's disease or syndrome (infantile cortical hyperostosis) 756.59
Caisson disease 993.3
Caked breast (puerperal, postpartum) 676.2
Cake kidney 753.3
Calabar swelling 125.2
Calcaneal spur 726.73
Calcaneoapophysitis 732.5
Calcaneonavicular bar 755.67
Calcareous —*see* condition
Calcicosis (occupational) 502
Calciferol (vitamin D) deficiency 268.9
  with
    osteomalacia 268.2
    rickets (*see also* Rickets) 268.0
Calcification
  adrenal (capsule) (gland) 255.41
    tuberculous (*see also* Tuberculosis) 017.6
  aorta 440.0
  artery (annular)—*see* Arteriosclerosis
  auricle (ear) 380.89
  bladder 596.8
    due to S. hematobium 120.0
  brain (cortex)—*see* Calcification, cerebral
  bronchus 519.19
  bursa 727.82
  cardiac (*see also* Degeneration, myocardial) 429.1
  cartilage (postinfectional) 733.99
  cerebral (cortex) 348.8
    artery 437.0
  cervix (uteri) 622.8

Calcification—*continued*
  choroid plexus 349.2
  conjunctiva 372.54
  corpora cavernosa (penis) 607.89
  cortex (brain)—*see* Calcification, cerebral
  dental pulp (nodular) 522.2
  dentinal papilla 520.4
  disc, intervertebral 722.90
    cervical, cervicothoracic 722.91
    lumbar, lumbosacral 722.93
    thoracic, thoracolumbar 722.92
  fallopian tube 620.8
  falx cerebri—*see* Calcification, cerebral
  fascia 728.89
  gallbladder 575.8
  general 275.40
  heart (*see also* Degeneration, myocardial) 429.1
    valve—*see* Endocarditis
  intervertebral cartilage or disc (postinfectional) 722.90
    cervical, cervicothoracic 722.91
    lumbar, lumbosacral 722.93
    thoracic, thoracolumbar 722.92
  intracranial—*see* Calcification, cerebral
  intraspinal ligament 728.89
  joint 719.80
    ankle 719.87
    elbow 719.82
    foot 719.87
    hand 719.84
    hip 719.85
    knee 719.86
    multiple sites 719.89
    pelvic region 719.85
    shoulder (region) 719.81
    specified site NEC 719.88
    wrist 719.83
  kidney 593.89
    tuberculous (*see also* Tuberculosis) 016.0
  larynx (senile) 478.79
  lens 366.8
  ligament 728.89
    intraspinal 728.89
    knee (medial collateral) 717.89
  lung 518.89
    active 518.89
    postinfectional 518.89
    tuberculous (*see also* Tuberculosis, pulmonary) 011.9
  lymph gland or node (postinfectional) 289.3
    tuberculous (*see also* Tuberculosis, lymph gland) 017.2
  mammographic 793.89
  massive (paraplegic) 728.10
  medial NEC (*see also* Arteriosclerosis, extremities) 440.20
  meninges (cerebral) 349.2
  metastatic 275.40
  Mönckeberg's—*see* Arteriosclerosis
  muscle 728.10
    heterotopic, postoperative 728.13
  myocardium, myocardial (*see also* Degeneration, myocardial) 429.1
  ovary 620.8
  pancreas 577.8
  penis 607.99
  periarticular 728.89
  pericardium (*see also* Pericarditis) 423.8

Calcification — *continued*
  pineal gland 259.8
  pleura 511.0
    postinfectional 518.89
    tuberculous (*see also* Tuberculosis, pleura) 012.0
  pulp (dental) (nodular) 522.2
  renal 593.89
  rider's bone 733.99
  sclera 379.16
  semilunar cartilage 717.89
  spleen 289.59
  subcutaneous 709.3
  suprarenal (capsule) (gland) 255.41
  tendon (sheath) 727.82
    with bursitis, synovitis or tenosynovitis 727.82
  trachea 519.19
  ureter 593.89
  uterus 621.8
  vitreous 379.29
Calcified — *see also* Calcification
  hematoma NEC 959.9
Calcinosis (generalized) (interstitial) (tumoral) (universalis) 275.49
  circumscripta 709.3
  cutis 709.3
  intervertebralis 275.49 [722.90]
  Raynaud's phenomenonsclerodactylytelangiectasis (CRST) 710.1
Calciphylaxis (*see also* Calcification, by site) 275.49
Calcium
  blood
    high (*see also* Hypercalcemia) 275.42
    low (*see also* Hypocalcemia) 275.41
  deposits — *see also* Calcification, by site
    in bursa 727.82
    in tendon (sheath) 727.82
      with bursitis, synovitis or tenosynovitis 727.82
  salts or soaps in vitreous 379.22
Calciuria 791.9
Calculi — *see* Calculus
Calculosis, intrahepatic — *see* Choledocholithiasis
Calculus, calculi, calculous 592.9
  ampulla of Vater — *see* Choledocholithiasis
  anuria (impacted) (recurrent) 592.0
  appendix 543.9
  bile duct (any) — *see* Choledocholithiasis
  biliary — *see* Cholelithiasis
  bilirubin, multiple — *see* Cholelithiasis
  bladder (encysted) (impacted) (urinary) 594.1
    diverticulum 594.0
  bronchus 518.89
  calyx (kidney) (renal) 592.0
    congenital 753.3
  cholesterol (pure) (solitary) — *see* Cholelithiasis
  common duct (bile) — *see* Choledocholithiasis
  conjunctiva 372.54
  cystic 594.1
    duct — *see* Cholelithiasis
  dental 523.6
    subgingival 523.6
    supragingival 523.6
  epididymis 608.89

Calculus, calculi, calculous — *continued*
  gallbladder — *see also* Cholelithiasis
    congenital 751.69
  hepatic (duct) — *see* Choledocholithiasis
  intestine (impaction) (obstruction) 560.39
  kidney (impacted) (multiple) (pelvis) (recurrent) (staghorn) 592.0
    congenital 753.3
  lacrimal (passages) 375.57
  liver (impacted) — *see* Choledocholithiasis
  lung 518.89
  mammographic 793.89
  nephritic (impacted) (recurrent) 592.0
  nose 478.19
  pancreas (duct) 577.8
  parotid gland 527.5
  pelvis, encysted 592.0
  prostate 602.0
  pulmonary 518.89
  renal (impacted) (recurrent) 592.0
    congenital 753.3
  salivary (duct) (gland) 527.5
  seminal vesicle 608.89
  staghorn 592.0
  Stensen's duct 527.5
  sublingual duct or gland 527.5
    congenital 750.26
  submaxillary duct, gland, or region 527.5
  suburethral 594.8
  tonsil 474.8
  tooth, teeth 523.6
  tunica vaginalis 608.89
  ureter (impacted) (recurrent) 592.1
  urethra (impacted) 594.2
  urinary (duct) (impacted) (passage) (tract) 592.9
    lower tract NEC 594.9
    specified site 594.8
  vagina 623.8
  vesical (impacted) 594.1
  Wharton's duct 527.5
Caliectasis 593.89
California
  disease 114.0
  encephalitis 062.5
Caligo cornea 371.03
Callositas, callosity (infected) 700
Callus (infected) 700
  bone 726.91
  excessive, following fracture — *see also* Late, effect (of), fracture
Calvé (-Perthes) disease (osteochondrosis, femoral capital) 732.1
Calvities (*see also* Alopecia) 704.00
Cameroon fever (*see also* Malaria) 084.6
Camptocormia 300.11
Camptodactyly (congenital) 755.59
Camurati-Engelmann disease (diaphyseal sclerosis) 756.59
Canal — *see* condition
Canaliculitis (lacrimal) (acute) 375.31
  Actinomyces 039.8
  chronic 375.41
Canavan's disease 330.0

INDEX TO DISEASES   **Carbunculus**

Cancer (M8000/3)—*see also* Neoplasm, by site, malignant

> *Note*—The term "cancer" when modified by an adjective or adjectival phrase indicating a morphological type should be coded in the same manner as "carcinoma" with that adjective or phrase. Thus, "squamous-cell cancer" should be coded in the same manner as "squamous-cell carcinoma," which appears in the list under "Carcinoma."

   bile duct type (M8160/3), liver 155.1
   hepatocellular (M8170/3) 155.0
Cancerous (M8000/3)—*see* Neoplasm, by site, malignant
Cancerphobia 300.29
Cancrum oris 528.1
Candidiasis, candidal 112.9
   with pneumonia 112.4
   balanitis 112.2
   congenital 771.7
   disseminated 112.5
   endocarditis 112.81
   esophagus 112.84
   intertrigo 112.3
   intestine 112.85
   lung 112.4
   meningitis 112.83
   mouth 112.0
   nails 112.3
   neonatal 771.7
   onychia 112.3
   otitis externa 112.82
   otomycosis 112.82
   paronychia 112.3
   perionyxis 112.3
   pneumonia 112.4
   pneumonitis 112.4
   skin 112.3
   specified site NEC 112.89
   systemic 112.5
   urogenital site NEC 112.2
   vagina 112.1
   vulva 112.1
   vulvovaginitis 112.1
Candidiosis —*see* Candidiasis
Candiru infection or infestation 136.8
Canities (premature) 704.3
   congenital 757.4
Canker (mouth) (sore) 528.2
   rash 034.1
Cannabinosis 504
Canton fever 081.9
Cap
   cradle 690.11
Capillariasis 127.5
Capillary —*see* condition
Caplan's syndrome 714.81
Caplan-Colinet syndrome 714.81
Capsule —*see* condition
Capsulitis (joint) 726.90
   adhesive (shoulder) 726.0
   hip 726.5
   knee 726.60
   labyrinthine 387.8
   thyroid 245.9
   wrist 726.4
Caput
   crepitus 756.0
   medusae 456.8
   succedaneum 767.19

Carapata disease 087.1
Carate —*see* Pinta
Carbohydrate-deficient glycoprotein syndrome (CDGS) 271.8
Carboxyhemoglobinemia 986
Carbuncle 680.9
   abdominal wall 680.2
   ankle 680.6
   anus 680.5
   arm (any part, above wrist) 680.3
   auditory canal, external 680.0
   axilla 680.3
   back (any part) 680.2
   breast 680.2
   buttock 680.5
   chest wall 680.2
   corpus cavernosum 607.2
   ear (any part) (external) 680.0
   eyelid 373.13
   face (any part, except eye) 680.0
   finger (any) 680.4
   flank 680.2
   foot (any part) 680.7
   forearm 680.3
   genital organ (male) 608.4
   gluteal (region) 680.5
   groin 680.2
   hand (any part) 680.4
   head (any part, except face) 680.8
   heel 680.7
   hip 680.6
   kidney (*see also* Abscess, kidney) 590.2
   knee 680.6
   labia 616.4
   lacrimal
      gland (*see also* Dacryoadenitis) 375.00
      passages (duct) (sac) (*see also* Dacryocystitis) 375.30
   leg, any part except foot 680.6
   lower extremity, any part except foot 680.6
   malignant 022.0
   multiple sites 680.9
   neck 680.1
   nose (external) (septum) 680.0
   orbit, orbital 376.01
   partes posteriores 680.5
   pectoral region 680.2
   penis 607.2
   perineum 680.2
   pinna 680.0
   scalp (any part) 680.8
   scrotum 608.4
   seminal vesicle 608.0
   shoulder 680.3
   skin NEC 680.9
   specified site NEC 680.8
   spermatic cord 608.4
   temple (region) 680.0
   testis 608.4
   thigh 680.6
   thumb 680.4
   toe (any) 680.7
   trunk 680.2
   tunica vaginalis 608.4
   umbilicus 680.2
   upper arm 680.3
   urethra 597.0
   vas deferens 608.4
   vulva 616.4
   wrist 680.4
Carbunculus (*see also* Carbuncle) 680.9

Carcinoid (tumor) (M8240/1)—*see also*
  Neoplasm, by site, uncertain behavior
  and struma ovarii (M9091/1) 236.2
  argentaffin (M8241/1)—*see* Neoplasm, by site
    uncertain behavior
    malignant (M8241/3)—*see* Neoplasm, by site,
      malignant
  benign (M9091/0) 220
  composite (M8244/3)—*see* Neoplasm, by site,
    malignant
  goblet cell (M8243/3)—*see* Neoplasm, by site,
    malignant
  malignant (M8240/1)—*see* Neoplasm, by site,
    uncertain behavior
  nonargentaffin (M8242/1)—*see also* Neoplasm,
    by site, uncertain behavior
    malignant (M8242/3)—*see* Neoplasm, by site,
      malignantstrumal (M9091/1) 236.2
  syndrome (intestinal) (metastatic) 259.2
  type bronchial adenoma (M8240/3)—*see*
    Neoplasm, lung, malignant
Carcinoidosis 259.2
Carcinoma (M8010/3)—*see also* Neoplasm, by
  site, malignant

> Note—Except where otherwise indicated, the
> morphological varieties of carcinoma in the list
> below should be coded by site as for
> "Neoplasm, malignant."

  with
    apocrine metaplasia (M8573/3)
    cartilaginous (and osseous) metaplasia
      (M8571/3)
    osseous (and cartilaginous) metaplasia
      (M8571/3)
    productive fibrosis (M8141/3)
    spindle cell metaplasia (M8572/3)
    squamous metaplasia (M8570/3)
  acidophil (M8280/3)
    specified site—*see* Neoplasm, by site,
      malignant
    unspecified site 194.3
  acidophil-basophil, mixed (M8281/3)
    specified site—*see* Neoplasm, by site,
      malignant
    unspecified site 194.3
  acinar (cell) (M8550/3)
  acinic cell (M8550/3)
  adenocystic (M8200/3)
  adenoid
    cystic (M8200/3)
    squamous cell (M8075/3)
  adenosquamous (M8560/3)
  adnexal (skin) (M8390/3)—*see* Neoplasm, skin,
    malignant
  adrenal cortical (M8370/3) 194.0
  alveolar (M8251/3)
    cell (M8250/3)—*see* Neoplasm, lung,
      malignant
  anaplastic type (M8021/3)
  apocrine (M8401/3)
    breast—*see* Neoplasm, breast, malignant
    specified site NEC—*see* Neoplasm, skin,
      malignant
    unspecified site 173.9
  basal cell (pigmented) (M8090/3)—*see also*
    Neoplasm, skin, malignant
    fibro-epithelial type (M8093/3)—*see*
      Neoplasm, skin, malignant
    morphea type (M8092/3)—*see* Neoplasm,
      skin, malignant

Carcinoma—*continued*
  multicentric (M8091/3)—*see* Neoplasm, skin,
    malignant
  basaloid (M8123/3)
  basal-squamous cell, mixed (M8094/3)—*see*
    Neoplasm, skin, malignant
  basophil (M8300/3)
    specified site—*see* Neoplasm, by site,
      malignant
    unspecified site 194.3
  basophil-acidophil, mixed (M8281/3)
    specified site—*see* Neoplasm, by site,
      malignant
    unspecified site 194.3
  basosquamous (M8094/3)—*see* Neoplasm, skin,
    malignant
  bile duct type (M8160/3)
    and hepatocellular, mixed (M8180/3) 155.0
    liver 155.1
    specified site NEC—*see* Neoplasm, by site,
      malignant
    unspecified site 155.1
  branchial or branchiogenic 146.8
  bronchial or bronchogenic—*see* Neoplasm,
    lung, malignant
  bronchiolar (terminal) (M8250/3)—*see*
    Neoplasm, lung, malignant
  bronchiolo-alveolar (M8250/3)—*see* Neoplasm,
    lung, malignant
  bronchogenic (epidermoid) 162.9
  C cell (M8510/3)
    specified site—*see* Neoplasm, by site,
      malignant
    unspecified site 193
  ceruminous (M8420/3) 173.2
  chorionic (M9100/3)
    specified site—*see* Neoplasm, by site,
      malignant
    unspecified site
      female 181
      male 186.9
  chromophobe (M8270/3)
    specified site—*see* Neoplasm, by site,
      malignant
    unspecified site 194.3
  clear cell (mesonephroid type) (M8310/3)
  cloacogenic (M8124/3)
    specified site—*see* Neoplasm, by site,
      malignant
    unspecified site 154.8
  colloid (M8480/3)
  cribriform (M8201/3)
  cylindroid type (M8200/3)
  diffuse type (M8145/3)
    specified site—*see* Neoplasm, by site,
      malignant
    unspecified site 151.9
  duct (cell) (M8500/3)
    with Paget's disease (M8541/3)—*see*
      Neoplasm, breast, malignant
    infiltrating (M8500/3)
      specified site—*see* Neoplasm, by site,
        malignant
      unspecified site 174.9
  ductal (M8500/3)
  ductular, infiltrating (M8521/3)
  embryonal (M9070/3)
    and teratoma, mixed (M9081/3)
    combined with choriocarcinoma
      (M9101/3)—*see* Neoplasm, by site,
      malignant

INDEX TO DISEASES   Carcinoma

Carcinoma—*continued*
  infantile type (M9071/3)
  liver 155.0
  polyembryonal type (M9072/3)
  endometrioid (M8380/3)
  eosinophil (M8280/3)
    specified site—*see* Neoplasm, by site, malignant
    unspecified site 194.3
  epidermoid (M8070/3)—*see also* Carcinoma, squamous cell
    and adenocarcinoma, mixed (M8560/3)
    in situ, Bowen's type (M8081/2)—*see* Neoplasm, skin, in situ
    intradermal—*see* Neoplasm, skin, in situ
  fibroepithelial type basal cell (M8093/3)—*see* Neoplasm, skin, malignant
  follicular (M8330/3)
    and papillary (mixed) (M8340/3) 193
    moderately differentiated type (M8332/3) 193
    pure follicle type (M8331/3) 193
    specified site—*see* Neoplasm, by site, malignant
    trabecular type (M8332/3) 193
    unspecified site 193
    well differentiated type (M8331/3) 193
  gelatinous (M8480/3)
  giant cell (M8031/3)
    and spindle cell (M8030/3)
  granular cell (M8320/3)
  granulosa cell (M8620/3) 183.0
  hepatic cell (M8170/3) 155.0
  hepatocellular (M8170/3) 155.0
    and bile duct, mixed (M8180/3) 155.0
  hepatocholangiolitic (M8180/3) 155.0
  Hurthle cell (thyroid) 193
  hypernephroid (M8311/3)
  in
    adenomatous
      polyp (M8210/3)
      polyposis coli (M8220/3) 153.9
    pleomorphic adenoma (M8940/3)
    polypoid adenoma (M8210/3)
    situ (M8010/3)—*see* Carcinoma, in situ
    tubular adenoma (M8210/3)
    villous adenoma (M8261/3)
  infiltrating duct (M8500/3)
    with Paget's disease (M8541/3)—*see* Neoplasm, breast, malignant
    specified site—*see* Neoplasm, by site, malignant
    unspecified site 174.9
  inflammatory (M8530/3)
    specified site—*see* Neoplasm, by site, malignant
    unspecified site 174.9
  in situ (M8010/2)—*see also* Neoplasm, by site, in situ
    epidermoid (M8070/2)—*see also* Neoplasm, by site, in situ
      with questionable stromal invasion (M8076/2)
        specified site—*see* Neoplasm, by site, in situ
        unspecified site 233.1
      Bowen's type (M8081/2)—*see* Neoplasm, skin, in situ

Carcinoma—*continued*
  intraductal (M8500/2)
    specified site—*see* Neoplasm, by site, in situ
    unspecified site 233.0
  lobular (M8520/2)
    specified site—*see* Neoplasm, by site, in situ
    unspecified site 233.0
  papillary (M8050/2)—*see* Neoplasm, by site, in situ
  squamous cell (M8070/2)—*see also* Neoplasm, by site, in situ
    with questionable stromal invasion (M8076/2)
      specified site—*see* Neoplasm, by site, in situ
      unspecified site 233.1
  transitional cell (M8120/2)—*see* Neoplasm, by site, in situ
  intestinal type (M8144/3)
    specified site—*see* Neoplasm, by site, malignant
    unspecified site 151.9
  intraductal (noninfiltrating) (M8500/2)
    papillary (M8503/2)
      specified site—*see* Neoplasm, by site, in situ
      unspecified site 233.0
    specified site—*see* Neoplasm, by site, in situ
    unspecified site 233.0
  intraepidermal (M8070/2)—*see also* Neoplasm, skin, in situ
    squamous cell, Bowen's type (M8081/2)—*see* Neoplasm, skin, in situ
  intraepithelial (M8010/2)—*see also* Neoplasm, by site, in situ
    squamous cell (M8072/2)—*see* Neoplasm, by site, in situ
  intraosseous (M9270/3) 170.1
    upper jaw (bone) 170.0
  islet cell (M8150/3)
    and exocrine, mixed (M8154/3)
      specified site—*see* Neoplasm, by site, malignant
      unspecified site 157.9
    pancreas 157.4
    specified site NEC—*see* Neoplasm, by site, malignant
    unspecified site 157.4
  juvenile, breast (M8502/3)—*see* Neoplasm, breast, malignant
  Kulchitsky's cell (carcinoid tumor of intestine) 259.2
  large cell (M8012/3)
    squamous cell, nonkeratinizing type (M8072/3)
  Leydig cell (testis) (M8650/3)
    specified site—*see* Neoplasm, by site, malignant
    unspecified site 186.9
      female 183.0
      male 186.9
  liver cell (M8170/3) 155.0
  lobular (infiltrating) (M8520/3)
    non-infiltrating (M8520/3)
      specified site—*see* Neoplasm, by site, in situ
      unspecified site 233.0
    specified site—*see* Neoplasm, by site, malignant
    unspecified site 174.9
  lymphoepithelial (M8082/3)
  medullary (M8510/3)
    with
      amyloid stroma (M8511/3)

Carcinoma—*continued*
  specified site—*see* Neoplasm, by site, malignant
  unspecified site 193
  lymphoid stroma (M8512/3)
    specified site—*see* Neoplasm, by site, malignant
    unspecified site 174.9
  mesometanephric (M9110/3)
  mesonephric (M9110/3)
  metastatic (M8010/6)—*see* Metastasis, cancer
  metatypical (M8095/3)—*see* Neoplasm, skin, malignant
  morphea type basal cell (M8092/3)—*see* Neoplasm, skin, malignant
  mucinous (M8480/3)
  mucin-producing (M8481/3)
  mucin-secreting (M8481/3)
  mucoepidermoid (M8430/3)
  mucoid (M8480/3)
    cell (M8300/3)
      specified site—*see* Neoplasm, by site, malignant
      unspecified site 194.3
  mucous (M8480/3)
  nonencapsulated sclerosing (M8350/3) 193
  noninfiltrating
    intracystic (M8504/2)—*see* Neoplasm, by site, in situ
    intraductal (M8500/2)
      papillary (M8503/2)
        specified site—*see* Neoplasm, by site, in situ
        unspecified site 233.0
      specified site—*see* Neoplasm, by site, in situ
      unspecified site 233.0
    lobular (M8520/2)
      specified site—*see* Neoplasm, by site, in situ
      unspecified site 233.0
  oat cell (M8042/3)
    specified site—*see* Neoplasm, by site, malignant
    unspecified site 162.9
  odontogenic (M9270/3) 170.1
    upper jaw (bone) 170.0
  onocytic (M8290/3)
  oxyphilic (M8290/3)
  papillary (M8050/3)
    and follicular (mixed) (M8340/3) 193
    epidermoid (M8052/3)
    intraductal (noninfiltrating) (M8503/2)
      specified site—*see* Neoplasm, by site, in situ
      unspecified site 233.0
    serous (M8460/3)
      specified site—*see* Neoplasm, by site, malignant
      surface (M8461/3)
        specified site—*see* Neoplasm, by site, malignant
        unspecified site 183.0
      unspecified site 183.0
    squamous cell (M8052/3)
    transitional cell (M8130/3)
  papillocystic (M8450/3)
    specified site—*see* Neoplasm, by site, malignant
    unspecified site 183.0
  parafollicular cell (M8510/3)
    specified site—*see* Neoplasm, by site, malignant
    unspecified site 193

Carcinoma—*continued*
  pleomorphic (M8022/3)
  polygonal cell (M8034/3)
  prickle cell (M8070/3)
  pseudoglandular, squamous cell (M8075/3)
  pseudomucinous (M8470/3)
    specified site—*see* Neoplasm, by site, malignant
    unspecified site 183.0
  pseudosarcomatous (M8033/3)
  regaud type (M8082/3)—*see* Neoplasm, nasopharynx, malignant
  renal cell (M8312/3) 189.0
  reserve cell (M8041/3)
  round cell (M8041/3)
  Schmincke (M8082/3)—*see* Neoplasm, nasopharynx, malignant
  Schneiderian (M8121/3)
    specified site—*see* Neoplasm, by site, malignant
    unspecified site 160.0
  scirrhous (M8141/3)
  sebaceous (M8410/3)—*see* Neoplasm, skin, malignant
  secondary (M8010/6)—*see* Neoplasm, by site, malignant, secondary
  secretory, breast (M8502/3)—*see* Neoplasm, breast, malignant
  serous (M8441/3)
    papillary (M8460/3)
      specified site—*see* Neoplasm, by site, malignant
      unspecified site 183.0
    surface, papillary (M8461/3)
      specified site—*see* Neoplasm, by site, malignant
      unspecified site 183.0
  Sertoli cell (M8640/3)
    specified site—*see* Neoplasm, by site, malignant
    unspecified site 186.9
  signet ring cell (M8490/3)
    metastatic (M8490/6)—*see* Neoplasm, by site, secondary
  simplex (M8231/3)
  skin appendage (M8390/3)—*see* Neoplasm, skin, malignant
  small cell (M8041/3)
    fusiform cell type (M8043/3)
    squamous cell, non-keratinizing type (M8073/3)
  solid (M8230/3)
    with amyloid stroma (M8511/3)
      specified site—*see* Neoplasm, by site, malignant
      unspecified site 193
  spheroidal cell (M8035/3)
  spindle cell (M8032/3)
    and giant cell (M8030/3)
  spinous cell (M8070/3)
  squamous (cell) (M8070/3)
    adenoid type (M8075/3)
    and adenocarcinoma, mixed (M8560/3)
    intraepidermal, Bowen's type—*see* Neoplasm, skin, in situ
    keratinizing type (large cell) (M8071/3)
    large cell, non-keratinizing type (M8072/3)
    microinvasive (M8076/3)
      specified site—*see* Neoplasm, by site, malignant
      unspecified site 180.9

INDEX TO DISEASES   **Cardiovascular**

Carcinoma—*continued*
  non-keratinizing type (M8072/3)
  papillary (M8052/3)
  pseudoglandular (M8075/3)
  small cell, non-keratinizing type (M8073/3)
  spindle cell type (M8074/3)
  verrucous (M8051/3)
  superficial spreading (M8143/3)
  sweat gland (M8400/3)—*see* Neoplasm, skin, malignant
  theca cell (M8600/3) 183.0
  thymic (M8580/3) 164.0
  trabecular (M8190/3)
  transitional (cell) (M8120/3)
    papillary (M8130/3)
    spindle cell type (M8122/3)
  tubular (M8211/3)
  undifferentiated type (M8020/3)
  urothelial (M8120/3)
  ventriculi 151.9
  verrucous (epidermoid) (squamous cell) (M8051/3)
  villous (M8262/3)
  water-clear cell (M8322/3) 194.1
  wolffian duct (M9110/3)
Carcinomaphobia 300.29
Carcinomatosis
  peritonei (M8010/6) 197.6
  specified site NEC (M8010/3)—*see* Neoplasm, by site, malignant
  unspecified site (M8010/6) 199.0
Carcinosarcoma (M8980/3)—*see also* Neoplasm, by site, malignant
  embryonal type (M8981/3)—*see* Neoplasm, by site, malignant
Cardia, cardial —*see* condition
Cardiac —*see also* condition
  death—*see* Disease, heart
  device
    defibrillator, automatic implantable V45.02
      in situ NEC V45.00
    pacemaker
      cardiac
        fitting or adjustment V53.3
        in situ V45.01
      carotid sinus
        fitting or adjustment V53.3
        in situ V45.09
  pacemaker—*see* Cardiac, device, pacemaker
  tamponade 423.3
Cardialgia (*see also* Pain, precordial) 786.51
Cardiectasis —*see* Hypertrophy, cardiac
Cardiochalasia 530.81
Cardiomalacia (*see also* Degeneration, myocardial) 429.1
Cardiomegalia glycogenica diffusa 271.0
Cardiomegaly (*see also* Hypertrophy, cardiac) 429.3
  congenital 746.89
  glycogen 271.0
  hypertensive (*see also* Hypertension, heart) 402.90
  idiopathic 429.3
Cardiomyoliposis (*see also* Degeneration, myocardial) 429.1
Cardiomyopathy (congestive) (constrictive) (familial) (infiltrative) (obstructive) (restrictive) (sporadic) 425.4
  alcoholic 425.5
  amyloid 277.39 *[425.7]*
  beriberi 265.0 *[425.7]*

Cardiomyopathy—*continued*
  cobalt-beer 425.5
  congenital 425.3
  due to
    amyloidosis 277.39 *[425.7]*
    beriberi 265.0 *[425.7]*
    cardiac glycogenesis 271.0 *[425.7]*
    Chagas' disease 086.0
    Friedreich's ataxia 334.0 *[425.8]*
    mucopolysaccharidosis 277.5 *[425.7]*
    myotonia atrophica 359.21 *[425.8]*
    progressive muscular dystrophy 359.1 *[425.8]*
    sarcoidosis 135 *[425.8]*
  glycogen storage 271.0 *[425.7]*
  hypertensive—*see* Hypertension, with, heart involvement
  hypertrophic
    nonobstructive 425.4
    obstructive 425.1
      congenital 746.84
  idiopathic (concentric) 425.4
  in
    Chagas' disease 086.0
    sarcoidosis 135 *[425.8]*
  ischemic 414.8
  metabolic NEC 277.9 *[425.7]*
    amyloid 277.39 *[425.7]*
    thyrotoxic (*see also* Thyrotoxicosis) 242.9 *[425.7]*
    thyrotoxicosis (*see also* Thyrotoxicosis) 242.9 *[425.7]*
  newborn 425.4
    congenital 425.3
  nutritional 269.9 *[425.7]*
    beriberi 265.0 *[425.7]*
  obscure of Africa 425.2
  peripartum 674.5
  postpartum 674.5
  primary 425.4
  secondary 425.9
  stress induced 429.83
  takotsubo 429.83
  thyrotoxic (*see also* Thyrotoxicosis) 242.9 *[425.7]*
  toxic NEC 425.9
  tuberculous (*see also* Tuberculosis) 017.9 *[425.8]*
Cardionephritis —*see* Hypertension, cardiorenal
Cardionephropathy —*see* Hypertension, cardiorenal
Cardionephrosis —*see* Hypertension, cardiorenal
Cardioneurosis 306.2
Cardiopathia nigra 416.0
Cardiopathy (*see also* Disease, heart) 429.9
  hypertensive (*see also* Hypertension, heart) 402.90
  idiopathic 425.4
  mucopolysaccharidosis 277.5 *[425.7]*
Cardiopericarditis (*see also* Pericarditis) 423.9
Cardiophobia 300.29
Cardioptosis 746.87
Cardiorenal —*see* condition
Cardiorrhexis (*see also* Infarct, myocardium) 410.9
Cardiosclerosis —*see* Arteriosclerosis, coronary
Cardiosis —*see* Disease, heart
Cardiospasm (esophagus) (reflex) (stomach) 530.0
  congenital 750.7
Cardiostenosis —*see* Disease, heart
Cardiosymphysis 423.1
Cardiothyrotoxicosis —*see* Hyperthyroidism
Cardiovascular —*see* condition

859

Carditis (acute) (bacterial) (chronic) (subacute) 429.89
  Coxsackie 074.20
  hypertensive (*see also* Hypertension, heart) 402.90
  meningococcal 036.40
  rheumatic—*see* Disease, heart, rheumatic
  rheumatoid 714.2
Care (of)
  child (routine) V20.1
  convalescent following V66.9
    chemotherapy V66.2
    medical NEC V66.5
    psychotherapy V66.3
    radiotherapy V66.1
    surgery V66.0
    surgical NEC V66.0
    treatment (for) V66.5
      combined V66.6
      fracture V66.4
      mental disorder NEC V66.3
      specified type NEC V66.5
  end-of-life care V66.7
  family member (handicapped) (sick)
    creating problem for family V61.49
    provided away from home for holiday relief V60.5
    unavailable, due to
      absence (person rendering care) (sufferer) V60.4
      inability (any reason) of person rendering care V60.4
  holiday relief V60.5
  hospice V66.7
  lack of (at or after birth) (infant) (child) 995.52
    adult 995.84
  lactation of mother V24.1
  palliative V66.7
  postpartum
    immediately after delivery V24.0
    routine follow-up V24.2
  prenatal V22.1
    first pregnancy V22.0
    high risk pregnancy V23.9
      specified problem NEC V23.8
  terminal V66.7
  unavailable, due to
    absence of person rendering care V60.4
    inability (any reason) of person rendering care V60.4
  well baby V20.1
Caries (bone) (*see also* Tuberculosis, bone) 015.9 *[730.8]*
  arrested 521.04
  cementum 521.03
  cerebrospinal (tuberculous) 015.0 *[730.88]*
  dental (acute) (chronic) (incipient) (infected) 521.00
    with pulp exposure 521.03
    extending to
      dentine 521.02
      pulp 521.03
    other specified NEC 521.09
    pit and fissure 521.06
    primary
      pit and fissure origin 521.06
      root surface 521.08
      smooth surface origin 521.07
    root surface 521.08
    smooth surface 521.07
  dentin (acute) (chronic) 521.02

Caries—*continued*
  enamel (acute) (chronic) (incipient) 521.01
  external meatus 380.89
  hip (*see also* Tuberculosis) 015.1 *[730.85]*
  initial 521.01
  knee 015.2 *[730.86]*
  labyrinth 386.8
  limb NEC 015.7 *[730.88]*
  mastoid (chronic) (process) 383.1
  middle ear 385.89
  nose 015.7 *[730.88]*
  orbit 015.7 *[730.88]*
  ossicle 385.24
  petrous bone 383.20
  sacrum (tuberculous) 015.0 *[730.88]*
  spine, spinal (column) (tuberculous) 015.0 *[730.88]*
  syphilitic 095.5
    congenital 090.0 *[730.8]*
  teeth (internal) 521.00
    initial 521.01
  vertebra (column) (tuberculous) 015.0 *[730.88]*
Carini's syndrome (ichthyosis congenita) 757.1
Carious teeth 521.00
Carneous mole 631
Carnosinemia 270.5
Carotid body or sinus syndrome 337.0
Carotidynia 337.0
Carotinemia (dietary) 278.3
Carotinosis (cutis) (skin) 278.3
Carpal tunnel syndrome 354.0
Carpenter's syndrome 759.89
Carpopedal spasm (*see also* Tetany) 781.7
Carpoptosis 736.05
Carrier (suspected) of
  amebiasis V02.2
  bacterial disease (meningococcal, staphylococcal, streptococcal) NEC V02.59
  cholera V02.0
  cystic fibrosis gene V83.81
  defective gene V83.89
  diphtheria V02.4
  dysentery (bacillary) V02.3
    amebic V02.2
  Endamoeba histolytica V02.2
  gastrointestinal pathogens NEC V02.3
  genetic defect V83.89
  gonorrhea V02.7
  group B streptococcus V02.51
  HAA (hepatitis Australian-antigen) V02.61
  hemophilia A (asymptomatic) V83.01
    symptomatic V83.02
  hepatitis V02.60
    Australian-antigen (HAA) V02.61
    B V02.61
    C V02.62
    serum V02.61
    specified type NEC V02.69
    viral V02.60
  infective organism NEC V02.9
  malaria V02.9
  paratyphoid V02.3
  Salmonella V02.3
    typhosa V02.1
  serum hepatitis V02.61
  Shigella V02.3
  Staphylococcus NEC V02.59
  Streptococcus NEC V02.52
    group B V02.51
  typhoid V02.1
  venereal disease NEC V02.8

INDEX TO DISEASES — Cataract

Carrión's disease (Bartonellosis) 088.0
Car sickness 994.6
Carter's
  relapsing fever (Asiatic) 087.0
Cartilage —*see* condition
Caruncle (inflamed)
  abscess, lacrimal (*see also* Dacryocystitis) 375.30
  conjunctiva 372.00
    acute 372.00
  eyelid 373.00
  labium (majus) (minus) 616.89
  lacrimal 375.30
  urethra (benign) 599.3
  vagina (wall) 616.89
Cascade stomach 537.6
Caseation lymphatic gland (*see also* Tuberculosis) 017.2
Caseous
  bronchitis—*see* Tuberculosis, pulmonary
  meningitis 013.0
  pneumonia—*see* Tuberculosis, pulmonary
Cassidy (-Scholte) syndrome (malignant carcinoid) 259.2
Castellani's bronchitis 104.8
Castleman's tumor or lymphoma (mediastinal lymph node hyperplasia) 785.6
Castration, traumatic 878.2
  complicated 878.3
Casts in urine 791.7
Cat's ear 744.29
Catalepsy 300.11
  catatonic (acute) (*see also* Schizophrenia) 295.2
  hysterical 300.11
  schizophrenic (*see also* Schizophrenia) 295.2
Cataphasia 307.0
Cataplexy (idiopathic) *see also* Narcolepsy
Cataract (anterior cortical) (anterior polar) (black) (capsular) (central) (cortical) (hypermature) (immature) (incipient) (mature) 366.9
  anterior
    and posterior axial embryonal 743.33
    pyramidal 743.31
    subcapsular polar
      infantile, juvenile, or presenile 366.01
      senile 366.13
  associated with
    calcinosis 275.40 *[366.42]*
    craniofacial dysostosis 756.0 *[366.44]*
    galactosemia 271.1 *[366.44]*
    hypoparathyroidism 252.1 *[366.42]*
    myotonic disorders 359.21 *[366.43]*
    neovascularization 366.33
  blue dot 743.39
  cerulean 743.39
  complicated NEC 366.30
  congenital 743.30
    capsular or subcapsular 743.31
    cortical 743.32
    nuclear 743.33
    specified type NEC 743.39
    total or subtotal 743.34
    zonular 743.32
  coronary (congenital) 743.39
    acquired 366.12
  cupuliform 366.14
  diabetic 250.5 *[366.41]*
  drug-induced 366.45
  due to
    chalcosis 360.24 *[366.34]*

Cataract—*continued*
  chronic choroiditis (*see also* Choroiditis) 363.20 *[366.32]*
  degenerative myopia 360.21 *[366.34]*
  glaucoma (*see also* Glaucoma) 365.9 *[366.31]*
  infection, intraocular NEC 366.32
  inflammatory ocular disorder NEC 366.32
  iridocyclitis, chronic 364.10 *[366.33]*
  pigmentary retinal dystrophy 362.74 *[366.34]*
  radiation 366.46
  electric 366.46
  glassblowers' 366.46
  heat ray 366.46
  heterochromic 366.33
  in eye disease NEC 366.30
  infantile (*see also* Cataract, juvenile) 366.00
  intumescent 366.12
  irradiational 366.46
  juvenile 366.00
    anterior subcapsular polar 366.01
    combined forms 366.09
    cortical 366.03
    lamellar 366.03
    nuclear 366.04
    posterior subcapsular polar 366.02
    specified NEC 366.09
    zonular 366.03
  lamellar 743.32
    infantile, juvenile, or presenile 366.03
  morgagnian 366.18
  myotonic 359.21 *[366.43]*
  myxedema 244.9 *[366.44]*
  nuclear 366.16
  posterior, polar (capsular) 743.31
    infantile, juvenile, or presenile 366.02
    senile 366.14
  presenile (*see also* Cataract, juvenile) 366.00
  punctate
    acquired 366.12
    congenital 743.39
  secondary (membrane) 366.50
    obscuring vision 366.53
    specified type, not obscuring vision 366.52
  senile 366.10
    anterior subcapsular polar 366.13
    combined forms 366.19
    cortical 366.15
    hypermature 366.18
    immature 366.12
    incipient 366.12
    mature 366.17
    nuclear 366.16
    posterior subcapsular polar 366.14
    specified NEC 366.19
    total or subtotal 366.17
  snowflake 250.5 *[366.41]*
  specified NEC 366.8
  subtotal (senile) 366.17
    congenital 743.34
  sunflower 360.24 *[366.34]*
  tetanic NEC 252.1 *[366.42]*
  total (mature) (senile) 366.17
    congenital 743.34
    localized 366.21
    traumatic 366.22
  toxic 366.45
  traumatic 366.20
    partially resolved 366.23
    total 366.22
  zonular (perinuclear) 743.32
    infantile, juvenile, or presenile 366.03

Cataracta

Cataracta 366.10
  brunescens 366.16
  cerulea 743.39
  complicata 366.30
  congenita 743.30
  coralliformis 743.39
  coronaria (congenital) 743.39
    acquired 366.12
  diabetic 250.5 *[366.41]*
  floriformis 360.24 *[366.34]*
  membranacea
    accreta 366.50
    congenita 743.39
  nigra 366.16
Catarrh, catarrhal (inflammation) (*see also* condition) 460
  acute 460
  asthma, asthmatic (*see also* Asthma) 493.9
  Bostock's (*see also* Fever, hay) 477.9
  bowel—*see* Enteritis
  bronchial 490
    acute 466.0
    chronic 491.0
    subacute 466.0
  cervix, cervical (canal) (uteri)—*see* Cervicitis
  chest (*see also* Bronchitis) 490
  chronic 472.0
  congestion 472.0
  conjunctivitis 372.03
  due to syphilis 095.9
    congenital 090.0
  enteric—*see* Enteritis
  epidemic 487.1
  Eustachian 381.50
  eye (acute) (vernal) 372.03
  fauces (*see also* Pharyngitis) 462
  febrile 460
  fibrinous acute 466.0
  gastroenteric—*see* Enteritis
  gastrointestinal—*see* Enteritis
  gingivitis 523.00
  hay (*see also* Fever, hay) 477.9
  infectious 460
  intestinal—*see* Enteritis
  larynx (*see also* Laryngitis, chronic) 476.0
  liver 070.1
    with hepatic coma 070.0
  lung (*see also* Bronchitis) 490
    acute 466.0
    chronic 491.0
  middle ear (chronic)—*see* Otitis media, chronic
  mouth 528.00
  nasal (chronic) (*see also* Rhinitis) 472.0
    acute 460
  nasobronchial 472.2
  nasopharyngeal (chronic) 472.2
    acute 460
  nose—*see* Catarrh, nasal
  ophthalmia 372.03
  pneumococcal, acute 466.0
  pulmonary (*see also* Bronchitis) 490
    acute 466.0
    chronic 491.0
  spring (eye) 372.13
  suffocating (*see also* Asthma) 493.9
  summer (hay) (*see also* Fever, hay) 477.9
  throat 472.1
  tracheitis 464.10
    with obstruction 464.11

Catarrh, catarrhal—*continued*
  tubotympanal 381.4
    acute (*see also* Otitis media, acute, nonsuppurative) 381.00
    chronic 381.10
  vasomotor (*see also* Fever, hay) 477.9
  vesical (bladder)—*see* Cystitis
Catarrhus aestivus (*see also* Fever, hay) 477.9
Catastrophe, cerebral (*see also* Disease, cerebrovascular, acute) 436
Catatonia, catatonic (acute) 781.99
  agitation 295.2
  dementia (praecox) 295.2
  due to or associated with physical condition 293.89
  excitation 295.2
  excited type 295.2
  in conditions classified elsewhere 293.89
  schizophrenia 295.2
  stupor 295.2
  with
    affective psychosis —*see* Psychosis, affective
Cat-scratch —*see also* Injury, superficial
  disease or fever 078.3
Cauda equina —*see also* condition syndrome 344.60
Cauliflower ear 738.7
Caul over face 768.9
Causalgia 355.9
  lower limb 355.71
  upper limb 354.4
Cause
  external, general effects NEC 994.9
  not stated 799.9
  unknown 799.9
Caustic burn —*see also* Burn, by site
  from swallowing caustic or corrosive substance—*see* Burn, internal organs
Cavare's disease (familial periodic paralysis) 359.3
Cave-in, injury
  crushing (severe) (*see also* Crush, by site) 869.1
  suffocation 994.7
Cavernitis (penis) 607.2
  lymph vessel—*see* Lymphangioma
Cavernositis 607.2
Cavernous —*see* condition
Cavitation of lung (*see also* Tuberculosis) 011.2
  nontuberculous 518.89
  primary, progressive 010.8
Cavity
  lung—*see* Cavitation of lung
  optic papilla 743.57
  pulmonary—*see* Cavitation of lung
  teeth 521.00
  vitreous (humor) 379.21
Cavovarus foot, congenital 754.59
Cavus foot (congenital) 754.71
  acquired 736.73
Cazenave's
  disease (pemphigus) NEC 694.4
  lupus (erythematosus) 695.4
CDGS (carbohydrate-deficient glycoprotein syndrome) 271.8
Cecitis —*see* Appendicitis
Cecocele —*see* Hernia
Cecum —*see* condition
Celiac
  artery compression syndrome 447.4
  disease 579.0
  infantilism 579.0

INDEX TO DISEASES

Cellulitis

Cell, cellular —*see also* condition
  anterior chamber (eye) (positive aqueous ray) 364.04
Cellulitis (diffuse) (with lymphangitis) (*see also* Abscess) 682.9
  abdominal wall 682.2
  anaerobic (*see also* Gas gangrene) 040.0
  ankle 682.6
  anus 566
  areola 611.0
  arm (any part, above wrist) 682.3
  auditory canal (external) 380.10
  axilla 682.3
  back (any part) 682.2
  breast 611.0
    postpartum 675.1
  broad ligament (*see also* Disease, pelvis, inflammatory) 614.4
    acute 614.3
  buttock 682.5
  cervical (neck region) 682.1
  cervix (uteri) (*see also* Cervicitis) 616.0
  cheek, external 682.0
    internal 528.3
  chest wall 682.2
  chronic NEC 682.9
  colostomy 569.61
  corpus cavernosum 607.2
  digit 681.9
  Douglas' cul-de-sac or pouch (chronic) (*see also* Disease, pelvis, inflammatory) 614.4
    acute 614.3
  drainage site (following operation) 998.59
  ear, external 380.10
  enterostomy 569.61
  erysipelar (*see also* Erysipelas) 035
  esophagostomy 530.86
  eyelid 373.13
  face (any part, except eye) 682.0
  finger (intrathecal) (periosteal) (subcutaneous) (subcuticular) 681.00
  flank 682.2
  foot (except toe) 682.7
  forearm 682.3
  gangrenous (*see also* Gangrene) 785.4
  genital organ NEC
    female—*see* Abscess, genital organ, female
    male 608.4
  glottis 478.71
  gluteal (region) 682.5
  gonococcal NEC 098.0
  groin 682.2
  hand (except finger or thumb) 682.4
  head (except face) NEC 682.8
  heel 682.7
  hip 682.6
  jaw (region) 682.0
  knee 682.6
  labium (majus) (minus) (*see also* Vulvitis) 616.10
  larynx 478.71
  leg, except foot 682.6
  lip 528.5
  mammary gland 611.0
  mouth (floor) 528.3
  multiple sites NEC 682.9
  nasopharynx 478.21
  navel 682.2
    newborn NEC 771.4
  neck (region) 682.1
  nipple 611.0

Cellulitis—*continued*
  nose 478.19
    external 682.0
  orbit, orbital 376.01
  palate (soft) 528.3
  pectoral (region) 682.2
  pelvis, pelvic
    with
      abortion—*see* Abortion, by type, with sepsis
      ectopic pregnancy (*see also* categories 633.0-633.9) 639.0
      molar pregnancy (*see also* categories 630-632) 639.0
    female (*see also* Disease, pelvis, inflammatory) 614.4
      acute 614.3
    following
      abortion 639.0
      ectopic or molar pregnancy 639.0
    male 567.21
  puerperal, postpartum, childbirth 670
  penis 607.2
  perineal, perineum 682.2
  perirectal 566
  peritonsillar 475
  periurethral 597.0
  periuterine (*see also* Disease, pelvis, inflammatory) 614.4
    acute 614.3
  pharynx 478.21
  phlegmonous NEC 682.9
  rectum 566
  retromammary 611.0
  retroperitoneal (*see also* Peritonitis) 567.238
  round ligament (*see also* Disease, pelvis, inflammatory) 614.4
    acute 614.3
  scalp (any part) 682.8
    dissecting 704.8
  scrotum 608.4
  seminal vesicle 608.0
  septic NEC 682.9
  shoulder 682.3
  specified sites NEC 682.8
  spermatic cord 608.4
  submandibular (region) (space) (triangle) 682.0
    gland 527.3
  submaxillary 528.3
    gland 527.3
  submental (pyogenic) 682.0
    gland 527.3
  suppurative NEC 682.9
  testis 608.4
  thigh 682.6
  thumb (intrathecal) (periosteal) (subcutaneous) (subcuticular) 681.00
  toe (intrathecal) (periosteal) (subcutaneous) (subcuticular) 681.10
  tonsil 475
  trunk 682.2
  tuberculous (primary) (*see also* Tuberculosis) 017.0
  tunica vaginalis 608.4
  umbilical 682.2
    newborn NEC 771.4
  vaccinal 999.39
  vagina—*see* Vaginitis
  vas deferens 608.4
  vocal cords 478.5
  vulva (*see also* Vulvitis) 616.10
  wrist 682.4

Cementoblastoma, benign (M9273/0) 213.1
  upper jaw (bone) 213.0
Cementoma (M9273/0) 213.1
  gigantiform (M9276/0) 213.1
    upper jaw (bone) 213.0
  upper jaw (bone) 213.0
Cementoperiostitis 523.40
Cephalgia, cephalalgia (*see also* Headache) 784.0
  histamine 346.2
  nonorganic origin 307.81
  psychogenic 307.81
  tension 307.81
Cephalhematocele, cephalematocele
  due to birth injury 767.19
  fetus or newborn 767.19
  traumatic (*see also* Contusion, head) 920
Cephalhematoma, cephalematoma (calcified)
  due to birth injury 767.19
  fetus or newborn 767.19
  traumatic (*see also* Contusion, head) 920
Cephalic —*see* condition
Cephalitis —*see* Encephalitis
Cephalocele 742.0
Cephaloma —*see* Neoplasm, by site, malignant
Cephalomenia 625.8
Cephalopelvic —*see* condition
Cercomoniasis 007.3
Cerebellitis —*see* Encephalitis
Cerebellum (cerebellar)—*see* condition
Cerebral —*see* condition
Cerebritis —*see* Encephalitis
Cerebrohepatorenal syndrome 759.89
Cerebromacular degeneration 330.1
Cerebromalacia (*see also* Softening, brain) 434.9
Cerebrosidosis 272.7
Cerebrospasticity —*see* Palsy, cerebral
Cerebrospinal —*see* condition
Cerebrum —*see* condition
Ceroid storage disease 272.7
Cerumen (accumulation) (impacted) 380.4
Cervical —*see also* condition
  auricle 744.43
  high risk human papillomavirus (HPV) DNA test positive 795.05
  intraepithelial glandular neoplasia 233.1
  low risk human papillomavirus (Hpv) DNA test positive 795.09
  rib 756.2
Cervicalgia 723.1
Cervicitis (acute) (chronic) (nonvenereal) (subacute) (with erosion or ectropion) 616.0
  with
    abortion—*see* Abortion, by type, with sepsis
    ectopic pregnancy (*see also* categories 633.0-633.9) 639.0
    molar pregnancy (*see also* categories 630-632) 639.0
    ulceration 616.0
  chlamydial 099.53
  complicating pregnancy or puerperium 646.6
    affecting fetus or newborn 760.8
  following
    abortion 639.0
    ectopic or molar pregnancy 639.0
  gonococcal (acute) 098.15
    chronic or duration of 2 months or more 098.35
  senile (atrophic) 616.0
  syphilitic 095.8
  trichomonal 131.09
  tuberculous (*see also* Tuberculosis) 016.7

Cervicoaural fistula 744.49
Cervicocolpitis (emphysematosa) (*see also* Cervicitis) 616.0
Cervix —*see* condition
Cesarean delivery, operation or section NEC 669.7
  affecting fetus or newborn 763.4
  post mortem, affecting fetus or newborn 761.6
  previous, affecting management of pregnancy 654.2
Céstan's syndrome 344.89
Céstan-Chenais paralysis 344.89
Céstan-Raymond syndrome 433.8
Cestode infestation NEC 123.9
  specified type NEC 123.8
Cestodiasis 123.9
CGF (congenital generalized fibromatosis) 759.89
Chaberts' disease 022.9
Chacaleh 266.2
Chafing 709.8
Chagas' disease (*see also* Trypanosomiasis, American) 086.2
  with heart involvement 086.0
Chagres fever 084.0
Chalasia (cardiac sphincter) 530.81
Chalazion 373.2
Chalazoderma 757.39
Chalcosis 360.24
  cornea 371.15
  crystalline lens 360.24 *[366.34]*
  retina 360.24
Chalicosis (occupational) (pulmonum) 502
Chancre (any genital site) (hard) (indurated) (infecting) (primary) (recurrent) 091.0
  congenital 090.0
  conjunctiva 091.2
  Ducrey's 099.0
  extragenital 091.2
  eyelid 091.2
  Hunterian 091.0
  lip (syphilis) 091.2
  mixed 099.8
  nipple 091.2
  Nisbet's 099.0
  of
    carate 103.0
    pinta 103.0
    yaws 102.0
  palate, soft 091.2
  phagedenic 099.0
  Ricord's 091.0
  Rollet's (syphilitic) 091.0
  seronegative 091.0
  seropositive 091.0
  simple 099.0
  soft 099.0
    bubo 099.0
    urethra 091.0
    yaws 102.0
Chancriform syndrome 114.1
Chancroid 099.0
  anus 099.0
  penis (Ducrey's bacillus) 099.0
  perineum 099.0
  rectum 099.0
  scrotum 099.0
  urethra 099.0
  vulva 099.0
Chandipura fever 066.8
Chandler's disease (osteochondritis dissecans, hip) 732.7

Change(s) (of)—*see also* Removal of
  arteriosclerotic—*see* Arteriosclerosis
  battery
    cardiac pacemaker V53.31
  bone 733.90
    diabetic 250.8 *[731.8]*
    in disease, unknown cause 733.90
  bowel habits 787.99
  cardiorenal (vascular) (*see also* Hypertension, cardiorenal) 404.90
  cardiovascular—*see* Disease, cardiovascular
  circulatory 459.9
  cognitive or personality change of other type, nonpsychotic 310.1
  color, teeth, tooth
    during formation 520.8
    extrinsic 523.6
    intrinsic posteruptive 521.7
  contraceptive device V25.42
  cornea, corneal
    degenerative NEC 371.40
    membrane NEC 371.30
    senile 371.41
  coronary (*see also* Ischemia, heart) 414.9
  degenerative
    chamber angle (anterior) (iris) 364.56
    ciliary body 364.57
    spine or vertebra (*see also* Spondylosis) 721.90
  dental pulp, regressive 522.2
  drains V58.49
  dressing
    wound V58.30
      nonsurgical V58.30
      surgical V58.31
  fixation device V54.89
    external V54.89
    internal V54.01
  heart—*see also* Disease, heart
  hip joint 718.95
  hyperplastic larynx 478.79
  hypertrophic
    nasal sinus (*see also* Sinusitis) 473.9
    turbinate, nasal 478.0
    upper respiratory tract 478.9
  inflammatory—*see* Inflammation
  joint (*see also* Derangement, joint) 718.90
    sacroiliac 724.6
  Kirschner wire V54.89
  knee 717.9
  macular, congenital 743.55
  malignant (M——/3)—*see also* Neoplasm, by site, malignant

Note—for malignant change occurring in a neoplasm, use the appropriate M code with behavior digit /3 e.g., malignant change in uterine fibroid—M8890/3. For malignant change occurring in a nonneoplastic condition (e.g., gastric ulcer) use the M code M8000/3.

  mental (status) NEC 780.97
    due to or associated with physical condition—*see* Syndrome, brain
  myocardium, myocardial—*see* Degeneration, myocardial
  of life (*see also* Menopause) 627.2
  pacemaker battery (cardiac) V53.31
  peripheral nerve 355.9
  personality (nonpsychotic) NEC 310.1
  plaster cast V54.89
  refractive, transient 367.81

Change(s) (of)—*continued*
  regressive, dental pulp 522.2
  retina 362.9
    myopic (degenerative) (malignant) 360.21
    vascular appearance 362.13
  sacroiliac joint 724.6
  scleral 379.19
    degenerative 379.16
  senile (*see also* Senility) 797
  sensory (*see also* Disturbance, sensation) 782.0
  skin texture 782.8
  spinal cord 336.9
  splint, external V54.89
  subdermal implantable contraceptive V25.5
  suture V58.32
  traction device V54.89
  trophic 355.9
    arm NEC 354.9
    leg NEC 355.8
    lower extremity NEC 355.8
    upper extremity NEC 354.9
  vascular 459.9
  vasomotor 443.9
  voice 784.49
    psychogenic 306.1
  wound packing V58.30
    nonsurgical V58.30
    surgical V58.31
Changing sleep-work schedule, affecting sleep 327.36
Changuinola fever 066.0
Chapping skin 709.8
Character
  depressive 301.12
Charcot's
  arthropathy 094.0 *[713.5]*
  cirrhosis—*see* Cirrhosis, biliary
  disease 094.0
    spinal cord 094.0
  fever (biliary) (hepatic) (intermittent)—*see* Choledocholithiasis
  joint (disease) 094.0 *[713.5]*
    diabetic 250.6 *[713.5]*
    syringomyelic 336.0 *[713.5]*
  syndrome (intermittent claudication) 443.9
    due to atherosclerosis 440.21
Charcot-Marie-Tooth disease, paralysis, or syndrome 356.1
CHARGE association (syndrome) 759.89
Charleyhorse (quadriceps) 843.8
  muscle, except quadriceps—*see* Sprain, by site
Charlouis' disease (*see also* Yaws) 102.9
Chauffeur's fracture—*see* Fracture, ulna, lower end
Cheadle (-Möller) (-Barlow) disease or syndrome (infantile scurvy) 267
Checking (of)
  contraceptive device (intrauterine) V25.42
  device
    fixation V54.89
      external V54.89
      internal V54.09
    traction V54.89
  Kirschner wire V54.89
  plaster cast V54.89
  splint, external V54.89
Checkup
  following treatment—*see* Examination
  health V70.0
  infant (not sick) V20.2

Checkup—*continued*
　newborn, routine
　　initial V20.2
　　subsequent V20.2
　pregnancy (normal) V22.1
　　first V22.0
　　high risk pregnancy V23.9
　　　specified problem NEC V23.8
Chédiak-Higashi (-Steinbrinck) anomaly, disease, or syndrome (congenital gigantism of peroxidase granules) 288.2
Cheek —*see also* condition
　biting 528.9
Cheese itch 133.8
Cheese washers' lung 495.8
Cheilitis 528.5
　actinic (due to sun) 692.72
　　chronic NEC 692.74
　　　due to radiation, except from sun 692.82
　　due to radiation, except from sun 692.82
　acute 528.5
　angular 528.5
　catarrhal 528.5
　chronic 528.5
　exfoliative 528.5
　gangrenous 528.5
　glandularis apostematosa 528.5
　granulomatosa 351.8
　infectional 528.5
　membranous 528.5
　Miescher's 351.8
　suppurative 528.5
　ulcerative 528.5
　vesicular 528.5
Cheilodynia 528.5
Cheilopalatoschisis (*see also* Cleft, palate, with cleft lip) 749.20
Cheilophagia 528.9
Cheiloschisis (*see also* Cleft, lip) 749.10
Cheilosis 528.5
　with pellagra 265.2
　angular 528.5
　due to
　　dietary deficiency 266.0
　　vitamin deficiency 266.0
Cheiromegaly 729.89
Cheiropompholyx 705.81
Cheloid (*see also* Keloid) 701.4
Chemical burn —*see also* Burn, by site
　from swallowing chemical—*see* Burn, internal organs
Chemodectoma (M8693/1)—*see* Paraganglioma, nonchromaffin
Chemoprophylaxis NEC V07.39
Chemosis, conjunctiva 372.73
Chemotherapy
　convalescence V66.2
　encounter (for) V58.11
　maintenance V58.11
　prophylactic NEC V07.39
　　fluoride V07.31
Cherubism 526.89
Chest —*see* condition
Cheyne-Stokes respiration (periodic) 786.04

Chiari's
　disease or syndrome (hepatic vein thrombosis) 453.0
　malformation
　　type I 348.4
　　type II (*see also* Spina bifida) 741.0
　　type III 742.0
　　type IV 742.2
　network 746.89
Chiari-Frommel syndrome 676.6
Chicago disease (North American blastomycosis) 116.0
Chickenpox (*see also* Varicella) 052.9
　exposure to V01.71
　vaccination and inoculation (prophylactic) V05.4
Chiclero ulcer 085.4
Chiggers 133.8
Chignon 111.2
　fetus or newborn (from vacuum extraction) 767.19
Chigoe disease 134.1
Chikungunya fever 066.3
Chilaiditi's syndrome (subphrenic displacement, colon) 751.4
Chilblains 991.5
　lupus 991.5
Child
　behavior causing concern V61.20
Childbed fever 670
Childbirth —*see also* Delivery
　puerperal complications—*see* Puerperal
Childhood, period of rapid growth V21.0
Chill (s) 780.99
　with fever 780.6
　congestive 780.99
　　in malarial regions 084.6
　septic—*see* Septicemia
　urethral 599.84
Chilomastigiasis 007.8
Chin —*see* condition
Chinese dysentery 004.9
Chiropractic dislocation (*see also* Lesion, nonallopathic, by site) 739.9
Chitral fever 066.0
Chlamydia, chlamydial -*see* condition
Chloasma 709.09
　cachecticorum 709.09
　eyelid 374.52
　　congenital 757.33
　　hyperthyroid 242.0
　gravidarum 646.8
　idiopathic 709.09
　skin 709.09
　symptomatic 709.09
Chloroma (M9930/3) 205.3
Chlorosis 280.9
　Egyptian (*see also* Ancylostomiasis) 126.9
　miners' (*see also* Ancylostomiasis) 126.9
Chlorotic anemia 280.9
Chocolate cyst (ovary) 617.1
Choked
　disk or disc—*see* Papilledema
　on food, phlegm, or vomitus NEC (*see also* Asphyxia, food) 933.1
　phlegm 933.1
　while vomiting NEC (*see also* Asphyxia, food) 933.1

INDEX TO DISEASES

Chokes (resulting from bends) 993.3
Choking sensation 784.99
Cholangiectasis (*see also* Disease, gallbladder) 575.8
Cholangiocarcinoma (M8160/3)
  and hepatocellular carcinoma, combined (M8180/3) 155.0
  liver 155.1
  specified site NEC—*see* Neoplasm, by site, malignant
  unspecified site 155.1
Cholangiohepatitis 575.8
  due to fluke infestation 121.1
Cholangiohepatoma (M8180/3) 155.0
Cholangiolitis (acute) (chronic) (extrahepatic) (gangrenous) 576.1
  intrahepatic 575.8
  paratyphoidal (*see also* Fever, paratyphoid) 002.9
  typhoidal 002.0
Cholangioma (M8160/0) 211.5
  malignant—*see* Cholangiocarcinoma
Cholangitis (acute) (ascending) (catarrhal) (chronic) (infective) (malignant) (primary) (recurrent) (sclerosing) (secondary) (stenosing) (suppurative) 576.1
  chronic nonsuppurative destructive 571.6
  nonsuppurative destructive (chronic) 571.6
Cholecystdocholithiasis —*see* Choledocholithiasis
Cholecystitis 575.10
  with
    calculus, stones in
      bile duct (common) (hepatic)—*see* Choledocholithiasis
      gallbladder—*see* Cholelithiasis
  acute and chronic 575.12
  chronic 575.11
  emphysematous (acute) (*see also* Cholecystitis, acute) 575.0
  gangrenous (*see also* Cholecystitis, acute) 575.0
  paratyphoidal, current (*see also* Fever, paratyphoid) 002.9
  suppurative (*see also* Cholecystitis, acute) 575.0
  typhoidal 002.0
Choledochitis (suppurative) 576.1
Choledocholith —*see* Choledocholithiasis
Choledocholithiasis 574.5

Note—Use the following fifth-digit subclassification with category 574:

0 without mention of obstruction
1 with obstruction

  with
    cholecystitis 574.4
      acute 574.3
      chronic 574.4
    cholelithiasis 574.9
      with
        cholecystitis 574.7
          acute 574.6
            and chronic 574.8
        chronic 574.7

Cholesterol

Cholelithiasis (impacted) (multiple) 574.2

Note—Use the following fifth-digit subclassification with category 574:

0 without mention of obstruction
1 with obstruction

  with
    cholecystitis 574.1
      acute 574.0
      chronic 574.1
    choledocholithiasis 574.9
      with
        cholecystitis 574.7
          acute 574.6
            and chronic 574.8
        chronic cholecystitis 574.7
Cholemia (*see also* Jaundice) 782.4
  familial 277.4
  Gilbert's (familial nonhemolytic) 277.4
Cholemic gallstone —*see* Cholelithiasis
Choleperitoneum, choleperitonitis (*see also* Disease, gallbladder) 567.81
Cholera (algid) (Asiatic) (asphyctic) (epidemic) (gravis) (Indian) (malignant) (morbus) (pestilential) (spasmodic) 001.9
  antimonial 985.4
  carrier (suspected) of V02.0
  classical 001.0
  contact V01.0
  due to
    Vibrio
      cholerae (Inaba, Ogawa, Hikojima serotypes) 001.0
      El Tor 001.1
  El Tor 001.1
  exposure to V01.0
  vaccination, prophylactic (against) V03.0
Cholerine (*see also* Cholera) 001.9
Cholestasis 576.8
  due to total parenteral nutrition (TPN) 573.8
Cholesteatoma (ear) 385.30
  attic (primary) 385.31
  diffuse 385.35
  external ear (canal) 380.21
  marginal (middle ear) 385.32
    with involvement of mastoid cavity 385.33
    secondary (with middle ear involvement) 385.33
  mastoid cavity 385.30
  middle ear (secondary) 385.32
    with involvement of mastoid cavity 385.33—
  postmastoidectomy cavity (recurrent) 383.32
  primary 385.31
  recurrent, postmastoidectomy cavity 383.32
  secondary (middle ear) 385.32
    with involvement of mastoid cavity 385.33
Cholesteatosis (middle ear) (*see also* Cholesteatoma) 385.30
  diffuse 385.35
Cholesteremia 272.0
Cholesterin
  granuloma, middle ear 385.82
  in vitreous 379.22
Cholesterol
  deposit
    retina 362.82
    vitreous 379.22
  elevated (high) 272.0
    with elevated (high) triglycerides 272.2
  imbibition of gallbladder (*see also* Disease, gallbladder) 575.6

Cholesterolemia 272.0
  essential 272.0
  familial 272.0
  hereditary 272.0
Cholesterosis, cholesterolosis (gallbladder) 575.6
  middle ear (*see also* Cholesteatoma) 385.30
  with
    cholecystitis—*see* Cholecystitis
    cholelithiasis—*see* Cholelithiasis
Cholocolic fistula (*see also* Fistula, gallbladder) 575.5
Choluria 791.4
Chondritis (purulent) 733.99
  auricle 380.03
  costal 733.6
    Tietze's 733.6
  patella, posttraumatic 717.7
  pinna 380.03
  posttraumatica patellae 717.7
  tuberculous (active) (*see also* Tuberculosis) 015.9
    intervertebral 015.0 *[730.88]*
Chondroangiopathia calcarea seu punctate 756.59
Chondroblastoma (M9230/0)—*see also*
    Neoplasm, bone, benign
  malignant (M9230/3)—*see* Neoplasm, bone, malignant
Chondrocalcinosis (articular) (crystal deposition) (dihydrate) (*see also* Arthritis, due to, crystals) 275.49 *[712.3]*
  due to
    calcium pyrophosphate 275.49 *[712.2]*
    dicalcium phosphate crystals 275.49 *[712.1]*
    pyrophosphate crystals 275.4 *[712.2]*
Chondrodermatitis nodularis helicis 380.00
Chondrodysplasia 756.4
  angiomatose 756.4
  calcificans congenita 756.59
  epiphysialis punctata 756.59
  hereditary deforming 756.4
  rhizomelic punctata 277.86
Chondrodystrophia (fetalis) 756.4
  calcarea 756.4
  calcificans congenita 756.59
  fetalis hypoplastica 756.59
  hypoplastica calcinosa 756.59
  punctata 756.59
  tarda 277.5
Chondrodystrophy (familial) (hypoplastic) 756.4
  myotonic (congenital) 359.23
Chondroectodermal dysplasia 756.55
Chondrolysis 733.99
Chondroma (M9220/0)—*see also* Neoplasm, cartilage, benign
  juxtacortical (M9221/0)—*see* Neoplasm, bone, benign
  periosteal (M9221/0)—*see* Neoplasm, bone, benign
Chondromalacia 733.92
  epiglottis (congenital) 748.3
  generalized 733.92
  knee 717.7
  larynx (congenital) 748.3
  localized, except patella 733.92
  patella, patellae 717.7
  systemic 733.92
  tibial plateau 733.92
  trachea (congenital) 748.3
Chondromatosis (M9220/1)—*see* Neoplasm, cartilage, uncertain behavior

Chondromyxosarcoma (M9220/3)—*see* Neoplasm, cartilage, malignant
Chondro-osteodysplasia (Morquio-Brailsford type) 277.5
Chondro-osteodystrophy 277.5
Chondro-osteodystrophy 277.5
Chondro-osteoma (M9210/0)—*see* Neoplasm, bone, benign
Chondropathia tuberosa 733.6
Chondrosarcoma (M9220/3)—*see also* Neoplasm, cartilage, malignant
  juxtacortical (M9221/3)—*see* Neoplasm, bone, malignant
  mesenchymal (M9240/3)—*see* Neoplasm, connective tissue, malignant
Chordae tendineae rupture (chronic) 429.5
Chordee (nonvenereal) 607.89
  congenital 752.63
  gonococcal 098.2
Chorditis (fibrinous) (nodosa) (tuberosa) 478.5
Chordoma (M9370/3)—*see* Neoplasm, by site, malignant
Chorea (gravis) (minor) (spasmodic) 333.5
  with
    heart involvement—*see* Chorea with rheumatic heart disease
    rheumatic heart disease (chronic, inactive, or quiescent) (conditions classifiable to 393-398)—*see also* Rheumatic heart condition involved
      active or acute (conditions classifiable to 391) 392.0
  acute—*see* Chorea, Sydenham's
  apoplectic (*see also* Disease, cerebrovascular, acute) 436
  chronic 333.4
  electric 049.8
  gravidarum—*see* Eclampsia, pregnancy
  habit 307.22
  hereditary 333.4
  Huntington's 333.4
  posthemiplegic 344.89
  pregnancy—*see* Eclampsia, pregnancy
  progressive 333.4
    chronic 333.4
    hereditary 333.4
  rheumatic (chronic) 392.9
    with heart disease or involvement—*see* Chorea, with rheumatic heart disease
  senile 333.5
  Sydenham's 392.9
    with heart involvement—*see* Chorea, with rheumatic heart disease
  nonrheumatic 333.5
  variabilis 307.23
Choreoathetosis (paroxysmal) 333.5
Chorioadenoma (destruens) (M9100/1) 236.1
Chorioamnionitis 658.4
  affecting fetus or newborn 762.7
Chorioangioma (M9120/0) 219.8
Choriocarcinoma (M9100/3)
  combined with
    embryonal carcinoma (M9101/3)—*see* Neoplasm, by site, malignant
    teratoma (M9101/3)—*see* Neoplasm, by site, malignant
  specified site—*see* Neoplasm, by site, malignant
  unspecified site
    female 181
    male 186.9

Chorioencephalitis, lymphocytic (acute) (serous) 049.0
Chorioepithelioma (M9100/3)—*see* Choriocarcinoma
Choriomeningitis (acute) (benign) (lymphocytic) (serous) 049.0
Chorionepithelioma (M9100/3)—*see* Choriocarcinoma
Chorionitis (*see also* Scleroderma) 710.1
Chorioretinitis 363.20
  disseminated 363.10
    generalized 363.13
    in
      neurosyphilis 094.83
      secondary syphilis 091.51
    peripheral 363.12
    posterior pole 363.11
    tuberculous (*see also* Tuberculosis) 017.3 *[363.13]*
  due to
    histoplasmosis (*see also* Histoplasmosis) 115.92
    toxoplasmosis (acquired) 130.2
      congenital (active) 771.2
  focal 363.00
    juxtapapillary 363.01
    peripheral 363.04
    posterior pole NEC 363.03
  juxtapapillaris, juxtapapillary 363.01
  progressive myopia (degeneration) 360.21
  syphilitic (secondary) 091.51
    congenital (early) 090.0 *[363.13]*
      late 090.5 *[363.13]*
    late 095.8 *[363.13]*
  tuberculous (*see also* Tuberculosis) 017.3 *[363.13]*
Choristoma —*see* Neoplasm, by site, benign
Choroid —*see* condition
Choroideremia, choroidermia (initial stage) (late stage) (partial or total atrophy) 363.55
Choroiditis (*see also* Chorioretinitis) 363.20
  leprous 030.9 *[363.13]*
  senile guttate 363.41
  sympathetic 360.11
  syphilitic (secondary) 091.51
    congenital (early) 090.0 *[363.13]*
      late 090.5 *[363.13]*
    late 095.8 *[363.13]*
  Tay's 363.41
  tuberculous (*see also* Tuberculosis) 017.3 *[363.13]*
Choroidopathy NEC 363.9
  degenerative (*see also* Degeneration, choroid) 363.40
  hereditary (*see also* Dystrophy, choroid) 363.50
  specified type NEC 363.8
Choroidoretinitis —*see* Chorioretinitis
Choroidosis, central serous 362.41
Choroidretinopathy, serous 362.41
Christian's syndrome (chronic histiocytosis X) 277.89
Christian-Weber disease (nodular nonsuppurative panniculitis) 729.30
Christmas disease 286.1
Chromaffinoma (M8700/0)—*see also* Neoplasm, by site, benign
  malignant (M8700/3)—*see* Neoplasm, by site, malignant
Chromatopsia 368.59
Chromhidrosis, chromidrosis 705.89
Chromoblastomycosis 117.2
Chromomycosis 117.2
Chromophytosis 111.0

Chromotrichomycosis 111.8
Chronic —*see* condition
Churg-Strauss syndrome 446.4
Chyle cyst, mesentery 457.8
Chylocele (nonfilarial) 457.8
  filarial (*see also* Infestation, filarial) 125.9
  tunica vaginalis (nonfilarial) 608.84
    filarial (*see also* Infestation, filarial) 125.9
Chylomicronemia (fasting) (with hyperprebetalipoproteinemia) 272.3
Chylopericardium (acute) 420.90
Chylothorax (nonfilarial) 457.8
  filarial (*see also* Infestation, filarial) 125.9
Chylous
  ascites 457.8
  cyst of peritoneum 457.8
  hydrocele 603.9
  hydrothorax (nonfilarial) 457.8
    filarial (*see also* Infestation, filarial) 125.9
Chyluria 791.1
  bilharziasis 120.0
  due to
    Brugia (malayi) 125.1
    Wuchereria (bancrofti) 125.0
      malayi 125.1
  filarial (*see also* Infestation, filarial) 125.9
  filariasis (*see also* Infestation, filarial) 125.9
  nonfilarial 791.1
Cicatricial (deformity)—*see* Cicatrix
Cicatrix (adherent) (contracted) (painful) (vicious) 709.2
  adenoid 474.8
  alveolar process 525.8
  anus 569.49
  auricle 380.89
  bile duct (*see also* Disease, biliary) 576.8
  bladder 596.8
  bone 733.99
  brain 348.8
  cervix (postoperative) (postpartal) 622.3
    in pregnancy or childbirth 654.6
      causing obstructed labor 660.2
  chorioretinal 363.30
    disseminated 363.35
    macular 363.32
    peripheral 363.34
    posterior pole NEC 363.33
  choroid—*see* Cicatrix, chorioretinal
  common duct (*see also* Disease, biliary) 576.8
  congenital 757.39
  conjunctiva 372.64
  cornea 371.00
    tuberculous (*see also* Tuberculosis) 017.3 *[371.05]*
  duodenum (bulb) 537.3
  esophagus 530.3
  eyelid 374.46
    with
      ectropion—*see* Ectropion
      entropion—*see* Entropion
  hypopharynx 478.29
  knee, semilunar cartilage 717.5
  lacrimal
    canaliculi 375.53
    duct
      acquired 375.56
      neonatal 375.55
    punctum 375.52
    sac 375.54
  larynx 478.79
  limbus (cystoid) 372.64
  lung 518.89

Cicatrix—*continued*
  macular 363.32
    disseminated 363.35
    peripheral 363.34
  middle ear 385.89
  mouth 528.9
  muscle 728.89
  nasolacrimal duct
    acquired 375.56
    neonatal 375.55
  nasopharynx 478.29
  palate (soft) 528.9
  penis 607.89
  prostate 602.8
  rectum 569.49
  retina 363.30
    disseminated 363.35
    macular 363.32
    peripheral 363.34
    posterior pole NEC 363.33
  semilunar cartilage—*see* Derangement, meniscus
  seminal vesicle 608.89
  skin 709.2
    infected 686.8
    postinfectional 709.2
    tuberculous (*see also* Tuberculosis) 017.0
  specified site NEC 709.2
  throat 478.29
  tongue 529.8
  tonsil (and adenoid) 474.8
  trachea 478.9
  tuberculous NEC (*see also* Tuberculosis) 011.9
  ureter 593.89
  urethra 599.84
  uterus 621.8
  vagina 623.4
    in pregnancy or childbirth 654.7
      causing obstructed labor 660.2
  vocal cord 478.5
  wrist, constricting (annular) 709.2
CIDP (chronic inflammatory demyelinating polyneuropathy) 357.81
CIN I [cervical intraepithelial neoplasia I] 622.11
CIN II [cervical intraepithelial neoplasia II] 622.12
CIN III [cervical intraepithelial neoplasia III] 233.1
Cinchonism
  correct substance properly administered 386.9
  overdose or wrong substance given or taken 961.4
Circine herpes 110.5
Circle of Willis —*see* condition
Circular —*see also* condition
  hymen 752.49
Circulating anticoagulants 286.5
  following childbirth 666.3
  postpartum 666.3
Circulation
  collateral (venous), any site 459.89
  defective 459.9
    congenital 747.9
    lower extremity 459.89
  embryonic 747.9
  failure 799.89
    fetus or newborn 779.89
    peripheral 785.59
  fetal, persistent 747.83
  heart, incomplete 747.9
Circulatory system —*see* condition
Circulus senilis 371.41

Circumcision
  in absence of medical indication V50.2
  ritual V50.2
  routine V50.2
Circumscribed —*see* condition
Circumvallata placenta —*see* Placenta, abnormal
Cirrhosis, cirrhotic 571.5
  with alcoholism 571.2
  alcoholic (liver) 571.2
  atrophic (of liver)—*see* Cirrhosis, portal
  Baumgarten-Cruveilhier 571.5
  biliary (cholangiolitic) (cholangitic) (cholestatic) (extrahepatic) (hypertrophic) (intrahepatic) (nonobstructive) (obstructive) (pericholangiolitic) (posthepatic) (primary) (secondary) (xanthomatous) 571.6
    due to
      clonorchiasis 121.1
      flukes 121.3
  brain 331.9
  capsular—*see* Cirrhosis, portal
  cardiac 571.5
    alcoholic 571.2
  central (liver)—*see* Cirrhosis, liver
  Charcot's 571.6
  cholangiolitic—*see* Cirrhosis, biliary
  cholangitic—*see* Cirrhosis, biliary
  cholestatic—*see* Cirrhosis, biliary
  clitoris (hypertrophic) 624.2
  coarsely nodular 571.5
  congestive (liver)—*see* Cirrhosis, cardiac
  Cruveilhier-Baumgarten 571.5
  cryptogenic (of liver) 571.5
    alcoholic 571.2
  dietary (*see also* Cirrhosis, portal) 571.5
  due to
    bronzed diabetes 275.0
    congestive hepatomegaly—*see* Cirrhosis, cardiac
    cystic fibrosis 277.00
    hemochromatosis 275.0
    hepatolenticular degeneration 275.1
    passive congestion (chronic)—*see* Cirrhosis, cardiac
    Wilson's disease 275.1
    xanthomatosis 272.2
  extrahepatic (obstructive)—*see* Cirrhosis, biliary
  fatty 571.8
    alcoholic 571.0
  florid 571.2
  Glisson's—*see* Cirrhosis, portal
  Hanot's (hypertrophic)—*see* Cirrhosis, biliary
  hepatic—*see* Cirrhosis, liver
  hepatolienal—*see* Cirrhosis, liver
  hobnail—*see* Cirrhosis, portal
  hypertrophic—*see also* Cirrhosis, liver
    biliary—*see* Cirrhosis, biliary
    Hanot's—*see* Cirrhosis, biliary
  infectious NEC—*see* Cirrhosis, portal
  insular—*see* Cirrhosis, portal
  intrahepatic (obstructive) (primary) (secondary)—*see* Cirrhosis, biliary
  juvenile (*see also* Cirrhosis, portal) 571.5
  kidney (*see also* Sclerosis, renal) 587
  Laennec's (of liver) 571.2
    nonalcoholic 571.5
  liver (chronic) (hepatolienal) (hypertrophic) (nodular) (splenomegalic) (unilobar) 571.5
    with alcoholism 571.2
    alcoholic 571.2

INDEX TO DISEASES — Cleft

Cirrhosis, cirrhotic—*continued*
  congenital (due to failure of obliteration of umbilical vein) 777.8
  cryptogenic 571.5
    alcoholic 571.2
  fatty 571.8
    alcoholic 571.0
  macronodular 571.5
    alcoholic 571.2
  micronodular 571.5
    alcoholic 571.2
  nodular, diffuse 571.5
    alcoholic 571.2
  pigmentary 275.0
  portal 571.5
    alcoholic 571.2
  postnecrotic 571.5
    alcoholic 571.2
    syphilitic 095.3
  lung (chronic) (*see also* Fibrosis, lung) 515
  macronodular (of liver) 571.5
    alcoholic 571.2
  malarial 084.9
  metabolic NEC 571.5
  micronodular (of liver) 571.5
    alcoholic 571.2
  monolobular—*see* Cirrhosis, portal
  multilobular—*see* Cirrhosis, portal
  nephritis (*see also* Sclerosis, renal) 587
  nodular—*see* Cirrhosis, liver
  nutritional (fatty) 571.5
  obstructive (biliary) (extrahepatic) (intrahepatic)—*see* Cirrhosis, biliary
  ovarian 620.8
  paludal 084.9
  pancreas (duct) 577.8
  pericholangiolitic—*see* Cirrhosis, biliary
  periportal—*see* Cirrhosis, portal
  pigment, pigmentary (of liver) 275.0
  portal (of liver) 571.5
    alcoholic 571.2
  posthepatitic (*see also* Cirrhosis, postnecrotic) 571.5
  postnecrotic (of liver) 571.5
    alcoholic 571.2
  primary (intrahepatic)—*see* Cirrhosis, biliary
  pulmonary (*see also* Fibrosis, lung) 515
  renal (*see also* Sclerosis, renal) 587
  septal (*see also* Cirrhosis, postnecrotic) 571.5
  spleen 289.51
  splenomegalic (of liver)—*see* Cirrhosis, liver
  stasis (liver)—*see* Cirrhosis, liver
  stomach 535.4
  Todd's (*see also* Cirrhosis, biliary) 571.6
  toxic (nodular)—*see* Cirrhosis, postnecrotic
  trabecular—*see* Cirrhosis, postnecrotic
  unilobar—*see* Cirrhosis, liver
  vascular (of liver)—*see* Cirrhosis, liver
  xanthomatous (biliary) (*see also* Cirrhosis, biliary) 571.6
    due to xanthomatosis (familial) (metabolic) (primary) 272.2
Cistern, subarachnoid 793.0
Citrullinemia 270.6
Citrullinuria 270.6
Ciuffini-Pancoast tumor (M8010/3) (carcinoma, pulmonary apex) 162.3
Civatte's disease or poikiloderma 709.09
Clam diggers' itch 120.3
Clap —*see* Gonorrhea
Clark's paralysis 343.9

Clarke-Hadfield syndrome (pancreatic infantilism) 577.8
Clastothrix 704.2
Claude's syndrome 352.6
Claude Bernard-Horner syndrome (*see also* Neuropathy, peripheral, autonomic) 337.9
Claudication, intermittent 443.9
  cerebral (artery) (*see also* Ischemia, cerebral, transient) 435.9
  due to atherosclerosis 440.21
  spinal cord (arteriosclerotic) 435.1
    syphilitic 094.89
  spinalis 435.1
  venous (axillary) 453.8
Claudicatio venosa intermittens 453.8
Claustrophobia 300.29
Clavus (infected) 700
Claw foot (congenital) 754.71
  acquired 736.74
Claw hand (acquired) 736.06
  congenital 755.59
Clawtoe (congenital) 754.71
  acquired 735.5
Clay eating 307.52
Clay shovelers' fracture —*see* Fracture, vertebra, cervical
Cleansing of artificial opening (*see also* Attention to artificial opening) V55.9
Cleft (congenital)—*see also* Imperfect, closure
  alveolar process 525.8
  branchial (persistent) 744.41
    cyst 744.42
  clitoris 752.49
  cricoid cartilage, posterior 748.3
  facial (*see also* Cleft, lip) 749.10
  lip 749.10
    with cleft palate 749.20
      bilateral (lip and palate) 749.24
        with unilateral lip or palate 749.25
        complete 749.23
        incomplete 749.24
      unilateral (lip and palate) 749.22
        with bilateral lip or palate 749.25
        complete 749.21
        incomplete 749.22
    bilateral 749.14
      with cleft palate, unilateral 749.25
      complete 749.13
      incomplete 749.14
    unilateral 749.12
      with cleft palate, bilateral 749.25
      complete 749.11
      incomplete 749.12
  nose 748.1
  palate 749.00
    with cleft lip 749.20
      bilateral (lip and palate) 749.24
        with unilateral lip or palate 749.25
        complete 749.23
        incomplete 749.24
      unilateral (lip and palate) 749.22
        with bilateral lip or palate 749.25
        complete 749.21
        incomplete 749.22
    bilateral 749.04
      with cleft lip, unilateral 749.25
      complete 749.03
      incomplete 749.04
    unilateral 749.02
      with cleft lip, bilateral 749.25
      complete 749.01

Cleft — *continued*
    incomplete 749.02
    penis 752.69
    posterior, cricoid cartilage 748.3
    scrotum 752.89
    sternum (congenital) 756.3
    thyroid cartilage (congenital) 748.3
    tongue 750.13
    uvula 749.02
        with cleft lip (*see also* Cleft, lip, with cleft palate) 749.20
    water 366.12
Cleft hand (congenital) 755.58
Cleidocranial dysostosis 755.59
Cleidotomy, fetal 763.89
Cleptomania 312.32
Clérambault's syndrome 297.8
    erotomania 302.89
Clergyman's sore throat 784.49
Click, clicking
    systolic syndrome 785.2
Clifford's syndrome (postmaturity) 766.22
Climacteric (*see also* Menopause) 627.2
    arthritis NEC (*see also* Arthritis, climacteric) 716.3
    depression (*see also* Psychosis, affective) 296.2
    disease 627.2
        recurrent episode 296.3
        single episode 296.2
    female (symptoms) 627.2
    male (symptoms) (syndrome) 608.89
    melancholia (*see also* Psychosis, affective) 296.2
        recurrent episode 296.3
        single episode 296.2
    paranoid state 297.2
    paraphrenia 297.2
    polyarthritis NEC 716.39
    male 608.89
    symptoms (female) 627.2
Clinical research investigation (control) (participant) V70.7
Clinodactyly 755.59
Clitoris —*see* condition
Cloaca, persistent 751.5
Clonorchiasis 121.1
Clonorchiosis 121.1
Clonorchis infection, liver 121.1
Clonus 781.0
Closed bite 524.20
Closed surgical procedure converted to open procedure
    arthroscopic V64.43
    laparoscopic V64.41
    thoracoscopic V64.42
Closure
    artificial opening (*see also* Attention to artificial opening) V55.9
    congenital, nose 748.0
    cranial sutures, premature 756.0
    defective or imperfect NEC—*see* Imperfect, closure
    fistula, delayed—*see* Fistula
    fontanelle, delayed 756.0
    foramen ovale, imperfect 745.5
    hymen 623.3
    interauricular septum, defective 745.5
    interventricular septum, defective 745.4
    lacrimal duct 375.56
        congenital 743.65
        neonatal 375.55

Closure—*continued*
    nose (congenital) 748.0
        acquired 738.0
    vagina 623.2
    valve—*see* Endocarditis
    vulva 624.8
Clot (blood)
    artery (obstruction) (occlusion) (*see also* Embolism) 444.9
    atrial appendage 429.89
    bladder 596.7
    brain (extradural or intradural) (*see also* Thrombosis, brain) 434.0
        late effect—*see* Late effect(s) (of) cerebrovascular disease
    circulation 444.9
    heart (*see also* Infarct, myocardium) 410.9
        without myocardial infarction 429.89
    vein (*see also* Thrombosis) 453.9
Clotting defect NEC (*see also* Defect, coagulation) 286.9
Clouded state 780.09
    epileptic (*see also* Epilepsy) 345.9
    paroxysmal (idiopathic) (*see also* Epilepsy) 345.9
Clouding
    corneal graft 996.51
Cloudy
    antrum, antra 473.0
    dialysis effluent 792.5
Clouston's (hidrotic) ectodermal dysplasia 757.31
Clubbing of fingers 781.5
Clubfinger 736.29
    acquired 736.29
    congenital 754.89
Clubfoot (congenital) 754.70
    acquired 736.71
    equinovarus 754.51
    paralytic 736.71
Club hand (congenital) 754.89
    acquired 736.07
Clubnail (acquired) 703.8
    congenital 757.5
Clump kidney 753.3
Clumsiness 781.3
    syndrome 315.4
Cluttering 307.0
Clutton's joints 090.5
Coagulation, intravascular (diffuse) (disseminated) (*see also* Fibrinolysis) 286.6
    newborn 776.2
Coagulopathy (*see also* Defect, coagulation) 286.9
    consumption 286.6
    intravascular (disseminated) NEC 286.6
    newborn 776.2
Coalition
    calcaneoscaphoid 755.67
    calcaneus 755.67
    tarsal 755.67
Coal miners'
    elbow 727.2
    lung 500
Coal workers' lung or pneumoconiosis 500
Coarctation
    aorta (postductal) (preductal) 747.10
    pulmonary artery 747.3
Coated tongue 529.3
Coats' disease 362.12
Cocainism (*see also* Dependence) 304.2
Coccidioidal granuloma 114.3

INDEX TO DISEASES — Colitis

Coccidioidomycosis 114.9
  with pneumonia 114.0
  cutaneous (primary) 114.1
  disseminated 114.3
  extrapulmonary (primary) 114.1
  lung 114.5
    acute 114.0
    chronic 114.4
    primary 114.0
  meninges 114.2
  primary (pulmonary) 114.0
    acute 114.0
  prostate 114.3
  pulmonary 114.5
    acute 114.0
    chronic 114.4
    primary 114.0
  specified site NEC 114.3
Coccidioidosis 114.9
  lung 114.5
    acute 114.0
    chronic 114.4
    primary 114.0
  meninges 114.2
Coccidiosis (colitis) (diarrhea) (dysentery) 007.2
Cocciuria 791.9
Coccus in urine 791.9
Coccydynia 724.79
Coccygodynia 724.79
Coccyx —*see* condition
Cochin-China
  diarrhea 579.1
    anguilluliasis 127.2
  ulcer 085.1
Cock's peculiar tumor 706.2
Cockayne's disease or syndrome (microcephaly and dwarfism) 759.89
Cockayne-Weber syndrome (epidermolysis bullosa) 757.39
Cocked-up toe 735.2
Codman's tumor (benign chondroblastoma) (M9230/0)—*see* Neoplasm, bone, benign
Coenurosis 123.8
Coffee workers' lung 495.8
Cogan's syndrome 370.52
  congenital oculomotor apraxia 379.51
  nonsyphilitic interstitial keratitis 370.52
Coiling, umbilical cord —*see* Complications, umbilical cord
Coitus, painful (female) 625.0
  male 608.89
  psychogenic 302.76
Cold 460
  with influenza, flu, or grippe 487.1
  abscess—*see also* Tuberculosis, abscess
  articular—*see* Tuberculosis, joint
  agglutinin
    disease (chronic) or syndrome 283.0
    hemoglobinuria 283.0
      paroxysmal (cold) (nocturnal) 283.2
  allergic (*see also* Fever, hay) 477.9
  bronchus or chest—*see* Bronchitis
    with grippe or influenza 487.1
  common (head) 460
    vaccination, prophylactic (against) V04.7
  deep 464.10
  effects of 991.9
    specified effect NEC 991.8
  excessive 991.9
    specified effect NEC 991.8
  exhaustion from 991.8

Cold —*continued*
  exposure to 991.9
    specified effect NEC 991.8
  grippy 487.1
  head 460
  injury syndrome (newborn) 778.2
  intolerance 780.99
  on lung—*see* Bronchitis
  rose 477.0
  sensitivity, autoimmune 283.0
  virus 460
Coldsore (*see also* Herpes, simplex) 054.9
Colibacillosis 041.4
  generalized 038.42
Colibacilluria 791.9
Colic (recurrent) 789.0
  abdomen 789.0
    (recurrent)psychogenic 307.89
  appendicular 543.9
  appendix 543.9
  bile duct—*see* Choledocholithiasis
  biliary—*see* Cholelithiasis
  bilious—*see* Cholelithiasis
  common duct—*see* Choledocholithiasis
  Devonshire NEC 984.9
    specified type of lead—*see* Table of drugs and chemicals
  flatulent 787.3
  gallbladder or gallstone—*see* Cholelithiasis
  gastric 536.8
  hepatic (duct)—*see* Choledocholithiasis
  hysterical 300.11
  infantile 789.0
  intestinal 789.0
  kidney 788.0
  lead NEC 984.9
    specified type of lead—*see* Table of drugs and chemicals
  liver (duct)—*see* Choledocholithiasis
  mucous 564.9
    psychogenic 316 [564.9]
  nephritic 788.0
  painter's NEC 984.9
  pancreas 577.8
  psychogenic 306.4
  renal 788.0
  saturnine NEC 984.9
    specified type of lead—*see* Table of drugs and chemicals
  spasmodic 789.0
  ureter 788.0
  urethral 599.84
    due to calculus 594.2
  uterus 625.8
    menstrual 625.3
  vermicular 543.9
  virus 460
  worm NEC 128.9
Colicystitis (*see also* Cystitis) 595.9
Colitis (acute) (catarrhal) (croupous) (cystica superficialis) (exudative) (hemorrhagic) (noninfectious) (phlegmonous) (presumed noninfectious) 558.9
  adaptive 564.9
  allergic 558.3
  amebic (*see also* Amebiasis) 006.9
    nondysenteric 006.2
  anthrax 022.2
  bacillary (*see also* Infection, Shigella) 004.9
  balantidial 007.0

Colitis

Colitis—*continued*
  chronic 558.9
    ulcerative (*see also* Colitis, ulcerative) 556.9
  coccidial 007.2
  dietetic 558.9
  due to radiation 558.1
  functional 558.9
  gangrenous 009.0
  giardial 007.1
  granulomatous 555.1
  gravis (*see also* Colitis, ulcerative) 556.9
  infectious (*see also* Enteritis, due to, specific organism) 009.0
    presumed 009.1
  ischemic 557.9
    acute 557.0
    chronic 557.1
    due to mesenteric artery insufficiency 557.1
  membranous 564.9
    psychogenic 316 *[564.9]*
  mucous 564.9
    psychogenic 316 *[564.9]*
  necrotic 009.0
  polyposa (*see also* Colitis, ulcerative) 556.9
  protozoal NEC 007.9
  pseudomembranous 008.45
  pseudomucinous 564.9
  regional 555.1
  segmental 555.1
  septic (*see also* Enteritis, due to, specific organism) 009.0
  spastic 564.9
    psychogenic 316 *[564.9]*
  staphylococcus 008.41
    food 005.0
  thromboulcerative 557.0
  toxic 558.2
  transmural 555.1
  trichomonal 007.3
  tuberculous (ulcerative) 014.8
  ulcerative (chronic) (idiopathic) (nonspecific) 556.9
    entero- 556.0
    fulminant 557.0
    ileo- 556.1
    left-sided 556.5
    procto- 556.2
    proctosigmoid 556.3
    psychogenic 316 *[556]*
    specified NEC 556.8
    universal 556.6

Collagen disease NEC 710.9
  nonvascular 710.9
  vascular (allergic) (*see also* Angiitis, hypersensitivity) 446.20

Collagenosis (*see also* Collagen disease) 710.9
  cardiovascular 425.4
  mediastinal 519.3

Collapse 780.2
  adrenal 255.8
  cardiorenal (*see also* Hypertension, cardiorenal) 404.90
  cardiorespiratory 785.51
    fetus or newborn 779.85
  cardiovascular (*see also* Disease, heart) 785.51
    fetus or newborn 779.85
  circulatory (peripheral) 785.59
    with
      abortion—*see* Abortion, by type, with shock
      ectopic pregnancy (*see also* categories 633.0-633.9) 639.5

INDEX TO DISEASES

Collapse—*continued*
      molar pregnancy (*see also* categories 630-632) 639.5
    during or after labor and delivery 669.1
    fetus or newborn 779.85
    following
      abortion 639.5
      ectopic or molar pregnancy 639.5
  during or after labor and delivery 669.1
    fetus or newborn 779.89
  external ear canal 380.50
    secondary to
      inflammation 380.53
      surgery 380.52
      trauma 380.51
  general 780.2
  heart—*see* Disease, heart
  heat 992.1
  hysterical 300.11
  labyrinth, membranous (congenital) 744.05
  lung (massive) (*see also* Atelectasis) 518.0
    pressure, during labor 668.0
  myocardial—*see* Disease, heart
  nervous (*see also* Disorder, mental, nonpsychotic) 300.9
  neurocirculatory 306.2
  nose 738.0
  postoperative (cardiovascular) 998.0
  pulmonary (*see also* Atelectasis) 518.0
    fetus or newborn 770.5
      partial 770.5
      primary 770.4
  thorax 512.8
    iatrogenic 512.1
    postoperative 512.1
  trachea 519.19
  valvular—*see* Endocarditis
  vascular (peripheral) 785.59
    with
      abortion—*see* Abortion, by type, with shock
      ectopic pregnancy (*see also* categories 633.0-633.9) 639.5
      molar pregnancy (*see also* categories 630-632) 639.5
    cerebral (*see also* Disease, cerebrovascular, acute) 436
    during or after labor and delivery 669.1
    fetus or newborn 779.89
    following
      abortion 639.5
      ectopic or molar pregnancy 639.5
  vasomotor 785.59
  vertebra 733.13

Collateral —*see also* condition
  circulation (venous) 459.89
  dilation, veins 459.89

Colles' fracture (closed) (reversed) (separation) 813.41
  open 813.51

Collet's syndrome 352.6

Collet-Sicard syndrome 352.6

Colliculitis urethralis (*see also* Urethritis) 597.89

Colliers'
  asthma 500
  lung 500
  phthisis (*see also* Tuberculosis) 011.4

Collodion baby (ichthyosis congenita) 757.1

Colloid milium 709.3

INDEX TO DISEASES   Complications

Coloboma NEC 743.49
  choroid 743.59
  fundus 743.52
  iris 743.46
  lens 743.36
  lids 743.62
  optic disc (congenital) 743.57
    acquired 377.23
  retina 743.56
  sclera 743.47
Coloenteritis —*see* Enteritis
Colon —*see* condition
Coloptosis 569.89
Color
  amblyopia NEC 368.59
    acquired 368.55
  blindness NEC (congenital) 368.59
    acquired 368.55
Colostomy
  attention to V55.3
  fitting or adjustment V53.5
  malfunctioning 569.62
  status V44.3
Colpitis (*see also* Vaginitis) 616.10
Colpocele 618.6
Colpocystitis (*see also* Vaginitis) 616.10
Colporrhexis 665.4
Colpospasm 625.1
Column, spinal, vertebral —*see* condition
Coma 780.01
  apoplectic (*see also* Disease, cerebrovascular, acute) 436
  diabetic (with ketoacidosis) 250.3
    hyperosmolar 250.2
  eclamptic (*see also* Eclampsia) 780.39
  epileptic 345.3
  hepatic 572.2
  hyperglycemic 250.2
  hyperosmolar (diabetic) (nonketotic) 250.2
  hypoglycemic 251.0
    diabetic 250.3
  insulin 250.3
    hyperosmolar 250.2
    non-diabetic 251.0
    organic hyperinsulinism 251.0
  Kussmaul's (diabetic) 250.3
  liver 572.2
  newborn 779.2
  prediabetic 250.2
  uremic—*see* Uremia
Combat fatigue (*see also* Reaction, stress, acute) 308.9
Combined —*see* condition
Comedo 706.1
Comedocarcinoma (M8501/3)—*see also* Neoplasm, breast, malignant
  noninfiltrating (M8501/2)
    specified site—*see* Neoplasm, by site, in situ
    unspecified site 233.0
Comedomastitis 610.4
Comedones 706.1
  lanugo 757.4
Comma bacillus, carrier (suspected) of V02.3
Comminuted fracture —*see* Fracture, by site
Common
  aortopulmonary trunk 745.0
  atrioventricular canal (defect) 745.69
  atrium 745.69
  cold (head) 460
    vaccination, prophylactic (against) V04.7
  truncus (arteriosus) 745.0
  ventricle 745.3

Commotio (current)
  cerebri (*see also* Concussion, brain) 850.9
    with skull fracture—*see* Fracture, skull, by site
  retinae 921.3
  spinalis—*see* Injury, spinal, by site
Commotion (current)
  brain (without skull fracture) (*see also* Concussion, brain) 850.9
    with skull fracture—*see* Fracture, skull, by site
  spinal cord—*see* Injury, spinal, by site
Communication
  abnormal—*see also* Fistula
    between
      base of aorta and pulmonary artery 745.0
      left ventricle and right atrium 745.4
      pericardial sac and pleural sac 748.8
      pulmonary artery and pulmonary vein 747.3
    congenital, between uterus and anterior abdominal wall 752.3
      bladder 752.3
      intestine 752.3
      rectum 752.3
  left ventricular-right atrial 745.4
  pulmonary artery-pulmonary vein 747.3
Compartment syndrome —*see* Syndrome, compartment
Compensation
  broken—*see* Failure, heart
  failure—*see* Failure, heart
  neurosis, psychoneurosis 300.11
Complaint —*see also* Disease
  bowel, functional 564.9
    psychogenic 306.4
  intestine, functional 564.9
    psychogenic 306.4
  kidney (*see also* Disease, renal) 593.9
  liver 573.9
  miners' 500
Complete —*see* condition
Complex
  cardiorenal (*see also* Hypertension, cardiorenal) 404.90
  castration 300.9
  Costen's 524.60
  ego-dystonic homosexuality 302.0
  Eisenmenger's (ventricular septal defect) 745.4
  homosexual, ego-dystonic 302.0
  hypersexual 302.89
  inferiority 301.9
  jumped process
    spine—*see* Dislocation, vertebra
  primary, tuberculosis (*see also* Tuberculosis) 010.0
  Taussig-Bing (transposition, aorta and overriding pulmonary artery) 745.11
Complications
  abortion NEC—*see* categories 634–639
  accidental puncture or laceration during a procedure 998.2
  amputation stump (late) (surgical) 997.60
    traumatic—*see* Amputation, traumatic
  anastomosis (and bypass)—*see also* Complications, due to (presence of) any device, implant, or graft classified to 996.0–996.5 NEC
    hemorrhage NEC 998.11
    intestinal (internal) NEC 997.4
      involving urinary tract 997.5
    mechanical—*see* Complications, mechanical, graft
    urinary tract (involving intestinal tract) 997.5

Complications — INDEX TO DISEASES

Complications—continued
 anesthesia, anesthetic NEC (see also Anesthesia, complication) 995.22
  in labor and delivery 668.9
   affecting fetus or newborn 763.5
   cardiac 668.1
   central nervous system 668.2
   pulmonary 668.0
   specified type NEC 668.8
 aortocoronary (bypass) graft 996.03
  atherosclerosis —see Arteriosclerosis, coronary
  embolism 996.72
  occlusion NEC 996.72
  thrombus 996.72
 arthroplasty (see also Complications, prosthetic joint) 996.49
 artificial opening
  cecostomy 569.60
  colostomy 569.6
  cystostomy 997.5
  enterostomy 569.60
  esophagostomy 530.87
   infection 530.86
   mechanical 530.87
  gastrostomy 536.40
  ileostomy 569.60
  jejunostomy 569.60
  nephrostomy 997.5
  tracheostomy 519.00
  ureterostomy 997.5
  urethrostomy 997.5
 bariatric surgery 997.4
 bile duct implant (prosthetic) NEC 996.79
  infection or inflammation 996.69
  mechanical 996.59
 bleeding (intraoperative) (postoperative) 998.11
 blood vessel graft 996.1
  aortocoronary 996.03
   atherosclerosis —see Arteriosclerosis, coronary
   embolism 996.72
   occlusion NEC 996.72
   thrombus 996.72
  atherosclerosis —see Arteriosclerosis, extremities
  embolism 996.74
  occlusion NEC 996.74
  thrombus 996.74
 bone growth stimulator NEC 996.78
  infection or inflammation 996.67
 bone marrow transplant 996.85
 breast implant (prosthetic) NEC 996.79
  infection or inflammation 996.69
  mechanical 996.54
 bypass—see also Complications, anastomosis
  aortocoronary 996.03
   atherosclerosis —see Arteriosclerosis, coronary
   embolism 996.72
   occlusion NEC 996.72
   thrombus 996.72
  carotid artery 996.1
   atherosclerosis —see Arteriosclerosis, extremities
   embolism 996.74
   occlusion NEC 996.74
   thrombus 996.74
 cardiac (see also Disease, heart) 429.9
  device, implant, or graft NEC 996.72
   infection or inflammation 996.61

Complications—continued
  long-term effect 429.4
  mechanical (see also Complications, mechanical, by type) 996.00
   valve prosthesis 996.71
   infection or inflammation 996.61
  postoperative NEC 997.1
   long-term effect 429.4
 cardiorenal (see also Hypertension, cardiorenal) 404.90
 carotid artery bypass graft 996.1
  atherosclerosis —see Arteriosclerosis, extremities
  embolism 996.74
  occlusion NEC 996.74
  thrombus 996.74
 cataract fragments in eye 998.82
 catheter device—see also Complications, due to (presence of) any device, implant, or graft classified to 996.0-996.5 NEC
  mechanical—see Complications, mechanical, catheter
 cecostomy 569.60
 cesarean section wound 674.3
 chemotherapy (antineoplastic) 995.29
 chin implant (prosthetic) NEC 996.79
  infection or inflammation 996.69
  mechanical 996.59
 colostomy (enterostomy) 569.60
  specified type NEC 569.69
 contraceptive device, intrauterine NEC 996.76
  infection 996.65
  inflammation 996.65
  mechanical 996.32
 cord (umbilical)—see Complications, umbilical cord
 cornea
  due to
   contact lens 371.82
 coronary (artery) bypass (graft) NEC 996.03
  atherosclerosis —see Arteriosclerosis, coronary
  embolism 996.72
  infection or inflammation 996.61
  mechanical 996.03
  occlusion NEC 996.72
  specified type NEC 996.72
  thrombus 996.72
 cystostomy 997.5
 delivery 669.9
  procedure (instrumental) (manual) (surgical) 669.4
  specified type NEC 669.8
 dialysis (hemodialysis) (peritoneal) (renal) NEC 999.9
  catheter NEC—see also Complications, due to (presence of) any device, implant or graft classified to 996.0-996.5 NEC
   infection or inflammation 996.62
    peritoneal 996.68
   mechanical 996.1
    peritoneal 996.56
 drug NEC 995.29
 due to (presence of) any device, implant, or graft classified to 996.0-996.5 NEC 996.70
  with infection or inflammation—see Complications, infection or inflammation, due to (presence of) any device, implant, or graft classified to 996.0-996.5 NEC
  arterial NEC 996.74
   coronary NEC 996.03
    atherosclerosis —see Arteriosclerosis, coronary

INDEX TO DISEASES

Complications

Complications—*continued*
    embolism 996.72
    occlusion NEC 996.72
    specified type NEC 996.72
    thrombus 996.72
    renal dialysis 996.73
  arteriovenous fistula or shunt NEC 996.74
  bone growth stimulator 996.78
  breast NEC 996.79
  cardiac NEC 996.72
    defibrillator 996.72
    pacemaker 996.72
    valve prosthesis 996.71
  catheter NEC 996.79
    spinal 996.75
    urinary, indwelling 996.76
    vascular NEC 996.74
      renal dialysis 996.73
    ventricular shunt 996.75
  coronary (artery) bypass (graft) NEC 996.03
    atherosclerosis —*see* Arteriosclerosis, coronary
    embolism 996.72
    occlusion NEC 996.72
    thrombus 996.72
  electrodes
    brain 996.75
    heart 996.72
  esophagostomy 530.87
  gastrointestinal NEC 996.79
  genitourinary NEC 996.76
  heart valve prosthesis NEC 996.71
  infusion pump 996.74
  insulin pump 996.57
  internal
    joint prosthesis 996.77
    orthopedic NEC 996.78
    specified type NEC 996.79
  intrauterine contraceptive device NEC 996.76
  joint prosthesis, internal NEC 996.77
  mechanical—*see* Complications, mechanical
  nervous system NEC 996.75
  ocular lens NEC 996.79
  orbital NEC 996.79
  orthopedic NEC 996.78
    joint, internal 996.77
  renal dialysis 996.73
  specified type NEC 996.79
  urinary catheter, indwelling 996.76
  vascular NEC 996.74
  ventricular shunt 996.75
  during dialysis NEC 999.9
  ectopic or molar pregnancy NEC 639.9
  electroshock therapy NEC 999.9
  enterostomy 569.60
    specified type NEC 569.69
  esophagostomy 530.87
    infection 530.86
    mechanical 530.87
  external (fixation) device with internal component(s) NEC 996.78
    infection or inflammation 996.67
    mechanical 996.49
  extracorporeal circulation NEC 999.9
  eye implant (prosthetic) NEC 996.79
    infection or inflammation 996.69
    mechanical
      ocular lens 996.53
      orbital globe 996.59
  gastrointestinal, postoperative NEC (*see also* Complications, surgical procedures) 997.4

Complications—*continued*
  gastrostomy 536.40
    specified type NEC 536.49
  genitourinary device, implant or graft NEC 996.76
    infection or inflammation 996.65
    urinary catheter, indwelling 996.64
    mechanical (*see also* Complications, mechanical, by type) 996.30
      specified NEC 996.39
  graft (bypass) (patch)—*see also* Complications, due to (presence of) any device, implant, or graft classified to 996.0-996.5 NEC
  bone marrow 996.85
  corneal NEC 996.79
    infection or inflammation 996.69
    rejection or reaction 996.51
  mechanical—*see* Complications, mechanical, graft
  organ (immune or nonimmune cause) (partial) (total) 996.80
    bone marrow 996.85
    heart 996.83
    intestines 996.87
    kidney 996.81
    liver 996.82
    lung 996.84
    pancreas 996.86
    specified NEC 996.89
  skin NEC 996.79
    infection or inflammation 996.69
    rejection 996.52
      artificial 996.55
      decellularized allodermis 996.55
  heart—*see also* Disease, heart
  transplant (immune or nonimmune cause) 996.83
  hematoma (intraoperative) (postoperative) 998.12
  hemorrhage (intraoperative) (postoperative) 998.11
  hyperalimentation therapy NEC 999.9
  immunization (procedure)—*see* Complications, vaccination
  implant—*see also* Complications, due to (presence of) any device, implant, or graft classified to 996.0-996.5 NEC
    dental placement, hemorrhagic 525.71
    mechanical—*see* Complications, mechanical, implant
  infection and inflammation
    due to (presence of) any device, implant, or graft classified to 996.0-996.5 NEC 996.60
      arterial NEC 996.62
        coronary 996.61
        renal dialysis 996.62
      arteriovenous fistula or shunt 996.62
      artificial heart 996.61
      bone growth stimulator 996.67
      breast 996.69
      cardiac 996.61
      catheter NEC 996.69
        central venous 999.31
        Hickman 999.31
        peripherally inserted central (PICC) 999.31
        peritoneal 996.68
        spinal 996.63
        triple lumen 999.31
        urinary, indwelling 996.64
        vascular (arterial) (dialysis) (peripheral venous) NEC 996.62
        ventricular shunt 996.63

Complications — INDEX TO DISEASES

Complications—*continued*
- central venous catheter 999.31
- coronary artery bypass 996.61
- electrodes
  - brain 996.63
  - heart 996.61
- gastrointestinal NEC 996.69
- genitourinary NEC 996.65
  - indwelling urinary catheter 996.64
- heart assist device 996.61
- heart valve 996.61
- Hickman catheter 999.31
- infusion pump 996.62
- insulin pump 996.69
- intrauterine contraceptive device 996.65
- joint prosthesis, internal 996.66
- ocular lens 996.69
- orbital (implant) 996.69
- orthopedic NEC 996.67
  - joint, internal 996.66
- peripherally inserted central catheter (PICC) 999.31
- specified type NEC 996.69
- triple lumen catheter 999.31
- urinary catheter, indwelling 996.64
- ventricular shunt 996.63
- infusion (procedure) 999.9
  - blood—*see* Complications, transfusion
  - infection NEC 999.39
  - sepsis NEC 999.39
- inhalation therapy NEC 999.9
- injection (procedure) 999.9
  - drug reaction (*see also* Reaction, drug) 995.27
  - infection NEC 999.39
  - sepsis NEC 999.39
  - serum (prophylactic) (therapeutic)—*see* Complications, vaccination
  - vaccine (any)—*see* Complications, vaccination
- inoculation (any)—*see* Complications, vaccination
- insulin pump 996.57
- internal device (catheter) (electronic) (fixation) (prosthetic) NEC—*see also* Complications, due to (presence of) any device, implant, or graft classified to 996.0-996.5 NEC
  - mechanical—*see* Complications, mechanical
- intestinal transplant (immune or nonimmune cause) 996.87
- intraoperative bleeding or hemorrhage 998.11
- intrauterine contraceptive device (*see also* Complications, contraceptive device) 996.76
  - infection or inflammation 996.65
  - with fetal damage affecting management of pregnancy 655.8
- jejunostomy 569.60
- kidney transplant (immune or nonimmune cause) 996.81
- labor 669.9
  - specified condition NEC 669.8
- liver transplant (immune or nonimmune cause) 996.82
- lumbar puncture 349.0
- mechanical
  - anastomosis—*see* Complications, mechanical, graft
  - artificial heart 996.09
  - bypass—*see* Complications, mechanical, graft
  - catheter NEC 996.59
    - cardiac 996.09
    - cystostomy 996.39
    - dialysis (hemodialysis) 996.1

Complications—*continued*
- peritoneal 996.56
- during a procedure 998.2
- urethral, indwelling 996.31
- colostomy 569.62
- device NEC 996.59
  - balloon (counterpulsation), intra-aortic 996.1
  - cardiac 996.00
    - automatic implantable defibrillator 996.04
    - long-term effect 429.4
    - specified NEC 996.09
  - contraceptive, intrauterine 996.32
  - counterpulsation, intra-aortic 996.1
  - fixation, external, with internal components 996.49
  - fixation, internal (nail, rod, plate) 996.40
  - genitourinary 996.30
    - specified NEC 996.39
  - insulin pump 996.57
  - nervous system 996.2
  - orthopedic, internal 996.40
    - prosthetic joint (*see also* Complications, mechanical device, orthopedic, prosthetic, joint) 996.47
  - prosthetic NEC 996.59
    - joint (*see also* Complications, prosthetic joint) 996.47
      - articular bearing surface wear 996.46
      - aseptic loosening 996.41
      - breakage 996.43
      - dislocation 996.42
      - failure 996.43
      - fracture 996.43
        - around prosthetic 996.44
        - peri-prosthetic 996.44
      - instability 996.42
      - loosening 996.41
      - peri-prosthetic osteolysis 996.45
      - subluxation 996.42
      - wear 996.46
  - umbrella, vena cava 996.1
  - vascular 996.1
- dorsal column stimulator 996.2
- electrode NEC 996.59
  - brain 996.2
  - cardiac 996.01
  - spinal column 996.2
- enterostomy 569.62
- esophagostomy 530.87
- fistula, arteriovenous, surgically created 996.1
- gastrostomy 536.42
- graft NEC 996.52
  - aortic (bifurcation) 996.1
  - aortocoronary bypass 996.03
  - blood vessel NEC 996.1
  - bone 996.49
  - cardiac 996.00
  - carotid artery bypass 996.1
  - cartilage 996.49
  - corneal 996.51
  - coronary bypass 996.03
  - decellularized allodermis 996.55
  - genitourinary 996.30
    - specified NEC 996.39
  - muscle 996.49
  - nervous system 996.2
  - organ (immune or nonimmune cause) 996.80
    - heart 996.83
    - intestines 996.87
    - kidney 996.81
    - liver 996.82

INDEX TO DISEASES — **Complications**

Complications—*continued*
    lung 996.84
    pancreas 996.86
    specified NEC 996.89
  orthopedic, internal 996.49
  peripheral nerve 996.2
  prosthetic NEC 996.59
  skin 996.52
    artificial 996.55
  specified NEC 996.59
  tendon 996.49
  tissue NEC 996.52
  tooth 996.59
  ureter, without mention of resection 996.39
  vascular 996.1
 heart valve prosthesis 996.02
  long-term effect 429.4
 implant NEC 996.59
  cardiac 996.00
    automatic implantable defibrillator 996.04
    long-term effect 429.4
    specified NEC 996.09
  electrode NEC 996.59
    brain 996.2
    cardiac 996.01
    spinal column 996.2
  genitourinary 996.30
  nervous system 996.2
  orthopedic, internal 996.49
  prosthetic NEC 996.59
    in
      bile duct 996.59
      breast 996.54
      chin 996.59
      eye
        ocular lens 996.53
        orbital globe 996.59
    vascular 996.1
 insulin pump 996.57
 nonabsorbable surgical material 996.59
 pacemaker NEC 996.59
  brain 996.2
  cardiac 996.01
  nerve (phrenic) 996.2
 patch—*see* Complications, mechanical, graft
 prosthesis NEC 996.59
  bile duct 996.59
  breast 996.54
  chin 996.59
  ocular lens 996.53
  reconstruction, vas deferens 996.39
 reimplant NEC 996.59
  extremity (*see also* Complications, reattached, extremity) 996.90
  organ (*see also* Complications, transplant, organ, by site) 996.80
 repair—*see* Complications, mechanical, graft
 respirator (ventilator) V46.14
 shunt NEC 996.59
  arteriovenous, surgically created 996.1
  ventricular (communicating) 996.2
 stent NEC 996.59
 tracheostomy 519.02
 vas deferens reconstruction 996.39
 ventilator (respirator) V46.14
medical care NEC 999.9
 cardiac NEC 997.1
 gastrointestinal NEC 997.4
 nervous system NEC 997.00
 peripheral vascular NEC 997.2
 respiratory NEC 997.3

Complications—*continued*
 urinary NEC 997.5
 vascular
  mesenteric artery 997.71
  other vessels 997.79
  peripheral vessels 997.2
  renal artery 997.72
nephrostomy 997.5
nervous system
 device, implant, or graft NEC 349.1
  mechanical 996.2
 postoperative NEC 997.00
obstetric 669.9
 procedure (instrumental) (manual) (surgical) 669.4
 specified NEC 669.8
 surgical wound 674.3
ocular lens implant NEC 996.79
 infection or inflammation 996.69
 mechanical 996.53
organ transplant—*see* Complications, transplant, organ, by site
orthopedic device, implant, or graft
 internal (fixation) (nail) (plate) (rod) NEC 996.78
  infection or inflammation 996.67
 joint prosthesis 996.77
  infection or inflammation 996.66
  mechanical 996.40
pacemaker (cardiac) 996.72
 infection or inflammation 996.61
 mechanical 996.01
pancreas transplant (immune or nonimmune cause) 996.86
perfusion NEC 999.9
perineal repair (obstetrical) 674.3
 disruption 674.2
pessary (uterus) (vagina)—*see* Complications, contraceptive device
phototherapy 990
postcystoscopic 997.5
postmastoidectomy NEC 383.30
postoperative—*see* Complications, surgical procedures
pregnancy NEC 646.9
 affecting fetus or newborn 761.9
prosthetic device, internal—*see also* Complications, due to (presence of) any device, implant, or graft classified to 996.0-996.5 NEC
 mechanical NEC (*see also* Complications, mechanical) 996.59
puerperium NEC (*see also* Puerperal) 674.9
puncture, spinal 349.0
pyelogram 997.5
radiation 990
radiotherapy 990
reattached
 body part, except extremity 996.99
 extremity (infection) (rejection) 996.90
  arm(s) 996.94
  digit(s) (hand) 996.93
    foot 996.95
  finger(s) 996.93
  foot 996.95
  forearm 996.91
  hand 996.92
  leg 996.96
  lower NEC 996.96
  toe(s) 996.95
  upper NEC 996.94

Complications—*continued*
  reimplant—*see also* Complications, due to (presence of) any device, implant, or graft classified to 996.0-996.5 NEC
    bone marrow 996.85
    extremity (*see also* Complications, reattached, extremity) 996.90
      due to infection 996.90
    mechanical—*see* Complications, mechanical, reimplant
    organ (immune or nonimmune cause) (partial) (total) (*see also* Complications, transplant, organ, by site) 996.80
    renal allograft 996.81
  renal dialysis—*see* Complications, dialysis
  respirator (ventilator), mechanical V46.14
  respiratory 519.9
    device, implant or graft NEC 996.79
      infection or inflammation 996.69
      mechanical 996.59
    distress syndrome, adult, following trauma or surgery 518.5
    insufficiency, acute, postoperative 518.5
    postoperative NEC 997.3
    therapy NEC 999.9
  sedation during labor and delivery 668.9
    affecting fetus or newborn 763.5
    cardiac 668.1
    central nervous system 668.2
    pulmonary 668.0
    specified type NEC 668.8
  seroma (intraoperative) (postoperative) (noninfected) 998.13
    infected 998.51
  shunt—*see also* Complications, due to (presence of) any device, implant, or graft classified to 996.0-996.5 NEC
    mechanical—*see* Complications, mechanical, shunt
  specified body system NEC
    device, implant, or graft—*see* Complications, due to (presence of) any device, implant, or graft classified to 996.0-996.5 NEC
    postoperative NEC 997.99
  spinal puncture or tap 349.0
  stoma, external
    gastrointestinal tract
      colostomy 569.60
      enterostomy 569.60
      esophagostomy 530.87
        infection 530.86
        mechanical 530.87
      gastrostomy 536.40
    urinary tract 997.5
  stomach banding 997.4
  stomach stapling 997.4
  surgical procedures 998.9
    accidental puncture or laceration 998.2
    amputation stump (late) 997.60
    anastomosis—*see* Complications, anastomosis
    burst stitches or sutures (external) 998.32
      internal 998.31
    cardiac 997.1
      long-term effect following cardiac surgery 429.4
    cataract fragments in eye 998.82
    catheter device—*see* Complications, catheter device
    cecostomy malfunction 569.62
    colostomy malfunction 569.62
    cystostomy malfunction 997.5

Complications—*continued*
    dehiscence (of incision) (external) 998.32
      internal 998.31
    dialysis NEC (*see also* Complications, dialysis) 999.9
    disruption
      anastomosis (internal)—*see* Complications, mechanical, graft
      internal suture (line) 998.31
      wound (external) 998.32
        internal 998.31
    dumping syndrome (postgastrectomy) 564.2
    elephantiasis or lymphedema 997.99
      postmastectomy 457.0
    emphysema (surgical) 998.81
    enterostomy malfunction 569.62
    esophagostomy malfunction 530.87
    evisceration 998.32
    fistula (persistent postoperative) 998.6
    foreign body inadvertently left in wound (sponge) (suture) (swab) 998.4
    from nonabsorbable surgical material (Dacron) (mesh) (permanent suture) (reinforcing) (Teflon)—*see* Complications, due to (presence of) any device, implant, or graft classified to 996.0-996.5 NEC
    gastrointestinal NEC 997.4
    gastrostomy malfunction 536.42
    hematoma 998.12
    hemorrhage 998.11
    ileostomy malfunction 569.62
    internal prosthetic device NEC (*see also* Complications, internal device) 996.70
      hemolytic anemia 283.19
      infection or inflammation 996.60
      malfunction—*see* Complications, mechanical
      mechanical complication—*see* Complications, mechanical
      thrombus 996.70
    jejunostomy malfunction 569.62
    nervous system NEC 997.00
    obstruction, internal anastomosis—*see* Complications, mechanical, graft
    other body system NEC 997.99
    peripheral vascular NEC 997.2
    postcardiotomy syndrome 429.4
    postcholecystectomy syndrome 576.0
    postcommissurotomy syndrome 429.4
    postgastrectomy dumping syndrome 564.2
    postmastectomy lymphedema syndrome 457.0
    postmastoidectomy 383.30
      cholesteatoma, recurrent 383.32
      cyst, mucosal 383.31
      granulation 383.33
      inflammation, chronic 383.33
    postvagotomy syndrome 564.2
    postvalvulotomy syndrome 429.4
    reattached extremity (infection) (rejection) (*see also* Complications, reattached, extremity) 996.90
    respiratory NEC 997.3
    seroma 998.13
    shock (endotoxic) (hypovolemic) (septic) 998.0
    shunt, prosthetic (thrombus)—*see also* Complications, due to (presence of) any device, implant, or graft classified to 996.0-996.5 NEC
      hemolytic anemia 283.19
    specified complication NEC 998.89

INDEX TO DISEASES — **Compression**

Complications—*continued*
  stitch abscess 998.59
  transplant—*see* Complications, graft
  ureterostomy malfunction 997.5
  urethrostomy malfunction 997.5
  urinary NEC 997.5
  vascular
    mesenteric artery 997.71
    other vessels 997.79
    peripheral vessels 997.2
    renal artery 997.72
  wound infection 998.59
  therapeutic misadventure NEC 999.9
    surgical treatment 998.9
  tracheostomy 519.00
  transfusion (blood) (lymphocytes) (plasma) NEC 999.8
    acute lung injury (TRALI) 518.7
    atrophy, liver, yellow, subacute (within 8 months of administration)—*see* Hepatitis, viral
    bone marrow 996.85
    embolism
      air 999.1
      thrombus 999.2
    hemolysis NEC 999.8
      bone marrow 996.85
    hepatitis (serum) (type B) (within 8 months after administration) *see* Hepatitis, viral
    incompatibility reaction (ABO) (blood group) 999.6
      Rh (factor) 999.7
    infection 999.39
    jaundice (serum) (within 8 months after administration) *see* Hepatitis, viral
    sepsis 999.39
    shock or reaction NEC 999.8
      bone marrow 996.85
    subacute yellow atrophy of liver (within 8 months after administration) *see* Hepatitis, viral
    thromboembolism 999.2
  transplant—*see also* Complications, due to (presence of) any device, implant, or graft classified to 996.0-996.5 NEC
    bone marrow 996.85
    organ (immune or nonimmune cause) (partial) (total) 996.80
      bone marrow 996.85
      heart 996.83
      intestines 996.87
      kidney 996.81
      liver 996.82
      lung 996.84
      pancreas 996.86
      specified NEC 996.89
  trauma NEC (early) 958.8
  ultrasound therapy NEC 999.9
  umbilical cord
    affecting fetus or newborn 762.6
    complicating delivery 663.9
      affecting fetus or newborn 762.6
      specified type NEC 663.8
  urethral catheter NEC 996.76
    infection or inflammation 996.64
    mechanical 996.31
  urinary, postoperative NEC 997.5
  vaccination 999.9
    anaphylaxis NEC 999.4
    cellulitis 999.39
    encephalitis or encephalomyelitis 323.51

Complications—*continued*
    hepatitis (serum) (type B) (within 8 months after administration) *see* Hepatitis, viral
    infection (general) (local) NEC 999.39
    jaundice (serum) (within 8 months after administration) *see* Hepatitis, viral
    meningitis 997.09 *[321.8]*
    myelitis 323.52
    protein sickness 999.5
    reaction (allergic) 999.5
      Herxheimer's 995.0
      serum 999.5
    sepsis 999.39
    serum intoxication, sickness, rash, or other serum reaction NEC 999.5
    shock (allergic) (anaphylactic) 999.4
    subacute yellow atrophy of liver (within 8 months after administration) *see* Hepatitis, viral
    vaccinia (generalized) 999.0
      localized 999.39
  vascular
    device, implant, or graft NEC 996.74
      infection or inflammation 996.62
      mechanical NEC 996.1
        cardiac (*see also* Complications, mechanical, by type) 996.00
    following infusion, perfusion, or transfusion 999.2
    postoperative NEC 997.2
      mesenteric artery 997.71
      other vessels 997.79
      peripheral vessels 997.2
      renal artery 997.72
  ventilation therapy NEC 999.9
  ventilator (respirator), mechanical V46.14
Compound presentation complicating delivery 652.8
  causing obstructed labor 660.0
Compressed air disease 993.3
Compression
  with injury—*see* specific injury
  arm NEC 354.9
  artery 447.1
    celiac, syndrome 447.4
  brachial plexus 353.0
  brain (stem) 348.4
    due to
      contusion, brain—*see* Contusion, brain
      injury NEC—*see also* Hemorrhage, brain, traumatic
      birth—*see* Birth, injury, brain
      laceration, brain—*see* Laceration, brain
    osteopathic 739.0
  bronchus 519.19
  by cicatrix—*see* Cicatrix
  cardiac 423.9
  cauda equina 344.60
    with neurogenic bladder 344.61
  celiac (artery) (axis) 447.4
  cerebral—*see* Compression, brain
  cervical plexus 353.2
  cord (umbilical)—*see* Compression, umbilical cord
  cranial nerve 352.9
    second 377.49
    third (partial) 378.51
      total 378.52
    fourth 378.53
    fifth 350.8
    sixth 378.54
    seventh 351.8

Compression — INDEX TO DISEASES

Compression—*continued*
  divers' squeeze 993.3
  duodenum (external) (*see also* Obstruction, duodenum) 537.3
  during birth 767.9
  esophagus 530.3
    congenital, external 750.3
  Eustachian tube 381.63
  facies (congenital) 754.0
  fracture—*see* Fracture, by site
  heart—*see* Disease, heart
  intestine (*see also* Obstruction, intestine) 560.9
    with hernia—*see* Hernia, by site, with obstruction
  laryngeal nerve, recurrent 478.79
  leg NEC 355.8
  lower extremity NEC 355.8
  lumbosacral plexus 353.1
  lung 518.89
  lymphatic vessel 457.1
  medulla—*see* Compression, brain
  nerve NEC—*see also* Disorder, nerve
    arm NEC 354.9
    autonomic nervous system (*see also* Neuropathy, peripheral, autonomic) 337.9
    axillary 353.0
    cranial NEC 352.9
    due to displacement of intervertebral disc 722.2
      with myelopathy 722.70
      cervical 722.0
        with myelopathy 722.71
      lumbar, lumbosacral 722.10
        with myelopathy 722.73
      thoracic, thoracolumbar 722.11
        with myelopathy 722.72
    iliohypogastric 355.79
    ilioinguinal 355.79
    leg NEC 355.8
    lower extremity NEC 355.8
    median (in carpal tunnel) 354.0
    obturator 355.79
    optic 377.49
    plantar 355.6
    posterior tibial (in tarsal tunnel) 355.5
    root (by scar tissue) NEC 724.9
      cervical NEC 723.4
      lumbar NEC 724.4
      lumbosacral 724.4
      thoracic 724.4
    saphenous 355.79
    sciatic (acute) 355.0
    sympathetic 337.9
    traumatic—*see* Injury, nerve
    ulnar 354.2
    upper extremity NEC 354.9
  peripheral—*see* Compression, nerve
  spinal (cord) (old or nontraumatic) 336.9
    by displacement of intervertebral disc—*see* Displacement, intervertebral disc
    nerve
      root NEC 724.9
        postoperative 722.80
          cervical region 722.81
          lumbar region 722.83
          thoracic region 722.82
        traumatic—*see* Injury, nerve, spinal
      traumatic—*see* Injury, nerve, spinal
    spondylogenic 721.91
      cervical 721.1
      lumbar, lumbosacral 721.42

Compression—*continued*
    thoracic 721.41
    traumatic—*see also* Injury, spinal, by site
      with fracture, vertebra—*see* Fracture, vertebra, by site, with spinal cord injury
    spondylogenic—*see* Compression, spinal cord, spondylogenic
  subcostal nerve (syndrome) 354.8
  sympathetic nerve NEC 337.9
  syndrome 958.5
  thorax 512.8
    iatrogenic 512.1
    postoperative 512.1
  trachea 519.19
    congenital 748.3
  ulnar nerve (by scar tissue) 354.2
  umbilical cord
    affecting fetus or newborn 762.5
      cord prolapsed 762.4
    complicating delivery 663.2
      cord around neck 663.1
      cord prolapsed 663.0
  upper extremity NEC 354.9
  ureter 593.3
  urethra—*see* Stricture, urethra
  vein 459.2
  vena cava (inferior) (superior) 459.2
  vertebral NEC—*see* Compression, spinal (cord)
Compulsion, compulsive
  eating 307.51
  neurosis (obsessive) 300.3
  personality 301.4
  states (mixed) 300.3
  swearing 300.3
    in Gilles de la Tourette's syndrome 307.23
  tics and spasms 307.22
  water drinking NEC (syndrome) 307.9
Concato's disease (pericardial polyserositis) 423.2
  peritoneal 568.82
  pleural—*see* Pleurisy
Concavity, chest wall 738.3
Concealed
  hemorrhage NEC 459.0
  penis 752.65
Concentric fading 368.12
Concern (normal) about sick person in family V61.49
Concrescence (teeth) 520.2
Concretio cordis 423.1
  rheumatic 393
Concretion —*see also* Calculus
  appendicular 543.9
  canaliculus 375.57
  clitoris 624.8
  conjunctiva 372.54
  eyelid 374.56
  intestine (impaction) (obstruction) 560.39
  lacrimal (passages) 375.57
  prepuce (male) 605
    female (clitoris) 624.8
  salivary gland (any) 527.5
  seminal vesicle 608.89
  stomach 537.89
  tonsil 474.8
Concussion (current) 850.9
  with
    loss of consciousness 850.5
      brief (less than one hour)
        30 minutes or less 850.11
        31-59 minutes 850.12

INDEX TO DISEASES

Concussion—*continued*
    moderate (1-24 hours) 850.2
    prolonged (more than 24 hours) (with complete recovery) (with return to pre-existing conscious level) 850.3
    without return to pre-existing conscious level 850.4
    mental confusion or disorientation (without loss of consciousness) 850.0
    with loss of consciousness—*see* Concussion, with, loss of consciousness
  without loss of consciousness 850.0
  blast (air) (hydraulic) (immersion) (underwater) 869.0
    with open wound into cavity 869.1
    abdomen or thorax—*see* Injury, internal, by site
    brain—*see* Concussion, brain
    ear (acoustic nerve trauma) 951.5
      with perforation, tympanic membrane—*see* Wound, open, ear drum
    thorax—*see* Injury, internal, intrathoracic organs NEC
  brain or cerebral (without skull fracture) 850.9
    with
      loss of consciousness 850.5
        brief (less than one hour)
          30 minutes or less 850.11
          31-59 minutes 850.12
        moderate (1-24 hours) 850.2
        prolonged (more than 24 hours) (with complete recovery) (with return to pre-existing conscious level) 850.3
        without return to pre-existing conscious level 850.4
      mental confusion or disorientation (without loss of consciousness) 850.0
        with loss of consciousness—*see* Concussion, brain, with, loss of consciousness
      skull fracture—*see* Fracture, skull, by site
    without loss of consciousness 850.0
  cauda equina 952.4
  cerebral—*see* Concussion, brain
  conus medullaris (spine) 952.4
  hydraulic—*see* Concussion, blast
  internal organs—*see* Injury, internal, by site
  labyrinth—*see* Injury, intracranial
  ocular 921.3
  osseous labyrinth—*see* Injury, intracranial
  spinal (cord)—*see also* Injury, spinal, by site
    due to
      broken
        back—*see* Fracture, vertebra, by site, with spinal cord injury
        neck—*see* Fracture, vertebra, cervical, with spinal cord injury
      fracture, fracture dislocation, or compression fracture of spine or vertebra—*see* Fracture, vertebra, by site, with spinal cord injury
  syndrome 310.2
  underwater blast—*see* Concussion, blast
Condition —*see also* Disease
  psychiatric 298.9
  respiratory NEC 519.9
    acute or subacute NEC 519.9
      due to
        external agent 508.9
          specified type NEC 508.8
        fumes or vapors (chemical) (inhalation) 506.3

Condition—*continued*
        radiation 508.0
    chronic NEC 519.9
      due to
        external agent 508.9
          specified type NEC 508.8
        fumes or vapors (chemical) (inhalation) 506.4
        radiation 508.1
      due to
        external agent 508.9
          specified type NEC 508.8
        fumes or vapors (chemical) (inhalation) 506.9
Conduct disturbance (*see also* Disturbance, conduct) 312.9
  adjustment reaction 309.3
  hyperkinetic 314.2
Condyloma NEC 078.10
  acuminatum 078.11
  gonorrheal 098.0
  latum 091.3
  syphilitic 091.3
    congenital 090.0
  venereal, syphilitic 091.3
Confinement —*see* Delivery
Conflagration —*see also* Burn, by site
  asphyxia (by inhalation of smoke, gases, fumes, or vapors) 987.9
  specified agent—*see* Table of drugs and chemicals
Conflict
  family V61.9
    specified circumstance NEC V61.8
  interpersonal NEC V62.81
  marital V61.10
    involving divorce or estrangement V61.0
  parent-child V61.20
  partner V61.10
Confluent —*see* condition
Confusion, confused (mental) (state) (*see also* State, confusional) 298.9
  acute 293.0
  epileptic 293.0
  postoperative 293.9
  psychogenic 298.2
  reactive (from emotional stress, psychological trauma) 298.2
  subacute 293.1
Confusional arousals 327.41
Congelation 991.9
Congenital —*see also* condition
  aortic septum 747.29
  generalized fibromatosis (CGF) 759.89
  intrinsic factor deficiency 281.0
  malformation—*see* Anomaly
Congestion, congestive
  asphyxia, newborn 768.9
  bladder 596.8
  bowel 569.89
  brain (*see also* Disease, cerebrovascular NEC) 437.8
    malarial 084.9
  breast 611.79
  bronchi 519.19
  bronchial tube 519.19
  catarrhal 472.0
  cerebral—*see* Congestion, brain
  cerebrospinal—*see* Congestion, brain
  chest 786.9
  chill 780.99
    malarial (*see also* Malaria) 084.6

Congestion, congestive—*continued*
circulatory NEC 459.9
conjunctiva 372.71
due to disturbance of circulation 459.9
duodenum 537.3
enteritis—*see* Enteritis
eye 372.71
fibrosis syndrome (pelvic) 625.5
gastroenteritis—*see* Enteritis
general 799.89
glottis 476.0
heart (*see also* Failure, heart) 428.0
hepatic 573.0
hypostatic (lung) 514
intestine 569.89
intracranial—*see* Congestion, brain
kidney 593.89
labyrinth 386.50
larynx 476.0
liver 573.0
lung 786.9
  active or acute (*see also* Pneumonia) 486
    congenital 770.0
  chronic 514
  hypostatic 514
  idiopathic, acute 518.5
  passive 514
malaria, malarial (brain) (fever) (*see also* Malaria) 084.6
medulla—*see* Congestion, brain
nasal 478.19
nose 478.19
orbit, orbital 376.33
  inflammatory (chronic) 376.10
    acute 376.00
ovary 620.8
pancreas 577.8
pelvic, female 625.5
pleural 511.0
prostate (active) 602.1
pulmonary—*see* Congestion, lung
renal 593.89
retina 362.89
seminal vesicle 608.89
spinal cord 336.1
spleen 289.51
  chronic 289.51
stomach 537.89
trachea 464.11
urethra 599.84
uterus 625.5
  with subinvolution 621.1
viscera 799.89
Congestive —*see* Congestion
Conical
  cervix 622.6
  cornea 371.60
  teeth 520.2
Conjoined twins 759.4
  causing disproportion (fetopelvic) 653.7
Conjugal maladjustment V61.10
  involving divorce or estrangement V61.0
Conjunctiva —*see* condition
Conjunctivitis (exposure) (infectious) (nondiphtheritic) (pneumococcal) (pustular) (staphylococcal) (streptococcal) NEC 372.30
  actinic 370.24
  acute 372.00
    atopic 372.05
    contagious 372.03
    follicular 372.02

Conjunctivitis—*continued*
  hemorrhagic (viral) 077.4
  adenoviral (acute) 077.3
  allergic (chronic) 372.14
    with hay fever 372.05
  anaphylactic 372.05
  angular 372.03
  Apollo (viral) 077.4
  atopic 372.05
  blennorrhagic (neonatorum) 098.40
  catarrhal 372.03
  chemical 372.01
    allergic 372.05
    meaning corrosion, *see* Burn, conjunctiva
  chlamydial 077.98
    due to
      Chlamydial trachomatis—*see* Trachoma
    paratrachoma 077.0
  chronic 372.10
    allergic 372.14
    follicular 372.12
    simple 372.11
    specified type NEC 372.14
    vernal 372.13
  diphtheritic 032.81
  due to
    dust 372.05
    enterovirus type 70 077.4
    erythema multiforme 695.1 *[372.33]*
    filariasis (*see also* Filariasis) 125.9 *[372.15]*
    mucocutaneous
      disease NEC 372.33
      leishmaniasis 085.5 *[372.15]*
    Reiter's disease 099.3 *[372.33]*
    syphilis 095.8 *[372.10]*
    toxoplasmosis (acquired) 130.1
      congenital (active) 771.2
    trachoma—*see* Trachoma
  dust 372.05
  eczematous 370.31
  epidemic 077.1
    hemorrhagic 077.4
  follicular (acute) 372.02
    adenoviral (acute) 077.3
  chronic 372.12
  glare 370.24
  gonococcal (neonatorum) 098.40
  granular (trachomatous) 076.1
    late effect 139.1
  hemorrhagic (acute) (epidemic) 077.4
  herpetic (simplex) 054.43
    zoster 053.21
  inclusion 077.0
  infantile 771.6
  influenzal 372.03
  Koch-Weeks 372.03
  light 372.05
  medicamentosa 372.05
  membranous 372.04
  meningococcic 036.89
  Morax-Axenfeld 372.02
  mucopurulent NEC 372.03
  neonatal 771.6
    gonococcal 098.40
  Newcastle's 077.8
  nodosa 360.14
  of Beal 077.3
  parasitic 372.15
    filariasis (*see also* Filariasis) 125.9 *[372.15]*
    mucocutaneous leishmaniasis 085.5 *[372.15]*
  Parinaud's 372.02

INDEX TO DISEASES

Conjunctivitis—*continued*
  petrificans 372.39
  phlyctenular 370.31
  pseudomembranous 372.04
    diphtheritic 032.81
  purulent 372.03
  Reiter's 099.3 *[372.33]*
  rosacea 695.3 *[372.31]*
  serous 372.01
    viral 077.99
  simple chronic 372.11
  specified NEC 372.39
  sunlamp 372.04
  swimming pool 077.0
  trachomatous (follicular) 076.1
    acute 076.0
    late effect 139.1
  traumatic NEC 372.39
  tuberculous (*see also* Tuberculosis) 017.3 *[370.31]*
  tularemic 021.3
  tularensis 021.3
  vernal 372.13
    limbar 372.13 *[370.32]*
  viral 077.99
    acute hemorrhagic 077.4
    specified NEC 077.8
Conjunctivochalasis 372.81
Conjunctoblepharitis —*see* Conjunctivitis
Conn (-Louis) syndrome (primary aldosteronism) 255.12
Connective tissue —*see* condition
Conradi (-Hünermann) syndrome or disease (chondrodysplasia calcificans congenita) 756.59
Consanguinity V19.7
Consecutive —*see* condition
Consolidated lung (base)—*see* Pneumonia, lobar
Constipation 564.00
  atonic 564.09
  drug induced
    correct substance properly administered 564.09
    overdose or wrong substance given or taken 977.9
      specified drug—*see* Table of drugs and chemicals
  neurogenic 564.09
  other specified NEC 564.09
  outlet dysfunction 564.02
  psychogenic 306.4
  simple 564.00
  slow transit 564.01
  spastic 564.09
Constitutional —*see also* condition
  arterial hypotension (*see also* Hypotension) 458.9
  obesity 278.00
    morbid 278.01
  psychopathic state 301.9
  short stature in childhood 783.43
  state, developmental V21.9
    specified development NEC V21.8
  substandard 301.6
Constitutionally substandard 301.6
Constriction
  anomalous, meningeal bands or folds 742.8
  aortic arch (congenital) 747.10
  asphyxiation or suffocation by 994.7
  bronchus 519.19
  canal, ear (*see also* Stricture, ear canal, acquired) 380.50
  duodenum 537.3
  gallbladder (*see also* Obstruction, gallbladder) 575.2
    congenital 751.69

Constriction—*continued*
  intestine (*see also* Obstruction, intestine) 560.9
  larynx 478.74
    congenital 748.3
  meningeal bands or folds, anomalous 742.8
  organ or site, congenital NEC—*see* Atresia
  prepuce (congenital) 605
  pylorus 537.0
    adult hypertrophic 537.0
    congenital or infantile 750.5
    newborn 750.5
  ring (uterus) 661.4
    affecting fetus or newborn 763.7
  spastic—*see also* Spasm
    ureter 593.3
    urethra—*see* Stricture, urethra
  stomach 537.89
  ureter 593.3
  urethra—*see* Stricture, urethra
  visual field (functional) (peripheral) 368.45
Constrictive —*see* condition
Consultation V65.9
  medical—*see also* Counseling, medical
  specified reason NEC V65.8
  without complaint or sickness V65.9
    feared complaint unfounded V65.5
    specified reason NEC V65.8
Consumption —*see* Tuberculosis
Contact
  with
    AIDS virus V01.79
    anthrax V01.81
    cholera V01.0
    communicable disease V01.9
      specified type NEC V01.89
      viral NEC V01.79
    Escherichia coli (E. coli) V01.83
    German measles V01.4
    gonorrhea V01.6
    HIV V01.79
    human immunodeficiency virus V01.79
    meningococcus V01.84
    parasitic disease NEC V01.89
    poliomyelitis V01.2
    rabies V01.5
    rubella V01.4
    SARS-associated coronavirus V01.82
    smallpox V01.3
    syphilis V01.6
    tuberculosis V01.1
    varicella V01.71
    venereal disease V01.6
    viral disease NEC V01.79
  dermatitis—*see* Dermatitis
Contamination, food (*see also* Poisoning, food) 005.9
Contraception, contraceptive
  advice NEC V25.09
    family planning V25.09
    fitting of diaphragm V25.02
    prescribing or use of
      oral contraceptive agent V25.01
      specified agent NEC V25.02
  counseling NEC V25.09
    emergency V25.03
    family planning V25.09
    fitting of diaphragm V25.02
    prescribing or use of
      oral contraceptive agent V25.01
        emergency V25.03
        postcoital V25.03
      specified agent NEC V25.02

Contraception, contraceptive—*continued*
  device (in situ) V45.59
    causing menorrhagia 996.76
    checking V25.42
    complications 996.32
    insertion V25.1
    intrauterine V45.51
    reinsertion V25.42
    removal V25.42
    subdermal V45.52
  fitting of diaphragm V25.02
  insertion
    intrauterine contraceptive device V25.1
    subdermal implantable V25.5
  maintenance V25.40
    examination V25.40
      intrauterine device V25.42
      oral contraceptive V25.41
      specified method NEC V25.49
      subdermal implantable V25.43
    intrauterine device V25.42
    oral contraceptive V25.41
    specified method NEC V25.49
    subdermal implantable V25.43
  management NEC V25.49
  prescription
    oral contraceptive agent V25.01
      emergency V25.03
      postcoital V25.03
      repeat V25.41
    specified agent NEC V25.02
      repeat V25.49
  sterilization V25.2
  surveillance V25.40
    intrauterine device V25.42
    oral contraceptive agent V25.41
    specified method NEC V25.49
    subdermal implantable V25.43
Contraction, contracture, contracted
  Achilles tendon (*see also* Short, tendon, Achilles) 727.81
  anus 564.89
  axilla 729.9
  bile duct (*see also* Disease, biliary) 576.8
  bladder 596.8
    neck or sphincter 596.0
  bowel (*see also* Obstruction, intestine) 560.9
  Braxton Hicks 644.1
  bronchus 519.19
  burn (old)—*see* Cicatrix
  cecum (*see also* Obstruction, intestine) 560.9
  cervix (*see also* Stricture, cervix) 622.4
    congenital 752.49
  cicatricial—*see* Cicatrix
  colon (*see also* Obstruction, intestine) 560.9
  conjunctiva trachomatous, active 076.1
    late effect 139.1
  Dupuytren's 728.6
  eyelid 374.41
  eye socket (after enucleation) 372.64
  face 729.9
  fascia (lata) (postural) 728.89
    Dupuytren's 728.6
    palmar 728.6
    plantar 728.71
  finger NEC 736.29
    congenital 755.59
    joint (*see also* Contraction, joint) 718.44

Contraction—*continued*
  flaccid, paralytic
    joint (*see also* Contraction, joint) 718.4
    muscle 728.85
    ocular 378.50
  gallbladder (*see also* Obstruction, gallbladder) 575.2
  hamstring 728.89
    tendon 727.81
  heart valve—*see* Endocarditis
  Hicks' 644.1
  hip (*see also* Contraction, joint) 718.4
  hourglass
    bladder 596.8
      congenital 753.8
    gallbladder (*see also* Obstruction, gallbladder) 575.2
      congenital 751.69
    stomach 536.8
      congenital 750.7
      psychogenic 306.4
    uterus 661.4
      affecting fetus or newborn 763.7
    hysterical 300.11
  infantile (*see also* Epilepsy) 345.6
  internal os (*see also* Stricture, cervix) 622.4
  intestine (*see also* Obstruction, intestine) 560.9
  joint (abduction) (acquired) (adduction) (flexion) (rotation) 718.40
    ankle 718.47
    congenital NEC 755.8
      generalized or multiple 754.89
        lower limb joints 754.89
      hip (*see also* Subluxation, congenital, hip) 754.32
      lower limb (including pelvic girdle) not involving hip 754.89
      upper limb (including shoulder girdle) 755.59
    elbow 718.42
    foot 718.47
    hand 718.44
    hip 718.45
    hysterical 300.11
    knee 718.46
    multiple sites 718.49
    pelvic region 718.45
    shoulder (region) 718.41
    specified site NEC 718.48
    wrist 718.43
  kidney (granular) (secondary) (*see also* Sclerosis, renal) 587
    congenital 753.3
    hydronephritic 591
    pyelonephritic (*see also* Pyelitis, chronic) 590.00
    tuberculous (*see also* Tuberculosis) 016.0
  ligament 728.89
    congenital 756.89
  liver—*see* Cirrhosis, liver
  muscle (postinfectional) (postural) NEC 728.85
    congenital 756.89
      sternocleidomastoid 754.1
    extraocular 378.60
    eye (extrinsic) (*see also* Strabismus) 378.9
      paralytic (*see also* Strabismus, paralytic) 378.50
    flaccid 728.85
    hysterical 300.11
    ischemic (Volkmann's) 958.6
    paralytic 728.85

INDEX TO DISEASES

Contraction—continued
- posttraumatic 958.6
- psychogenic 306.0
  - specified as conversion reaction 300.11
- myotonic 728.85
- neck (*see also* Torticollis) 723.5
  - congenital 754.1
  - psychogenic 306.0
- ocular muscle (*see also* Strabismus) 378.9
  - paralytic (*see also* Strabismus, paralytic) 378.50
- organ or site, congenital NEC—*see* Atresia
- outlet (pelvis)—*see* Contraction, pelvis
- palmar fascia 728.6
- paralytic
  - joint (*see also* Contraction, joint) 718.4
  - muscle 728.85
  - ocular (*see also* Strabismus, paralytic) 378.50
- pelvis (acquired) (general) 738.6
  - affecting fetus or newborn 763.1
  - complicating delivery 653.1
    - causing obstructed labor 660.1
    - generally contracted 653.1
      - causing obstructed labor 660.1
    - inlet 653.2
      - causing obstructed labor 660.1
    - midpelvic 653.8
      - causing obstructed labor 660.1
    - midplane 653.8
      - causing obstructed labor 660.1
    - outlet 653.3
      - causing obstructed labor 660.1
- plantar fascia 728.71
- premature
  - atrial 427.61
  - auricular 427.61
  - auriculoventricular 427.61
  - heart (junctional) (nodal) 427.60
  - supraventricular 427.61
  - ventricular 427.69
- prostate 602.8
- pylorus (*see also* Pylorospasm) 537.81
- rectosigmoid (*see also* Obstruction, intestine) 560.9
- rectum, rectal (sphincter) 564.89
  - psychogenic 306.4
- ring (Bandl's) 661.4
  - affecting fetus or newborn 763.7
- scar—*see* Cicatrix
- sigmoid (*see also* Obstruction, intestine) 560.9
- socket, eye 372.64
- spine (*see also* Curvature, spine) 737.9
- stomach 536.8
  - hourglass 536.8
    - congenital 750.7
    - psychogenic 306.4
  - psychogenic 306.4
- tendon (sheath) (*see also* Short, tendon) 727.81
- toe 735.8
- ureterovesical orifice (postinfectional) 593.3
- urethra 599.84
- uterus 621.8
  - abnormal 661.9
    - affecting fetus or newborn 763.7
  - clonic, hourglass or tetanic 661.4
    - affecting fetus or newborn 763.7
  - dyscoordinate 661.4
    - affecting fetus or newborn 763.7
  - hourglass 661.4
    - affecting fetus or newborn 763.7
  - hypotonic NEC 661.2
    - affecting fetus or newborn 763.7
  - incoordinate 661.4

Contraction—continued
- affecting fetus or newborn 763.7
- inefficient or poor 661.2
  - affecting fetus or newborn 763.7
- irregular 661.2
  - affecting fetus or newborn 763.7
- tetanic 661.4
  - affecting fetus or newborn 763.7
- vagina (outlet) 623.2
- vesical 596.8
  - neck or urethral orifice 596.0
- visual field, generalized 368.45
- Volkmann's (ischemic) 958.6

Contusion (skin surface intact) 924.9
- with
  - crush injury—*see* Crush
  - dislocation—*see* Dislocation, by site
  - fracture—*see* Fracture, by site
  - internal injury—*see also* Injury, internal, by site
    - heart—*see* Contusion, cardiac
    - kidney—*see* Contusion, kidney
    - liver—*see* Contusion, liver
    - lung—*see* Contusion, lung
    - spleen—*see* Contusion, spleen
  - intracranial injury—*see* Injury, intracranial
  - nerve injury—*see* Injury, nerve
  - open wound—*see* Wound, open, by site
- abdomen, abdominal (muscle) (wall) 922.2
  - organ(s) NEC 868.00
- adnexa, eye NEC 921.9
- ankle 924.21
  - with other parts of foot 924.20
- arm 923.9
  - lower (with elbow) 923.10
  - upper 923.03
    - with shoulder or axillary region 923.09
- auditory canal (external) (meatus) (and other part(s) of neck, scalp, or face, except eye) 920
- auricle, ear (and other part(s) of neck, scalp, or face except eye) 920
- axilla 923.02
  - with shoulder or upper arm 923.09
- back 922.31
- bone NEC 924.9
- brain (cerebral) (membrane) (with hemorrhage) 851.8

Note—Use the following fifth-digit subclassification with categories 851-854:

0 unspecified state of consciousness
1 with no loss of consciousness
2 with brief [less than one hour] loss of consciousness
3 with moderate [1-24 hours] loss of consciousness
4 with prolonged [more than 24 hours] loss of consciousness and return to pre-existing conscious level
5 with prolonged [more than 24 hours] loss of consciousness, without return to pre-existing conscious level
Use fifth-digit 5 to designate when a patient is unconscious and dies before regaining conciousness, regardless of the duration of the loss of conciousness
6 with loss of consciousness of unspecified duration
9 with concussion, unspecified

Contusion—*continued*
  with
    open intracranial wound 851.9
    skull fracture—*see* Fracture, skull, by site
  cerebellum 851.4
    with open intracranial wound 851.5
  cortex 851.0
    with open intracranial wound 851.1
  occipital lobe 851.4
    with open intracranial wound 851.5
  stem 851.4
    with open intracranial wound 851.5
  breast 922.0
  brow (and other part(s) of neck, scalp, or face, except eye) 920
  buttock 922.32
  canthus 921.1
  cardiac 861.01
    with open wound into thorax 861.11
  cauda equina (spine) 952.4
  cerebellum—*see* Contusion, brain, cerebellum
  cerebral—*see* Contusion, brain
  cheek(s) (and other part(s) of neck, scalp, or face, except eye) 920
  chest (wall) 922.1
  chin (and other part(s) of neck, scalp, or face, except eye) 920
  clitoris 922.4
  conjunctiva 921.1
  conus medullaris (spine) 952.4
  cornea 921.3
  corpus cavernosum 922.4
  cortex (brain) (cerebral)—*see* Contusion, brain, cortex
  costal region 922.1
  ear (and other part(s) of neck, scalp, or face except eye) 920
  elbow 923.11
    with forearm 923.10
  epididymis 922.4
  epigastric region 922.2
  eye NEC 921.9
  eyeball 921.3
  eyelid(s) (and periocular area) 921.1
  face (and neck, or scalp any part, except eye) 920
  femoral triangle 922.2
  fetus or newborn 772.6
  finger(s) (nail) (subungual) 923.3
  flank 922.2
  foot (with ankle) (excluding toe(s)) 924.20
  forearm (and elbow) 923.10
  forehead (and other part(s) of neck, scalp, or face, except eye) 920
  genital organs, external 922.4
  globe (eye) 921.3
  groin 922.2
  gum(s) (and other part(s) of neck, scalp, or face, except eye) 920
  hand(s) (except fingers alone) 923.20
  head (any part, except eye) (and face) (and neck) 920
  heart—*see* Contusion, cardiac
  heel 924.20
  hip 924.01
    with thigh 924.00
  iliac region 922.2
  inguinal region 922.2
  internal organs (abdomen, chest, or pelvis) NEC—*see* Injury, internal, by site
  interscapular region 922.33

Contusion—*continued*
  iris (eye) 921.3
  kidney 866.01
    with open wound into cavity 866.11
  knee 924.11
    with lower leg 924.10
  labium (majus) (minus) 922.4
  lacrimal apparatus, gland, or sac 921.1
  larynx (and other part(s) of neck, scalp, or face, except eye) 920
  late effect—*see* Late, effects (of), contusion
  leg 924.5
    lower (with knee) 924.10
  lens 921.3
  lingual (and other part(s) of neck, scalp, or face, except eye) 920
  lip(s) (and other part(s) of neck, scalp, or face, except eye) 920
  liver 864.01
    with
      laceration—*see* Laceration, liver
      open wound into cavity 864.11
  lower extremity 924.5
    multiple sites 924.4
  lumbar region 922.31
  lung 861.21
    with open wound into thorax 861.31
  malar region (and other part(s) of neck, scalp, or face, except eye) 920
  mandibular joint (and other part(s) of neck, scalp, or face, except eye) 920
  mastoid region (and other part(s) of neck, scalp, or face, except eye) 920
  membrane, brain—*see* Contusion, brain
  midthoracic region 922.1
  mouth (and other part(s) of neck, scalp, or face, except eye) 920
  multiple sites (not classifiable to same three-digit category) 924.8
    lower limb 924.4
    trunk 922.8
    upper limb 923.8
  muscle NEC 924.9
  myocardium—*see* Contusion, cardiac
  nasal (septum) (and other part(s) of neck, scalp, or face, except eye) 920
  neck (and scalp, or face any part, except eye) 920
  nerve—*see* Injury, nerve, by site
  nose (and other part(s) of neck, scalp, or face, except eye) 920
  occipital region (scalp) (and neck or face, except eye) 920
    lobe—*see* Contusion, brain, occipital lobe
  orbit (region) (tissues) 921.2
  palate (soft) (and other part(s) of neck, scalp, or face, except eye) 920
  parietal region (scalp) (and neck, or face, except eye) 920
    lobe—*see* Contusion, brain
  penis 922.4
  pericardium—*see* Contusion, cardiac
  perineum 922.4
  periocular area 921.1
  pharynx (and other part(s) of neck, scalp, or face, except eye) 920
  popliteal space (*see also* Contusion, knee) 924.11
  prepuce 922.4
  pubic region 922.4
  pudenda 922.4

INDEX TO DISEASES

Contusion—*continued*
  pulmonary—*see* Contusion, lung
  quadriceps femoralis 924.00
  rib cage 922.1
  sacral region 922.32
  salivary ducts or glands (and other part(s) of neck, scalp, or face, except eye) 920
  scalp (and neck, or face any part, except eye) 920
  scapular region 923.01
    with shoulder or upper arm 923.09
  sclera (eye) 921.3
  scrotum 922.4
  shoulder 923.00
    with upper arm or axillar regions 923.09
  skin NEC 924.9
  skull 920
  spermatic cord 922.4
  spinal cord—*see also* Injury, spinal, by site
    cauda equina 952.4
    conus medullaris 952.4
  spleen 865.01
    with open wound into cavity 865.11
  sternal region 922.1
  stomach—*see* Injury, internal, stomach
  subconjunctival 921.1
  subcutaneous NEC 924.9
  submaxillary region (and other part(s) of neck, scalp, or face, except eye) 920
  submental region (and other part(s) of neck, scalp, or face, except eye) 920
  subperiosteal NEC 924.9
  supraclavicular fossa (and other part(s) of neck, scalp, or face, except eye) 920
  supraorbital (and other part(s) of neck, scalp, or face, except eye) 920
  temple (region) (and other part(s) of neck, scalp, or face, except eye) 920
  testis 922.4
  thigh (and hip) 924.00
  thorax 922.1
    organ—*see* Injury, internal, intrathoracic
  throat (and other part(s) of neck, scalp, or face, except eye) 920
  thumb(s) (nail) (subungual) 923.3
  toe(s) (nail) (subungual) 924.3
  tongue (and other part(s) of neck, scalp, or face, except eye) 920
  trunk 922.9
    multiple sites 922.8
    specified site—*see* Contusion, by site
  tunica vaginalis 922.4
  tympanum (membrane) (and other part(s) of neck, scalp, or face, except eye) 920
  upper extremity 923.9
    multiple sites 923.8
  uvula (and other part(s) of neck, scalp, or face, except eye) 920
  vagina 922.4
  vocal cord(s) (and other part(s) of neck, scalp, or face, except eye) 920
  vulva 922.4
  wrist 923.21
    with hand(s), except finger(s) alone 923.20
Conus (any type) (congenital) 743.57
  acquired 371.60
  medullaris syndrome 336.8

Convalescence (following) V66.9
  chemotherapy V66.2
  medical NEC V66.5
  psychotherapy V66.3
  radiotherapy V66.1
  surgery NEC V66.0
  treatment (for) NEC V66.5
    combined V66.6
    fracture V66.4
    mental disorder NEC V66.3
    specified disorder NEC V66.5
Conversion
  closed surgical procedure to open procedure
    arthroscopic V64.43
    laparoscopic V64.41
    thoracoscopic V64.42
  hysteria, hysterical, any type 300.11
  neurosis, any 300.11
  reaction, any 300.11
Converter, tuberculosis (test reaction) 795.5
Convulsions (idiopathic) 780.39
  apoplectiform (*see also* Disease, cerebrovascular, acute) 436
  brain 780.39
  cerebral 780.39
  cerebrospinal 780.39
  due to trauma NEC—*see* Injury, intracranial
  eclamptic (*see also* Eclampsia) 780.39
  epileptic (*see also* Epilepsy) 345.9
  epileptiform (*see also* Seizure, epileptiform) 780.39
  epileptoid (*see also* Seizure, epileptiform) 780.39
  ether
    anesthetic
      correct substance properly administered 780.39
      overdose or wrong substance given 968.2
    other specified type—*see* Table of drugs and chemicals
  febrile (simple) 780.31
    complex 780.32
  generalized 780.39
  hysterical 300.11
  infantile 780.39
    epilepsy—*see* Epilepsy
  internal 780.39
  jacksonian (*see also* Epilepsy) 345.5
  myoclonic 333.2
  newborn 779.0
  paretic 094.1
  pregnancy (nephritic) (uremic)—*see* Eclampsia, pregnancy
  psychomotor (*see also* Epilepsy) 345.4
  puerperal, postpartum—*see* Eclampsia, pregnancy
  recurrent 780.39
    epileptic—*see* Epilepsy
  reflex 781.0
  repetitive 780.39
    epileptic—*see* Epilepsy
    salaam (*see also* Epilepsy) 345.6
  scarlatinal 034.1
  spasmodic 780.39
  tetanus, tetanic (*see also* Tetanus) 037
  thymic 254.8
  uncinate 780.39
  uremic 586
Convulsive —*see also* Convulsions
  disorder or state 780.39
    epileptic—*see* Epilepsy
  equivalent, abdominal (*see also* Epilepsy) 345.5

Cooke-Apert-Gallais syndrome (adrenogenital) 255.2
Cooley's anemia (erythroblastic) 282.49
Coolie itch 126.9
Cooper's
 disease 610.1
 hernia—*see* Hernia, Cooper's
Coordination disturbance 781.3
Copper wire arteries, retina 362.13
Copra itch 133.8
Coprolith 560.39
Coprophilia 302.89
Coproporphyria, hereditary 277.1
Coprostasis 560.39
 with hernia—*see also* Hernia, by site, with obstruction
 gangrenous—*see* Hernia, by site, with gangrene
Cor
 biloculare 745.7
 bovinum—*see* Hypertrophy, cardiac
 bovis—*see also* Hypertrophy, cardiac
 pulmonale (chronic) 416.9
  acute 415.0
 triatriatum, triatrium 746.82
 triloculare 745.8
  biatriatum 745.3
  biventriculare 745.69
Corbus' disease 607.1
Cord —*see also* condition
 around neck (tightly) (with compression)
  affecting fetus or newborn 762.5
  complicating delivery 663.1
   without compression 663.3
    affecting fetus or newborn 762.6
 bladder NEC 344.61
  tabetic 094.0
 prolapse
  affecting fetus or newborn 762.4
  complicating delivery 663.0
Cord's angiopathy (*see also* Tuberculosis) 017.3 *[362.18]*
Cordis ectopia 746.87
Corditis (spermatic) 608.4
Corectopia 743.46
Cori type glycogen storage disease —*see* Disease, glycogen storage
Cork-handlers' disease or lung 495.3
Corkscrew esophagus 530.5
Corlett's pyosis (impetigo) 684
Corn (infected) 700
Cornea—*see also* **condition**
 donor V59.5
 guttata (dystrophy) 371.57
 plana 743.41
Cornelia de Lange's syndrome (Amsterdam dwarf, mental retardation, and brachycephaly) 759.89
Cornual gestation or pregnancy —*see* Pregnancy, cornual
Cornu cutaneum 702.8
Coronary (artery)—*see also* condition
 arising from aorta or pulmonary trunk 746.85
Corpora —*see also* condition
 amylacea (prostate) 602.8
 cavernosa—*see* condition
Corpulence (*see also* Obesity) 278.0
Corpus —*see* condition
Corrigan's disease —*see* Insufficiency, aortic
Corrosive burn —*see* Burn, by site
Corsican fever (*see also* Malaria) 084.6

Cortical —*see also* condition
 blindness 377.75
 necrosis, kidney (bilateral) 583.6
Corticoadrenal —*see* condition
Corticosexual syndrome 255.2
Coryza (acute) 460
 with grippe or influenza 487.1
 syphilitic 095.8
  congenital (chronic) 090.0
Costen's syndrome or complex 524.60
Costiveness (*see also* Constipation) 564.00
Costochondritis 733.6
Cotard's syndrome (paranoia) 297.1
Cot death 798.0
Cotungo's disease 724.3
Cough 786.2
 with hemorrhage (*see also* Hemoptysis) 786.3
 affected 786.2
 bronchial 786.2
  with grippe or influenza 487.1
 chronic 786.2
 epidemic 786.2
 functional 306.1
 hemorrhagic 786.3
 hysterical 300.11
 laryngeal, spasmodic 786.2
 nervous 786.2
 psychogenic 306.1
 smokers' 491.0
 tea tasters' 112.89
Counseling NEC V65.40
 without complaint or sickness V65.49
 abuse victim NEC V62.89
  child V61.21
  partner V61.11
  spouse V61.11
 child abuse, maltreatment, or neglect V61.21
 contraceptive NEC V25.09
  device (intrauterine) V25.02
  maintenance V25.40
   intrauterine contraceptive device V25.42
   oral contraceptive (pill) V25.41
   specified type NEC V25.49
   subdermal implantable V25.43
  management NEC V25.9
  oral contraceptive (pill) V25.01
   emergency V25.03
   postcoital V25.03
  prescription NEC V25.02
   oral contraceptive (pill) V25.01
    emergency V25.03
    postcoital V25.03
   repeat prescription V25.41
  repeat prescription V25.40
  subdermal implantable V25.43
  surveillance V25.40
 dietary V65.3
 exercise V65.41
 expectant mother, pediatric pre-birth visit V65.11
 explanation of
  investigation finding NEC V65.49
  medication NEC V65.49
 family planning V25.09
  natural
   procreative V26.41
   to avoid pregnancy V25.04
 for nonattending third party V65.19
 genetic V26.33
 gonorrhea V65.45

INDEX TO DISEASES — Cranium

Counseling—*continued*
  health (advice) (education) (instruction) NEC V65.49
  HIV V65.44
  human immunodeficiency virus V65.44
  injury prevention V65.43
  insulin pump training V65.46
  marital V61.10
  medical (for) V65.9
    boarding school resident V60.6
    condition not demonstrated V65.5
    feared complaint and no disease found V65.5
    institutional resident V60.6
    on behalf of another V65.19
    person living alone V60.3
  natural family planning
    procreative V26.41
    to avoid pregnancy V25.04
  parent-child conflict V61.20
    specified problem NEC V61.29
  partner abuse
    perpetrator V61.12
    victim V61.11
  pediatric pre-birth visit for expectant mother V65.11
  perpetrator of
    child abuse V62.83
      parental V61.22
    partner abuse V61.12
    spouse abuse V61.12
  procreative V65.49
  sex NEC V65.49
    transmitted disease NEC V65.45
      HIV V65.44
  specified reason NEC V65.49
  spousal abuse
    perpetrator V61.12
    victim V61.11
  substance use and abuse V65.42
  syphilis V65.45
  victim (of)
    abuse NEC V62.89
    child abuse V61.21
    partner abuse V61.11
    spousal abuse V61.11
Coupled rhythm 427.89
Couvelaire uterus (complicating delivery)—*see* Placenta, separation
Cowper's gland —*see* condition
Cowperitis (*see also* Urethritis) 597.89
  gonorrheal (acute) 098.0
    chronic or duration of 2 months or over 098.2
Cowpox (abortive) 051.0
  due to vaccination 999.0
  eyelid 051.0 *[373.5]*
    postvaccination 999.0 *[373.5]*
Coxa
  plana 732.1
  valga (acquired) 736.31
    congenital 755.61
    late effect of rickets 268.1
  vara (acquired) 736.32
    congenital 755.62
    late effect of rickets 268.1
Coxae malum senilis 715.25
Coxalgia (nontuberculous) 719.45
  tuberculous (*see also* Tuberculosis) 015.1 *[730.85]*
Coxalgic pelvis 736.30
Coxitis 716.65

Coxsackie (infection) (virus) 079.2
  central nervous system NEC 048
  endocarditis 074.22
  enteritis 008.67
  meningitis (aseptic) 047.0
  myocarditis 074.23
  pericarditis 074.21
  pharyngitis 074.0
  pleurodynia 074.1
  specific disease NEC 074.8
Crabs, meaning pubic lice 132.2
Crack baby 760.75
Cracked
  nipple 611.2
    puerperal, postpartum 676.1
  puerperal, postpartum 676.1
  tooth 521.81
Cradle cap 690.11
Craft neurosis 300.89
Craigiasis 007.8
Cramp(s) 729.82
  abdominal 789.0
  bathing 994.1
  colic 789.0
    psychogenic 306.4
  due to immersion 994.1
  extremity (lower) (upper) NEC 729.82
  fireman 992.2
  heat 992.2
  hysterical 300.11
  immersion 994.1
  intestinal 789.0
    psychogenic 306.4
  linotypist's 300.89
    organic 333.84
  muscle (extremity) (general) 729.82
    due to immersion 994.1
    hysterical 300.11
  occupational (hand) 300.89
    organic 333.84
  psychogenic 307.89
  salt depletion 276.1
  sleep related leg 327.52
  stoker 992.2
  stomach 789.0
  telegraphers' 300.89
    organic 333.84
  typists' 300.89
    organic 333.84
  uterus 625.8
    menstrual 625.3
  writers' 333.84
    organic 333.84
    psychogenic 300.89
Cranial —*see* condition
Cranioclasis, fetal 763.89
Craniocleidodysostosis 755.59
Craniofenestria (skull) 756.0
Craniolacunia (skull) 756.0
Craniopagus 759.4
Craniopathy, metabolic 733.3
Craniopharyngeal —*see* condition
Craniopharyngioma (M9350/1) 237.0
Craniorachischisis (totalis) 740.1
Cranioschisis 756.0
Craniostenosis 756.0
Craniosynostosis 756.0
Craniotabes (cause unknown) 733.3
  rachitic 268.1
  syphilitic 090.5
Craniotomy, fetal 763.89
Cranium —*see* condition

Craw-craw

Craw-craw 125.3
CRBSI (catheter-related bloodstream infection) 999.31
Creaking joint 719.60
  ankle 719.67
  elbow 719.62
  foot 719.67
  hand 719.64
  hip 719.65
  knee 719.66
  multiple sites 719.69
  pelvic region 719.65
  shoulder (region) 719.61
  specified site NEC 719.68
  wrist 719.63
Creeping
  eruption 126.9
  palsy 335.21
  paralysis 335.21
Crenated tongue 529.8
Creotoxism 005.9
Crepitus
  caput 756.0
  joint 719.60
    ankle 719.67
    elbow 719.62
    foot 719.67
    hand 719.64
    hip 719.65
    knee 719.66
    multiple sites 719.69
    pelvic region 719.65
    shoulder (region) 719.61
    specified site NEC 719.68
    wrist 719.63
Crescent or conus choroid, congenital 743.57
Cretin, cretinism (athyrotic) (congenital) (endemic) (metabolic) (nongoitrous) (sporadic) 243
  goitrous (sporadic) 246.1
  pelvis (dwarf type) (male type) 243
    with disproportion (fetopelvic) 653.1
      affecting fetus or newborn 763.1
      causing obstructed labor 660.1
        affecting fetus or newborn 763.1
  pituitary 253.3
Cretinoid degeneration 243
Creutzfeldt-Jakob disease (syndrome) (new variant) 046.1
  with dementia
    with behavioral disturbance 046.1 *[294.11]*
    without behavioral disturbance 046.1 *[294.10]*
Crib death 798.0
Cribriform hymen 752.49
Cri-du-chat syndrome 758.31
Crigler-Najjar disease or syndrome (congenital hyperbilirubinemia) 277.4
Crimean hemorrhagic fever 065.0
Criminalism 301.7
Crisis
  abdomen 789.0
  addisonian (acute adrenocortical insufficiency) 255.41
  adrenal (cortical) 255.41
  asthmatic—*see* Asthma
  brain, cerebral (*see also* Disease, cerebrovascular, acute) 436
  celiac 579.0
  Dietl's 593.4

INDEX TO DISEASES

Crisis—*continued*
  emotional NEC 309.29
    acute reaction to stress 308.0
    adjustment reaction 309.9
    specific to childhood or adolescence 313.9
  gastric (tabetic) 094.0
  glaucomatocyclitic 364.22
  heart (*see also* Failure, heart) 428.9
  hypertensive—*see* Hypertension
  nitritoid
    correct substance properly administered 458.29
    overdose or wrong substance given or taken 961.1
  oculogyric 378.87
    psychogenic 306.7
  Pel's 094.0
  psychosexual identity 302.6
  rectum 094.0
  renal 593.81
  sickle cell 282.62
  stomach (tabetic) 094.0
  tabetic 094.0
  thyroid (*see also* Thyrotoxicosis) 242.9
  thyrotoxic (*see also* Thyrotoxicosis) 242.9
  vascular—*see* Disease, cerebrovascular, acute
Crocq's disease (acrocyanosis) 443.89
Crohn's disease (*see also* Enteritis, regional) 555.9
Cronkhite-Canada syndrome 211.3
Crooked septum, nasal 470
Cross
  birth (of fetus) complicating delivery 652.3
    with successful version 652.1
    causing obstructed labor 660.0
  bite, anterior or posterior 524.27
  eye (*see also* Esotropia) 378.00
Crossed ectopia of kidney 753.3
Crossfoot 754.50
Croup, croupus (acute) (angina) (catarrhal) (infective) (inflammatory) (laryngeal) (membranous) (nondiphtheritic) (pseudomembranous) 464.4
  asthmatic (*see also* Asthma) 493.9
  bronchial 466.0
  diphtheritic (membranous) 032.3
  false 478.75
  spasmodic 478.75
    diphtheritic 032.3
  stridulous 478.75
    diphtheritic 032.3
Crouzon's disease (craniofacial dysostosis) 756.0
Crowding, teeth 524.31
CRST syndrome (cutaneous systemic sclerosis) 710.1
Cruchet's disease (encephalitis lethargica) 049.8
Cruelty in children (*see also* Disturbance, conduct) 312.9
Crural ulcer (*see also* Ulcer, lower extremity) 707.10
Crush, crushed, crushing (injury) 929.9
  abdomen 926.19
    internal—*see* Injury, internal, abdomen
  ankle 928.21
    with other parts of foot 928.20
  arm 927.9
    lower (and elbow) 927.10
    upper 927.03
      with shoulder or axillary region 927.09

INDEX TO DISEASES   **Curvature**

Crush, crushed, crushing—*continued*
  axilla 927.02
    with shoulder or upper arm 927.09
  back 926.11
  breast 926.19
  buttock 926.12
  cheek 925.1
  chest—*see* Injury, internal, chest
  ear 925.1
  elbow 927.11
    with forearm 927.10
  face 925.1
  finger(s) 927.3
    with hand(s) 927.20
      and wrist(s) 927.21
  flank 926.19
  foot, excluding toe(s) alone (with ankle) 928.20
  forearm (and elbow) 927.10
  genitalia, external (female) (male) 926.0
    internal—*see* Injury, internal, genital organ NEC
  hand, except finger(s) alone (and wrist) 927.20
  head—*see* Fracture, skull, by site
  heel 928.20
  hip 928.01
    with thigh 928.00
  internal organ (abdomen, chest, or pelvis)—*see* Injury, internal, by site
  knee 928.11
    with leg, lower 928.10
  labium (majus) (minus) 926.0
  larynx 925.2
  late effect—*see* Late, effects (of), crushing
  leg 928.9
    lower 928.10
      and knee 928.11
    upper 928.00
  limb
    lower 928.9
      multiple sites 928.8
    upper 927.9
      multiple sites 927.8
  multiple sites NEC 929.0
  neck 925.2
  nerve—*see* Injury, nerve, by site
  nose 802.0
    open 802.1
  penis 926.0
  pharynx 925.2
  scalp 925.2
  scapular region 927.01
    with shoulder or upper arm 927.09
  scrotum 926.0
  shoulder 927.00
    with upper arm or axillary region 927.09
  skull or cranium—*see* Fracture, skull, by site
  spinal cord—*see* Injury, spinal, by site
  syndrome (complication of trauma) 958.5
  testis 926.0
  thigh (with hip) 928.00
  throat 925.2
  thumb(s) (and fingers) 927.3
  toe(s) 928.3
    with foot 928.20
      and ankle 928.21
  tonsil 925.2
  trunk 926.9
    chest—*see* Injury, internal, intrathoracic organs NEC
    internal organ—*see* Injury, internal, by site
    multiple sites 926.8
    specified site NEC 926.19

Crush, crushed, crushing—*continued*
  vulva 926.0
  wrist 927.21
    with hand(s), except fingers alone 927.20
Crusta lactea 690.11
Crusts 782.8
Crutch paralysis 953.4
Cruveilhier's disease 335.21
Cruveilhier-Baumgarten cirrhosis, disease, or syndrome 571.5
Cruz-Chagas disease (*see also* Trypanosomiasis) 086.2
Crying
  constant, continuous
    adolescent 780.95
    adult 780.95
    baby 780.92
    child 780.95
    infant 780.92
    newborn 780.92
  excessive
    adolescent 780.95
    adult 780.95
    baby 780.92
    child 780.95
    infant 780.92
    newborn 780.92
Cryoglobulinemia (mixed) 273.2
Crypt (anal) (rectal) 569.49
Cryptitis (anal) (rectal) 569.49
Cryptococcosis (European) (pulmonary) (systemic) 117.5
Cryptococcus 117.5
  epidermicus 117.5
  neoformans, infection by 117.5
Cryptopapillitis (anus) 569.49
Cryptophthalmos (eyelid) 743.06
Cryptorchid, cryptorchism, cryptorchidism 752.51
Cryptosporidiosis 007.4
Cryptotia 744.29
Crystallopathy
  calcium pyrophosphate (*see also* Arthritis) 275.49 *[712.2]*
  dicalcium phosphate (*see also* Arthritis) 275.49 *[712.1]*
  gouty 274.0
  pyrophosphate NEC (*see also* Arthritis) 275.49 *[712.2]*
  uric acid 274.0
Crystalluria 791.9
Csillag's disease (lichen sclerosus et atrophicus) 701.0
Cuban itch 050.1
Cubitus
  valgus (acquired) 736.01
    congenital 755.59
    late effect of rickets 268.1
  varus (acquired) 736.02
    congenital 755.59
    late effect of rickets 268.1
Cultural deprivation V62.4
Cupping of optic disc 377.14
Curling's ulcer —*see* Ulcer, duodenum
Curling esophagus 530.5
Curschmann (-Batten) (-Steinert) disease or syndrome 359.21
Curvature
  organ or site, congenital NEC—*see* Distortion
  penis (lateral) 752.69

Curvature—*continued*
  Pott's (spinal) (*see also* Tuberculosis) 015.0
    [737.43]
  radius, idiopathic, progressive (congenital)
    755.54
  spine (acquired) (angular) (idiopathic)
    (incorrect) (postural) 737.9
    congenital 754.2
    due to or associated with
      Charcot-Marie-Tooth disease 356.1 *[737.40]*
      mucopolysaccharidosis 277.5 *[737.40]*
      neurofibromatosis 237.71 *[737.40]*
      osteitis
        deformans 731.0 *[737.40]*
        fibrosa cystica 252.01 *[737.40]*
      osteoporosis (*see also* Osteoporosis) 733.00
        [737.40]
      poliomyelitis (*see also* Poliomyelitis) 138
        [737.40]
      tuberculosis (Pott's curvature) (*see also*
        Tuberculosis) 015.0 *[737.43]*
    kyphoscoliotic (*see also* Kyphoscoliosis)
      737.30
    kyphotic (*see also* Kyphosis) 737.10
    late effect of rickets 268.1 *[737.40]*
    Pott's 015.0 *[737.40]*
    scoliotic (*see also* Scoliosis) 737.30
    specified NEC 737.8
    tuberculous 015.0 *[737.40]*
Cushing's
  basophilism, disease, or syndrome (iatrogenic)
    (idiopathic) (pituitary basophilism) (pituitary
    dependent) 255.0
  ulcer—*see* Ulcer, peptic
Cushingoid due to steroid therapy
  correct substance properly administered 255.0
  overdose or wrong substance given or taken
    962.0
Cut (external)—*see* Wound, open, by site
Cutaneous —*see also* condition
  hemorrhage 782.7
  horn (cheek) (eyelid) (mouth) 702.8
  larva migrans 126.9
Cutis —*see also* condition
  hyperelastic 756.83
    acquired 701.8
  laxa 756.83
    senilis 701.8
  marmorata 782.61
  osteosis 709.3
  pendula 756.83
    acquired 701.8
  rhomboidalis nuchae 701.8
  verticis gyrata 757.39
    acquired 701.8
Cyanopathy, newborn 770.83
Cyanosis 782.5
  autotoxic 289.7
  common atrioventricular canal 745.69
  congenital 770.83
  conjunctiva 372.71
  due to
    endocardial cushion defect 745.60
    nonclosure, foramen botalli 745.5
    patent foramen botalli 745.5
    persistent foramen ovale 745.5
  enterogenous 289.7
  fetus or newborn 770.83
  ostium primum defect 745.61
  paroxysmal digital 443.0
  retina, retinal 362.10

Cycle
  anovulatory 628.0
  menstrual, irregular 626.4
Cyclencephaly 759.89
Cyclical vomiting 536.2
  psychogenic 306.4
Cyclitic membrane 364.74
Cyclitis (*see also* Iridocyclitis) 364.3
  acute 364.00
    primary 364.01
    recurrent 364.02
  chronic 364.10
    in
      sarcoidosis 135 *[364.11]*
      tuberculosis (*see also* Tuberculosis) 017.3
        [364.11]
  Fuchs' heterochromic 364.21
  granulomatous 364.10
  lens induced 364.23
  nongranulomatous 364.00
  posterior 363.21
  primary 364.01
  recurrent 364.02
  secondary (noninfectious) 364.04
    infectious 364.03
  subacute 364.00
    primary 364.01
    recurrent 364.02
Cyclokeratitis —*see* Keratitis
Cyclophoria 378.44
Cyclopia, cyclops 759.89
Cycloplegia 367.51
Cyclospasm 367.53
Cyclosporiasis 007.5
Cyclothymia 301.13
Cyclothymic personality 301.13
Cyclotropia 378.33
Cyesis —*see* Pregnancy
Cylindroma (M8200/3)—*see also* Neoplasm, by
  site, malignant
  eccrine dermal (M8200/0)—*see* Neoplasm, skin, benign
  skin (M8200/0)—*see* Neoplasm, skin, benign
Cylindruria 791.7
Cyllosoma 759.89
Cynanche
  diphtheritic 032.3
  tonsillaris 475
Cynorexia 783.6
Cyphosis —*see* Kyphosis
Cyprus fever (*see also* Brucellosis) 023.9
Cyriax's syndrome (slipping rib) 733.99
Cyst (mucus) (retention) (serous) (simple)

> *Note*—In general, cysts are not neoplastic and
> are classified to the appropriate category for
> disease of the specified anatomical site. This
> generalization does not apply to certain types of
> cysts which are neoplastic in nature, for
> example, dermoid, nor does it apply to cysts of
> certain structures, for example, branchial cleft,
> which are classified as developmental
> anomalies. The following listing includes some
> of the most frequently reported sites of cysts as
> well as qualifiers which indicate the type of cyst.
> The latter qualifiers usually are not repeated
> under the anatomical sites. Since the code
> assignment for a given site may vary depending
> upon the type of cyst, the coder should refer to
> the listings under the specified type of cyst
> before consideration is given to the site.

INDEX TO DISEASES   Cyst

Cyst —*continued*
   accessory, fallopian tube 752.11
   adenoid (infected) 474.8
   adrenal gland 255.8
      congenital 759.1
   air, lung 518.89
   allantoic 753.7
   alveolar process (jaw bone) 526.2
   amnion, amniotic 658.8
   anterior chamber (eye) 364.60
      exudative 364.62
      implantation (surgical) (traumatic) 364.61
      parasitic 360.13
   anterior nasopalatine 526.1
   antrum 478.19
   anus 569.49
   apical (periodontal) (tooth) 522.8
   appendix 543.9
   arachnoid, brain 348.0
   arytenoid 478.79
   auricle 706.2
   Baker's (knee) 727.51
      tuberculous (*see also* Tuberculosis) 015.2
   Bartholin's gland or duct 616.2
   bile duct (*see also* Disease, biliary) 576.8
   bladder (multiple) (trigone) 596.8
   Blessig's 362.62
   blood, endocardial (*see also* Endocarditis) 424.90
   blue dome 610.0
   bone (local) 733.20
      aneurysmal 733.22
      jaw 526.2
         developmental (odontogenic) 526.0
         fissural 526.1
         latent 526.89
      solitary 733.21
      unicameral 733.21
   brain 348.0
      congenital 742.4
      hydatid (*see also* Echinococcus) 122.9
      third ventricle (colloid) 742.4
   branchial (cleft) 744.42
   branchiogenic 744.42
   breast (benign) (blue dome) (pedunculated) (solitary) (traumatic) 610.0
      involution 610.4
      sebaceous 610.8
   broad ligament (benign) 620.8
      embryonic 752.11
   bronchogenic (mediastinal) (sequestration) 518.89
      congenital 748.4
   buccal 528.4
   bulbourethral gland (Cowper's) 599.89
   bursa, bursal 727.49
      pharyngeal 478.26
   calcifying odontogenic (M9301/0) 213.1
      upper jaw (bone) 213.0
   canal of Nuck (acquired) (serous) 629.1
      congenital 752.41
   canthus 372.75
   carcinomatous (M8010/3)—*see* Neoplasm, by site, malignant
   cartilage (joint)—*see* Derangement, joint
   cauda equina 336.8
   cavum septi pellucidi NEC 348.0
   celomic (pericardium) 746.89
   cerebellopontine (angle)—*see* Cyst, brain
   cerebellum—*see* Cyst, brain
   cerebral—*see* Cyst, brain

Cyst —*continued*
   cervical lateral 744.42
   cervix 622.8
      embryonal 752.41
      nabothian (gland) 616.0
   chamber, anterior (eye) 364.60
      exudative 364.62
      implantation (surgical) (traumatic) 364.61
      parasitic 360.13
   chiasmal, optic NEC (*see also* Lesion, chiasmal) 377.54
   chocolate (ovary) 617.1
   choledochal (congenital) 751.69
      acquired 576.8
   choledochus 751.69
   chorion 658.8
   choroid plexus 348.0
   chyle, mesentery 457.8
   ciliary body 364.60
      exudative 364.64
      implantation 364.61
      primary 364.63
   clitoris 624.8
   coccyx (*see also* Cyst, bone) 733.20
   colloid
      third ventricle (brain) 742.4
      thyroid gland—*see* Goiter
   colon 569.89
   common (bile) duct (*see also* Disease, biliary) 576.8
   congenital NEC 759.89
      adrenal glands 759.1
      epiglottis 748.3
      esophagus 750.4
      fallopian tube 752.11
      kidney 753.10
         multiple 753.19
         single 753.11
      larynx 748.3
      liver 751.62
      lung 748.4
      mediastinum 748.8
      ovary 752.0
      oviduct 752.11
      pancreas 751.7
      periurethral (tissue) 753.8
      prepuce NEC 752.69
         penis 752.69
      sublingual 750.26
      submaxillary gland 750.26
      thymus (gland) 759.2
      tongue 750.19
      ureterovesical orifice 753.4
      vulva 752.41
   conjunctiva 372.75
   cornea 371.23
   corpora quadrigemina 348.0
   corpus
      albicans (ovary) 620.2
      luteum (ruptured) 620.1
   Cowper's gland (benign) (infected) 599.89
   cranial meninges 348.0
   craniobuccal pouch 253.8
   craniopharyngeal pouch 253.8
   cystic duct (*see also* Disease, gallbladder) 575.8
   Cysticercus (any site) 123.1
   Dandy-Walker 742.3
      with spina bifida (*see also* Spina bifida) 741.0
   dental 522.8
      developmental 526.0
      eruption 526.0

895

Cyst INDEX TO DISEASES

Cyst —*continued*
   lateral periodontal 526.0
   primordial (keratocyst) 526.0
   root 522.8
  dentigerous 526.0
   mandible 526.0
   maxilla 526.0
  dermoid (M9084/0)—*see also* Neoplasm, by site, benign
   with malignant transformation (M9084/3) 183.0
   implantation
    external area or site (skin) NEC 709.8
    iris 364.61
    skin 709.8
    vagina 623.8
    vulva 624.8
   mouth 528.4
   oral soft tissue 528.4
   sacrococcygeal 685.1
    with abscess 685.0
  developmental of ovary, ovarian 752.0
  dura (cerebral) 348.0
   spinal 349.2
  ear (external) 706.2
  echinococcal (*see also* Echinococcus) 122.9
  embryonal
   cervix uteri 752.41
   genitalia, female external 752.41
   uterus 752.3
   vagina 752.41
  endometrial 621.8
   ectopic 617.9
  endometrium (uterus) 621.8
   ectopic—*see* Endometriosis
  enteric 751.5
  enterogenous 751.5
  epidermal (inclusion) (*see also* Cyst, skin) 706.2
  epidermoid (inclusion) (*see also* Cyst, skin) 706.2
   mouth 528.4
   not of skin—*see* Cyst, by site
   oral soft tissue 528.4
  epididymis 608.89
  epiglottis 478.79
  epiphysis cerebri 259.8
  epithelial (inclusion) (*see also* Cyst, skin) 706.2
  epoophoron 752.11
  eruption 526.0
  esophagus 530.89
  ethmoid sinus 478.19
  eye (retention) 379.8
   congenital 743.03
   posterior segment, congenital 743.54
  eyebrow 706.2
  eyelid (sebaceous) 374.84
   infected 373.13
   sweat glands or ducts 374.84
  falciform ligament (inflammatory) 573.8
  fallopian tube 620.8
  female genital organs NEC 629.89
  fimbrial (congenital) 752.11
  fissural (oral region) 526.1
  follicle (atretic) (graafian) (ovarian) 620.0
   nabothian (gland) 616.0
  follicular (atretic) (ovarian) 620.0
   dentigerous 526.0
  frontal sinus 478.19
  gallbladder or duct 575.8
  ganglion 727.43
  Gartner's duct 752.41

Cyst —*continued*
  gas, of mesentery 568.89
  gingiva 523.8
  gland of moll 374.84
  globulomaxillary 526.1
  graafian follicle 620.0
  granulosal lutein 620.2
  hemangiomatous (M9121/0) (*see also* Hemangioma) 228.00
  hydatid (*see also* Echinococcus) 122.9
   fallopian tube (Morgagni) 752.11
   liver NEC 122.8
   lung NEC 122.9
   Morgagni 752.89
    fallopian tube 752.11
   specified site NEC 122.9
  hymen 623.8
   embryonal 752.41
  hypopharynx 478.26
  hypophysis, hypophyseal (duct) (recurrent) 253.8
   cerebri 253.8
  implantation (dermoid)
   anterior chamber (eye) 364.61
   external area or site (skin) NEC 709.8
   iris 364.61
   vagina 623.8
   vulva 624.8
  incisor, incisive canal 526.1
  inclusion (epidermal) (epithelial) (epidermoid) (mucous) (squamous) (*see also* Cyst, skin) 706.2
   not of skin—*see* Neoplasm, by site, benign
  intestine (large) (small) 569.89
  intracranial—*see* Cyst, brain
  intraligamentous 728.89
   knee 717.89
  intrasellar 253.8
  iris (idiopathic) 364.60
   exudative 364.62
   implantation (surgical) (traumatic) 364.61
   miotic pupillary 364.55
   parasitic 360.13
  Iwanoff's 362.62
  jaw (bone) (aneurysmal) (extravasation) (hemorrhagic) (traumatic) 526.2
   developmental (odontogenic) 526.0
   fissural 526.1
  keratin 706.2
  kidney (congenital) 753.10
   acquired 593.2
   calyceal (*see also* Hydronephrosis) 591
   multiple 753.19
   pyelogenic (*see also* Hydronephrosis) 591
   simple 593.2
   single 753.11
   solitary (not congenital) 593.2
  labium (majus) (minus) 624.8
   sebaceous 624.8
  lacrimal
   apparatus 375.43
   gland or sac 375.12
  larynx 478.79
  lens 379.39
   congenital 743.39
  lip (gland) 528.5
  liver 573.8
   congenital 751.62
   hydatid (*see also* Echinococcus) 122.8
    granulosis 122.0
    multilocularis 122.5

INDEX TO DISEASES   **Cyst**

Cyst —*continued*
  lung 518.89
    congenital 748.4
    giant bullous 492.0
  lutein 620.1
  lymphangiomatous (M9173/0) 228.1
  lymphoepithelial
    mouth 528.4
    oral soft tissue 528.4
  macula 362.54
  malignant (M8000/3)—*see* Neoplasm, by site, malignant
  mammary gland (sweat gland) (*see also* Cyst, breast) 610.0
  mandible 526.2
    dentigerous 526.0
    radicular 522.8
  maxilla 526.2
    dentigerous 526.0
    radicular 522.8
  median
    anterior maxillary 526.1
    palatal 526.1
  mediastinum (congenital) 748.8
  meibomian (gland) (retention) 373.2
    infected 373.12
  membrane, brain 348.0
  meninges (cerebral) 348.0
    spinal 349.2
  meniscus knee 717.5
  mesentery, mesenteric (gas) 568.89
    chyle 457.8
    gas 568.89
  mesonephric duct 752.89
  mesothelial
    peritoneum 568.89
    pleura (peritoneal) 568.89
  milk 611.5
  miotic pupillary (iris) 364.55
  Morgagni (hydatid) 752.89
    fallopian tube 752.11
  mouth 528.4
  mullerian duct 752.89
  multilocular (ovary) (M8000/1) 239.5
  myometrium 621.8
  nabothian (follicle) (ruptured) 616.0
  nasal sinus 478.19
  nasoalveolar 528.4
  nasolabial 528.4
  nasopalatine (duct) 526.1
    anterior 526.1
  nasopharynx 478.26
  neoplastic (M8000/1)—*see also* Neoplasm, by site, unspecified nature
    benign (M8000/0)—*see* Neoplasm, by site, benign
    uterus 621.8
  nervous system—*see* Cyst, brain
  neuroenteric 742.59
  neuroepithelial ventricle 348.0
  nipple 610.0
  nose 478.19
    skin of 706.2
  odontogenic, developmental 526.0
  omentum (lesser) 568.89
    congenital 751.8
  oral soft tissue (dermoid) (epidermoid) (lymphoepithelial) 528.4
  ora serrata 361.19
  orbit 376.81

Cyst —*continued*
  ovary, ovarian (twisted) 620.2
    adherent 620.2
    chocolate 617.1
    corpus
      albicans 620.2
      luteum 620.1
    dermoid (M9084/0) 220
    developmental 752.0
    due to failure of involution NEC 620.2
    endometrial 617.1
    follicular (atretic) (graafian) (hemorrhagic) 620.0
    hemorrhagic 620.2
    in pregnancy or childbirth 654.4
      affecting fetus or newborn 763.89
      causing obstructed labor 660.2
        affecting fetus or newborn 763.1
    multilocular (M8000/1) 239.5
    pseudomucinous (M8470/0) 220
    retention 620.2
    serous 620.2
    theca lutein 620.2
    tuberculous (*see also* Tuberculosis) 016.6
    unspecified 620.2
  oviduct 620.8
  palatal papilla (jaw) 526.1
  palate 526.1
    fissural 526.1
    median (fissural) 526.1
  palatine, of papilla 526.1
  pancreas, pancreatic 577.2
    congenital 751.7
    false 577.2
    hemorrhagic 577.2
    true 577.2
  paranephric 593.2
  para ovarian 752.11
  paraphysis, cerebri 742.4
  parasitic NEC 136.9
  parathyroid (gland) 252.8
  paratubal (fallopian) 620.8
  paraurethral duct 599.89
  paroophoron 752.11
  parotid gland 527.6
    mucous extravasation or retention 527.6
  parovarian 752.11
  pars planus 364.60
    exudative 364.64
    primary 364.63
  pelvis, female
    in pregnancy or childbirth 654.4
      affecting fetus or newborn 763.89
      causing obstructed labor 660.2
        affecting fetus or newborn 763.1
  penis (sebaceous) 607.89
  periapical 522.8
  pericardial (congenital) 746.89
    acquired (secondary) 423.8
  pericoronal 526.0
  perineural (Tarlov's) 355.9
  periodontal 522.8
    lateral 526.0
  peripancreatic 577.2
  peripelvic (lymphatic) 593.2
  peritoneum 568.89
    chylous 457.8
  pharynx (wall) 478.26
  pilonidal (infected) (rectum) 685.1
    with abscess 685.0
    malignant (M9084/3) 173.5

897

Cyst — *INDEX TO DISEASES*

Cyst —*continued*
  pituitary (duct) (gland) 253.8
  placenta (amniotic)—*see* Placenta, abnormal
  pleura 519.8
  popliteal 727.51
  porencephalic 742.4
    acquired 348.0
  postanal (infected) 685.1
    with abscess 685.0
  posterior segment of eye, congenital 743.54
  postmastoidectomy cavity 383.31
  preauricular 744.47
  prepuce 607.89
    congenital 752.69
  primordial (jaw) 526.0
  prostate 600.3
  pseudomucinous (ovary) (M8470/0) 220
  pudenda (sweat glands) 624.8
  pupillary, miotic 364.55
    sebaceous 624.8
  radicular (residual) 522.8
  radiculodental 522.8
  ranular 527.6
  Rathke's pouch 253.8
  rectum (epithelium) (mucous) 569.49
  renal—*see* Cyst, kidney
  residual (radicular) 522.8
  retention (ovary) 620.2
  retina 361.19
    macular 362.54
    parasitic 360.13
    primary 361.13
    secondary 361.14
  retroperitoneal 568.89
  sacrococcygeal (dermoid) 685.1
    with abscess 685.0
  salivary gland or duct 527.6
    mucous extravasation or retention 527.6
  Sampson's 617.1
  sclera 379.19
  scrotum (sebaceous) 706.2
    sweat glands 706.2
  sebaceous (duct) (gland) 706.2
    breast 610.8
    eyelid 374.84
    genital organ NEC
      female 629.89
      male 608.89
    scrotum 706.2
  semilunar cartilage (knee) (multiple) 717.5
  seminal vesicle 608.89
  serous (ovary) 620.2
  sinus (antral) (ethmoidal) (frontal) (maxillary)
      (nasal) (sphenoidal) 478.19
  Skene's gland 599.89
  skin (epidermal) (epidermoid, inclusion)
      (epithelial) (inclusion) (retention)
      (sebaceous) 706.2
    breast 610.8
    eyelid 374.84
    genital organ NEC
      female 629.89
      male 608.89
    neoplastic 216.3
    scrotum 706.2
    sweat gland or duct 705.89
  solitary
    bone 733.21
    kidney 593.2
  spermatic cord 608.89
  sphenoid sinus 478.19

Cyst —*continued*
  spinal meninges 349.2
  spine (*see also* Cyst, bone) 733.20
  spleen NEC 289.59
    congenital 759.0
    hydatid (*see also* Echinococcus) 122.9
  spring water (pericardium) 746.89
  subarachnoid 348.0
    intrasellar 793.0
  subdural (cerebral) 348.0
    spinal cord 349.2
  sublingual gland 527.6
    mucous extravasation or retention 527.6
  submaxillary gland 527.6
    mucous extravasation or retention 527.6
  suburethral 599.89
  suprarenal gland 255.8
  suprasellar—*see* Cyst, brain
  sweat gland or duct 705.89
  sympathetic nervous system 337.9
  synovial 727.40
    popliteal space 727.51
  Tarlov's 355.9
  tarsal 373.2
  tendon (sheath) 727.42
  testis 608.89
  theca-lutein (ovary) 620.2
  Thornwaldt's, Tornwaldt's 478.26
  thymus (gland) 254.8
  thyroglossal (duct) (infected) (persistent) 759.2
  thyroid (gland) 246.2
    adenomatous—*see* Goiter, nodular
    colloid (*see also* Goiter) 240.9
  thyrolingual duct (infected) (persistent) 759.2
  tongue (mucous) 529.8
  tonsil 474.8
  tooth (dental root) 522.8
  tubo-ovarian 620.8
    inflammatory 614.1
  tunica vaginalis 608.89
  turbinate (nose) (*see also* Cyst, bone) 733.20
  Tyson's gland (benign) (infected) 607.89
  umbilicus 759.89
  urachus 753.7
  ureter 593.89
  ureterovesical orifice 593.89
    congenital 753.4
  urethra 599.84
  urethral gland (Cowper's) 599.89
  uterine
    ligament 620.8
      embryonic 752.11
    tube 620.8
  uterus (body) (corpus) (recurrent) 621.8
    embryonal 752.3
  utricle (ear) 386.8
    prostatic 599.89
  utriculus masculinus 599.89
  vagina, vaginal (squamous cell) (wall) 623.8
    embryonal 752.41
    implantation 623.8
    inclusion 623.8
  vallecula, vallecular 478.79
  ventricle, neuroepithelial 348.0
  verumontanum 599.89
  vesical (orifice) 596.8
  vitreous humor 379.29
  vulva (sweat glands) 624.8
    congenital 752.41
    implantation 624.8
    inclusion 624.8

Cyst —*continued*
    sebaceous gland 624.8
    vulvovaginal gland 624.8
    wolffian 752.89
Cystadenocarcinoma (M8440/3)—*see also* Neoplasm, by site, malignant
    bile duct type (M8161/3) 155.1
    endometrioid (M8380/3)—*see* Neoplasm, by site, malignant
    mucinous (M8470/3)
        papillary (M8471/3)
            specified site—*see* Neoplasm, by site, malignant
            unspecified site 183.0
        specified site—*see* Neoplasm, by site, malignant
        unspecified site 183.0
    papillary (M8450/3)
        mucinous (M8471/3)
            specified site—*see* Neoplasm, by site, malignant
            unspecified site 183.0
        pseudomucinous (M8471/3)
            specified site—*see* Neoplasm, by site, malignant
            unspecified site 183.0
        serous (M8460/3)
            specified site—*see* Neoplasm, by site, malignant
            unspecified site 183.0
        specified site—*see* Neoplasm, by site, malignant
        unspecified 183.0
    pseudomucinous (M8470/3)
        papillary (M8471/3)
            specified site—*see* Neoplasm, by site, malignant
            unspecified site 183.0
        specified site—*see* Neoplasm, by site, malignant
        unspecified site 183.0
    serous (M8441/3)
        papillary (M8460/3)
            specified site—*see* Neoplasm, by site, malignant
            unspecified site 183.0
        specified site—*see* Neoplasm, by site, malignant
        unspecified site 183.0
Cystadenofibroma (M9013/0)
    clear cell (M8313/0)—*see* Neoplasm, by site, benign
    endometrioid (M8381/0) 220
        borderline malignancy (M8381/1) 236.2
        malignant (M8381/3) 183.0
    mucinous (M9015/0)
        specified site—*see* Neoplasm, by site, benign
        unspecified site 220
    serous (M9014/0)
        specified site—*see* Neoplasm, by site, benign
        unspecified site 220
    specified site—*see* Neoplasm, by site, benign
    unspecified site 220
Cystadenoma (M8440/0)—*see also* Neoplasm, by site, benign
    bile duct (M8161/0) 211.5
    endometrioid (M8380/0)—*see also* Neoplasm, by site, benign
        borderline malignancy (M8380/1)—*see* Neoplasm, by site, uncertain behavior

Cystadenoma—*continued*
    malignant (M8440/3)—*see* Neoplasm, by site, malignant
    mucinous (M8470/0)
        borderline malignancy (M8470/1)
            specified site—*see* Neoplasm, uncertain behavior
            unspecified site 236.2
        papillary (M8471/0)
            borderline malignancy (M8471/1)
                specified site—*see* Neoplasm, by site, uncertain behavior
                unspecified site 236.2
            specified site—*see* Neoplasm, by site, benign
            unspecified site 220
        specified site—*see* Neoplasm, by site, benign
        unspecified site 220
    papillary (M8450/0)
        borderline malignancy (M8450/1)
            specified site—*see* Neoplasm, by site, uncertain behavior
            unspecified site 236.2
        lymphomatosum (M8561/0) 210.2
        mucinous (M8471/0)
            borderline malignancy (M8471/1)
                specified site—*see* Neoplasm, by site, uncertain behavior
                unspecified site 236.2
            specified site—*see* Neoplasm, by site, benign
            unspecified site 220
        pseudomucinous (M8471/0)
            borderline malignancy (M8471/1)
                specified site—*see* Neoplasm, by site, uncertain behavior
                unspecified site 236.2
            specified site—*see* Neoplasm, by site, benign
            unspecified site 220
        serous (M8460/0)
            borderline malignancy (M8460/1)
                specified site—*see* Neoplasm, by site, uncertain behavior
                unspecified site 236.2
            specified site—*see* Neoplasm, by site, benign
            unspecified site 220
        specified site—*see* Neoplasm, by site, benign
        unspecified site 220
    pseudomucinous (M8470/0)
        borderline malignancy (M8470/1)
            specified site—*see* Neoplasm, by site, uncertain behavior
            unspecified site 236.2
        papillary (M8471/0)
            borderline malignancy (M8471/1)
                specified site—*see* Neoplasm, by site, uncertain behavior
                unspecified site 236.2
            specified site—*see* Neoplasm, by site, benign
            unspecified site 220
        specified site—*see* Neoplasm, by site, benign
        unspecified site 220
    serous (M8441/0)
        borderline malignancy (M8441/1)
            specified site—*see* Neoplasm, by site, uncertain behavior
            unspecified site 236.2

Cystadenoma—*continued*
  papillary (M8460/0)
    borderline malignancy (M8460/1)
      specified site—*see* Neoplasm, by site, uncertain behavior
      unspecified site 236.2
    specified site—*see* Neoplasm, by site, benign
    unspecified site 220
  specified site—*see* Neoplasm, by site, benign
  unspecified site 220
  thyroid 226
Cystathioninemia 270.4
Cystathioninuria 270.4
Cystic —*see also* condition
  breast, chronic 610.1
  corpora lutea 620.1
  degeneration, congenital
    brain 742.4
    kidney (*see also* Cystic, disease, kidney) 753.10
  disease
    breast, chronic 610.1
    kidney, congenital 753.10
      medullary 753.16
      multiple 753.19
      polycystic—*see* Polycystic, kidney
      single 753.11
      specified NEC 753.19
    liver, congenital 751.62
    lung 518.89
      congenital 748.4
    pancreas, congenital 751.7
    semilunar cartilage 717.5
  duct—*see* condition
  eyeball, congenital 743.03
  fibrosis (pancreas) 277.00
    with
      manifestations
        gastrointestinal 277.03
        pulmonary 277.02
        specified NEC 277.09
      meconium ileus 277.01
      pulmonary exacerbation 277.02
  hygroma (M9173/0) 228.1
  kidney, congenital 753.10
    medullary 753.16
    multiple 753.19
    polycystic—*see* Polycystic, kidney
    single 753.11
    specified NEC 753.19
  liver, congenital 751.62
  lung 518.89
    congenital 748.4
  mass—*see* Cyst
  mastitis, chronic 610.1
  ovary 620.2
  pancreas, congenital 751.7
Cysticerciasis 123.1
Cysticercosis (mammary) (subretinal) 123.1
Cysticercus 123.1
  cellulosae infestation 123.1
Cystinosis (malignant) 270.0
Cystinuria 270.0
Cystitis (bacillary) (colli) (diffuse) (exudative) (hemorrhagic) (purulent) (recurrent) (septic) (suppurative) (ulcerative) 595.9
  with
    abortion—*see* Abortion, by type, with urinary tract infection

Cystitis—*continued*
    ectopic pregnancy (*see also* categories 633.0-633.9) 639.8
    fibrosis 595.1
    leukoplakia 595.1
    malakoplakia 595.1
    metaplasia 595.1
    molar pregnancy (*see also* categories 630-632) 639.8
  actinomycotic 039.8 *[595.4]*
  acute 595.0
    of trigone 595.3
  allergic 595.89
  amebic 006.8 *[595.4]*
  bilharzial 120.9 *[595.4]*
  blennorrhagic (acute) 098.11
    chronic or duration of 2 months or more 098.31
  bullous 595.89
  calculous 594.1
  chlamydial 099.53
  chronic 595.2
    interstitial 595.1
    of trigone 595.3
  complicating pregnancy, childbirth, or puerperium 646.6
    affecting fetus or newborn 760.1
  cystic(a) 595.81
  diphtheritic 032.84
  echinococcal
    granulosus 122.3 *[595.4]*
    multilocularis 122.6 *[595.4]*
  emphysematous 595.89
  encysted 595.81
  follicular 595.3
  following
    abortion 639.8
    ectopic or molar pregnancy 639.8
  gangrenous 595.89
  glandularis 595.89
  gonococcal (acute) 098.11
    chronic or duration of 2 months or more 098.31
  incrusted 595.89
  interstitial 595.1
  irradiation 595.82
  irritation 595.89
  malignant 595.89
  monilial 112.2
  of trigone 595.3
  panmural 595.1
  polyposa 595.89
  prostatic 601.3
  radiation 595.82
  Reiter's (abacterial) 099.3
  specified NEC 595.89
  subacute 595.2
  submucous 595.1
  syphilitic 095.8
  trichomoniasis 131.09
  tuberculous (*see also* Tuberculosis) 016.1
  ulcerative 595.1
Cystocele
  female (without uterine prolapse) 618.01
    with uterine prolapse 618.4
      complete 618.3
      incomplete 618.2
    lateral 618.02
    midline 618.01
    paravaginal 618.02

Cystocele—*continued*
  in pregnancy or childbirth 654.4
    affecting fetus or newborn 763.89
    causing obstructed labor 660.2
      affecting fetus or newborn 763.1
  male 596.8
Cystoid
  cicatrix limbus 372.64
  degeneration macula 362.53
Cystolithiasis 594.1
Cystoma (M8440/0)—*see also* Neoplasm, by site, benign
  endometrial, ovary 617.1
  mucinous (M8470/0)
    specified site—*see* Neoplasm, by site, benign
    unspecified site 220
  serous (M8441/0)
    specified site—*see* Neoplasm, by site, benign
    unspecified site 220
  simple (ovary) 620.2
Cystoplegia 596.53
Cystoptosis 596.8
Cystopyelitis (*see also* Pyelitis) 590.80
Cystorrhagia 596.8
Cystosarcoma phyllodes (M9020/1) 238.3
  benign (M9020/0) 217
  malignant (M9020/3)—*see* Neoplasm, breast, malignant
Cystostomy status V44.50
  appendico-vesicostomy V44.52
  cutaneous-vesicostomy V44.51
  specified type NEC V44.59
  with complication 997.5
Cystourethritis (*see also* Urethritis) 597.89
Cystourethrocele (*see also* Cystocele)
  female (without uterine prolapse) 618.09
    with uterine prolapse 618.4
      complete 618.3
      incomplete 618.2
  male 596.8
Cytomegalic inclusion disease 078.5
  congenital 771.1
Cytomycosis, reticuloendothelial (*see also* Histoplasmosis, American) 115.00
Cytopenia 289.9
  refractory
    with
      multilineage dysplasia (RCMD) 238.72
        and ringed sideroblasts (RCMD-RS) 238.72

INDEX TO DISEASES

INDEX TO DISEASES

D

Daae (-Finsen) **disease** (epidemic pleurodynia) 074.1
Dabney's grip 074.1
Da Costa's syndrome (neurocirculatory asthenia) 306.2
Dacryoadenitis, dacryadenitis 375.00
  acute 375.01
  chronic 375.02
Dacryocystitis 375.30
  acute 375.32
  chronic 375.42
  neonatal 771.6
  phlegmonous 375.33
  syphilitic 095.8
    congenital 090.0
  trachomatous, active 076.1
    late effect 139.1
  tuberculous (see also Tuberculosis) 017.3
Dacryocystoblennorrhea 375.42
Dacryocystocele 375.43
Dacryolith, dacryolithiasis 375.57
Dacryoma 375.43
Dacryopericystitis (acute) (subacute) 375.32
  chronic 375.42
Dacryops 375.11
Dacryosialadenopathy, atrophic 710.2
Dacryostenosis 375.56
  congenital 743.65
Dactylitis
  bone (see also Osteomyelitis) 730.2
  sickle-cell 282.62
    Hb-C 282.64
    Hb-SS 282.62
    specified NEC 282.69
  syphilitic 095.5
  tuberculous (see also Tuberculosis) 015.5
Dactylolysis spontanea 136.0
Dactylosymphysis (see also Syndactylism) 755.10
Damage
  arteriosclerotic—see Arteriosclerosis
  brain 348.9
    anoxic, hypoxic 348.1
      during or resulting from a procedure 997.01
    ischemic, in newborn 768.7
    child NEC 343.9
    due to birth injury 767.0
    minimal (child) (see also Hyperkinesia) 314.9
    newborn 767.0
  cardiac—see also Disease, heart
  cardiorenal (vascular) (see also Hypertension, cardiorenal) 404.90
  central nervous system—see Damage, brain
  cerebral NEC—see Damage, brain
  coccyx, complicating delivery 665.6
  coronary (see also Ischemia, heart) 414.9
  eye, birth injury 767.8
  heart—see also Disease, heart
    valve—see Endocarditis
  hypothalamus NEC 348.9
  liver 571.9
    alcoholic 571.3
    medication 995.20
  myocardium (see also Degeneration, myocardial) 429.1

Damage—continued
  pelvic
    joint or ligament, during delivery 665.6
    organ NEC
      with
        abortion—see Abortion, by type, with damage to pelvic organs
        ectopic pregnancy (see also categories 633.0-633.9) 639.2
        molar pregnancy (see also categories 630-632) 639.2
      during delivery 665.5
      following
        abortion 639.2
        ectopic or molar pregnancy 639.2
  renal (see also Disease, renal) 593.9
  skin, solar 692.79
    acute 692.72
    chronic 692.74
  subendocardium, subendocardial (see also Degeneration, myocardial) 429.1
  vascular 459.9
Dameshek's syndrome (erythroblastic anemia) 282.49
Dana-Putnam syndrome (subacute combined sclerosis with pernicious anemia) 281.0 *[336.2]*
Danbolt (-Closs) **syndrome** (acrodermatitis enteropathica) 686.8
Dandruff 690.18
Dandy fever 061
Dandy-Walker deformity or syndrome (atresia, foramen of Magendie) 742.3
  with spina bifida (see also Spina bifida) 741.0
Dangle foot 736.79
Danielssen's disease (anesthetic leprosy) 030.1
Danlos' syndrome 756.83
Darier's disease (congenital) (keratosis follicularis) 757.39
  due to vitamin A deficiency 264.8
  meaning erythema annulare centrifugum 695.0
Darier-Roussy sarcoid 135
Darling's
  disease (see also Histoplasmosis, American) 115.00
  histoplasmosis (see also Histoplasmosis, American) 115.00
Dartre 054.9
Darwin's tubercle 744.29
Davidson's anemia (refractory) 284.9
Davies' disease 425.0
Davies-Colley syndrome (slipping rib) 733.99
Dawson's encephalitis 046.2
Day blindness (see also Blindness, day) 368.60
Dead
  fetus
    retained (in utero) 656.4
      early pregnancy (death before 22 completed weeks gestation) 632
      late (death after 22 completed weeks gestation) 656.4
    syndrome 641.3
  labyrinth 386.50
  ovum, retained 631
Deaf and dumb NEC 389.7

INDEX TO DISEASES

Deaf mutism (acquired) (congenital) NEC 389.7
  endemic 243
  hysterical 300.11
  syphilitic, congenital 090.0
Deafness (acquired) (complete) (congenital) (hereditary) (middle ear) (partial) 389.9
  with
    blindness V49.85
    blue sclera and fragility of bone 756.51
  auditory fatigue 389.9
  aviation 993.0
    nerve injury 951.5
  boilermakers' 951.5
  central 389.14
    with conductive hearing loss 389.20
      bilateral 389.22
      unilateral 389.21
  conductive (air) 389.00
    with sensorineural hearing loss 389.20
      bilateral 389.22
      unilateral 389.21
    bilateral 389.06
    combined types 389.08
    external ear 389.01
    inner ear 389.04
    middle ear 389.03
    multiple types 389.08
    tympanic membrane 389.02
    unilateral 389.05
  emotional (complete) 300.11
  functional (complete) 300.11
  high frequency 389.8
  hysterical (complete) 300.11
  injury 951.5
  low frequency 389.8
  mental 784.69
  mixed conductive and sensorineural 389.20
    bilateral 389.22
    unilateral 389.21
  nerve
    with conductive hearing loss 389.20
      bilateral 389.22
      unilateral 389.21
    bilateral 389.12
    unilateral 389.13
  neural
    with conductive hearing loss 389.20
      bilateral 389.22
      unilateral 389.21
    bilateral 389.12
    unilateral 389.13
  noise-induced 388.12
    nerve injury 951.5
  nonspeaking 389.7
  perceptive 389.10
    with conductive hearing loss 389.20
      bilateral 389.22
      unilateral 389.21
    central 389.14
    neural
      bilateral 389.12
      unilateral 389.13
    sensorineural 389.10
      asymmetrical 389.16
      bilateral 389.18
      unilateral 389.15
    sensory
      bilateral 389.11
      unilateral 389.17
  psychogenic (complete) 306.7

Deafness—*continued*
  sensorineural (*see also* Deafness, perceptive) 389.10
    asymmetrical 389.16
    bilateral 389.18
    unilateral 389.15
  sensory
    with conductive hearing loss 389.20
      bilateral 389.22
      unilateral 389.21
    bilateral 389.11
    unilateral 389.17
  specified type NEC 389.8
  sudden NEC 388.2
  syphilitic 094.89
  transient ischemic 388.02
  transmission—*see* Deafness, conductive
  traumatic 951.5
  word (secondary to organic lesion) 784.69
    developmental 315.31
Death
  after delivery (cause not stated) (sudden) 674.9
  anesthetic
    due to
      correct substance properly administered 995.4
      overdose or wrong substance given 968.4
        specified anesthetic—*see* Table of drugs and chemicals
    during delivery 668.9
  brain 348.8
  cardiac (sudden) (SCD)—code to underlying condition
    family history of V17.41
    personal history of, successfully resuscitated V12.53
  cause unknown 798.2
  cot (infant) 798.0
  crib (infant) 798.0
  fetus, fetal (cause not stated) (intrauterine) 779.9
    early, with retention (before 22 completed weeks gestation) 632
    from asphyxia or anoxia (before labor) 768.0
      during labor 768.1
    late, affecting management of pregnancy (after 22 completed weeks gestation) 656.4
  from pregnancy NEC 646.9
  instantaneous 798.1
  intrauterine (*see also* Death, fetus) 779.9
    complicating pregnancy 656.4
  maternal, affecting fetus or newborn 761.6
  neonatal NEC 779.9
  sudden (cause unknown) 798.1
    cardiac (SCD)
      family history of V17.41
      personal history of, successfully resuscitated V12.53
    during delivery 669.9
      under anesthesia NEC 668.9
    infant, syndrome (SIDS) 798.0
    puerperal, during puerperium 674.9
  unattended (cause unknown) 798.9
  under anesthesia NEC
    due to
      correct substance properly administered 995.4
      overdose or wrong substance given 968.4
        specified anesthetic—*see* Table of drugs and chemicals
    during delivery 668.9
  violent 798.1

904

de Beurmann-Gougerot disease (sporotrichosis) 117.1
Debility (general) (infantile) (postinfectional) 799.3
  with nutritional difficulty 269.9
  congenital or neonatal NEC 779.9
  nervous 300.5
  old age 797
  senile 797
Débove's disease (splenomegaly) 789.2
Decalcification
  bone (*see also* Osteoporosis) 733.00
  teeth 521.89
Decapitation 874.9
  fetal (to facilitate delivery) 763.89
Decapsulation, kidney 593.89
Decay
  dental 521.00
  senile 797
  tooth, teeth 521.00
Decensus, uterus —*see* Prolapse, uterus
Deciduitis (acute)
  with
    abortion—*see* Abortion, by type, with sepsis
    ectopic pregnancy (*see also* categories 633.0-633.9) 639.0
    molar pregnancy (*see also* categories 630-632) 639.0
  affecting fetus or newborn 760.8
  following
    abortion 639.0
    ectopic or molar pregnancy 639.0
  in pregnancy 646.6
  puerperal, postpartum 670
Deciduoma malignum (M9100/3) 181
Deciduous tooth (retained) 520.6
Decline (general) (*see also* Debility) 799.3
Decompensation
  cardiac (acute) (chronic) (*see also* Disease, heart) 429.9
    failure—*see* Failure, heart
  cardiorenal (*see also* Hypertension, cardiorenal) 404.90
  cardiovascular (*see also* Disease, cardiovascular) 429.2
  heart (*see also* Disease, heart) 429.9
    failure—*see* Failure, heart
  hepatic 572.2
  myocardial (acute) (chronic) (*see also* Disease, heart) 429.9
    failure—*see* Failure, heart
  respiratory 519.9
Decompression sickness 993.3
Decrease, decreased
  blood
    platelets (*see also* Thrombocytopenia) 287.5
    pressure 796.3
      due to shock following
        injury 958.4
        operation 998.0
    white cell count 288.50
      specified NEC 288.59
  cardiac reserve—*see* Disease, heart
  estrogen 256.39
    postablative 256.2
  fetal movements 655.7
  fragility of erythrocytes 289.89
  function
    adrenal (cortex) 255.41
      medulla 255.5
    ovary in hypopituitarism 253.4

Decrease, decreased—*continued*
  parenchyma of pancreas 577.8
  pituitary (gland) (lobe) (anterior) 253.2
    posterior (lobe) 253.8
  functional activity 780.99
  glucose 790.29
  haptoglobin (serum) NEC 273.8
  leukocytes 288.50
  libido 799.81
  lymphocytes 288.51
  platelets (*see also* Thrombocytopenia) 287.5
  pulse pressure 785.9
  respiration due to shock following injury 958.4
  sexual desire 799.81
  tear secretion NEC 375.15
  tolerance
    fat 579.8
    salt and water 276.9
  vision NEC 369.9
  white blood cell count 288.50
Decubital gangrene 707.00 *[785.4]*
Decubiti (*see also* Decubitus) 707.00
Decubitus (ulcer) 707.00
  with gangrene 707.00 *[785.4]*
  ankle 707.06
  back
    lower 707.03
    upper 707.02
  buttock 707.05
  elbow 707.01
  head 707.09
  heel 707.07
  hip 707.04
  other site 707.09
  sacrum 707.03
  shoulder blades 707.02
Deepening acetabulum 718.85
Defect, defective 759.9
  3-beta-hydroxysteroid dehydrogenase 255.2
  11-hydroxylase 255.2
  21-hydroxylase 255.2
  abdominal wall, congenital 756.70
  aorticopulmonary septum 745.0
  aortic septal 745.0
  atrial septal (ostium secundum type) 745.5
    acquired 429.71
    ostium primum type 745.61
    sinus venosus 745.8
  atrioventricular
    canal 745.69
    septum 745.4
      acquired 429.71
  atrium secundum 745.5
    acquired 429.71
  auricular septal 745.5
    acquired 429.71
  bilirubin excretion 277.4
  biosynthesis, testicular androgen 257.2
  bridge 525.60
  bulbar septum 745.0
  butanol-insoluble iodide 246.1
  chromosome—*see* Anomaly, chromosome
  circulation (acquired) 459.9
    congenital 747.9
    newborn 747.9
  clotting NEC (*see also* Defect, coagulation) 286.9
  coagulation (factor) (*see also* Deficiency, coagulation factor) 286.9

Defect, defective —*continued*
    with
        abortion—*see* Abortion, by type, with hemorrhage
        ectopic pregnancy (*see also* categories 634-638) 639.1
        molar pregnancy (*see also* categories 630-632) 639.1
    acquired (any) 286.7
    antepartum or intrapartum 641.3
        affecting fetus or newborn 762.1
    causing hemorrhage of pregnancy or delivery 641.3
    complicating pregnancy, childbirth, or the puerperium 649.3
    due to
        liver disease 286.7
        vitamin K deficiency 286.7
    newborn, transient 776.3
    postpartum 666.3
    specified type NEC 286.9
    conduction (heart) 426.9
    bone (*see also* Deafness, conductive) 389.00
    congenital, organ or site NEC—*see also* Anomaly
    circulation 747.9
    Descemet's membrane 743.9
        specified type NEC 743.49
    diaphragm 756.6
    ectodermal 757.9
    esophagus 750.9
    pulmonic cusps—*see* Anomaly, heart valve
    respiratory system 748.9
        specified type NEC 748.8
    crown 525.60
    cushion endocardial 745.60
    dental restoration 525.60
    dentin (hereditary) 520.5
    Descemet's membrane (congenital) 743.9
        acquired 371.30
        specific type NEC 743.49
    deutan 368.52
    developmental—*see also* Anomaly, by site
        cauda equina 742.59
        left ventricle 746.9
            with atresia or hypoplasia of aortic orifice or valve, with hypoplasia of ascending aorta 746.7
            in hypoplastic left heart syndrome 746.7
        testis 752.9
        vessel 747.9
    diaphragm
        with elevation, eventration, or hernia—*see* Hernia, diaphragm
        congenital 756.6
            with elevation, eventration, or hernia 756.6
            gross (with elevation, eventration, or hernia) 756.6
    ectodermal, congenital 757.9
    Eisenmenger's (ventricular septal defect) 745.4
    endocardial cushion 745.60
        specified type NEC 745.69
    esophagus, congenital 750.9
    extensor retinaculum 728.9
    fibrin polymerization (*see also* Defect, coagulation) 286.3
    filling
        biliary tract 793.3
        bladder 793.5
        dental 525.60
        gallbladder 793.3

Defect, defective —*continued*
    kidney 793.5
    stomach 793.4
    ureter 793.5
    fossa ovalis 745.5
    gene, carrier (suspected) of V83.89
    Gerbode 745.4
    glaucomatous, without elevated tension 365.89
    Hageman (factor) (*see also* Defect, coagulation) 286.3
    hearing (*see also* Deafness) 389.9
    high grade 317
    homogentisic acid 270.2
    interatrial septal 745.5
        acquired 429.71
    interauricular septal 745.5
        acquired 429.71
    interventricular septal 745.4
        with pulmonary stenosis or atresia, dextroposition of aorta, and hypertrophy of right ventricle 745.2
        acquired 429.71
        in tetralogy of Fallot 745.2
    iodide trapping 246.1
    iodotyrosine dehalogenase 246.1
    kynureninase 270.2
    learning, specific 315.2
    major osseous 731.3
    mental (*see also* Retardation, mental) 319
    osseous, major 731.3
    osteochondral NEC 738.8
    ostium
        primum 745.61
        secundum 745.5
    pericardium 746.89
    peroxidase-binding 246.1
    placental blood supply—*see* Placenta, insufficiency
    platelet (qualitative) 287.1
        constitutional 286.4
    postural, spine 737.9
    protan 368.51
    pulmonic cusps, congenital 746.00
    renal pelvis 753.9
        obstructive 753.29
        specified type NEC 753.3
    respiratory system, congenital 748.9
        specified type NEC 748.8
    retina, retinal 361.30
        with detachment (*see also* Detachment, retina, with retinal defect) 361.00
        multiple 361.33
            with detachment 361.02
        nerve fiber bundle 362.85
        single 361.30
            with detachment 361.01
    septal (closure) (heart) NEC 745.9
        acquired 429.71
        atrial 745.5
        specified type NEC 745.8
    speech NEC 784.5
        developmental 315.39
        secondary to organic lesion 784.5
    Taussig-Bing (transposition, aorta and overriding pulmonary artery) 745.11
    teeth, wedge 521.20
    thyroid hormone synthesis 246.1
    tritan 368.53
    ureter 753.9
        obstructive 753.29

INDEX TO DISEASES

Defect, defective—*continued*
  vascular (acquired) (local) 459.9
    congenital (peripheral) NEC 747.60
      gastrointestinal 747.61
      lower limb 747.64
      renal 747.62
      specified NEC 747.69
      spinal 747.82
      upper limb 747.63
  ventricular septal 745.4
    with pulmonary stenosis or atresia, dextraposition of aorta, and hypertrophy of right ventricle 745.2
    acquired 429.71
    atrioventricular canal type 745.69
    between infundibulum and anterior portion 745.4
    in tetralogy of Fallot 745.2
    isolated anterior 745.4
  vision NEC 369.9
  visual field 368.40
    arcuate 368.43
    heteronymous, bilateral 368.47
    homonymous, bilateral 368.46
    localized NEC 368.44
    nasal step 368.44
    peripheral 368.44
    sector 368.43
  voice 784.40
  wedge, teeth (abrasion) 521.20
Defeminization syndrome 255.2
Deferentitis 608.4
  gonorrheal (acute) 098.14
    chronic or duration of 2 months or over 098.34
Defibrination syndrome (*see also* Fibrinolysis) 286.6
Deficiency, deficient
  3-beta-hydroxysteroid dehydrogenase 255.2
  6-phosphogluconic dehydrogenase (anemia) 282.2
  11-beta-hydroxylase 255.2
  17-alpha-hydroxylase 255.2
  18-hydroxysteroid dehydrogenase 255.2
  20-alpha-hydroxylase 255.2
  21-hydroxylase 255.2
  AAT (alpha-1 antitrypsin) 273.4
  abdominal muscle syndrome 756.79
  accelerator globulin (Ac G) (blood) (*see also* Defect, coagulation) 286.3
  AC globulin (congenital) (*see also* Defect, coagulation) 286.3
    acquired 286.7
  activating factor (blood) (*see also* Defect, coagulation) 286.3
  adenohypophyseal 253.2
  adenosine deaminase 277.2
  aldolase (hereditary) 271.2
  alpha-1-antitrypsin 273.4
  alpha-1-trypsin inhibitor 273.4
  alpha-fucosidase 271.8
  alpha-lipoprotein 272.5
  alpha-mannosidase 271.8
  amino acid 270.9
  anemia—*see* Anemia, deficiency
  aneurin 265.1
    with beriberi 265.0
  antibody NEC 279.00
  antidiuretic hormone 253.5

Deficiency, deficient—*continued*
  antihemophilic
    factor (A) 286.0
      B 286.1
      C 286.2
    globulin (AHG) NEC 286.0
  antithrombin III 289.81
  antitrypsin 273.4
  argininosuccinate synthetase or lyase 270.6
  ascorbic acid (with scurvy) 267
  autoprothrombin
    I (*see also* Defect, coagulation) 286.3
    II 286.1
    C (*see also* Defect, coagulation) 286.3
  bile salt 579.8
  biotin 266.2
  biotinidase 277.6
  bradykinase-1 277.6
  brancher enzyme (amylopectinosis) 271.0
  calciferol 268.9
    with
      osteomalacia 268.2
      rickets (*see also* Rickets) 268.0
  calcium 275.40
    dietary 269.3
  calorie, severe 261
  carbamyl phosphate synthetase 270.6
  cardiac (*see also* Insufficiency, myocardial) 428.0
  carnitine 277.81
    due to
      hemodialysis 277.83
      inborn errors of metabolism 277.82
      valproic acid therapy 277.83
    iatrogenic 277.83
    palmitoyltransferase (CPT1, CPT2) 277.85
    palmityl transferase (CPT1, CPT2) 277.85
    primary 277.81
    secondary 277.84
  carotene 264.9
  Carr factor (*see also* Defect, coagulation) 286.9
  central nervous system 349.9
  ceruloplasmin 275.1
  cevitamic acid (with scurvy) 267
  choline 266.2
  Christmas factor 286.1
  chromium 269.3
  citrin 269.1
  clotting (blood) (*see also* Defect, coagulation) 286.9
  coagulation factor NEC 286.9
    with
      abortion—*see* Abortion, by type, with hemorrhage
      ectopic pregnancy (*see also* categories 634-638) 639.1
      molar pregnancy (*see also* categories 630-632) 639.1
    acquired (any) 286.7
    antepartum or intrapartum 641.3
      affecting fetus or newborn 762.1
    complicating pregnancy, childbirth, or the puerperium 649.3
    due to
      liver disease 286.7
      vitamin K deficiency 286.7
    newborn, transient 776.3
    postpartum 666.3
    specified type NEC 286.3
  color vision (congenital) 368.59
    acquired 368.55

Deficiency, deficient—*continued*
  combined glucocorticoid and mineralocorticoid 255.41
  combined, two or more coagulation factors (*see also* Defect, coagulation) 286.9
  complement factor NEC 279.8
  contact factor (*see also* Defect, coagulation) 286.3
  copper NEC 275.1
  corticoadrenal 255.41
  craniofacial axis 756.0
  cyanocobalamin (vitamin B$_{12}$) 266.2
  debrancher enzyme (limit dextrinosis) 271.0
  desmolase 255.2
  diet 269.9
  dihydrofolate reductase 281.2
  dihydropteridine reductase 270.1
  disaccharidase (intestinal) 271.3
  disease NEC 269.9
  ear(s) V48.8
  edema 262
  endocrine 259.9
  enzymes, circulating NEC (*see also* Deficiency, by specific enzyme) 277.6
  ergosterol 268.9
    with
      osteomalacia 268.2
      rickets (*see also* Rickets) 268.0
  erythrocytic glutathione (anemia) 282.2
  eyelid(s) V48.8
  factor (*see also* Defect, coagulation) 286.9
    I (congenital) (fibrinogen) 286.3
      antepartum or intrapartum 641.3
        affecting fetus or newborn 762.1
      newborn, transient 776.3
      postpartum 666.3
    II (congenital) (prothrombin) 286.3
    V (congenital) (labile) 286.3
    VII (congenital) (stable) 286.3
    VIII (congenital) (functional) 286.0
      with
        functional defect 286.0
        vascular defect 286.4
    IX (Christmas) (congenital) (functional) 286.1
    X (congenital) (Stuart-Prower) 286.3
    XI (congenital) (plasma thromboplastin antecedent) 286.2
    XII (congenital) (Hageman) 286.3
    XIII (congenital) (fibrin stabilizing) 286.3
    Hageman 286.3
    multiple (congenital) 286.9
      acquired 286.7
  fibrinase (*see also* Defect, coagulation) 286.3
  fibrinogen (congenital) (*see also* Defect, coagulation) 286.3
    acquired 286.6
  fibrin stabilizing factor (congenital) (*see also* Defect, coagulation) 286.3
    acquired 286.7
  finger—*see* Absence, finger
  Fletcher factor (*see also* Defect, coagulation) 286.9
  fluorine 269.3
  folate, anemia 281.2
  folic acid (vitamin B$_c$) 266.2
    anemia 281.2
  follicle-stimulating hormone (FSH) 253.4
  fructokinase 271.2
  fructose-1, 6-diphosphate 271.2
  fructose-1-phosphate aldolase 271.2
  FSH (follicle-stimulating hormone) 253.4

Deficiency, deficient—*continued*
  fucosidase 271.8
  galactokinase 271.1
  galactose-1-phosphate uridyl transferase 271.1
  gamma globulin in blood 279.00
  glass factor (*see also* Defect, coagulation) 286.3
  glucocorticoid 255.41
  glucose-6-phosphatase 271.0
  glucose-6-phosphate dehydrogenase anemia 282.2
  glucuronyl transferase 277.4
  glutathione-reductase (anemia) 282.2
  glycogen synthetase 271.0
  growth hormone 253.3
  Hageman factor (congenital) (*see also* Defect, coagulation) 286.3
  head V48.0
  hemoglobin (*see also* Anemia) 285.9
  hepatophosphorylase 271.0
  hexose monophosphate (HMP) shunt 282.2
  HGH (human growth hormone) 253.3
  HG-PRT 277.2
  homogentisic acid oxidase 270.2
  hormone—*see also* Deficiency, by specific hormone
    anterior pituitary (isolated) (partial) NEC 253.4
      growth (human) 253.3
    follicle-stimulating 253.4
    growth (human) (isolated) 253.3
    human growth 253.3
    interstitial cell-stimulating 253.4
    luteinizing 253.4
    melanocyte-stimulating 253.4
    testicular 257.2
  human growth hormone 253.3
  humoral 279.00
    with
      hyper-IgM 279.05
        autosomal recessive 279.05
        X-linked 279.05
      increased IgM 279.05
    congenital hypogammaglobulinemia 279.04
      non-sex-linked 279.06
    selective immunoglobulin NEC 279.03
      IgA 279.01
      IgG 279.03
      IgM 279.02
        increased 279.05
      specified NEC 279.09
  hydroxylase 255.2
  hypoxanthine-guanine phosphoribosyltransferase (HG-PRT) 277.2
  ICSH (interstitial cell-stimulating hormone) 253.4
  immunity NEC 279.3
    cell-mediated 279.10
      with
        hyperimmunoglobulinemia 279.2
        thrombocytopenia and eczema 279.12
      specified NEC 279.19
    combined (severe) 279.2
      syndrome 279.2
    common variable 279.06
    humoral NEC 279.00
    IgA (secretory) 279.01
    IgG 279.03
    IgM 279.02
  immunoglobulin, selective NEC 279.03
    IgA 279.01
    IgG 279.03
    IgM 279.02

INDEX TO DISEASES   **Deficiency, deficient**

Deficiency, deficient—*continued*
  inositol (B complex) 266.2
  interferon 279.4
  internal organ V47.0
  interstitial cell-stimulating hormone (ICSH) 253.4
  intrinsic (urethral) sphincter (ISD) 599.82
  intrinsic factor (Castle's) (congenital) 281.0
  invertase 271.3
  iodine 269.3
  iron, anemia 280.9
  labile factor (congenital) (*see also* Defect, coagulation) 286.3
    acquired 286.7
  lacrimal fluid (acquired) 375.15
    congenital 743.64
  lactase 271.3
  Laki-Lorand factor (*see also* Defect, coagulation) 286.3
  lecithin-cholesterol acyltranferase 272.5
  LH (luteinizing hormone) 253.4
  limb V49.0
    lower V49.0
      congenital (*see also* Deficiency, lower limb, congenital) 755.30
    upper V49.0
      congenital (*see also* Deficiency, upper limb, congenital) 755.20
  lipocaic 577.8
  lipoid (high-density) 272.5
  lipoprotein (familial) (high density) 272.5
  liver phosphorylase 271.0
  long chain 3-hydroxyacyl CoA dehydrogenase (LCHAD) 277.85
  long chain/very long chain acyl CoA dehydrogenase (LCAD, VLCAD) 277.85
  lower limb V49.0
    congenital 755.30
      with complete absence of distal elements 755.31
      longitudinal (complete) (partial) (with distal deficiencies, incomplete) 755.32
        with complete absence of distal elements 755.31
        combined femoral, tibial, fibular (incomplete) 755.33
        femoral 755.34
        fibular 755.37
        metatarsal(s) 755.38
        phalange(s) 755.39
          meaning all digits 755.31
        tarsal(s) 755.38
        tibia 755.36
        tibiofibular 755.35
      transverse 755.31
  luteinizing hormone (LH) 253.4
  lysosomal alpha-1, 4 glucosidase 271.0
  magnesium 275.2
  mannosidase 271.8
  medium chain acyl CoA dehydrogenase (MCAD) 277.85
  melanocyte-stimulating hormone (MSH) 253.4
  menadione (vitamin K) 269.0
    newborn 776.0
  mental (familial) (hereditary) (*see also* Retardation, mental) 319
  methylenetetrahydrofolate reductase (MTHFR) 270.4
  mineral NEC 269.3
  mineralocorticoid 255.42
  molybdenum 269.3

Deficiency, deficient—*continued*
  moral 301.7
  multiple, syndrome 260
  myocardial (*see also* Insufficiency myocardial) 428.0
  myophosphorylase 271.0
  NADH (DPNH) -methemoglobin-reductase (congenital) 289.7
  NADH diaphorase or reductase (congenital) 289.7
  neck V48.1
  niacin (amide) (-tryptophan) 265.2
  nicotinamide 265.2
  nicotinic acid (amide) 265.2
  nose V48.8
  number of teeth (*see also* Anodontia) 520.0
  nutrition, nutritional 269.9
    specified NEC 269.8
  ornithine transcarbamylase 270.6
  ovarian 256.39
  oxygen (*see also* Anoxia) 799.02
  pantothenic acid 266.2
  parathyroid (gland) 252.1
  phenylalanine hydroxylase 270.1
  phosphoenolpyruvate carboxykinase 271.8
  phosphofructokinase 271.2
  phosphoglucomutase 271.0
  phosphohexosisomerase 271.0
  phosphomannomutase 271.8
  phosphomannose isomerase 271.8
  phosphomannosyl mutase 271.8
  phosphorylase kinase, liver 271.0
  pituitary (anterior) 253.2
    posterior 253.5
  placenta—*see* Placenta, insufficiency
  plasma
    cell 279.00
    protein (paraproteinemia) (pyroglobulinemia) 273.8
      gamma globulin 279.00
    thromboplastin
      antecedent (PTA) 286.2
      component (PTC) 286.1
  platelet NEC 287.1
    constitutional 286.4
  polyglandular 258.9
  potassium (K) 276.8
  proaccelerin (congenital) (*see also* Defect, congenital) 286.3
    acquired 286.7
  proconvertin factor (congenital) (*see also* Defect, coagulation) 286.3
    acquired 286.7
  prolactin 253.4
  protein 260
    anemia 281.4
    C 289.81
    plasma—*see* Deficiency, plasma, protein
    S 289.81
  prothrombin (congenital) (*see also* Defect, coagulation) 286.3
    acquired 286.7
  Prower factor (*see also* Defect, coagulation) 286.3
  PRT 277.2
  pseudocholinesterase 289.89
  psychobiological 301.6
  PTA 286.2
  PTC 286.1
  purine nucleoside phosphorylase 277.2
  pyracin (alpha) (beta) 266.1

Deficiency, deficient—*continued*
  pyridoxal 266.1
  pyridoxamine 266.1
  pyridoxine (derivatives) 266.1
  pyruvate carboxylase 271.8
  pyruvate dehydrogenase 271.8
  pyruvate kinase (PK) 282.3
  riboflavin (vitamin B_2) 266.0
  saccadic eye movements 379.57
  salivation 527.7
  salt 276.1
  secretion
    ovary 256.39
    salivary gland (any) 527.7
    urine 788.5
  selenium 269.3
  serum
    antitrypsin, familial 273.4
    protein (congenital) 273.8
  short chain acyl CoA dehydrogenase (SCAD) 277.85
  short stature homeobox gene (SHOX)
    with
      dyschondrosteosis 756.89
      short stature (idiopathic) 783.43
      Turner's syndrome 758.6
  smooth pursuit movements (eye) 379.58
  sodium (Na) 276.1
  SPCA (*see also* Defect, coagulation) 286.3
  specified NEC 269.8
  stable factor (congenital) (*see also* Defect, coagulation) 286.3
    acquired 286.7
  Stuart (-Prower) factor (*see also* Defect, coagulation) 286.3
  sucrase 271.3
  sucrase-isomaltase 271.3
  sulfite oxidase 270.0
  syndrome, multiple 260
  thiamine, thiaminic (chloride) 265.1
  thrombokinase (*see also* Defect, coagulation) 286.3
    newborn 776.0
  thrombopoieten 287.39
  thymolymphatic 279.2
  thyroid (gland) 244.9
  tocopherol 269.1
  toe—*see* Absence, toe
  tooth bud (*see also* Anodontia) 520.0
  trunk V48.1
  UDPG-glycogen transferase 271.0
  upper limb V49.0
    congenital 755.20
      with complete absence of distal elements 755.21
      longitudinal (complete) (partial) (with distal deficiencies, incomplete) 755.22
        carpal(s) 755.28
        combined humeral, radial, ulnar (incomplete) 755.23
        humeral 755.24
        metacarpal(s) 755.28
        phalange(s) 755.29
          meaning all digits 755.21
        radial 755.26
        radioulnar 755.25
        ulnar 755.27
      transverse (complete) (partial) 755.21
  vascular 459.9
  vasopressin 253.5
  viosterol (*see also* Deficiency, calciferol) 268.9

Deficiency, deficient—*continued*
  vitamin (multiple) NEC 269.2
    A 264.9
      with
        Bitôt's spot 264.1
        corneal 264.2
          with corneal ulceration 264.3
        keratomalacia 264.4
        keratosis, follicular 264.8
        night blindness 264.5
        scar of cornea, xerophthalmic 264.6
        specified manifestation NEC 264.8
        ocular 264.7
        xeroderma 264.8
        xerophthalmia 264.7
        xerosis
          conjunctival 264.0
            with Bitôt's spot 264.1
          corneal 264.2
            with corneal ulceration 264.3
    B (complex) NEC 266.9
      with
        beriberi 265.0
        pellagra 265.2
        specified type NEC 266.2
    B_1 NEC 265.1
      beriberi 265.0
    B_2 266.0
    B_6 266.1
    B_{12} 266.2
    B_c (folic acid) 266.2
    C (ascorbic acid) (with scurvy) 267
    D (calciferol) (ergosterol) 268.9
      with
        osteomalacia 268.2
        rickets (*see also* Rickets) 268.0
    E 269.1
    folic acid 266.2
    G 266.0
    H 266.2
    K 269.0
      of newborn 776.0
    nicotinic acid 265.2
    P 269.1
    PP 265.2
    specified NEC 269.1
    zinc 269.3
Deficient —*see also* Deficiency
  blink reflex 374.45
  craniofacial axis 756.0
  number of teeth (*see also* Anodontia) 520.0
  secretion of urine 788.5
Deficit
  neurologic NEC 781.99
    due to
      cerebrovascular lesion (*see also* Disease, cerebrovascular, acute) 436
      late effect—*see* Late effect(s) (of) cerebrovascular disease
      transient ischemic attack 435.9
    ischemic
      reversible (RIND) 434.91
        history of (personal) V12.54
      prolonged (PRIND) 434.91
        history of (personal) V12.54
  oxygen 799.02
Deflection
  radius 736.09
  septum (acquired) (nasal) (nose) 470
  spine—*see* Curvature, spine
  turbinate (nose) 470

INDEX TO DISEASES — Deformity

Defluvium
  capillorum (*see also* Alopecia) 704.00
  ciliorum 374.55
  unguium 703.8
Deformity 738.9
  abdomen, congenital 759.9
  abdominal wall
    acquired 738.8
    congenital 756.70
    muscle deficiency syndrome 756.79
  acquired (unspecified site) 738.9
    specified site NEC 738.8
  adrenal gland (congenital) 759.1
  alimentary tract, congenital 751.9
    lower 751.5
    specified type NEC 751.8
    upper (any part, except tongue) 750.9
      specified type NEC 750.8
      tongue 750.10
        specified type NEC 750.19
  ankle (joint) (acquired) 736.70
    abduction 718.47
    congenital 755.69
    contraction 718.47
    specified NEC 736.79
  anus (congenital) 751.5
    acquired 569.49
  aorta (congenital) 747.20
    acquired 447.8
    arch 747.21
      acquired 447.8
    coarctation 747.10
  aortic
    arch 747.21
      acquired 447.8
    cusp or valve (congenital) 746.9
      acquired (*see also* Endocarditis, aortic) 424.1
    ring 747.21
  appendix 751.5
  arm (acquired) 736.89
    congenital 755.50
  arteriovenous (congenital) (peripheral) NEC 747.60
    gastrointestinal 747.61
    lower limb 747.64
    renal 747.62
    specified NEC 747.69
    spinal 747.82
    upper limb 747.63
  artery (congenital) (peripheral) NEC (*see also* Deformity, vascular) 747.60
    acquired 447.8
    cerebral 747.81
    coronary (congenital) 746.85
      acquired (*see also* Ischemia, heart) 414.9
    retinal 743.9
    umbilical 747.5
  atrial septal (congenital) (heart) 745.5
  auditory canal (congenital) (external) (*see also* Deformity, ear) 744.3
    acquired 380.50
  auricle
    ear (congenital) (*see also* Deformity, ear) 744.3
      acquired 380.32
    heart (congenital) 746.9
  back (acquired)—*see* Deformity, spine
  Bartholin's duct (congenital) 750.9
  bile duct (congenital) 751.60
    acquired 576.8

Deformity—*continued*
    with calculus, choledocholithiasis, or stones—*see* Choledocholithiasis
  biliary duct or passage (congenital) 751.60
    acquired 576.8
    with calculus, choledocholithiasis, or stones—*see* Choledocholithiasis
  bladder (neck) (sphincter) (trigone) (acquired) 596.8
    congenital 753.9
  bone (acquired) NEC 738.9
    congenital 756.9
    turbinate 738.0
  boutonniere (finger) 736.21
  brain (congenital) 742.9
    acquired 348.8
    multiple 742.4
    reduction 742.2
    vessel (congenital) 747.81
  breast (acquired) 611.8
    congenital 757.9
  bronchus (congenital) 748.3
    acquired 519.19
  bursa, congenital 756.9
  canal of Nuck 752.9
  canthus (congenital) 743.9
    acquired 374.89
  capillary (acquired) 448.9
    congenital NEC (*see also* Deformity, vascular) 747.60
  cardiac—*see* Deformity, heart
  cardiovascular system (congenital) 746.9
  caruncle, lacrimal (congenital) 743.9
    acquired 375.69
  cascade, stomach 537.6
  cecum (congenital) 751.5
    acquired 569.89
  cerebral (congenital) 742.9
    acquired 348.8
  cervix (acquired) (uterus) 622.8
    congenital 752.40
  cheek (acquired) 738.19
    congenital 744.9
  chest (wall) (acquired) 738.3
    congenital 754.89
    late effect of rickets 268.1
  chin (acquired) 738.19
    congenital 744.9
  choroid (congenital) 743.9
    acquired 363.8
    plexus (congenital) 742.9
      acquired 349.2
  cicatricial—*see* Cicatrix
  cilia (congenital) 743.9
    acquired 374.89
  circulatory system (congenital) 747.9
  clavicle (acquired) 738.8
    congenital 755.51
  clitoris (congenital) 752.40
    acquired 624.8
  clubfoot—*see* Clubfoot
  coccyx (acquired) 738.6
    congenital 756.10
  colon (congenital) 751.5
    acquired 569.89
  concha (ear) (congenital) (*see also* Deformity, ear) 744.3
    acquired 380.32
  congenital, organ or site not listed (*see also* Anomaly) 759.9

Deformity—*continued*
  cornea (congenital) 743.9
    acquired 371.70
  coronary artery (congenital) 746.85
    acquired (*see also* Ischemia, heart) 414.9
  cranium (acquired) 738.19
    congenital (*see also* Deformity, skull,
      congenital) 756.0
  cricoid cartilage (congenital) 748.3
    acquired 478.79
  cystic duct (congenital) 751.60
    acquired 575.8
  Dandy-Walker 742.3
    with spina bifida (*see also* Spina bifida) 741.0
  diaphragm (congenital) 756.6
    acquired 738.8
  digestive organ(s) or system (congenital) NEC
    751.9
    specified type NEC 751.8
  ductus arteriosus 747.0
  duodenal bulb 537.89
  duodenum (congenital) 751.5
    acquired 537.89
  dura (congenital) 742.9
    brain 742.4
      acquired 349.2
    spinal 742.59
      acquired 349.2
  ear (congenital) 744.3
    acquired 380.32
    auricle 744.3
      causing impairment of hearing 744.02
    causing impairment of hearing 744.00
    external 744.3
      causing impairment of hearing 744.02
    internal 744.05
    lobule 744.3
    middle 744.03
      ossicles 744.04
    ossicles 744.04
  ectodermal (congenital) NEC 757.9
    specified type NEC 757.8
  ejaculatory duct (congenital) 752.9
    acquired 608.89
  elbow (joint) (acquired) 736.00
    congenital 755.50
    contraction 718.42
  endocrine gland NEC 759.2
  epididymis (congenital) 752.9
    acquired 608.89
    torsion 608.24
  epiglottis (congenital) 748.3
    acquired 478.79
  esophagus (congenital) 750.9
    acquired 530.89
  Eustachian tube (congenital) NEC 744.3
    specified type NEC 744.24
  extremity (acquired) 736.9
    congenital, except reduction deformity 755.9
      lower 755.60
      upper 755.50
    reduction—*see* Deformity, reduction
  eye (congenital) 743.9
    acquired 379.8
    muscle 743.9
  eyebrow (congenital) 744.89
  eyelid (congenital) 743.9
    acquired 374.89
    specified type NEC 743.62
  face (acquired) 738.19
    congenital (any part) 744.9

Deformity—*continued*
  due to intrauterine malposition and pressure
    754.0
  fallopian tube (congenital) 752.10
    acquired 620.8
  femur (acquired) 736.89
    congenital 755.60
  fetal
    with fetopelvic disproportion 653.7
      affecting fetus or newborn 763.1
    causing obstructed labor 660.1
      affecting fetus or newborn 763.1
    known or suspected, affecting management of
      pregnancy 655.9
  finger (acquired) 736.20
    boutonniere type 736.21
    congenital 755.50
    flexion contracture 718.44
    swan neck 736.22
  flexion (joint) (acquired) 736.9
    congenital NEC 755.9
    hip or thigh (acquired) 736.39
      congenital (*see also* Subluxation, congenital,
        hip) 754.32
  foot (acquired) 736.70
    cavovarus 736.75
      congenital 754.59
    congenital NEC 754.70
      specified type NEC 754.79
    valgus (acquired) 736.79
      congenital 754.60
        specified type NEC 754.69
    varus (acquired) 736.79
      congenital 754.50
        specified type NEC 754.59
  forearm (acquired) 736.00
    congenital 755.50
  forehead (acquired) 738.19
    congenital (*see also* Deformity, skull,
      congenital) 756.0
  frontal bone (acquired) 738.19
    congenital (*see also* Deformity, skull,
      congenital) 756.0
  gallbladder (congenital) 751.60
    acquired 575.8
  gastrointestinal tract (congenital) NEC 751.9
    acquired 569.89
    specified type NEC 751.8
  genitalia, genital organ(s) or system NEC
    congenital 752.9
    female (congenital) 752.9
      acquired 629.89
      external 752.40
      internal 752.9
    male (congenital) 752.9
      acquired 608.89
  globe (eye) (congenital) 743.9
    acquired 360.89
  gum (congenital) 750.9
    acquired 523.9
  gunstock 736.02
  hand (acquired) 736.00
    claw 736.06
    congenital 755.50
    minus (and plus) (intrinsic) 736.09
    pill roller (intrinsic) 736.09
    plus (and minus) (intrinsic) 736.09
    swan neck (intrinsic) 736.09
  head (acquired) 738.10
    congenital (*see also* Deformity, skull,
      congenital) 756.0

INDEX TO DISEASES

Deformity—*continued*
  specified NEC 738.19
  heart (congenital) 746.9
    auricle (congenital) 746.9
    septum 745.9
      auricular 745.5
      specified type NEC 745.8
      ventricular 745.4
    valve (congenital) NEC 746.9
      acquired—*see* Endocarditis
      pulmonary (congenital) 746.00
      specified type NEC 746.89
    ventricle (congenital) 746.9
  heel (acquired) 736.76
    congenital 755.67
  hepatic duct (congenital) 751.60
    acquired 576.8
      with calculus, choledocholithiasis, or
        stones—*see* Choledocholithiasis
  hip (joint) (acquired) 736.30
    congenital NEC 755.63
    flexion 718.45
      congenital (*see also* Subluxation, congenital, hip) 754.32
  hourglass—*see* Contraction, hourglass
  humerus (acquired) 736.89
    congenital 755.50
  hymen (congenital) 752.40
  hypophyseal (congenital) 759.2
  ileocecal (coil) (valve) (congenital) 751.5
    acquired 569.89
  ileum (intestine) (congenital) 751.5
    acquired 569.89
  ilium (acquired) 738.6
    congenital 755.60
  integument (congenital) 757.9
  intervertebral cartilage or disc (acquired)—*see also* Displacement, intervertebral disc
    congenital 756.10
  intestine (large) (small) (congenital) 751.5
    acquired 569.89
  iris (acquired) 364.75
    congenital 743.9
    prolapse 364.89
  ischium (acquired) 738.6
    congenital 755.60
  jaw (acquired) (congenital) NEC 524.9
    due to intrauterine malposition and pressure 754.0
  joint (acquired) NEC 738.8
    congenital 755.9
    contraction (abduction) (adduction) (extension) (flexion)—*see* Contraction, joint
  kidney(s) (calyx) (pelvis) (congenital) 753.9
    acquired 593.89
    vessel 747.62
      acquired 459.9
  Klippel-Feil (brevicollis) 756.16
  knee (acquired) NEC 736.6
    congenital 755.64
  labium (majus) (minus) (congenital) 752.40
    acquired 624.8
  lacrimal apparatus or duct (congenital) 743.9
    acquired 375.69
  larynx (muscle) (congenital) 748.3
    acquired 478.79
    web (glottic) (subglottic) 748.2
  leg (lower) (upper) (acquired) NEC 736.89
    congenital 755.60
    reduction—*see* Deformity, reduction, lower limb

Deformity—*continued*
  lens (congenital) 743.9
    acquired 379.39
  lid (fold) (congenital) 743.9
    acquired 374.89
  ligament (acquired) 728.9
    congenital 756.9
  limb (acquired) 736.9
    congenital, except reduction deformity 755.9
      lower 755.60
        reduction (*see also* Deformity, reduction, lower limb) 755.30
      upper 755.50
        reduction (*see also* Deformity, reduction, lower limb) 755.20
    specified NEC 736.89
  lip (congenital) NEC 750.9
    acquired 528.5
    specified type NEC 750.26
  liver (congenital) 751.60
    acquired 573.8
    duct (congenital) 751.60
      acquired 576.8
        with calculus, choledocholithiasis, or
          stones—*see* Choledocholithiasis
  lower extremity—*see* Deformity, leg
  lumbosacral (joint) (region) (congenital) 756.10
    acquired 738.5
  lung (congenital) 748.60
    acquired 518.89
    specified type NEC 748.69
  lymphatic system, congenital 759.9
  Madelung's (radius) 755.54
  maxilla (acquired) (congenital) 524.9
  meninges or membrane (congenital) 742.9
    brain 742.4
      acquired 349.2
    spinal (cord) 742.59
      acquired 349.2
  mesentery (congenital) 751.9
    acquired 568.89
  metacarpus (acquired) 736.00
    congenital 755.50
  metatarsus (acquired) 736.70
    congenital 754.70
  middle ear, except ossicles (congenital) 744.03
    ossicles 744.04
  mitral (leaflets) (valve) (congenital) 746.9
    acquired—*see* Endocarditis, mitral
    Ebstein's 746.89
    parachute 746.5
    specified type NEC 746.89
    stenosis, congenital 746.5
  mouth (acquired) 528.9
    congenital NEC 750.9
      specified type NEC 750.26
  multiple, congenital NEC 759.7
    specified type NEC 759.89
  muscle (acquired) 728.9
    congenital 756.9
      specified type NEC 756.89
      sternocleidomastoid (due to intrauterine malposition and pressure) 754.1
  musculoskeletal system, congenital NEC 756.9
    specified type NEC 756.9
  nail (acquired) 703.9
    congenital 757.9
  nasal—*see* Deformity, nose
  neck (acquired) NEC 738.2
    congenital (any part) 744.9
      sternocleidomastoid 754.1

Deformity—*continued*
  nervous system (congenital) 742.9
  nipple (congenital) 757.9
    acquired 611.8
  nose, nasal (cartilage) (acquired) 738.0
    bone (turbinate) 738.0
    congenital 748.1
      bent 754.0
      squashed 754.0
    saddle 738.0
      syphilitic 090.5
    septum 470
      congenital 748.1
    sinus (wall) (congenital) 748.1
      acquired 738.0
    syphilitic (congenital) 090.5
      late 095.8
  ocular muscle (congenital) 743.9
    acquired 378.60
  opticociliary vessels (congenital) 743.9
  orbit (congenital) (eye) 743.9
    acquired NEC 376.40
      associated with craniofacial deformities 376.44
      due to
        bone disease 376.43
        surgery 376.47
        trauma 376.47
  organ of Corti (congenital) 744.05
  ovary (congenital) 752.0
    acquired 620.8
  oviduct (congenital) 752.10
    acquired 620.8
  palate (congenital) 750.9
    acquired 526.89
    cleft (congenital) (*see also* Cleft, palate) 749.00
    hard, acquired 526.89
    soft, acquired 528.9
  pancreas (congenital) 751.7
    acquired 577.8
  parachute, mitral valve 746.5
  parathyroid (gland) 759.2
  parotid (gland) (congenital) 750.9
    acquired 527.8
  patella (acquired) 736.6
    congenital 755.64
  pelvis, pelvic (acquired) (bony) 738.6
    with disproportion (fetopelvic) 653.0
      affecting fetus or newborn 763.1
      causing obstructed labor 660.1
        affecting fetus or newborn 763.1
    congenital 755.60
    rachitic (late effect) 268.1
  penis (glans) (congenital) 752.9
    acquired 607.89
  pericardium (congenital) 746.9
    acquired—*see* Pericarditis
  pharynx (congenital) 750.9
    acquired 478.29
  Pierre Robin (congenital) 756.0
  pinna (acquired) 380.32
    congenital 744.3
  pituitary (congenital) 759.2
  pleural folds (congenital) 748.8
  portal vein (congenital) 747.40
  posture—*see* Curvature, spine
  prepuce (congenital) 752.9
    acquired 607.89
  prostate (congenital) 752.9
    acquired 602.8

Deformity—*continued*
  pulmonary valve—*see* Endocarditis, pulmonary
  pupil (congenital) 743.9
    acquired 364.75
  pylorus (congenital) 750.9
    acquired 537.89
  rachitic (acquired), healed or old 268.1
  radius (acquired) 736.00
    congenital 755.50
    reduction—*see* Deformity, reduction, upper limb
  rectovaginal septum (congenital) 752.40
    acquired 623.8
  rectum (congenital) 751.5
    acquired 569.49
  reduction (extremity) (limb) 755.4
    brain 742.2
    lower limb 755.30
      with complete absence of distal elements 755.31
      longitudinal (complete) (partial) (with distal deficiencies, incomplete) 755.32
        with complete absence of distal elements 755.31
        combined femoral, tibial, fibular (incomplete) 755.33
        femoral 755.34
        fibular 755.37
        metatarsal(s) 755.38
        phalange(s) 755.39
          meaning all digits 755.31
        tarsal(s) 755.38
        tibia 755.36
        tibiofibular 755.35
      transverse 755.31
    upper limb 755.20
      with complete absence of distal elements 755.21
      longitudinal (complete) (partial) (with distal deficiencies, incomplete) 755.22
        with complete absence of distal elements 755.21
        carpal(s) 755.28
        combined humeral, radial, ulnar (incomplete) 755.23
        humeral 755.24
        metacarpal(s) 755.28
        phalange(s) 755.29
          meaning all digits 755.21
        radial 755.26
        radioulnar 755.25
        ulnar 755.27
      transverse (complete) (partial) 755.21
  renal—*see* Deformity, kidney
  respiratory system (congenital) 748.9
    specified type NEC 748.8
  rib (acquired) 738.3
    congenital 756.3
    cervical 756.2
  rotation (joint) (acquired) 736.9
    congenital 755.9
    hip or thigh 736.39
      congenital (*see also* Subluxation, congenital, hip) 754.32
  sacroiliac joint (congenital) 755.69
    acquired 738.5
  sacrum (acquired) 738.5
    congenital 756.10
  saddle
    back 737.8
    nose 738.0
      syphilitic 090.5

INDEX TO DISEASES

Deformity

Deformity—continued
- salivary gland or duct (congenital) 750.9
  - acquired 527.8
- scapula (acquired) 736.89
  - congenital 755.50
- scrotum (congenital) 752.9
  - acquired 608.89
- sebaceous gland, acquired 706.8
- seminal tract or duct (congenital) 752.9
  - acquired 608.89
- septum (nasal) (acquired) 470
  - congenital 748.1
- shoulder (joint) (acquired) 736.89
  - congenital 755.50
    - specified type NEC 755.59
  - contraction 718.41
- sigmoid (flexure) (congenital) 751.5
  - acquired 569.89
- sinus of Valsalva 747.29
- skin (congenital) 757.9
  - acquired NEC 709.8
- skull (acquired) 738.19
  - congenital 756.0
    - with
      - anencephalus 740.0
      - encephalocele 742.0
      - hydrocephalus 742.3
        - with spina bifida (*see also* Spina bifida) 741.0
      - microcephalus 742.1
    - due to intrauterine malposition and pressure 754.0
- soft parts, organs or tissues (of pelvis)
  - in pregnancy or childbirth NEC 654.9
    - affecting fetus or newborn 763.89
    - causing obstructed labor 660.2
      - affecting fetus or newborn 763.1
- spermatic cord (congenital) 752.9
  - acquired 608.89
    - torsion 608.22
      - extravaginal 608.21
      - intravaginal 608.22
- spinal
  - column—*see* Deformity, spine
  - cord (congenital) 742.9
    - acquired 336.8
    - vessel (congenital) 747.82
  - nerve root (congenital) 742.9
    - acquired 724.9
  - vessel 747.82
- spine (acquired) NEC 738.5
  - congenital 756.10
    - due to intrauterine malposition and pressure 754.2
  - kyphoscoliotic (*see also* Kyphoscoliosis) 737.30
  - kyphotic (*see also* Kyphosis) 737.10
  - lordotic (*see also* Lordosis) 737.20
  - rachitic 268.1
  - scoliotic (*see also* Scoliosis) 737.30
- spleen
  - acquired 289.59
  - congenital 759.0
- Sprengel's (congenital) 755.52
- sternum (acquired) 738.3
  - congenital 756.3
- stomach (congenital) 750.9
  - acquired 537.89
- submaxillary gland (congenital) 750.9
  - acquired 527.8

Deformity—continued
- swan neck (acquired)
  - finger 736.22
  - hand 736.09
- talipes—*see* Talipes
- teeth, tooth NEC 520.9
- testis (congenital) 752.9
  - acquired 608.89
    - torsion 608.20
- thigh (acquired) 736.89
  - congenital 755.60
- thorax (acquired) (wall) 738.3
  - congenital 754.89
  - late effect of rickets 268.1
- thumb (acquired) 736.20
  - congenital 755.50
- thymus (tissue) (congenital) 759.2
- thyroid (gland) (congenital) 759.2
  - cartilage 748.3
    - acquired 478.79
- tibia (acquired) 736.89
  - congenital 755.60
  - saber 090.5
- toe (acquired) 735.9
  - congenital 755.66
  - specified NEC 735.8
- tongue (congenital) 750.10
  - acquired 529.8
- tooth, teeth NEC 520.9
- trachea (rings) (congenital) 748.3
  - acquired 519.19
- transverse aortic arch (congenital) 747.21
- tricuspid (leaflets) (valve) (congenital) 746.9
  - acquired—*see* Endocarditis, tricuspid
  - atresia or stenosis 746.1
  - specified type NEC 746.89
- trunk (acquired) 738.3
  - congenital 759.9
- ulna (acquired) 736.00
  - congenital 755.50
- upper extremity—*see* Deformity, arm
- urachus (congenital) 753.7
- ureter (opening) (congenital) 753.9
  - acquired 593.89
- urethra (valve) (congenital) 753.9
  - acquired 599.84
- urinary tract or system (congenital) 753.9
  - urachus 753.7
- uterus (congenital) 752.3
  - acquired 621.8
- uvula (congenital) 750.9
  - acquired 528.9
- vagina (congenital) 752.40
  - acquired 623.8
- valve, valvular (heart) (congenital) 746.9
  - acquired—*see* Endocarditis
  - pulmonary 746.00
  - specified type NEC 746.89
- vascular (congenital) (peripheral) NEC 747.60
  - acquired 459.9
  - gastrointestinal 747.61
  - lower limb 747.64
  - renal 747.62
  - specified site NEC 747.69
  - spinal 747.82
  - upper limb 747.63
- vas deferens (congenital) 752.9
  - acquired 608.89

Deformity—*continued*
  vein (congenital) NEC (*see also* Deformity, vascular) 747.60
    brain 747.81
    coronary 746.9
    great 747.40
  vena cava (inferior) (superior) (congenital) 747.40
  vertebra—*see* Deformity, spine
  vesicourethral orifice (acquired) 596.8
    congenital NEC 753.9
      specified type NEC 753.8
  vessels of optic papilla (congenital) 743.9
  visual field (contraction) 368.45
  vitreous humor (congenital) 743.9
    acquired 379.29
  vulva (congenital) 752.40
    acquired 624.8
  wrist (joint) (acquired) 736.00
    congenital 755.50
    contraction 718.43
    valgus 736.03
      congenital 755.59
    varus 736.04
      congenital 755.59
Degeneration, degenerative
  adrenal (capsule) (gland) 255.8
    with hypofunction 255.41
    fatty 255.8
    hyaline 255.8
    infectional 255.8
    lardaceous 277.39
  amyloid (any site) (general) 277.39
  anterior cornua, spinal cord 336.8
  aorta, aortic 440.0
    fatty 447.8
    valve (heart) (*see also* Endocarditis, aortic) 424.1
  arteriovascular—*see* Arteriosclerosis
  artery, arterial (atheromatous) (calcareous)—*see also* Arteriosclerosis
    amyloid 277.39
    lardaceous 277.39
    medial NEC (*see also* Arteriosclerosis, extremities) 440.20
  articular cartilage NEC (*see also* Disorder, cartilage, articular) 718.0
    elbow 718.02
    knee 717.5
    patella 717.7
    shoulder 718.01
    spine (*see also* Spondylosis) 721.90
  atheromatous—*see* Arteriosclerosis
  bacony (any site) 277.39
  basal nuclei or ganglia NEC 333.0
  bone 733.90
  brachial plexus 353.0
  brain (cortical) (progressive) 331.9
    arteriosclerotic 437.0
    childhood 330.9
      specified type NEC 330.8
    congenital 742.4
    cystic 348.0
      congenital 742.4
    familial NEC 331.89
    grey matter 330.8
    heredofamilial NEC 331.89
    in
      alcoholism 303.9 *[331.7]*
      beriberi 265.0 *[331.7]*
      cerebrovascular disease 437.9 *[331.7]*

Degeneration, degenerative—*continued*
    congenital hydrocephalus 742.3 *[331.7]*
      with spina bifida (*see also* Spina bifida) 741.0 *[331.7]*
    Fabry's disease 272.7 *[330.2]*
    Gaucher's disease 272.7 *[330.2]*
    Hunter's disease or syndrome 277.5 *[330.3]*
    lipidosis
      cerebral 330.1
      generalized 272.7 *[330.2]*
    mucopolysaccharidosis 277.5 *[330.3]*
    myxedema (*see also* Myxedema) 244.9 *[331.7]*
    neoplastic disease NEC (M8000/1) 239.9 *[331.7]*
    Niemann-Pick disease 272.7 *[330.2]*
    sphingolipidosis 272.7 *[330.2]*
    vitamin B_{12} deficiency 266.2 *[331.7]*
  motor centers 331.89
  senile 331.2
    specified type NEC 331.89
  breast—*see* Disease, breast
  Bruch's membrane 363.40
  bundle of His 426.50
    left 426.3
    right 426.4
  calcareous NEC 275.49
  capillaries 448.9
    amyloid 277.39
    fatty 448.9
    lardaceous 277.39
  cardiac (brown) (calcareous) (fatty) (fibrous) (hyaline) (mural) (muscular) (pigmentary) (senile) (with arteriosclerosis) (*see also* Degeneration, myocardial) 429.1
    valve, valvular—*see* Endocarditis
  cardiorenal (*see also* Hypertension, cardiorenal) 404.90
  cardiovascular (*see also* Disease, cardiovascular) 429.2
    renal (*see also* Hypertension, cardiorenal) 404.90
  cartilage (joint)—*see* Derangement, joint
  cerebellar NEC 334.9
    primary (hereditary) (sporadic) 334.2
  cerebral—*see* Degeneration, brain
  cerebromacular 330.1
  cerebrovascular 437.1
    due to hypertension 437.2
    late effect—*see* Late effect(s) (of) cerebrovascular disease
  cervical plexus 353.2
  cervix 622.8
    due to radiation (intended effect) 622.8
      adverse effect or misadventure 622.8
  changes, spine or vertebra (*see also* Spondylosis) 721.90
  chitinous 277.39
  chorioretinal 363.40
    congenital 743.53
    hereditary 363.50
  choroid (colloid) (drusen) 363.40
    hereditary 363.50
    senile 363.41
      diffuse secondary 363.42
  cochlear 386.8
  collateral ligament (knee) (medial) 717.82
    lateral 717.81
  combined (spinal cord) (subacute) 266.2 *[336.2]*
    with anemia (pernicious) 281.0 *[336.2]*
      due to dietary deficiency 281.1 *[336.2]*

INDEX TO DISEASES

Degeneration, degenerative—*continued*
  due to vitamin B$_{12}$ deficiency anemia (dietary) 281.1 *[336.2]*
  conjunctiva 372.50
    amyloid 277.39 *[372.50]*
  cornea 371.40
    calcerous 371.44
    familial (hereditary) (*see also* Dystrophy, cornea) 371.50
      macular 371.55
      reticular 371.54
    hyaline (of old scars) 371.41
    marginal (Terrien's) 371.48
    mosaic (shagreen) 371.41
    nodular 371.46
    peripheral 371.48
    senile 371.41
  cortical (cerebellar) (parenchymatous) 334.2
    alcoholic 303.9 *[334.4]*
    diffuse, due to arteriopathy 437.0
  corticostriatal-spinal 334.8
  cretinoid 243
  cruciate ligament (knee) (posterior) 717.84
    anterior 717.83
  cutis 709.3
    amyloid 277.39
  dental pulp 522.2
  disc disease—*see* Degeneration, intervertebral disc
  dorsolateral (spinal cord)—*see* Degeneration, combined
  endocardial 424.90
  extrapyramidal NEC 333.90
  eye NEC 360.40
    macular (*see also* Degeneration, macula) 362.50
      congenital 362.75
      hereditary 362.76
  fatty (diffuse) (general) 272.8
    liver 571.8
      alcoholic 571.0
    localized site—*see* Degeneration, by site, fatty
    placenta—*see* Placenta, abnormal
  globe (eye) NEC 360.40
    macular—*see* Degeneration, macula
  grey matter 330.8
  heart (brown) (calcareous) (fatty) (fibrous) (hyaline) (mural) (muscular) (pigmentary) (senile) (with arteriosclerosis) (*see also* Degeneration, myocardial) 429.1
    amyloid 277.39 *[425.7]*
    atheromatous—*see* Arteriosclerosis, coronary
    gouty 274.82
    hypertensive (*see also* Hypertension, heart) 402.90
    ischemic 414.9
    valve, valvular—*see* Endocarditis
  hepatolenticular (Wilson's) 275.1
  hepatorenal 572.4
  heredofamilial
    brain NEC 331.89
    spinal cord NEC 336.8
  hyaline (diffuse) (generalized) 728.9
    localized—*see also* Degeneration, by site
      cornea 371.41
      keratitis 371.41
  hypertensive vascular—*see* Hypertension
  infrapatellar fat pad 729.31
  internal semilunar cartilage 717.3
  intervertebral disc 722.6
    with myelopathy 722.70
    cervical, cervicothoracic 722.4

Degeneration, degenerative—*continued*
    with myelopathy 722.71
    lumbar, lumbosacral 722.52
      with myelopathy 722.73
    thoracic, thoracolumbar 722.51
      with myelopathy 722.72
  intestine 569.89
    amyloid 277.39
    lardaceous 277.39
  iris (generalized) (*see also* Atrophy, iris) 364.59
    pigmentary 364.53
    pupillary margin 364.54
  ischemic—*see* Ischemia
  joint disease (*see also* Osteoarthrosis) 715.9
    multiple sites 715.09
    spine (*see also* Spondylosis) 721.90
  kidney (*see also* Sclerosis, renal) 587
    amyloid 277.39 *[583.81]*
    cyst, cystic (multiple) (solitary) 593.2
      congenital (*see also* Cystic, disease, kidney) 753.10
    fatty 593.89
    fibrocystic (congenital) 753.19
    lardaceous 277.39 *[583.81]*
    polycystic (congenital) 753.12
      adult type (APKD) 753.13
      autosomal dominant 753.13
      autosomal recessive 753.14
      childhood type (CPKD) 753.14
      infantile type 753.14
    waxy 277.39 *[583.81]*
  Kuhnt-Junius (retina) 362.52
  labyrinth, osseous 386.8
  lacrimal passages, cystic 375.12
  lardaceous (any site) 277.39
  lateral column (posterior), spinal cord (*see also* Degeneration, combined) 266.2 *[336.2]*
  lattice 362.63
  lens 366.9
    infantile, juvenile, or presenile 366.00
    senile 366.10
  lenticular (familial) (progressive) (Wilson's) (with cirrhosis of liver) 275.1
    striate artery 437.0
  lethal ball, prosthetic heart valve 996.02
  ligament
    collateral (knee) (medial) 717.82
      lateral 717.81
    cruciate (knee) (posterior) 717.84
      anterior 717.83
  liver (diffuse) 572.8
    amyloid 277.39
    congenital (cystic) 751.62
    cystic 572.8
      congenital 751.62
    fatty 571.8
      alcoholic 571.0
    hypertrophic 572.8
    lardaceous 277.39
    parenchymatous, acute or subacute (*see also* Necrosis, liver) 570
    pigmentary 572.8
    toxic (acute) 573.8
    waxy 277.39
  lung 518.8
  lymph gland 289.3
    hyaline 289.3
    lardaceous 277.39
  macula (acquired) (senile) 362.50
    atrophic 362.51
    Best's 362.76

Degeneration, degenerative—*continued*
   congenital 362.75
   cystic 362.54
   cystoid 362.53
   disciform 362.52
   dry 362.51
   exudative 362.52
   familial pseudoinflammatory 362.77
   hereditary 362.76
   hole 362.54
   juvenile (Stargardt's) 362.75
   nonexudative 362.51
   pseudohole 362.54
   wet 362.52
  medullary—*see* Degeneration, brain
  membranous labyrinth, congenital (causing impairment of hearing) 744.05
  meniscus—*see* Derangement, joint
  microcystoid 362.62
  mitral—*see* Insufficiency, mitral
  Mönckeberg's (*see also* Arteriosclerosis, extremities) 440.20
  moral 301.7
  motor centers, senile 331.2
  mural (*see also* Degeneration, myocardial) 429.1
   heart, cardiac (*see also* Degeneration, myocardium) 429.1
   myocardium, myocardial (*see also* Degeneration, myocardial) 429.1
  muscle 728.9
   fatty 728.9
   fibrous 728.9
   heart (*see also* Degeneration, myocardial) 429.1
   hyaline 728.9
  muscular progressive 728.2
  myelin, central nervous system NEC 341.9
  myocardium, myocardial (brown) (calcareous) (fatty) (fibrous) (hyaline) (mural) (muscular) (pigmentary) (senile) (with arteriosclerosis) 429.1
   with rheumatic fever (conditions classifiable to 390) 398.0
    active, acute, or subacute 391.2
     with chorea 392.0
    inactive or quiescent (with chorea) 398.0
   amyloid 277.39 *[425.7]*
   congenital 746.89
   fetus or newborn 779.89
   gouty 274.82
   hypertensive (*see also* Hypertension, heart) 402.90
   ischemic 414.8
   rheumatic (*see also* Degeneration, myocardium, with rheumatic fever) 398.0
   syphilitic 093.82
  nasal sinus (mucosa) (*see also* Sinusitis) 473.9
   frontal 473.1
   maxillary 473.0
  nerve—*see* Disorder, nerve
  nervous system 349.89
   amyloid 277.39 *[357.4]*
   autonomic (*see also* Neuropathy, peripheral, autonomic) 337.9
   fatty 349.89
   peripheral autonomic NEC (*see also* Neuropathy, peripheral, autonomic) 337.9
  nipple 611.9
  nose 478.19
  oculoacoustiocerebral, congenital (progressive) 743.8

Degeneration, degenerative—*continued*
  olivopontocerebellar (familial) (hereditary) 333.0
  osseous labyrinth 386.8
  ovary 620.8
   cystic 620.2
   microcystic 620.2
  pallidal, pigmentary (progressive) 333.0
  pancreas 577.8
   tuberculous (*see also* Tuberculosis) 017.9
  papillary muscle 429.81
  paving stone 362.61
  penis 607.89
  peritoneum 568.89
  pigmentary (diffuse) (general)
   localized—*see* Degeneration, by site
   pallidal (progressive) 333.0
   secondary 362.65
  pineal gland 259.8
  pituitary (gland) 253.8
  placenta (fatty) (fibrinoid) (fibroid)—*see* Placenta, abnormal
  popliteal fat pad 729.31
  posterolateral (spinal cord) (*see also* Degeneration, combined) 266.2 *[336.2]*
  pulmonary valve (heart) (*see also* Endocarditis, pulmonary) 424.3
  pulp (tooth) 522.2
  pupillary margin 364.54
  renal (*see also* Sclerosis, renal) 587
   fibrocystic 753.19
   polycystic 753.12
    adult type (APKD) 753.13
    autosomal dominant 753.13
    autosomal recessive 753.14
    childhood type (CPKD) 753.14
    infantile type 753.14
  reticuloendothelial system 289.89
  retina (peripheral) 362.60
   with retinal defect (*see also* Detachment, retina, with retinal defect) 361.00
   cystic (senile) 362.50
   cystoid 362.53
   hereditary (*see also* Dystrophy, retina) 362.70
    cerebroretinal 362.71
    congenital 362.75
    juvenile (Stargardt's) 362.75
    macula 362.76
   Kuhnt-Junius 362.52
   lattice 362.63
   macular (*see also* Degeneration, macula) 362.50
   microcystoid 362.62
   palisade 362.63
   paving stone 362.61
   pigmentary (primary) 362.74
    secondary 362.65
   posterior pole (*see also* Degeneration, macula) 362.50
   secondary 362.66
   senile 362.60
    cystic 362.53
    reticular 362.64
  saccule, congenital (causing impairment of hearing) 744.05
  sacculocochlear 386.8
  senile 797
   brain 331.2
   cardiac, heart, or myocardium (*see also* Degeneration, myocardial) 429.1
   motor centers 331.2

Degeneration, degenerative—*continued*
  reticule 362.64
  retina, cystic 362.50
  vascular—*see* Arteriosclerosis
  silicone rubber poppet (prosthetic valve) 996.02
  sinus (cystic) (*see also* Sinusitis) 473.9
    polypoid 471.1
  skin 709.3
    amyloid 277.39
    colloid 709.3
  spinal (cord) 336.8
    amyloid 277.39
    column 733.90
    combined (subacute) (*see also* Degeneration, combined) 266.2 *[336.2]*
      with anemia (pernicious) 281.0 *[336.2]*
    dorsolateral (*see also* Degeneration, combined) 266.2 *[336.2]*
    familial NEC 336.8
    fatty 336.8
    funicular (*see also* Degeneration, combined) 266.2 *[336.2]*
    heredofamilial NEC 336.8
    posterolateral (*see also* Degeneration, combined) 266.2 *[336.2]*
    subacute combined—*see* Degeneration, combined
    tuberculous (*see also* Tuberculosis) 013.8
  spine 733.90
  spleen 289.59
    amyloid 277.39
    lardaceous 277.39
  stomach 537.89
    lardaceous 277.39
  strionigral 333.0
  sudoriparous (cystic) 705.89
  suprarenal (capsule) (gland) 255.8
    with hypofunction 255.41
  sweat gland 705.89
  synovial membrane (pulpy) 727.9
  tapetoretinal 362.74
    adult or presenile form 362.50
  testis (postinfectional) 608.89
  thymus (gland) 254.8
    fatty 254.8
    lardaceous 277.39
  thyroid (gland) 246.8
  tricuspid (heart) (valve)—*see* Endocarditis, tricuspid
  tuberculous NEC (*see also* Tuberculosis) 011.9
  turbinate 733.90
  uterus 621.8
    cystic 621.8
  vascular (senile)—*see also* Arteriosclerosis
    hypertensive—*see* Hypertension
  vitreoretinal (primary) 362.73
    secondary 362.66
  vitreous humor (with infiltration) 379.21
  wallerian NEC—*see* Disorder, nerve
  waxy (any site) 277.39
  Wilson's hepatolenticular 275.1
Deglutition
  paralysis 784.99
    hysterical 300.11
  pneumonia 507.0
Degos' disease or syndrome 447.8
Degradation disorder, branched-chain amino-acid 270.3
Dehiscence
  anastomosis—*see* Complications, anastomosis
  cesarean wound 674.1

Dehiscence—*continued*
  episiotomy 674.2
  operation wound 998.32
    internal 998.31
  perineal wound (postpartum) 674.2
  postoperative 998.32
    abdomen 998.32
      internal 998.31
    internal 998.31
  uterine wound 674.1
Dehydration (cachexia) 276.51
  newborn 775.5
  with
    hypernatremia 276.0
    hyponatremia 276.1
Deiters' nucleus syndrome 386.19
Déjérine's disease 356.0
Déjérine-Klumpke paralysis 767.6
Déjérine-Roussy syndrome 338.0
Déjérine-Sottas disease or neuropathy (hypertrophic) 356.0
Déjérine-Thomas atrophy or syndrome 333.0
de Lange's syndrome (Amsterdam dwarf, mental retardation, and brachycephaly) 759.89
Delay, delayed
  adaptation, cones or rods 368.63
  any plane in pelvis
    affecting fetus or newborn 763.1
    complicating delivery 660.1
  birth or delivery NEC 662.1
    affecting fetus or newborn 763.9
    second twin, triplet, or multiple mate 662.3
  closure—*see also* Fistula
    cranial suture 756.0
    fontanel 756.0
  coagulation NEC 790.92
  conduction (cardiac) (ventricular) 426.9
  delivery NEC 662.1
    second twin, triplet, etc. 662.3
      affecting fetus or newborn 763.89
  development
    in childhood 783.40
      physiological 783.40
    intellectual NEC 315.9
    learning NEC 315.2
    reading 315.00
    sexual 259.0
    speech 315.39
      and language due to hearing loss 315.34
      associated with hyperkinesis 314.1
    spelling 315.09
  gastric emptying 536.8
  menarche 256.39
    due to pituitary hypofunction 253.4
  menstruation (cause unknown) 626.8
  milestone in childhood 783.42
  motility—*see* Hypomotility
  passage of meconium (newborn) 777.1
  primary respiration 768.9
  puberty 259.0
  separation of umbilical cord 779.83
  sexual maturation, female 259.0
Del Castillo's syndrome (germinal aplasia) 606.0
Deleage's disease 359.89
Deletion syndrome
  5p 758.31
  22q11.2 758.32
  autosomal NEC 758.39
  constitutional 5q deletion 758.39
Delhi (boil) (button) (sore) 085.1

Delinquency (juvenile) 312.9
　group (*see also* Disturbance, conduct) 312.2
　neurotic 312.4
Delirium, delirious 780.09
　acute (psychotic) 293.0
　alcoholic 291.0
　　acute 291.0
　　chronic 291.1
　alcoholicum 291.0
　chronic (*see also* Psychosis) 293.89
　　due to or associated with physical
　　　condition—*see* Psychosis, organic
　due to conditions classified elsewhere 293.0
　drug-induced 292.81
　eclamptic (*see also* Eclampsia) 780.39
　exhaustion (*see also* Reaction, stress, acute)
　　　308.9
　hysterical 300.11
　in
　　presenile dementia 290.11
　　senile dementia 290.3
　induced by drug 292.81
　manic, maniacal (acute) (*see also* Psychosis,
　　　affective) 296.0
　　recurrent episode 296.1
　　single episode 296.0
　puerperal 293.9
　senile 290.3
　subacute (psychotic) 293.1
　thyroid (*see also* Thyrotoxicosis) 242.9
　traumatic—*see also* Injury, intracranial
　　with
　　　lesion, spinal cord—*see* Injury, spinal, by
　　　　site
　　　shock, spinal—*see* Injury, spinal, by site
　tremens (impending) 291.0
　uremic—*see* Uremia
　withdrawal
　　alcoholic (acute) 291.0
　　　chronic 291.1
　　drug 292.0
Delivery

> Note—Use the following fifth-digit
> subclassification with categories
> 640-648, 651-676:
>
> 0　unspecified as to episode of care
> 1　delivered, with or without mention of
> 　　antepartum condition
> 2　delivered, with mention of
> 　　postpartum complication
> 3　antepartum condition or complication
> 4　postpartum condition or
> 　　complication

　breech (assisted) (spontaneous) 652.2
　　affecting fetus or newborn 763.0
　　extraction NEC 669.6
　cesarean (for) 669.7
　　abnormal
　　　cervix 654.6
　　　pelvic organs or tissues 654.9
　　　pelvis (bony) (major) NEC 653.0
　　　presentation or position 652.9
　　　　in multiple gestation 652.6
　　　size, fetus 653.5
　　　soft parts (of pelvis) 654.9
　　　uterus, congenital 654.0
　　　vagina 654.7
　　　vulva 654.8
　　abruptio placentae 641.2

Delivery—*continued*
　acromion presentation 652.8
　affecting fetus or newborn 763.4
　anteversion, cervix or uterus 654.4
　atony, uterus 661.2
　　with hemorrhage 666.1
　bicornis or bicornuate uterus 654.0
　breech presentation 652.2
　brow presentation 652.4
　cephalopelvic disproportion (normally formed
　　fetus) 653.4
　chin presentation 652.4
　cicatrix of cervix 654.6
　contracted pelvis (general) 653.1
　　inlet 653.2
　　outlet 653.3
　cord presentation or prolapse 663.0
　cystocele 654.4
　deformity (acquired) (congenital)
　　pelvic organs or tissues NEC 654.9
　　pelvis (bony) NEC 653.0
　displacement, uterus NEC 654.4
　disproportion NEC 653.9
　distress
　　fetal 656.8
　　maternal 669.0
　eclampsia 642.6
　face presentation 652.4
　failed
　　forceps 660.7
　　trial of labor NEC 660.6
　　vacuum extraction 660.7
　　ventouse 660.7
　fetal deformity 653.7
　fetal-maternal hemorrhage 656.0
　fetus, fetal
　　distress 656.8
　　prematurity 656.8
　fibroid (tumor) (uterus) 654.1
　footling 652.8
　　with successful version 652.1
　hemorrhage (antepartum) (intrapartum) NEC
　　641.9
　hydrocephalic fetus 653.6
　incarceration of uterus 654.3
　incoordinate uterine action 661.4
　inertia, uterus 661.2
　　primary 661.0
　　secondary 661.1
　lateroversion, uterus or cervix 654.4
　mal lie 652.9
　malposition
　　fetus 652.9
　　　in multiple gestation 652.6
　　pelvic organs or tissues NEC 654.9
　　uterus NEC or cervix 654.4
　malpresentation NEC 652.9
　　in multiple gestation 652.6
　maternal
　　diabetes mellitus 648.0
　　heart disease NEC 648.6
　meconium in liquor 656.8
　　staining only 792.3
　oblique presentation 652.3
　oversize fetus 653.5
　pelvic tumor NEC 654.9
　placental insufficiency 656.5
　placenta previa 641.0
　　with hemorrhage 641.1
　poor dilation, cervix 661.0

INDEX TO DISEASES — Delivery

Delivery—*continued*
- pre-eclampsia 642.4
  - severe 642.5
- previous
  - cesarean delivery 654.2
  - surgery (to)
    - cervix 654.6
    - gynecological NEC 654.9
    - rectum 654.8
    - uterus NEC 654.9
      - from previous cesarean delivery 654.2
    - vagina 654.7
- prolapse
  - arm or hand 652.7
  - uterus 654.4
- prolonged labor 662.1
- rectocele 654.4
- retroversion, uterus or cervix 654.3
- rigid
  - cervix 654.6
  - pelvic floor 654.4
  - perineum 654.8
  - vagina 654.7
  - vulva 654.8
- sacculation, pregnant uterus 654.4
- scar(s)
  - cervix 654.6
  - cesarean delivery 654.2
  - uterus NEC 654.9
    - due to previous cesarean delivery 654.2
- Shirodkar suture in situ 654.5
- shoulder presentation 652.8
- stenosis or stricture, cervix 654.6
- transverse presentation or lie 652.3
- tumor, pelvic organs or tissues NEC 654.4
- umbilical cord presentation or prolapse 663.0
- completely normal case—*see* category 650
- complicated (by) NEC 669.9
  - abdominal tumor, fetal 653.7
    - causing obstructed labor 660.1
  - abnormal, abnormality of
    - cervix 654.6
      - causing obstructed labor 660.2
    - forces of labor 661.9
    - formation of uterus 654.0
    - pelvic organs or tissues 654.9
      - causing obstructed labor 660.2
    - pelvis (bony) (major) NEC 653.0
      - causing obstructed labor 660.1
    - presentation or position NEC 652.9
      - causing obstructed labor 660.0
    - size, fetus 653.5
      - causing obstructed labor 660.1
    - soft parts (of pelvis) 654.9
      - causing obstructed labor 660.2
    - uterine contractions NEC 661.9
    - uterus (formation) 654.0
      - causing obstructed labor 660.2
    - vagina 654.7
      - causing obstructed labor 660.2
  - abnormally formed uterus (any type) (congenital) 654.0
    - causing obstructed labor 660.2
  - acromion presentation 652.8
    - causing obstructed labor 660.0
  - adherent placenta 667.0
    - with hemorrhage 666.0
  - adhesions, uterus (to abdominal wall) 654.4
  - advanced maternal age NEC 659.6
    - multigravida 659.6
    - primigravida 659.5

Delivery—*continued*
- air embolism 673.0
- amnionitis 658.4
- amniotic fluid embolism 673.1
- anesthetic death 668.9
- annular detachment, cervix 665.3
- antepartum hemorrhage—*see* Delivery, complicated, hemorrhage
- anteversion, cervix or uterus 654.4
  - causing obstructed labor 660.2
- apoplexy 674.0
  - placenta 641.2
- arrested active phase 661.1
- asymmetrical pelvis bone 653.0
  - causing obstructed labor 660.1
- atony, uterus with hemorrhage (hypotonic) (inertia) 666.1
  - hypertonic 661.4
- Bandl's ring 661.4
- battledore placenta—*see* Placenta, abnormal
- bicornis or bicornuate uterus 654.0
  - causing obstructed labor 660.2
- birth injury to mother NEC 665.9
- bleeding (*see also* Delivery, complicated, hemorrhage) 641.9
- breech presentation (assisted) (buttocks) (complete) (frank) (spontaneous) 652.2
  - with successful version 652.1
- brow presentation 652.4
- cephalopelvic disproportion (normally formed fetus) 653.4
  - causing obstructed labor 660.1
- cerebral hemorrhage 674.0
- cervical dystocia 661.2
- chin presentation 652.4
  - causing obstructed labor 660.0
- cicatrix
  - cervix 654.6
    - causing obstructed labor 660.2
  - vagina 654.7
    - causing obstructed labor 660.2
- coagulation defect 649.3
- colporrhexis 665.4
  - with perineal laceration 664.0
- compound presentation 652.8
  - causing obstructed labor 660.0
- compression of cord (umbilical) 663.2
  - around neck 663.1
  - cord prolapsed 663.0
- contraction, contracted pelvis 653.1
  - causing obstructed labor 660.1
  - general 653.1
    - causing obstructed labor 660.1
  - inlet 653.2
    - causing obstructed labor 660.1
  - midpelvic 653.8
    - causing obstructed labor 660.1
  - midplane 653.8
    - causing obstructed labor 660.1
  - outlet 653.3
    - causing obstructed labor 660.1
- contraction ring 661.4
- cord (umbilical) 663.9
  - around neck, tightly or with compression 663.1
    - without compression 663.3
  - bruising 663.6
  - complication NEC 663.9
    - specified type NEC 663.8
  - compression NEC 663.2
  - entanglement NEC 663.3

921

Delivery—continued
    with compression 663.2
    forelying 663.0
    hematoma 663.6
    marginal attachment 663.8
    presentation 663.0
    prolapse (complete) (occult) (partial) 663.0
    short 663.4
    specified complication NEC 663.8
    thrombosis (vessels) 663.6
    vascular lesion 663.6
    velamentous insertion 663.8
  Couvelaire uterus 641.2
  cretin pelvis (dwarf type) (male type) 653.1
    causing obstructed labor 660.1
  crossbirth 652.3
    with successful version 652.1
    causing obstructed labor 660.0
  cyst (Gartner's duct) 654.7
  cystocele 654.4
    causing obstructed labor 660.2
  death of fetus (near term) 656.4
    early (before 22 completed weeks'
      gestation) 632
  deformity (acquired) (congenital)
    fetus 653.7
      causing obstructed labor 660.1
    pelvic organs or tissues NEC 654.9
      causing obstructed labor 660.2
    pelvis (bony) NEC 653.0
      causing obstructed labor 660.1
  delay, delayed
    delivery in multiple pregnancy 662.3
    due to locked mates 660.5
    following rupture of membranes
      (spontaneous) 658.2
      artificial 658.3
  depressed fetal heart tones 659.7
  diastasis recti 665.8
  dilatation
    bladder 654.4
      causing obstructed labor 660.2
    cervix, incomplete, poor or slow 661.0
  diseased placenta 656.7
  displacement uterus NEC 654.4
    causing obstructed labor 660.2
  disproportion NEC 653.9
    causing obstructed labor 660.1
  disruptio uteri—*see* Delivery, complicated,
    rupture, uterus
  distress
    fetal 656.8
    maternal 669.0
  double uterus (congenital) 654.0
    causing obstructed labor 660.2
  dropsy amnion 657
  dysfunction, uterus 661.9
    hypertonic 661.4
    hypotonic 661.2
      primary 661.0
      secondary 661.1
    incoordinate 661.4
  dystocia
    cervical 661.2
    fetal—*see* Delivery, complicated, abnormal,
      presentation
    maternal—*see* Delivery, complicated,
      prolonged labor
    pelvic—*see* Delivery, complicated,
      contraction pelvis
    positional 652.8

Delivery—continued
    shoulder girdle 660.4
  eclampsia 642.6
  ectopic kidney 654.4
    causing obstructed labor 660.2
  edema, cervix 654.6
    causing obstructed labor 660.2
  effusion, amniotic fluid 658.1
  elderly multigravida 659.6
  elderly primigravida 659.5
  embolism (pulmonary) 673.2
    air 673.0
    amniotic fluid 673.1
    blood-clot 673.2
    cerebral 674.0
    fat 673.8
    pyemic 673.3
    septic 673.3
  entanglement, umbilical cord 663.3
    with compression 663.2
    around neck (with compression) 663.1
  eversion, cervix or uterus 665.2
  excessive
    fetal growth 653.5
      causing obstructed labor 660.1
    size of fetus 653.5
      causing obstructed labor 660.1
  face presentation 652.4
    causing obstructed labor 660.0
    to pubes 660.3
  failure, fetal head to enter pelvic brim 652.5
    causing obstructed labor 660.0
  female genital mutilation 660.8
  fetal
    acid-base balance 656.8
    death (near term) NEC 656.4
      early (before 22 completed weeks'
        gestation) 632
    deformity 653.7
      causing obstructed labor 660.1
    distress 656.8
    heart rate or rhythm 659.7
    reduction of multiple fetuses reduced to
      single fetus 651.7
  fetopelvic disproportion 653.4
    causing obstructed labor 660.1
  fever during labor 659.2
  fibroid (tumor) (uterus) 654.1
    causing obstructed labor 660.2
  fibromyomata 654.1
    causing obstructed labor 660.2
  forelying umbilical cord 663.0
  fracture of coccyx 665.6
  hematoma 664.5
    broad ligament 665.7
    ischial spine 665.7
    pelvic 665.7
    perineum 664.5
    soft tissues 665.7
    subdural 674.0
    umbilical cord 663.6
    vagina 665.7
    vulva or perineum 664.5
  hemorrhage (uterine) (antepartum)
    (intrapartum) (pregnancy) 641.9
    accidental 641.2
    associated with
      afibrinogenemia 641.3
      coagulation defect 641.3
        hyperfibrinolysis 641.3
        hypofibrinogenemia 641.3

INDEX TO DISEASES

Delivery

Delivery—*continued*
  cerebral 674.0
  due to
    low-lying placenta 641.1
    placenta previa 641.1
    premature separation of placenta (normally implanted) 641.2
    retained placenta 666.0
    trauma 641.8
    uterine leiomyoma 641.8
  marginal sinus rupture 641.2
  placenta NEC 641.9
  postpartum (atonic) (immediate) (within 24 hours) 666.1
    with retained or trapped placenta 666.0
    third stage 666.0
    delayed 666.2
    secondary 666.2
  hourglass contraction, uterus 661.4
  hydramnios 657
  hydrocephalic fetus 653.6
    causing obstructed labor 660.1
  hydrops fetalis 653.7
    causing obstructed labor 660.1
  hypertension—*see* Hypertension, complicating pregnancy
  hypertonic uterine dysfunction 661.4
  hypotonic uterine dysfunction 661.2
  impacted shoulders 660.4
  incarceration, uterus 654.3
    causing obstructed labor 660.2
  incomplete dilation (cervix) 661.0
  incoordinate uterus 661.4
  indication NEC 659.9
    specified type NEC 659.8
  inertia, uterus 661.2
    hypertonic 661.4
    hypotonic 661.2
    primary 661.0
    secondary 661.1
  infantile
    genitalia 654.4
      causing obstructed labor 660.2
    uterus (os) 654.4
      causing obstructed labor 660.2
  injury (to mother) NEC 665.9
  intrauterine fetal death (near term) NEC 656.4
    early (before 22 completed weeks' gestation) 632
  inversion, uterus 665.2
  kidney, ectopic 654.4
    causing obstructed labor 660.2
  knot (true), umbilical cord 663.2
  labor, premature (before 37 completed weeks gestation) 644.2
  laceration 664.9
    anus (sphincter) (healed) (old) 654.8
      not associated with third-degree perineal laceration 664.6
      with mucosa 664.3
    bladder (urinary) 665.5
    bowel 665.5
    central 664.4
    cervix (uteri) 665.3
    fourchette 664.0
    hymen 664.0
    labia (majora) (minora) 664.0
    pelvic
      floor 664.1
      organ NEC 665.5
    perineum, perineal 664.4

Delivery—*continued*
    first degree 664.0
    second degree 664.1
    third degree 664.2
    fourth degree 664.3
    central 664.4
    extensive NEC 664.4
    muscles 664.1
    skin 664.0
    slight 664.0
  peritoneum 665.5
  periurethral tissue 664.8
  rectovaginal (septum) (without perineal laceration) 665.4
    with perineum 664.2
      with anal or rectal mucosa 664.3
  skin (perineum) 664.0
  specified site or type NEC 664.8
  sphincter ani (healed) (old) 654.8
    not associated with third-degree perineal laceration 664.6
    with mucosa 664.3
  urethra 665.5
  uterus 665.1
    before labor 665.0
  vagina, vaginal (deep) (high) (sulcus) (wall) (without perineal laceration) 665.4
    with perineum 664.0
    muscles, with perineum 664.1
  vulva 664.0
  lateroversion, uterus or cervix 654.4
    causing obstructed labor 660.2
  locked mates 660.5
  low implantation of placenta—*see* Delivery, complicated, placenta, previa
  mal lie 652.9
  malposition
    fetus NEC 652.9
      causing obstructed labor 660.0
    pelvic organs or tissues NEC 654.9
      causing obstructed labor 660.2
    placenta 641.1
      without hemorrhage 641.0
    uterus NEC or cervix 654.4
      causing obstructed labor 660.2
  malpresentation 652.9
    causing obstructed labor 660.0
  marginal sinus (bleeding) (rupture) 641.2
  maternal hypotension syndrome 669.2
  meconium in liquor 656.8
  membranes, retained—*see* Delivery, complicated, placenta, retained
  mentum presentation 652.4
    causing obstructed labor 660.0
  metrorrhagia (myopathia)—*see* Delivery, complicated, hemorrhage
  metrorrhexis—*see* Delivery, complicated, rupture, uterus
  multiparity (grand) 659.4
  myelomeningocele, fetus 653.7
    causing obstructed labor 660.1
  Nägele's pelvis 653.0
    causing obstructed labor 660.1
  nonengagement, fetal head 652.5
    causing obstructed labor 660.0
  oblique presentation 652.3
    causing obstructed labor 660.0
  obstetric
    shock 669.1
    trauma NEC 665.9

Delivery—*continued*
- obstructed labor 660.9
  - due to
    - abnormality pelvic organs or tissues (conditions classifiable to 654.0-654.9) 660.2
    - deep transverse arrest 660.3
    - impacted shoulders 660.4
    - locked twins 660.5
    - malposition and malpresentation of fetus (conditions classifiable to 652.0-652.9) 660.0
    - persistent occipitoposterior 660.3
    - shoulder dystocia 660.4
- occult prolapse of umbilical cord 663.0
- oversize fetus 653.5
  - causing obstructed labor 660.1
- pathological retraction ring, uterus 661.4
- pelvic
  - arrest (deep) (high) (of fetal head) (transverse) 660.3
  - deformity (bone)—*see also* Deformity, pelvis, with disproportion
    - soft tissue 654.9
      - causing obstructed labor 660.2
  - tumor NEC 654.9
    - causing obstructed labor 660.2
- penetration, pregnant uterus by instrument 665.1
- perforation—*see* Delivery, complicated, laceration
- persistent
  - hymen 654.8
    - causing obstructed labor 660.2
  - occipitoposterior 660.3
- placenta, placental
  - ablatio 641.2
  - abnormality 656.7
    - with hemorrhage 641.2
  - abruptio 641.2
  - accreta 667.0
    - with hemorrhage 666.0
  - adherent (without hemorrhage) 667.0
    - with hemorrhage 666.0
  - apoplexy 641.2
  - battledore 663.8
  - detachment (premature) 641.2
  - disease 656.7
  - hemorrhage NEC 641.9
  - increta (without hemorrhage) 667.0
    - with hemorrhage 666.0
  - low (implantation) 641.1
    - without hemorrhage 641.0
  - malformation 656.7
    - with hemorrhage 641.2
  - malposition 641.1
    - without hemorrhage 641.0
  - marginal sinus rupture 641.2
  - percreta 667.0
    - with hemorrhage 666.0
  - premature separation 641.2
  - previa (central) (lateral) (marginal) (partial) 641.1
    - without hemorrhage 641.0
  - retained (with hemorrhage) 666.0
    - without hemorrhage 667.0
  - rupture of marginal sinus 641.2
  - separation (premature) 641.2
  - trapped 666.0
    - without hemorrhage 667.0
  - vicious insertion 641.1

Delivery—*continued*
- polyhydramnios 657
- polyp, cervix 654.6
  - causing obstructed labor 660.2
- precipitate labor 661.3
- premature
  - labor (before 37 completed weeks gestation) 644.2
  - rupture, membranes 658.1
    - delayed delivery following 658.2
- presenting umbilical cord 663.0
- previous
  - cesarean delivery 654.2
  - surgery
    - cervix 654.6
      - causing obstructed labor 660.2
    - gynecological NEC 654.9
      - causing obstructed labor 660.2
    - perineum 654.8
    - rectum 654.8
    - uterus NEC 654.9
      - due to previous cesarean delivery 654.2
    - vagina 654.7
      - causing obstructed labor 660.2
    - vulva 654.8
- primary uterine inertia 661.0
- primipara, elderly or old 659.5
- prolapse
  - arm or hand 652.7
    - causing obstructed labor 660.0
  - cord (umbilical) 663.0
  - fetal extremity 652.8
  - foot or leg 652.8
    - causing obstructed labor 660.0
  - umbilical cord (complete) (occult) (partial) 663.0
  - uterus 654.4
    - causing obstructed labor 660.2
- prolonged labor 662.1
  - active phase 661.2
  - due to
    - cervical dystocia 661.2
    - contraction ring 661.4
    - tetanic uterus 661.4
    - uterine inertia 661.2
      - primary 661.0
      - secondary 661.1
  - first stage 662.0
  - latent phase 661.0
  - second stage 662.2
- pyrexia during labor 659.2
- rachitic pelvis 653.2
  - causing obstructed labor 660.1
- rectocele 654.4
  - causing obstructed labor 660.2
- retained membranes or portions of placenta 666.2
  - without hemorrhage 667.1
- retarded (prolonged) birth 662.1
- retention secundines (with hemorrhage) 666.2
  - without hemorrhage 667.1
- retroversion, uterus or cervix 654.3
  - causing obstructed labor 660.2
- rigid
  - cervix 654.6
    - causing obstructed labor 660.2
  - pelvic floor 654.4
    - causing obstructed labor 660.2
  - perineum or vulva 654.8
    - causing obstructed labor 660.2

Delivery—*continued*
   vagina 654.7
     causing obstructed labor 660.2
  Robert's pelvis 653.0
   causing obstructed labor 660.1
  rupture—*see also* Delivery, complicated, laceration
   bladder (urinary) 665.5
   cervix 665.3
   marginal sinus 641.2
   membranes, premature 658.1
   pelvic organ NEC 665.5
   perineum (without mention of other laceration)—*see* Delivery, complicated, laceration, perineum
   peritoneum 665.5
   urethra 665.5
   uterus (during labor) 665.1
    before labor 665.0
  sacculation, pregnant uterus 654.4
  sacral teratomas, fetal 653.7
   causing obstructed labor 660.1
  scar(s)
   cervix 654.6
    causing obstructed labor 660.2
   cesarean delivery 654.2
    causing obstructed labor 660.2
   perineum 654.8
    causing obstructed labor 660.2
   uterus NEC 654.9
    causing obstructed labor 660.2
    due to previous cesarean delivery 654.2
   vagina 654.7
    causing obstructed labor 660.2
   vulva 654.8
    causing obstructed labor 660.2
  scoliotic pelvis 653.0
   causing obstructed labor 660.1
  secondary uterine inertia 661.1
  secundines, retained—*see* Delivery, complicated, placenta, retained
  separation
   placenta (premature) 641.2
   pubic bone 665.6
   symphysis pubis 665.6
  septate vagina 654.7
   causing obstructed labor 660.2
  shock (birth) (obstetric) (puerperal) 669.1
  short cord syndrome 663.4
  shoulder
   girdle dystocia 660.4
   presentation 652.8
    causing obstructed labor 660.0
  Siamese twins 653.7
   causing obstructed labor 660.1
  slow slope active phase 661.2
  spasm
   cervix 661.4
   uterus 661.4
  spondylolisthesis, pelvis 653.3
   causing obstructed labor 660.1
  spondylolysis (lumbosacral) 653.3
   causing obstructed labor 660.1
  spondylosis 653.0
   causing obstructed labor 660.1
  stenosis or stricture
   cervix 654.6
    causing obstructed labor 660.2
   vagina 654.7
    causing obstructed labor 660.2
  sudden death, unknown cause 669.9

Delivery—*continued*
  tear (pelvic organ) (*see also* Delivery, complicated, laceration) 664.9
   anal sphincter (healed) (old) 654.8
    not associated with third-degree perineal laceration 664.6
  teratomas, sacral, fetal 653.7
   causing obstructed labor 660.1
  tetanic uterus 661.4
  tipping pelvis 653.0
   causing obstructed labor 660.1
  transverse
   arrest (deep) 660.3
   presentation or lie 652.3
    with successful version 652.1
    causing obstructed labor 660.0
  trauma (obstetrical) NEC 665.9
  tumor
   abdominal, fetal 653.7
    causing obstructed labor 660.1
   pelvic organs or tissues NEC 654.9
    causing obstructed labor 660.2
  umbilical cord (*see also* Delivery, complicated, cord) 663.9
   around neck tightly, or with compression 663.1
   entanglement NEC 663.3
    with compression 663.2
   prolapse (complete) (occult) (partial) 663.0
  unstable lie 652.0
   causing obstructed labor 660.0
  uterine
   inertia (*see also* Delivery, complicated, inertia, uterus) 661.2
   spasm 661.4
  vasa previa 663.5
  velamentous insertion of cord 663.8
  young maternal age 659.8
  delayed NEC 662.1
   following rupture of membranes (spontaneous) 658.2
   artificial 658.3
   second twin, triplet, etc. 662.3
  difficult NEC 669.9
   previous, affecting management of pregnancy or childbirth V23.49
   specified type NEC 669.8
  early onset (spontaneous) 644.2
  forceps NEC 669.5
   affecting fetus or newborn 763.2
  footling 652.8
   with successful version 652.1
  missed (at or near term) 656.4
  multiple gestation NEC 651.9
   with fetal loss and retention of one or more fetus(es) 651.6
   following (elective) fetal reduction 651.7
   specified type NEC 651.8
    with fetal loss and retention of one or more fetus(es) 651.6
    following (elective) fetal reduction 651.7
  nonviable infant 656.4
  normal—*see* category 650
  precipitate 661.3
   affecting fetus or newborn 763.6
  premature NEC (before 37 completed weeks gestation) 644.2
   previous, affecting management of pregnancy V23.41

Delivery—*continued*
  quadruplet NEC 651.2
    with fetal loss and retention of one or more fetus(es) 651.5
    following (elective) fetal reduction 651.7
  quintuplet NEC 651.8
    with fetal loss and retention of one or more fetus(es) 651.6
    following (elective) fetal reduction 651.7
  sextuplet NEC 651.8
    with fetal loss and retention of one or more fetus(es) 651.6
    following (elective) fetal reduction 651.7
  specified complication NEC 669.8
  stillbirth (near term) NEC 656.4
    early (before 22 completed weeks' gestation) 632
  term pregnancy (live birth) NEC—*see* category 650
  stillbirth NEC 656.4
  threatened premature 644.2
  triplets NEC 651.1
    with fetal loss and retention of one or more fetus(es) 651.4
    delayed delivery (one or more mates) 662.3
    following (elective) fetal reduction 651.7
    locked mates 660.5
  twins NEC 651.0
    with fetal loss and retention of one or more fetus(es) 651.3
    delayed delivery (one or more mates) 662.3
    following (elective) fetal reduction 651.7
    locked mates 660.5
  uncomplicated—*see* category 650
  vacuum extractor NEC 669.5
    affecting fetus or newborn 763.3
  ventouse NEC 669.5
    affecting fetus or newborn 763.3
Dellen, cornea 371.41
Delusions (paranoid) 297.9
  grandiose 297.1
  parasitosis 300.29
  systematized 297.1
Dementia 294.8
  alcohol-induced persisting (*see also* Psychosis, alcoholic) 291.2
  Alzheimer's—*see* Alzheimer's dementia
  arteriosclerotic (simple type) (uncomplicated) 290.40
    with
      acute confusional state 290.41
      delirium 290.41
      delusions 290.42
      depressed mood 290.43
      depressed type 290.43
      paranoid type 290.42
  Binswanger's 290.12
  catatonic (acute) (*see also* Schizophrenia) 295.2
  congenital (*see also* Retardation, mental) 319
  degenerative 290.9
    presenile-onset—*see* Dementia, presenile
    senile-onset—*see* Dementia, senile
  developmental (*see also* Schizophrenia) 295.9
  dialysis 294.8
    transient 293.9
  drug-induced persisting (*see also* Psychosis, drug) 292.82
  due to or associated with condition(s) classified elsewhere
    Alzheimer's
      with behavioral disturbance 331.0 *[294.11]*

Dementia—*continued*
    without behavioral disturbance 331.0 *[294.10]*
  cerebral lipidoses
    with behavioral disturbance 330.1 *[294.11]*
    without behavioral disturbance 330.1 *[294.10]*
  epilepsy
    with behavioral disturbance 345.9 *[294.11]*
    without behavioral disturbance 345.9 *[294.10]*
  hepatolenticular degeneration
    with behavioral disturbance 275.1 *[294.11]*
    without behavioral disturbance 275.1 *[294.10]*
  HIV
    with behavioral disturbance 042 *[294.11]*
    without behavioral disturbance 042 *[294.10]*
  Huntington's chorea
    with behavioral disturbance 333.4 *[294.11]*
    without behavioral disturbance 333.4 *[294.10]*
  Jakob-Creutzfeldt disease (new variant)
    with behavioral disturbance 046.1 *[294.11]*
    without behavioral disturbance 046.1 *[294.10]*
  Lewy bodies
    with behavioral disturbance 331.82 *[294.11]*
    without behavioral disturbance 331.82 *[294.10]*
  multiple sclerosis
    with behavioral disturbance 340 *[294.11]*
    without behavioral disturbance 340 *[294.10]*
  neurosyphilis
    with behavioral disturbance 094.9 *[294.11]*
    without behavioral disturbance 094.9 *[294.10]*
  Parkinsonism
    with behavioral disturbance 331.82 *[294.11]*
    without behavioral disturbance 331.82 *[294.10]*
  Pelizaeus-Merzbacher disease
    with behavioral disturbance 333.0 *[294.11]*
    without behavioral disturbance 333.0 *[294.10]*
  Pick's disease
    with behavioral disturbance 331.11 *[294.11]*
    without behavioral disturbance 331.11 *[294.10]*
  polyarteritis nodosa
    with behavioral disturbance 446.0 *[294.11]*
    without behavioral disturbance 446.0 *[294.10]*
  syphilis
    with behavioral disturbance 094.1 *[294.11]*
    without behavioral disturbance 094.1 *[294.10]*
  Wilson's disease
    with behavioral disturbance 275.1 *[294.11]*
    without behavioral disturbance 275.1 *[294.10]*
  frontal 331.19
    with behavioral disturbance 331.19 *[294.11]*
    without behavioral disturbance 331.19 *[294.10]*
  frontotemporal 331.19
    with behavioral disturbance 331.19 *[294.11]*
    without behavioral disturbance 331.19 *[294.10]*
  hebephrenic (acute) 295.1

INDEX TO DISEASES

Dementia—*continued*
  Heller's (infantile psychosis) (*see also*
    Psychosis, childhood) 299.1
  idiopathic 290.9
    presenile-onset—*see* Dementia, presenile
    senile-onset—*see* Dementia, senile
  in
    arteriosclerotic brain disease 290.40
    senility 290.0
  induced by drug 292.82
  infantile, infantilia (*see also* Psychosis,
    childhood) 299.0
  Lewy body 331.82
    with behavioral disturbance 331.82 *[294.11]*
    without behavioral disturbance 331.82 *[294.10]*
  multi-infarct (cerebrovascular) (*see also*
    Dementia, arteriosclerotic) 290.40
  old age 290.0
  paralytica, paralytic 094.1
    juvenilis 090.40
    syphilitic 094.1
      congenital 090.40
    tabetic form 094.1
  paranoid (*see also* Schizophrenia) 295.3
  paraphrenic (*see also* Schizophrenia) 295.3
  paretic 094.1
  praecox (*see also* Schizophrenia) 295.9
  presenile 290.10
    with
      acute confusional state 290.11
      delirium 290.11
      delusional features 290.12
      depressive features 290.13
    depressed type 290.13
    paranoid type 290.12
    simple type 290.10
    uncomplicated 290.10
  primary (acute) (*see also* Schizophrenia) 295.0
  progressive, syphilitic 094.1
  puerperal—*see* Psychosis, puerperal
  schizophrenic (*see also* Schizophrenia) 295.9
  senile 290.0
    with
      acute confusional state 290.3
      delirium 290.3
      delusional features 290.20
      depressive features 290.21
    depressed type 290.21
    exhaustion 290.0
    paranoid type 290.20
  simple type (acute) (*see also* Schizophrenia) 295.0
  simplex (acute) (*see also* Schizophrenia) 295.0
  syphilitic 094.1
  uremic—*see* Uremia
  vascular 290.40
    with
      delirium 290.41
      delusions 290.42
      depressed mood 290.43
Demerol dependence (*see also* Dependence)
  304.0
Demineralization, ankle (*see also* Osteoporosis)
  733.00
Demodex folliculorum (infestation) 133.8
de Morgan's spots (senile angiomas) 448.1
Demyelinating
  polyneuritis, chronic inflammatory 357.81
Demyelination, demyelinization
  central nervous system 341.9
    specified NEC 341.8
  corpus callosum (central) 341.8
  global 340

Dependence

Dengue (fever) 061
  sandfly 061
  vaccination, prophylactic (against) V05.1
  virus hemorrhagic fever 065.4
Dens
  evaginatus 520.2
  in dente 520.2
  invaginatus 520.2
Density
  increased, bone (disseminated) (generalized)
    (spotted) 733.99
  lung (nodular) 518.89
Dental —*see also* condition
  examination only V72.2
Dentia praecox 520.6
Denticles (in pulp) 522.2
Dentigerous cyst 526.0
Dentin
  irregular (in pulp) 522.3
  opalescent 520.5
  secondary (in pulp) 522.3
  sensitive 521.89
Dentinogenesis imperfecta 520.5
Dentinoma (M9271/0) 213.1
  upper jaw (bone) 213.0
Dentition 520.7
  abnormal 520.6
  anomaly 520.6
  delayed 520.6
  difficult 520.7
  disorder of 520.6
  precocious 520.6
  retarded 520.6
Denture sore (mouth) 528.9
Dependence

> Note—Use the following fifth-digit
> subclassification with category 304:
>
> 0 unspecified
> 1 continuous
> 2 episodic
> 3 in remission

  with
    withdrawal symptoms
      alcohol 291.81
      drug 292.0
  14-hydroxy-dihydromorphinone 304.0
  absinthe 304.6
  acemorphan 304.0
  acetanilid(e) 304.6
  acetophenetidin 304.6
  acetorphine 304.0
  acetyldihydrocodeine 304.0
  acetyldihydrocodeinone 304.0
  Adalin 304.1
  Afghanistan black 304.3
  agrypnal 304.1
  alcohol, alcoholic (ethyl) (methyl) (wood) 303.9
    maternal, with suspected fetal damage
      affecting management of pregnancy 655.4
  allobarbitone 304.1
  allonal 304.1
  allylisopropylacetylurea 304.1
  alphaprodine (hydrochloride) 304.0
  Alurate 304.1
  Alvodine 304.0
  amethocaine 304.6
  amidone 304.0
  amidopyrine 304.6

Dependence—*continued*
  aminopyrine 304.6
  amobarbital 304.1
  amphetamine(s) (type) (drugs classifiable to 969.7) 304.4
  amylene hydrate 304.6
  amylobarbitone 304.1
  amylocaine 304.6
  Amytal (sodium) 304.1
  analgesic (drug) NEC 304.6
    synthetic with morphine-like effect 304.0
  anesthetic (agent) (drug) (gas) (general) (local) NEC 304.6
  Angel dust 304.6
  anileridine 304.0
  antipyrine 304.6
  anxiolytic 304.1
  aprobarbital 304.1
  aprobarbitone 304.1
  atropine 304.6
  Avertin (bromide) 304.6
  barbenyl 304.1
  barbital(s) 304.1
  barbitone 304.1
  barbiturate(s) (compounds) (drugs classifiable to 967.0) 304.1
  barbituric acid (and compounds) 304.1
  benzedrine 304.4
  benzylmorphine 304.0
  Beta-chlor 304.1
  bhang 304.3
  blue velvet 304.0
  Brevital 304.1
  bromal (hydrate) 304.1
  bromide(s) NEC 304.1
  bromine compounds NEC 304.1
  bromisovalum 304.1
  bromoform 304.1
  Bromo-seltzer 304.1
  bromural 304.1
  butabarbital (sodium) 304.1
  butabarpal 304.1
  butallylonal 304.1
  butethal 304.1
  buthalitone (sodium) 304.1
  Butisol 304.1
  butobarbitone 304.1
  butyl chloral (hydrate) 304.1
  caffeine 304.4
  cannabis (indica) (sativa) (resin) (derivatives) (type) 304.3
  carbamazepine 304.6
  Carbrital 304.1
  carbromal 304.1
  carisoprodol 304.6
  Catha (edulis) 304.4
  chloral (betaine) (hydrate) 304.1
  chloralamide 304.1
  chloralformamide 304.1
  chloralose 304.1
  chlordiazepoxide 304.1
  Chloretone 304.1
  chlorobutanol 304.1
  chlorodyne 304.1
  chloroform 304.6
  Cliradon 304.0
  coca (leaf) and derivatives 304.2
  cocaine 304.2
    hydrochloride 304.2
    salt (any) 304.2
  codeine 304.0

Dependence—*continued*
  combination of drugs (excluding morphine or opioid type drug) NEC 304.8
  morphine or opioid type drug with any other drug 304.7
  croton-chloral 304.1
  cyclobarbital 304.1
  cyclobarbitone 304.1
  dagga 304.3
  Delvinal 304.1
  Demerol 304.0
  desocodeine 304.0
  desomorphine 304.0
  desoxyephedrine 304.4
  DET 304.5
  dexamphetamine 304.4
  dexedrine 304.4
  dextromethorphan 304.0
  dextromoramide 304.0
  dextronorpseudophedrine 304.4
  dextrorphan 304.0
  diacetylmorphine 304.0
  Dial 304.1
  diallylbarbituric acid 304.1
  diamorphine 304.0
  diazepam 304.1
  dibucaine 304.6
  dichloroethane 304.6
  diethyl barbituric acid 304.1
  diethylsulfone-diethylmethane 304.1
  difencloxazine 304.0
  dihydrocodeine 304.0
  dihydrocodeinone 304.0
  dihydrohydroxycodeinone 304.0
  dihydroisocodeine 304.0
  dihydromorphine 304.0
  dihydromorphinone 304.0
  dihydroxcodeinone 304.0
  Dilaudid 304.0
  dimenhydrinate 304.6
  dimethylmeperidine 304.0
  dimethyltriptamine 304.5
  Dionin 304.0
  diphenoxylate 304.6
  dipipanone 304.0
  d-lysergic acid diethylamide 304.5
  DMT 304.5
  Dolophine 304.0
  DOM 304.2
  Doriden 304.1
  dormiral 304.1
  Dormison 304.1
  Dromoran 304.0
  drug NEC 304.9
    analgesic NEC 304.6
    combination (excluding morphine or opioid type drug) NEC 304.8
      morphine or opioid type drug with any other drug 304.7
    complicating pregnancy, childbirth, or puerperium 648.3
      affecting fetus or newborn 779.5
    hallucinogenic 304.5
    hypnotic NEC 304.1
    narcotic NEC 304.9
    psychostimulant NEC 304.4
    sedative NEC 304.1
    soporific NEC 304.1
    specified type NEC 304.6
    suspected damage to fetus affecting management of pregnancy 655.5

INDEX TO DISEASES

Dependence

Dependence—*continued*
  synthetic, with morphine-like effect 304.0
    tranquilizing 304.1
 duboisine 304.6
 ectylurea 304.1
 Endocaine 304.6
 Equanil 304.1
 Eskabarb 304.1
 ethchlorvynol 304.1
 ether (ethyl) (liquid) (vapor) (vinyl) 304.6
 ethidene 304.6
 ethinamate 304.1
 ethoheptazine 304.6
 ethyl
  alcohol 303.9
  bromide 304.6
  carbamate 304.6
  chloride 304.6
  morphine 304.0
 ethylene (gas) 304.6
  dichloride 304.6
 ethylidene chloride 304.6
 etilfen 304.1
 etorphine 304.0
 etoval 304.1
 eucodal 304.0
 euneryl 304.1
 Evipal 304.1
 Evipan 304.1
 fentanyl 304.0
 ganja 304.3
 gardenal 304.1
 gardenpanyl 304.1
 gelsemine 304.6
 Gelsemium 304.6
 Gemonil 304.1
 glucochloral 304.1
 glue (airplane) (sniffing) 304.6
 glutethimide 304.1
 hallucinogenics 304.5
 hashish 304.3
 headache powder NEC 304.6
 Heavenly Blue 304.5
 hedonal 304.1
 hemp 304.3
 heptabarbital 304.1
 Heptalgin 304.0
 heptobarbitone 304.1
 heroin 304.0
  salt (any) 304.0
 hexethal (sodium) 304.1
 hexobarbital 304.1
 Hycodan 304.0
 hydrocodone 304.0
 hydromorphinol 304.0
 hydromorphinone 304.0
 hydromorphone 304.0
 hydroxycodeine 304.0
 hypnotic NEC 304.1
 Indian hemp 304.3
 inhalant 304.6
 intranarcon 304.1
 Kemithal 304.1
 ketobemidone 304.0
 khat 304.4
 kif 304.3
 Lactuca (virosa) extract 304.1
 lactucarium 304.1
 laudanum 304.0
 Lebanese red 304.3
 Leritine 304.0

Dependence—*continued*
 lettuce opium 304.1
 Levanil 304.1
 Levo-Dromoran 304.0
 levo-iso-methadone 304.0
 levorphanol 304.0
 Librium 304.1
 Lomotil 304.6
 Lotusate 304.1
 LSD (-25) (and derivatives) 304.5
 Luminal 304.1
 lysergic acid 304.5
  amide 304.5
 maconha 304.3
 magic mushroom 304.5
 marihuana 304.3
 MDA (methylene dioxyamphetamine) 304.4
 Mebaral 304.1
 Medinal 304.1
 Medomin 304.1
 megahallucinogenics 304.5
 meperidine 304.0
 mephobarbital 304.1
 meprobamate 304.1
 mescaline 304.5
 methadone 304.0
 methamphetamine(s) 304.4
 methaqualone 304.1
 metharbital 304.1
 methitural 304.1
 methobarbitone 304.1
 methohexital 304.1
 methopholine 304.6
 methyl
  alcohol 303.9
  bromide 304.6
  morphine 304.0
  sulfonal 304.1
 methylated spirit 303.9
 methylbutinol 304.6
 methyldihydromorphinone 304.0
 methylene
  chloride 304.6
  dichloride 304.6
  dioxyamphetamine (MDA) 304.4
 methylparafynol 304.1
 methylphenidate 304.4
 methyprylone 304.1
 metopon 304.0
 Miltown 304.1
 morning glory *see*ds 304.5
 morphinan(s) 304.0
 morphine (sulfate) (sulfite) (type) (drugs
   classifiable to 965.00-965.09) 304.0
 morphine or opioid type drug (drugs classifiable
   to 965.00-965.09) with any other drug 304.7
 morphinol(s) 304.0
 morphinon 304.0
 morpholinylethylmorphine 304.0
 mylomide 304.1
 myristicin 304.5
 narcotic (drug) NEC 304.9
 nealbarbital 304.1
 nealbarbitone 304.1
 Nembutal 304.1
 Neonal 304.1
 Neraval 304.1
 Neravan 304.1
 neurobarb 304.1
 nicotine 305.1
 Nisentil 304.0

929

Dependence—*continued*
nitrous oxide 304.6
Noctec 304.1
Noludar 304.1
nonbarbiturate sedatives and tranquilizers with similar effect 304.1
noptil 304.1
normorphine 304.0
noscapine 304.0
Novocaine 304.6
Numorphan 304.0
nunol 304.1
Nupercaine 304.6
Oblivon 304.1
on
  aspirator V46.0
  hemodialysis V45.1
  hyperbaric chamber V46.8
  iron lung V46.11
  machine (enabling) V46.9
    specified type NEC V46.8
  peritoneal dialysis V45.1
  Possum (Patient-Operated-Selector-Mechanism) V46.8
  renal dialysis machine V45.1
  respirator (ventilator) V46.11
    encounter
      during
        mechanical failure V46.14
        power failure V46.12
      for weaning V46.13
  supplemental oxygen V46.2
opiate 304.0
opioids 304.0
opioid type drug 304.0
  with any other drug 304.7
opium (alkaloids) (derivatives) (tincture) 304.0
ortal 304.1
Oxazepam 304.1
oxycodone 304.0
oxymorphone 304.0
Palfium 304.0
Panadol 304.6
pantopium 304.0
pantopon 304.0
papaverine 304.0
paracetamol 304.6
paracodin 304.0
paraldehyde 304.1
paregoric 304.0
Parzone 304.0
PCP (phencyclidine) 304.6
Pearly Gates 304.5
pentazocine 304.0
pentobarbital 304.1
pentobarbitone (sodium) 304.1
Pentothal 304.1
Percaine 304.6
Percodan 304.0
Perichlor 304.1
Pernocton 304.1
Pernoston 304.1
peronine 304.0
pethidine (hydrochloride) 304.0
petrichloral 304.1
peyote 304.5
Phanodorn 304.1
phenacetin 304.6
phenadoxone 304.0
phenaglycodol 304.1
phenazocine 304.0

Dependence—*continued*
phencyclidine 304.6
phenmetrazine 304.4
phenobal 304.1
phenobarbital 304.1
phenobarbitone 304.1
phenomorphan 304.0
phenonyl 304.1
phenoperidine 304.0
pholcodine 304.0
piminodine 304.0
Pipadone 304.0
Pitkin's solution 304.6
Placidyl 304.1
polysubstance 304.8
Pontocaine 304.6
pot 304.3
potassium bromide 304.1
Preludin 304.4
Prinadol 304.0
probarbital 304.1
procaine 304.6
propanal 304.1
propoxyphene 304.6
psilocibin 304.5
psilocin 304.5
psilocybin 304.5
psilocyline 304.5
psilocyn 304.5
psychedelic agents 304.5
psychostimulant NEC 304.4
psychotomimetic agents 304.5
pyrahexyl 304.3
Pyramidon 304.6
quinalbarbitone 304.1
racemoramide 304.0
racemorphan 304.0
Rela 304.6
scopolamine 304.6
secobarbital 304.1
Seconal 304.1
sedative NEC 304.1
  nonbarbiturate with barbiturate effect 304.1
Sedormid 304.1
sernyl 304.1
sodium bromide 304.1
Soma 304.6
Somnal 304.1
Somnos 304.1
Soneryl 304.1
soporific (drug) NEC 304.1
specified drug NEC 304.6
speed 304.4
spinocaine 304.6
Stovaine 304.6
STP 304.5
stramonium 304.6
Sulfonal 304.1
sulfonethylmethane 304.1
sulfonmethane 304.1
Surital 304.1
synthetic drug with morphine-like effect 304.0
talbutal 304.1
tetracaine 304.6
tetrahydrocannabinol 304.3
tetronal 304.1
THC 304.3
thebacon 304.0
thebaine 304.0
thiamil 304.1
thiamylal 304.1

INDEX TO DISEASES

Dependence—*continued*
  thiopental 304.1
  tobacco 305.1
  toluene, toluol 304.6
  tranquilizer NEC 304.1
    nonbarbiturate with barbiturate effect 304.1
  tribromacetaldehyde 304.6
  tribromethanol 304.6
  tribromomethane 304.6
  trichloroethanol 304.6
  trichoroethyl phosphate 304.1
  triclofos 304.1
  Trional 304.1
  Tuinal 304.1
  Turkish Green 304.3
  urethan(e) 304.6
  Valium 304.1
  Valmid 304.1
  veganin 304.0
  veramon 304.1
  Veronal 304.1
  versidyne 304.6
  vinbarbital 304.1
  vinbarbitone 304.1
  vinyl bitone 304.1
  vitamin B_6 266.1
  wine 303.9
  Zactane 304.6
Dependency
  passive 301.6
  reactions 301.6
Depersonalization (episode, in neurotic state)
    (neurotic) (syndrome) 300.6
Depletion
  carbohydrates 271.9
  complement factor 279.8
  extracellular fluid 276.52
  plasma 276.52
  potassium 276.8
    nephropathy 588.89
  salt or sodium 276.1
    causing heat exhaustion or prostration 992.4
    nephropathy 593.9
  volume 276.50
    extracellular fluid 276.52
    plasma 276.52
Deposit
  argentous, cornea 371.16
  bone, in Boeck's sarcoid 135
  calcareous, calcium—*see* Calcification
  cholesterol
    retina 362.82
    skin 709.3
    vitreous (humor) 379.22
  conjunctival 372.56
  cornea, corneal NEC 371.10
    argentous 371.16
    in
      cystinosis 270.0 *[371.15]*
      mucopolysaccharidosis 277.5 *[371.15]*
  crystalline, vitreous (humor) 379.22
  hemosiderin, in old scars of cornea 371.11
  metallic, in lens 366.45
  skin 709.3
  teeth, tooth (betel) (black) (green) (materia alba)
    (orange) (soft) (tobacco) 523.6
  urate, in kidney (*see also* Disease, renal) 593.9
Depraved appetite 307.52
Depression 311
  acute (*see also* Psychosis, affective) 296.2
    recurrent episode 296.3

Depressive reaction

Depression—*continued*
    single episode 296.2
  agitated (*see also* Psychosis, affective) 296.2
    recurrent episode 296.3
    single episode 296.2
  anaclitic 309.21
  anxiety 300.4
  arches 734
    congenital 754.61
  autogenous (*see also* Psychosis, affective) 296.2
    recurrent episode 296.3
    single episode 296.2
  basal metabolic rate (BMR) 794.7
  bone marrow 289.9
  central nervous system 799.1
    newborn 779.2
  cerebral 331.9
    newborn 779.2
  cerebrovascular 437.8
    newborn 779.2
  chest wall 738.3
  endogenous (*see also* Psychosis, affective) 296.2
    recurrent episode 296.3
    single episode 296.2
  functional activity 780.99
  hysterical 300.11
  involutional, climacteric, or menopausal (*see
      also* Psychosis, affective) 296.2
    recurrent episode 296.3
    single episode 296.2
  manic (*see also* Psychosis, affective) 296.80
  medullary 348.8
    newborn 779.2
  mental 300.4
  metatarsal heads—*see* Depression, arches
  metatarsus—*see* Depression, arches
  monopolar (*see also* Psychosis, affective) 296.2
    recurrent episode 296.3
    single episode 296.2
  nervous 300.4
  neurotic 300.4
  nose 738.0
  postpartum 648.4
  psychogenic 300.4
    reactive 298.0
  psychoneurotic 300.4
  psychotic (*see also* Psychosis, affective) 296.2
    reactive 298.0
    recurrent episode 296.3
    single episode 296.2
  reactive 300.4
    neurotic 300.4
    psychogenic 298.0
    psychoneurotic 300.4
    psychotic 298.0
  recurrent 296.3
  respiratory center 348.8
    newborn 770.89
  scapula 736.89
  senile 290.21
  situational (acute) (brief) 309.0
    prolonged 309.1
  skull 754.0
  sternum 738.3
  visual field 368.40
Depressive reaction —*see also* Reaction,
    depressive
  acute (transient) 309.0
    with anxiety 309.28
    prolonged 309.1
  situational (acute) 309.0
    prolonged 309.1

931

Deprivation
  cultural V62.4
  emotional V62.89
    affecting
      adult 995.82
      infant or child 995.51
  food 994.2
    specific substance NEC 269.8
  protein (familial) (kwashiorkor) 260
  sleep V69.4
  social V62.4
    affecting
      adult 995.82
      infant or child 995.51
  symptoms, syndrome
    alcohol 291.81
    drug 292.0
  vitamins (*see also* Deficiency, vitamin) 269.2
  water 994.3
de Quervain's
  disease (tendon sheath) 727.04
  thyroiditis (subacute granulomatous thyroiditis) 245.1
Derangement
  ankle (internal) 718.97
    current injury (*see also* Dislocation, ankle) 837.0
    recurrent 718.37
  cartilage (articular) NEC (*see also* Disorder, cartilage, articular) 718.0
    knee 717.9
      recurrent 718.36
    recurrent 718.3
  collateral ligament (knee) (medial) (tibial) 717.82
    current injury 844.1
      lateral (fibular) 844.0
    lateral (fibular) 717.81
      current injury 844.0
  cruciate ligament (knee) (posterior) 717.84
    anterior 717.83
      current injury 844.2
    current injury 844.2
  elbow (internal) 718.92
    current injury (*see also* Dislocation, elbow) 832.00
    recurrent 718.32
  gastrointestinal 536.9
  heart—*see* Disease, heart
  hip (joint) (internal) (old) 718.95
    current injury (*see also* Dislocation, hip) 835.00
    recurrent 718.35
  intervertebral disc—*see* Displacement, intervertebral disc
  joint (internal) 718.90
    ankle 718.97
    current injury—*see also* Dislocation, by site
      knee, meniscus or cartilage (*see also* Tear, meniscus) 836.2
    elbow 718.92
    foot 718.97
    hand 718.94
    hip 718.95
    knee 717.9
    multiple sites 718.99
    pelvic region 718.95
    recurrent 718.30
      ankle 718.37
      elbow 718.32
      foot 718.37

Derangement—*continued*
    hand 718.34
    hip 718.35
    knee 718.36
    multiple sites 718.39
    pelvic region 718.35
    shoulder (region) 718.31
    specified site NEC 718.38
    temporomandibular (old) 524.69
    wrist 718.33
  shoulder (region) 718.91
    specified site NEC 718.98
    spine NEC 724.9
    temporomandibular 524.69
    wrist 718.93
  knee (cartilage) (internal) 717.9
    current injury (*see also* Tear, meniscus) 836.2
    ligament 717.89
      capsular 717.85
      collateral—*see* Derangement, collateral ligament
      cruciate—*see* Derangement, cruciate ligament
      specified NEC 717.85
    recurrent 718.36
  low back NEC 724.9
  meniscus NEC (knee) 717.5
    current injury (*see also* Tear, meniscus) 836.2
    lateral 717.40
      anterior horn 717.42
      posterior horn 717.43
      specified NEC 717.49
    medial 717.3
      anterior horn 717.1
      posterior horn 717.2
    recurrent 718.3
    site other than knee—*see* Disorder, cartilage, articular
  mental (*see also* Psychosis) 298.9
  rotator cuff (recurrent) (tear) 726.10
    current 840.4
  sacroiliac (old) 724.6
    current—*see* Dislocation, sacroiliac
  semilunar cartilage (knee) 717.5
    current injury 836.2
      lateral 836.1
      medial 836.0
    recurrent 718.3
  shoulder (internal) 718.91
    current injury (*see also* Dislocation, shoulder) 831.00
    recurrent 718.31
  spine (recurrent) NEC 724.9
    current—*see* Dislocation, spine
  temporomandibular (internal) (joint) (old) 524.69
    current—*see* Dislocation, jaw
Dercum's disease or syndrome (adiposis dolorosa) 272.8
Derealization (neurotic) 300.6
Dermal —*see* condition
Dermaphytid —*see* Dermatophytosis
Dermatergosis —*see* Dermatitis
Dermatitis (allergic) (contact) (occupational) (venenata) 692.9
  ab igne 692.82
  acneiform 692.9
  actinic (due to sun) 692.70
    acute 692.72
    chronic NEC 692.74
    other than from sun NEC 692.82

INDEX TO DISEASES

Dermatitis

Dermatitis—*continued*
- ambustionis
  - due to
    - burn or scald—*see* Burn, by site
    - sunburn (*see also* Sunburn) 692.71
- amebic 006.6
- ammonia 691.0
- anaphylactoid NEC 692.9
- arsenical 692.4
- artefacta 698.4
  - psychogenic 316 *[698.4]*
- asthmatic 691.8
- atopic (allergic) (intrinsic) 691.8
  - psychogenic 316 *[691.8]*
- atrophicans 701.8
  - diffusa 701.8
  - maculosa 701.3
- berlock, berloque 692.72
- blastomycetic 116.0
- blister beetle 692.89
- Brucella NEC 023.9
- bullosa 694.9
  - striata pratensis 692.6
- bullous 694.9
  - mucosynechial, atrophic 694.60
    - with ocular involvement 694.61
  - seasonal 694.8
- calorica
  - due to
    - burn or scald—*see* Burn, by site
    - cold 692.89
    - sunburn (*see also* Sunburn) 692.71
- caterpillar 692.89
- cercarial 120.3
- combustionis
  - due to
    - burn or scald—*see* Burn, by site
    - sunburn (*see also* Sunburn) 692.71
- congelationis 991.5
- contusiformis 695.2
- diabetic 250.8
- diaper 691.0
- diphtheritica 032.85
- due to
  - acetone 692.2
  - acids 692.4
  - adhesive plaster 692.4
  - alcohol (skin contact) (substances classifiable to 980.0-980.9) 692.4
    - taken internally 693.8
  - alkalis 692.4
  - allergy NEC 692.9
  - ammonia (household) (liquid) 692.4
  - animal
    - dander (cat) (dog) 692.84
    - hair (cat) (dog) 692.84
  - arnica 692.3
  - arsenic 692.4
    - taken internally 693.8
  - blister beetle 692.89
  - cantharides 692.3
  - carbon disulphide 692.2
  - caterpillar 692.89
  - caustics 692.4
  - cereal (ingested) 693.1
    - contact with skin 692.5
  - chemical(s) NEC 692.4
    - internal 693.8
    - irritant NEC 692.4
    - taken internally 693.8
  - chlorocompounds 692.2

Dermatitis—*continued*
- coffee (ingested) 693.1
  - contact with skin 692.5
- cold weather 692.89
- cosmetics 692.81
- cyclohexanes 692.2
- dander, animal (cat) (dog) 692.84
- deodorant 692.81
- detergents 692.0
- dichromate 692.4
- drugs and medicinals (correct substance properly administered) (internal use) 693.0
  - external (in contact with skin) 692.3
    - wrong substance given or taken 976.9
      - specified substance—*see* Table of drugs and chemicals
  - wrong substance given or taken 977.9
    - specified substance—*see* Table of drugs and chemicals
- dyes 692.89
  - hair 692.89
- epidermophytosis—*see* Dermatophytosis
- esters 692.2
- external irritant NEC 692.9
  - specified agent NEC 692.89
- eye shadow 692.81
- fish (ingested) 693.1
  - contact with skin 692.5
- flour (ingested) 693.1
  - contact with skin 692.5
- food (ingested) 693.1
  - in contact with skin 692.5
- fruit (ingested) 693.1
  - contact with skin 692.5
- fungicides 692.3
- furs 692.84
- glycols 692.2
- greases NEC 692.1
- hair, animal (cat) (dog) 692.84
- hair dyes 692.89
- hot
  - objects and materials—*see* Burn, by site
  - weather or places 692.89
- hydrocarbons 692.2
- infrared rays, except from sun 692.82
  - solar NEC (*see also* Dermatitis, due to, sun) 692.70
- ingested substance 693.9
  - drugs and medicinals (*see also* Dermatitis, due to, drugs and medicinals) 693.0
  - food 693.1
  - specified substance NEC 693.8
- ingestion or injection of
  - chemical 693.8
  - drug (correct substance properly administered) 693.0
    - wrong substance given or taken 977.9
      - specified substance—*see* Table of drugs and chemicals
- insecticides 692.4
- internal agent 693.9
  - drugs and medicinals (*see also* Dermatitis, due to, drugs and medicinals) 693.0
  - food (ingested) 693.1
    - in contact with skin 692.5
  - specified agent NEC 693.8
- iodine 692.3
- iodoform 692.3
- irradiation 692.82
- jewelry 692.83
- keratolytics 692.3

933

Dermatitis

Dermatitis—*continued*
   ketones 692.2
   lacquer tree (Rhus verniciflua) 692.6
   light (sun) NEC (*see also* Dermatitis, due to, sun) 692.70
      other 692.82
   low temperature 692.89
   mascara 692.81
   meat (ingested) 693.1
      contact with skin 692.5
   mercury, mercurials 692.3
   metals 692.83
   milk (ingested) 693.1
      contact with skin 692.5
   Neomycin 692.3
   nylon 692.4
   oils NEC 692.1
   paint solvent 692.2
   pediculocides 692.3
   petroleum products (substances classifiable to 981) 692.4
   phenol 692.3
   photosensitiveness, photosensitivity (sun) 692.72
      other light 692.82
   plants NEC 692.6
   plasters, medicated (any) 692.3
   plastic 692.4
   poison
      ivy (Rhus toxicodendron) 692.6
      oak (Rhus diversiloba) 692.6
      plant or vine 692.6
      sumac (Rhus venenata) 692.6
      vine (Rhus radicans) 692.6
   preservatives 692.89
   primrose (primula) 692.6
   primula 692.6
   radiation 692.82
      sun NEC (*see also* Dermatitis, due to, sun) 692.70
      tanning bed 692.82
   radioactive substance 692.82
   radium 692.82
   ragweed (Senecio jacobae) 692.6
   Rhus (diversiloba) (radicans) (toxicodendron) (venenata) (verniciflua) 692.6
   rubber 692.4
   scabicides 692.3
   Senecio jacobae 692.6
   solar radiation—*see* Dermatitis, due to, sun
   solvents (any) (substances classifiable to 982.0-982.8) 692.2
      chlorocompound group 692.2
      cyclohexane group 692.2
      ester group 692.2
      glycol group 692.2
      hydrocarbon group 692.2
      ketone group 692.2
      paint 692.2
   specified agent NEC 692.89
   sun 692.70
      acute 692.72
      chronic NEC 692.74
      specified NEC 692.79
   sunburn (*see also* Sunburn) 692.71
   sunshine NEC (*see also* Dermatitis, due to, sun) 692.70
   tanning bed 692.82
   tetrachlorethylene 692.2
   toluene 692.2
   topical medications 692.3

Dermatitis—*continued*
   turpentine 692.2
   ultraviolet rays, except from sun 692.82
      sun NEC (*see also* Dermatitis, due to, sun) 692.70
   vaccine or vaccination (correct substance properly administered) 693.0
      wrong substance given or taken
         bacterial vaccine 978.8
            specified—*see* Table of drugs and chemicals
         other vaccines NEC 979.9
            specified—*see* Table of drugs and chemicals
   varicose veins (*see also* Varicose, vein, inflamed or infected) 454.1
   x-rays 692.82
  dyshydrotic 705.81
  dysmenorrheica 625.8
  eczematoid NEC 692.9
   infectious 690.8
  eczematous NEC 692.9
  epidemica 695.89
  erysipelatosa 695.81
  escharotica—*see* Burn, by site
  exfoliativa, exfoliative 695.89
   generalized 695.89
   infantum 695.81
   neonatorum 695.81
  eyelid 373.31
   allergic 373.32
   contact 373.32
   eczematous 373.31
   herpes (zoster) 053.20
      simplex 054.41
   infective 373.5
      due to
         actinomycosis 039.3 *[373.5]*
         herpes
            simplex 054.41
            zoster 053.20
         impetigo 684 *[373.5]*
         leprosy (*see also* Leprosy) 030.0 *[373.4]*
         lupus vulgaris (tuberculous) (*see also* Tuberculosis) 017.0 *[373.4]*
         mycotic dermatitis (*see also* Dermatomycosis) 111.9 *[373.5]*
         vaccinia 051.0 *[373.5]*
            postvaccination 999.0 *[373.5]*
         yaws (*see also* Yaws) 102.9 *[373.4]*
  facta, factitia 698.4
   psychogenic 316 *[698.4]*
  ficta 698.4
   psychogenic 316 *[698.4]*
  flexural 691.8
  follicularis 704.8
  friction 709.8
  fungus 111.9
   specified type NEC 111.8
  gangrenosa, gangrenous (infantum) (*see also* Gangrene) 785.4
  gestationis 646.8
  gonococcal 098.89
  gouty 274.89
  harvest mite 133.8
  heat 692.89
  herpetiformis (bullous) (erythematous) (pustular) (vesicular) 694.0
   juvenile 694.2
   senile 694.5
  hiemalis 692.89

INDEX TO DISEASES   Dermatosis

Dermatitis—*continued*
  hypostatic, hypostatica 454.1
    with ulcer 454.2
  impetiginous 684
  infantile (acute) (chronic) (intertriginous)
    (intrinsic) (seborrheic) 690.12
  infectiosa eczematoides 690.8
  infectious (staphylococcal) (streptococcal) 686.9
    eczematoid 690.8
  infective eczematoid 690.8
  Jacquet's (diaper dermatitis) 691.0
  leptus 133.8
  lichenified NEC 692.9
  lichenoid, chronic 701.0
  lichenoides purpurica pigmentosa 709.1
  meadow 692.6
  medicamentosa (correct substance properly
    administered) (internal use) (*see also*
    Dermatitis, due to, drugs or medicinals)
    693.0
    due to contact with skin 692.3
  mite 133.8
  multiformis 694.0
    juvenile 694.2
    senile 694.5
  napkin 691.0
  neuro 698.3
  neurotica 694.0
  nummular NEC 692.9
  osteatosis, osteatotic 706.8
  papillaris capillitii 706.1
  pellagrous 265.2
  perioral 695.3
  perstans 696.1
  photosensitivity (sun) 692.72
    other light 692.82
  pigmented purpuric lichenoid 709.1
  polymorpha dolorosa 694.0
  primary irritant 692.9
  pruriginosa 694.0
  pruritic NEC 692.9
  psoriasiform nodularis 696.2
  psychogenic 316
  purulent 686.00
  pustular contagious 051.2
  pyococcal 686.00
  pyocyaneus 686.09
  pyogenica 686.00
  radiation 692.82
  repens 696.1
  Ritter's (exfoliativa) 695.81
  Schamberg's (progressive pigmentary
    dermatosis) 709.09
  schistosome 120.3
  seasonal bullous 694.8
  seborrheic 690.10
    infantile 690.12
  sensitization NEC 692.9
  septic (*see also* Septicemia) 686.00
    gonococcal 098.89
  solar, solare NEC (*see also* Dermatitis, due to,
    sun) 692.70
  stasis 459.81
    due to
      postphlebitic syndrome 459.12
        with ulcer 459.13
      varicose veins—*see* Varicose
    ulcerated or with ulcer (varicose) 454.2
  sunburn (*see also* Sunburn) 692.71
  suppurative 686.00
  traumatic NEC 709.8

Dermatitis—*continued*
  trophoneurotica 694.0
  ultraviolet, except from sun 692.82
    due to sun NEC (*see also* Dermatitis, due to,
    sun) 692.70
  varicose 454.1
    with ulcer 454.2
  vegetans 686.8
  verrucosa 117.2
  xerotic 706.8
Dermatoarthritis, lipoid 272.8 *[713.0]*
Dermatochalasia, dermatochalasis 374.87
Dermatofibroma (lenticulare) (M8832/0)—*see
  also* Neoplasm, skin, benign
  protuberans (M8832/1)—*see* Neoplasm, skin,
    uncertain behavior
Dermatofibrosarcoma (protuberans) (M8832/3)
  see Neoplasm, skin, malignant
Dermatographia 708.3
Dermatolysis (congenital) (exfoliativa) 757.39
  acquired 701.8
  eyelids 374.34
  palpebrarum 374.34
  senile 701.8
Dermatomegaly NEC 701.8
Dermatomucomyositis 710.3
Dermatomycosis 111.9
  furfuracea 111.0
  specified type NEC 111.8
Dermatomyositis (acute) (chronic) 710.3
Dermatoneuritis of children 985.0
Dermatophiliasis 134.1
Dermatophytide —*see* Dermatophytosis
Dermatophytosis (Epidermophyton) (infection)
  (microsporum) (tinea) (Trichophyton) 110.9
  beard 110.0
  body 110.5
  deep seated 110.6
  fingernails 110.1
  foot 110.4
  groin 110.3
  hand 110.2
  nail 110.1
  perianal (area) 110.3
  scalp 110.0
  scrotal 110.8
  specified site NEC 110.8
  toenails 110.1
  vulva 110.8
Dermatopolyneuritis 985.0
Dermatorrhexis 756.83
  acquired 701.8
Dermatosclerosis (*see also* Scleroderma) 710.1
  localized 701.0
Dermatosis 709.9
  Andrews' 686.8
  atopic 691.8
  Bowen's (M8081/2)—*see* Neoplasm, skin, in situ
  bullous 694.9
    specified type NEC 694.8
  erythematosquamous 690.8
  exfoliativa 695.89
  factitial 698.4
  gonococcal 098.89
  herpetiformis 694.0
    juvenile 694.2
    senile 694.5
  hysterical 300.11
  linear IgA 694.8
  menstrual NEC 709.8
  neutrophilic, acute febrile 695.89

Dermatosis—*continued*
  occupational (*see also* Dermatitis) 692.9
  papulosa nigra 709.8
  pigmentary NEC 709.00
    progressive 709.09
    Schamberg's 709.09
    Siemens-Bloch 757.33
  progressive pigmentary 709.09
  psychogenic 316
  pustular subcorneal 694.1
  Schamberg's (progressive pigmentary) 709.09
  senile NEC 709.3
  Unna's (seborrheic dermatitis) 690.10
Dermographia 708.3
Dermographism 708.3
Dermoid (cyst) (M9084/0)—*see also* Neoplasm, by site, benign
  with malignant transformation (M9084/3) 183.0
Dermopathy
  infiltrative, with thyrotoxicosis 242.0
  senile NEC 709.3
Dermophytosis —*see* Dermatophytosis
Descemet's membrane —*see* condition
Descemetocele 371.72
Descending —*see* condition
Descensus uteri (complete) (incomplete) (partial) (without vaginal wall prolapse) 618.1
  with mention of vaginal wall prolapse—*see* Prolapse, uterovaginal
Desensitization to allergens V07.1
Desert
  rheumatism 114.0
  sore (*see also* Ulcer, skin) 707.9
Desertion (child) (newborn) 995.52
  adult 995.84
Desmoid (extra-abdominal) (tumor) (M8821/1)—*see also* Neoplasm, connective tissue, uncertain behavior
  abdominal (M8822/1)—*see* Neoplasm, connective tissue, uncertain behavior
Despondency 300.4
Desquamative dermatitis NEC 695.89
Destruction
  articular facet (*see also* Derangement, joint) 718.9
    vertebra 724.9
  bone 733.90
    syphilitic 095.5
  joint (*see also* Derangement, joint) 718.9
    sacroiliac 724.6
  kidney 593.89
  live fetus to facilitate birth NEC 763.89
  ossicles (ear) 385.24
  rectal sphincter 569.49
  septum (nasal) 478.19
  tuberculous NEC (*see also* Tuberculosis) 011.9
  tympanic membrane 384.82
  tympanum 385.89
  vertebral disc—*see* Degeneration, intervertebral disc
Destructiveness (*see also* Disturbance, conduct) 312.9
  adjustment reaction 309.3
Detachment
  cartilage—*see also* Sprain, by site
    knee—*see* Tear, meniscus
  cervix, annular 622.8
    complicating delivery 665.3
  choroid (old) (postinfectional) (simple) (spontaneous) 363.70

Detatchment—*continued*
  hemorrhagic 363.72
  serous 363.71
  knee, medial meniscus (old) 717.3
    current injury 836.0
  ligament—*see* Sprain, by site
  placenta (premature)—*see* Placenta, separation
  retina (recent) 361.9
    with retinal defect (rhegmatogenous) 361.00
      giant tear 361.03
      multiple 361.02
      partial
        with
          giant tear 361.03
          multiple defects 361.02
          retinal dialysis (juvenile) 361.04
          single defect 361.01
      retinal dialysis (juvenile) 361.04
      single 361.01
      subtotal 361.05
      total 361.05
    delimited (old) (partial) 361.06
    old
      delimited 361.06
      partial 361.06
      total or subtotal 361.07
    pigment epithelium (RPE) (serous) 362.42
      exudative 362.42
      hemorrhagic 362.43
    rhegmatogenous (*see also* Detachment, retina, with retinal defect) 361.00
    serous (without retinal defect) 361.2
    specified type NEC 361.89
    traction (with vitreoretinal organization) 361.81
  vitreous humor 379.21
Detergent asthma 507.8
Deterioration
  epileptic
    with behavioral disturbance 345.9 *[294.11]*
    without behavioral disturbance 345.9 *[294.10]*
  heart, cardiac (*see also* Degeneration, myocardial) 429.1
  mental (*see also* Psychosis) 298.9
  myocardium, myocardial (*see also* Degeneration, myocardial) 429.1
  senile (simple) 797
  transplanted organ—*see* Complications, transplant, organ, by site
de Toni-Fanconi syndrome (cystinosis) 270.0
Deuteranomaly 368.52
Deuteranopia (anomalous trichromat) (complete) (incomplete) 368.52
Deutschländer's disease —*see* Fracture, foot
Development
  abnormal, bone 756.9
  arrested 783.40
    bone 733.91
    child 783.40
    due to malnutrition (protein-calorie) 263.2
    fetus or newborn 764.9
    tracheal rings (congenital) 748.3
  defective, congenital—*see also* Anomaly
    cauda equina 742.59
    left ventricle 746.9
      with atresia or hypoplasia of aortic orifice or valve with hypoplasia of ascending aorta 746.7
      in hypoplastic left heart syndrome 746.7

INDEX TO DISEASES

Diabetes, diabetic

Development—*continued*
  delayed (*see also* Delay, development) 783.40
    arithmetical skills 315.1
    language (skills) 315.31
      and speech due to hearing loss 315.34
      expressive 315.31
      mixed receptive-expressive 315.32
    learning skill, specified NEC 315.2
    mixed skills 315.5
    motor coordination 315.4
    reading 315.00
    specified
      learning skill NEC 315.2
      type NEC, except learning 315.8
    speech 315.39
      and language due to hearing loss 315.34
      associated with hyperkinesia 314.1
      phonological 315.39
    spelling 315.09
    written expression 315.2
  imperfect, congenital—*see also* Anomaly
    heart 746.9
    lungs 748.60
  improper (fetus or newborn) 764.9
  incomplete (fetus or newborn) 764.9
    affecting management of pregnancy 656.5
    bronchial tree 748.3
    organ or site not listed—*see* Hypoplasia
    respiratory system 748.9
  sexual, precocious NEC 259.1
  tardy, mental (*see also* Retardation, mental) 319
Developmental —*see* condition
Devergie's disease (pityriasis rubra pilaris) 696.4
Deviation
  conjugate (eye) 378.87
    palsy 378.81
    spasm, spastic 378.82
  esophagus 530.89
  eye, skew 378.87
  mandible, opening and closing 524.53
  midline (jaw) (teeth) 524.29
    specified site NEC—*see* Malposition
  occlusal plane 524.76
  organ or site, congenital NEC—*see* Malposition, congenital
  septum (acquired) (nasal) 470
    congenital 754.0
  sexual 302.9
    bestiality 302.1
    coprophilia 302.89
    ego-dystonic
      homosexuality 302.0
      lesbianism 302.0
    erotomania 302.89
      Clérambault's 297.8
    exhibitionism (sexual) 302.4
    fetishism 302.81
      transvestic 302.3
    frotteurism 302.89
    homosexuality, ego-dystonic 302.0
      pedophilic 302.2
    lesbianism, ego-dystonic 302.0
    masochism 302.83
    narcissism 302.89
    necrophilia 302.89
    nymphomania 302.89
    pederosis 302.2
    pedophilia 302.2
    sadism 302.84
    sadomasochism 302.84
    satyriasis 302.89

Deviation—*continued*
    specified type NEC 302.89
    transvestic fetishism 302.3
    transvestism 302.3
    voyeurism 302.82
    zoophilia (erotica) 302.1
  teeth, midline 524.29
  trachea 519.19
  ureter (congenital) 753.4
Devic's disease 341.0
Device
  cerebral ventricle (communicating) in situ V45.2
  contraceptive—*see* Contraceptive, device
  drainage, cerebrospinal fluid V45.2
Devil's
  grip 074.1
  pinches (purpura simplex) 287.2
Devitalized tooth 522.9
Devonshire colic 984.9
  specified type of lead—*see* Table of drugs and chemicals
Dextraposition, aorta 747.21
  with ventricular septal defect, pulmonary stenosis or atresia, and hypertrophy of right ventricle 745.2
  in tetralogy of Fallot 745.2
Dextratransposition, aorta 745.11
Dextrinosis, limit (debrancher enzyme deficiency) 271.0
Dextrocardia (corrected) (false) (isolated) (secondary) (true) 746.87
  with
    complete transposition of viscera 759.3
    situs inversus 759.3
Dextroversion, kidney (left) 753.3
Dhobie itch 110.3
Diabetes, diabetic (brittle) (congenital) (familial) (mellitus) (poorly controlled) (severe) (slight) (without complication) 250.0

> Note—Use the following fifth-digit subclassification with category 250:
>
> 0 type II or unspecified type, not stated as uncontrolled
>   Fifth-digit 0 is for use for type II patients, even if the patient requires insulin
> 1 type I [juvenile type], not stated as uncontrolled
> 2 type II or unspecified type, uncontrolled
>   Fifth-digit 2 is for use for type II patients, even if the paiten requires insulin
> 3 type I [juvenile type], uncontrolled

  with
    coma (with ketoacidosis) 250.3
      hyperosmolar (nonketotic) 250.2
    complication NEC 250.9
      specified NEC 250.8
    gangrene 250.7 *[785.4]*
    hyperosmolarity 250.2
    ketosis, ketoacidosis 250.1
    osteomyelitis 250.8 *[731.8]*
    specified manifestations NEC 250.8
  acetonemia 250.1
  acidosis 250.1
  amyotrophy 250.6 *[353.1]*
  angiopathy, peripheral 250.7 *[443.81]*
  asymptomatic 790.29
  autonomic neuropathy (peripheral) 250.6 *[337.1]*
  bone change 250.8 *[731.8]*

Diabetes, diabetic—continued
  bronze, bronzed 275.0
  cataract 250.5 [366.41]
  chemical 790.29
    complicating pregnancy, childbirth, or puerperium 648.8
  coma (with ketoacidosis) 250.3
    hyperglycemic 250.3
    hyperosmolar (nonketotic) 250.2
    hypoglycemic 250.3
    insulin 250.3
  complicating pregnancy, childbirth, or puerperium (maternal) 648.0
    affecting fetus or newborn 775.0
  complication NEC 250.9
    specified NEC 250.8
  dorsal sclerosis 250.6 [340]
  dwarfism-obesity syndrome 258.1
  gangrene 250.7 [785.4]
  gastroparesis 250.6 [536.3]
  gestational 648.8
    complicating pregnancy, childbirth, or puerperium 648.8
  glaucoma 250.5 [365.44]
  glomerulosclerosis (intercapillary) 250.4 [581.81]
  glycogenosis, secondary 250.8 [259.8]
  hemochromatosis 275.0
  hyperosmolar coma 250.2
  hyperosmolarity 250.2
  hypertension-nephrosis syndrome 250.4 [581.81]
  hypoglycemia 250.8
  hypoglycemic shock 250.8
  insipidus 253.5
    nephrogenic 588.1
    pituitary 253.5
    vasopressin-resistant 588.1
  intercapillary glomerulosclerosis 250.4 [581.81]
  iritis 250.5 [364.42]
  ketosis, ketoacidosis 250.1
  Kimmelstiel (-Wilson) disease or syndrome (intercapillary glomerulosclerosis) 250.4 [581.81]
  Lancereaux's (diabetes mellitus with marked emaciation) 250.8 [261]
  latent (chemical) 790.29
    complicating pregnancy, childbirth, or puerperium 648.8
  lipoidosis 250.8 [272.7]
  macular edema 250.5 [362.07]
  maternal
    with manifest disease in the infant 775.1
    affecting fetus or newborn 775.0
  microaneurysms, retinal 250.5 [362.01]
  mononeuropathy 250.6 [355.9]
  neonatal, transient 775.1
  nephropathy 250.4 [583.81]
  nephrosis (syndrome) 250.4 [581.81]
  neuralgia 250.6 [357.2]
  neuritis 250.6 [357.2]
  neurogenic arthropathy 250.6 [713.5]
  neuropathy 250.6 [357.2]
  nonclinical 790.29
  osteomyelitis 250.8 [731.8]
  peripheral autonomic neuropathy 250.6 [337.1]
  phosphate 275.3
  polyneuropathy 250.6 [357.2]
  renal (true) 271.4
  retinal
    edema 250.5 [362.07]
    hemorrhage 250.5 [362.01]
    microaneurysms 250.5 [362.01]

Diabetes, diabetic—continued
  retinitis 250.5 [362.01]
  retinopathy 250.5 [362.01]
    background 250.5 [362.01]
    nonproliferative 250.5 [362.03]
      mild 250.5 [362.04]
      moderate 250.5 [362.05]
      severe 250.5 [362.06]
    proliferative 250.5 [362.02]
  steroid induced
    correct substance properly administered 251.8
    overdose or wrong substance given or taken 962.0
  stress 790.29
  subclinical 790.29
  subliminal 790.29
  sugar 250.0
  ulcer (skin) 250.8 [707.9]
    lower extremity 250.8 [707.10]
      ankle 250.8 [707.13]
      calf 250.8 [707.12]
      foot 250.8 [707.15]
      heel 250.8 [707.14]
      knee 250.8 [707.19]
      specified site NEC 250.8 [707.19]
      thigh 250.8 [707.11]
      toes 250.8 [707.15]
    specified site NEC 250.8 [707.8]
  xanthoma 250.8 [272.2]
Diacyclothrombopathia 287.1
Diagnosis deferred 799.9
Dialysis (intermittent) (treatment)
  anterior retinal (juvenile) (with detachment) 361.04
  extracorporeal V56.0
  hemodialysis V56.0
    status only V45.1
  peritoneal V56.8
    status only V45.1
  renal V56.0
    status only V45.1
  specified type NEC V56.8
Diamond-Blackfan anemia or syndrome (congenital hypoplastic anemia) 284.01
Diamond-Gardener syndrome (autoerythrocyte sensitization) 287.2
Diaper rash 691.0
Diaphoresis (excessive) NEC (see also Hyperhidrosis) 780.8
Diaphragm —see condition
Diaphragmalgia 786.52
Diaphragmitis 519.4
Diaphyseal aclasis 756.4
Diaphysitis 733.99
Diarrhea, diarrheal (acute) (autumn) (bilious) (bloody) (catarrhal) (choleraic) (chronic) (gravis) (green) (infantile) (lienteric) (noninfectious) (presumed noninfectious) (putrefactive) (secondary) (sporadic) (summer) (symptomatic) (thermic) 787.91
  achlorhydric 536.0
  allergic 558.3
  amebic (see also Amebiasis) 006.9
    with abscess—see Abscess, amebic
    acute 006.0
    chronic 006.1
    nondysenteric 006.2
  bacillary—see Dysentery, bacillary
  bacterial NEC 008.5
  balantidial 007.0
  bile salt-induced 579.8

INDEX TO DISEASES

Diarrhea, diarrheal—*continued*
  cachectic NEC 787.91
  chilomastix 007.8
  choleriformis 001.1
  coccidial 007.2
  Cochin-China 579.1
    anguilluliasis 127.2
    psilosis 579.1
  Dientamoeba 007.8
  dietetic 787.91
  due to
    achylia gastrica 536.8
    Aerobacter aerogenes 008.2
    Bacillus coli—*see* Enteritis, E. coli
    bacteria NEC 008.5
    bile salts 579.8
    Capillaria
      hepatica 128.8
      philippinensis 127.5
    Clostridium perfringens (C) (F) 008.46
    Enterobacter aerogenes 008.2
    enterococci 008.49
    Escherichia coli—*see* Enteritis, E. coli
    Giardia lamblia 007.1
    Heterophyes heterophyes 121.6
    irritating foods 787.91
    Metagonimus yokogawai 121.5
    Necator americanus 126.1
    Paracolobactrum arizonae 008.1
    Paracolon bacillus NEC 008.47
      Arizona 008.1
    Proteus (bacillus) (mirabilis) (Morganii) 008.3
    Pseudomonas aeruginosa 008.42
    S. japonicum 120.2
    specified organism NEC 008.8
      bacterial 008.49
      viral NEC 008.69
    Staphylococcus 008.41
    Streptococcus 008.49
      anaerobic 008.46
    Strongyloides stercoralis 127.2
    Trichuris trichiuria 127.3
    virus NEC (*see also* Enteritis, viral) 008.69
  dysenteric 009.2
    due to specified organism NEC 008.8
  dyspeptic 787.91
  endemic 009.3
  epidemic 009.3
  fermentative 787.91
  flagellate 007.9
  Flexner's (ulcerative) 004.1
  functional 564.5
    following gastrointestinal surgery 564.4
    psychogenic 306.4
  giardial 007.1
  Giardia lamblia 007.1
  hill 579.1
  hyperperistalsis (nervous) 306.4
  infectious 009.2
    presumed 009.3
  inflammatory 787.91
    due to specified organism NEC 008.8
  malarial (*see also* Malaria) 084.6
  mite 133.8
  mycotic 117.9
  nervous 306.4
  neurogenic 564.5
  parenteral NEC 009.2
  postgastrectomy 564.4
  postvagotomy 564.4
  prostaglandin induced 579.8

Diarrhea, diarrheal—*continued*
  protozoal NEC 007.9
  psychogenic 306.4
  septic 009.2
    due to specified organism NEC 008.8
  specified organism NEC 008.8
    bacterial 008.49
    viral NEC 008.69
  Staphylococcus 008.41
  Streptococcus 008.49
    anaerobic 088.46
  toxic 558.2
  travelers' 009.2
    due to specified organism NEC 008.8
  trichomonal 007.3
  tropical 579.1
  tuberculous 014.8
  ulcerative (chronic) (*see also* Colitis, ulcerative) 556.9
  viral (*see also* Enteritis, viral) 008.8
  zymotic NEC 009.2
Diastasis
  cranial bones 733.99
    congenital 756.0
  joint (traumatic)—*see* Dislocation, by site
  muscle 728.84
    congenital 756.89
  recti (abdomen) 728.84
    complicating delivery 665.8
    congenital 756.79
Diastema, teeth, tooth 524.30
Diastematomyelia 742.51
Diataxia, cerebral, infantile 343.0
Diathesis
  allergic V15.09
  bleeding (familial) 287.9
  cystine (familial) 270.0
  gouty 274.9
  hemorrhagic (familial) 287.9
    newborn NEC 776.0
  oxalic 271.8
  scrofulous (*see also* Tuberculosis) 017.2
  spasmophilic (*see also* Tetany) 781.7
  ulcer 536.9
  uric acid 274.9
Diaz's disease or osteochondrosis 732.5
Dibothriocephaliasis 123.4
  larval 123.5
Dibothriocephalus (infection) (infestation) (latus) 123.4
  larval 123.5
Dicephalus 759.4
Dichotomy, teeth 520.2
Dichromat, dichromata (congenital) 368.59
Dichromatopsia (congenital) 368.59
Dichuchwa 104.0
Dicroceliasis 121.8
Didelphys, didelphic (*see also* Double uterus) 752.2
Didymitis (*see also* Epididymitis) 604.90
Died —*see also* Death
  without
    medical attention (cause unknown) 798.9
    sign of disease 798.2
Dientamoeba diarrhea 007.8
Dietary
  inadequacy or deficiency 269.9
  surveillance and counseling V65.3
Dietl's crisis 593.4

Dieulafoy lesion (hemorrhagic)
  of
    duodenum 537.84
    esophagus 530.82
    intestine 569.86
    stomach 537.84
Dieulafoy's ulcer —*see* Ulcer, stomach
Difficult
  birth, affecting fetus or newborn 763.9
  delivery NEC 669.9
Difficulty
  feeding 783.3
    adult 783.3
    breast 676.8
    child 783.3
    elderly 783.3
    infant 783.3
    newborn 779.3
    nonorganic (infant) NEC 307.59
  mechanical, gastroduodenal stoma 537.89
  reading 315.00
    specific, spelling 315.09
  swallowing (*see also* Dysphagia) 787.20
  walking 719.7
Diffuse —*see* condition
Diffused ganglion 727.42
DiGeorge's syndrome (thymic hypoplasia) 279.11
Digestive —*see* condition
Di Guglielmo's disease or syndrome (M9841/3) 207.0
Diktyoma (M9051/3)—*see* Neoplasm, by site, malignant
Dilaceration, tooth 520.4
Dilatation
  anus 564.89
    venule—*see* Hemorrhoids
  aorta (focal) (general) (*see also* Aneurysm, aorta) 441.9
    congenital 747.29
    infectional 093.0
    ruptured 441.5
    syphilitic 093.0
  appendix (cystic) 543.9
  artery 447.8
  bile duct (common) (cystic) (congenital) 751.69
    acquired 576.8
  bladder (sphincter) 596.8
    congenital 753.8
    in pregnancy or childbirth 654.4
      causing obstructed labor 660.2
        affecting fetus or newborn 763.1
  blood vessel 459.89
  bronchus, bronchi 494.0
    with acute exacerbation 494.1
  calyx (due to obstruction) 593.89
  capillaries 448.9
  cardiac (acute) (chronic) (*see also* Hypertrophy, cardiac) 429.3
    congenital 746.89
      valve NEC 746.89
        pulmonary 746.09
    hypertensive (*see also* Hypertension, heart) 402.90
  cavum septi pellucidi 742.4
  cecum 564.89
    psychogenic 306.4
  cervix (uteri)—*see also* Incompetency, cervix
    incomplete, poor, slow
      affecting fetus or newborn 763.7
      complicating delivery 661.0

Dilatation—*continued*
    affecting fetus or newborn 763.7
  colon 564.7
    congenital 751.3
    due to mechanical obstruction 560.89
    psychogenic 306.4
  common bile duct (congenital) 751.69
    acquired 576.8
      with calculus, choledocholithiasis, or stones—*see* Choledocholithiasis
  cystic duct 751.69
    acquired (any bile duct) 575.8
  duct, mammary 610.4
  duodenum 564.89
  esophagus 530.89
    congenital 750.4
    due to
      achalasia 530.0
      cardiospasm 530.0
  Eustachian tube, congenital 744.24
  fontanel 756.0
  gallbladder 575.8
    congenital 751.69
  gastric 536.8
    acute 536.1
    psychogenic 306.4
  heart (acute) (chronic) (*see also* Hypertrophy, cardiac) 429.3
    congenital 746.89
    hypertensive (*see also* Hypertension, heart) 402.90
    valve—*see also* Endocarditis
      congenital 746.89
  ileum 564.89
    psychogenic 306.4
  inguinal rings—*see* Hernia, inguinal
  jejunum 564.89
    psychogenic 306.4
  kidney (calyx) (collecting structures) (cystic) (parenchyma) (pelvis) 593.89
  lacrimal passages 375.69
  lymphatic vessel 457.1
  mammary duct 610.4
  Meckel's diverticulum (congenital) 751.0
  meningeal vessels, congenital 742.8
  myocardium (acute) (chronic) (*see also* Hypertrophy, cardiac) 429.3
  organ or site, congenital NEC—*see* Distortion
  pancreatic duct 577.8
  pelvis, kidney 593.89
  pericardium—*see* Pericarditis
  pharynx 478.29
  prostate 602.8
  pulmonary
    artery (idiopathic) 417.8
      congenital 747.3
    valve, congenital 746.09
  pupil 379.43
  rectum 564.89
  renal 593.89
  saccule vestibularis, congenital 744.05
  salivary gland (duct) 527.8
  sphincter ani 564.89
  stomach 536.8
    acute 536.1
    psychogenic 306.4
  submaxillary duct 527.8
  trachea, congenital 748.3
  ureter (idiopathic) 593.89
    congenital 753.20
    due to obstruction 593.5

INDEX TO DISEASES

Dilatation—*continued*
  urethra (acquired) 599.84
  vasomotor 443.9
  vein 459.89
  ventricular, ventricle (acute) (chronic) (*see also* Hypertrophy, cardiac) 429.3
    cerebral, congenital 742.4
    hypertensive (*see also* Hypertension, heart) 402.90
  venule 459.89
    anus—*see* Hemorrhoids
  vesical orifice 596.8
Dilated, dilation —*see* Dilatation
Diminished
  hearing (acuity) (*see also* Deafness) 389.9
  pulse pressure 785.9
  vision NEC 369.9
  vital capacity 794.2
Diminuta taenia 123.6
Diminution, sense or sensation (cold) (heat) (tactile) (vibratory) (*see also* Disturbance, sensation) 782.0
Dimitri-Sturge-Weber disease (encephalocutaneous angiomatosis) 759.6
Dimple
  parasacral 685.1
    with abscess 685.0
  pilonidal 685.1
    with abscess 685.0
  postanal 685.1
    with abscess 685.0
Dioctophyma renale (infection) (infestation) 128.8
Dipetalonemiasis 125.4
Diphallus 752.69
Diphtheria, diphtheritic (gangrenous) (hemorrhagic) 032.9
  carrier (suspected) of V02.4
  cutaneous 032.85
  cystitis 032.84
  faucial 032.0
  infection of wound 032.85
  inoculation (anti) (not sick) V03.5
  laryngeal 032.3
  myocarditis 032.82
  nasal anterior 032.2
  nasopharyngeal 032.1
  neurological complication 032.89
  peritonitis 032.83
  specified site NEC 032.89
Diphyllobothriasis (intestine) 123.4
  larval 123.5
Diplacusis 388.41
Diplegia (upper limbs) 344.2
  brain or cerebral 437.8
  congenital 343.0
  facial 351.0
    congenital 352.6
  infantile or congenital (cerebral) (spastic) (spinal) 343.0
  lower limbs 344.1
  syphilitic, congenital 090.49
Diplococcus, diplococcal —*see* condition
Diplomyelia 742.59
Diplopia 368.2
  refractive 368.15
Dipsomania (*see also* Alcoholism) 303.9
  with psychosis (*see also* Psychosis, alcoholic) 291.9
Dipylidiasis 123.8
  intestine 123.8
Direction, teeth, abnormal 524.30

Dirt-eating child 307.52
Disability
  heart—*see* Disease, heart
  learning NEC 315.2
    special spelling 315.09
Disarticulation (*see also* Derangement, joint) 718.9
  meaning
    amputation
      status—*see* Absence, by site
      traumatic —*see* Amputation, traumatic
    dislocation, traumatic or congenital—*see* Dislocation
Disaster, cerebrovascular (*see also* Disease, cerebrovascular, acute) 436
Discharge
  anal NEC 787.99
  breast (female) (male) 611.79
  conjunctiva 372.89
  continued locomotor idiopathic (*see also* Epilepsy) 345.5
  diencephalic autonomic idiopathic (*see also* Epilepsy) 345.5
  ear 388.60
    blood 388.69
    cerebrospinal fluid 388.61
  excessive urine 788.42
  eye 379.93
  nasal 478.19
  nipple 611.79
  patterned motor idiopathic (*see also* Epilepsy) 345.5
  penile 788.7
  postnasal—*see* Sinusitis
  sinus, from mediastinum 510.0
  umbilicus 789.9
  urethral 788.7
    bloody 599.84
  vaginal 623.5
Discitis 722.90
  cervical, cervicothoracic 722.91
  lumbar, lumbosacral 722.93
  thoracic, thoracolumbar 722.92
Discogenic syndrome —*see* Displacement, intervertebral disc
Discoid
  kidney 753.3
  meniscus, congenital 717.5
  semilunar cartilage 717.5
Discoloration
  mouth 528.9
  nails 703.8
  teeth 521.7
    due to
      drugs 521.7
      metals (copper) (silver) 521.7
      pulpal bleeding 521.7
    during formation 520.8
    extrinsic 523.6
    intrinsic posteruptive 521.7
Discomfort
  chest 786.59
  visual 368.13
Discomycosis —*see* Actinomycosis
Discontinuity, ossicles, ossicular chain 385.23
Discrepancy
  centric occlusion
    maximum intercuspation 524.55
    of teeth 524.55
  leg length (acquired) 736.81
    congenital 755.30
  uterine size-date 649.6

Discrimination

Discrimination
political V62.4
racial V62.4
religious V62.4
sex V62.4
Disease, diseased —*see also* Syndrome
Abrami's (acquired hemolytic jaundice) 283.9
absorbent system 459.89
accumulation—*see* Thesaurismosis
acid-peptic 536.8
Acosta's 993.2
Adams-Stokes (-Morgagni) (syncope with heart block) 426.9
Addison's (bronze) (primary adrenal insufficiency) 255.41
anemia (pernicious) 281.0
tuberculous (*see also* Tuberculosis) 017.6
Addison-Gull—*see* Xanthoma
adenoids (and tonsils) (chronic) 474.9
adrenal (gland) (capsule) (cortex) 255.9
hyperfunction 255.3
hypofunction 255.41
specified type NEC 255.8
ainhum (dactylolysis spontanea) 136.0
akamushi (scrub typhus) 081.2
Akureyri (epidemic neuromyasthenia) 049.8
Albarrán's (colibacilluria) 791.9
Albers-Schönberg's (marble bones) 756.52
Albert's 726.71
Albright (-Martin) (-Bantam) 275.49
Alibert's (mycosis fungoides) (M9700/3) 202.1
Alibert-Bazin (M9700/3) 202.1
alimentary canal 569.9
alligator skin (ichthyosis congenital) 757.1
acquired 701.1
Almeida's (Brazilian blastomycosis) 116.1
Alpers' 330.8
alpine 993.2
altitude 993.2
alveoli, teeth 525.9
Alzheimer's—*see* Alzheimer's
amyloid (any site) 277.30
anarthritic rheumatoid 446.5
Anders' (adiposis tuberosa simplex) 272.8
Andersen's (glycogenosis IV) 271.0
Anderson's (angiokeratoma corporis diffusum) 272.7
Andes 993.2
Andrews' (bacterid) 686.8
angiospastic, angiospasmodic 443.9
cerebral 435.9
with transient neurologic deficit 435.9
vein 459.89
anterior
chamber 364.9
horn cell 335.9
specified type NEC 335.8
antral (chronic) 473.0
acute 461.0
anus NEC 569.49
aorta (nonsyphilitic) 447.9
syphilitic NEC 093.89
aortic (heart) (valve) (*see also* Endocarditis, aortic) 424.1
apollo 077.4
aponeurosis 726.90
appendix 543.9
aqueous (chamber) 364.9
arc-welders' lung 503
Armenian 277.31
Arnold-Chiari (*see also* Spina bifida) 741.0

INDEX TO DISEASES

Disease, diseased—*continued*
arterial 447.9
occlusive (*see also* Occlusion, by site) 444.22
with embolus or thrombus—*see* Occlusion, by site
due to stricture or stenosis 447.1
specified type NEC 447.8
arteriocardiorenal (*see also* Hypertension, cardiorenal) 404.90
arteriolar (generalized) (obliterative) 447.9
specified type NEC 447.8
arteriorenal—*see* Hypertension, kidney
arteriosclerotic—*see also* Arteriosclerosis
cardiovascular 429.2
coronary —*see* Arteriosclerosis, coronary
heart —*see* Arteriosclerosis, coronary
artery 447.9
cerebral 437.9
coronary —*see* Arteriosclerosis, coronary
specified type NEC 447.8
arthropod-borne NEC 088.9
specified type NEC 088.89
Asboe-Hansen's (incontinentia pigmenti) 757.33
atticoantral, chronic (with posterior or superior marginal perforation of ear drum) 382.2
auditory canal, ear 380.9
Aujeszky's 078.89
auricle, ear NEC 380.30
Australian X 062.4
autoimmune NEC 279.4
hemolytic (cold type) (warm type) 283.0
parathyroid 252.1
thyroid 245.2
aviators' (*see also* Effect, adverse, high altitude) 993.2
ax(e)-grinders' 502
Ayala's 756.89
Ayerza's (pulmonary artery sclerosis with pulmonary hypertension) 416.0
Azorean (of the nervous system) 334.8
Babington's (familial hemorrhagic telangiectasia) 448.0
back bone NEC 733.90
bacterial NEC 040.89
zoonotic NEC 027.9
specified type NEC 027.8
Baehr-Schiffrin (thrombotic thrombocytopenic purpura) 446.6
Baelz's (cheilitis glandularis apostematosa) 528.5
Baerensprung's (eczema marginatum) 110.3
Balfour's (chloroma) 205.3
balloon (*see also* Effect, adverse, high altitude) 993.2
Baló's 341.1
Bamberger (-Marie) (hypertrophic pulmonary osteoarthropathy) 731.2
Bang's (Brucella abortus) 023.1
Bannister's 995.1
Banti's (with cirrhosis) (with portal hypertension)—*see* Cirrhosis, liver
Barcoo (*see also* Ulcer, skin) 707.9
barium lung 503
Barlow (-Möller) (infantile scurvy) 267
barometer makers' 985.0
Barraquer (-Simons) (progressive lipodystrophy) 272.6
basal ganglia 333.90
degenerative NEC 333.0
specified NEC 333.89
Basedow's (exophthalmic goiter) 242.0

INDEX TO DISEASES

Disease, diseased—*continued*
  basement membrane NEC 583.89
    with
      pulmonary hemorrhage (Goodpasture's syndrome) 446.21 *[583.81]*
  Bateman's 078.0
    purpura (senile) 287.2
  Batten's 330.1 *[362.71]*
  Batten-Mayou (retina) 330.1 *[362.71]*
  Batten-Steinert 359.21
  Battey 031.0
  Baumgarten-Cruveilhier (cirrhosis of liver) 571.5
  bauxite-workers' 503
  Bayle's (dementia paralytica) 094.1
  Bazin's (primary) (*see also* Tuberculosis) 017.1
  Beard's (neurasthenia) 300.5
  Beau's (*see also* Degeneration, myocardial) 429.1
  Bechterew's (ankylosing spondylitis) 720.0
  Becker's
    idiopathic mural endomyocardial disease 425.2
    myotonia congenita, recessive form 359.22
  Begbie's (exophthalmic goiter) 242.0
  Behr's 362.50
  Beigel's (white piedra) 111.2
  Bekhterev's (ankylosing spondylitis) 720.0
  Bell's (*see also* Psychosis, affective) 296.0
  Bennett's (leukemia) 208.9
  Benson's 379.22
  Bergeron's (hysteroepilepsy) 300.11
  Berlin's 921.3
  Bernard-Soulier (thrombopathy) 287.1
  Bernhardt (-Roth) 355.1
  beryllium 503
  Besnier-Boeck (-Schaumann) (sarcoidosis) 135
  Best's 362.76
  Beurmann's (sporotrichosis) 117.1
  Bielschowsky (-Jansky) 330.1
  Biermer's (pernicious anemia) 281.0
  Biett's (discoid lupus erythematosus) 695.4
  bile duct (*see also* Disease, biliary) 576.9
  biliary (duct) (tract) 576.9
    with calculus, choledocholithiasis, or stones—*see* Choledocholithiasis
  Billroth's (meningocele) (*see also* Spina bifida) 741.9
  Binswanger's 290.12
  Bird's (oxaluria) 271.8
  bird fanciers' 495.2
  black lung 500
  bladder 596.9
    specified NEC 596.8
  bleeder's 286.0
  Bloch-Sulzberger (incontinentia pigmenti) 757.33
  Blocq's (astasia-abasia) 307.9
  blood (-forming organs) 289.9
    specified NEC 289.89
    vessel 459.9
  Bloodgood's 610.1
  Blount's (tibia vara) 732.4
  blue 746.9
  Bodechtel-Guttmann (subacute sclerosing panencephalitis) 046.2
  Boeck's (sarcoidosis) 135
  bone 733.90
    fibrocystic NEC 733.29
    jaw 526.2
    marrow 289.9
    Paget's (osteitis deformans) 731.0

Disease, diseased—*continued*
  specified type NEC 733.99
  von Recklinghausen's (osteitis fibrosa cystica) 252.01
  Bonfils'—*see* Disease, Hodgkin's
  Borna 062.9
  Bornholm (epidemic pleurodynia) 074.1
  Bostock's (*see also* Fever, hay) 477.9
  Bouchard's (myopathic dilatation of the stomach) 536.1
  Bouillaud's (rheumatic heart disease) 391.9
  Bourneville (-Brissaud) (tuberous sclerosis) 759.5
  Bouveret (-Hoffmann) (paroxysmal tachycardia) 427.2
  bowel 569.9
    functional 564.9
    psychogenic 306.4
  Bowen's (M8081/2)—*see* Neoplasm, skin, in situ
  Bozzolo's (multiple myeloma) (M9730/3) 203.0
  Bradley's (epidemic vomiting) 078.82
  Brailsford's 732.3
    radius, head 732.3
    tarsal, scaphoid 732.5
  Brailsford-Morquio (mucopolysaccharidosis IV) 277.5
  brain 348.9
    Alzheimer's 331.0
      with dementia—*see* Alzheimer's, dementia
    arterial, artery 437.9
    arteriosclerotic 437.0
    congenital 742.9
    degenerative—*see* Degeneration, brain
    inflammatory—*see also* Encephalitis
      late effect—*see* category 326
    organic 348.9
      arteriosclerotic 437.0
    parasitic NEC 123.9
    Pick's 331.11
      with dementia
        with behavioral disturbance 331.11 *[294.11]*
        without behavioral disturbance 331.11 *[294.10]*
    senile 331.2
  braziers' 985.8
  breast 611.9
    cystic (chronic) 610.1
    fibrocystic 610.1
    inflammatory 611.0
    Paget's (M8540/3) 174.0
    puerperal, postpartum NEC 676.3
    specified NEC 611.8
  Breda's (*see also* Yaws) 102.9
  Breisky's (kraurosis vulvae) 624.09
  Bretonneau's (diphtheritic malignant angina) 032.0
  Bright's (*see also* Nephritis) 583.9
    arteriosclerotic (*see also* Hypertension, kidney) 403.90
  Brill's (recrudescent typhus) 081.1
    flea-borne 081.0
    louse-borne 081.1
  Brill-Symmers (follicular lymphoma) (M9690/3) 202.0
  Brill-Zinsser (recrudescent typhus) 081.1
  Brinton's (leather bottle stomach) (M8142/3) 151.9
  Brion-Kayser (*see also* Fever, paratyphoid) 002.9

943

Disease, diseased—*continued*
  broad
    beta 272.2
    ligament, noninflammatory 620.9
      specified NEC 620.8
  Brocq's 691.8
    meaning
      atopic (diffuse) neurodermatitis 691.8
      dermatitis herpetiformis 694.0
      lichen simplex chronicus 698.3
      parapsoriasis 696.2
      prurigo 698.2
  Brocq-Duhring (dermatitis herpetiformis) 694.0
  Brodie's (joint) (*see also* Osteomyelitis) 730.1
  bronchi 519.19
  bronchopulmonary 519.19
  bronze (Addison's) 255.41
    tuberculous (*see also* Tuberculosis) 017.6
  Brown-Séquard 344.89
  Bruck's 733.99
  Bruck-de Lange (Amsterdam dwarf, mental retardation, and brachycephaly) 759.89
  Bruhl's (splenic anemia with fever) 285.8
  Bruton's (X-linked agammaglobulinemia) 279.04
  buccal cavity 528.9
  Buchanan's (juvenile osteochondrosis, iliac crest) 732.1
  Buchman's (osteochondrosis juvenile) 732.1
  Budgerigar-fanciers' 495.2
  Büdinger-Ludloff-Läwen 717.89
  Buerger's (thromboangiitis obliterans) 443.1
  Bürger-Grütz (essential familial hyperlipemia) 272.3
  Burns' (lower ulna) 732.3
  bursa 727.9
  Bury's (erythema elevatum diutinum) 695.89
  Buschke's 710.1
  Busquet's (*see also* Osteomyelitis) 730.1
  Busse-Buschke (cryptococcosis) 117.5
  C$_2$ (*see also* Alcoholism) 303.9
  Caffey's (infantile cortical hyperostosis) 756.59
  caisson 993.3
  calculus 592.9
  California 114.0
  Calvé (-Perthes) (osteochondrosis, femoral capital) 732.1
  Camurati-Engelmann (diaphyseal sclerosis) 756.59
  Canavan's 330.0
  capillaries 448.9
  Carapata 087.1
  cardiac-*see* Disease, heart
  cardiopulmonary, chronic 416.9
  cardiorenal (arteriosclerotic) (hepatic) (hypertensive) (vascular) (*see also* Hypertension, cardiorenal) 404.90
  cardiovascular (arteriosclerotic) 429.2
    congenital 746.9
    hypertensive (*see also* Hypertension, heart) 402.90
      benign 402.10
      malignant 402.00
    renal (*see also* Hypertension, cardiorenal) 404.90
    syphilitic (asymptomatic) 093.9
  carotid gland 259.8
  Carrión's (Bartonellosis) 088.0
  cartilage NEC 733.90
    specified NEC 733.99
  Castellani's 104.8

Disease, diseased—*continued*
  cat-scratch 078.3
  Cavare's (familial periodic paralysis) 359.3
  Cazenave's (pemphigus) 694.4
  cecum 569.9
  celiac (adult) 579.0
    infantile 579.0
  cellular tissue NEC 709.9
  central core 359.0
  cerebellar, cerebellum—*see* Disease, brain
  cerebral (*see also* Disease, brain) 348.9
    arterial, artery 437.9
    degenerative—*see* Degeneration, brain
  cerebrospinal 349.9
  cerebrovascular NEC 437.9
    acute 436
      embolic—*see* Embolism, brain
      late effect—*see* Late effect(s) (of) cerebrovascular disease
      puerperal, postpartum, childbirth 674.0
      thrombotic—*see* Thrombosis, brain
    arteriosclerotic 437.0
    embolic—*see* Embolism, brain
    ischemic, generalized NEC 437.1
    late effect—*see* Late effect(s) (of) cerebrovascular disease
    occlusive 437.1
    puerperal, postpartum, childbirth 674.0
    specified type NEC 437.8
    thrombotic—*see* Thrombosis, brain
  ceroid storage 272.7
  cervix (uteri)
    inflammatory 616.0
    noninflammatory 622.9
      specified NEC 622.8
  Chabert's 022.9
  Chagas' (*see also* Trypanosomiasis, American) 086.2
  Chandler's (osteochondritis dissecans, hip) 732.7
  Charcot's (joint) 094.0 *[713.5]*
    spinal cord 094.0
  Charcot-Marie-Tooth 356.1
  Charlouis' (*see also* Yaws) 102.9
  Cheadle (-Möller) (-Barlow) (infantile scurvy) 267
  Chédiak-Steinbrinck (-Higashi) (congenital gigantism of peroxidase granules) 288.2
  cheek, inner 528.9
  chest 519.9
  Chiari's (hepatic vein thrombosis) 453.0
  Chicago (North American blastomycosis) 116.0
  chignon (white piedra) 111.2
  chigoe, chigo (jigger) 134.1
  childhood granulomatous 288.1
  Chinese liver fluke 121.1
  chlamydial NEC 078.88
  cholecystic (*see also* Disease, gallbladder) 575.9
  choroid 363.9
    degenerative (*see also* Degeneration, choroid) 363.40
    hereditary (*see also* Dystrophy, choroid) 363.50
    specified type NEC 363.8
  Christian's (chronic histiocytosis X) 277.89
  Christian-Weber (nodular nonsuppurative panniculitis) 729.30
  Christmas 286.1
  ciliary body 364.9
    specified NEC 364.89
  circulatory (system) NEC 459.9

INDEX TO DISEASES

Disease, diseased—*continued*
  chronic, maternal, affecting fetus or newborn 760.3
  specified NEC 459.89
  syphilitic 093.9
    congenital 090.5
Civatte's (poikiloderma) 709.09
climacteric 627.2
  male 608.89
coagulation factor deficiency (congenital) (*see also* Defect, coagulation) 286.9
Coats' 362.12
coccidioidal pulmonary 114.5
  acute 114.0
  chronic 114.4
  primary 114.0
  residual 114.4
Cockayne's (microcephaly and dwarfism) 759.89
Cogan's 370.52
cold
  agglutinin 283.0
    or hemoglobinuria 283.0
      paroxysmal (cold) (nocturnal) 283.2
  hemagglutinin (chronic) 283.0
collagen NEC 710.9
  nonvascular 710.9
  specified NEC 710.8
  vascular (allergic) (*see also* Angiitis, hypersensitivity) 446.20
colon 569.9
  functional 564.9
    congenital 751.3
  ischemic 557.0
combined system (of spinal cord) 266.2 *[336.2]*
  with anemia (pernicious) 281.0 *[336.2]*
compressed air 993.3
Concato's (pericardial polyserositis) 423.2
  peritoneal 568.82
  pleural—*see* Pleurisy
congenital NEC 799.89
conjunctiva 372.9
  chlamydial 077.98
    specified NEC 077.8
  specified type NEC 372.89
  viral 077.99
    specified NEC 077.8
connective tissue, diffuse (*see also* Disease, collagen) 710.9
Conor and Bruch's (boutonneuse fever) 082.1
Conradi (-Hünermann) 756.59
Cooley's (erythroblastic anemia) 282.49
Cooper's 610.1
Corbus' 607.1
cork-handlers' 495.3
cornea (*see also* Keratopathy) 371.9
coronary (*see also* Ischemia, heart) 414.9
  congenital 746.85
  ostial, syphilitic 093.20
    aortic 093.22
    mitral 093.21
    pulmonary 093.24
    tricuspid 093.23
Corrigan's—*see* Insufficiency, aortic
Cotugno's 724.3
Coxsackie (virus) NEC 074.8
cranial nerve NEC 352.9
Creutzfeldt-Jakob (new variant) 046.1
  with dementia
    with behavioral disturbance 046.1 *[294.11]*
    without behavioral disturbance 046.1 *[294.10]*

Disease, diseased—*continued*
Crigler-Najjar (congenital hyperbilirubinemia) 277.4
Crocq's (acrocyanosis) 443.89
Crohn's (intestine) (*see also* Enteritis, regional) 555.9
Crouzon's (craniofacial dysostosis) 756.0
Cruchet's (encephalitis lethargica) 049.8
Cruveilhier's 335.21
Cruz-Chagas (*see also* Trypanosomiasis, American) 086.2
crystal deposition (*see also* Arthritis, due to, crystals) 712.9
Csillag's (lichen sclerosus et atrophicus) 701.0
Curschmann's 359.21
Cushing's (pituitary basophilism) 255.0
cystic
  breast (chronic) 610.1
  kidney, congenital (*see also* Cystic, disease, kidney) 753.10
  liver, congenital 751.62
  lung 518.89
    congenital 748.4
  pancreas 577.2
    congenital 751.7
  renal, congenital (*see also* Cystic, disease, kidney) 753.10
  semilunar cartilage 717.5
cysticercus 123.1
cystine storage (with renal sclerosis) 270.0
cytomegalic inclusion (generalized) 078.5
  with
    pneumonia 078.5 *[484.1]*
    congenital 771.1
Daae (-Finsen) (epidemic pleurodynia) 074.1
dancing 297.8
Danielssen's (anesthetic leprosy) 030.1
Darier's (congenital) (keratosis follicularis) 757.39
  erythema annulare centrifugum 695.0
  vitamin A deficiency 264.8
Darling's (histoplasmosis) (*see also* Histoplasmosis, American) 115.00
Davies' 425.0
de Beurmann-Gougerot (sporotrichosis) 117.1
Débove's (splenomegaly) 789.2
deer fly (*see also* Tularemia) 021.9
deficiency 269.9
degenerative—*see also* Degeneration
  disc—*see* Degeneration, intervertebral disc
Degos' 447.8
Déjérine (-Sottas) 356.0
Deleage's 359.89
demyelinating, demyelinizating (brain stem) (central nervous system) 341.9
  multiple sclerosis 340
  specified NEC 341.8
de Quervain's (tendon sheath) 727.04
  thyroid (subacute granulomatous thyroiditis) 245.1
Dercum's (adiposis dolorosa) 272.8
Deutschländer's—*see* Fracture, foot
Devergie's (pityriasis rubra pilaris) 696.4
Devic's 341.0
diaphorase deficiency 289.7
diaphragm 519.4
diarrheal, infectious 009.2
diatomaceous earth 502
Diaz's (osteochondrosis astragalus) 732.5
digestive system 569.9

Disease, diseased—*continued*
 Di Guglielmo's (erythemic myelosis) (M9841/3) 207.0
 Dimitri-Sturge-Weber (encephalocutaneous angiomatosis) 759.6
 disc, degenerative—*see* Degeneration, intervertebral disc
 discogenic (*see also* Disease, intervertebral disc) 722.90
 diverticular—*see* Diverticula
 Down's (mongolism) 758.0
 Dubini's (electric chorea) 049.8
 Dubois' (thymus gland) 090.5
 Duchenne's 094.0
  locomotor ataxia 094.0
  muscular dystrophy 359.1
  paralysis 335.22
  pseudohypertrophy, muscles 359.1
 Duchenne-Griesinger 359.1
 ductless glands 259.9
 Duhring's (dermatitis herpetiformis) 694.0
 Dukes (-Filatov) 057.8
 duodenum NEC 537.9
  specified NEC 537.89
 Duplay's 726.2
 Dupré's (meningism) 781.6
 Dupuytren's (muscle contracture) 728.6
 Durand-Nicolas-Favre (climatic bubo) 099.1
 Duroziez's (congenital mitral stenosis) 746.5
 Dutton's (trypanosomiasis) 086.9
 Eales' 362.18
 ear (chronic) (inner) NEC 388.9
  middle 385.9
   adhesive (*see also* Adhesions, middle ear) 385.10
   specified NEC 385.89
 Eberth's (typhoid fever) 002.0
 Ebstein's
  heart 746.2
  meaning diabetes 250.4 *[581.81]*
 Echinococcus (*see also* Echinococcus) 122.9
 ECHO virus NEC 078.89
 Economo's (encephalitis lethargica) 049.8
 Eddowes' (brittle bones and blue sclera) 756.51
 Edsall's 992.2
 Eichstedt's (pityriasis versicolor) 111.0
 Ellis-van Creveld (chondroectodermal dysplasia) 756.55
 endocardium—*see* Endocarditis
 endocrine glands or system NEC 259.9
  specified NEC 259.8
 endomyocardial, idiopathic mural 425.2
 Engel-von Recklinghausen (osteitis fibrosa cystica) 252.01
 Engelmann's (diaphyseal sclerosis) 756.59
 English (rickets) 268.0
 Engman's (infectious eczematoid dermatitis) 690.8
 enteroviral, enterovirus NEC 078.89
  central nervous system NEC 048
 epidemic NEC 136.9
 epididymis 608.9
 epigastric, functional 536.9
  psychogenic 306.4
 Erb (-Landouzy) 359.1
 Erb-Goldflam 358.00
 Erichsen's (railway spine) 300.16
 esophagus 530.9
  functional 530.5
  psychogenic 306.4
 Eulenburg's (congenital paramyotonia) 359.29

Disease, diseased—*continued*
 Eustachian tube 381.9
 Evans' (thrombocytopenic purpura) 287.32
 external auditory canal 380.9
 extrapyramidal NEC 333.90
 eye 379.90
  anterior chamber 364.9
  inflammatory NEC 364.3
  muscle 378.9
 eyeball 360.9
 eyelid 374.9
 eyeworm of Africa 125.2
 Fabry's (angiokeratoma corporis diffusum) 272.7
 facial nerve (seventh) 351.9
  newborn 767.5
 Fahr-Volhard (malignant nephrosclerosis) 403.00
 fallopian tube, noninflammatory 620.9
  specified NEC 620.8
 familial periodic 277.31
  paralysis 359.3
 Fanconi's (congenital pancytopenia) 284.09
 Farber's (disseminated lipogranulomatosis) 272.8
 fascia 728.9
  inflammatory 728.9
 Fauchard's (periodontitis) 523.40
 Favre-Durand-Nicolas (climatic bubo) 099.1
 Favre-Racouchot (elastoidosis cutanea nodularis) 701.8
 Fede's 529.0
 Feer's 985.0
 Felix's (juvenile osteochondrosis, hip) 732.1
 Fenwick's (gastric atrophy) 537.89
 Fernels' (aortic aneurysm) 441.9
 fibrocaseous, of lung (*see also* Tuberculosis, pulmonary) 011.9
 fibrocystic—*see also* Fibrocystic, disease
  newborn 277.01
 Fiedler's (leptospiral jaundice) 100.0
 fifth 057.0
 Filatoff's (infectious mononucleosis) 075
 Filatov's (infectious mononucleosis) 075
 file-cutters' 984.9
  specified type of lead—*see* Table of drugs and chemicals
 filterable virus NEC 078.89
 fish skin 757.1
  acquired 701.1
 Flajani (-Basedow) (exophthalmic goiter) 242.0
 Flatau-Schilder 341.1
 flax-dressers' 504
 Fleischner's 732.3
 flint 502
 fluke—*see* Infestation, fluke
 Følling's (phenylketonuria) 270.1
 foot and mouth 078.4
 foot process 581.3
 Forbes' (glycogenosis III) 271.0
 Fordyce's (ectopic sebaceous glands) (mouth) 750.26
 Fordyce-Fox (apocrine miliaria) 705.82
 Fothergill's
  meaning scarlatina anginosa 034.1
  neuralgia (*see also* Neuralgia, trigeminal) 350.1
 Fournier's 608.83
 fourth 057.8
 Fox (-Fordyce) (apocrine miliaria) 705.82
 Francis' (*see also* Tularemia) 021.9

INDEX TO DISEASES

Disease, diseased—*continued*
Franklin's (heavy chain) 273.2
Frei's (climatic bubo) 099.1
Freiberg's (flattening metatarsal) 732.5
Friedländer's (endarteritis obliterans)—*see* Arteriosclerosis
Friedreich's
  combined systemic or ataxia 334.0
  facial hemihypertrophy 756.0
  myoclonia 333.2
Fröhlich's (adiposogenital dystrophy) 253.8
Frommel's 676.6
frontal sinus (chronic) 473.1
  acute 461.1
Fuller's earth 502
fungus, fungous NEC 117.9
Gaisböck's (polycythemia hypertonica) 289.0
gallbladder 575.9
  congenital 751.60
Gamna's (siderotic splenomegaly) 289.51
Gamstorp's (adynamia episodica hereditaria) 359.3
Gandy-Nanta (siderotic splenomegaly) 289.51
gannister (occupational) 502
Garré's (*see also* Osteomyelitis) 730.1
gastric (*see also* Disease, stomach) 537.9
gastrointestinal (tract) 569.9
  amyloid 277.39
  functional 536.9
    psychogenic 306.4
Gaucher's (adult) (cerebroside lipidosis) (infantile) 272.7
Gayet's (superior hemorrhagic polioencephalitis) 265.1
Gee (-Herter) (-Heubner) (-Thaysen) (nontropical sprue) 579.0
generalized neoplastic (M8000/6) 199.0
genital organs NEC
  female 629.9
    specified NEC 629.89
  male 608.9
Gerhardt's (erythromelalgia) 443.82
Gerlier's (epidemic vertigo) 078.81
Gibert's (pityriasis rosea) 696.3
Gibney's (perispondylitis) 720.9
Gierke's (glycogenosis I) 271.0
Gilbert's (familial nonhemolytic jaundice) 277.4
Gilchrist's (North American blastomycosis) 116.0
Gilford (-Hutchinson) (progeria) 259.8
Gilles de la Tourette's (motor-verbal tic) 307.23
Giovannini's 117.9
gland (lymph) 289.9
Glanzmann's (hereditary hemorrhagic thrombasthenia) 287.1
glassblowers' 527.1
Glénard's (enteroptosis) 569.89
Glisson's (*see also* Rickets) 268.0
glomerular
  membranous, idiopathic 581.1
  minimal change 581.3
glycogen storage (Andersen's) (Cori types 1-7) (Forbes') (McArdle-Schmid-Pearson) (Pompe's) (types I-VII) 271.0
  cardiac 271.0 *[425.7]*
  generalized 271.0
  glucose-6-phosphatase deficiency 271.0
  heart 271.0 *[425.7]*
  hepatorenal 271.0
  liver and kidneys 271.0
  myocardium 271.0 *[425.7]*

Disease, diseased—*continued*
von Gierke's (glycogenosis I) 271.0
Goldflam-Erb 358.00
Goldscheider's (epidermolysis bullosa) 757.39
Goldstein's (familial hemorrhagic telangiectasia) 448.0
gonococcal NEC 098.0
Goodall's (epidemic vomiting) 078.82
Gordon's (exudative enteropathy) 579.8
Gougerot's (trisymptomatic) 709.1
Gougerot-Carteaud (confluent reticulate papillomatosis) 701.8
Gougerot-Hailey-Hailey (benign familial chronic pemphigus) 757.39
graft-versus-host (bone marrow) 996.85
  due to organ transplant NEC—*see* Complications, transplant, organ
grain-handlers' 495.8
Grancher's (splenopneumonia)—*see* Pneumonia
granulomatous (childhood) (chronic) 288.1
graphite lung 503
Graves' (exophthalmic goiter) 242.0
Greenfield's 330.0
green monkey 078.89
Griesinger's (*see also* Ancylostomiasis) 126.9
grinders' 502
Grisel's 723.5
Gruby's (tinea tonsurans) 110.0
Guertin's (electric chorea) 049.8
Guillain-Barré 357.0
Guinon's (motor-verbal tic) 307.23
Gull's (thyroid atrophy with myxedema) 244.8
Gull and Sutton's—*see* Hypertension, kidney
gum NEC 523.9
Günther's (congenital erythropoietic porphyria) 277.1
gynecological 629.9
  specified NEC 629.89
H 270.0
Haas' 732.3
Habermann's (acute parapsoriasis varioliformis) 696.2
Haff 985.1
Hageman (congenital factor XII deficiency) (*see also* Defect, congenital) 286.3
Haglund's (osteochondrosis os tibiale externum) 732.5
Hagner's (hypertrophic pulmonary osteoarthropathy) 731.2
Hailey-Hailey (benign familial chronic pemphigus) 757.39
hair (follicles) NEC 704.9
  specified type NEC 704.8
Hallervorden-Spatz 333.0
Hallopeau's (lichen sclerosus et atrophicus) 701.0
Hamman's (spontaneous mediastinal emphysema) 518.1
hand, foot, and mouth 074.3
Hand-Schüller-Christian (chronic histiocytosis X) 277.89
Hanot's—*see* Cirrhosis, biliary
Hansen's (leprosy) 030.9
  benign form 030.1
  malignant form 030.0
Harada's 363.22
Harley's (intermittent hemoglobinuria) 283.2
Hart's (pellagra-cerebellar ataxia renal aminoaciduria) 270.0
Hartnup (pellagra-cerebellar ataxia-renal aminoaciduria) 270.0

Disease, diseased—*continued*
Hashimoto's (struma lymphomatosa) 245.2
Hb—*see* Disease, hemoglobin
heart (organic) 429.9
  with
    acute pulmonary edema (*see also* Failure, ventricular, left) 428.1
    hypertensive 402.91
      with renal failure 404.92
      benign 402.11
        with renal failure 404.12
      malignant 402.01
        with renal failure 404.02
    kidney disease—*see* Hypertension, cardiorenal
    rheumatic fever (conditions classifiable to 390)
      active 391.9
        with chorea 392.0
      inactive or quiescent (with chorea) 398.90
  amyloid 277.39 *[425.7]*
  aortic (valve) (*see also* Endocarditis, aortic) 424.1
  arteriosclerotic or sclerotic (minimal) (senile)—*see* Arteriosclerosis, coronary
  artery, arterial —*see* Arteriosclerosis, coronary
  atherosclerotic —*see* Arteriosclerosis, coronary
  beer drinkers' 425.5
  beriberi 265.0 *[425.7]*
  black 416.0
  congenital NEC 746.9
    cyanotic 746.9
    maternal, affecting fetus or newborn 760.3
    specified type NEC 746.89
  congestive (*see also* Failure, heart) 428.0
  coronary 414.9
  cryptogenic 429.9
  due to
    amyloidosis 277.39 *[425.7]*
    beriberi 265.0 *[425.7]*
    cardiac glycogenosis 271.0 *[425.7]*
    Friedreich's ataxia 334.0 *[425.8]*
    gout 274.82
    mucopolysaccharidosis 277.5 *[425.7]*
    myotonia atrophica 359.21 *[425.8]*
    progressive muscular dystrophy 359.1 *[425.8]*
    sarcoidosis 135 *[425.8]*
  fetal 746.9
    inflammatory 746.89
  fibroid (*see also* Myocarditis) 429.0
  functional 427.9
    postoperative 997.1
    psychogenic 306.2
  glycogen storage 271.0 *[425.7]*
  gonococcal NEC 098.85
  gouty 274.82
  hypertensive (*see also* Hypertension, heart) 402.90
    benign 402.10
    malignant 402.00
  hyperthyroid (*see also* Hyperthyroidism) 242.9 *[425.7]*
  incompletely diagnosed—*see* Disease, heart
  ischemic (chronic) (*see also* Ischemia, heart) 414.9
    acute (*see also* Infarct, myocardium) 410.9
      without myocardial infarction 411.89
        with coronary (artery) occlusion 411.81

Disease, diseased—*continued*
  asymptomatic 412
    diagnosed on ECG or other special investigation but currently presenting no symptoms 412
  kyphoscoliotic 416.1
  mitral (*see also* Endocarditis, mitral) 394.9
  muscular (*see also* Degeneration, myocardial) 429.1
  postpartum 674.8
  psychogenic (functional) 306.2
  pulmonary (chronic) 416.9
    acute 415.0
    specified NEC 416.8
  rheumatic (chronic) (inactive) (old) (quiescent) (with chorea) 398.90
    active or acute 391.9
      with chorea (active) (rheumatic) (Sydenham's) 392.0
    specified type NEC 391.8
  maternal, affecting fetus or newborn 760.3
  rheumatoid—*see* Arthritis, rheumatoid
  sclerotic —*see* Arteriosclerosis, coronary
  senile (*see also* Myocarditis) 429.0
  specified type NEC 429.89
  syphilitic 093.89
    aortic 093.1
      aneurysm 093.0
    asymptomatic 093.89
    congenital 090.5
  thyroid (gland) (*see also* Hyperthyroidism) 242.9 *[425.7]*
  thyrotoxic (*see also* Thyrotoxicosis) 242.9 *[425.7]*
  tuberculous (*see also* Tuberculosis) 017.9 *[425.7]*
  valve, valvular (obstructive) (regurgitant)—*see also* Endocarditis
    congenital NEC (*see also* Anomaly, heart, valve) 746.9
    pulmonary 746.00
    specified type NEC 746.89
  vascular—*see* Disease, cardiovascular
heavy-chain (gamma G) 273.2
Heberden's 715.04
Hebra's
  dermatitis exfoliativa 695.89
  erythema multiforme exudativum 695.1
  pityriasis
    maculata et circinata 696.3
    rubra 695.89
      pilaris 696.4
  prurigo 698.2
Heerfordt's (uveoparotitis) 135
Heidenhain's 290.10
  with dementia 290.10
Heilmeyer-Schöner (M9842/3) 207.1
Heine-Medin (*see also* Poliomyelitis) 045.9
Heller's (*see also* Psychosis, childhood) 299.1
Heller-Döhle (syphilitic aortitis) 093.1
hematopoietic organs 289.9
hemoglobin (Hb) 282.7
  with thalassemia 282.49
  abnormal (mixed) NEC 282.7
    with thalassemia 282.49
  AS genotype 282.5
  Bart's 282.49
  C (Hb-C) 282.7
    with other abnormal hemoglobin NEC 282.7
    elliptocytosis 282.7

INDEX TO DISEASES

Disease, diseased—*continued*
- Hb-S (without crisis) 282.63
  - with
    - crisis 282.64
    - vaso-occlusive pain 282.64
  - sickle-cell (without crisis) 282.63
    - with
      - crisis 282.64
      - vaso-occlusive pain 282.64
  - thalassemia 282.49
- constant spring 282.7
- D (Hb-D) 282.7
  - with other abnormal hemoglobin NEC 282.7
  - Hb-S (without crisis) 282.68
    - with crisis 282.69
  - sickle-cell (without crisis) 282.68
    - with crisis 282.69
  - thalassemia 282.49
- E (Hb-E) 282.7
  - with other abnormal hemoglobin NEC 282.7
  - Hb-S (without crisis) 282.68
    - with crisis 282.69
  - sickle-cell (without crisis) 282.68
    - with crisis 282.69
  - thalassemia 282.49
- elliptocytosis 282.7
- F (Hb-F) 282.7
- G (Hb-G) 282.7
- H (Hb-H) 282.49
- hereditary persistence, fetal (HPFH) ("Swiss variety") 282.7
- high fetal gene 282.7
- I thalassemia 282.49
- M 289.7
- S—*see also* Disease, sickle-cell, Hb-S
  - thalassemia (without crisis) 282.41
    - with
      - crisis 282.42
      - vaso-occlusive pain 282.42
- spherocytosis 282.7
- unstable, hemolytic 282.7
- Zurich (Hb-Zurich) 282.7
- hemolytic (fetus) (newborn) 773.2
  - autoimmune (cold type) (warm type) 283.0
  - due to or with
    - incompatibility
      - ABO (blood group) 773.1
      - blood (group) (Duffy) (Kell) (Kidd) (Lewis) (M) (S) NEC 773.2
      - Rh (blood group) (factor) 773.0
    - Rh negative mother 773.0
  - unstable hemoglobin 282.7
- hemorrhagic 287.9
  - newborn 776.0
- Henoch (-Schönlein) (purpura nervosa) 287.0
- hepatic—*see* Disease, liver
- hepatolenticular 275.1
- heredodegenerative NEC
  - brain 331.89
  - spinal cord 336.8
- Hers' (glycogenosis VI) 271.0
- Herter (-Gee) (-Heubner) (nontropical sprue) 579.0
- Herxheimer's (diffuse idiopathic cutaneous atrophy) 701.8
- Heubner's 094.89
- Heubner-Herter (nontropical sprue) 579.0
- high fetal gene or hemoglobin thalassemia 282.49
- Hildenbrand's (typhus) 081.9

Disease, diseased—*continued*
- hip (joint) NEC 719.95
  - congenital 755.63
  - suppurative 711.05
  - tuberculous (*see also* Tuberculosis) 015.1 [730.85]
- Hippel's (retinocerebral angiomatosis) 759.6
- Hirschfeld's (acute diabetes mellitus) (*see also* Diabetes) 250.0
- Hirschsprung's (congenital megacolon) 751.3
- His (-Werner) (trench fever) 083.1
- HIV 042
- Hodgkin's (M9650/3) 201.9

> Note—Use the following fifth-digit subclassification with categories 201:
>
> 0 unspecified site
> 1 lymph nodes of head, face, and neck
> 2 intrathoracic lymph nodes
> 3 intra-abdominal lymph nodes
> 4 lymph nodes of axilla and upper limb
> 5 lymph nodes of inguinal region and lower limb
> 6 intrapelvic lymph nodes
> 7 spleen
> 8 lymph nodes of multiple sites

- lymphocytic
  - depletion (M9653/3) 201.7
    - diffuse fibrosis (M9654/3) 201.7
    - reticular type (M9655/3) 201.7
  - predominance (M9651/3) 201.4
- lymphocytic-histiocytic predominance (M9651/3) 201.4
- mixed cellularity (M9652/3) 201.6
- nodular sclerosis (M9656/3) 201.5
  - cellular phase (M9657/3) 201.5
- Hodgson's 441.9
  - ruptured 441.5
- Hoffa (-Kastert) (liposynovitis prepatellaris) 272.8
- Holla (*see also* Spherocytosis) 282.0
- homozygous-Hb-S 282.61
- hoof and mouth 078.4
- hookworm (*see also* Ancylostomiasis) 126.9
- Horton's (temporal arteritis) 446.5
- host-versus-graft (immune or nonimmune cause) 996.80
  - bone marrow 996.85
  - heart 996.83
  - intestines 996.87
  - kidney 996.81
  - liver 996.82
  - lung 996.84
  - pancreas 996.86
  - specified NEC 996.89
- HPFH (hereditary persistence of fetal hemoglobin) ("Swiss variety") 282.7
- Huchard's (continued arterial hypertension) 401.9
- Huguier's (uterine fibroma) 218.9
- human immunodeficiency (virus) 042
- hunger 251.1
- Hunt's
  - dyssynergia cerebellaris myoclonica 334.2
  - herpetic geniculate ganglionitis 053.11
- Huntington's 333.4
- Huppert's (multiple myeloma) (M9730/3) 203.0
- Hurler's (mucopolysaccharidosis I) 277.5

Disease, diseased—*continued*
  Hutchinson's, meaning
    angioma serpiginosum 709.1
    cheiropompholyx 705.81
    prurigo estivalis 692.72
  Hutchinson-Boeck (sarcoidosis) 135
  Hutchinson-Gilford (progeria) 259.8
  hyaline (diffuse) (generalized) 728.9
    membrane (lung) (newborn) 769
  hydatid (*see also* Echinococcus) 122.9
  Hyde's (prurigo nodularis) 698.3
  hyperkinetic (*see also* Hyperkinesia) 314.9
    heart 429.82
  hypertensive (*see also* Hypertension) 401.9
  hypophysis 253.9
    hyperfunction 253.1
    hypofunction 253.2
  Iceland (epidemic neuromyasthenia) 049.8
  I cell 272.7
  ill-defined 799.89
  immunologic NEC 279.9
  immunoproliferative 203.8
  inclusion 078.5
    salivary gland 078.5
  infancy, early NEC 779.9
  infective NEC 136.9
  inguinal gland 289.9
  internal semilunar cartilage, cystic 717.5
  intervertebral disc 722.90
    with myelopathy 722.70
    cervical, cervicothoracic 722.91
      with myelopathy 722.71
    lumbar, lumbosacral 722.93
      with myelopathy 722.73
    thoracic, thoracolumbar 722.92
      with myelopathy 722.72
  intestine 569.9
    functional 564.9
      congenital 751.3
      psychogenic 306.4
    lardaceous 277.39
    organic 569.9
    protozoal NEC 007.9
  iris 364.9
    specified NEC 364.89
  iron
    metabolism 275.0
    storage 275.0
  Isambert's (*see also* Tuberculosis, larynx) 012.3
  Iselin's (osteochondrosis, fifth metatarsal) 732.5
  Island (scrub typhus) 081.2
  itai-itai 985.5
  Jadassohn's (maculopapular erythroderma) 696.2
  Jadassohn-Pellizari's (anetoderma) 701.3
  Jakob-Creutzfeldt (new variant) 046.1
    with dementia
      with behavioral disturbance 046.1 *[294.11]*
      without behavioral disturbance 046.1 *[294.10]*
  Jaksch (-Luzet) (pseudoleukemia infantum) 285.8
  Janet's 300.89
  Jansky-Bielschowsky 330.1
  jaw NEC 526.9
    fibrocystic 526.2
  Jensen's 363.05
  Jeune's (asphyxiating thoracic dystrophy) 756.4
  jigger 134.1
  Johnson-Stevens (erythema multiforme exudativum) 695.1

Disease, diseased—*continued*
  joint NEC 719.9
    ankle 719.97
    Charcot 094.0 *[713.5]*
    degenerative (*see also* Osteoarthrosis) 715.9
      multiple 715.09
      spine (*see also* Spondylosis) 721.90
    elbow 719.92
    foot 719.97
    hand 719.94
    hip 719.95
    hypertrophic (chronic) (degenerative) (*see also* Osteoarthrosis) 715.9
      spine (*see also* Spondylosis) 721.90
    knee 719.96
    Luschka 721.90
    multiple sites 719.99
    pelvic region 719.95
    sacroiliac 724.6
    shoulder (region) 719.91
    specified site NEC 719.98
    spine NEC 724.9
      pseudarthrosis following fusion 733.82
      sacroiliac 724.6
    wrist 719.93
  Jourdain's (acute gingivitis) 523.00
  Jüngling's (sarcoidosis) 135
  Kahler (-Bozzolo) (multiple myeloma) (M9730/3) 203.0
  Kalischer's 759.6
  Kaposi's 757.33
    lichen ruber 697.8
      acuminatus 696.4
      moniliformis 697.8
    xeroderma pigmentosum 757.33
  Kaschin-Beck (endemic polyarthritis) 716.00
    ankle 716.07
    arm 716.02
      lower (and wrist) 716.03
      upper (and elbow) 716.02
    foot (and ankle) 716.07
    forearm (and wrist) 716.03
    hand 716.04
    leg 716.06
      lower 716.06
      upper 716.05
    multiple sites 716.09
    pelvic region (hip) (thigh) 716.05
    shoulder region 716.01
    specified site NEC 716.08
  Katayama 120.2
  Kawasaki 446.1
  Kedani (scrub typhus) 081.2
  kidney (functional) (pelvis) (*see also* Disease, renal) 593.9
    chronic 585.9
      requiring chronic dialysis 585.6
      stage
        I 585.1
        II (mild) 585.2
        III (moderate) 585.3
        IV (severe) 585.4
        V 585.5
    cystic (congenital) 753.10
      multiple 753.19
      single 753.11
      specified NEC 753.19
    fibrocystic (congenital) 753.19
    in gout 274.10
    polycystic (congenital) 753.12
      adult type (APKD) 753.13

INDEX TO DISEASES

Disease, diseased—*continued*
  autosomal dominant 753.13
  autosomal recessive 753.14
  childhood type (CPKD) 753.14
  infantile type 753.14
 Kienböck's (carpal lunate) (wrist) 732.3
 Kimmelstiel (-Wilson) (intercapillary glomerulosclerosis) 250.4 *[581.81]*
 Kinnier Wilson's (hepatolenticular degeneration) 275.1
 kissing 075
 Kleb's (*see also* Nephritis) 583.9
 Klinger's 446.4
 Klippel's 723.8
 Klippel-Feil (brevicollis) 756.16
 knight's 911.1
 Köbner's (epidermolysis bullosa) 757.39
 Koenig-Wichmann (pemphigus) 694.4
 Köhler's
  first (osteoarthrosis juvenilis) 732.5
  second (Freiberg's infraction, metatarsal head) 732.5
  patellar 732.4
  tarsal navicular (bone) (osteoarthrosis juvenilis) 732.5
 Köhler-Freiberg (infraction, metatarsal head) 732.5
 Köhler-Mouchet (osteoarthrosis juvenilis) 732.5
 Köhler-Pellegrini-Stieda (calcification, knee joint) 726.62
 Kok 759.89
 König's (osteochondritis dissecans) 732.7
 Korsakoff's (nonalcoholic) 294.0
  alcoholic 291.1
 Kostmann's (infantile genetic agranulocytosis) 288.01
 Krabbe's 330.0
 Kraepelin-Morel (*see also* Schizophrenia) 295.9
 Kraft-Weber-Dimitri 759.6
 Kufs' 330.1
 Kugelberg-Welander 335.11
 Kuhnt-Junius 362.52
 Kümmell's (-Verneuil) (spondylitis) 721.7
 Kundrat's (lymphosarcoma) 200.1
 kuru 046.0
 Kussmaul (-Meier) (polyarteritis nodosa) 446.0
 Kyasanur Forest 065.2
 Kyrle's (hyperkeratosis follicularis in cutem penetrans) 701.1
 labia
  inflammatory 616.10
  noninflammatory 624.9
   specified NEC 624.8
 labyrinth, ear 386.8
 lacrimal system (apparatus) (passages) 375.9
  gland 375.00
  specified NEC 375.89
 Lafora's 333.2
 Lagleyze-von Hippel (retinocerebral angiomatosis) 759.6
 Lancereaux-Mathieu (leptospiral jaundice) 100.0
 Landry's 357.0
 Lane's 569.89
 lardaceous (any site) 277.39
 Larrey-Weil (leptospiral jaundice) 100.0
 Larsen (-Johansson) (juvenile osteopathia patellae) 732.4
 larynx 478.70
 Lasègue's (persecution mania) 297.9
 Leber's 377.16

Disease, diseased—*continued*
 Lederer's (acquired infectious hemolytic anemia) 283.19
 Legg's (capital femoral osteochondrosis) 732.1
 Legg-Calvé-Perthes (capital femoral osteochondrosis) 732.1
 Legg-Calvé-Waldenström (femoral capital osteochondrosis) 732.1
 Legg-Perthes (femoral capital osteochondrosis) 732.1
 Legionnaires' 482.84
 Leigh's 330.8
 Leiner's (exfoliative dermatitis) 695.89
 Leloir's (lupus erythematosus) 695.4
 Lenegre's 426.0
 lens (eye) 379.39
 Leriche's (osteoporosis, posttraumatic) 733.7
 Letterer-Siwe (acute histiocytosis X) (M9722/3) 202.5
 Lev's (acquired complete heart block) 426.0
 Lewandowski's (*see also* Tuberculosis) 017.0
 Lewandowski-Lutz (epidermodysplasia verruciformis) 078.19
 Lewy body 331.82
  with dementia
   with behavioral disturbance 331.82 *[294.11]*
   without behavioral disturbance 331.82 *[294.10]*
 Leyden's (periodic vomiting) 536.2
 Libman-Sacks (verrucous endocarditis) 710.0 *[424.91]*
 Lichtheim's (subacute combined sclerosis with pernicious anemia) 281.0 *[336.2]*
 ligament 728.9
 light chain 203.0
 Lightwood's (renal tubular acidosis) 588.89
 Lignac's (cystinosis) 270.0
 Lindau's (retinocerebral angiomatosis) 759.6
 Lindau-von Hippel (angiomatosis retinocerebellosa) 759.6
 lip NEC 528.5
 lipidosis 272.7
 lipoid storage NEC 272.7
 Lipschütz's 616.50
 Little's—*see* Palsy, cerebral
 liver 573.9
  alcoholic 571.3
   acute 571.1
   chronic 571.3
  chronic 571.9
   alcoholic 571.3
  cystic, congenital 751.62
  drug-induced 573.3
  due to
   chemicals 573.3
   fluorinated agents 573.3
   hypersensitivity drugs 573.3
   isoniazids 573.3
  end stage NEC 572.8
   due to hepatitis —*see* Hepatitis
  fibrocystic (congenital) 751.62
  glycogen storage 271.0
  organic 573.9
  polycystic (congenital) 751.62
 Lobo's (keloid blastomycosis) 116.2
 Lobstein's (brittle bones and blue sclera) 756.51
 locomotor system 334.9
 Lorain's (pituitary dwarfism) 253.3
 Lou Gehrig's 335.20
 Lucas-Championnière (fibrinous bronchitis) 466.0
 Ludwig's (submaxillary cellulitis) 528.3

951

Disease, diseased — *continued*
  luetic—*see* Syphilis
  lumbosacral region 724.6
  lung NEC 518.89
    black 500
    congenital 748.60
    cystic 518.89
      congenital 748.4
    fibroid (chronic) (*see also* Fibrosis, lung) 515
    fluke 121.2
      Oriental 121.2
    in
      amyloidosis 277.39 *[517.8]*
      polymyositis 710.4 *[517.8]*
      sarcoidosis 135 *[517.8]*
      Sjögren's syndrome 710.2 *[517.8]*
      syphilis 095.1
      systemic lupus erythematosus 710.0 *[517.8]*
      systemic sclerosis 710.1 *[517.2]*
    interstitial (chronic) 515
      acute 136.3
    nonspecific, chronic 496
    obstructive (chronic) (COPD) 496
      with
        acute
          bronchitis 491.22
          exacerbation NEC 491.21
        alveolitis, allergic (*see also* Alveolitis, allergic) 495.9
        asthma (chronic) (obstructive) 493.2
        bronchiectasis 494.0
          with exacerbation (acute) 494.1
        bronchitis (chronic) 491.20
          with
            acute bronchitis 491.22
            exacerbation (acute) 491.21
          decompensated 491.21
            with exacerbation 491.21
        emphysema NEC 492.8
    diffuse (with fibrosis) 496
    polycystic 518.89
      asthma (chronic) (obstructive) 493.2
      congenital 748.4
    purulent (cavitary) 513.0
    restrictive 518.89
    rheumatoid 714.81
      diffuse interstitial 714.81
    specified NEC 518.89
  Lutembacher's (atrial septal defect with mitral stenosis) 745.5
  Lutz-Miescher (elastosis perforans serpiginosa) 701.1
  Lutz-Splendore-de Almeida (Brazilian blastomycosis) 116.1
  Lyell's (toxic epidermal necrolysis) 695.1
    due to drug
      correct substance properly administered 695.1
      overdose or wrong substance given or taken 977.9
        specific drug—*see* Table of drugs and chemicals
  Lyme 088.81
  lymphatic (gland) (system) 289.9
    channel (noninfective) 457.9
    vessel (noninfective) 457.9
      specified NEC 457.8
  lymphoproliferative (chronic) (M9970/1) 238.79
  Machado-Joseph 334.8
  Madelung's (lipomatosis) 272.8

Disease, diseased — *continued*
  Madura (actinomycotic) 039.9
    mycotic 117.4
  Magitot's 526.4
  Majocchi's (purpura annularis telangiectodes) 709.1
  malarial (*see also* Malaria) 084.6
  Malassez's (cystic) 608.89
  Malibu 919.8
    infected 919.9
  malignant (M8000/3)—*see also* Neoplasm, by site, malignant
    previous, affecting management of pregnancy V23.8
  Manson's 120.1
  maple bark 495.6
  maple syrup (urine) 270.3
  Marburg (virus) 078.89
  Marchiafava (-Bignami) 341.8
  Marfan's 090.49
    congenital syphilis 090.49
    meaning Marfan's syndrome 759.82
  Marie-Bamberger (hypertrophic pulmonary osteoarthropathy) (secondary) 731.2
    primary or idiopathic (acropachyderma) 757.39
    pulmonary (hypertrophic osteoarthropathy) 731.2
  Marie-Strümpell (ankylosing spondylitis) 720.0
  Marion's (bladder neck obstruction) 596.0
  Marsh's (exophthalmic goiter) 242.0
  Martin's 715.27
  mast cell 757.33
    systemic (M9741/3) 202.6
  mastoid (*see also* Mastoiditis) 383.9
    process 385.9
  maternal, unrelated to pregnancy NEC, affecting fetus or newborn 760.9
  Mathieu's (leptospiral jaundice) 100.0
  Mauclaire's 732.3
  Mauriac's (erythema nodosum syphiliticum) 091.3
  Maxcy's 081.0
  McArdle (-Schmid-Pearson) (glycogenosis V) 271.0
  mediastinum NEC 519.3
  Medin's (*see also* Poliomyelitis) 045.9
  Mediterranean (with hemoglobinopathy) 282.49
  medullary center (idiopathic) (respiratory) 348.8
  Meige's (chronic hereditary edema) 757.0
  Meleda 757.39
  Ménétrier's (hypertrophic gastritis) 535.2
  Ménière's (active) 386.00
    cochlear 386.02
    cochleovestibular 386.01
    inactive 386.04
    in remission 386.04
    vestibular 386.03
  meningeal—*see* Meningitis
  mental (*see also* Psychosis) 298.9
  Merzbacher-Pelizaeus 330.0
  mesenchymal 710.9
  mesenteric embolic 557.0
  metabolic NEC 277.9
  metal polishers' 502
  metastatic—*see* Metastasis
  Mibelli's 757.39
  microdrepanocytic 282.49
  microvascular —*code to condition*
  Miescher's 709.3

INDEX TO DISEASES

Disease, diseased—*continued*
Mikulicz's (dryness of mouth, absent or decreased lacrimation) 527.1
Milkman (-Looser) (osteomalacia with pseudofractures) 268.2
Miller's (osteomalacia) 268.2
Mills' 335.29
Milroy's (chronic hereditary edema) 757.0
Minamata 985.0
Minor's 336.1
Minot's (hemorrhagic disease, newborn) 776.0
Minot-von Willebrand-Jürgens (angiohemophilia) 286.4
Mitchell's (erythromelalgia) 443.82
mitral—*see* Endocarditis, mitral
Mljet (mal de Meleda) 757.39
Möbius', Moebius' 346.8
Moeller's 267
Möller (-Barlow) (infantile scurvy) 267
Mönckeberg's (*see also* arteriosclerosis, extremities) 440.20
Mondor's (thrombophlebitis of breast) 451.89
Monge's 993.2
Morel-Kraepelin (*see also* Schizophrenia) 295.9
Morgagni's (syndrome) (hyperostosis frontalis interna) 733.3
Morgagni-Adams-Stokes (syncope with heart block) 426.9
Morquio (-Brailsford) (-Ullrich) (mucopolysaccharidosis IV) 277.5
Morton's (with metatarsalgia) 355.6
Morvan's 336.0
motor neuron (bulbar) (mixed type) 335.20
Mouchet's (juvenile osteochondrosis, foot) 732.5
mouth 528.9
Moyamoya 437.5
Mucha's (acute parapsoriasis varioliformis) 696.2
mu-chain 273.2
mucolipidosis (I) (II) (III) 272.7
Münchmeyer's (exostosis luxurians) 728.11
Murri's (intermittent hemoglobinuria) 283.2
muscle 359.9
  inflammatory 728.9
  ocular 378.9
musculoskeletal system 729.9
mushroom workers' 495.5
Myà's (congenital dilation, colon) 751.3
mycotic 117.9
myeloproliferative (chronic) (M9960/1) 238.79
myocardium, myocardial (*see also* Degeneration, myocardial) 429.1
  hypertensive (*see also* Hypertension, heart) 402.90
  primary (idiopathic) 425.4
myoneural 358.9
Naegeli's 287.1
nail 703.9
  specified type NEC 703.8
Nairobi sheep 066.1
nasal 478.19
  cavity NEC 478.19
  sinus (chronic)—*see* Sinusitis
navel (newborn) NEC 779.89
  delayed separation of umbilical cord 779.83
nemaline body 359.0
neoplastic, generalized (M8000/6) 199.0
nerve—*see* Disorder, nerve
nervous system (central) 349.9

Disease, diseased—*continued*
  autonomic, peripheral (*see also* Neuropathy, peripheral, autonomic) 337.9
  congenital 742.9
  inflammatory—*see* Encephalitis
  parasympathetic (*see also* Neuropathy, peripheral, autonomic) 337.9
  peripheral NEC 355.9
  specified NEC 349.89
  sympathetic (*see also* Neuropathy, peripheral, autonomic) 337.9
  vegetative (*see also* Neuropathy, peripheral, autonomic) 337.9
Nettleship's (urticaria pigmentosa) 757.33
Neumann's (pemphigus vegetans) 694.4
neurologic (central) NEC (*see also* Disease, nervous system) 349.9
  peripheral NEC 355.9
neuromuscular system NEC 358.9
Newcastle 077.8
Nicolas (-Durand) -Favre (climatic bubo) 099.1
Niemann-Pick (lipid histiocytosis) 272.7
nipple 611.9
  Paget's (M8540/3) 174.0
Nishimoto (-Takeuchi) 437.5
nonarthropod-borne NEC 078.89
  central nervous system NEC 049.9
  enterovirus NEC 078.89
non-autoimmune hemolytic NEC 283.10
Nonne-Milroy-Meige (chronic hereditary edema) 757.0
Norrie's (congenital progressive oculoacousticocerebral degeneration) 743.8
nose 478.19
nucleus pulposus—*see* Disease, intervertebral disc
nutritional 269.9
  maternal, affecting fetus or newborn 760.4
oasthouse, urine 270.2
obliterative vascular 447.1
Odelberg's (juvenile osteochondrosis) 732.1
Oguchi's (retina) 368.61
Ohara's (*see also* Tularemia) 021.9
Ollier's (chondrodysplasia) 756.4
Opitz's (congestive splenomegaly) 289.51
Oppenheim's 358.8
Oppenheim-Urbach (necrobiosis lipoidica diabeticorum) 250.8 *[709.3]*
optic nerve NEC 377.49
orbit 376.9
  specified NEC 376.89
Oriental liver fluke 121.1
Oriental lung fluke 121.2
Ormond's 593.4
Osgood's tibia (tubercle) 732.4
Osgood-Schlatter 732.4
Osler (-Vaquez) (polycythemia vera) (M9950/1) 238.4
Osler-Rendu (familial hemorrhagic telangiectasia) 448.0
osteofibrocystic 252.01
Otto's 715.35
outer ear 380.9
ovary (noninflammatory) NEC 620.9
  cystic 620.2
  polycystic 256.4
  specified NEC 620.8
Owren's (congenital) (*see also* Defect, coagulation) 286.3
Paas' 756.59
Paget's (osteitis deformans) 731.0

953

Disease, diseased—*continued*
  with infiltrating duct carcinoma of the breast (M8541/3)—*see* Neoplasm, breast, malignant
  bone 731.0
    osteosarcoma in (M9184/3)—*see* Neoplasm, bone, malignant
  breast (M8540/3) 174.0
  extramammary (M8542/3)—*see also* Neoplasm, skin, malignant
    anus 154.3
    skin 173.5
  malignant (M8540/3)
    breast 174.0
    specified site NEC (M8542/3)—*see* Neoplasm, skin, malignant
    unspecified site 174.0
  mammary (M8540/3) 174.0
  nipple (M8540/3) 174.0
  palate (soft) 528.9
Paltauf-Sternberg 201.9
pancreas 577.9
  cystic 577.2
    congenital 751.7
  fibrocystic 277.00
Panner's 732.3
  capitellum humeri 732.3
  head of humerus 732.3
  tarsal navicular (bone) (osteochondrosis) 732.5
panvalvular—*see* Endocarditis, mitral
parametrium 629.9
parasitic NEC 136.9
  cerebral NEC 123.9
  intestinal NEC 129
  mouth 112.0
  skin NEC 134.9
  specified type—*see* Infestation
  tongue 112.0
parathyroid (gland) 252.9
  specified NEC 252.8
Parkinson's 332.0
parodontal 523.9
Parrot's (syphilitic osteochondritis) 090.0
Parry's (exophthalmic goiter) 242.0
Parson's (exophthalmic goiter) 242.0
Pavy's 593.6
Paxton's (white piedra) 111.2
Payr's (splenic flexure syndrome) 569.89
pearl-workers' (chronic osteomyelitis) (*see also* Osteomyelitis) 730.1
Pel-Ebstein—*see* Disease, Hodgkin's
Pelizaeus-Merzbacher 330.0
  with dementia
    with behavioral disturbance 330.0 *[294.11]*
    without behavioral disturbance 330.0 *[294.10]*
Pellegrini-Stieda (calcification, knee joint) 726.62
pelvis, pelvic
  female NEC 629.9
    specified NEC 629.89
  gonococcal (acute) 098.19
    chronic or duration of 2 months or over 098.39
  infection (*see also* Disease, pelvis, inflammatory) 614.9
  inflammatory (female) (PID) 614.9
    with
      abortion—*see* Abortion, by type, with sepsis

Disease, diseased—*continued*
    ectopic pregnancy (*see also* categories 633.0-633.9) 639.0
    molar pregnancy (*see also* categories 630-632) 639.0
  acute 614.3
  chronic 614.4
  complicating pregnancy 646.6
    affecting fetus or newborn 760.8
  following
    abortion 639.0
    ectopic or molar pregnancy 639.0
  peritonitis (acute) 614.5
    chronic NEC 614.7
  puerperal, postpartum, childbirth 670
  specified NEC 614.8
  organ, female NEC 629.9
    specified NEC 629.89
  peritoneum, female NEC 629.9
    specified NEC 629.89
penis 607.9
  inflammatory 607.2
peptic NEC 536.9
  acid 536.8
periapical tissues NEC 522.9
pericardium 423.9
  specified type NEC 423.8
perineum
  female
    inflammatory 616.9
      specified NEC 616.89
    noninflammatory 624.9
      specified NEC 624.8
  male (inflammatory) 682.2
periodic (familial) (Reimann's) NEC 277.31
  paralysis 359.3
periodontal NEC 523.9
  specified NEC 523.8
periosteum 733.90
peripheral
  arterial 443.9
  autonomic nervous system (*see also* Neuropathy, autonomic) 337.9
  nerve NEC (*see also* Neuropathy) 356.9
    multiple—*see* Polyneuropathy
  vascular 443.9
    specified type NEC 443.89
peritoneum 568.9
  pelvic, female 629.9
    specified NEC 629.89
Perrin-Ferraton (snapping hip) 719.65
persistent mucosal (middle ear) (with posterior or superior marginal perforation of ear drum) 382.2
Perthes' (capital femoral osteochondrosis) 732.1
Petit's (*see also* Hernia, lumbar) 553.8
Peutz-Jeghers 759.6
Peyronie's 607.85
Pfeiffer's (infectious mononucleosis) 075
pharynx 478.20
Phocas' 610.1
photochromogenic (acid-fast bacilli) (pulmonary) 031.0
  nonpulmonary 031.9
Pick's
  brain 331.11
    with dementia
      with behavioral disturbance 331.11 *[294.11]*
      without behavioral disturbance 331.11 *[294.10]*

INDEX TO DISEASES

Disease, diseased

Disease, diseased—*continued*
  cerebral atrophy 331.11
    with dementia
      with behavioral disturbance 331.11
        [294.11]
      without behavioral disturbance 331.11
        [294.10]
  lipid histiocytosis 272.7
  liver (pericardial pseudocirrhosis of liver) 423.2
  pericardium (pericardial pseudocirrhosis of liver) 423.2
  polyserositis (pericardial pseudocirrhosis of liver) 423.2
  Pierson's (osteochondrosis) 732.1
  pigeon fancier's or breeders' 495.2
  pineal gland 259.8
  pink 985.0
  Pinkus' (lichen nitidus) 697.1
  pinworm 127.4
  pituitary (gland) 253.9
    hyperfunction 253.1
    hypofunction 253.2
  pituitary snuff-takers' 495.8
  placenta
    affecting fetus or newborn 762.2
    complicating pregnancy or childbirth 656.7
  pleura (cavity) (*see also* Pleurisy) 511.0
  Plummer's (toxic nodular goiter) 242.3
  pneumatic
    drill 994.9
    hammer 994.9
  policeman's 729.2
  Pollitzer's (hidradenitis suppurativa) 705.83
  polycystic (congenital) 759.89
    kidney or renal 753.12
      adult type (APKD) 753.13
      autosomal dominant 753.13
      autosomal recessive 753.14
      childhood type (CPKD) 753.14
      infantile type 753.14
    liver or hepatic 751.62
    lung or pulmonary 518.89
      congenital 748.4
    ovary, ovaries 256.4
    spleen 759.0
  Pompe's (glycogenosis II) 271.0
  Poncet's (tuberculous rheumatism) (*see also* Tuberculosis) 015.9
  Posada-Wernicke 114.9
  Potain's (pulmonary edema) 514
  Pott's (*see also* Tuberculosis) 015.0 *[730.88]*
    osteomyelitis 015.0 *[730.88]*
    paraplegia 015.0 *[730.88]*
    spinal curvature 015.0 *[737.43]*
    spondylitis 015.0 *[720.81]*
  Potter's 753.0
  Poulet's 714.2
  pregnancy NEC (*see also* Pregnancy) 646.9
  Preiser's (osteoporosis) 733.09
  Pringle's (tuberous sclerosis) 759.5
  Profichet's 729.9
  prostate 602.9
    specified type NEC 602.8
  protozoal NEC 136.8
    intestine, intestinal NEC 007.9
  pseudo-Hurler's (mucolipidosis III) 272.7
  psychiatric (*see also* Psychosis) 298.9
  psychotic (*see also* Psychosis) 298.9
  Puente's (simple glandular cheilitis) 528.5
  puerperal NEC (*see also* Puerperal) 674.9

Disease, diseased—*continued*
  pulmonary—*see also* Disease, lung
    amyloid 277.39 *[517.8]*
    artery 417.9
    circulation, circulatory 417.9
      specified NEC 417.8
    diffuse obstructive (chronic) 496
      with
        acute bronchitis 491.22
        asthma (chronic) (obstructive) 493.2
        bronchitis (chronic) 491.20
          with exacerbation (acute) 491.21
          exacerbation NEC (acute) 491.21
    heart (chronic) 416.9
      specified NEC 416.8
    hypertensive (vascular) 416.0
      cardiovascular 416.0
    obstructive diffuse (chronic) 496
      decompensated 491.21
        with exacerbation 491.21
      with
        acute bronchitis 491.22
        asthma (chronic) (obstructive) 493.2
        bronchitis (chronic) 491.20
          with
            exacerbation (acute) 491.21
          acute 491.22
          exacerbation NEC (acute) 491.21
    valve (*see also* Endocarditis, pulmonary) 424.3
  pulp (dental) NEC 522.9
  pulseless 446.7
  Putnam's (subacute combined sclerosis with pernicious anemia) 281.0 *[336.2]*
  Pyle (-Cohn) (craniometaphyseal dysplasia) 756.89
  pyramidal tract 333.90
  Quervain's
    tendon sheath 727.04
    thyroid (subacute granulomatous thyroiditis) 245.1
  Quincke's—*see* Edema, angioneurotic
  Quinquaud (acne decalvans) 704.09
  rag sorters' 022.1
  Raynaud's (Paroxysmal digital cyanosis) 443.0
  reactive airway—*see* Asthma
  Recklinghausen's (M9540/1) 237.71
    bone (osteitis fibrosa cystica) 252.01
  Recklinghausen-Applebaum (hemochromatosis) 275.0
  Reclus' (cystic) 610.1
  rectum NEC 569.49
  Refsum's (heredopathia atactica polyneuritiformis) 356.3
  Reichmann's (gastrosuccorrhea) 536.8
  Reimann's (periodic) 277.31
  Reiter's 099.3
  renal (functional) (pelvis) (*see also* Disease, kidney) 593.9
    with
      edema (*see also* Nephrosis) 581.9
      exudative nephritis 583.89
      lesion of interstitial nephritis 583.89
      stated generalized cause—*see* Nephritis
    acute 593.9
    basement membrane NEC 583.89
      with
        pulmonary hemorrhage (Goodpasture's syndrome) 446.21 *[583.81]*
    chronic (*see also* Disease, kidney, chronic) 585.9

Disease, diseased—*continued*
  complicating pregnancy or puerperium NEC 646.2
    with hypertension—*see* Toxemia, of pregnancy
    affecting fetus or newborn 760.1
  cystic, congenital (*see also* Cystic, disease, kidney) 753.10
  diabetic 250.4 *[583.81]*
  due to
    amyloidosis 277.39 *[583.81]*
    diabetes mellitus 250.4 *[583.81]*
    systemic lupus erythematosis 710.0 *[583.81]*
  end-stage 585.6
  exudative 583.89
  fibrocystic (congenital) 753.19
  gonococcal 098.19 *[583.81]*
  gouty 274.10
  hypertensive (*see also* Hypertension, kidney) 403.90
  immune complex NEC 583.89
  interstitial (diffuse) (focal) 583.89
  lupus 710.0 *[583.81]*
  maternal, affecting fetus or newborn 760.1
    hypertensive 760.0
  phosphate-losing (tubular) 588.0
  polycystic (congenital) 753.12
    adult type (APKD) 753.13
    autosomal dominant 753.13
    autosomal recessive 753.14
    childhood type (CPKD) 753.14
    infantile type 753.14
  specified lesion or cause NEC (*see also* Glomerulonephritis) 583.89
  subacute 581.9
  syphilitic 095.4
  tuberculous (*see also* Tuberculosis) 016.0 *[583.81]*
  tubular (*see also* Nephrosis, tubular) 584.5
Rendu-Olser-Weber (familial hemorrhagic telangiectasia) 448.0
renovascular (arteriosclerotic) (*see also* Hypertension, kidney) 403.90
respiratory (tract) 519.9
  acute or subacute (upper) NEC 465.9
    due to fumes or vapors 506.3
    multiple sites NEC 465.8
    noninfectious 478.9
    streptococcal 034.0
  chronic 519.9
    arising in the perinatal period 770.7
    due to fumes or vapors 506.4
  due to
    aspiration of liquids or solids 508.9
    external agents NEC 508.9
      specified NEC 508.8
    fumes or vapors 506.9
      acute or subacute NEC 506.3
      chronic 506.4
  fetus or newborn NEC 770.9
  obstructive 496
  specified type NEC 519.8
  upper (acute) (infectious) NEC 465.9
    multiple sites NEC 465.8
    noninfectious NEC 478.9
    streptococcal 034.0
retina, retinal NEC 362.9
  Batten's or Batten-Mayou 330.1 *[362.71]*
  degeneration 362.89
  vascular lesion 362.17

Disease, diseased—*continued*
  rheumatic (*see also* Arthritis) 716.8
    heart—*see* Disease, heart, rheumatic
  rheumatoid (heart)—*see* Arthritis, rheumatoid
  rickettsial NEC 083.9
    specified type NEC 083.8
  Riedel's (ligneous thyroiditis) 245.3
  Riga (-Fede) (cachectic aphthae) 529.0
  Riggs' (compound periodontitis) 523.40
  Ritter's 695.81
  Rivalta's (cervicofacial actinomycosis) 039.3
  Robles' (onchocerciasis) 125.3 *[360.13]*
  Roger's (congenital interventricular septal defect) 745.4
  Rokitansky's (*see also* Necrosis, liver) 570
  Romberg's 349.89
  Rosenthal's (factor XI deficiency) 286.2
  Rossbach's (hyperchlorhydria) 536.8
    psychogenic 306.4
  Roth (-Bernhardt) 355.1
  Runeberg's (progressive pernicious anemia) 281.0
  Rust's (tuberculous spondylitis) (*see also* Tuberculosis) 015.0 *[720.81]*
  Rustitskii's (multiple myeloma) (M9730/3) 203.0
  Ruysch's (Hirschsprung's disease) 751.3
  Sachs (-Tay) 330.1
  sacroiliac NEC 724.6
  salivary gland or duct NEC 527.9
    inclusion 078.5
    streptococcal 034.0
    virus 078.5
  Sander's (paranoia) 297.1
  Sandhoff's 330.1
  sandworm 126.9
  Savill's (epidemic exfoliative dermatitis) 695.89
  Schamberg's (progressive pigmentary dermatosis) 709.09
  Schaumann's (sarcoidosis) 135
  Schenck's (sporotrichosis) 117.1
  Scheuermann's (osteochondrosis) 732.0
  Schilder (-Flatau) 341.1
  Schimmelbusch's 610.1
  Schlatter's tibia (tubercle) 732.4
  Schlatter-Osgood 732.4
  Schmorl's 722.30
    cervical 722.39
    lumbar, lumbosacral 722.32
    specified region NEC 722.39
    thoracic, thoracolumbar 722.31
  Scholz's 330.0
  Schönlein (-Henoch) (purpura rheumatica) 287.0
  Schottmüller's (*see also* Fever, paratyphoid) 002.9
  Schüller-Christian (chronic histiocytosis X) 277.89
  Schultz's (agranulocytosis) 288.09
  Schwalbe-Ziehen-Oppenheimer 333.6
  Schwartz-Jampel 359.23
  Schweninger-Buzzi (macular atrophy) 701.3
  sclera 379.19
  scrofulous (*see also* Tuberculosis) 017.2
  scrotum 608.9
  sebaceous glands NEC 706.9
  Secretan's (posttraumatic edema) 782.3
  semilunar cartilage, cystic 717.5
  seminal vesicle 608.9
  Senear-Usher (pemphigus erythematosus) 694.4
  serum NEC 999.5
  Sever's (osteochondrosis calcaneum) 732.5

INDEX TO DISEASES

Disease, diseased—*continued*
  sexually transmitted —*see* Disease, venereal
  Sézary's (reticulosis) (M9701/3) 202.2
  Shaver's (bauxite pneumoconiosis) 503
  Sheehan's (postpartum pituitary necrosis) 253.2
  shimamushi (scrub typhus) 081.2
  shipyard 077.1
  sickle-cell 282.60
    with
      crisis 282.62
      Hb-S disease 282.61
      other abnormal hemoglobin (Hb-D) (Hb-E) (Hb-G) (Hb-J) (Hb-K) (Hb-O) (Hb-P) (high fetal gene) (without crisis) 282.68
        with crisis 282.69
    elliptocytosis 282.60
    Hb-C (without crisis) 282.63
      with
        crisis 282.64
        vaso-occlusive pain 282.64
    Hb-S 282.61
      with
        crisis 282.62
        Hb-C (without crisis) 282.63
          with
            crisis 282.64
            vaso-occlusive pain 282.64
        other abnormal hemoglobin (Hb-D) (Hb-E) (Hb-G) (Hb-J) (Hb-K) (Hb-O) (Hb-P) (high fetal gene) (without crisis) 282.68
          with crisis 282.69
    spherocytosis 282.60
    thalassemia (without crisis) 282.41
      with
        crisis 282.42
        vaso-occlusive pain 282.42
  Siegal-Cattan-Mamou (periodic) 277.31
  silo fillers' 506.9
  Simian B 054.3
  Simmonds' (pituitary cachexia) 253.2
  Simons' (progressive lipodystrophy) 272.6
  Sinding-Larsen (juvenile osteopathia patellae) 732.4
  sinus—*see also* Sinusitis
    brain 437.9
    specified NEC 478.19
  Sirkari's 085.0
  sixth (*see also* Exanthem subitum) 058.10
  Sjögren (-Gougerot) 710.2
    with lung involvement 710.2 *[517.8]*
  Skevas-Zerfus 989.5
  skin NEC 709.9
    due to metabolic disorder 277.9
    specified type NEC 709.8
  sleeping (*see also* Narcolepsy) 347.00
    meaning sleeping sickness (*see also* Trypanosomiasis) 086.5
  small vessel 443.9
  Smith-Strang (oasthouse urine) 270.2
  Sneddon-Wilkinson (subcorneal pustular dermatosis) 694.1
  South African creeping 133.8
  Spencer's (epidemic vomiting) 078.82
  Spielmeyer-Stock 330.1
  Spielmeyer-Vogt 330.1
  spine, spinal 733.90
    combined system (*see also* Degeneration, combined) 266.2 *[336.2]*
      with pernicious anemia 281.0 *[336.2]*
    cord NEC 336.9
      congenital 742.9

Disease, diseased—*continued*
  demyelinating NEC 341.8
  joint (*see also* Disease, joint, spine) 724.9
    tuberculous 015.0 *[730.8]*
  spinocerebellar 334.9
    specified NEC 334.8
  spleen (organic) (postinfectional) 289.50
    amyloid 277.39
    lardaceous 277.39
    polycystic 759.0
    specified NEC 289.59
  sponge divers' 989.5
  Stanton's (melioidosis) 025
  Stargardt's 362.75
  Startle 759.89
  Steinert's 359.21
  Sternberg's—*see* Disease, Hodgkin's
  Stevens-Johnson (erythema multiforme exudativum) 695.1
  Sticker's (erythema infectiosum) 057.0
  Stieda's (calcification, knee joint) 726.62
  Still's (juvenile rheumatoid arthritis) 714.30
  Stiller's (asthenia) 780.79
  Stokes' (exophthalmic goiter) 242.0
  Stokes-Adams (syncope with heart block) 426.9
  Stokvis (-Talma) (enterogenous cyanosis) 289.7
  stomach NEC (organic) 537.9
    functional 536.9
      psychogenic 306.4
    lardaceous 277.39
  stonemasons' 502
  storage
    glycogen (*see also* Disease, glycogen storage) 271.0
    lipid 272.7
    mucopolysaccharide 277.5
  striatopallidal system 333.90
    specified NEC 333.89
  Strümpell-Marie (ankylosing spondylitis) 720.0
  Stuart's (congenital factor X deficiency) (*see also* Defect, coagulation) 286.3
  Stuart-Prower (congenital factor X deficiency) (*see also* Defect, coagulation) 286.3
  Sturge (-Weber) (-Dimitri) (encephalocutaneous angiomatosis) 759.6
  Stuttgart 100.89
  Sudeck's 733.7
  supporting structures of teeth NEC 525.9
  suprarenal (gland) (capsule) 255.9
    hyperfunction 255.3
    hypofunction 255.41
  Sutton's 709.09
  Sutton and Gull's—*see* Hypertension, kidney
  sweat glands NEC 705.9
    specified type NEC 705.89
  sweating 078.2
  Sweeley-Klionsky 272.4
  Swift (-Feer) 985.0
  swimming pool (bacillus) 031.1
  swineherd's 100.89
  Sylvest's (epidemic pleurodynia) 074.1
  Symmers (follicular lymphoma) (M9690/3) 202.0
  sympathetic nervous system (*see also* Neuropathy, peripheral, autonomic) 337.9
  synovium 727.9
  syphilitic—*see* Syphilis
  systemic tissue mast cell (M9741/3) 202.6
  Taenzer's 757.4
  Takayasu's (pulseless) 446.7
  Talma's 728.85

Disease, diseased—*continued*
  Tangier (familial high-density lipoprotein deficiency) 272.5
  Tarral-Besnier (pityriasis rubra pilaris) 696.4
  Tay-Sachs 330.1
  Taylor's 701.8
  tear duct 375.69
  teeth, tooth 525.9
    hard tissues 521.9
      specified NEC 521.89
    pulp NEC 522.9
  tendon 727.9
    inflammatory NEC 727.9
  terminal vessel 443.9
  testis 608.9
  Thaysen-Gee (nontropical sprue) 579.0
  Thomsen's 359.22
  Thomson's (congenital poikiloderma) 757.33
  Thornwaldt's, Tornwaldt's (pharyngeal bursitis) 478.29
  throat 478.20
    septic 034.0
  thromboembolic (*see also* Embolism) 444.9
  thymus (gland) 254.9
    specified NEC 254.8
  thyroid (gland) NEC 246.9
    heart (*see also* Hyperthyroidism) 242.9 *[425.7]*
    lardaceous 277.39
    specified NEC 246.8
  Tietze's 733.6
  Tommaselli's
    correct substance properly administered 599.7
    overdose or wrong substance given or taken 961.4
  tongue 529.9
  tonsils, tonsillar (and adenoids) (chronic) 474.9
    specified NEC 474.8
  tooth, teeth 525.9
    hard tissues 521.9
      specified NEC 521.89
    pulp NEC 522.9
  Tornwaldt's (pharyngeal bursitis) 478.29
  Tourette's 307.23
  trachea 519.19
  tricuspid—*see* Endocarditis, tricuspid
  triglyceride-storage, type I, II, III 272.7
  triple vessel (coronary arteries) —*see* Arteriosclerosis, coronary
  trisymptomatic, Gougerot's 709.1
  trophoblastic (*see also* Hydatidiform mole) 630
    previous, affecting management of pregnancy V23.1
  tsutsugamushi (scrub typhus) 081.2
  tube (fallopian), noninflammatory 620.9
    specified NEC 620.8
  tuberculous NEC (*see also* Tuberculosis) 011.9
  tubo-ovarian
    inflammatory (*see also* Salpingo-oophoritis) 614.2
    noninflammatory 620.9
      specified NEC 620.8
  tubotympanic, chronic (with anterior perforation of ear drum) 382.1
  tympanum 385.9
  Uhl's 746.84
  umbilicus (newborn) NEC 779.89
    delayed separation 779.83
  Underwood's (sclerema neonatorum) 778.1
  undiagnosed 799.9
  Unna's (seborrheic dermatitis) 690.18

Disease, diseased—*continued*
  unstable hemoglobin hemolytic 282.7
  Unverricht (-Lundborg) 333.2
  Urbach-Oppenheim (necrobiosis lipoidica diabeticorum) 250.8 *[709.3]*
  Urbach-Wiethe (lipoid proteinosis) 272.8
  ureter 593.9
  urethra 599.9
    specified type NEC 599.84
  urinary (tract) 599.9
    bladder 596.9
      specified NEC 596.8
    maternal, affecting fetus or newborn 760.1
  Usher-Senear (pemphigus erythematosus) 694.4
  uterus (organic) 621.9
    infective (*see also* Endometritis) 615.9
    inflammatory (*see also* Endometritis) 615.9
    noninflammatory 621.9
      specified type NEC 621.8
  uveal tract
    anterior 364.9
    posterior 363.9
  vagabonds' 132.1
  vagina, vaginal
    inflammatory 616.10
    noninflammatory 623.9
      specified NEC 623.8
  Valsuani's (progressive pernicious anemia, puerperal) 648.2
    complicating pregnancy or puerperium 648.2
  valve, valvular—*see* Endocarditis
  van Bogaert-Nijssen (-Peiffer) 330.0
  van Creveld-von Gierke (glycogenosis I) 271.0
  van den Bergh's (enterogenous cyanosis) 289.7
  van Neck's (juvenile osteochondrosis) 732.1
  Vaquez (-Osler) (polycythemia vera) (M9950/1) 238.4
  vascular 459.9
    arteriosclerotic—*see* Arteriosclerosis
    hypertensive—*see* Hypertension
    obliterative 447.1
      peripheral 443.9
    occlusive 459.9
    peripheral (occlusive) 443.9
      in diabetes mellitus 250.7 *[443.81]*
      specified type NEC 443.89
  vas deferens 608.9
  vasomotor 443.9
  vasospastic 443.9
  vein 459.9
  venereal 099.9
    fifth 099.1
    sixth 099.1
    chlamydial NEC 099.50
      anus 099.52
      bladder 099.53
      cervix 099.53
      epididymis 099.54
      genitourinary NEC 099.55
        lower 099.53
        specified NEC 099.54
      pelvic inflammatory disease 099.54
      perihepatic 099.56
      peritoneum 099.56
      pharynx 099.51
      rectum 099.52
      specified site NEC 099.59
      testis 099.54
      vagina 099.53
      vulva 099.53

INDEX TO DISEASES

Disease, diseased—*continued*
  complicating pregnancy, childbirth, or puerperium 647.2
  specified nature or type NEC 099.8
    chlamydial—*see* Disease, venereal, chlamydial
  Verneuil's (syphilitic bursitis) 095.7
  Verse's (calcinosis intervertebralis) 275.49 *[722.90]*
  vertebra, vertebral NEC 733.90
    disc—*see* Disease, Intervertebral disc
  vibration NEC 994.9
  Vidal's (lichen simplex chronicus) 698.3
  Vincent's (trench mouth) 101
  Virchow's 733.99
  virus (filterable) NEC 078.89
    arbovirus NEC 066.9
    arthropod-borne NEC 066.9
    central nervous system NEC 049.9
      specified type NEC 049.8
    complicating pregnancy, childbirth, or puerperium 647.6
    contact (with) V01.79
      varicella V01.71
    exposure to V01.79
      varicella V01.71
    Marburg 078.89
    maternal
      with fetal damage affecting management of pregnancy 655.3
    nonarthropod-borne NEC 078.89
      central nervous system NEC 049.9
      specified NEC 049.8
    vaccination, prophylactic (against) V04.89
  vitreous 379.29
  vocal cords NEC 478.5
  Vogt's (Cecile) 333.71
  Vogt-Spielmeyer 330.1
  Volhard-Fahr (malignant nephrosclerosis) 403.00
  Volkmann's
    acquired 958.6
  von Bechterew's (ankylosing spondylitis) 720.0
  von Economo's (encephalitis lethargica) 049.8
  von Eulenburg's (congenital paramyotonia) 359.29
  von Gierke's (glycogenosis I) 271.0
  von Graefe's 378.72
  von Hippel's (retinocerebral angiomatosis) 759.6
  von Hippel-Lindau (angiomatosis retinocerebellosa) 759.6
  von Jaksch's (pseudoleukemia infantum) 285.8
  von Recklinghausen's (M9540/1) 237.71
    bone (osteitis fibrosa cystica) 252.01
  von Recklinghausen-Applebaum (hemochromatosis) 275.0
  von Willebrand (-Jürgens) (angiohemophilia) 286.4
  von Zambusch's (lichen sclerosus et atrophicus) 701.0
  Voorhoeve's (dyschondroplasia) 756.4
  Vrolik's (osteogenesis imperfecta) 756.51
  vulva
    inflammatory 616.10
    noninflammatory 624.9
      specified NEC 624.8
  Wagner's (colloid milium) 709.3
  Waldenström's (osteochondrosis capital femoral) 732.1

Disease, diseased—*continued*
  Wallgren's (obstruction of splenic vein with collateral circulation) 459.89
  Wardrop's (with lymphangitis) 681.9
    finger 681.02
    toe 681.11
  Wassilieff's (leptospiral jaundice) 100.0
  wasting NEC 799.4
    due to malnutrition 261
    paralysis 335.21
  Waterhouse-Friderichsen 036.3
  waxy (any site) 277.39
  Weber-Christian (nodular nonsuppurative panniculitis) 729.30
  Wegner's (syphilitic osteochondritis) 090.0
  Weil's (leptospiral jaundice) 100.0
    of lung 100.0
  Weir Mitchell's (erythromelalgia) 443.82
  Werdnig-Hoffmann 335.0
  Werlhof's (*see also* Purpura, thrombocytopenic) 287.39
  Wermer's 258.01
  Werner's (progeria adultorum) 259.8
  Werner-His (trench fever) 083.1
  Werner-Schultz (agranulocytosis) 288.09
  Wernicke's (superior hemorrhagic polioencephalitis) 265.1
  Wernicke-Posadas 114.9
  Whipple's (intestinal lipodystrophy) 040.2
  whipworm 127.3
  white
    blood cell 288.9
      specified NEC 288.8
    spot 701.0
  White's (congenital) (keratosis follicularis) 757.39
  Whitmore's (melioidosis) 025
  Widal-Abrami (acquired hemolytic jaundice) 283.9
  Wilkie's 557.1
  Wilkinson-Sneddon (subcorneal pustular dermatosis) 694.1
  Willis' (diabetes mellitus) (*see also* Diabetes) 250.0
  Wilson's (hepatolenticular degeneration) 275.1
  Wilson-Brocq (dermatitis exfoliativa) 695.89
  winter vomiting 078.82
  Wise's 696.2
  Wohlfart-Kugelberg-Welander 335.11
  Woillez's (acute idiopathic pulmonary congestion) 518.5
  Wolman's (primary familial xanthomatosis) 272.7
  wool-sorters' 022.1
  Zagari's (xerostomia) 527.7
  Zahorsky's (exanthem subitum) 058.10
  Ziehen-Oppenheim 333.6
  zoonotic, bacterial NEC 027.9
    specified type NEC 027.8
Disfigurement (due to scar) 709.2
  head V48.6
  limb V49.4
  neck V48.7
  trunk V48.7
Disgerminoma —*see* Dysgerminoma
Disinsertion, retina 361.04
Disintegration, complete, of the body 799.89
  traumatic 869.1
Disk kidney 753.3
Dislocatable hip, congenita 1 (*see also* Dislocation, hip, congenital) 754.30

Dislocation

Dislocation (articulation) (closed) (displacement) (simple) (subluxation) 839.8

> Note—"Closed" includes simple, complete, partial, uncomplicated, and unspecified dislocation. "Open" includes dislocation specified as infected or compound and dislocation with foreign body. "Chronic," "habitual," "old," or "recurrent" dislocations should be coded as indicated under the entry "Dislocation, recurrent"; and "pathological" as indicated under the entry "Dislocation, pathological." For late effect of dislocation see Late, effect, dislocation.

with fracture—*see* Fracture, by site
acromioclavicular (joint) (closed) 831.04
   open 831.14
anatomical site (closed)
   specified NEC 839.69
      open 839.79
   unspecified or ill-defined 839.8
      open 839.9
ankle (scaphoid bone) (closed) 837.0
   open 837.1
arm (closed) 839.8
   open 839.9
astragalus (closed) 837.0
   open 837.1
atlanto-axial (closed) 839.01
   open 839.11
atlas (closed) 839.01
   open 839.11
axis (closed) 839.02
   open 839.12
back (closed) 839.8
   open 839.9
Bell-Daly 723.8
breast bone (closed) 839.61
   open 839.71
capsule, joint—*see* Dislocation, by site
carpal (bone)—*see* Dislocation, wrist
carpometacarpal (joint) (closed) 833.04
   open 833.14
cartilage (joint)—*see also* Dislocation, by site
   knee—*see* Tear, meniscus
cervical, cervicodorsal, or cervicothoracic (spine) (vertebra)—*see* Dislocation, vertebra, cervical
chiropractic (*see also* Lesion, nonallopathic) 739.9
chondrocostal—*see* Dislocation, costochondral
chronic—*see* Dislocation, recurrent
clavicle (closed) 831.04
   open 831.14
coccyx (closed) 839.41
   open 839.51
collar bone (closed) 831.04
   open 831.14
compound (open) NEC 839.9
congenital NEC 755.8
   hip (*see also* Dislocation, hip, congenital) 754.30
   lens 743.37
   rib 756.3
   sacroiliac 755.69
   spine NEC 756.19
   vertebra 756.19
coracoid (closed) 831.09
   open 831.19
costal cartilage (closed) 839.69
   open 839.79

Dislocation—*continued*
costochondral (closed) 839.69
   open 839.79
cricoarytenoid articulation (closed) 839.69
   open 839.79
cricothyroid (cartilage) articulation (closed) 839.69
   open 839.79
dorsal vertebrae (closed) 839.21
   open 839.31
ear ossicle 385.23
elbow (closed) 832.00
   anterior (closed) 832.01
      open 832.11
   congenital 754.89
   divergent (closed) 832.09
      open 832.19
   lateral (closed) 832.04
      open 832.14
   medial (closed) 832.03
      open 832.13
   open 832.10
   posterior (closed) 832.02
      open 832.12
   recurrent 718.32
   specified type NEC 832.09
      open 832.19
eye 360.81
   lateral 376.36
eyeball 360.81
   lateral 376.36
femur
   distal end (closed) 836.50
      anterior 836.52
         open 836.62
      lateral 836.53
         open 836.63
      medial 836.54
         open 836.64
      open 836.60
      posterior 836.51
         open 836.61
   proximal end (closed) 835.00
      anterior (pubic) 835.03
         open 835.13
      obturator 835.02
         open 835.12
      open 835.10
      posterior 835.01
         open 835.11
fibula
   distal end (closed) 837.0
      open 837.1
   proximal end (closed) 836.59
      open 836.69
finger(s) (phalanx) (thumb) (closed) 834.00
   interphalangeal (joint) 834.02
      open 834.12
   metacarpal (bone), distal end 834.01
      open 834.11
   metacarpophalangeal (joint) 834.01
      open 834.11
   open 834.10
   recurrent 718.34
foot (closed) 838.00
   open 838.10
   recurrent 718.37
forearm (closed) 839.8
   open 839.9
fracture—*see* Fracture, by site

INDEX TO DISEASES   **Dislocation**

Dislocation—*continued*
  glenoid (closed) 831.09
    open 831.19
  habitual—*see* Dislocation, recurrent
  hand (closed) 839.8
    open 839.9
  hip (closed) 835.00
    anterior 835.03
      obturator 835.02
        open 835.12
      open 835.13
    congenital (unilateral) 754.30
      with subluxation of other hip 754.35
      bilateral 754.31
    developmental 718.75
    open 835.10
    posterior 835.01
      open 835.11
    recurrent 718.35
  humerus (closed) 831.00
    distal end (*see also* Dislocation, elbow) 832.00
    open 831.10
    proximal end (closed) 831.00
      anterior (subclavicular) (subcoracoid)
        (subglenoid) (closed) 831.01
        open 831.11
      inferior (closed) 831.03
        open 831.13
      open 831.10
      posterior (closed) 831.02
        open 831.12
  implant—*see* Complications, mechanical
  incus 385.23
  infracoracoid (closed) 831.01
    open 831.11
  innominate (pubic junction) (sacral junction)
    (closed) 839.69
    acetabulum (*see also* Dislocation, hip) 835.00
    open 839.79
  interphalangeal (joint)
    finger or hand (closed) 834.02
      open 834.12
    foot or toe (closed) 838.06
      open 838.16
  jaw (cartilage) (meniscus) (closed) 830.0
    open 830.1
    recurrent 524.69
  joint NEC (closed) 839.8
    developmental 718.7
    open 839.9
    pathological—*see* Dislocation, pathological
    recurrent—*see* Dislocation, recurrent
  knee (closed) 836.50
    anterior 836.51
      open 836.61
    congenital (with genu recurvatum) 754.41
    habitual 718.36
    lateral 836.54
      open 836.64
    medial 836.53
      open 836.63
    old 718.36
    open 836.60
    posterior 836.52
      open 836.62
    recurrent 718.36
    rotatory 836.59
      open 836.69
  lacrimal gland 375.16
  leg (closed) 839.8
    open 839.9

Dislocation—*continued*
  lens (crystalline) (complete) (partial) 379.32
    anterior 379.33
    congenital 743.37
    ocular implant 996.53
    posterior 379.34
    traumatic 921.3
  ligament—*see* Dislocation, by site
  lumbar (vertebrae) (closed) 839.20
    open 839.30
  lumbosacral (vertebrae) (closed) 839.20
    congenital 756.19
    open 839.30
  mandible (closed) 830.0
    open 830.1
  maxilla (inferior) (closed) 830.0
    open 830.1
  meniscus (knee)—*see also* Tear, meniscus
    other sites—*see* Dislocation, by site
  metacarpal (bone)
    distal end (closed) 834.01
      open 834.11
    proximal end (closed) 833.05
      open 833.15
  metacarpophalangeal (joint) (closed) 834.01
    open 834.11
  metatarsal (bone) (closed) 838.04
    open 838.14
  metatarsophalangeal (joint) (closed) 838.05
    open 838.15
  midcarpal (joint) (closed) 833.03
    open 833.13
  midtarsal (joint) (closed) 838.02
    open 838.12
  Monteggia's—*see* Dislocation, hip
  multiple locations (except fingers only or toes
    only) (closed) 839.8
    open 839.9
  navicular (bone) foot (closed) 837.0
    open 837.1
  neck (*see also* Dislocation, vertebra, cervical)
    839.00
  Nélaton's—*see* Dislocation, ankle
  nontraumatic (joint)—*see* Dislocation,
    pathological
  nose (closed) 839.69
    open 839.79
  not recurrent, not current injury—*see*
    Dislocation, pathological
  occiput from atlas (closed) 839.01
    open 839.11
  old—*see* Dislocation, recurrent
  open (compound) NEC 839.9
  ossicle, ear 385.23
  paralytic (flaccid) (spastic)—*see* Dislocation,
    pathological
  patella (closed) 836.3
    congenital 755.64
    open 836.4
  pathological NEC 718.20
    ankle 718.27
    elbow 718.22
    foot 718.27
    hand 718.24
    hip 718.25
    knee 718.26
    lumbosacral joint 724.6
    multiple sites 718.29
    pelvic region 718.25
    sacroiliac 724.6
    shoulder (region) 718.21

Dislocation—*continued*
  specified site NEC 718.28
  spine 724.8
    sacroiliac 724.6
  wrist 718.23
 pelvis (closed) 839.69
    acetabulum (*see also* Dislocation, hip) 835.00
    open 839.79
 phalanx
    foot or toe (closed) 838.09
      open 838.19
    hand or finger (*see also* Dislocation, finger) 834.00
 postpoliomyelitic—*see* Dislocation, pathological
 prosthesis, internal—*see* Complications, mechanical
 radiocarpal (joint) (closed) 833.02
    open 833.12
 radioulnar (joint)
    distal end (closed) 833.01
      open 833.11
    proximal end (*see also* Dislocation, elbow) 832.00
 radius
    distal end (closed) 833.00
      open 833.10
    proximal end (closed) 832.01
      open 832.11
 recurrent (*see also* Derangement, joint, recurrent) 718.3
    elbow 718.32
    hip 718.35
    joint NEC 718.38
    knee 718.36
    lumbosacral (joint) 724.6
    patella 718.36
    sacroiliac 724.6
    shoulder 718.31
    temporomandibular 524.69
 rib (cartilage) (closed) 839.69
    congenital 756.3
    open 839.79
 sacrococcygeal (closed) 839.42
    open 839.52
 sacroiliac (joint) (ligament) (closed) 839.42
    congenital 755.69
    open 839.52
    recurrent 724.6
 sacrum (closed) 839.42
    open 839.52
 scaphoid (bone)
    ankle or foot (closed) 837.0
      open 837.1
    wrist (closed) (*see also* Dislocation, wrist) 833.00
      open 833.10
 scapula (closed) 831.09
    open 831.19
 semilunar cartilage, knee—*see* Tear, meniscus
 septal cartilage (nose) (closed) 839.69
    open 839.79
 septum (nasal) (old) 470
 sesamoid bone—*see* Dislocation, by site
 shoulder (blade) (ligament) (closed) 831.00
    anterior (subclavicular) (subcoracoid) (subglenoid) (closed) 831.01
      open 831.11
    chronic 718.31
    inferior 831.03
      open 831.13

Dislocation—*continued*
    open 831.10
    posterior (closed) 831.02
      open 831.12
    recurrent 718.31
 skull—*see* Injury, intracranial
 Smith's—*see* Dislocation, foot
 spine (articular process) (*see also* Dislocation, vertebra) (closed) 839.40
    atlanto-axial (closed) 839.01
      open 839.11
      recurrent 723.8
    cervical, cervicodorsal, cervicothoracic (closed) (*see also* Dislocation, vertebrae, cervical) 839.00
      open 839.10
      recurrent 723.8
    coccyx 839.41
      open 839.51
    congenital 756.19
    due to birth trauma 767.4
    open 839.50
    recurrent 724.9
    sacroiliac 839.42
      recurrent 724.6
    sacrum (sacrococcygeal) (sacroiliac) 839.42
      open 839.52
 spontaneous—*see* Dislocation, pathological
 sternoclavicular (joint) (closed) 839.61
    open 839.71
 sternum (closed) 839.61
    open 839.71
 subastragalar—*see* Dislocation, foot
 subglenoid (closed) 831.01
    open 831.11
 symphysis
    jaw (closed) 830.0
      open 830.1
    mandibular (closed) 830.0
      open 830.1
    pubis (closed) 839.69
      open 839.79
 tarsal (bone) (joint) 838.01
    open 838.11
 tarsometatarsal (joint) 838.03
    open 838.13
 temporomandibular (joint) (closed) 830.0
    open 830.1
    recurrent 524.69
 thigh
    distal end (*see also* Dislocation, femur, distal end) 836.50
    proximal end (*see also* Dislocation, hip) 835.00
 thoracic (vertebrae) (closed) 839.21
    open 839.31
 thumb(s) (*see also* Dislocation, finger) 834.00
 thyroid cartilage (closed) 839.69
    open 839.79
 tibia
    distal end (closed) 837.0
      open 837.1
    proximal end (closed) 836.50
      anterior 836.51
        open 836.61
      lateral 836.54
        open 836.64
      medial 836.53
        open 836.63
      open 836.60
      posterior 836.52

Dislocation—*continued*
    open 836.62
   rotatory 836.59
    open 836.69
  tibiofibular
   distal (closed) 837.0
    open 837.1
   superior (closed) 836.59
    open 836.69
  toe(s) (closed) 838.09
   open 838.19
  trachea (closed) 839.69
   open 839.79
  ulna
   distal end (closed) 833.09
    open 833.19
   proximal end—*see* Dislocation, elbow
  vertebra (articular process) (body) (closed)
    (traumatic) 839.40
   cervical, cervicodorsal or cervicothoracic
    (closed) 839.00
    first (atlas) 839.01
     open 839.11
    second (axis) 839.02
     open 839.12
    third 839.03
     open 839.13
    fourth 839.04
     open 839.14
    fifth 839.05
     open 839.15
    sixth 839.06
     open 839.16
    seventh 839.07
     open 839.17
    congenital 756.19
    multiple sites 839.08
     open 839.18
    open 839.10
   congenital 756.19
   dorsal 839.21
    open 839.31
    recurrent 724.9
   lumbar, lumbosacral 839.20
    open 839.30
   non-traumatic —*see* Displacement,
    intervertebral disc
   open NEC 839.50
   recurrent 724.9
   specified region NEC 839.49
    open 839.59
   thoracic 839.21
    open 839.31
  wrist (carpal bone) (scaphoid) (semilunar)
    (closed) 833.00
   carpometacarpal (joint) 833.04
    open 833.14
   metacarpal bone, proximal end 833.05
    open 833.15
   midcarpal (joint) 833.03
    open 833.13
   open 833.10
   radiocarpal (joint) 833.02
    open 833.12
   radioulnar (joint) 833.01
    open 833.11
   recurrent 718.33
   specified site NEC 833.09
    open 833.19
  xiphoid cartilage (closed) 839.61
   open 839.71

Dislodgement
  artificial skin graft 996.55
  decellularized allodermis graft 996.55
Disobedience, hostile (covert) (overt) (*see also*
    Disturbance, conduct) 312.0
Disorder —*see also* Disease
  academic underachievement, childhood and
    adolescence 313.83
  accommodation 367.51
   drug-induced 367.89
   toxic 367.89
  adjustment (*see also* Reaction, adjustment)
    309.9
   with
    anxiety 309.24
    anxiety and depressed mood 309.28
    depressed mood 309.0
    disturbance of conduct 309.3
    disturbance of emotions and conduct 309.4
  adrenal (capsule) (cortex) (gland) 255.9
   specified type NEC 255.8
  adrenogenital 255.2
  affective (*see also* Psychosis, affective) 296.90
   atypical 296.81
  aggressive, unsocialized (*see also* Disturbance,
    conduct) 312.0
  alcohol, alcoholic (*see also* Alcohol) 291.9
  allergic—*see* Allergy
  amino acid (metabolic) (*see also* Disturbance,
    metabolism, amino acid) 270.9
   albinism 270.2
   alkaptonuria 270.2
   argininosuccinicaciduria 270.6
   beta-amino-isobutyricaciduria 277.2
   cystathioninuria 270.4
   cystinosis 270.0
   cystinuria 270.0
   glycinuria 270.0
   homocystinuria 270.4
   imidazole 270.5
   maple syrup (urine) disease 270.3
   neonatal, transitory 775.89
   oasthouse urine disease 270.2
   ochronosis 270.2
   phenylketonuria 270.1
   phenylpyruvic oligophrenia 270.1
   purine NEC 277.2
   pyrimidine NEC 277.2
   renal transport NEC 270.0
   specified type NEC 270.8
   transport NEC 270.0
    renal 270.0
   xanthinuria 277.2
  amnestic (*see also* Amnestic syndrome) 294.08
   alcohol-induced persisting 291.1
   drug-induced persisting 292.83
   in conditions classified elsewhere 294.0
  anaerobic glycolysis with anemia 282.3
  anxiety (*see also* Anxiety) 300.00
   due to or associated with physical condition
    293.84
  arteriole 447.9
   specified type NEC 447.8
  artery 447.9
   specified type NEC 447.8
  articulation—*see* Disorder, joint
  Asperger's 299.8
  attachment of infancy or early childhood 313.89

Disorder — *continued*
  attention deficit 314.00
    with hyperactivity 314.01
    predominantly
      combined hyperactive/inattentive 314.01
      hyperactive/impulsive 314.01
      inattentive 314.00
    residual type 314.8
  auditory processing disorder 388.45
    acquired 388.45
    developmental 315.32
  autistic 299.0
  autoimmune NEC 279.4
    hemolytic (cold type) (warm type) 283.0
    parathyroid 252.1
    thyroid 245.2
  avoidant, childhood or adolescence 313.21
  balance
    acid-base 276.9
      mixed (with hypercapnia) 276.4
    electrolyte 276.9
    fluid 276.9
  behavior NEC (*see also* Disturbance, conduct) 312.9
    disruptive 312.9
  bilirubin excretion 277.4
  bipolar (affective) (alternating) 296.80

Note—Use the following fifth-digit subclassification with categories 296.0-296.6:

0   unspecified
1   mild
2   moderate
3   severe, without mention of psychotic behavior
4   severe, specified as with psychotic behavior
5   in partial or unspecified remission
6   in full remission

---

  atypical 296.7
  currently
    depressed 296.5
    hypomanic 296.4
    manic 296.4
  mixed 296.6
  specified type NEC 296.89
  type I 296.7
    most recent episode (or current)
      depressed 296.5
      hypomanic 296.4
      manic 296.4
      mixed 296.6
      unspecified 296.7
    single manic episode 296.0
  type II (recurrent major depressive episodes with hypomania) 296.89
  bladder 596.9
    functional NEC 596.59
    specified NEC 596.8
  bleeding 286.9
  bone NEC 733.90
    specified NEC 733.99
  brachial plexus 353.0
  branched-chain amino-acid degradation 270.3
  breast 611.9
    puerperal, postpartum 676.3
    specified NEC 611.8
  Briquet's 300.81
  bursa 727.9
    shoulder region 726.10

Disorder — *continued*
  carbohydrate metabolism, congenital 271.9
  cardiac, functional 427.9
    postoperative 997.1
    psychogenic 306.2
  cardiovascular, psychogenic 306.2
  cartilage NEC 733.90
    articular 718.00
      ankle 718.07
      elbow 718.02
      foot 718.07
      hand 718.04
      hip 718.05
      knee 717.9
      multiple sites 718.09
      pelvic region 718.05
      shoulder region 718.01
      specified
        site NEC 718.08
        type NEC 733.99
      wrist 718.03
  catatonic—*see* Catatonia
  central auditory processing 315.32
    acquired 388.45
    developmental 315.32
  cervical region NEC 723.9
  cervical root (nerve) NEC 353.2
  character NEC (*see also* Disorder, personality) 301.9
  ciliary body 364.9
    specified NEC 364.89
  coagulation (factor) (*see also* Defect, coagulation) 286.9
    factor VIII (congenital) (functional) 286.0
    factor IX (congenital) (functional) 286.1
    neonatal, transitory 776.3
  coccyx 724.70
    specified NEC 724.79
  cognitive 294.9
  colon 569.9
    functional 564.9
    congenital 751.3
  communication 307.9
  conduct (*see also* Disturbance, conduct) 312.9
    adjustment reaction 309.3
    adolescent onset type 312.82
    childhood onset type 312.81
    compulsive 312.30
      specified type NEC 312.39
    hyperkinetic 314.2
    onset unspecified 312.89
    socialized (type) 312.20
      aggressive 312.23
      unaggressive 312.21
    specified NEC 312.89
  conduction, heart 426.9
    specified NEC 426.89
  conflict
    sexual orientation 302.0
  congenital
    glycosylation (CDG) 271.8
  convulsive (secondary) (*see also* Convulsions) 780.39
    due to injury at birth 767.0
    idiopathic 780.39
  coordination 781.3
  cornea NEC 371.89
    due to contact lens 371.82
  corticosteroid metabolism NEC 255.2
  cranial nerve—*see* Disorder, nerve, cranial
  cyclothymic 301.13

INDEX TO DISEASES

Disorder—*continued*
  degradation, branched-chain amino acid 270.3
  delusional 297.1
  dentition 520.6
  depersonalization 300.6
  depressive NEC 311
    atypical 296.82
    major (*see also* Psychosis, affective) 296.2
      recurrent episode 296.3
      single episode 296.2
  development, specific 315.9
    associated with hyperkinesia 314.1
    coordination 315.4
    language 315.31
      and speech due to hearing loss 315.34
    learning 315.2
      arithmetical 315.1
      reading 315.00
    mixed 315.5
    motor coordination 315.4
    specified type NEC 315.8
    speech 315.39
      and language due to hearing loss 315.34
  diaphragm 519.4
  digestive 536.9
    fetus or newborn 777.9
      specified NEC 777.8
    psychogenic 306.4
  disintegrative, childhood 299.1
  dissociative 300.15
    identity 300.14
    nocturnal 307.47
  drug-related 292.9
  dysmorphic body 300.7
  dysthymic 300.4
  ear 388.9
    degenerative NEC 388.00
    external 380.9
      specified 380.89
      pinna 380.30
    specified type NEC 388.8
    vascular NEC 388.00
  eating NEC 307.50
  electrolyte NEC 276.9
    with
      abortion—*see* Abortion, by type, with metabolic disorder
      ectopic pregnancy (*see also* categories 633.0-633.9) 639.4
      molar pregnancy (*see also* categories 630-632) 639.4
    acidosis 276.2
      metabolic 276.2
      respiratory 276.2
    alkalosis 276.3
      metabolic 276.3
      respiratory 276.3
    following
      abortion 639.4
      ectopic or molar pregnancy 639.4
    neonatal, transitory NEC 775.5
  emancipation as adjustment reaction 309.22
  emotional (*see also* Disorder, mental, nonpsychotic) V40.9
  endocrine 259.9
    specified type NEC 259.8
  esophagus 530.9
    functional 530.5
    psychogenic 306.4
  explosive
    intermittent 312.34

Disorder—*continued*
  isolated 312.35
  expressive language 315.31
  eye 379.90
    globe—*see* Disorder, globe
    ill-defined NEC 379.99
    limited duction NEC 378.63
    specified NEC 379.8
  eyelid 374.9
    degenerative 374.50
    sensory 374.44
    specified type NEC 374.89
    vascular 374.85
  factitious (with combined psychological and physical signs and symptoms) (with predominantly physical signs and symptoms) 300.19
    with predominantly psychological signs and symptoms 300.16
  factor, coagulation (*see also* Defect, coagulation) 286.9
    VIII (congenital) (functional) 286.0
    IX (congenital) (functional) 286.1
  fascia 728.9
  fatty acid oxidation 277.85
  feeding —*see* Feeding
  female sexual arousal 302.72
  fluid NEC 276.9
  gastric (functional) 536.9
    motility 536.8
    psychogenic 306.4
    secretion 536.8
  gastrointestinal (functional) NEC 536.9
    newborn (neonatal) 777.9
      specified NEC 777.8
    psychogenic 306.4
  gender (child) 302.6
    adult 302.85
  gender identity (childhood) 302.6
    adolescents 302.85
    adults (-life) 302.85
  genitourinary system, psychogenic 306.50
  globe 360.9
    degenerative 360.20
      specified NEC 360.29
    specified type NEC 360.89
  hearing—*see also* Deafness
    conductive type (air) (*see also* Deafness, conductive) 389.00
    mixed conductive and sensorineural 389.20
      bilateral 389.22
      unilateral 389.21
    nerve
      bilateral 389.12
      unilateral 389.13
    perceptive (*see also* Deafness, perceptive) 389.10
    sensorineural type NEC (*see also* Deafness, sensorineural) 389.10
  heart action 427.9
    postoperative 997.1
  hematological, transient neonatal 776.9
    specified type NEC 776.8
  hematopoietic organs 289.9
  hemorrhagic NEC 287.9
    due to intrinsic circulating anticoagulants 286.5
    specified type NEC 287.8
  hemostasis (*see also* Defect, coagulation) 286.9
  homosexual conflict 302.0
  hypomanic (chronic) 301.11

965

Disorder—continued
identity
  childhood and adolescence 313.82
    gender 302.6
  gender 302.6
immune mechanism (immunity) 279.9
  single complement (C_1-C_9) 279.8
  specified type NEC 279.8
impulse control (see also Disturbance, conduct, compulsive) 312.30
infant sialic acid storage 271.8
integument, fetus or newborn 778.9
  specified type NEC 778.8
interactional psychotic (childhood) (see also Psychosis, childhood) 299.1
intermittent explosive 312.34
intervertebral disc 722.90
  cervical, cervicothoracic 722.91
  lumbar, lumbosacral 722.93
  thoracic, thoracolumbar 722.92
intestinal 569.9
  functional NEC 564.9
    congenital 751.3
    postoperative 564.4
  psychogenic 306.4
introverted, of childhood and adolescence 313.22
involuntary emotional expression (IEED) 310.8
iris 364.9
  specified NEC 364.89
iron, metabolism 275.0
isolated explosive 312.35
joint NEC 719.90
  ankle 719.97
  elbow 719.92
  foot 719.97
  hand 719.94
  hip 719.95
  knee 719.96
  multiple sites 719.99
  pelvic region 719.95
  psychogenic 306.0
  shoulder (region) 719.91
  specified site NEC 719.98
  temporomandibular 524.60
    sounds on opening or closing 524.64
    specified NEC 524.69
  wrist 719.93
kidney 593.9
  functional 588.9
    specified NEC 588.89
labyrinth, labyrinthine 386.9
  specified type NEC 386.8
lactation 676.9
language (developmental) (expressive) 315.31
  mixed receptive-expressive 315.32
learning 315.9
ligament 728.9
ligamentous attachments, peripheral—see also Enthesopathy
  spine 720.1
limb NEC 729.9
  psychogenic 306.0
lipid
  metabolism, congenital 272.9
  storage 272.7
lipoprotein deficiency (familial) 272.5
low back NEC 724.9
  psychogenic 306.0

Disorder—continued
lumbosacral
  plexus 353.1
  root (nerve) NEC 353.4
lymphoproliferative (chronic) NEC (M9970/1) 238.79
major depressive (see also Psychosis, affective) 296.2
  recurrent episode 296.3
  single episode 296.2
male erectile 607.84
  nonorganic origin 302.72
manic (see also Psychosis, affective) 296.0
  atypical 296.81
mathematics 315.1
meniscus NEC (see also Disorder, cartilage, articular) 718.0
menopausal 627.9
  specified NEC 627.8
menstrual 626.9
  psychogenic 306.52
  specified NEC 626.8
mental (nonpsychotic) 300.9
  affecting management of pregnancy, childbirth, or puerperium 648.4
  drug-induced 292.9
    hallucinogen persistent perception 292.89
    specified type NEC 292.89
  due to or associated with
    alcoholism 291.9
    drug consumption NEC 292.9
      specified type NEC 292.89
    physical condition NEC 293.9
  induced by drug 292.9
    specified type NEC 292.89
  neurotic (see also Neurosis) 300.9
  of infancy, childhood or adolescence 313.9
  persistent
    other
      due to conditions classified elsewhere 294.8
    unspecified
      due to conditions classified elsewhere 294.9
  presenile 310.1
    psychotic NEC 290.10
  previous, affecting management of pregnancy V23.8
  psychoneurotic (see also Neurosis) 300.9
  psychotic (see also Psychosis) 298.9
    brief 298.8
    senile 290.20
  specific, following organic brain damage 310.9
    cognitive or personality change of other type 310.1
    frontal lobe syndrome 310.0
    postconcussional syndrome 310.2
    specified type NEC 310.8
  transient
    in conditions classified elsewhere 293.9
metabolism NEC 277.9
  with
    abortion—see Abortion, by type, with metabolic disorder
    ectopic pregnancy (see also categories 633.0-633.9) 639.4
    molar pregnancy (see also categories 630-632) 639.4
  alkaptonuria 270.2
  amino acid (see also Disorder, amino acid) 270.9
    specified type NEC 270.8
  ammonia 270.6

INDEX TO DISEASES

Disorder—*continued*
  arginine 270.6
  argininosuccinic acid 270.6
  basal 794.7
  bilirubin 277.4
  calcium 275.40
  carbohydrate 271.9
    specified type NEC 271.8
  cholesterol 272.9
  citrulline 270.6
  copper 275.1
  corticosteroid 255.2
  cystine storage 270.0
  cystinuria 270.0
  fat 272.9
  fatty acid oxidation 277.85
  following
    abortion 639.4
    ectopic or molar pregnancy 639.4
  fructosemia 271.2
  fructosuria 271.2
  fucosidosis 271.8
  due to conditions classified elsewhere 294.8
  galactose-1-phosphate uridyl transferase 271.1
  glutamine 270.7
  glycine 270.7
  glycogen storage NEC 271.0
    hepatorenal 271.0
  hemochromatosis 275.0
  in labor and delivery 669.0
  iron 275.0
  lactose 271.3
  lipid 272.9
    specified type NEC 272.8
    storage 272.7
  lipoprotein—*see also* Hyperlipemia deficiency (familial) 272.5
  lysine 270.7
  magnesium 275.2
  mannosidosis 271.8
  mineral 275.9
    specified type NEC 275.8
  mitochondrial 277.87
  mucopolysaccharide 277.5
  nitrogen 270.9
  ornithine 270.6
  oxalosis 271.8
  pentosuria 271.8
  phenylketonuria 270.1
  phosphate 275.3
  phosphorus 275.3
  plasma protein 273.9
    specified type NEC 273.8
  porphyrin 277.1
  purine 277.2
  pyrimidine 277.2
  serine 270.7
  sodium 276.9
  specified type NEC 277.89
  steroid 255.2
  threonine 270.7
  urea cycle 270.6
  xylose 271.8
  micturition NEC 788.69
    psychogenic 306.53
  misery and unhappiness, of childhood and adolescence 313.1
  mitochondrial metabolism 277.87
  mitral valve 424.0
  mood (*see also* Disorder, bipolar) 296.90
    episodic 296.90

Disorder—*continued*
    specified NEC 296.99
    in conditions classified elsewhere 293.83
  motor tic 307.20
    chronic 307.22
    transient (childhood) 307.21
  movement NEC 333.90
    hysterical 300.11
    medication-induced 333.90
    periodic limb 327.51
    sleep related, unspecified 780.58
      other organic 327.59
    specified type NEC 333.99
    stereotypic 307.3
  mucopolysaccharide 277.5
  muscle 728.9
    psychogenic 306.0
    specified type NEC 728.3
  muscular attachments, peripheral—*see also* Enthesopathy
    spine 720.1
  musculoskeletal system NEC 729.9
    psychogenic 306.0
  myeloproliferative (chronic) NEC (M9960/1) 238.79
  myoneural 358.9
    due to lead 358.2
    specified type NEC 358.8
    toxic 358.2
  myotonic 359.29
  neck region NEC 723.9
  nerve 349.9
    abducens NEC 378.54
    accessory 352.4
    acoustic 388.5
    auditory 388.5
    auriculotemporal 350.8
    axillary 353.0
    cerebral—*see* Disorder, nerve, cranial
    cranial 352.9
      first 352.0
      second 377.49
      third
        partial 378.51
        total 378.52
      fourth 378.53
      fifth 350.9
      sixth 378.54
      seventh NEC 351.9
      eighth 388.5
      ninth 352.2
      tenth 352.3
      eleventh 352.4
      twelfth 352.5
      multiple 352.6
    entrapment—*see* Neuropathy, entrapment
    facial 351.9
      specified NEC 351.8
    femoral 355.2
    glossopharyngeal NEC 352.2
    hypoglossal 352.5
    iliohypogastric 355.79
    ilioinguinal 355.79
    intercostal 353.8
    lateral
      cutaneous of thigh 355.1
      popliteal 355.3
    lower limb NEC 355.8
    medial, popliteal 355.4
    median NEC 354.1
    obturator 355.79

Disorder—*continued*
  oculomotor
    partial 378.51
    total 378.52
  olfactory 352.0
  optic 377.49
    hypoplasia 377.43
    ischemic 377.41
    nutritional 377.33
    toxic 377.34
  peroneal 355.3
  phrenic 354.8
  plantar 355.6
  pneumogastric 352.3
  posterior tibial 355.5
  radial 354.3
  recurrent laryngeal 352.3
  root 353.9
    specified NEC 353.8
  saphenous 355.79
  sciatic NEC 355.0
  specified NEC 355.9
    lower limb 355.79
    upper limb 354.8
  spinal 355.9
  sympathetic NEC 337.9
  trigeminal 350.9
    specified NEC 350.8
  trochlear 378.53
  ulnar 354.2
  upper limb NEC 354.9
  vagus 352.3
nervous system NEC 349.9
  autonomic (peripheral) (*see also* Neuropathy, peripheral, autonomic) 337.9
  cranial 352.9
  parasympathetic (*see also* Neuropathy, peripheral, autonomic) 337.9
  specified type NEC 349.89
  sympathetic (*see also* Neuropathy, peripheral, autonomic) 337.9
  vegetative (*see also* Neuropathy, peripheral, autonomic) 337.9
neurohypophysis NEC 253.6
neurological NEC 781.99
  peripheral NEC 355.9
neuromuscular NEC 358.9
  hereditary NEC 359.1
  specified NEC 358.8
  toxic 358.2
neurotic 300.9
  specified type NEC 300.89
neutrophil, polymorphonuclear (functional) 288.1
nightmare 307.47
night terror 307.46
obsessive-compulsive 300.3
oppositional defiant, childhood and adolescence 313.81
optic
  chiasm 377.54
    associated with
      inflammatory disorders 377.54
      neoplasm NEC 377.52
        pituitary 377.51
      pituitary disorders 377.51
      vascular disorders 377.53
  nerve 377.49
  radiations 377.63
  tracts 377.63
orbit 376.9
  specified NEC 376.89

Disorder—*continued*
  orgasmic
    female 302.73
    male 302.74
  overanxious, of childhood and adolescence 313.0
  oxidation, fatty acid 277.85
  pancreas, internal secretion (other than diabetes mellitus) 251.9
    specified type NEC 251.8
  panic 300.01
    with agoraphobia 300.21
  papillary muscle NEC 429.81
  paranoid 297.9
    induced 297.3
    shared 297.3
  parathyroid 252.9
    specified type NEC 252.8
  paroxysmal, mixed 780.39
  pentose phosphate pathway with anemia 282.2
  periodic limb movement 327.51
  peroxisomal 277.86
  personality 301.9
    affective 301.10
    aggressive 301.3
    amoral 301.7
    anancastic, anankastic 301.4
    antisocial 301.7
    asocial 301.7
    asthenic 301.6
    avoidant 301.82
    borderline 301.83
    compulsive 301.4
    cyclothymic 301.13
    dependent-passive 301.6
    dyssocial 301.7
    emotional instability 301.59
    epileptoid 301.3
    explosive 301.3
    following organic brain damage 310.1
    histrionic 301.50
    hyperthymic 301.11
    hypomanic (chronic) 301.11
    hypothymic 301.12
    hysterical 301.50
    immature 301.89
    inadequate 301.6
    introverted 301.21
    labile 301.59
    moral deficiency 301.7
    narcissistic 301.81
    obsessional 301.4
    obsessive-compulsive 301.4
    overconscientious 301.4
    paranoid 301.0
    passive (-dependent) 301.6
    passive-aggressive 301.84
    pathological NEC 301.9
    pseudosocial 301.7
    psychopathic 301.9
    schizoid 301.20
      introverted 301.21
      schizotypal 301.22
    schizotypal 301.22
    seductive 301.59
    type A 301.4
    unstable 301.59
  pervasive developmental 299.9
    childhood-onset 299.8
    specified NEC 299.8
  phonological 315.39

INDEX TO DISEASES

Disorder

Disorder—*continued*
  pigmentation, choroid (congenital) 743.53
  pinna 380.30
    specified type NEC 380.39
  pituitary, thalamic 253.9
    anterior NEC 253.4
    iatrogenic 253.7
    postablative 253.7
    specified NEC 253.8
  pityriasis-like NEC 696.8
  platelets (blood) 287.1
  polymorphonuclear neutrophils (functional) 288.1
  porphyrin metabolism 277.1
  postmenopausal 627.9
    specified type NEC 627.8
  post-traumatic stress (PTSD) 309.81
    acute 309.81
    brief 309.81
    chronic 309.81
  premenstrual dysphoric (PMDD) 625.4
  psoriatic-like NEC 696.8
  psychic, with diseases classified elsewhere 316
  psychogenic NEC (*see also* condition) 300.9
    allergic NEC
      respiratory 306.1
    anxiety 300.00
      atypical 300.00
      generalized 300.02
    appetite 307.59
    articulation, joint 306.0
    asthenic 300.5
    blood 306.8
    cardiovascular (system) 306.2
    compulsive 300.3
    cutaneous 306.3
    depressive 300.4
    digestive (system) 306.4
    dysmenorrheic 306.52
    dyspneic 306.1
    eczematous 306.3
    endocrine (system) 306.6
    eye 306.7
    feeding 307.59
    functional NEC 306.9
    gastric 306.4
    gastrointestinal (system) 306.4
    genitourinary (system) 306.50
    heart (function) (rhythm) 306.2
    hemic 306.8
    hyperventilatory 306.1
    hypochondriacal 300.7
    hysterical 300.10
    intestinal 306.4
    joint 306.0
    learning 315.2
    limb 306.0
    lymphatic (system) 306.8
    menstrual 306.52
    micturition 306.53
    monoplegic NEC 306.0
    motor 307.9
    muscle 306.0
    musculoskeletal 306.0
    neurocirculatory 306.2
    obsessive 300.3
    occupational 300.89
    organ or part of body NEC 306.9
    organs of special sense 306.7
    paralytic NEC 306.0
    phobic 300.20
    physical NEC 306.9
    pruritic 306.3

Disorder—*continued*
    rectal 306.4
    respiratory (system) 306.1
    rheumatic 306.0
    sexual (function) 302.70
      specified type NEC 302.79
    sexual orientation conflict 302.0
    skin (allergic) (eczematous) (pruritic) 306.3
    sleep 307.40
      initiation or maintenance 307.41
        persistent 307.42
        transient 307.41
      movement 780.58
      sleep terror 307.46
      specified type NEC 307.49
    specified part of body NEC 306.8
    stomach 306.4
  psychomotor NEC 307.9
    hysterical 300.11
  psychoneurotic (*see also* Neurosis) 300.9
    mixed NEC 300.89
  psychophysiologic (*see also* Disorder, psychosomatic) 306.9
  psychosexual identity (childhood) 302.6
    adult-life 302.85
  psychosomatic NEC 306.9
    allergic NEC
      respiratory 306.1
    articulation, joint 306.0
    cardiovascular (system) 306.2
    cutaneous 306.3
    digestive (system) 306.4
    dysmenorrheic 306.52
    dyspneic 306.1
    endocrine (system) 306.6
    eye 306.7
    gastric 306.4
    gastrointestinal (system) 306.4
    genitourinary (system) 306.50
    heart (functional) (rhythm) 306.2
    hyperventilatory 306.1
    intestinal 306.4
    joint 306.0
    limb 306.0
    lymphatic (system) 306.8
    menstrual 306.52
    micturition 306.53
    monoplegic NEC 306.0
    muscle 306.0
    musculoskeletal 306.0
    neurocirculatory 306.2
    organs of special sense 306.7
    paralytic NEC 306.0
    pruritic 306.3
    rectal 306.4
    respiratory (system) 306.1
    rheumatic 306.0
    sexual (function) 302.70
      specified type NEC 302.79
    skin 306.3
    specified part of body NEC 306.8
    stomach 306.4
  psychotic (*see also* Psychosis) 298.9
    brief 298.8
  PTSD (post-traumatic stress disorder) 309.81
  purine metabolism NEC 277.2
  pyrimidine metabolism NEC 277.2
  reactive attachment of infancy or early childhood 313.89
  reading, developmental 315.00
  reflex 796.1

Disorder—*continued*
REM sleep behavior 327.42
renal function, impaired 588.9
   specified type NEC 588.89
renal transport NEC 588.89
respiration, respiratory NEC 519.9
   due to
      aspiration of liquids or solids 508.9
      inhalation of fumes or vapors 506.9
   psychogenic 306.1
retina 362.9
   specified type NEC 362.89
rumination 307.53
sacroiliac joint NEC 724.6
sacrum 724.6
schizo-affective (*see also* Schizophrenia) 295.7
schizoid, childhood or adolescence 313.22
schizophreniform 295.4
schizotypal personality 301.22
secretion, thyrocalcitonin 246.0
seizure 345.9
   recurrent 345.9
      epileptic—*see* Epilepsy
sense of smell 781.1
   psychogenic 306.7
separation anxiety 309.21
sexual (*see also* Deviation, sexual) 302.9
   aversion 302.79
   desire, hypoactive 302.71
   function, psychogenic 302.70
shyness, of childhood and adolescence 313.21
single complement (C_1-C_9) 279.8
skin NEC 709.9
   fetus or newborn 778.9
      specified type 778.8
   psychogenic (allergic) (eczematous) (pruritic) 306.3
   specified type NEC 709.8
   vascular 709.1
sleep 780.50
   alcohol induced 291.82
   arousal 307.46
      confusional 327.41
   circadian rhythm 327.30
      advanced sleep phase type 327.32
      alcohol induced 291.82
      delayed sleep phase type 327.31
      drug induced 292.85
      free running type 327.34
      in conditions classified elsewhere 327.37
      irregular sleep-wake type 327.33
      jet lag type 327.35
      other 327.39
      shift work type 327.36
   drug induced 292.85
   initiation or maintenance (*see also* Insomnia) 780.52
      nonorganic origin (transient) 307.41
      persistent 307.42
   nonorganic origin 307.40
      specified type NEC 307.49
   organic specified type NEC 327.8
   periodic limb movement 327.51
   specified NEC 780.59
   wake
      cycle—*see* Disorder, sleep, circadian rhythm
      schedule—*see* Disorder, sleep, circadian rhythm
   with apnea—*see* Apnea, sleep
social, of childhood and adolescence 313.22
soft tissue 729.9
somatization 300.81

Disorder—*continued*
somatoform (atypical) (undifferentiated) 300.82
   severe 300.81
   specified type NEC 300.89
speech NEC 784.5
   nonorganic origin 307.9
spine NEC 724.9
   ligamentous or muscular attachments, peripheral 720.1
steroid metabolism NEC 255.2
stomach (functional) (*see also* Disorder, gastric) 536.9
   psychogenic 306.4
storage, iron 275.0
stress (*see also* Reaction, stress, acute) 308.3
   posttraumatic
      acute 309.81
      brief 309.81
      chronic 309.81
substitution 300.11
suspected—*see* Observation
synovium 727.9
temperature regulation, fetus or newborn 778.4
temporomandibular joint NEC 524.60
   sounds on opening or closing 524.64
   specified NEC 524.69
tendon 727.9
   shoulder region 726.10
thoracic root (nerve) NEC 353.3
thyrocalcitonin secretion 246.0
thyroid (gland) NEC 246.9
   specified type NEC 246.8
tic 307.20
   chronic (motor or vocal) 307.22
   motor-verbal 307.23
   organic origin 333.1
   transient (of childhood) 307.21
tooth NEC 525.9
   development NEC 520.9
      specified type NEC 520.8
   eruption 520.6
   specified type NEC 525.8
Tourette's 307.23
transport, carbohydrate 271.9
   specified type NEC 271.8
tubular, phosphate-losing 588.0
tympanic membrane 384.9
unaggressive, unsocialized (*see also* Disturbance, conduct) 312.1
undersocialized, unsocialized—*see also* Disturbance, conduct
   aggressive (type) 312.0
   unaggressive (type) 312.1
vision, visual NEC 368.9
   binocular NEC 368.30
   cortex 377.73
      associated with
         inflammatory disorders 377.73
         neoplasms 377.71
         vascular disorders 377.72
   pathway NEC 377.63
      associated with
         inflammatory disorders 377.63
         neoplasms 377.61
         vascular disorders 377.62
vocal tic
   chronic 307.22
wakefulness (*see also* Hypersomnia) 780.54
   nonorganic origin (transient) 307.43
   persistent 307.44
written expression 315.2
Disorganized globe 360.29

INDEX TO DISEASES   **Disproportion**

Displacement, displaced

> *Note*—For acquired displacement of bones, cartilage, joints, tendons, due to injury, see also Dislocation. Displacements at ages under one year should be considered congenital, provided there is no indication the condition was acquired after birth.

   acquired traumatic of bond, cartilage, joint, tendon NEC (without fracture) *(see also* Dislocation) 839.8
      with fracture—*see* Fracture, by site
   adrenal gland (congenital) 759.1
   alveolus and teeth, vertical 524.75
   appendix, retrocecal (congenital) 751.5
   auricle (congenital) 744.29
   bladder (acquired) 596.8
      congenital 753.8
   brachial plexus (congenital) 742.8
   brain stem, caudal 742.4
   canaliculus lacrimalis 743.65
   cardia, through esophageal hiatus 750.6
   cerebellum, caudal 742.4
   cervix —*see* Displacement, uterus
   colon (congenital) 751.4
   device, implant, or graft—*see* Complications, mechanical
   epithelium
      columnar of cervix 622.10
      cuboidal, beyond limits of external os (uterus) 752.49
   esophageal mucosa into cardia of stomach, congenital 750.4
   esophagus (acquired) 530.89
      congenital 750.4
   eyeball (acquired) (old) 376.36
      congenital 743.8
      current injury 871.3
      lateral 376.36
   fallopian tube (acquired) 620.4
      congenital 752.19
      opening (congenital) 752.19
   gallbladder (congenital) 751.69
   gastric mucosa 750.7
      into
         duodenum 750.7
         esophagus 750.7
         Meckel's diverticulum, congenital 750.7
   globe (acquired) (lateral) (old) 376.36
      current injury 871.3
   graft
      artificial skin graft 996.55
      decellularized allodermis graft 996.55
   heart (congenital) 746.87
      acquired 429.89
   hymen (congenital) (upward) 752.49
   internal prosthesis NEC—*see* Complications, mechanical
   intervertebral disc (with neuritis, radiculitis, sciatica, or other pain) 722.2
      with myelopathy 722.70
      cervical, cervicodorsal, cervicothoracic 722.0
         with myelopathy 722.71
         due to major trauma—*see* Dislocation, vertebra, cervical
      due to trauma—*see* Dislocation, vertebra
      lumbar, lumbosacral 722.10
         with myelopathy 722.73
         due to major trauma—*see* Dislocation, vertebra, lumbar

Displacement, displaced—*continued*
   thoracic, thoracolumbar 722.11
      with myelopathy 722.72
      due to major trauma—*see* Dislocation, vertebra, thoracic
   intrauterine device 996.32
   kidney (acquired) 593.0
      congenital 753.3
   lacrimal apparatus or duct (congenital) 743.65
   macula (congenital) 743.55
   Meckel's diverticulum (congenital) 751.0
   nail (congenital) 757.5
      acquired 703.8
   opening of Wharton's duct in mouth 750.26
   organ or site, congenital NEC—*see* Malposition, congenital
   ovary (acquired) 620.4
      congenital 752.0
      free in peritoneal cavity (congenital) 752.0
      into hernial sac 620.4
   oviduct (acquired) 620.4
      congenital 752.19
   parathyroid (gland) 252.8
   parotid gland (congenital) 750.26
   punctum lacrimale (congenital) 743.65
   sacroiliac (congenital) (joint) 755.69
      current injury—*see* Dislocation, sacroiliac
      old 724.6
   spine (congenital) 756.19
   spleen, congenital 759.0
   stomach (congenital) 750.7
      acquired 537.89
   subglenoid (closed) 831.01
   sublingual duct (congenital) 750.26
   teeth, tooth 524.30
      horizontal 524.33
      vertical 524.34
   tongue (congenital) (downward) 750.19
   trachea (congenital) 748.3
   ureter or ureteric opening or orifice (congenital) 753.4
   uterine opening of oviducts or fallopian tubes 752.19
   uterus, uterine *(see also* Malposition, uterus) 621.6
      congenital 752.3
   ventricular septum 746.89
      with rudimentary ventricle 746.89
   xyphoid bone (process) 738.3

Disproportion 653.9
   affecting fetus or newborn 763.1
   caused by
      conjoined twins 653.7
      contraction, pelvis (general) 653.1
         inlet 653.2
         midpelvic 653.8
         midplane 653.8
         outlet 653.3
      fetal
         ascites 653.7
         hydrocephalus 653.6
         hydrops 653.7
         meningomyelocele 653.7
         sacral teratoma 653.7
         tumor 653.7
      hydrocephalic fetus 653.6
      pelvis, pelvic, abnormality (bony) NEC 653.0
      unusually large fetus 653.5
         causing obstructed labor 660.1
   cephalopelvic, normally formed fetus 653.4
      causing obstructed labor 660.1
   fetal NEC 653.5

971

Disproportion—*continued*
  causing obstructed labor 660.1
  fetopelvic, normally formed fetus 653.4
    causing obstructed labor 660.1
  mixed maternal and fetal origin, normally formed fetus 653.4
  pelvis, pelvic (bony) NEC 653.1
    causing obstructed labor 660.1
  specified type NEC 653.8
Disruption
  cesarean wound 674.1
  family V61.0
  gastrointestinal anastomosis 997.4
  ligament(s)—*see also* Sprain
    knee
      current injury—*see* Dislocation, knee
      old 717.89
        capsular 717.85
        collateral (medial) 717.82
          lateral 717.81
        cruciate (posterior) 717.84
          anterior 717.83
        specified site NEC 717.85
  marital V61.10
    involving divorce or estrangement V61.0
  operation wound (external) 998.32
    internal 998.31
  organ transplant, anastomosis site—*see* Complications, transplant, organ, by site
  ossicles, ossicular chain 385.23
    traumatic—*see* Fracture, skull, base
  parenchyma
    liver (hepatic)—*see* Laceration, liver, major
    spleen—*see* Laceration, spleen, parenchyma, massive
  phase-shift, of 24 hour sleep wake cycle, unspecified 780.55
    nonorganic origin 307.45
  sleep wake cycle (24 hour), unspecified 780.55
    circadian rhythm 327.33
    nonorganic origin 307.45
  suture line (external) 998.32
    internal 998.31
  wound
    cesarean operation 674.1
    episiotomy 674.2
    operation 998.32
      cesarean 674.1
      internal 998.31
    perineal (obstetric) 674.2
    uterine 674.1
Disruptio uteri —*see also* Rupture, uterus
  complicating delivery—*see* Delivery, complicated, rupture, uterus
Dissatisfaction with
  employment V62.2
  school environment V62.3
Dissecting —*see* condition
Dissection
  aorta 441.00
    abdominal 441.02
    thoracic 441.01
    thoracoabdominal 441.03
  artery, arterial
    carotid 443.21
    coronary 414.12
    iliac 443.22
    renal 443.23
    specified NEC 443.29
    vertebral 443.24
  vascular 459.9
  wound—*see* Wound, open, by site

Disseminated —*see* condition
Dissociated personality NEC 300.15
Dissociation
  auriculoventricular or atrioventricular (any degree) (AV) 426.89
    with heart block 426.0
  interference 426.89
  isorhythmic 426.89
  rhythm
    atrioventricular (AV) 426.89
    interference 426.89
Dissociative
  identity disorder 300.14
  reaction NEC 300.15
Dissolution, vertebra (*see also* Osteoporosis) 733.00
Distention
  abdomen (gaseous) 787.3
  bladder 596.8
  cecum 569.89
  colon 569.89
  gallbladder 575.8
  gaseous (abdomen) 787.3
  intestine 569.89
  kidney 593.89
  liver 573.9
  seminal vesicle 608.89
  stomach 536.8
    acute 536.1
    psychogenic 306.4
  ureter 593.5
  uterus 621.8
Distichia, distichiasis (eyelid) 743.63
Distoma hepaticum infestation 121.3
Distomiasis 121.9
  bile passages 121.3
    due to Clonorchis sinensis 121.1
  hemic 120.9
  hepatic (liver) 121.3
    due to Clonorchis sinensis (clonorchiasis) 121.1
  intestinal 121.4
  liver 121.3
    due to Clonorchis sinensis 121.1
  lung 121.2
  pulmonary 121.2
Distomolar (fourth molar) 520.1
  causing crowding 524.31
Disto-occlusion (division I) (division II) 524.22
Distortion (congenital)
  adrenal (gland) 759.1
  ankle (joint) 755.69
  anus 751.5
  aorta 747.29
  appendix 751.5
  arm 755.59
  artery (peripheral) NEC (*see also* Distortion, peripheral vascular system) 747.60
    cerebral 747.81
    coronary 746.85
    pulmonary 747.3
    retinal 743.58
    umbilical 747.5
  auditory canal 744.29
    causing impairment of hearing 744.02
  bile duct or passage 751.69
  bladder 753.8
  brain 742.4
  bronchus 748.3
  cecum 751.5
  cervix (uteri) 752.49

INDEX TO DISEASES   **Distress**

Distortion—*continued*
   chest (wall) 756.3
   clavicle 755.51
   clitoris 752.49
   coccyx 756.19
   colon 751.5
   common duct 751.69
   cornea 743.41
   cricoid cartilage 748.3
   cystic duct 751.69
   duodenum 751.5
   ear 744.29
      auricle 744.29
         causing impairment of hearing 744.02
      causing impairment of hearing 744.09
      external 744.29
         causing impairment of hearing 744.02
      inner 744.05
      middle, except ossicles 744.03
         ossicles 744.04
      ossicles 744.04
   endocrine (gland) NEC 759.2
   epiglottis 748.3
   Eustachian tube 744.24
   eye 743.8
      adnexa 743.69
   face bone(s) 756.0
   fallopian tube 752.19
   femur 755.69
   fibula 755.69
   finger(s) 755.59
   foot 755.67
   gallbladder 751.69
   genitalia, genital organ(s)
      female 752.89
         external 752.49
         internal NEC 752.89
      male 752.89
         penis 752.69
   glottis 748.3
   gyri 742.4
   hand bone(s) 755.59
   heart (auricle) (ventricle) 746.89
      valve (cusp) 746.89
   hepatic duct 751.69
   humerus 755.59
   hymen 752.49
   ileum 751.5
   intestine (large) (small) 751.5
      with anomalous adhesions, fixation or malrotation 751.4
   jaw NEC 524.89
   jejunum 751.5
   kidney 753.3
   knee (joint) 755.64
   labium (majus) (minus) 752.49
   larynx 748.3
   leg 755.69
   lens 743.36
   liver 751.69
   lumbar spine 756.19
      with disproportion (fetopelvic) 653.4
         affecting fetus or newborn 763.1
         causing obstructed labor 660.1
   lumbosacral (joint) (region) 756.19
   lung (fissures) (lobe) 748.69
   nerve 742.8
   nose 748.1
   organ
      of Corti 744.05
      or site not listed—*see* Anomaly, specified type NEC

Distortion—*continued*
   ossicles, ear 744.04
   ovary 752.0
   oviduct 752.19
   pancreas 751.7
   parathyroid (gland) 759.2
   patella 755.64
   peripheral vascular system NEC 747.60
      gastrointestinal 747.61
      lower limb 747.64
      renal 747.62
      spinal 747.82
      upper limb 747.63
   pituitary (gland) 759.2
   radius 755.59
   rectum 751.5
   rib 756.3
   sacroiliac joint 755.69
   sacrum 756.19
   scapula 755.59
   shoulder girdle 755.59
   site not listed—*see* Anomaly, specified type NEC
   skull bone(s) 756.0
      with
         anencephalus 740.0
         encephalocele 742.0
         hydrocephalus 742.3
            with spina bifida (*see also* Spina bifida) 741.0
         microcephalus 742.1
   spinal cord 742.59
   spine 756.19
   spleen 759.0
   sternum 756.3
   thorax (wall) 756.3
   thymus (gland) 759.2
   thyroid (gland) 759.2
      cartilage 748.3
   tibia 755.69
   toe(s) 755.66
   tongue 750.19
   trachea (cartilage) 748.3
   ulna 755.59
   ureter 753.4
      causing obstruction 753.20
   urethra 753.8
      causing obstruction 753.6
   uterus 752.3
   vagina 752.49
   vein (peripheral) NEC (*see also* Distortion, peripheral vascular system) 747.60
      great 747.49
      portal 747.49
      pulmonary 747.49
   vena cava (inferior) (superior) 747.49
   vertebra 756.19
   visual NEC 368.15
      shape or size 368.14
   vulva 752.49
   wrist (bones) (joint) 755.59
Distress
   abdomen 789.0
   colon 789.0
   emotional V40.9
   epigastric 789.0
   fetal (syndrome) 768.4
      affecting management of pregnancy or childbirth 656.8
      liveborn infant 768.4
      first noted
         before onset of labor 768.2
         during labor and delivery 768.3

Distress—*continued*
  stillborn infant (death before onset of labor) 768.0
    death during labor 768.1
  gastrointestinal (functional) 536.9
    psychogenic 306.4
  intestinal (functional) NEC 564.9
    psychogenic 306.4
  intrauterine (*see* Distress, fetal)
  leg 729.5
  maternal 669.0
  mental V40.9
  respiratory 786.09
    acute (adult) 518.82
    adult syndrome (following shock, surgery, or trauma) 518.5
      specified NEC 518.82
    fetus or newborn 770.89
    syndrome (idiopathic) (newborn) 769
  stomach 536.9
    psychogenic 306.4
Distribution vessel, atypical NEC 747.60
  coronary artery 746.85
  spinal 747.82
Districhiasis 704.2
Disturbance —*see also* Disease
  absorption NEC 579.9
    calcium 269.3
    carbohydrate 579.8
    fat 579.8
    protein 579.8
    specified type NEC 579.8
    vitamin (*see also* Deficiency, vitamin) 269.2
  acid-base equilibrium 276.9
  activity and attention, simple, with hyperkinesis 314.01
  amino acid (metabolic) (*see also* Disorder, amino acid) 270.9
    imidazole 270.5
    maple syrup (urine) disease 270.3
    transport 270.0
  assimilation, food 579.9
  attention, simple 314.00
    with hyperactivity 314.01
  auditory, nerve, except deafness 388.5
  behavior (*see also* Disturbance, conduct) 312.9
  blood clotting (hypoproteinemia) (mechanism) (*see also* Defect, coagulation) 286.9
  central nervous system NEC 349.9
  cerebral nerve NEC 352.9
  circulatory 459.9
  conduct 312.9

Note—*Use the following fifth-digit subclassification with categories 312.0-312.2:*

0   unspecified
1   mild
2   moderate
3   severe

    adjustment reaction 309.3
    adolescent onset type 312.82
    childhood onset type 312.81
    compulsive 312.30
      intermittent explosive disorder 312.34
      isolated explosive disorder 312.35
      kleptomania 312.32
      pathological gambling 312.31
      pyromania 312.33
    hyperkinetic 314.2
    intermittent explosive 312.34

Disturbance—*continued*
    isolated explosive 312.35
    memory (*see also* Amnesia) 780.99
    mixed with emotions 312.4
    socialized (type) 312.20
      aggressive 312.23
      unaggressive 312.21
    specified type NEC 312.89
    undersocialized, unsocialized
      aggressive (type) 312.0
      unaggressive (type) 312.1
  coordination 781.3
  cranial nerve NEC 352.9
  deep sensibility—*see* Disturbance, sensation
  digestive 536.9
    psychogenic 306.4
  electrolyte—*see* Imbalance, electrolyte
  emotions specific to childhood or adolescence 313.9
    with
      academic underachievement 313.83
      anxiety and fearfulness 313.0
      elective mutism 313.23
      identity disorder 313.82
      jealousy 313.3
      misery and unhappiness 313.1
      oppositional defiant disorder 313.81
      overanxiousness 313.0
      sensitivity 313.21
      shyness 313.21
      social withdrawal 313.22
      withdrawal reaction 313.22
    involving relationship problems 313.3
    mixed 313.89
    specified type NEC 313.89
  endocrine (gland) 259.9
    neonatal, transitory 775.9
      specified NEC 775.89
  equilibrium 780.4
  feeding (elderly) (infant) 783.3
    newborn 779.3
    nonorganic origin NEC 307.59
    psychogenic NEC 307.59
  fructose metabolism 271.2
  gait 781.2
    hysterical 300.11
  gastric (functional) 536.9
    motility 536.8
    psychogenic 306.4
    secretion 536.8
  gastrointestinal (functional) 536.9
    psychogenic 306.4
  habit, child 307.9
  hearing, except deafness 388.40
  heart, functional (conditions classifiable to 426, 427, 428)
    due to presence of (cardiac) prosthesis 429.4
    postoperative (immediate) 997.1
      long-term effect of cardiac surgery 429.4
    psychogenic 306.2
  hormone 259.9
  innervation uterus, sympathetic, parasympathetic 621.8
  keratinization NEC
    gingiva 523.10
    lip 528.5
    oral (mucosa) (soft tissue) 528.79
      residual ridge mucosa
        excessive 528.72
        minimal 528.71
    tongue 528.79

INDEX TO DISEASES   **Disturbance**

Disturbance—*continued*
  labyrinth, labyrinthine (vestibule) 386.9
  learning, specific NEC 315.2
  memory (*see also* Amnesia) 780.93
    mild, following organic brain damage 310.8
  mental (*see also* Disorder, mental) 300.9
    associated with diseases classified elsewhere 316
  metabolism (acquired) (congenital) (*see also* Disorder, metabolism) 277.9
    with
      abortion—*see* Abortion, by type, with metabolic disorder
      ectopic pregnancy (*see also* categories 633.0-633.9) 639.4
      molar pregnancy (*see also* categories 630-632) 639.4
    amino acid (*see also* Disorder, amino acid) 270.9
      aromatic NEC 270.2
      branched-chain 270.3
      specified type NEC 270.8
      straight-chain NEC 270.7
      sulfur-bearing 270.4
      transport 270.0
    ammonia 270.6
    arginine 270.6
    argininosuccinic acid 270.6
    carbohydrate NEC 271.9
    cholesterol 272.9
    citrulline 270.6
    cystathionine 270.4
    fat 272.9
    following
      abortion 639.4
      ectopic or molar pregnancy 639.4
    general 277.9
      carbohydrate 271.9
      iron 275.0
      phosphate 275.3
      sodium 276.9
    glutamine 270.7
    glycine 270.7
    histidine 270.5
    homocystine 270.4
    in labor or delivery 669.0
    iron 275.0
    isoleucine 270.3
    leucine 270.3
    lipoid 272.9
      specified type NEC 272.8
    lysine 270.7
    methionine 270.4
    neonatal, transitory 775.9
      specified type NEC 775.89
    nitrogen 788.9
    ornithine 270.6
    phosphate 275.3
    phosphatides 272.7
    serine 270.7
    sodium NEC 276.9
    threonine 270.7
    tryptophan 270.2
    tyrosine 270.2
    urea cycle 270.6
    valine 270.3
  motor 796.1
  nervous functional 799.2
  neuromuscular mechanism (eye) due to syphilis 094.84
  nutritional 269.9

Disturbance—*continued*
  nail 703.8
  ocular motion 378.87
    psychogenic 306.7
  oculogyric 378.87
    psychogenic 306.7
  oculomotor NEC 378.87
    psychogenic 306.7
  olfactory nerve 781.1
  optic nerve NEC 377.49
  oral epithelium, including tongue 528.79
    residual ridge mucosa
      excessive 528.72
      minimal 528.71
  personality (pattern) (trait) (*see also* Disorder, personality) 301.9
    following organic brain damage 310.1
  polyglandular 258.9
  psychomotor 307.9
  pupillary 379.49
  reflex 796.1
  rhythm, heart 427.9
    postoperative (immediate) 997.1
      long-term effect of cardiac surgery 429.4
    psychogenic 306.2
  salivary secretion 527.7
  sensation (cold) (heat) (localization) (tactile discrimination localization) (texture) (vibratory) NEC 782.0
    hysterical 300.11
    skin 782.0
    smell 781.1
    taste 781.1
  sensory (*see also* Disturbance, sensation) 782.0
    innervation 782.0
  situational (transient) (*see also* Reaction, adjustment) 309.9
    acute 308.3
  sleep 780.50
    initiation or maintenance (*see also* Insomnia) 780.52
      nonorganic origin 307.41
    nonorganic origin 307.40
      specified type NEC 307.49
    specified NEC 780.59
      nonorganic origin 307.49
    wakefulness (*see also* Hypersomnia) 780.54
      nonorganic origin 307.43
    with apnea—*see* Apnea, sleep
  sociopathic 301.7
  speech NEC 784.5
    developmental 315.39
      associated with hyperkinesis 314.1
    secondary to organic lesion 784.5
  stomach (functional) (*see also* Disturbance, gastric) 536.9
  sympathetic (nerve) (*see also* Neuropathy, peripheral, autonomic) 337.9
  temperature sense 782.0
    hysterical 300.11
  tooth
    eruption 520.6
    formation 520.4
    structure, hereditary NEC 520.5
  touch (*see also* Disturbance, sensation) 782.0
  vascular 459.9
    arteriosclerotic—*see* Arteriosclerosis
  vasomotor 443.9
  vasospastic 443.9
  vestibular labyrinth 386.9
  vision, visual NEC 368.9

Disturbance — *continued*
   psychophysical 368.16
   specified NEC 368.8
   subjective 368.10
   voice 784.40
   wakefulness (initiation or maintenance) (*see also* Hypersomnia) 780.54
     nonorganic origin 307.43
Disulfiduria, beta-mercaptolactate-cysteine 270.0
Disuse atrophy, bone 733.7
Ditthomska syndrome 307.81
Diuresis 788.42
Divers'
   palsy or paralysis 993.3
   squeeze 993.3
Diverticula, diverticulosis, diverticulum (acute) (multiple) (perforated) (ruptured) 562.10
   with diverticulitis 562.11
   aorta (Kommerell's) 747.21
   appendix (noninflammatory) 543.9
   bladder (acquired) (sphincter) 596.3
     congenital 753.8
   broad ligament 620.8
   bronchus (congenital) 748.3
     acquired 494.0
       with acute exacerbation 494.1
   calyx, calyceal (kidney) 593.89
   cardia (stomach) 537.1
   cecum 562.10
     with
       diverticulitis 562.11
         with hemorrhage 562.13
       hemorrhage 562.12
     congenital 751.5
   colon (acquired) 562.10
     with
       diverticulitis 562.11
         with hemorrhage 562.13
       hemorrhage 562.12
     congenital 751.5
   duodenum 562.00
     with
       diverticulitis 562.01
         with hemorrhage 562.03
       hemorrhage 562.02
     congenital 751.5
   epiphrenic (esophagus) 530.6
   esophagus (congenital) 750.4
     acquired 530.6
     epiphrenic 530.6
     pulsion 530.6
     traction 530.6
     Zenker's 530.6
   Eustachian tube 381.89
   fallopian tube 620.8
   gallbladder (congenital) 751.69
   gastric 537.1
   heart (congenital) 746.89
   ileum 562.00
     with
       diverticulitis 562.01
         with hemorrhage 562.03
       hemorrhage 562.02
   intestine (large) 562.10
     with
       diverticulitis 562.11
         with hemorrhage 562.13
       hemorrhage 562.12
     congenital 751.5
     small 562.00

Diverticula, diverticulosis — *continued*
   with
     diverticulitis 562.01
       with hemorrhage 562.03
     hemorrhage 562.02
     congenital 751.5
   jejunum 562.00
     with
       diverticulitis 562.01
         with hemorrhage 562.03
       hemorrhage 562.02
   kidney (calyx) (pelvis) 593.89
     with calculus 592.0
   Kommerell's 747.21
   laryngeal ventricle (congenital) 748.3
   Meckel's (displaced) (hypertrophic) 751.0
   midthoracic 530.6
   organ or site, congenital NEC — *see* Distortion
   pericardium (congenital) (cyst) 746.89
     acquired (true) 423.8
   pharyngoesophageal (pulsion) 530.6
   pharynx (congenital) 750.27
   pulsion (esophagus) 530.6
   rectosigmoid 562.10
     with
       diverticulitis 562.11
         with hemorrhage 562.13
       hemorrhage 562.12
     congenital 751.5
   rectum 562.10
     with
       diverticulitis 562.11
         with hemorrhage 562.13
       hemorrhage 562.12
   renal (calyces) (pelvis) 593.89
     with calculus 592.0
   Rokitansky's 530.6
   seminal vesicle 608.0
   sigmoid 562.10
     with
       diverticulitis 562.11
         with hemorrhage 562.13
       hemorrhage 562.12
     congenital 751.5
   small intestine 562.00
     with
       diverticulitis 562.01
         with hemorrhage 562.03
       hemorrhage 562.02
   stomach (cardia) (juxtacardia) (juxtapyloric) (acquired) 537.1
     congenital 750.7
   subdiaphragmatic 530.6
   trachea (congenital) 748.3
     acquired 519.19
   traction (esophagus) 530.6
   ureter (acquired) 593.89
     congenital 753.4
   ureterovesical orifice 593.89
   urethra (acquired) 599.2
     congenital 753.8
   ventricle, left (congenital) 746.89
   vesical (urinary) 596.3
     congenital 753.8
   Zenker's (esophagus) 530.6
Diverticulitis (acute) (*see also* Diverticula) 562.11
   with hemorrhage 562.13
   bladder (urinary) 596.3
   cecum (perforated) 562.11
     with hemorrhage 562.13

Diverticulitis—*continued*
  colon (perforated) 562.11
    with hemorrhage 562.13
  duodenum 562.01
    with hemorrhage 562.03
  esophagus 530.6
  ileum (perforated) 562.01
    with hemorrhage 562.03
  intestine (large) (perforated) 562.11
    with hemorrhage 562.13
    small 562.01
      with hemorrhage 562.03
  jejunum (perforated) 562.01
    with hemorrhage 562.03
  Meckel's (perforated) 751.0
  pharyngoesophageal 530.6
  rectosigmoid (perforated) 562.11
    with hemorrhage 562.13
  rectum 562.11
    with hemorrhage 562.13
  sigmoid (old) (perforated) 562.11
    with hemorrhage 562.13
  small intestine (perforated) 562.01
    with hemorrhage 562.03
  vesical (urinary) 596.3
Diverticulosis —*see* Diverticula
Division
  cervix uteri 622.8
    external os into two openings by frenum 752.49
  external (cervical) into two openings by frenum 752.49
  glans penis 752.69
  hymen 752.49
  labia minora (congenital) 752.49
  ligament (partial or complete) (current)—*see also* Sprain, by site
    with open wound—*see* Wound, open, by site
  muscle (partial or complete) (current)—*see also* Sprain, by site
    with open wound—*see* Wound, open, by site
  nerve—*see* Injury, nerve, by site
  penis glans 752.69
  spinal cord—*see* Injury, spinal, by site
  vein 459.9
    traumatic—*see* Injury, vascular, by site
Divorce V61.0
Dix-Hallpike neurolabyrinthitis 386.12
Dizziness 780.4
  hysterical 300.11
  psychogenic 306.9
Doan-Wiseman syndrome (primary splenic neutropenia) 289.53
Dog bite —*see* Wound, open, by site
Döhle-Heller aortitis 093.1
Döhle body-panmyelopathic syndrome 288.2
Dolichocephaly, dolichocephalus 754.0
Dolichocolon 751.5
Dolichostenomelia 759.82
Donohue's syndrome (leprechaunism) 259.8
Donor
  blood V59.01
    other blood components V59.09
    stem cells V59.02
    whole blood V59.01
  bone V59.2
    marrow V59.3
  cornea V59.5
  egg (oocyte) (ovum) V59.70
    age 35 and over V59.73
      anonymous recipient V59.73
      designated recipient V59.74

Donor—*continued*
  under age 35 V59.71
    anonymous recipient V59.71
    designated recipient V59.72
  heart V59.8
  kidney V59.4
  liver V59.6
  lung V59.8
  lymphocyte V59.8
  organ V59.9
    specified NEC V59.8
  potential, examination of V70.8
  skin V59.1
  specified organ or tissue NEC V59.8
  sperm V59.8
  stem cells V59.02
  tissue V59.9
    specified type NEC V59.8
Donovanosis (granuloma venereum) 099.2
DOPS (diffuse obstructive pulmonary syndrome) 496
Double
  albumin 273.8
  aortic arch 747.21
  auditory canal 744.29
  auricle (heart) 746.82
  bladder 753.8
  external (cervical) os 752.49
  kidney with double pelvis (renal) 753.3
  larynx 748.3
  meatus urinarius 753.8
  organ or site NEC—*see* Accessory
  orifice
    heart valve NEC 746.89
      pulmonary 746.09
  outlet, right ventricle 745.11
  pelvis (renal) with double ureter 753.4
  penis 752.69
  tongue 750.13
  ureter (one or both sides) 753.4
    with double pelvis (renal) 753.4
  urethra 753.8
  urinary meatus 753.8
  uterus (any degree) 752.2
    with doubling of cervix and vagina 752.2
    in pregnancy or childbirth 654.0
      affecting fetus or newborn 763.89
  vagina 752.49
    with doubling of cervix and uterus 752.2
  vision 368.2
  vocal cords 748.3
  vulva 752.49
  whammy (syndrome) 360.81
Douglas' pouch, cul-de-sac —*see* condition
Down's disease or syndrome (mongolism) 758.0
Down-growth, epithelial (anterior chamber) 364.61
Dracontiasis 125.7
Dracunculiasis 125.7
Dracunculosis 125.7
Drainage
  abscess (spontaneous)—*see* Abscess
  anomalous pulmonary veins to hepatic veins or right atrium 747.41
  stump (amputation) (surgical) 997.62
  suprapubic, bladder 596.8
Dream state, hysterical 300.13
Drepanocytic anemia (*see also* Disease, sickle cell) 282.60
Dresbach's syndrome (elliptocytosis) 282.1
Dreschlera (infection) 118
  hawaiiensis 117.8

Dressler's syndrome (postmyocardial infarction) 411.0
Dribbling (post-void) 788.35
Drift, ulnar 736.09
Drinking (alcohol)—*see also* Alcoholism
  excessive, to excess NEC (*see also* Abuse, drugs, nondependent) 305.0
    bouts, periodic 305.0
    continual 303.9
    episodic 305.0
    habitual 303.9
    periodic 305.0
Drip, postnasal (chronic) 784.91
  due to
    allergic rhinitis —*see* Rhinitis, allergic
    common cold 460
    gastroesophageal reflux —*see* Reflux, gastroesophageal
    nasopharyngitis —*see* Nasopharyngitis
    other known condition —*code to condition*
    sinusitis —*see* Sinusitis
Drivers' license examination V70.3
Droop
  Cooper's 611.8
  facial 781.94
Drop
  finger 736.29
  foot 736.79
  hematocrit (precipitous) 790.01
  toe 735.8
  wrist 736.05
Dropped
  dead 798.1
  heart beats 426.6
Dropsy, dropsical (*see also* Edema) 782.3
  abdomen 789.59
  amnion (*see also* Hydramnios) 657
  brain—*see* Hydrocephalus
  cardiac (*see also* Failure, heart) 428.0
  cardiorenal (*see also* Hypertension, cardiorenal) 404.90
  chest 511.9
  fetus or newborn 778.0
    due to isoimmunization 773.3
  gangrenous (*see also* Gangrene) 785.4
  heart (*see also* Failure, heart) 428.0
  hepatic—*see* Cirrhosis, liver
  infantile—*see* Hydrops, fetalis
  kidney (*see also* Nephrosis) 581.9
  liver—*see* Cirrhosis, liver
  lung 514
  malarial (*see also* Malaria) 084.9
  neonatorum—*see* Hydrops, fetalis
  nephritic 581.9
  newborn—*see* Hydrops, fetalis
  nutritional 269.9
  ovary 620.8
  pericardium (*see also* Pericarditis) 423.9
  renal (*see also* Nephrosis) 581.9
  uremic—*see* Uremia
Drowned, drowning 994.1
  lung 518.5
Drowsiness 780.09
Drug —*see also* condition
  addiction (*see also* listing under Dependence) 304.9
  adverse effect NEC, correct substance properly administered 995.20
  allergy 995.27
  dependence (*see also* listing under Dependence) 304.9

Drug—*continued*
  habit (*see also* listing under Dependence) 304.9
  hypersensitivity 995.27
  induced
    circadian rhythm sleep disorder 292.85
    hypersomnia 292.85
    insomnia 292.85
    mental disorder 292.9
      anxiety 292.89
      mood 292.84
      sexual 292.89
      sleep 292.85
      specified type 292.89
    parasomnia 292.85
    persisting
      amnestic disorder 292.83
      dementia 292.82
    psychotic disorder
      with
        delusions 292.11
        hallucinations 292.12
    sleep disorder 292.85
  intoxication 292.89
  overdose—*see* Table of drugs and chemicals
  poisoning—*see* Table of drugs and chemicals
  therapy (maintenance) status NEC
    chemotherapy, antineoplastic V58.11
    immunotherapy, antineoplastic V58.12
    long-term (current) use V58.69
      antibiotics V58.62
      anticoagulants V58.61
      anti-inflammatories, non-steroidal (NSAID) V58.64
      antiplatelets V58.63
      antithrombotics V58.63
      aspirin V58.66
      high-risk medications NEC V58.69
      insulin V58.67
      steroids V58.65
    wrong substance given or taken in error—*see* Table of drugs and chemicals
Drunkenness (*see also* Abuse, drugs, nondependent) 305.0
  acute in alcoholism (*see also* Alcoholism) 303.0
  chronic (*see also* Alcoholism) 303.9
  pathologic 291.4
  simple (acute) 305.0
    in alcoholism 303.0
  sleep 307.47
Drusen
  optic disc or papilla 377.21
  retina (colloid) (hyaloid degeneration) 362.57
    hereditary 362.77
Drusenfieber 075
Dry, dryness —*see also* condition
  eye 375.15
    syndrome 375.15
  larynx 478.79
  mouth 527.7
  nose 478.19
  skin syndrome 701.1
  socket (teeth) 526.5
  throat 478.29
DSAP (disseminated superficial actinic porokeratosis) 692.75
Duane's retraction syndrome 378.71
Duane-Stilling-Turk syndrome (ocular retraction syndrome) 378.71
Dubin-Johnson disease or syndrome 277.4
Dubini's disease (electric chorea) 049.8
Dubois' abscess or disease 090.5

Duchenne's
  disease 094.0
    locomotor ataxia 094.0
    muscular dystrophy 359.1
    pseudohypertrophy, muscles 359.1
  paralysis 335.22
  syndrome 335.22
Duchenne-Aran myelopathic muscular atrophy
  (nonprogressive) (progressive) 335.21
Duchenne-Griesinger disease 359.1
Ducrey's
  bacillus 099.0
  chancre 099.0
  disease (chancroid) 099.0
Duct, ductus —*see* condition
Duengero 061
Duhring's disease (dermatitis herpetiformis) 694.0
Dukes (-Filatov) disease 057.8
Dullness
  cardiac (decreased) (increased) 785.3
Dumb ague (*see also* Malaria) 084.6
Dumbness (*see also* Aphasia) 784.3
Dumdum fever 085.0
Dumping syndrome (postgastrectomy) 564.2
  nonsurgical 536.8
Duodenitis (nonspecific) (peptic) 535.60
  due to
    Strongyloides stercoralis 127.2
  with hemorrhage 535.61
Duodenocholangitis 575.8
Duodenum, duodenal —*see* condition
Duplay's disease, periarthritis, or syndrome 726.2
Duplex —*see also* Accessory
  kidney 753.3
  placenta—*see* Placenta, abnormal
  uterus 752.2
Duplication —*see also* Accessory
  anus 751.5
  aortic arch 747.21
  appendix 751.5
  biliary duct (any) 751.69
  bladder 753.8
  cecum 751.5
    and appendix 751.5
  clitoris 752.49
  cystic duct 751.69
  digestive organs 751.8
  duodenum 751.5
  esophagus 750.4
  fallopian tube 752.19
  frontonasal process 756.0
  gallbladder 751.69
  ileum 751.5
  intestine (large) (small) 751.5
  jejunum 751.5
  kidney 753.3
  liver 751.69
  nose 748.1
  pancreas 751.7
  penis 752.69
  respiratory organs NEC 748.9
  salivary duct 750.22
  spinal cord (incomplete) 742.51
  stomach 750.7
  ureter 753.4
  vagina 752.49
  vas deferens 752.89
  vocal cords 748.3
Dupré's disease or syndrome (meningism) 781.6

Dupuytren's
  contraction 728.6
  disease (muscle contracture) 728.6
  fracture (closed) 824.4
    ankle (closed) 824.4
      open 824.5
    fibula (closed) 824.4
      open 824.5
    open 824.5
    radius (closed) 813.42
      open 813.52
  muscle contracture 728.6
Durand-Nicolas-Favre disease (climatic bubo) 099.1
Duroziez's disease (congenital mitral stenosis) 746.5
Dust
  conjunctivitis 372.05
  reticulation (occupational) 504
Dutton's
  disease (trypanosomiasis) 086.9
  relapsing fever (West African) 087.1
Dwarf, dwarfism 259.4
  with infantilism (hypophyseal) 253.3
  achondroplastic 756.4
  Amsterdam 759.89
  bird-headed 759.89
  congenital 259.4
  constitutional 259.4
  hypophyseal 253.3
  infantile 259.4
  Levi type 253.3
  Lorain-Levi (pituitary) 253.3
  Lorain type (pituitary) 253.3
  metatropic 756.4
  nephrotic-glycosuric, with hypophosphatemic rickets 270.0
  nutritional 263.2
  ovarian 758.6
  pancreatic 577.8
  pituitary 253.3
  polydystrophic 277.5
  primordial 253.3
  psychosocial 259.4
  renal 588.0
    with hypertension—*see* Hypertension, kidney
  Russell's (uterine dwarfism and craniofacial dysostosis) 759.89
Dyke-Young anemia or syndrome (acquired macrocytic hemolytic anemia) (secondary) (symptomatic) 283.9
Dynia abnormality (*see also* Defect, coagulation) 286.9
Dysacousis 388.40
Dysadrenocortism 255.9
  hyperfunction 255.3
  hypofunction 255.41
Dysarthria 784.5
Dysautonomia (*see also* Neuropathy, peripheral, autonomic) 337.9
  familial 742.8
Dysbarism 993.3
Dysbasia 719.7
  angiosclerotica intermittens 443.9
    due to atherosclerosis 440.21
  hysterical 300.11
  lordotica (progressiva) 333.6
  nonorganic origin 307.9
  psychogenic 307.9
Dysbetalipoproteinemia (familial) 272.2
Dyscalculia 315.1
Dyschezia (*see also* Constipation) 564.00

Dyschondroplasia (with hemangiomata) 756.4
  Voorhoeve's 756.4
Dyschondrosteosis 756.59
Dyschromia 709.00
Dyscollagenosis 710.9
Dyscoria 743.41
Dyscraniopyophalangy 759.89
Dyscrasia
  blood 289.9
    with antepartum hemorrhage 641.3
    fetus or newborn NEC 776.9
    hemorrhage, subungual 287.8
    puerperal, postpartum 666.3
  ovary 256.8
  plasma cell 273.9
  pluriglandular 258.9
  polyglandular 258.9
Dysdiadochokinesia 781.3
Dysectasia, vesical neck 596.8
Dysendocrinism 259.9
Dysentery, dysenteric (bilious) (catarrhal)
    (diarrhea) (epidemic) (gangrenous)
    (hemorrhagic) (infectious) (sporadic)
    (tropical) (ulcerative) 009.0
  abscess, liver (*see also* Abscess, amebic) 006.3
  amebic (*see also* Amebiasis) 006.9
    with abscess—*see* Abscess, amebic
    acute 006.0
    carrier (suspected) of V02.2
    chronic 006.1
  arthritis (*see also* Arthritis, due to, dysentery)
      009.0 *[711.3]*
    bacillary 004.9 *[711.3]*
  asylum 004.9
  bacillary 004.9
    arthritis 004.9 *[711.3]*
    Boyd 004.2
    Flexner 004.1
    Schmitz (-Stutzer) 004.0
    Shiga 004.0
    Shigella 004.9
      group A 004.0
      group B 004.1
      group C 004.2
      group D 004.3
      specified type NEC 004.8
    Sonne 004.3
    specified type NEC 004.8
  bacterium 004.9
  balantidial 007.0
  Balantidium coli 007.0
  Boyd's 004.2
  Chilomastix 007.8
  Chinese 004.9
  choleriform 001.1
  coccidial 007.2
  Dientamoeba fragilis 007.8
  due to specified organism NEC—*see* Enteritis,
      due to, by organism
  Embadomonas 007.8
  Endolimax nana—*see* Dysentery, amebic
  Entamoba, entamebic—*see* Dysentery, amebic
  Flexner's 004.1
  Flexner-Boyd 004.2
  giardial 007.1
  Giardia lamblia 007.1
  Hiss-Russell 004.1
  lamblia 007.1
  leishmanial 085.0
  malarial (*see also* Malaria) 084.6
  metazoal 127.9

Dysentery, dysenteric—*continued*
  Monilia 112.89
  protozoal NEC 007.9
  Russell's 004.8
  salmonella 003.0
  schistosomal 120.1
  Schmitz (-Stutzer) 004.0
  Shiga 004.0
  Shigella NEC (*see also* Dysentery, bacillary)
      004.9
    boydii 004.2
    dysenteriae 004.0
      Schmitz 004.0
      Shiga 004.0
    flexneri 004.1
    Group A 004.0
    Group B 004.1
    Group C 004.2
    Group D 004.3
    Schmitz 004.0
    Shiga 004.0
    Sonnei 004.3
  Sonne 004.3
  strongyloidiasis 127.2
  trichomonal 007.3
  tuberculous (*see also* Tuberculosis) 014.8
  viral (*see also* Enteritis, viral) 008.8
Dysequilibrium 780.4
Dysesthesia 782.0
  hysterical 300.11
Dysfibrinogenemia (congenital) (*see also* Defect,
    coagulation) 286.3
Dysfunction
  adrenal (cortical) 255.9
    hyperfunction 255.3
    hypofunction 255.41
  associated with sleep stages or arousal from
      sleep 780.56
    nonorganic origin 307.47
  bladder NEC 596.59
  bleeding, uterus 626.8
  brain, minimal (*see also* Hyperkinesia) 314.9
  cerebral 348.30
  colon 564.9
    psychogenic 306.4
  colostomy or enterostomy 569.62
  cystic duct 575.8
  diastolic 429.9
    with heart failure—*see* Failure, heart
    due to
      cardiomyopathy—*see* Cardiomyopathy
      hypertension—*see* Hypertension, heart
  endocrine NEC 259.9
  endometrium 621.8
  enteric stoma 569.62
  enterostomy 569.62
  erectile 607.84
    nonorganic origin 302.72
  esophagostomy 530.87
  Eustachian tube 381.81
  gallbladder 575.8
  gastrointestinal 536.9
  gland, glandular NEC 259.9
  heart 427.9
    postoperative (immediate) 997.1
      long-term effect of cardiac surgery 429.4
  hemoglobin 289.89
  hepatic 573.9
  hepatocellular NEC 573.9
  hypophysis 253.9
    hyperfunction 253.1

INDEX TO DISEASES   **Dyshidrosis**

Dysfunction—*continued*
  hypofunction 253.2
  posterior lobe 253.6
    hypofunction 253.5
kidney (*see also* Disease, renal) 593.9
labyrinthine 386.50
  specified NEC 386.58
liver 573.9
  constitutional 277.4
minimal brain (child) (*see also* Hyperkinesia) 314.9
ovary, ovarian 256.9
  hyperfunction 256.1
    estrogen 256.0
  hypofunction 256.39
    postablative 256.2
  postablative 256.2
  specified NEC 256.8
papillary muscle 429.81
  with myocardial infarction 410.8
parathyroid 252.8
  hyperfunction 252.00
  hypofunction 252.1
pineal gland 259.8
pituitary (gland) 253.9
  hyperfunction 253.1
  hypofunction 253.2
  posterior 253.6
    hypofunction 253.5
placental—*see* Placenta, insufficiency
platelets (blood) 287.1
polyglandular 258.9
  specified NEC 258.8
psychosexual 302.70
  with
    dyspareunia (functional) (psychogenic) 302.76
    frigidity 302.72
    impotence 302.72
    inhibition
      orgasm
        female 302.73
        male 302.74
      sexual
        desire 302.71
        excitement 302.72
    premature ejaculation 302.75
    sexual aversion 302.79
    specified disorder NEC 302.79
    vaginismus 306.51
pylorus 537.9
rectum 564.9
  psychogenic 306.4
segmental (*see also* Dysfunction, somatic) 739.9
senile 797
sexual 302.70
sinoatrial node 427.81
somatic 739.9
  abdomen 739.9
  acromioclavicular 739.7
  cervical 739.1
  cervicothoracic 739.1
  costochondral 739.8
  costovertebral 739.8
  extremities
    lower 739.6
    upper 739.7
  head 739.0
  hip 739.5
  umbar, lumbosacral 739.3
  occipitocervical 739.0

Dysfunction—*continued*
  pelvic 739.5
  pubic 739.5
  rib cage 739.8
  sacral 739.4
  sacrococcygeal 739.4
  sacroiliac 739.4
  specified site NEC 739.9
  sternochondral 739.8
  sternoclavicular 739.7
  temporomandibular 739.0
  thoracic, thoracolumbar 739.2
stomach 536.9
  psychogenic 306.4
suprarenal 255.9
  hyperfunction 255.3
  hypofunction 255.41
symbolic NEC 784.60
  specified type NEC 784.69
systolic 429.9
  with heart failure—*see* Failure, heart
temporomandibular (joint) (joint-pain-syndrome) NEC 524.60
  sounds on opening or closing 524.64
  specified NEC 524.69
testicular 257.9
  hyperfunction 257.0
  hypofunction 257.2
  specified type NEC 257.8
thymus 254.9
thyroid 246.9
  complicating pregnancy, childbirth, or puerperium 648.1
  hyperfunction—*see* Hyperthyroidism
  hypofunction—*see* Hypothyroidism
uterus, complicating delivery 661.9
  affecting fetus or newborn 763.7
  hypertonic 661.4
  hypotonic 661.2
    primary 661.0
    secondary 661.1
velopharyngeal (acquired) 528.9
  congenital 750.29
ventricular 429.9
  with congestive heart failure (*see also* Failure, heart) 428.0
  due to
    cardiomyopathy—*see* Cardiomyopathy
    hypertension—*see* Hypertension, heart
  left, reversible following sudden emotional stress 429.83
vesicourethral NEC 596.59
vestibular 386.50
  specified type NEC 386.58
Dysgammaglobulinemia 279.06
Dysgenesis
  gonadal (due to chromosomal anomaly) 758.6
    pure 752.7
  kidney(s) 753.0
  ovarian 758.6
  renal 753.0
  reticular 279.2
  seminiferous tubules 758.6
  tidal platelet 287.31
Dysgerminoma (M9060/3)
  specified site—*see* Neoplasm, by site, malignant
  unspecified site
    female 183.0
    male 186.9
Dysgeusia 781.1
Dysgraphia 781.3
Dyshidrosis 705.81

Dysidrosis 705.81
Dysinsulinism 251.8
Dyskaryotic cervical smear 795.09
Dyskeratosis (*see also* Keratosis) 701.1
  bullosa hereditaria 757.39
  cervix 622.10
  congenital 757.39
  follicularis 757.39
    vitamin A deficiency 264.8
  gingiva 523.8
  oral soft tissue NEC 528.79
  tongue 528.79
  uterus NEC 621.8
Dyskinesia 781.3
  biliary 575.8
  esophagus 530.5
  hysterical 300.11
  intestinal 564.89
  neuroleptic-induced tardive 333.85
  nonorganic origin 307.9
  orofacial 333.82
    due to drugs 333.85
  psychogenic 307.9
  subacute, due to drugs 333.85
  tardive (oral) 333.85
Dyslalia 784.5
  developmental 315.39
Dyslexia 784.61
  developmental 315.02
  secondary to organic lesion 784.61
Dyslipidemia 272.4
Dysmaturity (*see also* Immaturity) 765.1
  lung 770.4
  pulmonary 770.4
Dysmenorrhea (essential) (exfoliative) (functional) (intrinsic) (membranous) (primary) (secondary) 625.3
  psychogenic 306.52
Dysmetabolic syndrome X 277.7
Dysmetria 781.3
Dysmorodystrophia mesodermalis congenita 759.82
Dysnomia 784.3
Dysorexia 783.0
  hysterical 300.11
Dysostosis
  cleidocranial, cleidocranialis 755.59
  craniofacial 756.0
  Fairbank's (idiopathic familial generalized osteophytosis) 756.50
  mandibularis 756.0
  mandibulofacial, incomplete 756.0
  multiplex 277.5
  orodigitofacial 759.89
Dyspareunia (female) 625.0
  male 608.89
  psychogenic 302.76
Dyspepsia (allergic) (congenital) (fermentative) (flatulent) (functional) (gastric) (gastrointestinal) (neurogenic) (occupational) (reflex) 536.8
  acid 536.8
  atonic 536.3
    psychogenic 306.4
  diarrhea 787.91
    psychogenic 306.4
  intestinal 564.89
    psychogenic 306.4
  nervous 306.4
  neurotic 306.4
  psychogenic 306.4

Dysphagia 787.20
  cervical 787.29
  functional 300.11
  hysterical 300.11
  nervous 300.11
  neurogenic 787.29
  oral phase 787.21
  oropharyngeal phase 787.22
  pharyngeal phase 787.23
  pharyngoesophageal phase 787.24
  psychogenic 306.4
  sideropenic 280.8
  spastica 530.5
  specified NEC 787.29
Dysphagocytosis, congenital 288.1
Dysphasia 784.5
Dysphonia 784.49
  clericorum 784.49
  functional 300.11
  hysterical 300.11
  psychogenic 306.1
  spastica 478.79
Dyspigmentation —*see also* Pigmentation
  eyelid (acquired) 374.52
Dyspituitarism 253.9
  hyperfunction 253.1
  hypofunction 253.2
  posterior lobe 253.6
Dysplasia —*see also* Anomaly
  artery
    fibromuscular NEC 447.8
      carotid 447.8
      renal 447.3
  bladder 596.8
  bone (fibrous) NEC 733.29
    diaphyseal, progressive 756.59
    jaw 526.89
    monostotic 733.29
    polyostotic 756.54
    solitary 733.29
  brain 742.9
  bronchopulmonary, fetus or newborn 770.7
  cervix (uteri) 622.10
    cervical intraepithelial neoplasia I [CIN 1] 622.11
    cervical intraepithelial neoplasia II [CIN II] 622.12
    cervical intraepithelial neoplasia III [CIN III] 233.1
    CIN I 622.11
    CIN II 622.12
    CIN III 233.1
    mild 622.11
    moderate 622.12
    severe 233.1
  chondroectodermal 756.55
  chondromatose 756.4
  colon 211.3
  craniocarpotarsal 759.89
  craniometaphyseal 756.89
  dentinal 520.5
  diaphyseal, progressive 756.59
  ectodermal (anhidrotic) (Bason) (Clouston's) (congenital) (Feinmesser) (hereditary) (hidrotic) (Marshall) (Robinson's) 757.31
  epiphysealis 756.9
    multiplex 756.56
    punctata 756.59
  epiphysis 756.9
    multiple 756.56

INDEX TO DISEASES

Dysplasia—*continued*
epithelial
epiglottis 478.79
uterine cervix 622.10
erythroid NEC 289.89
eye (*see also* Microphthalmos) 743.10
familial metaphyseal 756.89
fibromuscular, artery NEC 447.8
carotid 447.8
renal 447.3
fibrous
bone NEC 733.29
diaphyseal, progressive 756.59
jaw 526.89
monostotic 733.29
polyostotic 756.54
solitary 733.29
high grade, focal—*see* Neoplasm, by site, benign
hip (congenital) 755.63
with dislocation (*see also* Dislocation, hip, congenital) 754.30
hypohidrotic ectodermal 757.31
joint 755.8
kidney 753.15
leg 755.69
linguofacialis 759.89
lung 748.5
macular 743.55
mammary (benign) (gland) 610.9
cystic 610.1
specified type NEC 610.8
metaphyseal 756.9
familial 756.89
monostotic fibrous 733.29
muscle 756.89
myeloid NEC 289.89
nervous system (general) 742.9
neuroectodermal 759.6
oculoauriculovertebral 756.0
oculodentodigital 759.89
olfactogenital 253.4
osteo-onycho-arthro (hereditary) 756.89
periosteum 733.99
polyostotic fibrous 756.54
progressive diaphyseal 756.59
prostate 602.3
intraepithelial neoplasia I [PIN I] 602.3
intraepithelial neoplasia II [PIN II] 602.3
intraepithelial neoplasia III [PIN III] 233.4
renal 753.15
renofacialis 753.0
retinal NEC 743.56
retrolental 362.21
spinal cord 742.9
thymic, with immunodeficiency 279.2
vagina 623.0
severe 233.31
vocal cord 478.5
vulva 624.8
intraepithelial neoplasia I [VIN I] 624.01
intraepithelial neoplasia II [VIN II] 624.02
intraepithelial neoplasia III [VIN III] 233.32
mild 624.01
moderate 624.02
severe 233.32
VIN I 624.01
VIN II 624.02
VIN III 233.32
Dyspnea (nocturnal) (paroxysmal) 786.09
asthmatic (bronchial) (*see also* Asthma) 493.9
with bronchitis (*see also* Asthma) 493.9

Dyspnea—*continued*
chronic 493.2
cardiac (*see also* Failure, ventricular, left) 428.1
cardiac (*see also* Failure, ventricular, left) 428.1
functional 300.11
hyperventilation 786.01
hysterical 300.11
Monday morning 504
newborn 770.89
psychogenic 306.1
uremic—*see* Uremia
Dyspraxia 781.3
syndrome 315.4
Dysproteinemia 273.8
transient with copper deficiency 281.4
Dysprothrombinemia (constitutional) (*see also* Defect, coagulation) 286.3
Dysreflexia, autonomic 337.3
Dysrhythmia
cardiac 427.9
postoperative (immediate) 997.1
long-term effect of cardiac surgery 429.4
specified type NEC 427.89
cerebral or cortical 348.30
Dyssecretosis, mucoserous 710.2
Dyssocial reaction without manifest psychiatric disorder
adolescent V71.02
adult V71.01
child V71.02
Dyssomnia NEC 780.56
nonorganic origin 307.47
Dyssplenism 289.4
Dyssynergia
biliary (*see also* Disease, biliary) 576.8
cerebellaris myoclonica 334.2
detrusor sphincter (bladder) 596.55
ventricular 429.89
Dystasia, hereditary areflexic 334.3
Dysthymia 300.4
Dysthymic disorder 300.4
Dysthyroidism 246.9
Dystocia 660.9
affecting fetus or newborn 763.1
cervical 661.2
affecting fetus or newborn 763.7
contraction ring 661.4
affecting fetus or newborn 763.7
fetal 660.9
abnormal size 653.5
affecting fetus or newborn 763.1
deformity 653.7
maternal 660.9
affecting fetus or newborn 763.1
positional 660.0
affecting fetus or newborn 763.1
shoulder (girdle) 660.4
affecting fetus or newborn 763.1
uterine NEC 661.4
affecting fetus or newborn 763.7
Dystonia
acute
due to drugs 333.72
neuroleptic-induced acute 333.72
deformans progressiva 333.6
lenticularis 333.6
musculorum deformans 333.6
torsion (idiopathic) 333.6
acquired 333.79
fragments (of) 333.89
genetic 333.6
symptomatic 333.79

Dystonic
  movements 781.0
Dystopia kidney 753.3
Dystrophy, dystrophia 783.9
  adiposogenital 253.8
  asphyxiating thoracic 756.4
  Becker's type 359.22
  brevicollis 756.16
  Bruch's membrane 362.77
  cervical (sympathetic) NEC 337.0
  chondro-osseus with punctate epiphyseal
      dysplasia 756.59
  choroid (hereditary) 363.50
    central (areolar) (partial) 363.53
      total (gyrate) 363.54
    circinate 363.53
    circumpapillary (partial) 363.51
      total 363.52
    diffuse
      partial 363.56
      total 363.57
    generalized
      partial 363.56
      total 363.57
    gyrate
      central 363.54
      generalized 363.57
    helicoid 363.52
    peripapillary—*see* Dystrophy, choroid,
        circumpapillary
    serpiginous 363.54
  cornea (hereditary) 371.50
    anterior NEC 371.52
    Cogan's 371.52
    combined 371.57
    crystalline 371.56
    endothelial (Fuchs') 371.57
    epithelial 371.50
      juvenile 371.51
      microscopic cystic 371.52
    granular 371.53
    lattice 371.54
    macular 371.55
    marginal (Terrien's) 371.48
    Meesman's 371.51
    microscopic cystic (epithelial) 371.52
    nodular, Salzmann's 371.46
    polymorphous 371.58
    posterior NEC 371.58
    ring-like 371.52
    Salzmann's nodular 371.46
    stromal NEC 371.56
  dermatochondrocorneal 371.50
  Duchenne's 359.1
  due to malnutrition 263.9
  Erb's 359.1
  familial
    hyperplastic periosteal 756.59
    osseous 277.5
  foveal 362.77
  Fuchs', cornea 371.57
  Gowers' muscular 359.1
  hair 704.2
  hereditary, progressive muscular 359.1
  hypogenital, with diabetic tendency 759.81
  Landouzy-Déjérine 359.1
  Leyden-Möbius 359.1
  mesodermalis congenita 759.82
  muscular 359.1
    congenital (hereditary) 359.0
      myotonic 359.22

Dystrophy, dystrophia—*continued*
    distal 359.1
    Duchenne's 359.1
    Erb's 359.1
    fascioscapulohumeral 359.1
    Gowers' 359.1
    hereditary (progressive) 359.1
    Landouzy-Déjérine 359.1
    limb-girdle 359.1
    myotonic 359.21
    progressive (hereditary) 359.1
      Charcot-Marie-Tooth 356.1
    pseudohypertrophic (infantile) 359.1
  myocardium, myocardial (*see also*
      Degeneration, myocardial) 429.1
  myotonic 359.21
  myotonica 359.21
  nail 703.8
    congenital 757.5
  neurovascular (traumatic) (*see also* Neuropathy,
      peripheral, autonomic) 337.9
  nutritional 263.9
  ocular 359.1
  oculocerebrorenal 270.8
  oculopharyngeal 359.1
  ovarian 620.8
  papillary (and pigmentary) 701.1
  pelvicrural atrophic 359.1
  pigmentary (*see also* Acanthosis) 701.2
  pituitary (gland) 253.8
  polyglandular 258.8
  posttraumatic sympathetic—*see* Dystrophy,
      sympathetic
  progressive ophthalmoplegic 359.1
  retina, retinal (hereditary) 362.70
    albipunctate 362.74
    Bruch's membrane 362.77
    cone, progressive 362.75
    hyaline 362.77
    in
      Bassen-Kornzweig syndrome 272.5
          [362.72]
      cerebroretinal lipidosis 330.1 *[362.71]*
      Refsum's disease 356.3 *[362.72]*
      systemic lipidosis 272.7 *[362.71]*
    juvenile (Stargardt's) 362.75
    pigmentary 362.74
    pigment epithelium 362.76
    progressive cone (-rod) 362.75
    pseudoinflammatory foveal 362.77
    rod, progressive 362.75
    sensory 362.75
    vitelliform 362.76
  Salzmann's nodular 371.46
  scapuloperoneal 359.1
  skin NEC 709.9
  sympathetic (posttraumatic) (reflex) 337.20
    lower limb 337.22
    specified NEC 337.29
    upper limb 337.21
  tapetoretinal NEC 362.74
  thoracic asphyxiating 756.4
  unguium 703.8
    congenital 757.5
  vitreoretinal (primary) 362.73
    secondary 362.66
  vulva 624.09
Dysuria 788.1
  psychogenic 306.53

E

Eagle-Barrett syndrome 756.71
Eales' disease (syndrome) 362.18
Ear —*see also* condition
   ache 388.70
      otogenic 388.71
      referred 388.72
   lop 744.29
   piercing V50.3
   swimmers' acute 380.12
   tank 380.12
   tropical 111.8 *[380.15]*
   wax 380.4
Earache 388.70
   otogenic 388.71
   referred 388.72
Early satiety 780.94
Eaton-Lambert syndrome (*see also* Neoplasm, by site, malignant) 199.1 *[358.1]*
Eberth's disease (typhoid fever) 002.0
Ebstein's
   anomaly or syndrome (downward displacement, tricuspid valve into right ventricle) 746.2
   disease (diabetes) 250.4 *[581.81]*
Eccentro-osteochondrodysplasia 277.5
Ecchondroma (M9210/0)—*see* Neoplasm, bone, benign
Ecchondrosis (M9210/1) 238.0
Ecchordosis physaliphora 756.0
Ecchymosis (multiple) 459.89
   conjunctiva 372.72
   eye (traumatic) 921.0
   eyelids (traumatic) 921.1
   newborn 772.6
   spontaneous 782.7
   traumatic—*see* Contusion
Echinococciasis —*see* Echinococcus
Echinococcosis —*see* Echinococcus
Echinococcus (infection) 122.9
   granulosus 122.4
      liver 122.0
      lung 122.1
      orbit 122.3 *[376.13]*
      specified site NEC 122.3
      thyroid 122.2
   liver NEC 122.8
      granulosus 122.0
      multilocularis 122.5
   lung NEC 122.9
      granulosus 122.1
      multilocularis 122.6
   multilocularis 122.7
      liver 122.5
      specified site NEC 122.6
   orbit 122.9 *[376.13]*
      granulosus 122.3 *[376.13]*
      multilocularis 122.6 *[376.13]*
   specified site NEC 122.9
      granulosus 122.3
      multilocularis 122.6 *[376.13]*
   thyroid NEC 122.9
      granulosus 122.2
      multilocularis 122.6
Echinorhynchiasis 127.7
Echinostomiasis 121.8
Echolalia 784.69
ECHO virus infection NEC 079.1

Eclampsia, eclamptic (coma) (convulsions) (delirium) 780.39
   female, child-bearing age NEC—*see* Eclampsia, pregnancy
   gravidarum—*see* Eclampsia, pregnancy
   male 780.39
   not associated with pregnancy or childbirth 780.39
   pregnancy, childbirth or puerperium 642.6
      with pre-existing hypertension 642.7
      affecting fetus or newborn 760.0
   uremic 586
Eclipse blindness (total) 363.31
Economic circumstance affecting care V60.9
   specified type NEC V60.8
Economo's disease (encephalitis lethargica) 049.8
Ectasia, ectasis
   aorta (*see also* Aneurysm, aorta) 441.9
      ruptured 441.5
   breast 610.4
   capillary 448.9
   cornea (marginal) (postinfectional) 371.71
   duct (mammary) 610.4
   gastric antral vascular (GAVE) 537.82
      with hemorrhage 537.83
      without hemorrhage 537.82
   kidney 593.89
   mammary duct (gland) 610.4
   papillary 448.9
   renal 593.89
   salivary gland (duct) 527.8
   scar, cornea 371.71
   sclera 379.11
Ecthyma 686.8
   contagiosum 051.2
   gangrenosum 686.09
   infectiosum 051.2
Ectocardia 746.87
Ectodermal dysplasia, congenital 757.31
Ectodermosis erosiva pluriorificialis 695.1
Ectopic, ectopia (congenital) 759.89
   abdominal viscera 751.8
      due to defect in anterior abdominal wall 756.79
   ACTH syndrome 255.0
   adrenal gland 759.1
   anus 751.5
   auricular beats 427.61
   beats 427.60
   bladder 753.5
   bone and cartilage in lung 748.69
   brain 742.4
   breast tissue 757.6
   cardiac 746.87
   cerebral 742.4
   cordis 746.87
   endometrium 617.9
   gallbladder 751.69
   gastric mucosa 750.7
   gestation—*see* Pregnancy, ectopic
   heart 746.87
   hormone secretion NEC 259.3
   hyperparathyroidism 259.3
   kidney (crossed) (intrathoracic) (pelvis) 753.3
      in pregnancy or childbirth 654.4
         causing obstructed labor 660.2

Ectopic, ectopia—*continued*
  lens 743.37
  lentis 743.37
  mole—*see* Pregnancy, ectopic
  organ or site NEC—*see* Malposition, congenital
  ovary 752.0
  pancreas, pancreatic tissue 751.7
  pregnancy—*see* Pregnancy, ectopic
  pupil 364.75
  renal 753.3
  sebaceous glands of mouth 750.26
  secretion
    ACTH 255.0
    adrenal hormone 259.3
    adrenalin 259.3
    adrenocorticotropin 255.0
    antidiuretic hormone (ADH) 259.3
    epinephrine 259.3
    hormone NEC 259.3
    norepinephrine 259.3
    pituitary (posterior) 259.3
  spleen 759.0
  testis 752.51
  thyroid 759.2
  ureter 753.4
  ventricular beats 427.69
  vesicae 753.5
Ectrodactyly 755.4
  finger (*see also* Absence, finger, congenital) 755.29
  toe (*see also* Absence, toe, congenital) 755.39
Ectromelia 755.4
  lower limb 755.30
  upper limb 755.20
Ectropion 374.10
  anus 569.49
  cervix 622.0
    with mention of cervicitis 616.0
  cicatricial 374.14
  congenital 743.62
  eyelid 374.10
    cicatricial 374.14
    congenital 743.62
    mechanical 374.12
    paralytic 374.12
    senile 374.11
    spastic 374.13
  iris (pigment epithelium) 364.54
  lip (congenital) 750.26
    acquired 528.5
  mechanical 374.12
  paralytic 374.12
  rectum 569.49
  senile 374.11
  spastic 374.13
  urethra 599.84
  uvea 364.54
Eczema (acute) (allergic) (chronic) (erythematous) (fissum) (occupational) (rubrum) (squamous) 692.9
  asteatotic 706.8
  atopic 691.8
  contact NEC 692.9
  dermatitis NEC 692.9
  due to specified cause—*see* Dermatitis, due to
  dyshidrotic 705.81
  external ear 380.22
  flexural 691.8
  gouty 274.89
  herpeticum 054.0
  hypertrophicum 701.8
  hypostatic—*see* Varicose, vein
  impetiginous 684

Eczema—*continued*
  infantile (acute) (chronic) (due to any substance) (intertriginous) (seborrheic) 690.12
  intertriginous NEC 692.9
    infantile 690.12
  intrinsic 691.8
  lichenified NEC 692.9
  marginatum 110.3
  nummular 692.9
  pustular 686.8
  seborrheic 690.18
    infantile 690.12
  solare 692.72
  stasis (lower extremity) 454.1
    ulcerated 454.2
  vaccination, vaccinatum 999.0
  varicose (lower extremity)—*see* Varicose, vein
  verrucosum callosum 698.3
Eczematoid, exudative 691.8
Eddowes' syndrome (brittle bones and blue sclera) 756.51
Edema, edematous 782.3
  with nephritis (*see also* Nephrosis) 581.9
  allergic 995.1
  angioneurotic (allergic) (any site) (with urticaria) 995.1
    hereditary 277.6
  angiospastic 443.9
  Berlin's (traumatic) 921.3
  brain 348.5
    due to birth injury 767.8
    fetus or newborn 767.8
  cardiac (*see also* Failure, heart) 428.0
  cardiovascular (*see also* Failure, heart) 428.0
  cerebral—*see* Edema, brain
  cerebrospinal vessel—*see* Edema, brain
  cervix (acute) (uteri) 622.8
    puerperal, postpartum 674.8
  chronic hereditary 757.0
  circumscribed, acute 995.1
    hereditary 277.6
  complicating pregnancy (gestational) 646.1
    with hypertension—*see* Toxemia, of pregnancy
  conjunctiva 372.73
  connective tissue 782.3
  cornea 371.20
    due to contact lenses 371.24
    idiopathic 371.21
    secondary 371.22
  due to
    lymphatic obstruction—*see* Edema, lymphatic
    salt retention 276.0
  epiglottis—*see* Edema, glottis
  essential, acute 995.1
    hereditary 277.6
  extremities, lower—*see* Edema, legs
  eyelid NEC 374.82
  familial, hereditary (legs) 757.0
  famine 262
  fetus or newborn 778.5
  genital organs
    female 629.89
    male 608.86
  gestational 646.1
    with hypertension—*see* Toxemia, of pregnancy
  glottis, glottic, glottides (obstructive) (passive) 478.6
    allergic 995.1
    hereditary 277.6

INDEX TO DISEASES — **Effect, adverse**

Edema, edematous—*continued*
  due to external agent—*see* Condition, respiratory, acute, due to specified agent
  heart (*see also* Failure, heart) 428.0
    newborn 779.89
  heat 992.7
  hereditary (legs) 757.0
  inanition 262
  infectious 782.3
  intracranial 348.5
    due to injury at birth 767.8
  iris 364.89
  joint (*see also* Effusion, joint) 719.0
  larynx (*see also* Edema, glottis) 478.6
  legs 782.3
    due to venous obstruction 459.2
    hereditary 757.0
  localized 782.3
    due to venous obstruction 459.2
      lower extremity 459.2
  lower extremities—*see* Edema, legs
  lungs 514
    acute 518.4
      with heart disease or failure (*see also* Failure, ventricular, left) 428.1
        congestive 428.0
      chemical (due to fumes or vapors) 506.1
      due to
        external agent(s) NEC 508.9
          specified NEC 508.8
        fumes and vapors (chemical) (inhalation) 506.1
        radiation 508.0
    chemical (acute) 506.1
      chronic 506.4
    chronic 514
      chemical (due to fumes or vapors) 506.4
      due to
        external agent(s) NEC 508.9
          specified NEC 508.8
        fumes or vapors (chemical) (inhalation) 506.4
        radiation 508.1
    due to
      external agent 508.9
        specified NEC 508.8
    high altitude 993.2
    near drowning 994.1
    postoperative 518.4
    terminal 514
  lymphatic 457.1
    due to mastectomy operation 457.0
  macula 362.83
    cystoid 362.53
    diabetic 250.5 *[362.07]*
  malignant (*see also* Gangrene, gas) 040.0
  Milroy's 757.0
  nasopharynx 478.25
  neonatorum 778.5
  nutritional (newborn) 262
    with dyspigmentation, skin and hair 260
  optic disc or nerve—*see* Papilledema
  orbit 376.33
    circulatory 459.89
  palate (soft) (hard) 528.9
  pancreas 577.8
  penis 607.83
  periodic 995.1
    hereditary 277.6
  pharynx 478.25
  pitting 782.3

Edema, edematous—*continued*
  pulmonary—*see* Edema, lung
  Quincke's 995.1
    hereditary 277.6
  renal (*see also* Nephrosis) 581.9
  retina (localized) (macular) (peripheral) 362.83
    cystoid 362.53
    diabetic 250.5 *[362.07]*
  salt 276.0
  scrotum 608.86
  seminal vesicle 608.86
  spermatic cord 608.86
  spinal cord 336.1
  starvation 262
  stasis (*see also* Hypertension, venous) 459.30
  subconjunctival 372.73
  subglottic (*see also* Edema, glottis) 478.6
  supraglottic (*see also* Edema, glottis) 478.6
  testis 608.86
  toxic NEC 782.3
  traumatic NEC 782.3
  tunica vaginalis 608.86
  vas deferens 608.86
  vocal cord—*see* Edema, glottis
  vulva (acute) 624.8
Edentia (complete) (partial) (*see also* Absence, tooth) 520.0
  acquired (*see also* Edentulism) 525.40
    due to
      caries 525.13
      extraction 525.10
      periodontal disease 525.12
      specified NEC 525.19
      trauma 525.11
  causing malocclusion 524.30
  congenital (deficiency of tooth buds) 520.0
Edentulism 525.40
  complete 525.40
    class I 525.41
    class II 525.42
    class III 525.43
    class IV 525.44
  partial 525.50
    class I 525.51
    class II 525.52
    class III 525.53
    class IV 525.54
Edsall's disease 992.2
Educational handicap V62.3
Edwards' syndrome 758.2
Effect, adverse NEC
  abnormal gravitational (G) forces or states 994.9
  air pressure—*see* Effect, adverse, atmospheric pressure
  altitude (high)—*see* Effect, adverse, high altitude
  anesthetic
    in labor and delivery NEC 668.9
      affecting fetus or newborn 763.5
  antitoxin—*see* Complications, vaccination
  atmospheric pressure 993.9
    due to explosion 993.4
    high 993.3
    low—*see* Effect, adverse, high altitude
    specified effect NEC 993.8
  biological, correct substance properly administered (*see also* Effect, adverse, drug) 995.20
  blood (derivatives) (serum) (transfusion)—*see* Complications, transfusion
  chemical substance NEC 989.9

987

Effect, adverse—*continued*
  specified—*see* Table of drugs and chemicals
  cobalt, radioactive (*see also* Effect, adverse, radioactive substance) 990
  cold (temperature) (weather) 991.9
    chilblains 991.5
    frostbite—*see* Frostbite
    specified effect NEC 991.8
  drugs and medicinals 995.20
    correct substance properly administered 995.20
    overdose or wrong substance given or taken 977.9
    specified drug—*see* Table of drugs and chemicals
  electric current (shock) 994.8
    burn—*see* Burn, by site
  electricity (electrocution) (shock) 994.8
    burn—*see* Burn, by site
  exertion (excessive) 994.5
  exposure 994.9
    exhaustion 994.4
  external cause NEC 994.9
  fallout (radioactive) NEC 990
  fluoroscopy NEC 990
  foodstuffs
    allergic reaction (*see also* Allergy, food) 693.1
      anaphylactic shock due to food NEC 995.60
    noxious 988.9
      specified type NEC (*see also* Poisoning, by name of noxious foodstuff) 988.8
  gases, fumes, or vapors—*see* Table of drugs and chemicals
  glue (airplane) sniffing 304.6
  heat—*see* Heat
  high altitude NEC 993.2
    anoxia 993.2
    on
      fears 993.0
      sinuses 993.1
    polycythemia 289.0
  hot weather—*see* Heat
  hunger 994.2
  immersion, foot 991.4
  immunization—*see* Complications, vaccination
  immunological agents—*see* Complications, vaccination
  implantation (removable) of isotope or radium NEC 990
  infrared (radiation) (rays) NEC 990
    burn—*see* Burn, by site
    dermatitis or eczema 692.82
  infusion—*see* Complications, infusion
  ingestion or injection of isotope (therapeutic) NEC 990
  irradiation NEC (*see also* Effect, adverse, radiation) 990
  isotope (radioactive) NEC 990
  lack of care (child) (infant) (newborn) 995.52
    adult 995.84
  lightning 994.0
    burn—*see* Burn, by site
  Lirugin—*see* Complications, vaccination
  medicinal substance, correct, properly administered (*see also* Effect, adverse, drugs) 995.20
  mesothorium NEC 990
  motion 994.6
  noise, inner ear 388.10
  other drug, medicinal and biological substance 995.29

Effect, adverse—*continued*
  overheated places—*see* Heat
  polonium NEC 990
  psychosocial, of work environment V62.1
  radiation (diagnostic) (fallout) (infrared) (natural source) (therapeutic) (tracer) (ultraviolet) (x-ray) NEC 990
    with pulmonary manifestations
      acute 508.0
      chronic 508.1
    dermatitis or eczema 692.82
      due to sun NEC (*see also* Dermatitis, due to, sun) 692.70
    fibrosis of lungs 508.1
    maternal with suspected damage to fetus affecting management of pregnancy 655.6
    pneumonitis 508.0
  radioactive substance NEC 990
    dermatitis or eczema 692.82
  radioactivity NEC 990
  radiotherapy NEC 990
    dermatitis or eczema 692.82
  radium NEC 990
  reduced temperature 991.9
    frostbite—*see* Frostbite
    immersion, foot (hand) 991.4
    specified effect NEC 991.8
  roentgenography NEC 990
  roentgenoscopy NEC 990
  roentgen rays NEC 990
  serum (prophylactic) (therapeutic) NEC 999.5
  specified NEC 995.89
    external cause NEC 994.9
  strangulation 994.7
  submersion 994.1
  teletherapy NEC 990
  thirst 994.3
  transfusion—*see* Complications, transfusion
  ultraviolet (radiation) (rays) NEC 990
    burn—*see also* Burn, by site
      from sun (*see also* Sunburn) 692.71
    dermatitis or eczema 692.82
      due to sun NEC (*see also* Dermatitis, due to, sun) 692.70
  uranium NEC 990
  vaccine (any)—*see* Complications, vaccination
  weightlessness 994.9
  whole blood—*see also* Complications, transfusion
    overdose or wrong substance given (*see also* Table of drugs and chemicals) 964.7
  working environment V62.1
  x-rays NEC 990
    dermatitis or eczema 692.82
Effect, remote
  of cancer —*see* condition
Effects, late —*see* Late, effect (of)
Effluvium, telogen 704.02
Effort
  intolerance 306.2
  syndrome (aviators) (psychogenic) 306.2
Effusion
  Amniotic fluid (*see also* Rupture, membranes, premature) 658.1
  brain (serous) 348.5
  bronchial (*see also* Bronchitis) 490
  cerebral 348.5
  cerebrospinal (*see also* Meningitis) 322.9
    vessel 348.5
  chest—*see* Effusion, pleura
  intracranial 348.5

INDEX TO DISEASES — Elevation

Effusion—*continued*
  joint 719.00
    ankle 719.07
    elbow 719.02
    foot 719.07
    hand 719.04
    hip 719.05
    knee 719.06
    multiple sites 719.09
    pelvic region 719.05
    shoulder (region) 719.01
    specified site NEC 719.08
    wrist 719.03
  meninges (*see also* Meningitis) 322.9
  pericardium, pericardial (*see also* Pericarditis) 423.9
    acute 420.90
  peritoneal (chronic) 568.82
  pleura, pleurisy, pleuritic, pleuropericardial 511.9
    bacterial, nontuberculous 511.1
    fetus or newborn 511.9
    malignant 197.2
    nontuberculous 511.9
      bacterial 511.1
    pneumococcal 511.1
    staphylococcal 511.1
    streptococcal 511.1
    tuberculous (*see also* Tuberculosis, pleura) 012.0
      primary progressive 010.1
    traumatic 862.29
      with open wound 862.39
  pulmonary—*see* Effusion, pleura
  spinal (*see also* Meningitis) 322.9
  thorax, thoracic—*see* Effusion, pleura
Egg (oocyte) (ovum)
  donor V59.70
    age 35 and over V59.73
      anonymous recipient V59.73
      designated recipient V59.74
    under age 35 V59.71
      anonymous recipient V59.71
      designated recipient V59.72
Eggshell nails 703.8
  congenital 757.5
Ego-dystonic
  homosexuality 302.0
  lesbianism 302.0
  sexual orientation 302.0
Egyptian splenomegaly 120.1
Ehlers-Danlos syndrome 756.83
Ehrlichiosis 082.40
  chaffeensis 082.41
  specified type NEC 082.49
Eichstedt's disease (pityriasis versicolor) 111.0
Eisenmenger's complex or syndrome
  (ventricular septal defect) 745.4
Ejaculation, semen
  painful 608.89
    psychogenic 306.59
  premature 302.75
  retrograde 608.87
Ekbom syndrome (restless legs) 333.94
Ekman's syndrome (brittle bones and blue sclera) 756.51
Elastic skin 756.83
  acquired 701.8
Elastofibroma (M8820/0)—*see* Neoplasm, connective tissue, benign
Elastoidosis
  cutanea nodularis 701.8
  cutis cystica et comedonica 701.8

Elastoma 757.39
  juvenile 757.39
  Miescher's (elastosis perforans serpiginosa) 701.1
Elastomyofibrosis 425.3
Elastosis 701.8
  atrophicans 701.8
  perforans serpiginosa 701.1
  reactive perforating 701.1
  senilis 701.8
  solar (actinic) 692.74
Elbow —*see* condition
Electric
  current, electricity, effects (concussion) (fatal) (nonfatal) (shock) 994.8
  burn—*see* Burn, by site
  feet (foot) syndrome 266.2
Electrocution 994.8
Electrolyte imbalance 276.9
  with
    abortion—*see* Abortion, by type, with metabolic disorder
    ectopic pregnancy (*see also* categories 633.0-633.9) 639.4
    hyperemesis gravidarum (before 22 completed weeks gestation) 643.1
    molar pregnancy (*see also* categories 630-632) 639.4
  following
    abortion 639.4
    ectopic or molar pregnancy 639.4
Elephant man syndrome 237.71
Elephantiasis (nonfilarial) 457.1
  arabicum (*see also* Infestation, filarial) 125.9
  congenita hereditaria 757.0
  congenital (any site) 757.0
  due to
    Brugia (malayi) 125.1
    mastectomy operation 457.0
    Wuchereria (bancrofti) 125.0
      malayi 125.1
  eyelid 374.83
  filarial (*see also* Infestation, filarial) 125.9
  filariensis (*see also* Infestation, filarial) 125.9
  gingival 523.8
  glandular 457.1
  graecorum 030.9
  lymphangiectatic 457.1
  lymphatic vessel 457.1
    due to mastectomy operation 457.0
  neuromatosa 237.71
  postmastectomy 457.0
  scrotum 457.1
  streptococcal 457.1
  surgical 997.99
    postmastectomy 457.0
  telangiectodes 457.1
  vulva (nonfilarial) 624.8
Elevated —*see* Elevation
Elevation
  17-ketosteroids 791.9
  acid phosphatase 790.5
  alkaline phosphatase 790.5
  amylase 790.5
  antibody titers 795.79
  basal metabolic rate (BMR) 794.7
  blood pressure (*see also* Hypertension) 401.9
    reading (incidental) (isolated) (nonspecific), no diagnosis of hypertension 796.2
  blood sugar 790.29
  body temperature (of unknown origin) (*see also* Pyrexia) 780.6

989

Elevation—*continued*
  C-reactive protein (CRP) 790.95
  cancer antigen 125 [CA 125] 795.82
  carcinoembryonic antigen [CEA] 795.81
  cholesterol 272.0
    with triglycerides 272.2
  conjugate, eye 378.81
  CRP (C-reactive protein) 790.95
  diaphragm, congenital 756.6
  glucose
    fasting 790.21
    tolerance test 790.22
  immunoglobulin level 795.79
  indolacetic acid 791.9
  lactic acid dehydrogenase (LDH) level 790.4
  leukocytes 288.60
  lipase 790.5
  lipoprotein a level 272.8
  liver function test (LFT) 790.6
    alkaline phosphatase 790.5
    aminotransferase 790.4
    bilirubin 782.4
    hepatic enzyme NEC 790.5
    lactate dehydrogenase 790.4
  lymphocytes 288.61
  prostate specific antigen (PSA) 790.93
  renin 790.99
    in hypertension (*see also* Hypertension, renovascular) 405.91
  Rh titer 999.7
  scapula, congenital 755.52
  sedimentation rate 790.1
  SGOT 790.4
  SGPT 790.4
  transaminase 790.4
  triglycerides 272.1
    with cholesterol 272.2
  vanillylmandelic acid 791.9
  venous pressure 459.89
  VMA 791.9
  white blood cell count 288.60
    specified NEC 288.69
Elliptocytosis (congenital) (hereditary) 282.1
  Hb-C (disease) 282.7
  hemoglobin disease 282.7
  sickle-cell (disease) 282.60
    trait 282.5
Ellis-van Creveld disease or syndrome (chondroectodermal dysplasia) 756.55
Ellison-Zollinger syndrome (gastric hypersecretion with pancreatic islet cell tumor) 251.5
Elongation, elongated (congenital)—*see also* Distortion
  bone 756.9
  cervix (uteri) 752.49
    acquired 622.6
    hypertrophic 622.6
  colon 751.5
  common bile duct 751.69
  cystic duct 751.69
  frenulum, penis 752.69
  labia minora, acquired 624.8
  ligamentum patellae 756.89
  petiolus (epiglottidis) 748.3
  styloid bone (process) 733.99
  tooth, teeth 520.2
  uvula 750.26
    acquired 528.9
Elschnig bodies or pearls 366.51
El Tor cholera 001.1
Emaciation (due to malnutrition) 261

Emancipation disorder 309.22
Embadomoniasis 007.8
Embarrassment heart, cardiac —*see* Disease, heart
Embedded tooth, teeth 520.6
  root only 525.3
Embolic —*see* condition
Embolism 444.9
  with
    abortion—*see* Abortion, by type, with embolism
    ectopic pregnancy (*see also* categories 633.0-633.9) 639.6
    molar pregnancy (*see also* categories 630-632) 639.6
  air (any site) 958.0
    with
      abortion—*see* Abortion, by type, with embolism
      ectopic pregnancy (*see also* categories 633.0-633.9) 639.6
      molar pregnancy (*see also* categories 630-632) 639.6
    due to implanted device—*see* Complications, due to (presence of) any device, implant, or graft classified to 996.0-996.5 NEC
    following
      abortion 639.6
      ectopic or molar pregnancy 639.6
    infusion, perfusion, or transfusion 999.1
    in pregnancy, childbirth, or puerperium 673.0
    traumatic 958.0
  amniotic fluid (pulmonary) 673.1
    with
      abortion—*see* Abortion, by type, with embolism
      ectopic pregnancy (*see also* categories 633.0-633.9) 639.6
      molar pregnancy (*see also* categories 630-632) 639.6
    following
      abortion 639.6
      ectopic or molar pregnancy 639.6
  aorta, aortic 444.1
    abdominal 444.0
    bifurcation 444.0
    saddle 444.0
    thoracic 444.1
  artery 444.9
    auditory, internal 433.8
    basilar (*see also* Occlusion, artery, basilar) 433.0
    bladder 444.89
    carotid (common) (internal) (*see also* Occlusion, artery, carotid) 433.1
    cerebellar (anterior inferior) (posterior inferior) (superior) 433.8
    cerebral (*see also* Embolism, brain) 434.1
    choroidal (anterior) 433.8
    communicating posterior 433.8
    coronary (*see also* Infarct, myocardium) 410.9
      without myocardial infarction 411.81
    extremity 444.22
      lower 444.22
      upper 444.21
    hypophyseal 433.8
    mesenteric (with gangrene) 557.0
    ophthalmic (*see also* Occlusion, retina) 362.30
    peripheral 444.22
    pontine 433.8

INDEX TO DISEASES   **Embolism**

Embolism—*continued*
  precerebral NEC—*see* Occlusion, artery,
    precerebral
  pulmonary—*see* Embolism, pulmonary
  pyemic 449
    pulmonary 415.12
  renal 593.81
  retinal (*see also* Occlusion, retina) 362.30
  septic 449
    pulmonary 415.12
  specified site NEC 444.89
  vertebral (*see also* Occlusion, artery,
    vertebral) 433.2
  auditory, internal 433.8
  basilar (artery) (*see also* Occlusion, artery,
    basilar) 433.0
  birth, mother—*see* Embolism, obstetrical
  blood-clot
    with
      abortion—*see* Abortion, by type, with embolism
      ectopic pregnancy (*see also* categories
        633.0-633.9) 639.6
      molar pregnancy (*see also* categories
        630-632) 639.6
    following
      abortion 639.6
      ectopic or molar pregnancy 639.6
    in pregnancy, childbirth, or puerperium 673.2
  brain 434.1
    with
      abortion—*see* Abortion, by type, with embolism
      ectopic pregnancy (*see also* categories
        633.0-633.9) 639.6
      molar pregnancy (*see also* categories
        630-632) 639.6
    following
      abortion 639.6
      ectopic or molar pregnancy 639.6
    late effect—*see* Late effect(s) (of)
      cerebrovascular disease
    puerperal, postpartum, childbirth 674.0
  capillary 448.9
  cardiac (*see also* Infarct, myocardium) 410.9
  carotid (artery) (common) (internal) (*see also*
    Occlusion, artery, carotid) 433.1
  cavernous sinus (venous)—*see* Embolism,
    intracranial venous sinus
  cerebral (*see also* Embolism, brain) 434.1
  cholesterol—*see* Atheroembolism
  choroidal (anterior) (artery) 433.8
  coronary (artery or vein) (systemic) (*see also*
    Infarct, myocardium) 410.9
    without myocardial infarction 411.81
  due to (presence of) any device, implant, or graft
    classifiable to 996.0-996.5 —*see*
      Complications, due to (presence of) any
      device, implant, or graft classified to
      996.0-996.5 NEC
  encephalomalacia (*see also* Embolism, brain) 434.1
  extremities 444.22
    lower 444.22
    upper 444.21
  eye 362.30
  fat (cerebral) (pulmonary) (systemic) 958.1
    with
      abortion—*see* Abortion, by type, with embolism
      ectopic pregnancy (*see also* categories
        633.0-633.9) 639.6
      molar pregnancy (*see also* categories
        630-632) 639.6
    complicating delivery or puerperium 673.8

Embolism—*continued*
  following
    abortion 639.6
    ectopic or molar pregnancy 639.6
    in pregnancy, childbirth, or the puerperium 673.8
  femoral (artery) 444.22
    vein 453.8
      deep 453.41
  following
    abortion 639.6
    ectopic or molar pregnancy 639.6
    infusion, perfusion, or transfusion
      air 999.1
      thrombus 999.2
  heart (fatty) (*see also* Infarct, myocardium) 410.9
  hepatic (vein) 453.0
  iliac (artery) 444.81
  iliofemoral 444.81
  in pregnancy, childbirth, or puerperium
    (pulmonary)—*see* Embolism, obstetrical
  intestine (artery) (vein) (with gangrene) 557.0
  intracranial (*see also* Embolism, brain) 434.1
    venous sinus (any) 325
      late effect—*see* category 326
      nonpyogenic 437.6
        in pregnancy or puerperium 671.5
  kidney (artery) 593.81
  lateral sinus (venous)—*see* Embolism,
    intracranial venous sinus
  longitudinal sinus (venous)—*see* Embolism,
    intracranial venous sinus
  lower extremity 444.22
  lung (massive)—*see* Embolism, pulmonary
  meninges (*see also* Embolism, brain) 434.1
  mesenteric (artery) (with gangrene) 557.0
  multiple NEC 444.9
  obstetrical (pulmonary) 673.2
    air 673.0
    amniotic fluid (pulmonary) 673.1
    blood-clot 673.2
    cardiac 674.8
    fat 673.8
    heart 674.8
    pyemic 673.3
    septic 673.3
    specified NEC 674.8
  ophthalmic (*see also* Occlusion, retina) 362.30
  paradoxical NEC 444.9
  penis 607.82
  peripheral arteries NEC 444.22
    lower 444.22
    upper 444.21
  pituitary 253.8
  popliteal (artery) 444.22
  portal (vein) 452
  postoperative NEC 997.2
    cerebral 997.02
    mesenteric artery 997.71
    other vessels 997.79
    peripheral vascular 997.2
    pulmonary 415.11
      septic 415.12
    renal artery 997.72
  precerebral artery (*see also* Occlusion, artery,
    precerebral) 433.9
  puerperal—*see* Embolism, obstetrical
  pulmonary (artery) (vein) 415.1
    with
      abortion—*see* Abortion, by type, with
        embolism

Embolism INDEX TO DISEASES

Embolism—*continued*
    ectopic pregnancy (*see also* categories 633.0-633.9) 639.6
    molar pregnancy (*see also* categories 630-632) 639.6
    following
        abortion 639.6
        ectopic or molar pregnancy 639.6
    iatrogenic 415.11
    in pregnancy, childbirth, or puerperium—*see* Embolism, obstetrical
    postoperative 415.11
    septic 415.12
    pyemic (multiple) (*see also* Septicemia) 415.12
        with
        abortion—*see* Abortion, by type, with embolism
        ectopic pregnancy (*see also* categories 633.0-633.9) 639.6
        molar pregnancy (*see also* categories 630-632) 639.6
    Aerobacter aerogenes 415.12
    enteric gram-negative bacilli 415.12
    Enterobacter aerogenes 415.12
    Escherichia coli 415.12
    following
        abortion 639.6
        ectopic or molar pregnancy 639.6
    Hemophilus influenzae 415.12
    pneumococcal 415.12
    Proteus vulgaris 415.12
    Pseudomonas (aeruginosa) 415.12
    puerperal, postpartum, childbirth (any organism) 673.3
    Serratia 415.12
    specified organism NEC 415.12
    staphylococcal 415.12
        aureus 415.12
        specified organism NEC 415.12
    streptococcal 415.12
    renal (artery) 593.81
        vein 453.3
    retina, retinal (*see also* Occlusion, retina) 362.30
    saddle (aorta) 444.0
    septic 415.12
        arterial 449
    septicemic—*see* Embolism, pyemic
    sinus—*see* Embolism, intracranial venous sinus
    soap
        with
        abortion—*see* Abortion, by type, with embolism
        ectopic pregnancy (*see also* categories 633.0-633.9) 639.6
        molar pregnancy (*see also* categories 630-632) 639.6
    following
        abortion 639.6
        ectopic or molar pregnancy 639.6
    spinal cord (nonpyogenic) 336.1
        in pregnancy or puerperium 671.5
        pyogenic origin 324.1
            late effect—*see* category 326
    spleen, splenic (artery) 444.89
    thrombus (thromboembolism) following infusion, perfusion, or transfusion 999.2
    upper extremity 444.21
    vein 453.9
        with inflammation or phlebitis—*see* Thrombophlebitis
        cerebral (*see also* Embolism, brain) 434.1
        coronary (*see also* Infarct, myocardium) 410.9
            without myocardial infarction 411.81

Embolism—*continued*
    hepatic 453.0
    lower extremity 453.8
        deep 453.40
            calf 453.42
            distal (lower leg) 453.42
            femoral 453.41
            iliac 453.41
            lower leg 453.42
            peroneal 453.42
            popliteal 453.41
            proximal (upper leg) 453.41
            thigh 453.41
            tibial 453.42
    mesenteric (with gangrene) 557.0
    portal 452
    pulmonary—*see* Embolism, pulmonary
    renal 453.3
    specified NEC 453.8
        with inflammation or phlebitis—*see* Thrombophlebitis
    vena cava (inferior) (superior) 453.2
    vessels of brain (*see also* Embolism, brain) 434.1
Embolization —*see* Embolism
Embolus —*see* Embolism
Embryoma (M9080/1)—*see also* Neoplasm, by site, uncertain behavior
    benign (M9080/0)—*see* Neoplasm, by site, benign
    kidney (M8960/3) 189.0
    liver (M8970/3) 155.0
    malignant (M9080/3)—*see also* Neoplasm, by site, malignant
        kidney (M8960/3) 189.0
        liver (M8970/3) 155.0
        testis (M9070/3) 186.9
            undescended 186.0
    testis (M9070/3) 186.9
        undescended 186.0
Embryonic
    circulation 747.9
    heart 747.9
    vas deferens 752.89
Embryopathia NEC 759.9
Embryotomy, fetal 763.89
Embryotoxon 743.43
    interfering with vision 743.42
Emesis —*see also* Vomiting
    gravidarum—*see* Hyperemesis, gravidarum
Emissions, nocturnal (semen) 608.89
Emotional
    crisis—*see* Crisis, emotional
    disorder (*see also* Disorder, mental) 300.9
    instability (excessive) 301.3
    overlay—*see* Reaction, adjustment
    upset 300.9
Emotionality, pathological 301.3
Emotogenic disease (*see also* Disorder, psychogenic) 306.9
Emphysema (atrophic) (centriacinar) (centrilobular) (chronic) (diffuse) (essential) (hypertrophic) (interlobular) (lung) (obstructive) (panlobular) (paracicatricial) (paracinar) (postural) (pulmonary) (senile) (subpleural) (traction) (unilateral) (unilobular) (vesicular) 492.8
    with bronchitis
        chronic 491.20
            with
                acute bronchitis 491.22
                exacerbation (acute) 491.21

INDEX TO DISEASES

Emphysema—*continued*
   bullous (giant) 492.0
   cellular tissue 958.7
      surgical 998.81
   compensatory 518.2
   congenital 770.2
   conjunctiva 372.89
   connective tissue 958.7
      surgical 998.81
   due to fumes or vapors 506.4
   eye 376.89
   eyelid 374.85
      surgical 998.81
      traumatic 958.7
   fetus or newborn (interstitial) (mediastinal) (unilobular) 770.2
   heart 416.9
   interstitial 518.1
      congenital 770.2
      fetus or newborn 770.2
   laminated tissue 958.7
      surgical 998.81
   mediastinal 518.1
      fetus or newborn 770.2
   newborn (interstitial) (mediastinal) (unilobular) 770.2
   obstructive diffuse with fibrosis 492.8
   orbit 376.89
   subcutaneous 958.7
      due to trauma 958.7
      nontraumatic 518.1
      surgical 998.81
   surgical 998.81
   thymus (gland) (congenital) 254.8
   traumatic 958.7
   tuberculous (*see also* Tuberculosis, pulmonary) 011.9
Employment examination (certification) V70.5
Empty sella (turcica) syndrome 253.8
Empyema (chest) (diaphragmatic) (double) (encapsulated) (general) (interlobar) (lung) (medial) (necessitatis) (perforating chest wall) (pleura) (pneumococcal) (residual) (sacculated) (streptococcal) (supradiaphragmatic) 510.9
   with fistula 510.0
   accessory sinus (chronic) (*see also* Sinusitis) 473.9
   acute 510.9
      with fistula 510.0
   antrum (chronic) (*see also* Sinusitis, maxillary) 473.0
   brain (any part) (*see also* Abscess, brain) 324.0
   ethmoidal (sinus) (chronic) (*see also* Sinusitis, ethmoidal) 473.2
   extradural (*see also* Abscess, extradural) 324.9
   frontal (sinus) (chronic) (*see also* Sinusitis, frontal) 473.1
   gallbladder (*see also* Cholecystitis, acute) 575.0
   mastoid (process) (acute) (*see also* Mastoiditis, acute) 383.00
   maxilla, maxillary 526.4
   sinus (chronic) (*see also* Sinusitis, maxillary) 473.0
   nasal sinus (chronic) (*see also* Sinusitis) 473.9
   sinus (accessory) (nasal) (*see also* Sinusitis) 473.9
   sphenoidal (chronic) (sinus) (*see also* Sinusitis, sphenoidal) 473.3
   subarachnoid (*see also* Abscess, extradural) 324.9
   subdural (*see also* Abscess, extradural) 324.9
   tuberculous (*see also* Tuberculosis, pleura) 012.0
   ureter (*see also* Ureteritis) 593.89
   ventricular (*see also* Abscess, brain) 324.0
Enameloma 520.2

Encephalitis (bacterial) (chronic) (hemorrhagic) (idiopathic) (nonepidemic) (spurious) (subacute) 323.9
   acute—*see also* Encephalitis, viral
      disseminated (postinfectious) NEC 136.9 *[323.61]*
         postimmunization or postvaccination 323.51
      inclusional 049.8
      inclusion body 049.8
      necrotizing 049.8
   arboviral, arbovirus NEC 064
   arthropod-borne (*see also* Encephalitis, viral, arthropod-borne) 064
   Australian X 062.4
   Bwamba fever 066.3
   California (virus) 062.5
   Central European 063.2
   Czechoslovakian 063.2
   Dawson's (inclusion body) 046.2
   diffuse sclerosing 046.2
   due to
      actinomycosis 039.8 *[323.41]*
      cat-scratch disease 078.3 *[323.01]*
      human herpesvirus 6 058.21
      human herpesvirus 7 058.29
      human herpesvirus NEC 058.29
      infection classified elsewhere 136.9 *[323.41]*
      infectious mononucleosis 075 *[323.01]*
      malaria (*see also* Malaria) 084.6 *[323.2]*
      Negishi virus 064
      ornithosis 073.7 *[323.01]*
      prophylactic inoculation against smallpox 323.51
      rickettsiosis (*see also* Rickettsiosis) 083.9 *[323.1]*
      rubella 056.01
      toxoplasmosis (acquired) 130.0
         congenital (active) 771.2 *[323.41]*
      typhus (fever) (*see also* Typhus) 081.9 *[323.1]*
      vaccination (smallpox) 323.51
   Eastern equine 062.2
   endemic 049.8
   epidemic 049.8
   equine (acute) (infectious) (viral) 062.9
      Eastern 062.2
      Venezuelan 066.2
      Western 062.1
   Far Eastern 063.0
   following vaccination or other immunization procedure 323.51
   herpes 054.3
   human herpesvirus 6 058.21
   human herpesvirus 7 058.29
   human herpesvirus NEC 058.29
   Ilheus (virus) 062.8
   inclusion body 046.2
   infectious (acute) (virus) NEC 049.8
   influenzal 487.8 *[323.41]*
      lethargic 049.8
   Japanese (B type) 062.0
   La Crosse 062.5
   Langat 063.8
   late effect—*see* Late, effect, encephalitis
   lead 984.9 *[323.71]*
   lethargic (acute) (infectious) (influenzal) 049.8
   lethargica 049.8
   louping ill 063.1
   lupus 710.0 *[323.81]*
   lymphatica 049.0
   Mengo 049.8
   meningococcal 036.1
   mumps 072.2
   Murray Valley 062.4

Encephalitis — *continued*
  myoclonic 049.8
  Negishi virus 064
  otitic NEC 382.4 *[323.41]*
  parasitic NEC 123.9 *[323.41]*
  periaxialis (concentrica) (diffusa) 341.1
  postchickenpox 052.0
  postexanthematous NEC 057.9 *[323.62]*
  postimmunization 323.51
  postinfectious NEC 136.9 *[323.62]*
  postmeasles 055.0
  posttraumatic 323.81
  postvaccinal (smallpox) 323.51
  postvaricella 052.0
  postviral NEC 079.99 *[323.62]*
    postexanthematous 057.9 *[323.62]*
    specified NEC 057.8 *[323.62]*
  Powassan 063.8
  progressive subcortical (Binswanger's) 290.12
  Rasmussen 323.81
  Rio Bravo 049.8
  rubella 056.01
  Russian
    autumnal 062.0
    spring-summer type (taiga) 063.0
  saturnine 984.9 *[323.71]*
  Semliki Forest 062.8
  serous 048
  slow-acting virus NEC 046.8
  specified cause NEC 323.81
  St. Louis type 062.3
  subacute sclerosing 046.2
  subcorticalis chronica 290.12
  summer 062.0
  suppurative 324.0
  syphilitic 094.81
    congenital 090.41
  tick-borne 063.9
  torula, torular 117.5 *[323.41]*
  toxic NEC 989.9 *[323.71]*
  toxoplasmic (acquired) 130.0
    congenital (active) 771.2 *[323.41]*
  trichinosis 124 *[323.41]*
  Trypanosomiasis (*see also* Trypanosomiasis) 086.9 *[323.2]*
  tuberculous (*see also* Tuberculosis) 013.6
  type B (Japanese) 062.0
  type C 062.3
  van Bogaert's 046.2
  Venezuelan 066.2
  Vienna type 049.8
  viral, virus 049.9
    arthropod-borne NEC 064
      mosquito-borne 062.9
        Australian X disease 062.4
        California virus 062.5
        Eastern equine 062.2
        Ilheus virus 062.8
        Japanese (B type) 062.0
        Murray Valley 062.4
        specified type NEC 062.8
        St. Louis 062.3
        type B 062.0
        type C 062.3
        Western equine 062.1
      tick-borne 063.9
        biundulant 063.2
        Central European 063.2
        Czechoslovakian 063.2
        diphasic meningoencephalitis 063.2
        Far Eastern 063.0

Encephalitis — *continued*
    Langat 063.8
    louping ill 063.1
    Powassan 063.8
    Russian spring-summer (taiga) 063.0
    specified type NEC 063.8
    vector unknown 064
  slow acting NEC 046.8
  specified type NEC 049.8
  vaccination, prophylactic (against) V05.0
  von Economo's 049.8
  Western equine 062.1
  West Nile type 066.41
Encephalocele 742.0
  orbit 376.81
Encephalocystocele 742.0
Encephalomalacia (brain) (cerebellar) (cerebral) (cerebrospinal) (*see also* Softening, brain) 434.9
  due to
    hemorrhage (*see also* Hemorrhage, brain) 431
    recurrent spasm of artery 435.9
  embolic (cerebral) (*see also* Embolism, brain) 434.1
  subcorticalis chronicus arteriosclerotica 290.12
  thrombotic (*see also* Thrombosis, brain) 434.0
Encephalomeningitis —*see* Meningoencephalitis
Encephalomeningocele 742.0
Encephalomeningomyelitis —*see* Meningoencephalitis
Encephalomeningopathy (*see also* Meningoencephalitis) 349.9
Encephalomyelitis (chronic) (granulomatous) (hemorrhagic necrotizing, acute) (myalgic, benign) (*see also* Encephalitis) 323.9
  abortive disseminated 049.8
  acute disseminated (ADEM) (postinfectious) 136.9 *[323.61]*
    infectious 136.9 *[323.61]*
    noninfectious 323.81
    postimmunization 323.51
  due to
    cat-scratch disease 078.3 *[323.01]*
    infectious mononucleosis 075 *[323.01]*
    ornithosis 073.7 *[323.01]*
    vaccination (any) 323.51
  equine (acute) (infectious) 062.9
    Eastern 062.2
    Venezuelan 066.2
    Western 062.1
  funicularis infectiosa 049.8
  late effect—*see* Late, effect, encephalitis
  Munch-Peterson's 049.8
  postchickenpox 052.0
  postimmunization 323.51
  postmeasles 055.0
  postvaccinal (smallpox) 323.51
  rubella 056.01
  specified cause NEC 323.81
  syphilitic 094.81
  West Nile 066.41
Encephalomyelocele 742.0
Encephalomyelomeningitis —*see* Meningoencephalitis
Encephalomyeloneuropathy 349.9
Encephalomyelopathy 349.9
  subacute necrotizing (infantile) 330.8
Encephalomyeloradiculitis (acute) 357.0
Encephalomyeloradiculoneuritis (acute) 357.0
Encephalomyeloradiculopathy 349.9
Encephalomyocarditis 074.23

Encephalopathia hyperbilirubinemica newborn 774.7
due to isoimmunization (conditions classifiable to 773.0-773.2) 773.4
Encephalopathy (acute) 348.30
alcoholic 291.2
anoxic—*see* Damage, brain, anoxic
arteriosclerotic 437.0
   late effect—*see* Late effect(s) (of) cerebrovascular disease
bilirubin, newborn 774.7
   due to isoimmunization 773.4
congenital 742.9
demyelinating (callosal) 341.8
due to
   birth injury (intracranial) 767.8
   dialysis 294.8
      transient 293.9
   hyperinsulinism—*see* Hyperinsulinism
   influenza (virus) 487.8
   lack of vitamin (*see also* Deficiency, vitamin) 269.2
   nicotinic acid deficiency 291.2
   serum (nontherapeutic) (therapeutic) 999.5
   syphilis 094.81
   trauma (postconcussional) 310.2
      current (*see also* Concussion, brain) 850.9
         with skull fracture—*see* Fracture, skull, by site, with intracranial injury
   vaccination 323.51
hepatic 572.2
hyperbilirubinemic, newborn 774.7
   due to isoimmunization (conditions classifiable to 773.0-773.2) 773.4
hypertensive 437.2
hypoglycemic 251.2
hypoxic—*see also* Damage, brain, anoxic
   ischemic (HIE) 768.7
infantile cystic necrotizing (congenital) 341.8
lead 984.9 *[323.71]*
leukopolio 330.0
metabolic (*see also* Delirium) 348.31
   toxic 349.82
necrotizing
   hemorrhagic 323.61
   subacute 330.8
other specified type NEC 348.39
pellagrous 265.2
portal-systemic 572.2
postcontusional 310.2
posttraumatic 310.2
saturnine 984.9 *[323.71]*
septic 348.31
spongioform, subacute (viral) 046.1
subacute
   necrotizing 330.8
   spongioform 046.1
   viral, spongioform 046.1
subcortical progressive (Schilder) 341.1
   chronic (Binswanger's) 290.12
toxic 349.82
   metabolic 349.82
traumatic (postconcussional) 310.2
   current (*see also* Concussion, brain) 850.9
      with skull fracture—*see* Fracture, skull, by site, with intracranial injury
vitamin B deficiency NEC 266.9
Wernicke's (superior hemorrhagic polioencephalitis) 265.1

Enchephalorrhagia (*see also* Hemorrhage, brain) 432.9
healed or old V12.54
late effect—*see* Late effect(s) (of) cerebrovascular disease
Encephalosis, posttraumatic 310.2
Enchondroma (M9220/0)—*see also* Neoplasm, bone, benign
multiple, congenital 756.4
Enchondromatosis (cartilaginous) (congenital) (multiple) 756.4
Enchondroses, multiple (cartilaginous) (congenital) 756.4
Encopresis (*see also* Incontinence, feces) 787.6
nonorganic origin 307.7
Encounter for —*see also* Admission for
administrative purpose only V68.9
   referral of patient without examination or treatment V68.81
   specified purpose NEC V68.89
chemotherapy, antineoplastic V58.11
disability examination V68.01
end-of-life care V66.7
hospice care V66.7
immunotherapy, antineoplastic V58.12
palliative care V66.7
radiotherapy V58.0
respirator (ventilator) dependence
   during
      mechanical failure V46.14
      power failure V46.12
   for weaning V46.13
screening mammogram NEC V76.12
   for high-risk patient V76.11
paternity testing V70.4
terminal care V66.7
weaning from respirator (ventilator) V46.13
Encystment —*see* Cyst
End-of-life care V66.7
Endamebiasis —*see* Amebiasis
Endamoeba —*see* Amebiasis
Endarteritis (bacterial, subacute) (infective) (septic) 447.6
brain, cerebral or cerebrospinal 437.4
   late effect—*see* Late effect(s) (of) cerebrovascular disease
coronary (artery) —*see* Arteriosclerosis, coronary
deformans—*see* Arteriosclerosis
embolic (*see also* Embolism) 444.9
obliterans—*see also* Arteriosclerosis
   pulmonary 417.8
pulmonary 417.8
retina 362.18
senile—*see* Arteriosclerosis
syphilitic 093.89
   brain or cerebral 094.89
   congenital 090.5
   spinal 094.89
tuberculous (*see also* Tuberculosis) 017.9
Endemic —*see* condition
Endocarditis (chronic) (indeterminate) (interstitial) (marantis) (nonbacterial thrombotic) (residual) (sclerotic) (sclerous) (senile) (valvular) 424.90
with
   rheumatic fever (conditions classifiable to 390)
      active—*see* Endocarditis, acute, rheumatic
      inactive or quiescent (with chorea) 397.9
acute or subacute 421.9

Endocarditis—*continued*
   rheumatic (aortic) (mitral) (pulmonary)
     (tricuspid) 391.1
     with chorea (acute) (rheumatic)
      (Sydenham's) 392.0
  aortic (heart) (nonrheumatic) (valve) 424.1
   with
    mitral (valve) disease 396.9
     active or acute 391.1
      with chorea (acute) (rheumatic)
       (Sydenham's) 392.0
     rheumatic fever (conditions classifiable to
      390)
      active—*see* Endocarditis, acute, rheumatic
     inactive or quiescent (with chorea) 395.9
      with mitral disease 396.9
   acute or subacute 421.9
   arteriosclerotic 424.1
   congenital 746.89
   hypertensive 424.1
   rheumatic (chronic) (inactive) 395.9
    with mitral (valve) disease 396.9
     active or acute 391.1
      with chorea (acute) (rheumatic)
       (Sydenham's) 392.0
    active or acute 391.1
     with chorea (acute) (rheumatic)
      (Sydenham's) 392.0
   specified cause, except rheumatic 424.1
   syphilitic 093.22
  arteriosclerotic or due to arteriosclerosis 424.99
  atypical verrucous (Libman-Sacks) 710.0
   [424.91]
  bacterial (acute) (any valve) (chronic) (subacute)
   421.0
  blastomycotic 116.0 *[421.1]*
  candidal 112.81
  congenital 425.3
  constrictive 421.0
  Coxsackie 074.22
  due to
   blastomycosis 116.0 *[421.1]*
   candidiasis 112.81
   Coxsackie (virus) 074.22
   disseminated lupus erythematosus 710.0
    [424.91]
   histoplasmosis (*see also* Histoplasmosis) 115.94
   hypertension (benign) 424.99
   moniliasis 112.81
   prosthetic cardiac valve 996.61
   Q fever 083.0 *[421.1]*
   serratia marcescens 421.0
   typhoid (fever) 002.0 *[421.1]*
  fetal 425.3
  gonococcal 098.84
  hypertensive 424.99
  infectious or infective (acute) (any valve)
   (chronic) (subacute) 421.0
  lenta (acute) (any valve) (chronic) (subacute)
   421.0
  Libman-Sacks 710.0 *[424.91]*
  Loeffler's (parietal fibroplastic) 421.0
  malignant (acute) (any valve) (chronic)
   (subacute) 421.0
  meningococcal 036.42
  mitral (chronic) (double) (fibroid) (heart)
   (inactive) (valve) (with chorea) 394.9
   with
    aortic (valve) disease 396.9
     active or acute 391.1

Endocarditis—*continued*
     with chorea (acute) (rheumatic)
      (Sydenham's) 392.0
    rheumatic fever (conditions classifiable to
     390)
     active—*see* Endocarditis, acute, rheumatic
    inactive or quiescent (with chorea) 394.9
     with aortic valve disease 396.9
   active or acute 391.1
    bacterial 421.0
    with chorea (acute) (rheumatic)
     (Sydenham's) 392.0
   arteriosclerotic 424.0
   congenital 746.89
   hypertensive 424.0
   nonrheumatic 424.0
    acute or subacute 421.9
   syphilitic 093.21
  monilial 112.81
  mycotic (acute) (any valve) (chronic) (subacute)
   421.0
  pneumococcic (acute) (any valve) (chronic)
   (subacute) 421.0
  pulmonary (chronic) (heart) (valve) 424.3
   with
    rheumatic fever (conditions classifiable to
     390)
     active—*see* Endocarditis, acute, rheumatic
    inactive or quiescent (with chorea) 397.1
   acute or subacute 421.9
   rheumatic 391.1
    with chorea (acute) (rheumatic)
     (Sydenham's) 392.0
   arteriosclerotic or due to arteriosclerosis 424.3
   congenital 746.09
   hypertensive or due to hypertension (benign)
    424.3
   rheumatic (chronic) (inactive) (with chorea)
    397.1
    active or acute 391.1
     with chorea (acute) (rheumatic)
      (Sydenham's) 392.0
   syphilitic 093.24
  purulent (acute) (any valve) (chronic) (subacute)
   421.0
  rheumatic (chronic) (inactive) (with chorea)
   397.9
   active or acute (aortic) (mitral) (pulmonary)
    (tricuspid) 391.1
    with chorea (acute) (rheumatic)
     (Sydenham's) 392.0
  septic (acute) (any valve) (chronic) (subacute)
   421.0
  specified cause, except rheumatic 424.99
  streptococcal (acute) (any valve) (chronic)
   (subacute) 421.0
  subacute—*see* Endocarditis, acute
  suppurative (any valve) (acute) (chronic)
   (subacute) 421.0
  syphilitic NEC 093.20
  toxic (*see also* Endocarditis, acute) 421.9
  tricuspid (chronic) (heart) (inactive) (rheumatic)
   (valve) (with chorea) 397.0
   with
    rheumatic fever (conditions classifiable to
     390)
     active—*see* Endocarditis, acute, rheumatic
    inactive or quiescent (with chorea) 397.0
   active or acute 391.1
    with chorea (acute) (rheumatic)
     (Sydenham's) 392.0

INDEX TO DISEASES

Endocarditis—*continued*
  arteriosclerotic 424.2
  congenital 746.89
  hypertensive 424.2
  nonrheumatic 424.2
    acute or subacute 421.9
    specified cause, except rheumatic 424.2
  syphilitic 093.23
  tuberculous (*see also* Tuberculosis) 017.9
    [424.91]
  typhoid 002.0 *[421.1]*
  ulcerative (acute) (any valve) (chronic)
    (subacute) 421.0
  vegetative (acute) (any valve) (chronic)
    (subacute) 421.0
  verrucous (acute) (any valve) (chronic)
    (subacute) NEC 710.0 *[424.91]*
  nonbacterial 710.0 *[424.91]*
  nonrheumatic 710.0 *[424.91]*
Endocardium, endocardial —*see also* condition
  cushion defect 745.60
  specified type NEC 745.69
Endocervicitis (*see also* Cervicitis) 616.0
  due to
    intrauterine (contraceptive) device 996.65
  gonorrheal (acute) 098.15
    chronic or duration of 2 months or over 098.35
  hyperplastic 616.0
  syphilitic 095.8
  trichomonal 131.09
  tuberculous (*see also* Tuberculosis) 016.7
Endocrine —*see* condition
Endocrinopathy, pluriglandular 258.9
Endodontitis 522.0
Endomastoiditis (*see also* Mastoiditis) 383.9
Endometrioma 617.9
Endometriosis 617.9
  appendix 617.5
  bladder 617.8
  bowel 617.5
  broad ligament 617.3
  cervix 617.0
  colon 617.5
  cul-de-sac (Douglas') 617.3
  exocervix 617.0
  fallopian tube 617.2
  female genital organ NEC 617.8
  gallbladder 617.8
  in scar of skin 617.6
  internal 617.0
  intestine 617.5
  lung 617.8
  myometrium 617.0
  ovary 617.1
  parametrium 617.3
  pelvic peritoneum 617.3
  peritoneal (pelvic) 617.3
  rectovaginal septum 617.4
  rectum 617.5
  round ligament 617.3
  skin 617.6
  specified site NEC 617.8
  stromal (M8931/1) 236.0
  umbilicus 617.8
  uterus 617.0
    internal 617.0
  vagina 617.4
  vulva 617.8

Endometritis (nonspecific) (purulent) (septic)
    (suppurative) 615.9
  with
    abortion—*see* Abortion, by type, with sepsis
    ectopic pregnancy (*see also* categories
      633.0-633.9) 639.0
    molar pregnancy (*see also* categories 630-632)
      639.0
  acute 615.0
  blennorrhagic 098.16
    acute 098.16
    chronic or duration of 2 months or over 098.36
  cervix, cervical (*see also* Cervicitis) 616.0
    hyperplastic 616.0
  chronic 615.1
  complicating pregnancy 646.6
    affecting fetus or newborn 760.8
  decidual 615.9
  following
    abortion 639.0
    ectopic or molar pregnancy 639.0
  gonorrheal (acute) 098.16
    chronic or duration of 2 months or over 098.36
  hyperplastic (*see also* Hyperplasia,
    endometrium) 621.30
    cervix 616.0
  polypoid—*see* Endometritis, hyperplastic
  puerperal, postpartum, childbirth 670
  senile (atrophic) 615.9
  subacute 615.0
  tuberculous (*see also* Tuberculosis) 016.7
Endometrium —*see* condition
Endomyocardiopathy, South African 425.2
Endomyocarditis —*see* Endocarditis
Endomyofibrosis 425.0
Endomyometritis (*see also* Endometritis) 615.9
Endopericarditis —*see* Endocarditis
Endoperineuritis —*see* Disorder, nerve
Endophlebitis (*see also* Phlebitis) 451.9
  leg 451.2
    deep (vessels) 451.19
    superficial (vessels) 451.0
  portal (vein) 572.1
  retina 362.18
  specified site NEC 451.89
  syphilitic 093.89
Endophthalmia (*see also* Endophthalmitis) 360.00
  gonorrheal 098.42
Endophthalmitis (globe) (infective) (metastatic)
    (purulent) (subacute) 360.00
  acute 360.01
  bleb associated 379.63
  chronic 360.03
  parasitic 360.13
  phacoanaphylactic 360.19
  specified type NEC 360.19
  sympathetic 360.11
Endosalpingioma (M9111/1) 236.2
Endosalpingiosis 629.89
Endosteitis —*see* Osteomyelitis
Endothelioma, bone (M9260/3)—*see* Neoplasm,
    bone, malignant
Endotheliosis 287.8
  hemorrhagic infectional 287.8
Endotoxemia —*code to condition*
Endotoxic shock 785.52
Endotrachelitis (*see also* Cervicitis) 616.0
Enema rash 692.89
**Engel-von Recklinghausen disease or
    syndrome** (osteitis fibrosa cystica) 252.01

Engelmann's disease (diaphyseal sclerosis) 756.59
English disease (*see also* Rickets) 268.0
Engman's disease (infectious eczematoid dermatitis) 690.8
Engorgement
  breast 611.79
    newborn 778.7
    puerperal, postpartum 676.2
  liver 573.9
  lung 514
  pulmonary 514
  retina, venous 362.37
  stomach 536.8
  venous, retina 362.37
Enlargement, enlarged —*see also* Hypertrophy
  abdomen 789.3
  adenoids 474.12
    and tonsils 474.10
  alveolar process or ridge 525.8
  apertures of diaphragm (congenital) 756.6
  blind spot, visual field 368.42
  gingival 523.8
  heart, cardiac (*see also* Hypertrophy, cardiac) 429.3
  lacrimal gland, chronic 375.03
  liver (*see also* Hypertrophy, liver) 789.1
  lymph gland or node 785.6
  orbit 376.46
  organ or site, congenital NEC—*see* Anomaly, specified type NEC
  parathyroid (gland) 252.01
  pituitary fossa 793.0
  prostate (simple) (soft) 600.00
    with
      other lower urinary tract symptoms (LUTS) 600.01
      urinary
        obstruction 600.01
        retention 600.01
  sella turcica 793.0
  spleen (*see also* Splenomegaly) 789.2
    congenital 759.0
  thymus (congenital) (gland) 254.0
  thyroid (gland) (*see also* Goiter) 240.9
  tongue 529.8
  tonsils 474.11
    and adenoids 474.10
  uterus 621.2
Enophthalmos 376.50
  due to
    atrophy of orbital tissue 376.51
    surgery 376.52
    trauma 376.52
Enostosis 526.89
Entamebiasis —*see* Amebiasis
Entamebic —*see* Amebiasis
Entanglement, umbilical cord (s) 663.3
  with compression 663.2
  affecting fetus or newborn 762.5
  around neck with compression 663.1
  twins in monoamniotic sac 663.2
Enteralgia 789.0
Enteric —*see* condition
Enteritis (acute) (catarrhal) (choleraic) (chronic) (congestive) (diarrheal) (exudative) (follicular) (hemorrhagic) (infantile) (lienteric) (noninfectious) (perforative) (phlegmonous) (presumed noninfectious) (pseudomembranous) 558.9
  adaptive 564.9
  aertrycke infection 003.0

Enteritis—*continued*
  allergic 558.3
  amebic (*see also* Amebiasis) 006.9
    with abscess—*see* Abscess, amebic
    acute 006.0
      with abscess—*see* Abscess, amebic
      nondysenteric 006.2
    chronic 006.1
      with abscess—*see* Abscess, amebic
      nondysenteric 006.2
  anaerobic (cocci) (gram-negative) (gram-positive) (mixed) NEC 008.46
  bacillary NEC 004.9
  bacterial NEC 008.5
    specified NEC 008.49
  Bacteroides (fragilis) (melaninogeniscus) (oralis) 008.46
  Butyrivibrio (fibriosolvens) 008.46
  Campylobacter 008.43
  Candida 112.85
  Chilomastix 007.8
  choleriformis 001.1
  chronic 558.9
    ulcerative (*see also* Colitis, ulcerative) 556.9
  cicatrizing (chronic) 555.0
  Clostridium
    botulinum 005.1
    difficile 008.45
    haemolyticum 008.46
    novyi 008.46
    perfringens (C) (F) 008.46
    specified type NEC 008.46
  coccidial 007.2
  dietetic 558.9
  due to
    achylia gastrica 536.8
    adenovirus 008.62
    Aerobacter aerogenes 008.2
    anaerobes—*see* Enteritis, anaerobic 008.46
    Arizona (bacillus) 008.1
    astrovirus 008.66
    Bacillus coli—*see* Enteritis, E. coli 008.0
    bacteria NEC 008.5
      specified NEC 008.49
    Bacteroides 008.46
    Butyrivibrio (fibriosolvens) 008.46
    Calcivirus 008.65
    Campylobacter 008.43
    Clostridium—*see* Enteritis, Clostridium
    Cockle agent 008.64
    Coxsackie (virus) 008.67
    Ditchling agent 008.64
    ECHO virus 008.67
    Enterobacter aerogenes 008.2
    enterococci 008.49
    enterovirus NEC 008.67
    Escherichia coli—*see* Enteritis, E. coli
    Eubacterium 008.46
    Fusobacterium (nucleatum) 008.46
    gram-negative bacteria NEC 008.47
      anaerobic NEC 008.46
    Hawaii agent 008.63
    irritating foods 558.9
    Klebsiella aerogenes 008.47
    Marin County agent 008.66
    Montgomery County agent 008.63
    Norwalk-like agent 008.63
    Norwalk virus 008.63
    Otofuke agent 008.63
    Paracolobactrum arizonae 008.1

Enteritis—continued
   paracolon bacillus NEC 008.47
      Arizona 008.1
   Paramatta agent 008.64
   Peptococcus 008.46
   Peptostreptococcus 008.46
   Propionibacterium 008.46
   Proteus (bacillus) (mirabilis) (morganii) 008.3
   Pseudomonas aeruginosa 008.42
   radiation 558.1
   Rotavirus 008.61
   Sapporo agent 008.63
   small round virus (SRV) NEC 008.64
      featureless NEC 008.63
      structured NEC 008.63
   Snow Mountain (SM) agent 008.63
   specified
      bacteria NEC 008.49
      organism, nonbacterial NEC 008.8
      virus NEC 008.69
   Staphylococcus 008.41
   Streptococcus 008.49
      anaerobic 008.46
   Taunton agent 008.63
   Torovirus 008.69
   Treponema 008.46
   Veillonella 008.46
   virus 008.8
      specified type NEC 008.69
   Wollan (W) agent 008.64
   Yersinia enterocolitica 008.44
   dysentery—*see* Dysentery
   E. coli 008.00
      enterohemorrhagic 008.04
      enteroinvasive 008.03
      enteropathogenic 008.01
      enterotoxigenic 008.02
      specified type NEC 008.09
   el tor 001.1
   embadomonial 007.8
   epidemic 009.0
   Eubacterium 008.46
   fermentative 558.9
   fulminant 557.0
   Fusobacterium (nucleatum) 008.46
   gangrenous (*see also* Enteritis, due to, by organism) 009.0
   giardial 007.1
   gram-negative bacteria NEC 008.47
      anaerobic NEC 008.46
   infectious NEC (*see also* Enteritis, due to, by organism) 009.0
      presumed 009.1
   influenzal 487.8
   ischemic 557.9
      acute 557.0
      chronic 557.1
      due to mesenteric artery insufficiency 557.1
   membranous 564.9
   mucous 564.9
   myxomembranous 564.9
   necrotic (*see also* Enteritis, due to, by organism) 009.0
   necroticans 005.2
   necrotizing of fetus or newborn 777.5
   neurogenic 564.9
   newborn 777.8
      necrotizing 777.5
   parasitic NEC 129
   paratyphoid (fever) (*see also* Fever, paratyphoid) 002.9

Enteritis—continued
   Peptococcus 008.46
   Peptostreptococcus 008.46
   Propionibacterium 008.46
   protozoal NEC 007.9
   radiation 558.1
   regional (of) 555.9
      intestine
         large (bowel, colon, or rectum) 555.1
            with small intestine 555.2
         small (duodenum, ileum, or jejunum) 555.0
            with large intestine 555.2
   Salmonella infection 003.0
   salmonellosis 003.0
   segmental (*see also* Enteritis, regional) 555.9
   septic (*see also* Enteritis, due to, by organism) 009.0
   Shigella 004.9
   simple 558.9
   spasmodic 564.9
   spastic 564.9
   staphylococcal 008.41
      due to food 005.0
   streptococcal 008.49
      anaerobic 008.46
   toxic 558.2
   Treponema (denticola) (macrodentium) 008.46
   trichomonal 007.3
   tuberculous (*see also* Tuberculosis) 014.8
   typhosa 002.0
   ulcerative (chronic) (*see also* Colitis, ulcerative) 556.9
   Veillonella 008.46
   viral 008.8
      adenovirus 008.62
      enterovirus 008.67
      specified virus NEC 008.69
   Yersinia enterocolitica 008.44
   zymotic 009.0
Enteroarticular syndrome 099.3
Enterobiasis 127.4
Enterobius vermicularis 127.4
Enterocele (*see also* Hernia) 553.9
   pelvis, pelvic (acquired) (congenital) 618.6
   vagina, vaginal (acquired) (congenital) 618.6
Enterocolitis —*see also* Enteritis
   fetus or newborn 777.8
      necrotizing 777.5
   fulminant 557.0
   granulomatous 555.2
   hemorrhagic (acute) 557.0
      chronic 557.1
   necrotizing (acute) (membranous) 557.0
   primary necrotizing 777.5
   pseudomembranous 008.45
   radiation 558.1
      newborn 777.5
   ulcerative 556.0
Enterocystoma 751.5
Enterogastritis —*see* Enteritis
Enterogenous cyanosis 289.7
Enterolith, enterolithiasis (impaction) 560.39
   with hernia—*see also* Hernia, by site, with obstruction
      gangrenous—*see* Hernia, by site, with gangrene
Enteropathy 569.9
   exudative (of Gordon) 579.8
   gluten 579.0
   hemorrhagic, terminal 557.0
   protein-losing 579.8
Enteroperitonitis (*see also* Peritonitis) 567.9

Enteroptosis

Enteroptosis 569.89
Enterorrhagia 578.9
Enterospasm 564.9
    psychogenic 306.4
Enterostenosis (*see also* Obstruction, intestine) 560.9
Enterostomy status V44.4
    with complication 569.60
Enthesopathy 726.39
    ankle and tarsus 726.70
    elbow region 726.30
        specified NEC 726.39
    hip 726.5
    knee 726.60
    peripheral NEC 726.8
    shoulder region 726.10
        adhesive 726.0
    spinal 720.1
    wrist and carpus 726.4
Entrance, air into vein —*see* Embolism, air
Entrapment, nerve —*see* Neuropathy, entrapment
Entropion (eyelid) 374.00
    cicatricial 374.04
    congenital 743.62
    late effect of trachoma (healed) 139.1
    mechanical 374.02
    paralytic 374.02
    senile 374.01
    spastic 374.03
Enucleation of eye (current) (traumatic) 871.3
Enuresis 788.30
    habit disturbance 307.6
    nocturnal 788.36
        psychogenic 307.6
    nonorganic origin 307.6
    psychogenic 307.6
Enzymopathy 277.9
Eosinopenia 288.59
Eosinophilia 288.3
    allergic 288.3
    hereditary 288.3
    idiopathic 288.3
    infiltrative 518.3
    Loeffler's 518.3
    myalgia syndrome 710.5
    pulmonary (tropical) 518.3
    secondary 288.3
    tropical 518.3
Eosinophilic —*see also* condition
    fasciitis 728.89
    granuloma (bone) 277.89
    infiltration lung 518.3
Ependymitis (acute) (cerebral) (chronic) (granular) (*see also* Meningitis) 322.9
Ependymoblastoma (M9392/3)
    specified site—*see* Neoplasm, by site, malignant
    unspecified site 191.9
Ependymoma (epithelial) (malignant) (M9391/3)
    anaplastic type (M9392/3)
        specified site—*see* Neoplasm, by site, malignant
        unspecified site 191.9
    benign (M9391/0)
        specified site—*see* Neoplasm, by site, benign
        unspecified site 225.0
    myxopapillary (M9394/1) 237.5
    papillary (M9393/1) 237.5
    specified site—*see* Neoplasm, by site, malignant
    unspecified site 191.9
Ependymopathy 349.2
    spinal cord 349.2

INDEX TO DISEASES

Ephelides, ephelis 709.09
Ephemeral fever (*see also* Pyrexia) 780.6
Epiblepharon (congenital) 743.62
Epicanthus, epicanthic fold (congenital) (eyelid) 743.63
Epicondylitis (elbow) (lateral) 726.32
    medial 726.31
Epicystitis (*see also* Cystitis) 595.9
Epidemic —*see* condition
Epidermidalization, cervix —*see* condition
Epidermidization, cervix —*see* condition
Epidermis, epidermal —*see* condition
Epidermization, cervix —*see* condition
Epidermodysplasia verruciformis 078.19
Epidermoid
    cholesteatoma—*see* Cholesteatoma
    inclusion (*see also* Cyst, skin) 706.2
Epidermolysis
    acuta (combustiformis) (toxica) 695.1
    bullosa 757.39
    necroticans combustiformis 695.1
        due to drug
            correct substance properly administered 695.1
            overdose or wrong substance given or taken 977.9
            specified drug—*see* Table of drugs and chemicals
Epidermophytid —*see* Dermatophytosis
Epidermophytosis (infected)—*see* Dermatophytosis
Epidermosis, ear (middle) (*see also* Cholesteatoma) 385.30
Epididymis —*see* condition
Epididymitis (nonvenereal) 604.90
    with abscess 604.0
    acute 604.99
    blennorrhagic (acute) 098.0
        chronic or duration of 2 months or over 098.2
    caseous (*see also* Tuberculosis) 016.4
    chlamydial 099.54
    diphtheritic 032.89 *[604.91]*
    filarial 125.9 *[604.91]*
    gonococcal (acute) 098.0
        chronic or duration of 2 months or over 098.2
    recurrent 604.99
    residual 604.99
    syphilitic 095.8 *[604.91]*
    tuberculous (*see also* Tuberculosis) 016.4
Epididymo-orchitis (*see also* Epididymitis) 604.90
    with abscess 604.0
    chlamydial 099.54
    gonococcal (acute) 098.13
        chronic or duration of 2 months or over 098.33
Epidural —*see* condition
Epigastritis (*see also* Gastritis) 535.5
Epigastrium, epigastric —*see* condition
Epigastrocele (*see also* Hernia, epigastric) 553.29
Epiglottiditis (acute) 464.30
    with obstruction 464.31
    chronic 476.1
    viral 464.30
        with obstruction 464.31
Epiglottis —*see* condition
Epiglottitis (acute) 464.30
    with obstruction 464.31
    chronic 476.1
    viral 464.30
        with obstruction 464.31
Epignathus 759.4

INDEX TO DISEASES

Epilepsia
 partialis continua (*see also* Epilepsy) 345.7
 procursiva (*see also* Epilepsy) 345.8
Epilepsy, epileptic (idiopathic) 345.9

> *Note—use the following fifth-digit subclassification with categories 345.0, 345.1, 345.4-345.9*
>
> 0 without mention of intractable epilepsy
> 1 with intractable epilepsy

 abdominal 345.5
 absence (attack) 345.0
 akinetic 345.0
  psychomotor 345.4
 automatism 345.4
 autonomic diencephalic 345.5
 brain 345.9
 Bravais-Jacksonian 345.5
 cerebral 345.9
 climacteric 345.9
 clonic 345.1
 clouded state 345.9
 coma 345.3
 communicating 345.4
 complicating pregnancy, childbirth or the puerperium 649.4
 congenital 345.9
 convulsions 345.9
 cortical (focal) (motor) 345.5
 cursive (running) 345.8
 cysticercosis 123.1
 deterioration
  with behavioral disturbance 345.9 *[294.11]*
  without behavioral disturbance 345.9 *[294.10]*
 due to syphilis 094.89
 equivalent 345.5
 fit 345.9
 focal (motor) 345.5
 gelastic 345.8
 generalized 345.9
  convulsive 345.1
   flexion 345.1
  nonconvulsive 345.0
 grand mal (idiopathic) 345.1
 Jacksonian (motor) (sensory) 345.5
 Kojevnikoff's, Kojevnikov's, Kojewnikoff's 345.7
 laryngeal 786.2
 limbic system 345.4
 localization related (focal) (partial) and epileptic syndromes
  with
   complex partial seizures 345.4
   simple partial seizures 345.5
 major (motor) 345.1
 minor 345.0
 mixed (type) 345.9
 motor partial 345.5
 musicogenic 345.1
 myoclonus, myoclonic 345.1
  progressive (familial) 333.2
 nonconvulsive, generalized 345.0
 parasitic NEC 123.9
 partial (focalized) 345.5
  with
   impairment of consciousness 345.4
   memory and ideational disturbances 345.4
   abdominal type 345.5
   motor type 345.5
   psychomotor type 345.4

Episcleritis

Epilepsy, epileptic—*continued*
  psychosensory type 345.4
  secondarily generalized 345.4
  sensory type 345.5
  somatomotor type 345.5
  somatosensory type 345.5
  temporal lobe type 345.4
  visceral type 345.5
  visual type 345.5
  without impairment of consciousness 345.5
 peripheral 345.9
 petit mal 345.0
 photokinetic 345.8
 progressive myoclonic (familial) 333.2
 psychic equivalent 345.5
 psychomotor 345.4
 psychosensory 345.4
 reflex 345.1
 seizure 345.9
 senile 345.9
 sensory-induced 345.5
 sleep (*see also* Narcolepsy) 347.00
 somatomotor type 345.5
 somatosensory 345.5
 specified type NEC 345.8
 status (grand mal) 345.3
  focal motor 345.7
  petit mal 345.2
  psychomotor 345.7
  temporal lobe 345.7
 symptomatic 345.9
 temporal lobe 345.4
 tonic (-clonic) 345.1
 traumatic (injury unspecified) 907.0
  injury specified—*see* Late, effect (of) specified injury
 twilight 293.0
 uncinate (gyrus) 345.4
 Unverricht (-Lundborg) (familial myoclonic) 333.2
 visceral 345.5
 visual 345.5
Epileptiform
 convulsions 780.39
 seizure 780.39
Epiloia 759.5
Epimenorrhea 626.2
Epipharyngitis (*see also* Nasopharyngitis) 460
Epiphora 375.20
 due to
  excess lacrimation 375.21
  insufficient drainage 375.22
Epiphyseal arrest 733.91
 femoral head 732.2
Epiphyseolysis, epiphysiolysis (*see also* Osteochondrosis) 732.9
Epiphysitis (*see also* Osteochondrosis) 732.9
 juvenile 732.6
 marginal (Scheuermann's) 732.0
 os calcis 732.5
 syphilitic (congenital) 090.0
 vertebral (Scheuermann's) 732.0
Epiplocele (*see also* Hernia) 553.9
Epiploitis (*see also* Peritonitis) 567.9
Epiplosarcomphalocele (*see also* Hernia, umbilicus) 553.1
Episcleritis 379.00
 gouty 274.89 *[379.09]*
 nodular 379.02
 periodica fugax 379.01
  angioneurotic—*see* Edema, angioneurotic

Episcleritis—*continued*
specified NEC 379.09
staphylococcal 379.00
suppurative 379.00
syphilitic 095.0
tuberculous (*see also* Tuberculosis) 017.3 *[379.09]*
Episode
brain (*see also* Disease, cerebrovascular, acute) 436
cerebral (*see also* Disease, cerebrovascular, acute) 436
depersonalization (in neurotic state) 300.6
hyporesponsive 780.09
psychotic (*see also* Psychosis) 298.9
organic, transient 293.9
schizophrenic (acute) NEC (*see also* Schizophrenia) 295.4
Epispadias
female 753.8
male 752.62
Episplenitis 289.59
Epistaxis (multiple) 784.7
hereditary 448.0
vicarious menstruation 625.8
Epithelioma (malignant) (M8011/3)—*see also* Neoplasm, by site, malignant
adenoides cysticum (M8100/0)—*see* Neoplasm, skin, benign
basal cell (M8090/3)—*see* Neoplasm, skin, malignant
benign (M8011/0)—*see* Neoplasm, by site, benign
Bowen's (M8081/2)—*see* Neoplasm, skin, in situ
calcifying (benign) (Malherbe's) (M8110/0)—*see* Neoplasm, skin, benign
external site—*see* Neoplasm, skin, malignant
intraepidermal, Jadassohn (M8096/0)—*see* Neoplasm, skin, benign
squamous cell (M8070/3)—*see* Neoplasm, by site, malignant
Epitheliopathy
pigment, retina 363.15
posterior multifocal placoid (acute) 363.15
Epithelium, epithelial —*see* condition
Epituberculosis (allergic) (with atelectasis) (*see also* Tuberculosis) 010.8
Eponychia 757.5
Epstein's
nephrosis or syndrome (*see also* Nephrosis) 581.9
pearl (mouth) 528.4
Epstein-Barr infection (viral) 075
chronic 780.79 *[139.8]*
Epulis (giant cell) (gingiva) 523.8
Equinia 024
Equinovarus (congenital) 754.51
acquired 736.71
Equivalent
convulsive (abdominal) (*see also* Epilepsy) 345.5
epileptic (psychic) (*see also* Epilepsy) 345.5
Erb's
disease 359.1
palsy, paralysis (birth) (brachial) (newborn) 767.6
spinal (spastic) syphilitic 094.89
pseudohypertrophic muscular dystrophy 359.1
Erb (-Duchenne) paralysis (birth injury) (newborn) 767.6
Erb-Goldflam disease or syndrome 358.00

Erdheim's syndrome (acromegalic macrospondylitis) 253.0
Erection, painful (persistent) 607.3
Ergosterol deficiency (vitamin D) 268.9
with
osteomalacia 268.2
rickets (*see also* Rickets) 268.0
Ergotism (ergotized grain) 988.2
from ergot used as drug (migraine therapy)
correct substance properly administered 349.82
overdose or wrong substance given or taken 975.0
Erichsen's disease (railway spine) 300.16
Erlacher-Blount syndrome (tibia vara) 732.4
Erosio interdigitalis blastomycetica 112.3
Erosion
arteriosclerotic plaque—*see* Arteriosclerosis, by site
artery NEC 447.2
without rupture 447.8
bone 733.99
bronchus 519.19
cartilage (joint) 733.99
cervix (uteri) (acquired) (chronic) (congenital) 622.0
with mention of cervicitis 616.0
cornea (recurrent) (*see also* Keratitis) 371.42
traumatic 918.1
dental (idiopathic) (occupational) 521.30
extending into
dentine 521.32
pulp 521.33
generalized 521.35
limited to enamel 521.31
localized 521.34
duodenum, postpyloric—*see* Ulcer, duodenum
esophagus 530.89
gastric 535.4
intestine 569.89
lymphatic vessel 457.8
pylorus, pyloric (ulcer) 535.4
sclera 379.16
spine, aneurysmal 094.89
spleen 289.59
stomach 535.4
teeth (idiopathic) (occupational) (*see also* Erosion, dental) 521.30
due to
medicine 521.30
persistent vomiting 521.30
urethra 599.84
uterus 621.8
vertebra 733.99
Erotomania 302.89
Clérambault's 297.8
Error
in diet 269.9
refractive 367.9
astigmatism (*see also* Astigmatism) 367.20
drug-induced 367.89
hypermetropia 367.0
hyperopia 367.0
myopia 367.1
presbyopia 367.4
toxic 367.89
Eructation 787.3
nervous 306.4
psychogenic 306.4
Eruption
creeping 126.9
drug—*see* Dermatitis, due to, drug
Hutchinson, summer 692.72

Eruption—*continued*
  Kaposi's varicelliform 054.0
  napkin (psoriasiform) 691.0
  polymorphous
    light (sun) 692.72
    other source 692.82
  psoriasiform, napkin 691.0
  recalcitrant pustular 694.8
  ringed 695.89
  skin (*see also* Dermatitis) 782.1
    creeping (meaning hookworm) 126.9
    due to
      chemical(s) NEC 692.4
        internal use 693.8
      drug—*see* Dermatitis, due to, drug
      prophylactic inoculation or vaccination
        against disease—*see* Dermatitis, due to,
        vaccine
      smallpox vaccination NEC—*see* Dermatitis,
        due to, vaccine
    erysipeloid 027.1
    feigned 698.4
    Hutchinson, summer 692.72
    Kaposi's, varicelliform 054.0
    vaccinia 999.0
    lichenoid, axilla 698.3
    polymorphous, due to light 692.72
    toxic NEC 695.0
    vesicular 709.8
  teeth, tooth
    accelerated 520.6
    delayed 520.6
    difficult 520.6
    disturbance of 520.6
    in abnormal sequence 520.6
    incomplete 520.6
    late 520.6
    natal 520.6
    neonatal 520.6
    obstructed 520.6
    partial 520.6
    persistent primary 520.6
    premature 520.6
    prenatal 520.6
  vesicular 709.8
Erysipelas (gangrenous) (infantile) (newborn)
    (phlegmonous) (suppurative) 035
  external ear 035 *[380.13]*
  puerperal, postpartum, childbirth 670
Erysipelatoid (Rosenbach's) 027.1
Erysipeloid (Rosenbach's) 027.1
Erythema, erythematous (generalized) 695.9
  ab igne—*see* Burn, by site, first degree
  annulare (centrifugum) (rheumaticum) 695.0
  arthriticum epidemicum 026.1
  brucellum (*see also* Brucellosis) 023.9
  bullosum 695.1
  caloricum—*see* Burn, by site, first degree
  chronicum migrans 088.81
    chronicum 088.81
  circinatum 695.1
  diaper 691.0
  due to
    chemical (contact) NEC 692.4
      internal 693.8
    drug (internal use) 693.0
      contact 692.3
  elevatum diutinum 695.89
  endemic 265.2
  epidemic, arthritic 026.1
  figuratum perstans 695.0

Erythema, erythematous—*continued*
  gluteal 691.0
  gyratum (perstans) (repens) 695.1
  heat—*see* Burn, by site, first degree
  ichthyosiforme congenitum 757.1
  induratum (primary) (scrofulosorum) (*see also*
    Tuberculosis) 017.1
    nontuberculous 695.2
  infantum febrile 057.8
  infectional NEC 695.9
  infectiosum 057.0
  inflammation NEC 695.9
  intertrigo 695.89
  iris 695.1
  lupus (discoid) (localized) (*see also* Lupus,
    erythematosus) 695.4
  marginatum 695.0
    rheumaticum—*see* Fever, rheumatic
  medicamentosum—*see* Dermatitis, due to, drug
  migrans 529.1
  multiforme 695.1
    bullosum 695.1
    conjunctiva 695.1
    exudativum (Hebra) 695.1
    pemphigoides 694.5
  napkin 691.0
  neonatorum 778.8
  nodosum 695.2
    tuberculous (*see also* Tuberculosis) 017.1
  nummular, nummulare 695.1
  palmar 695.0
  palmaris hereditarium 695.0
  pernio 991.5
  perstans solare 692.72
  rash, newborn 778.8
  scarlatiniform (exfoliative) (recurrent) 695.0
  simplex marginatum 057.8
  solare (*see also* Sunburn) 692.71
  streptogenes 696.5
  toxic, toxicum NEC 695.0
    newborn 778.8
  tuberculous (primary) (*see also* Tuberculosis)
    017.0
  venenatum 695.0
Erythematosus —*see* condition
Erythematous —*see* condition
Erythermalgia (primary) 443.82
Erythralgia 443.82
Erythrasma 039.0
Erythredema 985.0
  polyneuritica 985.0
  polyneuropathy 985.0
Erythremia (acute) (M9841/3) 207.0
  chronic (M9842/3) 207.1
  secondary 289.0
Erythroblastopenia (acquired) 284.89
  congenital 284.01
Erythroblastophthisis 284.01
Erythroblastosis (fetalis) (newborn) 773.2
  due to
    ABO
      antibodies 773.1
      incompatibility, maternal/fetal 773.1
      isoimmunization 773.1
    Rh
      antibodies 773.0
      incompatibility, maternal/fetal 773.0
      isoimmunization 773.0
Erythrocyanosis (crurum) 443.89
Erythrocythemia —*see* Erythremia
Erythrocytopenia 285.9

Erythrocytosis (megalosplenic)
  familial 289.6
  oval, hereditary (*see also* Elliptocytosis) 282.1
  secondary 289.0
  stress 289.0
Erythroderma (*see also* Erythema) 695.9
  desquamativa (in infants) 695.89
  exfoliative 695.89
  ichthyosiform, congenital 757.1
  infantum 695.89
  maculopapular 696.2
  neonatorum 778.8
  psoriaticum 696.1
  secondary 695.9
Erythrodysesthesia, palmar plantar (PPE) 693.0
Erythrogenesis imperfecta 284.09
Erythroleukemia (M9840/3) 207.0
Erythromelalgia 443.82
Erythromelia 701.8
Erythropenia 285.9
Erythrophagocytosis 289.9
Erythrophobia 300.23
Erythroplakia
  oral mucosa 528.79
  tongue 528.79
Erythroplasia (Queyrat) (M8080/2)
  specified site—*see* Neoplasm, skin, in situ
  unspecified site 233.5
Erythropoiesis, idiopathic ineffective 285.0
Escaped beats, heart 427.60
  postoperative 997.1
Esoenteritis —*see* Enteritis
Esophagalgia 530.89
Esophagectasis 530.89
  due to cardiospasm 530.0
Esophagismus 530.5
Esophagitis (alkaline) (chemical) (chronic)
  (infectional) (necrotic) (postoperative) 530.10
  acute 530.12
  candidal 112.84
  reflux 530.11
  specified NEC 530.19
  tuberculous (*see also* Tuberculosis) 017.8
  ulcerative 530.19
Esophagocele 530.6
Esophagodynia 530.89
Esophagomalacia 530.89
Esophagoptosis 530.89
Esophagospasm 530.5
Esophagostenosis 530.3
Esophagostomiasis 127.7
Esophagostomy
  complication 530.87
    infection 530.86
    malfunctioning 530.87
    mechanical 530.87
Esophagotracheal —*see* condition
Esophagus —*see* condition
Esophoria 378.41
  convergence, excess 378.84
  divergence, insufficiency 378.85
Esotropia (nonaccommodative) 378.00
  accommodative 378.35
  alternating 378.05
    with
      A pattern 378.06
      specified noncomitancy NEC 378.08
      V pattern 378.07
      X pattern 378.08
      Y pattern 378.08
    intermittent 378.22

Esotropia—*continued*
  intermittent 378.20
    alternating 378.22
    monocular 378.21
  monocular 378.01
    with
      A pattern 378.02
      specified noncomitancy NEC 378.04
      V pattern 378.03
      X pattern 378.04
      Y pattern 378.04
    intermittent 378.21
Espundia 085.5
Essential —*see* condition
Esterapenia 289.89
Esthesioneuroblastoma (M9522/3) 160.0
Esthesioneurocytoma (M9521/3) 160.0
Esthesioneuroepithelioma (M9523/3) 160.0
Esthiomene 099.1
Estivo-autumnal
  fever 084.0
  malaria 084.0
Estrangement V61.0
Estriasis 134.0
Ethanolaminuria 270.8
Ethanolism (*see also* Alcoholism) 303.9
Ether dependence, dependency (*see also*
  Dependence) 304.6
Etherism (*see also* Dependence) 304.6
Ethmoid, ethmoidal —*see* condition
Ethmoiditis (chronic) (nonpurulent) (purulent)
  (*see also* Sinusitis, ethmoidal) 473.2
  influenzal 487.1
  Woakes' 471.1
Ethylism (*see also* Alcoholism) 303.9
Eulenburg's disease (congenital paramyotonia)
  359.29
Eunuchism 257.2
Eunuchoidism 257.2
  hypogonadotropic 257.2
European blastomycosis 117.5
Eustachian —*see* condition
Euthyroid sick syndrome 790.94
Euthyroidism 244.9
Evaluation
  fetal lung maturity 659.8
  for suspected condition (*see also* Observation) V71.9
    abuse V71.81
    exposure
      antrax V71.82
      biologic agent NEC V71.83
      SARS V71.83
    neglect V71.81
    newborn—*see* Observation, suspected,
      condition, newborn
    specified condition NEC V71.89
  mental health V70.2
  requested by authority V70.1
  nursing care V63.8
  social service V63.8
Evans' syndrome (thrombocytopenic purpura)
  287.32
Eventration
  colon into chest—*see* Hernia, diaphragm
  diaphragm (congenital) 756.6
Eversion
  bladder 596.8
  cervix (uteri) 622.0
    with mention of cervicitis 616.0
  foot NEC 736.79

INDEX TO DISEASES

Examination

Eversion—*continued*
   congenital 755.67
   lacrimal punctum 375.51
   punctum lacrimale (postinfectional) (senile) 375.51
   ureter (meatus) 593.89
   urethra (meatus) 599.84
   uterus 618.1
      complicating delivery 665.2
         affecting fetus or newborn 763.89
      puerperal, postpartum 674.8
Evidence
   of malignancy
      cytologic
         without histologic confirmation 795.06
Evisceration
   birth injury 767.8
   bowel (congenital)—*see* Hernia, ventral
   congenital (*see also* Hernia, ventral) 553.29
   operative wound 998.32
   traumatic NEC 869.1
      eye 871.3
Evulsion —*see* Avulsion
Ewing's
   angioendothelioma (M9260/3)—*see* Neoplasm, bone, malignant
   sarcoma (M9260/3)—*see* Neoplasm, bone, malignant
   tumor (M9260/3)—*see* Neoplasm, bone, malignant
Exaggerated lumbosacral angle (with impinging spine) 756.12
Examination (general) (routine) (of) (for) V70.9
   allergy V72.7
   annual V70.0
   cardiovascular preoperative V72.81
   cervical Papanicolaou smear V76.2
      as a part of routine gynecological examination V72.31
      to confirm findings of recent normal smear following initial abnormal smear V72.32
   child care (routine) V20.2
   clinical research investigation (normal control patient) (participant) V70.7
   dental V72.2
   developmental testing (child) (infant) V20.2
   donor (potential) V70.8
   ear V72.19
   eye V72.0
   following
      accident (motor vehicle) V71.4
      alleged rape or seduction (victim or culprit) V71.5
      inflicted injury (victim or culprit) NEC V71.6
      rape or seduction, alleged (victim or culprit) V71.5
      treatment (for) V67.9
         combined V67.6
         fracture V67.4
         involving high-risk medication NEC V67.51
         mental disorder V67.3
         specified condition NEC V67.59
   follow-up (routine) (following) V67.9
      cancer chemotherapy V67.2
      chemotherapy V67.2
      disease NEC V67.59
      high-risk medication NEC V67.51
      injury NEC V67.59
      population survey V70.6
      postpartum V24.2
      psychiatric V67.3
      psychotherapy V67.3

Examination—*continued*
      radiotherapy V67.1
      specified surgery NEC V67.09
      surgery V67.00
         vaginal pap smear V67.01
   gynecological V72.31
      for contraceptive maintenance V25.40
         intrauterine device V25.42
         pill V25.41
         specified method NEC V25.49
   health (of)
      armed forces personnel V70.5
      checkup V70.0
      child, routine V20.2
      defined subpopulation NEC V70.5
      inhabitants of institutions V70.5
      occupational V70.5
      pre-employment screening V70.5
      preschool children V70.5
         for admission to school V70.3
      prisoners V70.5
         for entrance into prison V70.3
      prostitutes V70.5
      refugees V70.5
      school children V70.5
      students V70.5
   hearing V72.19
      following failed hearing screening V72.11
   infant V20.2
   laboratory V72.6
   lactating mother V24.1
   medical (for) (of) V70.9
      administrative purpose NEC V70.3
      admission to
         old age home V70.3
         prison V70.3
         school V70.3
      adoption V70.3
      armed forces personnel V70.5
      at health care facility V70.0
      camp V70.3
      child, routine V20.2
      clinical research investigation (control) (normal comparison) (participant) V70.7
      defined subpopulation NEC V70.5
      donor (potential) V70.8
      driving license V70.3
      general V70.9
         routine V70.0
         specified reason NEC V70.8
      immigration V70.3
      inhabitants of institutions V70.5
      insurance certification V70.3
      marriage V70.3
      medicolegal reasons V70.4
      naturalization V70.3
      occupational V70.5
      population survey V70.6
      pre-employment V70.5
      preschool children V70.5
         for admission to school V70.3
      prison V70.3
      prisoners V70.5
         for entrance into prison V70.3
      prostitutes V70.5
      refugees V70.5
      school children V70.5
      specified reason NEC V70.8
      sport competition V70.3
      students V70.5
   medicolegal reason V70.4

Examination—*continued*
  pelvic (annual) (periodic) V72.31
  periodic (annual) (routine) V70.0
  postpartum
    immediately after delivery V24.0
    routine follow-up V24.2
  pregnancy (unconfirmed) (possible) V72.40
    negative result V72.41
    positive result V72.42
  prenatal V22.1
    first pregnancy V22.0
    high-risk pregnancy V23.9
      specified problem NEC V23.8
  preoperative V72.84
    cardiovascular V72.81
    respiratory V72.82
    specified NEC V72.83
  preprocedural V72.84
    cardiovascular V72.81
    general physical V72.83
    respiratory V72.82
    specified NEC V72.83
  psychiatric V70.2
    follow-up not needing further care V67.3
    requested by authority V70.1
  radiological NEC V72.5
  respiratory preoperative V72.82
  screening—*see* Screening
  sensitization V72.7
  skin V72.7
    hypersensitivity V72.7
  special V72.9
  specified type or reason NEC V72.85
    preoperative V72.83
    specified NEC V72.83
  teeth V72.2
  vaginal Papanicolaou smear V76.47
    following hysterectomy for malignant
      condition V67.01
  victim or culprit following
    alleged rape or seduction V71.5
    inflicted injury NEC V71.6
  vision V72.0
  well baby V20.2
Exanthem, exanthema (*see also* Rash) 782.1
  Boston 048
  epidemic, with meningitis 048
  lichenoid psoriasiform 696.2
  subitum 058.10
    due to
      human herpesvirus 6 058.11
      human herpesvirus 7 058.12
  viral, virus NEC 057.9
    specified type NEC 057.8
Excess, excessive, excessively
  alcohol level in blood 790.3
  carbohydrate tissue, localized 278.1
  carotene (dietary) 278.3
  cold 991.9
    specified effect NEC 991.8
  convergence 378.84
  crying 780.95
    of
      adolescent 780.95
      adult 780.95
      baby 780.92
      child 780.95
      infant (baby) 780.92
      newborn 780.92
  development, breast 611.1
  diaphoresis (*see also* Hyperhidrosis) 780.8

Excess, excessive, excessively—*continued*
  distance, interarch 524.28
  divergence 378.85
  drinking (alcohol) NEC (*see also* Abuse, drugs,
    nondependent) 305.0
    continual (*see also* Alcoholism) 303.9
    habitual (*see also* Alcoholism) 303.9
  eating 783.6
  eyelid fold (congenital) 743.62
  fat 278.02
    in heart (*see also* Degeneration, myocardial) 429.1
    tissue, localized 278.1
  foreskin 605
  gas 787.3
  gastrin 251.5
  glucagon 251.4
  heat (*see also* Heat) 992.9
  horizontal
    overjet 524.26
    overlap 524.26
  interarch distance 524.28
  intermaxillary vertical dimension 524.37
  interocclusal distance of teeth 524.37
  large
    colon 564.7
      congenital 751.3
    fetus or infant 766.0
      with obstructed labor 660.1
        affecting management of pregnancy 656.6
      causing disproportion 653.5
    newborn (weight of 4500 grams or more) 766.0
  long
    colon 751.5
    organ or site, congenital NEC—*see* Anomaly,
      specified type NEC
    umbilical cord (entangled)
      affecting fetus or newborn 762.5
      in pregnancy or childbirth 663.3
        with compression 663.2
  menstruation 626.2
  number of teeth 520.1
    causing crowding 524.31
  nutrients (dietary) NEC 783.6
  potassium (K) 276.7
  salivation (*see also* Ptyalism) 527.7
  secretion—*see also* Hypersecretion
    milk 676.6
    sputum 786.4
    sweat (*see also* Hyperhidrosis) 780.8
  short
    organ or site, congenital NEC—*see* Anomaly,
      specified type NEC
    umbilical cord
      affecting fetus or newborn 762.6
      in pregnancy or childbirth 663.4
  skin NEC 701.9
    eyelid 743.62
      acquired 374.30
  sodium (Na) 276.0
  spacing of teeth 524.32
  sputum 786.4
  sweating (*see also* Hyperhidrosis) 780.8
  tearing (ducts) (eye) (*see also* Epiphora) 375.20
  thirst 783.5
    due to deprivation of water 994.3
  tuberosity 524.07
  vitamin
    A (dietary) 278.2
      administered as drug (chronic) (prolonged
        excessive intake) 278.2
      reaction to sudden overdose 963.5

Excess, excessive, excessively—*continued*
  D (dietary) 278.4
    administered as drug (chronic) (prolonged excessive intake) 278.4
      reaction to sudden overdose 963.5
  weight 278.02
    gain 783.1
      of pregnancy 646.1
    loss 783.21
Excitability, abnormal, under minor stress 309.29
Excitation
  catatonic (*see also* Schizophrenia) 295.2
  psychogenic 298.1
  reactive (from emotional stress, psychological trauma) 298.1
Excitement
  manic (*see also* Psychosis, affective) 296.0
    recurrent episode 296.1
    single episode 296.0
  mental, reactive (from emotional stress, psychological trauma) 298.1
  state, reactive (from emotional stress, psychological trauma) 298.1
Excluded pupils 364.76
Excoriation (traumatic) (*see also* Injury, superficial, by site) 919.8
  neurotic 698.4
Excyclophoria 378.44
Excyclotropia 378.33
Exencephalus, exencephaly 742.0
Exercise
  breathing V57.0
  remedial NEC V57.1
  therapeutic NEC V57.1
Exfoliation, teeth due to systemic causes 525.0
Exfoliative —*see also* condition
  dermatitis 695.89
Exhaustion, exhaustive (physical NEC) 780.79
  battle (*see also* Reaction, stress, acute) 308.9
  cardiac (*see also* Failure, heart) 428.9
  delirium (*see also* Reaction, stress, acute) 308.9
  due to
    cold 991.8
    excessive exertion 994.5
    exposure 994.4
  fetus or newborn 779.89
  heart (*see also* Failure, heart) 428.9
  heat 992.5
    due to
      salt depletion 992.4
      water depletion 992.3
  manic (*see also* Psychosis, affective) 296.0
    recurrent episode 296.1
    single episode 296.0
  maternal, complicating delivery 669.8
    affecting fetus or newborn 763.89
  mental 300.5
  myocardium, myocardial (*see also* Failure, heart) 428.9
  nervous 300.5
  old age 797
  postinfectional NEC 780.79
  psychogenic 300.5
  psychosis (*see also* Reaction, stress, acute) 308.9
  senile 797
    dementia 290.0
Exhibitionism (sexual) 302.4
Exomphalos 756.79

Exophoria 378.42
  convergence, insufficiency 378.83
  divergence, excess 378.85
Exophthalmic
  cachexia 242.0
  goiter 242.0
  ophthalmoplegia 242.0 *[376.22]*
Exophthalmos 376.30
  congenital 743.66
  constant 376.31
  endocrine NEC 259.9 *[376.22]*
  hyperthyroidism 242.0 *[376.21]*
  intermittent NEC 376.34
  malignant 242.0 *[376.21]*
  pulsating 376.35
    endocrine NEC 259.9 *[376.22]*
  thyrotoxic 242.0 *[376.21]*
Exostosis 726.91
  cartilaginous (M9210/0)—*see* Neoplasm, bone, benign
  congenital 756.4
  ear canal, external 380.81
  gonococcal 098.89
  hip 726.5
  intracranial 733.3
  jaw (bone) 526.81
  luxurians 728.11
  multiple (cancellous) (congenital) (hereditary) 756.4
  nasal bones 726.91
  orbit, orbital 376.42
  osteocartilaginous (M9210/0)—*see* Neoplasm, bone, benign
  spine 721.8
    with spondylosis—*see* Spondylosis
  syphilitic 095.5
  wrist 726.4
Exotropia 378.10
  alternating 378.15
    with
      A pattern 378.16
      specified noncomitancy 378.18
      V pattern 378.17
      X pattern 378.18
      Y pattern 378.18
    intermittent 378.24
  intermittent 378.20
    alternating 378.24
    monocular 378.23
  monocular 378.11
    with
      A pattern 378.12
      specified noncomitancy NEC 378.14
      V pattern 378.13
      X pattern 378.14
      Y pattern 378.14
    intermittent 378.23
Explanation of
  investigation finding V65.4
  medication V65.4
Exposure 994.9
  cold 991.9
    specified effect NEC 991.8
  effects of 994.9
  exhaustion due to 994.4
  to
    AIDS virus V01.79
    anthrax V01.81
    asbestos V15.84
    body fluids (hazardous) V15.85
    cholera V01.0

Exposure—*continued*
  communicable disease V01.9
    specified type NEC V01.89
  Escherichia coli (E. coli) V01.83
  German measles V01.4
  gonorrhea V01.6
  hazardous body fluids V15.85
  HIV V01.79
  human immunodeficiency virus V01.79
  lead V15.86
  meningococcus V01.84
  parasitic disease V01.89
  poliomyelitis V01.2
  potentially hazardous body fluids V15.85
  rabies V01.5
  rubella V01.4
  SARS-associated coronavirus V01.82
  smallpox V01.3
  syphilis V01.6
  tuberculosis V01.1
  varicella V01.71
  venereal disease V01.6
  viral disease NEC V01.79
    varicella V01.71
Exsanguination, fetal 772.0
Exstrophy
  abdominal content 751.8
  bladder (urinary) 753.5
Extensive —*see* condition
Extra —*see also* Accessory
  rib 756.3
    cervical 756.2
Extraction
  with hook 763.89
  breech NEC 669.6
    affecting fetus or newborn 763.0
  cataract postsurgical V45.61
  manual NEC 669.8
    affecting fetus or newborn 763.89
Extrasystole 427.60
  atrial 427.61
  postoperative 997.1
  ventricular 427.69
Extrauterine gestation or pregnancy —*see* Pregnancy, ectopic
Extravasation
  blood 459.0
    lower extremity 459.0
  chyle into mesentery 457.8
  pelvicalyceal 593.4
  pyelosinus 593.4
  urine 788.8
    from ureter 788.8
Extremity —*see* condition
Extrophy —*see* Exstrophy
Extroversion
  bladder 753.5
  uterus 618.1
    complicating delivery 665.2
      affecting fetus or newborn 763.89
    postpartal (old) 618.1
Extruded tooth 524.34
Extrusion
  alveolus and teeth 524.75
  breast implant (prosthetic) 996.54
  device, implant, or graft—*see* Complications, mechanical
  eye implant (ball) (globe) 996.59
  intervertebral disc—*see* Displacement, intervertebral disc
  lacrimal gland 375.43

Extrusion—*continued*
  mesh (reinforcing) 996.59
  ocular lens implant 996.53
  prosthetic device NEC—*see* Complications, mechanical
  vitreous 379.26
Exudate, pleura —*see* Effusion, pleura
Exudates, retina 362.82
Exudative —*see* condition
Eye, eyeball, eyelid—*see* condition
Eyestrain 368.13
Eyeworm disease of Africa 125.2

F

Faber's anemia or syndrome (achlorhydric anemia) 280.9
Fabry's disease (angiokeratoma corporis diffusum) 272.7
Face, facial —*see* condition
Facet of cornea 371.44
Faciocephalalgia, autonomic (*see also* Neuropathy, peripheral, autonomic) 337.9
Facioscapulohumeral myopathy 359.1
Factitious disorder, illness —*see* Illness, factitious
Factor
  deficiency—*see* Deficiency, factor
  psychic, associated with diseases classified elsewhere 316
  risk—*see* Problem
Fahr-Volhard disease (malignant nephrosclerosis) 403.00
Failure, failed
  adenohypophyseal 253.2
  attempted abortion (legal) (*see also* Abortion, failed) 638.9
  bone marrow (anemia) 284.9
    acquired (secondary) 284.89
    congenital 284.09
    idiopathic 284.9
  cardiac (*see also* Failure, heart) 428.9
    newborn 779.89
  cardiorenal (chronic) 428.9
    hypertensive (*see also* Hypertension, cardiorenal) 404.93
  cardiorespiratory 799.1
    specified during or due to a procedure 997.1
      long-term effect of cardiac surgery 429.4
  cardiovascular (chronic) 428.9
  cerebrovascular 437.8
  cervical dilatation in labor 661.0
    affecting fetus or newborn 763.7
  circulation, circulatory 799.89
    fetus or newborn 779.89
    peripheral 785.50
  compensation—*see* Disease, heart
  congestive (*see also* Failure, heart) 428.0
  coronary (*see also* Insufficiency, coronary) 411.89
  dental implant 525.79
    due to
      lack of attached gingiva 525.72
      occlusal trauma (caused by poor prosthetic design) 525.72
      parafunctional habits 525.72
      periodontal infection (peri-implantitis) 525.72
      poor oral hygiene 525.72
    endosseous NEC 525.79
    osseointegration 525.71
      due to
        complications of systemic disease 525.71
        poor bone quality 525.71
      iatrogenic 525.71
    post-osseointegration
      biological 525.72
        iatrogenic 525.72
      due to complications of systemic disease 525.72
      mechanical 525.73
    pre-integration 525.71
    pre-osseointegration 525.71

Failure, failed—*continued*
    dental prosthesis causing loss of dental implant 525.73
  dental restoration
    marginal integrity 525.61
    periodontal anatomical integrity 525.65
  descent of head (at term) 652.5
    affecting fetus or newborn 763.1
    in labor 660.0
      affecting fetus or newborn 763.1
  device, implant, or graft—*see* Complications, mechanical
  engagement of head NEC 652.5
    in labor 660.0
  extrarenal 788.9
  fetal head to enter pelvic brim 652.5
    affecting fetus or newborn 763.1
    in labor 660.0
      affecting fetus or newborn 763.1
  forceps NEC 660.7
    affecting fetus or newborn 763.1
  fusion (joint) (spinal) 996.49
  growth in childhood 783.43
  heart (acute) (sudden) 428.9
    with
      abortion—*see* Abortion, by type, with specified complication NEC
      acute pulmonary edema (*see also* Failure, ventricular, left) 428.1
        with congestion (*see also* Failure, heart) 428.0
      decompensation (*see also* Failure, heart) 428.0
      dilation—*see* Disease, heart
      ectopic pregnancy (*see also* categories 633.0-633.9) 639.8
      molar pregnancy (*see also* categories 630-632) 639.8
    arteriosclerotic 440.9
    combined left-right sided 428.0
    combined systolic and diastolic 428.40
      acute 428.41
      acute on chronic 428.43
      chronic 428.42
    compensated (*see also* Failure, heart) 428.0
    complicating
      abortion—*see* Abortion, by type, with specified complication NEC
      delivery (cesarean) (instrumental) 669.4
      ectopic pregnancy (*see also* categories 633.0-633.9) 639.8
      molar pregnancy (*see also* categories 630-632) 639.8
      obstetric anesthesia or sedation 668.1
      surgery 997.1
    congestive (compensated) (decompensated) (*see also* Failure, heart) 428.0
      with rheumatic fever (conditions classifiable to 390)
        active 391.8
        inactive or quiescent (with chorea) 398.91
      fetus or newborn 779.89
      hypertensive (*see also* Hypertension, heart) 402.91
        with renal disease (*see also* Hypertension, cardiorenal) 404.91
          with renal failure 404.93
        benign 402.11
        malignant 402.01

Failure, failed—*continued*
  rheumatic (chronic) (inactive) (with chorea) 398.91
    active or acute 391.8
      with chorea (Sydenham's) 392.0
  decompensated (*see also* Failure, heart) 428.0
  degenerative (*see also* Degeneration, myocardial) 429.1
  diastolic 428.30
    acute 428.31
    acute or chronic 428.33
    chronic 428.32
  due to presence of (cardiac) prosthesis 429.4
  fetus or newborn 779.89
  following
    abortion 639.8
    cardiac surgery 429.4
    ectopic or molar pregnancy 639.8
  high output NEC 428.9
  hypertensive (*see also* Hypertension, heart) 402.91
    with renal disease (*see also* Hypertension, cardiorenal) 404.91
      with renal failure 404.93
    benign 402.11
    malignant 402.01
  left (ventricular) (*see also* Failure, ventricular, left) 428.1
    with right-sided failure (*see also* Failure, heart) 428.0
  low output (syndrome) NEC 428.9
  organic—*see* Disease, heart
  postoperative (immediate) 997.1
    long term effect of cardiac surgery 429.4
  rheumatic (chronic) (congestive) (inactive) 398.91
  right (secondary to left heart failure, conditions classifiable to 428.1) (ventricular) (*see also* Failure, heart) 428.0
  senile 797
  specified during or due to a procedure 997.1
    long-term effect of cardiac surgery 429.4
  systolic 428.20
    acute 428.21
    acute on chronic 428.23
    chronic 428.22
  thyrotoxic (*see also* Thyrotoxicosis) 242.9 [425.7]
  valvular—*see* Endocarditis
hepatic 572.8
  acute 570
  due to a procedure 997.4
hepatorenal 572.4
hypertensive heart (*see also* Hypertension, heart) 402.91
  benign 402.11
  malignant 402.01
induction (of labor) 659.1
  abortion (legal) (*see also* Abortion, failed) 638.9
  affecting fetus or newborn 763.89
  by oxytocic drugs 659.1
  instrumental 659.0
  mechanical 659.0
  medical 659.1
  surgical 659.0
initial alveolar expansion, newborn 770.4
involution, thymus (gland) 254.8
kidney—*see* Failure, renal
lactation 676.4
Leydig's cell, adult 257.2

Failure, failed—*continued*
  liver 572.8
    acute 570
  medullary 799.89
  mitral—*see* Endocarditis, mitral
  myocardium, myocardial (*see also* Failure, heart) 428.9
    chronic (*see also* Failure, heart) 428.0
    congestive (*see also* Failure, heart) 428.0
  ovarian (primary) 256.39
    iatrogenic 256.2
    postablative 256.2
    postirradiation 256.2
    postsurgical 256.2
  ovulation 628.0
  prerenal 788.9
  renal 586
    with
      abortion—*see* Abortion, by type, with renal failure
      ectopic pregnancy (*see also* categories 633.0-633.9) 639.3
      edema (*see also* Nephrosis) 581.9
      hypertension (*see also* Hypertension, kidney) 403.91
      hypertensive heart disease (conditions classifiable to 402) 404.92
        with heart failure 404.93
        benign 404.12
          with heart failure 404.13
        malignant 404.02
          with heart failure 404.03
      molar pregnancy (*see also* categories 630-632) 639.3
      tubular necrosis (acute) 584.5
    acute 584.9
      with lesion of
        necrosis
          cortical (renal) 584.6
          medullary (renal) (papillary) 584.7
          tubular 584.5
        specified pathology NEC 584.8
    chronic 585.9
      hypertensive or with hypertension (*see also* Hypertension, kidney) 403.91
    due to a procedure 997.5
    following
      abortion 639.3
      crushing 958.5
      ectopic or molar pregnancy 639.3
      labor and delivery (acute) 669.3
    hypertensive (*see also* Hypertension, kidney) 403.91
    puerperal, postpartum 669.3
  respiration, respiratory 518.81
    acute 518.81
    acute and chronic 518.84
    center 348.8
      newborn 770.84
    chronic 518.83
    due to trauma, surgery or shock 518.5
    newborn 770.84
  rotation
    cecum 751.4
    colon 751.4
    intestine 751.4
    kidney 753.3
  segmentation—*see also* Fusion
    fingers (*see also* Syndactylism, fingers) 755.11
    toes (*see also* Syndactylism, toes) 755.13

INDEX TO DISEASES   **Fat**

Failure, failed—*continued*
  seminiferous tubule, adult 257.2
  senile (general) 797
    with psychosis 290.20
  testis, primary (seminal) 257.2
  to progress 661.2
  to thrive
    adult 783.7
    child 783.41
  transplant 996.80
    bone marrow 996.85
    organ (immune or nonimmune cause) 996.80
      bone marrow 996.85
      heart 996.83
      intestines 996.87
      kidney 996.81
      liver 996.82
      lung 996.84
      pancreas 996.86
      specified NEC 996.89
    skin 996.52
      artificial 996.55
      decellularized allodermis 996.55
      temporary allograft or pigskin graft—*omit code*
  trial of labor NEC 660.6
    affecting fetus or newborn 763.1
  tubal ligation 998.89
  urinary 586
  vacuum extraction
    abortion—*see* Abortion, failed
    delivery NEC 660.7
      affecting fetus or newborn 763.1
  vasectomy 998.89
  ventouse NEC 660.7
    affecting fetus or newborn 763.1
  ventricular (*see also* Failure, heart) 428.9
    left 428.1
      with rheumatic fever (conditions classifiable to 390)
        active 391.8
          with chorea 392.0
        inactive or quiescent (with chorea) 398.91
      hypertensive (*see also* Hypertension, heart) 402.91
        benign 402.11
        malignant 402.01
      rheumatic (chronic) (inactive) (with chorea) 398.91
        active or acute 391.8
          with chorea 392.0
    right (*see also* Failure, heart) 428.0
  vital centers, fetus or newborn 779.8
  weight gain in childhood 783.41
Fainting (fit) (spell) 780.2
Falciform hymen 752.49
Fall, maternal, affecting fetus or newborn 760.5
Fallen arches 734
Falling, any organ or part —*see* Prolapse
Fallopian
  insufflation
    fertility testing V26.21
    following sterilization reversal V26.22
  tube—*see* condition
Fallot's
  pentalogy 745.2
  tetrad or tetralogy 745.2
  triad or trilogy 746.09
Fallout, radioactive (adverse effect) NEC 990

False —*see also* condition
  bundle branch block 426.50
  bursa 727.89
  croup 478.75
  joint 733.82
  labor (pains) 644.1
  opening, urinary, male 752.69
  passage, urethra (prostatic) 599.4
  positive
    serological test for syphilis 795.6
    Wassermann reaction 795.6
  pregnancy 300.11
Family, familial —*see also* condition
  disruption V61.0
  hemophagocytic
    lymphohistiocytosis 288.4
    reticulosis 288.4
  Li-fraumeni (syndrome) V84.01
  planning advice V25.09
    natural
      procreative V26.41
      to avoid pregnancy V25.04
  problem V61.9
    specified circumstance NEC V61.8
  retinoblastoma (syndrome) 190.5
Famine 994.2
  edema 262
Fanconi's anemia (congenital pancytopenia) 284.09
Fanconi (-de Toni) (-Debré) syndrome (cystinosis) 270.0
Farber (-Uzman) syndrome or disease (disseminated lipogranulomatosis) 272.8
Farcin 024
Farcy 024
Farmers'
  lung 495.0
  skin 692.74
Farsightedness 367.0
Fascia —*see* condition
Fasciculation 781.0
Fasciculitis optica 377.32
Fasciitis 729.4
  eosinophilic 728.89
  necrotizing 728.86
  nodular 728.79
  perirenal 593.4
  plantar 728.71
  pseudosarcomatous 728.79
  traumatic (old) NEC 728.79
    current—*see* Sprain, by site
Fasciola hepatica infestation 121.3
Fascioliasis 121.3
Fasciolopsiasis (small intestine) 121.4
Fasciolopsis (small intestine) 121.4
Fast pulse 785.0
Fat
  embolism (cerebral) (pulmonary) (systemic) 958.1
    with
      abortion—*see* Abortion, by type, with embolism
      ectopic pregnancy (*see also* categories 633.0-633.9) 639.6
      molar pregnancy (*see also* categories 630-632) 639.6
    complicating delivery or puerperium 673.8
    following
      abortion 639.6
      ectopic or molar pregnancy 639.6

Fat —continued
 in pregnancy, childbirth, or the puerperium 673.8
 excessive 278.02
  in heart (see also Degeneration, myocardial) 429.1
 general 278.02
 hernia, herniation 729.30
  eyelid 374.34
  knee 729.31
  orbit 374.34
  retro-orbital 374.34
  retropatellar 729.31
  specified site NEC 729.39
 indigestion 579.8
 in stool 792.1
 localized (pad) 278.1
  heart (see also Degeneration, myocardial) 429.1
  knee 729.31
  retropatellar 729.31
 necrosis—see also Fatty, degeneration
  breast (aseptic) (segmental) 611.3
  mesentery 567.82
  omentum 567.82
  peritoneum 567.82
 pad 278.1
Fatal syncope 798.1
Fatigue 780.79
 auditory deafness (see also Deafness) 389.9
 chronic, syndrome 780.71
 combat (see also Reaction, stress, acute) 308.9
 during pregnancy 646.8
 general 780.79
  psychogenic 300.5
 heat (transient) 992.6
 muscle 729.89
 myocardium (see also Failure, heart) 428.9
 nervous 300.5
 neurosis 300.5
 operational 300.89
 postural 729.89
 posture 729.89
 psychogenic (general) 300.5
 senile 797
 syndrome NEC 300.5
  chronic 780.71
 undue 780.79
 voice 784.49
Fatness 278.02
Fatty —see also condition
 apron 278.1
 degeneration (diffuse) (general) NEC 272.8
  localized—see Degeneration, by site, fatty
  placenta—see Placenta, abnormal
 heart (enlarged) (see also Degeneration, myocardial) 429.1
 infiltration (diffuse) (general) (see also Degeneration, by site, fatty) 272.8
  heart (enlarged) (see also Degeneration, myocardial) 429.1
 liver 571.8
  alcoholic 571.0
 necrosis—see Degeneration, fatty
 phanerosis 272.8
Fauces —see condition
Fauchard's disease (periodontitis) 523.40
Faucitis 478.29
Faulty —see also condition
 position of teeth 524.30
Favism (anemia) 282.2
Favre-Racouchot disease (elastoidosis cutanea nodularis) 701.8

Favus 110.9
 beard 110.0
 capitis 110.0
 corporis 110.5
 eyelid 110.8
 foot 110.4
 hand 110.2
 scalp 110.0
 specified site NEC 110.8
Fear, fearfulness (complex) (reaction) 300.20
 child 313.0
 of
  animals 300.29
  closed spaces 300.29
  crowds 300.29
  eating in public 300.23
  heights 300.29
  open spaces 300.22
   with panic attacks 300.21
  public speaking 300.23
  streets 300.22
   with panic attacks 300.21
  travel 300.22
   with panic attacks 300.21
  washing in public 300.23
 transient 308.0
Feared complaint unfounded V65.5
Febricula (continued) (simple) (see also Pyrexia) 780.6
Febrile (see also Pyrexia) 780.6
 convulsion (simple) 780.31
  complex 780.32
 seizure (simple) 780.31
  atypical 780.32
  complex 780.32
  complicated 780.32
Febris (see also Fever) 780.6
 aestiva (see also Fever, hay) 477.9
 flava (see also Fever, yellow) 060.9
 melitensis 023.0
 pestis (see also Plague) 020.9
 puerperalis 672
 recurrens (see also Fever, relapsing) 087.9
  pediculo vestimenti 087.0
 rubra 034.1
 typhoidea 002.0
 typhosa 002.0
Fecal —see condition
Fecalith (impaction) 560.39
 with hernia—see also Hernia, by site, with obstruction
  gangrenous—see Hernia, by site, with gangrene
 appendix 543.9
 congenital 777.1
Fede's disease 529.0
Feeble-minded 317
Feeble rapid pulse due to shock following injury 958.4
Feeding
 faulty (elderly) (infant) 783.3
  newborn 779.3
 formula check V20.2
 improper (elderly) (infant) 783.3
  newborn 779.3
 problem (elderly) (infant) 783.3
  newborn 779.3
  nonorganic origin 307.59
Feeling of foreign body in throat 784.99
Feer's disease 985.0
Feet —see condition

INDEX TO DISEASES   Fever

Feigned illness V65.2
Feil-Klippel syndrome (brevicollis) 756.16
Feinmesser's (hidrotic) ectodermal dysplasia 757.31
Felix's disease (juvenile osteochondrosis, hip) 732.1
Felon (any digit) (with lymphangitis) 681.01
   herpetic 054.6
Felty's syndrome (rheumatoid arthritis with splenomegaly and leukopenia) 714.1
Feminism in boys 302.6
Feminization, testicular 259.5
   with pseudohermaphroditism, male 259.5
Femoral hernia —*see* Hernia, femoral
Femora vara 736.32
Femur, femoral —*see* condition
Fenestrata placenta —*see* Placenta, abnormal
Fenestration, fenestrated —*see also* Imperfect, closure
   aorta-pulmonary 745.0
   aorticopulmonary 745.0
   aortopulmonary 745.0
   cusps, heart valve NEC 746.89
      pulmonary 746.09
   hymen 752.49
   pulmonic cusps 746.09
Fenwick's disease 537.89
Fermentation (gastric) (gastrointestinal) (stomach) 536.8
   intestine 564.89
      psychogenic 306.4
   psychogenic 306.4
Fernell's disease (aortic aneurysm) 441.9
Fertile eunuch syndrome 257.2
Fertility, meaning multiparity—*see* Multiparity
Fetal alcohol syndrome 760.71
Fetalis uterus 752.3
Fetid
   breath 784.99
   sweat 705.89
Fetishism 302.81
   transvestic 302.3
Fetomaternal hemorrhage
   affecting management of pregnancy 656.0
   fetus or newborn 772.0
Fetus, fetal —*see also* condition
   papyraceous 779.89
   type lung tissue 770.4
Fever 780.6
   with chills 780.6
      in malarial regions (*see also* Malaria) 084.6
   abortus NEC 023.9
   Aden 061
   African tick-borne 087.1
   American
      mountain tick 066.1
      spotted 082.0
   and ague (*see also* Malaria) 084.6
   aphthous 078.4
   arbovirus hemorrhagic 065.9
   Assam 085.0
   Australian A or Q 083.0
   Bangkok hemorrhagic 065.4
   biliary, Charcot's intermittent—*see* Choledocholithiasis
   bilious, hemoglobinuric 084.8
   blackwater 084.8
   blister 054.9
   Bonvale Dam 780.79
   boutonneuse 082.1

Fever—*continued*
   brain 323.9
      late effect—*see* category 326
   breakbone 061
   Bullis 082.8
   Bunyamwera 066.3
   Burdwan 085.0
   Bwamba (encephalitis) 066.3
   Cameroon (*see also* Malaria) 084.6
   Canton 081.9
   catarrhal (acute) 460
      chronic 472.0
   cat-scratch 078.3
   cerebral 323.9
      late effect—*see* category 326
   cerebrospinal (meningococcal) (*see also* Meningitis, cerebrospinal) 036.0
   Chagres 084.0
   Chandipura 066.8
   changuinola 066.0
   Charcot's (biliary) (hepatic) (intermittent)—*see* Choledocholithiasis
   Chikungunya (viral) 066.3
      hemorrhagic 065.4
   childbed 670
   Chitral 066.0
   Colombo (*see also* Fever, paratyphoid) 002.9
   Colorado tick (virus) 066.1
   congestive
      malarial (*see also* Malaria) 084.6
      remittent (*see also* Malaria) 084.6
   Congo virus 065.0
   continued 780.6
      malarial 084.0
   Corsican (*see also* Malaria) 084.6
   Crimean hemorrhagic 065.0
   Cyprus (*see also* Brucellosis) 023.9
   dandy 061
   deer fly (*see also* Tularemia) 021.9
   dehydration, newborn 778.4
   dengue (virus) 061
      hemorrhagic 065.4
   desert 114.0
   due to heat 992.0
   Dumdum 085.0
   enteric 002.0
   ephemeral (of unknown origin) (*see also* Pyrexia) 780.6
   epidemic, hemorrhagic of the Far East 065.0
   erysipelatous (*see also* Erysipelas) 035
   estivo-autumnal (malarial) 084.0
   etiocholanolone 277.31
   famine—*see also* Fever, relapsing
      meaning typhus—*see* Typhus
   Far Eastern hemorrhagic 065.0
   five day 083.1
   Fort Bragg 100.89
   gastroenteric 002.0
   gastromalarial (*see also* Malaria) 084.6
   Gibraltar (*see also* Brucellosis) 023.9
   glandular 075
   Guama (viral) 066.3
   Haverhill 026.1
   hay (allergic) (with rhinitis) 477.9
      with
         asthma (bronchial) (*see also* Asthma) 493.0
      due to
         dander, animal (cat) (dog) 477.2
         dust 477.8
         fowl 477.8
         hair, animal (cat) (dog) 477.2

Fever—*continued*
    pollen, any plant or tree 477.0
      specified allergen other than pollen 477.8
    heat (effects) 992.0
    hematuric, bilious 084.8
    hemoglobinuric (malarial) 084.8
      bilious 084.8
    hemorrhagic (arthropod-borne) NEC 065.9
      with renal syndrome 078.6
      arenaviral 078.7
      Argentine 078.7
      Bangkok 065.4
      Bolivian 078.7
      Central Asian 065.0
      chikungunya 065.4
      Crimean 065.0
      dengue (virus) 065.4
      Ebola 065.8
      epidemic 078.6
        of Far East 065.0
      Far Eastern 065.0
      Junin virus 078.7
      Korean 078.6
      Kyasanur forest 065.2
      Machupo virus 078.7
      mite-borne NEC 065.8
      mosquito-borne 065.4
      Omsk 065.1
      Philippine 065.4
      Russian (Yaroslav) 078.6
      Singapore 065.4
      Southeast Asia 065.4
      Thailand 065.4
      tick-borne NEC 065.3
    hepatic (*see also* Cholecystitis) 575.8
      intermittent (Charcot's)—*see*
        Choledocholithiasis
    herpetic (*see also* Herpes) 054.9
    Hyalomma tick 065.0
    icterohemorrhagic 100.0
    inanition 780.6
      newborn 778.4
    infective NEC 136.9
    intermittent (bilious) (*see also* Malaria) 084.6
      hepatic (Charcot)—*see* Choledocholithiasis
      of unknown origin (*see also* Pyrexia) 780.6
    pernicious 084.0
    iodide
      correct substance properly administered 780.6
      overdose or wrong substance given or taken 975.5
    Japanese river 081.2
    jungle yellow 060.0
    Junin virus, hemorrhagic 078.7
    Katayama 120.2
    Kedani 081.2
    Kenya 082.1
    Korean hemorrhagic 078.6
    Lassa 078.89
    Lone Star 082.8
    lung—*see* Pneumonia
    Machupo virus, hemorrhagic 078.7
    malaria, malarial (*see also* Malaria) 084.6
    Malta (*see also* Brucellosis) 023.9
    Marseilles 082.1
    marsh (*see also* Malaria) 084.6
    Mayaro (viral) 066.3
    Mediterranean (*see also* Brucellosis) 023.9
      familial 277.31
      tick 082.1
    meningeal—*see* Meningitis

Fever—*continued*
    metal fumes NEC 985.8
    Meuse 083.1
    Mexican—*see* Typhus, Mexican
    Mianeh 087.1
    miasmatic (*see also* Malaria) 084.6
    miliary 078.2
    milk, female 672
    mill 504
    mite-borne hemorrhagic 065.8
    Monday 504
    mosquito-borne NEC 066.3
      hemorrhagic NEC 065.4
    mountain 066.1
      meaning
        Rocky Mountain spotted 082.0
        undulant fever (*see also* Brucellosis) 023.9
      tick (American) 066.1
    Mucambo (viral) 066.3
    mud 100.89
    Neapolitan (*see also* Brucellosis) 023.9
    neutropenic 288.00
    nine-mile 083.0
    nonexanthematous tick 066.1
    North Asian tick-borne typhus 082.2
    Omsk hemorrhagic 065.1
    O'nyong-nyong (viral) 066.3
    Oropouche (viral) 066.3
    Oroya 088.0
    paludal (*see also* Malaria) 084.6
    Panama 084.0
    pappataci 066.0
    paratyphoid 002.9
      A 002.1
      B (Schottmüller's) 002.2
      C (Hirschfeld) 002.3
    parrot 073.9
    periodic 277.31
    pernicious, acute 084.0
    persistent (of unknown origin) (*see also* Pyrexia) 780.6
    petechial 036.0
    pharyngoconjunctival 077.2
      adenoviral type 3 077.2
    Philippine hemorrhagic 065.4
    phlebotomus 066.0
    Piry 066.8
    Pixuna (viral) 066.3
    Plasmodium ovale 084.3
    pleural (*see also* Pleurisy) 511.0
    pneumonic—*see* Pneumonia
    polymer fume 987.8
    postoperative 998.89
      due to infection 998.59
    pretibial 100.89
    puerperal, postpartum 672
    putrid—*see* Septicemia
    pyemic—*see* Septicemia
    Q 083.0
      with pneumonia 083.0 [484.8]
    quadrilateral 083.0
    quartan (malaria) 084.2
    Queensland (coastal) 083.0
      seven-day 100.89
    Quintan (A) 083.1
    quotidian 084.0
    rabbit (*see also* Tularemia) 021.9
    rat-bite 026.9
      due to
        Spirillum minor or minus 026.0
        Spirochaeta morsus muris 026.0

INDEX TO DISEASES Fever

Fever—*continued*
    Streptobacillus moniliformis 026.1
  recurrent—*see* Fever, relapsing
  relapsing 087.9
    Carter's (Asiatic) 087.0
    Dutton's (West African) 087.1
    Koch's 087.9
    louse-borne (epidemic) 087.0
    Novy's (American) 087.1
    Obermeyer's (European) 087.0
    spirillum NEC 087.9
    tick-borne (endemic) 087.1
  remittent (bilious) (congestive) (gastric) (*see also* Malaria) 084.6
  rheumatic (active) (acute) (chronic) (subacute) 390
    with heart involvement 391.9
      carditis 391.9
      endocarditis (aortic) (mitral) (pulmonary) (tricuspid) 391.1
      multiple sites 391.8
      myocarditis 391.2
      pancarditis, acute 391.8
      pericarditis 391.0
      specified type NEC 391.8
      valvulitis 391.1
    inactive or quiescent with cardiac hypertrophy 398.99
      carditis 398.90
      endocarditis 397.9
        aortic (valve) 395.9
          with mitral (valve) disease 396.9
        mitral (valve) 394.9
          with aortic (valve) disease 396.9
        pulmonary (valve) 397.1
        tricuspid (valve) 397.0
      heart conditions (classifiable to 429.3, 429.6, 429.9) 398.99
        failure (congestive) (conditions classifiable to 428.0, 428.9) 398.91
        left ventricular failure (conditions classifiable to 428.1) 398.91
        myocardial degeneration (conditions classifiable to 429.1) 398.0
        myocarditis (conditions classifiable to 429.0) 398.0
      pancarditis 398.99
      pericarditis 393
  Rift Valley (viral) 066.3
  Rocky Mountain spotted 082.0
  rose 477.0
  Ross river (viral) 066.3
  Russian hemorrhagic 078.6
  sandfly 066.0
  San Joaquin (valley) 114.0
  São Paulo 082.0
  scarlet 034.1
  septic—*see* Septicemia
  seven-day 061
    Japan 100.89
    Queensland 100.89
  shin bone 083.1
  Singapore hemorrhagic 065.4
  solar 061
  sore 054.9
  South African tick-bite 087.1
  Southeast Asia hemorrhagic 065.4
  spinal—*see* Meningitis
  spirillary 026.0
  splenic (*see also* Anthrax) 022.9

Fever—*continued*
  spotted (Rocky Mountain) 082.0
    American 082.0
    Brazilian 082.0
    Colombian 082.0
    meaning
      cerebrospinal meningitis 036.0
      typhus 082.9
  spring 309.23
  steroid
    correct substance properly administered 780.6
    overdose or wrong substance given or taken 962.0
  streptobacillary 026.1
  subtertian 084.0
  Sumatran mite 081.2
  sun 061
  swamp 100.89
  sweating 078.2
  swine 003.8
  sylvatic yellow 060.0
  Tahyna 062.5
  tertian—*see* Malaria, tertian
  Thailand hemorrhagic 065.4
  thermic 992.0
  three day 066.0
    with Coxsackie exanthem 074.8
  tick
    American mountain 066.1
    Colorado 066.1
    Kemerovo 066.1
    Mediterranean 082.1
    mountain 066.1
    nonexanthematous 066.1
    Quaranfil 066.1
  tick-bite NEC 066.1
  tick-borne NEC 066.1
    hemorrhagic NEC 065.3
  transitory of newborn 778.4
  trench 083.1
  tsutsugamushi 081.2
  typhogastric 002.0
  typhoid (abortive) (ambulant) (any site) (hemorrhagic) (infection) (intermittent) (malignant) (rheumatic) 002.0
  typhomalarial (*see also* Malaria) 084.6
  typhus—*see* Typhus
  undulant (*see also* Brucellosis) 023.9
  unknown origin (*see also* Pyrexia) 780.6
  uremic—*see* Uremia
  uveoparotid 135
  valley (Coccidioidomycosis) 114.0
  Venezuelan equine 066.2
  Volhynian 083.1
  Wesselsbron (viral) 066.3
  West
    African 084.8
    Nile (viral) 066.40
      with
        cranial nerve disorders 066.42
        encephalitis 066.41
        optic neuritis 066.42
        other complications 066.49
        other neurologic manifestations 066.42
        polyradiculitis 066.42
  Whitmore's 025
  Wolhynian 083.1
  worm 128.9
  Yaroslav hemorrhagic 078.6

Fever—*continued*
  yellow 060.9
    jungle 060.0
    sylvatic 060.0
    urban 060.1
  vaccination, prophylactic (against) V04.4
  Zika (viral) 066.3
Fibrillation
  atrial (established) (paroxysmal) 427.31
  auricular (atrial) (established) 427.31
  cardiac (ventricular) 427.41
  coronary (*see also* Infarct, myocardium) 410.9
  heart (ventricular) 427.41
  muscular 728.9
  postoperative 997.1
  ventricular 427.41
Fibrin
  ball or bodies, pleural (sac) 511.0
  chamber, anterior (eye) (gelatinous exudate) 364.04
Fibrinogenolysis (hemorrhagic)—*see* Fibrinolysis
Fibrinogenopenia (congenital) (hereditary) (*see also* Defect, coagulation) 286.3
  acquired 286.6
Fibrinolysis (acquired) (hemorrhagic) (pathologic) 286.6
  with
    abortion—*see* Abortion, by type, with hemorrhage, delayed or excessive
    ectopic pregnancy (*see also* categories 633.0-633.9) 639.1
    molar pregnancy (*see also* categories 630-632) 639.1
  antepartum or intrapartum 641.3
    affecting fetus or newborn 762.1
  following
    abortion 639.1
    ectopic or molar pregnancy 639.1
  newborn, transient 776.2
  postpartum 666.3
Fibrinopenia (hereditary) (*see also* Defect, coagulation) 286.3
  acquired 286.6
Fibrinopurulent —*see* condition
Fibrinous —*see* condition
Fibroadenoma (M9010/0)
  cellular intracanalicular (M9020/0) 217
  giant (intracanalicular) (M9020/0) 217
  intracanalicular (M9011/0)
    cellular (M9020/0) 217
    giant (M9020/0) 217
  specified site—*see* Neoplasm, by site, benign
  unspecified site 217
  juvenile (M9030/0) 217
  pericanalicular (M9012/0)
    specified site—*see* Neoplasm, by site, benign
    unspecified site 217
  phyllodes (M9020/0) 217
  prostate 600.20
    with
      other lower urinary tract symptoms (LUTS) 600.21
      urinary
        obstruction 600.21
        retention 600.21
  specified site—*see* Neoplasm, by site, benign
  unspecified site 217
Fibroadenosis, breast (chronic) (cystic) (diffuse) (periodic) (segmental) 610.2

Fibroangioma (M9160/0)—*see also* Neoplasm, by site, benign
  juvenile (M9160/0)
    specified site—*see* Neoplasm, by site, benign
    unspecified site 210.7
Fibrocellulitis progressiva ossificans 728.11
Fibrochondrosarcoma (M9220/3)—*see* Neoplasm, cartilage, malignant
Fibrocystic
  disease 277.00
    bone NEC 733.29
    breast 610.1
    jaw 526.2
    kidney (congenital) 753.19
    liver 751.62
    lung 518.89
      congenital 748.4
    pancreas 277.00
  kidney (congenital) 753.19
Fibrodysplasia ossificans multiplex (progressiva) 728.11
Fibroelastosis (cordis) (endocardial) (endomyocardial) 425.3
Fibroid (tumor) (M8890/0)—*see also* Neoplasm, connective tissue, benign
  disease, lung (chronic) (*see also* Fibrosis, lung) 515
  heart (disease) (*see also* Myocarditis) 429.0
  induration, lung (chronic) (*see also* Fibrosis, lung) 515
  in pregnancy or childbirth 654.1
    affecting fetus or newborn 763.89
    causing obstructed labor 660.2
      affecting fetus or newborn 763.1
  liver—*see* Cirrhosis, liver
  lung (*see also* Fibrosis, lung) 515
  pneumonia (chronic) (*see also* Fibrosis, lung) 515
  uterus (M8890/0) (*see also* Leiomyoma, uterus) 218.9
Fibrolipoma (M8851/0) (*see also* Lipoma, by site) 214.9
Fibroliposarcoma (M8850/3)—*see* Neoplasm, connective tissue, malignant
Fibroma (M8810/0)—*see also* Neoplasm, connective tissue, benign
  ameloblastic (M9330/0) 213.1
    upper jaw (bone) 213.0
  bone (nonossifying) 733.99
    ossifying (M9262/0)—*see* Neoplasm, bone, benign
  cementifying (M9274/0)—*see* Neoplasm, bone, benign
  chondromyxoid (M9241/0)—*see* Neoplasm, bone, benign
  desmoplastic (M8823/1)—*see* Neoplasm, connective tissue, uncertain behavior
  facial (M8813/0)—*see* Neoplasm, connective tissue, benign
  invasive (M8821/1)—*see* Neoplasm, connective tissue, uncertain behavior
  molle (M8851/0) (*see also* Lipoma, by site) 214.9
  myxoid (M8811/0)—*see* Neoplasm, connective tissue, benign
  nasopharynx, nasopharyngeal (juvenile) (M9160/0) 210.7
  nonosteogenic (nonossifying)—*see* Dysplasia, fibrous
  odontogenic (M9321/0) 213.1
    upper jaw (bone) 213.0

INDEX TO DISEASES   **Fibrosis, fibrotic**

Fibroma—*continued*
  ossifying (M9262/0)—*see* Neoplasm, bone, benign
  periosteal (M8812/0)—*see* Neoplasm, bone, benign
  prostate 600.20
    with
      other lower urinary tract symptoms (LUTS) 600.21
      urinary
        obstruction 600.21
        retention 600.21
  soft (M8851/0) (*see also* Lipoma, by site) 214.9
Fibromatosis 728.79
  abdominal (M8822/1)—*see* Neoplasm, connective tissue, uncertain behavior
  aggressive (M8821/1)—*see* Neoplasm, connective tissue, uncertain behavior
  congenital generalized (CGF) 759.89
  Dupuytren's 728.6
  gingival 523.8
  plantar fascia 728.71
  proliferative 728.79
  pseudosarcomatous (proliferative) (subcutaneous) 728.79
  subcutaneous pseudosarcomatous (proliferative) 728.79
Fibromyalgia 729.1
Fibromyoma (M8890/0)—*see also* Neoplasm, connective tissue, benign
  uterus (corpus) (*see also* Leiomyoma, uterus) 218.9
    in pregnancy or childbirth 654.1
      affecting fetus or newborn 763.89
      causing obstructed labor 660.2
        affecting fetus or newborn 763.1
Fibromyositis (*see also* Myositis) 729.1
  scapulohumeral 726.2
Fibromyxolipoma (M8852/0) (*see also* Lipoma, by site) 214.9
Fibromyxoma (M8811/0)—*see* Neoplasm, connective tissue, benign
Fibromyxosarcoma (M8811/3)—*see* Neoplasm, connective tissue, malignant
Fibro-odontoma, ameloblastic (M9290/0) 213.1
  upper jaw (bone) 213.0
Fibro-osteoma (M9262/0)—*see* Neoplasm, bone, benign
Fibroplasia, retrolental 362.21
Fibropurulent —*see* condition
Fibrosarcoma (M8810/3)—*see also* Neoplasm, connective tissue, malignant
  ameloblastic (M9330/3) 170.1
    upper jaw (bone) 170.0
  congenital (M8814/3)—*see* Neoplasm, connective tissue, malignant
  fascial (M8813/3)—*see* Neoplasm, connective tissue, malignant
  infantile (M8814/3)—*see* Neoplasm, connective tissue, malignant
  odontogenic (M9330/3) 170.1
    upper jaw (bone) 170.0
  periosteal (M8812/3)—*see* Neoplasm, bone, malignant
Fibrosclerosis
  breast 610.3
  corpora cavernosa (penis) 607.89
  familial multifocal NEC 710.8
  multifocal (idiopathic) NEC 710.8
  penis (corpora cavernosa) 607.89

Fibrosis, fibrotic
  adrenal (gland) 255.8
  alveolar (diffuse) 516.3
  amnion 658.8
  anal papillae 569.49
  anus 569.49
  appendix, appendiceal, noninflammatory 543.9
  arteriocapillary—*see* Arteriosclerosis
  bauxite (of lung) 503
  biliary 576.8
    due to Clonorchis sinensis 121.1
  bladder 596.8
    interstitial 595.1
    localized submucosal 595.1
    panmural 595.1
  bone, diffuse 756.59
  breast 610.3
  capillary—*see also* Arteriosclerosis
    lung (chronic) (*see also* Fibrosis, lung) 515
  cardiac (*see also* Myocarditis) 429.0
  cervix 622.8
  chorion 658.8
  corpus cavernosum 607.89
  cystic (of pancreas) 277.00
    with
      manifestations
        gastrointestinal 277.03
        pulmonary 277.02
        specified NEC 277.09
      meconium ileus 277.01
      pulmonary exacerbation 277.02
  due to (presence of) any device, implant, or graft—*see* Complications, due to (presence of) any device, implant, or graft classified to 996.0-996.5 NEC
  ejaculatory duct 608.89
  endocardium (*see also* Endocarditis) 424.90
  endomyocardial (African) 425.0
  epididymis 608.89
  eye muscle 378.62
  graphite (of lung) 503
  heart (*see also* Myocarditis) 429.0
  hepatic—*see also* Cirrhosis, liver
    due to Clonorchis sinensis 121.1
  hepatolienal—*see* Cirrhosis, liver
  hepatosplenic—*see* Cirrhosis, liver
  infrapatellar fat pad 729.31
  interstitial pulmonary, newborn 770.7
  intrascrotal 608.89
  kidney (*see also* Sclerosis, renal) 587
  liver—*see* Cirrhosis, liver
  lung (atrophic) (capillary) (chronic) (confluent) (massive) (perialveolar) (peribronchial) 515
    with
      anthracosilicosis (occupational) 500
      anthracosis (occupational) 500
      asbestosis (occupational) 501
      bagassosis (occupational) 495.1
      bauxite 503
      berylliosis (occupational) 503
      byssinosis (occupational) 504
      calcicosis (occupational) 502
      chalicosis (occupational) 502
      dust reticulation (occupational) 504
      farmers' lung 495.0
      gannister disease (occupational) 502
      graphite 503
      pneumonoconiosis (occupational) 505
      pneumosiderosis (occupational) 503
      siderosis (occupational) 503
      silicosis (occupational) 502

Fibrosis, fibrotic—*continued*
  tuberculosis (*see also* Tuberculosis) 011.4
  diffuse (idiopathic) (interstitial) 516.3
  due to
    bauxite 503
    fumes or vapors (chemical) (inhalation) 506.4
    graphite 503
  following radiation 508.1
  postinflammatory 515
  silicotic (massive) (occupational) 502
  tuberculous (*see also* Tuberculosis) 011.4
  lymphatic gland 289.3
  median bar 600.90
    with
      other lower urinary tract symptoms (LUTS) 600.91
      urinary
        obstruction 600.91
        retention 600.91
  mediastinum (idiopathic) 519.3
  meninges 349.2
  muscle NEC 728.2
    iatrogenic (from injection) 999.9
  myocardium, myocardial (*see also* Myocarditis) 429.0
  oral submucous 528.8
  ovary 620.8
  oviduct 620.8
  pancreas 577.8
    cystic 277.00
      with
        manifestations
          gastrointestinal 277.03
          pulmonary 277.02
          specified NEC 277.09
        meconium ileus 277.01
        pulmonary exacerbation 277.02
  penis 607.89
  periappendiceal 543.9
  periarticular (*see also* Ankylosis) 718.5
  pericardium 423.1
  perineum, in pregnancy or childbirth 654.8
    affecting fetus or newborn 763.89
    causing obstructed labor 660.2
      affecting fetus or newborn 763.1
  perineural NEC 355.9
    foot 355.6
  periureteral 593.89
  placenta—*see* Placenta, abnormal
  pleura 511.0
  popliteal fat pad 729.31
  preretinal 362.56
  prostate (chronic) 600.90
    with
      other lower urinary tract symptoms (LUTS) 600.91
      urinary
        obstruction 600.91
        retention 600.91
  pulmonary (chronic) (*see also* Fibrosis, lung) 515
    alveolar capillary block 516.3
    interstitial
      diffuse (idiopathic) 516.3
      newborn 770.7
  radiation—*see* Effect, adverse, radiation
  rectal sphincter 569.49
  retroperitoneal, idiopathic 593.4
  sclerosing mesenteric (idiopathic) 567.82
  scrotum 608.89
  seminal vesicle 608.89

Fibrosis, fibrotic—*continued*
  senile 797
  skin NEC 709.2
  spermatic cord 608.89
  spleen 289.59
    bilharzial (*see also* Schistosomiasis) 120.9
  subepidermal nodular (M8832/0)—*see* Neoplasm, skin, benign
  submucous NEC 709.2
    oral 528.8
    tongue 528.8
  syncytium—*see* Placenta, abnormal
  testis 608.89
    chronic, due to syphilis 095.8
  thymus (gland) 254.8
  tunica vaginalis 608.89
  ureter 593.89
  urethra 599.84
  uterus (nonneoplastic) 621.8
    bilharzial (*see also* Schistosomiasis) 120.9
    neoplastic (*see also* Leiomyoma, uterus) 218.9
  vagina 623.8
  valve, heart (*see also* Endocarditis) 424.90
  vas deferens 608.89
  vein 459.89
    lower extremities 459.89
  vesical 595.1
Fibrositis (periarticular) (rheumatoid) 729.0
  humeroscapular region 726.2
  nodular, chronic
    Jaccoud's 714.4
    rheumatoid 714.4
  ossificans 728.11
  scapulohumeral 726.2
Fibrothorax 511.0
Fibrotic —*see* Fibrosis
Fibrous —*see* condition
Fibroxanthoma (M8831/0)—*see also* Neoplasm, connective tissue, benign
  atypical (M8831/1)—*see* Neoplasm, connective tissue, uncertain behavior
  malignant (M8831/3)—*see* Neoplasm, connective tissue, malignant
Fibroxanthosarcoma (M8831/3)—*see* Neoplasm, connective tissue, malignant
Fiedler's
  disease (leptospiral jaundice) 100.0
  myocarditis or syndrome (acute isolated myocarditis) 422.91
Fiessinger-Leroy (-Reiter) syndrome 099.3
Fiessinger-Rendu syndrome (erythema muliforme exudativum) 695.1
Fifth disease (eruptive) 057.0
  venereal 099.1
Filaria, filarial —*see* Infestation, filarial
Filariasis (*see also* Infestation, filarial) 125.9
  bancroftian 125.0
  Brug's 125.1
  due to
    bancrofti 125.0
    Brugia (Wuchereria) (malayi) 125.1
    Loa loa 125.2
    malayi 125.1
    organism NEC 125.6
    Wuchereria (bancrofti) 125.0
      malayi 125.1
  Malayan 125.1
  ozzardi 125.5
  specified type NEC 125.6
Filatoff's, Filatov's, Filatow's disease (infectious mononucleosis) 075

INDEX TO DISEASES

Findings, abnormal

File-cutters' disease 984.9
  specified type of lead—*see* Table of drugs and chemicals
Filling defect
  biliary tract 793.3
  bladder 793.5
  duodenum 793.4
  gallbladder 793.3
  gastrointestinal tract 793.4
  intestine 793.4
  kidney 793.5
  stomach 793.4
  ureter 793.5
Filtering bleb, eye (postglaucoma) (status) V45.69
  with complication or rupture 997.99
  postcataract extraction (complication) 997.99
Fimbrial cyst (congenital) 752.11
Fimbriated hymen 752.49
Financial problem affecting care V60.2
Findings, abnormal, without diagnosis (examination) (laboratory test) 796.4
  17-ketosteroids, elevated 791.9
  acetonuria 791.6
  acid phosphatase 790.5
  albumin-globulin ratio 790.99
  albuminuria 791.0
  alcohol in blood 790.3
  alkaline phosphatase 790.5
  amniotic fluid 792.3
  amylase 790.5
  anisocytosis 790.09
  antenatal screening 796.5
  anthrax positive 795.31
  antibody titers, elevated 795.79
  anticardiolipin antibody 795.79
  antigen-antibody reaction 795.79
  antiphospholipid antibody 795.79
  bacteriuria 791.9
  ballistocardiogram 794.39
  bicarbonate 276.9
  bile in urine 791.4
  bilirubin 277.4
  bleeding time (prolonged) 790.92
  blood culture, positive 790.7
  blood gas level 790.91
  blood sugar level 790.29
    high 790.29
      fasting glucose 790.21
      glucose tolerance test 790.22
    low 251.2
  C-reactive protein (CRP) 790.95
  calcium 275.40
  cancer antigen 125 [CA 125] 795.82
  carbonate 276.9
  carcinoembryonic antigen [CEA] 795.81
  casts, urine 791.7
  catecholamines 791.9
  cells, urine 791.7
  cerebrospinal fluid (color) (content) (pressure) 792.0
  cervical
    high risk human papillomavirus (HPV) DNA test positive 795.05
    low risk human papillomavirus (HPV) DNA test positive 795.09
  chloride 276.9
  cholesterol 272.9
    high 272.0
      with high triglycerides 272.2
  chromosome analysis 795.2

Findings, abnormal —*continued*
  chyluria 791.1
  circulation time 794.39
  cloudy dialysis effluent 792.5
  cloudy urine 791.9
  coagulation study 790.92
  cobalt, blood 790.6
  color of urine (unusual) NEC 791.9
  copper, blood 790.6
  crystals, urine 791.9
  culture, positive NEC 795.39
    blood 790.7
    HIV V08
    human immunodeficiency virus V08
    nose 795.39
    skin lesion NEC 795.39
    spinal fluid 792.0
    sputum 795.39
    stool 792.1
    throat 795.39
    urine 791.9
    viral
      human immunodeficiency V08
    wound 795.39
  echocardiogram 793.2
  echoencephalogram 794.01
  echogram NEC—*see* Findings, abnormal, structure
  electrocardiogram (ECG) (EKG) 794.31
  electroencephalogram (EEG) 794.02
  electrolyte level, urinary 791.9
  electromyogram (EMG) 794.17
    ocular 794.14
  electro-oculogram (EOG) 794.12
  electroretinogram (ERG) 794.11
  enzymes, serum NEC 790.5
  fibrinogen titer coagulation study 790.92
  filling defect—*see* Filling defect
  function study NEC 794.9
    auditory 794.15
    bladder 794.9
    brain 794.00
    cardiac 794.30
    endocrine NEC 794.6
      thyroid 794.5
    kidney 794.4
    liver 794.8
    nervous system
      central 794.00
      peripheral 794.19
    oculomotor 794.14
    pancreas 794.9
    placenta 794.9
    pulmonary 794.2
    retina 794.11
    special senses 794.19
    spleen 794.9
    vestibular 794.16
  gallbladder, nonvisualization 793.3
  glucose 790.29
    elevated
      fasting 790.21
      tolerance test 790.22
  glycosuria 791.5
  heart
    shadow 793.2
    sounds 785.3
  hematinuria 791.2
  hematocrit
    drop (precipitous) 790.01
    elevated 282.7

1019

Findings, abnormal — *continued*
   low 285.9
  hematologic NEC 790.99
  hematuria 599.7
  hemoglobin
    elevated 282.7
    low 285.9
  hemoglobinuria 791.2
  histological NEC 795.4
  hormones 259.9
  immunoglobulins, elevated 795.79
  indolacetic acid, elevated 791.9
  iron 790.6
  karyotype 795.2
  ketonuria 791.6
  lactic acid dehydrogenase (LDH) 790.4
  lead 790.6
  lipase 790.5
  lipids NEC 272.9
  lithium, blood 790.6
  liver function test 790.6
  lung field (coin lesion) (shadow) 793.1
  magnesium, blood 790.6
  mammogram 793.80
    calcification 793.89
    caclulus 793.89
    microcalcification 793.81
  mediastinal shift 793.2
  melanin, urine 791.9
  microbiologic NEC 795.39
  mineral, blood NEC 790.6
  myoglobinuria 791.3
  nasal swab, anthrax 795.31
  neonatal screening 796.6
  nitrogen derivatives, blood 790.6
  nonvisualization of gallbladder 793.3
  nose culture, positive 795.39
  odor of urine (unusual) NEC 791.9
  oxygen saturation 790.91
  Papanicolaou (smear) 795.1
    cervix 795.00
      with
        atypical squamous cells
          cannot exclude high grade squamous
            intrepithelial lesion (ASC-H) 795.02
          of undetermined significance (ASC-US)
            795.01
        cytologic evidence of malignancy 795.06
        high grade squamous intraepithelial lesion
          (HGSIL) 795.04
        low grade squamous intraepithelial lesion
          (LGSIL) 795.03
    dyskaryotic 795.09
    nonspecific finding NEC 795.09
  other site 795.1
  peritoneal fluid 792.9
  phonocardiogram 794.39
  phosphorus 275.3
  pleural fluid 792.9
  pneumoencephalogram 793.0
  PO$_2$-oxygen ratio 790.91
  poikilocytosis 790.09
  potassium
    deficiency 276.8
    excess 276.7
  PPD 795.5
  prostate specific antigen (PSA) 790.93
  protein, serum NEC 790.99
  proteinuria 791.0
  prothrombin time (partial) (prolonged) (PT)
    (PTT) 790.92

Findings, abnormal — *continued*
  pyuria 791.9
  radiologic (x-ray) 793.99
    abdomen 793.6
    biliary tract 793.3
    breast 793.89
      abnormal mammogram NOS 793.80
      mammographic
        calcification 793.89
        calculus 793.89
        microcalcification 793.81
    gastrointestinal tract 793.4
    genitourinary organs 793.5
    head 793.0
    image test inconclusive due to excess body fat
      793.91
    intrathoracic organs NEC 793.2
    lung 793.1
    musculoskeletal 793.7
    placenta 793.99
    retroperitoneum 793.6
    skin 793.99
    skull 793.0
    subcutaneous tissue 793.99
  red blood cell 790.09
    count 790.09
    morphology 790.09
    sickling 790.09
    volume 790.09
  saliva 792.4
  scan NEC 794.9
    bladder 794.9
    bone 794.9
    brain 794.09
    kidney 794.4
    liver 794.8
    lung 794.2
    pancreas 794.9
    placental 794.9
    spleen 794.9
    thyroid 794.5
  sedimentation rate, elevated 790.1
  semen 792.2
  serological (for)
    human immunodeficiency virus (HIV)
      inconclusive 795.71
      positive V08
    syphilis—*see* Findings, serology for syphilis
  serology for syphilis
    false positive 795.6
    positive 097.1
      false 795.6
      follow-up of latent syphilis—*see* Syphilis,
        latent
      only finding—*see* Syphilis, latent
  serum 790.99
    blood NEC 790.99
    enzymes NEC 790.5
    proteins 790.99
  SGOT 790.4
  SGPT 790.4
  sickling of red blood cells 790.09
  skin test, positive 795.79
    tuberculin (without active tuberculosis) 795.5
  sodium 790.6
    deficiency 276.1
    excess 276.0
  spermatozoa 792.2
  spinal fluid 792.0
    culture, positive 792.0
  sputum culture, positive 795.39

INDEX TO DISEASES   **Fistula**

Findings, abnormal —*continued*
  for acid-fast bacilli 795.39
  stool NEC 792.1
    bloody 578.1
      occult 792.1
    color 792.1
    culture, positive 792.1
    occult blood 792.1
  stress test 794.39
  structure, body (echogram) (thermogram)
      (ultrasound) (x-ray) NEC 793.99
    abdomen 793.6
    breast 793.89
      abnormal mammogram 793.80
      mammographic
        calcification 793.89
        calculus 793.89
        microcalcification 793.81
    gastrointestinal tract 793.4
    genitourinary organs 793.5
    head 793.0
      echogram (ultrasound) 794.01
    intrathoracic organs NEC 793.2
    lung 793.1
    musculoskeletal 793.7
    placenta 793.99
    retroperitoneum 793.6
    skin 793.99
    subcutaneous tissue NEC 793.99
  synovial fluid 792.9
  thermogram—*see* Finding, abnormal, structure
  throat culture, positive 795.39
  thyroid (function) 794.5
    metabolism (rate) 794.5
    scan 794.5
    uptake 794.5
  total proteins 790.99
  toxicology (drugs) (heavy metals) 796.0
  transaminase (level) 790.4
  triglycerides 272.9
    high 272.1
      with high cholesterol 272.2
  tuberculin skin test (without active tuberculosis) 795.5
  tumor markers NEC 795.89
  ultrasound—*see also* Finding, abnormal, structure
    cardiogram 793.2
  uric acid, blood 790.6
  urine, urinary constituents 791.9
    acetone 791.6
    albumin 791.0
    bacteria 791.9
    bile 791.4
    blood 599.7
    casts or cells 791.7
    chyle 791.1
    culture, positive 791.9
    glucose 791.5
    hemoglobin 791.2
    ketone 791.6
    protein 791.0
    pus 791.9
    sugar 791.5
  vaginal fluid 792.9
  vanillylmandelic acid, elevated 791.9
  vectorcardiogram (VCG) 794.39
  ventriculogram (cerebral) 793.0
  VMA, elevated 791.9
  Wassermann reaction
    false positive 795.6

Findings, abnormal —*continued*
  positive 097.1
    follow-up of latent syphilis—*see* Syphilis, latent
    only finding—*see* Syphilis, latent
  white blood cell 288.9
    count 288.9
      elevated 288.60
      low 288.50
    differential 288.9
    morphology 288.9
  wound culture 795.39
  xerography 793.89
  zinc, blood 790.6
Finger —*see* condition
Finnish type nephrosis (congenital) 759.89
Fire, St. Anthony's (*see also* Erysipelas) 035
Fish
  hook stomach 537.89
  meal workers' lung 495.8
Fisher's syndrome 357.0
Fissure, fissured
  abdominal wall (congenital) 756.79
  anus, anal 565.0
    congenital 751.5
  buccal cavity 528.9
  clitoris (congenital) 752.49
  ear, lobule (congenital) 744.29
  epiglottis (congenital) 748.3
  larynx 478.79
    congenital 748.3
  lip 528.5
    congenital (*see also* Cleft, lip) 749.10
  nipple 611.2
    puerperal, postpartum 676.1
  palate (congenital) (*see also* Cleft, palate) 749.00
  postanal 565.0
  rectum 565.0
  skin 709.8
    streptococcal 686.9
  spine (congenital) (*see also* Spina bifida) 741.9
  sternum (congenital) 756.3
  tongue (acquired) 529.5
    congenital 750.13
Fistula (sinus) 686.9
  abdomen (wall) 569.81
    bladder 596.2
    intestine 569.81
    ureter 593.82
    uterus 619.2
  abdominorectal 569.81
  abdominosigmoidal 569.81
  abdominothoracic 510.0
  abdominouterine 619.2
    congenital 752.3
  abdominovesical 596.2
  accessory sinuses (*see also* Sinusitis) 473.9
  actinomycotic—*see* Actinomycosis
  alveolar
    antrum (*see also* Sinusitis, maxillary) 473.0
    process 522.7
  anorectal 565.1
  antrobuccal (*see also* Sinusitis, maxillary) 473.0
  antrum (*see also* Sinusitis, maxillary) 473.0
  anus, anal (infectional) (recurrent) 565.1
    congenital 751.5
    tuberculous (*see also* Tuberculosis) 014.8
  aortic sinus 747.29
  aortoduodenal 447.2
  appendix, appendicular 543.9

Fistula

Fistula—*continued*
arteriovenous (acquired) 447.0
　brain 437.3
　　congenital 747.81
　　　ruptured (*see also* Hemorrhage,
　　　　subarachnoid) 430
　　ruptured (*see also* Hemorrhage,
　　　subarachnoid) 430
　cerebral 437.3
　　congenital 747.81
　congenital (peripheral) 747.60
　　brain—*see* Fistula, arteriovenous, brain,
　　　congenital
　　coronary 746.85
　　gastrointestinal 747.61
　　lower limb 747.64
　　pulmonary 747.3
　　renal 747.62
　　specified NEC 747.69
　　upper limb 747.63
　coronary 414.19
　　congenital 746.85
　heart 414.19
　pulmonary (vessels) 417.0
　　congenital 747.3
　surgically created (for dialysis) V45.1
　　complication NEC 996.73
　　　atherosclerosis —*see* Arteriosclerosis,
　　　　extremities
　　　embolism 996.74
　　　infection or inflammation 996.62
　　　mechanical 996.1
　　　occlusion NEC 996.74
　　　thrombus 996.74
　traumatic—*see* Injury, blood vessel, by site
artery 447.2
aural 383.81
　congenital 744.49
auricle 383.81
　congenital 744.49
Bartholin's gland 619.8
bile duct (*see also* Fistula, biliary) 576.4
biliary (duct) (tract) 576.4
　congenital 751.69
bladder (neck) (sphincter) 596.2
　into seminal vesicle 596.2
bone 733.99
brain 348.8
　arteriovenous—*see* Fistula, arteriovenous,
　　brain
branchial (cleft) 744.41
branchiogenous 744.41
breast 611.0
　puerperal, postpartum 675.1
bronchial 510.0
bronchocutaneous, bronchomediastinal,
　bronchopleural, bronchopleuromediastinal
　(infective) 510.0
　tuberculous (*see also* Tuberculosis) 011.3
bronchoesophageal 530.89
　congenital 750.3
buccal cavity (infective) 528.3
canal, ear 380.89
carotid-cavernous
　congenital 747.81
　　with hemorrhage 430
　traumatic 900.82
　　with hemorrhage (*see also* Hemorrhage,
　　　brain, traumatic) 853.0
　　late effect 908.3
cecosigmoidal 569.81

Fistula—*continued*
cecum 569.81
cerebrospinal (fluid) 349.81
cervical, lateral (congenital) 744.41
cervicoaural (congenital) 744.49
cervicosigmoidal 619.1
cervicovesical 619.0
cervix 619.8
chest (wall) 510.0
cholecystocolic (*see also* Fistula, gallbladder)
　575.5
cholecystocolonic (*see also* Fistula, gallbladder)
　575.5
cholecystoduodenal (*see also* Fistula,
　gallbladder) 575.5
cholecystoenteric (*see also* Fistula, gallbladder)
　575.5
cholecystogastric (*see also* Fistula, gallbladder)
　575.5
cholecystointestinal (*see also* Fistula,
　gallbladder) 575.5
choledochoduodenal 576.4
cholocolic (*see also* Fistula, gallbladder) 575.5
coccyx 685.1
　with abscess 685.0
colon 569.81
colostomy 569.69
colovaginal (acquired) 619.1
common duct (bile duct) 576.4
congenital, NEC—*see* Anomaly, specified type
　NEC
cornea, causing hypotony 360.32
coronary, arteriovenous 414.19
　congenital 746.85
costal region 510.0
cul-de-sac, Douglas' 619.8
cutaneous 686.9
cystic duct (*see also* Fistula, gallbladder) 575.5
　congenital 751.69
dental 522.7
diaphragm 510.0
　bronchovisceral 510.0
　pleuroperitoneal 510.0
　pulmonoperitoneal 510.0
duodenum 537.4
ear (canal) (external) 380.89
enterocolic 569.81
enterocutaneous 569.81
enteroenteric 569.81
entero-uterine 619.1
　congenital 752.3
enterovaginal 619.1
　congenital 752.49
enterovesical 596.1
epididymis 608.89
　tuberculous (*see also* Tuberculosis) 016.4
esophagobronchial 530.89
　congenital 750.3
esophagocutaneous 530.89
esophagopleurocutaneous 530.89
esophagotracheal 530.84
　congenital 750.3
esophagus 530.89
　congenital 750.4
ethmoid (*see also* Sinusitis, ethmoidal) 473.2
eyeball (cornea) (sclera) 360.32
eyelid 373.11
fallopian tube (external) 619.2
fecal 569.81
　congenital 751.5
from periapical lesion 522.7

Fistula—*continued*
  frontal sinus (*see also* Sinusitis, frontal) 473.1
  gallbladder 575.5
    with calculus, cholelithiasis, stones (*see also* Cholelithiasis) 574.2
    congenital 751.69
  gastric 537.4
  gastrocolic 537.4
    congenital 750.7
    tuberculous (*see also* Tuberculosis) 014.8
  gastroenterocolic 537.4
  gastroesophageal 537.4
  gastrojejunal 537.4
  gastrojejunocolic 537.4
  genital
    organs
      female 619.9
        specified site NEC 619.8
      male 608.89
    tract-skin (female) 619.2
  hepatopleural 510.0
  hepatopulmonary 510.0
  horseshoe 565.1
  ileorectal 569.81
  ileosigmoidal 569.81
  ileostomy 569.69
  ileovesical 596.1
  ileum 569.81
  in ano 565.1
    tuberculous (*see also* Tuberculosis) 014.8
  inner ear (*see also* Fistula, labyrinth) 386.40
  intestine 569.81
  intestinocolonic (abdominal) 569.81
  intestinoureteral 593.82
  intestinouterine 619.1
  intestinovaginal 619.1
    congenital 752.49
  intestinovesical 596.1
  involving female genital tract 619.9
    digestive-genital 619.1
    genital tract-skin 619.2
    specified site NEC 619.8
    urinary-genital 619.0
  ischiorectal (fossa) 566
  jejunostomy 569.69
  jejunum 569.81
  joint 719.80
    ankle 719.87
    elbow 719.82
    foot 719.87
    hand 719.84
    hip 719.85
    knee 719.86
    multiple sites 719.89
    pelvic region 719.85
    shoulder (region) 719.81
    specified site NEC 719.88
    tuberculous—*see* Tuberculosis, joint
    wrist 719.83
  kidney 593.89
  labium (majus) (minus) 619.8
  labyrinth, labyrinthine NEC 386.40
    combined sites 386.48
    multiple sites 386.48
    oval window 386.42
    round window 386.41
    semicircular canal 386.43
  lacrimal, lachrymal (duct) (gland) (sac) 375.61
  lacrimonasal duct 375.61
  laryngotracheal 748.3
  larynx 478.79

Fistula—*continued*
  lip 528.5
    congenital 750.25
  lumbar, tuberculous (*see also* Tuberculosis) 015.0 *[730.8]*
  lung 510.0
  lymphatic (node) (vessel) 457.8
  mamillary 611.0
  mammary (gland) 611.0
    puerperal, postpartum 675.1
  mastoid (process) (region) 383.1
  maxillary (*see also* Sinusitis, maxillary) 473.0
  mediastinal 510.0
  mediastinobronchial 510.0
  mediastinocutaneous 510.0
  middle ear 385.89
  mouth 528.3
  nasal 478.19
    sinus (*see also* Sinusitis) 473.9
  nasopharynx 478.29
  nipple—*see* Fistula, breast
  nose 478.19
  oral (cutaneous) 528.3
    maxillary (*see also* Sinusitis, maxillary) 473.0
    nasal (with cleft palate) (*see also* Cleft, palate) 749.00
  orbit, orbital 376.10
  oro-antral (*see also* Sinusitis, maxillary) 473.0
  oval window (internal ear) 386.42
  oviduct (external) 619.2
  palate (hard) 526.89
    soft 528.9
  pancreatic 577.8
  pancreaticoduodenal 577.8
  parotid (gland) 527.4
    region 528.3
  pelvoabdominointestinal 569.81
  penis 607.89
  perianal 565.1
  pericardium (pleura) (sac) (*see also* Pericarditis) 423.8
  pericecal 569.81
  perineal—*see* Fistula, perineum
  perineorectal 569.81
  perineosigmoidal 569.81
  perineo-urethroscrotal 608.89
  perineum, perineal (with urethral involvement) NEC 599.1
    tuberculous (*see also* Tuberculosis) 017.9
    ureter 593.82
  perirectal 565.1
    tuberculous (*see also* Tuberculosis) 014.8
  peritoneum (*see also* Peritonitis) 567.22
  periurethral 599.1
  pharyngo-esophageal 478.29
  pharynx 478.29
    branchial cleft (congenital) 744.41
  pilonidal (infected) (rectum) 685.1
    with abscess 685.0
  pleura, pleural, pleurocutaneous, pleuroperitoneal 510.0
    stomach 510.0
    tuberculous (*see also* Tuberculosis) 012.0
  pleuropericardial 423.8
  postauricular 383.81
  postoperative, persistent 998.6
  preauricular (congenital) 744.46
  prostate 602.8
  pulmonary 510.0
    arteriovenous 417.0
      congenital 747.3

Fistula—*continued*
   tuberculous (*see also* Tuberculosis,
      pulmonary) 011.9
  pulmonoperitoneal 510.0
  rectolabial 619.1
  rectosigmoid (intercommunicating) 569.81
  rectoureteral 593.82
  rectourethral 599.1
    congenital 753.8
  rectouterine 619.1
    congenital 752.3
  rectovaginal 619.1
    congenital 752.49
    old, postpartal 619.1
    tuberculous (*see also* Tuberculosis) 014.8
  rectovesical 596.1
    congenital 753.8
  rectovesicovaginal 619.1
  rectovulvar 619.1
    congenital 752.49
  rectum (to skin) 565.1
    tuberculous (*see also* Tuberculosis) 014.8
  renal 593.89
  retroauricular 383.81
  round window (internal ear) 386.41
  salivary duct or gland 527.4
    congenital 750.24
  sclera 360.32
  scrotum (urinary) 608.89
    tuberculous (*see also* Tuberculosis) 016.5
  semicircular canals (internal ear) 386.43
  sigmoid 569.81
    vesicoabdominal 596.1
  sigmoidovaginal 619.1
    congenital 752.49
  skin 686.9
    ureter 593.82
    vagina 619.2
  sphenoidal sinus (*see also* Sinusitis, sphenoidal)
      473.3
  splenocolic 289.59
  stercoral 569.81
  stomach 537.4
  sublingual gland 527.4
    congenital 750.24
  submaxillary
    gland 527.4
      congenital 750.24
    region 528.3
  thoracic 510.0
    duct 457.8
  thoracicoabdominal 510.0
  thoracicogastric 510.0
  thoracicointestinal 510.0
  thoracoabdominal 510.0
  thoracogastric 510.0
  thorax 510.0
  thyroglossal duct 759.2
  thyroid 246.8
  trachea (congenital) (external) (internal) 748.3
  tracheoesophageal 530.84
    congenital 750.3
    following tracheostomy 519.09
  traumatic
    arteriovenous (*see also* Injury, blood vessel,
      by site) 904.9
    brain—*see* Injury, intracranial
  tuberculous—*see* Tuberculosis, by site
  typhoid 002.0
  umbilical 759.89
  umbilico-urinary 753.8

Fistula—*continued*
  urachal, urachus 753.7
  ureter (persistent) 593.82
  ureteroabdominal 593.82
  ureterocervical 593.82
  ureterorectal 593.82
  ureterosigmoido-abdominal 593.82
  ureterovaginal 619.0
  ureterovesical 596.2
  urethra 599.1
    congenital 753.8
    tuberculous (*see also* Tuberculosis) 016.3
  urethroperineal 599.1
  urethroperineovesical 596.2
  urethrorectal 599.1
    congenital 753.8
  urethroscrotal 608.89
  urethrovaginal 619.0
  urethrovesical 596.2
  urethrovesicovaginal 619.0
  urinary (persistent) (recurrent) 599.1
  uteroabdominal (anterior wall) 619.2
    congenital 752.3
  uteroenteric 619.1
  uterofecal 619.1
  uterointestinal 619.1
    congenital 752.3
  uterorectal 619.1
    congenital 752.3
  uteroureteric 619.0
  uterovaginal 619.8
  uterovesical 619.0
    congenital 752.3
  uterus 619.8
  vagina (wall) 619.8
    postpartal, old 619.8
  vaginocutaneous (postpartal) 619.2
  vaginoileal (acquired) 619.1
  vaginoperineal 619.2
  vesical NEC 596.2
  vesicoabdominal 596.2
  vesicocervicovaginal 619.0
  vesicocolic 596.1
  vesicocutaneous 596.2
  vesicoenteric 596.1
  vesicointestinal 596.1
  vesicometrorectal 619.1
  vesicoperineal 596.2
  vesicorectal 596.1
    congenital 753.8
  vesicosigmoidal 596.1
  vesicosigmoidovaginal 619.1
  vesicoureteral 596.2
  vesicoureterovaginal 619.0
  vesicourethral 596.2
  vesicourethrorectal 596.1
  vesicouterine 619.0
    congenital 752.3
  vesicovaginal 619.0
  vulvorectal 619.1
    congenital 752.49
Fit 780.39
  apoplectic (*see also* Disease, cerebrovascular,
      acute) 436
    late effect—*see* Late effect(s) (of)
      cerebrovascular disease
  epileptic (*see also* Epilepsy) 345.9
  fainting 780.2
  hysterical 300.11
  newborn 779.0

INDEX TO DISEASES

Fitting (of)
  artificial
    arm (complete) (partial) V52.0
    breast V52.4
    eye(s) V52.2
    leg(s) (complete) (partial) V52.1
  brain neuropacemaker V53.02
  cardiac pacemaker V53.31
  carotid sinus pacemaker V53.39
  cerebral ventricle (communicating) shunt V53.01
  colostomy belt V53.5
  contact lenses V53.1
  cystostomy device V53.6
  defibrillator, automatic implantable V53.32
  dentures V52.3
  device, unspecified type V53.90
    abdominal V53.5
    cardiac
      defibrillator, automatic implantable V53.32
      pacemaker V53.31
      specified NEC V53.39
    cerebral ventricle (communicating) shunt V53.01
    insulin pump V53.91
    intrauterine contraceptive V25.1
    nervous system V53.09
    orthodontic V53.4
    orthoptic V53.1
    other device V53.99
    prosthetic V52.9
      breast V52.4
      dental V52.3
      eye V52.2
      specified type NEC V52.8
    special senses V53.09
    substitution
      auditory V53.09
      nervous system V53.09
      visual V53.09
    urinary V53.6
  diaphragm (contraceptive) V25.02
  glasses (reading) V53.1
  growth rod V54.02
  hearing aid V53.2
  ileostomy device V53.5
  intestinal appliance or device NEC V53.5
  intrauterine contraceptive device V25.1
  neuropacemaker (brain) (peripheral nerve) (spinal cord) V53.02
  orthodontic device V53.4
  orthopedic (device) V53.7
    brace V53.7
    cast V53.7
    corset V53.7
    shoes V53.7
  pacemaker (cardiac) V53.31
    brain V53.02
    carotid sinus V53.39
    peripheral nerve V53.02
    spinal cord V53.02
  prosthesis V52.9
    arm (complete) (partial) V52.0
    breast V52.4
    dental V52.3
    eye V52.2
    leg (complete) (partial) V52.1
    specified type NEC V52.8
  spectacles V53.1
  wheelchair V53.8
Fitz's syndrome (acute hemorrhagic pancreatitis) 577.0

Fitz-Hugh and Curtis syndrome 098.86
  due to
    Chlamydia trachomatis 099.56
    Neisseria gonorrhoeae (gonococcal peritonitis) 098.86
Fixation
  joint—*see* Ankylosis
  larynx 478.79
  pupil 364.76
  stapes 385.22
    deafness (*see also* Deafness, conductive) 389.04
  uterus (acquired)—*see* Malposition, uterus
  vocal cord 478.5
Flaccid —*see* condition
  foot 736.79
  forearm 736.09
  palate, congenital 750.26
Flail
  chest 807.4
    newborn 767.3
  joint (paralytic) 718.80
    ankle 718.87
    elbow 718.82
    foot 718.87
    hand 718.84
    hip 718.85
    knee 718.86
    multiple sites 718.89
    pelvic region 718.85
    shoulder (region) 718.81
    specified site NEC 718.88
    wrist 718.83
Flajani (-Basedow) syndrome or disease (exophthalmic goiter) 242.0
Flap, liver 572.8
Flare, anterior chamber (aqueous) (eye) 364.04
Flashback phenomena (drug) (hallucinogenic) 292.89
Flat
  chamber (anterior) (eye) 360.34
  chest, congenital 754.89
  electroencephalogram (EEG) 348.8
  foot (acquired) (fixed type) (painful) (postural) (spastic) 734
    congenital 754.61
      rocker bottom 754.61
      vertical talus 754.61
    rachitic 268.1
    rocker bottom (congenital) 754.61
    vertical talus, congenital 754.61
  organ or site, congenital NEC—*see* Anomaly, specified type NEC
  pelvis 738.6
    with disproportion (fetopelvic) 653.2
      affecting fetus or newborn 763.1
      causing obstructed labor 660.1
        affecting fetus or newborn 763.1
    congenital 755.69
Flatau-Schilder disease 341.1
Flattening
  head, femur 736.39
  hip 736.39
  lip (congenital) 744.89
  nose (congenital) 754.0
    acquired 738.0
Flatulence 787.3
Flatus 787.3
  vaginalis 629.89
Flax dressers' disease 504
Flea bite —*see* Injury, superficial, by site

Fleischer

Fleischer (-Kayser) ring (corneal pigmentation) 275.1 *[371.14]*
Fleischner's disease 732.3
Fleshy mole 631
Flexibilitas cerea (*see also* Catalepsy) 300.11
Flexion
   cervix —*see* Flexion, uterus
   contracture, joint (*see also* Contraction, joint) 718.4
   deformity, joint (*see also* Contraction, joint) 736.9
      hip, congenital (*see also* Subluxation, congenital, hip) 754.32
   uterus (*see also* Malposition, uterus) 621.6
Flexner's
   bacillus 004.1
   diarrhea (ulcerative) 004.1
   dysentery 004.1
Flexner-Boyd dysentery 004.2
Flexure —*see* condition
Floater, vitreous 379.24
Floating
   cartilage (joint) (*see also* Disorder, cartilage, articular) 718.0
      knee 717.6
   gallbladder (congenital) 751.69
   kidney 593.0
      congenital 753.3
   liver (congenital) 751.69
   rib 756.3
   spleen 289.59
Flooding 626.2
Floor —*see* condition
Floppy
   infant NEC 781.99
   iris syndrome 364.81
   valve syndrome (mitral) 424.0
Flu —*see also* Influenza
   gastric NEC 008.8
Fluctuating blood pressure 796.4
Fluid
   abdomen 789.59
   chest (*see also* Pleurisy, with effusion) 511.9
   heart (*see also* Failure, heart) 428.0
   joint (*see also* Effusion, joint) 719.0
   loss (acute) 276.50
      with
         hypernatremia 276.0
         hyponatremia 276.1
   lung—*see also* Edema, lung
      encysted 511.8
   peritoneal cavity 789.59
      malignant 789.51
   pleural cavity (*see also* Pleurisy, with effusion) 511.9
   retention 276.6
Flukes NEC (*see also* Infestation, fluke) 121.9
   blood NEC (*see also* Infestation, Schistosoma) 120.9
   liver 121.3
Fluor (albus) (vaginalis) 623.5
   trichomonal (Trichomonas vaginalis) 131.00
Fluorosis (dental) (chronic) 520.3
Flushing 782.62
   menopausal 627.2
Flush syndrome 259.2
Flutter
   atrial or auricular 427.32
   heart (ventricular) 427.42
      atrial 427.32
   impure 427.32
   postoperative 997.1
   ventricular 427.42

INDEX TO DISEASES

Flux (bloody) (serosanguineous) 009.0
Focal —*see* condition
Fochier's abscess —*see* Abscess, by site
Focus, Assmann's (*see also* Tuberculosis) 011.0
Fogo selvagem 694.4
Foix-Alajouanine syndrome 336.1
Folds, anomalous —*see also* Anomaly, specified type NEC
   Bowman's membrane 371.31
   Descemet's membrane 371.32
   epicanthic 743.63
   heart 746.89
   posterior segment of eye, congenital 743.54
Folie à deux 297.3
Follicle
   cervix (nabothian) (ruptured) 616.0
   graafian, ruptured, with hemorrhage 620.0
   nabothian 616.0
Folliclis (primary) (*see also* Tuberculosis) 017.0
Follicular —*see also* condition
   cyst (atretic) 620.0
Folliculitis 704.8
   abscedens et suffodiens 704.8
   decalvans 704.09
   gonorrheal (acute) 098.0
      chronic or duration of 2 months or more 098.2
   keloid, keloidalis 706.1
   pustular 704.8
   ulerythematosa reticulata 701.8
Folliculosis, conjunctival 372.02
Folling's disease (phenylketonuria) 270.1
Follow-up (examination) (routine) (following) V67.9
   cancer chemotherapy V67.2
   chemotherapy V67.2
   fracture V67.4
   high-risk medication V67.51
   injury NEC V67.59
   postpartum
      immediately after delivery V24.0
      routine V24.2
   psychiatric V67.3
   psychotherapy V67.3
   radiotherapy V67.1
   specified condition NEC V67.59
   specified surgery NEC V67.09
   surgery V67.00
      vaginal pap smear V67.01
   treatment V67.9
      combined NEC V67.6
      fracture V67.4
      involving high-risk medication NEC V67.51
      mental disorder V67.3
      specified NEC V67.59
Fong's syndrome (hereditary osteoonychodysplasia) 756.89
Food
   allergy 693.1
   anaphylactic shock—*see* Anaphylactic shock, due to, food
   asphyxia (from aspiration or inhalation) (*see also* Asphyxia, food) 933.1
   choked on (*see also* Asphyxia, food) 933.1
   deprivation 994.2
      specified kind of food NEC 269.8
   intoxication (*see also* Poisoning, food) 005.9
   lack of 994.2
   poisoning (*see also* Poisoning, food) 005.9
   refusal or rejection NEC 307.59
   strangulation or suffocation (*see also* Asphyxia, food) 933.1
   toxemia (*see also* Poisoning, food) 005.9

INDEX TO DISEASES — Foreign body

Foot —*see also* condition
and mouth disease 078.4
process disease 581.3
Foramen ovale (nonclosure) (patent) (persistent) 745.5
Forbes' (glycogen storage) disease 271.0
Forbes-Albright syndrome (nonpuerperal amenorrhea and lactation associated with pituitary tumor) 253.1
Forced birth or delivery NEC 669.8
affecting fetus or newborn NEC 763.89
Forceps
delivery NEC 669.5
affecting fetus or newborn 763.2
Fordyce's disease (ectopic sebaceous glands) (mouth) 750.26
Fordyce-Fox disease (apocrine miliaria) 705.82
Forearm —*see* condition
Foreign body

> Note—For foreign body with open wound or other injury, see Wound, open, or the type of injury specified.

accidentally left during a procedure 998.4
anterior chamber (eye) 871.6
  magnetic 871.5
    retained or old 360.51
  retained or old 360.61
ciliary body (eye) 871.6
  magnetic 871.5
    retained or old 360.52
  retained or old 360.62
entering through orifice (current) (old)
  accessory sinus 932
  air passage (upper) 933.0
    lower 934.8
  alimentary canal 938
  alveolar process 935.0
  antrum (Highmore) 932
  anus 937
  appendix 936
  asphyxia due to (*see also* Asphyxia, food) 933.1
  auditory canal 931
  auricle 931
  bladder 939.0
  bronchioles 934.8
  bronchus (main) 934.1
  buccal cavity 935.0
  canthus (inner) 930.1
  cecum 936
  cervix (canal) uterine 939.1
  coil, ileocecal 936
  colon 936
  conjunctiva 930.1
  conjunctival sac 930.1
  cornea 930.0
  digestive organ or tract NEC 938
  duodenum 936
  ear (external) 931
  esophagus 935.1
  eye (external) 930.9
    combined sites 930.8
    intraocular—*see* Foreign body, by site
    specified site NEC 930.8
  eyeball 930.8
    intraocular—*see* Foreign body, intraocular
  eyelid 930.1
    retained or old 374.86
  frontal sinus 932

Foreign body—*continued*
  gastrointestinal tract 938
  genitourinary tract 939.9
  globe 930.8
    penetrating 871.6
      magnetic 871.5
        retained or old 360.50
      retained or old 360.60
  gum 935.0
  Highmore's antrum 932
  hypopharynx 933.0
  ileocecal coil 936
  ileum 936
  inspiration (of) 933.1
  intestine (large) (small) 936
  lacrimal apparatus, duct, gland, or sac 930.2
  larynx 933.1
  lung 934.8
  maxillary sinus 932
  mouth 935.0
  nasal sinus 932
  nasopharynx 933.0
  nose (passage) 932
  nostril 932
  oral cavity 935.0
  palate 935.0
  penis 939.3
  pharynx 933.0
  pyriform sinus 933.0
  rectosigmoid 937
    junction 937
  rectum 937
  respiratory tract 934.9
    specified part NEC 934.8
  sclera 930.1
  sinus 932
    accessory 932
    frontal 932
    maxillary 932
    nasal 932
    pyriform 933.0
  small intestine 936
  stomach (hairball) 935.2
  suffocation by (*see also* Asphyxia, food) 933.1
  swallowed 938
    tongue 933.0
  tear ducts or glands 930.2
  throat 933.0
  tongue 935.0
    swallowed 933.0
  tonsil, tonsillar 933.0
    fossa 933.0
  trachea 934.0
  ureter 939.0
  urethra 939.0
  uterus (any part) 939.1
  vagina 939.2
  vulva 939.2
  wind pipe 934.0
feeling of, in throat 784.99
granuloma (old) 728.82
  bone 733.99
  in operative wound (inadvertently left) 998.4
    due to surgical material intentionally left—*see* Complications, due to (presence of) any device, implant, or graft classified to 996.0-996.5 NEC
  muscle 728.82
  skin 709.4
  soft tissue 709.1
  subcutaneous tissue 709.4

Foreign body—*continued*
  in
    bone (residual) 733.99
    open wound—*see* Wound, open, by site
      complicated
    soft tissue (residual) 729.6
  inadvertently left in operation wound (causing
    adhesions, obstruction, or perforation) 998.4
  ingestion, ingested NEC 938
  inhalation or inspiration (*see also* Asphyxia,
    food) 933.1
  internal organ, not entering through an
    orifice—*see* Injury, internal, by site, with
    open wound
  intraocular (nonmagnetic) 871.6
    combined sites 871.6
      magnetic 871.5
        retained or old 360.59
      retained or old 360.69
    magnetic 871.5
      retained or old 360.50
    retained or old 360.60
    specified site NEC 871.6
      magnetic 871.5
        retained or old 360.59
      retained or old 360.69
  iris (nonmagnetic) 871.6
    magnetic 871.5
      retained or old 360.52
    retained or old 360.62
  lens (nonmagnetic) 871.6
    magnetic 871.5
      retained or old 360.53
    retained or old 360.63
  lid, eye 930.1
  ocular muscle 870.4
    retained or old 376.6
  old or residual
    bone 733.99
    eyelid 374.86
    middle ear 385.83
    muscle 729.6
      ocular 376.6
    retrobulbar 376.6
    skin 729.6
      with granuloma 709.4
    soft tissue 729.6
      with granuloma 709.4
    subcutaneous tissue 729.6
      with granuloma 709.4
  operation wound, left accidentally 998.4
  orbit 870.4
    retained or old 376.6
  posterior wall, eye 871.6
    magnetic 871.5
      retained or old 360.55
    retained or old 360.65
  respiratory tree 934.9
    specified site NEC 934.8
  retained (old) (nonmagnetic) (in)
    anterior chamber (eye) 360.61
      magnetic 360.51
    ciliary body 360.62
      magnetic 360.52
    eyelid 374.86
    globe 360.60
      magnetic 360.50
    intraocular 360.60
      magnetic 360.50
      specified site NEC 360.69
        magnetic 360.59

Foreign body—*continued*
  iris 360.62
    magnetic 360.52
  lens 360.63
    magnetic 360.53
  muscle 729.6
  orbit 376.6
  posterior wall of globe 360.65
    magnetic 360.55
  retina 360.65
    magnetic 360.55
  retrobulbar 376.6
  skin 729.6
    with granuloma 709.4
  soft tissue 729.6
    with granuloma 709.4
  subcutaneous tissue 729.6
    with granuloma 709.4
  vitreous 360.64
    magnetic 360.54
  retina 871.6
    magnetic 871.5
      retained or old 360.55
    retained or old 360.65
  superficial, without major open wound (*see also*
    Injury, superficial, by site) 919.6
  swallowed NEC 938
  throat, feeling of 784.99
  vitreous (humor) 871.6
    magnetic 871.5
      retained or old 360.54
    retained or old 360.64
Forking, aqueduct of Sylvius 742.3
  with spina bifida (*see also* Spina bifida) 741.0
Formation
  bone in scar tissue (skin) 709.3
  connective tissue in vitreous 379.25
  Elschnig pearls (postcataract extraction) 366.51
  hyaline in cornea 371.49
  sequestrum in bone (due to infection) (*see also*
    Osteomyelitis) 730.1
  valve
    colon, congenital 751.5
    ureter (congenital) 753.29
Formication 782.0
Fort Bragg fever 100.89
Fossa —*see also* condition
  pyriform—*see* condition
Foster-Kennedy syndrome 377.04
Fothergill's
  disease, meaning scarlatina anginosa 034.1
  neuralgia (*see also* Neuralgia, trigeminal) 350.1
Foul breath 784.99
Found dead (cause unknown) 798.9
Foundling V20.0
Fournier's disease (idiopathic gangrene) 608.83
Fourth
  cranial nerve—*see* condition
  disease 057.8
  molar 520.1
Foville's syndrome 344.89
Fox's
  disease (apocrine miliaria) 705.82
  impetigo (contagiosa) 684
Fox-Fordyce disease (apocrine miliaria) 705.82

INDEX TO DISEASES   **Fracture**

Fracture (abduction) (adduction) (avulsion) (compression) (crush) (dislocation) (oblique) (separation) (closed) 829.0

> *Note—For fracture of any of the following sites with fracture of other bones—see Fracture, multiple.*
>
> *"Closed" includes the following descriptions of fractures, with or without delayed healing, unless they are specified as open or compound:*
>
> *comminuted*
> *depressed*
> *elevated*
> *fissured*
> *greenstick*
> *impacted*
> *linear*
> *simple*
> *slipped epiphysis*
> *spiral*
> *unspecified*
>
> *"Open" includes the following descriptions of fractures, with or without delayed healing:*
>
> *compound*
> *infected*
> *missile*
> *puncture*
> *with foreign body*
>
> *For late effect of fracture, see Late, effect, fracture, by site.*

with
   internal injuries in same region (conditions classifiable to 860-869)—*see also* Injury, internal, by site
   pelvic region—*see* Fracture, pelvis
acetabulum (with visceral injury) (closed) 808.0
   open 808.1
acromion (process) (closed) 811.01
   open 811.11
alveolus (closed) 802.8
   open 802.9
ankle (malleolus) (closed) 824.8
   bimalleolar (Dupuytren's) (Pott's) 824.4
     open 824.5
   bone 825.21
     open 825.31
   lateral malleolus only (fibular) 824.2
     open 824.3
   medial malleolus only (tibial) 824.0
     open 824.1
   open 824.9
   pathologic 733.16
   talus 825.21
     open 825.31
   trimalleolar 824.6
     open 824.7
antrum—*see* Fracture, skull, base
arm (closed) 818.0
   and leg(s) (any bones) 828.0
     open 828.1
   both (any bones) (with rib(s)) (with sternum) 819.0
     open 819.1
   lower 813.80
     open 813.90
   open 818.1

Fracture—*continued*
   upper—*see* Fracture, humerus
astragalus (closed) 825.21
   open 825.31
atlas—*see* Fracture, vertebra, cervical, first
axis—*see* Fracture, vertebra, cervical, second
back—*see* Fracture, vertebra, by site
Barton's—*see* Fracture, radius, lower end
basal (skull)—*see* Fracture, skull, base
Bennett's (closed) 815.01
   open 815.11
bimalleolar (closed) 824.4
   open 824.5
bone (closed) NEC 829.0
   birth injury NEC 767.3
   open 829.1
   pathologic NEC (*see also* Fracture, pathologic) 733.10
   stress NEC (*see also* Fracture, stress) 733.95
boot top—*see* Fracture, fibula
boxers'—*see* Fracture, metacarpal bone(s)
breast bone—*see* Fracture, sternum
bucket handle (semilunar cartilage)—*see* Tear, meniscus
burst—*see* Fracture, traumatic, by site
bursting—*see* Fracture, phalanx, hand, distal
calcaneus (closed) 825.0
   open 825.1
capitate (bone) (closed) 814.07
   open 814.17
capitellum (humerus) (closed) 812.49
   open 812.59
carpal bone(s) (wrist NEC) (closed) 814.00
   open 814.10
   specified site NEC 814.09
     open 814.19
cartilage, knee (semilunar)—*see* Tear, meniscus
cervical—*see* Fracture, vertebra, cervical
chauffeur's—*see* Fracture, ulna, lower end
chisel—*see* Fracture, radius, upper end
clavicle (interligamentous part) (closed) 810.00
   acromial end 810.03
     open 810.13
   due to birth trauma 767.2
   open 810.10
   shaft (middle third) 810.02
     open 810.12
   sternal end 810.01
     open 810.11
clayshovelers'—*see* Fracture, vertebra, cervical
coccyx—*see also* Fracture, vertebra, coccyx
   complicating delivery 665.6
collar bone—*see* Fracture, clavicle
Colles' (reversed) (closed) 813.41
   open 813.51
comminuted—*see* Fracture, by site
compression—*see also* Fracture, by site
   nontraumatic—*see* Fracture, pathologic
congenital 756.9
coracoid process (closed) 811.02
   open 811.12
coronoid process (ulna) (closed) 813.02
   mandible (closed) 802.23
     open 802.33
   open 813.12
corpus cavernosum penis 959.13
costochondral junction—*see* Fracture, rib
costosternal junction—*see* Fracture, rib
cranium—*see* Fracture, skull, by site
cricoid cartilage (closed) 807.5
   open 807.6

1029

Fracture INDEX TO DISEASES

Fracture—*continued*
  cuboid (ankle) (closed) 825.23
    open 825.33
  cuneiform
    foot (closed) 825.24
      open 825.34
    wrist (closed) 814.03
      open 814.13
  dental implant 525.73
  dental restorative material
    with loss of material 525.64
    without loss of material 525.63
  due to
    birth injury—*see* Birth injury, fracture
    gunshot—*see* Fracture, by site, open
    neoplasm—*see* Fracture, pathologic
    osteoporosis—*see* Fracture, pathologic
  Dupuytren's (ankle) (fibula) (closed) 824.4
    open 824.5
    radius 813.42
      open 813.52
  Duverney's—*see* Fracture, ilium
  elbow—*see also* Fracture, humerus, lower end
    olecranon (process) (closed) 813.01
      open 813.11
    supracondylar (closed) 812.41
      open 812.51
  ethmoid (bone) (sinus)—*see* Fracture, skull, base
  face bone(s) (closed) NEC 802.8
    with
      other bone(s)—*see also* Fracture, multiple, skull
      skull—*see also* Fracture, skull
        involving other bones—*see* Fracture, multiple, skull
    open 802.9
  fatigue—*see* Fracture, march
  femur, femoral (closed) 821.00
    cervicotrochanteric 820.03
      open 820.13
    condyles, epicondyles 821.21
      open 821.31
    distal end—*see* Fracture, femur, lower end
    epiphysis (separation)
      capital 820.01
        open 820.11
      head 820.01
        open 820.11
      lower 821.22
        open 821.32
      trochanteric 820.01
        open 820.11
      upper 820.01
        open 820.11
    head 820.09
      open 820.19
    lower end or extremity (distal end) (closed) 821.20
      condyles, epicondyles 821.21
        open 821.31
      epiphysis (separation) 821.22
        open 821.32
      multiple sites 821.29
        open 821.39
      open 821.30
      specified site NEC 821.29
        open 821.39
      supracondylar 821.23
        open 821.33
      T-shaped 821.21

Fracture—*continued*
      open 821.31
    neck (closed) 820.8
      base (cervicotrochanteric) 820.03
        open 820.13
      extracapsular 820.20
        open 820.30
      intertrochanteric (section) 820.21
        open 820.31
      intracapsular 820.00
        open 820.10
      intratrochanteric 820.21
        open 821.31
      midcervical 820.02
        open 820.12
      open 820.9
      pathologic 733.14
        specified part NEC 733.15
      specified site NEC 820.09
        open 820.19
      transcervical 820.02
        open 820.12
      transtrochanteric 820.20
        open 820.30
    open 821.10
    pathologic 733.14
      specified part NEC 733.15
    peritrochanteric (section) 820.20
      open 820.30
    shaft (lower third) (middle third) (upper third) 821.01
      open 821.11
    subcapital 820.09
      open 820.19
    subtrochanteric (region) (section) 820.22
      open 820.32
    supracondylar 821.23
      open 821.33
    transepiphyseal 820.01
      open 820.11
    trochanter (greater) (lesser) (*see also* Fracture, femur, neck, by site) 820.20
      open 820.30
    T-shaped, into knee joint 821.21
      open 821.31
    upper end 820.8
      open 820.9
  fibula (closed) 823.81
    with tibia 823.82
      open 823.92
    distal end 824.8
      open 824.9
    epiphysis
      lower 824.8
        open 824.9
      upper—*see* Fracture, fibula, upper end
    head—*see* Fracture, fibula, upper end
    involving ankle 824.2
      open 824.3
    lower end or extremity 824.8
      open 824.9
    malleolus (external) (lateral) 824.2
      open 824.3
    open NEC 823.91
    pathologic 733.16
    proximal end—*see* Fracture, fibula, upper end
    shaft 823.21
      with tibia 823.22
        open 823.32
      open 823.31
    stress 733.93

1030

INDEX TO DISEASES Fracture

Fracture—*continued*
  torus 853.41
    with tibia 823.42
  upper end or extremity (epiphysis) (head) (proximal end) (styloid) 823.01
    with tibia 823.02
      open 823.12
    open 823.11
  finger(s), of one hand (closed) (*see also* Fracture, phalanx, hand) 816.00
    with
      metacarpal bone(s), of same hand 817.0
        open 817.1
      thumb of same hand 816.03
        open 816.13
    open 816.10
  foot, except toe(s) alone (closed) 825.20
    open 825.30
  forearm (closed) NEC 813.80
    lower end (distal end) (lower epiphysis) 813.40
      open 813.50
    open 813.90
    shaft 813.20
      open 813.30
    upper end (proximal end) (upper epiphysis) 813.00
      open 813.10
  fossa, anterior, middle, or posterior—*see* Fracture, skull, base
  frontal (bone)—*see also* Fracture, skull, vault
    sinus—*see* Fracture, skull base
  Galeazzi's—*see* Fracture, radius, lower end
  glenoid (cavity) (fossa) (scapula) (closed) 811.03
    open 811.13
  Gosselin's—*see* Fracture, ankle
  greenstick—*see* Fracture, by site
  grenade-throwers'—*see* Fracture, humerus, shaft
  gutter—*see* Fracture, skull, vault
  hamate (closed) 814.08
    open 814.18
  hand, one (closed) 815.00
    carpals 814.00
      open 814.10
      specified site NEC 814.09
        open 814.19
    metacarpals 815.00
      open 815.10
    multiple, bones of one hand 817.0
      open 817.1
    open 815.10
    phalanges (*see also* Fracture, phalanx, hand) 816.00
      open 816.10
  healing
    aftercare (*see also* Aftercare, fracture) V54.89
    change of cast V54.89
    complications—*see* condition
    convalescence V66.4
    removal of
      cast V54.89
      fixation device
        external V54.89
        internal V54.01
  heel bone (closed) 825.0
    open 825.1
  hip (closed) (*see also* Fracture, femur, neck) 820.8
    open 820.9

Fracture—*continued*
  pathologic 733.14
  humerus (closed) 812.20
    anatomical neck 812.02
      open 812.12
    articular process (*see also* Fracture, humerus, condyle(s) 812.44
      open 812.54
    capitellum 812.49
      open 812.59
    condyle(s) 812.44
      lateral (external) 812.42
        open 812.52
      medial (internal epicondyle) 812.43
        open 812.53
      open 812.54
    distal end—*see* Fracture, humerus, lower end
    epiphysis
      lower (*see also* Fracture, humerus, condyle(s)) 812.44
        open 812.54
      upper 812.09
        open 812.19
    external condyle 812.42
      open 812.52
    great tuberosity 812.03
      open 812.13
    head 812.09
      open 812.19
    internal epicondyle 812.43
      open 812.53
    lesser tuberosity 812.09
      open 812.19
    lower end or extremity (distal end) (*see also* Fracture, humerus, by site) 812.40
      multiple sites NEC 812.49
        open 812.59
      open 812.50
      specified site NEC 812.49
        open 812.59
    neck 812.01
      open 812.11
    open 812.30
    pathologic 733.11
    proximal end—*see* Fracture, humerus, upper end
    shaft 812.21
      open 812.31
    supracondylar 812.41
      open 812.51
    surgical neck 812.01
      open 812.11
    trochlea 812.49
      open 812.59
    T-shaped 812.44
      open 812.54
    tuberosity—*see* Fracture, humerus, upper end
    upper end or extremity (proximal end) (*see also* Fracture, humerus, by site) 812.00
      open 812.10
      specified site NEC 812.09
        open 812.19
  hyoid bone (closed) 807.5
    open 807.6
  hyperextension—*see* Fracture, radius, lower end
  ilium (with visceral injury) (closed) 808.41
    open 808.51
  impaction, impacted—*see* Fracture, by site
  incus—*see* Fracture, skull, base
  innominate bone (with visceral injury) (closed) 808.49

1031

Fracture

Fracture—*continued*
  open 808.59
  instep, of one foot (closed) 825.20
    with toe(s) of same foot 827.0
      open 827.1
    open 825.30
  insufficiency—*see* Fracture, pathologic, by site
  internal
    ear—*see* Fracture, skull, base
    semilunar cartilage, knee—*see* Tear, meniscus, medial
  intertrochanteric—*see* Fracture, femur, neck, intertrochanteric
  ischium (with visceral injury) (closed) 808.42
    open 808.52
  jaw (bone) (lower) (closed) (*see also* Fracture, mandible) 802.20
    angle 802.25
      open 802.35
    open 802.30
    upper—*see* Fracture, maxilla
  knee
    cap (closed) 822.0
      open 822.1
    cartilage (semilunar)—*see* Tear, meniscus
  labyrinth (osseous)—*see* Fracture, skull, base
  larynx (closed) 807.5
    open 807.6
  late effect—*see* Late, effects (of), fracture
  Le Fort's—*see* Fracture, maxilla
  leg (closed) 827.0
    with rib(s) or sternum 828.0
      open 828.1
    both (any bones) 828.0
      open 828.1
    lower—*see* Fracture, tibia
      open 827.1
    upper—*see* Fracture, femur
  limb
    lower (multiple) (closed) NEC 827.0
      open 827.1
    upper (multiple) (closed) NEC 818.0
      open 818.1
  long bones, due to birth trauma—*see* Birth injury, fracture
  lumbar—*see* Fracture, vertebra, lumbar
  lunate bone (closed) 814.02
    open 814.12
  malar bone (closed) 802.4
    open 802.5
  Malgaigne's (closed) 808.43
    open 808.53
  malleolus (closed)0 824.8
    bimalleolar 824.4
      open 824.5
    lateral 824.2
      and medial—*see also* Fracture, malleolus, bimalleolar
      with lip of tibia—*see* Fracture, malleolus, trimalleolar
      open 824.3
    medial (closed) 824.0
      and lateral—*see also* Fracture, malleolus, bimalleolar
      with lip of tibia—*see* Fracture, malleolus, trimalleolar
      open 824.1
    open 824.9
    trimalleolar (closed) 824.6
      open 824.7
  malleus—*see* Fracture, skull, base

Fracture—*continued*
  malunion 733.81
  mandible (closed) 802.20
    angle 802.25
      open 802.35
    body 802.28
      alveolar border 802.27
        open 802.37
      open 802.38
      symphysis 802.26
        open 802.36
    condylar process 802.21
      open 802.31
    coronoid process 802.23
      open 802.33
    multiple sites 802.29
      open 802.39
    open 802.30
    ramus NEC 802.24
      open 802.34
    subcondylar 802.22
      open 802.32
  manubrium—*see* Fracture, sternum
  march 733.95
    fibula 733.93
    metatarsals 733.94
    tibia 733.93
  maxilla, maxillary (superior) (upper jaw) (closed) 802.4
    inferior—*see* Fracture, mandible
    open 802.5
  meniscus, knee—*see* Tear, meniscus
  metacarpus, metacarpal (bone(s)), of one hand (closed) 815.00
    with phalanx, phalanges, hand (finger(s)) (thumb) of same hand 817.0
      open 817.1
    base 815.02
      first metacarpal 815.01
        open 815.11
      open 815.12
      thumb 815.01
        open 815.11
    multiple sites 815.09
      open 815.19
    neck 815.04
      open 815.14
    open 815.10
    shaft 815.03
      open 815.13
  metatarsus, metatarsal (bone(s)), of one foot (closed) 825.25
    with tarsal bone(s) 825.29
      open 825.39
    open 825.35
  Monteggia's (closed) 813.03
    open 813.13
  Moore's—*see* Fracture, radius, lower end
  multangular bone (closed)
    larger 814.05
      open 814.15
    smaller 814.06
      open 814.16

Fracture—*continued*
multiple (closed) 829.0

> Note—Multiple fractures of sites classifiable to the same three- or four-digit category are coded to that category, except for sites classifiable to 810-818 or 820-827 in different limbs.
>
> Multiple fractures of sites classifiable to different fourth-digit subdivisions within the same three-digit category should be dealt with according to coding rules.
>
> Multiple fractures of sites classifiable to different three-digit categories (identifiable from the listing under "Fracture"), and of sites classifiable to 810-818 or 820-827 in different limbs should be coded according to the following list, which should be referred to in the following priority order: skull or face bones, pelvis or vertebral column, legs, arms.

    arm (multiple bones in same arm except in hand alone) (sites classifiable to 810-817 with sites classifiable to a different three-digit category in 810-817 in same arm) (closed) 818.0
      open 818.1
    arms, both or arm(s) with rib(s) or sternum (sites classifiable to 810-818 with sites classifiable to same range of categories in other limb or to 807) (closed) 819.0
      open 819.1
    bones of trunk NEC (closed) 809.0
      open 809.1
    hand, metacarpal bone(s) with phalanx or phalanges of same hand (sites classifiable to 815 with sites classifiable to 816 in same hand) (closed) 817.0
      open 817.1
    leg (multiple bones in same leg) (sites classifiable to 820-826 with sites classifiable to a different three-digit category in that range in same leg) (closed) 827.0
      open 827.1
    legs, both or leg(s) with arm(s), rib(s), or sternum (sites classifiable to 820-827 with sites classifiable to same range of categories in other leg or to 807 or 810-819) (closed) 828.0
      open 828.1
    open 829.1
    pelvis with other bones except skull or face bones (sites classifiable to 808 with sites classifiable to 805-807 or 810-829) (closed) 809.0
      open 809.1
    skull, specified or unspecified bones, or face bone(s) with any other bone(s) (sites classifiable to 800-803 with sites classifiable to 805-829) (closed) 804.0

Fracture—*continued*

> Note—Use the following fifth-digit subclassification with categories 800, 801, 803, and 804:
>
> 0 unspecified state of consciousness
> 1 with no loss of consciousness
> 2 with brief [less than one hour] loss of consciousness
> 3 with moderate [1-24 hours] loss of consciousness
> 4 with prolonged [more than 24 hours] loss of consciousness and return to pre-existing conscious level
> 5 with prolonged [more than 24 hours] loss of consciousness, without return to pre-existing conscious level
> Use fifth-digit 5 to designate when a patient is unconcious and dies before regaining conciousness, regardless of the duration of the loss of conciousness
> 6 with loss of consciousness of unspecified duration
> 9 with concussion, unspecified

    with
      contusion, cerebral 804.1
      epidural hemorrhage 804.2
      extradural hemorrhage 804.2
      hemorrhage (intracranial) NEC 804.3
      intracranial injury NEC 804.4
      laceration, cerebral 804.1
      subarachnoid hemorrhage 804.2
      subdural hemorrhage 804.2
    open 804.5
      with
        contusion, cerebral 804.6
        epidural hemorrhage 804.7
        extradural hemorrhage 804.7
        hemorrhage (intracranial) NEC 804.8
        intracranial injury NEC 804.9
        laceration, cerebral 804.6
        subarachnoid hemorrhage 804.7
        subdural hemorrhage 804.7
    vertebral column with other bones, except skull or face bones (sites classifiable to 805 or 806 with sites classifiable to 807-808 or 810-829) (closed) 809.0
      open 809.1
  nasal (bone(s)) (closed) 802.0
    open 802.1
    sinus—*see* Fracture, skull, base
  navicular
    carpal (wrist) (closed) 814.01
      open 814.11
    tarsal (ankle) (closed) 825.22
      open 825.32
  neck—*see* Fracture, vertebra, cervical
  neural arch—*see* Fracture, vertebra, by site
  nonunion 733.82
  nose, nasal (bone) (septum) (closed) 802.0
    open 802.1
  occiput—*see* Fracture, skull, base
  odontoid process—*see* Fracture, vertebra, cervical
  olecranon (process) (ulna) (closed) 813.01
    open 813.11
  orbit, orbital (bone) (region) (closed) 802.8
    floor (blow-out) 802.6
      open 802.7

Fracture — *continued*
   open 802.9
   roof—*see* Fracture, skull, base
   specified part NEC 802.8
      open 802.9
  os
    calcis (closed) 825.0
      open 825.1
    magnum (closed) 814.07
      open 814.17
    pubis (with visceral injury) (closed) 808.2
      open 808.3
    triquetrum (closed) 814.03
      open 814.13
  osseous
    auditory meatus—*see* Fracture, skull, base
    labyrinth—*see* Fracture, skull, base
    ossicles, auditory (incus) (malleus)
      (stapes)—*see* Fracture, skull, base
  osteoporotic—*see* Fracture, pathologic
  palate (closed) 802.8
    open 802.9
  paratrooper—*see* Fracture, tibia, lower end
  parietal bone—*see* Fracture, skull, vault
  parry—*see* Fracture, Monteggia's
  patella (closed) 822.0
    open 822.1
  pathologic (cause unknown) 733.10
    ankle 733.16
    femur (neck) 733.14
      specified NEC 733.15
    fibula 733.16
    hip 733.14
    humerus 733.11
    radius 733.12
    specified site NEC 733.19
    tibia 733.16
    ulna 733.12
    vertebrae (collapse) 733.13
    wrist 733.12
  pedicle (of vertebral arch)—*see* Fracture,
    vertebra, by site
  pelvis, pelvic (bone(s)) (with visceral injury)
    (closed) 808.8
    multiple (with disruption of pelvic circle)
      808.43
      open 808.53
    open 808.9
    rim (closed) 808.49
      open 808.59
  peritrochanteric (closed) 820.20
    open 820.30
  phalanx, phalanges, of one
    foot (closed) 826.0
      with bone(s) of same lower limb 827.0
        open 827.1
      open 826.1
    hand (closed) 816.00
      with metacarpal bone(s) of same hand 817.0
        open 817.1
      distal 816.02
        open 816.12
      middle 816.01
        open 816.11
      multiple sites NEC 816.03
        open 816.13
      open 816.10
      proximal 816.01
        open 816.11
  pisiform (closed) 814.04
    open 814.14

Fracture — *continued*
  pond—Fracture, skull, vault
  Pott's (closed) 824.4
    open 824.5
  prosthetic device, internal—*see* Complications,
    mechanical
  pubis (with visceral injury) (closed) 808.2
    open 808.3
  Quervain's (closed) 814.01
    open 814.11
  radius (alone) (closed) 813.81
    with ulna NEC 813.83
      open 813.93
    distal end—*see* Fracture, radius, lower end
    epiphysis
      lower—*see* Fracture, radius, lower end
      upper—*see* Fracture, radius, upper end
    head—*see* Fracture, radius, upper end
    lower end or extremity (distal end) (lower
      epiphysis) 813.42
      with ulna (lower end) 813.44
        open 813.54
      open 813.52
      torus 813.45
    neck—*see* Fracture, radius, upper end
    open NEC 813.91
    pathologic 733.12
    proximal end—*see* Fracture, radius, upper end
    shaft (closed) 813.21
      with ulna (shaft) 813.23
        open 813.33
      open 813.31
    upper end 813.07
      with ulna (upper end) 813.08
        open 813.18
      epiphysis 813.05
        open 813.15
      head 813.05
        open 813.15
      multiple sites 813.07
        open 813.17
      neck 813.06
        open 813.16
      open 813.17
      specified site NEC 813.07
        open 813.17
  ramus
    inferior or superior (with visceral injury)
      (closed) 808.2
      open 808.3
    ischium—*see* Fracture, ischium
  mandible 802.24
    open 802.34
  rib(s) (closed) 807.0

Note—Use the following fifth-digit subclassification with categories 807.0-807.1:

0 *rib(s), unspecified*
1 *one rib*
2 *two ribs*
3 *three ribs*
4 *four ribs*
5 *five ribs*
6 *six ribs*
7 *seven ribs*
8 *eight or more ribs*
9 *multiple ribs, unspecified*

---

    with flail chest (open) 807.4
    open 807.1
  root, tooth 873.63

INDEX TO DISEASES — Fracture

Fracture—*continued*
   complicated 873.73
   sacrum—*see* Fracture, vertebra, sacrum
   scaphoid
      ankle (closed) 825.22
         open 825.32
      wrist (closed) 814.01
         open 814.11
   scapula (closed) 811.00
      acromial, acromion (process) 811.01
         open 811.11
      body 811.09
         open 811.19
      coracoid process 811.02
         open 811.12
      glenoid (cavity) (fossa) 811.03
         open 811.13
      neck 811.03
         open 811.13
      open 811.10
   semilunar
      bone, wrist (closed) 814.02
         open 814.12
      cartilage (interior) (knee)—*see* Tear, meniscus
   sesamoid bone—*see* Fracture, by site
   Shepherd's (closed) 825.21
      open 825.31
   shoulder—*see also* Fracture, humerus, upper end
      blade—*see* Fracture, scapula
   silverfork—*see* Fracture, radius, lower end
   sinus (ethmoid) (frontal) (maxillary) (nasal) (sphenoidal)—*see* Fracture, skull, base
      maxillary—*see* Fracture, maxilla
   Skillern's—*see* Fracture, radius, shaft
   skull (multiple NEC) (with face bones) (closed) 803.0

Note—Use the following fifth-digit subclassification with categories 800, 801, 803, and 804:

0 unspecified state of consciousness
1 with no loss of consciousness
2 with brief [less than one hour] loss of consciousness
3 with moderate [1-24 hours] loss of consciousness
4 with prolonged [more than 24 hours] loss of consciousness and return to pre-existing conscious level
5 with prolonged [more than 24 hours] loss of consciousness, without return to pre-existing conscious level
Use fifth-digit 5 to designate when a patient is unconscious and dies before regaining consciousness, regardless of the duration of the loss of consciousness
6 with loss of consciousness of unspecified duration
9 with concussion, unspecified

---

      with
         contusion, cerebral 803.1
         epidural hemorrhage 803.2
         extradural hemorrhage 803.2
         hemorrhage (intracranial) NEC 803.3
         intracranial injury NEC 803.4
         laceration, cerebral 803.1
         other bones—*see* Fracture, multiple, skull
         subarachnoid hemorrhage 803.2

Fracture—*continued*
         subdural hemorrhage 803.2
      base (antrum) (ethmoid bone) (fossa) (internal ear) (nasal sinus) (occiput) (sphenoid) (temporal bone) (closed) 801.0
         with
            contusion, cerebral 801.1
            epidural hemorrhage 801.2
            extradural hemorrhage 801.2
            hemorrhage (intracranial) NEC 801.3
            intracranial injury NEC 801.4
            laceration, cerebral 801.1
            subarachnoid hemorrhage 801.2
            subdural hemorrhage 801.2
         open 801.5
            with
                contusion, cerebral 801.6
                epidural hemorrhage 801.7
                extradural hemorrhage 801.7
                hemorrhage (intracranial) NEC 801.8
                intracranial injury NEC 801.9
                laceration, cerebral 801.6
                subarachnoid hemorrhage 801.7
                subdural hemorrhage 801.7
      birth injury 767.3
      face bones—*see* Fracture, face bones
      open 803.5
         with
            contusion, cerebral 803.6
            epidural hemorrhage 803.7
            extradural hemorrhage 803.7
            hemorrhage (intracranial) NEC 803.8
            intracranial injury NEC 803.9
            laceration, cerebral 803.6
            subarachnoid hemorrhage 803.7
            subdural hemorrhage 803.7
      vault (frontal bone) (parietal bone) (vertex) (closed) 800.0
         with
            contusion, cerebral 800.1
            epidural hemorrhage 800.2
            extradural hemorrhage 800.2
            hemorrhage (intracranial) NEC 800.3
            intracranial injury NEC 800.4
            laceration, cerebral 800.1
            subarachnoid hemorrhage 800.2
            subdural hemorrhage 800.2
      open 800.5
         with
            contusion, cerebral 800.6
            epidural hemorrhage 800.7
            extradural hemorrhage 800.7
            hemorrhage (intracranial) NEC 800.8
            intracranial injury NEC 800.9
            laceration, cerebral 800.6
            subarachnoid hemorrhage 800.7
            subdural hemorrhage 800.7
   Smith's 813.41
      open 813.51
   sphenoid (bone) (sinus)—*see* Fracture, skull, base
   spine—*see also* Fracture, vertebra, by site
      due to birth trauma 767.4
   spinous process—*see* Fracture, vertebra, by site
   spontaneous—*see* Fracture, pathologic
   sprinters'—*see* Fracture, ilium
   stapes—*see* Fracture, skull, base
   stave—*see also* Fracture, metacarpus, metacarpal bone(s)
      spine—*see* Fracture, tibia, upper end
   sternum (closed) 807.2

Fracture INDEX TO DISEASES

Fracture—*continued*
  with flail chest (open) 807.4
  open 807.3
Stieda's—*see* Fracture, femur, lower end
stress 733.95
  fibula 733.93
  metatarsals 733.94
  specified site NEC 733.95
  tibia 733.93
styloid process
  metacarpal (closed) 815.02
    open 815.12
  radius—*see* Fracture, radius, lower end
  temporal bone—*see* Fracture, skull, base
  ulna—*see* Fracture, ulna, lower end
supracondylar, elbow 812.41
  open 812.51
symphysis pubis (with visceral injury) (closed) 808.2
  open 808.3
talus (ankle bone) (closed) 825.21
  open 825.31
tarsus, tarsal bone(s) (with metatarsus) of one foot (closed) NEC 825.29
  open 825.39
temporal bone (styloid)—*see* Fracture, skull, base
tendon—*see* Sprain, by site
thigh—*see* Fracture, femur, shaft
thumb (and finger(s)) of one hand (closed) (*see also* Fracture, phalanx, hand) 816.00
  with metacarpal bone(s) of same hand 817.0
    open 817.1
  metacarpal(s)—*see* Fracture, metacarpus
  open 816.10
thyroid cartilage (closed) 807.5
  open 807.6
tibia (closed) 823.80
  with fibula 823.82
    open 823.92
  condyles—*see* Fracture, tibia, upper end
  distal end 824.8
    open 824.9
  epiphysis
    lower 824.8
      open 824.9
    upper—*see* Fracture, tibia, upper end
  head (involving knee joint)—*see* Fracture, tibia, upper end
  intercondyloid eminence—*see* Fracture, tibia, upper end
  involving ankle 824.0
    open 824.1
  lower end or extremity (anterior lip) (posterior lip) 824.8
    open 824.9
  malleolus (internal) (medial) 824.0
    open 824.1
  open NEC 823.90
  pathologic 733.16
  proximal end—*see* Fracture, tibia, upper end
  shaft 823.20
    with fibula 823.22
      open 823.32
    open 823.30
  spine—*see* Fracture, tibia, upper end
  stress 733.93
  torus 823.40
    with tibia 823.42
  tuberosity—*see* Fracture, tibia, upper end

Fracture—*continued*
  upper end or extremity (condyle) (epiphysis) (head) (spine) (proximal end) (tuberosity) 823.00
    with fibula 823.02
      open 823.12
    open 823.10
toe(s), of one foot (closed) 826.0
  with bone(s) of same lower limb 827.0
    open 827.1
  open 826.1
tooth (root) 873.63
  complicated 873.73
torus
  fibula 823.41
    with tibia 823.42
  radius 813.45
  tibia 823.40
    with fibula 823.42
trachea (closed) 807.5
  open 807.6
transverse process—*see* Fracture, vertebra, by site
trapezium (closed) 814.05
  open 814.15
trapezoid bone (closed) 814.06
  open 814.16
trimalleolar (closed) 824.6
  open 824.7
triquetral (bone) (closed) 814.03
  open 814.13
trochanter (greater) (lesser) (closed) (*see also* Fracture, femur, neck, by site) 820.20
  open 820.30
trunk (bones) (closed) 809.0
  open 809.1
tuberosity (external)—*see* Fracture, by site
ulna (alone) (closed) 813.82
  with radius NEC 813.83
    open 813.93
  coronoid process (closed) 813.02
    open 813.12
  distal end—*see* Fracture, ulna, lower end
  epiphysis
    lower—*see* Fracture, ulna, lower end
    upper—*see* Fracture, ulna, upper, end
  head—*see* Fracture, ulna, lower end
  lower end (distal end) (head) (lower epiphysis) (styloid process) 813.43
    with radius (lower end) 813.44
      open 813.54
    open 813.53
  olecranon process (closed) 813.01
    open 813.11
  open NEC 813.92
  pathologic 733.12
  proximal end—*see* Fracture, ulna, upper end
  shaft 813.22
    with radius (shaft) 813.23
      open 813.33
    open 813.32
  styloid process—*see* Fracture, ulna, lower end
  transverse—*see* Fracture, ulna, by site
  upper end (epiphysis) 813.04
    with radius (upper end) 813.08
      open 813.18
    multiple sites 813.04
      open 813.14
    open 813.14
    specified site NEC 813.04
      open 813.14

INDEX TO DISEASES

Fracture—*continued*
  unciform (closed) 814.08
    open 814.18
  vertebra, vertebral (back) (body) (column)
    (neural arch) (pedicle) (spine) (spinous
    process) (transverse process) (closed) 805.8
    with
      hematomyelia—*see* Fracture, vertebra, by
        site, with spinal cord injury
      injury to
        cauda equina—*see* Fracture, vertebra,
          sacrum, with spinal cord injury
        nerve—*see* Fracture, vertebra, by site, with
          spinal cord injury
      paralysis—*see* Fracture, vertebra, by site,
        with spinal cord injury
      paraplegia—*see* Fracture, vertebra, by site,
        with spinal cord injury
      quadriplegia—*see* Fracture, vertebra, by site,
        with spinal cord injury
      spinal concussion—*see* Fracture, vertebra,
        by site, with spinal cord injury
      spinal cord injury (closed) NEC 806.8

Note—Use the following fifth-digit subclassification with categories 806.0-806.3:

C_1-C_4 *or unspecified level and* D_1-D_6 (T_1-T_6) *or unspecified level with:*

0 *unspecified spinal cord injury*
1 *complete lesion of cord*
2 *anterior cord syndrome*
3 *central cord syndrome*
4 *specified injury NEC*

C_5-C_7 *level and* D_7-D_{12} *level with:*

5 *unspecified spinal cord injury*
6 *complete lesion of cord*
7 *anterior cord syndrome*
8 *central cord syndrome*
9 *specified injury NEC*

---

        cervical 806.0
          open 806.1
        dorsal, dorsolumbar 806.2
          open 806.3
          open 806.9
        thoracic, thoracolumbar 806.2
          open 806.3
    atlanto-axial—*see* Fracture, vertebra, cervical
    cervical (hangman) (teardrop) (closed) 805.00
      with spinal cord injury—*see* Fracture,
        vertebra, with spinal cord injury, cervical
      first (atlas) 805.01
        open 805.11
      second (axis) 805.02
        open 805.12
      third 805.03
        open 805.13
      fourth 805.04
        open 805.14
      fifth 805.05
        open 805.15
      sixth 805.06
        open 805.16
      seventh 805.07
        open 805.17
      multiple sites 805.08
        open 805.18

Fracture—*continued*
      open 805.10
    chronic 733.13
    coccyx (closed) 805.6
      with spinal cord injury (closed) 806.60
        cauda equina injury 806.62
          complete lesion 806.61
            open 806.71
          open 806.72
        open 806.70
        specified type NEC 806.69
          open 806.79
      open 805.7
    collapsed 733.13
    compression, not due to trauma 733.13
    dorsal (closed) 805.2
      with spinal cord injury—*see* Fracture,
        vertebra, with spinal cord injury, dorsal
      open 805.3
    dorsolumbar (closed) 805.2
      with spinal cord injury—*see* Fracture,
        vertebra, with spinal cord injury, dorsal
      open 805.3
    due to osteoporosis 733.13
    fetus or newborn 767.4
    lumbar (closed) 805.4
      with spinal cord injury (closed) 806.4
        open 806.5
      open 805.5
    nontraumatic 733.13
    open NEC 805.9
    pathologic 733.13
    sacrum (closed) 805.6
      with spinal cord injury 806.60
        cauda equina injury 806.62
          complete lesion 806.61
            open 806.71
          open 806.72
        open 806.70
        specified type NEC 806.69
          open 806.79
      open 805.7
    site unspecified (closed) 805.8
      with spinal cord injury (closed) 806.8
        open 806.9
      open 805.9
    stress (any site) 733.95
    thoracic (closed) 805.2
      with spinal cord injury—*see* Fracture,
        vertebra, with spinal cord injury,
        thoracic
      open 805.3
  vertex—*see* Fracture, skull, vault
  vomer (bone) 802.0
    open 802.1
  Wagstaffe's—*see* Fracture, ankle
  wrist (closed) 814.00
    open 814.10
    pathologic 733.12
  xiphoid (process)—*see* Fracture, sternum
  zygoma (zygomatic arch) (closed) 802.4
    open 802.5
Fragile X syndrome 759.83
Fragilitas
  crinium 704.2
  hair 704.2
  ossium 756.51
    with blue sclera 756.51
  unguium 703.8
    congenital 757.5

Fragility
  bone 756.51
    with deafness and blue sclera 756.51
  capillary (hereditary) 287.8
  hair 704.2
  nails 703.8
Fragmentation —*see* Fracture, by site
Frambesia, frambesial (tropica) (*see also* Yaws) 102.9
  initial lesion or ulcer 102.0
  primary 102.0
Frambeside
  gummatous 102.4
  of early yaws 102.2
Frambesioma 102.1
Franceschetti's syndrome (mandibulofacial dysostosis) 756.0
Francis' disease (*see also* Tularemia) 021.9
Frank's essential thrombocytopenia (*see also* Purpura, thrombocytopenic) 287.39
Franklin's disease (heavy chain) 273.2
Fraser's syndrome 759.89
Freckle 709.09
  malignant melanoma in (M8742/3)—*see* Melanoma
  melanotic (of Hutchinson) (M8742/2)—*see* Neoplasm, skin, in situ
Freeman-Sheldon syndrome 759.89
Freezing 991.9
  specified effect NEC 991.8
Frei's disease (climatic bubo) 099.1
Freiberg's
  disease (osteochondrosis, second metatarsal) 732.5
  infraction of metatarsal head 732.5
  osteochondrosis 732.5
Fremitus, friction, cardiac 785.3
Frenulum lingua 750.0
Frenum
  external os 752.49
  tongue 750.0
Frequency (urinary) NEC 788.41
  micturition 788.41
  nocturnal 788.43
  psychogenic 306.53
Frey's syndrome (auriculotemporal syndrome) 705.22
Friction
  burn (*see also* Injury, superficial, by site) 919.0
  fremitus, cardiac 785.3
  precordial 785.3
  sounds, chest 786.7
Friderichsen-Waterhouse syndrome or disease 036.3
Friedländer's
  B (bacillus) NEC (*see also* condition) 041.3
  sepsis or septicemia 038.49
  disease (endarteritis obliterans)—*see* Arteriosclerosis
Friedreich's
  ataxia 334.0
  combined systemic disease 334.0
  disease 333.2
    combined systemic 334.0
  myoclonia 333.2
  sclerosis (spinal cord) 334.0
Friedrich-Erb-Arnold syndrome (acropachyderma) 757.39
Frigidity 302.72
  psychic or psychogenic 302.72
Fröhlich's disease or syndrome (adiposogenital dystrophy) 253.8

Froin's syndrome 336.8
Frommel's disease 676.6
Frommel-Chiari syndrome 676.6
Frontal —*see also* condition
  lobe syndrome 310.0
Frostbite 991.3
  face 991.0
  foot 991.2
  hand 991.1
  specified site NEC 991.3
Frotteurism 302.89
Frozen 991.9
  pelvis 620.8
  shoulder 726.0
Fructosemia 271.2
Fructosuria (benign) (essential) 271.2
Fuchs'
  black spot (myopic) 360.21
  corneal dystrophy (endothelial) 371.57
  heterochromic cyclitis 364.21
Fucosidosis 271.8
Fugue 780.99
  dissociative 300.13
  hysterical (dissociative) 300.13
  reaction to exceptional stress (transient) 308.1
Fukuhara syndrome 277.87
Fuller Albright's syndrome (osteitis fibrosa disseminata) 756.59
Fuller's earth disease 502
Fulminant, fulminating —*see* condition
Functional —*see* condition
Functioning
  borderline intellectual V62.89
Fundus —*see also* condition
  flavimaculatus 362.76
Fungemia 117.9
Fungus, fungous
  cerebral 348.8
  disease NEC 117.9
  infection—*see* Infection, fungus
  testis (*see also* Tuberculosis) 016.5 [608.81]
Funiculitis (acute) 608.4
  chronic 608.4
  endemic 608.4
  gonococcal (acute) 098.14
    chronic or duration of 2 months or over 098.34
  tuberculous (*see also* Tuberculosis) 016.5
F.U.O. (*see also* Pyrexia) 780.6
Funnel
  breast (acquired) 738.3
    congenital 754.81
    late effect of rickets 268.1
  chest (acquired) 738.3
    congenital 754.81
    late effect of rickets 268.1
  pelvis (acquired) 738.6
    with disproportion (fetopelvic) 653.3
      affecting fetus or newborn 763.1
      causing obstructed labor 660.1
        affecting fetus or newborn 763.1
    congenital 755.69
    tuberculous (*see also* Tuberculosis) 016.9
Furfur 690.18
  microsporon 111.0
Furor, paroxysmal (idiopathic) (*see also* Epilepsy) 345.8
Furriers' lung 495.8
Furrowed tongue 529.5
  congenital 750.13
Furrowing nail (s) (transverse) 703.8
  congenital 757.5

Furuncle 680.9
  abdominal wall 680.2
  ankle 680.6
  anus 680.5
  arm (any part, above wrist) 680.3
  auditory canal, external 680.0
  axilla 680.3
  back (any part) 680.2
  breast 680.2
  buttock 680.5
  chest wall 680.2
  corpus cavernosum 607.2
  ear (any part) 680.0
  eyelid 373.13
  face (any part, except eye) 680.0
  finger (any) 680.4
  flank 680.2
  foot (any part) 680.7
  forearm 680.3
  gluteal (region) 680.5
  groin 680.2
  hand (any part) 680.4
  head (any part, except face) 680.8
  heel 680.7
  hip 680.6
  kidney (*see also* Abscess, kidney) 590.2
  knee 680.6
  labium (majus) (minus) 616.4
  lacrimal
    gland (*see also* Dacryoadenitis) 375.00
    passages (duct) (sac) (*see also* Dacryocystitis) 375.30
  leg, any part except foot 680.6
  malignant 022.0
  multiple sites 680.9
  neck 680.1
  nose (external) (septum) 680.0
  orbit 376.01
  partes posteriores 680.5
  pectoral region 680.2
  penis 607.2
  perineum 680.2
  pinna 680.0
  scalp (any part) 680.8
  scrotum 608.4
  seminal vesicle 608.0
  shoulder 680.3
  skin NEC 680.9
  specified site NEC 680.8
  spermatic cord 608.4
  temple (region) 680.0
  testis 604.90
  thigh 680.6
  thumb 680.4
  toe (any) 680.7
  trunk 680.2
  tunica vaginalis 608.4
  umbilicus 680.2
  upper arm 680.3
  vas deferens 608.4
  vulva 616.4
  wrist 680.4
Furunculosis (*see also* Furuncle) 680.9
  external auditory meatus 680.0 *[380.13]*
Fusarium (infection) 118
Fusion, fused (congenital)
  anal (with urogenital canal) 751.5
  aorta and pulmonary artery 745.0
  astragaloscaphoid 755.67
  atria 745.5
  atrium and ventricle 745.69

Fusion, fused—*continued*
  auditory canal 744.02
  auricles, heart 745.5
  binocular, with defective stereopsis 368.33
  bone 756.9
  cervical spine—*see* Fusion, spine
  choanal 748.0
  commissure, mitral valve 746.5
  cranial sutures, premature 756.0
  cusps, heart valve NEC 746.89
    mitral 746.5
    tricuspid 746.89
  ear ossicles 744.04
  fingers (*see also* Syndactylism, fingers) 755.11
  hymen 752.42
  hymeno-urethral 599.89
    causing obstructed labor 660.1
      affecting fetus or newborn 763.1
  joint (acquired)—*see also* Ankylosis
    congenital 755.8
  kidneys (incomplete) 753.3
  labium (majus) (minus) 752.49
  larynx and trachea 748.3
  limb 755.8
    lower 755.69
    upper 755.59
  lobe, lung 748.5
  lumbosacral (acquired) 724.6
    congenital 756.15
    surgical V45.4
  nares (anterior) (posterior) 748.0
  nose, nasal 748.0
  nostril(s) 748.0
  organ or site NEC—*see* Anomaly, specified type NEC
  ossicles 756.9
    auditory 744.04
  pulmonary valve segment 746.02
  pulmonic cusps 746.02
  ribs 756.3
  sacroiliac (acquired) (joint) 724.6
    congenital 755.69
    surgical V45.4
  skull, imperfect 756.0
  spine (acquired) 724.9
    arthrodesis status V45.4
    congenital (vertebra) 756.15
    postoperative status V45.4
  sublingual duct with submaxillary duct at opening in mouth 750.26
  talonavicular (bar) 755.67
  teeth, tooth 520.2
  testes 752.89
  toes (*see also* Syndactylism, toes) 755.13
  trachea and esophagus 750.3
  twins 759.4
  urethral-hymenal 599.89
  vagina 752.49
  valve cusps—*see* Fusion, cusps, heart valve
  ventricles, heart 745.4
  vertebra (arch)—*see* Fusion, spine
  vulva 752.49
Fusospirillosis (mouth) (tongue) (tonsil) 101
Fussy infant (baby) 780.91

G

Gafsa boil 085.1
Gain, weight (abnormal) (excessive) (see also Weight, gain) 783.1
Gaisböck's disease or syndrome (polycythemia hypertonica) 289.0
Gait
  abnormality 781.2
    hysterical 300.11
  ataxic 781.2
    hysterical 300.11
  disturbance 781.2
    hysterical 300.11
  paralytic 781.2
  scissor 781.2
  spastic 781.2
  staggering 781.2
    hysterical 300.11
Galactocele (breast) (infected) 611.5
  puerperal, postpartum 676.8
Galactophoritis 611.0
  puerperal, postpartum 675.2
Galactorrhea 676.6
  not associated with childbirth 611.6
Galactosemia (classic) (congenital) 271.1
Galactosuria 271.1
Galacturia 791.1
  bilharziasis 120.0
Galen's vein —*see* condition
Gallbladder —*see also* condition
  acute (*see also* Disease, gallbladder) 575.0
Gall duct —*see* condition
Gallop rhythm 427.89
Gallstone (cholemic) (colic) (impacted)—*see also* Cholelithiasis
  causing intestinal obstruction 560.31
Gambling, pathological 312.31
Gammaloidosis 277.39
Gammopathy 273.9
  macroglobulinemia 273.3
  monoclonal (benign) (essential) (idiopathic) (with lymphoplasmacytic dyscrasia) 273.1
Gamna's disease (siderotic splenomegaly) 289.51
Gampsodactylia (congenital) 754.71
Gamstorp's disease (adynamia episodica hereditaria) 359.3
Gandy-Nanta disease (siderotic splenomegaly) 289.51
Gang activity without manifest psychiatric disorder V71.09
  adolescent V71.02
  adult V71.01
  child V71.02
Gangliocytoma (M9490/0)—*see* Neoplasm, connective tissue, benign
Ganglioglioma (M9505/1)—*see* Neoplasm, by site, uncertain behavior
Ganglion 727.43
  joint 727.41
  of yaws (early) (late) 102.6
  periosteal (*see also* Periostitis) 730.3
  tendon sheath (compound) (diffuse) 727.42
  tuberculous (*see also* Tuberculosis) 015.9
Ganglioneuroblastoma (M9490/3)—*see* Neoplasm, connective tissue, malignant
Ganglioneuroma (M9490/0)—*see also* Neoplasm, connective tissue, benign

Ganglioneuroma—*continued*
  malignant (M9490/3)—*see* Neoplasm, connective tissue, malignant
Ganglioneuromatosis (M9491/0)—*see* Neoplasm, connective tissue, benign
Ganglionitis
  fifth nerve (*see also* Neuralgia, trigeminal) 350.1
  gasserian 350.1
  geniculate 351.1
    herpetic 053.11
    newborn 767.5
  herpes zoster 053.11
  herpetic geniculate (Hunt's syndrome) 053.11
Gangliosidosis 330.1
Gangosa 102.5
Gangrene, gangrenous (anemia) (artery) (cellulitis) (dermatitis) (dry) (infective) (moist) (pemphigus) (septic) (skin) (stasis) (ulcer) 785.4
  with
    arteriosclerosis (native artery) 440.24
      bypass graft 440.30
        autologous vein 440.31
        nonautologous biological 440.32
    diabetes (mellitus) 250.7 *[785.4]*
  abdomen (wall) 785.4
  adenitis 683
  alveolar 526.5
  angina 462
    diphtheritic 032.0
  anus 569.49
  appendices epiploicae—*see* Gangrene, mesentery
  appendix—*see* Appendicitis, acute
  arteriosclerotic —*see* Arteriosclerosis, with, gangrene
  auricle 785.4
  Bacillus welchii (*see also* Gangrene, gas) 040.0
  bile duct (*see also* Cholangitis) 576.8
  bladder 595.89
  bowel—*see* Gangrene, intestine
  cecum—*see* Gangrene, intestine
  Clostridium perfringens or welchii (*see also* Gangrene, gas) 040.0
  colon—*see* Gangrene, intestine
  connective tissue 785.4
  cornea 371.40
  corpora cavernosa (infective) 607.2
    noninfective 607.89
  cutaneous, spreading 785.4
  decubital (*see also* Decubitus) 707.00 *[785.4]*
  diabetic (any site) 250.7 *[785.4]*
  dropsical 785.4
  emphysematous (*see also* Gangrene, gas) 040.0
  epidemic (ergotized grain) 988.2
  epididymis (infectional) (*see also* Epididymitis) 604.99
  erysipelas (*see also* Erysipelas) 035
  extremity (lower) (upper) 785.4
  gallbladder or duct (*see also* Cholecystitis, acute) 575.0
  gas (bacillus) 040.0
    with
      abortion—*see* Abortion, by type, with sepsis
      ectopic pregnancy (*see also* categories 633.0-633.9) 639.0

Gangrene, gangrenous — continued
    molar pregnancy (*see also* categories 630-632) 639.0
    following
        abortion 639.0
        ectopic or molar pregnancy 639.0
        puerperal, postpartum, childbirth 670
    glossitis 529.0
    gum 523.8
    hernia — *see* Hernia, by site, with gangrene
    hospital noma 528.1
    intestine, intestinal (acute) (hemorrhagic) (massive) 557.0
        with
            hernia — *see* Hernia, by site, with gangrene
            mesenteric embolism or infarction 557.0
            obstruction (*see also* Obstruction, intestine) 560.9
    laryngitis 464.00
        with obstruction 464.01
    liver 573.8
    lung 513.0
        spirochetal 104.8
    lymphangitis 457.2
    Meleney's (cutaneous) 686.09
    mesentery 557.0
        with
            embolism or infarction 557.0
            intestinal obstruction (*see also* Obstruction, intestine) 560.9
    mouth 528.1
    noma 528.1
    orchitis 604.90
    ovary (*see also* Salpingo-oophoritis) 614.2
    pancreas 577.0
    penis (infectional) 607.2
        noninfective 607.89
    perineum 785.4
    pharynx 462
        septic 034.0
    pneumonia 513.0
    Pott's 440.24
    presenile 443.1
    pulmonary 513.0
    pulp, tooth 522.1
    quinsy 475
    Raynaud's (symmetric gangrene) 443.0 *[785.4]*
    rectum 569.49
    retropharyngeal 478.24
    rupture — *see* Hernia, by site, with gangrene
    scrotum 608.4
        noninfective 608.83
    senile 440.24
    sore throat 462
    spermatic cord 608.4
        noninfective 608.89
    spine 785.4
    spirochetal NEC 104.8
    spreading cutaneous 785.4
    stomach 537.89
    stomatitis 528.1
    symmetrical 443.0 *[785.4]*
    testis (infectional) (*see also* Orchitis) 604.99
        noninfective 608.89
    throat 462
        diphtheritic 032.0
    thyroid (gland) 246.8
    tonsillitis (acute) 463
    tooth (pulp) 522.1
    tuberculous NEC (*see also* Tuberculosis) 011.9
    tunica vaginalis 608.4

Gangrene, gangrenous — continued
    noninfective 608.89
    umbilicus 785.4
    uterus (*see also* Endometritis) 615.9
    uvulitis 528.3
    vas deferens 608.4
        noninfective 608.89
    vulva (*see also* Vulvitis) 616.10
Gannister disease (occupational) 502
    with tuberculosis — *see* Tuberculosis, pulmonary
Ganser's syndrome, hysterical 300.16
Gardner-Diamond syndrome (autoerythrocyte sensitization) 287.2
Gargoylism 277.5
Garré's
    disease (*see also* Osteomyelitis) 730.1
    osteitis (sclerosing) (*see also* Osteomyelitis) 730.1
    osteomyelitis (*see also* Osteomyelitis) 730.1
Garrod's pads, knuckle 728.79
Gartner's duct
    cyst 752.41
    persistent 752.41
Gas 787.3
    asphyxia, asphyxiation, inhalation, poisoning, suffocation NEC 987.9
        specified gas — *see* Table of drugs and chemicals
    bacillus gangrene or infection — *see* Gas, gangrene
    cyst, mesentery 568.89
    excessive 787.3
    gangrene 040.0
        with
            abortion — *see* Abortion, by type, with sepsis
            ectopic pregnancy (*see also* categories 633.0-633.9) 639.0
            molar pregnancy (*see also* categories 630-632) 639.0
        following
            abortion 639.0
            ectopic or molar pregnancy 639.0
            puerperal, postpartum, childbirth 670
    on stomach 787.3
    pains 787.3
Gastradenitis 535.0
Gastralgia 536.8
    psychogenic 307.89
Gastrectasis, gastrectasia 536.1
    psychogenic 306.4
Gastric — *see* condition
Gastrinoma (M8153/1)
    malignant (M8153/3)
        pancreas 157.4
        specified site NEC — *see* Neoplasm, by site, malignant
        unspecified site 157.4
    specified site — *see* Neoplasm, by site, uncertain behavior
    unspecified site 235.5
Gastritis 535.5

Note — Use the following fifth-digit subclassification for category 535:

0 *without mention of hemorrhage*
1 *with hemorrhage*

    acute 535.0
    alcoholic 535.3
    allergic 535.4

INDEX TO DISEASES   **Genital**

Gastritis—*continued*
  antral 535.4
  atrophic 535.1
  atrophic-hyperplastic 535.1
  bile-induced 535.4
  catarrhal 535.0
  chronic (atrophic) 535.1
  cirrhotic 535.4
  corrosive (acute) 535.4
  dietetic 535.4
  due to diet deficiency 269.9 *[535.4]*
  eosinophilic 535.4
  erosive 535.4
  follicular 535.4
    chronic 535.1
  giant hypertrophic 535.2
  glandular 535.4
    chronic 535.1
  hypertrophic (mucosa) 535.2
    chronic giant 211.1
  irritant 535.4
  nervous 306.4
  phlegmonous 535.0
  psychogenic 306.4
  sclerotic 535.4
  spastic 536.8
  subacute 535.0
  superficial 535.4
  suppurative 535.0
  toxic 535.4
  tuberculous (*see also* Tuberculosis) 017.9
Gastrocarcinoma (M8010/3) 151.9
Gastrocolic —*see* condition
Gastrocolitis —*see* Enteritis
Gastrodisciasis 121.8
Gastroduodenitis (*see also* Gastritis) 535.5
  catarrhal 535.0
  infectional 535.0
  virus, viral 008.8
    specified type NEC 008.69
Gastrodynia 536.8
Gastroenteritis (acute) (catarrhal) (congestive) (hemorrhagic) (noninfectious) (*see also* Enteritis) 558.9
  aertrycke infection 003.0
  allergic 558.3
  chronic 558.9
    ulcerative (*see also* Colitis, ulcerative) 556.9
  dietetic 558.9
  due to
    food poisoning (*see also* Poisoning, food) 005.9
    radiation 558.1
  epidemic 009.0
  functional 558.9
  infectious (*see also* Enteritis, due to, by organism) 009.0
    presumed 009.1
  salmonella 003.0
  septic (*see also* Enteritis, due to, by organism) 009.0
  toxic 558.2
  tuberculous (*see also* Tuberculosis) 014.8
  ulcerative (*see also* Colitis, ulcerative) 556.9
  viral NEC 008.8
    specified type NEC 008.69
  zymotic 009.0
Gastroenterocolitis —*see* Enteritis
Gastroenteropathy, protein-losing 579.8
Gastroenteroptosis 569.89
Gastroesophageal laceration-hemorrhage syndrome 530.7
Gastroesophagitis 530.19

Gastrohepatitis (*see also* Gastritis) 535.5
Gastrointestinal —*see* condition
Gastrojejunal —*see* condition
Gastrojejunitis (*see also* Gastritis) 535.5
Gastrojejunocolic —*see* condition
Gastroliths 537.89
Gastromalacia 537.89
Gastroparalysis 536.3
  diabetic 250.6 *[337.1]*
Gastroparesis 536.3
  diabetic 250.6 *[536.3]*
Gastropathy 537.9
  congestive portal 537.89
  erythematous 535.5
  exudative 579.8
  portal hypertension 537.89
Gastroptosis 537.5
Gastrorrhagia 578.0
Gastrorrhea 536.8
  psychogenic 306.4
Gastroschisis (congenital) 756.79
  acquired 569.89
Gastrospasm (neurogenic) (reflex) 536.8
  neurotic 306.4
  psychogenic 306.4
Gastrostaxis 578.0
Gastrostenosis 537.89
Gastrostomy
  attention to V55.1
  complication 536.40
    specified type 536.49
  infection 536.41
  malfunctioning 536.42
  status V44.1
Gastrosuccorrhea (continuous) (intermittent) 536.8
  neurotic 306.4
  psychogenic 306.4
Gaucher's
  disease (adult) (cerebroside lipidosis) (infantile) 272.7
  hepatomegaly 272.7
  splenomegaly (cerebroside lipidosis) 272.7
GAVE (gastric antral vascular ectasia) 537.82
  with hemorrhage 537.83
  without hemorrhage 537.82
Gayet's disease (superior hemorrhagic polioencephalitis) 265.1
Gayet-Wernicke's syndrome (superior hemorrhagic polioencephalitis) 265.1
Gee (-Herter) (-Heubner) (-Thaysen) disease or syndrome (nontropical sprue) 579.0
Gélineau's syndrome (*see also* Narcolepsy) 347.00
Gemination, teeth 520.2
Gemistocytoma (M9411/3)
  specified site—*see* Neoplasm, by site, malignant
  unspecified site 191.9
General, generalized —*see* condition
Genetic
  susceptibility to
    MEN (multiple endocrine neoplasia) V84.81
    neoplasia
      multiple endocrine [MEN] V84.81
    neoplasm
      malignant, of
        breast V84.01
        endometrium V84.04
        other V84.09
        ovary V84.02
        prostate V84.03
      specified disease NEC V84.89
Genital —*see* condition

Genito-anorectal syndrome   **INDEX TO DISEASES**

Genito-anorectal syndrome 099.1
Genitourinary system —*see* condition
Genu
  congenital 755.64
  extrorsum (acquired) 736.42
    congenital 755.64
    late effects of rickets 268.1
  introrsum (acquired) 736.41
    congenital 755.64
    late effects of rickets 268.1
  rachitic (old) 268.1
  recurvatum (acquired) 736.5
    congenital 754.40
      with dislocation of knee 754.41
    late effects of rickets 268.1
  valgum (acquired) (knock-knee) 736.41
    congenital 755.64
    late effects of rickets 268.1
  varum (acquired) (bowleg) 736.42
    congenital 755.64
    late effects of rickets 268.1
Geographic tongue 529.1
Geophagia 307.52
Geotrichosis 117.9
  intestine 117.9
  lung 117.9
  mouth 117.9
Gephyrophobia 300.29
Gerbode defect 745.4
Gerhardt's
  disease (erythromelalgia) 443.82
  syndrome (vocal cord paralysis) 478.30
Gerlier's disease (epidemic vertigo) 078.81
German measles 056.9
  exposure to V01.4
Germinoblastoma (diffuse) (M9614/3) 202.8
  follicular (M9692/3) 202.0
Germinoma (M9064/3)—*see* Neoplasm, by site, malignant
Gerontoxon 371.41
Gerstmann's syndrome (finger agnosia) 784.69
Gestation (period)—*see also* Pregnancy
  ectopic NEC (*see also* Pregnancy, ectopic) 633.90
    with intrauterine pregnancy 633.91
Gestational proteinuria 646.2
  with hypertension—*see* Toxemia, of pregnancy
Ghon tubercle primary infection (*see also* Tuberculosis) 010.0
Ghost
  teeth 520.4
  vessels, cornea 370.64
Ghoul hand 102.3
Gianotti Crosti syndrome 057.8
  due to known virus—*see* Infection, virus
  due to unknown virus 057.8
Giant
  cell
    epulis 523.8
    peripheral (gingiva) 523.8
    tumor, tendon sheath 727.02
  colon (congenital) 751.3
  esophagus (congenital) 750.4
  kidney 753.3
  urticaria 995.1
    hereditary 277.6
Giardia lamblia infestation 007.1
Giardiasis 007.1
Gibert's disease (pityriasis rosea) 696.3
Gibraltar fever —*see* Brucellosis

Giddiness 780.4
  hysterical 300.11
  psychogenic 306.9
Gierke's disease (glycogenosis I) 271.0
Gigantism (cerebral) (hypophyseal) (pituitary) 253.0
Gilbert's disease or cholemia (familial nonhemolytic jaundice) 277.4
Gilchrist's disease (North American blastomycosis) 116.0
Gilford (-Hutchinson) disease or syndrome (progeria) 259.8
Gilles de la Tourette's disease (motor-verbal tic) 307.23
Gillespie's syndrome (dysplasia oculodentodigitalis) 759.89
Gingivitis 523.10
  acute 523.00
    necrotizing 101
    non-plaque induced 523.01
    plaque induced 523.00
  catarrhal 523.00
  chronic 523.10
    non-plaque induced 523.11
  desquamative 523.10
  expulsiva 523.40
  hyperplastic 523.10
  marginal, simple 523.10
  necrotizing, acute 101
  non-plaque induced 523.11
  pellagrous 265.2
  plaque induced 523.10
  ulcerative 523.10
    acute necrotizing 101
  Vincent's 101
Gingivoglossitis 529.0
Gingivopericementitis 523.40
Gingivosis 523.10
Gingivostomatitis 523.10
  herpetic 054.2
Giovannini's disease 117.9
GISA (glycopeptide intermediate staphylococcus aureus) V09.8
Gland, glandular —*see* condition
Glanders 024
Glanzmann (-Naegeli) disease or thrombasthenia 287.1
Glassblowers' disease 527.1
Glaucoma (capsular) (inflammatory) (noninflammatory) (primary) 365.9
  with increased episcleral venous pressure 365.82
  absolute 360.42
  acute 365.22
    narrow angle 365.22
    secondary 365.60
  angle closure 365.20
    acute 365.22
    chronic 365.23
    intermittent 365.21
    interval 365.21
    residual stage 365.24
    subacute 365.21
  border line 365.00
  chronic 365.11
    noncongestive 365.11
    open angle 365.11
    simple 365.11
  closed angle—*see* Glaucoma, angle closure
  congenital 743.20
    associated with other eye anomalies 743.22

INDEX TO DISEASES Globinuria

Glaucoma—*continued*
  simple 743.21
  congestive—*see* Glaucoma, narrow angle
  corticosteroid-induced (glaucomatous stage) 365.31
    residual stage 365.32
  hemorrhagic 365.60
  hypersecretion 365.81
  in or with
    aniridia 743.45 *[365.42]*
    Axenfeld's anomaly 743.44 *[365.41]*
    concussion of globe 921.3 *[365.65]*
    congenital syndromes NEC 759.89 *[365.44]*
    dislocation of lens
      anterior 379.33 *[365.59]*
      posterior 379.34 *[365.59]*
    disorder of lens NEC 365.59
    epithelial down-growth 364.61 *[365.64]*
    glaucomatocyclitic crisis 364.22 *[365.62]*
    hypermature cataract 366.18 *[365.51]*
    hyphema 364.41 *[365.63]*
    inflammation, ocular 365.62
    iridocyclitis 364.3 *[365.62]*
    iris
      anomalies NEC 743.46 *[365.42]*
      atrophy, essential 364.51 *[365.42]*
      bombé 364.74 *[365.61]*
      rubeosis 364.42 *[365.63]*
    microcornea 743.41 *[365.43]*
    neurofibromatosis 237.71 *[365.44]*
    ocular
      cysts NEC 365.64
      disorders NEC 365.60
      trauma 365.65
      tumors NEC 365.64
    postdislocation of lens
      anterior 379.33 *[365.59]*
      posterior 379.34 *[365.59]*
    pseudoexfoliation of capsule 366.11 *[365.52]*
    pupillary block or seclusion 364.74 *[365.61]*
    recession of chamber angle 364.77 *[365.65]*
    retinal vein occlusion 362.35 *[365.63]*
    Rieger's anomaly or syndrome 743.44 *[365.41]*
    rubeosis of iris 364.42 *[365.63]*
    seclusion of pupil 364.74 *[365.61]*
    spherophakia 743.36 *[365.59]*
    Sturge-Weber (-Dimitri) syndrome 759.6 *[365.44]*
    systemic syndrome NEC 365.44
    tumor of globe 365.64
    vascular disorders NEC 365.63
  infantile 365.14
    congenital 743.20
      associated with other eye anomalies 743.22
      simple 743.21
  juvenile 365.14
  low tension 365.12
  malignant 365.83
  narrow angle (primary) 365.20
    acute 365.22
    chronic 365.23
    intermittent 365.21
    interval 365.21
    residual stage 365.24
    subacute 365.21
  newborn 743.20
    associated with other eye anomalies 743.22
    simple 743.21
  noncongestive (chronic) 365.11
  nonobstructive (chronic) 365.11

Glaucoma—*continued*
  obstructive 365.60
    due to lens changes 365.59
  open angle 365.10
    with
      borderline intraocular pressure 365.01
      cupping of optic discs 365.01
      primary 365.11
      residual stage 365.15
  phacolytic 365.51
    with hypermature cataract 366.18 *[365.51]*
  pigmentary 365.13
  postinfectious 365.60
  pseudoexfoliation 365.52
    with pseudoexfoliation of capsule 366.11 *[365.52]*
  secondary NEC 365.60
  simple (chronic) 365.11
  simplex 365.11
  steroid responders 365.03
  suspect 365.00
  syphilitic 095.8
  traumatic NEC 365.65
    newborn 767.8
  tuberculous (*see also* Tuberculosis) 017.3 *[365.62]*
  wide angle (*see also* Glaucoma, open angle) 365.10
Glaucomatous flecks (subcapsular) 366.31
Glazed tongue 529.4
Gleet 098.2
Glénard's disease or syndrome (enteroptosis) 569.89
Glinski-Simmonds syndrome (pituitary cachexia) 253.2
Glioblastoma (multiforme) (M9440/3)
  with sarcomatous component (M9442/3)
    specified site—*see* Neoplasm, by site, malignant
    unspecified site 191.9
  giant cell (M9441/3)
    specified site—*see* Neoplasm, by site, malignant
    unspecified site 191.9
  specified site—*see* Neoplasm, by site, malignant
  unspecified site 191.9
Glioma (malignant) (M9380/3)
  astrocytic (M9400/3)
    specified site—*see* Neoplasm, by site, malignant
    unspecified site 191.9
  mixed (M9382/3)
    specified site—*see* Neoplasm, by site, malignant
    unspecified site 191.9
  nose 748.1
  specified site NEC—*see* Neoplasm, by site, malignant
  subependymal (M9383/1) 237.5
  unspecified site 191.9
Gliomatosis cerebri (M9381/3) 191.0
Glioneuroma (M9505/1)—*see* Neoplasm, by site, uncertain behavior
Gliosarcoma (M9380/3)
  specified site—*see* Neoplasm, by site, malignant
  unspecified site 191.9
Gliosis (cerebral) 349.89
  spinal 336.0
Glisson's
  cirrhosis—*see* Cirrhosis, portal
  disease (*see also* Rickets) 268.0
Glissonitis 573.3
Globinuria 791.2

1045

Globus

Globus 306.4
  hystericus 300.11
Glomangioma (M8712/0) (see also Hemangioma) 228.00
Glomangiosarcoma (M8710/3)—see Neoplasm, connective tissue, malignant
Glomerular nephritis (see also Nephritis) 583.9
Glomerulitis (see also Nephritis) 583.9
Glomerulonephritis (see also Nephritis) 583.9
  with
    edema (see also Nephrosis) 581.9
    lesion of
      exudative nephritis 583.89
      interstitial nephritis (diffuse) (focal) 583.89
      necrotizing glomerulitis 583.4
        acute 580.4
        chronic 582.4
      renal necrosis 583.9
        cortical 583.6
        medullary 583.7
      specified pathology NEC 583.89
        acute 580.89
        chronic 582.89
    necrosis, renal 583.9
      cortical 583.6
      medullary (papillary) 583.7
    specified pathology or lesion NEC 583.89
  acute 580.9
    with
      exudative nephritis 580.89
      interstitial nephritis (diffuse) (focal) 580.89
      necrotizing glomerulitis 580.4
    extracapillary with epithelial crescents 580.4
    poststreptococcal 580.0
    proliferative (diffuse) 580.0
    rapidly progressive 580.4
    specified pathology NEC 580.89
  arteriolar (see also Hypertension, kidney) 403.90
  arteriosclerotic (see also Hypertension, kidney) 403.90
  ascending (see also Pyelitis) 590.80
  basement membrane NEC 583.89
    with
      pulmonary hemorrhage (Goodpasture's syndrome) 446.21 [583.81]
  chronic 582.9
    with
      exudative nephritis 582.89
      interstitial nephritis (diffuse) (focal) 582.89
      necrotizing glomerulitis 582.4
      specified pathology or lesion NEC 582.89
    endothelial 582.2
    extracapillary with epithelial crescents 582.4
    hypocomplementemic persistent 582.2
    lobular 582.2
    membranoproliferative 582.2
    membranous 582.1
      and proliferative (mixed) 582.2
      sclerosing 582.1
    mesangiocapillary 582.2
    mixed membranous and proliferative 582.2
    proliferative (diffuse) 582.0
    rapidly progressive 582.4
    sclerosing 582.1
  cirrhotic—see Sclerosis, renal
  desquamative—see Nephrosis
  due to or associated with
    amyloidosis 277.39 [583.81]
      with nephrotic syndrome 277.39 [581.81]
      chronic 277.39 [582.81]

INDEX TO DISEASES

Glomerulonephritis—continued
  diabetes mellitus 250.4 [583.81]
    with nephrotic syndrome 250.4 [581.81]
  diphtheria 032.89 [580.81]
  gonococcal infection (acute) 098.19 [583.81]
    chronic or duration or 2 months or over 098.39 [583.81]
  infectious hepatitis 070.9 [580.81]
  malaria (with nephrotic syndrome) 084.9 [581.81]
  mumps 072.79 [580.81]
  polyarteritis (nodosa) (with nephrotic syndrome) 446.0 [581.81]
  specified pathology NEC 583.89
    acute 580.89
    chronic 582.89
  streptotrichosis 039.8 [583.81]
  subacute bacterial endocarditis 421.0 [580.81]
  syphilis (late) 095.4
    congenital 090.5 [583.81]
    early 091.69 [583.81]
  systemic lupus erythematosus 710.0 [583.81]
    with nephrotic syndrome 710.0 [581.81]
    chronic 710.0 [582.81]
  tuberculosis (see also Tuberculosis) 016.0 [583.81]
  typhoid fever 002.0 [580.81]
extracapillary with epithelial crescents 583.4
  acute 580.4
  chronic 582.4
exudative 583.89
  acute 580.89
  chronic 582.89
focal (see also Nephritis) 583.9
  embolic 580.4
granular 582.89
granulomatous 582.89
hydremic (see also Nephrosis) 581.9
hypocomplementemic persistent 583.2
  with nephrotic syndrome 581.2
  chronic 582.2
immune complex NEC 583.89
infective (see also Pyelitis) 590.80
interstitial (diffuse) (focal) 583.89
  with nephrotic syndrome 581.89
  acute 580.89
  chronic 582.89
latent or quiescent 582.9
lobular 583.2
  with nephrotic syndrome 581.2
  chronic 582.2
membranoproliferative 583.2
  with nephrotic syndrome 581.2
  chronic 582.2
membranous 583.1
  with nephrotic syndrome 581.1
  and proliferative (mixed) 583.2
    with nephrotic syndrome 581.2
    chronic 582.2
  chronic 582.1
  sclerosing 582.1
    with nephrotic syndrome 581.1
mesangiocapillary 583.2
  with nephrotic syndrome 581.2
  chronic 582.2
minimal change 581.3
mixed membranous and proliferative 583.2
  with nephrotic syndrome 581.2
  chronic 582.2
necrotizing 583.4
  acute 580.4

INDEX TO DISEASES

Glomerulonephritis—*continued*
  chronic 582.4
  nephrotic (*see also* Nephrosis) 581.9
  old—*see* Glomerulonephritis, chronic
  parenchymatous 581.89
  poststreptococcal 580.0
  proliferative (diffuse) 583.0
    with nephrotic syndrome 581.0
    acute 580.0
    chronic 582.0
  purulent (*see also* Pyelitis) 590.80
  quiescent—*see* Nephritis, chronic
  rapidly progressive 583.4
    acute 580.4
    chronic 582.4
  sclerosing membranous (chronic) 582.1
    with nephrotic syndrome 581.1
  septic (*see also* Pyelitis) 590.80
  specified pathology or lesion NEC 583.89
    with nephrotic syndrome 581.89
    acute 580.89
    chronic 582.89
  suppurative (acute) (disseminated) (*see also* Pyelitis) 590.80
  toxic—*see* Nephritis, acute
  tubal, tubular—*see* Nephrosis, tubular
  type II (Ellis)—*see* Nephrosis
  vascular—*see* Hypertension, kidney
Glomerulosclerosis (*see also* Sclerosis, renal) 587
  focal 582.1
    with nephrotic syndrome 581.1
  intercapillary (nodular) (with diabetes) 250.4 *[581.81]*
Glossagra 529.6
Glossalgia 529.6
Glossitis 529.0
  areata exfoliativa 529.1
  atrophic 529.4
  benign migratory 529.1
  gangrenous 529.0
  Hunter's 529.4
  median rhomboid 529.2
  Moeller's 529.4
  pellagrous 265.2
Glossocele 529.8
Glossodynia 529.6
  exfoliativa 529.4
Glossoncus 529.8
Glossophytia 529.3
Glossoplegia 529.8
Glossoptosis 529.8
Glossopyrosis 529.6
Glossotrichia 529.3
Glossy skin 701.9
Glottis —*see* condition
Glottitis —*see* Glossitis
Glucagonoma (M8152/0)
  malignant (M8152/3)
    pancreas 157.4
    specified site NEC—*see* Neoplasm, by site, malignant
    unspecified site 157.4
  pancreas 211.7
  specified site NEC—*see* Neoplasm, by site, benign
  unspecified site 211.7
Glucoglycinuria 270.7
Glue ear syndrome 381.20
Glue sniffing (airplane glue) (*see also* Dependence) 304.6
Glycinemia (with methylmalonic acidemia) 270.7

Goiter

Glycinuria (renal) (with ketosis) 270.0
Glycogen
  infiltration (*see also* Disease, glycogen storage) 271.0
  storage disease (*see also* Disease, glycogen storage) 271.0
Glycogenosis (*see also* Disease, glycogen storage) 271.0
  cardiac 271.0 *[425.7]*
  Cori, types I-VII 271.0
  diabetic, secondary 250.8 *[259.8]*
  diffuse (with hepatic cirrhosis) 271.0
  generalized 271.0
  glucose-6-phosphatase deficiency 271.0
  hepatophosphorylase deficiency 271.0
  hepatorenal 271.0
  myophosphorylase deficiency 271.0
Glycopenia 251.2
Glycopeptide
  intermediate staphylococcus aureus (GISA) V09.8
  resistent
    enterococcus V09.8
    staphylococcus aureus (GRSA) V09.8
Glycoprolinuria 270.8
Glycosuria 791.5
  renal 271.4
Gnathostoma (spinigerum) (infection) (infestation) 128.1
  wandering swellings from 128.1
Gnathostomiasis 128.1
Goiter (adolescent) (colloid) (diffuse) (dipping) (due to iodine deficiency) (endemic) (euthyroid) (heart) (hyperplastic) (internal) (intrathoracic) (juvenile) (mixed type) (nonendemic) (parenchymatous) (plunging) (sporadic) (subclavicular) (substernal) 240.9
  with
    hyperthyroidism (recurrent) (*see also* Goiter, toxic) 242.0
    thyrotoxicosis (*see also* Goiter, toxic) 242.0
  adenomatous (*see also* Goiter, nodular) 241.9
  cancerous (M8000/3) 193
  complicating pregnancy, childbirth, or puerperium 648.1
  congenital 246.1
  cystic (*see also* Goiter, nodular) 241.9
  due to enzyme defect in synthesis of thyroid hormone (butane-insoluble iodine) (coupling) (deiodinase) (iodide trapping or organification) (iodotyrosine dehalogenase) (peroxidase) 246.1
  dyshormonogenic 246.1
  exophthalmic (*see also* Goiter, toxic) 242.0
  familial (with deaf-mutism) 243
  fibrous 245.3
  lingual 759.2
  lymphadenoid 245.2
  malignant (M8000/3) 193
  multinodular (nontoxic) 241.1
    toxic or with hyperthyroidism (*see also* Goiter, toxic) 242.2
  nodular (nontoxic) 241.9
    with
      hyperthyroidism (*see also* Goiter, toxic) 242.3
      thyrotoxicosis (*see also* Goiter, toxic) 242.3
    endemic 241.9
    exophthalmic (diffuse) (*see also* Goiter, toxic) 242.0
    multinodular (nontoxic) 241.1

Goiter—*continued*
  sporadic 241.9
  toxic (*see also* Goiter, toxic) 242.3
  uninodular (nontoxic) 241.0
  nontoxic (nodular) 241.9
    multinodular 241.1
    uninodular 241.0
  pulsating (*see also* Goiter, toxic) 242.0
  simple 240.0
  toxic 242.0

Note—Use the following fifth-digit subclassification with category 242:

0 without mention of thyrotoxic crisis or storm
1 with mention of thyrotoxic crisis or storm

---

    adenomatous 242.3
      multinodular 242.2
      uninodular 242.1
    multinodular 242.2
    nodular 242.3
      multinodular 242.2
      uninodular 242.1
    uninodular 242.1
  uninodular (nontoxic) 241.0
    toxic or with hyperthyroidism (*see also* Goiter, toxic) 242.1
Goldberg (-Maxwell) (-Morris) **syndrome** (testicular feminization) 259.5
Goldblatt's
  hypertension 440.1
  kidney 440.1
Goldenhar's syndrome (oculoauriculovertebral dysplasia) 756.0
Goldflam-Erb disease or syndrome 358.00
Goldscheider's disease (epidermolysis bullosa) 757.39
Goldstein's disease (familial hemorrhagic telangiectasia) 448.0
Golfer's elbow 726.32
Goltz-Gorlin syndrome (dermal hypoplasia) 757.39
Gonadoblastoma (M9073/1)
  specified site—*see* Neoplasm, by site uncertain behavior
  unspecified site
    female 236.2
    male 236.4
Gonecystitis (*see also* Vesiculitis) 608.0
Gongylonemiasis 125.6
  mouth 125.6
Goniosynechiae 364.73
Gonococcemia 098.89
Gonococcus, gonococcal (disease) (infection) (*see also* condition) 098.0
  anus 098.7
  bursa 098.52
  chronic NEC 098.2
  complicating pregnancy, childbirth, or puerperium 647.1
    affecting fetus or newborn 760.2
  conjunctiva, conjunctivitis (neonatorum) 098.40
  dermatosis 098.89
  endocardium 098.84
  epididymo-orchitis 098.13
    chronic or duration of 2 months or over 098.33
  eye (newborn) 098.40
  fallopian tube (chronic) 098.37
    acute 098.17

Gonococcus, gonococcal—*continued*
  genitourinary (acute) (organ) (system) (tract) (*see also* Gonorrhea) 098.0
    lower 098.0
      chronic 098.2
    upper 098.10
      chronic 098.30
  heart NEC 098.85
  joint 098.50
  keratoderma 098.81
  keratosis (blennorrhagica) 098.81
  lymphatic (gland) (node) 098.89
  meninges 098.82
  orchitis (acute) 098.13
    chronic or duration of 2 months or over 098.33
  pelvis (acute) 098.19
    chronic or duration of 2 months or over 098.39
  pericarditis 098.83
  peritonitis 098.86
  pharyngitis 098.6
  pharynx 098.6
  proctitis 098.7
  pyosalpinx (chronic) 098.37
    acute 098.17
  rectum 098.7
  septicemia 098.89
  skin 098.89
  specified site NEC 098.89
  synovitis 098.51
  tendon sheath 098.51
  throat 098.6
  urethra (acute) 098.0
    chronic or duration of 2 months or over 098.2
  vulva (acute) 098.0
    chronic or duration of 2 months or over 098.2
Gonocytoma (M9073/1)
  specified site—*see* Neoplasm, by site, uncertain behavior
  unspecified site
    female 236.2
    male 236.4
Gonorrhea 098.0
  acute 098.0
  Bartholin's gland (acute) 098.0
    chronic or duration of 2 months or over 098.2
  bladder (acute) 098.11
    chronic or duration of 2 months or over 098.31
  carrier (suspected of) V02.7
  cervix (acute) 098.15
    chronic or duration of 2 months or over 098.35
  chronic 098.2
  complicating pregnancy, childbirth, or puerperium 647.1
    affecting fetus or newborn 760.2
  conjunctiva, conjunctivitis (neonatorum) 098.40
  contact V01.6
  Cowper's gland (acute) 098.0
    chronic or duration of 2 months or over 098.2
  duration of two months or over 098.2
  exposure to V01.6
  fallopian tube (chronic) 098.37
    acute 098.17
  genitourinary (acute) (organ) (system) (tract) 098.0
    chronic 098.2
    duration of two months or over 098.2
  kidney (acute) 098.19
    chronic or duration of 2 months or over 098.39
  ovary (acute) 098.19
    chronic or duration of 2 months or over 098.39

Gonorrhea—*continued*
  pelvis (acute) 098.19
    chronic or duration of 2 months or over 098.39
  penis (acute) 098.0
    chronic or duration of 2 months or over 098.2
  prostate (acute) 098.12
    chronic or duration of 2 months or over 098.32
  seminal vesicle (acute) 098.14
    chronic or duration of 2 months or over 098.34
  specified site NEC—*see* Gonococcus
  spermatic cord (acute) 098.14
    chronic or duration of 2 months or over 098.34
  urethra (acute) 098.0
    chronic or duration of 2 months or over 098.2
  vagina (acute) 098.0
    chronic or duration of 2 months or over 098.2
  vas deferens (acute) 098.14
    chronic or duration of 2 months or over 098.34
  vulva (acute) 098.0
    chronic or duration of 2 months or over 098.2
Goodpasture's syndrome (pneumorenal) 446.21
Good's syndrome 279.06
Gopalan's syndrome (burning feet) 266.2
Gordon's disease (exudative enteropathy) 579.8
Gorlin-Chaudhry-Moss syndrome 759.89
Gougerot's syndrome (trisymptomatic) 709.1
Gougerot-Blum syndrome (pigmented purpuric lichenoid dermatitis) 709.1
Gougerot-Carteaud disease or syndrome (confluent reticulate papillomatosis) 701.8
Gougerot-Hailey-Hailey disease (benign familial chronic pemphigus) 757.39
Gougerot (-Houwer) -Sjögren syndrome (keratoconjunctivitis sicca) 710.2
Gouley's syndrome (constrictive pericarditis) 423.2
Goundou 102.6
Gout, gouty 274.9
  with specified manifestations NEC 274.89
  arthritis (acute) 274.0
  arthropathy 274.0
  degeneration, heart 274.82
  diathesis 274.9
  eczema 274.89
  episcleritis 274.89 *[379.09]*
  external ear (tophus) 274.81
  glomerulonephritis 274.10
  iritis 274.89 *[364.11]*
  joint 274.0
  kidney 274.10
  lead 984.9
    specified type of lead—*see* Table of drugs and chemicals
  nephritis 274.10
  neuritis 274.89 *[357.4]*
  phlebitis 274.89 *[451.9]*
  rheumatic 714.0
  saturnine 984.9
    specified type of lead—*see* Table of drugs and chemicals
  spondylitis 274.0
  synovitis 274.0
  syphilitic 095.8
  tophi 274.0
    ear 274.81
    heart 274.82
    specified site NEC 274.82
Gowers'
  muscular dystrophy 359.1
  syndrome (vasovagal attack) 780.2
Gowers-Paton-Kennedy syndrome 377.04

Gradenigo's syndrome 383.02
Graft-versus-host disease (bone marrow) 996.85
  due to organ transplant NEC—*see* Complications, transplant, organ
Graham Steell's murmur (pulmonic regurgitation) (*see also* Endocarditis, pulmonary) 424.3
Grain-handlers' disease or lung 495.8
Grain mite (itch) 133.8
Grand
  mal (idiopathic) (*see also* Epilepsy) 345.1
    hysteria of Charcot 300.11
    nonrecurrent or isolated 780.39
  multipara
    affecting management of labor and delivery 659.4
    status only (not pregnant) V61.5
Granite workers' lung 502
Granular —*see also* condition
  inflammation, pharynx 472.1
  kidney (contracting) (*see also* Sclerosis, renal) 587
  liver—*see* Cirrhosis, liver
  nephritis—*see* Nephritis
Granulation tissue, abnormal —*see also* Granuloma
  abnormal or excessive 701.5
  postmastoidectomy cavity 383.33
  postoperative 701.5
  skin 701.5
Granulocytopenia, granulocytopenic (primary) 288.00
  malignant 288.09
Granuloma NEC 686.1
  abdomen (wall) 568.89
    skin (pyogenicum) 686.1
      from residual foreign body 709.4
  annulare 695.89
  anus 569.49
  apical 522.6
  appendix 543.9
  aural 380.23
  beryllium (skin) 709.4
    lung 503
  bone (*see also* Osteomyelitis) 730.1
    eosinophilic 277.89
    from residual foreign body 733.99
  canaliculus lacrimalis 375.81
  cerebral 348.8
  cholesterin, middle ear 385.82
  coccidioidal (progressive) 114.3
    lung 114.4
    meninges 114.2
    primary (lung) 114.0
  colon 569.89
  conjunctiva 372.61
  dental 522.6
  ear, middle (cholesterin) 385.82
    with otitis media—*see* Otitis media
  eosinophilic 277.89
    bone 277.89
    lung 277.89
    oral mucosa 528.9
  exuberant 701.5
  eyelid 374.89
  facial
    lethal midline 446.3
    malignant 446.3
  faciale 701.8
  fissuratum (gum) 523.8
  foot NEC 686.1
  foreign body (in soft tissue) NEC 728.82

Granuloma INDEX TO DISEASES

Granuloma—*continued*
  bone 733.99
    in operative wound 998.4
    muscle 728.82
    skin 709.4
    subcutaneous tissue 709.4
  fungoides 202.1
  gangraenescens 446.3
  giant cell (central) (jaw) (reparative) 526.3
    gingiva 523.8
    peripheral (gingiva) 523.8
  gland (lymph) 289.3
  Hodgkin's (M9661/3) 201.1
  ileum 569.89
  infectious NEC 136.9
  inguinale (Donovan) 099.2
    venereal 099.2
  intestine 569.89
  iridocyclitis 364.10
  jaw (bone) 526.3
    reparative giant cell 526.3
  kidney (*see also* Infection, kidney) 590.9
  lacrimal sac 375.81
  larynx 478.79
  lethal midline 446.3
  lipid 277.89
  lipoid 277.89
  liver 572.8
  lung (infectious) (*see also* Fibrosis, lung) 515
    coccidioidal 114.4
    eosinophilic 277.89
  lymph gland 289.3
  Majocchi's 110.6
  malignant, face 446.3
  mandible 526.3
  mediastinum 519.3
  midline 446.3
  monilial 112.3
  muscle 728.82
    from residual foreign body 728.82
  nasal sinus (*see also* Sinusitis) 473.9
  operation wound 998.59
    foreign body 998.4
    stitch (external) 998.89
      internal organ 998.89
    talc 998.7
  oral mucosa, eosinophilic or pyogenic 528.9
  orbit, orbital 376.11
  paracoccidioidal 116.1
  penis, venereal 099.2
  periapical 522.6
  peritoneum 568.89
    due to ova of helminths NEC (*see also* Helminthiasis) 128.9
  postmastoidectomy cavity 383.33
  postoperative–*see* Granuloma, operation wound
  prostate 601.8
  pudendi (ulcerating) 099.2
  pudendorum (ulcerative) 099.2
  pulp, internal (tooth) 521.49
  pyogenic, pyogenicum (skin) 686.1
    maxillary alveolar ridge 522.6
    oral mucosa 528.9
  rectum 569.49
  reticulohistiocytic 277.89
  rubrum nasi 705.89
  sarcoid 135
  Schistosoma 120.9
  septic (skin) 686.1
  silica (skin) 709.4

Granuloma—*continued*
  sinus (accessory) (infectional) (nasal) (*see also* Sinusitis) 473.9
  skin (pyogenicum) 686.1
    from foreign body or material 709.4
  sperm 608.89
  spine
    syphilitic (epidural) 094.89
    tuberculous (*see also* Tuberculosis) 015.0 [730.88]
  stitch (postoperative) 998.89
    internal wound 998.89
  suppurative (skin) 686.1
  suture (postoperative) 998.89
    internal wound 998.89
  swimming pool 031.1
  talc 728.82
    in operation wound 998.7
  telangiectaticum (skin) 686.1
  tracheostomy 519.09
  trichophyticum 110.6
  tropicum 102.4
  umbilicus 686.1
    newborn 771.4
  urethra 599.84
  uveitis 364.10
  vagina 099.2
  venereum 099.2
  vocal cords 478.5
  Wegener's (necrotizing respiratory granulomatosis) 446.4
Granulomatosis NEC 686.1
  disciformis chronica et progressiva 709.3
  infantiseptica 771.2
  lipoid 277.89
  lipophagic, intestinal 040.2
  miliary 027.0
  necrotizing, respiratory 446.4
  progressive, septic 288.1
  Wegener's (necrotizing respiratory) 446.4
Granulomatous tissue —*see* Granuloma
Granulosis rubra nasi 705.89
Graphite fibrosis (of lung) 503
Graphospasm 300.89
  organic 333.84
Grating scapula 733.99
Gravel (urinary) (*see also* Calculus) 592.9
Graves' disease (exophthalmic goiter) (*see also* Goiter, toxic) 242.0
Gravis —*see* condition
Grawitz's tumor (hypernephroma) (M8312/3) 189.0
Grayness, hair (premature) 704.3
  congenital 757.4
Gray or grey syndrome (chloramphenicol) (newborn) 779.4
Greenfield's disease 330.0
Green sickness 280.9
Greenstick fracture —*see* Fracture, by site
Greig's syndrome (hypertelorism) 756.0
Grief 309.0
Griesinger's disease (*see also* Ancylostomiasis) 126.9
Grinder's
  asthma 502
  lung 502
  phthisis (*see also* Tuberculosis) 011.4
Grinding, teeth 306.8
Grip
  Dabney's 074.1
  devil's 074.1

INDEX TO DISEASES

Grippe, grippal —*see also* Influenza
  Balkan 083.0
  intestinal 487.8
  summer 074.8
Grippy cold 487.1
Grisel's disease 723.5
Groin —*see* condition
Grooved
  nails (transverse) 703.8
  tongue 529.5
    congenital 750.13
Ground itch 126.9
Growing pains, children 781.99
Growth (fungoid) (neoplastic) (new)
    (M8000/1)—*see also* Neoplasm, by site,
    unspecified nature
  adenoid (vegetative) 474.12
  benign (M8000/0)—*see* Neoplasm, by site,
    benign
  fetal, poor 764.9
    affecting management of pregnancy 656.5
  malignant (M8000/3)—*see* Neoplasm, by site
    malignant
  rapid, childhood V21.0
  secondary (M8000/6)—*see* Neoplasm, by site,
    malignant, secondary
GRSA (glycopeptide resistant staphylococcus
    aureus) V09.8
Gruber's hernia —*see* Hernia, Gruber's
Gruby's disease (tinea tonsurans) 110.0
G-trisomy 758.0
Guama fever 066.3
Gubler (-Millard) paralysis or syndrome 344.89
Guérin-Stern syndrome (arthrogryposis
    multiplex congenita) 754.89
Guertin's disease (electric chorea) 049.8
Guillain-Barré disease or syndrome 357.0
Guinea worms (infection) (infestation) 125.7
Guinon's disease (motor-verbal tic) 307.23
Gull's disease (thyroid atrophy with myxedema)
    244.8
Gull and Sutton's disease —*see* Hypertension,
    kidney
Gum —*see* condition
Gumboil 522.7
Gumma (syphilitic) 095.9
  artery 093.89
    cerebral or spinal 094.89
  bone 095.5
    of yaws (late) 102.6
  brain 094.89
  cauda equina 094.89
  central nervous system NEC 094.9
  ciliary body 095.8 *[364.11]*
  congenital 090.5
    testis 090.5
  eyelid 095.8 *[373.5]*
  heart 093.89
  intracranial 094.89
  iris 095.8 *[364.11]*
  kidney 095.4
  larynx 095.8
  leptomeninges 094.2
  liver 095.3
  meninges 094.2
  myocardium 093.82
  nasopharynx 095.8
  neurosyphilitic 094.9
  nose 095.8
  orbit 095.8

Gumma—*continued*
  palate (soft) 095.8
  penis 095.8
  pericardium 093.81
  pharynx 095.8
  pituitary 095.8
  scrofulous (*see also* Tuberculosis) 017.0
  skin 095.8
  specified site NEC 095.8
  spinal cord 094.89
  tongue 095.8
  tonsil 095.8
  trachea 095.8
  tuberculous (*see also* Tuberculosis) 017.0
  ulcerative due to yaws 102.4
  ureter 095.8
  yaws 102.4
    bone 102.6
Gunn's syndrome (jaw-winking syndrome)
    742.8
Gunshot wound —*see also* Wound, open, by site
  fracture—*see* Fracture, by site, open
  internal organs (abdomen, chest, or pelvis)—*see*
      Injury, internal, by site, with open wound
  intracranial—*see* Laceration, brain, with open
      intracranial wound
Günther's disease or syndrome (congenital
    erythropoietic porphyria) 277.1
Gustatory hallucination 780.1
Gynandrism 752.7
Gynandroblastoma (M8632/1)
  specified site—*see* Neoplasm, by site, uncertain
    behavior
  unspecified site
    female 236.2
    male 236.4
Gynandromorphism 752.7
Gynatresia (congenital) 752.49
Gynecoid pelvis, male 738.6
Gynecological examination V72.31
  for contraceptive maintenance V25.40
Gynecomastia 611.1
Gynephobia 300.29
Gyrate scalp 757.39

H

Haas' disease (osteochondrosis head of humerus) 732.3
Habermann's disease (acute parapsoriasis varioliformis) 696.2
Habit, habituation
 chorea 307.22
 disturbance, child 307.9
 drug (*see also* Dependence) 304.9
 laxative (*see also* Abuse, drugs, nondependent) 305.9
 spasm 307.20
  chronic 307.22
  transient (of childhood) 307.21
 tic 307.20
  chronic 307.22
  transient (of childhood) 307.21
 use of
  nonprescribed drugs (*see also* Abuse, drugs, nondependent) 305.9
  patent medicines (*see also* Abuse, drugs, nondependent) 305.9
 vomiting 536.2
Hadfield-Clarke syndrome (pancreatic infantilism) 577.8
Haff disease 985.1
Hageman factor defect, deficiency, or disease (*see also* Defect, coagulation) 286.3
Haglund's disease (osteochondrosis os tibiale externum) 732.5
Haglund-Läwen-Fründ syndrome 717.89
Hagner's disease (hypertrophic pulmonary osteoarthropathy) 731.2
Hag teeth, tooth 524.39
Hailey-Hailey disease (benign familial chronic pemphigus) 757.39
Hair —*see also* condition
 plucking 307.9
Hairball in stomach 935.2
Hairy black tongue 529.3
Half vertebra 756.14
Halitosis 784.99
Hallermann-Streiff syndrome 756.0
Hallervorden-Spatz disease or syndrome 333.0
Hallopeau's
 acrodermatitis (continua) 696.1
 disease (lichen sclerosis et atrophicus) 701.0
Hallucination (auditory) (gustatory) (olfactory) (tactile) 780.1
 alcohol-induced 291.3
 drug-induced 292.12
 visual 368.16
Hallucinosis 298.9
 alcohol-induced (acute) 291.3
 drug-induced 292.12
Hallus —*see* Hallux
Hallux 735.9
 limitus 735.8
 malleus (acquired) 735.3
 rigidus (acquired) 735.2
  congenital 755.66
  late effects of rickets 268.1
 valgus (acquired) 735.0
  congenital 755.66
 varus (acquired) 735.1
  congenital 755.66
Halo, visual 368.15
Hamartoblastoma 759.6

Hamartoma 759.6
 epithelial (gingival), odontogenic, central, or peripheral (M9321/0) 213.1
 upper jaw (bone) 213.0
 vascular 757.32
Hamartosis, hamartoses NEC 759.6
Hamman's disease or syndrome (spontaneous mediastinal emphysema) 518.1
Hamman-Rich syndrome (diffuse interstitial pulmonary fibrosis) 516.3
Hammer toe (acquired) 735.4
 congenital 755.66
 late effects of rickets 268.1
Hand —*see* condition
Hand-Schüller-Christian disease or syndrome (chronic histiocytosis x) 277.89
Hand-foot syndrome 693.0
Hanging (asphyxia) (strangulation) (suffocation) 994.7
Hangnail (finger) (with lymphangitis) 681.02
Hangover (alcohol) (*see also* Abuse, drugs, nondependent) 305.0
Hanot's cirrhosis or disease —*see* Cirrhosis, biliary
Hanot-Chauffard (-Troisier) syndrome (bronze diabetes) 275.0
Hansen's disease (leprosy) 030.9
 benign form 030.1
 malignant form 030.0
Harada's disease or syndrome 363.22
Hard chancre 091.0
Hard firm prostate 600.10
 with
  urinary
   obstruction 600.11
   retention 600.11
Hardening
 artery—*see* Arteriosclerosis
 brain 348.8
 liver 571.8
Hare's syndrome (M8010/3) (carcinoma, pulmonary apex) 162.3
Harelip (*see also* Cleft, lip) 749.10
Harkavy's syndrome 446.0
Harlequin (fetus) 757.1
 color change syndrome 779.89
Harley's disease (intermittent hemoglobinuria) 283.2
Harris'
 lines 733.91
 syndrome (organic hyperinsulinism) 251.1
Hart's disease or syndrome (pellagra-cerebellar ataxia-renal aminoaciduria) 270.0
Hartmann's pouch (abnormal sacculation of gallbladder neck) 575.8
 of intestine V44.3
  attention to V55.3
Hartnup disease (pellagra-cerebellar ataxia-renal aminoaciduria) 270.0
Harvester lung 495.0
Hashimoto's disease or struma (struma lymphomatosa) 245.2
Hassall-Henle bodies (corneal warts) 371.41
Haut mal (*see also* Epilepsy) 345.1
Haverhill fever 026.1
Hawaiian wood rose dependence 304.5
Hawkins' keloid 701.4

Hay
  asthma (see also Asthma) 493.0
    fever (allergic) (with rhinitis) 477.9
      with asthma (bronchial) (see also Asthma) 493.0
      allergic, due to grass, pollen, ragweed, or tree 477.0
      conjunctivitis 372.05
      due to
        dander, animal (cat) (dog) 477.2
        dust 477.8
        fowl 477.8
        hair, animal (cat) (dog) 477.2
        pollen 477.0
        specified allergen other than pollen 477.8
Hayem-Faber syndrome (achlorhydric anemia) 280.9
Hayem-Widal syndrome (acquired hemolytic jaundice) 283.9
Haygarth's nodosities 715.04
Hazard-Crile tumor (M8350/3) 193
Hb (abnormal)
  disease—see Disease, hemoglobin
  trait—see Trait
H disease 270.0
Head —see also condition
  banging 307.3
Headache 784.0
  allergic 346.2
  cluster 346.2
  due to
    loss, spinal fluid 349.0
    lumbar puncture 349.0
    saddle block 349.0
  emotional 307.81
  histamine 346.2
  lumbar puncture 349.0
  menopausal 627.2
  migraine 346.9
  nonorganic origin 307.81
  postspinal 349.0
  psychogenic 307.81
  psychophysiologic 307.81
  sick 346.1
  spinal 349.0
    complicating labor and delivery 668.8
    postpartum 668.8
  spinal fluid loss 349.0
  tension 307.81
  vascular 784.0
    migraine type 346.9
  vasomotor 346.9
Health
  advice V65.4
  audit V70.0
  checkup V70.0
  education V65.4
  hazard (see also History of) V15.9
    falling V15.88
    specified cause NEC V15.89
  instruction V65.4
  services provided because of (of)
    boarding school residence V60.6
    holiday relief for person providing home care V60.5
    inadequate
      housing V60.1
      resources V60.2
    lack of housing V60.0
    no care available in home V60.4
    person living alone V60.3
    poverty V60.3

Health—continued
    residence in institution V60.6
    specified cause NEC V60.8
    vacation relief for person providing home care V60.5
Healthy
  donor (see also Donor) V59.9
  infant or child
    accompanying sick mother V65.0
    receiving care V20.1
  person
    accompanying sick relative V65.0
    admitted for sterilization V25.2
    receiving prophylactic inoculation or vaccination (see also Vaccination, prophylactic) V05.9
Hearing
  conservation and treatment V72.12
  examination V72.19
    following failed hearing screening V72.11
Heart —see condition
Heartburn 787.1
  psychogenic 306.4
Heat (effects) 992.9
  apoplexy 992.0
  burn—see also Burn, by site
    from sun (see also Sunburn) 692.71
  collapse 992.1
  cramps 992.2
  dermatitis or eczema 692.89
  edema 992.7
  erythema—see Burn, by site
  excessive 992.9
    specified effect NEC 992.8
  exhaustion 992.5
    anhydrotic 992.3
    due to
      salt (and water) depletion 992.4
      water depletion 992.3
  fatigue (transient) 992.6
  fever 992.0
  hyperpyrexia 992.0
  prickly 705.1
  prostration—see Heat, exhaustion
  pyrexia 992.0
  rash 705.1
  specified effect NEC 992.8
  stroke 992.0
  sunburn (see also Sunburn) 692.71
  syncope 992.1
Heavy-chain disease 273.2
Heavy-for-dates (fetus or infant) 766.1
  4500 grams or more 766.0
  exceptionally 766.0
Hebephrenia, hebephrenic (acute) (see also Schizophrenia) 295.1
  dementia (praecox) (see also Schizophrenia) 295.1
  schizophrenia (see also Schizophrenia) 295.1
Heberden's
  disease or nodes 715.04
  syndrome (angina pectoris) 413.9
Hebra's disease
  dermatitis exfoliativa 695.89
  erythema multiforme exudativum 695.1
  pityriasis 695.89
    maculata et circinata 696.3
    rubra 695.89
      pilaris 696.4
  prurigo 698.2
Hebra, nose 040.1

Hedinger's syndrome (malignant carcinoid) 259.2
Heel —*see* condition
Heerfordt's disease or syndrome (uveoparotitis) 135
Hegglin's anomaly or syndrome 288.2
Heidenhain's disease 290.10
  with dementia 290.10
Heilmeyer-Schöner disease (M9842/3) 207.1
Heine-Medin disease (*see also* Poliomyelitis) 045.9
Heinz-body anemia, congenital 282.7
Heller's disease or syndrome (infantile psychosis) (*see also* Psychosis, childhood) 299.1
H.E.L.L.P. 642.5
Helminthiasis (*see also* Infestation, by specific parasite) 128.9
  Ancylostoma (*see also* Ancylostoma) 126.9
  intestinal 127.9
    mixed types (types classifiable to more than one of the titles 120.0-127.7) 127.8
    specified type 127.7
  mixed types (intestinal) (types classifiable to more than one of the titles 120.0-127.7) 127.8
  Necator americanus 126.1
  specified type NEC 128.8
  Trichinella 124
Heloma 700
Hemangioblastoma (M9161/1)—*see also* Neoplasm, connective tissue, uncertain behavior
  malignant (M9161//3)—*see* Neoplasm, connective tissue, malignant
Hemangioblastomatosis, cerebelloretinal 759.6
Hemangioendothelioma (M9130/1)—*see also* Neoplasm, by site, uncertain behavior
  benign (M9130/0) 228.00
  bone (diffuse) (M9130/3)—*see* Neoplasm, bone, malignant
  malignant (M9130/3)—*see* Neoplasm, connective tissue, malignant
  nervous system (M9130/0) 228.09
Hemangioendotheliosarcoma (M9130/3)—*see* Neoplasm, connective tissue, malignant
Hemangiofibroma (M9160/0)—*see* Neoplasm, by site, benign
Hemangiolipoma (M8861/0)—*see* Lipoma
Hemangioma (M9120/0) 228.00
  arteriovenous (M9123/0)—*see* Hemangioma, by site
  brain 228.02
  capillary (M9131/0)—*see* Hemangioma, by site
  cavernous (M9121/0)—*see* Hemangioma, by site
  central nervous system NEC 228.09
  choroid 228.09
  heart 228.09
  infantile (M9131/0)—*see* Hemangioma, by site
  intra-abdominal structures 228.04
  intracranial structures 228.02
  intramuscular (M9132/0)—*see* Hemangioma, by site
  iris 228.09
  juvenile (M9131/0)—*see* Hemangioma, by site
  malignant (M9120/3)—*see* Neoplasm, connective tissue, malignant
  meninges 228.09
    brain 228.02
    spinal cord 228.09
  peritoneum 228.04
  placenta—*see* Placenta, abnormal

Hemangioma—*continued*
  plexiform (M9131/0)—*see* Hemangioma, by site
  racemose (M9123/0)—*see* Hemangioma, by site
  retina 228.03
  retroperitoneal tissue 228.04
  sclerosing (M8832/0)—*see* Neoplasm, skin, benign
  simplex (M9131/0)—*see* Hemangioma, by site
  skin and subcutaneous tissue 228.01
  specified site NEC 228.09
  spinal cord 228.09
  venous (M9122/0)—*see* Hemangioma, by site
  verrucous keratotic (M9142/0)—*see* Hemangioma, by site
Hemangiomatosis (systemic) 757.32
  involving single site—*see* Hemangioma
Hemangiopericytoma (M9150/1)—*see also* Neoplasm, connective tissue, uncertain behavior
  benign (M9150/0)—*see* Neoplasm, connective tissue, benign
  malignant (M9150/3)—*see* Neoplasm, connective tissue, malignant
Hemangiosarcoma (M9120/3)—*see* Neoplasm, connective tissue, malignant
Hemarthrosis (nontraumatic) 719.0
  ankle 719.17
  elbow 719.12
  foot 719.17
  hand 719.14
  hip 719.15
  knee 719.16
  multiple sites 719.19
  pelvic region 719.15
  shoulder (region) 719.11
  specified site NEC 719.18
  traumatic—*see* Sprain, by site
  wrist 719.13
Hematemesis 578.0
  with ulcer—*see* Ulcer, by site, with hemorrhage
  due to S. japonicum 120.2
  Goldstein's (familial hemorrhagic telangiectasia) 448.0
  newborn 772.4
    due to swallowed maternal blood 777.3
Hematidrosis 705.89
Hematinuria (*see also* Hemoglobinuria) 791.2
  malarial 084.8
  paroxysmal 283.2
Hematite miners' lung 503
Hematobilia 576.8
Hematocele (congenital) (diffuse) (idiopathic) 608.83
  broad ligament 620.7
  canal of Nuck 629.0
  cord, male 608.83
  fallopian tube 620.8
  female NEC 629.0
  ischiorectal 569.89
  male NEC 608.83
  ovary 629.0
  pelvis, pelvic
    female 629.0
      with ectopic pregnancy (*see also* Pregnancy, ectopic) 633.90
      with intrauterine pregnancy 633.91
    male 608.83
  periuterine 629.0
  retrouterine 629.0
  scrotum 608.83

Hematocele—*continued*
  spermatic cord (diffuse) 608.83
  testis 608.84
  traumatic—*see* Injury, internal, pelvis
  tunica vaginalis 608.83
  uterine ligament 629.0
  uterus 621.4
  vagina 623.6
  vulva 624.5
Hematocephalus 742.4
Hematochezia (*see also* Melena) 578.1
Hematochyluria (*see also* Infestation, filarial) 125.9
Hematocolpos 626.8
Hematocornea 371.12
Hematogenous —*see* condition
Hematoma (skin surface intact) (traumatic)—*see also* Contusion

> Note—*Hematomas are coded according to origin and the nature and site of the hematoma or the accompanying injury. Hematomas of unspecified origin are coded as injuries of the sites involved, except:*
> (a) *hematomas of genital organs which are coded as diseases of the organ involved unless they complicate pregnancy or delivery*
> (b) *hematomas of the eye which are coded as diseases of the eye.*
>
> *For late effect of hematoma classifiable to 920-924 see Late, effect, contusion*

  with
    crush injury—*see* Crush
    fracture—*see* Fracture, by site
    injury of internal organs—*see also* Injury, internal, by site
      kidney—*see* Hematoma, kidney, traumatic
      liver—*see* Hematoma, liver, traumatic
      spleen—*see* Hematoma, spleen
    nerve injury—*see* Injury, nerve
    open wound—*see* Wound, open, by site
    skin surface intact—*see* Contusion
  abdomen (wall)—*see* Contusion, abdomen
  amnion 658.8
  aorta, dissecting 441.00
    abdominal 441.02
    thoracic 441.01
    thoracoabdominal 441.03
  arterial (complicating trauma) 904.9
    specified site—*see* Injury, blood vessel, by site
  auricle (ear) 380.31
  birth injury 767.8
    skull 767.19

Hematoma—*continued*
  brain (traumatic) 853.0

> Note—*Use the following fifth-digit subclassification with categories 851-854:*
>
> 0 unspecified state of consciousness
> 1 with no loss of consciousness
> 2 with brief [less than one hour] loss of consciousness
> 3 with moderate [1-24 hours] loss of consciousness
> 4 with prolonged [more than 24 hours] loss of consciousness and return to pre-existing conscious level
> 5 with prolonged [more than 24 hours] loss of consciousness, without return to pre-existing conscious level
> *Use fifth-digit 5 to designate when a patient is unconscious and dies before regaining consciousness, regardless of the duration of the loss of consciousness*
> 6 with loss of consciousness of unspecified duration
> 9 with concussion, unspecified

  with
    cerebral
      contusion—*see* Contusion, brain
      laceration—*see* Laceration, brain
    open intracranial wound 853.1
    skull fracture—*see* Fracture, skull, by site
  extradural or epidural 852.4
    with open intracranial wound 852.5
    fetus or newborn 767.0
    nontraumatic 432.0
  fetus or newborn NEC 767.0
  nontraumatic (*see also* Hemorrhage, brain) 431
    epidural or extradural 432.0
    newborn NEC 772.8
    subarachnoid, arachnoid, or meningeal (*see also* Hemorrhage, subarachnoid) 430
    subdural (*see also* Hemorrhage, subdural) 432.1
  subarachnoid, arachnoid, or meningeal 852.0
    with open intracranial wound 852.1
    fetus or newborn 772.2
    nontraumatic (*see also* Hemorrhage, subarachnoid) 430
  subdural 852.2
    with open intracranial wound 852.3
    fetus or newborn (localized) 767.0
    nontraumatic (*see also* Hemorrhage, subdural) 432.1
  breast (nontraumatic) 611.8
  broad ligament (nontraumatic) 620.7
    complicating delivery 665.7
    traumatic—*see* Injury, internal, broad ligament
  calcified NEC 959.9
  capitis 920
    due to birth injury 767.19
    newborn 767.19
  cerebral—*see* Hematoma, brain
  cesarean section wound 674.3
  chorion—*see* Placenta, abnormal
  complicating delivery (perineum) (vulva) 664.5
    pelvic 665.7
    vagina 665.7
  corpus
    cavernosum (nontraumatic) 607.82

INDEX TO DISEASES

Hematoma—*continued*
  luteum (nontraumatic) (ruptured) 620.1
  dura (mater)—*see* Hematoma, brain, subdural
  epididymis (nontraumatic) 608.83
  epidural (traumatic)—*see also* Hematoma, brain, extradural
    spinal—*see* Injury, spinal, by site
  episiotomy 674.3
  external ear 380.31
  extradural—*see also* Hematoma, brain, extradural
    fetus or newborn 767.0
    nontraumatic 432.0
      fetus or newborn 767.0
  fallopian tube 620.8
  genital organ (nontraumatic)
    female NEC 629.89
    male NEC 608.83
    traumatic (external site) 922.4
      internal—*see* Injury, internal, genital organ
  graafian follicle (ruptured) 620.0
  internal organs (abdomen, chest, or pelvis)—*see also* Injury, internal, by site
    kidney—*see* Hematoma, kidney, traumatic
    liver—*see* Hematoma, liver, traumatic
    spleen—*see* Hematoma, spleen
  intracranial—*see* Hematoma, brain
  kidney, cystic 593.81
    traumatic 866.01
      with open wound into cavity 866.11
  labia (nontraumatic) 624.5
  lingual (and other parts of neck, scalp, or face, except eye) 920
  liver (subcapsular) 573.8
    birth injury 767.8
    fetus or newborn 767.8
    traumatic NEC 864.01
      with
        laceration—*see* Laceration, liver
        open wound into cavity 864.11
  mediastinum—*see* Injury, internal, mediastinum
  meninges, meningeal (brain)—*see also* Hematoma, brain, subarachnoid
    spinal—*see* Injury, spinal, by site
  mesosalpinx (nontraumatic) 620.8
    traumatic—*see* Injury, internal, pelvis
  muscle (traumatic)—*see* Contusion, by site
  nasal (septum) (and other part(s) of neck, scalp, or face, except eye) 920
  obstetrical surgical wound 674.3
  orbit, orbital (nontraumatic) 376.32
    traumatic 921.2
  ovary (corpus luteum) (nontraumatic) 620.1
    traumatic—*see* Injury, internal, ovary
  pelvis (female) (nontraumatic) 629.89
    complicating delivery 665.7
    male 608.83
    traumatic—*see also* Injury, internal, pelvis
      specified organ NEC (*see also* Injury, internal, pelvis) 867.6
  penis (nontraumatic) 607.82
  pericranial (and neck, or face any part, except eye) 920
    due to injury at birth 767.19
  perineal wound (obstetrical) 674.3
    complicating delivery 664.5
  perirenal, cystic 593.81
  pinna 380.31
  placenta—*see* Placenta, abnormal
  postoperative 998.12
  retroperitoneal (nontraumatic) 568.81

Hematoma—*continued*
    traumatic—*see* Injury, internal, retroperitoneum
  retropubic, male 568.81
  scalp (and neck, or face any part, except eye) 920
    fetus or newborn 767.19
  scrotum (nontraumatic) 608.83
    traumatic 922.4
  seminal vesicle (nontraumatic) 608.83
    traumatic—*see* Injury, internal, seminal vesicle
  spermatic cord—*see also* Injury, internal, spermatic cord
    nontraumatic 608.83
  spinal (cord) (meninges)—*see also* Injury, spinal, by site
    fetus or newborn 767.4
    nontraumatic 336.1
  spleen 865.01
    with
      laceration—*see* Laceration, spleen
      open wound into cavity 865.11
  sternocleidomastoid, birth injury 767.8
  sternomastoid, birth injury 767.8
  subarachnoid—*see also* Hematoma, brain, subarachnoid
    fetus or newborn 772.2
    nontraumatic (*see also* Hemorrhage, subarachnoid) 430
    newborn 772.2
  subdural—*see also* Hematoma, brain, subdural
    fetus or newborn (localized) 767.0
    nontraumatic (*see also* Hemorrhage, subdural) 432.1
  subperiosteal (syndrome) 267
    traumatic—*see* Hematoma, by site
  superficial, fetus or newborn 772.6
  syncytium—*see* Placenta, abnormal
  testis (nontraumatic) 608.83
    birth injury 767.8
    traumatic 922.4
  tunica vaginalis (nontraumatic) 608.83
  umbilical cord 663.6
    affecting fetus or newborn 762.6
  uterine ligament (nontraumatic) 620.7
    traumatic—*see* Injury, internal, pelvis
  uterus 621.4
    traumatic—*see* Injury, internal, pelvis
  vagina (nontraumatic) (ruptured) 623.6
    complicating delivery 665.7
    traumatic 922.4
  vas deferens (nontraumatic) 608.83
    traumatic—*see* Injury, internal, vas deferens
  vitreous 379.23
  vocal cord 920
  vulva (nontraumatic) 624.5
    complicating delivery 664.5
    fetus or newborn 767.8
    traumatic 922.4
Hematometra 621.4
Hematomyelia 336.1
  with fracture of vertebra (*see also* Fracture, vertebra, by site, with spinal cord injury) 806.8
  fetus or newborn 767.4
Hematomyelitis 323.9
  late effect—*see* category 326
Hematoperitoneum (*see also* Hemoperitoneum) 568.81

Hematopneumothorax (see also Hemothorax) 511.8
Hematopoiesis, cyclic 288.02
Hematoporphyria (acquired) (congenital) 277.1
Hematoporphyrinuria (acquired) (congenital) 277.1
Hematorachis, hematorrhachis 336.1
  fetus or newborn 767.4
Hematosalpinx 620.8
  with
    ectopic pregnancy (see also categories 633.0-633.9) 639.2
    molar pregnancy (see also categories 630-632) 639.2
  infectional (see also Salpingo-oophoritis) 614.2
Hematospermia 608.82
Hematothorax (see also Hemothorax) 511.8
Hematotympanum 381.03
Hematuria (benign) (essential) (idiopathic) 599.7
  due to S. hematobium 120.0
  endemic 120.0
  intermittent 599.7
  malarial 084.8
  paroxysmal 599.7
  sulfonamide
    correct substance properly administered 599.7
    overdose or wrong substance given or taken 961.0
  tropical (bilharziasis) 120.0
  tuberculous (see also Tuberculosis) 016.9
Hematuric bilious fever 084.8
Hemeralopia 368.10
  acquired 286.5
Hemiabiotrophy 799.89
Hemi-akinesia 781.8
Hemianalgesia (see also Disturbance, sensation) 782.0
Hemianencephaly 740.0
Hemianesthesia (see also Disturbance, sensation) 782.0
Hemianopia, hemianopsia (altitudinal) (homonymous) 368.46
  binasal 368.47
  bitemporal 368.47
  heteronymous 368.47
  syphilitic 095.8
Hemiasomatognosia 307.9
Hemiathetosis 781.0
Hemiatrophy 799.89
  cerebellar 334.8
  face 349.89
    progressive 349.89
  fascia 728.9
  leg 728.2
  tongue 529.8
Hemiballism (us) 333.5
Hemiblock (cardiac) (heart) (left) 426.2
Hemicardia 746.89
Hemicephalus, hemicephaly 740.0
Hemichorea 333.5
Hemicrania 346.9
  congenital malformation 740.0
Hemidystrophy —see Hemiatrophy
Hemiectromelia 755.4
Hemihypalgesia (see also Disturbance, sensation) 782.0
Hemihypertrophy (congenital) 759.89
  cranial 756.0
Hemihypesthesia (see also Disturbance, sensation) 782.0
Hemi-inattention 781.8

Hemimelia 755.4
  lower limb 755.30
    paraxial (complete) (incomplete) (intercalary) (terminal) 755.32
    fibula 755.37
    tibia 755.36
    transverse (complete) (partial) 755.31
  upper limb 755.20
    paraxial (complete) (incomplete) (intercalary) (terminal) 755.22
    radial 755.26
    ulnar 755.27
    transverse (complete) (partial) 755.21
Hemiparalysis (see also Hemiplegia) 342.9
Hemiparesis (see also Hemiplegia) 342.9
Hemiparesthesia (see also Disturbance, sensation) 782.0
Hemiplegia 342.9
  acute (see also Disease, cerebrovascular, acute) 436
  alternans facialis 344.89
  apoplectic (see also Disease, cerebrovascular, acute) 436
    late effect or residual
      affecting
        dominant side 438.21
        nondominant side 438.22
        unspecified side 438.20
  arteriosclerotic 437.0
    late effect or residual
      affecting
        dominant side 438.21
        nondominant side 438.22
        unspecified side 438.20
  ascending (spinal) NEC 344.89
  attack (see also Disease, cerebrovascular, acute) 436
  brain, cerebral (current episode) 437.8
    congenital 343.1
  cerebral—see Hemiplegia, brain
  congenital (cerebral) (spastic) (spinal) 343.1
  conversion neurosis (hysterical) 300.11
  cortical—see Hemiplegia, brain
  due to
    arteriosclerosis 437.0
      late effect or residual
        affecting
          dominant side 438.21
          nondominant side 438.22
          unspecified side 438.20
    cerebrovascular lesion (see also Disease, cerebrovascular, acute) 436
      late effect
        affecting
          dominant side 438.21
          nondominant side 438.22
          unspecified side 438.20
  embolic (current) (see also Embolism, brain) 434.1
    late effect
      affecting
        dominant side 438.21
        nondominant side 438.22
        unspecified side 438.20
  flaccid 342.0
  hypertensive (current episode) 437.8
  infantile (postnatal) 343.4
  late effect
    birth injury, intracranial or spinal 343.4
    cerebrovascular lesion—see Late effect(s) (of) cerebrovascular disease

Hemiplegia—*continued*
  viral encephalitis 139.0
  middle alternating NEC 344.89
  newborn NEC 767.0
  seizure (current episode) (*see also* Disease, cerebrovascular, acute) 436
  spastic 342.1
    congenital or infantile 343.1
    specified NEC 342.8
  thrombotic (current) (*see also* Thrombosis, brain) 434.0
  late effect—*see* late effect(s) (of) cerebrovascular disease
Hemisection, spinal cord —*see* Fracture, vertebra, by site, with spinal cord injury
Hemispasm 781.0
  facial 781.0
Hemispatial neglect 781.8
Hemisporosis 117.9
Hemitremor 781.0
Hemivertebra 756.14
Hemobilia 576.8
Hemocholecyst 575.8
Hemochromatosis (acquired) (diabetic) (hereditary) (liver) (myocardium) (primary idiopathic) (secondary) 275.0
  with refractory anemia 238.72
Hemodialysis V56.0
Hemoglobin —*see also* condition
  abnormal (disease)—*see* Disease, hemoglobin
  AS genotype 282.5
  fetal, hereditary persistence 282.7
  high-oxygen-affinity 289.0
  low NEC 285.9
  S (Hb-S), heterozygous 282.5
Hemoglobinemia 283.2
  due to blood transfusion NEC 999.8
    bone marrow 996.85
  paroxysmal 283.2
Hemoglobinopathy (mixed) (*see also* Disease, hemoglobin) 282.7
  with thalassemia 282.49
  sickle-cell 282.60
    with thalassemia (without crisis) 282.41
    with
      crisis 282.42
      vaso-occlusive pain 282.42
Hemoglobinuria, hemoglobinuric 791.2
  with anemia, hemolytic, acquired (chronic) NEC 283.2
  cold (agglutinin) (paroxysmal) (with Raynaud's syndrome) 283.2
  due to
    exertion 283.2
    hemolysis (from external causes) NEC 283.2
  exercise 283.2
  fever (malaria) 084.8
  infantile 791.2
  intermittent 283.2
  malarial 084.8
  march 283.2
  nocturnal (paroxysmal) 283.2
  paroxysmal (cold) (nocturnal) 283.2
Hemolymphangioma (M9175/0) 228.1
Hemolysis
  fetal—*see* Jaundice, fetus or newborn
  intravascular (disseminated) NEC 286.6
  with
    abortion—*see* Abortion, by type, with hemorrhage, delayed or excessive

Hemolysis—*continued*
  ectopic pregnancy (*see also* categories 633.0-633.9) 639.1
  hemorrhage of pregnancy 641.3
    affecting fetus or newborn 762.1
  molar pregnancy (*see also* categories 630-632) 639.1
  acute 283.2
  following
    abortion 639.1
    ectopic or molar pregnancy 639.1
  neonatal—*see* Jaundice, fetus or newborn
  transfusion NEC 999.8
    bone marrow 996.85
Hemolytic —*see also* condition
  anemia—*see* Anemia, hemolytic
  uremic syndrome 283.11
Hemometra 621.4
Hemopericardium (with effusion) 423.0
  newborn 772.8
  traumatic (*see also* Hemothorax, traumatic) 860.2
    with open wound into thorax 860.3
Hemoperitoneum 568.81
  infectional (*see also* Peritonitis) 567.29
  traumatic—*see* Injury, internal, peritoneum
Hemophagocytic syndrome 288.4
  infection-associated 288.4
Hemophilia (familial) (hereditary) 286.0
  A 286.0
    carrier (asymptomatic) V83.01
    symptomatic V83.02
  B (Leyden) 286.1
  C 286.2
  calcipriva (*see also* Fibrinolysis) 286.7
  classical 286.0
  nonfamilial 286.7
  secondary 286.5
  vascular 286.4
Hemophilus influenzae NEC 041.5
  arachnoiditis (basic) (brain) (spinal) 320.0
    late effect—*see* category 326
  bronchopneumonia 482.2
  cerebral ventriculitis 320.0
    late effect—*see* category 326
  cerebrospinal inflammation 320.0
    late effect—*see* category 326
  infection NEC 041.5
  leptomeningitis 320.0
    late effect—*see* category 326
  meningitis (cerebral) (cerebrospinal) (spinal) 320.0
    late effect—*see* category 326
  meningomyelitis 320.0
    late effect—*see* category 326
  pachymeningitis (adhesive) (fibrous) (hemorrhagic) (hypertrophic) (spinal) 320.0
    late effect—*see* category 326
  pneumonia (broncho-) 482.2
Hemophthalmos 360.43
Hemopneumothorax (*see also* Hemothorax) 511.8
  traumatic 860.4
    with open wound into thorax 860.5
Hemoptysis 786.3
  due to Paragonimus (westermani) 121.2
  newborn 770.3
  tuberculous (*see also* Tuberculosis, pulmonary) 011.9

Hemorrhage, hemorrhagic (nontraumatic) 459.0
  abdomen 459.0
  accidental (antepartum) 641.2
    affecting fetus or newborn 762.1
  adenoid 474.8
  adrenal (capsule) (gland) (medulla) 255.41
    newborn 772.5
  after labor—*see* Hemorrhage, postpartum
  alveolar
    lung, newborn 770.3
    process 525.8
  alveolus 525.8
  amputation stump (surgical) 998.11
    secondary, delayed 997.69
  anemia (chronic) 280.0
    acute 285.1
  antepartum—*see* Hemorrhage, pregnancy
  anus (sphincter) 569.3
  apoplexy (stroke) 432.9
  arachnoid—*see* Hemorrhage, subarachnoid
  artery NEC 459.0
    brain (*see also* Hemorrhage, brain) 431
      middle meningeal—*see* Hemorrhage, subarachnoid
  basilar (ganglion) (*see also* Hemorrhage, brain) 431
  bladder 596.8
  blood dyscrasia 289.9
  bowel 578.9
    newborn 772.4
  brain (miliary) (nontraumatic) 431
    with
      birth injury 767.0
    arachnoid—*see* Hemorrhage, subarachnoid
    due to
      birth injury 767.0
      rupture of aneurysm (congenital) (*see also* Hemorrhage, subarachnoid) 430
        mycotic 431
        syphilis 094.89
    epidural or extradural—*see* Hemorrhage, extradural
    fetus or newborn (anoxic) (hypoxic) (due to birth trauma) (nontraumatic) 767.0
      intraventricular 772.10
        grade I 772.11
        grade II 772.12
        grade III 772.13
        grade IV 772.14
    iatrogenic 997.02
    postoperative 997.02
    puerperal, postpartum, childbirth 674.0
    stem 431
    subarachnoid, arachnoid or meningeal—*see* Hemorrhage, subarachnoid
    subdural—*see* Hemorrhage, subdural

Hemorrhage, hemorrhagic—*continued*
  traumatic NEC 853.0

> Note—Use the following fifth-digit subclassification with categories 851-854:
>
> 0 *unspecified state of consciousness*
> 1 *with no loss of consciousness*
> 2 *with brief [less than one hour] loss of consciousness*
> 3 *with moderate [1-24 hours] loss of consciousness*
> 4 *with prolonged [more than 24 hours] loss of consciousness and return to pre-existing conscious level*
> 5 *with prolonged [more than 24 hours] loss of consciousness, without return to pre-existing conscious level*
> *Use fifth-digit 5 to designate when a patient is unconscious and dies before regaining consciousness, regardless of the duration of the loss of consciousness*
> 6 *with loss of consciousness of unspecified duration*
> 9 *with concussion, unspecified*

  with
    cerebral
      contusion—*see* Contusion, brain
      laceration—*see* Laceration, brain
    open intracranial wound 853.1
    skull fracture—*see* Fracture, skull, by site
  extradural or epidural 852.4
    with open intracranial wound 852.5
  subarachnoid 852.0
    with open intracranial wound 852.1
  subdural 852.2
    with open intracranial wound 852.3
  breast 611.79
  bronchial tube—*see* Hemorrhage, lung
  bronchopulmonary—*see* Hemorrhage, lung
  bronchus (cause unknown) (*see also* Hemorrhage, lung) 786.3
  bulbar (*see also* Hemorrhage, brain) 431
  bursa 727.89
  capillary 448.9
    primary 287.8
  capsular—*see* Hemorrhage, brain
  cardiovascular 429.89
  cecum 578.9
  cephalic (*see also* Hemorrhage, brain) 431
  cerebellar (*see also* Hemorrhage, brain) 431
  cerebellum (*see also* Hemorrhage, brain) 431
  cerebral (*see also* Hemorrhage, brain) 431
    fetus or newborn (anoxic) (traumatic) 767.0
  cerebromeningeal (*see also* Hemorrhage, brain) 431
  cerebrospinal (*see also* Hemorrhage, brain) 431
  cerebrovascular accident—*see* Hemorrhage, brain
  cerebrum (*see also* Hemorrhage, brain) 431
  cervix (stump) (uteri) 622.8
  cesarean section wound 674.3
  chamber, anterior (eye) 364.41
  childbirth—*see* Hemorrhage, complicating, delivery
  choroid 363.61
    expulsive 363.62
  ciliary body 364.41
  cochlea 386.8
  colon—*see* Hemorrhage, intestine

Hemorrhage, hemorrhagic—*continued*
  complicating
    delivery 641.9
      affecting fetus or newborn 762.1
      associated with
        afibrinogenemia 641.3
          affecting fetus or newborn 763.89
        coagulation defect 641.3
          affecting fetus or newborn 763.89
        hyperfibrinolysis 641.3
          affecting fetus or newborn 763.89
        hypofibrinogenemia 641.3
          affecting fetus or newborn 763.89
      due to
        low-lying placenta 641.1
          affecting fetus or newborn 762.0
        placenta previa 641.1
          affecting fetus or newborn 762.0
        premature separation of placenta 641.2
          affecting fetus or newborn 762.1
        retained
          placenta 666.0
          secundines 666.2
        trauma 641.8
          affecting fetus or newborn 763.89
        uterine leiomyoma 641.8
          affecting fetus or newborn 763.89
    surgical procedure 998.11
  complication(s)
    of dental implant placement 525.71
  concealed NEC 459.0
  congenital 772.9
  conjunctiva 372.72
    newborn 772.8
  cord, newborn 772.0
    slipped ligature 772.3
    stump 772.3
  corpus luteum (ruptured) 620.1
  cortical (*see also* Hemorrhage, brain) 431
  cranial 432.9
  cutaneous 782.7
    newborn 772.6
  cyst, pancreas 577.2
  cystitis—*see* Cystitis
  delayed
    with
      abortion—*see* Abortion, by type, with hemorrhage, delayed or excessive
      ectopic pregnancy (*see also* categories 633.0-633.9) 639.1
      molar pregnancy (*see also* categories 630-632) 639.1
    following
      abortion 639.1
      ectopic or molar pregnancy 639.1
    postpartum 666.2
  diathesis (familial) 287.9
    newborn 776.0
  disease 287.9
    newborn 776.0
    specified type NEC 287.8
  disorder 287.9
    due to intrinsic circulating anticoagulants 286.5
    specified type NEC 287.8
  due to
    any device, implant, or graft (presence of) classifiable to 996.0-996.5—*see* Complications, due to (presence of) any device, implant, or graft classified to 996.0—996.5 NEC

Hemorrhage, hemorrhagic—*continued*
    intrinsic circulating anticoagulant 286.5
  duodenum, duodenal 537.89
    ulcer—*see* Ulcer, duodenum, with hemorrhage
  dura mater—*see* Hemorrhage, subdural
  endotracheal—*see* Hemorrhage, lung
  epicranial subaponeurotic (massive) 767.11
  epidural—*see* Hemorrhage, extradural
  episiotomy 674.3
  esophagus 530.82
    varix (*see also* Varix, esophagus, bleeding) 456.0
  excessive
    with
      abortion—*see* Abortion, by type, with hemorrhage, delayed or excessive
      ectopic pregnancy (*see also* categories 633.0-633.9) 639.1
      molar pregnancy (*see also* categories 630-632) 639.1
    following
      abortion 639.1
      ectopic or molar pregnancy 639.1
  external 459.0
  extradural (traumatic)—*see also* Hemorrhage, brain, traumatic, extradural
    birth injury 767.0
    fetus or newborn (anoxic) (traumatic) 767.0
    nontraumatic 432.0
  eye 360.43
    chamber (anterior) (aqueous) 364.41
    fundus 362.81
  eyelid 374.81
  fallopian tube 620.8
  fetomaternal 772.0
    affecting management of pregnancy or puerperium 656.0
  fetus, fetal 772.0
    from
      cut end of co-twin's cord 772.0
      placenta 772.0
      ruptured cord 772.0
      vasa previa 772.0
    into
      co-twin 772.0
      mother's circulation 772.0
        affecting management of pregnancy or puerperium 656.0
  fever (*see also* Fever, hemorrhagic) 065.9
    with renal syndrome 078.6
    arthropod-borne NEC 065.9
    Bangkok 065.4
    Crimean 065.0
    dengue virus 065.4
    epidemic 078.6
    Junin virus 078.7
    Korean 078.6
    Machupo virus 078.7
    mite-borne 065.8
    mosquito-borne 065.4
    Philippine 065.4
    Russian (Yaroslav) 078.6
    Singapore 065.4
    southeast Asia 065.4
    Thailand 065.4
    tick-borne NEC 065.3
  fibrinogenolysis (*see also* Fibrinolysis) 286.6
  fibrinolytic (acquired) (*see also* Fibrinolysis) 286.6
  fontanel 767.19
  from tracheostomy stoma 519.09
  fundus, eye 362.81

Hemorrhage, hemorrhagic—*continued*
  funis
    affecting fetus or newborn 772.0
    complicating delivery 663.8
  gastric (*see also* Hemorrhage, stomach) 578.9
  gastroenteric 578.9
    newborn 772.4
  gastrointestinal (tract) 578.9
    newborn 772.4
  genitourinary (tract) NEC 599.89
  gingiva 523.8
  globe 360.43
  gravidarum—*see* Hemorrhage, pregnancy
  gum 523.8
  heart 429.89
  hypopharyngeal (throat) 784.8
  intermenstrual 626.6
    irregular 626.6
    regular 626.5
  internal (organs) 459.0
    capsule (*see also* Hemorrhage, brain) 431
    ear 386.8
    newborn 772.8
  intestine 578.9
    congenital 772.4
    newborn 772.4
  into
    bladder wall 596.7
    bursa 727.89
    corpus luysii (*see also* Hemorrhage, brain) 431
  intra-abdominal 459.0
    during or following surgery 998.11
  intra-alveolar, newborn (lung) 770.3
  intracerebral (*see also* Hemorrhage, brain) 431
  intracranial NEC 432.9
    puerperal, postpartum, childbirth 674.0
    traumatic—*see* Hemorrhage, brain, traumatic
  intramedullary NEC 336.1
  intraocular 360.43
  intraoperative 998.11
  intrapartum—*see* Hemorrhage, complicating, delivery
  intrapelvic
    female 629.89
    male 459.0
  intraperitoneal 459.0
  intrapontine (*see also* Hemorrhage, brain) 431
  intrauterine 621.4
    complicating delivery—*see* Hemorrhage, complicating, delivery
    in pregnancy or childbirth—*see* Hemorrhage, pregnancy
    postpartum (*see also* Hemorrhage, postpartum) 666.1
  intraventricular (*see also* Hemorrhage, brain) 431
    fetus or newborn (anoxic) (traumatic) 772.10
      grade I 772.11
      grade II 772.12
      grade III 772.13
      grade IV 772.14
  intravesical 596.7
  iris (postinfectional) (postinflammatory) (toxic) 364.41
  joint (nontraumatic) 719.10
    ankle 719.17
    elbow 719.12
    foot 719.17
    forearm 719.13
    hand 719.14
    hip 719.15
    knee 719.16

Hemorrhage, hemorrhagic—*continued*
    lower leg 719.16
    multiple sites 719.19
    pelvic region 719.15
    shoulder (region) 719.11
    specified site NEC 719.18
    thigh 719.15
    upper arm 719.12
    wrist 719.13
  kidney 593.81
  knee (joint) 719.16
  labyrinth 386.8
  leg NEC 459.0
  lenticular striate artery (*see also* Hemorrhage, brain) 431
  ligature, vessel 998.11
  liver 573.8
  lower extremity NEC 459.0
  lung 786.3
    newborn 770.3
    tuberculous (*see also* Tuberculosis, pulmonary) 011.9
  malaria 084.8
  marginal sinus 641.2
  massive subaponeurotic, birth injury 767.11
  maternal, affecting fetus or newborn 762.1
  mediastinum 786.3
  medulla (*see also* Hemorrhage, brain) 431
  membrane (brain) (*see also* Hemorrhage, subarachnoid) 430
    spinal cord—*see* Hemorrhage, spinal cord
  meninges, meningeal (brain) (middle) (*see also* Hemorrhage, subarachnoid) 430
    spinal cord—*see* Hemorrhage, spinal cord
  mesentery 568.81
  metritis 626.8
  midbrain (*see also* Hemorrhage, brain) 431
  mole 631
  mouth 528.9
  mucous membrane NEC 459.0
    newborn 772.8
  muscle 728.89
  nail (subungual) 703.8
  nasal turbinate 784.7
    newborn 772.8
  nasopharynx 478.29
  navel, newborn 772.3
  newborn 772.9
    adrenal 772.5
    alveolar (lung) 770.3
    brain (anoxic) (hypoxic) (due to birth trauma) 767.0
    cerebral (anoxic) (hypoxic) (due to birth trauma) 767.0
    conjunctiva 772.8
    cutaneous 772.6
    diathesis 776.0
    due to vitamin K deficiency 776.0
    epicranial subaponeurotic (massive) 767.11
    gastrointestinal 772.4
    internal (organs) 772.8
    intestines 772.4
    intra-alveolar (lung) 770.3
    intracranial (from any perinatal cause) 767.0
    intraventricular (from any perinatal cause) 772.10
      grade I 772.11
      grade II 772.12
      grade III 772.13
      grade IV 772.14
    lung 770.3
    pulmonary (massive) 770.3

INDEX TO DISEASES

Hemorrhage, hemorrhagic—*continued*
  spinal cord, traumatic 767.4
  stomach 772.4
  subaponeurotic (massive) 767.11
  subarachnoid (from any perinatal cause) 772.2
  subconjunctival 772.8
  subgaleal 767.11
  umbilicus 772.0
    slipped ligature 772.3
    vasa previa 772.0
  nipple 611.79
  nose 784.7
    newborn 772.8
  obstetrical surgical wound 674.3
  omentum 568.89
    newborn 772.4
  optic nerve (sheath) 377.42
  orbit 376.32
  ovary 620.1
  oviduct 620.8
  pancreas 577.8
  parathyroid (gland) (spontaneous) 252.8
  parturition—*see* Hemorrhage, complicating, delivery
  penis 607.82
  pericardium, pericarditis 423.0
  perineal wound (obstetrical) 674.3
  peritoneum, peritoneal 459.0
  peritonsillar tissue 474.8
    after operation on tonsils 998.11
    due to infection 475
  petechial 782.7
  pituitary (gland) 253.8
  placenta NEC 641.9
    affecting fetus or newborn 762.1
    from surgical or instrumental damage 641.8
      affecting fetus or newborn 762.1
    previa 641.1
      affecting fetus or newborn 762.0
  pleura—*see* Hemorrhage, lung
  polioencephalitis, superior 265.1
  polymyositis—*see* Polymyositis
  pons (*see also* Hemorrhage, brain) 431
  pontine (*see also* Hemorrhage, brain) 431
  popliteal 459.0
  postcoital 626.7
  postextraction (dental) 998.11
  postmenopausal 627.1
  postnasal 784.7
  postoperative 998.11
  postpartum (atonic) (following delivery of placenta) 666.1
    delayed or secondary (after 24 hours) 666.2
    retained placenta 666.0
    third stage 666.0
  pregnancy (concealed) 641.9
    accidental 641.2
      affecting fetus or newborn 762.1
    affecting fetus or newborn 762.1
    before 22 completed weeks gestation 640.9
      affecting fetus or newborn 762.1
    due to
      abruptio placenta 641.2
        affecting fetus or newborn 762.1
      afibrinogenemia or other coagulation defect (conditions classifiable to 286.0-286.9) 641.3
        affecting fetus or newborn 762.1
      coagulation defect 641.3
        affecting fetus or newborn 762.1
      hyperfibrinolysis 641.3

Hemorrhage, hemorrhagic—*continued*
        affecting fetus or newborn 762.1
      hypofibrinogenemia 641.3
        affecting fetus or newborn 762.1
      leiomyoma, uterus 641.8
        affecting fetus or newborn 762.1
      low-lying placenta 641.1
        affecting fetus or newborn 762.1
      marginal sinus (rupture) 641.2
        affecting fetus or newborn 762.1
      placenta previa 641.1
        affecting fetus or newborn 762.0
      premature separation of placenta (normally implanted) 641.2
        affecting fetus or newborn 762.1
      threatened abortion 640.0
        affecting fetus or newborn 762.1
      trauma 641.8
        affecting fetus or newborn 762.1
    early (before 22 completed weeks gestation) 640.9
      affecting fetus or newborn 762.1
    previous, affecting management of pregnancy or childbirth V23.49
    unavoidable—*see* Hemorrhage, pregnancy, due to placenta previa
  prepartum (mother)—*see* Hemorrhage, pregnancy
  preretinal, cause unspecified 362.81
  prostate 602.1
  puerperal (*see also* Hemorrhage, postpartum) 666.1
  pulmonary—*see also* Hemorrhage, lung
    newborn (massive) 770.3
    renal syndrome 446.21
  purpura (primary) (*see also* Purpura, thrombocytopenic) 287.39
  rectum (sphincter) 569.3
  recurring, following initial hemorrhage at time of injury 958.2
  renal 593.81
    pulmonary syndrome 446.21
  respiratory tract (*see also* Hemorrhage, lung) 786.3
  retina, retinal (deep) (superficial) (vessels) 362.81
    diabetic 250.5 *[362.01]*
    due to birth injury 772.8
  retrobulbar 376.89
  retroperitoneal 459.0
  retroplacental (*see also* Placenta, separation) 641.2
  scalp 459.0
    due to injury at birth 767.19
  scrotum 608.83
  secondary (nontraumatic) 459.0
    following initial hemorrhage at time of injury 958.2
  seminal vesicle 608.83
  skin 782.7
    newborn 772.6
  spermatic cord 608.83
  spinal (cord) 336.1
    aneurysm (ruptured) 336.1
      syphilitic 094.89
    due to birth injury 767.4
    fetus or newborn 767.4
  spleen 289.59
  spontaneous NEC 459.0
    petechial 782.7
  stomach 578.9

Hemorrhage, hemorrhagic—*continued*
 newborn 772.4
 ulcer—*see* Ulcer, stomach, with hemorrhage
 subaponeurotic, newborn 767.11
  massive (birth injury) 767.11
 subarachnoid (nontraumatic) 430
  fetus or newborn (anoxic) (traumatic) 772.2
  puerperal, postpartum, childbirth 674.0
  traumatic—*see* Hemorrhage, brain, traumatic, subarachnoid
 subconjunctival 372.72
  due to birth injury 772.8
  newborn 772.8
 subcortical (*see also* Hemorrhage, brain) 431
 subcutaneous 782.7
 subdiaphragmatic 459.0
 subdural (nontraumatic) 432.1
  due to birth injury 767.0
  fetus or newborn (anoxic) (hypoxic) (due to birth trauma) 767.0
  puerperal, postpartum, childbirth 674.0
  spinal 336.1
  traumatic—*see* Hemorrhage, brain, traumatic, subdural
 subgaleal 767.11
 subhyaloid 362.81
 subperiosteal 733.99
 subretinal 362.81
 subtentorial (*see also* Hemorrhage, subdural) 432.1
 subungual 703.8
  due to blood dyscrasia 287.8
 suprarenal (capsule) (gland) 255.41
  fetus or newborn 772.5
 tentorium (traumatic)—*see also* Hemorrhage, brain, traumatic
  fetus or newborn 767.0
  nontraumatic—*see* Hemorrhage, subdural
 testis 608.83
 thigh 459.0
 third stage 666.0
 thorax—*see* Hemorrhage, lung
 throat 784.8
 thrombocythemia 238.71
 thymus (gland) 254.8
 thyroid (gland) 246.3
  cyst 246.3
 tongue 529.8
 tonsil 474.8
  postoperative 998.11
 tooth socket (postextraction) 998.11
 trachea—*see* Hemorrhage, lung
 traumatic—*see also* nature of injury
  brain—*see* Hemorrhage, brain, traumatic
  recurring or secondary (following initial hemorrhage at time of injury) 958.2
 tuberculous NEC (*see also* Tuberculosis, pulmonary) 011.9
 tunica vaginalis 608.83
 ulcer—*see* Ulcer, by site, with hemorrhage
 umbilicus, umbilical cord 772.0
  after birth, newborn 772.3
  complicating delivery 663.8
   affecting fetus or newborn 772.0
  slipped ligature 772.3
  stump 772.3
 unavoidable (due to placenta previa) 641.1
  affecting fetus or newborn 762.0
 upper extremity 459.0
 urethra (idiopathic) 599.84
 uterus, uterine (abnormal) 626.9

Hemorrhage, hemorrhagic—*continued*
 climacteric 627.0
 complicating delivery—*see* Hemorrhage, complicating, delivery
 due to
  intrauterine contraceptive device 996.76
   perforating uterus 996.32
 functional or dysfunctional 626.8
 in pregnancy—*see* Hemorrhage, pregnancy
 intermenstrual 626.6
  irregular 626.6
  regular 626.5
 postmenopausal 627.1
 postpartum (*see also* Hemorrhage, postpartum) 666.1
 prepubertal 626.8
 pubertal 626.3
 puerperal (immediate) 666.1
 vagina 623.8
 vasa previa 663.5
  affecting fetus or newborn 772.0
 vas deferens 608.83
 ventricular (*see also* Hemorrhage, brain) 431
 vesical 596.8
 viscera 459.0
  newborn 772.8
 vitreous (humor) (intraocular) 379.23
 vocal cord 478.5
 vulva 624.8
Hemorrhoids (anus) (rectum) (without complication) 455.6
 bleeding, prolapsed, strangulated, or ulcerated NEC 455.8
 external 455.5
 internal 455.2
 complicated NEC 455.8
 complicating pregnancy and puerperium 671.8
 external 455.3
  with complication NEC 455.5
  bleeding, prolapsed, strangulated, or ulcerated 455.5
  thrombosed 455.4
 internal 455.0
  with complication NEC 455.2
  bleeding, prolapsed, strangulated, or ulcerated 455.2
  thrombosed 455.1
 residual skin tag 455.9
 sentinel pile 455.9
 thrombosed NEC 455.7
  external 455.4
  internal 455.1
Hemosalpinx 620.8
Hemosiderosis 275.0
 dietary 275.0
 pulmonary (idiopathic) 275.0 [516.1]
 transfusion NEC 999.8
  bone marrow 996.85
Hemospermia 608.82
Hemothorax 511.8
 bacterial, nontuberculous 511.1
 newborn 772.8
 nontuberculous 511.8
  bacterial 511.1
 pneumococcal 511.1
 postoperative 998.11
 staphylococcal 511.1
 streptococcal 511.1
 traumatic 860.2
  with
   open wound into thorax 860.3

INDEX TO DISEASES — Hepatitis

Hemothorax—*continued*
  pneumothorax 860.4
    with open wound into thorax 860.5
  tuberculous (*see also* Tuberculosis, pleura) 012.0
Hemotympanum 385.89
Hench-Rosenberg syndrome (palindromic arthritis) (*see also* Rheumatism, palindromic) 719.3
Henle's warts 371.41
Henoch (-Schönlein)
  disease or syndrome (allergic purpura) 287.0
  purpura (allergic) 287.0
Henpue, henpuye 102.6
Heparitinuria 277.5
Hepar lobatum 095.3
Hepatalgia 573.8
Hepatic —*see also* condition
  flexure syndrome 569.89
Hepatitis 573.3
  acute (*see also* Necrosis, liver) 570
    alcoholic 571.1
    infective 070.1
      with hepatic coma 070.0
  alcoholic 571.1
  amebic—*see* Abscess, liver, amebic
  anicteric (acute)—*see* Hepatitis, viral
  antigen-associated (HAA) *see* Hepatitis, viral, type B
  Australian antigen (positive) *see* Hepatitis, viral, type B
  autoimmune 571.49
  catarrhal (acute) 070.1
    with hepatic coma 070.0
    chronic 571.40
    newborn 070.1
      with hepatic coma 070.0
  chemical 573.3
  cholangiolitic 573.8
  cholestatic 573.8
  chronic 571.40
    active 571.49
      viral—*see* Hepatitis, viral
    aggressive 571.49
    persistent 571.41
    viral—*see* Hepatitis, viral
  cytomegalic inclusion virus 078.5 *[573.1]*
  diffuse 573.3
  "dirty needle"—*see* Hepatitis, viral
    with hepatic coma 070.2
  drug-induced 573.3
  due to
    Coxsackie 074.8 *[573.1]*
    cytomegalic inclusion virus 078.5 *[573.1]*
    infectious mononucleosis 075 *[573.1]*
    malaria 084.9 *[573.2]*
    mumps 072.71
    secondary syphilis 091.62
    toxoplasmosis (acquired) 130.5
      congenital (active) 771.2
  epidemic—*see* Hepatitis, viral, type A
  fetus or newborn 774.4
  fibrous (chronic) 571.49
    acute 570
  from injection, inoculation, or transfusion (blood) (other substance) (plasma) (serum) (onset within 8 months after administration) *see* Hepatitis, viral
  fulminant (viral) (*see also* Hepatitis, viral) 070.9
    with hepatic coma 070.6
    type A 070.1
      with hepatic coma 070.0

Hepatitis—*continued*
  type B—*see* Hepatitis, viral, Type B
  giant cell (neonatal) 774.4
  hemorrhagic 573.8
  history of
    B V12.09
    C V12.09
  homologous serum—*see* Hepatitis, viral
  hypertrophic (chronic) 571.49
    acute 570
  nfectious, infective (acute) (chronic) (subacute) 070.1
    with hepatic coma 070.0
  inoculation—*see* Hepatitis, viral
  interstitial (chronic) 571.49
    acute 570
  lupoid 571.49
  malarial 084.9 *[573.2]*
  malignant (*see also* Necrosis, liver) 570
  neonatal (toxic) 774.4
  newborn 774.4
  parenchymatous (acute) (*see also* Necrosis, liver) 570
  peliosis 573.3
  persistent, chronic 571.41
  plasma cell 571.49
  postimmunization—*see* Hepatitis, viral
  postnecrotic 571.49
  posttransfusion—*see* Hepatitis, viral
  recurrent 571.49
  septic 573.3
  serum—*see* Hepatitis, viral
    carrier (suspected) of V02.61
  subacute (*see also* Necrosis, liver) 570
  suppurative (diffuse) 572.0
  syphilitic (late) 095.3
    congenital (early) 090.0 *[573.2]*
      late 090.5 *[573.2]*
    secondary 091.62
  toxic (noninfectious) 573.3
    fetus or newborn 774.4
  tuberculous (*see also* Tuberculosis) 017.9
  viral (acute) (anicteric) (cholangiolitic) (cholestatic) (chronic) (subacute) 070.9
    with hepatic coma 070.6
    AU-SH type virus—*see* Hepatitis, viral, type B
    Australian antigen—*see* Hepatitis, viral, type B
    B-antigen—*see* Hepatitis, viral, type B
    Coxsackie 074.8 *[573.1]*
    cytomegalic inclusion 078.5 *[573.1]*
    IH (virus)—*see* Hepatitis, viral, type A
    infectious hepatitis virus—*see* Hepatitis, viral, type A
    serum hepatitis virus—*see* Hepatitis, viral, type B
    SH—*see* Hepatitis, viral, type B
    specified type NEC 070.59
      with hepatic coma 070.49
    type A 070.1
      with hepatic coma 070.0
    type B (acute) 070.30
      with
        hepatic coma 070.20
          with hepatitis delta 070.21
        hepatitis delta 070.31
          with hepatic coma 070.21
    carrier status V02.61

Hepatitis

Hepatitis—*continued*
- chronic 070.32
  - with
    - hepatic coma 070.22
      - with hepatitis delta 070.23
    - hepatitis delta 070.33
      - with hepatic coma 070.23
- type C
  - with hepatic coma 070.41
  - acute 070.51
    - with hepatic coma 070.41
  - carrier status V02.62
  - chronic 070.54
    - with hepatic coma 070.44
  - in remission 070.54
  - unspecified 070.70
    - with hepatic coma 070.71
- type delta (with hepatitis B carrier state) 070.52
  - with
    - active hepatitis B disease—*see* Hepatitis, viral, type B
    - hepatic coma 070.42
- type E 070.53
  - with hepatic coma 070.43
- vaccination and inoculation (prophylactic) V05.3
- Waldenström's (lupoid hepatitis) 571.49

Hepatization, lung (acute)—*see also* Pneumonia, lobar
- chronic (*see also* Fibrosis, lung) 515

Hepatoblastoma (M8970/3) 155.0
Hepatocarcinoma (M8170/3) 155.0
Hepatocholangiocarcinoma (M8180/3) 155.0
Hepatocholangioma, benign (M8180/0) 211.5
Hepatocholangitis 573.8
Hepatocystitis (*see also* Cholecystitis) 575.10
Hepatodystrophy 570
Hepatolenticular degeneration 275.1
Hepatolithiasis —*see* Choledocholithiasis
Hepatoma (malignant) (M8170/3) 155.0
- benign (M8170/0) 211.5
- congenital (M8970/3) 155.0
- embryonal (M8970/3) 155.0

Hepatomegalia glycogenica diffusa 271.0
Hepatomegaly (*see also* Hypertrophy, liver) 789.1
- congenital 751.69
  - syphilitic 090.0
- due to Clonorchis sinensis 121.1
- Gaucher's 272.7
- syphilitic (congenital) 090.0

Hepatoptosis 573.8
Hepatorrhexis 573.8
Hepatosis, toxic 573.8
Hepatosplenomegaly 571.8
- due to S. japonicum 120.2
- hyperlipemic (Burger-Grutz type) 272.3

Herald patch 696.3
Hereditary —*see* condition
Heredodegeneration 330.9
- macular 362.70

Heredopathia ataxica polyneuritiformis 356.3
Heredosyphilis (*see also* Syphilis, congenital) 090.9
Hermaphroditism (true) 752.7
- with specified chromosomal anomaly—*see* Anomaly, chromosomes, sex

Hernia, hernial (acquired) (recurrent) 553.9
- with
  - gangrene (obstructed) NEC 551.9
  - obstruction NEC 552.9
    - and gangrene 551.9
- abdomen (wall)—*see* Hernia, ventral
- abdominal, specified site NEC 553.8
  - with
    - gangrene (obstructed) 551.8
    - obstruction 552.8
      - and gangrene 551.8
- appendix 553.8
  - with
    - gangrene (obstructed) 551.8
    - obstruction 552.8
      - and gangrene 551.8
- bilateral (inguinal)—*see* Hernia, inguinal
- bladder (sphincter)
  - congenital (female) (male) 756.71
  - female (*see also* Cystocele, female) 618.01
  - male 596.8
- brain 348.4
  - congenital 742.0
- broad ligament 553.8
- cartilage, vertebral—*see* Displacement, intervertebral disc
- cerebral 348.4
  - congenital 742.0
  - endaural 742.0
- ciliary body 364.89
  - traumatic 871.1
- colic 553.9
  - with
    - gangrene (obstructed) 551.9
    - obstruction 552.9
      - and gangrene 551.9
- colon 553.9
  - with
    - gangrene (obstructed) 551.9
    - obstruction 552.9
      - and gangrene 551.9
- colostomy (stoma) 569.69
- Cooper's (retroperitoneal) 553.8
  - with
    - gangrene (obstructed) 551.8
    - obstruction 552.8
      - and gangrene 551.8
- crural—*see* Hernia, femoral
- diaphragm, diaphragmatic 553.3
  - with
    - gangrene (obstructed) 551.3
    - obstruction 552.3
      - and gangrene 551.3
  - congenital 756.6
  - due to gross defect of diaphragm 756.6
  - traumatic 862.0
    - with open wound into cavity 862.1
- direct (inguinal)—*see* Hernia, inguinal
- disc, intervertebral—*see* Displacement, intervertebral disc
- diverticulum, intestine 553.9
  - with
    - gangrene (obstructed) 551.9
    - obstruction 552.9
      - and gangrene 551.9
- double (inguinal)—*see* Hernia, inguinal
- due to adhesion with obstruction 560.81
- duodenojejunal 553.8
  - with
    - gangrene (obstructed) 551.8
    - obstruction 552.8
      - and gangrene 551.8
- en glissade—*see* Hernia, inguinal

INDEX TO DISEASES   Hernia, hernial

Hernia, hernial—*continued*
  enterostomy (stoma) 569.69
  epigastric 553.29
    with
      gangrene (obstruction) 551.29
      obstruction 552.29
        and gangrene 551.29
    recurrent 553.21
      with
        gangrene (obstructed) 551.21
        obstruction 552.21
          and gangrene 551.21
  esophageal hiatus (sliding) 553.3
    with
      gangrene (obstructed) 551.3
      obstruction 552.3
        and gangrene 551.3
    congenital 750.6
  external (inguinal)—*see* Hernia, inguinal
  fallopian tube 620.4
  fascia 728.89
  fat 729.30
    eyelid 374.34
    orbital 374.34
    pad 729.30
      eye, eyelid 374.34
      knee 729.31
      orbit 374.34
      popliteal (space) 729.31
      specified site NEC 729.39
  femoral (unilateral) 553.00
    with
      gangrene (obstructed) 551.00
      obstruction 552.00
        with gangrene 551.00
    bilateral 553.02
      gangrenous (obstructed) 551.02
      obstructed 552.02
        with gangrene 551.02
      recurrent 553.03
        gangrenous (obstructed) 551.03
        obstructed 552.03
          with gangrene 551.03
    recurrent (unilateral) 553.01
      bilateral 553.03
        gangrenous (obstructed) 551.03
        obstructed 552.03
          with gangrene 551.03
      gangrenous (obstructed) 551.01
      obstructed 552.01
        with gangrene 551.01
  foramen
    Bochdalek 553.3
      with
        gangrene (obstructed) 551.3
        obstruction 552.3
          and gangrene 551.3
      congenital 756.6
    magnum 348.4
    Morgagni, morgagnian 553.3
      with
        gangrene 551.3
        obstruction 552.3
          and gangrene 551.3
      congenital 756.6
  funicular (umbilical) 553.1
    with
      gangrene (obstructed) 551.1
      obstruction 552.1
        and gangrene 551.1
    spermatic cord—*see* Hernia, inguinal

Hernia, hernial—*continued*
  gangrenous—*see* Hernia, by site, with gangrene
  gastrointestinal tract 553.9
    with
      gangrene (obstructed) 551.9
      obstruction 552.9
        and gangrene 551.9
  gluteal—*see* Hernia, femoral
  Gruber's (internal mesogastric) 553.8
    with
      gangrene (obstructed) 551.8
      obstruction 552.8
        and gangrene 551.8
  Hesselbach's 553.8
    with
      gangrene (obstructed) 551.8
      obstruction 552.8
        and gangrene 551.8
  hiatal (esophageal) (sliding) 553.3
    with
      gangrene (obstructed) 551.3
      obstruction 552.3
        and gangrene 551.3
    congenital 750.6
  incarcerated (*see also* Hernia, by site, with obstruction) 552.9
    gangrenous (*see also* Hernia, by site, with gangrene) 551.9
  incisional 553.21
    with
      gangrene (obstructed) 551.21
      obstruction 552.21
        and gangrene 551.21
    lumbar—*see* Hernia, lumbar
    recurrent 553.21
      with
        gangrene (obstructed) 551.21
        obstruction 552.21
          and gangrene 551.21
  indirect (inguinal)—*see* Hernia, inguinal
  infantile—*see* Hernia, inguinal
  infrapatellar fat pad 729.31
  inguinal (direct) (double) (encysted) (external) (funicular) (indirect) (infantile) (internal) (interstitial) (oblique) (scrotal) (sliding) 550.9

Note—Use the following fifth-digit subclassification with category 550:

0 unilateral or unspecified (not specified as recurrent)
1 unilateral or unspecified, recurrent
2 bilateral (not specified as recurrent)
3 bilateral, recurrent

---

    with
      gangrene (obstructed) 550.0
      obstruction 550.1
        and gangrene 550.0
  internal 553.8
    with
      gangrene (obstructed) 551.8
      obstruction 552.8
        and gangrene 551.8
    inguinal—*see* Hernia, inguinal
  interstitial 553.9
    with
      gangrene (obstructed) 551.9
      obstruction 552.9
        and gangrene 551.9
    inguinal—*see* Hernia, inguinal

Hernia, hernial—*continued*
  intervertebral cartilage or disc—*see*
    Displacement, intervertebral disc
  intestine, intestinal 553.9
    with
      gangrene (obstructed) 551.9
      obstruction 552.9
        and gangrene 551.9
  intra-abdominal 553.9
    with
      gangrene (obstructed) 551.9
      obstruction 552.9
        and gangrene 551.9
  intraparietal 553.9
    with
      gangrene (obstructed) 551.9
      obstruction 552.9
        and gangrene 551.9
  iris 364.89
    traumatic 871.1
  irreducible (*see also* Hernia, by site, with obstruction) 552.9
    gangrenous (with obstruction) (*see also* Hernia, by site, with gangrene) 551.9
  ischiatic 553.8
    with
      gangrene (obstructed) 551.8
      obstruction 552.8
        and gangrene 551.8
  ischiorectal 553.8
    with
      gangrene (obstructed) 551.8
      obstruction 552.8
        and gangrene 551.8
  lens 379.32
    traumatic 871.1
  linea
    alba—*see* Hernia, epigastric
    semilunaris—*see* Hernia, spigelian
  Littre's (diverticular) 553.9
    with
      gangrene (obstructed) 551.9
      obstruction 552.9
        and gangrene 551.9
  lumbar 553.8
    with
      gangrene (obstructed) 551.8
      obstruction 552.8
        and gangrene 551.8
    intervertebral disc 722.10
  lung (subcutaneous) 518.89
    congenital 748.69
  mediastinum 519.3
  mesenteric (internal) 553.8
    with
      gangrene (obstructed) 551.8
      obstruction 552.8
        and gangrene 551.8
  mesocolon 553.8
    with
      gangrene (obstructed) 551.8
      obstruction 552.8
        and gangrene 551.8
  muscle (sheath) 728.89
  nucleus pulposus—*see* Displacement, intervertebral disc
  oblique (inguinal)—*see* Hernia, inguinal
  obstructive (*see also* Hernia, by site, with obstruction) 552.9
    gangrenous (with obstruction) (*see also* Hernia, by site, with gangrene) 551.9

Hernia, hernial—*continued*
  obturator 553.8
    with
      gangrene (obstructed) 551.8
      obstruction 552.8
        and gangrene 551.8
  omental 553.8
    with
      gangrene (obstructed) 551.8
      obstruction 552.8
        and gangrene 551.8
  orbital fat (pad) 374.34
  ovary 620.4
  oviduct 620.4
  paracolostomy (stoma) 569.69
  paraduodenal 553.8
    with
      gangrene (obstructed) 551.8
      obstruction 552.8
        and gangrene 551.8
  paraesophageal 553.3
    with
      gangrene (obstructed) 551.3
      obstruction 552.3
        and gangrene 551.3
    congenital 750.6
  parahiatal 553.3
    with
      gangrene (obstructed) 551.3
      obstruction 552.3
        and gangrene 551.3
  paraumbilical 553.1
    with
      gangrene (obstructed) 551.1
      obstruction 552.1
        and gangrene 551.1
  parietal 553.9
    with
      gangrene (obstructed) 551.9
      obstruction 552.9
        and gangrene 551.9
  perineal 553.8
    with
      gangrene (obstructed) 551.8
      obstruction 552.8
        and gangrene 551.8
  peritoneal sac, lesser 553.8
    with
      gangrene (obstructed) 551.8
      obstruction 552.8
        and gangrene 551.8
  popliteal fat pad 729.31
  postoperative 553.21
    with
      gangrene (obstructed) 551.21
      obstruction 552.21
        and gangrene 551.21
  pregnant uterus 654.4
  prevesical 596.8
  properitoneal 553.8
    with
      gangrene (obstructed) 551.8
      obstruction 552.8
        and gangrene 551.8
  pudendal 553.8
    with
      gangrene (obstructed) 551.8
      obstruction 552.8
        and gangrene 551.8
  rectovaginal 618.6
  retroperitoneal 553.8

INDEX TO DISEASES

Hernia, hernial—*continued*
  with
    gangrene (obstructed) 551.8
    obstruction 552.8
      and gangrene 551.8
  Richter's (parietal) 553.9
    with
      gangrene (obstructed) 551.9
      obstruction 552.9
        and gangrene 551.9
  Rieux's, Riex's (retrocecal) 553.8
    with
      gangrene (obstructed) 551.8
      obstruction 552.8
        and gangrene 551.8
  sciatic 553.8
    with
      gangrene (obstructed) 551.8
      obstruction 552.8
        and gangrene 551.8
  scrotum, scrotal—*see* Hernia, inguinal
  sliding (inguinal)—*see also* Hernia, inguinal
  hiatus—*see* Hernia, hiatal
  spigelian 553.29
    with
      gangrene (obstructed) 551.29
      obstruction 552.29
        and gangrene 551.29
  spinal (*see also* Spina bifida) 741.9
    with hydrocephalus 741.0
  strangulated (*see also* Hernia, by site, with
    obstruction) 552.9
    gangrenous (with obstruction) (*see also*
      Hernia, by site, with gangrene) 551.9
  supraumbilicus (linea alba)—*see* Hernia,
    epigastric
  tendon 727.9
  testis (nontraumatic) 550.9
    meaning
      scrotal hernia 550.9
      symptomatic late syphilis 095.8
  Treitz's (fossa) 553.8
    with
      gangrene (obstructed) 551.8
      obstruction 552.8
        and gangrene 551.8
  tunica
    albuginea 608.89
    vaginalis 752.89
  umbilicus, umbilical 553.1
    with
      gangrene (obstructed) 551.1
      obstruction 552.1
        and gangrene 551.1
  ureter 593.89
    with obstruction 593.4
  uterus 621.8
    pregnant 654.4
  vaginal (posterior) 618.6
  Velpeau's (femoral) (*see also* Hernia, femoral)
    553.00
  ventral 553.20
    with
      gangrene (obstructed) 551.20
      obstruction 552.20
        and gangrene 551.20
    recurrent 553.21
      with
        gangrene (obstructed) 551.21
        obstruction 552.21
          and gangrene 551.21

Hernia, hernial—*continued*
  vesical
    congenital (female) (male) 756.71
    female (*see also* Cystocele, female) 618.01
    male 596.8
  vitreous (into anterior chamber) 379.21
    traumatic 871.1
Herniation —*see also* Hernia
  brain (stem) 348.4
  cerebral 348.4
  gastric mucosa (into duodenal bulb) 537.89
  mediastinum 519.3
  nucleus pulposus—*see* Displacement,
    intervertebral disc
Herpangina 074.0
Herpes, herpetic 054.9
  auricularis (zoster) 053.71
    simplex 054.73
  blepharitis (zoster) 053.20
    simplex 054.41
  circinate 110.5
  circinatus 110.5
    bullous 694.5
  conjunctiva (simplex) 054.43
    zoster 053.21
  cornea (simplex) 054.43
    disciform (simplex) 054.43
    zoster 053.21
  encephalitis 054.3
  eye (zoster) 053.29
    simplex 054.40
  eyelid (zoster) 053.20
    simplex 054.41
  febrilis 054.9
  fever 054.9
  geniculate ganglionitis 053.11
  genital, genitalis 054.10
    specified site NEC 054.19
  gestationis 646.8
  gingivostomatitis 054.2
  iridocyclitis (simplex) 054.44
    zoster 053.22
  iris (any site) 695.1
  iritis (simplex) 054.44
  keratitis (simplex) 054.43
    dendritic 054.42
    disciform 054.43
    interstitial 054.43
      zoster 053.21
  keratoconjunctivitis (simplex) 054.43
    zoster 053.21
  labialis 054.9
    meningococcal 036.89
  lip 054.9
  meningitis (simplex) 054.72
    zoster 053.0
  ophthalmicus (zoster) 053.20
    simplex 054.40
  otitis externa (zoster) 053.71
    simplex 054.73
  penis 054.13
  perianal 054.10
  pharyngitis 054.79
  progenitalis 054.10
  scrotum 054.19
  septicemia 054.5
  simplex 054.9
    complicated 054.8
      ophthalmic 054.40
        specified NEC 054.49
      specified NEC 054.79

Herpes, herpetic—*continued*
  congenital 771.2
  external ear 054.73
  keratitis 054.43
    dendritic 054.42
  meningitis 054.72
  myelitis 054.74
  neuritis 054.79
  specified complication NEC 054.79
    ophthalmic 054.49
  visceral 054.71
  stomatitis 054.2
  tonsurans 110.0
    maculosus (of Hebra) 696.3
  visceral 054.71
  vulva 054.12
  vulvovaginitis 054.11
  whitlow 054.6
  zoster 053.9
    auricularis 053.71
    complicated 053.8
      specified NEC 053.79
    conjunctiva 053.21
    cornea 053.21
    ear 053.71
    eye 053.29
    geniculate 053.11
    keratitis 053.21
      interstitial 053.21
    myelitis 053.14
    neuritis 053.10
    ophthalmicus(a) 053.20
    oticus 053.71
    otitis externa 053.71
    specified complication NEC 053.79
    specified site NEC 053.9
  zosteriform, intermediate type 053.9
Herrick's
  anemia (hemoglobin S disease) 282.61
  syndrome (hemoglobin S disease) 282.61
Hers' disease (glycogenosis VI) 271.0
Herter's infantilism (nontropical sprue) 579.0
Herter (-Gee) disease or syndrome (nontropical sprue) 579.0
Herxheimer's disease (diffuse idiopathic cutaneous atrophy) 701.8
Herxheimer's reaction 995.0
Hesitancy, urinary 788.64
Hesselbach's hernia —*see* Hernia, Hesselbach's
Heterochromia (congenital) 743.46
  acquired 364.53
  cataract 366.33
  cyclitis 364.21
  hair 704.3
  iritis 364.21
  retained metallic foreign body 360.62
    magnetic 360.52
  uveitis 364.21
Heterophoria 378.40
  alternating 378.45
  vertical 378.43
Heterophyes, small intestine 121.6
Heterophyiasis 121.6
Heteropsia 368.8
Heterotopia, heterotopic —*see also* Malposition, congenital
  cerebralis 742.4
  pancreas, pancreatic 751.7
  spinalis 742.59

Heterotropia 378.30
  intermittent 378.20
    vertical 378.31
  vertical (constant) (intermittent) 378.31
Heubner's disease 094.89
Heubner-Herter disease or syndrome (nontropical sprue) 579.0
Hexadactylism 755.00
Heyd's syndrome (hepatorenal) 572.4
HGSIL (high grade squamous intrepithelial lesion) (cytologic finding) (Pap smear finding) 795.04
  biopsy finding —code to CIN II or CIN III
Hibernoma (M8880/0)—*see* Lipoma
Hiccough 786.8
  epidemic 078.89
  psychogenic 306.1
Hiccup (*see also* Hiccough) 786.8
Hicks (-Braxton) contractures 644.1
Hidden penis 752.65
Hidradenitis (axillaris) (suppurative) 705.83
Hidradenoma (nodular) (M8400/0)—*see also* Neoplasm, skin, benign
  clear cell (M8402/0)—*see* Neoplasm, skin, benign
  papillary (M8405/0)—*see* Neoplasm, skin, benign
Hidrocystoma (M8404/0)—*see* Neoplasm, skin, benign
HIE (hypoxic-ischemic encephalopathy) 768.7
High
  A$_2$ anemia 282.49
  altitude effects 993.2
    anoxia 993.2
    on
      ears 993.0
      sinuses 993.1
    polycythemia 289.0
  arch
    foot 755.67
    palate 750.26
  artery (arterial) tension (*see also* Hypertension) 401.9
    without diagnosis of hypertension 796.2
  basal metabolic rate (BMR) 794.7
  blood pressure (*see also* Hypertension) 401.9
    incidental reading (isolated) (nonspecific), no diagnosis of hypertension 796.2
  cholesterol 272.0
    with high triglycerides 272.2
  compliance bladder 596.4
  diaphragm (congenital) 756.6
  frequency deafness (congenital) (regional) 389.8
  head at term 652.5
  output failure (cardiac) (*see also* Failure, heart) 428.9
  oxygen-affinity hemoglobin 289.0
  palate 750.26
  risk
    behavior —*see* Problem
    cervical, human papillomavirus (HPV) DNA test positive 795.05
    family situation V61.9
      specified circumstance NEC V61.8
    individual NEC V62.89
    infant NEC V20.1
    patient taking drugs (prescribed) V67.51
      nonprescribed (*see also* Abuse, drugs, nondependent) 305.9
    pregnancy V23.9

INDEX TO DISEASES

High—*continued*
  inadequate prenatal care V23.7
  specified problem NEC V23.8
  temperature (of unknown origin) (*see also* Pyrexia) 780.6
  thoracic rib 756.3
  triglycerides 272.1
    with high cholesterol 272.2
Hildenbrand's disease (typhus) 081.9
Hilger's syndrome 337.0
Hill diarrhea 579.1
Hilliard's lupus (*see also* Tuberculosis) 017.0
Hilum —*see* condition
Hip —*see* condition
Hippel's disease (retinocerebral angiomatosis) 759.6
Hippus 379.49
Hirschfeld's disease (acute diabetes mellitus) (*see also* Diabetes) 250.0
Hirschsprung's disease or megacolon (congenital) 751.3
Hirsuties (*see also* Hypertrichosis) 704.1
Hirsutism (*see also* Hypertrichosis) 704.1
Hirudiniasis (external) (internal) 134.2
His-Werner disease (trench fever) 083.1
Hiss-Russell dysentery 004.1
Histamine cephalgia 346.2
Histidinemia 270.5
Histidinuria 270.5
Histiocytic syndromes 288.4
Histiocytoma (M8832/0)—*see also* Neoplasm, skin, benign
  fibrous (M8830/0)—*see also* Neoplasm, skin, benign
    atypical (M8830/1)—*see* Neoplasm, connective tissue, uncertain behavior
    malignant (M8830/0)—*see* Neoplasm, connective tissue, malignant
Histiocytosis (acute) (chronic) (subacute) 277.89
  acute differentiated progressive (M9722/3) 202.5
  cholesterol 277.89
  essential 277.89
  lipid, lipoid (essential) 272.7
  lipochrome (familial) 288.1
  malignant (M9720/3) 202.3
  X (chronic) 277.89
    acute (progressive) (M9722/3) 202.5
Histoplasmosis 115.90
  with
    endocarditis 115.94
    meningitis 115.91
    pericarditis 115.93
    pneumonia 115.95
    retinitis 115.92
    specified manifestation NEC 115.99
  African (due to Histoplasma duboisii) 115.10
    with
      endocarditis 115.14
      meningitis 115.11
      pericarditis 115.13
      pneumonia 115.15
      retinitis 115.12
      specified manifestation NEC 115.19
  American (due to Histoplasma capsulatum) 115.00
    with
      endocarditis 115.04
      meningitis 115.01
      pericarditis 115.03
      pneumonia 115.05
      retinitis 115.02
      specified manifestation NEC 115.09

Histoplasmosis—*continued*
  Darling's—*see* Histoplasmosis, American
  large form (*see also* Histoplasmosis, African) 115.10
  lung 115.05
  small form (*see also* Histoplasmosis, American) 115.00
History (personal) of
  abuse
    emotional V15.42
    neglect V15.42
    physical V15.41
    sexual V15.41
  affective psychosis V11.1
  alcoholism V11.3
    specified as drinking problem (*see also* Abuse, drugs, nondependent) 305.0
  allergy to
    analgesic agent NEC V14.6
    anesthetic NEC V14.4
    antibiotic agent NEC V14.1
      penicillin V14.0
    anti-infective agent NEC V14.3
    diathesis V15.09
    drug V14.9
      specified type NEC V14.8
    eggs V15.03
    food additives V15.05
    insect bite V15.06
    latex V15.07
    medicinal agents V14.9
      specified type NEC V14.8
    milk products V15.02
    narcotic agent NEC V14.5
    nuts V15.05
      peanuts V15.01
    penicillin V14.0
    radiographic dye V15.08
    seafood V15.04
    serum V14.7
    specified food NEC V15.05
    specified nonmedicinal agents NEC V15.09
    spider bite V15.06
    sulfa V14.2
    sulfonamides V14.2
    therapeutic agent NEC V15.09
    vaccine V14.7
  anemia V12.3
  arrest, sudden cardiac V12.53
  arthritis V13.4
  attack, transient ischemic (TIA) V12.54
  benign neoplasm of brain V12.41
  blood disease V12.3
  calculi, urinary V13.01
  cardiovascular disease V12.50
    myocardial infarction 412
  child abuse V15.41
  cigarette smoking V15.82
  circulatory system disease V12.50
    myocardial infarction 412
  congenital malformation V13.69
  contraception V15.7
  death, sudden, successfully resuscitated V12.53
  deficit
    prolonged reversible ischemic neurologic (PRIND) V12.54
    reversible ischemic neurologic (RIND) V12.54
  diathesis, allergic V15.09
  digestive system disease V12.70
    peptic ulcer V12.71
    polyps, colonic V12.72

History — INDEX TO DISEASES

History—*continued*
  specified NEC V12.79
  disease (of) V13.9
    blood V12.3
    blood-forming organs V12.3
    cardiovascular system V12.50
    circulatory system V12.50
      specified NEC V12.59
    digestive system V12.70
      peptic ulcer V12.71
      polyps, colonic V12.72
      specified NEC V12.79
    infectious V12.00
      malaria V12.03
      poliomyelitis V12.02
      specified NEC V12.09
      tuberculosis V12.01
    parasitic V12.00
      specified NEC V12.09
    respiratory system V12.60
      pneumonia V12.61
      specified NEC V12.69
    skin V13.3
    specified site NEC V13.8
    subcutaneous tissue V13.3
    trophoblastic V13.1
      affecting management of pregnancy V23.1
  disorder (of) V13.9
    endocrine V12.2
    genital system V13.29
    hematological V12.3
    immunity V12.2
    mental V11.9
      affective type V11.1
      manic-depressive V11.1
      neurosis V11.2
      schizophrenia V11.0
      specified type NEC V11.8
    metabolic V12.2
    musculoskeletal NEC V13.5
    nervous system V12.40
      specified type NEC V12.49
    obstetric V13.29
      affecting management of current pregnancy V23.49
      pre-term labor V13.21
    sense organs V12.40
      specified type NEC V12.49
    specified site NEC V13.8
    urinary system V13.00
      calculi V13.01
      infection V13.02
      nephrotic syndrome V13.03
      specified NEC V13.09
  drug use
    nonprescribed (*see also* Abuse, drugs, nondependent) 305.9
    patent (*see also* Abuse, drugs, nondependent) 305.9
  dysplasia
    cervical (conditions classifiable to 622.10-622.12) V13.22
  effect NEC of external cause V15.89
  embolism (pulmonary) V12.51
  emotional abuse V15.42
  encephalitis V12.42
  endocrine disorder V12.2
  extracorporeal membrane oxygenation (ECMO) V15.87
  falling V15.88

History—*continued*
  family
    allergy V19.6
    anemia V18.2
    arteriosclerosis V17.49
    arthritis V17.7
    asthma V17.5
    blindness V19.0
    blood disorder NEC V18.3
    cardiovascular disease V17.49
    carrier, genetic disease V18.9
    cerebrovascular disease V17.1
    chronic respiratory condition NEC V17.6
    colonic polyps V18.51
    congenital anomalies V19.5
    consanguinity V19.7
    coronary artery disease V17.3
    cystic fibrosis V18.19
    deafness V19.2
    diabetes mellitus V18.0
    digestive disorders V18.59
    disease or disorder (of)
      allergic V19.6
      blood NEC V18.3
      cardiovascular NEC V17.49
      cerebrovascular V17.1
      colonic polyps V18.51
      coronary artery V17.3
      death, sudden cardiac (SCD) V17.41
      digestive V18.59
      ear NEC V19.3
      endocrine V18.19
        multiple neoplasia [MEN] syndrome V18.11
      eye NEC V19.1
      genitourinary NEC V18.7
      hypertensive V17.49
      infectious V18.8
      ischemic heart V17.3
      kidney V18.69
        polycystic V18.61
      mental V17.0
      metabolic V18.19
      musculoskeletal NEC V17.89
        osteoporosis V17.81
      neurological NEC V17.2
      parasitic V18.8
      psychiatric condition V17.0
      skin condition V19.4
    ear disorder NEC V19.3
    endocrine disease V18.19
      multiple neoplasia [MEN] syndrome V18.11
    epilepsy V17.2
    eye disorder NEC V19.1
    genetic disease carrier V18.9
    genitourinary disease NEC V18.7
    glomerulonephritis V18.69
    gout V18.19
    hay fever V17.6
    hearing loss V19.2
    hematopoietic neoplasia V16.7
    Hodgkin's disease V16.7
    Huntington's chorea V17.2
    hydrocephalus V19.5
    hypertension V17.49
    infarction, myocardial V17.3
    infectious disease V18.8
    ischemic heart disease V17.3
    kidney disease V18.69
      polycystic V18.61
    leukemia V16.6

INDEX TO DISEASES

History—*continued*
  lymphatic malignant neoplasia NEC V16.7
  malignant neoplasm (of) NEC V16.9
    anorectal V16.0
    anus V16.0
    appendix V16.0
    bladder V16.52
    bone V16.8
    brain V16.8
    breast V16.3
      male V16.8
    bronchus V16.1
    cecum V16.0
    cervix V16.49
    colon V16.0
    duodenum V16.0
    esophagus V16.0
    eye V16.8
    gallbladder V16.0
    gastrointestinal tract V16.0
    genital organs V16.40
    hemopoietic NEC V16.7
    ileum V16.0
    ilium V16.8
    intestine V16.0
    intrathoracic organs NEC V16.2
    kidney V16.51
    larynx V16.2
    liver V16.0
    lung V16.1
    lymphatic NEC V16.7
    ovary V16.41
    oviduct V16.41
    pancreas V16.0
    penis V16.49
    prostate V16.42
    rectum V16.0
    respiratory organs NEC V16.2
    skin V16.8
    specified site NEC V16.8
    stomach V16.0
    testis V16.43
    trachea V16.1
    ureter V16.59
    urethra V16.59
    urinary organs V16.59
    uterus V16.49
    vagina V16.49
    vulva V16.49
  MEN (multiple endocrine neoplasia syndrome) V18.11
  mental retardation V18.4
  metabolic disease NEC V18.19
  mongolism V19.5
  multiple
    endocrine neoplasia [MEN] syndrome V18.11
    myeloma V16.7
  musculoskeletal disease NEC V17.89
    osteoporosis V17.81
  myocardial infarction V17.3
  nephritis V18.69
  nephrosis V18.69
  osteoporosis V17.81
  parasitic disease V18.8
  polycystic kidney disease V18.61
  psychiatric disorder V17.0
  psychosis V17.0
  retardation, mental V18.4
  retinitis pigmentosa V19.1
  schizophrenia V17.0

History—*continued*
  skin conditions V19.4
  specified condition NEC V19.8
  stroke (cerebrovascular) V17.1
  sudden cardiac death (SCD) V17.41
  visual loss V19.0
  genital system disorder V13.29
    pre-term labor V13.21
  health hazard V15.9
    falling V15.88
    specified cause NEC V15.89
  hepatitis
    B V12.09
    C V12.09
  Hodgkin's disease V10.72
  hypospadias V13.61
  immunity disorder V12.2
  infarction, cerebral, without residual deficits V12.54
  infection
    central nervous system V12.42
    urinary (tract) V13.02
  infectious disease V12.00
    malaria V12.03
    poliomyelitis V12.02
    specified NEC V12.09
    tuberculosis V12.01
  injury NEC V15.5
  insufficient prenatal care V23.7
  irradiation V15.3
  leukemia V10.60
    lymphoid V10.61
    monocytic V10.63
    myeloid V10.62
    specified type NEC V10.69
  little or no prenatal care V23.7
  low birth weight (*see also* Status, low birth weight) V21.30
  lymphosarcoma V10.71
  malaria V12.03
  malignant neoplasm (of) V10.9
    accessory sinus V10.22
    adrenal V10.88
    anus V10.06
    bile duct V10.09
    bladder V10.51
    bone V10.81
    brain V10.85
    breast V10.3
    bronchus V10.11
    cervix uteri V10.41
    colon V10.05
    connective tissue NEC V10.89
    corpus uteri V10.42
    digestive system V10.00
      specified part NEC V10.09
    duodenum V10.09
    endocrine gland NEC V10.88
    epididymis V10.48
    esophagus V10.03
    eye V10.84
    fallopian tube V10.44
    female genital organ V10.40
      specified site NEC V10.44
    gallbladder V10.09
    gastrointestinal tract V10.00
    gum V10.02
    hematopoietic NEC V10.79
    hypopharynx V10.02
    ileum V10.09
    intrathoracic organs NEC V10.20

History   **INDEX TO DISEASES**

History—*continued*
- jejunum V10.09
- kidney V10.52
- large intestine V10.05
- larynx V10.21
- lip V10.02
- liver V10.07
- lung V10.11
- lymphatic NEC V10.79
- lymph glands or nodes NEC V10.79
- male genital organ V10.45
  - specified site NEC V10.49
- mediastinum V10.29
- melanoma (of skin) V10.82
- middle ear V10.22
- mouth V10.02
  - specified part NEC V10.02
- nasal cavities V10.22
- nasopharynx V10.02
- nervous system NEC V10.86
- nose V10.22
- oropharynx V10.02
- ovary V10.43
- pancreas V10.09
- parathyroid V10.88
- penis V10.49
- pharynx V10.02
- pineal V10.88
- pituitary V10.88
- placenta V10.44
- pleura V10.29
- prostate V10.46
- rectosigmoid junction V10.06
- rectum V10.06
- renal pelvis V10.53
- respiratory organs NEC V10.20
- salivary gland V10.02
- skin V10.83
  - melanoma V10.82
- small intestine NEC V10.09
- soft tissue NEC V10.89
- specified site NEC V10.89
- stomach V10.04
- testis V10.47
- thymus V10.29
- thyroid V10.87
- tongue V10.01
- trachea V10.12
- ureter V10.59
- urethra V10.59
- urinary organ V10.50
- uterine adnexa V10.44
- uterus V10.42
- vagina V10.44
- vulva V10.44
- manic-depressive psychosis V11.1
- meningitis V12.42
- mental disorder V11.9
  - affective type V11.1
  - manic-depressive V11.1
  - neurosis V11.2
  - schizophrenia V11.0
  - specified type NEC V11.8
- metabolic disorder V12.2
- musculoskeletal disorder NEC V13.5
- myocardial infarction 412
- neglect (emotional) V15.42
- nephrotic syndrome V13.03
- nervous system disorder V12.40
  - specified type NEC V12.49
- neurosis V11.2

History—*continued*
- noncompliance with medical treatment V15.81
- nutritional deficiency V12.1
- obstetric disorder V13.29
  - affecting management of current pregnancy V23.49
  - pre-term labor V23.41
  - pre-term labor V13.41
- parasitic disease V12.00
  - specified NEC V12.09
- perinatal problems V13.7
  - low birth weight (*see also* Status, low birth weight) V21.30
- physical abuse V15.41
- poisoning V15.6
- poliomyelitis V12.02
- polyps, colonic V12.72
- poor obstetric V23.49
  - affecting management of current pregnancy V23.49
  - pre-term labor V23.41
  - pre-term labor V13.41
- prolonged reversible ischemic neurologic deficits (PRIND) V12.54
- psychiatric disorder V11.9
  - affective type V11.1
  - manic-depressive V11.1
  - neurosis V11.2
  - schizophrenia V11.0
  - specified type NEC V11.8
- psychological trauma V15.49
  - emotional abuse V15.42
  - neglect V15.42
  - physical abuse V15.41
  - rape V15.41
- psychoneurosis V11.2
- radiation therapy V15.3
- rape V15.41
- respiratory system disease V12.60
  - pneumonia V12.61
  - specified NEC V12.69
- reticulosarcoma V10.71
- reversible ischemic neurologic deficit (RIND) V12.54
- schizophrenia V11.0
- skin disease V13.3
- smoking (tobacco) V15.82
- stroke without residual deficits V12.54
- subcutaneous tissue disease V13.3
- sudden
  - cardiac
    - arrest V12.53
    - death (successfully resuscitated) V12.53
- surgery (major) to
  - great vessels V15.1
  - heart V15.1
  - major organs NEC V15.2
- syndrome, nephrotic V13.03
- thrombophlebitis V12.52
- thrombosis V12.51
- tobacco use V15.82
- trophoblastic disease V13.1
  - affecting management of pregnancy V23.1
- tuberculosis V12.01
- ulcer, peptic V12.71
- urinary system disorder V13.00
  - calculi V13.01
  - infection V13.02
  - nephrotic syndrome V13.03
  - specified NEC V13.09

1074

INDEX TO DISEASES

HIV infection (disease) (illness)—*see* Human immunodeficiency virus (disease) (illness) (infection)
Hives (bold) (*see also* Urticaria) 708.9
Hoarseness 784.49
Hobnail liver —*see* Cirrhosis, portal
Hobo, hoboism V60.0
Hodgkin's
  disease (M9650/3) 201.9
    lymphocytic
      depletion (M9653/3) 201.7
        diffuse fibrosis (M9654/3) 201.7
        reticular type (M9655/3) 201.7
      predominance (M9651/3) 201.4
    lymphocytic-histiocytic predominance (M9651/3) 201.4
    mixed cellularity (M9652/3) 201.6
    nodular sclerosis (M9656/3) 201.5
      cellular phase (M9657/3) 201.5
  granuloma (M9661/3) 201.1
  lymphogranulomatosis (M9650/3) 201.9
  lymphoma (M9650/3) 201.9
  lymphosarcoma (M9650/3) 201.9
  paragranuloma (M9660/3) 201.0
  sarcoma (M9662/3) 201.2
Hodgson's disease (aneurysmal dilatation of aorta) 441.9
  ruptured 441.5
Hodi-potsy 111.0
Hoffa -(Kastert) disease or syndrome (liposynovitis prepatellaris) 272.8
Hoffmann's syndrome 244.9 *[359.5]*
Hoffmann-Bouveret syndrome (paroxysmal tachycardia) 427.2
Hole
  macula 362.54
  optic disc, crater-like 377.22
  retina (macula) 362.54
    round 361.31
      with detachment 361.01
Holla disease (*see also* Spherocytosis) 282.0
Holländer-Simons syndrome (progressive lipodystrophy) 272.6
Hollow foot (congenital) 754.71
  acquired 736.73
Holmes' syndrome (visual disorientation) 368.16
Holoprosencephaly 742.2
  due to
    trisomy 13 758.1
    trisomy 18 758.2
Holthouse's hernia —*see* Hernia, inguinal
Homesickness 309.89
Homocystinemia 270.4
Homocystinuria 270.4
Homologous serum jaundice (prophylactic) (therapeutic)—*see* Hepatitis, viral
Homosexuality —*omit code*
  ego-dystonic 302.0
  pedophilic 302.2
  problems with 302.0
Homozygous Hb-S disease 282.61
Honeycomb lung 518.89
  congenital 748.4
Hong Kong ear 117.3
HOOD (hereditary osteo-onychodysplasia) 756.89
Hooded
  clitoris 752.49
  penis 752.69
Hookworm (anemia) (disease) (infestation)—*see* Ancylostomiasis
Hoppe-Goldflam syndrome 358.00

Hordeolum (external) (eyelid) 373.11
  internal 373.12
Horn
  cutaneous 702.8
    cheek 702.8
    eyelid 702.8
    penis 702.8
  iliac 756.89
  nail 703.8
    congenital 757.5
  papillary 700
Horner's
  syndrome (*see also* Neuropathy, peripheral, autonomic) 337.9
    traumatic 954.0
  teeth 520.4
Horseshoe kidney (congenital) 753.3
Horton's
  disease (temporal arteritis) 446.5
  headache or neuralgia 346.2
Hospice care V66.7
Hospitalism (in children) NEC 309.83
Hourglass contraction, contracture
  bladder 596.8
  gallbladder 575.2
    congenital 751.69
  stomach 536.8
    congenital 750.7
    psychogenic 306.4
  uterus 661.4
    affecting fetus or newborn 763.7
Household circumstance affecting care V60.9
  specified type NEC V60.8
Housemaid's knee 727.2
Housing circumstance affecting care V60.9
  specified type NEC V60.8
Huchard's disease (continued arterial hypertension) 401.9
Hudson-Stähli lines 371.11
Huguier's disease (uterine fibroma) 218.9
Hum, venous —*omit code*
Human bite (open wound)—*see also* Wound, open, by site
  intact skin surface—*see* Contusion
Human immunodeficiency virus (disease) (illness) 042
  infection V08
    with symptoms, symptomatic 042
Human immunodeficiency virus-2 infection 079.53
Human immunovirus (disease) (illness) (infection)—*see* Human immunodeficiency virus (disease) (illness) (infection)
Human papillomavirus 079.4
  cervical
    high risk, DNA test positive 795.05
    low risk, DNA test positive 795.09
Human parovirus 079.83
Human T-cell lymphotrophic virus I infection 079.51
Human T-cell lymphotrophic virus II infection 079.52
Human T-cell lymphotropic virus-III (disease) (illness) (infection)—*see* Human immunodeficiency virus (disease) (illness) (infection)
HTLV-I infection 079.51
HTLV-II infection 079.52
HTLV-III (disease) (illness) (infection)—*see* Human immunodeficiency virus (disease) (illness) (infection)

HTLV-III/LAV
(disease) (illness) (infection)—*see* Human immunodeficiency virus (disease) (illness) (infection)
Humpback (acquired) 737.9
 congenital 756.19
Hunchback (acquired) 737.9
 congenital 756.19
Hunger 994.2
 air, psychogenic 306.1
 disease 251.1
Hunner's ulcer (*see also* Cystitis) 595.1
Hunt's
 neuralgia 053.11
 syndrome (herpetic geniculate ganglionitis) 053.11
 dyssynergia cerebellaris myoclonica 334.2
Hunter's glossitis 529.4
Hunter (-Hurler) syndrome (mucopolysaccharidosis II) 277.5
Hunterian chancre 091.0
Huntington's
 chorea 333.4
 disease 333.4
Huppert's disease (multiple myeloma) (M9730/3) 203.0
Hurler (-Hunter) disease or syndrome (mucopolysaccharidosis II) 277.5
Hürthle cell
 adenocarcinoma (M8290/3) 193
 adenoma (M8290/0) 226
 carcinoma (M8290/3) 193
 tumor (M8290/0) 226
Hutchinson's
 disease meaning
  angioma serpiginosum 709.1
  cheiropompholyx 705.81
  prurigo estivalis 692.72
   summer eruption, or summer prurigo 692.72
  incisors 090.5
  melanotic freckle (M8742/2)—*see also* Neoplasm, skin, in situ
   malignant melanoma in (M8742/3)—*see* Melanoma
  teeth or incisors (congenital syphilis) 090.5
Hutchinson-Boeck disease or syndrome (sarcoidosis) 135
Hutchinson-Gilford disease or syndrome (progeria) 259.8
Hyaline
 degeneration (diffuse) (generalized) 728.9
  localized—*see* Degeneration, by site
 membrane (disease) (lung) (newborn) 769
Hyalinosis cutis et mucosae 272.8
Hyalin plaque, sclera, senile 379.16
Hyalitis (asteroid) 379.22
 syphilitic 095.8
Hydatid
 cyst or tumor—*see also* Echinococcus
  fallopian tube 752.11
 mole—*see* Hydatidiform mole
 Morgagni (congenital) 752.89
  fallopian tube 752.11
Hydatidiform mole (benign) (complicating pregnancy) (delivered) (undelivered) 630
 invasive (M9100/1) 236.1
 malignant (M9100/1) 236.1
 previous, affecting management of pregnancy V23.1
Hydatidosis —*see* Echinococcus
Hyde's disease (prurigo nodularis) 698.3

Hydradenitis 705.83
Hydradenoma (M8400/0)—*see* Hidradenoma
Hydralazine lupus or syndrome
 correct substance properly administered 695.4
 overdose or wrong substance given or taken 972.6
Hydramnios 657
 affecting fetus or newborn 761.3
Hydrancephaly 742.3
 with spina bifida (*see also* Spina bifida) 741.0
Hydranencephaly 742.3
 with spina bifida (*see also* Spina bifida) 741.0
Hydrargyrism NEC 985.0
Hydrarthrosis (*see also* Effusion, joint) 719.0
 gonococcal 098.50
 intermittent (*see also* Rheumatism, palindromic) 719.3
 of yaws (early) (late) 102.6
 syphilitic 095.8
  congenital 090.5
Hydremia 285.9
Hydrencephalocele (congenital) 742.0
Hydrencephalomeningocele (congenital) 742.0
Hydroa 694.0
 aestivale 692.72
 gestationis 646.8
 herpetiformis 694.0
 pruriginosa 694.0
 vacciniforme 692.72
Hydroadenitis 705.83
Hydrocalycosis (*see also* Hydronephrosis) 591
 congenital 753.29
Hydrocalyx (*see also* Hydronephrosis) 591
Hydrocele (calcified) (chylous) (idiopathic) (infantile) (inguinal canal) (recurrent) (senile) (spermatic cord) (testis) (tunica vaginalis) 603.9
 canal of Nuck (female) 629.1
  male 603.9
 congenital 778.6
 encysted 603.0
  congenital 778.6
 female NEC 629.89
 infected 603.1
 round ligament 629.89
 specified type NEC 603.8
  congenital 778.6
 spinalis (*see also* Spina bifida) 741.9
 vulva 624.8
Hydrocephalic fetus
 affecting management of pregnancy 655.0
 causing disproportion 653.6
  with obstructed labor 660.1
   affecting fetus or newborn 763.1
Hydrocephalus (acquired) (external) (internal) (malignant) (noncommunicating) (obstructive) (recurrent) 331.4
 aqueduct of Sylvius stricture 742.3
  with spina bifida (*see also* Spina bifida) 741.0
 chronic 742.3
  with spina bifida (*see also* Spina bifida) 741.0
 communicating 331.3
 congenital (external) (internal) 742.3
  with spina bifida (*see also* Spina bifida) 741.0
 due to
  stricture of aqueduct of Sylvius 742.3
   with spina bifida (*see also* Spina bifida) 741.0
  toxoplasmosis (congenital) 771.2
 fetal affecting management of pregnancy 655.0

Hydrocephalus—*continued*
  foramen Magendie block (acquired) 331.3
    congenital 742.3
      with spina bifida (*see also* Spina bifida) 741.0
    newborn 742.3
      with spina bifida (*see also* Spina bifida) 741.0
    normal pressure 331.5
      idiopathic (INPH) 331.5
      secondary 331.3
    otitic 348.2
    syphilitic, congenital 090.49
    tuberculous (*see also* Tuberculosis) 013.8
Hydrocolpos (congenital) 623.8
Hydrocystoma (M8404/0)—*see* Neoplasm, skin, benign
Hydroencephalocele (congenital) 742.0
Hydroencephalomeningocele (congenital) 742.0
Hydrohematopneumothorax (*see also* Hemothorax) 511.8
Hydromeningitis —*see* Meningitis
Hydromeningocele (spinal) (*see also* Spina bifida) 741.9
  cranial 742.0
Hydrometra 621.8
Hydrometrocolpos 623.8
Hydromicrocephaly 742.1
Hydromphalus (congenital) (since birth) 757.39
Hydromyelia 742.53
Hydromyelocele (*see also* Spina bifida) 741.9
Hydronephrosis 591
  atrophic 591
  congenital 753.29
  due to S. hematobium 120.0
  early 591
  functionless (infected) 591
  infected 591
  intermittent 591
  primary 591
  secondary 591
  tuberculous (*see also* Tuberculosis) 016.0
Hydropericarditis (*see also* Pericarditis) 423.9
Hydropericardium (*see also* Pericarditis) 423.9
Hydroperitoneum 789.59
Hydrophobia 071
Hydrophthalmos (*see also* Buphthalmia) 743.20
Hydropneumohemothorax (*see also* Hemothorax) 511.8
Hydropneumopericarditis (*see also* Pericarditis) 423.9
Hydropneumopericardium (*see also* Pericarditis) 423.9
Hydropneumothorax 511.8
  nontuberculous 511.8
    bacterial 511.1
    pneumococcal 511.1
    staphylococcal 511.1
    streptococcal 511.1
    traumatic 860.0
      with open wound into thorax 860.1
    tuberculous (*see also* Tuberculosis, pleural) 012.0
Hydrops 782.3
  abdominis 789.59
  amnii (complicating pregnancy) (*see also* Hydramnios) 657
  articulorum intermittens (*see also* Rheumatism, palindromic) 719.3
  cardiac (*see also* Failure, heart) 428.0
  congenital—*see* Hydrops, fetalis

Hydrops—*continued*
  endolymphatic (*see also* Disease, Ménière's) 386.00
  fetal(is) or newborn 778.0
    due to isoimmunization 773.3
    not due to isoimmunization 778.0
  gallbladder 575.3
  idiopathic (fetus or newborn) 778.0
  joint (*see also* Effusion, joint) 719.0
  labyrinth (*see also* Disease, Ménière's) 386.00
  meningeal NEC 331.4
  nutritional 262
  pericardium—*see* Pericarditis
  pleura (*see also* Hydrothorax) 511.8
  renal (*see also* Nephrosis) 581.9
  spermatic cord (*see also* Hydrocele) 603.9
Hydropyonephrosis (*see also* Pyelitis) 590.80
  chronic 590.00
Hydrorachis 742.53
Hydrorrhea (nasal) 478.19
  gravidarum 658.1
  pregnancy 658.1
Hydrosadenitis 705.83
Hydrosalpinx (fallopian tube) (follicularis) 614.1
Hydrothorax (double) (pleural) 511.8
  chylous (nonfilarial) 457.8
    filaria (*see also* Infestation, filarial) 125.9
  nontuberculous 511.8
    bacterial 511.1
    pneumococcal 511.1
    staphylococcal 511.1
    streptococcal 511.1
  traumatic 862.29
    with open wound into thorax 862.39
  tuberculous (*see also* Tuberculosis, pleura) 012.0
Hydroureter 593.5
  congenital 753.22
Hydroureteronephrosis (*see also* Hydronephrosis) 591
Hydrourethra 599.84
Hydroxykynureninuria 270.2
Hydroxyprolinemia 270.8
Hydroxyprolinuria 270.8
Hygroma (congenital) (cystic) (M9173/0) 228.1
  prepatellar 727.3
  subdural—*see* Hematoma, subdural
Hymen —*see* condition
Hymenolepiasis (diminuta) (infection) (infestation) (nana) 123.6
Hymenolepis (diminuta) (infection) (infestation) (nana) 123.6
Hypalgesia (*see also* Disturbance, sensation) 782.0
Hyperabduction syndrome 447.8
Hyperacidity, gastric 536.8
  psychogenic 306.4
Hyperactive, hyperactivity 314.01
  basal cell, uterine cervix 622.10
  bladder 596.51
  bowel (syndrome) 564.9
    sounds 787.5
  cervix epithelial (basal) 622.10
  child 314.01
  colon 564.9
  gastrointestinal 536.8
    psychogenic 306.4
  intestine 564.9
  labyrinth (unilateral) 386.51
    with loss of labyrinthine reactivity 386.58
    bilateral 386.52

Hyeractive, hyperactivity—*continued*
  nasal mucous membrane 478.19
  stomach 536.8
  thyroid (gland) (*see also* Thyrotoxicosis) 242.9
Hyperacusis 388.42
Hyperadrenalism (cortical) 255.3
  medullary 255.6
Hyperadrenocorticism 255.3
  congenital 255.2
  iatrogenic
    correct substance properly administered 255.3
    overdose or wrong substance given or taken 962.0
Hyperaffectivity 301.11
Hyperaldosteronism (atypical) (hyperplastic) (normoaldosteronal) (normotensive) (primary) 255.10
  secondary 255.14
Hyperalgesia (*see also* Disturbance, sensation) 782.0
Hyperalimentation 783.6
  carotene 278.3
  specified NEC 278.8
  vitamin A 278.2
  vitamin D 278.4
Hyperaminoaciduria 270.9
  arginine 270.6
  citrulline 270.6
  cystine 270.0
  glycine 270.0
  lysine 270.7
  ornithine 270.6
  renal (types I, II, III) 270.0
Hyperammonemia (congenital) 270.6
Hyperamnesia 780.99
Hyperamylasemia 790.5
Hyperaphia 782.0
Hyperazotemia 791.9
Hyperbetalipoproteinemia (acquired) (essential) (familial) (hereditary) (primary) (secondary) 272.0
  with pre-betalipoproteinemia 272.2
Hyperbilirubinemia 782.4
  congenital 277.4
  constitutional 277.4
  neonatal (transient) (*see also* Jaundice, fetus or newborn) 774.6
  of prematurity 774.2
Hyperbilirubinemica encephalopathia, newborn 774.7
  due to isoimmunization 773.4
Hypercalcemia, hypercalcemic (idiopathic) 275.42
  nephropathy 588.89
Hypercalcinuria 275.40
Hypercapnia 786.09
  with mixed acid-base disorder 276.4
  fetal, affecting newborn 770.89
Hypercarotinemia 278.3
Hypercementosis 521.5
Hyperchloremia 276.9
Hyperchlorhydria 536.8
  neurotic 306.4
  psychogenic 306.4
Hypercholesterinemia —*see* Hypercholesterolemia
Hypercholesterolemia 272.0
  with hyperglyceridemia, endogenous 272.2
  essential 272.0
  familial 272.0
  hereditary 272.0
  primary 272.0
  pure 272.0

Hypercholesterolosis 272.0
Hyperchylia gastricsa 536.8
  psychogenic 306.4
Hyperchylomicronemia (familial) (with hyperbetalipoproteinemia) 272.3
Hypercoagulation syndrome (primary) 289.81
  secondary 289.82
Hypercorticosteronism
  correct substance properly administered 255.3
  overdose or wrong substance given or taken 962.0
Hypercortisonism
  correct substance properly administered 255.3
  overdose or wrong substance given or taken 962.0
Hyperdynamic beta-adrenergic state or syndrome (circulatory) 429.82
Hyperekplexia 759.89
Hyperelectrolytemia 276.9
Hyperemesis 536.2
  arising during pregnancy—*see* Hyperemesis, gravidarum
  gravidarum (mild) (before 22 completed weeks gestation) 643.0
    with
      carbohydrate depletion 643.1
      dehydration 643.1
      electrolyte imbalance 643.1
      metabolic disturbance 643.1
    affecting fetus or newborn 761.8
    severe (with metabolic disturbance) 643.1
  psychogenic 306.4
Hyperemia (acute) 780.99
  anal mucosa 569.49
  bladder 596.7
  cerebral 437.8
  conjunctiva 372.71
  ear, internal, acute 386.30
  enteric 564.89
  eye 372.71
  eyelid (active) (passive) 374.82
  intestine 564.89
  iris 364.41
  kidney 593.81
  labyrinth 386.30
  liver (active) (passive) 573.8
  lung 514
  ovary 620.8
  passive 780.99
  pulmonary 514
  renal 593.81
  retina 362.89
  spleen 289.59
  stomach 537.89
Hyperesthesia (body surface) (*see also* Disturbance, sensation) 782.0
  larynx (reflex) 478.79
    hysterical 300.11
  pharynx (reflex) 478.29
Hyperestrinism 256.0
Hyperestrogenism 256.0
Hyperestrogenosis 256.0
Hyperexplexia 759.89
Hyperextension, joint 718.80
  ankle 718.87
  elbow 718.82
  foot 718.87
  hand 718.84
  hip 718.85
  knee 718.86

Hypermaturity (fetus or newborn)
post-term infant 766.21
prolonged gestation infant 766.22
Hypermenorrhea 626.2
Hypermetabolism 794.7
Hypermethioninemia 270.4
Hypermetropia (congenital) 367.0
Hypermobility
cecum 564.9
coccyx 724.71
colon 564.9
  psychogenic 306.4
ileum 564.89
joint (acquired) 718.80
  ankle 718.87
  elbow 718.82
  foot 718.87
  hand 718.84
  hip 718.85
  knee 718.86
  multiple sites 718.89
  pelvic region 718.85
  shoulder (region) 718.81
  specified site NEC 718.88
  wrist 718.83
kidney, congenital 753.3
meniscus (knee) 717.5
scapula 718.81
stomach 536.8
  psychogenic 306.4
syndrome 728.5
testis, congenital 752.52
urethral 599.81
Hypermotility
gastrointestinal 536.8
intestine 564.9
  psychogenic 306.4
stomach 536.8
Hypernasality 784.49
Hypernatremia 276.0
with water depletion 276.0
Hypernephroma (M8312/3) 189.0
Hyperopia 367.0
Hyperorexia 783.6
Hyperornithinemia 270.6
Hyperosmia (*see also* Disturbance, sensation) 781.1
Hyperosmolality 276.0
Hyperosteogenesis 733.99
Hyperostosis 733.99
calvarial 733.3
cortical 733.3
  infantile 756.59
frontal, internal of skull 733.3
interna frontalis 733.3
monomelic 733.99
skull 733.3
  congenital 756.0
vertebral 721.8
  with spondylosis—*see* Spondylosis
  ankylosing 721.6
Hyperovarianism 256.1
Hyperovarism, hyperovaria 256.1
Hyperoxaluria (primary) 271.8
Hyperoxia 987.8

Hyperparathyroidism 252.00
ectopic 259.3
other 252.08
primary 252.01
secondary (of renal origin) 588.81
  non-renal 252.02
tertiary 252.08
Hyperpathia (*see also* Disturbance, sensation) 782.0
psychogenic 307.80
Hyperperistalsis 787.4
psychogenic 306.4
Hyperpermeability, capillary 448.9
Hyperphagia 783.6
Hyperphenylalaninemia 270.1
Hyperphoria 378.40
alternating 378.45
Hyperphosphatemia 275.3
Hyperpiesia (*see also* Hypertension) 401.9
Hyperpiesis (*see also* Hypertension) 401.9
Hyperpigmentation —*see* Pigmentation
Hyperpinealism 259.8
Hyperpipecolatemia 270.7
Hyperpituitarism 253.1
Hyperplasia, hyperplastic
adenoids (lymphoid tissue) 474.12
  and tonsils 474.10
adrenal (capsule) (cortex) (gland) 255.8
  with
    sexual precocity (male) 255.2
    virilism, adrenal 255.2
    virilization (female) 255.2
  congenital 255.2
  due to excess ACTH (ectopic) (pituitary) 255.0
  medulla 255.8
alpha cells (pancreatic)
  with
    gastrin excess 251.5
    glucagon excess 251.4
appendix (lymphoid) 543.0
artery, fibromuscular NEC 447.8
  carotid 447.8
  renal 447.3
bone 733.99
  marrow 289.9
breast (*see also* Hypertrophy, breast) 611.1
carotid artery 447.8
cementation, cementum (teeth) (tooth) 521.5
cervical gland 785.6
cervix (uteri) 622.10
  basal cell 622.10
  congenital 752.49
  endometrium 622.10
  polypoid 622.10
chin 524.05
clitoris, congenital 752.49
dentin 521.5
endocervicitis 616.0
endometrium, endometrial (adenomatous) (atypical) (cystic) (glandular) (polypoid) (uterus) 621.30
  with atypia 621.33
  without atypia
    complex 621.32
    simple 621.31
  cervix 622.10
epithelial 709.8
  focal, oral, including tongue 528.79
  mouth (focal) 528.79
  nipple 611.8
  skin 709.8

Hyperextension, joint—*continued*
  multiple sites 718.89
  pelvic region 718.85
  shoulder (region) 718.81
  specified site NEC 718.88
  wrist 718.83
Hyperfibrinolysis —*see* Fibrinolysis
Hyperfolliculinism 256.0
Hyperfructosemia 271.2
Hyperfunction
  adrenal (cortex) 255.3
    androgenic, acquired benign 255.3
    medulla 255.6
    virilism 255.2
  corticoadrenal NEC 255.3
  labyrinth—*see* Hyperactive, labyrinth
  medulloadrenal 255.6
  ovary 256.1
    estrogen 256.0
  pancreas 577.8
  parathyroid (gland) 252.00
  pituitary (anterior) (gland) (lobe) 253.1
  testicular 257.0
Hypergammaglobulinemia 289.89
  monoclonal, benign (BMH) 273.1
  polyclonal 273.0
  Waldenström's 273.0
Hyperglobulinemia 273.8
Hyperglycemia 790.29
  maternal
    affecting fetus or newborn 775.0
    manifest diabetes in infant 775.1
  postpancreatectomy (complete) (partial) 251.3
Hyperglyceridemia 272.1
  endogenous 272.1
  essential 272.1
  familial 272.1
  hereditary 272.1
  mixed 272.3
  pure 272.1
Hyperglycinemia 270.7
Hypergonadism
  ovarian 256.1
  testicular (infantile) (primary) 257.0
Hyperheparinemia (*see also* Circulating anticoagulants) 286.5
Hyperhidrosis, hyperidrosis 705.21
  axilla 705.21
  face 705.21
  focal (localized) 705.21
    primary 705.21
      axilla 705.21
      face 705.21
      palms 705.21
      soles 705.21
    secondary 705.22
      axilla 705.22
      face 705.22
      palms 705.22
      soles 705.22
  generalized 780.8
  palms 705.21
  psychogenic 306.3
  secondary 780.8
  soles 705.21
Hyperhistidinemia 270.5
Hyperinsulinism (ectopic) (functional) (organic) NEC 251.1
  iatrogenic 251.0
  reactive 251.2
  spontaneous 251.2

Hyperinsulism—*continued*
  therapeutic misadventure (from administration of insulin) 962.3
Hyperiodemia 276.9
Hyperirritability (cerebral), in newborn 779.1
Hyperkalemia 276.7
Hyperkeratosis (*see also* Keratosis) 701.1
  cervix 622.2
  congenital 757.39
  cornea 371.89
  due to yaws (early) (late) (palmar or plantar) 102.3
  eccentrica 757.39
  figurata centrifuga atrophica 757.39
  follicularis 757.39
    in cutem penetrans 701.1
  limbic (cornea) 371.89
  palmoplantaris climacterica 701.1
  pinta (carate) 103.1
  senile (with pruritus) 702.0
  tongue 528.79
  universalis congenita 757.1
  vagina 623.1
  vocal cord 478.5
  vulva 624.09
Hyperkinesia, hyperkinetic (disease) (reaction) (syndrome) 314.9
  with
    attention deficit —*see* Disorder, attention deficit
    conduct disorder 314.2
    developmental delay 314.1
    simple disturbance of activity and attention 314.01
    specified manifestation NEC 314.8
  heart (disease) 429.82
  of childhood or adolescence NEC 314.9
Hyperlacrimation (*see also* Epiphora) 375.20
Hyperlipemia (*see also* Hyperlipidemia) 272.4
Hyperlipidemia 272.4
  carbohydrate-induced 272.1
  combined 272.4
  endogenous 272.1
  exogenous 272.3
  fat-induced 272.3
  group
    A 272.0
    B 272.1
    C 272.2
    D 272.3
  mixed 272.2
  specified type NEC 272.4
Hyperlipidosis 272.7
  hereditary 272.7
Hyperlipoproteinemia (acquired) (essential) (familial) (hereditary) (primary) (secondary) 272.4
  Fredrickson type
    I 272.3
    IIa 272.0
    IIb 272.2
    III 272.2
    IV 272.1
    V 272.3
  low-density-lipoid-type (LDL) 272.0
  very-low-density-lipoid-type [VLDL] 272.1
Hyperlucent lung, unilateral 492.8
Hyperluteinization 256.1
Hyperlysinemia 270.7
Hypermagnesemia 275.2
  neonatal 775.5

INDEX TO DISEASES — Hypersecretion

Hyperplasia, hyperplastic—*continued*
    tongue (focal) 528.79
    vaginal wall 623.0
  erythroid 289.9
  fascialis ossificans (progressiva) 728.11
  fibromuscular, artery NEC 447.8
    carotid 447.8
    renal 447.3
  genital
    female 629.89
    male 608.89
  gingiva 523.8
  glandularis
    cystica uteri 621.30
    endometrium (uterus) 621.30
    interstitialis uteri 621.30
  granulocytic 288.69
  gum 523.8
  hymen, congenital 752.49
  islands of Langerhans 251.1
  islet cell (pancreatic) 251.9
    alpha cells
      with excess
        gastrin 251.5
        glucagon 251.4
    beta cells 251.1
  juxtaglomerular (complex) (kidney) 593.89
  kidney (congenital) 753.3
  liver (congenital) 751.69
  lymph node (gland) 785.6
  lymphoid (diffuse) (nodular) 785.6
    appendix 543.0
    intestine 569.89
  mandibular 524.02
    alveolar 524.72
    unilateral condylar 526.89
  Marchand multiple nodular (liver)—*see* Cirrhosis, postnecrotic
  maxillary 524.01
    alveolar 524.71
  medulla, adrenal 255.8
  myometrium, myometrial 621.2
  nose (lymphoid) (polypoid) 478.19
  oral soft tissue (inflammatory) (irritative) (mucosa) NEC 528.9
    gingiva 523.8
    tongue 529.8
  organ or site, congenital NEC—*see* Anomaly, specified type NEC
  ovary 620.8
  palate, papillary 528.9
  pancreatic islet cells 251.9
    alpha
      with excess
        gastrin 251.5
        glucagon 251.4
    beta 251.1
  parathyroid (gland) 252.01
  persistent, vitreous (primary) 743.51
  pharynx (lymphoid) 478.29
  prostate 600.90
    with
      other lower urinary tract symptoms (LUTS) 600.91
      urinary
        obstruction 600.91
        retention 600.91
    adenofibromatous 600.20
      with
        other lower urinary tract symptoms (LUTS) 600.21

Hyperplasia, hyperplastic—*continued*
    urinary
      obstruction 600.21
      retention 600.21
    nodular 600.10
      with
        urinary
          obstruction 600.11
          retention 600.11
  renal artery (fibromuscular) 447.3
  reticuloendothelial (cell) 289.9
  salivary gland (any) 527.1
  Schimmelbusch's 610.1
  suprarenal (capsule) (gland) 255.8
  thymus (gland) (persistent) 254.0
  thyroid (*see also* Goiter) 240.9
    primary 242.0
    secondary 242.2
  tonsil (lymphoid tissue) 474.11
    and adenoids 474.10
  urethrovaginal 599.89
  uterus, uterine (myometrium) 621.2
    endometrium (*see also* Hyperplasia, endometrium) 621.30
  vitreous (humor), primary persistent 743.51
  vulva 624.3
  zygoma 738.11
Hyperpnea (*see also* Hyperventilation) 786.01
Hyperpotassemia 276.7
Hyperprebetalipoproteinemia 272.1
  with chylomicronemia 272.3
  familial 272.1
Hyperprolactinemia 253.1
Hyperprolinemia 270.8
Hyperproteinemia 273.8
Hyperprothrombinemia 289.89
Hyperpselaphesia 782.0
Hyperpyrexia 780.6
  heat (effects of) 992.0
  malarial (*see also* Malaria) 084.6
  malignant, due to anesthetic 995.86
  rheumatic—*see* Fever, rheumatic
  unknown origin (*see also* Pyrexia) 780.6
Hyperreactor, vascular 780.2
Hyperreflexia 796.1
  bladder, autonomic 596.54
    with cauda equina 344.61
  detrusor 344.61
Hypersalivation (*see also* Ptyalism) 527.7
Hypersarcosinemia 270.8
Hypersecretion
  ACTH 255.3
  androgens (ovarian) 256.1
  calcitonin 246.0
  corticoadrenal 255.3
  cortisol 255.0
  estrogen 256.0
  gastric 536.8
    psychogenic 306.4
  gastrin 251.5
  glucagon 251.4
  hormone
    ACTH 255.3
    anterior pituitary 253.1
    growth NEC 253.0
    ovarian androgen 256.1
    testicular 257.0
    thyroid stimulating 242.8
  insulin—*see* Hyperinsulinism
  lacrimal glands (*see also* Epiphora) 375.20
  medulloadrenal 255.6

Hypersecretion—*continued*
  milk 676.6
  ovarian androgens 256.1
  pituitary (anterior) 253.1
  salivary gland (any) 527.7
  testicular hormones 257.0
  thyrocalcitonin 246.0
  upper respiratory 478.9
Hypersegmentation, hereditary 288.2
  eosinophils 288.2
  neutrophil nuclei 288.2
Hypersensitive, hypersensitiveness, hypersensitivity —*see also* Allergy
  angiitis 446.20
    specified NEC 446.29
  carotid sinus 337.0
  colon 564.9
    psychogenic 306.4
  DNA (deoxyribonucleic acid) NEC 287.2
  drug (*see also* Allergy, drug) 995.27
  esophagus 530.89
  insect bites—*see* Injury, superficial, by site
  labyrinth 386.58
  pain (*see also* Disturbance, sensation) 782.0
  pneumonitis NEC 495.9
  reaction (*see also* Allergy) 995.3
    upper respiratory tract NEC 478.8
  stomach (allergic) (nonallergic) 536.8
    psychogenic 306.4
Hypersomatotropism (classic) 253.0
Hypersomnia, unspecified 780.54
  with sleep apnea, unspecified 780.53
  alcohol induced 291.82
  drug induced 291.85
  due to
    medical condition classified elsewhere 327.14
      mental disorder 327.15
  idiopathic
    with long sleep time 327.11
    without long sleep time 327.12
  menstrual related 327.13
  nonorganic origin 307.43
    persistent (primary) 307.44
    transient 307.43
  organic 327.10
    other 327.19
  primary 307.44
  recurrent 327.13
Hypersplenia 289.4
Hypersplenism 289.4
Hypersteatosis 706.3
Hyperstimulation, ovarian 256.1
Hypersuprarenalism 255.3
Hypersusceptibility —*see* Allergy
Hyper-TBG-nemia 246.8
Hypertelorism 756.0
  orbit, orbital 376.41

"H" listing resumes after Hypertension table...

Hypertension, hypertensive

	Malignant	Benign	Unspecified
(arterial) (arteriolar) (crisis) (degeneration) (disease) (essential) (fluctuating) (idiopathic) (intermittent) (labile) (low renin) (orthostatic) (paroxysmal) (primary) (systemic) (uncontrolled) (vascular)	401.0	401.1	401.9
with			
chronic kidney disease			
stage I through stage IV, or unspecified	403.00	403.10	403.90
stage V or end stage renal disease	403.01	403.11	403.91
heart involvement (conditions classifiable to 429.0-429.3, 429.8, 429.9 due to hypertension) (*see also* Hypertension, heart)	402.00	402.10	402.90
with kidney involvement—*see* Hypertension, cardiorenal			
renal involvement (only conditions classifiable to 585, 586, 587) (excludes conditions classifiable to 584) (*see also* Hypertension, kidney)	403.00	403.10	403.90
with heart involvement—*see* Hypertension, cardiorenal			
failure (and sclerosis) (*see also* Hypertension, kidney)	403.01	403.11	403.91
sclerosis without failure (*see also* Hypertension, kidney)	403.00	403.10	403.90
accelerated (*see also* Hypertension, by type, malignant)	401.0	—	—
antepartum—*see* Hypertension complicating pregnancy, childbirth, or the puerperium			
cardiorenal (disease)	404.00	404.10	404.90
with			
chronic kidney disease			
stage I through stage IV, or unspecified	404.00	404.10	404.90
and heart failure	404.01	404.11	404.91
stage V or end stage renal disease	404.02	404.12	404.92
and heart failure	404.03	404.13	404.93
heart failure	404.01	404.11	404.91
and chronic kidney disease	404.01	404.11	404.91
stage I through stage IV or unspecified	404.01	404.11	404.91
stage V or end stage renal disease	404.03	404.13	404.93
cardiovascular disease (arteriosclerotic) (sclerotic)	402.00	402.10	402.90
with			
heart failure	402.01	402.11	402.91
renal involvement (conditions classifiable to 403) (*see also* Hypertension, cardiorenal)	404.00	404.10	404.90
cardiovascular renal (disease) (sclerosis) (*see also* Hypertension, cardiorenal)	404.00	404.10	404.90
cerebrovascular disease NEC	437.2	437.2	437.2
complicating pregnancy, childbirth, or the puerperium	642.2	642.0	642.9
with			
albuminuria (and edema) (mild)	—	—	642.4
severe	—	—	642.5
chronic kidney disease	642.2	642.2	642.2
and heart disease	642.2	642.2	642.2
edema (mild)	—	—	642.4
severe	—	—	642.5
heart disease	642.2	642.2	642.2
and chronic kidney disease	642.2	642.2	642.2
renal disease	642.2	642.2	642.2
and heart disease	642.2	642.2	642.2
chronic	642.2	642.0	642.0
with pre-eclampsia or eclampsia	642.7	642.7	642.7
fetus or newborn	760.0	760.0	760.0
essential	—	642.0	642.0
with pre-eclampsia or eclampsia	—	642.7	642.7
fetus or newborn	760.0	760.0	760.0
fetus or newborn	760.0	760.0	760.0
gestational	—	—	642.3
pre-existing	642.2	642.0	642.0
with pre-eclampsia or eclampsia	642.7	642.7	642.7
fetus or newborn	760.0	760.0	760.0
secondary to renal disease	642.1	642.1	642.1
with pre-eclampsia or eclampsia	642.7	642.7	642.7
fetus or newborn	760.0	760.0	760.0
transient	—	—	642.3
due to			
aldosteronism, primary	405.09	405.19	405.99
brain tumor	405.09	405.19	405.99
bulbar poliomyelitis	405.09	405.19	405.99
calculus			
kidney	405.09	405.19	405.99
ureter	405.09	405.19	405.99
coarctation, aorta	405.09	405.19	405.99
Cushing's disease	405.09	405.19	405.99
glomerulosclerosis (*see also* Hypertension, kidney)	403.00	403.10	403.90

Hypertension, hypertensive   **INDEX TO DISEASES**

	Malignant	Benign	Unspecified
periarteritis nodosa	405.09	405.19	405.99
pheochromocytoma	405.09	405.19	405.99
polycystic kidney(s)	405.09	405.19	405.99
polycythemia	405.09	405.19	405.99
porphyria	405.09	405.19	405.99
pyelonephritis	405.09	405.19	405.99
renal (artery)			
aneurysm	405.01	405.11	405.91
anomaly	405.01	405.11	405.91
embolism	405.01	405.11	405.91
fibromuscular hyperplasia	405.01	405.11	405.91
occlusion	405.01	405.11	405.91
stenosis	405.01	405.11	405.91
thrombosis	405.01	405.11	405.91
encephalopathy	437.2	437.2	437.2
gestational (transient) NEC	—	—	642.3
Goldblatt's	440.1	440.1	440.1
heart (disease) (conditions classifiable to 429.0-429.3, 429.8, 429.9 due to hypertension)	402.00	402.10	402.90
with			
heart failure	402.01	402.11	402.91
hypertensive kidney disease (conditions classifiable to 403) (*see also* Hypertension, cardiorenal)	404.00	404.10	404.90
renal sclerosis (*see also* Hypertension, cardiorenal)	404.00	404.10	404.90
intracranial, benign	—	348.2	—
intraocular	—	—	365.04
kidney	403.00	403.10	403.90
with			
chronic kidney disease			
stage I through stage IV, or unspecified	403.00	403.10	403.90
stage V or end stage renal disease	403.01	403.11	403.91
heart involvement (conditions classifiable to 429.0-429.3, 429.8, 429.9 due to hypertension) (*see also* Hypertension cardiorenal)	404.00	404.10	404.90
hypertensive heart (disease) (conditions classifiable to 402) (*see also* Hypertension, cardiorenal)	404.00	404.10	404.90
lesser circulation	—	—	416.0
necrotizing	401.0	—	—
ocular	—	—	365.04
portal (due to chronic liver disease)	—	—	572.3
postoperative	—	—	997.91
psychogenic	—	—	306.2
puerperal, postpartum—*see* Hypertension, complicating pregnancy, childbirth, or the puerperium			
pulmonary (artery)	—	—	416.8
idiopathic	—	—	416.0
primary	—	—	416.0
of newborn	—	—	747.83
with cor pulmonale (chronic)	—	—	416.8
acute	—	—	415.0
secondary	—	—	416.8
renal (disease) (*see also* Hypertension, kidney)	403.00	403.10	403.90
renovascular NEC	405.01	405.11	405.91
secondary NEC	405.09	405.19	405.99
due to			
aldosteronism, primary	405.09	405.19	405.99
brain tumor	405.09	405.19	405.99
bulbar poliomyelitis	405.09	405.19	405.99
calculus			
kidney	405.09	405.19	405.99
ureter	405.09	405.19	405.99
coarctation, aorta	405.09	405.19	405.99
Cushing's disease	405.09	405.19	405.99
glomerulosclerosis (*see also* Hypertension, kidney)	403.00	403.10	403.90
periarteritis nodosa	405.09	405.19	405.99
pheochromocytoma	405.09	405.19	405.99
polycystic kidney(s)	405.09	405.19	405.99
polycythemia	405.09	405.19	405.99
porphyria	405.09	405.19	405.99
pyelonephritis	405.09	405.19	405.99
renal (artery)			
aneurysm	405.01	405.11	405.91
anomaly	405.01	405.11	405.91
embolism	405.01	405.11	405.91
fibromuscular hyperplasia	405.01	405.11	405.91
occlusion	405.01	405.11	405.91
stenosis	405.01	405.11	405.91
thrombosis	405.01	405.11	405.91
transient	—	—	796.2

INDEX TO DISEASES — Hypertension, hypertensive

	Malignant	Benign	Unspecified
of pregnancy	—	—	642.3
venous, chronic (asymptomatic) (idiopathic)	—	—	459.30
with			
complication, NEC	—	—	459.39
due to			
deep vein thrombosis (*see also* Syndrome, postphlebetic)	—	—	459.10
inflammation	—	—	459.32
with ulcer	—	—	459.33
ulcer	—	—	459.31
with inflammation	—	—	459.33

Hyperthecosis, ovary 256.8
Hyperthermia (of unknown origin) (*see also* Pyrexia) 780.6
   malignant (due to anesthesia) 995.86
   newborn 778.4
Hyperthymergasia (*see also* Psychosis, affective) 296.0
   reactive (from emotional stress, psychological trauma) 298.1
   recurrent episode 296.1
   single episode 296.0
Hyperthymism 254.8
Hyperthyroid (recurrent)—*see* Hyperthyroidism
Hyperthyroidism (latent) (preadult) (recurrent) (without goiter) 242.9

> Note—Use the following fifth-digit subclassification with category 242:
>
> 0 without mention of thyrotoxic crisis or storm
> 1 with mention of thyrotoxic crisis or storm

   with
     goiter (diffuse) 242.0
       adenomatous 242.3
         multinodular 242.2
         uninodular 242.1
       nodular 242.3
         multinodular 242.2
         uninodular 242.1
     thyroid nodule 242.1
   complicating pregnancy, childbirth, or puerperium 648.1
   neonatal (transient) 775.3
Hypertonia —Hypertonicity
Hypertonicity
   bladder 596.51
   fetus or newborn 779.89
   gastrointestinal (tract) 536.8
   infancy 779.89
     due to electrolyte imbalance 779.89
   muscle 728.85
   stomach 536.8
     psychogenic 306.4
   uterus, uterine (contractions) 661.4
     affecting fetus or newborn 763.7
Hypertony —*see* Hypertonicity
Hypertransaminemia 790.4
Hypertrichosis 704.1
   congenital 757.4
   eyelid 374.54
   lanuginosa 757.4
     acquired 704.1
Hypertriglyceridemia, essential 272.1
Hypertrophy, hypertrophic
   adenoids (infectional) 474.12
     and tonsils (faucial) (infective) (lingual) (lymphoid) 474.10
   adrenal 255.8
   alveolar process or ridge 525.8
   anal papillae 569.49
   apocrine gland 705.82
   artery NEC 447.8
     carotid 447.8
     congenital (peripheral) NEC 747.60
     gastrointestinal 747.61
     lower limb 747.64
     renal 747.62
     specified NEC 747.69
     spinal 747.82
   arthritis (chronic) (*see also* Osteoarthrosis) 715.9

Hypertrophy, hypertrophic—*continued*
   spine (*see also* Spondylosis) 721.90
   arytenoid 478.79
   asymmetrical (heart) 429.9
   auricular—*see* Hypertrophy, cardiac
   Bartholin's gland 624.8
   bile duct 576.8
   bladder (sphincter) (trigone) 596.8
   blind spot, visual field 368.42
   bone 733.99
   brain 348.8
   breast 611.1
     cystic 610.1
     fetus or newborn 778.7
     fibrocystic 610.1
     massive pubertal 611.1
     puerperal, postpartum 676.3
     senile (parenchymatous) 611.1
   cardiac (chronic) (idiopathic) 429.3
     with
       rheumatic fever (conditions classifiable to 390)
         active 391.8
           with chorea 392.0
         inactive or quiescent (with chorea) 398.99
     congenital NEC 746.89
     fatty (*see also* Degeneration, myocardial) 429.1
     hypertensive (*see also* Hypertension, heart) 402.90
     rheumatic (with chorea) 398.99
       active or acute 391.8
         with chorea 392.0
     valve (*see also* Endocarditis) 424.90
       congenital NEC 746.89
   cartilage 733.99
   cecum 569.89
   cervix (uteri) 622.6
     congenital 752.49
     elongation 622.6
   clitoris (cirrhotic) 624.2
     congenital 752.49
   colon 569.89
     congenital 751.3
   conjunctiva, lymphoid 372.73
   cornea 371.89
   corpora cavernosa 607.89
   duodenum 537.89
   endometrium (uterus) (*see also* Hyperplasia, endometrium) 621.30
     cervix 622.6
   epididymis 608.89
   esophageal hiatus (congenital) 756.6
     with hernia—*see* Hernia, diaphragm
   eyelid 374.30
   falx, skull 733.99
   fat pad 729.30
     infrapatellar 729.31
     knee 729.31
     orbital 374.34
     popliteal 729.31
     prepatellar 729.31
     retropatellar 729.31
     specified site NEC 729.39
   foot (congenital) 755.67
   frenum, frenulum (tongue) 529.8
     linguae 529.8
     lip 528.5
   gallbladder or cystic duct 575.8
   gastric mucosa 535.2
   gingiva 523.8

INDEX TO DISEASES   **Hypertrophy, hypertrophic**

Hypertrophy, hypertrophic—*continued*
gland, glandular (general) NEC 785.6
gum (mucous membrane) 523.8
heart (idiopathic)—*see also* Hypertrophy,
    cardiac
    valve—*see also* Endocarditis
        congenital NEC 746.89
hemifacial 754.0
hepatic—*see* Hypertrophy, liver
hiatus (esophageal) 756.6
hilus gland 785.6
hymen, congenital 752.49
ileum 569.89
infrapatellar fat pad 729.31
intestine 569.89
jejunum 569.89
kidney (compensatory) 593.1
    congenital 753.3
labial frenulum 528.5
labium (majus) (minus) 624.3
lacrimal gland, chronic 375.03
ligament 728.9
    spinal 724.8
linguae frenulum 529.8
lingual tonsil (infectional) 474.11
lip (frenum) 528.5
    congenital 744.81
liver 789.1
    acute 573.8
    cirrhotic—*see* Cirrhosis, liver
    congenital 751.69
    fatty—*see* Fatty, liver
lymph gland 785.6
    tuberculous—*see* Tuberculosis, lymph gland
mammary gland—*see* Hypertrophy, breast
maxillary frenulum 528.5
Meckel's diverticulum (congenital) 751.0
medial meniscus, acquired 717.3
median bar 600.90
    with
        other lower urinary tract symptoms (LUTS)
            600.91
        urinary
            obstruction 600.91
            retention 600.91
mediastinum 519.3
meibomian gland 373.2
meniscus, knee, congenital 755.64
metatarsal head 733.99
metatarsus 733.99
mouth 528.9
mucous membrane
    alveolar process 523.8
    nose 478.19
    turbinate (nasal) 478.0
muscle 728.9
muscular coat, artery NEC 447.8
    carotid 447.8
    renal 447.3
myocardium (*see also* Hypertrophy, cardiac)
    429.3
    idiopathic 425.4
myometrium 621.2
nail 703.8
    congenital 757.5
nasal 478.19
    alae 478.19
    bone 738.0
    cartilage 478.19
    mucous membrane (septum) 478.19
    sinus (*see also* Sinusitis) 473.9

Hypertrophy, hypertrophic—*continued*
    turbinate 478.0
nasopharynx, lymphoid (infectional) (tissue)
    (wall) 478.29
neck, uterus 622.6
nipple 611.1
normal aperture diaphragm (congenital) 756.6
nose (*see also* Hypertrophy, nasal) 478.19
orbit 376.46
organ or site, congenital NEC—*see* Anomaly,
    specified type NEC
osteoarthropathy (pulmonary) 731.2
ovary 620.8
palate (hard) 526.89
    soft 528.9
pancreas (congenital) 751.7
papillae
    anal 569.49
    tongue 529.3
parathyroid (gland) 252.01
parotid gland 527.1
penis 607.89
phallus 607.89
    female (clitoris) 624.2
pharyngeal tonsil 474.12
pharyngitis 472.1
pharynx 478.29
    lymphoid (infectional) (tissue) (wall) 478.29
pituitary (fossa) (gland) 253.8
popliteal fat pad 729.31
preauricular (lymph) gland (Hampstead) 785.6
prepuce (congenital) 605
    female 624.2
prostate (asymptomatic) (early) (recurrent)
    600.90
    with
        other lower urinary tract symptoms (LUTS)
            600.91
        urinary
            obstruction 600.91
            retention 600.91
    adenofibromatous 600.20
        with
            other lower urinary tract symptoms
                (LUTS) 600.21
            urinary
                obstruction 600.21
                retention 600.21
    benign 600.00
        with
            other lower urinary tract symptoms
                (LUTS) 600.01
            urinary
                obstruction 600.01
                retention 600.01
    congenital 752.89
psuedoedematous hypodermal 757.0
pseudomuscular 359.1
pylorus (muscle) (sphincter) 537.0
    congenital 750.5
    infantile 750.5
rectal sphincter 569.49
rectum 569.49
renal 593.1
rhinitis (turbinate) 472.0
salivary duct or gland 527.1
    congenital 750.26
scaphoid (tarsal) 733.99
scar 701.4
scrotum 608.89
sella turcica 253.8

Hypertrophy, hypertrophic—*continued*
  seminal vesicle 608.89
  sigmoid 569.89
  skin condition NEC 701.9
  spermatic cord 608.89
  spinal ligament 724.8
  spleen—*see* Splenomegaly
  spondylitis (spine) (*see also* Spondylosis) 721.90
  stomach 537.89
  subaortic stenosis (idiopathic) 425.1
  sublingual gland 527.1
    congenital 750.26
  submaxillary gland 527.1
  suprarenal (gland) 255.8
  tendon 727.9
  testis 608.89
    congenital 752.89
  thymic, thymus (congenital) (gland) 254.0
  thyroid (gland) (*see also* Goiter) 240.9
    primary 242.0
    secondary 242.2
  toe (congenital) 755.65
    acquired 735.8
  tongue 529.8
    congenital 750.15
    frenum 529.8
    papillae (foliate) 529.3
  tonsil (faucial) (infective) (lingual) (lymphoid) 474.11
    and adenoids 474.10
    with
      adenoiditis 474.01
        tonsillitis 474.00
          and adenoiditis 474.02
  tunica vaginalis 608.89
  turbinate (mucous membrane) 478.0
  ureter 593.89
  urethra 599.84
  uterus 621.2
    puerperal, postpartum 674.8
  uvula 528.9
  vagina 623.8
  vas deferens 608.89
  vein 459.89
  ventricle, ventricular (heart) (left) (right)—*see also* Hypertrophy, cardiac
    congenital 746.89
    due to hypertension (left) (right) (*see also* Hypertension, heart) 402.90
      benign 402.10
      malignant 402.00
    right with ventricular septal defect, pulmonary stenosis or atresia, and dextraposition of aorta 745.2
  verumontanum 599.89
  vesical 596.8
  vocal cord 478.5
  vulva 624.3
    stasis (nonfilarial) 624.3
Hypertropia (intermittent) (periodic) 378.31
Hypertyrosinemia 270.2
Hyperuricemia 790.6
Hypervalinemia 270.3
Hyperventilation (tetany) 786.01
  hysterical 300.11
  psychogenic 306.1
  syndrome 306.1
Hyperviscidosis 277.00
Hyperviscosity (of serum) (syndrome) NEC 273.3
  polycythemic 289.0
  sclerocythemic 282.8

Hypervitaminosis (dietary) NEC 278.8
  A (dietary) 278.2
  D (dietary) 278.4
  from excessive administration or use of vitamin preparations (chronic) 278.8
    reaction to sudden overdose 963.5
    vitamin A 278.2
      reaction to sudden overdose 963.5
    vitamin D 278.4
      reaction to sudden overdose 963.5
    vitamin K
      correct substance properly administered 278.8
      overdose or wrong substance given or taken 964.3
Hypervolemia 276.6
Hypesthesia (*see also* Disturbance, sensation) 782.0
  cornea 371.81
Hyphema (anterior chamber) (ciliary body) (iris) 364.41
  traumatic 921.3
Hyphemia —*see* Hyphema
Hypoacidity, gastric 536.8
  psychogenic 306.4
Hypoactive labyrinth (function)—*see* Hypofunction, labyrinth
Hypoadrenalism 255.41
  tuberculous (*see also* Tuberculosis) 017.6
Hypoadrenocorticism 255.41
  pituitary 253.4
Hypoalbuminemia 273.8
Hypoaldosteronism 255.42
Hypoalphalipoproteinemia 272.5
Hypobarism 993.2
Hypobaropathy 993.2
Hypobetalipoproteinemia (familial) 272.5
Hypocalcemia 275.41
  cow's milk 775.4
  dietary 269.3
  neonatal 775.4
  phosphate-loading 775.4
Hypocalcification, teeth 520.4
Hypochloremia 276.9
Hypochlorhydria 536.8
  neurotic 306.4
  psychogenic 306.4
Hypocholesteremia 272.5
Hypochondria (reaction) 300.7
Hypochondriac 300.7
Hypochondriasis 300.7
Hypochromasia blood cells 280.9
Hypochromic anemia 280.9
  due to blood loss (chronic) 280.0
    acute 285.1
  microcytic 280.9
Hypocoagulability (*see also* Defect, coagulation) 286.9
Hypocomplementemia 279.8
Hypocythemia (progressive) 284.9
Hypodontia (*see also* Anodontia) 520.0
Hypoeosinophilia 288.59
Hypoesthesia (*see also* Disturbance, sensation) 782.0
  cornea 371.81
  tactile 782.0
Hypoestrinism 256.39
Hypoestrogenism 256.39
Hypoferremia 280.9
  due to blood loss (chronic) 280.0

Hypofertility
  female 628.9
  male 606.1
Hypofibrinogenemia 286.3
  acquired 286.6
  congenital 286.3
Hypofunction
  adrenal (gland) 255.41
    cortex 255.41
    medulla 255.5
    specified NEC 255.5
  cerebral 331.9
  corticoadrenal NEC 255.41
  intestinal 564.89
  labyrinth (unilateral) 386.53
    with loss of labyrinthine reactivity 386.55
    bilateral 386.54
      with loss of labyrinthine reactivity 386.56
  Leydig cell 257.2
  ovary 256.39
    postablative 256.2
  pituitary (anterior) (gland) (lobe) 253.2
    posterior 253.5
  testicular 257.2
    iatrogenic 257.1
    postablative 257.1
    postirradiation 257.1
    postsurgical 257.1
Hypogammaglobulinemia 279.00
  acquired primary 279.06
  non-sex-linked, congenital 279.06
  sporadic 279.06
  transient of infancy 279.09
Hypogenitalism (congenital) (female) (male) 752.89
  penis 752.69
Hypoglycemia (spontaneous) 251.2
  coma 251.0
    diabetic 250.3
  diabetic 250.8
  due to insulin 251.0
    therapeutic misadventure 962.3
  familial (idiopathic) 251.2
  following gastrointestinal surgery 579.3
  infantile (idiopathic) 251.2
  in infant of diabetic mother 775.0
  leucine-induced 270.3
  neonatal 775.6
  reactive 251.2
  specified NEC 251.1
Hypoglycemic shock 251.0
  diabetic 250.8
  due to insulin 251.0
  functional (syndrome) 251.1
Hypogonadism
  female 256.39
  gonadotrophic (isolated) 253.4
  hypogonadotropic (isolated) (with anosmia) 253.4
  isolated 253.4
  male 257.2
    hereditary familial (Reifenstein's syndrome) 259.5
  ovarian (primary) 256.39
  pituitary (secondary) 253.4
  testicular (primary) (secondary) 257.2
Hypohidrosis 705.0
Hypohidrotic ectodermal dysplasia 757.31
Hypoidrosis 705.0
Hypoinsulinemia, postsurgical 251.3
  postpancreatectomy (complete) (partial) 251.3
Hypokalemia 276.8
Hypokinesia 780.99

Hypoleukia splenica 289.4
Hypoleukocytosis 288.50
Hypolipidemia 272.5
Hypolipoproteinemia 272.5
Hypomagnesemia 275.2
  neonatal 775.4
Hypomania, hypomanic reaction (see also Psychosis, affective) 296.0
  recurrent episode 296.1
  single episode 296.0
Hypomastia (congenital) 757.6
Hypomenorrhea 626.1
Hypometabolism 783.9
Hypomotility
  gastrointestinal tract 536.8
    psychogenic 306.4
  intestine 564.89
    psychogenic 306.4
  stomach 536.8
    psychogenic 306.4
Hyponasality 784.49
Hyponatremia 276.1
Hypo-ovarianism 256.39
Hypo-ovarism 256.39
Hypoparathyroidism (idiopathic) (surgically induced) 252.1
  neonatal 775.4
Hypopharyngitis 462
Hypophoria 378.40
Hypophosphatasia 275.3
Hypophosphatemia (acquired) (congenital) (familial) 275.3
  renal 275.3
Hypophyseal, hypophysis —see also condition
  dwarfism 253.3
  gigantism 253.0
  syndrome 253.8
Hypophyseothalamic syndrome 253.8
Hypopiesis —see Hypotension
Hypopigmentation 709.00
  eyelid 374.53
Hypopinealism 259.8
Hypopituitarism (juvenile) (syndrome) 253.2
  due to
    hormone therapy 253.7
    hypophysectomy 253.7
    radiotherapy 253.7
  postablative 253.7
  postpartum hemorrhage 253.2
Hypoplasia, hypoplasis 759.89
  adrenal (gland) 759.1
  alimentary tract 751.8
    lower 751.2
    upper 750.8
  anus, anal (canal) 751.2
  aorta 747.22
  aortic
    arch (tubular) 747.10
    orifice or valve with hypoplasia of ascending aorta and defective development of left ventricle (with mitral valve atresia) 746.7
  appendix 751.2
  areola 757.6
  arm (see also Absence, arm, congenital) 755.20
  artery (congenital) (peripheral) NEC 747.60
    brain 747.81
    cerebral 747.81
    coronary 746.85
    gastrointestinal 747.61
    lower limb 747.64

Hypoplasia, hypoplasis—*continued*
  pulmonary 747.3
  renal 747.62
  retinal 743.58
  specified NEC 747.69
  spinal 747.82
  umbilical 747.5
  upper limb 747.63
auditory canal 744.29
  causing impairment of hearing 744.02
biliary duct (common) or passage 751.61
bladder 753.8
bone NEC 756.9
  face 756.0
  malar 756.0
  mandible 524.04
    alveolar 524.74
  marrow 284.9
    acquired (secondary) 284.89
    congenital 284.09
    idiopathic 284.9
  maxilla 524.03
    alveolar 524.73
  skull (*see also* Hypoplasia, skull) 756.0
brain 742.1
  gyri 742.2
  specified part 742.2
breast (areola) 757.6
bronchus (tree) 748.3
cardiac 746.89
  valve—*see* Hypoplasia, heart, valve
  vein 746.89
carpus (*see also* Absence, carpal, congenital) 755.28
cartilaginous 756.9
cecum 751.2
cementum 520.4
  hereditary 520.5
cephalic 742.1
cerebellum 742.2
cervix (uteri) 752.49
chin 524.06
clavicle 755.51
coccyx 756.19
colon 751.2
corpus callosum 742.2
cricoid cartilage 748.3
dermal, focal (Goltz) 757.39
digestive organ(s) or tract NEC 751.8
  lower 751.2
  upper 750.8
ear 744.29
  auricle 744.23
  lobe 744.29
  middle, except ossicles 744.03
    ossicles 744.04
  ossicles 744.04
enamel of teeth (neonatal) (postnatal) (prenatal) 520.4
  hereditary 520.5
endocrine (gland) NEC 759.2
endometrium 621.8
epididymis 752.89
epiglottis 748.3
erythroid, congenital 284.01
erythropoietic, chronic acquired 284.81
esophagus 750.3
Eustachian tube 744.24
eye (*see also* Microphthalmos) 743.10
  lid 743.62

Hypoplasia, hypoplasis—*continued*
face 744.89
  bone(s) 756.0
fallopian tube 752.19
femur (*see also* Absence, femur, congenital) 755.34
fibula (*see also* Absence, fibula, congenital) 755.37
finger (*see also* Absence, finger, congenital) 755.29
focal dermal 757.39
foot 755.31
gallbladder 751.69
genitalia, genital organ(s)
  female 752.89
    external 752.49
    internal NEC 752.89
  in adiposogenital dystrophy 253.8
  male 752.89
    penis 752.69
glottis 748.3
hair 757.4
hand 755.21
heart 746.89
  left (complex) (syndrome) 746.7
  valve NEC 746.89
    pulmonary 746.01
humerus (*see also* Absence, humerus, congenital) 755.24
hymen 752.49
intestine (small) 751.1
  large 751.2
iris 743.46
jaw 524.09
kidney(s) 753.0
labium (majus) (minus) 752.49
labyrinth, membranous 744.05
lacrimal duct (apparatus) 743.65
larynx 748.3
leg (*see also* Absence, limb, congenital, lower) 755.30
limb 755.4
  lower (*see also* Absence, limb, congenital, lower) 755.30
  upper (*see also* Absence, limb, congenital, upper) 755.20
liver 751.69
lung (lobe) 748.5
mammary (areolar) 757.6
mandibular 524.04
  alveolar 524.74
  unilateral condylar 526.89
maxillary 524.03
  alveolar 524.73
medullary 284.9
megakaryocytic 287.30
metacarpus (*see also* Absence, metacarpal, congenital) 755.28
metatarsus (*see also* Absence, metatarsal, congenital) 755.38
muscle 756.89
  eye 743.69
myocardium (congenital) (Uhl's anomaly) 746.84
nail(s) 757.5
nasolacrimal duct 743.65
nervous system NEC 742.8
neural 742.8
nose, nasal 748.1
ophthalmic (*see also* Microphthalmos) 743.10

INDEX TO DISEASES   Hypotension

Hypoplasia, hypoplasis—*continued*
optic nerve 377.43
organ
   of Corti 744.05
   or site NEC—*see* Anomaly, by site
osseous meatus (ear) 744.03
ovary 752.0
oviduct 752.19
pancreas 751.7
parathyroid (gland) 759.2
parotid gland 750.26
patella 755.64
pelvis, pelvic girdle 755.69
penis 752.69
peripheral vascular system (congenital) NEC 747.60
   gastrointestinal 747.61
   lower limb 747.64
   renal 747.62
   specified NEC 747.69
   spinal 747.82
   upper limb 747.63
pituitary (gland) 759.2
pulmonary 748.5
   arteriovenous 747.3
   artery 747.3
   valve 746.01
punctum lacrimale 743.65
radioulnar (*see also* Absence, radius, congenital, with ulna) 755.25
radius (*see also* Absence, radius, congenital) 755.26
rectum 751.2
respiratory system NEC 748.9
rib 756.3
sacrum 756.19
scapula 755.59
shoulder girdle 755.59
skin 757.39
skull (bone) 756.0
   with
      anencephalus 740.0
      encephalocele 742.0
      hydrocephalus 742.3
         with spina bifida (*see also* Spina bifida) 741.0
      microcephalus 742.1
spinal (cord) (ventral horn cell) 742.59
   vessel 747.82
spine 756.19
spleen 759.0
sternum 756.3
tarsus (*see also* Absence, tarsal, congenital) 755.38
testis, testicle 752.89
thymus (gland) 279.11
thyroid (gland) 243
   cartilage 748.3
tibiofibular (*see also* Absence, tibia, congenital, with fibula) 755.35
toe (*see also* Absence, toe, congenital) 755.39
tongue 750.16
trachea (cartilage) (rings) 748.3
Turner's (tooth) 520.4
ulna (*see also* Absence, ulna, congenital) 755.27
umbilical artery 747.5
ureter 753.29
uterus 752.3
vagina 752.49
vascular (peripheral) NEC (*see also* Hypoplasia, peripheral vascular system) 747.60

Hypoplasia, hypoplasis—*continued*
brain 747.81
vein(s) (peripheral) NEC (*see also* Hypoplasia, peripheral vascular system 747.60
   brain 747.81
   cardiac 746.89
   great 747.49
   portal 747.49
   pulmonary 747.49
   vena cava (inferior) (superior) 747.49
vertebra 756.19
vulva 752.49
zonule (ciliary) 743.39
zygoma 738.12
Hypopotassemia 276.8
Hypoproaccelerinemia (*see also* Defect, coagulation) 286.3
Hypoproconvertinemia (congenital) (*see also* Defect, coagulation) 286.3
Hypoproteinemia (essential) (hypermetabolic) (idiopathic) 273.8
Hypoproteinosis 260
Hypoprothrombinemia (congenital) (hereditary) (idiopathic) (*see also* Defect, coagulation) 286.3
   acquired 286.7
   newborn 776.3
Hypopselaphesia 782.0
Hypopyon (anterior chamber) (eye) 364.05
   iritis 364.05
   ulcer (cornea) 370.04
Hypopyrexia 780.99
Hyporeflex 796.1
Hyporeninemia, extreme 790.99
   in primary aldosteronism 255.10
Hyporesponsive episode 780.09
Hyposecretion
   ACTH 253.4
   ovary 256.39
      postablative 256.2
   salivary gland (any) 527.7
Hyposegmentation of neutrophils, hereditary 288.2
Hyposiderinemia 280.9
Hyposmolality 276.1
   syndrome 276.1
Hyposomatotropism 253.3
Hyposomnia, unspecified (*see also* Insomnia) 780.52
   with sleep apnea, unspecified 780.51
Hypospadias (male) 752.61
   female 753.8
Hypospermatogenesis 606.1
Hyposphagma 372.72
Hyposplenism 289.59
Hypostasis, pulmonary 514
Hypostatic —*see* condition
Hyposthenuria 593.89
Hyposuprarenalism 255.41
Hypo-TBG-nemia 246.8
Hypotension (arterial) (constitutional) 458.9
   chronic 458.1
   iatrogenic 458.29
   maternal, syndrome (following labor and delivery) 669.2
   of hemodialysis 458.21
   orthostatic (chronic) 458.0
      dysautonomic-dyskinetic syndrome 333.0
   permanent idiopathic 458.1
   postoperative 458.29

Hypotension—*continued*
  postural 458.0
  specified type NEC 458.8
  transient 796.3
Hypothermia (accidental) 991.6
  anesthetic 995.89
  newborn NEC 778.3
  not associated with low environmental
    temperature 780.99
Hypothymergasia (*see also* Psychosis, affective)
  296.2
  recurrent episode 296.3
  single episode 296.2
Hypothyroidism (acquired) 244.9
  complicating pregnancy, childbirth, or
    puerperium 648.1
  congenital 243
  due to
    ablation 244.1
      radioactive iodine 244.1
      surgical 244.0
    iodine (administration) (ingestion) 244.2
      radioactive 244.1
    irradiation therapy 244.1
    p-aminosalicylic acid (PAS) 244.3
    phenylbutazone 244.3
    resorcinol 244.3
    specified cause NEC 244.8
    surgery 244.0
  goitrous (sporadic) 246.1
  iatrogenic NEC 244.3
  iodine 244.2
  pituitary 244.8
  postablative NEC 244.1
  postsurgical 244.0
  primary 244.9
  secondary NEC 244.8
  specified cause NEC 244.8
  sporadic goitrous 246.1
Hypotonia, hypotonicity, hypotony 781.3
  benign congenital 358.8
  bladder 596.4
  congenital 779.89
    benign 358.8
  eye 360.30
    due to
      fistula 360.32
      ocular disorder NEC 360.33
    following loss of aqueous or vitreous 360.33
    primary 360.31
  infantile muscular (benign) 359.0
  muscle 728.9
  uterus, uterine (contractions)—*see* Inertia,
    uterus
Hypotrichosis 704.09
  congenital 757.4
  lid (congenital) 757.4
    acquired 374.55
  postinfectional NEC 704.09
Hypotropia 378.32
Hypoventilation 786.09
  congenital central alveolar syndrome 327.25
  idiopathic sleep related nonobstructive alveolar
    327.24
  sleep related, in conditions classifiable
    elsewhere 327.26
Hypovitaminosis (*see also* Deficiency, vitamin)
  269.2
Hypovolemia 276.52
  surgical shock 998.0
  traumatic (shock) 958.4

Hypoxemia (*see also* Anoxia) 799.02
  sleep related, in conditions classifiable
    elsewhere 327.26
Hypoxia (*see also* Anoxia) 799.02
  cerebral 348.1
    during or resulting from a procedure 997.01
    newborn 770.88
      mild or moderate 768.6
      severe 768.5
  fetal, affecting newborn 770.88
  intrauterine—*see* Distress, fetal
  myocardial (*see also* Insufficiency, coronary)
    411.89
    arteriosclerotic —*see* Arteriosclerosis,
      coronary
  newborn 770.88
  sleep related 327.24
Hypoxic-ischemic encephalopathy (HIE) 768.7
Hypsarrhythmia (*see also* Epilepsy) 345.6
Hysteralgia, pregnant uterus 646.8
Hysteria, hysterical 300.10
  anxiety 300.20
  Charcot's gland 300.11
  conversion (any manifestation) 300.11
  dissociative type NEC 300.15
  psychosis, acute 298.1
Hysteroepilepsy 300.11
Hysterotomy, affecting fetus or newborn
  763.89

I

Iatrogenic syndrome of excess cortisol 255.0
Iceland disease (epidemic neuromyasthenia) 049.8
Ichthyosis (congenita) 757.1
   acquired 701.1
   fetalis gravior 757.1
   follicularis 757.1
   hystrix 757.39
   lamellar 757.1
   lingual 528.6
   palmaris and plantaris 757.39
   simplex 757.1
   vera 757.1
   vulgaris 757.1
Ichthyotoxism 988.0
   bacterial (*see also* Poisoning, food) 005.9
Icteroanemia, hemolytic (acquired) 283.9
   congenital (*see also* Spherocytosis) 282.0
Icterus (*see also* Jaundice) 782.4
   catarrhal—*see* Icterus, infectious
   conjunctiva 782.4
      newborn 774.6
   epidemic—*see* Icterus, infectious
   febrilis—*see* Icterus, infectious
   fetus or newborn—*see* Jaundice, fetus or newborn
   gravis (*see also* Necrosis, liver) 570
      complicating pregnancy 646.7
         affecting fetus or newborn 760.8
      fetus or newborn NEC 773.0
      obstetrical 646.7
         affecting fetus or newborn 760.8
   hematogenous (acquired) 283.9
   hemolytic (acquired) 283.9
      congenital (*see also* Spherocytosis) 282.0
   hemorrhagic (acute) 100.0
      leptospiral 100.0
      newborn 776.0
      spirochetal 100.0
   infectious 070.1
      with hepatic coma 070.0
      leptospiral 100.0
      spirochetal 100.0
   intermittens juvenilis 277.4
   malignant (*see also* Necrosis, liver) 570
   neonatorum (*see also* Jaundice, fetus or newborn) 774.6
   pernicious (*see also* Necrosis, liver) 570
   spirochetal 100.0
Ictus solaris, solis 992.0
Ideation
   suicidal V62.84
Identity disorder 313.82
   dissociative 300.14
   gender role (child) 302.6
      adult 302.85
   psychosexual (child) 302.6
      adult 302.85
Idioglossia 307.9
Idiopathic —*see* condition
Idiosyncrasy (*see also* Allergy) 995.3
   drug, medicinal substance, and biological—*see* Allergy, drug
Idiot, idiocy (congenital) 318.2
   amaurotic (Bielschowsky) (-Jansky) (family) (infantile (late)) (juvenile (late)) (Vogt-Spielmeyer) 330.1
   microcephalic 742.1

Idiot, idiocy—*continued*
   Mongolian 758.0
   oxycephalic 756.0
Id reaction (due to bacteria) 692.89
IEED (involuntary emotional expression disorder) 310.8
IFIS (intraoperative floppy iris syndrome) 364.81
IgE asthma 493.0
Ileitis (chronic) (*see also* Enteritis) 558.9
   infectious 009.0
   noninfectious 558.9
   regional (ulcerative) 555.0
      with large intestine 555.2
   segmental 555.0
      with large intestine 555.2
   terminal (ulcerative) 555.0
      with large intestine 555.2
Ileocolitis (*see also* Enteritis) 558.9
   infectious 009.0
   regional 555.2
   ulcerative 556.1
Ileostomy status V44.2
   with complication 569.60
Ileotyphus 002.0
Ileum —*see* condition
Ileus (adynamic) (bowel) (colon) (inhibitory) (intestine) (neurogenic) (paralytic) 560.1
   arteriomesenteric duodenal 537.2
   due to gallstone (in intestine) 560.31
   duodenal, chronic 537.2
   following gastrointestinal surgery 997.4
   gallstone 560.31
   mechanical (*see also* Obstruction, intestine) 560.9
   meconium 777.1
      due to cystic fibrosis 277.01
   myxedema 564.89
   postoperative 997.4
   transitory, newborn 777.4
Iliac —*see* condition
Iliotibial band friction syndrome 728.89
Ill, louping 063.1
Illegitimacy V61.6
Illness —*see also* Disease
   factitious 300.19
      with
         combined psychological and physical signs and symptoms 300.19
         physical symptoms 300.19
      predominantly
         physical signs and symptoms 300.19
         psychological symptoms 300.16
      chronic (with physical symptoms) 301.51
   heart—*see* Disease, heart
   manic-depressive (*see also* Psychosis, affective) 296.80
   mental (*see also* Disorder, mental) 300.9
Imbalance 781.2
   autonomic (*see also* Neuropathy, peripheral, autonomic) 337.9
   electrolyte 276.9
      with
         abortion—*see* Abortion, by type, with metabolic disorder
         ectopic pregnancy (*see also* categories 633.0-633.9) 639.4
         hyperemesis gravidarum (before 22 completed weeks gestation) 643.1

Imbalance—continued
  molar pregnancy (see also categories
    630-632) 639.4
  following
    abortion 639.4
    ectopic or molar pregnancy 639.4
  neonatal, transitory NEC 775.5
  endocrine 259.9
  eye muscle NEC 378.9
    heterophoria—see Heterophoria
  glomerulotubular NEC 593.89
  hormone 259.9
  hysterical (see also Hysteria) 300.10
  labyrinth NEC 386.50
  posture 729.9
  sympathetic (see also Neuropathy, peripheral,
    autonomic) 337.9
Imbecile, imbecility 318.0
  moral 301.7
  old age 290.9
  senile 290.9
  specified IQ—see IQ
  unspecified IQ 318.0
Imbedding, intrauterine device 996.32
Imbibition, cholesterol (gallbladder) 575.6
Imerslund (-Gräsbeck) syndrome (anemia due to familial selective vitamin B_{12} malabsorption) 281.1
Iminoacidopathy 270.8
Iminoglycinuria, familial 270.8
Immature —see also Immaturity
  personality 301.89
Immaturity 765.1
  extreme 765.0
  fetus or infant light-for-dates—see
    Light-for-dates
  lung, fetus or newborn 770.4
  organ or site NEC—see Hypoplasia
  pulmonary, fetus or newborn 770.4
  reaction 301.89
  sexual (female) (male) 259.0
Immersion 994.1
  foot 991.4
  hand 991.4
Immobile, immobility
  intestine 564.89
  joint—see Ankylosis
  syndrome (paraplegic) 728.3
Immunization
  ABO
    affecting management of pregnancy 656.2
    fetus or newborn 773.1
  complication—see Complications, vaccination
  Rh factor
    affecting management of pregnancy 656.1
    fetus or newborn 773.0
    from transfusion 999.7
Immunodeficiency 279.3
  with
    adenosine-deaminase deficiency 279.2
    defect, predominant
      B-cell 279.00
      T-cell 279.10
    hyperimmunoglobulinemia 279.2
    lymphopenia, hereditary 279.2
    thrombocytopenia and eczema 279.12
    thymic
      aplasia 279.2
      dysplasia 279.2
  autosomal recessive, Swiss-type 279.2
  common variable 279.06

Immunodeficiency—continued
  severe combined (SCID) 279.2
  to Rh factor
    affecting management of pregnancy 656.1
    fetus or newborn 773.0
  X-linked, with increased IgM 279.05
Immunotherapy, prophylactic V07.2
  antineoplastic V58.12
Impaction, impacted
  bowel, colon, rectum 560.30
    with hernia—see also Hernia, by site, with
      obstruction
      gangrenous—see Hernia, by site, with
        gangrene
    by
      calculus 560.39
      gallstone 560.31
    fecal 560.39
    specified type NEC 560.39
  calculus—see Calculus
  cerumen (ear) (external) 380.4
  cuspid 520.6
  dental 520.6
  fecal, feces 560.39
    with hernia—see also Hernia, by site, with
      obstruction
      gangrenous—see Hernia, by site, with
        gangrene
  fracture—see Fracture, by site
  gallbladder—see Cholelithiasis
  gallstone(s)—see Cholelithiasis
    in intestine (any part) 560.31
  intestine(s) 560.30
    with hernia—see also Hernia, by site, with
      obstruction
      gangrenous—see Hernia, by site, with
        gangrene
    by
      calculus 560.39
      gallstone 560.31
    fecal 560.39
    specified type NEC 560.39
  intrauterine device (IUD) 996.32
  molar 520.6
  shoulder 660.4
    affecting fetus or newborn 763.1
  tooth, teeth 520.6
  turbinate 733.99
Impaired, impairment (function)
  arm V49.1
    movement, involving
      musculoskeletal system V49.1
      nervous system V49.2
  auditory discrimination 388.43
  back V48.3
  body (entire) V49.89
  cognitive, mild, so stated 331.83
  combined visual hearing V49.85
  dual sensory V49.85
  glucose
    fasting 790.21
    tolerance test (oral) 790.22
  hearing (see also Deafness) 389.9
    combined with visual impairment V49.85
  heart—see Disease, heart
  kidney (see also Disease, renal) 593.9
    disorder resulting from 588.9
      specified NEC 588.89
  leg V49.1
    movement, involving
      musculoskeletal system V49.1

INDEX TO DISEASES

Imperfect

Impaired, impairment—*continued*
  nervous system V49.2
 limb V49.1
  movement, involving
    musculoskeletal system V49.1
    nervous system V49.2
 liver 573.8
 mastication 524.9
 mild cognitive, so stated 331.83
 mobility
  ear ossicles NEC 385.22
  incostapedial joint 385.22
  malleus 385.21
 myocardium, myocardial (*see also*
    Insufficiency, myocardial) 428.0
 neuromusculoskeletal NEC V49.89
  back V48.3
  head V48.2
  limb V49.2
  neck V48.3
  spine V48.3
  trunk V48.3
 rectal sphincter 787.99
 renal (*see also* Disease, renal) 593.9
  disorder resulting from 588.9
  specified NEC 588.89
 spine V48.3
 vision NEC 369.9
  both eyes NEC 369.3
  combined with hearing impairment V49.85
  moderate 369.74
   both eyes 369.25
    with impairment of lesser eye (specified as)
     blind, not further specified 369.15
     low vision, not further specified 369.23
     near-total 369.17
     profound 369.18
     severe 369.24
     total 369.16
   one eye 369.74
    with vision of other eye (specified as)
     near-normal 369.75
     normal 369.76
  near-total 369.64
   both eyes 369.04
    with impairment of lesser eye (specified as)
     blind, not further specified 369.02
     total 369.03
   one eye 369.64
    with vision of other eye (specified as)
     near-normal 369.65
     normal 369.66
  one eye 369.60
   with low vision of other eye 369.10
  profound 369.67
   both eyes 369.08
    with impairment of lesser eye (specified as)
     blind, not further specified 369.05
     near-total 369.07
     total 369.06
   one eye 369.67
    with vision of other eye (specified as)
     near-normal 369.68
     normal 369.69
  severe 369.71
   both eyes 369.22
    with impairment of lesser eye (specified as)
     blind, not further specified 369.11

Impaired, impairment—*continued*
   low vision, not further specified 369.21
   near-total 369.13
   profound 369.14
   total 369.12
  one eye 369.71
   with vision of other eye (specified as)
    near-normal 369.72
    normal 369.73
  total
   both eyes 369.01
   one eye 369.61
    with vision of other eye (specified as)
     near-normal 369.62
     normal 369.63
Impaludism —*see* Malaria
Impediment, speech NEC 784.5
 psychogenic 307.9
 secondary to organic lesion 784.5
Impending
 cerebrovascular accident or attack 435.9
 coronary syndrome 411.1
 delirium tremens 291.0
 myocardial infarction 411.1
Imperception, auditory (acquired) (congenital) 389.9
Imperfect
 aeration, lung (newborn) 770.5
 closure (congenital)
  alimentary tract NEC 751.8
   lower 751.5
   upper 750.8
  atrioventricular ostium 745.69
  atrium (secundum) 745.5
   primum 745.61
  branchial cleft or sinus 744.41
  choroid 743.59
  cricoid cartilage 748.3
  cusps, heart valve NEC 746.89
   pulmonary 746.09
  ductus
   arteriosus 747.0
   Botalli 747.0
  ear drum 744.29
   causing impairment of hearing 744.03
  endocardial cushion 745.60
  epiglottis 748.3
  esophagus with communication to bronchus or trachea 750.3
  Eustachian valve 746.89
  eyelid 743.62
  face, facial (*see also* Cleft, lip) 749.10
  foramen
   Botalli 745.5
   ovale 745.5
  genitalia, genital organ(s) or system
   female 752.89
    external 752.49
    internal NEC 752.89
    uterus 752.3
   male 752.89
    penis 752.69
  glottis 748.3
  heart valve (cusps) NEC 746.89
  interatrial ostium or septum 745.5
  interauricular ostium or septum 745.5
  interventricular ostium or septum 745.4
  iris 743.46
  kidney 753.3
  larynx 748.3
  lens 743.36

1095

Imperfect—*continued*
  lip (*see also* Cleft, lip) 749.10
  nasal septum or sinus 748.1
  nose 748.1
  omphalomesenteric duct 751.0
  optic nerve entry 743.57
  organ or site NEC—*see* Anomaly, specified type, by site
  ostium
    interatrial 745.5
    interauricular 745.5
    interventricular 745.4
  palate (*see also* Cleft, palate) 749.00
  preauricular sinus 744.46
  retina 743.56
  roof of orbit 742.0
  sclera 743.47
  septum
    aortic 745.0
    aorticopulmonary 745.0
    atrial (secundum) 745.5
      primum 745.61
    between aorta and pulmonary artery 745.0
    heart 745.9
    interatrial (secundum) 745.5
      primum 745.61
    interauricular (secundum) 745.5
      primum 745.61
    interventricular 745.4
      with pulmonary stenosis or atresia, dextraposition of aorta, and hypertrophy of right ventricle 745.2
      in tetralogy of Fallot 745.2
    nasal 748.1
    ventricular 745.4
      with pulmonary stenosis or atresia, dextraposition of aorta, and hypertrophy of right ventricle 745.2
      in tetralogy of Fallot 745.2
  skull 756.0
    with
      anencephalus 740.0
      encephalocele 742.0
      hydrocephalus 742.3
        with spina bifida (*see also* Spina bifida) 741.0
      microcephalus 742.1
  spine (with meningocele) (*see also* Spina bifida) 741.90
  thyroid cartilage 748.3
  trachea 748.3
  tympanic membrane 744.29
    causing impairment of hearing 744.03
  uterus (with communication to bladder, intestine, or rectum) 752.3
  uvula 749.02
    with cleft lip (*see also* Cleft, palate, with cleft lip) 749.20
  vitelline duct 751.0
  development—*see* Anomaly, by site
  erection 607.84
  fusion—*see* Imperfect, closure
  inflation lung (newborn) 770.5
  intestinal canal 751.5
  poise 729.9
  rotation—*see* Malrotation
  septum, ventricular 745.4
Imperfectly descended testis 752.51

Imperforate (congenital)—*see also* Atresia
  anus 751.2
  bile duct 751.61
  cervix (uteri) 752.49
  esophagus 750.3
  hymen 752.42
  intestine (small) 751.1
    large 751.2
  jejunum 751.1
  pharynx 750.29
  rectum 751.2
  salivary duct 750.23
  urethra 753.6
  urinary meatus 753.6
  vagina 752.49
Impervious (congenital)—*see also* Atresia
  anus 751.2
  bile duct 751.61
  esophagus 750.3
  intestine (small) 751.1
    large 751.2
  rectum 751.2
  urethra 753.6
Impetiginization of other dermatoses 684
Impetigo (any organism) (any site) (bullous) (circinate) (contagiosa) (neonatorum) (simplex) 684
  Bockhart's (superficial folliculitis) 704.8
  external ear 684 [380.13]
  eyelid 684 [373.5]
  Fox's (contagiosa) 684
  furfuracea 696.5
  herpetiformis 694.3
    nonobstetrical 694.3
  staphylococcal infection 684
  ulcerative 686.8
  vulgaris 684
Impingement, soft tissue between teeth 524.89
  anterior 524.81
  posterior 524.82
Implant, endometrial 617.9
Implantation
  anomalous—*see also* Anomaly, specified type, by site
    ureter 753.4
  cyst
    external area or site (skin) NEC 709.8
    iris 364.61
    vagina 623.8
    vulva 624.8
  dermoid (cyst)
    external area or site (skin) NEC 709.8
    iris 364.61
    vagina 623.8
    vulva 624.8
  placenta, low or marginal—*see* Placenta previa
Impotence (sexual) 607.84
  organic origin NEC 607.84
  psychogenic 302.72
Impoverished blood 285.9
Impression, basilar 756.0
Imprisonment V62.5
Improper
  development, infant 764.9
Improperly tied umbilical cord (causing hemorrhage) 772.3
Impulses, obsessional 300.3
Impulsive neurosis 300.3
Inaction, kidney (*see also* Disease, renal) 593.9
Inactive —*see* condition

INDEX TO DISEASES   Incompatibility

Inadequate, inadequacy
  aesthetics of dental restoration 525.67
  biologic 301.6
  cardiac and renal—*see* Hypertension,
      cardiorenal
  constitutional 301.6
  development
    child 783.40
    fetus 764.9
      affecting management of pregnancy 656.5
    genitalia
      after puberty NEC 259.0
      congenital—*see* Hypoplasia, genitalia
    lungs 748.5
    organ or site NEC—*see* Hypoplasia, by site
  dietary 269.9
  distance, interarch 524.28
  education V62.3
  environment
    economic problem V60.2
    household condition NEC V60.1
    poverty V60.2
    unemployment V62.0
  functional 301.6
  household care, due to
    family member
      handicapped or ill V60.4
      temporarily away from home V60.4
        on vacation V60.5
    technical defects in home V60.1
    temporary absence from home of person
        rendering care V60.4
  housing (heating) (space) V60.1
  interarch distance 524.28
  material resources V60.2
  mental (*see also* Retardation, mental) 319
  nervous system 799.2
  personality 301.6
  prenatal care in current pregnancy V23.7
  pulmonary
    function 786.09
      newborn 770.89
    ventilation, newborn 770.89
    respiration 786.09
      newborn 770.89
  sample, Papanicolaou smear 795.08
  social 301.6
Inanition 263.9
  with edema 262
  due to
    deprivation of food 994.2
    malnutrition 263.9
  fever 780.6
Inappropriate secretion
  ACTH 255.0
  antidiuretic hormone (ADH) (excessive) 253.6
    deficiency 253.5
  ectopic hormone NEC 259.3
  pituitary (posterior) 253.6
Inattention after or at birth 995.52
Inborn errors of metabolism —*see* Disorder,
    metabolism
Incarceration, incarcerated
  bubonocele—*see also* Hernia, inguinal, with
      obstruction
    gangrenous—*see* Hernia, inguinal, with
        gangrene
  colon (by hernia)—*see also* Hernia, by site, with
      obstruction
    gangrenous—*see* Hernia, by site, with
        gangrene

Incarceration, incarcerated—*continued*
  enterocele 552.9
    gangrenous 551.9
  epigastrocele 552.29
    gangrenous 551.29
  epiplocele 552.9
    gangrenous 551.9
  exomphalos 552.1
    gangrenous 551.1
  fallopian tube 620.8
  hernia—*see also* Hernia, by site, with
      obstruction
    gangrenous—*see* Hernia, by site, with
        gangrene
  iris, in wound 871.1
  lens, in wound 871.1
  merocele (*see also* Hernia, femoral, with
      obstruction) 552.00
  Omentum (by hernia)—*see also* Hernia, by site,
      with obstruction
    gangrenous—*see* Hernia, by site, with
        gangrene
  omphalocele 756.79
  rupture (meaning hernia) (*see also* Hernia, by
      site, with obstruction) 552.9
    gangrenous (*see also* Hernia, by site, with
        gangrene) 551.9
  sarcoepiplocele 552.9
    gangrenous 551.9
  sarcoepiplomphalocele 552.1
    with gangrene 551.1
  uterus 621.8
    gravid 654.3
      causing obstructed labor 660.2
      affecting fetus or newborn 763.1
Incident, cerebrovascular (*see also* Disease,
    cerebrovascular, acute) 436
Incineration (entire body) (from fire,
    conflagration, electricity, or lightning)—*see*
    Burn, multiple, specified sites
Incised wound
  external—*see* Wound, open, by site
  internal organs (abdomen, chest, or pelvis)—*see*
      Injury, internal, by site, with open wound
Incision, incisional
  hernia—*see* Hernia, incisional
  surgical, complication—*see* Complications,
      surgical procedures
  traumatic
    external—*see* Wound, open, by site
    internal organs (abdomen, chest or
        pelvis)—*see* Injury, internal, by site, with
        open wound
Inclusion
  azurophilic leukocytic 288.2
  blennorrhea (neonatal) (newborn) 771.6
  cyst—*see* Cyst, skin
  gallbladder in liver (congenital) 751.69
Incompatibility
  ABO
    affecting management of pregnancy 656.2
    fetus or newborn 773.1
    infusion or transfusion reaction 999.6
  blood (group) (Duffy) (E) (K(ell)) (Kidd)
      (Lewis) (M) (N) (P) (S) NEC
    affecting management of pregnancy 656.2
    fetus or newborn 773.2
    infusion or transfusion reaction 999.6
  contour of existing restoration of tooth
    with oral health 525.65

1097

Incompatibility—*continued*
  marital V61.10
    involving divorce or estrangement V61.0
  Rh (blood group) (factor)
    affecting management of pregnancy 656.1
    fetus or newborn 773.0
    infusion or transfusion reaction 999.7
  Rhesus—*see* Incompatibility, Rh
Incompetency, incompetence, incompetent
  annular
    aortic (valve) (*see also* Insufficiency, aortic) 424.1
    mitral (valve)—(*see also* Insufficiency, mitral) 424.0
    pulmonary valve (heart) (*see also* Endocarditis, pulmonary) 424.3
  aortic (valve) (*see also* Insufficiency, aortic) 424.1
    syphilitic 093.22
  cardiac (orifice) 530.0
    valve—*see* Endocarditis
  cervix, cervical (os) 622.5
    in pregnancy 654.5
      affecting fetus or newborn 761.0
  esophagogastric (junction) (sphincter) 530.0
  heart valve, congenital 746.89
  mitral (valve)—*see* Insufficiency, mitral
  papillary muscle (heart) 429.81
  pelvic fundus
    pubocervical tissue 618.81
    rectovaginal tissue 618.82
  pulmonary valve (heart) (*see also* Endocarditis, pulmonary) 424.3
    congenital 746.09
  tricuspid (annular) (rheumatic) (valve) (*see also* Endocarditis, tricuspid) 397.0
  valvular—*see* Endocarditis
  vein, venous (saphenous) (varicose) (*see also* Varicose, vein) 454.9
  velopharyngeal (closure)
    acquired 528.9
    congenital 750.29
Incomplete —*see also* condition
  bladder emptying 788.21
  expansion lungs (newborn) 770.5
  gestation (liveborn)—*see* Immaturity
  rotation—*see* Malrotation
Incontinence 788.30
  without sensory awareness 788.34
  anal sphincter 787.6
  continuous leakage 788.37
  feces 787.6
    due to hysteria 300.11
    nonorganic origin 307.7
  hysterical 300.11
  mixed (male) (female) (urge and stress) 788.33
  overflow 788.38
  paradoxical 788.39
  rectal 787.6
  specified NEC 788.39
  stress (female) 625.6
    male NEC 788.32
  urethral sphincter 599.84
  urge 788.31
    and stress (male) (female) 788.33
  urine 788.30
    active 788.30
    male 788.30
      stress 788.32
        and urge 788.33
    neurogenic 788.39

Incontinence—*continued*
  nonorganic origin 307.6
  stress (female) 625.6
    male NEC 788.32
  urge 788.31
    and stress 788.33
Incontinentia pigmenti 757.33
Incoordinate
  uterus (action) (contractions) 661.4
    affecting fetus or newborn 763.7
Incoordination
  esophageal-pharyngeal (newborn) 787.24
  muscular 781.3
  papillary muscle 429.81
Increase, increased
  abnormal, in development 783.9
  androgens (ovarian) 256.1
  anticoagulants (antithrombin) (anti-VIIIa) (anti-IXa) (anti-Xa) (anti-XIa) 286.5
    postpartum 666.3
  cold sense (*see also* Disturbance, sensation) 782.0
  estrogen 256.0
  function
    adrenal (cortex) 255.3
      medulla 255.6
    pituitary (anterior) (gland) (lobe) 253.1
      posterior 253.6
  heat sense (*see also* Disturbance, sensation) 782.0
  intracranial pressure 781.99
    injury at birth 767.8
  light reflex of retina 362.13
  permeability, capillary 448.9
  pressure
    intracranial 781.99
      injury at birth 767.8
    intraocular 365.00
  pulsations 785.9
  pulse pressure 785.9
  sphericity, lens 743.36
  splenic activity 289.4
  venous pressure 459.89
    portal 572.3
Incrustation, cornea, lead or zinc 930.0
Incyclophoria 378.44
Incyclotropia 378.33
Indeterminate sex 752.7
India rubber skin 756.83
Indicanuria 270.2
Indigestion (bilious) (functional) 536.8
  acid 536.8
  catarrhal 536.8
  due to decomposed food NEC 005.9
  fat 579.8
  nervous 306.4
  psychogenic 306.4
Indirect —*see* condition
Indolent bubo NEC 099.8
Induced
  abortion—*see* Abortion, induced
  birth, affecting fetus or newborn 763.89
  delivery—*see* Delivery
  labor—*see* Delivery
Induration, indurated
  brain 348.8
  breast (fibrous) 611.79
    puerperal, postpartum 676.3
  broad ligament 620.8
  chancre 091.0
    anus 091.1
    congenital 090.0

Induration, indurated—*continued*
  extragenital NEC 091.2
  corpora cavernosa (penis) (plastic) 607.89
  liver (chronic) 573.8
    acute 573.8
  lung (black) (brown) (chronic) (fibroid) (*see also* Fibrosis, lung) 515
    essential brown 275.0 *[516.1]*
  penile 607.89
  phlebitic—*see* Phlebitis
  skin 782.8
  stomach 537.89
Induratio penis plastica 607.89
Industrial —*see* condition
Inebriety (*see also* Abuse, drugs, nondependent) 305.0
Inefficiency
  kidney (*see also* Disease, renal) 593.9
  thyroid (acquired) (gland) 244.9
Inelasticity, skin 782.8
Inequality, leg (acquired) (length) 736.81
  congenital 755.30
Inertia
  bladder 596.4
    neurogenic 596.54
      with cauda equina syndrome 344.61
  stomach 536.8
    psychogenic 306.4
  uterus, uterine 661.2
    affecting fetus or newborn 763.7
    primary 661.0
    secondary 661.1
  vesical 596.4
    neurogenic 596.54
      with cauda equina 344.61
Infant —*see also* condition
  excessive crying of 780.92
  fussy (baby) 780.91
  held for adoption V68.89
  newborn—*see* Newborn
  post-term (gestation period over 40 completed weeks to 42 completed weeks) 766.21
  prolonged gestation of (period over 42 completed weeks) 766.22
  syndrome of diabetic mother 775.0
"Infant Hercules" syndrome 255.2
Infantile —*see also* condition
  genitalia, genitals 259.0
    in pregnancy or childbirth NEC 654.4
      affecting fetus or newborn 763.89
      causing obstructed labor 660.2
        affecting fetus or newborn 763.1
  heart 746.9
  kidney 753.3
  lack of care 995.52
  macula degeneration 362.75
  melanodontia 521.05
  os, uterus (*see also* Infantile, genitalia) 259.0
  pelvis 738.6
    with disproportion (fetopelvic) 653.1
      affecting fetus or newborn 763.1
      causing obstructed labor 660.1
        affecting fetus or newborn 763.1
  penis 259.0
  testis 257.2
  uterus (*see also* Infantile, genitalia) 259.0
  vulva 752.49
Infantilism 259.9
  with dwarfism (hypophyseal) 253.3
  Brissaud's (infantile myxedema) 244.9
  celiac 579.0

Infantilism—*continued*
  Herter's (nontropical sprue) 579.0
  hypophyseal 253.3
  hypothalamic (with obesity) 253.8
  idiopathic 259.9
  intestinal 579.0
  pancreatic 577.8
  pituitary 253.3
  renal 588.0
  sexual (with obesity) 259.0
Infants, healthy liveborn —*see* Newborn
Infarct, infarction
  adrenal (capsule) (gland) 255.41
  amnion 658.8
  anterior (with contiguous portion of intraventricular septum) NEC (*see also* Infarct, myocardium) 410.1
  appendices epiploicae 557.0
  bowel 557.0
  brain (stem) 434.91
    embolic (*see also* Embolism, brain) 434.11
    healed or old, without residuals V12.54
    iatrogenic 997.02
    postoperative 997.02
    puerperal, postpartum, childbirth 674.0
    thrombotic (*see also* Thrombosis, brain) 434.01
  breast 611.8
  Brewer's (kidney) 593.81
  cardiac (*see also* Infarct, myocardium) 410.9
  cerebellar (*see also* Infarct, brain) 434.91
    embolic (*see also* Embolism, brain) 434.11
  cerebral (*see also* Infarct, brain) 434.91
    aborted 434.91
    embolic (*see also* Embolism, brain) 434.11
    thrombotic (*see also* Infarct, brain) 434.01
  chorion 658.8
  colon (acute) (agnogenic) (embolic) (hemorrhagic) (nonocclusive) (nonthrombotic) (occlusive) (segmental) (thrombotic) (with gangrene) 557.0
  coronary artery (*see also* Infarct, myocardium) 410.9
  cortical 434.91
  embolic (*see also* Embolism) 444.9
  fallopian tube 620.8
  gallbladder 575.8
  heart (*see also* Infarct, myocardium) 410.9
  hepatic 573.4
  hypophysis (anterior lobe) 253.8
  impending (myocardium) 411.1
  intestine (acute) (agnogenic) (embolic) (hemorrhagic) (nonocclusive) (nonthrombotic) (occlusive) (thrombotic) (with gangrene) 557.0
  kidney 593.81
  liver 573.4
  lung (embolic) (thrombotic) 415.19
    with
      abortion—*see* Abortion, by type, with, embolism
      ectopic pregnancy (*see also* categories 633.0-633.9) 639.6
      molar pregnancy (*see also* categories 630-632) 639.6
    following
      abortion 639.6
      ectopic or molar pregnancy 639.6
    iatrogenic 415.11
    in pregnancy, childbirth, or puerperium—*see* Embolism, obstetrical

Infarct, infarction   **INDEX TO DISEASES**

Infarct, infarction—*continued*
   postoperative 415.11
   septic 415.12
  lymph node or vessel 457.8
  medullary (brain)—*see* Infarct, brain
  meibomian gland (eyelid) 374.85
  mesentery, mesenteric (embolic) (thrombotic)
    (with gangrene) 557.0
  midbrain—*see* Infarct, brain
  myocardium, myocardial (acute or with a stated
    duration of 8 weeks or less) (with
    hypertension) 410.9

---

*Note—use the following fifth-digit
subclassification with category 410*

0 *episode unspecified*
1 *initial episode*
2 *subsequent episode without recurrence*

---

    with symptoms after 8 weeks from date of
      infarction 414.8
    anterior (wall) (with contiguous portion of
      intraventricular septum) NEC 410.1
    anteroapical (with contiguous portion of
      intraventricular septum) 410.1
    anterolateral (wall) 410.0
    anteroseptal (with contiguous portion of
      intraventricular septum) 410.1
    apical-lateral 410.5
    atrial 410.8
    basal-lateral 410.5
    chronic (with symptoms after 8 weeks from
      date of infarction) 414.8
    diagnosed on ECG, but presenting no
      symptoms 412
    diaphragmatic wall (with contiguous portion
      of intraventricular septum) 410.4
    healed or old, currently presenting no
      symptoms 412
    high lateral 410.5
    impending 411.1
    inferior (wall) (with contiguous portion of
      intraventricular septum) 410.4
    inferolateral (wall) 410.2
    inferoposterior wall 410.3
    intraoperative 997.1
    lateral wall 410.5
    non-Q wave 410.7
    non-ST elevation (NSTEMI) 410.7
    nontransmural 410.7
    papillary muscle 410.8
    past (diagnosed on ECG or other special
      investigation, but currently presenting no
      symptoms) 412
      with symptoms NEC 414.8
    posterior (strictly) (true) (wall) 410.6
    posterobasal 410.6
    posteroinferior 410.3
    posterolateral 410.5
    postprocedural 997.1
    previous, currently presenting no symptoms
      412
    Q-wave (see also Infarct, myocardium, by
      site) 410.9
    septal 410.8
    specified site NEC 410.8
    ST elevation (STEMI) 410.9
      anterior (wall) 410.1
      anterolateral (wall) 410.0
      inferior (wall) 410.4
      inferolateral (wall) 410.2

Infarct, infarction—*continued*
    inferoposterior (wall) 410.3
    lateral (wall) 410.5
    posterior (strictly) (true) (wall) 410.6
    specified site NEC 410.8
    subendocardial 410.7
    syphilitic 093.82
    non-ST elevation myocardial infarction
      (NSTEMI) 410.7
    nontransmural 410.7
  omentum 557.0
  ovary 620.8
  pancreas 577.8
  papillary muscle (*see also* Infarct, myocardium)
    410.8
  parathyroid gland 252.8
  pituitary (gland) 253.8
  placenta (complicating pregnancy) 656.7
    affecting fetus or newborn 762.2
  pontine—*see* Infarct, brain
  posterior NEC (*see also* Infarct, myocardium)
    410.6
  prostate 602.8
  pulmonary (artery) (hemorrhagic) (vein) 415.19
    with
      abortion—*see* Abortion, by type, with
        embolism
      ectopic pregnancy (*see also* categories
        633.0-633.9) 639.6
      molar pregnancy (*see also* categories
        630-632) 639.6
    following
      abortion 639.6
      ectopic or molar pregnancy 639.6
    iatrogenic 415.11
    in pregnancy, childbirth, or puerperium—*see*
      Embolism, obstetrical
    postoperative 415.11
    septic 415.12
  renal 593.81
    embolic or thrombotic 593.81
  retina, retinal 362.84
    with occlusion—*see* Occlusion, retina
  spinal (acute) (cord) (embolic) (nonembolic) 336.1
  spleen 289.59
    embolic or thrombotic 444.89
  subchorionic—*see* Infarct, placenta
  subendocardial (*see also* Infarct, myocardium)
    410.7
  suprarenal (capsule) (gland) 255.41
  syncytium—*see* Infarct, placenta
  testis 608.83
  thrombotic (*see also* Thrombosis) 453.9
    artery, arterial—*see* Embolism
  thyroid (gland) 246.3
  ventricle (heart) (*see also* Infarct, myocardium)
    410.9
Infecting —*see* condition
Infection, infected, infective (opportunistic)
  136.9
  with lymphangitis—*see* Lymphangitis
  abortion—*see* Abortion, by type, with sepsis
  abscess (skin)—*see* Abscess, by site
  Absidia 117.7
  Acanthocheilonema (perstans) 125.4
    streptocerca 125.6
  accessory sinus (chronic) (*see also* Sinusitis)
    473.9
  Achorion—*see* Dermatophytosis
  Acremonium falciforme 117.4
  acromioclavicular (joint) 711.91

INDEX TO DISEASES

Infection, infected, infective—*continued*
  actinobacillus
    lignieresii 027.8
    mallei 024
    muris 026.1
  actinomadura—*see* Actinomycosis
  Actinomyces (israelii)—*see also* Actinomycosis
    muris-ratti 026.1
  Actinomycetales (actinomadura) (Actinomyces) (Nocardia) (Streptomyces)—*see* Actinomycosis
  actinomycotic NEC (*see also* Actinomycosis) 039.9
  adenoid (chronic) 474.01
    acute 463
    and tonsil (chronic) 474.02
    acute or subacute 463
  adenovirus NEC 079.0
    in diseases classified elsewhere—*see* category 079
    unspecified nature or site 079.0
  Aerobacter aerogenes NEC 041.85
    enteritis 008.2
  aerogenes capsulatus (*see also* Gangrene, gas) 040.0
  aertrycke (*see also* Infection, Salmonella) 003.9
  ajellomyces dermatitidis 116.0
  alimentary canal NEC (*see also* Enteritis, due to, by organism) 009.0
  Allescheria boydii 117.6
  Alternaria 118
  alveolus, alveolar (process) (pulpal origin) 522.4
  ameba, amebic (histolytica) (*see also* Amebiasis) 006.9
    acute 006.0
    chronic 006.1
    free-living 136.2
    hartmanni 007.8
    specified
      site NEC 006.8
      type NEC 007.8
  amniotic fluid or cavity 658.4
    affecting fetus or newborn 762.7
  anaerobes (cocci) (gram-negative) (gram positive) (mixed) NEC 041.84
  anal canal 569.49
  Ancylostoma braziliense 126.2
  Angiostrongylus cantonensis 128.8
  anisakiasis 127.1
  Anisakis larva 127.1
  anthrax (*see also* Anthrax) 022.9
  antrum (chronic) (*see also* Sinusitis, maxillary) 473.0
  anus (papillae) (sphincter) 569.49
  arbor virus NEC 066.9
  arbovirus NEC 066.9
  argentophil-rod 027.0
  Ascaris lumbricoides 127.0
  ascomycetes 117.4
  Aspergillus (flavus) (fumigatus) (terreus) 117.3
  atypical
    acid-fast (bacilli) (*see also* Mycobacterium, atypical) 031.9
    mycobacteria (*see also* Mycobacterium, atypical) 031.9
  auditory meatus (circumscribed) (diffuse) (external) (*see also* Otitis, externa) 380.10
  auricle (ear) (*see also* Otitis, externa) 380.10
  axillary gland 683
  Babesiasis 088.82
  Babesiosis 088.82

Infection, infected, infective—*continued*
  Bacillus NEC 041.89
    abortus 023.1
    anthracis (*see also* Anthrax) 022.9
    cereus (food poisoning) 005.89
    coli—*see* Infection, Escherichia coli
    coliform NEC 041.85
    Ducrey's (any location) 099.0
    Flexner's 004.1
    Friedländer's NEC 041.3
    fusiformis 101
    gas (gangrene) (*see also* Gangrene, gas) 040.0
    mallei 024
    melitensis 023.0
    paratyphoid, paratyphosus 002.9
      A 002.1
      B 002.2
      C 002.3
    Schmorl's 040.3
    Shiga 004.0
    suipestifer (*see also* Infection, Salmonella) 003.9
    swimming pool 031.1
    typhosa 002.0
    welchii (*see also* Gangrene, gas) 040.0
    Whitmore's 025
  bacterial NEC 041.9
    specified NEC 041.89
      anaerobic NEC 041.84
      gram-negative NEC 041.85
        anaerobic NEC 041.84
  Bacterium
    paratyphosum 002.9
      A 002.1
      B 002.2
      C 002.3
    typhosum 002.0
  Bacteroides (fragilis) (melaninogenicus) (oralis) NEC 041.82
  balantidium coli 007.0
  Bartholin's gland 616.89
  Basidiobolus 117.7
  Bedsonia 079.98
    specified NEC 079.88
  bile duct 576.1
  bladder (*see also* Cystitis) 595.9
  Blastomyces, blastomycotic 116.0
    brasiliensis 116.1
    dermatitidis 116.0
    European 117.5
    Loboi 116.2
    North American 116.0
    South American 116.1
  bleb
    postprocedural 379.60
      stage 1 379.61
      stage 2 379.62
      stage 3 379.63
  blood stream—*see also* Septicemia
    catheter-related (CRBSI) 999.31
  bone 730.9
    specified—*see* Osteomyelitis
  Bordetella 033.9
    bronchiseptica 033.8
    parapertussis 033.1
    pertussis 033.0
  Borrelia
    bergdorfi 088.81
    vincentii (mouth) (pharynx) (tonsil) 101
  brain (*see also* Encephalitis) 323.9
    late effect—*see* category 326

Infection, infected, infective — *continued*
  membranes—(*see also* Meningitis) 322.9
    septic 324.0
      late effect—*see* category 326
    meninges (*see also* Meningitis) 320.9
  branchial cyst 744.42
  breast 611.0
    puerperal, postpartum 675.2
      with nipple 675.9
        specified type NEC 675.8
      nonpurulent 675.2
      purulent 675.1
  bronchus (*see also* Bronchitis) 490
    fungus NEC 117.9
  Brucella 023.9
    abortus 023.1
    canis 023.3
    melitensis 023.0
    mixed 023.8
    suis 023.2
  Brugia (Wuchereria) malayi 125.1
  bursa—*see* Bursitis
  buttocks (skin) 686.9
  Candida (albicans) (tropicalis) (*see also* Candidiasis) 112.9
    congenital 771.7
  Candiru 136.8
  Capillaria
    hepatica 128.8
    philippinensis 127.5
  cartilage 733.99
  cat liver fluke 121.0
  catheter-related bloodstream (CRBSI) 999.31
  cellulitis—*see* Cellulitis, by site
  Cephalosporum falciforme 117.4
  Cercomonas hominis (intestinal) 007.3
  cerebrospinal (*see also* Meningitis) 322.9
    late effect—*see* category 326
  cervical gland 683
  cervix (*see also* Cervicitis) 616.0
  cesarean section wound 674.3
  Chilomastix (intestinal) 007.8
  Chlamydia 079.98
    specified NEC 079.88
  Cholera (*see also* Cholera) 001.9
  chorionic plate 658.8
  Cladosporium
    bantianum 117.8
    carrionii 117.2
    mansoni 111.1
    trichoides 117.8
    wernecki 111.1
  Clonorchis (sinensis) (liver) 121.1
  Clostridium (haemolyticum) (novyi) NEC 041.84
    botulinum 005.1
    histolyticum (*see also* Gangrene, gas) 040.0
    oedematiens (*see also* Gangrene, gas) 040.0
    perfringens 041.83
      due to food 005.2
    septicum (*see also* Gangrene, gas) 040.0
    sordelii (*see also* Gangrene, gas) 040.0
    welchii (*see also* Gangrene, gas) 040.0
      due to food 005.2
  Coccidioides (immitis) (*see also* Coccidioidomycosis) 114.9
  coccus NEC 041.89
  colon (*see also* Enteritis, due to, by organism) 009.0
    bacillus—*see* Infection, Escherichia coli
  colostomy or enterostomy 569.61
  common duct 576.1

Infection, infected, infective — *continued*
  complicating pregnancy, childbirth, or puerperium NEC 647.9
    affecting fetus or newborn 760.2
  Condiobolus 117.7
  congenital NEC 771.89
    Candida albicans 771.7
    chronic 771.2
    Cytomegalovirus 771.1
    hepatitis, viral 771.2
    Herpes simplex 771.2
    listeriosis 771.2
    malaria 771.2
    poliomyelitis 771.2
    rubella 771.0
    toxoplasmosis 771.2
    tuberculosis 771.2
    urinary (tract) 771.82
    vaccinia 771.2
  coronavirus 079.89
    SARS-associated 079.82
  corpus luteum (*see also* Salpingo-oophoritis) 614.2
  Corynebacterium diphtheriae—*see* Diphtheria
  Coxsackie (*see also* Coxsackie) 079.2
    endocardium 074.22
    heart NEC 074.20
    in diseases classified elsewhere—*see* category 079
    meninges 047.0
    myocardium 074.23
    pericardium 074.21
    pharynx 074.0
    specified disease NEC 074.8
    unspecified nature or site 079.2
  Cryptococcus neoformans 117.5
  Cryptosporidia 007.4
  Cunninghamella 117.7
  cyst—*see* Cyst
  Cysticercus cellulosae 123.1
  cytomegalovirus 078.5
    congenital 771.1
  dental (pulpal origin) 522.4
  deuteromycetes 117.4
  Dicrocoelium dendriticum 121.8
  Dipetalonema (perstans) 125.4
    streptocerca 125.6
  diphtherial—*see* Diphtheria
  Diphyllobothrium (adult) (latum) (pacificum) 123.4
    larval 123.5
  Diplogonoporus (grandis) 123.8
  Dipylidium (caninum) 123.8
  Dirofilaria 125.6
  dog tapeworm 123.8
  Dracunculus medinensis 125.7
  Dreschlera 118
    hawaiiensis 117.8
  Ducrey's bacillus (any site) 099.0
  due to or resulting from
    central venous catheter 999.31
    device, implant, or graft (any) (presence of)—*see* Complications, infection and inflammation, due to (presence of) any device, implant, or graft classified to 996.0-996.5 NEC
    injection, inoculation, infusion, transfusion, or vaccination (prophylactic) (therapeutic) 999.39
  injury NEC—*see* Wound, open, by site, complicated
  surgery 998.59

INDEX TO DISEASES

Infection, infected, infective

Infection, infected, infective—*continued*
  duodenum 535.6
  ear—*see also* Otitis
    external (*see also* Otitis, externa) 380.10
    inner (*see also* Labyrinthitis) 386.30
    middle —*see* Otitis, media
  Eaton's agent NEC 041.81
  Eberthella typhosa 002.0
  Ebola 078.89
  echinococcosis 122.9
  Echinococcus (*see also* Echinococcus) 122.9
  Echinostoma 121.8
  ECHO virus 079.1
    in diseases classified elsewhere—*see* category 079
    unspecified nature or site 079.1
  Ehrlichiosis 082.40
    chaffeensis 082.41
    specified type NEC 082.49
  Endamoeba—*see* Infection, ameba
  endocardium (*see also* Endocarditis) 421.0
  endocervix (*see also* Cervicitis) 616.0
  Entamoeba—*see* Infection, ameba
  enteric (*see also* Enteritis, due to, by organism) 009.0
  Enterobacter aerogenes NEC 041.85
  Enterobacter sakazakii 041.85
  Enterobius vermicularis 127.4
  enterococcus NEC 041.04
  enterovirus NEC 079.89
    central nervous system NEC 048
    enteritis 008.67
    meningitis 047.9
  Entomophthora 117.7
  Epidermophyton—*see* Dermatophytosis
  epidermophytosis—*see* Dermatophytosis
  episiotomy 674.3
  Epstein-Barr virus 075
    chronic 780.79 *[139.8]*
  erysipeloid 027.1
  Erysipelothrix (insidiosa) (rhusiopathiae) 027.1
  erythema infectiosum 057.0
  Escherichia coli NEC 041.4
    enteritis—*see* Enteritis, E. coli
    generalized 038.42
    intestinal—*see* Enteritis, E. coli
  esophagostomy 530.86
  ethmoidal (chronic) (sinus) (*see also* Sinusitis, ethmoidal) 473.2
  Eubacterium 041.84
  Eustachian tube (ear) 381.50
    acute 381.51
    chronic 381.52
  exanthema subitum (*see also* Exanthem subitum) 058.10
  external auditory canal (meatus) (*see also* Otitis, externa) 380.10
  eye NEC 360.00
  eyelid 373.9
    specified NEC 373.8
  fallopian tube (*see also* Salpingo-oophoritis) 614.2
  fascia 728.89
  Fasciola
    gigantica 121.3
    hepatica 121.3
  Fasciolopsis (buski) 121.4
  fetus (intra-amniotic)—*see* Infection, congenital
  filarial—*see* Infestation, filarial
  finger (skin) 686.9
    abscess (with lymphangitis) 681.00

Infection, infected, infective—*continued*
    pulp 681.01
    cellulitis (with lymphangitis) 681.00
    distal closed space (with lymphangitis) 681.00
    nail 681.02
    fungus 110.1
  fish tapeworm 123.4
    larval 123.5
  flagellate, intestinal 007.9
  fluke—*see* Infestation, fluke
  focal
    teeth (pulpal origin) 522.4
    tonsils 474.00
    and adenoids 474.02
  Fonsecaea
    compactum 117.2
    pedrosoi 117.2
  food (*see also* Poisoning, food) 005.9
  foot (skin) 686.9
    fungus 110.4
  Francisella tularensis (*see also* Tularemia) 021.9
  frontal sinus (chronic) (*see also* Sinusitis, frontal) 473.1
  fungus NEC 117.9
    beard 110.0
    body 110.5
    dermatiacious NEC 117.8
    foot 110.4
    groin 110.3
    hand 110.2
    nail 110.1
    pathogenic to compromised host only 118
    perianal (area) 110.3
    scalp 110.0
    scrotum 110.8
    skin 111.9
      foot 110.4
      hand 110.2
    toenails 110.1
    trachea 117.9
  Fusarium 118
  Fusobacterium 041.84
  gallbladder (*see also* Cholecystitis, acute) 575.0
  Gardnerella vaginalis 041.89
  gas bacillus (*see also* Gas, gangrene) 040.0
  gastric (*see also* Gastritis) 535.5
  Gastrodiscoides hominis 121.8
  gastroenteric (*see also* Enteritis, due to, by organism) 009.0
  gastrointestinal (*see also* Enteritis, due to, by organism) 009.0
  gastrostomy 536.41
  generalized NEC (*see also* Septicemia) 038.9
  genital organ or tract NEC
    female 614.9
      with
        abortion—*see* Abortion, by type, with sepsis
        ectopic pregnancy (*see also* categories 633.0-633.9) 639.0
        molar pregnancy (*see also* categories 630-632) 639.0
      complicating pregnancy 646.6
        affecting fetus or newborn 760.8
      following
        abortion 639.0
        ectopic or molar pregnancy 639.0
      puerperal, postpartum, childbirth 670
        minor or localized 646.6
          affecting fetus or newborn 760.8
    male 608.4

1103

Infection, infected, infective—*continued*
  genitourinary tract NEC 599.0
  Ghon tubercle, primary (*see also* Tuberculosis) 010.0
  Giardia lamblia 007.1
  gingival (chronic) 523.10
    acute 523.00
    Vincent's 101
  glanders 024
  Glenosporopsis amazonica 116.2
  Gnathostoma spinigerum 128.1
  Gongylonema 125.6
  gonococcal NEC (*see also* Gonococcus) 098.0
  gram-negative bacilli NEC 041.85
    anaerobic 041.84
  guinea worm 125.7
  gum (*see also* Infection, gingival) 523.10
  Hantavirus 079.81
  heart 429.89
  Helicobacter pylori (H. pylori) 041.86
  helminths NEC 128.9
    intestinal 127.9
      mixed (types classifiable to more than one category in 120.0-127.7) 127.8
      specified type NEC 127.7
    specified type NEC 128.8
  Hemophilus influenzae NEC 041.5
    generalized 038.41
  Herpes (simplex) (*see also* Herpes, simplex) 054.9
    congenital 771.2
    zoster (*see also* Herpes, zoster) 053.9
      eye NEC 053.29
  Heterophyes heterophyes 121.6
  Histoplasma (*see also* Histoplasmosis) 115.90
    capsulatum (*see also* Histoplasmosis, American) 115.00
    duboisii (*see also* Histoplasmosis, African) 115.10
  HIV V08
    with symptoms, symptomatic 042
  hookworm (*see also* Ancylostomiasis) 126.9
  human herpesvirus 6 058.81
  human herpesvirus 7 058.82
  human herpesvirus 8 058.89
  human herpesvirus NEC 058.89
  human immunodeficiency virus V08
    with symptoms, symptomatic 042
  human papillomavirus 079.4
  hydrocele 603.1
  hydronephrosis 591
  Hymenolepis 123.6
  hypopharynx 478.29
  inguinal glands 683
    due to soft chancre 099.0
  intestine, intestinal (*see also* Enteritis, due to, by organism) 009.0
  intrauterine (*see also* Endometritis) 615.9
    complicating delivery 646.6
  isospora belli or hominis 007.2
  Japanese B encephalitis 062.0
  jaw (bone) (acute) (chronic) (lower) (subacute) (upper) 526.4
  joint—*see* Arthritis, infectious or infective
  Kaposi's sarcoma-associated herpesvirus 058.89
  kidney (cortex) (hematogenous) 590.9
    with
      abortion—*see* Abortion, by type, with urinary tract infection
      calculus 592.0

Infection, infected, infective—*continued*
  ectopic pregnancy (*see also* categories 633.0-633.9) 639.8
  molar pregnancy (*see also* categories 630-632) 639.8
  complicating pregnancy or puerperium 646.6
    affecting fetus or newborn 760.1
  following
    abortion 639.8
    ectopic or molar pregnancy 639.8
  pelvis and ureter 590.3
  Klebsiella pneumoniae NEC 041.3
  knee (skin) NEC 686.9
    joint—*see* Arthritis, infectious
  Koch's (*see also* Tuberculosis, pulmonary) 011.9
  labia (majora) (minora) (*see also* Vulvitis) 616.10
  lacrimal
    gland (*see also* Dacryoadenitis) 375.00
    passages (duct) (sac) (*see also* Dacryocystitis) 375.30
  larynx NEC 478.79
  leg (skin) NEC 686.9
  Leishmania (*see also* Leishmaniasis) 085.9
    braziliensis 085.5
    donovani 085.0
    Ethiopica 085.3
    furunculosa 085.1
    infantum 085.0
    mexicana 085.4
    tropica (minor) 085.1
      major 085.2
  Leptosphaeria senegalensis 117.4
  leptospira (*see also* Leptospirosis) 100.9
    Australis 100.89
    Bataviae 100.89
    pyrogenes 100.89
    specified type NEC 100.89
  leptospirochetal NEC (*see also* Leptospirosis) 100.9
  Leptothrix—*see* Actinomycosis
  Listeria monocytogenes (listeriosis) 027.0
    congenital 771.2
  liver fluke—*see* Infestation, fluke, liver
  Loa loa 125.2
    eyelid 125.2 [373.6]
  Loboa loboi 116.2
  local, skin (staphylococcal) (streptococcal) NEC 686.9
    abscess—*see* Abscess, by site
    cellulitis—*see* Cellulitis, by site
    ulcer (*see also* Ulcer, skin) 707.9
  Loefflerella
    mallei 024
    whitmori 025
  lung 518.89
    atypical Mycobacterium 031.0
    tuberculous (*see also* Tuberculosis, pulmonary) 011.9
    basilar 518.89
    chronic 518.89
    fungus NEC 117.9
    spirochetal 104.8
    virus—*see* Pneumonia, virus
  lymph gland (axillary) (cervical) (inguinal) 683
    mesenteric 289.2
  lymphoid tissue, base of tongue or posterior pharynx, NEC 474.00
  madurella
    grisea 117.4

1104

INDEX TO DISEASES

Infection, infected, infective—*continued*
mycetomii 117.4
major
with
abortion—*see* Abortion, by type, with sepsis
ectopic pregnancy (*see also* categories 633.0-633.9) 639.0
molar pregnancy (*see also* categories 630-632) 639.0
following
abortion 639.0
ectopic or molar pregnancy 639.0
puerperal, postpartum, childbirth 670
malarial—*see* Malaria
Malassezia furfur 111.0
Malleomyces
mallei 024
pseudomallei 025
mammary gland 611.0
puerperal, postpartum 675.2
Mansonella (ozzardi) 125.5
mastoid (suppurative)—*see* Mastoiditis
maxilla, maxillary 526.4
sinus (chronic) (*see also* Sinusitis, maxillary) 473.0
mediastinum 519.2
medina 125.7
meibomian
cyst 373.12
gland 373.12
melioidosis 025
meninges (*see also* Meningitis) 320.9
meningococcal (*see also* condition) 036.9
brain 036.1
cerebrospinal 036.0
endocardium 036.42
generalized 036.2
meninges 036.0
meningococcemia 036.2
specified site NEC 036.89
mesenteric lymph nodes or glands NEC 289.2
Metagonimus 121.5
metatarsophalangeal 711.97
microorganism resistant to drugs—*see* Resistance (to), drugs by microorganisms
Microsporidia 136.8
microsporum, microsporic—*see* Dermatophytosis
Mima polymorpha NEC 041.85
mixed flora NEC 041.89
Monilia (*see also* Candidiasis) 112.9
neonatal 771.7
monkeypox 057.8
Monosporium apiospermum 117.6
mouth (focus) NEC 528.9
parasitic 112.0
Mucor 117.7
muscle NEC 728.89
mycelium NEC 117.9
mycetoma
actinomycotic NEC (*see also* Actinomycosis) 039.9
mycotic NEC 117.4
Mycobacterium, mycobacterial (*see also* Mycobacterium) 031.9
mycoplasma NEC 041.81
mycotic NEC 117.9
pathogenic to compromised host only 118
skin NEC 111.9
systemic 117.9
myocardium NEC 422.90

Infection, infected, infective—*continued*
nail (chronic) (with lymphangitis) 681.9
finger 681.02
fungus 110.1
ingrowing 703.0
toe 681.11
fungus 110.1
nasal sinus (chronic) (*see also* Sinusitis) 473.9
nasopharynx (chronic) 478.29
acute 460
navel 686.9
newborn 771.4
Neisserian—*see* Gonococcus
Neotestudina rosatii 117.4
newborn, generalized 771.89
nipple 611.0
puerperal, postpartum 675.0
with breast 675.9
specified type NEC 675.8
Nocardia—*see* Actinomycosis
nose 478.19
nostril 478.19
obstetrical surgical wound 674.3
Oesophagostomum (apiostomum) 127.7
Oestrus ovis 134.0
Oidium albicans (*see also* Candidiasis) 112.9
Onchocerca (volvulus) 125.3
eye 125.3 [360.13]
eyelid 125.3 [373.6]
operation wound 998.59
Opisthorchis (felineus) (tenuicollis) (viverrini) 121.0
orbit 376.00
chronic 376.10
ovary (*see also* Salpingo-oophoritis) 614.2
Oxyuris vermicularis 127.4
pancreas 577.0
Paracoccidioides brasiliensis 116.1
Paragonimus (westermani) 121.2
parainfluenza virus 079.89
parameningococcus NEC 036.9
with meningitis 036.0
parasitic NEC 136.9
paratyphoid 002.9
Type A 002.1
Type B 002.2
Type C 002.3
paraurethral ducts 597.89
parotid gland 527.2
Pasteurella NEC 027.2
multocida (cat-bite) (dog-bite) 027.2
pestis (*see also* Plague) 020.9
pseudotuberculosis 027.2
septica (cat-bite) (dog-bite) 027.2
tularensis (*see also* Tularemia) 021.9
pelvic, female (*see also* Disease, pelvis, inflammatory) 614.9
penis (glans) (retention) NEC 607.2
herpetic 054.13
Peptococcus 041.84
Peptostreptococcus 041.84
periapical (pulpal origin) 522.4
peridental 523.30
perineal wound (obstetrical) 674.3
periodontal 523.31
periorbital 376.00
chronic 376.10
perirectal 569.49
perirenal (*see also* Infection, kidney) 590.9
peritoneal (*see also* Peritonitis) 567.9
periureteral 593.89

1105

Infection, infected, infective—*continued*
  periurethral 597.89
  Petriellidium boydii 117.6
  pharynx 478.29
    Coxsackie virus 074.0
    phlegmonous 462
    posterior, lymphoid 474.00
  Phialophora
    gougerotii 117.8
    jeanselmei 117.8
    verrucosa 117.2
  Piedraia hortai 111.3
  pinna, acute 380.11
  pinta 103.9
    intermediate 103.1
    late 103.2
    mixed 103.3
    primary 103.0
  pinworm 127.4
  pityrosporum furfur 111.0
  pleuropneumonia-like organisms NEC (PPLO) 041.81
  pneumococcal NEC 041.2
    generalized (purulent) 038.2
  Pneumococcus NEC 041.2
  postoperative wound 998.59
  posttraumatic NEC 958.3
  postvaccinal 999.39
  prepuce NEC 607.1
  Propionibacterium 041.84
  prostate (capsule) (*see also* Prostatitis) 601.9
  Proteus (mirabilis) (morganii) (vulgaris) NEC 041.6
    enteritis 008.3
  protozoal NEC 136.8
    intestinal NEC 007.9
  Pseudomonas NEC 041.7
    mallei 024
    pneumonia 482.1
    pseudomallei 025
  psittacosis 073.9
  puerperal, postpartum (major) 670
    minor 646.6
  pulmonary—*see* Infection, lung
  purulent—*see* Abscess
  putrid, generalized—*see* Septicemia
  pyemic—*see* Septicemia
  Pyrenochaeta romeroi 117.4
  Q fever 083.0
  rabies 071
  rectum (sphincter) 569.49
  renal (*see also* Infection, kidney) 590.9
    pelvis and ureter 590.3
  resistant to drugs—*see* Resistance (to), drugs by microorganisms
  respiratory 519.8
    chronic 519.8
    influenzal (acute) (upper) 487.1
    lung 518.89
    rhinovirus 460
    syncytial virus 079.6
    upper (acute) (infectious) NEC 465.9
      with flu, grippe, or influenza 487.1
      influenzal 487.1
      multiple sites NEC 465.8
      streptococcal 034.0
      viral NEC 465.9
  respiratory syncytial virus (RSV) 079.6

Infection, infected, infective—*continued*
  resulting from presence of shunt or other internal prosthetic device—*see* Complications, infection and inflammation, due to (presence of) any device, implant, or graft classified to 996.0-996.5 NEC
  retroperitoneal 567.39
  retrovirus 079.50
    human immunodeficiency virus type 2 [HIV-2] 079.53
    human T-cell lymphotrophic virus type I [HTLV-I] 079.51
    human T-cell lymphotrophic virus type II [HTLV-II] 079.52
    specified NEC 079.59
  Rhinocladium 117.1
  Rhinosporidium (*see* beri) 117.0
  rhinovirus
    in diseases classified elsewhere—*see* category 079
    unspecified nature or site 079.3
  Rhizopus 117.7
  rickettsial 083.9
  rickettsialpox 083.2
  rubella (*see also* Rubella) 056.9
    congenital 771.0
  Saccharomyces (*see also* Candidiasis) 112.9
  Saksenaea 117.7
  salivary duct or gland (any) 527.2
  Salmonella (aertrycke) (callinarum) (choleraesuis) (enteritidis) (suipestifer) (typhimurium) 003.9
    with
      arthritis 003.23
      gastroenteritis 003.0
      localized infection 003.20
        specified type NEC 003.29
      meningitis 003.21
      osteomyelitis 003.24
      pneumonia 003.22
      septicemia 003.1
      specified manifestation NEC 003.8
    due to food (poisoning) (any serotype) (*see also* Poisoning, food, due to, Salmonella)
    hirschfeldii 002.3
    localized 003.20
      specified type NEC 003.29
    paratyphi 002.9
      A 002.1
      B 002.2
      C 002.3
    schottmuelleri 002.2
    specified type NEC 003.8
    typhi 002.0
    typhosa 002.0
  saprophytic 136.8
  Sarcocystis, lindemanni 136.5
  SARS-associated coronavirus 079.82
  scabies 133.0
  Schistosoma—*see* Infestation, Schistosoma
  Schmorl's bacillus 040.3
  scratch or other superficial injury—*see* Injury, superficial, by site
  scrotum (acute) NEC 608.4
  secondary, burn or open wound (dislocation) (fracture) 958.3
  seminal vesicle (*see also* Vesiculitis) 608.0
  septic
    generalized—*see* Septicemia
    localized, skin (*see also* Abscess) 682.9
  septicemic—*see* Septicemia

INDEX TO DISEASES

Infection, infected, infective—*continued*
  seroma 998.51
  Serratia (marcescens) 041.85
    generalized 038.44
  sheep liver fluke 121.3
  Shigella 004.9
    boydii 004.2
    dysenteriae 004.0
    Flexneri 004.1
    group
      A 004.0
      B 004.1
      C 004.2
      D 004.3
    Schmitz (-Stutzer) 004.0
    Schmitzii 004.0
    Shiga 004.0
    Sonnei 004.3
    specified type NEC 004.8
  Sin Nombre virus 079.81
  sinus (*see also* Sinusitis) 473.9
    pilonidal 685.1
      with abscess 685.0
    skin NEC 686.9
  Skene's duct or gland (*see also* Urethritis) 597.89
  skin (local) (staphylococcal) (streptococcal) NEC 686.9
    abscess—*see* Abscess, by site
    cellulitis—*see* Cellulitis, by site
    due to fungus 111.9
      specified type NEC 111.8
    mycotic 111.9
      specified type NEC 111.8
    ulcer (*see also* Ulcer, skin) 707.9
  slow virus 046.9
    specified condition NEC 046.8
  Sparganum (mansoni) (proliferum) 123.5
  spermatic cord NEC 608.4
  sphenoidal (chronic) (sinus) (*see also* Sinusitis, sphenoidal) 473.3
  Spherophorus necrophorus 040.3
  spinal cord NEC (*see also* Encephalitis) 323.9
    abscess 324.1
      late effect—*see* category 326
    late effect—*see* category 326
    meninges—*see* Meningitis
    streptococcal 320.2
  Spirillum
    minus or minor 026.0
    morsus muris 026.0
    obermeieri 087.0
  spirochetal NEC 104.9
    lung 104.8
    specified nature or site NEC 104.8
  spleen 289.59
  Sporothrix schenckii 117.1
  Sporotrichum (schenckii) 117.1
  Sporozoa 136.8
  staphylococcal NEC 041.10
    aureus 041.11
    food poisoning 005.0
    generalized (purulent) 038.10
      aureus 038.11
      specified organism NEC 038.19
    pneumonia 482.40
      aureus 482.41
      specified type NEC 482.49
    septicemia 038.10
      aureus 038.11
      specified organism NEC 038.19
    specified NEC 041.19

Infection, infected, infective—*continued*
  steatoma 706.2
  Stellantchasmus falcatus 121.6
  Streptobacillus moniliformis 026.1
  streptococcal NEC 041.00
    generalized (purulent) 038.0
    group
      A 041.01
      B 041.02
      C 041.03
      D [enterococcus] 041.04
      G 041.05
    pneumonia—*see* Pneumonia, streptococcal 482.3
    septicemia 038.0
    sore throat 034.0
    specified NEC 041.09
  Streptomyces—*see* Actinomycosis
  streptotrichosis—*see* Actinomycosis
  Strongyloides (stercoralis) 127.2
  stump (amputation) (posttraumatic) (surgical) 997.62
    traumatic—*see* Amputation, traumatic, by site, complicated
  subcutaneous tissue, local NEC 686.9
  submaxillary region 528.9
  suipestifer (*see also* Infection, Salmonella) 003.9
  swimming pool bacillus 031.1
  syphilitic—*see* Syphilis
  systemic—*see* Septicemia
  Taenia—*see* Infestation, Taenia
  Taeniarhynchus saginatus 123.2
  tapeworm—*see* Infestation, tapeworm
  tendon (sheath) 727.89
  Ternidens diminutus 127.7
  testis (*see also* Orchitis) 604.90
  thigh (skin) 686.9
  threadworm 127.4
  throat 478.29
    pneumococcal 462
    staphylococcal 462
    streptococcal 034.0
    viral NEC (*see also* Pharyngitis) 462
  thumb (skin) 686.9
    abscess (with lymphangitis) 681.00
      pulp 681.01
    cellulitis (with lymphangitis) 681.00
    nail 681.02
  thyroglossal duct 529.8
  toe (skin) 686.9
    abscess (with lymphangitis) 681.10
    cellulitis (with lymphangitis) 681.10
    nail 681.11
    fungus 110.1
  tongue NEC 529.0
    parasitic 112.0
  tonsil (faucial) (lingual) (pharyngeal) 474.00
    acute or subacute 463
    and adenoid 474.02
    tag 474.00
  tooth, teeth 522.4
    periapical (pulpal origin) 522.4
    peridental 523.30
    periodontal 523.31
    pulp 522.0
    socket 526.5
  Torula histolytica 117.5
  Toxocara (cani) (cati) (felis) 128.0
  Toxoplasma gondii (*see also* Toxoplasmosis) 130.9
  trachea, chronic 491.8
    fungus 117.9

Infection, infected, infective—*continued*
  traumatic NEC 958.3
  trematode NEC 121.9
  trench fever 083.1
  Treponema
    denticola 041.84
    macrodenticum 041.84
    pallidum (*see also* Syphilis) 097.9
  Trichinella (spiralis) 124
  Trichomonas 131.9
    bladder 131.09
    cervix 131.09
    hominis 007.3
    intestine 007.3
    prostate 131.03
    specified site NEC 131.8
    urethra 131.02
    urogenitalis 131.00
    vagina 131.01
    vulva 131.01
  Trichophyton, trichophytid—*see* Dermatophytosis
  Trichosporon (beigelii) cutaneum 111.2
  Trichostrongylus 127.6
  Trichuris (trichiuria) 127.3
  Trombicula (irritans) 133.8
  Trypanosoma (*see also* Trypanosomiasis) 086.9
    cruzi 086.2
  tubal (*see also* Salpingo-oophoritis) 614.2
  tuberculous NEC (*see also* Tuberculosis) 011.9
  tubo-ovarian (*see also* Salpingo-oophoritis) 614.2
  tunica vaginalis 608.4
  tympanic membrane—*see* Myringitis
  typhoid (abortive) (ambulant) (bacillus) 002.0
  typhus 081.9
    flea-borne (endemic) 081.0
    louse-borne (epidemic) 080
    mite-borne 081.2
    recrudescent 081.1
    tick-borne 082.9
      African 082.1
      North Asian 082.2
  umbilicus (septic) 686.9
    newborn NEC 771.4
  ureter 593.89
  urethra (*see also* Urethritis) 597.80
  urinary (tract) NEC 599.0
    with
      abortion—*see* Abortion, by type, with urinary tract infection
      ectopic pregnancy (*see also* categories 633.0-633.9) 639.8
      molar pregnancy (*see also* categories 630-632) 639.8
    candidal 112.2
    complicating pregnancy, childbirth, or puerperium 646.6
      affecting fetus or newborn 760.1
      asymptomatic 646.5
        affecting fetus or newborn 760.1
    diplococcal (acute) 098.0
      chronic 098.2
    due to Trichomonas (vaginalis) 131.00
    following
      abortion 639.8
      ectopic or molar pregnancy 639.8
    gonococcal (acute) 098.0
      chronic or duration of 2 months or over 098.2
    newborn 771.82

Infection, infected, infective—*continued*
  trichomonal 131.00
  tuberculous (*see also* Tuberculosis) 016.3
  uterus, uterine (*see also* Endometritis) 615.9
  utriculus masculinus NEC 597.89
  vaccination 999.39
  vagina (granulation tissue) (wall) (*see also* Vaginitis) 616.10
  varicella 052.9
  varicose veins—*see* Varicose, veins
  variola 050.9
    major 050.0
    minor 050.1
  vas deferens NEC 608.4
  Veillonella 041.84
  verumontanum 597.89
  vesical (*see also* Cystitis) 595.9
  Vibrio
    cholerae 001.0
      El Tor 001.1
    parahaemolyticus (food poisoning) 005.4
    vulnificus 041.85
  Vincent's (gums) (mouth) (tonsil) 101
  virus, viral 079.99
    adenovirus
      in diseases classified elsewhere—*see* category 079
      unspecified nature or site 079.0
    central nervous system NEC 049.9
      enterovirus 048
        meningitis 047.9
        specified type NEC 047.8
      slow virus 046.9
        specified condition NEC 046.8
    chest 519.8
    conjunctivitis 077.99
      specified type NEC 077.8
    coronavirus 079.89
      SARS-associated 079.82
    Coxsackie (*see also* Infection, Coxsackie) 079.2
    Ebola 065.8
    ECHO
      in diseases classified elsewhere—*see* category 079
      unspecified nature or site 079.1
    encephalitis 049.9
      arthropod-borne NEC 064
      tick-borne 063.9
        specified type NEC 063.8
    enteritis NEC (*see also* Enteritis, viral) 008.8
    exanthem NEC 057.9
    Hantavirus 079.81
    human papilloma 079.4
    in diseases classified elsewhere—*see* category 079
    intestine (*see also* Enteritis, viral) 008.8
    lung—*see* Pneumonia, viral
    respiratory syncytial virus (RSV) 079.6
    rhinovirus
      in diseases classified elsewhere—*see* category 079
      unspecified nature or site 079.3
    salivary gland disease 078.5
    slow 046.9
      specified condition NEC 046.8
    specified type NEC 079.89
      in diseases classified elsewhere—*see* category 079
      unspecified nature or site 079.99
    warts 078.10
  vulva (*see also* Vulvitis) 616.10

INDEX TO DISEASES

Infestation

Infection, infected, infective—*continued*
  whipworm 127.3
  Whitmore's bacillus 025
  wound (local) (posttraumatic) NEC 958.3
    with
      dislocation—*see* Dislocation, by site, open
      fracture—*see* Fracture, by site, open
      open wound—*see* Wound, open, by site, complicated
    postoperative 998.59
    surgical 998.59
  Wuchereria 125.0
    bancrofti 125.0
    malayi 125.1
  yaws—*see* Yaws
  yeast (*see also* Candidiasis) 112.9
  yellow fever (*see also* Fever, yellow) 060.9
  Yersinia pestis (*see also* Plague) 020.9
  Zeis' gland 373.12
  zoonotic bacterial NEC 027.9
  Zopfia senegalensis 117.4
Infective, infectious —*see* condition
Inferiority complex 301.9
  constitutional psychopathic 301.9
Infertility
  female 628.9
    age related 628.8
    associated with
      adhesions, peritubal 614.6 *[628.2]*
      anomaly
        cervical mucus 628.4
        congenital
          cervix 628.4
          fallopian tube 628.2
          uterus 628.3
          vagina 628.4
      anovulation 628.0
      dysmucorrhea 628.4
      endometritis, tuberculous (*see also* Tuberculosis) 016.7 *[628.3]*
      Stein-Leventhal syndrome 256.4 *[628.0]*
    due to
      adiposogenital dystrophy 253.8 *[628.1]*
      anterior pituitary disorder NEC 253.4 *[628.1]*
        hyperfunction 253.1 *[628.1]*
      cervical anomaly 628.4
      fallopian tube anomaly 628.2
      ovarian failure 256.39 *[628.0]*
      Stein-Leventhal syndrome 256.4 *[628.0]*
      uterine anomaly 628.3
      vaginal anomaly 628.4
    nonimplantation 628.3
    origin
      cervical 628.4
      pituitary-hypothalamus NEC 253.8 *[628.1]*
        anterior pituitary NEC 253.4 *[628.1]*
          hyperfunction NEC 253.1 *[628.1]*
        dwarfism 253.3 *[628.1]*
        panhypopituitarism 253.2 *[628.1]*
      specified NEC 628.8
    tubal (block) (occlusion) (stenosis) 628.2
      adhesions 614.6 *[628.2]*
    uterine 628.3
    vaginal 628.4
    previous, requiring supervision of pregnancy V23.0
  male 606.9
    absolute 606.0
    due to
      azoospermia 606.0

Infertility—*continued*
      drug therapy 606.8
      extratesticular cause NEC 606.8
      germinal cell
        aplasia 606.0
        desquamation 606.1
      hypospermatogenesis 606.1
      infection 606.8
      obstruction, afferent ducts 606.8
      oligospermia 606.1
      radiation 606.8
      spermatogenic arrest (complete) 606.0
        incomplete 606.1
      systemic disease 606.8
Infestation 134.9
  Acanthocheilonema (perstans) 125.4
    streptocerca 125.6
  Acariasis 133.9
    demodex folliculorum 133.8
    Sarcoptes scabiei 133.0
    trombiculae 133.8
  Agamofilaria streptocerca 125.6
  Ancylostoma, Ankylostoma 126.9
    americanum 126.1
    braziliense 126.2
    canium 126.8
    ceylanicum 126.3
    duodenale 126.0
    new world 126.1
    old world 126.0
  Angiostrongylus cantonensis 128.8
  anisakiasis 127.1
  Anisakis larva 127.1
  arthropod NEC 134.1
  Ascaris lumbricoides 127.0
  Bacillus fusiformis 101
  Balantidium coli 007.0
  beef tapeworm 123.2
  Bothriocephalus (latus) 123.4
    larval 123.5
  broad tapeworm 123.4
    larval 123.5
  Brugia malayi 125.1
  Candiru 136.8
  Capillaria
    hepatica 128.8
    philippinensis 127.5
  cat liver fluke 121.0
  Cercomonas hominis (intestinal) 007.3
  cestodes 123.9
    specified type NEC 123.8
  chigger 133.8
  chigoe 134.1
  Chilomastix 007.8
  Clonorchis (sinensis) (liver) 121.1
  coccidia 007.2
  complicating pregnancy, childbirth, or puerperium 647.9
    affecting fetus or newborn 760.8
  Cysticercus cellulosae 123.1
  Demodex folliculorum 133.8
  Dermatobia (hominis) 134.0
  Dibothriocephalus (latus) 123.4
    larval 123.5
  Dicrocoelium dendriticum 121.8
  Diphyllobothrium (adult) (intestinal) (latum) (pacificum) 123.4
    larval 123.5
  Diplogonoporus (grandis) 123.8
  Dipylidium (caninum) 123.8
  Distoma hepaticum 121.3

Infestation—*continued*
  dog tapeworm 123.8
  Dracunculus medinensis 125.7
  dragon worm 125.7
  dwarf tapeworm 123.6
  Echinococcus (*see also* Echinococcus) 122.9
  Echinostoma ilocanum 121.8
  Embadomonas 007.8
  Endamoeba (histolytica)—*see* Infection, ameba
  Entamoeba (histolytica)—*see* Infection, ameba
  Enterobius vermicularis 127.4
  Epidermophyton—*see* Dermatophytosis
  eyeworm 125.2
  Fasciola
    gigantica 121.3
    hepatica 121.3
  Fasciolopsis (buski) (small intestine) 121.4
  filarial 125.9
    due to
      Acanthocheilonema (perstans) 125.4
        streptocerca 125.6
      Brugia (Wuchereria) malayi 125.1
      Dracunculus medinensis 125.7
      guinea worms 125.7
      Mansonella (ozzardi) 125.5
      Onchocerca volvulus 125.3
        eye 125.3 *[360.13]*
        eyelid 125.3 *[373.6]*
      Wuchereria (bancrofti) 125.0
        malayi 125.1
    specified type NEC 125.6
  fish tapeworm 123.4
    larval 123.5
  fluke 121.9
    blood NEC (*see also* Schistosomiasis) 120.9
    cat liver 121.0
    intestinal (giant) 121.4
    liver (sheep) 121.3
      cat 121.0
      Chinese 121.1
      clonorchiasis 121.1
      fascioliasis 121.3
      Oriental 121.1
    lung (oriental) 121.2
    sheep liver 121.3
  fly larva 134.0
  Gasterophilus (intestinalis) 134.0
  Gastrodiscoides hominis 121.8
  Giardia lamblia 007.1
  Gnathostoma (spinigerum) 128.1
  Gongylonema 125.6
  guinea worm 125.7
  helminth NEC 128.9
    intestinal 127.9
      mixed (types classifiable to more than one
        category in 120.0-127.7) 127.8
      specified type NEC 127.7
    specified type NEC 128.8
  Heterophyes heterophyes (small intestine) 121.6
  hookworm (*see also* Infestation, ancylostoma)
    126.9
  Hymenolepis (diminuta) (nana) 123.6
  intestinal NEC 129
  leeches (aquatic) (land) 134.2
  Leishmania—*see* Leishmaniasis
  lice (*see also* infestation, pediculus) 132.9
  Linguatulidae, linguatula (pentastoma) (serrata)
    134.1
  Loa loa 125.2
    eyelid 125.2 *[373.6]*

Infestation—*continued*
  louse (*see also* Infestation, pediculus) 132.9
    body 132.1
    head 132.0
    pubic 132.2
  maggots 134.0
  Mansonella (ozzardi) 125.5
  medina 125.7
  Metagonimus yokogawai (small intestine) 121.5
  Microfilaria streptocerca 125.3
    eye 125.3 *[360.13]*
    eyelid 125.3 *[373.6]*
  Microsporon furfur 111.0
  microsporum—*see* Dermatophytosis
  mites 133.9
    scabic 133.0
    specified type NEC 133.8
  Monilia (albicans) (*see also* Candidiasis) 112.9
    vagina 112.1
    vulva 112.1
    mouth 112.0
  Necator americanus 126.1
  nematode (intestinal) 127.9
    Ancylostoma (*see also* Ancylostoma) 126.9
    Ascaris lumbricoides 127.0
    conjunctiva NEC 128.9
    Dioctophyma 128.8
    Enterobius vermicularis 127.4
    Gnathostoma spinigerum 128.1
    Oesophagostomum (apiostomum) 127.7
    Physaloptera 127.4
    specified type NEC 127.7
    Strongyloides stercoralis 127.2
    Ternidens diminutus 127.7
    Trichinella spiralis 124
    Trichostrongylus 127.6
    Trichuris (trichiuria) 127.3
  Oesophagostomum (apiostomum) 127.7
  Oestrus ovis 134.0
  Onchocerca (volvulus) 125.3
    eye 125.3 *[360.13]*
    eyelid 125.3 *[373.6]*
  Opisthorchis (felineus) (tenuicollis) (viverrini)
    121.0
  Oxyuris vermicularis 127.4
  Paragonimus (westermani) 121.2
  parasite, parasitic NEC 136.9
    eyelid 134.9 *[373.6]*
    intestinal 129
    mouth 112.0
    orbit 376.13
    skin 134.9
    tongue 112.0
  pediculus 132.9
    capitis (humanus) (any site) 132.0
    corporis (humanus) (any site) 132.1
    eyelid 132.0 *[373.6]*
    mixed (classifiable to more than one category
      in 132.0-132.2) 132.3
    pubis (any site) 132.2
  phthirus (pubis) (any site) 132.2
    with any infestation classifiable to 132.0 and
      132.1 132.3
  pinworm 127.4
  pork tapeworm (adult) 123.0
  protozoal NEC 136.8
  pubic louse 132.2
  rat tapeworm 123.6
  red bug 133.8
  roundworm (large) NEC 127.0
  sand flea 134.1

INDEX TO DISEASES   **Inflammation, inflamed, inflammatory**

Infestation—*continued*
  saprophytic NEC 136.8
  Sarcoptes scabiei 133.0
  scabies 133.0
  Schistosoma 120.9
    bovis 120.8
    cercariae 120.3
    hematobium 120.0
    intercalatum 120.8
    japonicum 120.2
    mansoni 120.1
    mattheii 120.8
    specified
      site—*see* Schistosomiasis
      type NEC 120.8
    spindale 120.8
  screw worms 134.0
  skin NEC 134.9
  Sparganum (mansoni) (proliferum) 123.5
    larval 123.5
  specified type NEC 134.8
  Spirometra larvae 123.5
  Sporozoa NEC 136.8
  Stellantchasmus falcatus 121.6
  Strongyloides 127.2
  Strongylus (gibsoni) 127.7
  Taenia 123.3
    diminuta 123.6
    Echinococcus (*see also* Echinococcus) 122.9
    mediocanellata 123.2
    nana 123.6
    saginata (mediocanellata) 123.2
    solium (intestinal form) 123.0
      larval form 123.1
  Taeniarhynchus saginatus 123.2
  tapeworm 123.9
    beef 123.2
    broad 123.4
      larval 123.5
    dog 123.8
    dwarf 123.6
    fish 123.4
      larval 123.5
    pork 123.0
    rat 123.6
  Ternidens diminutus 127.7
  Tetranychus molestissimus 133.8
  threadworm 127.4
  tongue 112.0
  Toxocara (cani) (cati) (felis) 128.0
  trematode(s) NEC 121.9
  Trichina spiralis 124
  Trichinella spiralis 124
  Trichocephalus 127.3
  Trichomonas 131.9
    bladder 131.09
    cervix 131.09
    intestine 007.3
    prostate 131.03
    specified site NEC 131.8
    urethra (female) (male) 131.02
    urogenital 131.00
    vagina 131.01
    vulva 131.01
  Trichophyton—*see* Dermatophytosis
  Trichostrongylus instabilis 127.6
  Trichuris (trichiuria) 127.3
  Trombicula (irritans) 133.8
  Trypanosoma—*see* Trypanosomiasis
  Tunga penetrans 134.1
  Uncinaria americana 126.1

Infestation—*continued*
  whipworm 127.3
  worms NEC 128.9
    intestinal 127.9
  Wuchereria 125.0
    bancrofti 125.0
    malayi 125.1
Infiltrate, infiltration
  with an iron compound 275.0
  amyloid (any site) (generalized) 277.39
  calcareous (muscle) NEC 275.49
    localized—*see* Degeneration, by site
  calcium salt (muscle) 275.49
  corneal (*see also* Edema, cornea) 371.20
    eyelid 373.9
  fatty (diffuse) (generalized) 272.8
    localized—*see* Degeneration, by site, fatty
  glycogen, glycogenic (*see also* Disease,
      glycogen storage) 271.10
  heart, cardiac
    fatty (*see also* Degeneration, myocardial)
      429.1
    glycogenic 271.0 *[425.7]*
  inflammatory in vitreous 379.29
  kidney (*see also* Disease, renal) 593.9
  leukemic (M9800/3)—*see* Leukemia
  liver 573.8
    fatty—*see* Fatty, liver
    glycogen (*see also* Disease, glycogen storage)
      271.0
  lung (*see also* Infiltrate, pulmonary) 518.3
    eosinophilic 518.3
    x-ray finding only 793.1
  lymphatic (*see also* Leukemia, lymphatic) 204.9
    gland, pigmentary 289.3
  muscle, fatty 728.9
  myelogenous (*see also* Leukemia, myeloid)
    205.9
  myocardium, myocardial
    fatty (*see also* Degeneration, myocardial)
      429.1
    glycogenic 271.0 *[425.7]*
  pulmonary 518.3
    with
      eosinophilia 518.3
      pneumonia—*see* Pneumonia, by type
    x-ray finding only 793.1
  Ranke's primary (*see also* Tuberculosis) 010.0
  skin, lymphocyctic (benign) 709.8
  thymus (gland) (fatty) 254.8
  urine 788.8
  vitreous humor 379.29
Infirmity 799.89
  senile 797
Inflammation, inflamed, inflammatory (with
    exudation)
  abducens (nerve) 378.54
  accessory sinus (chronic) (*see also* Sinusitis)
    473.9
  adrenal (gland) 255.8
  alimentary canal—*see* Enteritis
  alveoli (teeth) 526.5
    scorbutic 267
  amnion—*see* Amnionitis
  anal canal 569.49
  antrum (chronic) (*see also* Sinusitis, maxillary)
    473.0
  anus 569.49
  appendix (*see also* Appendicitis) 541
  arachnoid—*see* Meningitis

Inflammation—*continued*
  areola 611.0
    puerperal, postpartum 675.0
  areolar tissue NEC 686.9
  artery—*see* Arteritis
  auditory meatus (external) (*see also* Otitis, externa) 380.10
  Bartholin's gland 616.89
  bile duct or passage 576.1
  bladder (*see also* Cystitis) 595.9
  bleb
    postprocedural 379.60
      stage 1 379.61
      stage 2 379.62
      stage 3 379.63
  bone—*see* Osteomyelitis
  bowel (*see also* Enteritis) 558.9
  brain (*see also* Encephalitis) 323.9
    late effect—*see* category 326
    membrane—*see* Meningitis
  breast 611.0
    puerperal, postpartum 675.2
  broad ligament (*see also* Disease, pelvis, inflammatory) 614.4
    acute 614.3
  bronchus—*see* Bronchitis
  bursa—*see* Bursitis
  capsule
    liver 573.3
    spleen 289.59
  catarrhal (*see also* Catarrh) 460
    vagina 616.10
  cecum (*see also* Appendicitis) 541
  cerebral (*see also* Encephalitis) 323.9
    late effect—*see* category 326
    membrane—*see* Meningitis
  cerebrospinal (*see also* Meningitis) 322.9
    late effect—*see* category 326
    meningococcal 036.0
    tuberculous (*see also* Tuberculosis) 013.6
  cervix (uteri) (*see also* Cervicitis) 616.0
  chest 519.9
  choroid NEC (*see also* Choroiditis) 363.20
  cicatrix (tissue)—*see* Cicatrix
  colon (*see also* Enteritis) 558.9
    granulomatous 555.1
    newborn 558.9
  connective tissue (diffuse) NEC 728.9
  cornea (*see also* Keratitis) 370.9
    with ulcer (*see also* Ulcer, cornea) 370.00
  corpora cavernosa (penis) 607.2
  cranial nerve—*see* Disorder, nerve, cranial
  diarrhea—*see* Diarrhea
  disc (intervertebral) (space) 722.90
    cervical, cervicothoracic 722.91
    lumbar, lumbosacral 722.93
    thoracic, thoracolumbar 722.93
  Douglas' cul-de-sac or pouch (chronic) (*see also* Disease, pelvis, inflammatory) 614.4
    acute 614.3
  due to (presence of) any device, implant, or graft classifiable to 996.0-996.5—*see* Complications, infection and inflammation, due to (presence of) any device, implant, or graft classified to 996.0-996.5 NEC
  duodenum 535.6
  dura mater—*see* Meningitis
  ear—*see also* Otitis
    external (*see also* Otitis, externa) 380.10
    inner (*see also* Labyrinthitis) 386.30
    middle—*see* Otitis media

Inflammation—*continued*
  esophagus 530.10
  ethmoidal (chronic) (sinus) (*see also* Sinusitis, ethmoidal) 473.2
  Eustachian tube (catarrhal) 381.50
    acute 381.51
    chronic 381.52
  extrarectal 569.49
  eye 379.99
  eyelid 373.9
    specified NEC 373.8
  fallopian tube (*see also* Salpingo-oophoritis) 614.2
  fascia 728.9
  fetal membranes (acute) 658.4
    affecting fetus or newborn 762.7
  follicular, pharynx 472.1
  frontal (chronic) (sinus) (*see also* Sinusitis, frontal) 473.1
  gallbladder (*see also* Cholecystitis, acute) 575.0
  gall duct (*see also* Cholecystitis) 575.10
  gastrointestinal (*see also* Enteritis) 558.9
  genital organ (diffuse) (internal)
    female 614.9
      with
        abortion—*see* Abortion, by type, with sepsis
        ectopic pregnancy (*see also* categories 633.0-633.9) 639.0
        molar pregnancy (*see also* categories 630-632) 639.0
      complicating pregnancy, childbirth, or puerperium 646.6
        affecting fetus or newborn 760.8
      following
        abortion 639.0
        ectopic or molar pregnancy 639.0
    male 608.4
  gland (lymph) (*see also* Lymphadenitis) 289.3
  glottis (*see also* Laryngitis) 464.00
    with obstruction 464.01
  granular, pharynx 472.1
  gum 523.10
  heart (*see also* Carditis) 429.89
  hepatic duct 576.8
  hernial sac—*see* Hernia, by site
  ileum (*see also* Enteritis) 558.9
    terminal or regional 555.0
    with large intestine 555.2
  intervertebral disc 722.90
    cervical, cervicothoracic 722.91
    lumbar, lumbosacral 722.93
    thoracic, thoracolumbar 722.92
  intestine (*see also* Enteritis) 558.9
  jaw (acute) (bone) (chronic) (lower) (suppurative) (upper) 526.4
  jejunum—*see* Enteritis
  joint NEC (*see also* Arthritis) 716.9
    sacroiliac 720.2
  kidney (*see also* Nephritis) 583.9
  knee (joint) 716.66
    tuberculous (active) (*see also* Tuberculosis) 015.2
  labium (majus) (minus) (*see also* Vulvitis) 616.10
  lacrimal
    gland (*see also* Dacryoadenitis) 375.00
    passages (duct) (sac) (*see also* Dacryocystitis) 375.30
  larynx (*see also* Laryngitis) 464.00
    with obstruction 464.01

INDEX TO DISEASES

Inflammation

Inflammation—*continued*
  diphtheritic 032.3
  leg NEC 686.9
  lip 528.5
  liver (capsule) (*see also* Hepatitis) 573.3
    acute 570
    chronic 571.40
    suppurative 572.0
  lung (acute) (*see also* Pneumonia) 486
    chronic (interstitial) 518.89
  lymphatic vessel (*see also* Lymphangitis) 457.2
  lymph node or gland (*see also* Lymphadenitis) 289.3
  mammary gland 611.0
    puerperal, postpartum 675.2
  maxilla, maxillary 526.4
    sinus (chronic) (*see also* Sinusitis, maxillary) 473.0
  membranes of brain or spinal cord—*see* Meningitis
  meninges—*see* Meningitis
  mouth 528.00
  muscle 728.9
  myocardium (*see also* Myocarditis) 429.0
  nasal sinus (chronic) (*see also* Sinusitis) 473.9
  nasopharynx—*see* Nasopharyngitis
  navel 686.9
    newborn NEC 771.4
  nerve NEC 729.2
  nipple 611.0
    puerperal, postpartum 675.0
  nose 478.19
    suppurative 472.0
  oculomotor nerve 378.51
  optic nerve 377.30
  orbit (chronic) 376.10
    acute 376.00
    chronic 376.10
  ovary (*see also* Salpingo-oophoritis) 614.2
  oviduct (*see also* Salpingo-oophoritis) 614.2
  pancreas—*see* Pancreatitis
  parametrium (chronic) (*see also* Disease, pelvis, inflammatory) 614.4
    acute 614.3
  parotid region 686.9
    gland 527.2
  pelvis, female (*see also* Disease, pelvis, inflammatory) 614.9
  penis (corpora cavernosa) 607.2
  perianal 569.49
  pericardium (*see also* Pericarditis) 423.9
  perineum (female) (male) 686.9
  perirectal 569.49
  peritoneum (*see also* Peritonitis) 567.9
  periuterine (*see also* Disease, pelvis, inflammatory) 614.9
  perivesical (*see also* Cystitis) 595.9
  petrous bone (*see also* Petrositis) 383.20
  pharynx (*see also* Pharyngitis) 462
    follicular 472.1
    granular 472.1
  pia mater—*see* Meningitis
  pleura—*see* Pleurisy
  postmastoidectomy cavity 383.30
    chronic 383.33
  prostate (*see also* Prostatitis) 601.9
  rectosigmoid—*see* Rectosigmoiditis
  rectum (*see also* Proctitis) 569.49
  respiratory, upper (*see also* Infection, respiratory, upper) 465.9

Inflammation—*continued*
  chronic, due to external agent—*see* Condition, respiratory, chronic, due to, external agent
  due to
    fumes or vapors (chemical) (inhalation) 506.2
    radiation 508.1
  retina (*see also* Retinitis) 363.20
  retrocecal (*see also* Appendicitis) 541
  retroperitoneal (*see also* Peritonitis) 567.9
  salivary duct or gland (any) (suppurative) 527.2
  scorbutic, alveoli, teeth 267
  scrotum 608.4
  sigmoid—*see* Enteritis
  sinus (*see also* Sinusitis) 473.9
  Skene's duct or gland (*see also* Urethritis) 597.89
  skin 686.9
  spermatic cord 608.4
  sphenoidal (sinus) (*see also* Sinusitis, sphenoidal) 473.3
  spinal
    cord (*see also* Encephalitis) 323.9
      late effect—*see* category 326
    membrane—*see* Meningitis
    nerve—*see* Disorder, nerve
  spine (*see also* Spondylitis) 720.9
  spleen (capsule) 289.59
  stomach—*see* Gastritis
  stricture, rectum 569.49
  subcutaneous tissue NEC 686.9
  suprarenal (gland) 255.8
  synovial (fringe) (membrane)—*see* Bursitis
  tendon (sheath) NEC 726.90
  testis (*see also* Orchitis) 604.90
  thigh 686.9
  throat (*see also* Sore throat) 462
  thymus (gland) 254.8
  thyroid (gland) (*see also* Thyroiditis) 245.9
  tongue 529.0
  tonsil—*see* Tonsillitis
  trachea—*see* Tracheitis
  trochlear nerve 378.53
  tubal (*see also* Salpingo-oophoritis) 614.2
  tuberculous NEC (*see also* Tuberculosis) 011.9
  tubo-ovarian (*see also* Salpingo-oophoritis) 614.2
  tunica vaginalis 608.4
  tympanic membrane—*see* Myringitis
  umbilicus, umbilical 686.9
    newborn NEC 771.4
  uterine ligament (*see also* Disease, pelvis, inflammatory) 614.4
    acute 614.3
  uterus (catarrhal) (*see also* Endometritis) 615.9
  uveal tract (anterior) (*see also* Iridocyclitis) 364.3
    posterior—*see* Chorioretinitis
    sympathetic 360.11
  vagina (*see also* Vaginitis) 616.10
  vas deferens 608.4
  vein (*see also* Phlebitis) 451.9
    thrombotic 451.9
      cerebral (*see also* Thrombosis, brain) 434.0
      leg 451.2
        deep (vessels) NEC 451.19
        superficial (vessels) 451.0
      lower extremity 451.2
        deep (vessels) NEC 451.19
        superficial (vessels) 451.0
  vocal cord 478.5
  vulva (*see also* Vulvitis) 616.10

Inflation, lung imperfect (newborn) 770.5
Influenza, influenzal 487.1
  with
    bronchitis 487.1
    bronchopneumonia 487.0
    cold (any type) 487.1
    digestive manifestations 487.8
    hemoptysis 487.1
    involvement of
      gastrointestinal tract 487.8
      nervous system 487.8
    laryngitis 487.1
    manifestations NEC 487.8
      respiratory 487.1
        pneumonia 487.0
    pharyngitis 487.1
    pneumonia (any form classifiable to 480-483, 485-486) 487.0
    respiratory manifestations NEC 487.1
    sinusitis 487.1
    sore throat 487.1
    tonsillitis 487.1
    tracheitis 487.1
    upper respiratory infection (acute) 487.1
  abdominal 487.8
  Asian 487.1
  bronchial 487.1
  bronchopneumonia 487.0
  catarrhal 487.1
  due to identified avian influenza virus 488
  epidemic 487.1
  gastric 487.8
  intestinal 487.8
  laryngitis 487.1
  maternal affecting fetus or newborn 760.2
    manifest influenza in infant 771.2
  pharyngitis 487.1
  pneumonia (any form) 487.0
  respiratory (upper) 487.1
  stomach 487.8
  vaccination, prophylactic (against) V04.81
Influenza-like disease 487.1
Infraction, Freiberg's (metatarsal head) 732.5
Infraeruption, teeth 524.34
Infusion complication, misadventure or reaction —*see* Complication, infusion
Ingestion
  chemical—*see* Table of drugs and chemicals
  drug or medicinal substance
    overdose or wrong substance given or taken 977.9
      specified drug—*see* Table of drugs and chemicals
  foreign body NEC (*see also* Foreign body) 938
Ingrowing
  hair 704.8
  nail (finger) (toe) (infected) 703.0
Inguinal —*see also* condition
  testis 752.51
Inhalation
  carbon monoxide 986
  flame
    mouth 947.0
    lung 947.1
  food or foreign body (*see also* Asphyxia, food or foreign body) 933.1
  gas, fumes, or vapor (noxious) 987.9
    specified agent—*see* Table of drugs and chemicals
  liquid or vomitus (*see also* Asphyxia, food or foreign body) 933.1

Inhalation—*continued*
  lower respiratory tract NEC 934.9
  meconium (fetus or newborn) 770.11
    with respiratory symptoms 770.12
  mucus (*see also* Asphyxia, mucus) 933.1
  oil (causing suffocation) (*see also* Asphyxia, food or foreign body) 933.1
  pneumonia—*see* Pneumonia, aspiration
  smoke 987.9
  steam 987.9
  stomach contents or secretions (*see also* Asphyxia, food or foreign body) 933.1
    in labor and deliver 668.0
Inhibition, inhibited
  academic as adjustment reaction 309.23
  orgasm
    female 302.73
    male 302.74
  sexual
    desire 302.71
    excitement 302.72
  work as adjustment reaction 309.23
Inhibitor, systemic lupus erythematosus (presence of) 286.5
Iniencephalus, iniencephaly 740.2
Injected eye 372.74
Injury 959.9

Note—For abrasion, insect bite (nonvenomous), blister, or scratch, see Injury, superficial. For laceration, traumatic rupture, tear, or penetrating wound of internal organs, such as heart, lung, liver, kidney, pelvic organs, whether or not accompanied by open wound in the same region, see Injury, internal. For nerve injury, see Injury, nerve. For late effect of injuries classifiable to 850-854, 860-869, 900-919, 950-959, see Late, effect, injury, by type.

  abdomen, abdominal (viscera)—*see also* Injury, internal, abdomen
    muscle or wall 959.12
  acoustic, resulting in deafness 951.5
  adenoid 959.09
  adrenal (gland)—*see* Injury, internal, adrenal
  alveolar (process) 959.09
  ankle (and foot) (and knee) (and leg, except thigh) 959.7
  anterior chamber, eye 921.3
  anus 959.19
  aorta (thoracic) 901.0
    abdominal 902.0
  appendix—*see* Injury, internal, appendix
  arm, upper (and shoulder) 959.2
  artery (complicating trauma) (*see also* Injury, blood vessel, by site) 904.9
    cerebral or meningeal (*see also* Hemorrhage, brain, traumatic, subarachnoid) 852.0
  auditory canal (external) (meatus) 959.09
  auricle, auris, ear 959.09
  axilla 959.2
  back 959.19
  bile duct—*see* Injury, internal, bile duct
  birth—*see also* Birth, injury
    canal NEC, complicating delivery 665.9
  bladder (sphincter)—*see* Injury, internal, bladder
  blast (air) (hydraulic) (immersion) (underwater) NEC 869.0
    with open wound into cavity NEC 869.1
    abdomen or thorax—*see* Injury, internal, by site

INDEX TO DISEASES — Injury

Injury—*continued*
  brain—*see* Concussion, brain
  ear (acoustic nerve trauma) 951.5
    with perforation of tympanic
      membrane—*see* Wound, open, ear, drum
  blood vessel NEC 904.9
    abdomen 902.9
      multiple 902.87
      specified NEC 902.89
    aorta (thoracic) 901.0
      abdominal 902.0
    arm NEC 903.9
    axillary 903.00
      artery 903.01
      vein 903.02
    azygos vein 901.89
    basilic vein 903.1
    brachial (artery) (vein) 903.1
    bronchial 901.89
    carotid artery 900.00
      common 900.01
      external 900.02
      internal 900.03
    celiac artery 902.20
      specified branch NEC 902.24
    cephalic vein (arm) 903.1
    colica dextra 902.26
    cystic
      artery 902.24
      vein 902.39
    deep plantar 904.6
    digital (artery) (vein) 903.5
    due to accidental puncture or laceration during
      procedure 998.2
    extremity
      lower 904.8
        multiple 904.7
        specified NEC 904.7
      upper 903.9
        multiple 903.8
        specified NEC 903.8
    femoral
      artery (superficial) 904.1
        above profunda origin 904.0
        common 904.0
      vein 904.2
    gastric
      artery 902.21
      vein 902.39
    head 900.9
      intracranial—*see* Injury, intracranial
      multiple 900.82
      specified NEC 900.89
    hemiazygos vein 901.89
    hepatic
      artery 902.22
      vein 902.11
    hypogastric 902.59
      artery 902.51
      vein 902.52
    ileocolic
      artery 902.26
      vein 902.31
    iliac 902.50
      artery 902.53
      specified branch NEC 902.59
      vein 902.54
    innominate
      artery 901.1
      vein 901.3
    intercostal (artery) (vein) 901.81

Injury—*continued*
    jugular vein (external) 900.81
      internal 900.1
    leg NEC 904.8
    mammary (artery) (vein) 901.82
    mesenteric
      artery 902.20
        inferior 902.27
        specified branch NEC 902.29
        superior (trunk) 902.25
          branches, primary 902.26
      vein 902.39
        inferior 902.32
        superior (and primary subdivisions) 902.31
    neck 900.9
      multiple 900.82
      specified NEC 900.89
    ovarian 902.89
      artery 902.81
      vein 902.82
    palmar artery 903.4
    pelvis 902.9
      multiple 902.87
      specified NEC 902.89
    plantar (deep) (artery) (vein) 904.6
    popliteal 904.40
      artery 904.41
      vein 904.42
    portal 902.33
    pulmonary 901.40
      artery 901.41
      vein 901.42
    radial (artery) (vein) 903.2
    renal 902.40
      artery 902.41
      specified NEC 902.49
      vein 902.42
    saphenous
      artery 904.7
      vein (greater) (lesser) 904.3
    splenic
      artery 902.23
      vein 902.34
    subclavian
      artery 901.1
      vein 901.3
    suprarenal 902.49
    thoracic 901.9
      multiple 901.83
      specified NEC 901.89
    tibial 904.50
      artery 904.50
        anterior 904.51
        posterior 904.53
      vein 904.50
        anterior 904.52
        posterior 904.54
    ulnar (artery) (vein) 903.3
    uterine 902.59
      artery 902.55
      vein 902.56
    vena cava
      inferior 902.10
        specified branches NEC 902.19
      superior 901.2
  brachial plexus 953.4
    newborn 767.6
  brain NEC (*see also* Injury, intracranial) 854.0
  breast 959.19
  broad ligament—*see* Injury, internal, broad
    ligament

1115

Injury—continued
- bronchus, bronchi—*see* Injury, internal, bronchus
- brow 959.09
- buttock 959.19
- canthus, eye 921.1
- cathode ray 990
- cauda equina 952.4
  - with fracture, vertebra—*see* Fracture, vertebra, sacrum
- cavernous sinus (*see also* Injury, intracranial) 854.0
- cecum—*see* Injury, internal, cecum
- celiac ganglion or plexus 954.1
- cerebellum (*see also* Injury, intracranial) 854.0
- cervix (uteri)—*see* Injury, internal, cervix
- cheek 959.09
- chest—*see* Injury, internal, chest
  - wall 959.11
- childbirth—*see also* Birth, injury
  - maternal NEC 665.9
- chin 959.09
- choroid (eye) 921.3
- clitoris 959.14
- coccyx 959.19
  - complicating delivery 665.6
- colon—*see* Injury, internal, colon
- common duct—*see* Injury, internal, common duct
- conjunctiva 921.1
  - superficial 918.2
- cord
  - spermatic—*see* Injury, internal, spermatic cord
  - spinal—*see* Injury, spinal, by site
- cornea 921.3
  - abrasion 918.1
  - due to contact lens 371.82
  - penetrating—*see* Injury, eyeball, penetrating
  - superficial 918.1
  - due to contact lens 371.82
- cortex (cerebral) (*see also* Injury, intracranial) 854.0
  - visual 950.3
- costal region 959.11
- costochondral 959.11
- cranial
  - bones—*see* Fracture, skull, by site
  - cavity (*see also* Injury, intracranial) 854.0
  - nerve—*see* Injury, nerve, cranial
- crushing—*see* Crush
- cutaneous sensory nerve
  - lower limb 956.4
  - upper limb 955.5
- delivery—*see also* Birth, injury
  - maternal NEC 665.9
- Descemet's membrane—*see* Injury, eyeball, penetrating
- diaphragm—*see* Injury, internal, diaphragm
- diffuse axonal—*see* Injury, intracranial
- duodenum—*see* Injury, internal, duodenum
- ear (auricle) (canal) (drum) (external) 959.09
- elbow (and forearm) (and wrist) 959.3
- epididymis 959.14
- epigastric region 959.12
- epiglottis 959.09
- epiphyseal, current—*see* Fracture, by site
- esophagus—*see* Injury, internal, esophagus
- Eustachian tube 959.09
- extremity (lower) (upper) NEC 959.8

Injury—continued
- eye 921.9
  - penetrating eyeball—*see* Injury, eyeball, penetrating
  - superficial 918.9
- eyeball 921.3
  - penetrating 871.7
    - with
      - partial loss (of intraocular tissue) 871.12
      - prolapse or exposure (of intraocular tissue) 871.1
    - without prolapse 871.0
    - foreign body (nonmagnetic) 871.6
      - magnetic 871.5
  - superficial 918.9
- eyebrow 959.09
- eyelid(s) 921.1
  - laceration—*see* Laceration, eyelid
  - superficial 918.0
- face (and neck) 959.09
- fallopian tube—*see* Injury, internal, fallopian tube
- finger(s) (nail) 959.5
- flank 959.19
- foot (and ankle) (and knee) (and leg except thigh) 959.7
- forceps NEC 767.9
  - scalp 767.19
- forearm (and elbow) (and wrist) 959.3
- forehead 959.09
- gallbladder—*see* Injury, internal, gallbladder
- gasserian ganglion 951.2
- gastrointestinal tract—*see* Injury, internal, gastrointestinal tract
- genital organ(s)
  - with
    - abortion—*see* Abortion, by type, with, damage to pelvic organs
    - ectopic pregnancy (*see also* categories 633.0-633.9) 639.2
    - molar pregnancy (*see also* categories 630-632) 639.2
  - external 959.14
    - fracture of corpus cavernosum penis 959.13
  - following
    - abortion 639.2
    - ectopic or molar pregnancy 639.2
  - internal—*see* Injury, internal, genital organs
  - obstetrical trauma NEC 665.9
    - affecting fetus or newborn 763.89
- gland
  - lacrimal 921.1
    - laceration 870.8
  - parathyroid 959.09
  - salivary 959.09
  - thyroid 959.09
- globe (eye) (*see also* Injury, eyeball) 921.3
- grease gun—*see* Wound, open, by site, complicated
- groin 959.19
- gum 959.09
- hand(s) (except fingers) 959.4
- head NEC 959.01
  - with
    - loss of consciousness 850.5
    - skull fracture—*see* Fracture, skull, by site
- heart—*see* Injury, internal, heart
- heel 959.7
- hip (and thigh) 959.6
- hymen 959.14
- hyperextension (cervical) (vertebra) 847.0

INDEX TO DISEASES   **Injury**

Injury—*continued*
  ileum—*see* Injury, internal, ileum
  iliac region 959.19
  infrared rays NEC 990
  instrumental (during surgery) 998.2
    birth injury—*see* Birth, injury
    nonsurgical (*see also* Injury, by site) 959.9
    obstetrical 665.9
      affecting fetus or newborn 763.89
      bladder 665.5
      cervix 665.3
      high vaginal 665.4
      perineal NEC 664.9
      urethra 665.5
      uterus 665.5
  internal 869.0

> *Note—For injury of internal organ(s) by foreign body entering through a natural orifice (e.g., inhaled, ingested, or swallowed)—see Foreign body, entering through orifice.*
>
> *For internal injury of any of the following sites with internal injury of any other of the sites—see Injury, internal, multiple.*

    with
      fracture
        pelvis—*see* Fracture, pelvis
        specified site, except pelvis—*see* Injury, internal, by site
      open wound into cavity 869.1
    abdomen, abdominal (viscera) NEC 868.00
      with
        fracture, pelvis—*see* Fracture, pelvis
        open wound into cavity 868.10
      specified site NEC 868.09
        with open wound into cavity 868.19
    adrenal (gland) 868.01
      with open wound into cavity 868.11
    aorta (thoracic) 901.0
      abdominal 902.0
    appendix 863.85
      with open wound into cavity 863.95
    bile duct 868.02
      with open wound into cavity 868.12
    bladder (sphincter) 867.0
      with
        abortion—*see* Abortion, by type, with, damage to pelvic organs
        ectopic pregnancy (*see also* categories 633.0-633.9) 639.2
        molar pregnancy (*see also* categories 630-632) 639.2
        open wound into cavity 867.1
      following
        abortion 639.2
        ectopic or molar pregnancy 639.2
      obstetrical trauma 665.5
        affecting fetus or newborn 763.89
    blood vessel—*see* Injury, blood vessel, by site
    broad ligament 867.6
      with open wound into cavity 867.7
    bronchus, bronchi 862.21
      with open wound into cavity 862.31
    cecum 863.89
      with open wound into cavity 863.99
    cervix (uteri) 867.4
      with
        abortion—*see* Abortion, by type, with damage to pelvic organs

Injury—*continued*
        ectopic pregnancy (*see also* categories 633.0-633.9) 639.2
        molar pregnancy (*see also* categories 630-632) 639.2
        open wound into cavity 867.5
      following
        abortion 639.2
        ectopic or molar pregnancy 639.2
      obstetrical trauma 665.3
        affecting fetus or newborn 763.89
    chest (*see also* Injury, internal, intrathoracic organs) 862.8
      with open wound into cavity 862.9
    colon 863.40
      with
        open wound into cavity 863.50
      rectum 863.46
        with open wound into cavity 863.56
      ascending (right) 863.41
        with open wound into cavity 863.51
      descending (left) 863.43
        with open wound into cavity 863.53
      multiple sites 863.46
        with open wound into cavity 863.56
      sigmoid 863.44
        with open wound into cavity 863.54
      specified site NEC 863.49
        with open wound into cavity 863.59
      transverse 863.42
        with open wound into cavity 863.52
    common duct 868.02
      with open wound into cavity 868.12
    complicating delivery 665.9
      affecting fetus or newborn 763.89
    diaphragm 862.0
      with open wound into cavity 862.1
    duodenum 863.21
      with open wound into cavity 863.31
    esophagus (intrathoracic) 862.22
      with open wound into cavity 862.32
      cervical region 874.4
        complicated 874.5
    fallopian tube 867.6
      with open wound into cavity 867.7
    gallbladder 868.02
      with open wound into cavity 868.12
    gastrointestinal tract NEC 863.80
      with open wound into cavity 863.90
    genital organ NEC 867.6
      with open wound into cavity 867.7
    heart 861.00
      with open wound into thorax 861.10
    ileum 863.29
      with open wound into cavity 863.39
    intestine NEC 863.89
      with open wound into cavity 863.99
      large NEC 863.40
        with open wound into cavity 863.50
      small NEC 863.20
        with open wound into cavity 863.30
    intra-abdominal (organ) 868.00
      with open wound into cavity 868.10
      multiple sites 868.09
        with open wound into cavity 868.19
      specified site NEC 868.09
        with open wound into cavity 868.19
    intrathoracic organs (multiple) 862.8
      with open wound into cavity 862.9
      diaphragm (only)—*see* Injury, internal, diaphragm

1117

Injury — *continued*
- heart (only)—*see* Injury, internal, heart
- lung (only)—*see* Injury, internal, lung
- specified site NEC 862.29
  - with open wound into cavity 862.39
- intrauterine (*see also* Injury, internal, uterus) 867.4
  - with open wound into cavity 867.5
- jejunum 863.29
  - with open wound into cavity 863.39
- kidney (subcapsular) 866.00
  - with
    - disruption of parenchyma (complete) 866.03
      - with open wound into cavity 866.13
    - hematoma (without rupture of capsule) 866.01
      - with open wound into cavity 866.11
    - laceration 866.02
      - with open wound into cavity 866.12
    - open wound into cavity 866.10
- liver 864.00
  - with
    - contusion 864.01
      - with open wound into cavity 864.11
    - hematoma 864.01
      - with open wound into cavity 864.11
    - laceration 864.05
      - with open wound into cavity 864.15
      - major (disruption of hepatic parenchyma) 864.04
        - with open wound into cavity 864.14
      - minor (capsule only) 864.02
        - with open wound into cavity 864.12
      - moderate (involving parenchyma) 864.03
        - with open wound into cavity 864.13
      - multiple 864.04
      - stellate 864.04
        - with open wound in cavity 864.14
    - open wound into cavity 864.10
- lung 861.20
  - with open wound into thorax 861.30
  - hemopneumothorax—*see* Hemopneumothorax, traumatic
  - hemothorax—*see* Hemothorax, traumatic
  - pneumohemothorax—*see* Pneumohemothorax, traumatic
  - pneumothorax—*see* Pneumothorax, traumatic
  - transfusion related, acute (TRALI) 518.7
- mediastinum 862.29
  - with open wound into cavity 862.39
- mesentery 863.89
  - with open wound into cavity 863.99
- mesosalpinx 867.6
  - with open wound into cavity 867.7
- multiple 869.0

> *Note—Multiple internal injuries of sites classifiable to the same three- or four-digit category should be classified to that category. Multiple injuries classifiable to different fourth-digit subdivisions of 861 (heart and lung injuries) should be dealt with according to coding rules.*

- with open wound into cavity 869.1
- intra-abdominal organ (sites classifiable to 863-868)
  - with
    - intrathoracic organ(s) (sites classifiable to 861-862) 869.0

Injury — *continued*
- with open wound into cavity 869.1
- other intra-abdominal organ(s) (sites classifiable to 863-868, except where classifiable to the same three-digit category) 868.09
  - with open wound into cavity 868.19
- intrathoracic organ (sites classifiable to 861-862)
  - with
    - intra-abdominal organ(s) (sites classifiable to 863-868) 869.0
      - with open wound into cavity 869.1
    - other intrathoracic organ(s) (sites classifiable to 861-862, except where classifiable to the same three-digit category) 862.8
      - with open wound into cavity 862.9
- myocardium—*see* Injury, internal, heart
- ovary 867.6
  - with open wound into cavity 867.7
- pancreas (multiple sites) 863.84
  - with open wound into cavity 863.94
- body 863.82
  - with open wound into cavity 863.92
- head 863.81
  - with open wound into cavity 863.91
- tail 863.83
  - with open wound into cavity 863.93
- pelvis, pelvic (organs) (viscera) 867.8
  - with
    - fracture, pelvis—*see* Fracture, pelvis
    - open wound into cavity 867.9
  - specified site NEC 867.6
    - with open wound into cavity 867.7
- peritoneum 868.03
  - with open wound into cavity 868.13
- pleura 862.29
  - with open wound into cavity 862.39
- prostate 867.6
  - with open wound into cavity 867.7
- rectum 863.45
  - with
    - colon 863.46
      - with open wound into cavity 863.56
    - open wound into cavity 863.55
- retroperitoneum 868.04
  - with open wound into cavity 868.14
- round ligament 867.6
  - with open wound into cavity 867.7
- seminal vesicle 867.6
  - with open wound into cavity 867.7
- spermatic cord 867.6
  - with open wound into cavity 867.7
- scrotal—*see* Wound, open, spermatic cord
- spleen 865.00
  - with
    - disruption of parenchyma (massive) 865.04
      - with open wound into cavity 865.14
    - hematoma (without rupture of capsule) 865.01
      - with open wound into cavity 865.11
    - open wound into cavity 865.10
    - tear, capsular 865.02
      - with open wound into cavity 865.12
      - extending into parenchyma 865.03
        - with open wound into cavity 865.13
- stomach 863.0
  - with open wound into cavity 863.1

INDEX TO DISEASES

Injury

Injury—continued
  suprarenal gland (multiple) 868.01
    with open wound into cavity 868.11
  thorax, thoracic (cavity) (organs) (multiple)
    (*see also* Injury, internal, intrathoracic
    organs) 862.8
    with open wound into cavity 862.9
  thymus (gland) 862.29
    with open wound into cavity 862.39
  trachea (intrathoracic) 862.29
    with open wound into cavity 862.39
    cervical region (*see also* Wound, open,
      trachea) 874.02
  ureter 867.2
    with open wound into cavity 867.3
  urethra (sphincter) 867.0
    with
      abortion—*see* Abortion, by type, with,
        damage to pelvic organs
      ectopic pregnancy (*see also* categories
        633.0-633.9) 639.2
      molar pregnancy (*see also* categories
        630-632) 639.2
      open wound into cavity 867.1
    following
      abortion 639.2
      ectopic or molar pregnancy 639.2
    obstetrical trauma 665.5
      affecting fetus or newborn 763.89
  uterus 867.4
    with
      abortion—*see* Abortion, by type, with,
        damage to pelvic organs
      ectopic pregnancy (*see also* categories
        633.0-633.9) 639.2
      molar pregnancy (*see also* categories
        630-632) 639.2
      open wound into cavity 867.5
    following
      abortion 639.2
      ectopic or molar pregnancy 639.2
    obstetrical trauma NEC 665.5
      affecting fetus or newborn 763.89
  vas deferens 867.6
    with open wound into cavity 867.7
  vesical (sphincter) 867.0
    with open wound into cavity 867.1
  viscera (abdominal) (*see also* Injury, internal,
    multiple) 868.00
    with
      fracture, pelvis—*see* Fracture, pelvis
      open wound into cavity 868.10
    thoracic NEC (*see also* Injury, internal,
      intrathoracic organs) 862.8
      with open wound into cavity 862.9
  interscapular region 959.19
  intervertebral disc 959.19
  intestine—*see* Injury, internal, intestine
  intra-abdominal (organs) NEC—*see* Injury,
    internal, intra-abdominal

Injury—continued
  intracranial 854.0

> Note—Use the following fifth-digit subclassification with categories 851-854:
>
> 0 unspecifidd state of consciousness
> 1 with no loss of consciousness
> 2 with brief [less than one hour] loss of consciousness
> 3 with moderate [1-24 hours] loss of consciousness
> 4 with prolonged [more than 24 hours] loss of consciousness and return to pre-existing conscious level
> 5 with prolonged [more than 24 hours] loss of consciousness, without return to pre-existing conscious level
>
> Use fifth-digit 5 to designate when a patient is unconscious and dies before regaining consciousness, regardless of the duration of the loss of consciousness
>
> 6 with loss of consciousness of unspecified duration
> 9 with concussion, unspecified

    with
      open intracranial wound 854.1
      skull fracture—*see* Fracture, skull, by site
    contusion 851.8
      with open intracranial wound 851.9
      brain stem 851.4
        with open intracranial wound 851.5
      cerebellum 851.4
        with open intracranial wound 851.5
      cortex (cerebral) 851.0
        with open intracranial wound 851.2
    hematoma—*see* Injury, intracranial,
      hemorrhage
    hemorrhage 853.0
      with
        laceration—*see* Injury, intracranial,
          laceration
        open intracranial wound 853.1
      extradural 852.4
        with open intracranial wound 852.5
      subarachnoid 852.0
        with open intracranial wound 852.1
      subdural 852.2
        with open intracranial wound 852.3
    laceration 851.8
      with open intracranial wound 851.9
      brain stem 851.6
        with open intracranial wound 851.7
      cerebellum 851.6
        with open intracranial wound 851.7
      cortex (cerebral) 851.2
        with open intracranial wound 851.3
  intraocular—*see* Injury, eyeball, penetrating
  intrathoracic organs (multiple)—*see* Injury,
    internal, intrathoracic organs
  intrauterine—*see* Injury, internal, intrauterine
  iris 921.3
    penetrating—*see* Injury, eyeball, penetrating
  jaw 959.09
  jejunum—*see* Injury, internal, jejunum

Injury — INDEX TO DISEASES

Injury—*continued*
  joint NEC 959.9
    old or residual 718.80
      ankle 718.87
      elbow 718.82
      foot 718.87
      hand 718.84
      hip 718.85
      knee 718.86
      multiple sites 718.89
      pelvic region 718.85
      shoulder (region) 718.81
      specified site NEC 718.88
      wrist 718.83
  kidney—*see* Injury, internal, kidney
  knee (and ankle) (and foot) (and leg, except thigh) 959.7
  labium (majus) (minus) 959.14
  labyrinth, ear 959.09
  lacrimal apparatus, gland, or sac 921.1
    laceration 870.8
  larynx 959.09
  late effect—*see* Late, effects (of), injury
  leg except thigh (and ankle) (and foot) (and knee) 959.7
    upper or thigh 959.6
  lens, eye 921.3
    penetrating—*see* Injury, eyeball, penetrating
  lid, eye—*see* Injury, eyelid
  lip 959.09
  liver—*see* Injury, internal, liver
  lobe, parietal—*see* Injury, intracranial
  lumbar (region) 959.19
    plexus 953.5
  lumbosacral (region) 959.19
    plexus 953.5
  lung—*see* Injury, internal, lung
  malar region 959.09
  mastoid region 959.09
  maternal, during pregnancy, affecting fetus or newborn 760.5
  maxilla 959.09
  mediastinum—*see* Injury, internal, mediastinum
  membrane
    brain (*see also* Injury, intracranial) 854.0
    tympanic 959.09
  meningeal artery—*see* Hemorrhage, brain, traumatic, subarachnoid
  meninges (cerebral)—*see* Injury, intracranial
  mesenteric
    artery—*see* Injury, blood vessel, mesenteric, artery
    plexus, inferior 954.1
    vein—*see* Injury, blood vessel, mesenteric, vein
  mesentery—*see* Injury, internal, mesentery
  mesosalpinx—*see* Injury, internal, mesosalpinx
  middle ear 959.09
  midthoracic region 959.11
  mouth 959.09
  multiple (sites not classifiable to the same four-digit category in 959.0-959.7) 959.8
    internal 869.0
      with open wound into cavity 869.1
  musculocutaneous nerve 955.4
  nail
    finger 959.5
    toe 959.7
  nasal (septum) (sinus) 959.09
  nasopharynx 959.09
  neck (and face) 959.09

Injury—*continued*
  nerve 957.9
    abducens 951.3
    abducent 951.3
    accessory 951.6
    acoustic 951.5
    ankle and foot 956.9
    anterior crural, femoral 956.1
    arm (*see also* Injury, nerve, upper limb) 955.9
    auditory 951.5
    axillary 955.0
    brachial plexus 953.4
    cervical sympathetic 954.0
    cranial 951.9
      first or olfactory 951.8
      second or optic 950.0
      third or oculomotor 951.0
      fourth or trochlear 951.1
      fifth or trigeminal 951.2
      sixth or abducens 951.3
      seventh or facial 951.4
      eighth, acoustic, or auditory 951.5
      ninth or glossopharyngeal 951.8
      tenth, pneumogastric, or vagus 951.8
      eleventh or accessory 951.6
      twelfth or hypoglossal 951.7
      newborn 767.7
    cutaneous sensory
      lower limb 956.4
      upper limb 955.5
    digital (finger) 955.6
      toe 956.5
    facial 951.4
      newborn 767.5
    femoral 956.1
    finger 955.9
    foot and ankle 956.9
    forearm 955.9
    glossopharyngeal 951.8
    hand and wrist 955.9
    head and neck, superficial 957.0
    hypoglossal 951.7
    involving several parts of body 957.8
    leg (*see also* Injury, nerve, lower limb) 956.9
    lower limb 956.9
      multiple 956.8
      specified site NEC 956.5
    lumbar plexus 953.5
    lumbosacral plexus 953.5
    median 955.1
      forearm 955.1
      wrist and hand 955.1
    multiple (in several parts of body) (sites not classifiable to the same three-digit category) 957.8
    musculocutaneous 955.4
    musculospiral 955.3
      upper arm 955.3
    oculomotor 951.0
    olfactory 951.8
    optic 950.0
    pelvic girdle 956.9
      multiple sites 956.8
      specified site NEC 956.5
    peripheral 957.9
      multiple (in several regions) (sites not classifiable to the same three-digit category) 957.8
      specified site NEC 957.1
    peroneal 956.3
      ankle and foot 956.3

INDEX TO DISEASES

Injury

Injury—*continued*
   lower leg 956.3
   plantar 956.5
   plexus 957.9
     celiac 954.1
     mesenteric, inferior 954.1
     spinal 953.9
       brachial 953.4
       lumbosacral 953.5
       multiple sites 953.8
     sympathetic NEC 954.1
   pneumogastric 951.8
   radial 955.3
     wrist and hand 955.3
   sacral plexus 953.5
   sciatic 956.0
     thigh 956.0
   shoulder girdle 955.9
     multiple 955.8
     specified site NEC 955.7
   specified site NEC 957.1
   spinal 953.9
     plexus—*see* Injury, nerve, plexus, spinal
     root 953.9
       cervical 953.0
       dorsal 953.1
       lumbar 953.2
       multiple sites 953.8
       sacral 953.3
   splanchnic 954.1
   sympathetic NEC 954.1
     cervical 954.0
   thigh 956.9
   tibial 956.5
     ankle and foot 956.2
     lower leg 956.5
     posterior 956.2
   toe 956.9
   trigeminal 951.2
   trochlear 951.1
   trunk, excluding shoulder and pelvic girdles 954.9
     specified site NEC 954.8
     sympathetic NEC 954.1
   ulnar 955.2
     forearm 955.2
     wrist (and hand) 955.2
   upper limb 955.9
     multiple 955.8
     specified site NEC 955.7
   vagus 951.8
   wrist and hand 955.9
  nervous system, diffuse 957.8
  nose (septum) 959.09
  obstetrical NEC 665.9
   affecting fetus or newborn 763.89
  occipital (region) (scalp) 959.09
   lobe (*see also* Injury, intracranial) 854.0
  optic 950.9
   chiasm 950.1
   cortex 950.3
   nerve 950.0
   pathways 950.2
  orbit, orbital (region) 921.2
   penetrating 870.3
     with foreign body 870.4
  ovary—*see* Injury, internal, ovary
  paint-gun—*see* Wound, open, by site, complicated
  palate (soft) 959.09
  pancreas—*see* Injury, internal, pancreas

Injury—*continued*
  parathyroid (gland) 959.09
  parietal (region) (scalp) 959.09
   lobe—*see* Injury, intracranial
  pelvic
   floor 959.19
     complicating delivery 664.1
       affecting fetus or newborn 763.89
   joint or ligament, complicating delivery 665.6
     affecting fetus or newborn 763.89
   organs—*see also* Injury, internal, pelvis
     with
       abortion—*see* Abortion, by type, with damage to pelvic organs
       ectopic pregnancy (*see also* categories 633.0-633.9) 639.2
       molar pregnancy (*see also* categories 633.0-633.9) 639.2
     following
       abortion 639.2
       ectopic or molar pregnancy 639.2
     obstetrical trauma 665.5
       affecting fetus or newborn 763.89
  pelvis 959.19
  penis 959.14
   fracture of corpus cavernosum 959.13
  perineum 959.14
  peritoneum—*see* Injury, internal, peritoneum
  periurethral tissue
   with
     abortion—*see* Abortion, by type, with damage to pelvic organs
     ectopic pregnancy (*see also* categories 633.0-633.9) 639.2
     molar pregnancy (*see also* categories 630-632) 639.2
   complicating delivery 665.5
     affecting fetus or newborn 763.89
   following
     abortion 639.2
     ectopic or molar pregnancy 639.2
  phalanges
   foot 959.7
   hand 959.5
  pharynx 959.09
  pleura—*see* Injury, internal, pleura
  popliteal space 959.7
  post-cardiac surgery (syndrome) 429.4
  prepuce 959.14
  prostate—*see* Injury, internal, prostate
  pubic region 959.19
  pudenda 959.14
  radiation NEC 990
  radioactive substance or radium NEC 990
  rectovaginal septum 959.14
  rectum—*see* Injury, internal, rectum
  retina 921.3
   penetrating—*see* Injury, eyeball, penetrating
  retroperitoneal—*see* Injury, internal, retroperitoneum
  roentgen rays NEC 990
  round ligament—*see* Injury, internal, round ligament
  sacral (region) 959.19
   plexus 953.5
  sacroiliac ligament NEC 959.19
  sacrum 959.19
  salivary ducts or glands 959.09
  scalp 959.09
   due to birth trauma 767.19
   fetus or newborn 767.19

Injury—*continued*
  scapular region 959.2
  sclera 921.3
    penetrating—*see* Injury, eyeball, penetrating
    superficial 918.2
  scrotum 959.14
  seminal vesicle—*see* Injury, internal, seminal vesicle
  shoulder (and upper arm) 959.2
  sinus
    cavernous (*see also* Injury, intracranial) 854.0
    nasal 959.09
  skeleton NEC, birth injury 767.3
  skin NEC 959.9
  skull—*see* Fracture, skull, by site
  soft tissue (of external sites) (severe)—*see* Wound, open, by site
  specified site NEC 959.8
  spermatic cord—*see* Injury, internal, spermatic cord
  spinal (cord) 952.9
    with fracture, vertebra—*see* Fracture, vertebra, by site, with spinal cord injury
    cervical (C_1-C_4) 952.00
      with
        anterior cord syndrome 952.02
        central cord syndrome 952.03
        complete lesion of cord 952.01
        incomplete lesion NEC 952.04
        posterior cord syndrome 952.04
      C_5-C_7 level 952.05
        with
          anterior cord syndrome 952.07
          central cord syndrome 952.08
          complete lesion of cord 952.06
          incomplete lesion NEC 952.09
          posterior cord syndrome 952.09
        specified type NEC 952.09
      specified type NEC 952.04
    dorsal (D_1-D_6) (T_1-T_6) (thoracic) 952.10
      with
        anterior cord syndrome 952.12
        central cord syndrome 952.13
        complete lesion of cord 952.11
        incomplete lesion NEC 952.14
        posterior cord syndrome 952.14
      D_7-D_{12} level (T_7-T_{12}) 952.15
        with
          anterior cord syndrome 952.17
          central cord syndrome 952.18
          complete lesion of cord 952.16
          incomplete lesion NEC 952.19
          posterior cord syndrome 952.19
        specified type NEC 952.19
      specified type NEC 952.14
    lumbar 952.2
    multiple sites 952.8
    nerve (root) NEC—*see* Injury, nerve, spinal, root
    plexus 953.9
      brachial 953.4
      lumbosacral 953.5
      multiple sites 953.8
    sacral 952.3
    thoracic (*see also* Injury, spinal, dorsal) 952.10
  spleen—*see* Injury, internal, spleen
  stellate ganglion 954.1
  sternal region 959.11
  stomach—*see* Injury, internal, stomach
  subconjunctival 921.1

Injury—*continued*
  subcutaneous 959.9
  subdural—*see* Injury, intracranial
  submaxillary region 959.09
  submental region 959.09
  subungual
    fingers 959.5
    toes 959.7
  superficial 919

Note—Use the following fourth-digit subdivisions with categories 910-919:

.0 *Abrasion or friction burn without mention of infection*
.1 *Abrasion or friction burn, infected*
.2 *Blister without mention of infection*
.3 *Blister, infected*
.4 *Insect bite, nonvenomous, without mention of infection*
.5 *Insect bite, nonvenomous, infected*
.6 *Superficial foreign body (splinter) without major open wound and without mention of infection*
.7 *Superficial foreign body (splinter) without major open wound, infected*
.8 *Other and unspecified superficial injury without mention of infection*
.9 *Other and unspecified superficial injury, infected*

For late effects of superficial injury, see category 906.2.

---

  abdomen, abdominal (muscle) (wall) (and other part(s) of trunk) 911
  ankle (and hip, knee, leg, or thigh) 916
  anus (and other part(s) of trunk) 911
  arm 913
    upper (and shoulder) 912
  auditory canal (external) (meatus) (and other part(s) of face, neck, or scalp, except eye) 910
  axilla (and upper arm) 912
  back (and other part(s) of trunk) 911
  breast (and other part(s) of trunk) 911
  brow (and other part(s) of face, neck or scalp, except eye) 910
  buttock (and other part(s) of trunk) 911
  canthus, eye 918.0
  cheek(s) (and other part(s) of face, neck, or scalp, except eye) 910
  chest wall (and other part(s) of trunk) 911
  chin (and other part(s) of face, neck, or scalp, except eye) 910
  clitoris (and other part(s) of trunk) 911
  conjunctiva 918.2
  cornea 918.1
    due to contact lens 371.82
  costal region (and other part(s) of trunk) 911
  ear(s) (auricle) (canal) (drum) (external) (and other part(s) of face, neck, or scalp, except eye) 910
  elbow (and forearm) (and wrist) 913
  epididymis (and other part(s) of trunk) 911
  epigastric region (and other part(s) of trunk) 911
  epiglottis (and other part(s) of face, neck, or scalp, except eye) 910
  eye(s) (and adnexa) NEC 918.9
  eyelid(s) (and periocular area) 918.0

INDEX TO DISEASES   **Injury**

Injury—*continued*
    face (any part(s), except eye) (and neck or scalp) 910
    finger(s) (nail) (any) 915
    flank (and other part(s) of trunk) 911
    foot (phalanges) (and toe(s)) 917
    forearm (and elbow) (and wrist) 913
    forehead (and other part(s) of face, neck, or scalp, except eye) 910
    globe (eye) 918.9
    groin (and other part(s) of trunk) 911
    gum(s) (and other part(s) of face, neck, or scalp, except eye) 910
    hand(s) (except fingers alone) 914
    head (and other part(s) of face, neck, or scalp, except eye) 910
    heel (and foot or toe) 917
    hip (and ankle, knee, leg, or thigh) 916
    iliac region (and other part(s) of trunk) 911
    interscapular region (and other part(s) of trunk) 911
    iris 918.9
    knee (and ankle, hip, leg, or thigh) 916
    labium (majus) (minus) (and other part(s) of trunk) 911
    lacrimal (apparatus) (gland) (sac) 918.0
    leg (lower) (upper) (and ankle, hip, knee, or thigh) 916
    lip(s) (and other part(s) of face, neck, or scalp, except eye) 910
    lower extremity (except foot) 916
    lumbar region (and other part(s) of trunk) 911
    malar region (and other part(s) of face, neck, or scalp, except eye) 910
    mastoid region (and other part(s) of face, neck, or scalp, except eye) 910
    midthoracic region (and other part(s) of trunk) 911
    mouth (and other part(s) of face, neck, or scalp, except eye) 910
    multiple sites (not classifiable to the same three-digit category) 919
    nasal (septum) (and other part(s) of face, neck, or scalp, except eye) 910
    neck (and face or scalp, any part(s), except eye) 910
    nose (septum) (and other part(s) of face, neck, or scalp, except eye) 910
    occipital region (and other part(s) of face, neck, or scalp, except eye) 910
    orbital region 918.0
    palate (soft) (and other part(s) of face, neck, or scalp, except eye) 910
    parietal region (and other part(s) of face, neck, or scalp, except eye) 910
    penis (and other part(s) of trunk) 911
    perineum (and other part(s) of trunk) 911
    periocular area 918.0
    pharynx (and other part(s) of face, neck, or scalp, except eye) 910
    popliteal space (and ankle, hip, leg, or thigh) 916
    prepuce (and other part(s) of trunk) 911
    pubic region (and other part(s) of trunk) 911
    pudenda (and other part(s) of trunk) 911
    sacral region (and other part(s) of trunk) 911
    salivary (ducts) (glands) (and other part(s) of face, neck, or scalp, except eye) 910
    scalp (and other part(s) of face or neck, except eye) 910
    scapular region (and upper arm) 912

Injury—*continued*
    sclera 918.2
    scrotum (and other part(s) of trunk) 911
    shoulder (and upper arm) 912
    skin NEC 919
    specified site(s) NEC 919
    sternal region (and other part(s) of trunk) 911
    subconjunctival 918.2
    subcutaneous NEC 919
    submaxillary region (and other part(s) of face, neck, or scalp, except eye) 910
    submental region (and other part(s) of face, neck, or scalp, except eye) 910
    supraclavicular fossa (and other part(s) of face, neck or scalp, except eye) 910
    supraorbital 918.0
    temple (and other part(s) of face, neck, or scalp, except eye) 910
    temporal region (and other part(s) of face, neck, or scalp, except eye) 910
    testis (and other part(s) of trunk) 911
    thigh (and ankle, hip, knee, or leg) 916
    thorax, thoracic (external) (and other part(s) of trunk) 911
    throat (and other part(s) of face, neck, or scalp, except eye) 910
    thumb(s) (nail) 915
    toe(s) (nail) (subungual) (and foot) 917
    tongue (and other part(s) of face, neck, or scalp, except eye) 910
    tooth, teeth (*see also* Abrasion, dental) 521.20
    trunk (any part(s)) 911
    tunica vaginalis (and other part(s) of trunk) 911
    tympanum, tympanic membrane (and other part(s) of face, neck, or scalp, except eye) 910
    upper extremity NEC 913
    uvula (and other part(s) of face, neck, or scalp, except eye) 910
    vagina (and other part(s) of trunk) 911
    vulva (and other part(s) of trunk) 911
    wrist (and elbow) (and forearm) 913
    supraclavicular fossa 959.19
    supraorbital 959.09
    surgical complication (external or internal site) 998.2
    symphysis pubis 959.19
        complicating delivery 665.6
            affecting fetus or newborn 763.89
    temple 959.09
    temporal region 959.09
    testis 959.14
    thigh (and hip) 959.6
    thorax, thoracic (external) 959.11
        cavity—*see* Injury, internal, thorax
        internal—*see* Injury, internal, intrathoracic organs
    throat 959.09
    thumb(s) (nail) 959.5
    thymus—*see* Injury, internal, thymus
    thyroid (gland) 959.09
    toe (nail) (any) 959.7
    tongue 959.09
    tonsil 959.09
    tooth NEC 873.63
        complicated 873.73
    trachea—*see* Injury, internal, trachea
    trunk 959.19
    tunica vaginalis 959.14
    tympanum, tympanic membrane 959.09

Injury—*continued*
  ultraviolet rays NEC 990
  ureter—*see* Injury, internal, ureter
  urethra (sphincter)—*see* Injury, internal, urethra
  uterus—*see* Injury, internal, uterus
  uvula 959.09
  vagina 959.14
  vascular—*see* Injury, blood vessel
  vas deferens—*see* Injury, internal, vas deferens
  vein (*see also* Injury, blood vessel, by site) 904.9
  vena cava
    inferior 902.10
    superior 901.2
  vesical (sphincter)—*see* Injury, internal, vesical
  viscera (abdominal)—*see* Injury, internal, viscera
    with fracture, pelvis—*see* Fracture, pelvis
  visual 950.9
    cortex 950.3
  vitreous (humor) 871.2
  vulva 959.14
  whiplash (cervical spine) 847.0
  wringer—*see* Crush, by site
  wrist (and elbow) (and forearm) 959.3
  x-ray NEC 990
Inoculation —*see also* Vaccination
  complication or reaction—*see* Complication, vaccination
INPH (idiopathic normal pressure hydrocephalus) 331.5
Insanity, insane (*see also* Psychosis) 298.9
  adolescent (*see also* Schizophrenia) 295.9
  alternating (*see also* Psychosis, affective, circular) 296.7
  confusional 298.9
    acute 293.0
    subacute 293.1
  delusional 298.9
  paralysis, general 094.1
    progressive 094.1
  paresis, general 094.1
  senile 290.20
Insect
  bite—*see* Injury, superficial, by site
  venomous, poisoning by 989.5
Insemination, artificial V26.1
Insensitivity
  adrenocorticotropin hormone (ACTH) 255.41
  androgen 259.5
    partial 259.5
Insertion
  cord (umbilical) lateral or velamentous 663.8
    affecting fetus or newborn 762.6
  intrauterine contraceptive device V25.1
  placenta, vicious—*see* Placenta, previa
  subdermal implantable contraceptive V25.5
  velamentous, umbilical cord 663.8
    affecting fetus or newborn 762.6
Insolation 992.0
  meaning sunstroke 992.0
Insomnia, unspecified 780.52
  with sleep apnea, unspecified 780.51
  adjustment 307.41
  alcohol induced 291.82
  behavioral, of childhood V69.5
  drug induced 292.85
  due to
    medical condition classified elsewhere 327.01
    mental disorder 327.02
  idiopathic 307.42

Insomnia—*continued*
  nonorganic origin 307.41
    persistent (primary) 307.42
    transient 307.41
  organic 327.00
    other 327.09
  paradoxical 307.42
  primary 307.42
  psychophysiological 307.42
  subjective complaint 307.49
Inspiration
  food or foreign body (*see also* Asphyxia, food or foreign body) 933.1
  mucus (*see also* Asphyxia, mucus) 933.1
Inspissated bile syndrome, newborn 774.4
Instability
  detrusor 596.59
  emotional (excessive) 301.3
  joint (posttraumatic) 718.80
    ankle 718.87
    elbow 718.82
    foot 718.87
    hand 718.84
    hip 718.85
    knee 718.86
    lumbosacral 724.6
    multiple sites 718.89
    pelvic region 718.85
    sacroiliac 724.6
    shoulder (region) 718.81
    specified site NEC 718.88
    wrist 718.83
  lumbosacral 724.6
  nervous 301.89
  personality (emotional) 301.59
  thyroid, paroxysmal 242.9
  urethral 599.83
  vasomotor 780.2
Insufficiency, insufficient
  accommodation 367.4
  adrenal (gland) (acute) (chronic) 255.41
    medulla 255.5
    primary 255.41
    specified NEC 255.5
  adrenocortical 255.41
  anterior (occlusal) guidance 524.54
  anus 569.49
  aortic (valve) 424.1
    with
      mitral (valve) disease 396.1
        insufficiency, incompetence, or regurgitation 396.3
        stenosis or obstruction 396.1
      stenosis or obstruction 424.1
        with mitral (valve) disease 396.8
    congenital 746.4
    rheumatic 395.1
      with
        mitral (valve) disease 396.1
          insufficiency, incompetence, or regurgitation 396.3
          stenosis or obstruction 396.1
        stenosis or obstruction 395.2
          with mitral (valve) disease 396.8
    specified cause NEC 424.1
    syphilitic 093.22
  arterial 447.1
    basilar artery 435.0
    carotid artery 435.8
    cerebral 437.1
    coronary (acute or subacute) 411.89

INDEX TO DISEASES

Insufficiency, insufficient—*continued*
  mesenteric 557.1
  peripheral 443.9
  precerebral 435.9
  vertebral artery 435.1
  vertibrobasilar 435.3
 arteriovenous 459.9
 basilar artery 435.0
 biliary 575.8
 cardiac (*see also* Insufficiency, myocardial) 428.0
  complicating surgery 997.1
  due to presence of (cardiac) prosthesis 429.4
  postoperative 997.1
   long-term effect of cardiac surgery 429.4
  specified during or due to a procedure 997.1
   long-term effect of cardiac surgery 429.4
 cardiorenal (*see also* Hypertension, cardiorenal) 404.90
 cardiovascular (*see also* Disease, cardiovascular) 429.2
  renal (*see also* Hypertension, cardiorenal) 404.90
 carotid artery 435.8
 cerebral (vascular) 437.9
 cerebrovascular 437.9
  with transient focal neurological signs and symptoms 435.9
  acute 437.1
   with transient focal neurological signs and symptoms 435.9
 circulatory NEC 459.9
  fetus or newborn 779.89
 convergence 378.83
 coronary (acute or subacute) 411.89
  chronic or with a stated duration of over 8 weeks 414.8
 corticoadrenal 255.41
 dietary 269.9
 divergence 378.85
 food 994.2
 gastroesophageal 530.89
 gonadal
  ovary 256.39
  testis 257.2
 gonadotropic hormone secretion 253.4
 heart—*see also* Insufficiency, myocardial
  fetus or newborn 779.89
  valve (*see also* Endocarditis) 424.90
   congenital NEC 746.89
 hepatic 573.8
 idiopathic autonomic 333.0
 interocclusal distance of teeth (ridge) 524.36
 kidney
  acute 593.9
  chronic 585.9
 labyrinth, labyrinthine (function) 386.53
  bilateral 386.54
  unilateral 386.53
 lacrimal 375.15
 liver 573.8
 lung (acute) (*see also* Insufficiency, pulmonary) 518.82
  following trauma, surgery, or shock 518.5
  newborn 770.89
 mental (congenital) (*see also* Retardation, mental) 319
 mesenteric 557.1
 mitral (valve) 424.0
  with
   aortic (valve) disease 396.3

Insufficiency, insufficient—*continued*
   insufficiency, incompetence, or regurgitation 396.3
   stenosis or obstruction 396.2
  obstruction or stenosis 394.2
   with aortic valve disease 396.8
  congenital 746.6
  rheumatic 394.1
   with
    aortic (valve) disease 396.3
     insufficiency, incompetence, or regurgitation 396.3
     stenosis or obstruction 396.2
    obstruction or stenosis 394.2
     with aortic valve disease 396.8
   active or acute 391.1
    with chorea, rheumatic (Sydenham's) 392.0
  specified cause, except rheumatic 424.0
 muscle
  heart—*see* Insufficiency, myocardial
  ocular (*see also* Strabismus) 378.9
 myocardial, myocardium (with arteriosclerosis) 428.0
  with rheumatic fever (conditions classifiable to 390)
   active, acute, or subacute 391.2
    with chorea 392.0
   inactive or quiescent (with chorea) 398.0
  congenital 746.89
  due to presence of (cardiac) prosthesis 429.4
  fetus or newborn 779.89
  following cardiac surgery 429.4
  hypertensive (*see also* Hypertension, heart) 402.91
   benign 402.11
   malignant 402.01
  postoperative 997.1
   long-term effect of cardiac surgery 429.4
  rheumatic 398.0
   active, acute, or subacute 391.2
    with chorea (Sydenham's) 392.0
  syphilitic 093.82
 nourishment 994.2
 organic 799.89
 ovary 256.39
  postablative 256.2
 pancreatic 577.8
 parathyroid (gland) 252.1
 peripheral vascular (arterial) 443.9
 pituitary (anterior) 253.2
  posterior 253.5
 placental—*see* Placenta, insufficiency
 platelets 287.5
 prenatal care in current pregnancy V23.7
 progressive pluriglandular 258.9
 pseudocholinesterase 289.89
 pulmonary (acute) 518.82
  following
   shock 518.5
   surgery 518.5
   trauma 518.5
  newborn 770.89
  valve (*see also* Endocarditis, pulmonary) 424.3
   congenital 746.09
 pyloric 537.0
 renal 593.9
  acute 593.9
  chronic 585.9
  due to a procedure 997.5

Insufficiency, insufficient—*continued*
  respiratory 786.09
    acute 518.82
      following shock, surgery, or trauma 518.5
    newborn 770.89
  rotation—*see* Malrotation
  suprarenal 255.41
    medulla 255.5
  tarso-orbital fascia, congenital 743.66
  tear film 375.15
  testis 257.2
  thyroid (gland) (acquired)—*see also* Hypothyroidism
    congenital 243
  tricuspid (*see also* Endocarditis, tricuspid) 397.0
    congenital 746.89
    syphilitic 093.23
  urethral sphincter 599.84
  valve, valvular (heart) (*see also* Endocarditis) 424.90
  vascular 459.9
    intestine NEC 557.9
    mesenteric 557.1
    peripheral 443.9
    renal (*see also* Hypertension, kidney) 403.90
  velopharyngeal
    acquired 528.9
    congenital 750.29
  venous (peripheral) 459.81
  ventricular—*see* Insufficiency, myocardial
  vertebral artery 435.1
  vertibrobasilar artery 435.3
  weight gain during pregnancy 646.8
  zinc 269.3
Insufflation
  fallopian
    fertility testing V26.21
    following sterilization reversal V26.22
  meconium 770.11
    with respiratory symptoms 770.12
Insular —*see* condition
Insulinoma (M8151/0)
  malignant (M8151/3)
    pancreas 157.4
    specified site—*see* Neoplasm, by site, malignant
    unspecified site 157.4
  pancreas 211.7
  specified site—*see* Neoplasm, by site, benign
  unspecified site 211.7
Insuloma —*see* Insulinoma
Insult
  brain 437.9
    acute 436
  cerebral 437.9
    acute 436
  cerebrovascular 437.9
    acute 436
  vascular NEC 437.9
    acute 436
Insurance examination (certification) V70.3
Intemperance (*see also* Alcoholism) 303.9
Interception of pregnancy (menstrual extraction) V25.3
Interference
  balancing side 524.56
  non-working side 524.56
Intermenstrual
  bleeding 626.6
    irregular 626.6
    regular 626.5

Intermenstrual—*continued*
  hemorrhage 626.6
    irregular 626.6
    regular 626.5
  ain(s) 625.2
Intermittent— *see* condition
Internal —*see* condition
Interproximal wear 521.10
Interruption
  aortic arch 747.11
  bundle of His 426.50
  fallopian tube (for sterilization) V25.2
  phase-shift, sleep cycle 307.45
  repeated REM-sleep 307.48
  sleep
    due to perceived environmental disturbances 307.48
    phase-shift, of 24-hour sleep-wake cycle 307.45
    repeated REM-sleep type 307.48
  vas deferens (for sterilization) V25.2
Intersexuality 752.7
Interstitial —*see* condition
Intertrigo 695.89
  labialis 528.5
Intervertebral disc —*see* condition
Intestine, intestinal —*see also* condition
  flu 487.8
Intolerance
  carbohydrate NEC 579.8
  cardiovascular exercise, with pain (at rest) (with less than ordinary activity) (with ordinary activity) V47.2
  cold 780.99
  disaccharide (hereditary) 271.3
  drug
    correct substance properly administered 995.27
    wrong substance given or taken in error 977.9
      specified drug—*see* Table of drugs and chemicals
  effort 306.2
  fat NEC 579.8
  foods NEC 579.8
  fructose (hereditary) 271.2
  glucose (-galactose) (congenital) 271.3
  gluten 579.0
  lactose (hereditary) (infantile) 271.3
  lysine (congenital) 270.7
  milk NEC 579.8
  protein (familial) 270.7
  starch NEC 579.8
  sucrose (-isomaltose) (congenital) 271.3
Intoxicated NEC (*see also* Alcoholism) 305.0
Intoxication
  acid 276.2
  acute
    alcoholic 305.0
      with alcoholism 303.0
      hangover effects 305.0
    caffeine 305.9
    hallucinogenic (*see also* Abuse, drugs, nondependent) 305.3
  alcohol (acute) 305.0
    with alcoholism 303.0
    hangover effects 305.0
    idiosyncratic 291.4
    pathological 291.4
  alimentary canal 558.2
  ammonia (hepatic) 572.2
  caffeine 305.9

Intoxication—*continued*
  chemical—*see also* Table of drugs and
      chemicals
    via placenta or breast milk 760.70
      alcohol 760.71
      anticonvulsants 760.77
      antifungals 760.74
      anti-infective agents 760.74
      antimetabolics 760.78
      cocaine 760.75
      "crack" 760.75
      hallucinogenic agents NEC 760.73
      medicinal agents NEC 760.79
      narcotics 760.72
      obstetric anesthetic or analgesic drug 763.5
      specified agent NEC 760.79
      suspected, affecting management of
          pregnancy 655.5
  cocaine, through placenta or breast milk 760.75
  delirium
    alcohol 291.0
    drug 292.81
  drug 292.89
    with delirium 292.81
    correct substance properly administered (*see
        also* Allergy, drug) 995.27
    newborn 779.4
    obstetric anesthetic or sedation 668.9
      affecting fetus or newborn 763.5
    overdose or wrong substance given or
        taken—*see* Table of drugs and chemicals
    pathologic 292.2
    specific to newborn 779.4
    via placenta or breast milk 760.70
      alcohol 760.71
      anticonvulsants 760.77
      antifungals 760.74
      anti-infective agents 760.74
      antimetabolics 760.78
      cocaine 760.75
      "crack" 760.75
      hallucinogenic agents 760.73
      medicinal agents NEC 760.79
      narcotics 760.72
      obstetric anesthetic or analgesic drug 763.5
      specified agent NEC 760.79
      suspected, affecting management of
          pregnancy 655.5
  enteric—*see* Intoxication, intestinal
  fetus or newborn, via placenta or breast milk
      760.70
    alcohol 760.71
    anticonvulsants 760.77
    antifungals 760.74
    anti-infective agents 760.74
    antimetabolics 760.78
    cocaine 760.75
    "crack" 760.75
    hallucinogenic agents 760.73
    medicinal agents NEC 760.79
    narcotics 760.72
    obstetric anesthetic or analgesic drug 763.5
    specified agent NEC 760.79
    suspected, affecting management of pregnancy
        655.5
  food—*see* Poisoning, food
  gastrointestinal 558.2
  hallucinogenic (acute) 305.3
  hepatocerebral 572.2
  idiosyncratic alcohol 291.4

Intoxication—*continued*
  intestinal 569.89
    due to putrefaction of food 005.9
  methyl alcohol (*see also* Alcoholism) 305.0
    with alcoholism 303.0
  non-foodborne due to toxins of Clostridium
      botulinum [*C. botulinum*] —*see* Botulism
  pathologic 291.4
    drug 292.2
  potassium (K) 276.7
  septic
    with
      abortion—*see* Abortion, by type, with sepsis
      ectopic pregnancy (*see also* categories
          633.0-633.9) 639.0
      molar pregnancy (*see also* categories
          630-632) 639.0
    during labor 659.3
    following
      abortion 639.0
      ectopic or molar pregnancy 639.0
    generalized—*see* Septicemia
    puerperal, postpartum, childbirth 670
  serum (prophylactic) (therapeutic) 999.5
  uremic—*see* Uremia
  water 276.6
Intracranial —*see* condition
Intrahepatic gallbladder 751.69
Intraligamentous —*see also* condition
  pregnancy—*see* Pregnancy, cornual
Intraocular —*see also* condition
  sepsis 360.00
Intrathoracic —*see also* condition
  kidney 753.3
  stomach—*see* Hernia, diaphragm
Intrauterine contraceptive device
  checking V25.42
  insertion V25.1
  in situ V45.51
  management V25.42
  prescription V25.02
    repeat V25.42
  reinsertion V25.42
  removal V25.42
Intraventricular —*see* condition
Intrinsic deformity —*see* Deformity
Intruded tooth 524.34
Intrusion, repetitive, of sleep (due to
    environmental disturbances) (with atypical
    polysomnographic features) 307.48
Intumescent, lens (eye) NEC 366.9
  senile 366.12
Intussusception (colon) (enteric) (intestine)
    (rectum) 560.0
  appendix 543.9
  congenital 751.5
  fallopian tube 620.8
  ileocecal 560.0
  ileocolic 560.0
  ureter (with obstruction) 593.4
Invagination
  basilar 756.0
  colon or intestine 560.0
Invalid (since birth) 799.89
Invalidism (chronic) 799.89
Inversion
  albumin-globulin (A-G) ratio 273.8
  bladder 596.8
  cecum (*see also* Intussusception) 560.0
  cervix 622.8

Inversion—*continued*
  nipple 611.79
    congenital 757.6
    puerperal, postpartum 676.3
  optic papilla 743.57
  organ or site, congenital NEC—*see* Anomaly, specified type NEC
  sleep rhythm 327.39
    nonorganic origin 307.45
  testis (congenital) 752.51
  uterus (postinfectional) (postpartal, old) 621.7
    chronic 621.7
    complicating delivery 665.2
      affecting fetus or newborn 763.89
  vagina—*see* Prolapse, vagina
Investigation
  allergens V72.7
  clinical research (control) (normal comparison) (participant) V70.7
Inviability —*see* Immaturity
Involuntary movement, abnormal 781.0
Involution, involutional —*see also* condition
  breast, cystic or fibrocystic 610.1
  depression (*see also* Psychosis, affective) 296.2
    recurrent episode 296.3
    single episode 296.2
  melancholia (*see also* Psychosis, affective) 296.2
    recurrent episode 296.3
    single episode 296.2
  ovary, senile 620.3
  paranoid state (reaction) 297.2
  paraphrenia (climacteric) (menopause) 297.2
  psychosis 298.8
  thymus failure 254.8
IQ
  under 20 318.2
  20-34 318.1
  35-49 318.0
  50-70 317
IRDS 769
Irideremia 743.45
Iridis rubeosis 364.42
  diabetic 250.5 *[364.42]*
Iridochoroiditis (panuveitis) 360.12
Iridocyclitis NEC 364.3
  acute 364.00
    primary 364.01
    recurrent 364.02
  chronic 364.10
    in
      lepromatous leprosy 030.0 *[364.11]*
      sarcoidosis 135 *[364.11]*
      tuberculosis (*see also* Tuberculosis) 017.3 *[364.11]*
  due to allergy 364.04
  endogenous 364.01
  gonococcal 098.41
  granulomatous 364.10
  herpetic (simplex) 054.44
    zoster 053.22
  hypopyon 364.05
  lens induced 364.23
  nongranulomatous 364.00
  primary 364.01
  recurrent 364.02
  rheumatic 364.10
  secondary 364.04
    infectious 364.03
    noninfectious 364.04
  subacute 364.00
    primary 364.01

Iridocyclitis—*continued*
    recurrent 364.02
  sympathetic 360.11
  syphilitic (secondary) 091.52
  tuberculous (chronic) (*see also* Tuberculosis) 017.3 *[364.11]*
Iridocyclochoroiditis (panuveitis) 360.12
Iridodialysis 364.76
Iridodonesis 364.89
Iridoplegia (complete) (partial) (reflex) 379.49
Iridoschisis 364.52
Iris —*see* condition
Iritis 364.3
  acute 364.00
    primary 364.01
    recurrent 364.02
  chronic 364.10
    in
      sarcoidosis 135 *[364.11]*
      tuberculosis (*see also* Tuberculosis) 017.3 *[364.11]*
  diabetic 250.5 *[364.42]*
  due to
    allergy 364.04
    herpes simplex 054.44
    leprosy 030.0 *[364.11]*
  endogenous 364.01
  gonococcal 098.41
  gouty 274.89 *[364.11]*
  granulomatous 364.10
  hypopyon 364.05
  lens induced 364.23
  nongranulomatous 364.00
  papulosa 095.8 *[364.11]*
  primary 364.01
  recurrent 364.02
  rheumatic 364.10
  secondary 364.04
    infectious 364.03
    noninfectious 364.04
  subacute 364.00
    primary 364.01
    recurrent 364.02
  sympathetic 360.11
  syphilitic (secondary) 091.52
    congenital 090.0 *[364.11]*
    late 095.8 *[364.11]*
  tuberculous (*see also* Tuberculosis) 017.3 *[364.11]*
  uratic 274.89 *[364.11]*
Iron
  deficiency anemia 280.9
  metabolism disease 275.0
  storage disease 275.0
Iron-miners' lung 503
Irradiated enamel (tooth, teeth) 521.89
Irradiation
  burn—*see* Burn, by site
  effects, adverse 990
Irreducible, irreducibility —*see* condition
Irregular, irregularity
  action, heart 427.9
  alveolar process 525.8
  bleeding NEC 626.4
  breathing 786.09
  colon 569.89
  contour of cornea 743.41
    acquired 371.70
  dentin in pulp 522.3
  eye movements NEC 379.59
  menstruation (cause unknown) 626.4
  periods 626.4

INDEX TO DISEASES

Irregular, irregularity—*continued*
prostate 602.9
pupil 364.75
respiratory 786.09
septum (nasal) 470
shape, organ or site, congenital NEC—*see* Distortion
sleep-wake rhythm (non-24-hour) 327.39
   nonorganic origin 307.45
vertebra 733.99

Irritability (nervous) 799.2
bladder 596.8
   neurogenic 596.54
      with cauda equina syndrome 344.61
bowel (syndrome) 564.1
bronchial (*see also* Bronchitis) 490
cerebral, newborn 779.1
colon 564.1
   psychogenic 306.4
duodenum 564.89
heart (psychogenic) 306.2
ileum 564.89
jejunum 564.89
myocardium 306.2
rectum 564.89
stomach 536.9
   psychogenic 306.4
sympathetic (nervous system) (*see also* Neuropathy, peripheral, autonomic) 337.9
urethra 599.84
ventricular (heart) (psychogenic) 306.2

Irritable —*see* Irritability

Irritation
anus 569.49
axillary nerve 353.0
bladder 596.8
brachial plexus 353.0
brain (traumatic) (*see also* Injury, intracranial) 854.0
   nontraumatic—*see* Encephalitis
bronchial (*see also* Bronchitis) 490
cerebral (traumatic) (*see also* Injury, intracranial) 854.0
   nontraumatic—*see* Encephalitis
cervical plexus 353.2
cervix (*see also* Cervicitis) 616.0
choroid, sympathetic 360.11
cranial nerve—*see* Disorder, nerve, cranial
digestive tract 536.9
   psychogenic 306.4
gastric 536.9
   psychogenic 306.4
gastrointestinal (tract) 536.9
   functional 536.9
   psychogenic 306.4
globe, sympathetic 360.11
intestinal (bowel) 564.9
labyrinth 386.50
lumbosacral plexus 353.1
meninges (traumatic) (*see also* Injury, intracranial) 854.0
   nontraumatic—*see* Meningitis
myocardium 306.2
nerve—*see* Disorder, nerve
nervous 799.2
nose 478.19
penis 607.89
perineum 709.9
peripheral
   autonomic nervous system (*see also* Neuropathy, peripheral, autonomic) 337.9

Irritation—*continued*
nerve—*see* Disorder, nerve
peritoneum (*see also* Peritonitis) 567.9
pharynx 478.29
plantar nerve 355.6
spinal (cord) (traumatic)—*see also* Injury, spinal, by site
   nerve—*see also* Disorder, nerve
      root NEC 724.9
      traumatic—*see* Injury, nerve, spinal
   nontraumatic—*see* Myelitis
stomach 536.9
   psychogenic 306.4
sympathetic nerve NEC (*see also* Neuropathy, peripheral, autonomic) 337.9
ulnar nerve 354.2
vagina 623.9

Isambert's disease 012.3

Ischemia, ischemic 459.9
basilar artery (with transient neurologic deficit) 435.0
bone NEC 733.40
bowel (transient) 557.9
   acute 557.0
   chronic 557.1
   due to mesenteric artery insufficiency 557.1
brain—*see also* Ischemia, cerebral
   recurrent focal 435.9
cardiac (*see also* Ischemia, heart) 414.9
cardiomyopathy 414.8
carotid artery (with transient neurologic deficit) 435.8
cerebral (chronic) (generalized) 437.1
   arteriosclerotic 437.0
   intermittent (with transient neurologic deficit) 435.9
   newborn 779.2
   puerperal, postpartum, childbirth 674.0
   recurrent focal (with transient neurologic deficit) 435.9
   transient (with transient neurologic deficit) 435.9
colon 557.9
   acute 557.0
   chronic 557.1
   due to mesenteric artery insufficiency 557.1
coronary (chronic) (*see also* Ischemia, heart) 414.9
heart (chronic or with a stated duration of over 8 weeks) 414.9
   acute or with a stated duration of 8 weeks or less (*see also* Infarct, myocardium) 410.9
      without myocardial infarction 411.89
         with coronary (artery) occlusion 411.81
   subacute 411.89
intestine (transient) 557.9
   acute 557.0
   chronic 557.1
   due to mesenteric artery insufficiency 557.1
kidney 593.81
labyrinth 386.50
muscles, leg 728.89
myocardium, myocardial (chronic or with a stated duration of over 8 weeks) 414.8
   acute (*see also* Infarct, myocardium) 410.9
      without myocardial infarction 411.89
         with coronary (artery) occlusion 411.81
renal 593.81
retina, retinal 362.84
small bowel 557.9
   acute 557.0

Ischemia, ischemic—*continued*
  chronic 557.1
  due to mesenteric artery insufficiency 557.1
  spinal cord 336.1
  subendocardial (*see also* Insufficiency, coronary) 411.89
  vertebral artery (with transient neurologic deficit) 435.1
Ischialgia (*see also* Sciatica) 724.3
Ischiopagus 759.4
Ischium, ischial —*see* condition
Ischomenia 626.8
Ischuria 788.5
Iselin's disease or osteochondrosis 732.5
Islands of
  parotid tissue in
    lymph nodes 750.26
    neck structures 750.26
  submaxillary glands in
    fascia 750.26
    lymph nodes 750.26
    neck muscles 750.26
Islet cell tumor, pancreas (M8150/0) 211.7
Isoimmunization NEC (*see also* Incompatibility) 656.2
  anti-E 656.2
  fetus or newborn 773.2
    ABO blood groups 773.1
    Rhesus (Rh) factor 773.0
Isolation V07.0
  social V62.4
Isosporosis 007.2
Issue
  medical certificate NEC V68.09
    cause of death V68.09
    disability examination V68.01
    fitness V68.09
    incapacity V68.09
  repeat prescription NEC V68.1
    appliance V68.1
    contraceptive V25.40
      device NEC V25.49
        intrauterine V25.42
        specified type NEC V25.49
      pill V25.41
    glasses V68.1
    medicinal substance V68.1
Itch (*see also* Pruritus) 698.9
  bakers' 692.89
  barbers' 110.0
  bricklayers' 692.89
  cheese 133.8
  clam diggers' 120.3
  coolie 126.9
  copra 133.8
  Cuban 050.1
  dew 126.9
  dhobie 110.3
  eye 379.99
  filarial (*see also* Infestation, filarial) 125.9
  grain 133.8
  grocers' 133.8
  ground 126.9
  harvest 133.8
  jock 110.3
  Malabar 110.9
    beard 110.0
    foot 110.4
    scalp 110.0
  meaning scabies 133.0
  Norwegian 133.0

Itch —*continued*
  perianal 698.0
  poultrymen's 133.8
  sarcoptic 133.0
  scrub 134.1
  seven year V61.10
    meaning scabies 133.0
  straw 133.8
  swimmers' 120.3
  washerwoman's 692.4
  water 120.3
  winter 698.8
Itsenko-Cushing syndrome (pituitary basophilism) 255.0
Ivemark's syndrome (asplenia with congenital heart disease) 759.0
Ivory bones 756.52
Ixodes 134.8
Ixodiasis 134.8

J

Jaccoud's nodular fibrositis, chronic (Jaccoud's syndrome) 714.4
Jackson's
  membrane 751.4
  paralysis or syndrome 344.89
  veil 751.4
Jacksonian
  epilepsy (*see also* Epilepsy) 345.5
  seizures (focal) (*see also* Epilepsy) 345.5
Jacob's ulcer (M8090/3)—*see* Neoplasm, skin, malignant, by site
Jacquet's dermatitis (diaper dermatitis) 691.0
Jadassohn's
  blue nevus (M8780/0)—*see* Neoplasm, skin, benign
  disease (maculopapular erythroderma) 696.2
  intraepidermal epithelioma (M8096/0)—*see* Neoplasm, skin, benign
Jadassohn-Lewandowski syndrome (pachyonychia congenita) 757.5
Jadassohn-Pellizari's disease (anetoderma) 701.3
Jadassohn-Tièche nevus (M8780/0)—*see* Neoplasm, skin, benign
Jaffe-Lichtenstein (-Uehlinger) syndrome 252.01
Jahnke's syndrome (encephalocutaneous angiomatosis) 759.6
Jakob-Creutzfeldt disease (syndrome) (new variant) 046.1
  with dementia
    with behavioral disturbance 046.1 [294.11]
    without behavioral disturbance 046.1 [294.10]
Jaksch (-Luzet) disease or syndrome (pseudoleukemia infantum) 285.8
Jamaican
  neuropathy 349.82
  paraplegic tropical ataxic-spastic syndrome 349.82
Janet's disease (psychasthenia) 300.89
Janiceps 759.4
Jansky-Bielschowsky amaurotic familial idiocy 330.1
Japanese
  B type encephalitis 062.0
  river fever 081.2
  seven-day fever 100.89
Jaundice (yellow) 782.4
  acholuric (familial) (splenomegalic) (*see also* Spherocytosis) 282.0
    acquired 283.9
  breast milk 774.39
  catarrhal (acute) 070.1
    with hepatic coma 070.0
    chronic 571.9
    epidemic—*see* Jaundice, epidemic
  cholestatic (benign) 782.4
  chronic idiopathic 277.4
  epidemic (catarrhal) 070.1
    with hepatic coma 070.0
    leptospiral 100.0
    spirochetal 100.0
  febrile (acute) 070.1
    with hepatic coma 070.0
    leptospiral 100.0
    spirochetal 100.0
  fetus or newborn 774.6
    due to or associated with

Jaundice—*continued*
  ABO
    antibodies 773.1
    incompatibility, maternal/fetal 773.1
    isoimmunization 773.1
  absence or deficiency of enzyme system for bilirubin conjugation (congenital) 774.39
  blood group incompatibility NEC 773.2
  breast milk inhibitors to conjugation 774.39
    associated with preterm delivery 774.2
  bruising 774.1
  Crigler-Najjar syndrome 277.4 [774.31]
  delayed conjugation 774.30
    associated with preterm delivery 774.2
    development 774.39
  drugs or toxins transmitted from mother 774.1
  G-6-PD deficiency 282.2 [774.0]
  galactosemia 271.1 [774.5]
  Gilbert's syndrome 277.4 [774.31]
  hepatocellular damage 774.4
  hereditary hemolytic anemia (*see also* Anemia, hemolytic) 282.9 [774.0]
  hypothyroidism, congenital 243 [774.31]
  incompatibility, maternal/fetal NEC 773.2
  infection 774.1
  inspissated bile syndrome 774.4
  isoimmunization NEC 773.2
  mucoviscidosis 277.01 [774.5]
  obliteration of bile duct, congenital 751.61 [774.5]
  polycythemia 774.1
  preterm delivery 774.2
  red cell defect 282.9 [774.0]
  Rh
    antibodies 773.0
    incompatibility, maternal/fetal 773.0
    isoimmunization 773.0
  spherocytosis (congenital) 282.0 [774.0]
  swallowed maternal blood 774.1
  physiological NEC 774.6
  from injection, inoculation, infusion, or transfusion (blood) (plasma) (serum) (other substance) (onset within 8 months after administration)—*see* Hepatitis, viral
  Gilbert's (familial nonhemolytic) 277.4
  hematogenous 283.9
  hemolytic (acquired) 283.9
    congenital (*see also* Spherocytosis) 282.0
  hemorrhagic (acute) 100.0
    leptospiral 100.0
    newborn 776.0
    spirochetal 100.0
  hepatocellular 573.8
  homologous (serum)—*see* Hepatitis, viral
  idiopathic, chronic 277.4
  infectious (acute) (subacute) 070.1
    with hepatic coma 070.0
    leptospiral 100.0
    spirochetal 100.0
  leptospiral 100.0
  malignant (*see also* Necrosis, liver) 570
  newborn (physiological) (*see also* Jaundice, fetus or newborn) 774.6
  nonhemolytic, congenital familial (Gilbert's) 277.4
  nuclear, newborn (*see also* Kernicterus of newborn) 774.7

Jaundice—*continued*
  obstructive NEC (*see also* Obstruction, biliary) 576.8
  postimmunization—*see* Hepatitis, viral
  posttransfusion—*see* Hepatitis, viral
  regurgitation (*see also* Obstruction, biliary) 576.8
  serum (homologous) (prophylactic) (therapeutic)—*see* Hepatitis, viral
  spirochetal (hemorrhagic) 100.0
  symptomatic 782.4
    newborn 774.6
Jaw —*see* condition
Jaw-blinking 374.43
  congenital 742.8
Jaw-winking phenomenon or syndrome 742.8
Jealousy
  alcoholic 291.5
  childhood 313.3
  sibling 313.3
Jejunitis (*see also* Enteritis) 558.9
Jejunostomy status V44.4
Jejunum, jejunal —*see* condition
Jensen's disease 363.05
Jericho boil 085.1
Jerks, myoclonic 333.2
Jervell-Lange-Nielsen syndrome 426.82
Jeune's disease or syndrome (asphyxiating thoracic dystrophy) 756.4
Jigger disease 134.1
Job's syndrome (chronic granulomatous disease) 288.1
Jod-Basedow phenomenon 242.8
Johnson-Stevens disease (erythema multiforme exudativum) 695.1
Joint —*see also* condition
  Charcot's 094.0 *[713.5]*
  false 733.82
  flail—*see* Flail, joint
  mice—*see* Loose, body, joint, by site
  sinus to bone 730.9
  von Gies' 095.8
Jordan's anomaly or syndrome 288.2
Josephs-Diamond-Blackfan anemia (congenital hypoplastic) 284.01
Joubert syndrome 759.89
Jumpers' knee 727.2
Jungle yellow fever 060.0
Jüngling's disease (sarcoidosis) 135
Junin virus hemorrhagic fever 078.7
Juvenile —*see also* condition
  delinquent 312.9
    group (*see also* Disturbance, conduct) 312.2
    neurotic 312.4

K

Kabuki syndrome 759.89
Kahler (-Bozzolo) **disease** (multiple myeloma) (M9730/3) 203.0
Kakergasia 300.9
Kakke 265.0
Kala-azar (Indian) (infantile) (Mediterranean) (Sudanese) 085.0
Kalischer's syndrome (encephalocutaneous angiomatosis) 759.6
Kallmann's syndrome (hypogonadotropic hypogonadism with anosmia) 253.4
Kanner's syndrome (autism) (*see also* Psychosis, childhood) 299.0
Kaolinosis 502
Kaposi's
  disease 757.33
    lichen ruber 696.4
      acuminatus 696.4
      moniliformis 697.8
    xeroderma pigmentosum 757.33
  sarcoma (M9140/3) 176.9
    adipose tissue 176.1
    aponeurosis 176.1
    artery 176.1
    associated herpesvirus infection 058.89
    blood vessel 176.1
    bursa 176.1
    connective tissue 176.1
    external genitalia 176.8
    fascia 176.1
    fatty tissue 176.1
    fibrous tissue 176.1
    gastrointestinal tract NEC 176.3
    ligament 176.1
    lung 176.4
    lymph
      gland(s) 176.5
      node(s) 176.5
    lymphatic(s) NEC 176.1
    muscle (skeletal) 176.1
    oral cavity NEC 176.8
    palate 176.2
    scrotum 176.8
    skin 176.0
    soft tissue 176.1
    specified site NEC 176.8
    subcutaneous tissue 176.1
    synovia 176.1
    tendon (sheath) 176.1
    vein 176.1
    vessel 176.1
    viscera NEC 176.9
    vulva 176.8
  varicella-like eruption 054.0
  vaccinia 999.0
Kartagener's syndrome or triad (sinusitis, bronchiectasis, situs inversus) 759.3
Kasabach-Merritt syndrome (capillary hemangioma associated with thrombocytopenic purpura) 287.39
Kaschin-Beck disease (endemic polyarthritis)—*see* Disease, Kaschin-Beck
Kast's syndrome (dyschondroplasia with hemangiomas) 756.4
Katatonia (*see also* Schizophrenia) 295.2
Katayama disease or fever 120.2
Kathisophobia 781.0
Kawasaki disease 446.1

Kayser-Fleischer ring (cornea) (pseudosclerosis) 275.1 *[371.14]*
Kaznelson's syndrome (congenital hypoplastic anemia) 284.01
Kearns-Sayre syndrome 277.87
Kedani fever 081.2
Kelis 701.4
Kelly (-Patterson) **syndrome** (sideropenic dysphagia) 280.8
Keloid, cheloid 701.4
  Addison's (morphea) 701.0
  cornea 371.00
  Hawkins' 701.4
  scar 701.4
Keloma 701.4
Kenya fever 082.1
Keratectasia 371.71
  congenital 743.41
Keratinization NEC
  alveolar ridge mucosa
    excessive 528.72
    minimal 528.71
Keratitis (nodular) (nonulcerative) (simple) (zonular) NEC 370.9
  with ulceration (*see also* Ulcer, cornea) 370.00
  actinic 370.24
  arborescens 054.42
  areolar 370.22
  bullosa 370.8
  deep—*see* Keratitis, interstitial
  dendritic(a) 054.42
  desiccation 370.34
  diffuse interstitial 370.52
  disciform(is) 054.43
    varicella 052.7 *[370.44]*
  epithelialis vernalis 372.13 *[370.32]*
  exposure 370.34
  filamentary 370.23
  gonococcal (congenital) (prenatal) 098.43
  herpes, herpetic (simplex) NEC 054.43
    zoster 053.21
  hypopyon 370.04
  in
    chickenpox 052.7 *[370.44]*
    exanthema (*see also* Exanthem) 057.9 *[370.44]*
    paravaccinia (*see also* Paravaccinia) 051.9 *[370.44]*
    smallpox (*see also* Smallpox) 050.9 *[370.44]*
    vernal conjunctivitis 372.13 *[370.32]*
  interstitial (nonsyphilitic) 370.50
    with ulcer (*see also* Ulcer, cornea) 370.00
    diffuse 370.52
    herpes, herpetic (simplex) 054.43
      zoster 053.21
    syphilitic (congenital) (hereditary) 090.3
    tuberculous (*see also* Tuberculosis) 017.3 *[370.59]*
  lagophthalmic 370.34
  macular 370.22
  neuroparalytic 370.35
  neurotrophic 370.35
  nummular 370.22
  oyster-shuckers' 370.8
  parenchymatous—*see* Keratitis, interstitial
  petrificans 370.8
  phlyctenular 370.31

Keratitis—continued
  postmeasles 055.71
  punctata, punctate 370.21
    leprosa 030.0 [370.21]
    profunda 090.3
    superficial (Thygeson's) 370.21
  purulent 370.8
  pustuliformis profunda 090.3
  rosacea 695.3 [370.49]
  sclerosing 370.54
  specified type NEC 370.8
  stellate 370.22
  striate 370.22
  superficial 370.20
    with conjunctivitis (see also
        Keratoconjunctivitis) 370.40
    punctate (Thygeson's) 370.21
  suppurative 370.8
  syphilitic (congenital) (prenatal) 090.3
  trachomatous 076.1
    late effect 139.1
  tuberculous (phlyctenular) (see also
      Tuberculosis) 017.3 [370.31]
  ulcerated (see also Ulcer, cornea) 370.00
  vesicular 370.8
  welders' 370.24
  xerotic (see also Keratomalacia) 371.45
    vitamin A deficiency 264.4
Keratoacanthoma 238.2
Keratocele 371.72
Keratoconjunctivitis (see also Keratitis) 370.40
  adenovirus type 8 077.1
  epidemic 077.1
  exposure 370.34
  gonococcal 098.43
  herpetic (simplex) 054.43
    zoster 053.21
  in
    chickenpox 052.7 [370.44]
    exanthema (see also Exanthem) 057.9
        [370.44]
    paravaccinia (see also Paravaccinia) 051.9
        [370.44]
    smallpox (see also Smallpox) 050.9 [370.44]
  infectious 077.1
  neurotrophic 370.35
  phlyctenular 370.31
  postmeasles 055.71
  shipyard 077.1
  sicca (Sjögren's syndrome) 710.2
    not in Sjögren's syndrome 370.33
  specified type NEC 370.49
  tuberculous (phlyctenular) (see also
      Tuberculosis) 017.3 [370.31]
Keratoconus 371.60
  acute hydrops 371.62
  congenital 743.41
  stable 371.61
Keratocyst (dental) 526.0
Keratoderma, keratodermia (congenital)
    (palmaris et plantaris) (symmetrical) 757.39
  acquired 701.1
  blennorrhagica 701.1
    gonococcal 098.81
  climacterium 701.1
  eccentrica 757.39
  gonorrheal 098.81
  punctata 701.1
  tylodes, progressive 701.1
Keratodermatocele 371.72

Keratoglobus 371.70
  congenital 743.41
    associated with buphthalmos 743.22
Keratohemia 371.12
Keratoiritis (see also Iridocyclitis) 364.3
  syphilitic 090.3
  tuberculous (see also Tuberculosis) 017.3
      [364.11]
Keratolysis exfoliativa (congenital) 757.39
  acquired 695.89
  neonatorum 757.39
Keratoma 701.1
  congenital 757.39
  malignum congenitale 757.1
  palmaris et plantaris hereditarium 757.39
  senile 702.0
Keratomalacia 371.45
  vitamin A deficiency 264.4
Keratomegaly 743.41
Keratomycosis 111.1
  nigricans (palmaris) 111.1
Keratopathy 371.40
  band (see also Keratitis) 371.43
  bullous (see also Keratitis) 371.23
  degenerative (see also Degeneration, cornea)
      371.40
  hereditary (see also Dystrophy, cornea) 371.50
  discrete colliquative 371.49
Keratoscleritis, tuberculous (see also
    Tuberculosis) 017.3 [370.31]
Keratosis 701.1
  actinic 702.0
  arsenical 692.4
  blennorrhagica 701.1
    gonococcal 098.81
  congenital (any type) 757.39
  ear (middle) (see also Cholesteatoma) 385.30
  female genital (external) 629.89
  follicular, vitamin A deficiency 264.8
  follicularis 757.39
    acquired 701.1
    congenital (acneiformis) (Siemens') 757.39
    spinulosa (decalvans) 757.39
    vitamin A deficiency 264.8
  gonococcal 098.81
  larynx, laryngeal 478.79
  male genital (external) 608.89
  middle ear (see also Cholesteatoma) 385.30
  nigricans 701.2
    congenital 757.39
  obturans 380.21
  oral epithelium
    residual ridge mucosa
      excessive 528.72
      minimal 528.71
  palmaris et plantaris (symmetrical) 757.39
  penile 607.89
  pharyngeus 478.29
  pilaris 757.39
    acquired 701.1
  punctata (palmaris et plantaris) 701.1
  scrotal 608.89
  seborrheic 702.19
    inflamed 702.11
  senilis 702.0
  solar 702.0
  suprafollicularis 757.39
  tonsillaris 478.29
  vagina 623.1
  vegetans 757.39
  vitamin A deficiency 264.8
Kerato-uveitis (see also Iridocyclitis) 364.3

INDEX TO DISEASES

Keraunoparalysis 994.0
Kerion (celsi) 110.0
Kernicterus of newborn (not due to isoimmunization) 774.7
   due to isoimmunization (conditions classifiable to 773.0-773.2) 773.4
Ketoacidosis 276.2
   diabetic 250.1
Ketonuria 791.6
   branched-chain, intermittent 270.3
Ketosis 276.2
   diabetic 250.1
Kidney —*see* condition
Kienböck's
   disease 732.3
      adult 732.8
   osteochondrosis 732.3
Kimmelstiel (-Wilson) disease or syndrome (intercapillary glomerulosclerosis) 250.4 [581.81]
Kink, kinking
   appendix 543.9
   artery 447.1
   cystic duct, congenital 751.61
   hair (acquired) 704.2
   ileum or intestine (*see also* Obstruction, intestine) 560.9
   Lane's (*see also* Obstruction, intestine) 560.9
   organ or site, congenital NEC—*see* Anomaly, specified type NEC, by site
   ureter (pelvic junction) 593.3
      congenital 753.20
   vein(s) 459.2
      caval 459.2
      peripheral 459.2
Kinnier Wilson's disease (hepatolenticular degeneration) 275.1
Kissing
   osteophytes 721.5
   spine 721.5
   vertebra 721.5
Klauder's syndrome (erythema multiforme exudativum) 695.1
Kleb's disease (*see also* Nephritis) 583.9
Klein-Waardenburg syndrome (ptosisepicanthus) 270.2
Kleine-Levin syndrome 327.13
Kleptomania 312.32
Klinefelter's syndrome 758.7
Klinger's disease 446.4
Klippel's disease 723.8
Klippel-Feil disease or syndrome (brevicollis) 756.16
Klippel-Trenaunay syndrome 759.89
Klumpke (-Déjérine) palsy, paralysis (birth) (newborn) 767.6
Klüver-Bucy (-Terzian) syndrome 310.0
Knee —*see* condition
Knifegrinders' rot (*see also* Tuberculosis) 011.4
Knock-knee (acquired) 736.41
   congenital 755.64
Knot
   intestinal, syndrome (volvulus) 560.2
   umbilical cord (true) 663.2
      affecting fetus or newborn 762.5
Knots, surfer 919.8
   infected 919.9
Knotting (of)
   hair 704.2
   intestine 560.2
Knuckle pads (Garrod's) 728.79

Köbner's disease (epidermolysis bullosa) 757.39
Koch's
   infection (*see also* Tuberculosis, pulmonary) 011.9
   relapsing fever 087.9
Koch-Weeks conjunctivitis 372.03
Koenig-Wichman disease (pemphigus) 694.4
Köhler's disease (osteochondrosis) 732.5
   first (osteochondrosis juvenilis) 732.5
   second (Freiburg's infarction, metatarsal head) 732.5
   patellar 732.4
   tarsal navicular (bone) (osteoarthosis juvenilis) 732.5
Köhler-Mouchet disease (osteoarthrosis juvenilis) 732.5
Köhler-Pellegrini-Stieda disease or syndrome (calcification, knee joint) 726.62
Koilonychia 703.8
   congenital 757.5
Kojevnikov's, Kojewnikoff's epilepsy (*see also* Epilepsy) 345.7
König's
   disease (osteochondritis dissecans) 732.7
   syndrome 564.89
Koniophthisis (*see also* Tuberculosis) 011.4
Koplik's spots 055.9
Kopp's asthma 254.8
Korean hemorrhagic fever 078.6
Korsakoff (-Wernicke) disease, psychosis, or syndrome (nonalcoholic) 294.0
   alcoholic 291.1
Korsakov's disease —*see* Korsakoff's disease
Korsakow's disease —*see* Korsakoff's disease
Kostmann's disease or syndrome (infantile genetic agranulocytosis) 288.01
Krabbe's
   disease (leukodystrophy) 330.0
   syndrome
      congenital muscle hypoplasia 756.89
      cutaneocerebral angioma 759.6
Kraepelin-Morel disease (*see also* Schizophrenia) 295.9
Kraft-Weber-Dimitri disease 759.6
Kraurosis
   ani 569.49
   penis 607.0
   vagina 623.8
   vulva 624.09
Kreotoxism 005.9
Krukenberg's
   spindle 371.13
   tumor (M8490/6) 198.6
Kufs' disease 330.1
Kugelberg-Welander disease 335.11
Kuhnt-Junius degeneration or disease 362.52
Kulchitsky's cell carcinoma (carcinoid tumor of intestine) 259.2
Kümmell's disease or spondylitis 721.7
Kundrat's disease (lymphosarcoma) 200.1
Kunekune —*see* Dermatophytosis
Kunkel syndrome (lupoid hepatitis) 571.49
Kupffer cell sarcoma (M9124/3) 155.0
Kuru 046.0
Kussmaul's
   coma (diabetic) 250.3
   disease (polyarteritis nodosa) 446.0
   respiration (air hunger) 786.09
Kwashiorkor (marasmus type) 260
Kyasanur Forest disease 065.2

Kyphoscoliosis, kyphoscoliotic (acquired) (see also Scoliosis) 737.30
  congenital 756.19
  due to radiation 737.33
  heart (disease) 416.1
  idiopathic 737.30
    infantile
      progressive 737.32
      resolving 737.31
  late effect of rickets 268.1 *[737.43]*
  specified NEC 737.39
  thoracogenic 737.34
  tuberculous (see also Tuberculosis) 015.0
    [737.43]
Kyphosis, kyphotic (acquired) (postural) 737.10
  adolescent postural 737.0
  congenital 756.19
  dorsalis juvenilis 732.0
  due to or associated with
    Charcot-Marie-Tooth disease 356.1 *[737.41]*
    mucopolysaccharidosis 277.5 *[737.41]*
    neurofibromatosis 237.71 *[737.41]*
    osteitis
      deformans 731.0 *[737.41]*
      fibrosa cystica 252.01 *[737.41]*
    osteoporosis (see also Osteoporosis) 733.0
      [737.41]
    poliomyelitis (see also Poliomyelitis) 138
      [737.41]
    radiation 737.11
    tuberculosis (see also Tuberculosis) 015.0
      [737.41]
  Kümmell's 721.7
  late effect of rickets 268.1 *[737.41]*
  Morquio-Brailsford type (spinal) 277.5 *[737.41]*
  pelvis 738.6
  postlaminectomy 737.12
  specified cause NEC 737.19
  syphilitic, congenital 090.5 *[737.41]*
  tuberculous (see also Tuberculosis) 015.0
    [737.41]
Kyrle's disease (hyperkeratosis follicularis in cutem penetrans) 701.1

L

Labia, labium —*see* condition
Labiated hymen 752.49
Labile
  blood pressure 796.2
  emotions, emotionality 301.3
  vasomotor system 443.9
Labioglossal paralysis 335.22
Labium leporinum (*see also* Cleft, lip) 749.10
Labor (*see also* Delivery)
  with complications—*see* Delivery, complicated
  abnormal NEC 661.9
    affecting fetus or newborn 763.7
  arrested active phase 661.1
    affecting fetus or newborn 763.7
  desultory 661.2
    affecting fetus or newborn 763.7
  dyscoordinate 661.4
    affecting fetus or newborn 763.7
  early onset (22-36 weeks gestation) 644.2
  failed
    induction 659.1
      mechanical 659.0
      medical 659.1
      surgical 659.0
    trial (vaginal delivery) 660.6
  false 644.1
  forced or induced, affecting fetus or newborn 763.89
  hypertonic 661.4
    affecting fetus or newborn 763.7
  hypotonic 661.2
    affecting fetus or newborn 763.7
    primary 661.0
      affecting fetus or newborn 763.7
    secondary 661.1
      affecting fetus or newborn 763.7
  incoordinate 661.4
    affecting fetus or newborn 763.7
  irregular 661.2
    affecting fetus or newborn 763.7
  long—*see* Labor, prolonged
  missed (at or near term) 656.4
  obstructed NEC 660.9
    affecting fetus or newborn 763.1
    due to female genital mutilation 660.8
    specified cause NEC 660.8
      affecting fetus or newborn 763.1
  pains, spurious 644.1
  precipitate 661.3
    affecting fetus or newborn 763.6
  premature 644.2
    threatened 644.0
  prolonged or protracted 662.1
    affecting fetus or newborn 763.89
    first stage 662.0
      affecting fetus or newborn 763.89
    second stage 662.2
      affecting fetus or newborn 763.89
  threatened NEC 644.1
  undelivered 644.1
Labored breathing (*see also* Hyperventilation) 786.09

Labyrinthitis (inner ear) (destructive) (latent) 386.30
  circumscribed 386.32
  diffuse 386.31
  focal 386.32
  purulent 386.33
  serous 386.31
  suppurative 386.33
  syphilitic 095.8
  toxic 386.34
  viral 386.35
Laceration —*see also* Wound, open, by site
  accidental, complicating surgery 998.2
  Achilles tendon 845.09
    with open wound 892.2
  anus (sphincter) 879.6
    with
      abortion—*see* Abortion, by type, with damage to pelvic organs
      ectopic pregnancy (*see also* categories 633.0-633.9) 639.2
      molar pregnancy (*see also* categories 630-632) 639.2
    complicated 879.7
    complicating delivery (healed) (old) 654.8
      with laceration of anal or rectal mucosa 664.3
      not associated with third-degree perineal laceration 664.6
    following
      abortion 639.2
      ectopic or molar pregnancy 639.2
    nontraumatic, nonpuerperal (healed) (old) 569.43
  bladder (urinary)
    with
      abortion—*see* Abortion, by type, with damage to pelvic organs
      ectopic pregnancy (*see also* categories 633.0-633.9) 639.2
      molar pregnancy (*see also* categories 630-632) 639.2
    following
      abortion 639.2
      ectopic or molar pregnancy 639.2
    obstetrical trauma 665.5
  blood vessel—*see* Injury, blood vessel, by site
  bowel
    with
      abortion—*see* Abortion, by type, with damage to pelvic organs
      ectopic pregnancy (*see also* categories 633.0-633.9) 639.2
      molar pregnancy (*see also* categories 630-632) 639.2
    following
      abortion 639.2
      ectopic or molar pregnancy 639.2
    obstetrical trauma 665.5
  brain (with hemorrhage) (cerebral) (membrane) 851.8

Laceration

Laceration—*continued*

> Note—Use the following fifth-digit subclassification with categories 851-854:
>
> 0 unspecified state of consciousness
> 1 with no loss of consciousness
> 2 with brief [less than one hour] loss of consciousness
> 3 with moderate [1-24 hours] loss of consciousness
> 4 with prolonged [more than 24 hours] loss of consciousness and return to pre-existing conscious level
> 5 with prolonged [more than 24 hours] loss of consciousness, without return to pre-existing conscious level
>
> Use fifth-digit 5 to designate when a patient is unconscious and dies before regaining consciousness, regardless of the duration of the loss of consciousness
>
> 6 with loss of consciousness of unspecified duration
> 9 with concussion, unspecified

with
  open intracranial wound 851.9
  skull fracture—*see* Fracture, skull, by site
cerebellum 851.6
  with open intracranial wound 851.7
cortex 851.2
  with open intracranial wound 851.3
during birth 767.0
stem 851.6
  with open intracranial wound 851.7
broad ligament
  with
    abortion—*see* Abortion, by type, with damage to pelvic organs
    ectopic pregnancy (*see also* categories 633.0-633.9) 639.2
    molar pregnancy (*see also* categories 630-632) 639.2
  following
    abortion 639.2
    ectopic or molar pregnancy 639.2
  nontraumatic 620.6
  obstetrical trauma 665.6
  syndrome (nontraumatic) 620.6
capsule, joint—*see* Sprain, by site
cardiac—*see* Laceration, heart
causing eversion of cervix uteri (old) 622.0
central, complicating delivery 664.4
cerebellum—*see* Laceration, brain, cerebellum
cerebral—*see also* Laceration, brain
  during birth 767.0
cervix (uteri)
  with
    abortion—*see* Abortion, by type, with damage to pelvic organs
    ectopic pregnancy (*see also* categories 633.0-633.9) 639.2
    molar pregnancy (*see also* categories 630-632) 639.2
  following
    abortion 639.2
    ectopic or molar pregnancy 639.2
  nonpuerperal, nontraumatic 622.3
  obstetrical trauma (current) 665.3
  old (postpartal) 622.3
  traumatic—*see* Injury, internal, cervix
chordae heart 429.5

Laceration—*continued*
complicated 879.9
cornea—*see* Laceration, eyeball
  superficial 918.1
cortex (cerebral)—*see* Laceration, brain, cortex
esophagus 530.89
eye(s)—*see* Laceration, ocular
eyeball NEC 871.4
  with prolapse or exposure of intraocular tissue 871.1
  penetrating—*see* Penetrating wound, eyeball
  specified as without prolapse of intraocular tissue 871.0
eyelid NEC 870.8
  full thickness 870.1
    involving lacrimal passages 870.2
  skin (and periocular area) 870.0
  penetrating—*see* Penetrating wound, orbit
fourchette
  with
    abortion—*see* Abortion, by type, with damage to pelvic organs
    ectopic pregnancy (*see also* categories 633.0-633.9) 639.2
    molar pregnancy (*see also* categories 630-632) 639.2
  complicating delivery 664.0
  following
    abortion 639.2
    ectopic or molar pregnancy 639.2
heart (without penetration of heart chambers) 861.02
  with
    open wound into thorax 861.12
    penetration of heart chambers 861.03
      with open wound into thorax 861.13
hernial sac—*see* Hernia, by site
internal organ (abdomen) (chest) (pelvis)
  NEC—*see* Injury, internal, by site
kidney (parenchyma) 866.02
  with
    complete disruption of parenchyma (rupture) 866.03
    with open wound into cavity 866.13
    open wound into cavity 866.12
labia
  complicating delivery 664.0
ligament—*see also* Sprain, by site
  with open wound—*see* Wound, open, by site
liver 864.05
  with open wound into cavity 864.15
  major (disruption of hepatic parenchyma) 864.04
    with open wound into cavity 864.14
  minor (capsule only) 864.02
    with open wound into cavity 864.12
  moderate (involving parenchyma without major disruption) 864.03
    with open wound into cavity 864.13
  multiple 864.04
    with open wound into cavity 864.14
  stellate 864.04
    with open wound into cavity 864.14
lung 861.22
  with open wound into thorax 861.32
meninges—*see* Laceration, brain
meniscus (knee) (*see also* Tear, meniscus) 836.2
  old 717.5
  site other than knee—*see also* Sprain, by site
  old NEC (*see also* Disorder, cartilage, articular) 718.0

INDEX TO DISEASES — Laceration

Laceration—*continued*
  muscle—*see also* Sprain, by site
    with open wound—*see* Wound, open, by site
  myocardium—*see* Laceration, heart
  nerve—*see* Injury, nerve, by site
  ocular NEC (*see also* Laceration, eyeball) 871.4
    adnexa NEC 870.8
      penetrating 870.3
        with foreign body 870.4
    orbit (eye) 870.8
      penetrating 870.3
        with foreign body 870.4
  pelvic
    floor (muscles)
      with
        abortion—*see* Abortion, by type, with damage to pelvic organs
        ectopic pregnancy (*see also* categories 633.0-633.9) 639.2
        molar pregnancy (*see also* categories 630-632) 639.2
      complicating delivery 664.1
      following
        abortion 639.2
        ectopic or molar pregnancy 639.2
      nonpuerperal 618.7
      old (postpartal) 618.7
    organ NEC
      with
        abortion—*see* Abortion, by type, with damage to pelvic organs
        ectopic pregnancy (*see also* categories 633.0-633.9) 639.2
        molar pregnancy (*see also* categories 630-632) 639.2
      complicating delivery 665.5
        affecting fetus or newborn 763.89
      following
        abortion 639.2
        ectopic or molar pregnancy 639.2
      obstetrical trauma 665.5
  perineum, perineal (old) (postpartal) 618.7
    with
      abortion—*see* Abortion, by type, with damage to pelvic floor
      ectopic pregnancy (*see also* categories 633.0-633.9) 639.2
      molar pregnancy (*see also* categories 630-632) 639.2
    complicating delivery 664.4
      first degree 664.0
      second degree 664.1
      third degree 664.2
      fourth degree 664.3
      central 664.4
      involving
        anal sphincter (healed) (old) 654.8
          not associated with third-degree perineal laceration 664.6
        fourchette 664.0
        hymen 664.0
        labia 664.0
        pelvic floor 664.1
        perineal muscles 664.1
        rectovaginal septum 664.2
          with anal mucosa 664.3
        skin 664.0
        sphincter (anal) (healed) (old) 654.8
          not associated with third-degree perineal laceration 664.6
          with anal mucosa 664.3

Laceration—*continued*
      vagina 664.0
      vaginal muscles 664.1
      vulva 664.0
    secondary 674.2
    following
      abortion 639.2
      ectopic or molar pregnancy 639.2
    male 879.6
      complicated 879.7
    muscles, complicating delivery 664.1
    nonpuerperal, current injury 879.6
      complicated 879.7
    secondary (postpartal) 674.2
  peritoneum
    with
      abortion—*see* Abortion, by type, with damage to pelvic organs
      ectopic pregnancy (*see also* categories 633.0-633.9) 639.2
      molar pregnancy (*see also* categories 630-632) 639.2
    following
      abortion 639.2
      ectopic or molar pregnancy 639.2
    obstetrical trauma 665.5
  periurethral tissue
    with
      abortion—*see* Abortion, by type, with damage to pelvic organs
      ectopic pregnancy (*see also* categories 633.0-633.9) 639.2
      molar pregnancy (*see also* categories 630-632) 639.2
    following
      abortion 639.2
      ectopic or molar pregnancy 639.2
    obstetrical trauma 665.5
  rectovaginal (septum)
    with
      abortion—*see* Abortion, by type, with damage to pelvic organs
      ectopic pregnancy (*see also* categories 633.0-633.9) 639.2
      molar pregnancy (*see also* categories 630-632) 639.2
    complicating delivery 665.4
      with perineum 664.2
        involving anal or rectal mucosa 664.3
    following
      abortion 639.2
      ectopic or molar pregnancy 639.2
    nonpuerperal 623.4
    old (postpartal) 623.4
  spinal cord (meninges)—*see also* Injury, spinal, by site
    due to injury at birth 767.4
    fetus or newborn 767.4
  spleen 865.09
    with
      disruption of parenchyma (massive) 865.04
        with open wound into cavity 865.14
      open wound into cavity 865.19
    capsule (without disruption of parenchyma) 865.02
      with open wound into cavity 865.12
    parenchyma 865.03
      with open wound into cavity 865.13
    massive disruption (rupture) 865.04
      with open wound into cavity 865.14

Laceration—*continued*
  tendon 848.9
    with open wound—*see* Wound, open, by site
    Achilles 845.09
      with open wound 892.2
    lower limb NEC 844.9
      with open wound NEC 894.2
    upper limb NEC 840.9
      with open wound NEC 884.2
  tentorium cerebelli—*see* Laceration, brain, cerebellum
  tongue 873.64
    complicated 873.74
  urethra
    with
      abortion—*see* Abortion, by type, with damage to pelvic organs
      ectopic pregnancy (*see also* categories 633.0- 633.9) 639.2
      molar pregnancy (*see also* categories 630-632) 639.2
    following
      abortion 639.2
      ectopic or molar pregnancy 639.2
    nonpuerperal, nontraumatic 599.84
    obstetrical trauma 665.5
  uterus
    with
      abortion—*see* Abortion, by type, with damage to pelvic organs
      ectopic pregnancy (*see also* categories 633.0-633.9) 639.2
      molar pregnancy (*see also* categories 630-632) 639.2
    following
      abortion 639.2
      ectopic or molar pregnancy 639.2
    nonpuerperal, nontraumatic 621.8
    obstetrical trauma NEC 665.5
    old (postpartal) 621.8
  vagina
    with
      abortion—*see* Abortion, by type, with damage to pelvic organs
      ectopic pregnancy (*see also* categories 633.0-633.9) 639.2
      molar pregnancy (*see also* categories 630-632) 639.2
      perineal involvement, complicating delivery 664.0
    complicating delivery 665.4
      first degree 664.0
      second degree 664.1
      third degree 664.2
      fourth degree 664.3
      high 665.4
      muscles 664.1
      sulcus 665.4
      wall 665.4
    following
      abortion 639.2
      ectopic or molar pregnancy 639.2
    nonpuerperal, nontraumatic 623.4
    old (postpartal) 623.4
  valve, heart—*see* Endocarditis
  vulva
    with
      abortion—*see* Abortion, by type, with damage to pelvic organs
      ectopic pregnancy (*see also* categories 633.0-633.9) 639.2

Laceration—*continued*
    molar pregnancy (*see also* categories 630-632) 639.2
    complicating delivery 664.0
    following
      abortion 639.2
      ectopic or molar pregnancy 639.2
    nonpuerperal, nontraumatic 624.4
    old (postpartal) 624.4
Lachrymal —*see* condition
Lachrymonasal duct —*see* condition
Lack of
  adequate intermaxillary vertical dimension 524.36
  appetite (*see also* Anorexia) 783.0
  care
    in home V60.4
    of adult 995.84
    of infant (at or after birth) 995.52
  coordination 781.3
  development—*see also* Hypoplasia
    physiological in childhood 783.40
  education V62.3
  energy 780.79
  financial resources V60.2
  food 994.2
    in environment V60.8
  growth in childhood 783.43
  heating V60.1
  housing (permanent) (temporary) V60.0
    adequate V60.1
  material resources V60.2
  medical attention 799.89
  memory (*see also* Amnesia) 780.93
    mild, following organic brain damage 310.1
  ovulation 628.0
  person able to render necessary care V60.4
  physical exercise V69.0
  physiologic development in childhood 783.40
  posterior occlusal support 524.57
  prenatal care in current pregnancy V23.7
  shelter V60.0
  sleep V69.4
  water 994.3
Lacrimal —*see* condition
Lacrimation, abnormal (*see also* Epiphora) 375.20
Lacrimonasal duct —*see* condition
Lactation, lactating (breast) (puerperal) (postpartum)
  defective 676.4
  disorder 676.9
    specified type NEC 676.8
  excessive 676.6
  failed 676.4
  mastitis NEC 675.2
  mother (care and/or examination) V24.1
  nonpuerperal 611.6
  suppressed 676.5
Lacticemia 271.3
  excessive 276.2
Lactosuria 271.3
Lacunar skull 756.0
Laennec's cirrhosis (alcoholic) 571.2
  nonalcoholic 571.5
Lafora's disease 333.2
Lag, lid (nervous) 374.41
Lagleyze-von Hippel disease (retinocerebral angiomatosis) 759.6

INDEX TO DISEASES   **Laryngotracheitis**

Lagophthalmos (eyelid) (nervous) 374.20
  cicatricial 374.23
  keratitis (*see also* Keratitis) 370.34
  mechanical 374.22
  paralytic 374.21
La grippe —*see* Influenza
Lahore sore 085.1
Lakes, venous (cerebral) 437.8
Laki-Lorand factor deficiency (*see also* Defect, coagulation) 286.3
Lalling 307.9
Lambliasis 007.1
Lame back 724.5
Lancereaux's diabetes (diabetes mellitus with marked emaciation) 250.8 *[261]*
Landouzy-Déjérine dystrophy (fascioscapulohumeral atrophy) 359.1
Landry's disease or paralysis 357.0
Landry-Guillain-Barré syndrome 357.0
Lane's
  band 751.4
  disease 569.89
  kink (*see also* Obstruction, intestine) 560.9
Langdon Down's syndrome (mongolism) 758.0
Language abolition 784.69
Lanugo (persistent) 757.4
Laparoscopic surgical procedure converted to open procedure V64.41
Lardaceous
  degeneration (any site) 277.39
  disease 277.39
  kidney 277.39 *[583.81]*
  liver 277.39
Large
  baby (regardless of gestational age) 766.1
    exceptionally (weight of 4500 grams or more) 766.0
    of diabetic mother 775.0
  ear 744.22
  fetus—*see also* Oversize, fetus
    causing disproportion 653.5
      with obstructed labor 660.1
    for dates
      fetus or newborn (regardless of gestational age) 766.1
        affecting management of pregnancy 656.6
        exceptionally (weight of 4500 grams or more) 766.0
  physiological cup 743.57
  stature 783.9
  waxy liver 277.39
  white kidney—*see* Nephrosis
Larsen's syndrome (flattened facies and multiple congenital dislocations) 755.8
Larsen-Johansson disease (juvenile osteopathia patellae) 732.4
Larva migrans
  cutaneous NEC 126.9
    ancylostoma 126.9
  of Diptera in vitreous 128.0
  visceral NEC 128.0
Laryngeal —*see also* condition
  syncope 786.2
Laryngismus (acute) (infectious) (stridulous) 478.75
  congenital 748.3
  diphtheritic 032.3

Laryngitis (acute) (edematous) (fibrinous) (gangrenous) (infective) (infiltrative) (malignant) (membranous) (phlegmonous) (pneumococcal) (pseudomembranous) (septic) (subglottic) (suppurative) (ulcerative) (viral) 464.00
  with
    influenza, flu, or grippe 487.1
    obstruction 464.01
    tracheitis (*see also* Laryngotracheitis) 464.20
      with obstruction 464.21
      acute 464.20
        with obstruction 464.21
      chronic 476.1
  atrophic 476.0
  Borrelia vincentii 101
  catarrhal 476.0
  chronic 476.0
    with tracheitis (chronic) 476.1
    due to external agent—*see* Condition, respiratory, chronic, due to
  diphtheritic (membranous) 032.3
  due to external agent—*see* Inflammation, respiratory, upper, due to
  H. influenzae 464.00
    with obstruction 464.01
  Hemophilus influenzae 464.00
    with obstruction 464.01
  hypertrophic 476.0
  influenzal 487.1
  pachydermic 478.79
  sicca 476.0
  spasmodic 478.75
    acute 464.00
      with obstruction 464.01
  streptococcal 034.0
  stridulous 478.75
  syphilitic 095.8
    congenital 090.5
  tuberculous (*see also* Tuberculosis, larynx) 012.3
  Vincent's 101
Laryngocele (congenital) (ventricular) 748.3
Laryngofissure 478.79
  congenital 748.3
Laryngomalacia (congenital) 748.3
Laryngopharyngitis (acute) 465.0
  chronic 478.9
    due to external agent—*see* Condition, respiratory, chronic, due to
  due to external agent—*see* Inflammation, respiratory, upper, due to
  septic 034.0
Laryngoplegia (*see also* Paralysis, vocal cord) 478.30
Laryngoptosis 478.79
Laryngospasm 478.75
  due to external agent—*see* Condition, respiratory, acute, due to
Laryngostenosis 478.74
  congenital 748.3
Laryngotracheitis (acute) (infectional) (viral) (*see also* Laryngitis) 464.20
  with obstruction 464.21
  atrophic 476.1
  Borrelia vincentii 101
  catarrhal 476.1
  chronic 476.1
    due to external agent—*see* Condition, respiratory, chronic, due to
  diphtheritic (membranous) 032.3

1141

Laryngotracheitis—*continued*
due to external agent—*see* Inflammation, respiratory, upper, due to
H. influenzae 464.20
with obstruction 464.21
hypertrophic 476.1
influenzal 487.1
pachydermic 478.75
sicca 476.1
spasmodic 478.75
acute 464.20
with obstruction 464.21
streptococcal 034.0
stridulous 478.75
syphilitic 095.8
congenital 090.5
tuberculous (*see also* Tuberculosis, larynx) 012.3
Vincent's 101
Laryngotracheobronchitis (*see also* Bronchitis) 490
acute 466.0
chronic 491.8
viral 466.0
Laryngotracheobronchopneumonitis —*see* Pneumonia, broncho-
Larynx, laryngeal —*see* condition
Lasègue's disease (persecution mania) 297.9
Lassa fever 078.89
Lassitude (*see also* Weakness) 780.79
Late —*see also* condition
infant
post-term (gestation period over 40 completed weeks to 42 completed weeks) 766.21
prolonged gestation (period over 42 completed weeks) 766.22
Late effect(s) (of) —*see also* condition
abscess
intracranial or intraspinal (conditions classifiable to 324)–*see* category 326
adverse effect of drug, medicinal or biological substance 909.5
allergic reaction 909.9
amputation
postoperative (late) 997.60
traumatic (injury classifiable to 885-887 and 895-897) 905.9
burn (injury classifiable to 948-949) 906.9
extremities NEC (injury classifiable to 943 or 945) 906.7
hand or wrist (injury classifiable to 944) 906.6
eye (injury classifiable to 940) 906.5
face, head, and neck (injury classifiable to 941) 906.5
specified site NEC (injury classifiable to 942 and 946-947) 906.8
cerebrovascular disease (conditions classifiable to 430-437) 438.9
with
alterations of sensations 438.6
aphasia 438.11
apraxia 438.81
ataxia 438.84
cognitive deficits 438.0
disturbances of vision 438.7
dysphagia 438.82
dysphasia 438.12
facial droop 438.83
facial weakness 438.83

Late effect(s) (of)—*continued*
hemiplegia/hemiparesis
affecting
dominant side 438.21
nondominant side 438.22
unspecified side 438.20
monoplegia of lower limb
affecting
dominant side 438.41
nondominant side 438.42
unspecified side 438.40
monoplegia of upper limb
affecting
dominant side 438.31
nondominant side 438.32
unspecified side 438.30
paralytic syndrome NEC
affecting
bilateral 438.53
dominant side 438.51
nondominant side 438.52
unspecified side 438.50
speech and language deficit 438.10
specified type NEC 438.19
vertigo 438.85
specified type NEC 438.89
childbirth complication(s) 677
complication(s) of
childbirth 677
delivery 677
pregnancy 677
puerperium 677
surgical and medical care (conditions classifiable to 996-999) 909.3
trauma (conditions classifiable to 958) 908.6
contusion (injury classifiable to 920-924) 906.3
crushing (injury classifiable to 925-929) 906.4
delivery complication(s) 677
dislocation (injury classifiable to 830-839) 905.6
encephalitis or encephalomyelitis (conditions classifiable to 323)—*see* category 326
in infectious diseases 139.8
viral (conditions classifiable to 049.8, 049.9, 062-064) 139.0
external cause NEC (conditions classifiable to 995) 909.9
certain conditions classifiable to categories 991-994 909.4
foreign body in orifice (injury classifiable to 930-939) 908.5
fracture (multiple) (injury classifiable to 828-829) 905.5
extremity
lower (injury classifiable to 821-827) 905.4
neck of femur (injury classifiable to 820) 905.3
upper (injury classifiable to 810-819) 905.2
face and skull (injury classifiable to 800-804) 905.0
skull and face (injury classifiable to 800-804) 905.0
spine and trunk (injury classifiable to 805 and 807-809) 905.1
with spinal cord lesion (injury classifiable to 806) 907.2
infection
pyogenic, intracranial—*see* category 326
infectious diseases (conditions classifiable to 001-136) NEC 139.8
injury (injury classifiable to 959) 908.9
blood vessel 908.3

INDEX TO DISEASES   Leakage

Late effect(s) (of)—*continued*
    abdomen and pelvis (injury classifiable to 902) 908.4
    extremity (injury classifiable to 903-904) 908.3
    head and neck (injury classifiable to 900) 908.3
        intracranial (injury classifiable to 850-854) 907.0
            with skull fracture 905.0
        thorax (injury classifiable to 901) 908.4
    internal organ NEC (injury classifiable to 867 and 869) 908.2
        abdomen (injury classifiable to 863-866 and 868) 908.1
        thorax (injury classifiable to 860-862) 908.0
    intracranial (injury classifiable to 850-854) 907.0
        with skull fracture (injury classifiable to 800-801 and 803-804) 905.0
    nerve NEC (injury classifiable to 957) 907.9
        cranial (injury classifiable to 950-951) 907.1
        peripheral NEC (injury classifiable to 957) 907.9
            lower limb and pelvic girdle (injury classifiable to 956) 907.5
            upper limb and shoulder girdle (injury classifiable to 955) 907.4
        roots and plexus(es), spinal (injury classifiable to 953) 907.3
        trunk (injury classifiable to 954) 907.3
    pregnancy complication(s) 677
    puerperal complication(s) 677
    spinal
        cord (injury classifiable to 806 and 952) 907.2
        nerve root(s) and plexus(es) (injury classifiable to 953) 907.3
    superficial (injury classifiable to 910-919) 906.2
    tendon (tendon injury classifiable to 840-848, 880-884 with .2, and 890-894 with .2) 905.8
  meningitis
    bacterial (conditions classifiable to 320)—*see* category 326
    unspecified cause (conditions classifiable to 322)—*see* category 326
  myelitis (*see also* Late, effect(s) (of), encephalitis)—*see* category 326
  parasitic diseases (conditions classifiable to 001-136 NEC) 139.8
  phlebitis or thrombophlebitis of intracranial venous sinuses (conditions classifiable to 325)—*see* category 326
  poisoning due to drug, medicinal or biological substance (conditions classifiable to 960-979) 909.0
  poliomyelitis, acute (conditions classifiable to 045) 138
  radiation (conditions classifiable to 990) 909.2
  rickets 268.1
  sprain and strain without mention of tendon injury (injury classifiable to 840-848, except tendon injury) 905.7
  tendon involvement 905.8
  toxic effect of
    drug, medicinal or biological substance (conditions classifiable to 960-979) 909.0
    nonmedical substance (conditions classifiable to 980-989) 909.1

Late effect(s) (of)—*continued*
  trachoma (conditions classifiable to 076) 139.1
  tuberculosis 137.0
    bones and joints (conditions classifiable to 015) 137.3
    central nervous system (conditions classifiable to 013) 137.1
    genitourinary (conditions classifiable to 016) 137.2
    pulmonary (conditions classifiable to 010-012) 137.0
    specified organs NEC (conditions classifiable to 014, 017-018) 137.4
  viral encephalitis (conditions classifiable to 049.8, 049.9, 062-064) 139.0
  wound, open
    extremity (injury classifiable to 880-884 and 890-894, except .2) 906.1
        tendon (injury classifiable to 880-884 with .2 and 890-894 with .2) 905.8
    head, neck, and trunk (injury classifiable to 870-879) 906.0
Latent —*see* condition
Lateral —*see* condition
Laterocession —*see* Lateroversion
Lateroflexion —*see* Lateroversion
Lateroversion
  cervix—*see* Lateroversion, uterus
  uterus, uterine (cervix) (postinfectional) (postpartal, old) 621.6
    congenital 752.3
    in pregnancy or childbirth 654.4
        affecting fetus or newborn 763.89
Lathyrism 988.2
Launois' syndrome (pituitary gigantism) 253.0
Launois-Bensaude's lipomatosis 272.8
Launois-Cléret syndrome (adiposogenital dystrophy) 253.8
Laurence-Moon-Biedl syndrome (obesity, polydactyly, and mental retardation) 759.89
LAV (disease) (illness) (infection)—*see* Human immunodeficiency virus (disease) (illness) (infection)
LAV/HTLV-III (disease) (illness) (infection)—*see* Human immunodeficiency virus (disease) (illness) (infection)
Lawford's syndrome (encephalocutaneous angiomatosis) 759.6
Lax, laxity —*see also* Relaxation
  ligament 728.4
  skin (acquired) 701.8
    congenital 756.83
Laxative habit (*see also* Abuse, drugs, nondependent) 305.9
Lazy leukocyte syndrome 288.09
LCAD (long chain/very long chain acyl CoA dehydrogenase deficiency, VLCAD) 277.85
LCHAD (long chain 3-hydroxyacyl CoA dehydrogenase deficiency) 277.85
Lead —*see also* condition
  exposure to V15.86
  incrustation of cornea 371.15
  poisoning 984.9
    specified type of lead—*see* Table of drugs and chemicals
Lead miner's lung 503
Leakage
  amniotic fluid 658.1
    with delayed delivery 658.2
        affecting fetus or newborn 761.1
  bile from drainage tube (T tube) 997.4

Leakage—*continued*
  blood (microscopic), fetal, into maternal circulation 656.0
    affecting management of pregnancy or puerperium 656.0
  device, implant, or graft—*see* Complications, mechanical
  spinal fluid at lumbar puncture site 997.09
  urine, continuous 788.37
Leaky heart —*see* Endocarditis
Learning defect, specific NEC (strephosymbolia) 315.2
Leather bottle stomach (M8142/3) 151.9
Leber's
  congenital amaurosis 362.76
  optic atrophy (hereditary) 377.16
Lederer's anemia or disease (acquired infectious hemolytic anemia) 283.19
Lederer-Brill syndrome (acquired infectious hemolytic anemia) 283.19
Leeches (aquatic) (land) 134.2
Left-sided neglect 781.8
Leg —*see* condition
Legal investigation V62.5
Legg (-Calvé) -Perthes disease or syndrome (osteochondrosis, femoral capital) 732.1
Legionnaires' disease 482.84
Leigh's disease 330.8
Leiner's disease (exfoliative dermatitis) 695.89
Leiofibromyoma (M8890/0)—*see also* Leiomyoma
  uterus (cervix) (corpus) (*see also* Leiomyoma, uterus) 218.9
Leiomyoblastoma (M8891/1)—*see* Neoplasm, connective tissue, uncertain behavior
Leiomyofibroma (M8890/0)—*see also* Neoplasm, connective tissue, benign
  uterus (cervix) (corpus) (*see also* Leiomyoma, uterus) 218.9
Leiomyoma (M8890/0)—*see also* Neoplasm, connective tissue, benign
  bizarre (M8893/0)—*see* Neoplasm, connective tissue, benign
  cellular (M8892/1)—*see* Neoplasm, connective tissue, uncertain behavior
  epithelioid (M8891/1)—*see* Neoplasm, connective tissue, uncertain behavior
  prostate (polypoid) 600.20
    with
      other lower urinary tract symptoms (LUTS) 600.21
      urinary
        obstruction 600.21
        retention 600.21
  uterus (cervix) (corpus) 218.9
    interstitial 218.1
    intramural 218.1
    submucous 218.0
    subperitoneal 218.2
    subserous 218.2
  vascular (M8894/0)—*see* Neoplasm, connective tissue, benign
Leiomyomatosis (intravascular) (M8890/1)—*see* Neoplasm, connective tissue, uncertain behavior
Leiomyosarcoma (M8890/3)—*see also* Neoplasm, connective tissue, malignant
  epithelioid (M8891/3)—*see* Neoplasm, connective tissue, malignant

Leishmaniasis 085.9
  American 085.5
    cutaneous 085.4
    mucocutaneous 085.5
  Asian desert 085.2
  Brazilian 085.5
  cutaneous 085.9
    acute necrotizing 085.2
    American 085.4
    Asian desert 085.2
    diffuse 085.3
    dry form 085.1
    Ethiopian 085.3
    eyelid 085.5 *[373.6]*
    late 085.1
    lepromatous 085.3
    recurrent 085.1
    rural 085.2
    ulcerating 085.1
    urban 085.1
    wet form 085.2
    zoonotic form 085.2
  dermal—*see also* Leishmaniasis, cutaneous
    post kala-azar 085.0
  eyelid 085.5 *[373.6]*
  infantile 085.0
  Mediterranean 085.0
  mucocutaneous (American) 085.5
  naso-oral 085.5
  nasopharyngeal 085.5
  Old World 085.1
  tegumentaria diffusa 085.4
  vaccination, prophylactic (against) V05.2
  visceral (Indian) 085.0
Leishmanoid, dermal —*see also* Leishmaniasis, cutaneous
  post kala-azar 085.0
Leloir's disease 695.4
Lemiere syndrome 451.89
Lenegre's disease 426.0
Lengthening, leg 736.81
Lennox-Gastaut syndrome 345.0
  with tonic seizures 345.1
Lennox's syndrome (*see also* Epilepsy) 345.0
Lens —*see* condition
Lenticonus (anterior) (posterior) (congenital) 743.36
Lenticular degeneration, progressive 275.1
Lentiglobus (posterior) (congenital) 743.36
Lentigo (congenital) 709.09
  juvenile 709.09
  Maligna (M8742/2)—*see also* Neoplasm, skin, in situ
    melanoma (M8742/3)—*see* Melanoma
  senile 709.09
Leonine leprosy 030.0
Leontiasis
  ossium 733.3
  syphilitic 095.8
    congenital 090.5
Léopold-Lévi's syndrome (paroxysmal thyroid instability) 242.9
Lepore hemoglobin syndrome 282.49
Lepothrix 039.0
Lepra 030.9
  Willan's 696.1
Leprechaunism 259.8
Lepromatous leprosy 030.0
Leprosy 030.9
  anesthetic 030.1
  beriberi 030.1

INDEX TO DISEASES — Lesion(s)

Leprosy—*continued*
  borderline (group B) (infiltrated) (neuritic) 030.3
  cornea (*see also* Leprosy, by type) 030.9
    [371.89]
  dimorphous (group B) (infiltrated)
    (lepromatous) (neuritic) (tuberculoid) 030.3
  eyelid 030.0 *[373.4]*
  indeterminate (group I) (macular) (neuritic)
    (uncharacteristic) 030.2
  leonine 030.0
  lepromatous (diffuse) (infiltrated) (macular)
    (neuritic) (nodular) (type L) 030.0
  macular (early) (neuritic) (simple) 030.2
  maculoanesthetic 030.1
  mixed 030.0
  neuro 030.1
  nodular 030.0
  primary neuritic 030.3
  specified type or group NEC 030.8
  tubercular 030.1
  tuberculoid (macular) (maculoanesthetic)
    (major) (minor) (neuritic) (type T) 030.1
Leptocytosis, hereditary 282.49
Leptomeningitis (chronic) (circumscribed)
  (hemorrhagic) (nonsuppurative) (*see also*
  Meningitis) 322.9
  aseptic 047.9
    adenovirus 049.1
    Coxsackie virus 047.0
    ECHO virus 047.1
    enterovirus 047.9
    lymphocytic choriomeningitis 049.0
  epidemic 036.0
  late effect—*see* category 326
  meningococcal 036.0
  pneumococcal 320.1
  syphilitic 094.2
  tuberculous (*see also* Tuberculosis, meninges)
    013.0
Leptomeningopathy (*see also* Meningitis) 322.9
Leptospiral —*see* condition
Leptospirochetal —*see* condition
Leptospirosis 100.9
  autumnalis 100.89
  canicula 100.89
  grippotyphosa 100.89
  hebdomidis 100.89
  icterohemorrhagica 100.0
  nanukayami 100.89
  pomona 100.89
  Weil's disease 100.0
Leptothricosis —*see* Actinomycosis
Leptothrix infestation —*see* Actinomycosis
Leptotricosis —*see* Actinomycosis
Leptus dermatitis 133.8
Léri's pleonosteosis 756.89
Léri-Weill syndrome 756.59
Leriche syndrome (aortic bifurcation occlusion)
  444.0
Lermoyez's syndrome (*see also* Disease,
  Ménière's) 386.00
Lesbianism —*omit code*
  egodystonic 302.0
  problems with 302.0
Lesch-Nyhan syndrome (hypoxanthine-guanine-
  phosphoribosyltransferase deficiency) 277.2
Lesion(s)
  abducens nerve 378.54
  alveolar process 525.8
  anorectal 569.49
  aortic (valve)—*see* Endocarditis, aortic

Lesion(s)—*continued*
  auditory nerve 388.5
  basal ganglion 333.90
  bile duct (*see also* Disease, biliary) 576.8
  bladder 596.9
  bone 733.90
  brachial plexus 353.0
  brain 348.8
    congenital 742.9
    vascular (*see also* Lesion, cerebrovascular)
      437.9
      degenerative 437.1
      healed or old without residuals V12.54
      hypertensive 437.2
      late effect—*see* Late effect(s) (of)
        cerebrovascular disease
  buccal 528.9
  calcified—*see* Calcification
  canthus 373.9
  carate—*see* Pinta, lesions
  cardia 537.89
  cardiac—*see also* Disease, heart congenital 746.9
    valvular—*see* Endocarditis
  cauda equina 344.60
    with neurogenic bladder 344.61
  cecum 569.89
  cerebral—*see* Lesion, brain
  cerebrovascular (*see also* Disease,
    cerebrovascular NEC) 437.9
    degenerative 437.1
    healed or old without residuals V12.54
    hypertensive 437.2
    specified type NEC 437.8
  cervical root (nerve) NEC 353.2
  chiasmal 377.54
    associated with
      inflammatory disorders 377.54
      neoplasm NEC 377.52
      pituitary 377.51
      pituitary disorders 377.51
      vascular disorders 377.53
  chorda tympani 351.8
  coin, lung 793.1
  colon 569.89
  congenital—*see* Anomaly
  conjunctiva 372.9
  coronary artery (*see also* Ischemia, heart) 414.9
  cranial nerve 352.9
    first 352.0
    second 377.49
    third
      partial 378.51
      total 378.52
    fourth 378.53
    fifth 350.9
    sixth 378.54
    seventh 351.9
    eighth 388.5
    ninth 352.2
    tenth 352.3
    eleventh 352.4
    twelfth 352.5
  cystic—*see* Cyst
  degenerative—*see* Degeneration
  dermal (skin) 709.9
  Dieulafoy (hemorrhagic)
    of
      duodenum 537.84
      intestine 569.86
      stomach 537.84
  duodenum 537.89
    with obstruction 537.3

Lesion(s)

Lesion(s)—*continued*
- eyelid 373.9
- gasserian ganglion 350.8
- gastric 537.89
- gastroduodenal 537.89
- gastrointestinal 569.89
- glossopharyngeal nerve 352.2
- heart (organic)—*see also* Disease, heart
  - vascular—*see* Disease, cardiovascular
- helix (ear) 709.9
- high grade myelodysplastic syndrome 238.73
- hyperchromic, due to pinta (carate) 103.1
- hyperkeratotic (*see also* Hyperkeratosis) 701.1
- hypoglossal nerve 352.5
- hypopharynx 478.29
- hypothalamic 253.9
- ileocecal coil 569.89
- ileum 569.89
- iliohypogastric nerve 355.79
- ilioinguinal nerve 355.79
- in continuity—*see* Injury, nerve, by site
- inflammatory—*see* Inflammation
- intestine 569.89
- intracerebral—*see* Lesion, brain
- intrachiasmal (optic) (*see also* Lesion, chiasmal) 377.54
- intracranial, space-occupying NEC 784.2
- joint 719.90
  - ankle 719.97
  - elbow 719.92
  - foot 719.97
  - hand 719.94
  - hip 719.95
  - knee 719.96
  - multiple sites 719.99
  - pelvic region 719.95
  - sacroiliac (old) 724.6
  - shoulder (region) 719.91
  - specified site NEC 719.98
  - wrist 719.93
- keratotic (*see also* Keratosis) 701.1
- kidney (*see also* Disease, renal) 593.9
- laryngeal nerve (recurrent) 352.3
- leonine 030.0
- lip 528.5
- liver 573.8
- low grade myelodysplastic syndrome 238.72
- lumbosacral
  - plexus 353.1
  - root (nerve) NEC 353.4
- lung 518.89
  - coin 793.1
- maxillary sinus 473.0
- mitral—*see* Endocarditis, mitral
- motor cortex 348.8
- nerve (*see also* Disorder, nerve) 355.9
- nervous system 349.9
  - congenital 742.9
- nonallopathic NEC 739.9
  - in region (of)
    - abdomen 739.9
    - acromioclavicular 739.7
    - cervical, cervicothoracic 739.1
    - costochondral 739.8
    - costovertebral 739.8
    - extremity
      - lower 739.6
      - upper 739.7
    - head 739.0
    - hip 739.5
    - lower extremity 739.6

INDEX TO DISEASES

Lesion(s)—*continued*
- lumbar, lumbosacral 739.3
- occipitocervical 739.0
- pelvic 739.5
- pubic 739.5
- rib cage 739.8
- sacral, sacrococcygeal, sacroiliac 739.4
- sternochondral 739.8
- sternoclavicular 739.7
- thoracic, thoracolumbar 739.2
- upper extremity 739.7
- nose (internal) 478.19
- obstructive—*see* Obstruction
- obturator nerve 355.79
- occlusive
  - artery—*see* Embolism, artery
  - organ or site NEC—*see* Disease, by site
- osteolytic 733.90
- paramacular, of retina 363.32
- peptic 537.89
- periodontal, due to traumatic occlusion 523.8
- perirectal 569.49
- peritoneum (granulomatous) 568.89
- pigmented (skin) 709.00
- pinta—*see* Pinta, lesions
- polypoid—*see* Polyp
- prechiasmal (optic) (*see also* Lesion, chiasmal) 377.54
- primary—*see also* Syphilis, primary
  - carate 103.0
  - pinta 103.0
  - yaws 102.0
- pulmonary 518.89
  - valve (*see also* Endocarditis, pulmonary) 424.3
- pylorus 537.89
- radiation NEC 990
- radium NEC 990
- rectosigmoid 569.89
- retina, retinal—*see also* Retinopathy
  - vascular 362.17
- retroperitoneal 568.89
- romanus 720.1
- sacroiliac (joint) 724.6
- salivary gland 527.8
  - benign lymphoepithelial 527.8
- saphenous nerve 355.79
- secondary—*see* Syphilis, secondary
- sigmoid 569.89
- sinus (accessory) (nasal) (*see also* Sinusitis) 473.9
- skin 709.9
  - suppurative 686.00
- SLAP (superior glenoid labrum) 840.7
- space-occupying, intracranial NEC 784.2
- spinal cord 336.9
  - congenital 742.9
  - traumatic (complete) (incomplete) (transverse)—*see also* Injury, spinal, by site
    - with
      - broken
        - back—*see* Fracture, vertebra, by site, with spinal cord injury
        - neck—*see* Fracture, vertebra, cervical, with spinal cord injury
      - fracture, vertebra—*see* Fracture, vertebra, by site, with spinal cord injury
- spleen 289.50
- stomach 537.89
- superior glenoid labrum (SLAP) 840.7

INDEX TO DISEASES

Leukemia, leukemic

Lesion(s)—*continued*
  syphilitic—*see* Syphilis
  tertiary—*see* Syphilis, tertiary
  thoracic root (nerve) 353.3
  tonsillar fossa 474.9
  tooth, teeth 525.8
    white spot 521.01
  traumatic NEC (*see also* nature and site of injury) 959.9
  tricuspid (valve)—*see* Endocarditis, tricuspid
  trigeminal nerve 350.9
  ulcerated or ulcerative—*see* Ulcer
  uterus NEC 621.9
  vagina 623.8
  vagus nerve 352.3
  valvular—*see* Endocarditis
  vascular 459.9
    affecting central nervous system (*see also* Lesion, cerebrovascular) 437.9
    following trauma (*see also* Injury, blood vessel, by site) 904.9
    retina 362.17
    traumatic—*see* Injury, blood vessel, by site
  umbilical cord 663.6
    affecting fetus or newborn 762.6
  visual
    cortex NEC (*see also* Disorder, visual, cortex) 377.73
    pathway NEC (*see also* Disorder, visual, pathway) 377.63
  warty—*see* Verruca
  white spot, on teeth 521.01
  x-ray NEC 990
Lethargic —*see* condition
Lethargy 780.79
Letterer-Siwe disease (acute histiocytosis X) (M9722/3) 202.5
Leucinosis 270.3
Leucocoria 360.44
Leucosarcoma (M9850/3) 207.8
Leukasmus 270.2
Leukemia, leukemic (congenital) (M9800/3) 208.9

> Note—Use the following fifth-digit subclassification for categories 203-208:
>
> 0 without mention of remission
> 1 with remission

  acute NEC (M9801/3) 208.0
  aleukemic NEC (M9804/3) 208.8
    granulocytic (M9864/3) 205.8
  basophilic (M9870/3) 205.1
  blast (cell) (M9801/3) 208.0
  blastic (M9801/3) 208.0
    granulocytic (M9861/3) 205.0
  chronic NEC (M9803/3) 208.1
  compound (M9810/3) 207.8
  eosinophilic (M9880/3) 205.1
  giant cell (M9910/3) 207.2
  granulocytic (M9860/3) 205.9
    acute (M9861/3) 205.0
    aleukemic (M9864/3) 205.8
    blastic (M9861/3) 205.0
    chronic (M9863/3) 205.1
    subacute (M9862/3) 205.2
    subleukemic (M9864/3) 205.8
  hairy cell (M9940/3) 202.4
  hemoblastic (M9801/3) 208.0
  histiocytic (M9890/3) 206.9
  lymphatic (M9820/3) 204.9
    acute (M9821/3) 204.0

Leukemia, leukemic—*continued*
    aleukemic (M9824/3) 204.8
    chronic (M9823/3) 204.1
    subacute (M9822/3) 204.2
    subleukemic (M9824/3) 204.8
  lymphoblastic (M9821/3) 204.0
  lymphocytic (M9820/3) 204.9
    acute (M9821/3) 204.0
    aleukemic (M9824/3) 204.8
    chronic (M9823/3) 204.1
    subacute (M9822/3) 204.2
    subleukemic (M9824/3) 204.8
  lymphogenous (M9820/3)—*see* Leukemia, lymphoid
  lymphoid (M9820/3) 204.9
    acute (M9821/3) 204.0
    aleukemic (M9824/3) 204.8
    blastic (M9821/3) 204.0
    chronic (M9823/3) 204.1
    subacute (M9822/3) 204.2
    subleukemic (M9824/3) 204.8
  lymphosarcoma cell (M9850/3) 207.8
  mast cell (M9900/3) 207.8
  megakaryocytic (M9910/3) 207.2
  megakaryocytoid (M9910/3) 207.2
  mixed (cell) (M9810/3) 207.8
  monoblastic (M9891/3) 206.0
  monocytic (Schilling-type) (M9890/3) 206.9
    acute (M9891/3) 206.0
    aleukemic (M9894/3) 206.8
    chronic (M9893/3) 206.1
    Naegeli-type (M9863/3) 205.1
    subacute (M9892/3) 206.2
    subleukemic (M9894/3) 206.8
  monocytoid (M9890/3) 206.9
    acute (M9891/3) 206.0
    aleukemic (M9894/3) 206.8
    chronic (M9893/3) 206.1
    myelogenous (M9863/3) 205.1
    subacute (M9892/3) 206.2
    subleukemic (M9894/3) 206.8
  monomyelocytic (M9860/3)—*see* Leukemia, myelomonocytic
  myeloblastic (M9861/3) 205.0
  myelocytic (M9863/3) 205.1
    acute (M9861/3) 205.0
  myelogenous (M9860/3) 205.9
    acute (M9861/3) 205.0
    aleukemic (M9864/3) 205.8
    chronic (M9863/3) 205.1
    monocytoid (M9863/3) 205.1
    subacute (M9862/3) 205.2
    subleukemic (M9864) 205.8
  myeloid (M9860/3) 205.9
    acute (M9861/3) 205.0
    aleukemic (M9864/3) 205.8
    chronic (M9863/3) 205.1
    subacute (M9862/3) 205.2
    subleukemic (M9864/3) 205.8
  myelomonocytic (M9860/3) 205.9
    acute (M9861/3) 205.0
    chronic (M9863/3) 205.1
  Naegeli-type monocytic (M9863/3) 205.1
  neutrophilic (M9865/3) 205.1
  plasma cell (M9830/3) 203.1
  plasmacytic (M9830/3) 203.1
  prolymphocytic (M9825/3)—*see* Leukemia, lymphoid
  promyelocytic, acute (M9866/3) 205.0
  Schilling-type monocytic (M9890/3)—*see* Leukemia, monocytic

Leukemia, leukemic—*continued*
   stem cell (M9801/3) 208.0
   subacute NEC (M9802/3) 208.2
   subleukemic NEC (M9804/3) 208.8
   thrombocytic (M9910/3) 207.2
   undifferentiated (M9801/3) 208.0
Leukemoid reaction (basophilic) (lymphocytic) (monocytic) (myelocytic) (neutrophilic) 288.62
Leukoclastic vasculitis 446.29
Leukocoria 360.44
Leukocythemia —*see* Leukemia
Leukocytopenia 288.50
Leukocytosis 288.60
   basophilic 288.8
   eosinophilic 288.3
   lymphocytic 288.8
   monocytic 288.8
   neutrophilic 288.8
Leukoderma 709.09
   syphilitic 091.3
      late 095.8
Leukodermia (*see also* Leukoderma) 709.09
Leukodystrophy (cerebral) (globoid cell) (metachromatic) (progressive) (sudanophilic) 330.0
Leukoedema, mouth or tongue 528.79
Leukoencephalitis
   acute hemorrhagic (postinfectious) NEC 136.9 *[323.61]*
      postimmunization or postvaccinal 323.51
   subacute sclerosing 046.2
   van Bogaert's 046.2
   van Bogaert's (sclerosing) 046.2
Leukoencephalopathy (*see also* Encephalitis) 323.9
   acute necrotizing hemorrhagic (postinfectious) 136.9 *[323.61]*
      postimmunization or postvaccinal 323.51
   metachromatic 330.0
   multifocal (progressive) 046.3
   progressive multifocal 046.3
Leukoerythroblastosis 289.9
Leukoerythrosis 289.0
Leukokeratosis (*see also* Leukoplakia) 702.8
   mouth 528.6
   nicotina palati 528.79
   tongue 528.6
Leukokoria 360.44
Leukokraurosis vulva, vulvae 624.09
Leukolymphosarcoma (M9850/3) 207.8
Leukoma (cornea) (interfering with central vision) 371.03
   adherent 371.04
Leukomalacia, periventricular 779.7
Leukomelanopathy, hereditary 288.2
Leukonychia (punctata) (striata) 703.8
   congenital 757.5
Leukopathia
   unguium 703.8
      congenital 757.5
Leukopenia 288.50
   basophilic 288.59
   cyclic 288.02
   eosinophilic 288.59
   familial 288.59
   malignant (see also Agranulocytosis) 288.09
   periodic 288.02
   transitory neonatal 776.7
Leukopenic —*see* condition

Leukoplakia 702.8
   anus 569.49
   bladder (postinfectional) 596.8
   buccal 528.6
   cervix (uteri) 622.2
   esophagus 530.83
   gingiva 528.6
   kidney (pelvis) 593.89
   larynx 478.79
   lip 528.6
   mouth 528.6
   oral soft tissue (including tongue) (mucosa) 528.6
   palate 528.6
   pelvis (kidney) 593.89
   penis (infectional) 607.0
   rectum 569.49
   syphilitic 095.8
   tongue 528.6
   tonsil 478.29
   ureter (postinfectional) 593.89
   urethra (postinfectional) 599.84
   uterus 621.8
   vagina 623.1
   vesical 596.8
   vocal cords 478.5
   vulva 624.09
Leukopolioencephalopathy 330.0
Leukorrhea (vagina) 623.5
   due to trichomonas (vaginalis) 131.00
   trichomonal (Trichomonas vaginalis) 131.00
Leukosarcoma (M9850/3) 207.8
Leukosis (M9800/3)—*see* Leukemia
Lev's disease or syndrome (acquired complete heart block) 426.0
Levi's syndrome (pituitary dwarfism) 253.3
Levocardia (isolated) 746.87
   with situs inversus 759.3
Levulosuria 271.2
Lewandowski's disease (primary) (*see also* Tuberculosis) 017.0
Lewandowski-Lutz disease (epidermodysplasia verruciformis) 078.19
Lewy body dementia 331.82
Lewy body disease 331.82
Leyden's disease (periodic vomiting) 536.2
Leyden's-Möbius dystrophy 359.1
Leydig cell
   carcinoma (M8650/3)
      specified site—*see* Neoplasm, by site, malignant
      unspecified site
         female 183.0
         male 186.9
   tumor (M8650/1)
      benign (M8650/0)
         specified site—*see* Neoplasm, by site, benign
         unspecified site
            female 220
            male 222.0
      malignant (M8650/3)
         specified site—*see* Neoplasm, by site, malignant
         unspecified site
            female 183.0
            male 186.9
      specified site—*see* Neoplasm, by site, uncertain behavior
      unspecified site
         female 236.2
         male 236.4

INDEX TO DISEASES

Leydig-Sertoli cell tumor (M8631/0)
  specified site—*see* Neoplasm, by site, benign
  unspecified site
    female 220
    male 222.0
LGSIL (low grade squamous intraepithelial lesion) 795.03
Liar, pathologic 301.7
Libman-Sacks disease or syndrome 710.0 *[424.91]*
Lice (infestation) 132.9
  body (pediculus corporis) 132.1
  crab 132.2
  head (pediculus capitis) 132.0
  mixed (classifiable to more than one of the categories 132.0-132.2) 132.3
  pubic (pediculus pubis) 132.2
Lichen 697.9
  albus 701.0
  annularis 695.89
  atrophicus 701.0
  corneus obtusus 698.3
  myxedematous 701.8
  nitidus 697.1
  pilaris 757.39
    acquired 701.1
  planopilaris 697.0
  planus (acute) (chronicus) (hypertrophic) (verrucous) 697.0
  morphoeicus 701.0
  sclerosus (et atrophicus) 701.0
  ruber 696.4
    acuminatus 696.4
    moniliformis 697.8
    obtusus corneus 698.3
    of Wilson 697.0
    planus 697.0
    sclerosus (et atrophicus) 701.0
  scrofulosus (primary) (*see also* Tuberculosis) 017.0
  simplex (Vidal's) 698.3
    chronicus 698.3
    circumscriptus 698.3
  spinulosus 757.39
    mycotic 117.9
  striata 697.8
  urticatus 698.2
Lichenification 698.3
  nodular 698.3
Lichenoides tuberculosis (primary) (*see also* Tuberculosis) 017.0
Lichtheim's disease or syndrome (subacute combined sclerosis with pernicious anemia) 281.0 *[336.2]*
Lien migrans 289.59
Lientery (*see also* Diarrhea) 787.91
  infectious 009.2
Life circumstance problem NEC V62.89
Li-Fraumeni cancer syndrome V84.01
Ligament —*see* condition
Light-for-dates (infant) 764.0
  with signs of fetal malnutrition 764.1
  affecting management of pregnancy 656.5
Light-headedness 780.4
Lightning (effects) (shock) (stroke) (struck by) 994.0
  burn—*see* Burn, by site
  foot 266.2
Lightwood's disease or syndrome (renal tubular acidosis) 588.89
Lignac's disease (cystinosis) 270.0
Lignac (-de Toni) (-Fanconi) (-Debré) syndrome (cystinosis) 270.0

Lipogranuloma, sclerosing

Lignac (-Fanconi) syndrome (cystinosis) 270.0
Ligneous thyroiditis 245.3
Likoff's syndrome (angina in menopausal women) 413.9
Limb —*see* condition
Limitation of joint motion (*see also* Stiffness, joint) 719.5
  sacroiliac 724.6
Limit dextrinosis 271.0
Limited
  cardiac reserve—*see* Disease, heart
  duction, eye NEC 378.63
  mandibular range of motion 524.52
Lindau's disease (retinocerebral angiomatosis) 759.6
Lindau (-von Hippel) disease (angiomatosis retinocerebellosa) 759.6
Linea corneae senilis 371.41
Lines
  Beau's (transverse furrows on fingernails) 703.8
  Harris' 733.91
  Hudson-Stähli 371.11
  Stähli's 371.11
Lingua
  geographical 529.1
  nigra (villosa) 529.3
  plicata 529.5
    congenital 750.13
  tylosis 528.6
Lingual (tongue)—*see also* condition
  thyroid 759.2
Linitis (gastric) 535.4
  plastica (M8142/3) 151.9
Lioderma essentialis (cum melanosis et telangiectasia) 757.33
Lip —*see also* condition
  biting 528.9
Lipalgia 272.8
Lipedema —*see* Edema
Lipemia (*see also* Hyperlipidemia) 272.4
  retina, retinalis 272.3
Lipidosis 272.7
  cephalin 272.7
  cerebral (infantile) (juvenile) (late) 330.1
  cerebroretinal 330.1 *[362.71]*
  cerebroside 272.7
  cerebrospinal 272.7
  chemically-induced 272.7
  cholesterol 272.7
  diabetic 250.8 *[272.7]*
  dystopic (hereditary) 272.7
  glycolipid 272.7
  hepatosplenomegalic 272.3
  hereditary, dystopic 272.7
  sulfatide 330.0
Lipoadenoma (M8324/0)—*see* Neoplasm, by site, benign
Lipoblastoma (M8881/0)—*see* Lipoma, by site
Lipoblastomatosis (M8881/0)—*see* Lipoma, by site
Lipochondrodystrophy 277.5
Lipochrome histiocytosis (familial) 288.1
Lipodystrophia progressiva 272.6
Lipodystrophy (progressive) 272.6
  insulin 272.6
  intestinal 040.2
  mesenteric 567.82
Lipofibroma (M8851/0)—*see* Lipoma, by site
Lipoglycoproteinosis 272.8
Lipogranuloma, sclerosing 709.8

1149

Lipogranulomatosis (disseminated) 272.8
  kidney 272.8
Lipoid —*see* condition
  histiocytosis 272.7
    essential 272.7
  nephrosis (*see also* Nephrosis) 581.3
  proteinosis of Urbach 272.8
Lipoidemia (*see also* Hyperlipidemia) 272.4
Lipoidosis (*see also* Lipidosis) 272.7
Lipoma (M8850/0) 214.9
  breast (skin) 214.1
  face 214.0
  fetal (M8881/0)—*see also* Lipoma, by site
    fat cell (M8880/0)—*see* Lipoma, by site
  infiltrating (M8856/0)—*see* Lipoma, by site
  intra-abdominal 214.3
  intramuscular (M8856/0)—*see* Lipoma, by site
  intrathoracic 214.2
  kidney 214.3
  mediastinum 214.2
  muscle 214.8
  peritoneum 214.3
  retroperitoneum 214.3
  skin 214.1
    face 214.0
  spermatic cord 214.4
  spindle cell (M8857/0)—*see* Lipoma, by site
  stomach 214.3
  subcutaneous tissue 214.1
    face 214.0
  thymus 214.2
  thyroid gland 214.2
Lipomatosis (dolorosa) 272.8
  epidural 214.8
  fetal (M8881/0)—*see* Lipoma, by site
  Launois-Bensaude's 272.8
Lipomyohemangioma (M8860/0)
  specified site—*see* Neoplasm, connective tissue, benign
  unspecified site 223.0
Lipomyoma (M8860/0)
  specified site—*see* Neoplasm, connective tissue, benign
  unspecified site 223.0
Lipomyxoma (M8852/0)—*see* Lipoma, by site
Lipomyxosarcoma (M8852/3)—*see* Neoplasm, connective tissue, malignant
Lipophagocytosis 289.89
Lipoproteinemia (alpha) 272.4
  broad-beta 272.2
  floating-beta 272.2
  hyper-pre-beta 272.1
Lipoproteinosis (Rössle-Urbach-Wiethe) 272.8
Liposarcoma (M8850/3)—*see also* Neoplasm, connective tissue, malignant
  differentiated type (M8851/3)—*see* Neoplasm, connective tissue, malignant
  embryonal (M8852/3)—*see* Neoplasm, connective tissue, malignant
  mixed type (M8855/3)—*see* Neoplasm, connective tissue, malignant
  myxoid (M8852/3)—*see* Neoplasm, connective tissue, malignant
  pleomorphic (M8854/3)—*see* Neoplasm, connective tissue, malignant
  round cell (M8853/3)—*see* Neoplasm, connective tissue, malignant
  well differentiated type (M8851/3)—*see* Neoplasm, connective tissue, malignant
Liposynovitis prepatellaris 272.8

Lipping
  cervix 622.0
  spine (*see also* Spondylosis) 721.90
  vertebra (*see also* Spondylosis) 721.90
Lip pits (mucus), congenital 750.25
Lipschütz disease or ulcer 616.50
Lipuria 791.1
  bilharziasis 120.0
Liquefaction, vitreous humor 379.21
Lisping 307.9
Lissauer's paralysis 094.1
Lissencephalia, lissencephaly 742.2
Listerellose 027.0
Listeriose 027.0
Listeriosis 027.0
  congenital 771.2
  fetal 771.2
  suspected fetal damage affecting management of pregnancy 655.4
Listlessness 780.79
Lithemia 790.6
Lithiasis —*see also* Calculus
  hepatic (duct)—*see* Choledocholithiasis
  urinary 592.9
Lithopedion 779.9
  affecting management of pregnancy 656.8
Lithosis (occupational) 502
  with tuberculosis—*see* Tuberculosis, pulmonary
Lithuria 791.9
Litigation V62.5
Little
  league elbow 718.82
  stroke syndrome 435.9
Little's disease —*see* Palsy, cerebral
Littre's
  gland—*see* condition
  hernia—*see* Hernia, Littre's
Littritis (*see also* Urethritis) 597.89
Livedo 782.61
  annularis 782.61
  racemose 782.61
  reticularis 782.61
Live flesh 781.0
Liver —*see also* condition
  donor V59.6
Livida, asphyxia
  newborn 768.6
Living
  alone V60.3
  with handicapped person V60.4
Lloyd's syndrome 258.1
Loa loa 125.2
Loasis 125.2
Lobe, lobar —*see* condition
Lobo's disease or blastomycosis 116.2
Lobomycosis 116.2
Lobotomy syndrome 310.0
Lobstein's disease (brittle bones and blue sclera) 756.51
Lobster-claw hand 755.58
Lobulation (congenital)—*see also* Anomaly, specified type NEC, by site
  kidney, fetal 753.3
  liver, abnormal 751.69
  spleen 759.0
Lobule, lobular —*see* condition
Local, localized —*see* condition
Locked bowel or intestine (*see also* Obstruction, intestine) 560.9
Locked twins 660.5
  affecting fetus or newborn 763.1

INDEX TO DISEASES

Locked-in state 344.81
Locking
  joint (*see also* Derangement, joint) 718.90
    knee 717.9
Lockjaw (*see also* Tetanus) 037
Locomotor ataxia (progressive) 094.0
Löffler's
  endocarditis 421.0
  eosinophilia or syndrome 518.3
  pneumonia 518.3
  syndrome (eosinophilic pneumonitis) 518.3
Löfgren's syndrome (sarcoidosis) 135
Loiasis 125.2
  eyelid 125.2 *[373.6]*
Loneliness V62.89
Lone star fever 082.8
Long labor 662.1
  affecting fetus or newborn 763.89
  first stage 662.0
  second stage 662.2
Long-term (current) drug use V58.69
  antibiotics V58.62
  anticoagulants V58.61
  anti-inflammatories, non-steroidal (NSAID) V58.64
  antiplatelets/antithrombotics V58.63
    aspirin V58.66
  high-risk medications NEC V58.69
  insulin V58.67
  pain killers V58.69
    anti-inflammatory non-steroidal (NSAID) V58.64
    aspirin V58.66
  steroids V58.65
  tamoxifen V58.69
Longitudinal stripes or grooves, nails 703.8
  congenital 757.5
Loop
  intestine (*see also* Volvulus) 560.2
  intrascleral nerve 379.29
  vascular on papilla (optic) 743.57
Loose —*see also* condition
  body
    in tendon sheath 727.82
    joint 718.10
      ankle 718.17
      elbow 718.12
      foot 718.17
      hand 718.14
      hip 718.15
      knee 717.6
      multiple sites 718.19
      pelvic region 718.15
      prosthetic implant—*see* Complications, mechanical
      shoulder (region) 718.11
      specified site NEC 718.18
      wrist 718.13
    cartilage (joint) (*see also* Loose, body, joint) 718.1
      knee 717.6
    facet (vertebral) 724.9
    prosthetic implant—*see* Complications, mechanical
    sesamoid, joint (*see also* Loose, body, joint) 718.1
  tooth, teeth 525.8
Loosening epiphysis 732.9
Looser (-Debray) -Milkman syndrome (osteomalacia with pseudofractures) 268.2
Lop ear (deformity) 744.29

Lorain's disease or syndrome (pituitary dwarfism) 253.3
Lorain-Levi syndrome (pituitary dwarfism) 253.3
Lordosis (acquired) (postural) 737.20
  congenital 754.2
  due to or associated with
    Charcot-Marie-Tooth disease 356.1 *[737.42]*
    mucopolysaccharidosis 277.5 *[737.42]*
    neurofibromatosis 237.71 *[737.42]*
    osteitis
      deformans 731.0 *[737.42]*
      fibrosa cystica 252.01 *[737.42]*
    osteoporosis (*see also* Osteoporosis) 733.00 *[737.42]*
    poliomyelitis (*see also* Poliomyelitis) 138 *[737.42]*
    tuberculosis (*see also* Tuberculosis) 015.0 *[737.42]*
  late effect of rickets 268.1 *[737.42]*
  postlaminectomy 737.21
  postsurgical NEC 737.22
  rachitic 268.1 *[737.42]*
  specified NEC 737.29
  tuberculous (*see also* Tuberculosis) 015.0 *[737.42]*
Loss
  appetite 783.0
    hysterical 300.11
    nonorganic origin 307.59
    psychogenic 307.59
  blood—*see* Hemorrhage
  central vision 368.41
  consciousness 780.09
    transient 780.2
  control, sphincter, rectum 787.6
    nonorganic origin 307.7
  ear ossicle, partial 385.24
  elasticity, skin 782.8
  extremity or member, traumatic, current—*see* Amputation, traumatic
  fluid (acute) 276.50
    with
      hypernatremia 276.0
      hyponatremia 276.1
    fetus or newborn 775.5
  hair 704.00
  hearing—*see also* Deafness
    central 389.14
    conductive (air) 389.00
      with sensorineural hearing loss 389.20
        bilateral 389.22
        unilateral 389.21
      bilateral 389.06
      combined types 389.08
      external ear 389.01
      inner ear 389.04
      middle ear 389.03
      multiple types 389.08
      tympanic membrane 389.02
      unilateral 389.05
    mixed conductive and sensorineural 389.20
      bilateral 389.22
      unilateral 389.21
    mixed type 389.20
      bilateral 389.22
      unilateral 389.21
    nerve
      bilateral 389.12
      unilateral 389.13

1151

Loss —*continued*
  neural
    bilateral 389.12
    unilateral 389.13
  noise-induced 388.12
  perceptive NEC (*see also* Loss, hearing, sensorineural) 389.10
  sensorineural 389.10
    with conductive hearing loss 389.20
      bilateral 389.22
      unilateral 389.21
    asymmetrical 389.16
    bilateral 389.18
    central 389.14
    neural
      bilateral 389.12
      unilateral 389.13
    sensory
      bilateral 389.11
      unilateral 389.17
    unilateral 389.15
  sensory
    bilateral 389.11
    unilateral 389.17
  specified type NEC 389.8
  sudden NEC 388.2
height 781.91
labyrinthine reactivity (unilateral) 386.55
  bilateral 386.56
memory (*see also* Amnesia) 780.93
  mild, following organic brain damage 310.1
mind (*see also* Psychosis) 298.9
occusal vertical dimension 524.37
organ or part—*see* Absence, by site, acquired
sensation 782.0
sense of
  smell (*see also* Disturbance, sensation) 781.1
  taste (*see also* Disturbance, sensation) 781.1
  touch (*see also* Disturbance, sensation) 781.1
sight (acquired) (complete) (congenital)—*see* Blindness
spinal fluid
  headache 349.0
substance of
  bone (*see also* Osteoporosis) 733.00
  cartilage 733.99
    ear 380.32
  vitreous (humor) 379.26
tooth, teeth
  acquired 525.10
    due to
      caries 525.13
      extraction 525.10
      periodontal disease 525.12
      specified NEC 525.19
      trauma 525.11
vision, visual (*see also* Blindness) 369.9
  both eyes (*see also* Blindness, both eyes) 369.3
  complete (*see also* Blindness, both eyes) 369.00
  one eye 369.8
  sudden 368.11
  transient 368.12
vitreous 379.26
voice (*see also* Aphonia) 784.41
weight (cause unknown) 783.21
Lou Gehrig's disease 335.20
Louis-Bar syndrome (ataxia-telangiectasia) 334.8
Louping ill 063.1
Lousiness —*see* Lice

Low
  back syndrome 724.2
  basal metabolic rate (BMR) 794.7
  birthweight 765.1
    extreme (less than 1000 grams) 765.0
    for gestational age 764.0
    status (*see also* Status, low birth weight) V21.30
  bladder compliance 596.52
  blood pressure (*see also* Hypotension) 458.9
    reading (incidental) (isolated) (nonspecific) 796.3
  cardiac reserve—*see* Disease, heart
  compliance bladder 596.52
  frequency deafness—*see* Disorder, hearing
  function—*see also* Hypofunction
    kidney (*see also* Disease, renal) 593.9
    liver 573.9
  hemoglobin 285.9
  implantation, placenta—*see* Placenta, previa
  insertion, placenta—*see* Placenta, previa
  lying
    kidney 593.0
    organ or site, congenital—*see* Malposition, congenital
    placenta—*see* Placenta, previa
  output syndrome (cardiac) (*see also* Failure, heart) 428.9
  platelets (blood) (*see also* Thrombocytopenia) 287.5
  reserve, kidney (*see also* Disease, renal) 593.9
  risk
    cervical, human papillomavirus (HPV) DNA test positive 795.09
  salt syndrome 593.9
  tension glaucoma 365.12
  vision 369.9
    both eyes 369.20
    one eye 369.70
Lowe (-Terrey-MacLachlan) syndrome (oculocerebrorenal dystrophy) 270.8
Lower extremity —*see* condition
Lown (-Ganong)-Levine syndrome (short P-R interval, normal QRS complex, and paroxysmal supraventricular tachycardia) 426.81
LSD reaction (*see also* Abuse, drugs, nondependent) 305.3
L-shaped kidney 753.3
Lucas-Championnière disease (fibrinous bronchitis) 466.0
Lucey-Driscoll syndrome (jaundice due to delayed conjugation) 774.30
Ludwig's
  angina 528.3
  disease (submaxillary cellulitis) 528.3
Lues (venerea), luetic—*see* Syphilis
Luetscher's syndrome (dehydration) 276.51
Lumbago 724.2
  due to displacement, intervertebral disc 722.10
Lumbalgia 724.2
  due to displacement, intervertebral disc 722.10
Lumbar —*see* condition
Lumbarization, vertebra 756.15
Lumbermen's itch 133.8
Lump —*see also* Mass
  abdominal 789.3
  breast 611.72
  chest 786.6
  epigastric 789.3
  head 784.2

INDEX TO DISEASES — Lymphadenitis

Lump—*continued*
  kidney 753.3
  liver 789.1
  lung 786.6
  mediastinal 786.6
  neck 784.2
  nose or sinus 784.2
  pelvic 789.3
  skin 782.2
  substernal 786.6
  throat 784.2
  umbilicus 789.3
Lunacy (*see also* Psychosis) 298.9
Lunatomalacia 732.3
Lung —*see also* condition
  donor V59.8
  drug addict's 417.8
  mainliners' 417.8
  vanishing 492.0
Lupoid (miliary) of Boeck 135
Lupus 710.0
  anticoagulant 289.81
  Cazenave's (erythematosus) 695.4
  discoid (local) 695.4
  disseminated 710.0
  erythematodes (discoid) (local) 695.4
  erythematosus (discoid) (local) 695.4
    disseminated 710.0
    eyelid 373.34
    systemic 710.0
      with
        encephalitis 710.0 *[323.81]*
        lung involvement 710.0 *[517.8]*
        inhibitor (presence of) 286.5
  exedens 017.0
  eyelid (*see also* Tuberculosis) 017.0 *[373.4]*
    Hilliard's 017.0
  hydralazine
    correct substance properly administered 695.4
    overdose or wrong substance given or taken 972.6
  miliaris disseminatus faciei 017.0
  nephritis 710.0 *[583.81]*
    acute 710.0 *[580.81]*
    chronic 710.0 *[582.81]*
  nontuberculous, not disseminated 695.4
  pernio (Besnier) 135
  tuberculous (*see also* Tuberculosis) 017.0
    eyelid (*see also* Tuberculosis) 017.0 *[373.4]*
  vulgaris 017.0
Luschka's joint disease 721.90
Luteinoma (M8610/0) 220
Lutembacher's disease or syndrome (atrial septal defect with mitral stenosis) 745.5
Luteoma (M8610/0) 220
Lutz-Miescher disease (elastosis perforans serpiginosa) 701.1
Lutz-Splendore-de Almeida disease (Brazilian blastomycosis) 116.1
Luxatio
  bulbi due to birth injury 767.8
  coxae congenita (*see also* Dislocation, hip, congenital) 754.30
  erecta—*see* Dislocation, shoulder
  imperfecta—*see* Sprain, by site
  perinealis—*see* Dislocation, hip
Luxation —*see also* Dislocation, by site
  eyeball 360.81
    due to birth injury 767.8
    lateral 376.36

Luxation—*continued*
  genital organs (external) NEC—*see* Wound, open, genital organs
  globe (eye) 360.81
    lateral 376.36
  lacrimal gland (postinfectional) 375.16
  lens (old) (partial) 379.32
    congenital 743.37
    syphilitic 090.49 *[379.32]*
    Marfan's disease 090.49
    spontaneous 379.32
  penis—*see* Wound, open, penis
  scrotum—*see* Wound, open, scrotum
  testis—*see* Wound, open, testis
L-xyloketosuria 271.8
Lycanthropy (*see also* Psychosis) 298.9
Lyell's disease or syndrome (toxic epidermal necrolysis) 695.1
  due to drug
    correct substance properly administered 695.1
    overdose or wrong substance given or taken 977.9
    specified drug—*see* Table of drugs and chemicals
Lyme disease 088.81
Lymph
  gland or node—*see* condition
  scrotum (*see also* Infestation, filarial) 125.9
Lymphadenitis 289.3
  with
    abortion—*see* Abortion, by type, with sepsis
    ectopic pregnancy (*see also* categories 633.0-633.9) 639.0
    molar pregnancy (*see also* categories 630-632) 639.0
  acute 683
    mesenteric 289.2
  any site, except mesenteric 289.3
    acute 683
    chronic 289.1
    mesenteric (acute) (chronic) (nonspecific) (subacute) 289.2
    subacute 289.1
      mesenteric 289.2
  breast, puerperal, postpartum 675.2
  chancroidal (congenital) 099.0
  chronic 289.1
    mesenteric 289.2
  dermatopathic 695.89
  due to
    anthracosis (occupational) 500
    Brugia (Wuchereria) malayi 125.1
    diphtheria (toxin) 032.89
    lymphogranuloma venereum 099.1
    Wuchereria bancrofti 125.0
  following
    abortion 639.0
    ectopic or molar pregnancy 639.0
  generalized 289.3
  gonorrheal 098.89
  granulomatous 289.1
  infectional 683
  mesenteric (acute) (chronic) (nonspecific) (subacute) 289.2
    due to Bacillus typhi 002.0
    tuberculous (*see also* Tuberculosis) 014.8
  mycobacterial 031.8
  purulent 683
  pyogenic 683
  regional 078.3
  septic 683

1153

Lymphadenitis

Lymphadenitis—*continued*
  streptococcal 683
  subacute, unspecified site 289.1
  suppurative 683
  syphilitic (early) (secondary) 091.4
    late 095.8
  tuberculous—*see* Tuberculosis, lymph gland
  venereal 099.1
Lymphadenoid goiter 245.2
Lymphadenopathy (general) 785.6
  due to toxoplasmosis (acquired) 130.7
    congenital (active) 771.2
Lymphadenopathy-associated virus (disease)
  (illness) (infection)—*see* Human
  Immunodeficiency virus (disease) (illness)
  (infection)
Lymphadenosis 785.6
  acute 075
Lymphangiectasis 457.1
  conjunctiva 372.89
  postinfectional 457.1
  scrotum 457.1
Lymphangiectatic elephantiasis, nonfilarial
  457.1
Lymphangioendothelioma (M9170/0) 228.1
  malignant (M9170/3)—*see* Neoplasm,
    connective tissue, malignant
Lymphangioma (M9170/0) 228.1
  capillary (M9171/0) 228.1
  cavernous (M9172/0) 228.1
  cystic (M9173/0) 228.1
  malignant (M9170/3)—*see* Neoplasm,
    connective tissue, malignant
Lymphangiomyoma (M9174/0) 228.1
Lymphangiomyomatosis (M9174/1)—*see*
  Neoplasm, connective tissue, uncertain
  behavior
Lymphangiosarcoma (M9170/3)—*see*
  Neoplasm, connective tissue, malignant
Lymphangitis 457.2
  with
    abortion—*see* Abortion, by type, with sepsis
    abscess—*see* Abscess, by site
    cellulitis—*see* Abscess, by site
    ectopic pregnancy (*see also* categories
      633.0-633.9) 639.0
    molar pregnancy (*see also* categories 630-632)
      639.0
  acute (with abscess or cellulitis) 682.9
    specified site—*see* Abscess, by site
  breast, puerperal, postpartum 675.2
  chancroidal 099.0
  chronic (any site) 457.2
  due to
    Brugia (Wuchereria) malayi 125.1
    Wuchereria bancrofti 125.0
  following
    abortion 639.0
    ectopic or molar pregnancy 639.0
  gangrenous 457.2
  penis
    acute 607.2
    gonococcal (acute) 098.0
      chronic or duration of 2 months or more
        098.2
  puerperal, postpartum, childbirth 670
  strumous, tuberculous (*see also* Tuberculosis)
    017.2
  subacute (any site) 457.2
  tuberculous—*see* Tuberculosis, lymph gland
Lymphatic (vessel)—*see* condition

Lymphatism 254.8
  scrofulous (*see also* Tuberculosis) 017.2
Lymphectasia 457.1
Lymphedema (*see also* Elephantiasis) 457.1
  acquired (chronic) 457.1
  chronic hereditary 757.0
  congenital 757.0
  idiopathic hereditary 757.0
  praecox 457.1
  secondary 457.1
  surgical NEC 997.99
    postmastectomy (syndrome) 457.0
Lymph-hemangioma (M9120/0)—*see*
  Hemangioma, by site
Lymphoblastic —*see* condition
Lymphoblastoma (diffuse) (M9630/3) 200.1
  giant follicular (M9690/3) 202.0
  macrofollicular (M9690/3) 202.0
Lymphoblastosis, acute benign 075
Lymphocele 457.8
Lymphocythemia 288.51
Lymphocytic —*see also* condition
  chorioencephalitis (acute) (serous) 049.0
  choriomeningitis (acute) (serous) 049.0
Lymphocytoma (diffuse) (malignant) (M9620/3)
  200.1
Lymphocytomatosis (M9620/3) 200.1
Lymphocytopenia 288.51
Lymphocytosis (symptomatic) 288.61
  infectious (acute) 078.89
Lymphoepithelioma (M8082/3)—*see* Neoplasm,
  by site, malignant
Lymphogranuloma (malignant) (M9650/3) 201.9
  inguinale 099.1
  venereal (any site) 099.1
    with stricture of rectum 099.1
  venereum 099.1
Lymphogranulomatosis (malignant) (M9650/3)
  201.9
  benign (Boeck's sarcoid) (Schaumann's) 135
  Hodgkin's (M9650/3) 201.9
Lymphohistiocytosis, familial hemophagocytic
  288.4
Lymphoid —*see* condition
Lympholeukoblastoma (M9850/3) 207.8
Lympholeukosarcoma (M9850/3) 207.8
Lymphoma (malignant) (M9590/3) 202.8

> *Note*—Use the following fifth-digit
> subclassification with categories 200-202:
>
> 0 unspecifidd site
> 1 lymph nodes of head, face and neck
> 2 intrathoracic lymph nodes
> 3 intra-abdominal lymph nodes
> 4 lymph nodes of axilla and upper limb
> 5 lymph nodes of inguinal region and
>   lower limb
> 6 intrapelvic lymph nodes
> 7 spleen
> 8 lymph nodes of multiple sites

  wenign (M9580/0)—*see* Neoplasm, by site, benign
  Burkitt's type (lymphoblastic) (undifferentiated)
    (M9750/3) 200.2
  Castleman's (mediastinal lymph node hyperplasia)
    785.6
  centroblastic-centrocytic
    diffuse (M9614/3) 202.8
    follicular (M9692/3) 202.0
  centroblastic type (diffuse) (M9632/3) 202.8

Lymphoma—*continued*
  follicular (M9697/3) 202.0
  centrocytic (M9622/3) 202.8
  compound (M9613/3) 200.8
  convoluted cell type (lymphoblastic) (M9602/3)
    202.8
  diffuse NEC (M9590/3) 202.8
    large B cell 202.8
  follicular (giant) (M9690/3) 202.0
    center cell (diffuse) (M9615/3) 202.8
      cleaved (diffuse) (M9623/3) 202.8
        follicular (M9695/3) 202.0
      non-cleaved (diffuse) (M9633/3) 202.8
        follicular (M9698/3) 202.0
    centroblastic-centrocytic (M9692/3) 202.0
    centroblastic type (M9697/3) 202.0
    lymphocytic
      intermediate differentiation (M9694/3) 202.0
      poorly differentiated (M9696/3) 202.0
    mixed (cell type) (lymphocytic-histiocytic)
      (small cell and large cell) (M9691/3) 202.0
  germinocytic (M9622/3) 202.8
  giant, follicular or follicle (M9690/3) 202.0
  histiocytic (diffuse) (M9640/3) 200.0
    nodular (M9642/3) 200.0
    pleomorphic cell type (M9641/3) 200.0
  Hodgkin's (M9650/3) (*see also* Disease,
    Hodgkin's) 201.9
  immunoblastic (type) (M9612/3) 200.8
  large cell (M9640/3) 200.7
    anaplastic 200.6
    nodular (M9642/3) 200.0
    pleomorphic cell type (M9641/3) 200.0
  lymphoblastic (diffuse) (M9630/3) 200.1
    Burkitt's type (M9750/3) 200.2
    convoluted cell type (M9602/3) 202.8
  lymphocytic (cell type) (diffuse) (M9620/3) 200.1
    with plasmacytoid differentiation, diffuse
      (M9611/3) 200.8
    intermediate differentiation (diffuse)
      (M9621/3) 200.1
      follicular (M9694/3) 202.0
      nodular (M9694/3) 202.0
    nodular (M9690/3) 202.0
    poorly differentiated (diffuse) (M9630/3) 200.1
      follicular (M9696/3) 202.0
      nodular (M9696/3) 202.0
    well differentiated (diffuse) (M9620/3) 200.1
      follicular (M9693/3) 202.0
      nodular (M9693/3) 202.0
  lymphocytic-histiocytic, mixed (diffuse)
    (M9613/3) 200.8
    follicular (M9691/3) 202.0
    nodular (M9691/3) 202.0
  lymphoplasmacytoid type (M9611/3) 200.8
  lymphosarcoma type (M9610/3) 200.1
  macrofollicular (M9690/3) 202.0
  mantle cell 200.4
  marginal zone 200.3
    extranodal B-cell 200.3
    nodal B-cell 200.3
    splenic B-cell 200.3
  mixed cell type (diffuse) (M9613/3) 200.8
    follicular (M9691/3) 202.0
    nodular (M9691/3) 202.0
  nodular (M9690/3) 202.0
    histiocytic (M9642/3) 200.0
    lymphocytic (M9690.3) 202.0
      intermediate differentiation (M9694/3) 202.0
      poorly differentiated (M9696/3) 202.0

Lymphoma—*continued*
  mixed (cell type) (lymphocytic-histiocytic)
    (small cell and large cell) (M9691/3) 202.0
  non-Hodgkin's type NEC (M9591/3) 202.8
  peripheral T-cell 202.7
  primary central nervous system 200.5
  reticulum cell (type) (M9640/3) 200.0
  small cell and large cell, mixed (diffuse)
    (M9613/3) 200.8
    follicular (M9691/3) 202.0
    nodular (9691/3) 202.0
  stem cell (type) (M9601/3) 202.8
  T-cell 202.1
    peripheral 202.7
  undifferentiated (cell type) (non-Burkitt's)
    (M9600/3) 202.8
    Burkitt's type (M9750/3) 200.2
Lymphomatosis (M9590/3)—*see also*
  Lymphoma
  granulomatous 099.1
Lymphopathia
  venereum 099.1
  veneris 099.1
Lymphopenia 288.51
  familial 279.2
Lymphoreticulosis, benign (of inoculation)
  078.3
Lymphorrhea 457.8
Lymphosarcoma (M9610/3) 200.1
  diffuse (M9610/3) 200.1
    with plasmacytoid differentiation (M9611/3)
      200.8
    lymphoplasmacytic (M9611/3) 200.8
  follicular (giant) (M9690/3) 202.0
    lymphoblastic (M9696/3) 202.0
    lymphocytic, intermediate differentiation
      (M9694/3) 202.0
    mixed cell type (M9691/3) 202.0
  giant follicular (M9690/3) 202.0
  Hodgkin's (M9650/3) 201.9
  immunoblastic (M9612/3) 200.8
  lymphoblastic (diffuse) (M9630/3) 200.1
    follicular (M9696/3) 202.0
    nodular (M9696/3) 202.0
  lymphocytic (diffuse) (M9620/3) 200.1
    intermediate differentiation (diffuse)
      (M9621/3) 200.1
      follicular (M9694/3) 202.0
      nodular (M9694/3) 202.0
  mixed cell type (diffuse) (M9613/3) 200.8
    follicular (M9691/3) 202.0
    nodular (M9691/3) 202.0
  nodular (M9690/3) 202.0
    lymphoblastic (M9696/3) 202.0
    lymphocytic, intermediate differentiation
      (M9694/3) 202.0
    mixed cell type (M9691/3) 202.0
  prolymphocytic (M9631/3) 200.1
  reticulum cell (M9640/3) 200.0
Lymphostasis 457.8
Lypemania (*see also* Melancholia) 296.2
Lyssa 071

INDEX TO DISEASES

M

Macacus ear 744.29
Maceration
   fetus (cause not stated) 779.9
   wet feet, tropical (syndrome) 991.4
Machado-Joseph disease 334.8
Machupo virus hemorrhagic fever 078.7
Macleod's syndrome (abnormal transradiancy, one lung) 492.8
Macrocephalia, macrocephaly 756.0
Macrocheilia (congenital) 744.81
Macrochilia (congenital) 744.81
Macrocolon (congenital) 751.3
Macrocornea 743.41
   associated with buphthalmos 743.22
Macrocytic —*see* condition
Macrocytosis 289.89
Macrodactylia, macrodactylism (fingers) (thumbs) 755.57
   toes 755.65
Macrodontia 520.2
Macroencephaly 742.4
Macrogenia 524.05
Macrogenitosomia (female) (male) (praecox) 255.2
Macrogingivae 523.8
Macroglobulinemia (essential) (idiopathic) (monoclonal) (primary) (syndrome) (Waldenström's) 273.3
Macroglossia (congenital) 750.15
   acquired 529.8
Macrognathia, macrognathism (congenital) 524.00
   mandibular 524.02
     alveolar 524.72
   maxillary 524.01
     alveolar 524.71
Macrogyria (congenital) 742.4
Macrohydrocephalus (*see also* Hydrocephalus) 331.4
Macromastia (*see also* Hypertrophy, breast) 611.1
Macrophage activation syndrome 288.4
Macropsia 368.14
Macrosigmoid 564.7
   congenital 751.3
Macrospondylitis, acromegalic 253.0
Macrostomia (congenital) 744.83
Macrotia (external ear) (congenital) 744.22
Macula
   cornea, corneal
     congenital 743.43
       interfering with vision 743.42
     interfering with central vision 371.03
     not interfering with central vision 371.02
   degeneration (*see also* Degeneration, macula) 362.50
   hereditary (*see also* Dystrophy, retina) 362.70
   edema, cystoid 362.53
Maculae ceruleae 132.1
Macules and papules 709.8
Maculopathy, toxic 362.55
Madarosis 374.55
Madelung's
   deformity (radius) 755.54
   disease (lipomatosis) 272.8
   lipomatosis 272.8

Madness (*see also* Psychosis) 298.9
   myxedema (acute) 293.0
   subacute 293.1
Madura
   disease (actinomycotic) 039.9
     mycotic 117.4
   foot (actinomycotic) 039.4
     mycotic 117.4
Maduromycosis (actinomycotic) 039.9
   mycotic 117.4
Maffucci's syndrome (dyschondroplasia with hemangiomas) 756.4
Magenblase syndrome 306.4
Main en griffe (acquired) 736.06
   congenital 755.59
Maintenance
   chemotherapy regimen or treatment V58.11
   dialysis regimen or treatment
     extracorporeal (renal) V56.0
     peritoneal V56.8
     renal V56.0
   drug therapy or regimen
     chemotherapy, antineoplastic V58.11
     immunotherapy, antineoplastic V58.12
   external fixation NEC V54.89
   radiotherapy V58.0
   traction NEC V54.89
Majocchi's
   disease (purpura annularis telangiectodes) 709.1
   granuloma 110.6
Major —*see* condition
Mal
   cerebral (idiopathic) (*see also* Epilepsy) 345.9
   comital (*see also* Epilepsy) 345.9
   de los pintos (*see also* Pinta) 103.9
   de Meleda 757.39
   de mer 994.6
   lie—*see* Presentation, fetal
   perforant (*see also* Ulcer, lower extremity) 707.15
Malabar itch 110.9
   beard 110.0
   foot 110.4
   scalp 110.0
Malabsorption 579.9
   calcium 579.8
   carbohydrate 579.8
   disaccharide 271.3
   drug-induced 579.8
   due to bacterial overgrowth 579.8
   fat 579.8
   folate, congenital 281.2
   galactose 271.1
   glucose-galactose (congenital) 271.3
   intestinal 579.9
   isomaltose 271.3
   lactose (hereditary) 271.3
   methionine 270.4
   monosaccharide 271.8
   postgastrectomy 579.3
   postsurgical 579.3
   protein 579.8
   sucrose (-isomaltose) (congenital) 271.3
   syndrome 579.9
     postgastrectomy 579.3
     postsurgical 579.3
Malacia, bone 268.2
   juvenile (*see also* Rickets) 268.0

Malacia, bone—*continued*
  Kienböck's (juvenile) (lunate) (wrist) 732.3
    adult 732.8
Malacoplakia
  bladder 596.8
  colon 569.89
  pelvis (kidney) 593.89
  ureter 593.89
  urethra 599.84
Malacosteon 268.2
  juvenile (*see also* Rickets) 268.0
Maladaptation —*see* Maladjustment
Maladie de Roger 745.4
Maladjustment
  conjugal V61.10
    involving divorce or estrangement V61.0
  educational V62.3
  family V61.9
    specified circumstance NEC V61.8
  marital V61.10
    involving divorce or estrangement V61.0
  occupational V62.2
  simple, adult (*see also* Reaction, adjustment) 309.9
  situational acute (*see also* Reaction, adjustment) 309.9
  social V62.4
Malaise 780.79
Malakoplakia —*see* Malacoplakia
Malaria, malarial (fever) 084.6
  algid 084.9
  any type, with
    algid malaria 084.9
    blackwater fever 084.8
    fever
      blackwater 084.8
      hemoglobinuric (bilious) 084.8
    hemoglobinuria, malarial 084.8
    hepatitis 084.9 *[573.2]*
    nephrosis 084.9 *[581.81]*
    pernicious complication NEC 084.9
      cardiac 084.9
      cerebral 084.9
  cardiac 084.9
  carrier (suspected) of V02.9
  cerebral 084.9
  complicating pregnancy, childbirth, or puerperium 647.4
  congenital 771.2
  congestion, congestive 084.6
    brain 084.9
  continued 084.0
  estivo-autumnal 084.0
  falciparum (malignant tertian) 084.0
  hematinuria 084.8
  hematuria 084.8
  hemoglobinuria 084.8
  hemorrhagic 084.6
  induced (therapeutically) 084.7
    accidental—*see* Malaria, by type
  liver 084.9 *[573.2]*
  malariae (quartan) 084.2
  malignant (tertian) 084.0
  mixed infections 084.5
  monkey 084.4
  ovale 084.3
  pernicious, acute 084.0
  Plasmodium, P.
    falciparum 084.0
    malariae 084.2
    ovale 084.3

Malaria, malarial—*continued*
  vivax 084.1
  quartan 084.2
  quotidian 084.0
  recurrent 084.6
    induced (therapeutically) 084.7
      accidental—*see* Malaria, by type
  remittent 084.6
  specified types NEC 084.4
  spleen 084.6
  subtertian 084.0
  tertian (benign) 084.1
    malignant 084.0
  tropical 084.0
  typhoid 084.6
  vivax (benign tertian) 084.1
Malassez's disease (testicular cyst) 608.89
Malassimilation 579.9
Maldescent, testis 752.51
Maldevelopment —*see also* Anomaly, by site
  brain 742.9
  colon 751.5
  hip (joint) 755.63
    congenital dislocation (*see also* Dislocation, hip, congenital) 754.30
  mastoid process 756.0
  middle ear, except ossicles 744.03
    ossicles 744.04
  newborn (not malformation) 764.9
  ossicles, ear 744.04
  spine 756.10
  toe 755.66
Male type pelvis 755.69
  with disproportion (fetopelvic) 653.2
    affecting fetus or newborn 763.1
    causing obstructed labor 660.1
      affecting fetus or newborn 763.1
Malformation (congenital)—*see also* Anomaly
  bone 756.9
  bursa 756.9
  Chiari
    type I 348.4
    type II (*see also* Spina bifida) 741.0
    type III 742.0
    type IV 742.2
  circulatory system NEC 747.9
    specified type NEC 747.89
  cochlea 744.05
  digestive system NEC 751.9
    lower 751.5
    specified type NEC 751.8
    upper 750.9
  eye 743.9
  gum 750.9
  heart NEC 746.9
    specified type NEC 746.89
    valve 746.9
  internal ear 744.05
  joint NEC 755.9
    specified type NEC 755.8
  Mondini's (congenital) (malformation, cochlea) 744.05
  muscle 756.9
  nervous system (central) 742.9
  pelvic organs or tissues
    in pregnancy or childbirth 654.9
      affecting fetus or newborn 763.89
      causing obstructed labor 660.2
        affecting fetus or newborn 763.1
  placenta (*see also* Placenta, abnormal) 656.7
  respiratory organs 748.9

INDEX TO DISEASES   Malposition

Malformation—*continued*
  specified type NEC 748.8
  Rieger's 743.44
  sense organs NEC 742.9
    specified type NEC 742.8
  skin 757.9
    specified type NEC 757.8
  spinal cord 742.9
  teeth, tooth NEC 520.9
  tendon 756.9
  throat 750.9
  umbilical cord (complicating delivery) 663.9
    affecting fetus or newborn 762.6
  umbilicus 759.9
  urinary system NEC 753.9
    specified type NEC 753.8
Malfunction —*see also* Dysfunction
  arterial graft 996.1
  cardiac pacemaker 996.01
  catheter device—*see* Complications, mechanical, catheter
  colostomy 569.62
    valve 569.62
  cystostomy 997.5
  device, implant, or graft NEC—*see* Complications, mechanical
  enteric stoma 569.62
  enterostomy 569.62
  esophagostomy 530.87
  gastroenteric 536.8
  gastrostomy 536.42
  ileostomy
    valve 569.62
  nephrostomy 997.5
  pacemaker—*see* Complications, mechanical, pacemaker
  prosthetic device, internal—*see* Complications, mechanical
  tracheostomy 519.02
  valve
    colostomy 569.62
    ileostomy 569.62
  vascular graft or shunt 996.1
Malgaigne's fracture (closed) 808.43
  open 808.53
Malherbe's
  calcifying epithelioma (M8110/0)—*see* Neoplasm, skin, benign
  tumor (M8110/0)—*see* Neoplasm, skin, benign
Malibu disease 919.8
  infected 919.9
Malignancy (M8000/3)—*see* Neoplasm, by site, malignant
Malignant —*see* condition
Malingerer, malingering V65.2
Mallet, finger (acquired) 736.1
  congenital 755.59
  late effect of rickets 268.1
Malleus 024
Mallory's bodies 034.1
Mallory-Weiss syndrome 530.7
Malnutrition (calorie) 263.9
  complicating pregnancy 648.9
  degree
    first 263.1
    second 263.0
    third 262
    mild 263.1
    moderate 263.0
    severe 261
      protein-calorie 262

Malnutrition—*continued*
  fetus 764.2
    "light-for-dates" 764.1
  following gastrointestinal surgery 579.3
  intrauterine or fetal 764.2
    fetus or infant "light-for-dates" 764.1
  lack of care, or neglect (child) (infant) 995.52
    adult 995.84
  malignant 260
  mild 263.1
  moderate 263.0
  protein 260
  protein-calorie 263.9
    severe 262
    specified type NEC 263.8
  severe 261
    protein-calorie NEC 262
Malocclusion (teeth) 524.4
  angle's class I 524.21
  angle's class II 524.22
  angle's class III 524.23
  due to
    abnormal swallowing 524.59
    accessory teeth (causing crowding) 524.31
    dentofacial abnormality NEC 524.89
    impacted teeth (causing crowding) 520.6
    missing teeth 524.30
    mouth breathing 524.59
    sleep posture 524.59
    supernumerary teeth (causing crowding) 524.31
    thumb sucking 524.59
    tongue, lip, or finger habits 524.59
  temporomandibular (joint) 524.69
Malposition
  cardiac apex (congenital) 746.87
  cervix—*see* Malposition, uterus
  congenital
    adrenal (gland) 759.1
    alimentary tract 751.8
      lower 751.5
      upper 750.8
    aorta 747.21
    appendix 751.5
    arterial trunk 747.29
    artery (peripheral) NEC (*see also* Malposition, congenital, peripheral vascular system) 747.60
      coronary 746.85
      pulmonary 747.3
    auditory canal 744.29
      causing impairment of hearing 744.02
    auricle (ear) 744.29
      causing impairment of hearing 744.02
      cervical 744.43
    biliary duct or passage 751.69
    bladder (mucosa) 753.8
      exteriorized or extroverted 753.5
    brachial plexus 742.8
    brain tissue 742.4
    breast 757.6
    bronchus 748.3
    cardiac apex 746.87
    cecum 751.5
    clavicle 755.51
    colon 751.5
    digestive organ or tract NEC 751.8
      lower 751.5
      upper 750.8
    ear (auricle) (external) 744.29
      ossicles 744.04

Malposition—*continued*
- endocrine (gland) NEC 759.2
- epiglottis 748.3
- Eustachian tube 744.24
- eye 743.8
- facial features 744.89
- fallopian tube 752.19
- finger(s) 755.59
  - supernumerary 755.01
- foot 755.67
- gallbladder 751.69
- gastrointestinal tract 751.8
- genitalia, genital organ(s) or tract
  - female 752.89
    - external 752.49
    - internal NEC 752.89
  - male 752.89
    - penis 752.69
    - scrotal transposition 752.81
- glottis 748.3
- hand 755.59
- heart 746.87
  - dextrocardia 746.87
    - with complete transposition of viscera 759.3
- hepatic duct 751.69
- hip (joint) (*see also* Dislocation, hip, congenital) 754.30
- intestine (large) (small) 751.5
  - with anomalous adhesions, fixation, or malrotation 751.4
- joint NEC 755.8
- kidney 753.3
- larynx 748.3
- limb 755.8
  - lower 755.69
  - upper 755.59
- liver 751.69
- lung (lobe) 748.69
- nail(s) 757.5
- nerve 742.8
- nervous system NEC 742.8
- nose, nasal (septum) 748.1
- organ or site NEC—*see* Anomaly, specified type NEC, by site
- ovary 752.0
- pancreas 751.7
- parathyroid (gland) 759.2
- patella 755.64
- peripheral vascular system 747.60
  - gastrointestinal 747.61
  - lower limb 747.64
  - renal 747.62
  - specified NEC 747.69
  - spinal 747.82
  - upper limb 747.63
- pituitary (gland) 759.2
- respiratory organ or system NEC 748.9
- rib (cage) 756.3
  - supernumerary in cervical region 756.2
- scapula 755.59
- shoulder 755.59
- spinal cord 742.59
- spine 756.19
- spleen 759.0
- sternum 756.3
- stomach 750.7
- symphysis pubis 755.69
- testis (undescended) 752.51
- thymus (gland) 759.2
- thyroid (gland) (tissue) 759.2

Malposition—*continued*
- cartilage 748.3
- toe(s) 755.66
  - supernumerary 755.02
- tongue 750.19
- trachea 748.3
- uterus 752.3
- vein(s) (peripheral) NEC (*see also* Malposition, congenital, peripheral vascular system) 747.60
  - great 747.49
  - portal 747.49
  - pulmonary 747.49
  - vena cava (inferior) (superior) 747.49
- device, implant, or graft—*see* Complications, mechanical
- fetus NEC (*see also* Presentation, fetal) 652.9
  - with successful version 652.1
  - affecting fetus or newborn 763.1
  - before labor, affecting fetus or newborn 761.7
  - causing obstructed labor 660.0
  - in multiple gestation (one fetus or more) 652.6
    - with locking 660.5
    - causing obstructed labor 660.0
- gallbladder (*see also* Disease, gallbladder) 575.8
- gastrointestinal tract 569.89
  - congenital 751.8
- heart (*see also* Malposition, congenital, heart) 746.87
- intestine 569.89
  - congenital 751.5
- pelvic organs or tissues
  - in pregnancy or childbirth 654.4
    - affecting fetus or newborn 763.89
    - causing obstructed labor 660.2
      - affecting fetus or newborn 763.1
- placenta—*see* Placenta, previa
- stomach 537.89
  - congenital 750.7
- tooth, teeth 524.30
  - with impaction 520.6
- uterus (acquired) (acute) (adherent) (any degree) (asymptomatic) (postinfectional) (postpartal, old) 621.6
  - anteflexion or anteversion (*see also* Anteversion, uterus) 621.6
  - congenital 752.3
  - flexion 621.6
    - lateral (*see also* Lateroversion, uterus) 621.6
  - in pregnancy or childbirth 654.4
    - affecting fetus or newborn 763.89
    - causing obstructed labor 660.2
      - affecting fetus or newborn 763.1
  - inversion 621.6
  - lateral (flexion) (version) (*see also* Lateroversion, uterus) 621.6
  - lateroflexion (*see also* Lateroversion, uterus) 621.6
  - lateroversion (*see also* Lateroversion, uterus) 621.6
  - retroflexion or retroversion (*see also* Retroversion, uterus) 621.6

Malposture 729.7

Malpresentation, fetus (*see also* Presentation, fetal) 652.9

Malrotation
- cecum 751.4
- colon 751.4
- intestine 751.4
- kidney 753.3

MALT (mucosa associated lymphoid tissue) 200.3

Malt workers' lung 495.4

INDEX TO DISEASES

Malta fever (*see also* Brucellosis) 023.9
Maltosuria 271.3
Maltreatment (of)
  adult 995.80
    emotional 995.82
    multiple forms 995.85
    neglect (nutritional) 995.84
    physical 995.81
    psychological 995.82
    sexual 995.83
  child 995.50
    emotional 995.51
    multiple forms 995.59
    neglect (nutritional) 995.52
    psychological 995.51
    physical 995.54
      shaken infant syndrome 995.55
    sexual 995.53
  spouse (*see also* Maltreatment, adult) 995.80
Malum coxae senilis 715.25
Malunion, fracture 733.81
Mammillitis (*see also* Mastitis) 611.0
  puerperal, postpartum 675.2
Mammitis (*see also* Mastitis) 611.0
  puerperal, postpartum 675.2
Mammographic
  calcification 793.89
  calculus 793.89
  microcalcification 793.81
Mammoplasia 611.1
Management
  contraceptive V25.9
    specified type NEC V25.8
  procreative V26.9
    specified type NEC V26.89
Mangled NEC (*see also* nature and site of injury) 959.9
Mania (monopolar) (*see also* Psychosis, affective) 296.0
  alcoholic (acute) (chronic) 291.9
  Bell's—*see* Mania, chronic
  chronic 296.0
    recurrent episode 296.1
    single episode 296.0
  compulsive 300.3
  delirious (acute) 296.0
    recurrent episode 296.1
    single episode 296.0
  epileptic (*see also* Epilepsy) 345.4
  hysterical 300.10
  inhibited 296.89
  puerperal (after delivery) 296.0
    recurrent episode 296.1
    single episode 296.0
  recurrent episode 296.1
  senile 290.8
  single episode 296.0
  stupor 296.89
  stuporous 296.89
  unproductive 296.89
Manic-depressive insanity, psychosis reaction, or syndrome (*see also* Psychosis, affective) 296.80
  circular (alternating) 296.7
    currently
      depressed 296.5
      episode unspecified 296.7
      hypomanic, previously depressed 296.4
      manic 296.4
    mixed 296.6
  depressed (type), depressive 296.2
    atypical 296.82

Manic-depressive insanity—*continued*
    recurrent episode 296.3
    single episode 296.2
  hypomanic 296.0
    recurrent episode 296.1
    single episode 296.0
  manic 296.0
    atypical 296.81
    recurrent episode 296.1
    single episode 296.0
  mixed NEC 296.89
  perplexed 296.89
  stuporous 296.89
Manifestations, rheumatoid
  lungs 714.81
  pannus—*see* Arthritis, rheumatoid
  subcutaneous nodules—*see* Arthritis, rheumatoid
Mankowsky's syndrome (familial dysplastic osteopathy) 731.2
Mannoheptulosuria 271.8
Mannosidosis 271.8
Manson's
  disease (schistosomiasis) 120.1
  pyosis (pemphigus contagiosus) 684
  schistosomiasis 120.1
Mansonellosis 125.5
Manual —*see* condition
Maple bark disease 495.6
Maple bark-strippers' lung 495.6
Maple syrup (urine) disease or syndrome 270.3
Marable's syndrome (celiac artery compression) 447.4
Marasmus 261
  brain 331.9
  due to malnutrition 261
  intestinal 569.89
  nutritional 261
  senile 797
  tuberculous NEC (*see also* Tuberculosis) 011.9
Marble
  bones 756.52
  skin 782.61
Marburg disease (virus) 078.89
March
  foot 733.94
  hemoglobinuria 283.2
Marchand multiple nodular hyperplasia (liver) 571.5
Marchesani (-Weill) syndrome (brachymorphism and ectopia lentis) 759.89
Marchiafava (-Bignami) disease or syndrome 341.8
Marchiafava-Micheli syndrome (paroxysmal nocturnal hemoglobinuria) 283.2
Marcus Gunn's syndrome (jaw-winking syndrome) 742.8
Marfan's
  congenital syphilis 090.49
  disease 090.49
  syndrome (arachnodactyly) 759.82
    meaning congenital syphilis 090.49
    with luxation of lens 090.49 [379.32]
Marginal
  implantation, placenta—*see* Placenta, previa
  placenta—*see* Placenta, previa
  sinus (hemorrhage) (rupture) 641.2
    affecting fetus or newborn 762.1
Marie's
  cerebellar ataxia 334.2
  syndrome (acromegaly) 253.0

Marie-Bamberger disease or syndrome
  (hypertrophic) (pulmonary) (secondary) 731.2
  idiopathic (acropachyderma) 757.39
  primary (acropachyderma) 757.39
Marie-Charcot-Tooth neuropathic atrophy, muscle 356.1
Marie-Strümpell arthritis or disease
  (ankylosing spondylitis) 720.0
Marihuana, marijuana
  abuse (see also Abuse, drugs, nondependent) 305.2
  dependence (see also Dependence) 304.3
Marion's disease (bladder neck obstruction) 596.0
Marital conflict V61.10
Mark
  port wine 757.32
  raspberry 757.32
  strawberry 757.32
  stretch 701.3
  tattoo 709.09
Maroteaux-Lamy syndrome
  (mucopolysaccharidosis VI) 277.5
Marriage license examination V70.3
Marrow (bone)
  arrest 284.9
  megakaryocytic 287.30
  poor function 289.9
Marseilles fever 082.1
Marsh's disease (exophthalmic goiter) 242.0
Marshall's (hidrotic) ectodermal dysplasia 757.31
Marsh fever (see also Malaria) 084.6
Martin's disease 715.27
Martin-Albright syndrome
  (pseudohypoparathyroidism) 275.49
Martorell-Fabre syndrome (pulseless disease) 446.7
Masculinization, female with adrenal hyperplasia 255.2
Masculinovoblastoma (M8670/0) 220
Masochism 302.83
Masons' lung 502
Mass
  abdominal 789.3
  anus 787.99
  bone 733.90
  breast 611.72
  cheek 784.2
  chest 786.6
  cystic—see Cyst
  ear 388.8
  epigastric 789.3
  eye 379.92
  female genital organ 625.8
  gum 784.2
  head 784.2
  intracranial 784.2
  joint 719.60
    ankle 719.67
    elbow 719.62
    foot 719.67
    hand 719.64
    hip 719.65
    knee 719.66
    multiple sites 719.69
    pelvic region 719.65
    shoulder (region) 719.61
    specified site NEC 719.68
    wrist 719.63
  kidney (see also Disease, kidney) 593.9

Mass—continued
  lung 786.6
  lymph node 785.6
  malignant (M8000/3)—see Neoplasm, by site, malignant
  mediastinal 786.6
  mouth 784.2
  muscle (limb) 729.89
  neck 784.2
  nose or sinus 784.2
  palate 784.2
  pelvis, pelvic 789.3
  penis 607.89
  perineum 625.8
  rectum 787.99
  scrotum 608.89
  skin 782.2
  specified organ NEC—see Disease of specified organ or site
  splenic 789.2
  substernal 786.6
    thyroid (see also Goiter) 240.9
  superficial (localized) 782.2
  testes 608.89
  throat 784.2
  tongue 784.2
  umbilicus 789.3
  uterus 625.8
  vagina 625.8
  vulva 625.8
Massive —see condition
Mastalgia 611.71
  psychogenic 307.89
Mast cell
  disease 757.33
    systemic (M9741/3) 202.6
  leukemia (M9900/3) 207.8
  sarcoma (M9742/3) 202.6
  tumor (M9740/1) 238.5
    malignant (M9740/3) 202.6
Masters-Allen syndrome 620.6
Mastitis (acute) (adolescent) (diffuse)
    (interstitial) (lobular) (nonpuerperal)
    (nonsuppurative) (parenchymatous)
    (phlegmonous) (simple) (subacute)
    (suppurative) 611.0
  chronic (cystic) (fibrocystic) 610.1
  cystic 610.1
    Schimmelbusch's type 610.1
  fibrocystic 610.1
  infective 611.0
  lactational 675.2
  lymphangitis 611.0
  neonatal (noninfective) 778.7
    infective 771.5
  periductal 610.4
  plasma cell 610.4
  puerperal, postpartum, (interstitial)
      (nonpurulent) (parenchymatous) 675.2
    purulent 675.1
    stagnation 676.2
  puerperalis 675.2
  retromammary 611.0
    puerperal, postpartum 675.1
  submammary 611.0
    puerperal, postpartum 675.1
Mastocytoma (M9740/1) 238.5
  malignant (M9740/3) 202.6
Mastocytosis 757.33
  malignant (M9741/3) 202.6
  systemic (M9741/3) 202.6

Mastodynia 611.71
  psychogenic 307.89
Mastoid —see condition
Mastoidalgia (see also Otalgia) 388.70
Mastoiditis (coalescent) (hemorrhagic) (pneumococcal) (streptococcal) (suppurative) 383.9
  acute or subacute 383.00
    with
      Gradenigo's syndrome 383.02
      petrositis 383.02
      specified complication NEC 383.02
      subperiosteal abscess 383.01
  chronic (necrotic) (recurrent) 383.1
  tuberculous (see also Tuberculosis) 015.6
Mastopathy, mastopathia 611.9
  chronica cystica 610.1
  diffuse cystic 610.1
  estrogenic 611.8
  ovarian origin 611.8
Mastoplasia 611.1
Masturbation 307.9
Maternal condition, affecting fetus or newborn
  acute yellow atrophy of liver 760.8
  albuminuria 760.1
  anesthesia or analgesia 763.5
  blood loss 762.1
  chorioamnionitis 762.7
  circulatory disease, chronic (conditions classifiable to 390-459, 745-747) 760.3
  congenital heart disease (conditions classifiable to 745-746) 760.3
  cortical necrosis of kidney 760.1
  death 761.6
  diabetes mellitus 775.0
    manifest diabetes in the infant 775.1
  disease NEC 760.9
    circulatory system, chronic (conditions classifiable to 390-459, 745-747) 760.3
    genitourinary system (conditions classifiable to 580-599) 760.1
    respiratory (conditions classifiable to 490-519, 748) 760.3
  eclampsia 760.0
  hemorrhage NEC 762.1
  hepatitis acute, malignant, or subacute 760.8
  hyperemesis (gravidarum) 761.8
  hypertension (arising during pregnancy) (conditions classifiable to 642) 760.0
  infection
    disease classifiable to 001-136 760.2
    genital tract NEC 760.8
    urinary tract 760.1
  influenza 760.2
    manifest influenza in the infant 771.2
  injury (conditions classifiable to 800-996) 760.5
  malaria 760.2
    manifest malaria in infant or fetus 771.2
  malnutrition 760.4
  necrosis of liver 760.8
  nephritis (conditions classifiable to 580-583) 760.1
  nephrosis (conditions classifiable to 581) 760.1
  noxious substance transmitted via breast milk or placenta 760.70
    alcohol 760.71
    anticonvulsants 760.77
    antifungals 760.74
    anti-infective agents 760.74
    antimetabolics 760.78
    cocaine 760.75

Maternal condition—continued
    "crack" 760.75
    diethylstilbestrol [DES] 760.76
    hallucinogenic agents 760.73
    medicinal agents NEC 760.79
    narcotics 760.72
    obstetric anesthetic or analgesic drug 760.72
    specified agent NEC 760.79
  nutritional disorder (conditions classifiable to 260-269) 760.4
  operation unrelated to current delivery 760.6
  pre-eclampsia 760.0
  pyelitis or pyelonephritis, arising during pregnancy (conditions classifiable to 590) 760.1
  renal disease or failure 760.1
  respiratory disease, chronic (conditions classifiable to 490-519, 748) 760.3
  rheumatic heart disease (chronic) (conditions classifiable to 393-398) 760.3
  rubella (conditions classifiable to 056) 760.2
    manifest rubella in the infant or fetus 771.0
  surgery unrelated to current delivery 760.6
    to uterus or pelvic organs 763.89
  syphilis (conditions classifiable to 090-097) 760.2
    manifest syphilis in the infant or fetus 090.0
  thrombophlebitis 760.3
  toxemia (of pregnancy) 760.0
    pre-eclamptic 760.0
  toxoplasmosis (conditions classifiable to 130) 760.2
    manifest toxoplasmosis in the infant or fetus 771.2
  transmission of chemical substance through the placenta 760.70
    alcohol 760.71
    anticonvulsants 760.77
    antifungals 760.74
    anti-infective agents 760.74
    antimetabolics 760.78
    cocaine 760.75
    "crack" 760.75
    diethylstilbestrol [DES] 760.76
    hallucinogenic agents 760.73
    narcotics 760.72
    specified substance NEC 760.79
  uremia 760.1
  urinary tract conditions (conditions classifiable to 580-599) 760.1
  vomiting (pernicious) (persistent) (vicious) 761.8
Maternity —see Delivery
Matheiu's disease (leptospiral jaundice) 100.0
Mauclaire's disease or osteochondrosis 732.3
Maxcy's disease 081.0
Maxilla, maxillary —see condition
May (-Hegglin) anomaly or syndrome 288.2
Mayaro fever 066.3
Mazoplasia 610.8
MBD (minimal brain dysfunction), child (see also Hyperkinesia) 314.9
MCAD (medium chain acyl CoA dehydrogenase deficiency) 277.85
McArdle (-Schmid-Pearson) disease or syndrome (glycogenosis V) 271.0
McCune-Albright syndrome (osteitis fibrosa disseminata) 756.59
MCLS (mucocutaneous lymph node syndrome) 446.1
McQuarrie's syndrome (idiopathic familial hypoglycemia) 251.2

Measles

Measles (black) (hemorrhagic) (suppressed) 055.9
  with
    encephalitis 055.0
    keratitis 055.71
    keratoconjunctivitis 055.71
    otitis media 055.2
    pneumonia 055.1
  complication 055.8
    specified type NEC 055.79
  encephalitis 055.0
  French 056.9
  German 056.9
  keratitis 055.71
  keratoconjunctivitis 055.71
  liberty 056.9
  otitis media 055.2
  pneumonia 055.1
  specified complications NEC 055.79
  vaccination, prophylactic (against) V04.2
Meatitis, urethral (*see also* Urethritis) 597.89
Meat poisoning —*see* Poisoning, food
Meatus, meatal —*see* condition
Meat-wrappers' asthma 506.9
Meckel's
  diverticulitis 751.0
  diverticulum (displaced) (hypertrophic) 751.0
Meconium
  aspiration 770.11
    with
      pneumonia 770.12
      pneumonitis 770.12
      respiratory symptoms 770.12
    below vocal cords 770.11
      with respiratory symptoms 770.12
    syndrome 770.12
  delayed passage in newborn 777.1
  ileus 777.1
    due to cystic fibrosis 277.01
  in liquor 792.3
    noted during delivery 656.8
  insufflation 770.11
    with respiratory symptoms 770.12
  obstruction
    fetus or newborn 777.1
      in mucoviscidosis 277.01
  passage of 792.3
    noted during delivery 763.84
  peritonitis 777.6
  plug syndrome (newborn) NEC 777.1
  staining 779.84
Median —*see also* condition
  arcuate ligament syndrome 447.4
  bar (prostate) 600.90
    with
      other lower urinary tract symptoms (LUTS) 600.91
      urinary
        obstruction 600.91
        retention 600.91
  vesical orifice 600.90
    with
      other lower urinary tract symptoms (LUTS) 600.91
      urinary
        obstruction 600.91
        retention 600.91
  rhomboid glossitis 529.2
Mediastinal shift 793.2

Mediastinitis (acute) (chronic) 519.2
  actinomycotic 039.8
  syphilitic 095.8
  tuberculous (*see also* Tuberculosis) 012.8
Mediastinopericarditis (*see also* Pericarditis) 423.9
  acute 420.90
  chronic 423.8
    rheumatic 393
  rheumatic, chronic 393
Mediastinum, mediastinal —*see* condition
Medical services provided for —*see* Health, services provided because (of)
Medicine poisoning (by overdose) (wrong substance given or taken in error) 977.9
  specified drug or substance—*see* Table of drugs and chemicals
Medin's disease (poliomyelitis) 045.9
Mediterranean
  anemia (with other hemoglobinopathy) 282.49
  disease or syndrome (hemipathic) 282.49
  fever (*see also* Brucellosis) 023.9
    familial 277.31
  kala-azar 085.0
  leishmaniasis 085.0
  tick fever 082.1
Medulla —*see* condition
Medullary
  cystic kidney 753.16
  sponge kidney 753.17
Medullated fibers
  optic (nerve) 743.57
  retina 362.85
Medulloblastoma (M9470/3)
  desmoplastic (M9471/3) 191.6
  specified site—*see* Neoplasm, by site, malignant
  unspecified site 191.6
Medulloepithelioma (M9501/3)—*see also* Neoplasm, by site, malignant
  teratoid (M9502/3)—*see* Neoplasm, by site, malignant
Medullomyoblastoma (M9472/3)
  specified site—*see* Neoplasm, by site, malignant
  unspecified site 191.6
Meekeren-Ehlers-Danlos syndrome 756.83
Megacaryocytic —*see* condition
Megacolon (acquired) (functional) (not Hirschsprung's disease) 564.7
  aganglionic 751.3
  congenital, congenitum 751.3
  Hirschsprung's (disease) 751.3
  psychogenic 306.4
  toxic (*see also* Colitis, ulcerative) 556.9
Megaduodenum 537.3
Megaesophagus (functional) 530.0
  congenital 750.4
Megakaryocytic —*see* condition
Megalencephaly 742.4
Megalerythema (epidermicum) (infectiosum) 057.0
Megalia, cutis et ossium 757.39
Megaloappendix 751.5
Megalocephalus, megalocephaly NEC 756.0
Megalocornea 743.41
  associated with buphthalmos 743.22
Megalocytic anemia 281.9
Megalodactylia (fingers) (thumbs) 755.57
  toes 755.65
Megaloduodenum 751.5
Megaloesophagus (functional) 530.0
  congenital 750.4
Megalogastria (congenital) 750.7

Megalomania 307.9
Megalophthalmos 743.8
Megalopsia 368.14
Megalosplenia (*see also* Splenomegaly) 789.2
Megaloureter 593.89
  congenital 753.22
Megarectum 569.49
Megasigmoid 564.7
  congenital 751.3
Megaureter 593.89
  congenital 753.22
Megrim 346.9
Meibomian
  cyst 373.2
    infected 373.12
  gland—*see* condition
  infarct (eyelid) 374.85
  stye 373.11
Meibomitis 373.12
Meige
  Milroy disease (chronic hereditary edema) 757.0
  syndrome (blepharospasm-oromandibular dystonia) 333.82
Melalgia, nutritional 266.2
Melancholia (*see also* Psychosis, affective) 296.90
  climacteric 296.2
    recurrent episode 296.3
    single episode 296.2
  hypochondriac 300.7
  intermittent 296.2
    recurrent episode 296.3
    single episode 296.2
  involutional 296.2
    recurrent episode 296.3
    single episode 296.2
  menopausal 296.2
    recurrent episode 296.3
    single episode 296.2
  puerperal 296.2
  reactive (from emotional stress, psychological trauma) 298.0
  recurrent 296.3
  senile 290.21
  stuporous 296.2
    recurrent episode 296.3
    single episode 296.2
Melanemia 275.0
Melanoameloblastoma (M9363/0)—*see* Neoplasm, bone, benign
Melanoblastoma (M8720/3)—*see* Melanoma
Melanoblastosis
  Block-Sulzberger 757.33
  cutis linearis sive systematisata 757.33
Melanocarcinoma (M8720/3)—*see* Melanoma
Melanocytoma, eyeball (M8726/0) 224.0
Melanoderma, melanodermia 709.09
  Addison's (primary adrenal insufficiency) 255.41
Melanodontia, infantile 521.05
Melanodontoclasia 521.05
Melanoepithelioma (M8720/3)—*see* Melanoma
Melanoma (malignant) (M8720/3) 172.9

> Note—Except where otherwise indicated, the morphological varieties of melanoma in the list below should be coded by site as for "Melanoma (malignant)." Internal sites should be coded to malignant neoplasm of those sites.

  abdominal wall 172.5
  ala nasi 172.3

Melanoma—*continued*
  amelanotic (M8730/3)—*see* Melanoma, by site
  ankle 172.7
  anus, anal 154.3
    canal 154.2
  arm 172.6
  auditory canal (external) 172.2
  auricle (ear) 172.2
  auricular canal (external) 172.2
  axilla 172.5
  axillary fold 172.5
  back 172.5
  balloon cell (M8722/3)—*see* Melanoma, by site
  benign (M8720/0)—*see* Neoplasm, skin, benign
  breast (female) (male) 172.5
  brow 172.3
  buttock 172.5
  canthus (eye) 172.1
  cheek (external) 172.3
  chest wall 172.5
  chin 172.3
  choroid 190.6
  conjunctiva 190.3
  ear (external) 172.2
  epithelioid cell (M8771/3)—*see also* Melanoma, by site
    and spindle cell, mixed (M8775/3)—*see* Melanoma, by site
  external meatus (ear) 172.2
  eye 190.9
  eyebrow 172.3
  eyelid (lower) (upper) 172.1
  face NEC 172.3
  female genital organ (external) NEC 184.4
  finger 172.6
  flank 172.5
  foot 172.7
  forearm 172.6
  forehead 172.3
  foreskin 187.1
  gluteal region 172.5
  groin 172.5
  hand 172.6
  heel 172.7
  helix 172.2
  hip 172.7
  in
    giant pigmented nevus (M8761/3)—*see* Melanoma, by site
    Hutchinson's melanotic freckle (M8742/3)—*see* Melanoma, by site
    junctional nevus (M8740/3)—*see* Melanoma, by site
    precancerous melanosis (M8741/3)—*see* Melanoma, by site
  interscapular region 172.5
  iris 190.0
  jaw 172.3
  juvenile (M8770/0)—*see* Neoplasm, skin, benign
  knee 172.7
  labium
    majus 184.1
    minus 184.2
  lacrimal gland 190.2
  leg 172.7
  lip (lower) (upper) 172.0
  liver 197.7
  lower limb NEC 172.7
  male genital organ (external) NEC 187.9
  meatus, acoustic (external) 172.2

Melanoma — INDEX TO DISEASES

Melanoma—*continued*
  meibomian gland 172.1
  metastatic
    of or from specified site—*see* Melanoma, by site
    site not of skin—*see* Neoplasm, by site, malignant, secondary
    to specified site—*see* Neoplasm, by site, malignant, secondary
    unspecified site 172.9
  nail 172.9
    finger 172.6
    toe 172.7
  neck 172.4
  nodular (M8721/3)—*see* Melanoma, by site
  nose, external 172.3
  orbit 190.1
  penis 187.4
  perianal skin 172.5
  perineum 172.5
  pinna 172.2
  popliteal (fossa) (space) 172.7
  prepuce 187.1
  pubes 172.5
  pudendum 184.4
  retina 190.5
  scalp 172.4
  scrotum 187.7
  septum nasal (skin) 172.3
  shoulder 172.6
  skin NEC 172.8
  spindle cell (M8772/3)—*see also* Melanoma, by site
    type A (M8773/3) 190.0
    type B (M8774/3) 190.0
  submammary fold 172.5
  superficial spreading (M8743/3)—*see* Melanoma, by site
  temple 172.3
  thigh 172.7
  toe 172.7
  trunk NEC 172.5
  umbilicus 172.5
  upper limb NEC 172.6
  vagina vault 184.0
  vulva 184.4
Melanoplakia 528.9
Melanosarcoma (M8720/3)—*see also* Melanoma
  epithelioid cell (M8771/3)—*see* Melanoma
Melanosis 709.09
  addisonian (primary adrenal insufficiency) 255.41
    tuberculous (*see also* Tuberculosis) 017.6
  adrenal 255.41
  colon 569.89
  conjunctiva 372.55
    congenital 743.49
  corii degenerativa 757.33
  cornea (presenile) (senile) 371.12
    congenital 743.43
      interfering with vision 743.42
    prenatal 743.43
      interfering with vision 743.42
  eye 372.55
    congenital 743.49
  jute spinners' 709.09
  lenticularis progressiva 757.33
  liver 573.8
  precancerous (M8741/2)—*see also* Neoplasm, skin, in situ
    malignant melanoma in (M8741/3)—*see* Melanoma
  Riehl's 709.09

Melanosis—*continued*
  sclera 379.19
    congenital 743.47
  suprarenal 255.41
  tar 709.09
  toxic 709.09
Melanuria 791.9
MELAS syndrome (mitochondrial encephalopathy, lactic acidosis and stroke-like episodes) 277.87
Melasma 709.09
  adrenal (gland) 255.41
  suprarenal (gland) 255.41
Melena 578.1
  due to
    swallowed maternal blood 777.3
    ulcer—*see* Ulcer, by site, with hemorrhage
  newborn 772.4
    due to swallowed maternal blood 777.3
Meleney's
  gangrene (cutaneous) 686.09
  ulcer (chronic undermining) 686.09
Melioidosis 025
Melitensis, febris 023.0
Melitococcosis 023.0
Melkersson (-Rosenthal) syndrome 351.8
Mellitus, diabetes —*see* Diabetes
Melorheostosis (bone) (leri) 733.99
Meloschisis 744.83
Melotia 744.29
Membrana
  capsularis lentis posterior 743.39
  epipapillaris 743.57
Membranacea placenta —*see* Placenta, abnormal
Membranaceous uterus 621.8
Membrane, membranous —*see also* condition
  folds, congenital—*see* Web
  Jackson's 751.4
  over face (causing asphyxia), fetus or newborn 768.9
  premature rupture—*see* Rupture, membranes, premature
  pupillary 364.74
    persistent 743.46
  retained (complicating delivery) (with hemorrhage) 666.2
    without hemorrhage 667.1
  secondary (eye) 366.50
  unruptured (causing asphyxia) 768.9
  vitreous humor 379.25
Membranitis, fetal 658.4
  affecting fetus or newborn 762.7
Memory disturbance, loss or lack (*see also* Amnesia) 780.93
  mild, following organic brain damage 310.1
MEN (multiple endocrine neoplasia) syndrome
  type 1 258.01
  type IIA 258.02
  type IIB 258.03
Menadione (vitamin K) deficiency 269.0
Menarche, precocious 259.1
Mendacity, pathologic 301.7
Mende's syndrome (ptosis-epicanthus) 270.2
Mendelson's syndrome (resulting from a procedure) 997.3
  obstetric 668.0
Ménétrier's disease or syndrome (hypertrophic gastritis) 535.2

INDEX TO DISEASES — Meningitis

Ménière's disease, syndrome, or vertigo 386.00
  cochlear 386.02
  cochleovestibular 386.01
  inactive 386.04
  in remission 386.04
  vestibular 386.03
Meninges, meningeal —*see* condition
Meningioma (M9530/0)—*see also* Neoplasm, meninges, benign
  angioblastic (M9535/0)—*see* Neoplasm, meninges, benign
  angiomatous (M9534/0)—*see* Neoplasm, meninges, benign
  endotheliomatous (M9531/0)—*see* Neoplasm, meninges, benign
  fibroblastic (M9532/0)—*see* Neoplasm, meninges, benign
  fibrous (M9532/0)—*see* Neoplasm, meninges, benign
  hemangioblastic (M9535/0)—*see* Neoplasm, meninges, benign
  hemangiopericytic (M9536/0)—*see* Neoplasm, meninges, benign
  malignant (M9530/3)—*see* Neoplasm, meninges, malignant
  meningiothelial (M9531/0)—*see* Neoplasm, meninges, benign
  meningotheliomatous (M9531/0)—*see* Neoplasm, meninges, benign
  mixed (M9537/0)—*see* Neoplasm, meninges, benign
  multiple (M9530/1) 237.6
  papillary (M9538/1) 237.6
  psammomatous (M9533/0)—*see* Neoplasm, meninges, benign
  syncytial (M9531/0)—*see* Neoplasm, meninges, benign
  transitional (M9537/0)—*see* Neoplasm, meninges, benign
Meningiomatosis (diffuse) (M9530/1) 237.6
Meningism (*see also* Meningismus) 781.6
Meningismus (infectional) (pneumococcal) 781.6
  due to serum or vaccine 997.09 *[321.8]*
  influenzal NEC 487.8
Meningitis (basal) (basic) (basilar) (brain) (cerebral) (cervical) (congestive) (diffuse) (hemorrhagic) (infantile) (membranous) (metastatic) (nonspecific) (pontine) (progressive) (simple) (spinal) (subacute) (sympathetica) (toxic) 322.9
  abacterial NEC (*see also* Meningitis, aseptic) 047.9
  actinomycotic 039.8 *[320.7]*
  adenoviral 049.1
  Aerobacter aerogenes 320.82
  anaerobes (cocci) (gram-negative) (gram-positive) (mixed) (NEC) 320.81
  arbovirus NEC 066.9 *[321.2]*
    specified type NEC 066.8 *[321.2]*
  aseptic (acute) NEC 047.9
    adenovirus 049.1
    Coxsackie virus 047.0
    due to
      adenovirus 049.1
      Coxsackie virus 047.0
      ECHO virus 047.1
      enterovirus 047.9
      mumps 072.1
      poliovirus (*see also* Poliomyelitis) 045.2 *[321.2]*
    ECHO virus 047.1
    herpes (simplex) virus 054.72
      zoster 053.0
    leptospiral 100.81

Meningitis—*continued*
  lymphocytic choriomeningitis 049.0
  noninfective 322.0
  Bacillus pyocyaneus 320.89
  bacterial NEC 320.9
    anaerobic 320.81
    gram-negative 320.82
      anaerobic 320.81
    Bacteroides (fragilis) (oralis) (melaninogenicus) 320.81
  cancerous (M8000/6) 198.4
  candidal 112.83
  carcinomatous (M8010/6) 198.4
  caseous (*see also* Tuberculosis, meninges) 013.0
  cerebrospinal (acute) (chronic) (diplococcal) (endemic) (epidemic) (fulminant) (infectious) (malignant) (meningococcal) (sporadic) 036.0
    carrier (suspected) of V02.59
  chronic NEC 322.2
  clear cerebrospinal fluid NEC 322.0
  Clostridium (haemolyticum) (novyi) NEC 320.81
  coccidioidomycosis 114.2
  Coxsackie virus 047.0
  cryptococcal 117.5 *[321.0]*
  diplococcal 036.0
    gram-negative 036.0
    gram-positive 320.1
  Diplococcus pneumoniae 320.1
  due to
    actinomycosis 039.8 *[320.7]*
    adenovirus 049.1
    coccidiomycosis 114.2
    enterovirus 047.9
      specified NEC 047.8
    histoplasmosis (*see also* Histoplasmosis) 115.91
    Listerosis 027.0 *[320.7]*
    Lyme disease 088.81 *[320.7]*
    moniliasis 112.83
    mumps 072.1
    neurosyphilis 094.2
    nonbacterial organisms NEC 321.8
    oidiomycosis 112.83
    poliovirus (*see also* Poliomyelitis) 045.2 *[321.2]*
    preventive immunization, inoculation, or vaccination 997.09 *[321.8]*
    sarcoidosis 135 *[321.4]*
    sporotrichosis 117.1 *[321.1]*
    syphilis 094.2
      acute 091.81
      congenital 090.42
      secondary 091.81
    trypanosomiasis (*see also* Trypanosomiasis) 086.9 *[321.3]*
    whooping cough 033.9 *[320.7]*
  E. coli 320.82
  ECHO virus 047.1
  endothelial-leukocytic, benign, recurrent 047.9
  Enterobacter aerogenes 320.82
  enteroviral 047.9
    specified type NEC 047.8
  enterovirus 047.9
    specified NEC 047.8
  eosinophilic 322.1
  epidemic NEC 036.0
  Escherichia coli (E. coli) 320.82
  Eubacterium 320.81
  fibrinopurulent NEC 320.9
    specified type NEC 320.89
  Friedländer (bacillus) 320.82
  fungal NEC 117.9 *[321.1]*

1167

Meningitis—continued
Fusobacterium 320.81
gonococcal 098.82
gram-negative bacteria NEC 320.82
  anaerobic 320.81
  cocci 036.0
    specified NEC 320.82
gram-negative cocci NEC 036.0
  specified NEC 320.82
gram-positive cocci NEC 320.9
H. influenzae 320.0
herpes (simplex) virus 054.72
  zoster 053.0
infectious NEC 320.9
influenzal 320.0
Klebsiella pneumoniae 320.82
late effect—see Late, effect, meningitis
leptospiral (aseptic) 100.81
Listerella (monocytogenes) 027.0 [320.7]
Listeria monocytogenes 027.0 [320.7]
lymphocytic (acute) (benign) (serous) 049.0
  choriomeningitis virus 049.0
meningococcal (chronic) 036.0
Mima polymorpha 320.82
Mollaret's 047.9
monilial 112.83
mumps (virus) 072.1
mycotic NEC 117.9 [321.1]—
Neisseria 036.0
neurosyphilis 094.2
nonbacterial NEC (see also Meningitis, aseptic) 047.9
nonpyogenic NEC 322.0
oidiomycosis 112.83
ossificans 349.2
Peptococcus 320.81
Peptostreptococcus 320.81
pneumococcal 320.1
poliovirus (see also Poliomyelitis) 045.2 [321.2]
Proprionibacterium 320.81
Proteus morganii 320.82
Pseudomonas (aeruginosa) (pyocyaneus) 320.82
purulent NEC 320.9
  specified organism NEC 320.89
pyogenic NEC 320.9
  specified organism NEC 320.89
Salmonella 003.21
septic NEC 320.9
  specified organism NEC 320.89
serosa circumscripta NEC 322.0
serous NEC (see also Meningitis, aseptic) 047.9
  lymphocytic 049.0
  syndrome 348.2
Serratia (marcescens) 320.82
specified organism NEC 320.89
sporadic cerebrospinal 036.0
sporotrichosis 117.1 [321.1]
staphylococcal 320.3
sterile 997.09
streptococcal (acute) 320.2
suppurative 320.9
  specified organism NEC 320.89
syphilitic 094.2
  acute 091.81
  congenital 090.42
  secondary 091.81
torula 117.5 [321.0]
traumatic (complication of injury) 958.8
Treponema (denticola) (macrodenticum) 320.81
trypanosomiasis 086.1 [321.3]
tuberculous (see also Tuberculosis, meninges) 013.0
typhoid 002.0 [320.7]

Meningitis—continued
Veillonella 320.81
Vibrio vulnificus 320.82
viral, virus NEC (see also Meningitis, aseptic) 047.9
Wallgren's (see also Meningitis, aseptic) 047.9
Meningocele (congenital) (spinal) (see also Spina bifida) 741.9
acquired (traumatic) 349.2
cerebral 742.0
cranial 742.0
Meningocerebritis —see Meningoencephalitis
Meningococcemia (acute) (chronic) 036.2
Meningococcus, meningococcal (see also condition) 036.9
adrenalitis, hemorrhagic 036.3
carditis 036.40
carrier (suspected) of V02.59
cerebrospinal fever 036.0
encephalitis 036.1
endocarditis 036.42
exposure to V01.84
infection NEC 036.9
meningitis (cerebrospinal) 036.0
myocarditis 036.43
optic neuritis 036.81
pericarditis 036.41
septicemia (chronic) 036.2
Meningoencephalitis (see also Encephalitis) 323.9
acute NEC 048
bacterial, purulent, pyogenic, or septic—see Meningitis
chronic NEC 094.1
diffuse NEC 094.1
diphasic 063.2
due to
  actinomycosis 039.8 [320.7]
  blastomycosis NEC (see also Blastomycosis) 116.0 [323.41]
  free-living amebae 136.2
  Listeria monocytogenes 027.0 [320.7]
  Lyme disease 088.81 [320.7]
  mumps 072.2
  Naegleria (amebae) (gruberi) (organisms) 136.2
  rubella 056.01
  sporotrichosis 117.1 [321.1]
  toxoplasmosis (acquired) 130.0
    congenital (active) 771.2 [323.41]
  Trypanosoma 086.1 [323.2]
epidemic 036.0
herpes 054.3
herpetic 054.3
H. influenzae 320.0
infectious (acute) 048
influenzal 320.0
late effect—see category 326
Listeria monocytogenes 027.0 [320.7]
lymphocytic (serous) 049.0
mumps 072.2
parasitic NEC 123.9 [323.41]
pneumococcal 320.1
primary amebic 136.2
rubella 056.01
serous 048
  lymphocytic 049.0
specific 094.2
staphylococcal 320.3
streptococcal 320.2
syphilitic 094.2

INDEX TO DISEASES

Meningoencephalitis—*continued*
  toxic NEC 989.9 *[323.71]*
    due to
      carbon tetrachloride 987.8 *[323.71]*
      hydroxyquinoline derivatives poisoning 961.3 *[323.71]*
      lead 984.9 *[323.71]*
      mercury 985.0 *[323.71]*
      thallium 985.8 *[323.71]*
  toxoplasmosis (acquired) 130.0
  trypanosomic 086.1 *[323.2]*
  tuberculous (*see also* Tuberculosis, meninges) 013.0
  virus NEC 048
Meningoencephalocele 742.0
  syphilitic 094.89
  congenital 090.49
Meningoencephalomyelitis (*see also* Meningoencephalitis) 323.9
  acute NEC 048
    disseminated (postinfectious) 136.9 *[323.61]*
      postimmunization or postvaccination 323.51
  due to
    actinomycosis 039.8 *[320.7]*
    torula 117.5 *[323.41]*
    toxoplasma or toxoplasmosis (acquired) 130.0
      congenital (active) 771.2 *[323.41]*
  late effect—*see* category 326
Meningoencephalomyelopathy (*see also* Meningoencephalomyelitis) 349.9
Meningoencephalopathy (*see also* Meningoencephalitis) 348.39
Meningoencephalopoliomyelitis (*see also* Poliomyelitis, bulbar) 045.0
  late effect 138
Meningomyelitis (*see also* Meningoencephalitis) 323.9
  blastomycotic NEC (*see also* Blastomycosis) 116.0 *[323.41]*
  due to
    actinomycosis 039.8 *[320.7]*
    blastomycosis (*see also* Blastomycosis) 116.0 *[323.41]*
    Meningococcus 036.0
    sporotrichosis 117.1 *[323.41]*
    torula 117.5 *[323.41]*
  late effect—*see* category 326
  lethargic 049.8
  meningococcal 036.0
  syphilitic 094.2
  tuberculous (*see also* Tuberculosis, meninges) 013.0
Meningomyelocele (*see also* Spina bifida) 741.9
  syphilitic 094.89
Meningomyeloneuritis —*see* Meningoencephalitis
Meningoradiculitis —*see* Meningitis
Meningovascular —*see* condition
Meniscocytosis 282.60
Menkes' syndrome —*see* Syndrome, Menkes'
Menolipsis 626.0
Menometrorrhagia 626.2
Menopause, menopausal (symptoms) (syndrome) 627.2
  arthritis (any site) NEC 716.3
  artificial 627.4
  bleeding 627.0
  crisis 627.2
  depression (*see also* Psychosis, affective) 296.2
    agitated 296.2
      recurrent episode 296.3

Menopause, menopausal—*continued*
    single episode 296.2
    psychotic 296.2
      recurrent episode 296.3
      single episode 296.2
    recurrent episode 296.3
    single episode 296.2
  melancholia (*see also* Psychosis, affective) 296.2
    recurrent episode 296.3
    single episode 296.2
  paranoid state 297.2
  paraphrenia 297.2
  postsurgical 627.4
  premature 256.31
    postirradiation 256.2
    postsurgical 256.2
  psychoneurosis 627.2
  psychosis NEC 298.8
  surgical 627.4
  toxic polyarthritis NEC 716.39
Menorrhagia (primary) 626.2
  climacteric 627.0
  menopausal 627.0
  postclimacteric 627.1
  postmenopausal 627.1
  preclimacteric 627.0
  premenopausal 627.0
  puberty (menses retained) 626.3
Menorrhalgia 625.3
Menoschesis 626.8
Menostaxis 626.2
Menses, retention 626.8
Menstrual —*see* Menstruation
  cycle, irregular 626.4
  disorders NEC 626.9
  extraction V25.3
  fluid, retained 626.8
  molimen 625.4
  period, normal V65.5
  regulation V25.3
Menstruation
  absent 626.0
  anovulatory 628.0
  delayed 626.8
  difficult 625.3
  disorder 626.9
    psychogenic 306.52
    specified NEC 626.8
  during pregnancy 640.8
  excessive 626.2
  frequent 626.2
  infrequent 626.1
  irregular 626.4
  latent 626.8
  membranous 626.8
  painful (primary) (secondary) 625.3
    psychogenic 306.52
  passage of clots 626.2
  precocious 626.8
  protracted 626.8
  retained 626.8
  retrograde 626.8
  scanty 626.1
  suppression 626.8
  vicarious (nasal) 625.8
Mentagra (*see also* Sycosis) 704.8
Mental —*see also* condition
  deficiency (*see also* Retardation, mental) 319
  deterioration (*see also* Psychosis) 298.9
  disorder (*see also* Disorder, mental) 300.9
  exhaustion 300.5

Mental—*continued*
　insufficiency (congenital) (*see also* Retardation, mental) 319
　observation without need for further medical care NEC V71.09
　retardation (*see also* Retardation, mental) 319
　subnormality (*see also* Retardation, mental) 319
　　mild 317
　　moderate 318.0
　　profound 318.2
　　severe 318.1
　upset (*see also* Disorder, mental) 300.9
Meralgia paresthetica 355.1
Mercurial —*see* condition
Mercurialism NEC 985.0
Merergasia 300.9
Merkel cell tumor —*see* Neoplasm, by site, malignant
Merocele (*see also* Hernia, femoral) 553.00
Meromelia 755.4
　lower limb 755.30
　　intercalary 755.32
　　　femur 755.34
　　　　tibiofibular (complete) (incomplete) 755.33
　　　fibula 755.37
　　　metatarsal(s) 755.38
　　　tibia 755.36
　　　tibiofibular 755.35
　　terminal (complete) (partial) (transverse) 755.31
　　　longitudinal 755.32
　　　　metatarsal(s) 755.38
　　　　phalange(s) 755.39
　　　　tarsal(s) 755.38
　　　transverse 755.31
　upper limb 755.20
　　intercalary 755.22
　　　carpal(s) 755.28
　　　humeral 755.24
　　　　radioulnar (complete) (incomplete) 755.23
　　　metacarpal(s) 755.28
　　　phalange(s) 755.29
　　　radial 755.26
　　　radioulnar 755.25
　　　ulnar 755.27
　　terminal (complete) (partial) (transverse) 755.21
　　　longitudinal 755.22
　　　　carpal(s) 755.28
　　　　metacarpal(s) 755.28
　　　　phalange(s) 755.29
　　　transverse 755.21
Merosmia 781.1
MERRF syndrome (myoclonus with epilepsy and with ragged red fibers) 277.87
Merycism (*see also* Rumination)—*see also* Vomiting
　psychogenic 307.53
Merzbacher-Pelizaeus disease 330.0
Mesaortitis —*see* Aortitis
Mesarteritis —*see* Arteritis
Mesencephalitis (*see also* Encephalitis) 323.9
　late effect—*see* category 326
Mesenchymoma (M8990/1)—*see also* Neoplasm, connective tissue, uncertain behavior
　benign (M8990/0)—*see* Neoplasm, connective tissue, benign
　malignant (M8990/3)—*see* Neoplasm, connective tissue, malignant

Mesenteritis
　retractile 567.82
　sclerosing 567.82
Mesentery, mesenteric —*see* condition
Mesiodens, mesiodentes 520.1
　causing crowding 524.31
Mesio-occlusion 524.23
Mesocardia (with asplenia) 746.87
Mesocolon —*see* condition
Mesonephroma (malignant) (M9110/3)—*see also* Neoplasm, by site, malignant
　benign (M9110/0)—*see* Neoplasm, by site, benign
Mesophlebitis —*see* Phlebitis
Mesostromal dysgenesis 743.51
Mesothelioma (malignant) (M9050/3)—*see also* Neoplasm, by site, malignant
　benign (M9050/0)—*see* Neoplasm, by site, benign
　biphasic type (M9053/3)—*see also* Neoplasm, by site, malignant
　　benign (M9053/0)—*see* Neoplasm, by site, benign
　epithelioid (M9052/3)—*see also* Neoplasm, by site, malignant
　　benign (M9052/0)—*see* Neoplasm, by site, benign
　fibrous (M9051/3)—*see also* Neoplasm, by site, malignant
　　benign (M9051/0)—*see* Neoplasm, by site, benign
Metabolic syndrome 277.7
Metabolism disorder 277.9
　specified type NEC 277.89
Metagonimiasis 121.5
Metagonimus infestation (small intestine) 121.5
Metal
　pigmentation (skin) 709.00
　polishers' disease 502
Metalliferous miners' lung 503
Metamorphopsia 368.14
Metaplasia
　bone, in skin 709.3
　breast 611.8
　cervix—*omit code*
　endometrium (squamous) 621.8
　esophagus 530.85
　intestinal, of gastric mucosa 537.89
　kidney (pelvis) (squamous) (*see also* Disease, renal) 593.89
　myelogenous 289.89
　myeloid 289.89
　　agnogenic 238.76
　　megakaryocytic 238.76
　spleen 289.59
　squamous cell
　　amnion 658.8
　　bladder 596.8
　　cervix—*see* condition
　　trachea 519.19
　　tracheobronchial tree 519.19
　uterus 621.8
　　cervix—*see* condition
Metastasis, metastatic
　abscess—*see* Abscess
　calcification 275.40
　cancer, neoplasm, or disease
　　from specified site (M8000/3)—*see* Neoplasm, by site, malignant
　　to specified site (M8000/6)—*see* Neoplasm, by site, secondary
　deposits (in) (M8000/6)—*see* Neoplasm, by site, secondary

Metastasis, metastatic—*continued*
  pneumonia 038.8 *[484.8]*
  spread (to) (M8000/6)—*see* Neoplasm, by site, secondary
Metatarsalgia 726.70
  anterior 355.6
  due to Freiberg's disease 732.5
  Morton's 355.6
Metatarsus, metatarsal —*see also* condition
  adductus varus (congenital) 754.53
  abductus valgus (congenital) 764.60
  primus varus 754.52
  valgus (adductus) (congenital) 754.60
  varus (abductus) (congenital) 754.53
    primus 754.52
Methemoglobinemia 289.7
  acquired (with sulfhemoglobinemia) 289.7
  congenital 289.7
  enzymatic 289.7
  Hb-M disease 289.7
  hereditary 289.7
  toxic 289.7
Methemoglobinuria (*see also* Hemoglobinuria) 791.2
Methicillin-resistant staphylococcus aureus (MRSA) V09.0
Methioninemia 270.4
Metritis (catarrhal) (septic) (suppurative) (*see also* Endometritis) 615.9
  blennorrhagic 098.16
    chronic or duration of 2 months or over 098.36
  cervical (*see also* Cervicitis) 616.0
  gonococcal 098.16
    chronic or duration of 2 months or over 098.36
  hemorrhagic 626.8
  puerperal, postpartum, childbirth 670
  tuberculous (*see also* Tuberculosis) 016.7
Metropathia hemorrhagica 626.8
Metroperitonitis (*see also* Peritonitis, pelvic, female) 614.5
Metrorrhagia 626.6
  arising during pregnancy—*see* Hemorrhage, pregnancy
  postpartum NEC 666.2
  primary 626.6
  psychogenic 306.59
  puerperal 666.2
Metrorrhexis —*see* Rupture, uterus
Metrosalpingitis (*see also* Salpingo-oophoritis) 614.2
Metrostaxis 626.6
Metrovaginitis (*see also* Endometritis) 615.9
  gonococcal (acute) 098.16
    chronic or duration of 2 months or over 098.36
Mexican fever —*see* Typhus, Mexican
Meyenburg-Altherr-Uehlinger syndrome 733.99
Meyer-Schwickerath and Weyers syndrome (dysplasia oculodentodigitalis) 759.89
Meynert's amentia (nonalcoholic) 294.0
  alcoholic 291.1
Mibelli's disease 757.39
Mice, joint (*see also* Loose, body, joint) 718.1
  knee 717.6
Micheli-Rietti syndrome (thalassemia minor) 282.49
Michotte's syndrome 721.5
Micrencephalon, micrencephaly 742.1
Microalbuminuria 791.0
Microaneurysm, retina 362.14
  diabetic 250.5 *[362.01]*

Microangiopathy 443.9
  diabetic (peripheral) 250.7 *[443.81]*
    retinal 250.5 *[362.01]*
  peripheral 443.9
    diabetic 250.7 *[443.81]*
  retinal 362.18
    diabetic 250.5 *[362.01]*
  thrombotic 446.6
    Moschcowitz's (thrombotic thrombocytopenic purpura) 446.6
Microcalcification, mammographic 793.81
Microcephalus, microcephalic, microcephaly 742.1
  due to toxoplasmosis (congenital) 771.2
Microcheilia 744.82
Microcolon (congenital) 751.5
Microcornea (congenital) 743.41
Microcytic —*see* condition
Microdeletions NEC 758.33
Microdontia 520.2
Microdrepanocytosis (thalassemia-Hb-S disease) 282.49
Microembolism
  atherothrombotic—*see also* Atheroembolism
  retina 362.33
Microencephalon 742.1
Microfilaria streptocerca infestation 125.3
Microgastria (congenital) 750.7
Microgenia 524.06
Microgenitalia (congenital) 752.89
  penis 752.64
Microglioma (M9710/3)
  specified site—*see* Neoplasm, by site, malignant
  unspecified site 191.9
Microglossia (congenital) 750.16
Micrognathia, micrognathism (congenital) 524.00
  mandibular 524.04
    alveolar 524.74
  maxillary 524.03
    alveolar 524.73
Microgyria (congenital) 742.2
Microinfarct, heart (*see also* Insufficiency, coronary) 411.89
Microlithiasis, alveolar, pulmonary 516.2
Micromyelia (congenital) 742.59
Micropenis 752.64
Microphakia (congenital) 743.36
Microphthalmia (congenital) (*see also* Microphthalmos) 743.10
Microphthalmos (congenital) 743.10
  associated with eye and adnexal anomalies NEC 743.12
  due to toxoplasmosis (congenital) 771.2
  isolated 743.11
  simple 743.11
  syndrome 759.89
Micropsia 368.14
Microsporidiosis 136.8
Microsporon furfur infestation 111.0
Microsporosis (*see also* Dermatophytosis) 110.9
  nigra 111.1
Microstomia (congenital) 744.84
Microthelia 757.6
Microthromboembolism —*see* Embolism
Microtia (congenital) (external ear) 744.23
Microtropia 378.34
Micturition
  disorder NEC 788.69
    psychogenic 306.53
  frequency 788.41

Micturition—*continued*
    psychogenic 306.53
    nocturnal 788.43
    painful 788.1
        psychogenic 306.53
Middle
    ear—*see* condition
    lobe (right) syndrome 518.0
Midplane —*see* condition
Miescher's disease 709.3
    cheilitis 351.8
    granulomatosis disciformis 709.3
Miescher-Leder syndrome or granulomatosis 709.3
Mieten's syndrome 759.89
Migraine (idiopathic) 346.9
    with aura 346.0
    abdominal (syndrome) 346.2
    allergic (histamine) 346.2
    atypical 346.1
    basilar 346.2
    classical 346.0
    common 346.1
    hemiplegic 346.8
    lower-half 346.2
    menstrual 625.4
    ophthalmic 346.8
    ophthalmoplegic 346.8
    retinal 346.2
    variant 346.2
Migrant, social V60.0
Migratory, migrating —*see also* condition
    person V60.0
    testis, congenital 752.52
Mikulicz's disease or syndrome (dryness of mouth, absent or decreased lacrimation) 527.1
Milian atrophia blanche 701.3
Miliaria (crystallina) (rubra) (tropicalis) 705.1
    apocrine 705.82
Miliary —*see* condition
Milium (*see also* Cyst, sebaceous) 706.2
    colloid 709.3
    eyelid 374.84
Milk
    crust 690.11
    excess secretion 676.6
    fever, female 672
    poisoning 988.8
    retention 676.2
    sickness 988.8
    spots 423.1
Milkers' nodes 051.1
Milk-leg (deep vessels) 671.4
    complicating pregnancy 671.3
    nonpuerperal 451.19
    puerperal, postpartum, childbirth 671.4
Milkman (-Looser) disease or syndrome (osteomalacia with pseudofractures) 268.2
Milky urine (*see also* Chyluria) 791.1
Millar's asthma (laryngismus stridulus) 478.75
Millard-Gubler paralysis or syndrome 344.89
Millard-Gubler-Foville paralysis 344.89
Miller-Dieker syndrome 758.33
Miller's disease (osteomalacia) 268.2
Miller Fisher's syndrome 357.0
Milles' syndrome (encephalocutaneous angiomatosis) 759.6
Mills' disease 335.29
Millstone makers' asthma or lung 502
Milroy's disease (chronic hereditary edema) 757.0

Miners' —*see also* condition
    asthma 500
    elbow 727.2
    knee 727.2
    lung 500
    nystagmus 300.89
    phthisis (*see also* Tuberculosis) 011.4
    tuberculosis (*see also* Tuberculosis) 011.4
Minkowski-Chauffard syndrome (*see also* Spherocytosis) 282.0
Minor —*see* condition
Minor's disease 336.1
Minot's disease (hemorrhagic disease, newborn) 776.0
Minot-von Willebrand (-Jürgens) disease or syndrome (angiohemophilia) 286.4
Minus (and plus) hand (intrinsic) 736.09
Miosis (persistent) (pupil) 379.42
Mirizzi's syndrome (hepatic duct stenosis) (*see also* Obstruction, biliary) 576.2
    with calculus, cholelithiasis, or stones—*see* Choledocholithiasis
Mirror writing 315.09
    secondary to organic lesion 784.69
Misadventure (prophylactic) (therapeutic) (*see also* Complications) 999.9
    administration of insulin 962.3
    infusion—*see* Complications, infusion
    local applications (of fomentations, plasters, etc.) 999.9
        burn or scald—*see* Burn, by site
    medical care (early) (late) NEC 999.9
        adverse effect of drugs or chemicals—*see* Table of drugs and chemicals
        burn or scald—*see* Burn, by site
    radiation NEC 990
    radiotherapy NEC 990
    surgical procedure (early) (late)—*see* Complications, surgical procedure
    transfusion—*see* Complications, transfusion
    vaccination or other immunological procedure—*see* Complications, vaccination
Misanthropy 301.7
Miscarriage —*see* Abortion, spontaneous
Mischief, malicious, child (*see also* Disturbance, conduct) 312.0
Misdirection
    aqueous 365.83
Mismanagement, feeding 783.3
Misplaced, misplacement
    kidney (*see also* Disease, renal) 593.0
        congenital 753.3
    organ or site, congenital NEC—*see* Malposition, congenital
Missed
    abortion 632
    delivery (at or near term) 656.4
    labor (at or near term) 656.4
Missing —*see also* Absence
    teeth (acquired) 525.10
        congenital (*see also* Anodontia) 520.0
        due to
            caries 525.13
            extraction 525.10
            periodontal disease 525.12
            trauma 525.11
        specified NEC 525.19
    vertebrae (congenital) 756.13
Misuse of drugs NEC (*see also* Abuse, drug, nondependent) 305.9
Mitchell's disease (erythromelalgia) 443.82

Mite (s)
  diarrhea 133.8
  grain (itch) 133.8
  hair follicle (itch) 133.8
  in sputum 133.8
Mitochondrial encephalopathy, lactic acidosis and stroke-like episodes (MELAS syndrome) 277.87
Mitochondrial neurogastrointestinal encephalopathy syndrome (MNGIE) 277.87
Mitral —*see* condition
Mittelschmerz 625.2
Mixed —*see* condition
Mljet disease (mal de Meleda) 757.39
Mobile, mobility
  cecum 751.4
  coccyx 733.99
  excessive—*see* Hypermobility
  gallbladder 751.69
  kidney 593.0
    congenital 753.3
  organ or site, congenital NEC—*see* Malposition, congenital
  spleen 289.59
Mobitz heart block (atrioventricular) 426.10
  type I (Wenckebach's) 426.13
  type II 426.12
Möbius'
  disease 346.8
  syndrome
    congenital oculofacial paralysis 352.6
    ophthalmoplegic migraine 346.8
Moeller (-Barlow) disease (infantile scurvy) 267
  glossitis 529.4
Mohr's syndrome (Types I and II) 759.89
Mola destruens (M9100/1) 236.1
Molarization, premolars 520.2
Molar pregnancy 631
  hydatidiform (delivered) (undelivered) 630
Mold (s) in vitreous 117.9
Molding, head (during birth)—*omit code*
Mole (pigmented) (M8720/0)—*see also* Neoplasm, skin, benign
  blood 631
  Breus' 631
  cancerous (M8720/3)—*see* Melanoma
  carneous 631
  destructive (M9100/1) 236.1
  ectopic—*see* Pregnancy, ectopic
  fleshy 631
  hemorrhagic 631
  hydatid, hydatidiform (benign) (complicating pregnancy) (delivered) (undelivered) (*see also* Hydatidiform mole) 630
    invasive (M9100/1) 236.1
    malignant (M9100/1) 236.1
    previous, affecting management of pregnancy V23.1
  invasive (hydatidiform) (M9100/1) 236.1
  malignant
    meaning
      malignant hydatidiform mole (M9100/1) 236.1
      melanoma (M8720/3)—*see* Melanoma
    nonpigmented (M8730/0)—*see* Neoplasm, skin, benign
  pregnancy NEC 631
  skin (M8720/0)—*see* Neoplasm, skin, benign
  tubal—*see* Pregnancy, tubal
  vesicular (*see also* Hydatidiform mole) 630
Molimen, molimina (menstrual) 625.4
Mollaret's meningitis 047.9
Mollities (cerebellar) (cerebral) 437.8
  ossium 268.2
Molluscum
  contagiosum 078.0
  epitheliale 078.0
  fibrosum (M8851/0)—*see* Lipoma, by site
  pendulum (M8851/0)—*see* Lipoma, by site
Mönckeberg's arteriosclerosis, degeneration disease, or sclerosis (*see also* Arteriosclerosis, extremities) 440.20
Monday fever 504
Monday morning dyspnea or asthma 504
Mondini's malformation (cochlea) 744.05
Mondor's disease (thrombophlebitis of breast) 451.89
Mongolian, mongolianism, mongolism mongoloid 758.0
  spot 757.33
Monilethrix (congenital) 757.4
Monilia infestation —*see* Candidiasis
Moniliasis —*see also* Candidiasis
  neonatal 771.7
  vulvovaginitis 112.1
Monkeypox 057.8
Monoarthritis 716.60
  ankle 716.67
  arm 716.62
    lower (and wrist) 716.63
    upper (and elbow) 716.62
  foot (and ankle) 716.67
  forearm (and wrist) 716.63
  hand 716.64
  leg 716.66
    lower 716.66
    upper 716.65
  pelvic region (hip) (thigh) 716.65
  shoulder (region) 716.61
  specified site NEC 716.68
Monoblastic —*see* condition
Monochromatism (cone) (rod) 368.54
Monocytic —*see* condition
Monocytopenia 288.59
Monocytosis (symptomatic) 288.63
Monofixation syndrome 378.34
Monomania (*see also* Psychosis) 298.9
Mononeuritis 355.9
  cranial nerve—*see* Disorder, nerve, cranial
  femoral nerve 355.2
  lateral
    cutaneous nerve of thigh 355.1
    popliteal nerve 355.3
  lower limb 355.8
    specified nerve NEC 355.79
  medial popliteal nerve 355.4
  median nerve 354.1
  multiplex 354.5
  plantar nerve 355.6
  posterior tibial nerve 355.5
  radial nerve 354.3
  sciatic nerve 355.0
  ulnar nerve 354.2
  upper limb 354.9
    specified nerve NEC 354.8
  vestibular 388.5
Mononeuropathy (*see also* Mononeuritis) 355.9
  diabetic NEC 250.6 *[355.9]*
    lower limb 250.6 *[355.8]*
    upper limb 250.6 *[354.9]*
  iliohypogastric nerve 355.79
  ilioinguinal nerve 355.79

Mononeuropathy INDEX TO DISEASES

Mononeuropathy—*continued*
  obturator nerve 355.79
  saphenous nerve 355.79
Mononucleosis, infectious 075
  with hepatitis 075 *[573.1]*
Monoplegia 344.5
  brain (current episode) (*see also* Paralysis, brain) 437.8
    fetus or newborn 767.8
  cerebral (current episode) (*see also* Paralysis, brain) 437.8
  congenital or infantile (cerebral) (spastic) (spinal) 343.3
  embolic (current) (*see also* Embolism, brain) 434.1
    late effect—*see* Late effect(s) (of) cerebrovascular disease
  infantile (cerebral) (spastic) (spinal) 343.3
  lower limb 344.30
    affecting
      dominant side 344.31
      nondominant side 344.32
    due to late effect of cerebrovascular accident—*see* Late effect(s) (of) cerebrovascular accident
  newborn 767.8
  psychogenic 306.0
    specified as conversion reaction 300.11
  thrombotic (current) (*see also* Thrombosis, brain) 434.0
    late effect—*see* Late effect(s) (of) cerebrovascular disease
  transient 781.4
  upper limb 344.40
    affecting
      dominant side 344.41
      nondominant side 344.42
    due to late effect of cerebrovascular accident—*see* Late effect(s) (of) cerebrovascular accident
Monorchism, monorchidism 752.89
Monteggia's fracture (closed) 813.03
  open 813.13
Mood swings
  brief compensatory 296.99
  rebound 296.99
Moore's syndrome (*see also* Epilepsy) 345.5
Mooren's ulcer (cornea) 370.07
Mooser-Neill reaction 081.0
Mooser bodies 081.0
Moral
  deficiency 301.7
  imbecility 301.7
Morax-Axenfeld conjunctivitis 372.03
Morbilli (*see also* Measles) 055.9
Morbus
  anglicus, anglorum 268.0
  Beigel 111.2
  caducus (*see also* Epilepsy) 345.9
  caeruleus 746.89
  celiacus 579.0
  comitialis (*see also* Epilepsy) 345.9
  cordis—*see* Disease, heart
    valvulorum—*see* Endocarditis
  coxae 719.95
    tuberculous (*see also* Tuberculosis) 015.1
  hemorrhagicus neonatorum 776.0
  maculosus neonatorum 772.6
  renum 593.0
  senilis (*see also* Osteoarthrosis) 715.9
Morel-Kraepelin disease (*see also* Schizophrenia) 295.9

Morel-Moore syndrome (hyperostosis frontalis interna) 733.3
Morel-Morgagni syndrome (hyperostosis frontalis interna) 733.3
Morgagni
  cyst, organ, hydatid, or appendage 752.89
    fallopian tube 752.11
  disease or syndrome (hyperostosis frontalis interna) 733.3
Morgagni-Adams-Stokes syndrome (syncope with heart block) 426.9
Morgagni-Stewart-Morel syndrome (hyperostosis frontalis interna) 733.3
Moria (*see also* Psychosis) 298.9
Morning sickness 643.0
Moron 317
Morphea (guttate) (linear) 701.0
Morphine dependence (*see also* Dependence) 304.0
Morphinism (*see also* Dependence) 304.0
Morphinomania (*see also* Dependence) 304.0
Morphoea 701.0
Morquio (-Brailsford) (-Ullrich) disease or syndrome (mucopolysaccharidosis IV) 277.5
  kyphosis 277.5
Morris syndrome (testicular feminization) 259.5
Morsus humanus (open wound)—*see also* Wound, open, by site
  skin surface intact—*see* Contusion
Mortification (dry) (moist) (*see also* Gangrene) 785.4
Morton's
  disease 355.6
  foot 355.6
  metatarsalgia (syndrome) 355.6
  neuralgia 355.6
  neuroma 355.6
  syndrome (metatarsalgia) (neuralgia) 355.6
  toe 355.6
Morvan's disease 336.0
Mosaicism, mosaic (chromosomal) 758.9
  autosomal 758.5
  sex 758.81
Moschcowitz's syndrome (thrombotic thrombocytopenic purpura) 446.6
Mother yaw 102.0
Motion sickness (from travel, any vehicle) (from roundabouts or swings) 994.6
Mottled teeth (enamel) (endemic) (nonendemic) 520.3
Mottling enamel (endemic) (nonendemic) (teeth) 520.3
Mouchet's disease 732.5
Mould (s) (in vitreous) 117.9
Moulders'
  bronchitis 502
  tuberculosis (*see also* Tuberculosis) 011.4
Mounier-Kuhn syndrome 748.3
  with
    acute exacerbation 494.1
    bronchiectasis 494.0
      with (acute) exacerbation 494.1
  acquired 519.19
    with bronchiectasis 494.0
      with (acute) exacerbation 494.1
Mountain
  fever—*see* Fever, mountain
  sickness 993.2
    with polycythemia, acquired 289.0
    acute 289.0
  tick fever 066.1

1174

INDEX TO DISEASES

Mouse, joint (*see also* Loose, body, joint) 718.1
   knee 717.6
Mouth —*see* condition
Movable
   coccyx 724.71
   kidney (*see also* Disease, renal) 593.0
     congenital 753.3
   organ or site, congenital NEC—*see* Malposition, congenital
   spleen 289.59
Movement
   abnormal (dystonic) (involuntary) 781.0
   decreased fetal 655.7
   paradoxical facial 374.43
Moya Moya disease 437.5
Mozart's ear 744.29
MRSA (methicillin-resistant staphylococcus aureus) V09.0
Mucha's disease (acute parapsoriasis varioliformis) 696.2
Mucha-Haberman syndrome (acute parapsoriasis varioliformis) 696.2
Mu-chain disease 273.2
Mucinosis (cutaneous) (papular) 701.8
Mucocele
   appendix 543.9
   buccal cavity 528.9
   gallbladder (*see also* Disease, gallbladder) 575.3
   lacrimal sac 375.43
   orbit (eye) 376.81
   salivary gland (any) 527.6
   sinus (accessory) (nasal) 478.19
   turbinate (bone) (middle) (nasal) 478.19
   uterus 621.8
Mucocutaneous lymph node syndrome (acute) (febrile) (infantile) 446.1
Mucoenteritis 564.9
Mucolipidosis I, II, III 272.7
Mucopolysaccharidosis (types 1-6) 277.5
   cardiopathy 277.5 *[425.7]*
Mucormycosis (lung) 117.7
Mucosa associated lymphoid tissue (MALT) 200.3
Mucositis —*see also* Inflammation, by site 528.00
   cervix (ulcerative) 616.81
   due to
     antineoplastic therapy (ulcerative) 528.01
     other drugs (ulcerative) 528.02
     specified NEC 528.09
   gastrointestinal (ulcerative) 538
   nasal (ulcerative) 478.11
   necroticans agranulocytica (*see also* Agranulocytosis) 288.09
   ulcerative 528.00
   vagina (ulcerative) 616.81
   vulva (ulcerative) 616.81
Mucous —*see also* condition
   patches (syphilitic) 091.3
     congenital 090.0
Mucoviscidosis 277.00
   with meconium obstruction 277.01
Mucus
   asphyxia or suffocation (*see also* Asphyxia, mucus) 933.1
     newborn 770.18
   in stool 792.1
   plug (*see also* Asphyxia, mucus) 933.1
     aspiration, of newborn 770.17
     tracheobronchial 519.19
       newborn 770.18
Muguet 112.0

Mulberry molars 090.5
Mullerian mixed tumor (M8950/3)—*see* Neoplasm, by site, malignant
Multicystic kidney 753.19
Multilobed placenta —*see* Placenta, abnormal
Multinodular prostate 600.10
   with
     urinary
       obstruction 600.11
       retention 600.11
Multiparity V61.5
   affecting
     fetus or newborn 763.89
     management of
       labor and delivery 659.4
       pregnancy V23.3
   requiring contraceptive management (*see also* Contraception) V25.9
Multipartita placenta —*see* Placenta, abnormal
Multiple, multiplex —*see also* condition
   birth
     affecting fetus or newborn 761.5
     healthy liveborn—*see* Newborn, multiple
   digits (congenital) 755.00
     fingers 755.01
     toes 755.02
   organ or site NEC—*see* Accessory
   personality 300.14
   renal arteries 747.62
Mumps 072.9
   with complication 072.8
     specified type NEC 072.79
   encephalitis 072.2
   hepatitis 072.71
   meningitis (aseptic) 072.1
   meningoencephalitis 072.2
   oophoritis 072.79
   orchitis 072.0
   pancreatitis 072.3
   polyneuropathy 072.72
   vaccination, prophylactic (against) V04.6
Mumu (*see also* Infestation, filarial) 125.9
Münchausen syndrome 301.51
Münchmeyer's disease or syndrome (exostosis luxurians) 728.11
Mural —*see* condition
Murmur (cardiac) (heart) (nonorganic) (organic) 785.2
   abdominal 787.5
   aortic (valve) (*see also* Endocarditis, aortic) 424.1
   benign—*omit code*
   cardiorespiratory 785.2
   diastolic—*see* condition
   Flint (*see also* Endocarditis, aortic) 424.1
   functional—*omit code*
   Graham Steell (pulmonic regurgitation) (*see also* Endocarditis, pulmonary) 424.3
   innocent—*omit code*
   insignificant—*omit code*
   midsystolic 785.2
   mitral (valve)—*see* stenosis, mitral
   physiologic—*see* condition
   presystolic, mitral—*see* Insufficiency, mitral
   pulmonic (valve) (*see also* Endocarditis, pulmonary) 424.3
   Still's (vibratory)—*omit code*
   systolic (valvular)—*see* condition
   tricuspid (valve)—*see* Endocarditis, tricuspid
   valvular—*see* condition
   vibratory—*omit code*
   undiagnosed 785.2
Murri's disease (intermittent hemoglobinuria) 283.2

Muscae volitantes 379.24
Muscle, muscular —*see* condition
Musculoneuralgia 729.1
Mushrooming hip 718.95
Mushroom workers' (pickers') lung 495.5
Mutation
  factor V leiden 289.81
  prothrombin gene 289.81
Mutism (*see also* Aphasia) 784.3
  akinetic 784.3
  deaf (acquired) (congenital) 389.7
  hysterical 300.11
  selective (elective) 313.23
    adjustment reaction 309.83
Myà's disease (congenital dilation, colon) 751.3
Myalgia (intercostal) 729.1
  eosinophilia syndrome 710.5
  epidemic 074.1
    cervical 078.89
  psychogenic 307.89
  traumatic NEC 959.9
Myasthenia 358.00
  cordis—*see* Failure, heart
  gravis 358.00
    with exacerbation (acute) 358.01
    in crisis 358.01
    neonatal 775.2
    pseudoparalytica 358.00
  stomach 536.8
    psychogenic 306.4
  syndrome in
    botulism 005.1 *[358.1]*
    diabetes mellitus 250.6 *[358.1]*
    hypothyroidism (*see also* Hypothyroidism) 244.9 *[358.1]*
    malignant neoplasm NEC 199.1 *[358.1]*
    pernicious anemia 281.0 *[358.1]*
    thyrotoxicosis (*see also* Thyrotoxicosis) 242.9 *[358.1]*
Myasthenic 728.87
Mycelium infection NEC 117.9
Mycetismus 988.1
Mycetoma (actinomycotic) 039.9
  bone 039.8
    mycotic 117.4
  foot 039.4
    mycotic 117.4
  madurae 039.9
    mycotic 117.4
  maduromycotic 039.9
    mycotic 117.4
  nocardial 039.9
Mycobacteriosis —*see* Mycobacterium
Mycobacterium, mycobacterial (infection) 031.9
  acid-fast (bacilli) 031.9
  anonymous (*see also* Mycobacterium, atypical) 031.9
  atypical (acid-fast bacilli) 031.9
    cutaneous 031.1
    pulmonary 031.0
      tuberculous (*see also* Tuberculosis, pulmonary) 011.9
    specified site NEC 031.8
  avium 031.0
    intracellulare complex bacteremia (MAC) 031.2
  balnei 031.1
  Battey 031.0
  cutaneous 031.1
  disseminated 031.2
    avium-intracellulare complex (DMAC) 031.2

Mycobacterium, mycobacterial—*continued*
  fortuitum 031.1
  intracellulare (battey bacillus) 031.0
  kakerifu 031.8
  kansasii 031.0
  kasongo 031.8
  leprae—*see* Leprosy
  luciflavum 031.0
  marinum 031.1
  pulmonary 031.0
    tuberculous (*see also* Tuberculosis, pulmonary) 011.9
  scrofulaceum 031.1
  tuberculosis (human, bovine)—*see also* Tuberculosis
    avian type 031.0
  ulcerans 031.1
  xenopi 031.0
Mycosis, mycotic 117.9
  cutaneous NEC 111.9
  ear 111.8 *[380.15]*
  fungoides (M9700/3) 202.1
  mouth 112.0
  pharynx 117.9
  skin NEC 111.9
  stomatitis 112.0
  systemic NEC 117.9
  tonsil 117.9
  vagina, vaginitis 112.1
Mydriasis (persistent) (pupil) 379.43
Myelatelia 742.59
Myelinoclasis, perivascular, acute (postinfectious) NEC 136.9 *[323.61]*
  postimmunization or postvaccinal 323.51
Myelinosis, central pontine 341.8
Myelitis (ascending) (cerebellar) (childhood) (chronic) (descending) (diffuse) (disseminated) (pressure) (progressive) (spinal cord) (subacute) (*see also* Encephalitis) 323.9
  acute (transverse) 341.20
    idiopathic 341.22
    in conditions classified elsewhere 341.21
  due to
    infection classified elsewhere 136.9 *[323.42]*
    specified cause NEC 323.82
    vaccination (any) 323.52
    viral diseases classified elsewhere 323.02
  herpes simplex 054.74
  herpes zoster 053.14
  late effect—*see* category 326
  optic neuritis in 341.0
  postchickenpox 052.2
  postimmunization 323.52
  postinfectious 136.9 *[323.63]*
  postvaccinal 323.52
  postvaricella 052.2
  syphilitic (transverse) 094.89
  toxic 989.9 *[323.72]*
  transverse 323.82
    acute 341.20
      idiopathic 341.22
      in conditions classified elsewhere 341.21
    idiopathic 341.22
  tuberculous (*see also* Tuberculosis) 013.6
  virus 049.9
Myeloblastic —*see* condition
Myelocele (*see also* Spina bifida) 741.9
  with hydrocephalus 741.0
Myelocystocele (*see also* Spina bifida) 741.9
Myelocytic —*see* condition
Myelocytoma 205.1

Myelodysplasia (spinal cord) 742.59
  meaning myelodysplastic syndrome—*see* Syndrome, myelodysplastic
Myeloencephalitis —*see* Encephalitis
Myelofibrosis 289.83
  with myeloid metaplasia 238.76
  idiopathic (chronic) 238.76
  megakaryocytic 238.79
  primary 238.76
  secondary 289.83
Myelogenous —*see* condition
Myeloid —*see* condition
Myelokathexis 288.09
Myeloleukodystrophy 330.0
Myelolipoma (M8870/0)—*see* Neoplasm, by site, benign
Myeloma (multiple) (plasma cell) (plasmacytic) (M9730/3) 203.0
  monostotic (M9731/1) 238.6
  solitary (M9731/1) 238.6
Myelomalacia 336.8
Myelomata, multiple (M9730/3) 203.0
Myelomatosis (M9730/3) 203.0
Myelomeningitis —*see* Meningoencephalitis
Myelomeningocele (spinal cord) (*see also* Spina bifida) 741.9
  fetal, causing fetopelvic disproportion 653.7
Myelo-osteo-musculodysplasia hereditaria 756.89
Myelopathic —*see* condition
Myelopathy (spinal cord) 336.9
  cervical 721.1
  diabetic 250.6 *[336.3]*
  drug-induced 336.8
  due to or with
    carbon tetrachloride 987.8 *[323.72]*
    degeneration or displacement, intervertebral disc 722.70
      cervical, cervicothoracic 722.71
      lumbar, lumbosacral 722.73
      thoracic, thoracolumbar 722.72
    hydroxyquinoline derivatives 961.3 *[323.72]*
    infection—*see* Encephalitis
    intervertebral disc disorder 722.70
      cervical, cervicothoracic 722.71
      lumbar, lumbosacral 722.73
      thoracic, thoracolumbar 722.72
    lead 984.9 *[323.72]*
    mercury 985.0 *[323.72]*
    neoplastic disease (*see also* Neoplasm, by site) 239.9 *[336.3]*
    pernicious anemia 281.0 *[336.3]*
    spondylosis 721.91
      cervical 721.1
      lumbar, lumbosacral 721.42
      thoracic 721.41
    thallium 985.8 *[323.72]*
  lumbar, lumbosacral 721.42
  necrotic (subacute) 336.1
  radiation-induced 336.8
  spondylogenic NEC 721.91
    cervical 721.1
    lumbar, lumbosacral 721.42
    thoracic 721.41
  thoracic 721.41
  toxic NEC 989.9 *[323.72]*
  transverse (*see also* Myelitis) 323.82
  vascular 336.1
Myelophthisis 284.2
Myeloproliferative disease (M9960/1) 238.79
Myeloradiculitis (*see also* Polyneuropathy) 357.0

Myeloradiculodysplasia (spinal) 742.59
Myelosarcoma (M9930/3) 205.3
Myelosclerosis 289.89
  with myeloid metaplasia (M9961/1) 238.76
  disseminated, of nervous system 340
  megakaryocytic (M9961/1) 238.79
Myelosis (M9860/3) (*see also* Leukemia, myeloid) 205.9
  acute (M9861/3) 205.0
  aleukemic (M9864/3) 205.8
  chronic (M9863/3) 205.1
  erythremic (M9840/3) 207.0
    acute (M9841/3) 207.0
  megakaryocytic (M9920/3) 207.2
  nonleukemic (chronic) 288.8
  subacute (M9862/3) 205.2
Myesthenia —*see* Myasthenia
Myiasis (cavernous) 134.0
  orbit 134.0 *[376.13]*
Myoadenoma, prostate 600.20
  with
    other lower urinary tract symptoms (LUTS) 600.21
    urinary
      obstruction 600.21
      retention 600.21
Myoblastoma
  granular cell (M9580/0)—*see also* Neoplasm, connective tissue, benign
  malignant (M9580/3)—*see* Neoplasm, connective tissue, malignant
  tongue (M9580/0) 210.1
Myocardial —*see* condition
Myocardiopathy (congestive) (constrictive) (familial) (hypertrophic nonobstructive) (idiopathic) (infiltrative) (obstructive) (primary) (restrictive) (sporadic) 425.4
  alcoholic 425.5
  amyloid 277.39 *[425.7]*
  beriberi 265.0 *[425.7]*
  cobalt-beer 425.5
  due to
    amyloidosis 277.39 *[425.7]*
    beriberi 265.0 *[425.7]*
    cardiac glycogenosis 271.0 *[425.7]*
    Chagas' disease 086.0
    Friedreich's ataxia 334.0 *[425.8]*
    influenza 487.8 *[425.8]*
    mucopolysaccharidosis 277.5 *[425.7]*
    myotonia atrophica 359.21 *[425.8]*
    progressive muscular dystrophy 359.1 *[425.8]*
    sarcoidosis 135 *[425.8]*
  glycogen storage 271.0 *[425.7]*
  hypertrophic obstructive 425.1
  metabolic NEC 277.9 *[425.7]*
  nutritional 269.9 *[425.7]*
  obscure (African) 425.2
  peripartum 674.5
  postpartum 674.5
  secondary 425.9
  thyrotoxic (*see also* Thyrotoxicosis) 242.9 *[425.7]*
  toxic NEC 425.9
Myocarditis (fibroid) (interstitial) (old) (progressive) (senile) (with arteriosclerosis) 429.0
  with
    rheumatic fever (conditions classifiable to 390) 398.0
      active (*see also* Myocarditis, acute, rheumatic) 391.2

Myocarditis—*continued*
    inactive or quiescent (with chorea) 398.0
  active (nonrheumatic) 422.90
    rheumatic 391.2
      with chorea (acute) (rheumatic)
        (Sydenham's) 392.0
  acute or subacute (interstitial) 422.90
    due to Streptococcus (beta-hemolytic) 391.2
    idiopathic 422.91
    rheumatic 391.2
      with chorea (acute) (rheumatic)
        (Sydenham's) 392.0
    specified type NEC 422.99
  aseptic of newborn 074.23
  bacterial (acute) 422.92
  chagasic 086.0
  chronic (interstitial) 429.0
  congenital 746.89
  constrictive 425.4
  Coxsackie (virus) 074.23
  diphtheritic 032.82
  due to or in
    Coxsackie (virus) 074.23
    diphtheria 032.82
    epidemic louse-borne typhus 080 *[422.0]*
    influenza 487.8 *[422.0]*
    Lyme disease 088.81 *[422.0]*
    scarlet fever 034.1 *[422.0]*
    toxoplasmosis (acquired) 130.3
    tuberculosis (*see also* Tuberculosis) 017.9
      [422.0]
    typhoid 002.0 *[422.0]*
    typhus NEC 081.9 *[422.0]*
  eosinophilic 422.91
  epidemic of newborn 074.23
  Fiedler's (acute) (isolated) (subacute) 422.91
  giant cell (acute) (subacute) 422.91
  gonococcal 098.85
  granulomatous (idiopathic) (isolated)
    (nonspecific) 422.91
  hypertensive (*see also* Hypertension, heart)
    402.90
  idiopathic 422.91
    granulomatous 422.91
  infective 422.92
  influenzal 487.8 *[422.0]*
  isolated (diffuse) (granulomatous) 422.91
  malignant 422.99
  meningococcal 036.43
  nonrheumatic, active 422.90
  parenchymatous 422.90
  pneumococcal (acute) (subacute) 422.92
  rheumatic (chronic) (inactive) (with chorea)
    398.0
    active or acute 391.2
      with chorea (acute) (rheumatic)
        (Sydenham's) 392.0
  septic 422.92
  specific (giant cell) (productive) 422.91
  staphylococcal (acute) (subacute) 422.92
  suppurative 422.92
  syphilitic (chronic) 093.82
  toxic 422.93
    rheumatic (*see also* Myocarditis, acute
      rheumatic) 391.2
  tuberculous (*see also* Tuberculosis) 017.9
    [422.0]
  typhoid 002.0 *[422.0]*
  valvular—*see* Endocarditis
  viral, except Coxsackie 422.91
    Coxsackie 074.23
    of newborn (Coxsackie) 074.23

Myocardium, myocardial —*see* condition
Myocardosis (*see also* Cardiomyopathy) 425.4
Myoclonia (essential) 333.2
  epileptica 333.2
  Friedrich's 333.2
  massive 333.2
Myoclonic
  epilepsy, familial (progressive) 333.2
  jerks 333.2
Myoclonus (familial essential) (multifocal)
  (simplex) 333.2
  with epilepsy and with ragged red fibers
    (MERRF syndrome) 277.87
  facial 351.8
  massive (infantile) 333.2
  pharyngeal 478.29
Myodiastasis 728.84
Myoendocarditis —*see also* Endocarditis
  acute or subacute 421.9
Myoepithelioma (M8982/0)—*see* Neoplasm, by
  site, benign
Myofascitis (acute) 729.1
  low back 724.2
Myofibroma (M8890/0)—*see also* Neoplasm,
  connective tissue, benign
  uterus (cervix) (corpus) (*see also* Leiomyoma)
    218.9
Myofibromatosis
  infantile 759.89
Myofibrosis 728.2
  heart (*see also* Myocarditis) 429.0
  humeroscapular region 726.2
  scapulohumeral 726.2
Myofibrositis (*see also* Myositis) 729.1
  scapulohumeral 726.2
Myogelosis (occupational) 728.89
Myoglobinuria 791.3
Myoglobulinuria, primary 791.3
Myokymia —*see also* Myoclonus
  facial 351.8
Myolipoma (M8860/0)
  specified site—*see* Neoplasm, connective tissue,
    benign
  unspecified site 223.0
Myoma (M8895/0)—*see also* Neoplasm,
  connective tissue, benign
  cervix (stump) (uterus) (*see also* Leiomyoma)
    218.9
  malignant (M8895/3)—*see* Neoplasm,
    connective tissue, malignant
  prostate 600.20
    with
      other lower urinary tract symptoms (LUTS)
        600.21
      urinary
        obstruction 600.21
        retention 600.21
  uterus (cervix) (corpus) (*see also* Leiomyoma)
    218.9
    in pregnancy or childbirth 654.1
      affecting fetus or newborn 763.89
      causing obstructed labor 660.2
        affecting fetus or newborn 763.1
Myomalacia 728.9
  cordis, heart (*see also* Degeneration,
    myocardial) 429.1
Myometritis (*see also* Endometritis) 615.9
Myometrium —*see* condition
Myonecrosis, clostridial 040.0

Myopathy 359.9
　alcoholic 359.4
　amyloid 277.39 *[359.6]*
　benign congenital 359.0
　central core 359.0
　centronuclear 359.0
　congenital (benign) 359.0
　critical illness 359.81
　distal 359.1
　due to drugs 359.4
　endocrine 259.9 *[359.5]*
　　specified type NEC 259.8 *[359.5]*
　extraocular muscles 376.82
　facioscapulohumeral 359.1
　in
　　Addison's disease 255.41 *[359.5]*
　　amyloidosis 277.39 *[359.6]*
　　cretinism 243 *[359.5]*
　　Cushing's syndrome 255.0 *[359.5]*
　　disseminated lupus erythematosus 710.0 *[359.6]*
　　giant cell arteritis 446.5 *[359.6]*
　　hyperadrenocorticism NEC 255.3 *[359.5]*
　　hyperparathyroidism 252.01 *[359.5]*
　　hypopituitarism 253.2 *[359.5]*
　　hypothyroidism (*see also* Hypothyroidism) 244.9 *[359.5]*
　　malignant neoplasm NEC (M8000/3) 199.1 *[359.6]*
　　myxedema (*see also* Myxedema) 244.9 *[359.5]*
　　polyarteritis nodosa 446.0 *[359.6]*
　　rheumatoid arthritis 714.0 *[359.6]*
　　sarcoidosis 135 *[359.6]*
　　scleroderma 710.1 *[359.6]*
　　Sjögren's disease 710.2 *[359.6]*
　　thyrotoxicosis (*see also* Thyrotoxicosis) 242.9 *[359.5]*
　inflammatory 359.89
　intensive care (ICU) 359.81
　limb-girdle 359.1
　myotubular 359.0
　necrotizing, acute 359.81
　nemaline 359.0
　ocular 359.1
　oculopharyngeal 359.1
　of critical illness 359.81
　primary 359.89
　progressive NEC 359.89
　proximal myotonic (PROMM) 359.21
　quadriplegic, acute 359.81
　rod body 359.0
　scapulohumeral 359.1
　specified type NEC 359.89
　toxic 359.4
Myopericarditis (*see also* Pericarditis) 423.9
Myopia (axial) (congenital) (increased curvature or refraction, nucleus of lens) 367.1
　degenerative, malignant 360.21
　malignant 360.21
　progressive high (degenerative) 360.21
Myosarcoma (M8895/3)—*see* Neoplasm, connective tissue, malignant
Myosis (persistent) 379.42
　stromal (endolymphatic) (M8931/1) 236.0
Myositis 729.1
　clostridial 040.0
　due to posture 729.1
　epidemic 074.1
　fibrosa or fibrous (chronic) 728.2
　　Volkmann's (complicating trauma) 958.6
　infective 728.0
　interstitial 728.81

Myositis—*continued*
　multiple—*see* Polymyositis
　occupational 729.1
　orbital, chronic 376.12
　ossificans 728.12
　　circumscribed 728.12
　　progressive 728.11
　　traumatic 728.12
　progressive fibrosing 728.11
　purulent 728.0
　rheumatic 729.1
　rheumatoid 729.1
　suppurative 728.0
　syphilitic 095.6
　traumatic (old) 729.1
Myospasia impulsiva 307.23
Myotonia (acquisita) (intermittens) 728.85
　atrophica 359.21
　congenita 359.22
　　acetazolamide responsive 359.22
　　dominant form 359.22
　　recessive form 359.22
　drug-induced 359.24
　dystrophica 359.21
　fluctuans 359.29
　levior 359.29
　permanens 359.29
Myotonic pupil 379.46
Myriapodiasis 134.1
Myringitis
　with otitis media—*see* Otitis media
　acute 384.00
　　specified type NEC 384.09
　bullosa hemorrhagica 384.01
　bullous 384.01
　chronic 384.1
Mysophobia 300.29
Mytilotoxism 988.0
Myxadenitis labialis 528.5
Myxedema (adult) (idiocy) (infantile) (juvenile) (thyroid gland) (*see also* Hypothyroidism) 244.9
　circumscribed 242.9
　congenital 243
　cutis 701.8
　localized (pretibial) 242.9
　madness (acute) 293.0
　　subacute 293.1
　papular 701.8
　pituitary 244.8
　postpartum 674.8
　pretibial 242.9
　primary 244.9
Myxochondrosarcoma (M9220/3)—*see* Neoplasm, cartilage, malignant
Myxofibroma (M8811/0)—*see also* Neoplasm, connective tissue, benign
　odontogenic (M9320/0) 213.1
　upper jaw (bone) 213.0
Myxofibrosarcoma (M8811/3)—*see* Neoplasm, connective tissue, malignant
Myxolipoma (M8852/0) (*see also* Lipoma, by site) 214.9
Myxoliposarcoma (M8852/3)—*see* Neoplasm, connective tissue, malignant
Myxoma (M8840/0)—*see also* Neoplasm, connective tissue, benign
　odontogenic (M9320/0) 213.1
　upper jaw (bone) 213.0
Myxosarcoma (M8840/3)—*see* Neoplasm, connective tissue, malignant

N

Naegeli's
 disease (hereditary hemorrhagic thrombasthenia) 287.1
 leukemia, monocytic (M9863/3) 205.1
 syndrome (incontinentia pigmenti) 757.33
Naffziger's syndrome 353.0
Naga sore (*see also* Ulcer, skin) 707.9
Nägele's pelvis 738.6
 with disproportion (fetopelvic) 653.0
  affecting fetus or newborn 763.1
  causing obstructed labor 660.1
   affecting fetus or newborn 763.1
Nager-de Reynier syndrome (dysostosis mandibularis) 756.0
Nail —*see also* condition
 biting 307.9
 patella syndrome (hereditary osteo-onychodysplasia) 756.89
Nanism, nanosomia (*see also* Dwarfism) 259.4
 hypophyseal 253.3
 pituitary 253.3
 renis, renalis 588.0
Nanukayami 100.89
Napkin rash 691.0
Narcissism 301.81
Narcolepsy 347.00
 with cataplexy 347.01
 in conditions classified elsewhere 347.10
  with cataplexy 347.11
Narcosis
 carbon dioxide (respiratory) 786.09
 due to drug
  correct substance properly administered 780.09
  overdose or wrong substance given or taken 977.9
   specified drug—*see* Table of drugs and chemicals
Narcotism (chronic) (*see also* listing under Dependence) 304.9
 acute
  correct substance properly administered 349.82
  overdose or wrong substance given or taken 967.8
   specified drug—*see* Table of drugs and chemicals
NARP syndrome (Neuropathy, ataxia and retinitis pigmentosa) 277.87
Narrow
 anterior chamber angle 365.02
 pelvis (inlet) (outlet)—*see* Contraction, pelvis
Narrowing
 artery NEC 447.1
  auditory, internal 433.8
  basilar 433.0
   with other precerebral artery 433.3
    bilateral 433.3
  carotid 433.1
   with other precerebral artery 433.3
    bilateral 433.3
  cerebellar 433.8
  choroidal 433.8
  communicating posterior 433.8
  coronary —*see also* Arteriosclerosis, coronary
   congenital 746.85
    due to syphilis 090.5

Narrowing—*continued*
  hypophyseal 433.8
  pontine 433.8
  precerebral NEC 433.9
   multiple or bilateral 433.3
   specified NEC 433.8
  vertebral 433.2
   with other precerebral artery 433.3
    bilateral 433.3
 auditory canal (external) (*see also* Stricture, ear canal, acquired) 380.50
 cerebral arteries 437.0
 cicatricial—*see* Cicatrix
 congenital—*see* Anomaly, congenital
 coronary artery—*see* Narrowing, artery, coronary
 ear, middle 385.22
 Eustachian tube (*see also* Obstruction, Eustachian tube) 381.60
 eyelid 374.46
  congenital 743.62
 intervertebral disc or space NEC—*see* Degeneration, intervertebral disc
 joint space, hip 719.85
 larynx 478.74
 lids 374.46
  congenital 743.62
 mesenteric artery (with gangrene) 557.0
 palate 524.89
 palpebral fissure 374.46
 retinal artery 362.13
 ureter 593.3
 urethra (*see also* Stricture, urethra) 598.9
Narrowness, abnormal, eyelid 743.62
Nasal —*see* condition
Nasolacrimal —*see* condition
Nasopharyngeal —*see also* condition
 bursa 478.29
 pituitary gland 759.2
 torticollis 723.5
Nasopharyngitis (acute) (infective) (subacute) 460
 chronic 472.2
 due to external agent—*see* Condition, respiratory, chronic, due to
 due to external agent—*see* Condition, respiratory, due to
 septic 034.0
 streptococcal 034.0
 suppurative (chronic) 472.2
 ulcerative (chronic) 472.2
Nasopharynx, nasopharyngeal —*see* condition
Natal tooth, teeth 520.6
Nausea (*see also* Vomiting) 787.02
 epidemic 078.82
 gravidarum—*see* Hyperemesis, gravidarum
 marina 994.6
 with vomiting 787.01
Naval —*see* condition
Neapolitan fever (*see also* Brucellosis) 023.9
Nearsightedness 367.1
Near-syncope 780.2
Nebécourt's syndrome 253.3
Nebula, cornea (eye) 371.01
 congenital 743.43
  interfering with vision 743.42
Necator americanus infestation 126.1
Necatoriasis 126.1

Neck
Neck —*see* condition
Necrencephalus (*see also* Softening, brain) 437.8
Necrobacillosis 040.3
Necrobiosis 799.89
  brain or cerebral (*see also* Softening, brain) 437.8
  lipoidica 709.3
    diabeticorum 250.8 *[709.3]*
Necrodermolysis 695.1
Necrolysis, toxic epidermal 695.1
  due to drug
    correct substance properly administered 695.1
    overdose or wrong substance given or taken 977.9
    specified drug—*see* Table of drugs and chemicals
Necrophilia 302.89
Necrosis, necrotic
  adrenal (capsule) (gland) 255.8
  antrum, nasal sinus 478.19
  aorta (hyaline) (*see also* Aneurysm, aorta) 441.9
    cystic medial 441.00
      abdominal 441.02
      thoracic 441.01
      thoracoabdominal 441.03
    ruptured 441.5
  arteritis 446.0
  artery 447.5
  aseptic, bone 733.40
    femur (head) (neck) 733.42
      medial condyle 733.43
    humoral head 733.41
    jaw 733.45
    medial femoral condyle 733.43
    specified site NEC 733.49
    talus 733.44
  avascular, bone NEC (*see also* Necrosis, aseptic, bone) 733.40
  bladder (aseptic) (sphincter) 596.8
  bone (*see also* Osteomyelitis) 730.1
    acute 730.0
    aseptic or avascular 733.40
      femur (head) (neck) 733.42
        medial condyle 733.43
      humoral head 733.41
      jaw 733.45
      medial femoral condyle 733.43
      specified site NEC 733.49
      talus 733.44
    ethmoid 478.19
    ischemic 733.40
    jaw 526.4
      aseptic 733.45
    marrow 289.89
    Paget's (osteitis deformans) 731.0
    tuberculous—*see* Tuberculosis, bone
  brain (softening) (*see also* Softening, brain) 437.8
  breast (aseptic) (fat) (segmental) 611.3
  bronchus, bronchi 519.19
  central nervous system NEC (*see also* Softening, brain) 437.8
  cerebellar (*see also* Softening, brain) 437.8
  cerebral (softening) (*see also* Softening, brain) 437.8
  cerebrospinal (softening) (*see also* Softening, brain) 437.8
  colon 557.0
  cornea (*see also* Keratitis) 371.40
  cortical, kidney 583.6
  cystic medial (aorta) 441.00
    abdominal 441.02

INDEX TO DISEASES

Necrosis, necrotic— *continued*
    thoracic 441.01
    thoracoabdominal 441.03
  dental 521.09
    pulp 522.1
  due to swallowing corrosive substance—*see* Burn, by site
  ear (ossicle) 385.24
  esophagus 530.89
  ethmoid (bone) 478.19
  eyelid 374.50
  fat, fatty (generalized) (*see also* Degeneration, fatty) 272.8
    abdominal wall 567.82
    breast (aseptic) (segmental) 611.3
    intestine 569.89
    localized—*see* Degeneration, by site, fatty
    mesentery 567.82
    omentum 567.82
    pancreas 577.8
    peritoneum 567.82
    skin (subcutaneous) 709.3
      newborn 778.1
  femur (aseptic) (avascular) 733.42
    head 733.42
    medial condyle 733.43
    neck 733.42
  gallbladder (*see also* Cholecystitis, acute) 575.0
  gangrenous 785.4
  gastric 537.89
  glottis 478.79
  heart (myocardium)—*see* Infarct, myocardium
  hepatic (*see also* Necrosis, liver) 570
  hip (aseptic) (avascular) 733.42
  intestine (acute) (hemorrhagic) (massive) 557.0
  ischemic 785.4
  jaw 526.4
    aseptic 733.45
  kidney (bilateral) 583.9
    acute 584.9
    cortical 583.6
      acute 584.6
        with
          abortion—*see* Abortion, by type, with renal failure
          ectopic pregnancy (*see also* categories 633.0-633.9) 639.3
          molar pregnancy (*see also* categories 630-632) 639.3
        complicating pregnancy 646.2
          affecting fetus or newborn 760.1
        following labor and delivery 669.3
    medullary (papillary) (*see also* Pyelitis) 590.80
      in
        acute renal failure 584.7
        nephritis, nephropathy 583.7
    papillary (*see also* Pyelitis) 590.80
      in
        acute renal failure 584.7
        nephritis, nephropathy 583.7
    tubular 584.5
      with
        abortion—*see* Abortion, by type, with renal failure
        ectopic pregnancy (*see also* categories 633.0-633.9) 639.3
        molar pregnancy (*see also* categories 630-632) 639.3
      complicating
        abortion 639.3
        ectopic or molar pregnancy 639.3

INDEX TO DISEASES   **Neoplasia**

Necrosis, necrotic—*continued*
    pregnancy 646.2
        affecting fetus or newborn 760.1
    following labor and delivery 669.3
    traumatic 958.5
  larynx 478.79
  liver (acute) (congenital) (diffuse) (massive) (subacute) 570
    with
      abortion—*see* Abortion, by type, with specified complication NEC
      ectopic pregnancy (*see also* categories 633.0-633.9) 639.8
      molar pregnancy (*see also* categories 630-632) 639.8
    complicating pregnancy 646.7
      affecting fetus or newborn 760.8
    following
      abortion 639.8
      ectopic or molar pregnancy 639.8
    obstetrical 646.7
    postabortal 639.8
    puerperal, postpartum 674.8
    toxic 573.3
  lung 513.0
  lymphatic gland 683
  mammary gland 611.3
  mastoid (chronic) 383.1
  mesentery 557.0
    fat 567.82
  mitral valve—*see* Insufficiency, mitral
  myocardium, myocardial—*see* Infarct, myocardium
  nose (septum) 478.19
  omentum 557.0
    with mesenteric infarction 557.0
    fat 567.82
  orbit, orbital 376.10
  ossicles, ear (aseptic) 385.24
  ovary (*see also* Salpingo-oophoritis) 614.2
  pancreas (aseptic) (duct) (fat) 577.8
    acute 577.0
    infective 577.0
  papillary, kidney (*see also* Pyelitis) 590.80
  perineum 624.8
  peritoneum 557.0
    with mesenteric infarction 557.0
    fat 567.82
  pharynx 462
    in granulocytopenia 288.09
  phosphorus 983.9
  pituitary (gland) (postpartum) (Sheehan) 253.2
  placenta (*see also* Placenta, abnormal) 656.7
  pneumonia 513.0
  pulmonary 513.0
  pulp (dental) 522.1
  pylorus 537.89
  radiation—*see* Necrosis, by site
  radium—*see* Necrosis, by site
  renal—*see* Necrosis, kidney
  sclera 379.19
  scrotum 608.89
  skin or subcutaneous tissue 709.8
    due to burn—*see* Burn, by site
    gangrenous 785.4
  spine, spinal (column) 730.18
    acute 730.18
    cord 336.1
  spleen 289.59
  stomach 537.89
  stomatitis 528.1

Necrosis, necrotic—*continued*
  subcutaneous fat 709.3
    fetus or newborn 778.1
  subendocardial—*see* Infarct, myocardium
  suprarenal (capsule) (gland) 255.8
  teeth, tooth 521.09
  testis 608.89
  thymus (gland) 254.8
  tonsil 474.8
  trachea 519.19
  tuberculous NEC—*see* Tuberculosis
  tubular (acute) (anoxic) (toxic) 584.5
    due to a procedure 997.5
  umbilical cord, affecting fetus or newborn 762.6
  vagina 623.8
  vertebra (lumbar) 730.18
    acute 730.18
    tuberculous (*see also* Tuberculosis) 015.0 *[730.8]*
  vesical (aseptic) (bladder) 596.8
  vulva 624.8
  x-ray—*see* Necrosis, by site
Necrospermia 606.0
Necrotizing angiitis 446.0
Negativism 301.7
Neglect (child) (newborn) NEC 995.52
  adult 995.84
  after or at birth 995.52
  hemispatial 781.8
  left-sided 781.8
  sensory 781.8
  visuospatial 781.8
Negri bodies 071
Neill-Dingwall syndrome (microcephaly and dwarfism) 759.89
Neisserian infection NEC—*see* Gonococcus
Nematodiasis NEC (*see also* Infestation, Nematode) 127.9
  ancylostoma (*see also* Ancylostomiasis) 126.9
Neoformans cryptococcus infection 117.5
Neonatal —*see also* condition
  adrenoleukodystrophy 277.86
  teeth, tooth 520.6
Neonatorum —*see* condition
Neoplasia
  multiple endocine [MEN]
    type I 258.01
    type II A 258.02
    type II B 258.03
  vaginal intraepithelial I [VAIN I] 623.0
  vaginal intraepithelial II [VAIN II] 623.0
  vaginal intraepithelial III [VAIN III] 233.31
  vulvar intraepithelial I [VIN I] 624.01
  vulvar intraepithelial II [VIN II] 624.02
  vulvar intraepithelial III [VIN III] 233.32

"N" listing resumes after "Neoplasm, neoplastic" table...

Neoplasms INDEX TO DISEASES

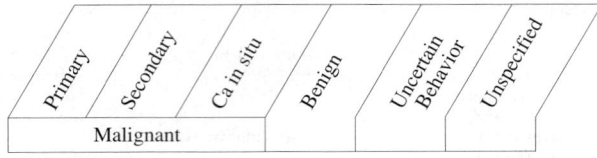

	Malignant			Benign	Uncertain Behavior	Unspecified
	Primary	Secondary	Ca in situ			
Neoplasm, neoplastic	199.1	199.1	234.9	229.9	238.9	239.9

Note—1. The list below gives the code numbers for neoplasms by anatomical site. For each site there are six possible code numbers according to whether the neoplasm in question is malignant, benign, in situ, of uncertain behavior, or of unspecified nature. The description of the neoplasm will often indicate which of the six columns is appropriate; e.g., malignant melanoma of skin, benign fibroadenoma of breast, carcinoma in situ of cervix uteri.

Where such descriptors are not present, the remainder of the Index should be consulted where guidance is given to the appropriate column for each morphological (histological) variety listed; e.g., Mesonephroma—see Neoplasm, malignant; Embryoma—see also Neoplasm, uncertain behavior; Disease, Bowen's—see Neoplasm, skin, in situ. However, the guidance in the Index can be overridden if one of the descriptors mentioned above is present; e.g., malignant adenoma of colon is coded to 153.9 and not to 211.3 as the adjective "malignant" overrides the Index entry "Adenoma—see also Neoplasm, benign."

*Note—2. Sites marked with the sign * (e.g., face NEC*) should be classified to malignant neoplasm of skin of these sites if the variety of neoplasm is a squamous cell carcinoma or an epidermoid carcinoma and to benign neoplasm of skin of these sites if the variety of neoplasm is a papilloma (any type).*

abdomen, abdominal	195.2	198.89	234.8	229.8	238.8	239.8
cavity	195.2	198.89	234.8	229.8	238.8	239.8
organ	195.2	198.89	234.8	229.8	238.8	239.8
viscera	195.2	198.89	234.8	229.8	238.8	239.8
wall	173.5	198.2	232.5	216.5	238.2	239.2
connective tissue	171.5	198.89	—	215.5	238.1	239.2
abdominopelvic	195.8	198.89	234.8	229.8	238.8	239.8
accessory sinus—*see* Neoplasm, sinus						
acoustic nerve	192.0	198.4	—	225.1	237.9	239.7
acromion (process)	170.4	198.5	—	213.4	238.0	239.2
adenoid (pharynx) (tissue)	147.1	198.89	230.0	210.7	235.1	239.0
adipose tissue (*see also* Neoplasm,						
connective tissue)	171.9	198.89	—	215.9	238.1	239.2
adnexa (uterine)	183.9	198.82	233.39	221.8	236.3	239.5
adrenal (cortex) (gland)						
(medulla)	194.0	198.7	234.8	227.0	237.2	239.7
ala nasi (external)	173.3	198.2	232.3	216.3	238.2	239.2
alimentary canal or						
tract NEC	159.9	197.8	230.9	211.9	235.5	239.0
alveolar	143.9	198.89	230.0	210.4	235.1	239.0
mucosa	143.9	198.89	230.0	210.4	235.1	239.0
lower	143.1	198.89	230.0	210.4	235.1	239.0
upper	143.0	198.89	230.0	210.4	235.1	239.0
ridge or process	170.1	198.5	—	213.1	238.0	239.2
carcinoma	143.9	—	—	—	—	—
lower	143.1	—	—	—	—	—
upper	143.0	—	—	—	—	—
lower	170.1	198.5	—	213.1	238.0	239.2
mucosa	143.9	198.89	230.0	210.4	235.1	239.0
lower	143.1	198.89	230.0	210.4	235.1	239.0
upper	143.0	198.89	230.0	210.4	235.1	239.0
upper	170.0	198.5	—	213.0	238.0	239.2
sulcus	145.1	198.89	230.0	210.4	235.1	239.0
alveolus	143.9	198.89	230.0	210.4	235.1	239.0
lower	143.1	198.89	230.0	210.4	235.1	239.0
upper	143.0	198.89	230.0	210.4	235.1	239.0
ampulla of Vater	156.2	197.8	230.8	211.5	235.3	239.0
ankle NEC*	195.5	198.89	232.7	229.8	238.8	239.8
anorectum, anorectal						
(junction)	154.8	197.5	230.7	211.4	235.2	239.0
antecubital fossa or space*	195.4	198.89	232.6	229.8	238.8	239.8
antrum (Highmore)						
(maxillary)	160.2	197.3	231.8	212.0	235.9	239.1

1184

INDEX TO DISEASES   Neoplasms

	Malignant Primary	Malignant Secondary	Ca in situ	Benign	Uncertain Behavior	Unspecified
pyloric	151.2	197.8	230.2	211.1	235.2	239.0
tympanicum	160.1	197.3	231.8	212.0	235.9	239.1
anus, anal	154.3	197.5	230.6	211.4	235.5	239.0
canal	154.2	197.5	230.5	211.4	235.5	239.0
contiguous sites with rectosigmoid junction or rectum	154.8	—	—	—	—	—
margin	173.5	198.2	232.5	216.5	238.2	239.2
skin	173.5	198.2	232.5	216.5	238.2	239.2
sphincter	154.2	197.5	230.5	211.4	235.5	239.0
aorta (thoracic)	171.4	198.89	—	215.4	238.1	239.2
abdominal	171.5	198.89	—	215.5	238.1	239.2
aortic body	194.6	198.89	—	227.6	237.3	239.7
aponeurosis	171.9	198.89	—	215.9	238.1	239.2
palmar	171.2	198.89	—	215.2	238.1	239.2
plantar	171.3	198.89	—	215.3	238.1	239.2
appendix	153.5	197.5	230.3	211.3	235.2	239.0
arachnoid (cerebral)	192.1	198.4	—	225.2	237.6	239.7
spinal	192.3	198.4	—	225.4	237.6	239.7
areola (female)	174.0	198.81	233.0	217	238.3	239.3
male	175.0	198.81	233.0	217	238.3	239.3
arm NEC*	195.4	198.89	232.6	229.8	238.8	239.8
artery—see Neoplasm, connective tissue						
aryepiglottic fold	148.2	198.89	230.0	210.8	235.1	239.0
hypopharyngeal aspect	148.2	198.89	230.0	210.8	235.1	239.0
laryngeal aspect	161.1	197.3	231.0	212.1	235.6	239.1
marginal zone	148.2	198.89	230.0	210.8	235.1	239.0
arytenoid (cartilage)	161.3	197.3	231.0	212.1	235.6	239.1
fold—see Neoplasm, aryepiglottic						
atlas	170.2	198.5	—	213.2	238.0	239.2
atrium, cardiac	164.1	198.89	—	212.7	238.8	239.8
auditory						
canal (external) (skin)	173.2	198.2	232.2	216.2	238.2	239.2
internal	160.1	197.3	231.8	212.0	235.9	239.1
nerve	192.0	198.4	—	225.1	237.9	239.7
tube	160.1	197.3	231.8	212.0	235.9	239.1
opening	147.2	198.89	230.0	210.7	235.1	239.0
auricle, ear	173.2	198.2	232.2	216.2	238.2	239.2
cartilage	171.0	198.89	—	215.0	238.1	239.2
auricular canal (external)	173.2	198.2	232.2	216.2	238.2	239.2
internal	160.1	197.3	231.8	212.0	235.9	239.1
autonomic nerve or nervous system NEC	171.9	198.89	—	215.9	238.1	239.2
axilla, axillary	195.1	198.89	234.8	229.8	238.8	239.8
fold	173.5	198.2	232.5	216.5	238.2	239.2
back NEC*	195.8	198.89	232.5	229.8	238.8	239.8
Bartholin's gland	184.1	198.82	233.32	221.2	236.3	239.5
basal ganglia	191.0	198.3	—	225.0	237.5	239.6
basis pedunculi	191.7	198.3	—	225.0	237.5	239.6
bile or biliary (tract)	156.9	197.8	230.8	211.5	235.3	239.0
canaliculi (biliferi) (intrahepatic)	155.1	197.8	230.8	211.5	235.3	239.0
canals, interlobular	155.1	197.8	230.8	211.5	235.3	239.0
contiguous sites	156.8	—	—	—	—	—
duct or passage (common) (cyst) (extrahepatic)	156.1	197.8	230.8	211.5	235.3	239.0
contiguous sites with gallbladder	156.8	—	—	—	—	—
interlobular	155.1	197.8	230.8	211.5	235.3	239.0
intrahepatic	155.1	197.8	230.8	211.5	235.3	239.0
and extrahepatic	156.9	197.8	230.8	211.5	235.3	239.0
bladder (urinary)	188.9	198.1	233.7	223.3	236.7	239.4
contiguous sites	188.8	—	—	—	—	—
dome	188.1	198.1	233.7	223.3	236.7	239.4

Neoplasms   **INDEX TO DISEASES**

	Malignant Primary	Malignant Secondary	Ca in situ	Benign	Uncertain Behavior	Unspecified
neck	188.5	198.1	233.7	223.3	236.7	239.4
orifice	188.9	198.1	233.7	223.3	236.7	239.4
ureteric	188.6	198.1	233.7	223.3	236.7	239.4
urethral	188.5	198.1	233.7	223.3	236.7	239.4
sphincter	188.8	198.1	233.7	223.3	236.7	239.4
trigone	188.0	198.1	233.7	223.3	236.7	239.4
urachus	188.7	—	233.7	223.3	236.7	239.4
wall	188.9	198.1	233.7	223.3	236.7	239.4
anterior	188.3	198.1	233.7	223.3	236.7	239.4
lateral	188.2	198.1	233.7	223.3	236.7	239.4
posterior	188.4	198.1	233.7	223.3	236.7	239.4
blood vessel—*see* Neoplasm, connective tissue						
bone (periosteum)	170.9	198.5	—	213.9	238.0	239.2

Note—Carcinomas and adenocarcinomas, of any type other than intraosseous or odontogenic, of the sites listed under "Neoplasm, bone" should be considered as constituting metastatic spread from an unspecified primary site and coded to 198.5 for morbidity coding and to 199.1 for underlying cause of death coding.

acetabulum	170.6	198.5	—	213.6	238.0	239.2
acromion (process)	170.4	198.5	—	213.4	238.0	239.2
ankle	170.8	198.5	—	213.8	238.0	239.2
arm NEC	170.4	198.5	—	213.4	238.0	239.2
astragalus	170.8	198.5	—	213.8	238.0	239.2
atlas	170.2	198.5	—	213.2	238.0	239.2
axis	170.2	198.5	—	213.2	238.0	239.2
back NEC	170.2	198.5	—	213.2	238.0	239.2
calcaneus	170.8	198.5	—	213.8	238.0	239.2
calvarium	170.0	198.5	—	213.0	238.0	239.2
carpus (any)	170.5	198.5	—	213.5	238.0	239.2
cartilage NEC	170.9	198.5	—	213.9	238.0	239.2
clavicle	170.3	198.5	—	213.3	238.0	239.2
clivus	170.0	198.5	—	213.0	238.0	239.2
coccygeal vertebra	170.6	198.5	—	213.6	238.0	239.2
coccyx	170.6	198.5	—	213.6	238.0	239.2
costal cartilage	170.3	198.5	—	213.3	238.0	239.2
costovertebral joint	170.3	198.5	—	213.3	238.0	239.2
cranial	170.0	198.5	—	213.0	238.0	239.2
cuboid	170.8	198.5	—	213.8	238.0	239.2
cuneiform	170.9	198.5	—	213.9	238.0	239.2
ankle	170.8	198.5	—	213.8	238.0	239.2
wrist	170.5	198.5	—	213.5	238.0	239.2
digital	170.9	198.5	—	213.9	238.0	239.2
finger	170.5	198.5	—	213.5	238.0	239.2
toe	170.8	198.5	—	213.8	238.0	239.2
elbow	170.4	198.5	—	213.4	238.0	239.2
ethmoid (labyrinth)	170.0	198.5	—	213.0	238.0	239.2
face	170.0	198.5	—	213.0	238.0	239.2
lower jaw	170.1	198.5	—	213.1	238.0	239.2
femur (any part)	170.7	198.5	—	213.7	238.0	239.2
fibula (any part)	170.7	198.5	—	213.7	238.0	239.2
finger (any)	170.5	198.5	—	213.5	238.0	239.2
foot	170.8	198.5	—	213.8	238.0	239.2
forearm	170.4	198.5	—	213.4	238.0	239.2
frontal	170.0	198.5	—	213.0	238.0	239.2
hand	170.5	198.5	—	213.5	238.0	239.2
heel	170.8	198.5	—	213.8	238.0	239.2
hip	170.6	198.5	—	213.6	238.0	239.2
humerus (any part)	170.4	198.5	—	213.4	238.0	239.2
hyoid	170.0	198.5	—	213.0	238.0	239.2
ilium	170.6	198.5	—	213.6	238.0	239.2
innominate	170.6	198.5	—	213.6	238.0	239.2
intervertebral cartilage or disc	170.2	198.5	—	213.2	238.0	239.2

INDEX TO DISEASES   Neoplasms

	Malignant			Benign	Uncertain Behavior	Unspecified
	Primary	Secondary	Ca in situ			

	Primary	Secondary	Ca in situ	Benign	Uncertain Behavior	Unspecified
ischium	170.6	198.5	—	213.6	238.0	239.2
jaw (lower)	170.1	198.5	—	213.1	238.0	239.2
upper	170.0	198.5	—	213.0	238.0	239.2
knee	170.7	198.5	—	213.7	238.0	239.2
leg NEC	170.7	198.5	—	213.7	238.0	239.2
limb NEC	170.9	198.5	—	213.9	238.0	239.2
lower (long bones)	170.7	198.5	—	213.7	238.0	239.2
short bones	170.8	198.5	—	213.8	238.0	239.2
upper (long bones)	170.4	198.5	—	213.4	238.0	239.2
short bones	170.5	198.5	—	213.5	238.0	239.2
long	170.9	198.5	—	213.9	238.0	239.2
lower limbs NEC	170.7	198.5	—	213.7	238.0	239.2
upper limbs NEC	170.4	198.5	—	213.4	238.0	239.2
malar	170.0	198.5	—	213.0	238.0	239.2
mandible	170.1	198.5	—	213.1	238.0	239.2
marrow NEC	202.9	198.5	—	—	—	238.79
mastoid	170.0	198.5	—	213.0	238.0	239.2
maxilla, maxillary (superior)	170.0	198.5	—	213.0	238.0	239.2
inferior	170.1	198.5	—	213.1	238.0	239.2
metacarpus (any)	170.5	198.5	—	213.5	238.0	239.2
metatarsus (any)	170.8	198.5	—	213.8	238.0	239.2
navicular (ankle)	170.8	198.5	—	213.8	238.0	239.2
hand	170.5	198.5	—	213.5	238.0	239.2
nose, nasal	170.0	198.5	—	213.0	238.0	239.2
occipital	170.0	198.5	—	213.0	238.0	239.2
orbit	170.0	198.5	—	213.0	238.0	239.2
parietal	170.0	198.5	—	213.0	238.0	239.2
patella	170.8	198.5	—	213.8	238.0	239.2
pelvic	170.6	198.5	—	213.6	238.0	239.2
phalanges	170.9	198.5	—	213.9	238.0	239.2
foot	170.8	198.5	—	213.8	238.0	239.2
hand	170.5	198.5	—	213.5	238.0	239.2
pubic	170.6	198.5	—	213.6	238.0	239.2
radius (any part)	170.4	198.5	—	213.4	238.0	239.2
rib	170.3	198.5	—	213.3	238.0	239.2
sacral vertebra	170.6	198.5	—	213.6	238.0	239.2
sacrum	170.6	198.5	—	213.6	238.0	239.2
scaphoid (of hand)	170.5	198.5	—	213.5	238.0	239.2
of ankle	170.8	198.5	—	213.8	238.0	239.2
scapula (any part)	170.4	198.5	—	213.4	238.0	239.2
sella turcica	170.0	198.5	—	213.0	238.0	239.2
short	170.9	198.5	—	213.9	238.0	239.2
lower limb	170.8	198.5	—	213.8	238.0	239.2
upper limb	170.5	198.5	—	213.5	238.0	239.2
shoulder	170.4	198.5	—	213.4	238.0	239.2
skeleton, skeletal NEC	170.9	198.5	—	213.9	238.0	239.2
skull	170.0	198.5	—	213.0	238.0	239.2
sphenoid	170.0	198.5	—	213.0	238.0	239.2
spine, spinal (column)	170.2	198.5	—	213.2	238.0	239.2
coccyx	170.6	198.5	—	213.6	238.0	239.2
sacrum	170.6	198.5	—	213.6	238.0	239.2
sternum	170.3	198.5	—	213.3	238.0	239.2
tarsus (any)	170.8	198.5	—	213.8	238.0	239.2
temporal	170.0	198.5	—	213.0	238.0	239.2
thumb	170.5	198.5	—	213.5	238.0	239.2
tibia (any part)	170.7	198.5	—	213.7	238.0	239.2
toe (any)	170.8	198.5	—	213.8	238.0	239.2
trapezium	170.5	198.5	—	213.5	238.0	239.2
trapezoid	170.5	198.5	—	213.5	238.0	239.2
turbinate	170.0	198.5	—	213.0	238.0	239.2
ulna (any part)	170.4	198.5	—	213.4	238.0	239.2
unciform	170.5	198.5	—	213.5	238.0	239.2

Neoplasms   **INDEX TO DISEASES**

	Malignant Primary	Malignant Secondary	Ca in situ	Benign	Uncertain Behavior	Unspecified
vertebra (column)	170.2	198.5	—	213.2	238.0	239.2
coccyx	170.6	198.5	—	213.6	238.0	239.2
sacrum	170.6	198.5	—	213.6	238.0	239.2
vomer	170.0	198.5	—	213.0	238.0	239.2
wrist	170.5	198.5	—	213.5	238.0	239.2
xiphoid process	170.3	198.5	—	213.3	238.0	239.2
zygomatic	170.0	198.5	—	213.0	238.0	239.2
book-leaf (mouth)	145.8	198.89	230.0	210.4	235.1	239.0
bowel—*see* Neoplasm, intestine						
brachial plexus	171.2	198.89	—	215.2	238.1	239.2
brain NEC	191.9	198.3	—	225.0	237.5	239.6
basal ganglia	191.0	198.3	—	225.0	237.5	239.6
cerebellopontine angle	191.6	198.3	—	225.0	237.5	239.6
cerebellum NOS	191.6	198.3	—	225.0	237.5	239.6
cerebrum	191.0	198.3	—	225.0	237.5	239.6
choroid plexus	191.5	198.3	—	225.0	237.5	239.6
contiguous sites	191.8	—	—	—	—	—
corpus callosum	191.8	198.3	—	225.0	237.5	239.6
corpus striatum	191.0	198.3	—	225.0	237.5	239.6
cortex (cerebral)	191.0	198.3	—	225.0	237.5	239.6
frontal lobe	191.1	198.3	—	225.0	237.5	239.6
globus pallidus	191.0	198.3	—	225.0	237.5	239.6
hippocampus	191.2	198.3	—	225.0	237.5	239.6
hypothalamus	191.0	198.3	—	225.0	237.5	239.6
internal capsule	191.0	198.3	—	225.0	237.5	239.6
medulla oblongata	191.7	198.3	—	225.0	237.5	239.6
meninges	192.1	198.4	—	225.2	237.6	239.7
midbrain	191.7	198.3	—	225.0	237.5	239.6
occipital lobe	191.4	198.3	—	225.0	237.5	239.6
parietal lobe	191.3	198.3	—	225.0	237.5	239.6
peduncle	191.7	198.3	—	225.0	237.5	239.6
pons	191.7	198.3	—	225.0	237.5	239.6
stem	191.7	198.3	—	225.0	237.5	239.6
tapetum	191.8	198.3	—	225.0	237.5	239.6
temporal lobe	191.2	198.3	—	225.0	237.5	239.6
thalamus	191.0	198.3	—	225.0	237.5	239.6
uncus	191.2	198.3	—	225.0	237.5	239.6
ventricle (floor)	191.5	198.3	—	225.0	237.5	239.6
branchial (cleft) (vestiges)	146.8	198.89	230.0	210.6	235.1	239.0
breast (connective tissue) (female) (glandular tissue) (soft parts)	174.9	198.81	233.0	217	238.3	239.3
areola	174.0	198.81	233.0	217	238.3	239.3
male	175.0	198.81	233.0	217	238.3	239.3
axillary tail	174.6	198.81	233.0	217	238.3	239.3
central portion	174.1	198.81	233.0	217	238.3	239.3
contiguous sites	174.8	—	—	—	—	—
ectopic sites	174.8	198.81	233.0	217	238.3	239.3
inner	174.8	198.81	233.0	217	238.3	239.3
lower	174.8	198.81	233.0	217	238.3	239.3
lower-inner quadrant	174.3	198.81	233.0	217	238.3	239.3
lower-outer quadrant	174.5	198.81	233.0	217	238.3	239.3
male	175.9	198.81	233.0	217	238.3	239.3
areola	175.0	198.81	233.0	217	238.3	239.3
ectopic tissue	175.9	198.81	233.0	217	238.3	239.3
nipple	175.0	198.81	233.0	217	238.3	239.3
mastectomy site (skin)	173.5	198.2	—	—	—	—
specified as breast tissue	174.8	198.81	—	—	—	—
midline	174.8	198.81	233.0	217	238.3	239.3
nipple	174.0	198.81	233.0	217	238.3	239.3
male	175.0	198.81	233.0	217	238.3	239.3
outer	174.8	198.81	233.0	217	238.3	239.3
skin	173.5	198.2	232.5	216.5	238.2	239.2

INDEX TO DISEASES — Neoplasms

	Malignant Primary	Malignant Secondary	Ca in situ	Benign	Uncertain Behavior	Unspecified
tail (axillary)	174.6	198.81	233.0	217	238.3	239.3
upper	174.8	198.81	233.0	217	238.3	239.3
upper-inner quadrant	174.2	198.81	233.0	217	238.3	239.3
upper-outer quadrant	174.4	198.81	233.0	217	238.3	239.3
broad ligament	183.3	198.82	233.39	221.0	236.3	239.5
bronchiogenic, bronchogenic (lung)	162.9	197.0	231.2	212.3	235.7	239.1
bronchiole	162.9	197.0	231.2	212.3	235.7	239.1
bronchus	162.9	197.0	231.2	212.3	235.7	239.1
carina	162.2	197.0	231.2	212.3	235.7	239.1
contiguous sites with lung or trachea	162.8	—	—	—	—	—
lower lobe of lung	162.5	197.0	231.2	212.3	235.7	239.1
main	162.2	197.0	231.2	212.3	235.7	239.1
middle lobe of lung	162.4	197.0	231.2	212.3	235.7	239.1
upper lobe of lung	162.3	197.0	231.2	212.3	235.7	239.1
brow	173.3	198.2	232.3	216.3	238.2	239.2
buccal (cavity)	145.9	198.89	230.0	210.4	235.1	239.0
commissure	145.0	198.89	230.0	210.4	235.1	239.0
groove (lower) (upper)	145.1	198.89	230.0	210.4	235.1	239.0
mucosa	145.0	198.89	230.0	210.4	235.1	239.0
sulcus (lower) (upper)	145.1	198.89	230.0	210.4	235.1	239.0
bulbourethral gland	189.3	198.1	233.9	223.81	236.99	239.5
bursa—see Neoplasm, connective tissue						
buttock NEC*	195.3	198.89	232.5	229.8	238.8	239.8
calf*	195.5	198.89	232.7	229.8	238.8	239.8
calvarium	170.0	198.5	—	213.0	238.0	239.2
calyx, renal	189.1	198.0	233.9	223.1	236.91	239.5
canal						
anal	154.2	197.5	230.5	211.4	235.5	239.0
auditory (external)	173.2	198.2	232.2	216.2	238.2	239.2
auricular (external)	173.2	198.2	232.2	216.2	238.2	239.2
canaliculi, biliary (biliferi) (intrahepatic)	155.1	197.8	230.8	211.5	235.3	239.0
canthus (eye) (inner) (outer)	173.1	198.2	232.1	216.1	238.2	239.2
capillary—see Neoplasm, connective tissue						
caput coli	153.4	197.5	230.3	211.3	235.2	239.0
cardia (gastric)	151.0	197.8	230.2	211.1	235.2	239.0
cardiac orifice (stomach)	151.0	197.8	230.2	211.1	235.2	239.0
cardio-esophageal junction	151.0	197.8	230.2	211.1	235.2	239.0
cardio-esophagus	151.0	197.8	230.2	211.1	235.2	239.0
carina (bronchus)	162.2	197.0	231.2	212.3	235.7	239.1
carotid (artery)	171.0	198.89	—	215.0	238.1	239.2
body	194.5	198.89	—	227.5	237.3	239.7
carpus (any bone)	170.5	198.5	—	213.5	238.0	239.2
cartilage (articular) (joint) NEC—see also Neoplasm, bone	170.9	198.5	—	213.9	238.0	239.2
arytenoid	161.3	197.3	231.0	212.1	235.6	239.1
auricular	171.0	198.89	—	215.0	238.1	239.2
bronchi	162.2	197.3	—	212.3	235.7	239.1
connective tissue—see Neoplasm, connective tissue						
costal	170.3	198.5	—	213.3	238.0	239.2
cricoid	161.3	197.3	231.0	212.1	235.6	239.1
cuneiform	161.3	197.3	231.0	212.1	235.6	239.1
ear (external)	171.0	198.89	—	215.0	238.1	239.2
ensiform	170.3	198.5	—	213.3	238.0	239.2
epiglottis	161.1	197.3	231.0	212.1	235.6	239.1
anterior surface	146.4	198.89	230.0	210.6	235.1	239.0
eyelid	171.0	198.89	—	215.0	238.1	239.2

Neoplasms INDEX TO DISEASES

	Malignant			Benign	Uncertain Behavior	Unspecified
	Primary	Secondary	Ca in situ			

intervertebral	170.2	198.5	—	213.2	238.0	239.2
larynx, laryngeal	161.3	197.3	231.0	212.1	235.6	239.1
nose, nasal	160.0	197.3	231.8	212.0	235.9	239.1
pinna	171.0	198.89	—	215.0	238.1	239.2
rib	170.3	198.5	—	213.3	238.0	239.2
semilunar (knee)	170.7	198.5	—	213.7	238.0	239.2
thyroid	161.3	197.3	231.0	212.1	235.6	239.1
trachea	162.0	197.3	231.1	212.2	235.7	239.1
cauda equina	192.2	198.3	—	225.3	237.5	239.7
cavity						
buccal	145.9	198.89	230.0	210.4	235.1	239.0
nasal	160.0	197.3	231.8	212.0	235.9	239.1
oral	145.9	198.89	230.0	210.4	235.1	239.0
peritoneal	158.9	197.6	—	211.8	235.4	239.0
tympanic	160.1	197.3	231.8	212.0	235.9	239.1
cecum	153.4	197.5	230.3	211.3	235.2	239.0
central						
nervous system—*see* Neoplasm, nervous system						
white matter	191.0	198.3	—	225.0	237.5	239.6
cerebellopontine (angle)	191.6	198.3	—	225.0	237.5	239.6
cerebellum, cerebellar	191.6	198.3	—	225.0	237.5	239.6
cerebrum, cerebral (cortex) (hemisphere)						
(white matter)	191.0	198.3	—	225.0	237.5	239.6
meninges	192.1	198.4	—	225.2	237.6	239.7
peduncle	191.7	198.3	—	225.0	237.5	239.6
ventricle (any)	191.5	198.3	—	225.0	237.5	239.6
cervical region	195.0	198.89	234.8	229.8	238.8	239.8
cervix (cervical) (uteri)						
(uterus)	180.9	198.82	233.1	219.0	236.0	239.5
canal	180.0	198.82	233.1	219.0	236.0	239.5
contiguous sites	180.8	—	—	—	—	—
endocervix (canal) (gland)	180.0	198.82	233.1	219.0	236.0	239.5
exocervix	180.1	198.82	233.1	219.0	236.0	239.5
external os	180.1	198.82	233.1	219.0	236.0	239.5
internal os	180.0	198.82	233.1	219.0	236.0	239.5
nabothian gland	180.0	198.82	233.1	219.0	236.0	239.5
squamocolumnar junction	180.8	198.82	233.1	219.0	236.0	239.5
stump	180.8	198.82	233.1	219.0	236.0	239.5
cheek	195.0	198.89	234.8	229.8	238.8	239.8
external	173.3	198.2	232.3	216.3	238.2	239.2
inner aspect	145.0	198.89	230.0	210.4	235.1	239.0
internal	145.0	198.89	230.0	210.4	235.1	239.0
mucosa	145.0	198.89	230.0	210.4	235.1	239.0
chest (wall) NEC	195.1	198.89	234.8	229.8	238.8	239.8
chiasma opticum	192.0	198.4	—	225.1	237.9	239.7
chin	173.3	198.2	232.3	216.3	238.2	239.2
choana	147.3	198.89	230.0	210.7	235.1	239.0
cholangiole	155.1	197.8	230.8	211.5	235.3	239.0
choledochal duct	156.1	197.8	230.8	211.5	235.3	239.0
choroid	190.6	198.4	234.0	224.6	238.8	239.8
plexus	191.5	198.3	—	225.0	237.5	239.6
ciliary body	190.0	198.4	234.0	224.0	238.8	239.8
clavicle	170.3	198.5	—	213.3	238.0	239.2
clitoris	184.3	198.82	233.32	221.2	236.3	239.5
clivus	170.0	198.5	—	213.0	238.0	239.2
cloacogenic zone	154.8	197.5	230.7	211.4	235.5	239.0
coccygeal						
body or glomus	194.6	198.89	—	227.6	237.3	239.7
vertebra	170.6	198.5	—	213.6	238.0	239.2
coccyx	170.6	198.5	—	213.6	238.0	239.2
colon—*see also* Neoplasm,						

INDEX TO DISEASES   Neoplasms

	Malignant			Benign	Uncertain Behavior	Unspecified
	Primary	Secondary	Ca in situ			

intestine, large and rectum	154.0	197.5	230.4	211.4	235.2	239.0
column, spinal—*see* Neoplasm, spine						
columnella	173.3	198.2	232.3	216.3	238.2	239.2
commissure						
labial, lip	140.6	198.89	230.0	210.4	235.1	239.0
laryngeal	161.0	197.3	231.0	212.1	235.6	239.1
common (bile) duct	156.1	197.8	230.8	211.5	235.3	239.0
concha	173.2	198.2	232.2	216.2	238.2	239.2
nose	160.0	197.3	231.8	212.0	235.9	239.1
conjunctiva	190.3	198.4	234.0	224.3	238.8	239.8
connective tissue NEC	171.9	198.89	—	215.9	238.1	239.2

> *Note*—For neoplasms of connective tissue (blood vessel, bursa, fasica, ligament, muscle, peripheral nerves, sympathetic and parasympathetic nerves, and ganglia, synovia, tendon, etc.) or of morphological types that indicate connective tissue, code according to the list under "Neoplasm, connective tissue;" for sites that do not appear in this list, code to neoplasm of that site; e.g.: liposarcoma, shoulder 171.2; leiomyosarcoma, stomach 151.9; neurofibroma, chest wall 215.4.
>
> Morphological types that indicate connective tissue appear in their proper palce in the alphabetic index with the instruction "see Neoplasm, connective tissue..."

abdomen	171.5	198.89	—	215.5	238.1	239.2
abdominal wall	171.5	198.89	—	215.5	238.1	239.2
ankle	171.3	198.89	—	215.3	238.1	239.2
antecubital fossa or space	171.2	198.89	—	215.2	238.1	239.2
arm	171.2	198.89	—	215.2	238.1	239.2
auricle (ear)	171.0	198.89	—	215.0	238.1	239.2
axilla	171.4	198.89	—	215.4	238.1	239.2
back	171.7	198.89	—	215.7	238.1	239.2
breast (female) (*see also* Neoplasm, breast)	174.9	198.81	233.0	217	238.3	239.3
male	175.9	198.81	233.0	217	238.3	239.3
buttock	171.6	198.89	—	215.6	238.1	239.2
calf	171.3	198.89	—	215.3	238.1	239.2
cervical region	171.0	198.89	—	215.0	238.1	239.2
cheek	171.0	198.89	—	215.0	238.1	239.2
chest (wall)	171.4	198.89	—	215.4	238.1	239.2
chin	171.0	198.89	—	215.0	238.1	239.2
contiguous sites	171.8	—	—	—	—	—
diaphragm	171.4	198.89	—	215.4	238.1	239.2
ear (external)	171.0	198.89	—	215.0	238.1	239.2
elbow	171.2	198.89	—	215.2	238.1	239.2
extrarectal	171.6	198.89	—	215.6	238.1	239.2
extremity	171.8	198.89	—	215.8	238.1	239.2
lower	171.3	198.89	—	215.3	238.1	239.2
upper	171.2	198.89	—	215.2	238.1	239.2
eyelid	171.0	198.89	—	215.0	238.1	239.2
face	171.0	198.89	—	215.0	238.1	239.2
finger	171.2	198.89	—	215.2	238.1	239.2
flank	171.7	198.89	—	215.7	238.1	239.2
foot	171.3	198.89	—	215.3	238.1	239.2
forearm	171.2	198.89	—	215.2	238.1	239.2
forehead	171.0	198.89	—	215.0	238.1	239.2
gastric	171.5	198.89	—	215.5	238.1	—
gastrointestinal	171.5	198.89	—	215.5	238.1	—
gluteal region	171.6	198.89	—	215.6	238.1	239.2
great vessels NEC	171.4	198.89	—	215.4	238.1	239.2
groin	171.6	198.89	—	215.6	238.1	239.2
hand	171.2	198.89	—	215.2	238.1	239.2
head	171.0	198.89	—	215.0	238.1	239.2
heel	171.3	198.89	—	215.3	238.1	239.2
hip	171.3	198.89	—	215.3	238.1	239.2
hypochondrium	171.5	198.89	—	215.5	238.1	239.2
iliopsoas muscle	171.6	198.89	—	215.5	238.1	239.2

Neoplasms   INDEX TO DISEASES

	Malignant Primary	Malignant Secondary	Ca in situ	Benign	Uncertain Behavior	Unspecified
infraclavicular region	171.4	198.89	—	215.4	238.1	239.2
inguinal (canal) (region)	171.6	198.89	—	215.6	238.1	239.2
intestine	171.5	198.89	—	215.5	238.1	—
intrathoracic	171.4	198.89	—	215.4	238.1	239.2
ischorectal fossa	171.6	198.89	—	215.6	238.1	239.2
jaw	143.9	198.89	230.0	210.4	235.1	239.0
knee	171.3	198.89	—	215.3	238.1	239.2
leg	171.3	198.89	—	215.3	238.1	239.2
limb NEC	171.9	198.89	—	215.8	238.1	239.2
lower	171.3	198.89	—	215.3	238.1	239.2
upper	171.2	198.89	—	215.2	238.1	239.2
nates	171.6	198.89	—	215.6	238.1	239.2
neck	171.0	198.89	—	215.0	238.1	239.2
orbit	190.1	198.4	234.0	224.1	238.8	239.8
pararectal	171.6	198.89	—	215.6	238.1	239.2
para-urethral	171.6	198.89	—	215.6	238.1	239.2
paravaginal	171.6	198.89	—	215.6	238.1	239.2
pelvis (floor)	171.6	198.89	—	215.6	238.1	239.2
pelvo-abdominal	171.8	198.89	—	215.8	238.1	239.2
perineum	171.6	198.89	—	215.6	238.1	239.2
perirectal (tissue)	171.6	198.89	—	215.6	238.1	239.2
periurethral (tissue)	171.6	198.89	—	215.6	238.1	239.2
popliteal fossa or space	171.3	198.89	—	215.3	238.1	239.2
presacral	171.6	198.89	—	215.6	238.1	239.2
psoas muscle	171.5	198.89	—	215.5	238.1	239.2
pterygoid fossa	171.0	198.89	—	215.0	238.1	239.2
rectovaginal septum or wall	171.6	198.89	—	215.6	238.1	239.2
rectovesical	171.6	198.89	—	215.6	238.1	239.2
retroperitoneum	158.0	197.6	—	211.8	235.4	239.0
sacrococcygeal region	171.6	198.89	—	215.6	238.1	239.2
scalp	171.0	198.89	—	215.0	238.1	239.2
scapular region	171.4	198.89	—	215.4	238.1	239.2
shoulder	171.2	198.89	—	215.2	238.1	239.2
skin (dermis) NEC	173.9	198.2	232.9	216.9	238.2	239.2
stomach	171.5	198.89	—	215.5	238.1	—
submental	171.0	198.89	—	215.0	238.1	239.2
supraclavicular region	171.0	198.89	—	215.0	238.1	239.2
temple	171.0	198.89	—	215.0	238.1	239.2
temporal region	171.0	198.89	—	215.0	238.1	239.2
thigh	171.3	198.89	—	215.3	238.1	239.2
thoracic (duct) (wall)	171.4	198.89	—	215.4	238.1	239.2
thorax	171.4	198.89	—	215.4	238.1	239.2
thumb	171.2	198.89	—	215.2	238.1	239.2
toe	171.3	198.89	—	215.3	238.1	239.2
trunk	171.7	198.89	—	215.7	238.1	239.2
umbilicus	171.5	198.89	—	215.5	238.1	239.2
vesicorectal	171.6	198.89	—	215.6	238.1	239.2
wrist	171.2	198.89	—	215.2	238.1	239.2
conus medullaris	192.2	198.3	—	225.3	237.5	239.7
cord (true) (vocal)	161.0	197.3	231.0	212.1	235.6	239.1
false	161.1	197.3	231.0	212.1	235.6	239.1
spermatic	187.6	198.82	233.6	222.8	236.6	239.5
spinal (cervical) (lumbar) (thoracic)	192.2	198.3	—	225.3	237.5	239.7
cornea (limbus)	190.4	198.4	234.0	224.4	238.8	239.8
corpus						
albicans	183.0	198.6	233.39	220	236.2	239.5
callosum, brain	191.8	198.3	—	225.0	237.5	239.6
cavernosum	187.3	198.82	233.5	222.1	236.6	239.5
gastric	151.4	197.8	230.2	211.1	235.2	239.0
penis	187.3	198.82	233.5	222.1	236.6	239.5
striatum, cerebrum	191.0	198.3	—	225.0	237.5	239.6

INDEX TO DISEASES — Neoplasms

	Malignant — Primary	Malignant — Secondary	Ca in situ	Benign	Uncertain Behavior	Unspecified
uteri	182.0	198.82	233.2	219.1	236.0	239.5
isthmus	182.1	198.82	233.2	219.1	236.0	239.5
cortex						
adrenal	194.0	198.7	234.8	227.0	237.2	239.7
cerebral	191.0	198.3	—	225.0	237.5	239.6
costal cartilage	170.3	198.5	—	213.3	238.0	239.2
costovertebral joint	170.3	198.5	—	213.3	238.0	239.2
Cowper's gland	189.3	198.1	233.9	223.81	236.99	239.5
cranial (fossa, any)	191.9	198.3	—	225.0	237.5	239.6
meninges	192.1	198.4	—	225.2	237.6	239.7
nerve (any)	192.0	198.4	—	225.1	237.9	239.7
craniobuccal pouch	194.3	198.89	234.8	227.3	237.0	239.7
craniopharyngeal (duct) (pouch)	194.3	198.89	234.8	227.3	237.0	239.7
cricoid	148.0	198.89	230.0	210.8	235.1	239.0
cartilage	161.3	197.3	231.0	212.1	235.6	239.1
cricopharynx	148.0	198.89	230.0	210.8	235.1	239.0
crypt of Morgagni	154.8	197.5	230.7	211.4	235.2	239.0
crystalline lens	190.0	198.4	234.0	224.0	238.8	239.8
cul-de-sac (Douglas')	158.8	197.6	—	211.8	235.4	239.0
cuneiform cartilage	161.3	197.3	231.0	212.1	235.6	239.1
cutaneous—see Neoplasm, skin						
cutis—see Neoplasm, skin						
cystic (bile) duct (common)	156.1	197.8	230.8	211.5	235.3	239.0
dermis—see Neoplasm, skin						
diaphragm	171.4	198.89	—	215.4	238.1	239.2
digestive organs, system, tube, tract NEC	159.9	197.8	230.9	211.9	235.5	239.0
contiguous sites with peritoneum	159.8	—	—	—	—	—
disc, intervertebral	170.2	198.5	—	213.2	238.0	239.2
disease, generalized	199.0	199.0	234.9	229.9	238.9	199.0
disseminated	199.0	199.0	234.9	229.9	238.9	199.0
Douglas' cul-de-sac or pouch	158.8	197.6	—	211.8	235.4	239.0
duodenojejunal junction	152.8	197.4	230.7	211.2	235.2	239.0
duodenum	152.0	197.4	230.7	211.2	235.2	239.0
dura (cranial) (mater)	192.1	198.4	—	225.2	237.6	239.7
cerebral	192.1	198.4	—	225.2	237.6	239.7
spinal	192.3	198.4	—	225.4	237.6	239.7
ear (external)	173.2	198.2	232.2	216.2	238.2	239.2
auricle or auris	173.2	198.2	232.2	216.2	238.2	239.2
canal, external	173.2	198.2	232.2	216.2	238.2	239.2
cartilage	171.0	198.89	—	215.0	238.1	239.2
external meatus	173.2	198.2	232.2	216.2	238.2	239.2
inner	160.1	197.3	231.8	212.0	235.9	239.8
lobule	173.2	198.2	232.2	216.2	238.2	239.2
middle	160.1	197.3	231.8	212.0	235.9	239.8
contiguous sites with accessory sinuses or nasal cavities	160.8	—	—	—	—	—
skin	173.2	198.2	232.2	216.2	238.2	239.2
earlobe	173.2	198.2	232.2	216.2	238.2	239.2
ejaculatory duct	187.8	198.82	233.6	222.8	236.6	239.5
elbow NEC*	195.4	198.89	232.6	229.8	238.8	239.8
endocardium	164.1	198.89	—	212.7	238.8	239.8
endocervix (canal) (gland)	180.0	198.82	233.1	219.0	236.0	239.5
endocrine gland NEC	194.9	198.89	—	227.9	237.4	239.7
pluriglandular NEC	194.8	198.89	234.8	227.8	237.4	239.7
endometrium (gland) (stroma)	182.0	198.82	233.2	219.1	236.0	239.5
ensiform cartilage	170.3	198.5	—	213.3	238.0	239.2
enteric—see Neoplasm, intestine						
ependyma (brain)	191.5	198.3	—	225.0	237.5	239.6

Neoplasms   **INDEX TO DISEASES**

	Malignant Primary	Malignant Secondary	Ca in situ	Benign	Uncertain Behavior	Unspecified
epicardium	164.1	198.89	—	212.7	238.8	239.8
epididymis	187.5	198.82	233.6	222.3	236.6	239.5
epidural	192.9	198.4	—	225.9	237.9	239.7
epiglottis	161.1	197.3	231.0	212.1	235.6	239.1
anterior aspect or surface	146.4	198.89	230.0	210.6	235.1	239.0
cartilage	161.3	197.3	231.0	212.1	235.6	239.1
free border (margin)	146.4	198.89	230.0	210.6	235.1	239.0
junctional region	146.5	198.89	230.0	210.6	235.1	239.0
posterior (laryngeal) surface	161.1	197.3	231.0	212.1	235.6	239.1
suprahyoid portion	161.1	197.3	231.0	212.1	235.6	239.1
esophagogastric junction	151.0	197.8	230.2	211.1	235.2	239.0
esophagus	150.9	197.8	230.1	211.0	235.5	239.0
abdominal	150.2	197.8	230.1	211.0	235.5	239.0
cervical	150.0	197.8	230.1	211.0	235.5	239.0
contiguous sites	150.8	—	—	—	—	—
distal (third)	150.5	197.8	230.1	211.0	235.5	239.0
lower (third)	150.5	197.8	230.1	211.0	235.5	239.0
middle (third)	150.4	197.8	230.1	211.0	235.5	239.0
proximal (third)	150.3	197.8	230.1	211.0	235.5	239.0
specified part NEC	150.8	197.8	230.1	211.0	235.5	239.0
thoracic	150.1	197.8	230.1	211.0	235.5	239.0
upper (third)	150.3	197.8	230.1	211.0	235.5	239.0
ethmoid (sinus)	160.3	197.3	231.8	212.0	235.9	239.1
bone or labyrinth	170.0	198.5	—	213.0	238.0	239.2
Eustachian tube	160.1	197.3	231.8	212.0	235.9	239.1
exocervix	180.1	198.82	233.1	219.0	236.0	239.5
external						
meatus (ear)	173.2	198.2	232.2	216.2	238.2	239.2
os, cervix uteri	180.1	198.82	233.1	219.0	236.0	239.5
extradural	192.9	198.4	—	225.9	237.9	239.7
extrahepatic (bile) duct	156.1	197.8	230.8	211.5	235.3	239.0
contiguous sites with gallbladder	156.8	—	—	—	—	—
extraocular muscle	190.1	198.4	234.0	224.1	238.8	239.8
extrarectal	195.3	198.89	234.8	229.8	238.8	239.8
extremity*	195.8	198.89	232.8	229.8	238.8	239.8
lower*	195.5	198.89	232.7	229.8	238.8	239.8
upper*	195.4	198.89	232.6	229.8	238.8	239.8
eye NEC	190.9	198.4	234.0	224.9	238.8	239.8
contiguous sites	190.8	—	—	—	—	—
specified sites NEC	190.8	198.4	234.0	224.8	238.8	239.8
eyeball	190.0	198.4	234.0	224.0	238.8	239.8
eyebrow	173.3	198.2	232.3	216.3	238.2	239.2
eyelid (lower) (skin) (upper)	173.1	198.2	232.1	216.1	238.2	239.2
cartilage	171.0	198.89	—	215.0	238.1	239.2
face NEC*	195.0	198.89	232.3	229.8	238.8	239.8
fallopian tube (accessory)	183.2	198.82	233.39	221.0	236.3	239.5
falx (cerebelli) (cerebri)	192.1	198.4	—	225.2	237.6	239.7
fascia—*see also* Neoplasm, connective tissue						
palmar	171.2	198.89	—	215.2	238.1	239.2
plantar	171.3	198.89	—	215.3	238.1	239.2
fatty tissue—*see* Neoplasm, connective tissue						
fauces, faucial NEC	146.9	198.89	230.0	210.6	235.1	239.0
pillars	146.2	198.89	230.0	210.6	235.1	239.0
tonsil	146.0	198.89	230.0	210.5	235.1	239.0
femur (any part)	170.7	198.5	—	213.7	238.0	239.2
fetal membrane	181	198.82	233.2	219.8	236.1	239.5
fibrous tissue—*see* Neoplasm, connective tissue						
fibula (any part)	170.7	198.5	—	213.7	238.0	239.2
filum terminale	192.2	198.3	—	225.3	237.5	239.7
finger NEC*	195.4	198.89	232.6	229.8	238.8	239.8
flank NEC*	195.8	198.89	232.5	229.8	238.8	239.8

INDEX TO DISEASES — Neoplasms

	Malignant Primary	Malignant Secondary	Ca in situ	Benign	Uncertain Behavior	Unspecified
follicle, nabothian	180.0	198.82	233.1	219.0	236.0	239.5
foot NEC*	195.5	198.89	232.7	229.8	238.8	239.8
forearm NEC*	195.4	198.89	232.6	229.8	238.8	239.8
forehead (skin)	173.3	198.2	232.3	216.3	238.2	239.2
foreskin	187.1	198.82	233.5	222.1	236.6	239.5
fornix						
pharyngeal	147.3	198.89	230.0	210.7	235.1	239.0
vagina	184.0	198.82	233.31	221.1	236.3	239.5
fossa (of)						
anterior (cranial)	191.9	198.3	—	225.0	237.5	239.6
cranial	191.9	198.3	—	225.0	237.5	239.6
ischiorectal	195.3	198.89	234.8	229.8	238.8	239.8
middle (cranial)	191.9	198.3	—	225.0	237.5	239.6
pituitary	194.3	198.89	234.8	227.3	237.0	239.7
posterior (cranial)	191.9	198.3	—	225.0	237.5	239.6
pterygoid	171.0	198.89	—	215.0	238.1	239.2
pyriform	148.1	198.89	230.0	210.8	235.1	239.0
Rosenmüller	147.2	198.89	230.0	210.7	235.1	239.0
tonsillar	146.1	198.89	230.0	210.6	235.1	239.0
fourchette	184.4	198.82	233.32	221.2	236.3	239.5
frenulum						
labii—*see* Neoplasm, lip, internal						
linguae	141.3	198.89	230.0	210.1	235.1	239.0
frontal						
bone	170.0	198.5	—	213.0	238.0	239.2
lobe, brain	191.1	198.3	—	225.0	237.5	239.6
meninges	192.1	198.4	—	225.2	237.6	239.7
pole	191.1	198.3	—	225.0	237.5	239.6
sinus	160.4	197.3	231.8	212.0	235.9	239.1
fundus						
stomach	151.3	197.8	230.2	211.1	235.2	239.0
uterus	182.0	198.82	233.2	219.1	236.0	239.5
gall duct (extrahepatic)	156.1	197.8	230.8	211.5	235.3	239.0
intrahepatic	155.1	197.8	230.8	211.5	235.3	239.0
gallbladder	156.0	197.8	230.8	211.5	235.3	239.0
contiguous sites with extrahepatic bile ducts	156.8	—	—	—	—	—
ganglia (*see also* Neoplasm, connective tissue)	171.9	198.89	—	215.9	238.1	239.2
basal	191.0	198.3	—	225.0	237.5	239.6
ganglion (*see also* Neoplasm, connective tissue)	171.9	198.89	—	215.9	238.1	239.2
cranial nerve	192.0	198.4	—	225.1	237.9	239.7
Gartner's duct	184.0	198.82	233.31	221.1	236.3	239.5
gastric—*see* Neoplasm, stomach						
gastrocolic	159.8	197.8	230.9	211.9	235.5	239.0
gastroesophageal junction	151.0	197.8	230.2	211.1	235.2	239.0
gastrointestinal (tract) NEC	159.9	197.8	230.9	211.9	235.5	239.0
generalized	199.0	199.0	234.9	229.9	238.9	199.0
genital organ or tract						
female NEC	184.9	198.82	233.39	221.9	236.3	239.5
contiguous sites	184.8	—	—	—	—	—
specified site NEC	184.8	198.82	233.39	221.8	236.3	239.5
male NEC	187.9	198.82	233.6	222.9	236.6	239.5
contiguous sites	187.8	—	—	—	—	—
specified site NEC	187.8	198.82	233.6	222.8	236.6	239.5
genitourinary tract						
female	184.9	198.82	233.39	221.9	236.3	239.5
male	187.9	198.82	233.6	222.9	236.6	239.5
gingiva (alveolar) (marginal)	143.9	198.89	230.0	210.4	235.1	239.0
lower	143.1	198.89	230.0	210.4	235.1	239.0
mandibular	143.1	198.89	230.0	210.4	235.1	239.0
maxillary	143.0	198.89	230.0	210.4	235.1	239.0

Neoplasms   **INDEX TO DISEASES**

	Malignant Primary	Malignant Secondary	Ca in situ	Benign	Uncertain Behavior	Unspecified
upper	143.0	198.89	230.0	210.4	235.1	239.0
gland, glandular (lymphatic) (system)—*see also* Neoplasm, lymph gland						
endocrine NEC	194.9	198.89	—	227.9	237.4	239.7
salivary—*see* Neoplasm, salivary, gland						
glans penis	187.2	198.82	233.5	222.1	236.6	239.5
globus pallidus	191.0	198.3	—	225.0	237.5	239.6
glomus						
coccygeal	194.6	198.89	—	227.6	237.3	239.7
jugularis	194.6	198.89	—	227.6	237.3	239.7
glosso-epiglottic fold(s)	146.4	198.89	230.0	210.6	235.1	239.0
glossopalatine fold	146.2	198.89	230.0	210.6	235.1	239.0
glossopharyngeal sulcus	146.1	198.89	230.0	210.6	235.1	239.0
glottis	161.0	197.3	231.0	212.1	235.6	239.1
gluteal region*	195.3	198.89	232.5	229.8	238.8	239.8
great vessels NEC	171.4	198.89	—	215.4	238.1	239.2
groin NEC*	195.3	198.89	232.5	229.8	238.8	239.8
gum	143.9	198.89	230.0	210.4	235.1	239.0
contiguous sites	143.8	—	—	—	—	—
lower	143.1	198.89	230.0	210.4	235.1	239.0
upper	143.0	198.89	230.0	210.4	235.1	239.0
hand NEC*	195.4	198.89	232.6	229.8	238.8	239.8
head NEC*	195.0	198.89	232.4	229.8	238.8	239.8
heart	164.1	198.89	—	212.7	238.8	239.8
contiguous sites with mediastinum or thymus	164.8	—	—	—	—	—
heel NEC*	195.5	198.89	232.7	229.8	238.8	239.8
helix	173.2	198.2	232.2	216.2	238.2	239.2
hematopoietic, hemopoietic tissue NEC	202.8	198.89	—	—	—	238.79
hemisphere, cerebral	191.0	198.3	—	225.0	237.5	239.6
hemorrhoidal zone	154.2	197.5	230.5	211.4	235.5	239.0
hepatic	155.2	197.7	230.8	211.5	235.3	239.0
duct (bile)	156.1	197.8	230.8	211.5	235.3	239.0
flexure (colon)	153.0	197.5	230.3	211.3	235.2	239.0
primary	155.0	—	—	—	—	—
hilus of lung	162.2	197.0	231.2	212.3	235.7	239.1
hip NEC*	195.5	198.89	232.7	229.8	238.8	239.8
hippocampus, brain	191.2	198.3	—	225.0	237.5	239.6
humerus (any part)	170.4	198.5	—	213.4	238.0	239.2
hymen	184.0	198.82	233.31	221.1	236.3	239.5
hypopharynx, hypopharyngeal NEC	148.9	198.89	230.0	210.8	235.1	239.0
contiguous sites	148.8	—	—	—	—	—
postcricoid region	148.0	198.89	230.0	210.8	235.1	239.0
posterior wall	148.3	198.89	230.0	210.8	235.1	239.0
pyriform fossa (sinus)	148.1	198.89	230.0	210.8	235.1	239.0
specified site NEC	148.8	198.89	230.0	210.8	235.1	239.0
wall	148.9	198.89	230.0	210.8	235.1	239.0
posterior	148.3	198.89	230.0	210.8	235.1	239.0
hypophysis	194.3	198.89	234.8	227.3	237.0	239.7
hypothalamus	191.0	198.3	—	225.0	237.5	239.6
ileocecum, ileocecal (coil, junction, valve)	153.4	197.5	230.3	211.3	235.2	239.0
ileum	152.2	197.4	230.7	211.2	235.2	239.0
ilium	170.6	198.5	—	213.6	238.0	239.2
immunoproliferative NEC	203.8	—	—	—	—	—
infraclavicular (region)*	195.1	198.89	232.5	229.8	238.8	239.8
inguinal (region)*	195.3	198.89	232.5	229.8	238.8	239.8
insula	191.0	198.3	—	225.0	237.5	239.6

INDEX TO DISEASES — Neoplasms

	Malignant			Benign	Uncertain Behavior	Unspecified
	Primary	Secondary	Ca in situ			

	Primary	Secondary	Ca in situ	Benign	Uncertain Behavior	Unspecified
insular tissue (pancreas)	157.4	197.8	230.9	211.7	235.5	239.0
brain	191.0	198.3	—	225.0	237.5	239.6
interarytenoid fold	148.2	198.89	230.0	210.8	235.1	239.0
hypopharyngeal aspect	148.2	198.89	230.0	210.8	235.1	239.0
laryngeal aspect	161.1	197.3	231.0	212.1	235.6	239.1
marginal zone	148.2	198.89	230.0	210.8	235.1	239.0
interdental papillae	143.9	198.89	230.0	210.4	235.1	239.0
lower	143.1	198.89	230.0	210.4	235.1	239.0
upper	143.0	198.89	230.0	210.4	235.1	239.0
internal						
capsule	191.0	198.3	—	225.0	237.5	239.6
os (cervix)	180.0	198.82	233.1	219.0	236.0	239.5
intervertebral cartilage						
or disc	170.2	198.5	—	213.2	238.0	239.2
intestine, intestinal	159.0	197.8	230.7	211.9	235.2	239.0
large	153.9	197.5	230.3	211.3	235.2	239.0
appendix	153.5	197.5	230.3	211.3	235.2	239.0
caput coli	153.4	197.5	230.3	211.3	235.2	239.0
cecum	153.4	197.5	230.3	211.3	235.2	239.0
colon	153.9	197.5	230.3	211.3	235.2	239.0
and rectum	154.0	197.5	230.4	211.4	235.2	239.0
ascending	153.6	197.5	230.3	211.3	235.2	239.0
caput	153.4	197.5	230.3	211.3	235.2	239.0
contiguous sites	153.8	—	—	—	—	—
descending	153.2	197.5	230.3	211.3	235.2	239.0
distal	153.2	197.5	230.3	211.3	235.2	239.0
left	153.2	197.5	230.3	211.3	235.2	239.0
pelvic	153.3	197.5	230.3	211.3	235.2	239.0
right	153.6	197.5	230.3	211.3	235.2	239.0
sigmoid (flexure)	153.3	197.5	230.3	211.3	235.2	239.0
transverse	153.1	197.5	230.3	211.3	235.2	239.0
contiguous sites	153.8	—	—	—	—	—
hepatic flexure	153.0	197.5	230.3	211.3	235.2	239.0
ileocecum, ileocecal						
(coil, valve)	153.4	197.5	230.3	211.3	235.2	239.0
sigmoid flexure (lower)						
(upper)	153.3	197.5	230.3	211.3	235.2	239.0
splenic flexure	153.7	197.5	230.3	211.3	235.2	239.0
small	152.9	197.4	230.7	211.2	235.2	239.0
contiguous sites	152.8	—	—	—	—	—
duodenum	152.0	197.4	230.7	211.2	235.2	239.0
ileum	152.2	197.4	230.7	211.2	235.2	239.0
jejunum	152.1	197.4	230.7	211.2	235.2	239.0
tract NEC	159.0	197.8	230.7	211.9	235.2	239.0
intra-abdominal	195.2	198.89	234.8	229.8	238.8	239.8
intracranial NEC	191.9	198.3	—	225.0	237.5	239.6
intrahepatic (bile) duct	155.1	197.8	230.8	211.5	235.3	239.0
intraocular	190.0	198.4	234.0	224.0	238.8	239.8
intraorbital	190.1	198.4	234.0	224.1	238.8	239.8
intrasellar	194.3	198.89	234.8	227.3	237.0	239.7
intrathoracic (cavity)						
(organs NEC)	195.1	198.89	234.8	229.8	238.8	239.8
contiguous sites with respiratory						
organs	165.8	—	—	—	—	—
iris	190.0	198.4	234.0	224.0	238.8	239.8
ischiorectal (fossa)	195.3	198.89	234.8	229.8	238.8	239.8
ischium	170.6	198.5	—	213.6	238.0	239.2
island of Reil	191.0	198.3	—	225.0	237.5	239.6
islands or islets of Langerhans	157.4	197.8	230.9	211.7	235.5	239.0
isthmus uteri	182.1	198.82	233.2	219.1	236.0	239.5
jaw	195.0	198.89	234.8	229.8	238.8	239.8
bone	170.1	198.5	—	213.1	238.0	239.2
carcinoma	143.9	—	—	—	—	—

1197

Neoplasms

INDEX TO DISEASES

	Malignant Primary	Malignant Secondary	Ca in situ	Benign	Uncertain Behavior	Unspecified
lower	143.1	—	—	—	—	—
upper	143.0	—	—	—	—	—
lower	170.1	198.5	—	213.1	238.0	239.2
upper	170.0	198.5	—	213.0	238.0	239.2
carcinoma (any type) (lower) (upper)	195.0	—	—	—	—	—
skin	173.3	198.2	232.3	216.3	238.2	239.2
soft tissues	143.9	198.89	230.0	210.4	235.1	239.0
lower	143.1	198.89	230.0	210.4	235.1	239.0
upper	143.0	198.89	230.0	210.4	235.1	239.0
jejunum	152.1	197.4	230.7	211.2	235.2	239.0
joint NEC (see also Neoplasm, bone)	170.9	198.5	—	213.9	238.0	239.2
acromioclavicular	170.4	198.5	—	213.4	238.0	239.2
bursa or synovial membrane—see Neoplasm, connective tissue						
costovertebral	170.3	198.5	—	213.3	238.0	239.2
sternocostal	170.3	198.5	—	213.3	238.0	239.2
temporomandibular	170.1	198.5	—	213.1	238.0	239.2
junction						
anorectal	154.8	197.5	230.7	211.4	235.5	239.0
cardioesophageal	151.0	197.8	230.2	211.1	235.2	239.0
esophagogastric	151.0	197.8	230.2	211.1	235.2	239.0
gastroesophageal	151.0	197.8	230.2	211.1	235.2	239.0
hard and soft palate	145.5	198.89	230.0	210.4	235.1	239.0
ileocecal	153.4	197.5	230.3	211.3	235.2	239.0
pelvirectal	154.0	197.5	230.4	211.4	235.2	239.0
pelviureteric	189.1	198.0	233.9	223.1	236.91	239.5
rectosigmoid	154.0	197.5	230.4	211.4	235.2	239.0
squamocolumnar, of cervix	180.8	198.82	233.1	219.0	236.0	239.5
kidney (parenchyma)	189.0	198.0	233.9	223.0	236.91	239.5
calyx	189.1	198.0	233.9	223.1	236.91	239.5
hilus	189.1	198.0	233.9	223.1	236.91	239.5
pelvis	189.1	198.0	233.9	223.1	236.91	239.5
knee NEC*	195.5	198.89	232.7	229.8	238.8	239.8
labia (skin)	184.4	198.82	233.32	221.2	236.3	239.5
majora	184.1	198.82	233.32	221.2	236.3	239.5
minora	184.2	198.82	233.32	221.2	236.3	239.5
labial—see also Neoplasm, lip						
sulcus (lower) (upper)	145.1	198.89	230.0	210.4	235.1	239.0
labium (skin)	184.4	198.82	233.32	221.2	236.3	239.5
majus	184.1	198.82	233.32	221.2	236.3	239.5
minus	184.2	198.82	233.32	221.2	236.3	239.5
lacrimal						
canaliculi	190.7	198.4	234.0	224.7	238.8	239.8
duct (nasal)	190.7	198.4	234.0	224.7	238.8	239.8
gland	190.2	198.4	234.0	224.2	238.8	239.8
punctum	190.7	198.4	234.0	224.7	238.8	239.8
sac	190.7	198.4	234.0	224.7	238.8	239.8
Langerhans, islands or islets	157.4	197.8	230.9	211.7	235.5	239.0
laryngopharynx	148.9	198.89	230.0	210.8	235.1	239.0
larynx, laryngeal NEC	161.9	197.3	231.0	212.1	235.6	239.1
aryepiglottic fold	161.1	197.3	231.0	212.1	235.6	239.1
cartilage (arytenoid) (cricoid) (cuneiform) (thyroid)	161.3	197.3	231.0	212.1	235.6	239.1
commissure (anterior) (posterior)	161.0	197.3	231.0	212.1	235.6	239.1
contiguous sites	161.8	—	—	—	—	—
extrinsic NEC	161.1	197.3	231.0	212.1	235.6	239.1
meaning hypopharynx	148.9	198.89	230.0	210.8	235.1	239.0
interarytenoid fold	161.1	197.3	231.0	212.1	235.6	239.1
intrinsic	161.0	197.3	231.0	212.1	235.6	239.1

INDEX TO DISEASES — Neoplasms

	Malignant			Benign	Uncertain Behavior	Unspecified
	Primary	Secondary	Ca in situ			
ventricular band	161.1	197.3	231.0	212.1	235.6	239.1
leg NEC*	195.5	198.89	232.7	229.8	238.8	239.8
lens, crystalline	190.0	198.4	234.0	224.0	238.8	239.8
lid (lower) (upper)	173.1	198.2	232.1	216.1	238.2	239.2
ligament—*see also* Neoplasm, connective tissue						
broad	183.3	198.82	233.39	221.0	236.3	239.5
Mackenrodt's	183.8	198.82	233.39	221.8	236.3	239.5
non-uterine—*see* Neoplasm, connective tissue						
round	183.5	198.82	—	221.0	236.3	239.5
sacro-uterine	183.4	198.82	—	221.0	236.3	239.5
uterine	183.4	198.82	—	221.0	236.3	239.5
utero-ovarian	183.8	198.82	233.39	221.8	236.3	239.5
uterosacral	183.4	198.82	—	221.0	236.3	239.5
limb*	195.8	198.89	232.8	229.8	238.8	239.8
lower*	195.5	198.89	232.7	229.8	238.8	239.8
upper*	195.4	198.89	232.6	229.8	238.8	239.8
limbus of cornea	190.4	198.4	234.0	224.4	238.8	239.8
lingual NEC (*see also* Neoplasm, tongue)	141.9	198.89	230.0	210.1	235.1	239.0
lingula, lung	162.3	197.0	231.2	212.3	235.7	239.1
lip (external) (lipstick area) (vermillion border)	140.9	198.89	230.0	210.0	235.1	239.0
buccal aspect—*see* Neoplasm, lip, internal						
commissure	140.6	198.89	230.0	210.4	235.1	239.0
contiguous sites	140.8	—	—	—	—	—
with oral cavity or pharynx	149.8	—	—	—	—	—
frenulum—*see* Neoplasm, lip, internal						
inner aspect—*see* Neoplasm, lip, internal						
internal (buccal) (frenulum) (mucosa) (oral)	140.5	198.89	230.0	210.0	235.1	239.0
lower	140.4	198.89	230.0	210.0	235.1	239.0
upper	140.3	198.89	230.0	210.0	235.1	239.0
lower	140.1	198.89	230.0	210.0	235.1	239.0
internal (buccal) (frenulum) (mucosa) (oral)	140.4	198.89	230.0	210.0	235.1	239.0
mucosa—*see* Neoplasm, lip, internal						
oral aspect—*see* Neoplasm, lip, internal						
skin (commissure) (lower) (upper)	173.0	198.2	232.0	216.0	238.2	239.2
upper	140.0	198.89	230.0	210.0	235.1	239.0
internal (buccal) (frenulum) (mucosa) (oral)	140.3	198.89	230.0	210.0	235.1	239.0
liver	155.2	197.7	230.8	211.5	235.3	239.0
primary	155.0	—	—	—	—	—
lobe						
azygos	162.3	197.0	231.2	212.3	235.7	239.1
frontal	191.1	198.3	—	225.0	237.5	239.6
lower	162.5	197.0	231.2	212.3	235.7	239.1
middle	162.4	197.0	231.2	212.3	235.7	239.1
occipital	191.4	198.3	—	225.0	237.5	239.6
parietal	191.3	198.3	—	225.0	237.5	239.6
temporal	191.2	198.3	—	225.0	237.5	239.6
upper	162.3	197.0	231.2	212.3	235.7	239.1
lumbosacral plexus	171.6	198.4	—	215.6	238.1	239.2
lung	162.9	197.0	231.2	212.3	235.7	239.1
azygos lobe	162.3	197.0	231.2	212.3	235.7	239.1
carina	162.2	197.0	231.2	212.3	235.7	239.1
contiguous sites with bronchus or trachea	162.8	—	—	—	—	—
hilus	162.2	197.0	231.2	212.3	235.7	239.1

Neoplasms — INDEX TO DISEASES

	Malignant			Benign	Uncertain Behavior	Unspecified
	Primary	Secondary	Ca in situ			
lingula	162.3	197.0	231.2	212.3	235.7	239.1
lobe NEC	162.9	197.0	231.2	212.3	235.7	239.1
lower lobe	162.5	197.0	231.2	212.3	235.7	239.1
main bronchus	162.2	197.0	231.2	212.3	235.7	239.1
middle lobe	162.4	197.0	231.2	212.3	235.7	239.1
upper lobe	162.3	197.0	231.2	212.3	235.7	239.1
lymph, lymphatic						
channel NEC (*see also* Neoplasm,						
connective tissue)	171.9	198.89	—	215.9	238.1	239.2
gland (secondary)	—	196.9	—	229.0	238.8	239.8
abdominal	—	196.2	—	229.0	238.8	239.8
aortic	—	196.2	—	229.0	238.8	239.8
arm	—	196.3	—	229.0	238.8	239.8
auricular (anterior)						
(posterior)	—	196.0	—	229.0	238.8	239.8
axilla, axillary	—	196.3	—	229.0	238.8	239.8
brachial	—	196.3	—	229.0	238.8	239.8
bronchial	—	196.1	—	229.0	238.8	239.8
bronchopulmonary	—	196.1	—	229.0	238.8	239.8
celiac	—	196.2	—	229.0	238.8	239.8
cervical	—	196.0	—	229.0	238.8	239.8
cervicofacial	—	196.0	—	229.0	238.8	239.8
Cloquet	—	196.5	—	229.0	238.8	239.8
colic	—	196.2	—	229.0	238.8	239.8
common duct	—	196.2	—	229.0	238.8	239.8
cubital	—	196.3	—	229.0	238.8	239.8
diaphragmatic	—	196.1	—	229.0	238.8	239.8
epigastric, inferior	—	196.6	—	229.0	238.8	239.8
epitrochlear	—	196.3	—	229.0	238.8	239.8
esophageal	—	196.1	—	229.0	238.8	239.8
face	—	196.0	—	229.0	238.8	239.8
femoral	—	196.5	—	229.0	238.8	239.8
gastric	—	196.2	—	229.0	238.8	239.8
groin	—	196.5	—	229.0	238.8	239.8
head	—	196.0	—	229.0	238.8	239.8
hepatic	—	196.2	—	229.0	238.8	239.8
hilar (pulmonary)	—	196.1	—	229.0	238.8	239.8
splenic	—	196.2	—	229.0	238.8	239.8
hypogastric	—	196.6	—	229.0	238.8	239.8
ileocolic	—	196.2	—	229.0	238.8	239.8
iliac	—	196.6	—	229.0	238.8	239.8
infraclavicular	—	196.3	—	229.0	238.8	239.8
inguina, inguinal	—	196.5	—	229.0	238.8	239.8
innominate	—	196.1	—	229.0	238.8	239.8
intercostal	—	196.1	—	229.0	238.8	239.8
intestinal	—	196.2	—	229.0	238.8	239.8
intrabdominal	—	196.2	—	229.0	238.8	239.8
intrapelvic	—	196.6	—	229.0	238.8	239.8
intrathoracic	—	196.1	—	229.0	238.8	239.9
jugular	—	196.0	—	229.0	238.8	239.8
leg	—	196.5	—	229.0	238.8	239.8
limb						
lower	—	196.5	—	229.0	238.8	239.8
upper	—	196.3	—	229.0	238.8	239.8
lower limb	—	196.5	—	229.0	238.8	238.9
lumbar	—	196.2	—	229.0	238.8	239.8
mandibular	—	196.0	—	229.0	238.8	239.8
mediastinal	—	196.1	—	229.0	238.8	239.8
mesenteric (inferior)						
(superior)	—	196.2	—	229.0	238.8	239.8
midcolic	—	196.2	—	229.0	238.8	239.8
multiple sites in categories						
196.0-196.6	—	196.8	—	229.0	238.8	239.8

INDEX TO DISEASES — Neoplasms

	Malignant Primary	Malignant Secondary	Ca in situ	Benign	Uncertain Behavior	Unspecified
neck	—	196.0	—	229.0	238.8	239.8
obturator	—	196.6	—	229.0	238.8	239.8
occipital	—	196.0	—	229.0	238.8	239.8
pancreatic	—	196.2	—	229.0	238.8	239.8
para-aortic	—	196.2	—	229.0	238.8	239.8
paracervical	—	196.6	—	229.0	238.8	239.8
parametrial	—	196.6	—	229.0	238.8	239.8
parasternal	—	196.1	—	229.0	238.8	239.8
parotid	—	196.0	—	229.0	238.8	239.8
pectoral	—	196.3	—	229.0	238.8	239.8
pelvic	—	196.6	—	229.0	238.8	239.8
peri-aortic	—	196.2	—	229.0	238.8	239.8
peripancreatic	—	196.2	—	229.0	238.8	239.8
popliteal	—	196.5	—	229.0	238.8	239.8
porta hepatis	—	196.2	—	229.0	238.8	239.8
portal	—	196.2	—	229.0	238.8	239.8
preauricular	—	196.0	—	229.0	238.8	239.8
prelaryngeal	—	196.0	—	229.0	238.8	239.8
presymphysial	—	196.6	—	229.0	238.8	239.8
pretracheal	—	196.0	—	229.0	238.8	239.8
primary (any site) NEC	202.9	—	—	—	—	—
pulmonary (hiler)	—	196.1	—	229.0	238.8	239.8
pyloric	—	196.2	—	229.0	238.8	239.8
retroperitoneal	—	196.2	—	229.0	238.8	239.8
retropharyngeal	—	196.0	—	229.0	238.8	239.8
Rosenmüller's	—	196.5	—	229.0	238.8	239.8
sacral	—	196.6	—	229.0	238.8	239.8
scalene	—	196.0	—	229.0	238.8	239.8
site NEC	—	196.9	—	229.0	238.8	239.8
splenic (hilar)	—	196.2	—	229.0	238.8	239.8
subclavicular	—	196.3	—	229.0	238.8	239.8
subinguinal	—	196.5	—	229.0	238.8	239.8
sublingual	—	196.0	—	229.0	238.8	239.8
submandibular	—	196.0	—	229.0	238.8	239.8
submaxillary	—	196.0	—	229.0	238.8	239.8
submental	—	196.0	—	229.0	238.8	239.8
subscapular	—	196.3	—	229.0	238.8	239.8
supraclavicular	—	196.0	—	229.0	238.8	239.8
thoracic	—	196.1	—	229.0	238.8	239.8
tibial	—	196.5	—	229.0	238.8	239.8
tracheal	—	196.1	—	229.0	238.8	239.8
tracheobronchial	—	196.1	—	229.0	238.8	239.8
upper limb	—	196.3	—	229.0	238.8	239.8
Virchow's	—	196.0	—	229.0	238.8	239.8
node—*see also* Neoplasm, lymph gland primary NEC	202.9	—	—	—	—	—
vessel (*see also* Neoplasm, connective tissue)	171.9	198.89	—	215.9	238.1	239.2
Mackenrodt's ligament	183.8	198.82	233.39	221.8	236.3	239.5
malar	170.0	198.5	—	213.0	238.0	239.2
region—*see* Neoplasm, cheek						
mammary gland—*see* Neoplasm, breast						
mandible	170.1	198.5	—	213.1	238.0	239.2
alveolar mucosa	143.1	198.89	230.0	210.4	235.1	239.0
ridge or process	170.1	198.5	—	213.1	238.0	239.2
carcinoma	143.1	—	—	—	—	—
carcinoma	143.1	—	—	—	—	—
marrow (bone) NEC	202.9	198.5	—	—	—	238.79
mastectomy site (skin)	173.5	198.2	—	—	—	—
specified as breast tissue	174.8	198.81	—	—	—	—

1201

Neoplasms   INDEX TO DISEASES

	Malignant Primary	Malignant Secondary	Ca in situ	Benign	Uncertain Behavior	Unspecified
mastoid (air cells) (antrum) (cavity)	160.1	197.3	231.8	212.0	235.9	239.1
bone or process	170.0	198.5	—	213.0	238.0	239.2
maxilla, maxillary (superior)	170.0	198.5	—	213.0	238.0	239.2
alveolar						
mucosa	143.0	198.89	230.0	210.4	235.1	239.0
ridge or process	170.0	198.5	—	213.0	238.0	239.2
carcinoma	143.0	—	—	—	—	—
antrum	160.2	197.3	231.8	212.0	235.9	239.1
carcinoma	143.0	—	—	—	—	—
inferior—*see* Neoplasm, mandible						
sinus	160.2	197.3	231.8	212.0	235.9	239.1
meatus						
external (ear)	173.2	198.2	232.2	216.2	238.2	239.2
Meckel's diverticulum	152.3	197.4	230.7	211.2	235.2	239.0
mediastinum, mediastinal	164.9	197.1	—	212.5	235.8	239.8
anterior	164.2	197.1	—	212.5	235.8	239.8
contiguous sites with heart and thymus	164.8	—	—	—	—	—
posterior	164.3	197.1	—	212.5	235.8	239.8
medulla						
adrenal	194.0	198.7	234.8	227.0	237.2	239.7
oblongata	191.7	198.3	—	225.0	237.5	239.6
meibomian gland	173.1	198.2	232.1	216.1	238.2	239.2
melanoma —*see* Melanoma						
meninges (brain) (cerebral) (cranial) (intracranial)	192.1	198.4	—	225.2	237.6	239.7
spinal (cord)	192.3	198.4	—	225.4	237.6	239.7
meniscus, knee joint (lateral) (medial)	170.7	198.5	—	213.7	238.0	239.2
mesentery, mesenteric	158.8	197.6	—	211.8	235.4	239.0
mesoappendix	158.8	197.6	—	211.8	235.4	239.0
mesocolon	158.8	197.6	—	211.8	235.4	239.0
mesopharynx—*see* Neoplasm, oropharynx						
mesosalpinx	183.3	198.82	233.39	221.0	236.3	239.5
mesovarium	183.3	198.82	233.39	221.0	236.3	239.5
metacarpus (any bone)	170.5	198.5	—	213.5	238.0	239.2
metastatic NEC—*see also* Neoplasm, by site, secondary	—	199.1	—	—	—	—
metatarsus (any bone)	170.8	198.5	—	213.8	238.0	239.2
midbrain	191.7	198.3	—	225.0	237.5	239.6
milk duct—*see* Neoplasm, breast						
mons						
pubis	184.4	198.82	233.32	221.2	236.3	239.5
veneris	184.4	198.82	233.32	221.2	236.3	239.5
motor tract	192.9	198.4	—	225.9	237.9	239.7
brain	191.9	198.3	—	225.0	237.5	239.6
spinal	192.2	198.3	—	225.3	237.5	239.7
mouth	145.9	198.89	230.0	210.4	235.1	239.0
contiguous sites	145.8	—	—	—	—	—
floor	144.9	198.89	230.0	210.3	235.1	239.0
anterior portion	144.0	198.89	230.0	210.3	235.1	239.0
contiguous sites	144.8	—	—	—	—	—
lateral portion	144.1	198.89	230.0	210.3	235.1	239.0
roof	145.5	198.89	230.0	210.4	235.1	239.0
specified part NEC	145.8	198.89	230.0	210.4	235.1	239.0
vestibule	145.1	198.89	230.0	210.4	235.1	239.0
mucosa						
alveolar (ridge or process)	143.9	198.89	230.0	210.4	235.1	239.0
lower	143.1	198.89	230.0	210.4	235.1	239.0
upper	143.0	198.89	230.0	210.4	235.1	239.0
buccal	145.0	198.89	230.0	210.4	235.1	239.0
cheek	145.0	198.89	230.0	210.4	235.1	239.0

1202

INDEX TO DISEASES — Neoplasms

	Malignant Primary	Malignant Secondary	Ca in situ	Benign	Uncertain Behavior	Unspecified
lip—*see* Neoplasm, lip, internal						
nasal	160.0	197.3	231.8	212.0	235.9	239.1
oral	145.0	198.89	230.0	210.4	235.1	239.0
Müllerian duct						
female	184.8	198.82	233.39	221.8	236.3	239.5
male	187.8	198.82	233.6	222.8	236.6	239.5
multiple sites NEC	199.0	199.0	234.9	229.9	238.9	199.0
muscle—*see also* Neoplasm, connective tissue						
extraocular	190.1	198.4	234.0	224.1	238.8	239.8
myocardium	164.1	198.89	—	212.7	238.8	239.8
myometrium	182.0	198.82	233.2	219.1	236.0	239.5
myopericardium	164.1	198.89	—	212.7	238.8	239.8
nabothian gland (follicle)	180.0	198.82	233.1	219.0	236.0	239.5
nail	173.9	198.2	232.9	216.9	238.2	239.2
finger	173.6	198.2	232.6	216.6	238.2	239.2
toe	173.7	198.2	232.7	216.7	238.2	239.2
nares, naris (anterior) (posterior)	160.0	197.3	231.8	212.0	235.9	239.1
nasal—*see* Neoplasm, nose						
nasolabial groove	173.3	198.2	232.3	216.3	238.2	239.2
nasolacrimal duct	190.7	198.4	234.0	224.7	238.8	239.8
nasopharynx, nasopharyngeal	147.9	198.89	230.0	210.7	235.1	239.0
contiguous sites	147.8	—	—	—	—	—
floor	147.3	198.89	230.0	210.7	235.1	239.0
roof	147.0	198.89	230.0	210.7	235.1	239.0
specified site NEC	147.8	198.89	230.0	210.7	235.1	239.0
wall	147.9	198.89	230.0	210.7	235.1	239.0
anterior	147.3	198.89	230.0	210.7	235.1	239.0
lateral	147.2	198.89	230.0	210.7	235.1	239.0
posterior	147.1	198.89	230.0	210.7	235.1	239.0
superior	147.0	198.89	230.0	210.7	235.1	239.0
nates	173.5	198.2	232.5	216.5	238.2	239.2
neck NEC*	195.0	198.89	234.8	229.8	238.8	239.8
nerve (autonomic) (ganglion) (parasympathetic) (peripheral) (sympathetic)—*see also* Neoplasm, connective tissue						
abducens	192.0	198.4	—	225.1	237.9	239.7
accessory (spinal)	192.0	198.4	—	225.1	237.9	239.7
acoustic	192.0	198.4	—	225.1	237.9	239.7
auditory	192.0	198.4	—	225.1	237.9	239.7
brachial	171.2	198.89	—	215.2	238.1	239.2
cranial (any)	192.0	198.4	—	225.1	237.9	239.7
facial	192.0	198.4	—	225.1	237.9	239.7
femoral	171.3	198.89	—	215.3	238.1	239.2
glossopharyngeal	192.0	198.4	—	225.1	237.9	239.7
hypoglossal	192.0	198.4	—	225.1	237.9	239.7
intercostal	171.4	198.89	—	215.4	238.1	239.2
lumbar	171.7	198.89	—	215.7	238.1	239.2
median	171.2	198.89	—	215.2	238.1	239.2
obturator	171.3	198.89	—	215.3	238.1	239.2
oculomotor	192.0	198.4	—	225.1	237.9	239.7
olfactory	192.0	198.4	—	225.1	237.9	239.7
optic	192.0	198.4	—	225.1	237.9	239.7
peripheral NEC	171.9	198.89	—	215.9	238.1	239.2
radial	171.2	198.89	—	215.2	238.1	239.2
sacral	171.6	198.89	—	215.6	238.1	239.2
sciatic	171.3	198.89	—	215.3	238.1	239.2
spinal NEC	171.9	198.89	—	215.9	238.1	239.2
trigeminal	192.0	198.4	—	225.1	237.9	239.7
trochlear	192.0	198.4	—	225.1	237.9	239.7
ulnar	171.2	198.89	—	215.2	238.1	239.2

Neoplasms INDEX TO DISEASES

	Malignant			Benign	Uncertain Behavior	Unspecified
	Primary	Secondary	Ca in situ			

vagus	192.0	198.4	—	225.1	237.9	239.7
nervous system (central)						
NEC	192.9	198.4	—	225.9	237.9	239.7
autonomic NEC	171.9	198.89	—	215.9	238.1	239.2
brain—*see also* Neoplasm, brain						
membrane or meninges	192.1	198.4	—	225.2	237.6	239.7
contiguous sites	192.8	—	—	—	—	—
parasympathetic NEC	171.9	198.89	—	215.9	238.1	239.2
sympathetic NEC	171.9	198.89	—	215.9	238.1	239.2
nipple (female)	174.9	198.81	233.0	217	238.3	239.3
male	175.9	198.81	233.0	217	238.3	239.3
nose, nasal	195.0	198.89	234.8	229.8	238.8	239.8
ala (external)	173.3	198.2	232.3	216.3	238.2	239.2
bone	170.0	198.5	—	213.0	238.0	239.2
cartilage	160.0	197.3	231.8	212.0	235.9	239.1
cavity	160.0	197.3	231.8	212.0	235.9	239.1
contiguous sites with accessory						
sinuses or middle ear	160.8	—	—	—	—	—
choana	147.3	198.89	230.0	210.7	235.1	239.0
external (skin)	173.3	198.2	232.3	216.3	238.2	239.2
fossa	160.0	197.3	231.8	212.0	235.9	239.1
internal	160.0	197.3	231.8	212.0	235.9	239.1
mucosa	160.0	197.3	231.8	212.0	235.9	239.1
septum	160.0	197.3	231.8	212.0	235.9	239.1
posterior margin	147.3	198.89	230.0	210.7	235.1	239.0
sinus—*see* Neoplasm, sinus						
skin	173.3	198.2	232.3	216.3	238.2	239.2
turbinate (mucosa)	160.0	197.3	231.8	212.0	235.9	239.1
bone	170.0	198.5	—	213.0	238.0	239.2
vestibule	160.0	197.3	231.8	212.0	235.9	239.1
nostril	160.0	197.3	231.8	212.0	235.9	239.1
nucleus pulposus	170.2	198.5	—	213.2	238.0	239.2
occipital						
bone	170.0	198.5	—	213.0	238.0	239.2
lobe or pole, brain	191.4	198.3	—	225.0	237.5	239.6
odontogenic—*see* Neoplasm,						
jaw bone						
oesophagus—*see* Neoplasm,						
esophagus						
olfactory nerve or bulb	192.0	198.4	—	225.1	237.9	239.7
olive (brain)	191.7	198.3	—	225.0	237.5	239.6
omentum	158.8	197.6	—	211.8	235.4	239.0
operculum (brain)	191.0	198.3	—	225.0	237.5	239.6
optic nerve, chiasm, or tract	192.0	198.4	—	225.1	237.9	239.7
oral (cavity)	145.9	198.89	230.0	210.4	235.1	239.0
contiguous sites with lip						
or pharynx	149.8	—	—	—	—	—
ill-defined	149.9	198.89	230.0	210.4	235.1	239.0
mucosa	145.9	198.89	230.0	210.4	235.1	239.0
orbit	190.1	198.4	234.0	224.1	238.8	239.8
bone	170.0	198.5	—	213.0	238.0	239.2
eye	190.1	198.4	234.0	224.1	238.8	239.8
soft parts	190.1	198.4	234.0	224.1	238.8	239.8
organ of Zuckerkandl	194.6	198.89	—	227.6	237.3	239.7
oropharynx	146.9	198.89	230.0	210.6	235.1	239.0
branchial cleft (vestige)	146.8	198.89	230.0	210.6	235.1	239.0
contiguous sites	146.8	—	—	—	—	—
junctional region	146.5	198.89	230.0	210.6	235.1	239.0
lateral wall	146.6	198.89	230.0	210.6	235.1	239.0
pillars of fauces	146.2	198.89	230.0	210.6	235.1	239.0
posterior wall	146.7	198.89	230.0	210.6	235.1	239.0
specified part NEC	146.8	198.89	230.0	210.6	235.1	239.0
vallecula	146.3	198.89	230.0	210.6	235.1	239.0

INDEX TO DISEASES — Neoplasms

	Malignant Primary	Malignant Secondary	Ca in situ	Benign	Uncertain Behavior	Unspecified
os						
external	180.1	198.82	233.1	219.0	236.0	239.5
internal	180.0	198.82	233.1	219.0	236.0	239.5
ovary	183.0	198.6	233.39	220	236.2	239.5
oviduct	183.2	198.82	233.39	221.0	236.3	239.5
palate	145.5	198.89	230.0	210.4	235.1	239.0
hard	145.2	198.89	230.0	210.4	235.1	239.0
junction of hard and soft palate	145.5	198.89	230.0	210.4	235.1	239.0
soft	145.3	198.89	230.0	210.4	235.1	239.0
nasopharyngeal surface	147.3	198.89	230.0	210.7	235.1	239.0
posterior surface	147.3	198.89	230.0	210.7	235.1	239.0
superior surface	147.3	198.89	230.0	210.7	235.1	239.0
palatoglossal arch	146.2	198.89	230.0	210.6	235.1	239.0
palatopharyngeal arch	146.2	198.89	230.0	210.6	235.1	239.0
pallium	191.0	198.3	—	225.0	237.5	239.6
palpebra	173.1	198.2	232.1	216.1	238.2	239.2
pancreas	157.9	197.8	230.9	211.6	235.5	239.0
body	157.1	197.8	230.9	211.6	235.5	239.0
contiguous sites	157.8	—	—	—	—	—
duct (of Santorini) (of Wirsung)	157.3	197.8	230.9	211.6	235.5	239.0
ectopic tissue	157.8	197.8	230.9	211.6	235.5	239.0
head	157.0	197.8	230.9	211.6	235.5	239.0
islet cells	157.4	197.8	230.9	211.7	235.5	239.0
neck	157.8	197.8	230.9	211.6	235.5	239.0
tail	157.2	197.8	230.9	211.6	235.5	239.0
para-aortic body	194.6	198.89	—	227.6	237.3	239.7
paraganglion NEC	194.6	198.89	—	227.6	237.3	239.7
parametrium	183.4	198.82	—	221.0	236.3	239.5
paranephric	158.0	197.6	—	211.8	235.4	239.0
pararectal	195.3	198.89	—	229.8	238.8	239.8
parasagittal (region)	195.0	198.89	234.8	229.8	238.8	239.8
parasellar	192.9	198.4	—	225.9	237.9	239.7
parathyroid (gland)	194.1	198.89	234.8	227.1	237.4	239.7
paraurethral	195.3	198.89	—	229.8	238.8	239.8
gland	189.4	198.1	233.9	223.89	236.99	239.5
paravaginal	195.3	198.89	—	229.8	238.8	239.8
parenchyma, kidney	189.0	198.0	233.9	223.0	236.91	239.5
parietal						
bone	170.0	198.5	—	213.0	238.0	239.2
lobe, brain	191.3	198.3	—	225.0	237.5	239.6
paroophoron	183.3	198.82	233.39	221.0	236.3	239.5
parotid (duct) (gland)	142.0	198.89	230.0	210.2	235.0	239.0
parovarium	183.3	198.82	233.39	221.0	236.3	239.5
patella	170.8	198.5	—	213.8	238.0	239.2
peduncle, cerebral	191.7	198.3	—	225.0	237.5	239.6
pelvirectal junction	154.0	197.5	230.4	211.4	235.2	239.0
pelvis, pelvic	195.3	198.89	234.8	229.8	238.8	239.8
bone	170.6	198.5	—	213.6	238.0	239.2
floor	195.3	198.89	234.8	229.8	238.8	239.8
renal	189.1	198.0	233.9	223.1	236.91	239.5
viscera	195.3	198.89	234.8	229.8	238.8	239.8
wall	195.3	198.89	234.8	229.8	238.8	239.8
pelvo-abdominal	195.8	198.89	234.8	229.8	238.8	239.8
penis	187.4	198.82	233.5	222.1	236.6	239.5
body	187.3	198.82	233.5	222.1	236.6	239.5
corpus (cavernosum)	187.3	198.82	233.5	222.1	236.6	239.5
glans	187.2	198.82	233.5	222.1	236.6	239.5
skin NEC	187.4	198.82	233.5	222.1	236.6	239.5
periadrenal (tissue)	158.0	197.6	—	211.8	235.4	239.0
perianal (skin)	173.5	198.2	232.5	216.5	238.2	239.2
pericardium	164.1	198.89	—	212.7	238.8	239.8

Neoplasms

INDEX TO DISEASES

	Malignant Primary	Malignant Secondary	Ca in situ	Benign	Uncertain Behavior	Unspecified
perinephric	158.0	197.6	—	211.8	235.4	239.0
perineum	195.3	198.89	234.8	229.8	238.8	239.8
periodontal tissue NEC	143.9	198.89	230.0	210.4	235.1	239.0
periosteum—*see* Neoplasm, bone						
peripancreatic	158.0	197.6	—	211.8	235.4	239.0
peripheral nerve NEC	171.9	198.89	—	215.9	238.1	239.2
perirectal (tissue)	195.3	198.89	—	229.8	238.8	239.8
perirenal (tissue)	158.0	197.6	—	211.8	235.4	239.0
peritoneum, peritoneal						
(cavity)	158.9	197.6	—	211.8	235.4	239.0
contiguous sites	158.8	—	—	—	—	—
with digestive organs	159.8	—	—	—	—	—
parietal	158.8	197.6	—	211.8	235.4	239.0
pelvic	158.8	197.6	—	211.8	235.4	239.0
specified part NEC	158.8	197.6	—	211.8	235.4	239.0
peritonsillar (tissue)	195.0	198.89	234.8	229.8	238.8	239.8
periurethral tissue	195.3	198.89	—	229.8	238.8	239.8
phalanges	170.9	198.5	—	213.9	238.0	239.2
foot	170.8	198.5	—	213.8	238.0	239.2
hand	170.5	198.5	—	213.5	238.0	239.2
pharynx, pharyngeal	149.0	198.89	230.0	210.9	235.1	239.0
bursa	147.1	198.89	230.0	210.7	235.1	239.0
fornix	147.3	198.89	230.0	210.7	235.1	239.0
recess	147.2	198.89	230.0	210.7	235.1	239.0
region	149.0	198.89	230.0	210.9	235.1	239.0
tonsil	147.1	198.89	230.0	210.7	235.1	239.0
wall (lateral) (posterior)	149.0	198.89	230.0	210.9	235.1	239.0
pia mater (cerebral) (cranial)	192.1	198.4	—	225.2	237.6	239.7
spinal	192.3	198.4	—	225.4	237.6	239.7
pillars of fauces	146.2	198.89	230.0	210.6	235.1	239.0
pineal (body) (gland)	194.4	198.89	234.8	227.4	237.1	239.7
pinna (ear) NEC	173.2	198.2	232.2	216.2	238.2	239.2
cartilage	171.0	198.89	—	215.0	238.1	239.2
piriform fossa or sinus	148.1	198.89	230.0	210.8	235.1	239.0
pituitary (body) (fossa)						
(gland) (lobe)	194.3	198.89	234.8	227.3	237.0	239.7
placenta	181	198.82	233.2	219.8	236.1	239.5
pleura, pleural (cavity)	163.9	197.2	—	212.4	235.8	239.1
contiguous sites	163.8	—	—	—	—	—
parietal	163.0	197.2	—	212.4	235.8	239.1
visceral	163.1	197.2	—	212.4	235.8	239.1
plexus						
brachial	171.2	198.89	—	215.2	238.1	239.2
cervical	171.0	198.89	—	215.0	238.1	239.2
choroid	191.5	198.3	—	225.0	237.5	239.6
lumbosacral	171.6	198.89	—	215.6	238.1	239.2
sacral	171.6	198.89	—	215.6	238.1	239.2
pluri-endocrine	194.8	198.89	234.8	227.8	237.4	239.7
pole						
frontal	191.1	198.3	—	225.0	237.5	239.6
occipital	191.4	198.3	—	225.0	237.5	239.6
pons (varolii)	191.7	198.3	—	225.0	237.5	239.6
popliteal fossa or space*	195.5	198.89	234.8	229.8	238.8	239.8
postcricoid (region)	148.0	198.89	230.0	210.8	235.1	239.0
posterior fossa (cranial)	191.9	198.3	—	225.0	237.5	239.6
postnasal space	147.9	198.89	230.0	210.7	235.1	239.0
prepuce	187.1	198.82	233.5	222.1	236.6	239.5
prepylorus	151.1	197.8	230.2	211.1	235.2	239.0
presacral (region)	195.3	198.89	—	229.8	238.8	239.8
prostate (gland)	185	198.82	233.4	222.2	236.5	239.5
utricle	189.3	198.1	233.9	223.81	236.99	239.5
pterygoid fossa	171.0	198.89	—	215.0	238.1	239.2
pubic bone	170.6	198.5	—	213.6	238.0	239.2

INDEX TO DISEASES — Neoplasms

	Malignant Primary	Malignant Secondary	Ca in situ	Benign	Uncertain Behavior	Unspecified
pudenda, pudendum (female)	184.4	198.82	233.32	221.2	236.3	239.5
pulmonary	162.9	197.0	231.2	212.3	235.7	239.1
putamen	191.0	198.3	—	225.0	237.5	239.6
pyloric						
antrum	151.2	197.8	230.2	211.1	235.2	239.0
canal	151.1	197.8	230.2	211.1	235.2	239.0
pylorus	151.1	197.8	230.2	211.1	235.2	239.0
pyramid (brain)	191.7	198.3	—	225.0	237.5	239.6
pyriform fossa or sinus	148.1	198.89	230.0	210.8	235.1	239.0
radius (any part)	170.4	198.5	—	213.4	238.0	239.2
Rathke's pouch	194.3	198.89	234.8	227.3	237.0	239.7
rectosigmoid (colon)						
(junction)	154.0	197.5	230.4	211.4	235.2	239.0
contiguous sites with						
anus or rectum	154.8	—	—	—	—	—
rectouterine pouch	158.8	197.6	—	211.8	235.4	239.0
rectovaginal septum or wall	195.3	198.89	234.8	229.8	238.8	239.8
rectovesical septum	195.3	198.89	234.8	229.8	238.8	239.8
rectum (ampulla)	154.1	197.5	230.4	211.4	235.2	239.0
and colon	154.0	197.5	230.4	211.4	235.2	239.0
contiguous sites with anus or						
rectosigmoid junction	154.8	—	—	—	—	—
renal	189.0	198.0	233.9	223.0	236.91	239.5
calyx	189.1	198.0	233.9	223.1	236.91	239.5
hilus	189.1	198.0	233.9	223.1	236.91	239.5
parenchyma	189.0	198.0	233.9	223.0	236.91	239.5
pelvis	189.1	198.0	233.9	223.1	236.91	239.5
respiratory						
organs or system NEC	165.9	197.3	231.9	212.9	235.9	239.1
contiguous sites with						
intrathoracic organs	165.8	—	—	—	—	—
specified sites NEC	165.8	197.3	231.8	212.8	235.9	239.1
tract NEC	165.9	197.3	231.9	212.9	235.9	239.1
upper	165.0	197.3	231.9	212.9	235.9	239.1
retina	190.5	198.4	234.0	224.5	238.8	239.8
retrobulbar	190.1	198.4	—	224.1	238.8	239.8
retrocecal	158.0	197.6	—	211.8	235.4	239.0
retromolar (area) (triangle)						
(trigone)	145.6	198.89	230.0	210.4	235.1	239.0
retro-orbital	195.0	198.89	234.8	229.8	238.8	239.8
retroperitoneal (space)						
(tissue)	158.0	197.6	—	211.8	235.4	239.0
contiguous sites	158.8	—	—	—	—	—
retroperitoneum	158.0	197.6	—	211.8	235.4	239.0
contiguous sites	158.8	—	—	—	—	—
retropharyngeal	149.0	198.89	230.0	210.9	235.1	239.0
retrovesical (septum)	195.3	198.89	234.8	229.8	238.8	239.8
rhinencephalon	191.0	198.3	—	225.0	237.5	239.6
rib	170.3	198.5	—	213.3	238.0	239.2
Rosenmüller's fossa	147.2	198.89	230.0	210.7	235.1	239.0
round ligament	183.5	198.82	—	221.0	236.3	239.5
sacrococcyx, sacrococcygeal	170.6	198.5	—	213.6	238.0	239.2
region	195.3	198.89	234.8	229.8	238.8	239.8
sacrouterine ligament	183.4	198.82	—	221.0	236.3	239.5
sacrum, sacral (vertebra)	170.6	198.5	—	213.6	238.0	239.2
salivary gland or duct						
(major)	142.9	198.89	230.0	210.2	235.0	239.0
contiguous sites	142.8	—	—	—	—	—
minor NEC	145.9	198.89	230.0	210.4	235.1	239.0
parotid	142.0	198.89	230.0	210.2	235.0	239.0
pluriglandular	142.8	198.89	230.0	210.2	235.0	239.0
sublingual	142.2	198.89	230.0	210.2	235.0	239.0
submandibular	142.1	198.89	230.0	210.2	235.0	239.0

1207

Neoplasms INDEX TO DISEASES

	Malignant Primary	Malignant Secondary	Ca in situ	Benign	Uncertain Behavior	Unspecified
submaxillary	142.1	198.89	230.0	210.2	235.0	239.0
salpinx (uterine)	183.2	198.82	233.39	221.0	236.3	239.5
Santorini's duct	157.3	197.8	230.9	211.6	235.5	239.0
scalp	173.4	198.2	232.4	216.4	238.2	239.2
scapula (any part)	170.4	198.5	—	213.4	238.0	239.2
scapular region	195.1	198.89	234.8	229.8	238.8	239.8
scar NEC (*see also* Neoplasm, skin)	173.9	198.2	232.9	216.9	238.2	239.2
sciatic nerve	171.3	198.89	—	215.3	238.1	239.2
sclera	190.0	198.4	234.0	224.0	238.8	239.8
scrotum (skin)	187.7	198.82	233.6	222.4	236.6	239.5
sebaceous gland—*see* Neoplasm, skin						
sella turcica	194.3	198.89	234.8	227.3	237.0	239.7
bone	170.0	198.5	—	213.0	238.0	239.2
semilunar cartilage (knee)	170.7	198.5	—	213.7	238.0	239.2
seminal vesicle	187.8	198.82	233.6	222.8	236.6	239.5
septum						
nasal	160.0	197.3	231.8	212.0	235.9	239.1
posterior margin	147.3	198.89	230.0	210.7	235.1	239.0
rectovaginal	195.3	198.89	234.8	229.8	238.8	239.8
rectovesical	195.3	198.89	234.8	229.8	238.8	239.8
urethrovaginal	184.9	198.82	233.39	221.9	236.3	239.5
vesicovaginal	184.9	198.82	233.39	221.9	236.3	239.5
shoulder NEC*	195.4	198.89	232.6	229.8	238.8	239.8
sigmoid flexure (lower) (upper)	153.3	197.5	230.3	211.3	235.2	239.0
sinus (accessory)	160.9	197.3	231.8	212.0	235.9	239.1
bone (any)	170.0	198.5	—	213.0	238.0	239.2
contiguous sites with middle ear or nasal cavities	160.8	—	—	—	—	—
ethmoidal	160.3	197.3	231.8	212.0	235.9	239.1
frontal	160.4	197.3	231.8	212.0	235.9	239.1
maxillary	160.2	197.3	231.8	212.0	235.9	239.1
nasal, paranasal NEC	160.9	197.3	231.8	212.0	235.9	239.1
pyriform	148.1	198.89	230.0	210.8	235.1	239.0
sphenoidal	160.5	197.3	231.8	212.0	235.9	239.1
skeleton, skeletal NEC	170.9	198.5	—	213.9	238.0	239.2
Skene's gland	189.4	198.1	233.9	223.89	236.99	239.5
skin NEC	173.9	198.2	232.9	216.9	238.2	239.2
abdominal wall	173.5	198.2	232.5	216.5	238.2	239.2
ala nasi	173.3	198.2	232.3	216.3	238.2	239.2
ankle	173.7	198.2	232.7	216.7	238.2	239.2
antecubital space	173.6	198.2	232.6	216.6	238.2	239.2
anus	173.5	198.2	232.5	216.5	238.2	239.2
arm	173.6	198.2	232.6	216.6	238.2	239.2
auditory canal (external)	173.2	198.2	232.2	216.2	238.2	239.2
auricle (ear)	173.2	198.2	232.2	216.2	238.2	239.2
auricular canal (external)	173.2	198.2	232.2	216.2	238.2	239.2
axilla, axillary fold	173.5	198.2	232.5	216.5	238.2	239.2
back	173.5	198.2	232.5	216.5	238.2	239.2
breast	173.5	198.2	232.5	216.5	238.2	239.2
brow	173.3	198.2	232.3	216.3	238.2	239.2
buttock	173.5	198.2	232.5	216.5	238.2	239.2
calf	173.7	198.2	232.7	216.7	238.2	239.2
canthus (eye) (inner) (outer)	173.1	198.2	232.1	216.1	238.2	239.2
cervical region	173.4	198.2	232.4	216.4	238.2	239.2
cheek (external)	173.3	198.2	232.3	216.3	238.2	239.2
chest (wall)	173.5	198.2	232.5	216.5	238.2	239.2
chin	173.3	198.2	232.3	216.3	238.2	239.2
clavicular area	173.5	198.2	232.5	216.5	238.2	239.2
clitoris	184.3	198.82	233.32	221.2	236.3	239.5
columnella	173.3	198.2	232.3	216.3	238.2	239.2

INDEX TO DISEASES — Neoplasms

	Malignant Primary	Malignant Secondary	Ca in situ	Benign	Uncertain Behavior	Unspecified
concha	173.2	198.2	232.2	216.2	238.2	239.2
contiguous sites	173.8	—	—	—	—	—
ear (external)	173.2	198.2	232.2	216.2	238.2	239.2
elbow	173.6	198.2	232.6	216.6	238.2	239.2
eyebrow	173.3	198.2	232.3	216.3	238.2	239.2
eyelid	173.1	198.2	232.1	216.1	238.2	239.2
face NEC	173.3	198.2	232.3	216.3	238.2	239.2
female genital organs (external)	184.4	198.82	233.30	221.2	236.3	239.5
clitoris	184.3	198.82	233.32	221.2	236.3	239.5
labium NEC	184.4	198.82	233.32	221.2	236.3	239.5
majus	184.1	198.82	233.32	221.2	236.3	239.5
minus	184.2	198.82	233.32	221.2	236.3	239.5
pudendum	184.4	198.82	233.32	221.2	236.3	239.5
vulva	184.4	198.82	233.32	221.2	236.3	239.5
finger	173.6	198.2	232.6	216.6	238.2	239.2
flank	173.5	198.2	232.5	216.5	238.2	239.2
foot	173.7	198.2	232.7	216.7	238.2	239.2
forearm	173.6	198.2	232.6	216.6	238.2	239.2
forehead	173.3	198.2	232.3	216.3	238.2	239.2
glabella	173.3	198.2	232.3	216.3	238.2	239.2
gluteal region	173.5	198.2	232.5	216.5	238.2	239.2
groin	173.5	198.2	232.5	216.5	238.2	239.2
hand	173.6	198.2	232.6	216.6	238.2	239.2
head NEC	173.4	198.2	232.4	216.4	238.2	239.2
heel	173.7	198.2	232.7	216.7	238.2	239.2
helix	173.2	198.2	232.2	216.2	238.2	239.2
hip	173.7	198.2	232.7	216.7	238.2	239.2
infraclavicular region	173.5	198.2	232.5	216.5	238.2	239.2
inguinal region	173.5	198.2	232.5	216.5	238.2	239.2
jaw	173.3	198.2	232.3	216.3	238.2	239.2
knee	173.7	198.2	232.7	216.7	238.2	239.2
labia						
majora	184.1	198.82	233.32	221.2	236.3	239.5
minora	184.2	198.82	233.32	221.2	236.3	239.5
leg	173.7	198.2	232.7	216.7	238.2	239.2
lid (lower) (upper)	173.1	198.2	232.1	216.1	238.2	239.2
limb NEC	173.9	198.2	232.9	216.9	238.2	239.5
lower	173.7	198.2	232.7	216.7	238.2	239.2
upper	173.6	198.2	232.6	216.6	238.2	239.2
lip (lower) (upper)	173.0	198.2	232.0	216.0	238.2	239.2
male genital organs	187.9	198.82	233.6	222.9	236.6	239.5
penis	187.4	198.82	233.5	222.1	236.6	239.5
prepuce	187.1	198.82	233.5	222.1	236.6	239.5
scrotum	187.7	198.82	233.6	222.4	236.6	239.5
mastectomy site	173.5	198.2	—	—	—	—
specified as breast tissue	174.8	198.81	—	—	—	—
meatus, acoustic (external)	173.2	198.2	232.2	216.2	238.2	239.2
melanoma —see Melanoma						
nates	173.5	198.2	232.5	216.5	238.2	239.2
neck	173.4	198.2	232.4	216.4	238.2	239.2
nose (external)	173.3	198.2	232.3	216.3	238.2	239.2
palm	173.6	198.2	232.6	216.6	238.2	239.2
palpebra	173.1	198.2	232.1	216.1	238.2	239.2
penis NEC	187.4	198.82	233.5	222.1	236.6	239.5
perianal	173.5	198.2	232.5	216.5	238.2	239.2
perineum	173.5	198.2	232.5	216.5	238.2	239.2
pinna	173.2	198.2	232.2	216.2	238.2	239.2
plantar	173.7	198.2	232.7	216.7	238.2	239.2
popliteal fossa or space	173.7	198.2	232.7	216.7	238.2	239.2
prepuce	187.1	198.82	233.5	222.1	236.6	239.5
pubes	173.5	198.2	232.5	216.5	238.2	239.2
sacrococcygeal region	173.5	198.2	232.5	216.5	238.2	239.2

Neoplasms

INDEX TO DISEASES

	Malignant Primary	Malignant Secondary	Ca in situ	Benign	Uncertain Behavior	Unspecified
scalp	173.4	198.2	232.4	216.4	238.2	239.2
scapular region	173.5	198.2	232.5	216.5	238.2	239.2
scrotum	187.7	198.82	233.6	222.4	236.6	239.5
shoulder	173.6	198.2	232.6	216.6	238.2	239.2
sole (foot)	173.7	198.2	232.7	216.7	238.2	239.2
specified sites NEC	173.8	198.2	232.8	216.8	232.8	239.2
submammary fold	173.5	198.2	232.5	216.5	238.2	239.2
supraclavicular region	173.4	198.2	232.4	216.4	238.2	239.2
temple	173.3	198.2	232.3	216.3	238.2	239.2
thigh	173.7	198.2	232.7	216.7	238.2	239.2
thoracic wall	173.5	198.2	232.5	216.5	238.2	239.2
thumb	173.6	198.2	232.6	216.6	238.2	239.2
toe	173.7	198.2	232.7	216.7	238.2	239.2
tragus	173.2	198.2	232.2	216.2	238.2	239.2
trunk	173.5	198.2	232.5	216.5	238.2	239.2
umbilicus	173.5	198.2	232.5	216.5	238.2	239.2
vulva	184.4	198.82	233.32	221.2	236.3	239.5
wrist	173.6	198.2	232.6	216.6	238.2	239.2
skull	170.0	198.5	—	213.0	238.0	239.2
soft parts or tissues—*see* Neoplasm, connective tissue						
specified site NEC	195.8	198.89	234.8	229.8	238.8	239.8
spermatic cord	187.6	198.82	233.6	222.8	236.6	239.5
sphenoid	160.5	197.3	231.8	212.0	235.9	239.1
bone	170.0	198.5	—	213.0	238.0	239.2
sinus	160.5	197.3	231.8	212.0	235.9	239.1
sphincter						
anal	154.2	197.5	230.5	211.4	235.5	239.0
of Oddi	156.1	197.8	230.8	211.5	235.3	239.0
spine, spinal (column)	170.2	198.5	—	213.2	238.0	239.2
bulb	191.7	198.3	—	225.0	237.5	239.6
coccyx	170.6	198.5	—	213.6	238.0	239.2
cord (cervical) (lumbar) (sacral) (thoracic)	192.2	198.3	—	225.3	237.5	239.7
dura mater	192.3	198.4	—	225.4	237.6	239.7
lumbosacral	170.2	198.5	—	213.2	238.0	239.2
membrane	192.3	198.4	—	225.4	237.6	239.7
meninges	192.3	198.4	—	225.4	237.6	239.7
nerve (root)	171.9	198.89	—	215.9	238.1	239.2
pia mater	192.3	198.4	—	225.4	237.6	239.7
root	171.9	198.89	—	215.9	238.1	239.2
sacrum	170.6	198.5	—	213.6	238.0	239.2
spleen, splenic NEC	159.1	197.8	230.9	211.9	235.5	239.0
flexure (colon)	153.7	197.5	230.3	211.3	235.2	239.0
stem, brain	191.7	198.3	—	225.0	237.5	239.6
Stensen's duct	142.0	198.89	230.0	210.2	235.0	239.0
sternum	170.3	198.5	—	213.3	238.0	239.2
stomach	151.9	197.8	230.2	211.1	235.2	239.0
antrum (pyloric)	151.2	197.8	230.2	211.1	235.2	239.0
body	151.4	197.8	230.2	211.1	235.2	239.0
cardia	151.0	197.8	230.2	211.1	235.2	239.0
cardiac orifice	151.0	197.8	230.2	211.1	235.2	239.0
contiguous sites	151.8	—		—		—
corpus	151.4	197.8	230.2	211.1	235.2	239.0
fundus	151.3	197.8	230.2	211.1	235.2	239.0
greater curvature NEC	151.6	197.8	230.2	211.1	235.2	239.0
lesser curvature NEC	151.5	197.8	230.2	211.1	235.2	239.0
prepylorus	151.1	197.8	230.2	211.1	235.2	239.0
pylorus	151.1	197.8	230.2	211.1	235.2	239.0
wall NEC	151.9	197.8	230.2	211.1	235.2	239.0
anterior NEC	151.8	197.8	230.2	211.1	235.2	239.0
posterior NEC	151.8	197.8	230.2	211.1	235.2	239.0
stroma, endometrial	182.0	198.82	233.2	219.1	236.0	239.5

INDEX TO DISEASES — Neoplasms

	Malignant Primary	Malignant Secondary	Ca in situ	Benign	Uncertain Behavior	Unspecified
stump, cervical	180.8	198.82	233.1	219.0	236.0	239.5
subcutaneous (nodule) (tissue) NEC—*see* Neoplasm, connective tissue						
subdural	192.1	198.4	—	225.2	237.6	239.7
subglottis, subglottic	161.2	197.3	231.0	212.1	235.6	239.1
sublingual	144.9	198.89	230.0	210.3	235.1	239.0
gland or duct	142.2	198.89	230.0	210.2	235.0	239.0
submandibular gland	142.1	198.89	230.0	210.2	235.0	239.0
submaxillary gland or duct	142.1	198.89	230.0	210.2	235.0	239.0
submental	195.0	198.89	234.8	229.8	238.8	239.8
subpleural	162.9	197.0	—	212.3	235.7	239.1
substernal	164.2	197.1	—	212.5	235.8	239.8
sudoriferous, sudoriparous gland, site unspecified	173.9	198.2	232.9	216.9	238.2	239.2
specified site—*see* Neoplasm, skin						
supraclavicular region	195.0	198.89	234.8	229.8	238.8	239.8
supraglottis	161.1	197.3	231.0	212.1	235.6	239.1
suprarenal (capsule) (cortex) (gland) (medulla)	194.0	198.7	234.8	227.0	237.2	239.7
suprasellar (region)	191.9	198.3	—	225.0	237.5	239.6
sweat gland (apocrine) (eccrine), site unspecified	173.9	198.2	232.9	216.9	238.2	239.2
specified site—*see* Neoplasm, skin						
sympathetic nerve or nervous system NEC	171.9	198.89	—	215.9	238.1	239.2
symphysis pubis	170.6	198.5	—	213.6	238.0	239.2
synovial membrane—*see* Neoplasm, connective tissue						
tapetum, brain	191.8	198.3	—	225.0	237.5	239.6
tarsus (any bone)	170.8	198.5	—	213.8	238.0	239.2
temple (skin)	173.3	198.2	232.3	216.3	238.2	239.2
temporal						
bone	170.0	198.5	—	213.0	238.0	239.2
lobe or pole	191.2	198.3	—	225.0	237.5	239.6
region	195.0	198.89	234.8	229.8	238.8	239.8
skin	173.3	198.2	232.3	216.3	238.2	239.2
tendon (sheath)—*see* Neoplasm, connective tissue						
tentorium (cerebelli)	192.1	198.4	—	225.2	237.6	239.7
testis, testes (descended) (scrotal)	186.9	198.82	233.6	222.0	236.4	239.5
ectopic	186.0	198.82	233.6	222.0	236.4	239.5
retained	186.0	198.82	233.6	222.0	236.4	239.5
undescended	186.0	198.82	233.6	222.0	236.4	239.5
thalamus	191.0	198.3	—	225.0	237.5	239.6
thigh NEC*	195.5	198.89	234.8	229.8	238.8	239.8
thorax, thoracic (cavity) (organs NEC)	195.1	198.89	234.8	229.8	238.8	239.8
duct	171.4	198.89	—	215.4	238.1	239.2
wall NEC	195.1	198.89	234.8	229.8	238.8	239.8
throat	149.0	198.89	230.0	210.9	235.1	239.0
thumb NEC*	195.4	198.89	232.6	229.8	238.8	239.8
thymus (gland)	164.0	198.89	—	212.6	235.8	239.8
contiguous sites with heart and mediastinum	164.8	—	—	—	—	—
thyroglossal duct	193	198.89	234.8	226	237.4	239.7
thyroid (gland)	193	198.89	234.8	226	237.4	239.7
cartilage	161.3	197.3	231.0	212.1	235.6	239.1
tibia (any part)	170.7	198.5	—	213.7	238.0	239.2
toe NEC*	195.5	198.89	232.7	229.8	238.8	239.8
tongue	141.9	198.89	230.0	210.1	235.1	239.0
anterior (two-thirds) NEC	141.4	198.89	230.0	210.1	235.1	239.0

Neoplasms

INDEX TO DISEASES

	Malignant — Primary	Malignant — Secondary	Ca in situ	Benign	Uncertain Behavior	Unspecified
dorsal surface	141.1	198.89	230.0	210.1	235.1	239.0
ventral surface	141.3	198.89	230.0	210.1	235.1	239.0
base (dorsal surface)	141.0	198.89	230.0	210.1	235.1	239.0
border (lateral)	141.2	198.89	230.0	210.1	235.1	239.0
contiguous sites	141.8	—	—	—	—	—
dorsal surface NEC	141.1	198.89	230.0	210.1	235.1	239.0
fixed part NEC	141.0	198.89	230.0	210.1	235.1	239.0
foramen cecum	141.1	198.89	230.0	210.1	235.1	239.0
frenulum linguae	141.3	198.89	230.0	210.1	235.1	239.0
junctional zone	141.5	198.89	230.0	210.1	235.1	239.0
margin (lateral)	141.2	198.89	230.0	210.1	235.1	239.0
midline NEC	141.1	198.89	230.0	210.1	235.1	239.0
mobile part NEC	141.4	198.89	230.0	210.1	235.1	239.0
posterior (third)	141.0	198.89	230.0	210.1	235.1	239.0
root	141.0	198.89	230.0	210.1	235.1	239.0
surface (dorsal)	141.1	198.89	230.0	210.1	235.1	239.0
base	141.0	198.89	230.0	210.1	235.1	239.0
ventral	141.3	198.89	230.0	210.1	235.1	239.0
tip	141.2	198.89	230.0	210.1	235.1	239.0
tonsil	141.6	198.89	230.0	210.1	235.1	239.0
tonsil	146.0	198.89	230.0	210.5	235.1	239.0
fauces, faucial	146.0	198.89	230.0	210.5	235.1	239.0
lingual	141.6	198.89	230.0	210.1	235.1	239.0
palatine	146.0	198.89	230.0	210.5	235.1	239.0
pharyngeal	147.1	198.89	230.0	210.7	235.1	239.0
pillar (anterior) (posterior)	146.2	198.89	230.0	210.6	235.1	239.0
tonsillar fossa	146.1	198.89	230.0	210.6	235.1	239.0
tooth socket NEC	143.9	198.89	230.0	210.4	235.1	239.0
trachea (cartilage) (mucosa)	162.0	197.3	231.1	212.2	235.7	239.1
contiguous sites with bronchus or lung	162.8	—	—	—	—	—
tracheobronchial	162.8	197.3	231.1	212.2	235.7	239.1
contiguous sites with lung	162.8	—	—	—	—	—
tragus	173.2	198.2	232.2	216.2	238.2	239.2
trunk NEC*	195.8	198.89	232.5	229.8	238.8	239.8
tubo-ovarian	183.8	198.82	233.39	221.8	236.3	239.5
tunica vaginalis	187.8	198.82	233.6	222.8	236.6	239.5
turbinate (bone)	170.0	198.5	—	213.0	238.0	239.2
nasal	160.0	197.3	231.8	212.0	235.9	239.1
tympanic cavity	160.1	197.3	231.8	212.0	235.9	239.1
ulna (any part)	170.4	198.5	—	213.4	238.0	239.2
umbilicus, umbilical	173.5	198.2	232.5	216.5	238.2	239.2
uncus, brain	191.2	198.3	—	225.0	237.5	239.6
unknown site or unspecified	199.1	199.1	234.9	229.9	238.9	239.9
urachus	188.7	198.1	233.7	223.3	236.7	239.4
ureter, ureteral	189.2	198.1	233.9	223.2	236.91	239.5
orifice (bladder)	188.6	198.1	233.7	223.3	236.7	239.4
ureter-bladder (junction)	188.6	198.1	233.7	223.3	236.7	239.4
urethra, urethral (gland)	189.3	198.1	233.9	223.81	236.99	239.5
orifice, internal	188.5	198.1	233.7	223.3	236.7	239.4
urethrovaginal (septum)	184.9	198.82	233.39	221.9	236.3	239.5
urinary organ or system NEC	189.9	198.1	233.9	223.9	236.99	239.5
bladder—see Neoplasm, bladder						
contiguous sites	189.8	—	—	—	—	—
specified sites NEC	189.8	198.1	233.9	223.89	236.99	239.5
utero-ovarian	183.8	198.82	233.39	221.8	236.3	239.5
ligament	183.3	198.82	—	221.0	236.3	239.5
uterosacral ligament	183.4	198.82	—	221.0	236.3	239.5
uterus, uteri, uterine	179	198.82	233.2	219.9	236.0	239.5
adnexa NEC	183.9	198.82	233.39	221.8	236.3	239.5
contiguous sites	183.8	—	—	—	—	—
body	182.0	198.82	233.2	219.1	236.0	239.5
contiguous sites	182.8	—	—	—	—	—

INDEX TO DISEASES — Neoplasms

	Malignant Primary	Malignant Secondary	Ca in situ	Benign	Uncertain Behavior	Unspecified
cervix	180.9	198.82	233.1	219.0	236.0	239.5
cornu	182.0	198.82	233.2	219.1	236.0	239.5
corpus	182.0	198.82	233.2	219.1	236.0	239.5
endocervix (canal) (gland)	180.0	198.82	233.1	219.0	236.0	239.5
endometrium	182.0	198.82	233.2	219.1	236.0	239.5
exocervix	180.1	198.82	233.1	219.0	236.0	239.5
external os	180.1	198.82	233.1	219.0	236.0	239.5
fundus	182.0	198.82	233.2	219.1	236.0	239.5
internal os	180.0	198.82	233.1	219.0	236.0	239.5
isthmus	182.1	198.82	233.2	219.1	236.0	239.5
ligament	183.4	198.82	—	221.0	236.3	239.5
broad	183.3	198.82	233.39	221.0	236.3	239.5
round	183.5	198.82	—	221.0	236.3	239.5
lower segment	182.1	198.82	233.2	219.1	236.0	239.5
myometrium	182.0	198.82	233.2	219.1	236.0	239.5
squamocolumnar junction	180.8	198.82	233.1	219.0	236.0	239.5
tube	183.2	198.82	233.39	221.0	236.3	239.5
utricle, prostatic	189.3	198.1	233.9	223.81	236.99	239.5
uveal tract	190.0	198.4	234.0	224.0	238.8	239.8
uvula	145.4	198.89	230.0	210.4	235.1	239.0
vagina, vaginal (fornix) (vault) (wall)	184.0	198.82	233.31	221.1	236.3	239.5
vaginovesical	184.9	198.82	233.39	221.9	236.3	239.5
septum	194.9	198.82	233.39	221.9	236.3	239.5
vallecula (epiglottis)	146.3	198.89	230.0	210.6	235.1	239.0
vascular—see Neoplasm, connective tissue						
vas deferens	187.6	198.82	233.6	222.8	236.6	239.5
Vater's ampulla	156.2	197.8	230.8	211.5	235.3	239.0
vein, venous—see Neoplasm, connective tissue						
vena cava (abdominal) (inferior)	171.5	198.89	—	215.5	238.1	239.2
superior	171.4	198.89	—	215.4	238.1	239.2
ventricle (cerebral) (floor) (fourth) (lateral) (third)	191.5	198.3	—	225.0	237.5	239.6
cardiac (left) (right)	164.1	198.89	—	212.7	238.8	239.8
ventricular band of larynx	161.1	197.3	231.0	212.1	235.6	239.1
ventriculus—see Neoplasm, stomach						
vermillion border—see Neoplasm, lip						
vermis, cerebellum	191.6	198.3	—	225.0	237.5	239.6
vertebra (column)	170.2	198.5	—	213.2	238.0	239.2
coccyx	170.6	198.5	—	213.6	238.0	239.2
sacrum	170.6	198.5	—	213.6	238.0	239.2
vesical—see Neoplasm, bladder						
vesicle, seminal	187.8	198.82	233.6	222.8	236.6	239.5
vesicocervical tissue	184.9	198.82	233.39	221.9	236.3	239.5
vesicorectal	195.3	198.89	234.8	229.8	238.8	239.8
vesicovaginal	184.9	198.82	233.39	221.9	236.3	239.5
septum	184.9	198.82	233.39	221.9	236.3	239.5
vessel (blood)—see Neoplasm, connective tissue						
vestibular gland, greater	184.1	198.82	233.32	221.2	236.3	239.5
vestibule mouth	145.1	198.89	230.0	210.4	235.1	239.0
nose	160.0	197.3	231.8	212.0	235.9	239.1
Virchow's gland	—	196.0	—	229.0	238.8	239.8
viscera NEC	195.8	198.89	234.8	229.8	238.8	239.8
vocal cords (true)	161.0	197.3	231.0	212.1	235.6	239.1
false	161.1	197.3	231.0	212.1	235.6	239.1
vomer	170.0	198.5	—	213.0	238.0	239.2

Neoplasms

INDEX TO DISEASES

| | Malignant ||| Benign | Uncertain Behavior | Unspecified |
	Primary	Secondary	Ca in situ			
vulva	184.4	198.82	233.32	221.2	236.3	239.5
vulvovaginal gland	184.4	198.82	233.32	221.2	236.3	239.5
Waldeyer's ring	149.1	198.89	230.0	210.9	235.1	239.0
Wharton's duct	142.1	198.89	230.0	210.2	235.0	239.0
white matter (central) (cerebral)	191.0	198.3	—	225.0	237.5	239.6
windpipe	162.0	197.3	231.1	212.2	235.7	239.1
Wirsung's duct	157.3	197.8	230.9	211.6	235.5	239.0
wolffian (body) (duct)						
female	184.8	198.82	233.39	221.8	236.3	239.5
male	187.8	198.82	233.6	222.8	236.6	239.5
womb—*see* Neoplasm, uterus						
wrist NEC*	195.4	198.89	232.6	229.8	238.8	239.8
xiphoid process	170.3	198.5	—	213.3	238.0	239.2
Zuckerkandl's organ	194.6	198.89	—	227.6	237.3	239.7

INDEX TO DISEASES   **Nephritis, nephritic**

Neovascularization
  choroid 362.16
  ciliary body 364.42
  cornea 370.60
    deep 370.63
    localized 370.61
  iris 364.42
  retina 362.16
  subretinal 362.16
Nephralgia 788.0
Nephritis, nephritic (albuminuric) (azotemic) (congenital) (degenerative) (diffuse) (disseminated) (epithelial) (familial) (focal) (granulomatous) (hemorrhagic) (infantile) (nonsuppurative, excretory) (uremic) 583.9
  with
    edema—see Nephrosis
    lesion of
      glomerulonephritis
        hypocomplementemic persistent 583.2
          with nephrotic syndrome 581.2
          chronic 582.2
        lobular 583.2
          with nephrotic syndrome 581.2
          chronic 582.2
        membranoproliferative 583.2
          with nephrotic syndrome 581.2
          chronic 582.2
        membranous 583.1
          with nephrotic syndrome 581.1
          chronic 582.1
        mesangiocapillary 583.2
          with nephrotic syndrome 581.2
          chronic 582.2
        mixed membranous and proliferative 583.2
          with nephrotic syndrome 581.2
          chronic 582.2
        proliferative (diffuse) 583.0
          with nephrotic syndrome 581.0
          acute 580.0
          chronic 582.0
        rapidly progressive 583.4
          acute 580.4
          chronic 582.4
      interstitial nephritis (diffuse) (focal) 583.89
        with nephrotic syndrome 581.89
        acute 580.89
        chronic 582.89
      necrotizing glomerulitis 583.4
        acute 580.4
        chronic 582.4
      renal necrosis 583.9
        cortical 583.6
        medullary 583.7
      specified pathology NEC 583.89
        with nephrotic syndrome 581.89
        acute 580.89
        chronic 582.89
  necrosis, renal 583.9
    cortical 583.6
    medullary (papillary) 583.7
  nephrotic syndrome (see also Nephrosis) 581.9
  papillary necrosis 583.7
  specified pathology NEC 583.89
  acute 580.9
    extracapillary with epithelial crescents 580.4
    hypertensive (see also Hypertension, kidney) 403.90
    necrotizing 580.4
    poststreptococcal 580.0
    proliferative (diffuse) 580.0

Nephritis, nephritic—continued
  rapidly progressive 580.4
  specified pathology NEC 580.89
  amyloid 277.39 *[583.81]*
    chronic 277.39 *[582.81]*
  arteriolar (see also Hypertension, kidney) 403.90
  arteriosclerotic (see also Hypertension, kidney) 403.90
  ascending (see also Pyelitis) 590.80
  atrophic 582.9
  basement membrane NEC 583.89
    with
      pulmonary hemorrhage (Goodpasture's syndrome) 446.21 *[583.81]*
  calculous, calculus 592.0
  cardiac (see also Hypertension, kidney) 403.90
  cardiovascular (see also Hypertension, kidney) 403.90
  chronic 582.9
    arteriosclerotic (see also Hypertension, kidney) 403.90
    hypertensive (see also Hypertension, kidney) 403.90
  cirrhotic (see also Sclerosis, renal) 587
  complicating pregnancy, childbirth, or puerperium 646.2
    with hypertension 642.1
      affecting fetus or newborn 760.0
    affecting fetus or newborn 760.1
  croupous 580.9
  desquamative—see Nephrosis
  due to
    amyloidosis 277.39 *[583.81]*
      chronic 277.39 *[582.81]*
    arteriosclerosis (see also Hypertension, kidney) 403.90
    diabetes mellitus 250.4 *[583.81]*
      with nephrotic syndrome 250.4 *[581.81]*
    diphtheria 032.89 *[580.81]*
    gonococcal infection (acute) 098.19 *[583.81]*
      chronic or duration of 2 months or over 098.39 *[583.81]*
    gout 274.10
    infectious hepatitis 070.9 *[580.81]*
    mumps 072.79 *[580.81]*
    specified kidney pathology NEC 583.89
      acute 580.89
      chronic 582.89
    streptotrichosis 039.8 *[583.81]*
    subacute bacterial endocarditis 421.0 *[580.81]*
    systemic lupus erythematosus 710.0 *[583.81]*
      chronic 710.0 *[582.81]*
    typhoid fever 002.0 *[580.81]*
  endothelial 582.2
  end stage (chronic) (terminal) NEC 585.6
  epimembranous 581.1
  exudative 583.89
    with nephrotic syndrome 581.89
    acute 580.89
    chronic 582.89
  gonococcal (acute) 098.19 *[583.81]*
    chronic or duration of 2 months or over 098.39 *[583.81]*
  gouty 274.10
  hereditary (Alport's syndrome) 759.89
  hydremic—see Nephrosis
  hypertensive (see also Hypertension, kidney) 403.90
  hypocomplementemic persistent 583.2
    with nephrotic syndrome 581.2

1215

Nephritis, nephritic—*continued*
  chronic 582.2
  immune complex NEC 583.89
  infective (*see also* Pyelitis) 590.80
  interstitial (diffuse) (focal) 583.89
    with nephrotic syndrome 581.89
    acute 580.89
    chronic 582.89
  latent or quiescent—*see* Nephritis, chronic
  lead 984.9
    specified type of lead—*see* Table of drugs and chemicals
  lobular 583.2
    with nephrotic syndrome 581.2
    chronic 582.2
  lupus 710.0 *[583.81]*
    acute 710.0 *[580.81]*
    chronic 710.0 *[582.81]*
  membranoproliferative 583.2
    with nephrotic syndrome 581.2
    chronic 582.2
  membranous 583.1
    with nephrotic syndrome 581.1
    chronic 582.1
  mesangiocapillary 583.2
    with nephrotic syndrome 581.2
    chronic 582.2
  minimal change 581.3
  mixed membranous and proliferative 583.2
    with nephrotic syndrome 581.2
    chronic 582.2
  necrotic, necrotizing 583.4
    acute 580.4
    chronic 582.4
  nephrotic—*see* Nephrosis
  old—*see* Nephritis, chronic
  parenchymatous 581.89
  polycystic 753.12
    adult type (APKD) 753.13
    autosomal dominant 753.13
    autosomal recessive 753.14
    childhood type (CPKD) 753.14
    infantile type 753.14
  poststreptococcal 580.0
  pregnancy—*see* Nephritis, complicating pregnancy
  proliferative 583.0
    with nephrotic syndrome 581.0
    acute 580.0
    chronic 582.0
  purulent (*see also* Pyelitis) 590.80
  rapidly progressive 583.4
    acute 580.4
    chronic 582.4
  salt-losing or salt-wasting (*see also* Disease, renal) 593.9
  saturnine 984.9
    specified type of lead—*see* Table of drugs and chemicals
  septic (*see also* Pyelitis) 590.80
  specified pathology NEC 583.89
    acute 580.89
    chronic 582.89
  staphylococcal (*see also* Pyelitis) 590.80
  streptotrichosis 039.8 *[583.81]*
  subacute (*see also* Nephrosis) 581.9
  suppurative (*see also* Pyelitis) 590.80
  syphilitic (late) 095.4
    congenital 090.5 *[583.81]*
    early 091.69 *[583.81]*
  terminal (chronic) (end-stage) NEC 585.6

Nephritis, nephritic—*continued*
  toxic—*see* Nephritis, acute
  tubal, tubular—*see* Nephrosis, tubular
  tuberculous (*see also* Tuberculosis) 016.0 *[583.81]*
  type II (Ellis)—*see* Nephrosis
  vascular—*see* Hypertension, kidney
  war 580.9
Nephroblastoma (M8960/3) 189.0
  epithelial (M8961/3) 189.0
  mesenchymal (M8962/3) 189.0
Nephrocalcinosis 275.49
Nephrocystitis, pustular (*see also* Pyelitis) 590.80
Nephrolithiasis (congenital) (pelvis) (recurrent) 592.0
  uric acid 274.11
Nephroma (M8960/3) 189.0
  mesoblastic (M8960/1) 236.9
Nephronephritis (*see also* Nephrosis) 581.9
Nephronopthisis 753.16
Nephropathy (*see also* Nephritis) 583.9
  with
    exudative nephritis 583.89
    interstitial nephritis (diffuse) (focal) 583.89
    medullary necrosis 583.7
    necrosis 583.9
      cortical 583.6
      medullary or papillary 583.7
    papillary necrosis 583.7
    specified lesion or cause NEC 583.89
  analgesic 583.89
    with medullary necrosis, acute 584.7
  arteriolar (*see also* Hypertension, kidney) 403.90
  arteriosclerotic (*see also* Hypertension, kidney) 403.90
  complicating pregnancy 646.2
  diabetic 250.4 *[583.81]*
  gouty 274.10
    specified type NEC 274.19
  hereditary amyloid 277.31
  hypercalcemic 588.89
  hypertensive (*see also* Hypertension, kidney) 403.90
  hypokalemic (vacuolar) 588.89
  IgA 583.9
  obstructive 593.89
    congenital 753.20
  phenacetin 584.7
  phosphate-losing 588.0
  potassium depletion 588.89
  proliferative (*see also* Nephritis, proliferative) 583.0
  protein-losing 588.89
  salt-losing or salt-wasting (*see also* Disease, renal) 593.9
  sickle-cell (*see also* Disease, sickle-cell) 282.60 *[583.81]*
  toxic 584.5
  vasomotor 584.5
  water-losing 588.89
Nephroptosis (*see also* Disease, renal) 593.0
  congenital (displaced) 753.3
Nephropyosis (*see also* Abscess, kidney) 590.2
Nephrorrhagia 593.81
Nephrosclerosis (arteriolar) (arteriosclerotic) (chronic) (hyaline) (*see also* Hypertension, kidney) 403.90
  gouty 274.10
  hyperplastic (arteriolar) (*see also* Hypertension, kidney) 403.90
  senile (*see also* Sclerosis, renal) 587

INDEX TO DISEASES

Neuralgia, neuralgic

Nephrosis, nephrotic (Epstein's) (syndrome) 581.9
  with
    lesion of
      focal glomerulosclerosis 581.1
      glomerulonephritis
        endothelial 581.2
        hypocomplementemic persistent 581.2
        lobular 581.2
        membranoproliferative 581.2
        membranous 581.1
        mesangiocapillary 581.2
        minimal change 581.3
        mixed membranous and proliferative 581.2
        proliferative 581.0
      segmental hyalinosis 581.1
      specified pathology NEC 581.89
  acute—*see* Nephrosis, tubular
  anoxic—*see* Nephrosis, tubular
  arteriosclerotic (*see also* Hypertension, kidney) 403.90
  chemical—*see* Nephrosis, tubular
  cholemic 572.4
  complicating pregnancy, childbirth, or puerperium—*see* Nephritis, complicating pregnancy
  diabetic 250.4 *[581.81]*
  Finnish type (congenital) 759.89
  hemoglobinuric—*see* Nephrosis, tubular
  in
    amyloidosis 277.39 *[581.81]*
    diabetes mellitus 250.4 *[581.81]*
    epidemic hemorrhagic fever 078.6
    malaria 084.9 *[581.81]*
    polyarteritis 446.0 *[581.81]*
    systemic lupus erythematosus 710.0 *[581.81]*
  ischemic—*see* Nephrosis, tubular
  lipoid 581.3
  lower nephron—*see* Nephrosis, tubular
  lupoid 710.0 *[581.81]*
  lupus 710.0 *[581.81]*
  malarial 084.9 *[581.81]*
  minimal change 581.3
  necrotizing—*see* Nephrosis, tubular
  osmotic (sucrose) 588.89
  polyarteritic 446.0 *[581.81]*
  radiation 581.9
  specified lesion or cause NEC 581.89
  syphilitic 095.4
  toxic—*see* Nephrosis, tubular
  tubular (acute) 584.5
    due to a procedure 997.5
    radiation 581.9
Nephrosonephritis hemorrhagic (endemic) 078.6
Nephrostomy status V44.6
  with complication 997.5
Nerve —*see* condition
Nerves 799.2
Nervous (*see also* condition) 799.2
  breakdown 300.9
  heart 306.2
  stomach 306.4
  tension 799.2
Nervousness 799.2
Nesidioblastoma (M8150/0)
  pancreas 211.7
  specified site NEC—*see* Neoplasm, by site, benign
  unspecified site 211.7
Netherton's syndrome (ichthyosiform erythroderma) 757.1

Nettle rash 708.8
Nettleship's disease (urticaria pigmentosa) 757.33
Neumann's disease (pemphigus vegetans) 694.4
Neuralgia, neuralgic (acute) (*see also* Neuritis) 729.2
  accessory (nerve) 352.4
  acoustic (nerve) 388.5
  ankle 355.8
  anterior crural 355.8
  anus 787.99
  arm 723.4
  auditory (nerve) 388.5
  axilla 353.0
  bladder 788.1
  brachial 723.4
  brain—*see* Disorder, nerve, cranial
  broad ligament 625.9
  cerebral—*see* Disorder, nerve, cranial
  ciliary 346.2
  cranial nerve—*see also* Disorder, nerve, cranial
    fifth or trigeminal (*see also* Neuralgia, trigeminal) 350.1
  ear 388.71
    middle 352.1
  facial 351.8
  finger 354.9
  flank 355.8
  foot 355.8
  forearm 354.9
  Fothergill's (*see also* Neuralgia, trigeminal) 350.1
    postherpetic 053.12
  glossopharyngeal (nerve) 352.1
  groin 355.8
  hand 354.9
  heel 355.8
  Horton's 346.2
  Hunt's 053.11
  hypoglossal (nerve) 352.5
  iliac region 355.8
  infraorbital (*see also* Neuralgia, trigeminal) 350.1
  inguinal 355.8
  intercostal (nerve) 353.8
    postherpetic 053.19
  jaw 352.1
  kidney 788.0
  knee 355.8
  loin 355.8
  malarial (*see also* Malaria) 084.6
  mastoid 385.89
  maxilla 352.1
  median thenar 354.1
  metatarsal 355.6
  middle ear 352.1
  migrainous 346.2
  Morton's 355.6
  nerve, cranial—*see* Disorder, nerve, cranial
  nose 352.0
  occipital 723.8
  olfactory (nerve) 352.0
  ophthalmic 377.30
    postherpetic 053.19
  optic (nerve) 377.30
  penis 607.9
  perineum 355.8
  pleura 511.0
  postherpetic NEC 053.19
    geniculate ganglion 053.11
    ophthalmic 053.19
    trifacial 053.12

Neuralgia, neuralgic—*continued*
   trigeminal 053.12
   pubic region 355.8
   radial (nerve) 723.4
   rectum 787.99
   sacroiliac joint 724.3
   sciatic (nerve) 724.3
   scrotum 608.9
   seminal vesicle 608.9
   shoulder 354.9
   Sluder's 337.0
   specified nerve NEC—*see* Disorder, nerve
   spermatic cord 608.9
   sphenopalatine (ganglion) 337.0
   subscapular (nerve) 723.4
   suprascapular (nerve) 723.4
   testis 608.89
   thenar (median) 354.1
   thigh 355.8
   tongue 352.5
   trifacial (nerve) (*see also* Neuralgia, trigeminal) 350.1
   trigeminal (nerve) 350.1
     postherpetic 053.12
   tympanic plexus 388.71
   ulnar (nerve) 723.4
   vagus (nerve) 352.3
   wrist 354.9
   writers' 300.89
     organic 333.84
Neurapraxia —*see* Injury, nerve
Neurasthenia 300.5
   cardiac 306.2
   gastric 306.4
   heart 306.2
   postfebrile 780.79
   postviral 780.79
Neurilemmoma (M9560/0)—*see also* Neoplasm, connective tissue, benign
   acoustic (nerve) 225.1
   malignant (M9560/3)—*see also* Neoplasm, connective tissue, malignant
     acoustic (nerve) 192.0
Neurilemmosarcoma (M9560/3)—*see* Neoplasm, connective tissue, malignant
Neurilemoma —*see* Neurilemmoma
Neurinoma (M9560/0)—*see* Neurilemmoma
Neurinomatosis (M9560/1)—*see also* Neoplasm, connective tissue, uncertain behavior
   centralis 759.5
Neuritis (*see also* Neuralgia) 729.2
   abducens (nerve) 378.54
   accessory (nerve) 352.4
   acoustic (nerve) 388.5
     syphilitic 094.86
   alcoholic 357.5
     with psychosis 291.1
   amyloid, any site 277.39 [357.4]
   anterior crural 355.8
   arising during pregnancy 646.4
   arm 723.4
   ascending 355.2
   auditory (nerve) 388.5
   brachial (nerve) NEC 723.4
     due to displacement, intervertebral disc 722.0
   cervical 723.4
   chest (wall) 353.8
   costal region 353.8
   cranial nerve—*see also* Disorder, nerve, cranial
     first or olfactory 352.0
     second or optic 377.30

Neuritis—*continued*
     third or oculomotor 378.52
     fourth or trochlear 378.53
     fifth or trigeminal (*see also* Neuralgia, trigeminal) 350.1
     sixth or abducens 378.54
     seventh or facial 351.8
       newborn 767.5
     eighth or acoustic 388.5
     ninth or glossopharyngeal 352.1
     tenth or vagus 352.3
     eleventh or accessory 352.4
     twelfth or hypoglossal 352.5
   Déjérine-Sottas 356.0
   diabetic 250.6 [357.2]
   diphtheritic 032.89 [357.4]
   due to
     beriberi 265.0 [357.4]
     displacement, prolapse, protrusion, or rupture of intervertebral disc 722.2
       cervical 722.0
       lumbar, lumbosacral 722.10
       thoracic, thoracolumbar 722.11
     herniation, nucleus pulposus 722.2
       cervical 722.0
       lumbar, lumbosacral 722.10
       thoracic, thoracolumbar 722.11
   endemic 265.0 [357.4]
   facial (nerve) 351.8
     newborn 767.5
   general—*see* Polyneuropathy
   geniculate ganglion 351.1
     due to herpes 053.11
   glossopharyngeal (nerve) 352.1
   gouty 274.89 [357.4]
   hypoglossal (nerve) 352.5
   ilioinguinal (nerve) 355.8
   in diseases classified elsewhere—*see* Polyneuropathy, in
   infectious (multiple) 357.0
   intercostal (nerve) 353.8
   interstitial hypertrophic progressive NEC 356.9
   leg 355.8
   lumbosacral NEC 724.4
   median (nerve) 354.1
     thenar 354.1
   multiple (acute) (infective) 356.9
     endemic 265.0 [357.4]
   multiplex endemica 265.0 [357.4]
   nerve root (*see also* Radiculitis) 729.2
   oculomotor (nerve) 378.52
   olfactory (nerve) 352.0
   optic (nerve) 377.30
     in myelitis 341.0
     meningococcal 036.81
   pelvic 355.8
   peripheral (nerve)—*see also* Neuropathy, peripheral
     complicating pregnancy or puerperium 646.4
     specified nerve NEC—*see* Mononeuritis
   pneumogastric (nerve) 352.3
   postchickenpox 052.7
   postherpetic 053.19
   progressive hypertrophic interstitial NEC 356.9
   puerperal, postpartum 646.4
   radial (nerve) 723.4
   retrobulbar 377.32
     syphilitic 094.85
   rheumatic (chronic) 729.2
   sacral region 355.8
   sciatic (nerve) 724.3

INDEX TO DISEASES

Neuritis—*continued*
  due to displacement of intervertebral disc 722.10
  serum 999.5
  specified nerve NEC—*see* Disorder, nerve
  spinal (nerve) 355.9
    root (*see also* Radiculitis) 729.2
  subscapular (nerve) 723.4
  suprascapular (nerve) 723.4
  syphilitic 095.8
  thenar (median) 354.1
  thoracic NEC 724.4
  toxic NEC 357.7
  trochlear (nerve) 378.53
  ulnar (nerve) 723.4
  vagus (nerve) 352.3
Neuroangiomatosis, encephalofacial 759.6
Neuroastrocytoma (M9505/1)—*see* Neoplasm, by site, uncertain behavior
Neuro-avitaminosis 269.2
Neuroblastoma (M9500/3)
  olfactory (M9522/3) 160.0
  specified site—*see* Neoplasm, by site, malignant
  unspecified site 194.0
Neurochorioretinitis (*see also* Chorioretinitis) 363.20
Neurocirculatory asthenia 306.2
Neurocytoma (M9506/0)—*see* Neoplasm, by site, benign
Neurodermatitis (circumscribed) (circumscripta) (local) 698.3
  atopic 691.8
  diffuse (Brocq) 691.8
  disseminated 691.8
  nodulosa 698.3
Neuroencephalomyelopathy, optic 341.0
Neuroepithelioma (M9503/3)—*see also* Neoplasm, by site, malignant
  olfactory (M9521/3) 160.0
Neurofibroma (M9540/0)—*see also* Neoplasm, connective tissue, benign
  melanotic (M9541/0)—*see* Neoplasm, connective tissue, benign
  multiple (M9540/1) 237.70
    Type 1 237.71
    Type 2 237.72
  plexiform (M9550/0)—*see* Neoplasm, connective tissue, benign
Neurofibromatosis (multiple) (M9540/1) 237.70
  acoustic 237.72
  malignant (M9540/3)—*see* Neoplasm, connective tissue, malignant
  Type 1 237.71
  Type 2 237.72
  von Recklinghausen's 237.71
Neurofibrosarcoma (M9540/3)—*see* Neoplasm, connective tissue, malignant
Neurogenic —*see also* condition
  bladder (atonic) (automatic) (autonomic) (flaccid) (hypertonic) (hypotonic) (inertia) (infranuclear) (irritable) (motor) (nonreflex) (nuclear) (paralysis) (reflex) (sensory) (spastic) (supranuclear) (uninhibited) 596.54
    with cauda equina syndrome 344.61
  bowel 564.81
  heart 306.2
Neuroglioma (M9505/1)—*see* Neoplasm, by site, uncertain behavior
Neurolabyrinthitis (of Dix and Hallpike) 386.12
Neurolathyrism 988.2
Neuroleprosy 030.1
Neuroleptic malignant syndrome 333.92

Neuropathy, neuropathic

Neurolipomatosis 272.8
Neuroma (M9570/0)—*see also* Neoplasm, connective tissue, benign
  acoustic (nerve) (M9560/0) 225.1
  amputation (traumatic)—*see also* Injury, nerve, by site
    surgical complication (late) 997.61
  appendix 211.3
  auditory nerve 225.1
  digital 355.6
    toe 355.6
  interdigital (toe) 355.6
  intermetatarsal 355.6
  Morton's 355.6
  multiple 237.70
    Type 1 237.71
    Type 2 237.72
  nonneoplastic 355.9
    arm NEC 354.9
    leg NEC 355.8
    lower extremity NEC 355.8
    specified site NEC—*see* Mononeuritis, by site
    upper extremity NEC 354.9
  optic (nerve) 225.1
  plantar 355.6
  plexiform (M9550/0)—*see* Neoplasm, connective tissue, benign
  surgical (nonneoplastic) 355.9
    arm NEC 354.9
    leg NEC 355.8
    lower extremity NEC 355.8
    upper extremity NEC 354.9
  traumatic—*see also* Injury, nerve, by site
    old—*see* Neuroma, nonneoplastic
Neuromyalgia 729.1
Neuromyasthenia (epidemic) 049.8
Neuromyelitis 341.8
  ascending 357.0
  optica 341.0
Neuromyopathy NEC 358.9
Neuromyositis 729.1
Neuronevus (M8725/0)—*see* Neoplasm, skin, benign
Neuronitis 357.0
  ascending (acute) 355.2
  vestibular 386.12
Neuroparalytic —*see* condition
Neuropathy, axtaxia and retinitis pigmentosa (NARP syndrome) 277.87
Neuropathy, neuropathic (*see also* Disorder, nerve) 355.9
  acute motor 357.82
  alcoholic 357.5
    with psychosis 291.1
  arm NEC 354.9
  ataxia and retinitis pigmentosa (NARP syndrome) 277.87
  autonomic (peripheral)—*see* Neuropathy, peripheral, autonomic
  axillary nerve 353.0
  brachial plexus 353.0
  cervical plexus 353.2
  chronic
    progressive segmentally demyelinating 357.89
    relapsing demyelinating 357.89
  congenital sensory 356.2
  Déjérine-Sottas 356.0
  diabetic 250.6 *[357.2]*
  entrapment 355.9
    iliohypogastric nerve 355.79

Neuropathy, neuropathic—*continued*
    ilioinguinal nerve 355.79
    lateral cutaneous nerve of thigh 355.1
    median nerve 354.0
    obturator nerve 355.79
    peroneal nerve 355.3
    posterior tibial nerve 355.5
    saphenous nerve 355.79
    ulnar nerve 354.2
  facial nerve 351.9
  hereditary 356.9
    peripheral 356.0
    sensory (radicular) 356.2
  hypertrophic
    Charcot-Marie-Tooth 356.1
    Déjérine-Sottas 356.0
    interstitial 356.9
    Refsum 356.3
  intercostal nerve 354.8
  ischemic—*see* Disorder, nerve
  Jamaican (ginger) 357.7
  leg NEC 355.8
  lower extremity NEC 355.8
  lumbar plexus 353.1
  median nerve 354.1
  motor
    acute 357.82
  multiple (acute) (chronic) (*see also* Polyneuropathy) 356.9
  optic 377.39
    ischemic 377.41
    nutritional 377.33
    toxic 377.34
  peripheral (nerve) (*see also* Polyneuropathy) 356.9
    arm NEC 354.9
    autonomic 337.9
      amyloid 277.39 *[337.1]*
      idiopathic 337.0
      in
        amyloidosis 277.39 *[337.1]*
        diabetes (mellitus) 250.6 *[337.1]*
        diseases classified elsewhere 337.1
        gout 274.89 *[337.1]*
        hyperthyroidism 242.9 *[337.1]*
    due to
      antitetanus serum 357.6
      arsenic 357.7
      drugs 357.6
      lead 357.7
      organophosphate compounds 357.7
      toxic agent NEC 357.7
    hereditary 356.0
    idiopathic 356.9
      progressive 356.4
      specified type NEC 356.8
    in diseases classified elsewhere—*see* Polyneuropathy, in
    leg NEC 355.8
    lower extremity NEC 355.8
    upper extremity NEC 354.9
  plantar nerves 355.6
  progressive hypertrophic interstitial 356.9
  radicular NEC 729.2
    brachial 723.4
    cervical NEC 723.4
    hereditary sensory 356.2
    lumbar 724.4
    lumbosacral 724.4
    thoracic NEC 724.4
  sacral plexus 353.1

Neuropathy, neuropathic—*continued*
  sciatic 355.0
  spinal nerve NEC 355.9
    root (*see also* Radiculitis) 729.2
  toxic 357.7
  trigeminal sensory 350.8
  ulnar nerve 354.2
  upper extremity NEC 354.9
  uremic 585.9 *[357.4]*
  vitamin B$_{12}$ 266.2 *[357.4]*
    with anemia (pernicious) 281.0 *[357.4]*
      due to dietary deficiency 281.1 *[357.4]*
Neurophthisis —*see also* Disorder, nerve
  peripheral 356.9
    diabetic 250.6 *[357.2]*
Neuropraxia —*see* Injury,nerve
Neuroretinitis 363.05
  syphilitic 094.85
Neurosarcoma 9M9540/3)—sde Neoplasm, connective tissue, malignant
Neurosclerosis —*see* Disorder, nerve
Neurosis, neurotic 300.9
  accident 300.16
  anancastic, anankastic 300.3
  anxiety (state) 300.00
    generalized 300.02
    panic type 300.01
  asthenic 300.5
  bladder 306.53
  cardiac (reflex) 306.2
  cardiovascular 306.2
  climacteric, unspecified type 627.2
  colon 306.4
  compensation 300.16
  compulsive, compulsion 300.3
  conversion 300.11
  craft 300.89
  cutaneous 306.3
  depersonalization 300.6
  depressive (reaction) (type) 300.4
  endocrine 306.6
  environmental 300.89
  fatigue 300.5
  functional (*see also* Disorder, psychosomatic) 306.9
  gastric 306.4
  gastrointestinal 306.4
  genitourinary 306.50
  heart 306.2
  hypochondriacal 300.7
  hysterical 300.10
    conversion type 300.11
    dissociative type 300.15
  impulsive 300.3
  incoordination 306.0
    larynx 306.1
    vocal cord 306.1
  intestine 306.4
  larynx 306.1
    hysterical 300.11
    sensory 306.1
  menopause, unspecified type 627.2
  mixed NEC 300.89
  musculoskeletal 306.0
  obsessional 300.3
    phobia 300.3
  obsessive-compulsive 300.3
  occupational 300.89
  ocular 306.7
  oral 307.0
  organ (*see also* Disorder, psychosomatic) 306.9

INDEX TO DISEASES

Nevus

Neurosis, neurotic—*continued*
  pharynx 306.1
  phobic 300.20
  posttraumatic (acute) (situational) 309.81
    chronic 309.81
  psychasthenic (type) 300.89
  railroad 300.16
  rectum 306.4
  respiratory 306.1
  rumination 306.4
  senile 300.89
  sexual 302.70
  situational 300.89
  specified type NEC 300.89
  state 300.9
    with depersonalization episode 300.6
  stomach 306.4
  vasomotor 306.2
  visceral 306.4
  war 300.16
Neurospongioblastosis diffusa 759.5
Neurosyphilis (arrested) (early) (inactive) (late) (latent) (recurrent) 094.9
  with ataxia (cerebellar) (locomotor) (spastic) (spinal) 094.0
  acute meningitis 094.2
  aneurysm 094.89
  arachnoid (adhesive) 094.2
  arteritis (any artery) 094.89
  asymptomatic 094.3
  congenital 090.40
  dura (mater) 094.89
  general paresis 094.1
  gumma 094.9
  hemorrhagic 094.9
  juvenile (asymptomatic) (meningeal) 090.40
  leptomeninges (aseptic) 094.2
  meningeal 094.2
  meninges (adhesive) 094.2
  meningovascular (diffuse) 094.2
  optic atrophy 094.84
  parenchymatous (degenerative) 094.1
  paresis (*see also* Paresis, general) 094.1
  paretic (*see also* Paresis, general) 094.1
  relapse 094.9
  remission in (sustained) 094.9
  serological 094.3
  specified nature or site NEC 094.89
  tabes (dorsalis) 094.0
    juvenile 090.40
  tabetic 094.0
    juvenile 090.40
  taboparesis 094.1
    juvenile 090.40
  thrombosis 094.89
  vascular 094.89
Neurotic (*see also* Neurosis) 300.9
  excoriation 698.4
  psychogenic 306.3
Neurotmesis —*see* Injury, nerve, by site
Neurotoxemia —*see* Toxemia
Neutro-oclusion 524.21
Neutropenia, neutropenic (idiopathic) (pernicious) (primary) 288.00
  chronic 288.09
    hypoplastic 288.09
  congenital (nontransient) 288.01
  cyclic 288.02
  drug induced 288.03
  due to infection 288.04
  fever 288.00

Neutropenia, neutropenic—*continued*
  genetic 288.01
  immune 288.09
  infantile 288.01
  malignant 288.09
  neonatal, transitory (isoimmune) (maternal transfer) 776.7
  periodic 288.02
  splenic 289.53
  splenomegaly 289.53
  toxic 288.09
Neutrophilia, hereditary giant 288.2
Nevocarcinoma (M8720/3)—*see* Melanoma
Nevus (M8720/0)—*see also* Neoplasm, skin, benign

> Note—Except where otherwise indicated, the varieties of nevus in the list below that are followed by a morphology code number (M-__-/0) should be coded by site as for "Neoplasm, skin, benign."

  acanthotic 702.8
  achromic (M8730/0)
  amelanotic (M8730/0)
  anemic, anemicus 709.09
  angiomatous (M9120/0) (*see also* Hemangioma) 228.00
  araneus 448.1
  avasculosus 709.09
  balloon cell (M8722/0)
  bathing trunk (M8761/1) 238.2
  blue (M8780/0)
    cellular (M8790/0)
    giant (M8790/0)
    Jadassohn's (M8780/0)
    malignant (M8780/3)—*see* Melanoma
  capillary (M9131/0) (*see also* Hemangioma) 228.00
  cavernous (M9121/0) (*see also* Hemangioma) 228.00
  cellular (M8720/0)
    blue (M8790/0)
  comedonicus 757.33
  compound (M8760/0)
  conjunctiva (M8720/0) 224.3
  dermal (M8750/0)
    and epidermal (M8760/0)
  epithelioid cell (and spindle cell) (M8770/0)
  flammeus 757.32
    osteohypertrophic 759.89
  hairy (M8720/0)
  halo (M8723/0)
  hemangiomatous (M9120/0) (*see also* Hemangioma) 228.00
  intradermal (M8750/0)
  intraepidermal (M8740/0)
  involuting (M8724/0)
  Jadassohn's (blue) (M8780/0)
  junction, junctional (M8740/0)
    malignant melanoma in (M8740/3)—*see* Melanoma
  juvenile (M8770/0)
  lymphatic (M9170/0) 228.1
  magnocellular (M8726/0)
    specified site—*see* Neoplasm, by site, benign
    unspecified site 224.0
  malignant (M8720/3)—*see* Melanoma
  meaning hemangioma (M9120/0) (*see also* Hemangioma) 228.00
  melanotic (pigmented) (M8720/0)
  multiplex 759.5

Nevus—continued
  nonneoplastic 448.1
  nonpigmented (M8730/0)
  nonvascular (M8720/0)
  oral mucosa, white sponge 750.26
  osteohypertrophic, flammeus 759.89
  papillaris (M8720/0)
  papillomatosus (M8720/0)
  pigmented (M8720/0)
    giant (M8761/1)—see also Neoplasm, skin, uncertain behavior
      malignant melanoma in (M8761/3)—see Melanoma
  systematicus 757.33
  pilosus (M8720/0)
  port wine 757.32
  sanguineous 757.32
  sebaceous (senile) 702.8
  senile 448.1
  spider 448.1
  spindle cell (and epithelioid cell) (M8770/0)
  stellar 448.1
  strawberry 757.32
  syringocystadenomatous papilliferous (M8406/0)
  unius lateris 757.33
  Unna's 757.32
  vascular 757.32
  verrucous 757.33
  white sponge (oral mucosa) 750.26
Newborn (infant) (liveborn)
  affected by maternal abuse of drugs (gestational) (via placenta) (via breast milk) (see also Noxious, substances transmitted through placenta or breast milk (affecting fetus or newborn)) 760.70
  apnea 770.81
    obstructive 770.82
    specified NEC 770.82
  cardiomyopathy 425.4
    congenital 425.3
  convulsion 779.0
  electrolyte imbalance NEC (transitory) 775.5
  gestation
    24 completed weeks 765.22
    25-26 completed weeks 765.23
    27-28 completed weeks 765.24
    29-30 completed weeks 765.25
    31-32 completed weeks 765.26
    33-34 completed weeks 765.27
    35-36 completed weeks 765.28
    37 or more completed weeks 765.29
    less than 24 completed weeks 765.21
    unspecified completed weeks 765.20
  infection 771.89
    candida 771.7
    mastitis 771.5
    specified NEC 771.89
    urinary tract 771.82
  mastitis 771.5
  multiple NEC
    born in hospital (without mention of cesarean delivery or section) V37.00
      with cesarean delivery or section V37.01
    born outside hospital
      hospitalized V37.1
      not hospitalized V37.2
    mates all liveborn
      born in hospital (without mention of cesarean delivery or section) V34.00
        with cesarean delivery or section V34.01

Newborn—continued
    born outside hospital
      hospitalized V34.1
      not hospitalized V34.2
    mates all stillborn
      born in hospital (without mention of cesarean delivery or section) V35.00
        with cesarean delivery or section V35.01
      born outside hospital
        hospitalized V35.1
        not hospitalized V35.2
    mates liveborn and stillborn
      born in hospital (without mention of cesarean delivery or section) V36.00
        with cesarean delivery or section V36.01
      born outside hospital
        hospitalized V36.1
        not hospitalized V36.2
  omphalitis 771.4
  seizure 779.0
  sepsis 771.81
  single
    born in hospital (without mention of cesarean delivery or section) V30.00
      with cesarean delivery or section V30.01
    born outside hospital
      hospitalized V30.1
      not hospitalized V30.2
  specified condition NEC 779.89
  twin NEC
    born in hospital (without mention of cesarean delivery or section) V33.00
      with cesarean delivery or section V33.01
    born outside hospital
      hospitalized V33.1
      not hospitalized V33.2
    mate liveborn
      born in hospital V31.0
      born outside hospital
        hospitalized V31.1
        not hospitalized V31.2
    mate stillborn
      born in hospital V32.0
      born outside hospital
        hospitalized V32.1
        not hospitalized V32.2
  unspecified as to single or multiple birth
    born in hospital (without mention of cesarean delivery or section) V39.00
      with cesarean delivery or section V39.01
    born outside hospital
      hospitalized V39.1
      not hospitalized V39.2
Newcastle's conjunctivitis or disease 077.8
Nezelof's syndrome (pure alymphocytosis) 279.13
Niacin (amide) deficiency 265.2
Nicolas-Durand-Favre disease (climatic bubo) 099.1
Nicolas-Favre disease (climatic bubo) 099.1
Nicotinic acid (amide) deficiency 265.2
Niemann-Pick disease (lipid histiocytosis) (splenomegaly) 272.7
Night
  blindness (see also Blindness, night) 368.60
    congenital 368.61
    vitamin A deficiency 264.5
  cramps 729.82
  sweats 780.8
  terrors, child 307.46
Nightmare 307.47
  REM-sleep type 307.47
Nipple —see condition

INDEX TO DISEASES

Nonviability

Nisbet's chancre 099.0
Nishimoto (-Takeuchi) disease 437.5
Nitritoid crisis or reaction —*see* Crisis, nitritoid
Nitrogen retention, extrarenal 788.9
Nitrosohemoglobinemia 289.89
Njovera 104.0
No
 diagnosis 799.9
 disease (found) V71.9
 room at the inn V65.0
Nocardiasis —*see* Nocardiosis
Nocardiosis 039.9
 with pneumonia 039.1
 lung 039.1
 specified type NEC 039.8
Nocturia 788.43
 psychogenic 306.53
Nocturnal —*see also* condition
 dyspnea (paroxysmal) 786.09
 emissions 608.89
 enuresis 788.36
  psychogenic 307.6
 frequency (micturition) 788.43
  psychogenic 306.53
Nodal rhythm disorder 427.89
Nodding of head 781.0
Node (s)—*see also* Nodule
 Heberden's 715.04
 larynx 478.79
 lymph—*see* condition
 milkers' 051.1
 Osler's 421.0
 rheumatic 729.89
 Schmorl's 722.30
  lumbar, lumbosacral 722.32
  specified region NEC 722.39
  thoracic, thoracolumbar 722.31
 singers' 478.5
 skin NEC 782.2
 tuberculous—*see* Tuberculosis, lymph gland
 vocal cords 478.5
Nodosities, Haygarth's 715.04
Nodule(s), nodular
 actinomycotic (*see also* Actinomycosis) 039.9
 arthritic—*see* Arthritis, nodosa
 cutaneous 782.2
 Haygarth's 715.04
 inflammatory—*see* Inflammation
 juxta-articular 102.7
  syphilitic 095.7
  yaws 102.7
 larynx 478.79
 lung, solitary 518.89
  emphysematous 492.8
 milkers' 051.1
 prostate 600.10
  with
   urinary
    obstruction 600.11
    retention 600.11
 rheumatic 729.89
 rheumatoid—*see* Arthritis rheumatoid
 scrotum (inflammatory) 608.4
 singers' 478.5
 skin NEC 782.2
 solitary, lung 518.89
  emphysematous 492.8
 subcutaneous 782.2

Nodule(s), nodular—*continued*
 thyroid (gland) (nontoxic) (uninodular) 241.0
  with
   hyperthyroidism 242.1
   thyrotoxicosis 242.1
  toxic or with hyperthyroidism 242.1
 vocal cords 478.5
Noma (gangrenous) (hospital) (infective) 528.1
 auricle (*see also* Gangrene) 785.4
 mouth 528.1
 pudendi (*see also* Vulvitis) 616.10
 vulvae (*see also* Vulvitis) 616.10
Nomadism V60.0
Non-adherence
 artificial skin graft 996.55
 decellularized allodermis graft 996.55
Non-autoimmune hemolytic anemia NEC 283.10
Nonclosure —*see also* Imperfect, closure
 ductus
  arteriosus 747.0
  Botalli 747.0
 Eustachian valve 746.89
 foramen
  Botalli 745.5
  ovale 745.5
Noncompliance with medical treatment V15.81
Nondescent (congenital)—*see also* Malposition, congenital
 cecum 751.4
 colon 751.4
 testis 752.51
Nondevelopment
 brain 742.1
  specified part 742.2
 heart 746.89
 organ or site, congenital NEC—*see* Hypoplasia
Nonengagement
 head NEC 652.5
  in labor 660.1
 affecting fetus or newborn 763.1
Nonexanthematous tick fever 066.1
Nonexpansion, lung (newborn) NEC 770.4
Nonfunctioning
 cystic duct (*see also* Disease, gallbladder) 575.8
 gallbladder (*see also* Disease, gallbladder) 575.8
 kidney (*see also* Disease, renal) 593.9
 labyrinth 386.58
Nonhealing
 stump (surgical) 997.60
 wound, surgical 998.83
Nonimplantation of ovum, causing infertility 628.3
Noninsufflation, fallopian tube 628.2
Nonne-Milroy-Meige syndrome (chronic hereditary edema) 757.0
Nonovulation 628.0
Nonpatent fallopian tube 628.2
Nonpneumatization, lung NEC 770.4
Nonreflex bladder 596.54
 with cauda equina 344.61
Nonretention of food —*see also* Vomiting
Nonrotation —*see* Malrotation
Nonsecretion, urine (*see also* Anuria) 788.5
 newborn 753.3
Nonunion
 fracture 733.82
 organ or site, congenital NEC—*see* Imperfect, closure
 symphysis pubis, congenital 755.69
 top sacrum, congenital 756.19
Nonviability 765.0

1223

Nonvisualization, gallbladder 793.3
Nonvitalized tooth 522.9
Non-working side interference 524.56
Normal
  delivery—*see* category 650
  menses V65.5
  state (feared complaint unfounded) V65.5
Normoblastosis 289.89
Normocytic anemia (infectional) 285.9
  due to blood loss (chronic) 280.0
    acute 285.1
Norrie's disease (congenital) (progressive oculoacousticocerebral degeneration) 743.8
North American blastomycosis 116.0
Norwegian itch 133.0
Nose, nasal —*see* condition
Nosebleed 784.7
Nosomania 298.9
Nosophobia 300.29
Nostalgia 309.89
Notch of iris 743.46
Notched lip, congenital (*see also* Cleft, lip) 749.10
Notching nose, congenital (tip) 748.1
Nothnagel's
  syndrome 378.52
  vasomotor acroparesthesia 443.89
Novy's relapsing fever (American) 087.1
Noxious
  foodstuffs, poisoning by
    fish 988.0
    fungi 988.1
    mushrooms 988.1
    plants (food) 988.2
    shellfish 988.0
    specified type NEC 988.8
    toadstool 988.1
  substances transmitted through placenta or breast milk (affecting fetus or newborn) 760.70
    acetretin 760.78
    alcohol 760.71
    aminopterin 760.78
    antiandrogens 760.79
    anticonvulsant 760.77
    antifungal 760.74
    anti-infective agents 760.74
    antimetabolic 760.78
    atorvastatin 760.78
    carbamazepine 760.77
    cocaine 760.75
    "crack" 760.75
    diethylstilbestrol (DES) 760.76
    divalproex sodium 760.77
    endocrine disrupting chemicals 760.79
    estrogens 760.79
    etretinate 760.78
    fluconazole 760.74
    fluvastatin 760.78
    hallucinogenic agents NEC 760.73
    hormones 760.79
    lithium 760.79
    lovastatin 760.78
    medicinal agents NEC 760.79
    methotrexate 760.78
    misoprostil 760.79
    narcotics 760.72
    obstetric anesthetic or analgesic 763.5
    phenobarbital 760.77
    phenytoin 760.77
    pravastatin 760.78

Noxious—*continued*
    progestins 760.79
    retinoic acid 760.78
    simvastatin 760.78
    solvents 760.79
    specified agent NEC 760.79
    statins 760.78
    suspected, affecting management of pregnancy 655.5
    tetracycline 760.74
    thalidomide 760.79
    trimethadione 760.77
    valproate 760.77
    valproic acid 760.77
    vitamin A 760.78
Nuchal hitch (arm) 652.8
Nucleus pulposus —*see* condition
Numbness 782.0
Nuns' knee 727.2
Nursemaid's
  elbow 832.0
  shoulder 831.0
Nutmeg liver 573.8
Nutrition, deficient or insufficient (particular kind of food) 269.9
  due to
    insufficient food 994.2
    lack of
      care (child) (infant) 995.52
        adult 995.84
      food 994.2
Nyctalopia (*see also* Blindness, night) 368.60
  vitamin A deficiency 264.5
Nycturia 788.43
  psychogenic 306.53
Nymphomania 302.89
Nystagmus 379.50
  associated with vestibular system disorders 379.54
  benign paroxysmal positional 386.11
  central positional 386.2
  congenital 379.51
  deprivation 379.53
  dissociated 379.55
  latent 379.52
  miners' 300.89
  positional
    benign paroxysmal 386.11
    central 386.2
  specified NEC 379.56
  vestibular 379.54
  visual deprivation 379.53

O

Oasthouse urine disease 270.2
Obermeyer's relapsing fever (European) 087.0
Obesity (constitutional) (exogenous) (familial) (nutritional) (simple) 278.00
  adrenal 255.8
  complicating pregnancy, childbirth, or the puerperium 649.1
  due to hyperalimentation 278.00
  endocrine NEC 259.9
  endogenous 259.9
  Fröhlich's (adiposogenital dystrophy) 253.8
  glandular NEC 259.9
  hypothyroid (*see also* Hypothyroidism) 244.9
  morbid 278.01
  of pregnancy 649.1
  pituitary 253.8
  severe 278.01
  thyroid (*see also* Hypothyroidism) 244.9
Oblique —*see also* condition
  lie before labor, affecting fetus or newborn 761.7
Obliquity, pelvis 738.6
Obliteration
  abdominal aorta 446.7
  appendix (lumen) 543.9
  artery 447.1
  ascending aorta 446.7
  bile ducts 576.8
    with calculus, choledocholithiasis, or stones—*see* Choledocholithiasis
    congenital 751.61
      jaundice from 751.61 *[774.5]*
  common duct 576.8
    with calculus, choledocholithiasis, or stones—*see* Choledocholithiasis
    congenital 751.61
  cystic duct 575.8
    with calculus, choledocholithiasis, or stones—*see* Choledocholithiasis
  disease, arteriolar 447.1
  endometrium 621.8
  eye, anterior chamber 360.34
  fallopian tube 628.2
  lymphatic vessel 457.1
    postmastectomy 457.0
  organ or site, congenital NEC—*see* Atresia
  placental blood vessels—*see* Placenta, abnormal
  supra-aortic branches 446.7
  ureter 593.89
  urethra 599.84
  vein 459.9
  vestibule (oral) 525.8
Observation (for) V71.9
  without need for further medical care V71.9
  accident NEC V71.4
    at work V71.3
  criminal assault V71.6
  deleterious agent ingestion V71.89
  disease V71.9
    cardiovascular V71.7
    heart V71.7
    mental V71.09
    specified condition NEC V71.89
  foreign body ingestion V71.89
  growth and development variations V21.8
  injuries (accidental) V71.4
    inflicted NEC V71.6
      during alleged rape or seduction V71.5

Observation—*continued*
  malignant neoplasm, suspected V71.1
  postpartum
    immediately after delivery V24.0
    routine follow-up V24.2
  pregnancy
    high-risk V23.9
      specified problem NEC V23.8
    normal (without complication) V22.1
      with nonobstetric complication V22.2
      first V22.0
  rape or seduction, alleged V71.5
    injury during V71.5
  suicide attempt, alleged V71.89
  suspected (undiagnosed) (unproven)
    abuse V71.81
    cardiovascular disease V71.7
    child or wife battering victim V71.6
    concussion (cerebral) V71.6
    condition NEC V71.89
      infant—*see* Observation, suspected, condition, newborn
      newborn V29.9
        cardiovascular disease V29.8
        congenital anomaly V29.8
        genetic V29.3
        infectious V29.0
        ingestion foreign object V29.8
        injury V29.8
        metabolic V29.3
        neoplasm V29.8
        neurological V29.1
        poison, poisoning V29.8
        respiratory V29.2
        specified NEC V29.8
    exposure
      anthrax V71.82
      biological agent NEC V71.83
      SARS V71.83
    infectious disease not requiring isolation V71.89
    malignant neoplasm V71.1
    mental disorder V71.09
    neglect V71.81
    neoplasm
      benign V71.89
      malignant V71.1
    specified condition NEC V71.89
    tuberculosis V71.2
  tuberculosis, suspected V71.2
Obsession, obsessional 300.3
  ideas and mental images 300.3
  impulses 300.3
  neurosis 300.3
  phobia 300.3
  psychasthenia 300.3
  ruminations 300.3
  state 300.3
  syndrome 300.3
Obsessive-compulsive 300.3
  neurosis 300.3
  personality 301.4
  reaction 300.3
Obstetrical trauma NEC (complicating delivery) 665.9
  with
    abortion—*see* Abortion, by type, with damage to pelvic organs

Obstetrical trauma—*continued*
   ectopic pregnancy (*see also* categories 633.0-633.9) 639.2
   molar pregnancy (*see also* categories 630-632) 639.2
   affecting fetus or newborn 763.89
   following
     abortion 639.2
     ectopic or molar pregnancy 639.2
Obstipation (*see also* Constipation) 564.00
   psychogenic 306.4
Obstruction, obstructed, obstructive
   airway NEC 519.8
     with
       allergic alveolitis NEC 495.9
       asthma NEC (*see also* Asthma) 493.9
       bronchiectasis 494.0
         with acute exacerbation 494.1
       bronchitis (*see also* Bronchitis, with, obstruction) 491.20
       emphysema NEC 492.8
     chronic 496
       with
         allergic alveolitis NEC 495.5
         asthma NEC (*see also* Asthma) 493.2
         bronchiectasis 494.0
           with acute exacerbation 494.1
         bronchitis (*see also* Bronchitis, chronic, obstructive) 491.20
         emphysema NEC 492.8
     due to
       bronchospasm 519.11
       foreign body 934.9
       inhalation of fumes or vapors 506.9
       laryngospasm 478.75
   alimentary canal (*see also* Obstruction, intestine) 560.9
   ampulla of Vater 576.2
     with calculus, cholelithiasis, or stones—*see* Choledocholithiasis
   aortic (heart) (valve) (*see also* Stenosis, aortic) 424.1
     rheumatic (*see also* Stenosis, aortic, rheumatic) 395.0
   aortoiliac 444.0
   aqueduct of Sylvius 331.4
     congenital 742.3
       with spina bifida (*see also* Spina bifida) 741.0
   Arnold-Chiari (*see also* Spina bifida) 741.0
   artery (*see also* Embolism, artery) 444.9
     basilar (complete) (partial) (*see also* Occlusion, artery, basilar) 433.0
     carotid (complete) (partial) (*see also* Occlusion, artery, carotid) 433.1
     precerebral—*see* Occlusion, artery, precerebral NEC
     retinal (central) (*see also* Occlusion, retina) 362.30
     vertebral (complete) (partial) (*see also* Occlusion, artery, vertebral) 433.2
   asthma (chronic) (with obstructive pulmonary disease) 493.2
   band (intestinal) 560.81
   bile duct or passage (*see also* Obstruction, biliary) 576.2
     congenital 751.61
       jaundice from 751.61 *[774.5]*
   biliary (duct) (tract) 576.2
     with calculus 574.51
       with cholecystitis (chronic) 574.41
         acute 574.31
     congenital 751.61

Obstruction, obstructed—*continued*
     jaundice from 751.61 *[774.5]*
   gallbladder 575.2
     with calculus 574.21
       with cholecystitis (chronic) 574.11
         acute 574.01
   bladder neck (acquired) 596.0
     congenital 753.6
   bowel (*see also* Obstruction, intestine) 560.9
   bronchus 519.19
   canal, ear (*see also* Stricture, ear canal, acquired) 380.50
   cardia 537.89
   caval veins (inferior) (superior) 459.2
   cecum (*see also* Obstruction, intestine) 560.9
   circulatory 459.9
   colon (*see also* Obstruction, intestine) 560.9
     sympathicotonic 560.89
   common duct (*see also* Obstruction, biliary) 576.2
     congenital 751.61
   coronary (*see also* Arteriosclerosis, coronary)
     acute (*see also* Infarct, myocardium) 410.9
     without myocardial infarction 411.81
   cystic duct (*see also* Obstruction, gallbladder) 575.2
     congenital 751.61
   device, implant, or graft—*see* Complications, due to (presence of) any device, implant, or graft classified to 996.0-996.5 NEC
   due to foreign body accidentally left in operation wound 998.4
   duodenum 537.3
     congenital 751.1
     due to
       compression NEC 537.3
       cyst 537.3
       intrinsic lesion or disease NEC 537.3
       scarring 537.3
       torsion 537.3
       ulcer 532.91
       volvulus 537.3
   ejaculatory duct 608.89
   endocardium 424.90
     arteriosclerotic 424.99
     specified cause, except rheumatic 424.99
   esophagus 530.3
   Eustachian tube (complete) (partial) 381.60
     cartilaginous
       extrinsic 381.63
       intrinsic 381.62
     due to
       cholesteatoma 381.61
       osseous lesion NEC 381.61
       polyp 381.61
     osseous 381.61
   fallopian tube (bilateral) 628.2
   fecal 560.39
     with hernia—*see also* Hernia, by site, with obstruction
       gangrenous—*see* Hernia, by site, with gangrene
   foramen of Monro (congenital) 742.3
     with spina bifida (*see also* Spina bifida) 741.0
   foreign body—*see* Foreign body
   gallbladder 575.2
     with calculus, cholelithiasis, or stones 574.21
       with cholecystitis (chronic) 574.11
         acute 574.01
     congenital 751.69
       jaundice from 751.69 *[774.5]*

INDEX TO DISEASES

Obstruction, obstructed

Obstruction, obstructed—*continued*
  gastric outlet 537.0
  gastrointestinal (*see also* Obstruction, intestine) 560.9
  glottis 478.79
  hepatic 573.8
    duct (*see also* Obstruction, biliary) 576.2
      congenital 751.61
    icterus (*see also* Obstruction, biliary) 576.8
      congenital 751.61
  ileocecal coil (*see also* Obstruction, intestine) 560.9
  ileum (*see also* Obstruction, intestine) 560.9
  iliofemoral (artery) 444.81
  internal anastomosis—*see* Complications, mechanical, graft
  intestine (mechanical) (neurogenic) (paroxysmal) (postinfectional) (reflex) 560.9
    with
      adhesions (intestinal) (peritoneal) 560.81
      hernia—*see also* Hernia, by site, with obstruction
        gangrenous—*see* Hernia, by site, with gangrene
    adynamic (*see also* Ileus) 560.1
    by gallstone 560.31
    congenital or infantile (small) 751.1
      large 751.2
    due to
      Ascaris lumbricoides 127.0
      mural thickening 560.89
      procedure 997.4
        involving urinary tract 997.5
    impaction 560.39
    infantile—*see* Obstruction, intestine, congenital
    newborn
      due to
        fecaliths 777.1
        inspissated milk 777.2
        meconium (plug) 777.1
          in mucoviscidosis 277.01
        transitory 777.4
    specified cause NEC 560.89
    transitory, newborn 777.4
    volvulus 560.2
  intracardiac ball valve prosthesis 996.02
  jaundice (*see also* Obstruction, biliary) 576.8
    congenital 751.61
  jejunum (*see also* Obstruction, intestine) 560.9
  kidney 593.89
  labor 660.9
    affecting fetus or newborn 763.1
    by
      bony pelvis (conditions classifiable to 653.0-653.9) 660.1
      deep transverse arrest 660.3
      impacted shoulder 660.4
      locked twins 660.5
      malposition (fetus) (conditions classifiable to 652.0-652.9) 660.0
        head during labor 660.3
      persistent occipitoposterior position 660.3
      soft tissue, pelvic (conditions classifiable to 654.0-654.9) 660.2
  lacrimal
    canaliculi 375.53
    congenital 743.65
    punctum 375.52
    sac 375.54
  lacrimonasal duct 375.56

Obstruction, obstructed—*continued*
    congenital 743.65
    neonatal 375.55
  lacteal, with steatorrhea 579.2
  laryngitis (*see also* Laryngitis) 464.01
  larynx 478.79
    congenital 748.3
  liver 573.8
    cirrhotic (*see also* Cirrhosis, liver) 571.5
  lung 518.89
    with
      asthma—*see* Asthma
      bronchitis (chronic) 491.20
      emphysema NEC 492.8
    airway, chronic 496
    chronic NEC 496
      with
        asthma (chronic) (obstructive) 493.2
    disease, chronic 496
      with
        asthma (chronic) (obstructive) 493.2
    emphysematous 492.8
  lymphatic 457.1
  meconium
    fetus or newborn 777.1
      in mucoviscidosis 277.01
    newborn due to fecaliths 777.1
  mediastinum 519.3
  mitral (rheumatic)—*see* Stenosis, mitral
  nasal 478.19
    duct 375.56
      neonatal 375.55
    sinus—*see* Sinusitis
  nasolacrimal duct 375.56
    congenital 743.65
    neonatal 375.55
  nasopharynx 478.29
  nose 478.19
  organ or site, congenital NEC—*see* Atresia
  pancreatic duct 577.8
  parotid gland 527.8
  pelviureteral junction (*see also* Obstruction, ureter) 593.4
  pharynx 478.29
  portal (circulation) (vein) 452
  prostate 600.90
    with
      other lower urinary tract symptoms (LUTS) 600.91
      urinary
        obstruction 600.91
        retention 600.91
    valve (urinary) 596.0
  pulmonary
    valve (heart) (*see also* Endocarditis, pulmonary) 424.3
    vein, isolated 747.49
  pyemic—*see* Septicemia
  pylorus (acquired) 537.0
    congenital 750.5
    infantile 750.5
  rectosigmoid (*see also* Obstruction, intestine) 560.9
  rectum 569.49
  renal 593.89
  respiratory 519.8
    chronic 496
  retinal (artery) (vein) (central) (*see also* Occlusion, retina) 362.30
  salivary duct (any) 527.8
    with calculus 527.5

Obstruction, obstructed—*continued*
  sigmoid (*see also* Obstruction, intestine) 560.9
  sinus (accessory) (nasal) (*see also* Sinusitis) 473.9
  Stensen's duct 527.8
  stomach 537.89
    acute 536.1
    congenital 750.7
  submaxillary gland 527.8
    with calculus 527.5
  thoracic duct 457.1
  thrombotic—*see* Thrombosis
  tooth eruption 520.6
  trachea 519.19
  tracheostomy airway 519.09
  tricuspid—*see* Endocarditis, tricuspid
  upper respiratory, congenital 748.8
  ureter (functional) 593.4
    congenital 753.20
    due to calculus 592.1
  ureteropelvic junction, congenital 753.21
  ureterovesical junction, congenital 753.22
  urethra 599.60
    congenital 753.6
  urinary (moderate) 599.60
    organ or tract (lower) 599.60
      due to
        benign prostatic hypertrophy (BPH)—*see* category 600
      specified NEC 599.69
        due to
          benign prostatic hypertrophy (BPH)—*see* category 600
    prostatic valve 596.0
    specified NEC 599.69
      due to
        benign prostatic hypertrophy (BPH)—*see* category 600
  uropathy 599.60
  uterus 621.8
  vagina 623.2
  valvular—*see* Endocarditis
  vascular graft or shunt 996.1
    atherosclerosis —*see* Arteriosclerosis, coronary
    embolism 996.74
    occlusion NEC 996.74
    thrombus 996.74
  vein, venous 459.2
    caval (inferior) (superior) 459.2
    thrombotic—*see* Thrombosis
  vena cava (inferior) (superior) 459.2
  ventricular shunt 996.2
  vesical 596.0
  vesicourethral orifice 596.0
  vessel NEC 459.9
Obturator —*see* condition
Occlusal
  plane deviation 524.76
  wear, teeth 521.10
Occlusion
  anus 569.49
    congenital 751.2
    infantile 751.2
  aortoiliac (chronic) 444.0
  aqueduct of Sylvius 331.4
    congenital 742.3
      with spina bifida (*see also* Spina bifida) 741.0
  arteries of extremities, lower 444.22
    without thrombus or embolus (*see also* Arteriosclerosis, extremities) 440.20

Occlusion—*continued*
    due to stricture or stenosis 447.1
    upper 444.21
      without thrombus or embolus (*see also* Arteriosclerosis, extremities) 440.20
      due to stricture or stenosis 447.1
  artery NEC (*see also* Embolism, artery) 444.9
    auditory, internal 433.8
    basilar 433.0
      with other precerebral artery 433.3
      bilateral 433.3
    brain or cerebral (*see also* Infarct, brain) 434.9
    carotid 433.1
      with other precerebral artery 433.3
      bilateral 433.3
    cerebellar (anterior inferior) (posterior inferior) (superior) 433.8
    cerebral (*see also* Infarct, brain) 434.9
    choroidal (anterior) 433.8
    chronic total
      coronary 414.2
      extremity(ies) 440.4
    complete
      coronary 414.2
      extremity(ies) 440.4
    communicating posterior 433.8
    coronary (thrombotic) (*see also* Infarct, myocardium) 410.9
      acute 410.9
        without myocardial infarction 411.81
      chronic total 414.2
      complete 414.2
      healed or old 412
      total 414.2
    extremity(ies)
      chronic total 440.4
      complete 440.4
      total 440.4
    hypophyseal 433.8
    iliac 444.81
    mesenteric (embolic) (thrombotic) (with gangrene) 557.0
    pontine 433.8
    precerebral NEC 433.9
      late effect—*see* Late effect(s) (of) cerebrovascular disease
      multiple or bilateral 433.3
      puerperal, postpartum, childbirth 674.0
      specified NEC 433.8
    renal 593.81
    retinal—*see* Occlusion, retina, artery
    spinal 433.8
    vertebral 433.2
      with other precerebral artery 433.3
      bilateral 433.3
  basilar (artery)—*see* Occlusion, artery, basilar
  bile duct (any) (*see also* Obstruction, biliary) 576.2
  bowel (*see also* Obstruction, intestine) 560.9
  brain (artery) (vascular) (*see also* Infarct, brain) 434.9
  breast (duct) 611.8
  carotid (artery) (common) (internal)—*see* Occlusion, artery, carotid
  cerebellar (anterior inferior) (artery) (posterior inferior) (superior) 433.8
  cerebral (artery) (*see also* Infarct, brain) 434.9
  cerebrovascular (*see also* Infarct, brain) 434.9
    diffuse 437.0
  cervical canal (*see also* Stricture, cervix) 622.4
    by falciparum malaria 084.0

INDEX TO DISEASES

Occlusion—*continued*
  cervix (uteri) (*see also* Stricture, cervix) 622.4
  choanal 748.0
  choroidal (artery) 433.8
  colon (*see also* Obstruction, intestine) 560.9
  communicating posterior artery 433.8
  coronary (artery) (thrombotic) (*see also* Infarct, myocardium) 410.9
    acute 410.9
      without myocardial infarction 411.81
    healed or old 412
    without myocardial infarction 411.81
  cystic duct (*see also* Obstruction, gallbladder) 575.2
    congenital 751.69
  disto
    division I 524.22
    division II 524.22
  embolic—*see* Embolism
  fallopian tube 628.2
    congenital 752.19
  gallbladder (*see also* Obstruction, gallbladder) 575.2
    congenital 751.69
      jaundice from 751.69 *[774.5]*
  gingiva, traumatic 523.8
  hymen 623.3
    congenital 752.42
  hypophyseal (artery) 433.8
  iliac artery 444.81
  intestine (*see also* Obstruction, intestine) 560.9
  kidney 593.89
  lacrimal apparatus—*see* Stenosis, lacrimal
  lung 518.89
  lymph or lymphatic channel 457.1
  mammary duct 611.8
  mesenteric artery (embolic) (thrombotic) (with gangrene) 557.0
  nose 478.1
    congenital 748.0
  organ or site, congenital NEC—*see* Atresia
  oviduct 628.2
    congenital 752.19
  periodontal, traumatic 523.8
  peripheral arteries (lower extremity) 444.22
    without thrombus or embolus (*see also* Arteriosclerosis, extremities) 440.20
    due to stricture or stenosis 447.1
    upper extremity 444.21
      without thrombus or embolus (*see also* Arteriosclerosis, extremities) 440.20
      due to stricture or stenosis 447.1
  pontine (artery) 433.8
  posterior lingual, of mandibular teeth 524.29
  precerebral artery—*see* Occlusion, artery, precerebral NEC
  puncta lacrimalia 375.52
  pupil 364.74
  pylorus (*see also* Stricture, pylorus) 537.0
  renal artery 593.81
  retina, retinal (vascular) 362.30
    artery, arterial 362.30
      branch 362.32
      central (total) 362.31
      partial 362.33
      transient 362.34
      tributary 362.32
    vein 362.30
      branch 362.36
      central (total) 362.35
      incipient 362.37

Occlusion—*continued*
    partial 362.37
    tributary 362.36
  spinal artery 433.8
  stent
    coronary 996.72
  teeth (mandibular) (posterior lingual) 524.29
  thoracic duct 457.1
  tubal 628.2
  ureter (complete) (partial) 593.4
    congenital 753.29
  urethra (*see also* Stricture, urethra) 598.9
    congenital 753.6
  uterus 621.8
  vagina 623.2
  vascular NEC 459.9
  vein—*see* Thrombosis
  vena cava (inferior) (superior) 453.2
  ventricle (brain) NEC 331.4
  vertebral (artery)—*see* Occlusion, artery, vertebral
  vessel (blood) NEC 459.9
  vulva 624.8
Occlusio pupillae 364.74
Occupational
  problems NEC V62.2
  therapy V57.21
Ochlophobia 300.29
Ochronosis (alkaptonuric) (congenital) (endogenous) 270.2
  with chloasma of eyelid 270.2
Ocular muscle —*see also* condition
  myopathy 359.1
  torticollis 781.93
Oculoauriculovertebral dysplasia 756.0
Oculogyric
  crisis or disturbance 378.87
    psychogenic 306.7
Oculomotor syndrome 378.81
Oddi's sphincter spasm 576.5
Odelberg's disease (juvenile osteochondrosis) 732.1
Odontalgia 525.9
Odontoameloblastoma (M9311/0) 213.1
  upper jaw (bone) 213.0
Odontoclasia 521.05
Odontoclasis 873.63
  complicated 873.73
Odontodysplasia, regional 520.4
Odontogenesis imperfecta 520.5
Odontoma (M9280/0) 213.1
  ameloblastic (M9311/0) 213.1
    upper jaw (bone) 213.0
  calcified (M9280/0) 213.1
    upper jaw (bone) 213.0
  complex (M9282/0) 213.1
    upper jaw (bone) 213.0
  compound (M9281/0) 213.1
    upper jaw (bone) 213.0
  fibroameloblastic (M9290/0) 213.1
    upper jaw (bone) 213.0
  follicular 526.0
    upper jaw (bone) 213.0
Odontomyelitis (closed) (open) 522.0
Odontonecrosis 521.09
Odontorrhagia 525.8
Odontosarcoma, ameloblastic (M9290/3) 170.1
  upper jaw (bone) 170.0
Odynophagia 787.20
Oesophagostomiasis 127.7
Oesophagostomum infestation 127.7

Oestriasis 134.0
Ogilvie's syndrome (sympathicotonic colon obstruction) 560.89
Oguchi's disease (retina) 368.61
Ohara's disease (*see also* Tularemia) 021.9
Oidiomycosis (*see also* Candidiasis) 112.9
Oidiomycotic meningitis 112.83
Oidium albicans infection (*see also* Candidiasis) 112.9
Old age 797
  dementia (of) 290.0
Olfactory —*see* condition
Oligemia 285.9
Oligergasia (*see also* Retardation, mental) 319
Oligoamnios 658.0
  affecting fetus or newborn 761.2
Oligoastrocytoma, mixed (M9382/3)
  specified site—*see* Neoplasm, by site, malignant
  unspecified site 191.9
Oligocythemia 285.9
Oligodendroblastoma (M9460/3)
  specified site—*see* Neoplasm, by site, malignant
  unspecified site 191.9
Oligodendroglioma (M9450/3)
  anaplastic type (M9451/3)
    specified site—*see* Neoplasm, by site, malignant
    unspecified site 191.9
  specified site—*see* Neoplasm, by site, malignant
  unspecified site 191.9
Oligodendroma —*see* Oligodendroglioma
Oligodontia (*see also* Anodontia) 520.0
Oligoencephalon 742.1
Oligohydramnios 658.0
  affecting fetus or newborn 761.2
  due to premature rupture of membranes 658.1
    affecting fetus or newborn 761.2
Oligohydrosis 705.0
Oligomenorrhea 626.1
Oligophrenia (*see also* Retardation, mental) 319
  phenylpyruvic 270.1
Oligospermia 606.1
Oligotrichia 704.09
  congenita 757.4
Oliguria 788.5
  with
    abortion—*see* Abortion, by type, with renal failure
    ectopic pregnancy (*see also* categories 633.0-633.9) 639.3
    molar pregnancy (*see also* categories 630-632) 639.3
  complicating
    abortion 639.3
    ectopic or molar pregnancy 639.3
    pregnancy 646.2
      with hypertension—*see* Toxemia, of pregnancy
  due to a procedure 997.5
  following labor and delivery 669.3
  heart or cardiac—*see* Failure, heart
  puerperal, postpartum 669.3
  specified due to a procedure 997.5
Ollier's disease (chondrodysplasia) 756.4
Omentitis (*see also* Peritonitis) 567.9
Omentocele (*see also* Hernia, omental) 553.8
Omentum, omental —*see* condition
Omphalitis (congenital) (newborn) 771.4
  not of newborn 686.9
  tetanus 771.3
Omphalocele 756.79

Omphalomesenteric duct, persistent 751.0
Omphalorrhagia, newborn 772.3
Omsk hemorrhagic fever 065.1
Onanism 307.9
Onchocerciasis 125.3
  eye 125.3 [360.13]
Onchocercosis 125.3
Oncocytoma (M8290/0)—*see* Neoplasm, by site, benign
Ondine's curse 348.8
Oneirophrenia (*see also* Schizophrenia) 295.4
Onychauxis 703.8
  congenital 757.5
Onychia (with lymphangitis) 681.9
  dermatophytic 110.1
  finger 681.02
  toe 681.11
Onychitis (with lymphangitis) 681.9
  finger 681.02
  toe 681.11
Onychocryptosis 703.0
Onychodystrophy 703.8
  congenital 757.5
Onychogryphosis 703.8
Onychogryposis 703.8
Onycholysis 703.8
Onychomadesis 703.8
Onychomalacia 703.8
Onychomycosis 110.1
  finger 110.1
  toe 110.1
Onycho-osteodysplasia 756.89
Onychophagy 307.9
Onychoptosis 703.8
Onychorrhexis 703.8
  congenital 757.5
Onychoschizia 703.8
Onychotrophia (*see also* Atrophy, nail) 703.8
O'nyong-nyong fever 066.3
Onyxis (finger) (toe) 703.0
Onyxitis (with lymphangitis) 681.9
  finger 681.02
  toe 681.11
Oocyte (egg) (ovum)
  donor V59.70
    age 35 and over V59.73
      anonymous recipient V59.73
      designated recipient V59.74
    under age 35 V59.71
      anonymous recipient V59.71
      designated recipient V59.72
Oophoritis (cystic) (infectional) (interstitial) (*see also* Salpingo-oophoritis) 614.2
  complicating pregnancy 646.6
  fetal (acute) 752.0
  gonococcal (acute) 098.19
    chronic or duration of 2 months or over 098.39
  tuberculous (*see also* Tuberculosis) 016.6
Opacity, opacities
  cornea 371.00
    central 371.03
    congenital 743.43
      interfering with vision 743.42
    degenerative (*see also* Degeneration, cornea) 371.40
    hereditary (*see also* Dystrophy, cornea) 371.50
    inflammatory (*see also* Keratitis) 370.9
    late effect of trachoma (healed) 139.1
    minor 371.01
    peripheral 371.02

INDEX TO DISEASES — Osgood-Schlatter

Opacity, opacities—*continued*
  enamel (fluoride) (nonfluoride) (teeth) 520.3
  lens (*see also* Cataract) 366.9
  snowball 379.22
  vitreous (humor) 379.24
    congenital 743.51
Opalescent dentin (hereditary) 520.5
Open, opening
  abnormal, organ or site, congenital—*see* Imperfect, closure
  angle with
    borderline intraocular pressure 365.01
    cupping of discs 365.01
  bite
    anterior 524.24
    posterior 524.25
  false—*see* Imperfect, closure
  margin on tooth restoration 525.61
  restoration margins 525.61
  wound—*see* Wound, open, by site
Operation
  causing mutilation of fetus 763.89
  destructive, on live fetus, to facilitate birth 763.89
  for delivery, fetus or newborn 763.89
  maternal, unrelated to current delivery, affecting fetus or newborn 760.6
Operational fatigue 300.89
Operative —*see* condition
Operculitis (chronic) 523.40
  acute 523.30
Operculum, retina 361.32
  with detachment 361.01
Ophiasis 704.01
Ophthalmia (*see also* Conjunctivitis) 372.30
  actinic rays 370.24
  allergic (acute) 372.05
    chronic 372.14
  blennorrhagic (neonatorum) 098.40
  catarrhal 372.03
  diphtheritic 032.81
  Egyptian 076.1
  electric, electrica 370.24
  gonococcal (neonatorum) 098.40
  metastatic 360.11
  migraine 346.8
  neonatorum, newborn 771.6
    gonococcal 098.40
  nodosa 360.14
  phlyctenular 370.31
    with ulcer (*see also* Ulcer, cornea) 370.00
  sympathetic 360.11
Ophthalmitis —*see* Ophthalmia
Ophthalmocele (congenital) 743.66
Ophthalmoneuromyelitis 341.0
Ophthalmopathy, infiltrative with thyrotoxicosis 242.0
Ophthalmoplegia (*see also* Strabismus) 378.9
  anterior internuclear 378.86
  ataxia-areflexia syndrome 357.0
  bilateral 378.9
  diabetic 250.5 *[378.86]*
  exophthalmic 242.0 *[376.22]*
  external 378.55
    progressive 378.72
    total 378.56
  interna(l) (complete) (total) 367.52
  internuclear 378.86
  migraine 346.8
  painful 378.55
  Parinaud's 378.81
  progressive external 378.72

Ophthalmoplegia—*continued*
  supranuclear, progressive 333.0
  total (external) 378.56
    internal 367.52
  unilateral 378.9
Opisthognathism 524.00
Opisthorchiasis (felineus) (tenuicollis) (viverrini) 121.0
Opisthotonos, opisthotonus 781.0
Opitz's disease (congestive splenomegaly) 289.51
Opiumism (*see also* Dependence) 304.0
Oppenheim's disease 358.8
Oppenheim-Urbach disease or syndrome (necrobiosis lipoidica diabeticorum) 250.8 *[709.3]*
Opsoclonia 379.59
Optic nerve —*see* condition
Orbit —*see* condition
Orchioblastoma (M9071/3) 186.9
Orchitis (nonspecific) (septic) 604.90
  with abscess 604.0
  blennorrhagic (acute) 098.13
    chronic or duration of 2 months or over 098.33
  diphtheritic 032.89 *[604.91]*
  filarial 125.9 *[604.91]*
  gangrenous 604.99
  gonococcal (acute) 098.13
    chronic or duration of 2 months or over 098.33
  mumps 072.0
  parotidea 072.0
  suppurative 604.99
  syphilitic 095.8 *[604.91]*
  tuberculous (*see also* Tuberculosis) 016.5 *[608.81]*
Orf 051.2
Organic —*see also* condition
  heart—*see* Disease, heart
  insufficiency 799.89
Oriental
  bilharziasis 120.2
  schistosomiasis 120.2
  sore 085.1
Orientation
  ego-dystonic sexual 302.0
Orifice —*see* condition
Origin, both great vessels from right ventricle 745.11
Ormond's disease or syndrome 593.4
Ornithosis 073.9
  with
    complication 073.8
      specified NEC 073.7
    pneumonia 073.0
    pneumonitis (lobular) 073.0
Orodigitofacial dysostosis 759.89
Oropouche fever 066.3
Orotaciduria, oroticaciduria (congenital) (hereditary) (pyrimidine deficiency) 281.4
Oroya fever 088.0
Orthodontics V58.5
  adjustment V53.4
  aftercare V58.5
  fitting V53.4
Orthopnea 786.02
Orthoptic training V57.4
Os, uterus —*see* condition
Osgood-Schlatter
  disease 732.4
  osteochondrosis 732.4

Osler's

Osler's
  disease (M9950/1) (polycythemia vera) 238.4
  nodes 421.0
Osler-Rendu disease (familial hemorrhagic telangiectasia) 448.0
Osler-Vaquez disease (M9950/1) (polycythemia vera) 238.4
Osler-Weber-Rendu syndrome (familial hemorrhagic telangiectasia) 448.0
Osmidrosis 705.89
Osseous —*see* condition
Ossification
  artery—*see* Arteriosclerosis
  auricle (ear) 380.39
  bronchus 519.19
  cardiac (*see also* Degeneration, myocardial) 429.1
  cartilage (senile) 733.99
  coronary —*see* Arteriosclerosis, coronary
  diaphragm 728.10
  ear 380.39
    middle (*see also* Otosclerosis) 387.9
  falx cerebri 349.2
  fascia 728.10
  fontanel
    defective or delayed 756.0
    premature 756.0
  heart (*see also* Degeneration, myocardial) 429.1
    valve—*see* Endocarditis
  larynx 478.79
  ligament
    posterior longitudinal 724.8
      cervical 723.7
  meninges (cerebral) 349.2
    spinal 336.8
  multiple, eccentric centers 733.99
  muscle 728.10
    heterotopic, postoperative 728.13
  myocardium, myocardial (*see also* Degeneration, myocardial) 429.1
  penis 607.81
  periarticular 728.89
  sclera 379.16
  tendon 727.82
  trachea 519.19
  tympanic membrane (*see also* Tympanosclerosis) 385.00
  vitreous (humor) 360.44
Osteitis (*see also* Osteomyelitis) 730.2
  acute 730.0
  alveolar 526.5
  chronic 730.1
  condensans (ilii) 733.5
  deformans (Paget's) 731.0
    due to or associated with malignant neoplasm (*see also* Neoplasm, bone, malignant) 170.9 *[731.1]*
  due to yaws 102.6
  fibrosa NEC 733.29
    cystica (generalisata) 252.01
    disseminata 756.59
    osteoplastica 252.01
  fragilitans 756.51
  Garré's (sclerosing) 730.1
  infectious (acute) (subacute) 730.0
    chronic or old 730.1
  jaw (acute) (chronic) (lower) (neonatal) (suppurative) (upper) 526.4
  parathyroid 252.01
  petrous bone (*see also* Petrositis) 383.20
  pubis 733.5
  sclerotic, nonsuppurative 730.1

Osteitis—*continued*
  syphilitic 095.5
  tuberculosa
    cystica (of Jüngling) 135
    multiplex cystoides 135
Osteoarthritica spondylitis (spine) (*see also* Spondylosis) 721.90
Osteoarthritis (*see also* Osteoarthrosis) 715.9
  distal interphalangeal 715.9
  hyperplastic 731.2
  interspinalis (*see also* Spondylosis) 721.90
  spine, spinal NEC (*see also* Spondylosis) 721.90
Osteoarthropathy (*see also* Osteoarthrosis) 715.9
  chronic idiopathic hypertrophic 757.39
  familial idiopathic 757.39
  hypertrophic pulmonary 731.2
    secondary 731.2
  idiopathic hypertrophic 757.39
  primary hypertrophic 731.2
  pulmonary hypertrophic 731.2
  secondary hypertrophic 731.2
Osteoarthrosis (degenerative) (hypertrophic) (rheumatoid) 715.9

> *Note*—*Use the following fifth-digit subclassification with category 715:*
>
> 0 *site unspecified*
> 1 *shoulder region*
> 2 *upper arm*
> 3 *forearm*
> 4 *hand*
> 5 *pelvic region and thigh*
> 6 *lower leg*
> 7 *ankle and foot*
> 8 *other specified sites except spine*
> 9 *multiple sites*

  deformans alkaptonurica 270.2
  generalized 715.09
  juvenilis (Köhler's) 732.5
  localized 715.3
    idiopathic 715.1
    primary 715.1
    secondary 715.2
  multiple sites, not specified as generalized 715.89
  polyarticular 715.09
  spine (*see also* Spondylosis) 721.90
  temperomandibular joint 524.69
Osteoblastoma (M9200/0)—*see* Neoplasm, bone, benign
Osteochondritis (*see also* Osteochondrosis) 732.9
  dissecans 732.7
    hip 732.7
  ischiopubica 732.1
  multiple 756.59
  syphilitic (congenital) 090.0
Osteochondrodermodysplasia 756.59
Osteochondrodystrophy 277.5
  deformans 277.5
  familial 277.5
  fetalis 756.4
Osteochondrolysis 732.7
Osteochondroma (M9210/0)—*see also* Neoplasm, bone, benign
  multiple, congenital 756.4
Osteochondromatosis (M9210/1) 238.0
  synovial 727.82
Osteochondromyxosarcoma (M9180/3)—*see* Neoplasm, bone, malignant
Osteochondropathy NEC 732.9

INDEX TO DISEASES   **Osteomalacosis**

Osteochondrosarcoma (M9180/3)—*see*
  Neoplasm, bone, malignant
Osteochondrosis 732.9
  acetabulum 732.1
  adult spine 732.8
  astragalus 732.5
  Blount's 732.4
  Buchanan's (juvenile osteochondrosis of iliac
    crest) 732.1
  Buchman's (juvenile osteochondrosis) 732.1
  Burns' 732.3
  calcaneus 732.5
  capitular epiphysis (femur) 732.1
  carpal
    lunate (wrist) 732.3
    scaphoid 732.3
  coxae juvenilis 732.1
  deformans juvenilis (coxae) (hip) 732.1
    Scheuermann's 732.0
    spine 732.0
    tibia 732.4
    vertebra 732.0
  Diaz's (astragalus) 732.5
  dissecans (knee) (shoulder) 732.7
  femoral capital epiphysis 732.1
  femur (head) (juvenile) 732.1
  foot (juvenile) 732.5
  Freiberg's (disease) (second metatarsal) 732.5
  Haas' 732.3
  Haglund's (os tibiale externum) 732.5
  hand (juvenile) 732.3
  head of
    femur 732.1
    humerus (juvenile) 732.3
  hip (juvenile) 732.1
  humerus (juvenile) 732.3
  iliac crest (juvenile) 732.1
  ilium (juvenile) 732.1
  ischiopubic synchondrosis 732.1
  Iselin's (osteochondrosis fifth metatarsal) 732.5
  juvenile, juvenilis 732.6
    arm 732.3
    capital femoral epiphysis 732.1
    capitellum humeri 732.3
    capitular epiphysis 732.1
    carpal scaphoid 732.3
    clavicle, sternal epiphysis 732.6
    coxae 732.1
    deformans 732.1
    foot 732.5
    hand 732.3
    hip and pelvis 732.1
    lower extremity, except foot 732.4
    lunate, wrist 732.3
    medial cuneiform bone 732.5
    metatarsal (head) 732.5
    metatarsophalangeal 732.5
    navicular, ankle 732.5
    patella 732.4
    primary patellar center (of Köhler) 732.4
    specified site NEC 732.6
    spine 732.0
    tarsal scaphoid 732.5
    tibia (epiphysis) (tuberosity) 732.4
    upper extremity 732.3
    vertebra (body) (Calvé) 732.0
      epiphyseal plates (of Scheuermann) 732.0
  Kienböck's (disease) 732.3
  Köhler's (disease) (navicular, ankle) 732.5
    patellar 732.4
    tarsal navicular 732.5

Osteochondrosis—*continued*
  Legg-Calvé-Perthes (disease) 732.1
  lower extremity (juvenile) 732.4
  lunate bone 732.3
  Mauclaire's 732.3
  metacarpal heads (of Mauclaire) 732.3
  metatarsal (fifth) (head) (second) 732.5
  navicular, ankle 732.5
  os calcis 732.5
  Osgood-Schlatter 732.4
  os tibiale externum 732.5
  Panner's 732.3
  patella (juvenile) 732.4
  patellar center
    primary (of Köhler) 732.4
    secondary (of Sinding-Larsen) 732.4
  pelvis (juvenile) 732.1
  Pierson's 732.1
  radial head (juvenile) 732.3
  Scheuermann's 732.0
  Sever's (calcaneum) 732.5
  Sinding-Larsen (secondary patellar center) 732.4
  spine (juvenile) 732.0
    adult 732.8
  symphysis pubis (of Pierson) (juvenile) 732.1
  syphilitic (congenital) 090.0
  tarsal (navicular) (scaphoid) 732.5
  tibia (proximal) (tubercle) 732.4
  tuberculous—*see* Tuberculosis, bone
  ulna 732.3
  upper extremity (juvenile) 732.3
  van Neck's (juvenile osteochondrosis) 732.1
  vertebral (juvenile) 732.0
    adult 732.8
Osteoclastoma (M9250/1) 238.0
  malignant (M9250/3)—*see* Neoplasm, bone,
    malignant
Osteocopic pain 733.90
Osteodynia 733.90
Osteodystrophy
  azotemic 588.0
  chronica deformans hypertrophica 731.0
  congenital 756.50
    specified type NEC 756.59
  deformans 731.0
  fibrosa localisata 731.0
  parathyroid 252.01
  renal 588.0
Osteofibroma (M9262/0)—*see* Neoplasm, bone,
  benign
Osteofibrosarcoma (M9182/3)—*see* Neoplasm,
  bone, malignant
Osteogenesis imperfecta 756.51
Osteogenic —*see* condition
Osteoma (M9180/0)—*see also* Neoplasm, bone,
  benign
  osteoid (M9191/0)—*see also* Neoplasm, bone,
    benign
    giant (M9200/0)—*see* Neoplasm, bone, benign
Osteomalacia 268.2
  chronica deformans hypertrophica 731.0
  due to vitamin D deficiency 268.2
  infantile (*see also* Rickets) 268.0
  juvenile (*see also* Rickets) 268.0
  pelvis 268.2
  vitamin D-resistant 275.3
Osteomalacic bone 268.2
Osteomalacosis 268.2

Osteomyelitis   INDEX TO DISEASES

Osteomyelitis (general) (infective) (localized) (neonatal) (purulent) (pyogenic) (septic) (staphylococcal) (streptococcal) (suppurative) (with periostitis) 730.2

> *Note—Use the following fifth-digit subclassification with category 730:*
>
> 0 site unspecified
> 1 shoulder region
> 2 upper arm
> 3 forearm
> 4 hand
> 5 pelvic region and thigh
> 6 lower leg
> 7 ankle and foot
> 8 other specified sites
> 9 multiple sites

  acute or subacute 730.0
  chronic or old 730.1
  due to or associated with
    diabetes mellitus 250.8 *[731.8]*
    tuberculosis (*see also* Tuberculosis, bone) 015.9 *[730.8]*
      limb bones 015.5 *[730.8]*
      specified bones NEC 015.7 *[730.8]*
      spine 015.0 *[730.8]*
    typhoid 002.0 *[730.8]*
  Garré's 730.1
  jaw (acute) (chronic) (lower) (neonatal) (suppurative) (upper) 526.4
  nonsuppurating 730.1
  orbital 376.03
  petrous bone (*see also* Petrositis) 383.20
  Salmonella 003.24
  sclerosing, nonsuppurative 730.1
  sicca 730.1
  syphilitic 095.5
    congenital 090.0 *[730.8]*
  tuberculous—*see* Tuberculosis, bone
  typhoid 002.0 *[730.8]*
Osteomyelofibrosis 289.89
Osteomyelosclerosis 289.89
Osteonecrosis 733.40
  meaning osteomyelitis 730.1
Osteo-onycho-arthro dysplasia 756.89
Osteo-onychodysplasia, hereditary 756.89
Osteopathia
  condensans disseminata 756.53
  hyperostotica multiplex infantilis 756.59
  hypertrophica toxica 731.2
  striata 756.4
Osteopathy resulting from poliomyelitis (*see also* Poliomyelitis) 045.9 *[730.7]*
  familial dysplastic 731.2
Osteopecilia 756.53
Osteopenia 733.90
Osteoperiostitis (*see also* Osteomyelitis) 730.2
  ossificans toxica 731.2
  toxica ossificans 731.2
Osteopetrosis (familial) 756.52
Osteophyte —*see* Exostosis
Osteophytosis —*see* Exostosis
Osteopoikilosis 756.53
Osteoporosis (generalized) 733.00
  circumscripta 731.0
  disuse 733.03
  drug-induced 733.09
  idiopathic 733.02
  postmenopausal 733.01

Osteoporosis—*continued*
  posttraumatic 733.7
  screening V82.81
  senile 733.01
  specified type NEC 733.09
Osteoporosis-osteomalacia syndrome 268.2
Osteopsathyrosis 756.51
Osteoradionecrosis, jaw 526.89
Osteosarcoma (M9180/3)—*see also* Neoplasm, bone, malignant
  chondroblastic (M9181/3)—*see* Neoplasm, bone, malignant
  fibroblastic (M9182/3)—*see* Neoplasm, bone, malignant
  in Paget's disease of bone (M9184/3)—*see* Neoplasm, bone, malignant
  juxtacortical (M9190/3)—*see* Neoplasm, bone, malignant
  parosteal (M9190/3)—*see* Neoplasm, bone, malignant
  telangiectatic (M9183/3)—*see* Neoplasm, bone, malignant
Osteosclerosis 756.52
  fragilis (generalisata) 756.52
Osteosclerotic anemia 289.89
Osteosis
  acromegaloid 757.39
  cutis 709.3
  parathyroid 252.01
  renal fibrocystic 588.0
Österreicher-Turner syndrome 756.89
Ostium
  atrioventriculare commune 745.69
  primum (arteriosum) (defect) (persistent) 745.61
  secundum (arteriosum) (defect) (patent) (persistent) 745.5
Ostrum-Furst syndrome 756.59
Otalgia 388.70
  otogenic 388.71
  referred 388.72
Othematoma 380.31
Otitic hydrocephalus 348.2
Otitis 382.9
  with effusion 381.4
    purulent 382.4
    secretory 381.4
    serous 381.4
    suppurative 382.4
  acute 382.9
  adhesive (*see also* Adhesions, middle ear) 385.10
  chronic 382.9
    with effusion 381.3
    mucoid, mucous (simple) 381.20
    purulent 382.3
    secretory 381.3
    serous 381.10
    suppurative 382.3
  diffuse parasitic 136.8
  externa (acute) (diffuse) (hemorrhagica) 380.10
    actinic 380.22
    candidal 112.82
    chemical 380.22
    chronic 380.23
      mycotic—*see* Otitis, externa, mycotic
      specified type NEC 380.23
    circumscribed 380.10
    contact 380.22

INDEX TO DISEASES   **Otitis**

Otitis—*continued*
  due to
    erysipelas 035 *[380.13]*
    impetigo 684 *[380.13]*
    seborrheic dermatitis 690.10 *[380.13]*
  eczematoid 380.22
  furuncular 680.0 *[380.13]*
  infective 380.10
    chronic 380.16
  malignant 380.14
  mycotic (chronic) 380.15
    due to
      aspergillosis 117.3 *[380.15]*
      moniliasis 112.82
      otomycosis 111.8 *[380.15]*
  reactive 380.22
  specified type NEC 380.22
  tropical 111.8 *[380.15]*
  insidiosa (*see also* Otosclerosis) 387.9
  interna (*see also* Labyrinthitis) 386.30
  media (hemorrhagic) (staphylococcal) (streptococcal) 382.9
    acute 382.9
      with effusion 381.00
        allergic 381.04
          mucoid 381.05
          sanguineous 381.06
          serous 381.04
        catarrhal 381.00
        exudative 381.00
        mucoid 381.02
          allergic 381.05
      necrotizing 382.00
        with spontaneous rupture of ear drum 382.01
        in
          influenza 487.8 *[382.02]*
          measles 055.2
          scarlet fever 034.1 *[382.02]*
      nonsuppurative 381.00
      purulent 382.00
        with spontaneous rupture of ear drum 382.01
      sanguineous 381.03
        allergic 381.06
      secretory 381.01
      seromucinous 381.02
      serous 381.01
        allergic 381.04
      suppurative 382.00
        with spontaneous rupture of ear drum 382.01
        due to
          influenza 487.8 *[382.02]*
          scarlet fever 034.1 *[382.02]*
      transudative 381.00
    adhesive (*see also* Adhesions, middle ear) 385.10
    allergic 381.4
      acute 381.04
        mucoid 381.05
        sanguineous 381.06
        serous 381.04
      chronic 381.3
    catarrhal 381.4
      acute 381.00
      chronic (simple) 381.10
    chronic 382.9
      with effusion 381.3
      adhesive (*see also* Adhesions, middle ear) 385.10

Otitis—*continued*
    allergic 381.3
    atticoantral, suppurative (with posterior or superior marginal perforation of ear drum) 382.2
    benign suppurative (with anterior perforation of ear drum) 382.1
    catarrhal 381.10
    exudative 381.3
    mucinous 381.20
    mucoid, mucous (simple) 381.20
    mucosanguineous 381.29
    nonsuppurative 381.3
    purulent 382.3
    secretory 381.3
    seromucinous 381.3
    serosanguineous 381.19
    serous (simple) 381.10
    suppurative 382.3
      atticoantral (with posterior or superior marginal perforation of ear drum) 382.2
      benign (with anterior perforation of ear drum) 382.1
      tuberculous (*see also* Tuberculosis) 017.4
      tubotympanic 382.1
    transudative 381.3
  exudative 381.4
    acute 381.00
    chronic 381.3
  fibrotic (*see also* Adhesions, middle ear) 385.10
  mucoid, mucous 381.4
    acute 381.02
    chronic (simple) 381.20
  mucosanguineous, chronic 381.29
  nonsuppurative 381.4
    acute 381.00
    chronic 381.3
  postmeasles 055.2
  purulent 382.4
    acute 382.00
      with spontaneous rupture of ear drum 382.01
    chronic 382.3
  sanguineous, acute 381.03
    allergic 381.06
  secretory 381.4
    acute or subacute 381.01
    chronic 381.3
  seromucinous 381.4
    acute or subacute 381.02
    chronic 381.3
  serosanguineous, chronic 381.19
  serous 381.4
    acute or subacute 381.01
    chronic (simple) 381.10
  subacute—*see* Otitis, media, acute
  suppurative 382.4
    acute 382.00
      with spontaneous rupture of ear drum 382.01
    chronic 382.3
      atticoantral 382.2
      benign 382.1
      tuberculous (*see also* Tuberculosis) 017.4
      tubotympanic 382.1
  transudative 381.4
    acute 381.00
    chronic 381.3
  tuberculous (*see also* Tuberculosis) 017.4
  postmeasles 055.2

Otoconia 386.8
Otolith syndrome 386.19
Otomycosis 111.8 *[380.15]*
  in
    aspergillosis 117.3 *[380.15]*
    moniliasis 112.82
Otopathy 388.9
Otoporosis (*see also* Otosclerosis) 387.9
Otorrhagia 388.69
  traumatic—*see* nature of injury
Otorrhea 388.60
  blood 388.69
  cerebrospinal (fluid) 388.61
Otosclerosis (general) 387.9
  cochlear (endosteal) 387.2
  involving
    otic capsule 387.2
    oval window
      nonobliterative 387.0
      obliterative 387.1
    round window 387.2
  nonobliterative 387.0
  obliterative 387.1
  specified type NEC 387.8
Otospongiosis (*see also* Otosclerosis) 387.9
Otto's disease or pelvis 715.35
Outburst, aggressive (*see also* Disturbance, conduct) 312.0
  in children or adolescents 313.9
Outcome of delivery
  multiple birth NEC V27.9
    all liveborn V27.5
    all stillborn V27.7
    some liveborn V27.6
    unspecified V27.9
  single V27.9
    liveborn V27.0
    stillborn V27.1
  twins V27.9
    both liveborn V27.2
    both stillborn V27.4
    one liveborn, one stillborn V27.3
Outlet —*see also* condition
  syndrome (thoracic) 353.0
Outstanding ears (bilateral) 744.29
Ovalocytosis (congenital) (hereditary) (*see also* Elliptocytosis) 282.1
Ovarian —*see also* condition
  pregnancy—*see* Pregnancy, ovarian
  remnant syndrome 620.8
  vein syndrome 593.4
Ovaritis (cystic) (*see also* Salpingo-oophoritis) 614.2
Ovary, ovarian —*see* condition
Overactive —*see also* Hyperfunction
  bladder 596.51
  eye muscle (*see also* Strabismus) 378.9
  hypothalamus 253.8
  thyroid (*see also* Thyrotoxicosis) 242.9
Overactivity, child 314.01
Overbite (deep) (excessive) (horizontal) (vertical) 524.29
Overbreathing (*see also* Hyperventilation) 786.01
Overconscientious personality 301.4
Overdevelopment —*see also* Hypertrophy
  breast (female) (male) 611.1
  nasal bones 738.0
  prostate, congenital 752.89
Overdistention —*see* Distention

Overdose overdosage (drug) 977.9
  specified drug or substance—*see* Table of drugs and chemicals
Overeating 783.6
  with obesity 278.0
  nonorganic origin 307.51
Overexertion (effects) (exhaustion) 994.5
Overexposure (effects) 994.9
  exhaustion 994.4
Overfeeding (*see also* Overeating) 783.6
Overfill, endodontic 526.62
Overgrowth, bone NEC 733.99
Overhanging
  tooth restoration 525.62
  unrepairable, dental restorative materials 525.62
Overheated (effects) (places)—*see* Heat
Overinhibited child 313.0
Overjet 524.29
  excessive horizontal 524.26
Overlaid, overlying (suffocation) 994.7
Overlap
  excessive horizontal 524.26
Overlapping toe (acquired) 735.8
  congenital (fifth toe) 755.66
Overload
  fluid 276.6
  potassium (K) 276.7
  sodium (Na) 276.0
Overnutrition (*see also* Hyperalimentation) 783.6
Overproduction —*see also* Hypersecretion
  ACTH 255.3
  cortisol 255.0
  growth hormone 253.0
  thyroid-stimulating hormone (TSH) 242.8
Overriding
  aorta 747.21
  finger (acquired) 736.29
    congenital 755.59
  toe (acquired) 735.8
    congenital 755.66
Oversize
  fetus (weight of 4500 grams or more) 766.0
    affecting management of pregnancy 656.6
    causing disproportion 653.5
      with obstructed labor 660.1
        affecting fetus or newborn 763.1
Overstimulation, ovarian 256.1
Overstrained 780.79
  heart—*see* Hypertrophy, cardiac
Overweight (*see also* Obesity) 278.02
Overwork 780.79
Oviduct —*see* condition
Ovotestis 752.7
Ovulation (cycle)
  failure or lack of 628.0
  pain 625.2
Ovum
  blighted 631
  donor V59.70
    age 35 and over V59.73
      anonymous recipient V59.73
      designated recipient V59.74
    under age 35 V59.71
      anonymous recipient V59.71
      designated recipient V59.72
  dropsical 631
  pathologic 631
Owren's disease or syndrome (parahemophilia) (*see also* Defect, coagulation) 286.3
Oxalosis 271.8

Oxaluria 271.8
Ox heart —*see* Hypertrophy, cardiac
OX syndrome 758.6
Oxycephaly, oxycephalic 756.0
　syphilitic, congenital 090.0
Oxyuriasis 127.4
Oxyuris vermicularis (infestation) 127.4
Ozena 472.0

INDEX TO DISEASES

INDEX TO DISEASES

P

Pacemaker syndrome 429.4
Pachyderma, pachydermia 701.8
 laryngis 478.5
 laryngitis 478.79
 larynx (verrucosa) 478.79
Pachydermatitis 701.8
Pachydermatocele (congenital) 757.39
 acquired 701.8
Pachydermatosis 701.8
Pachydermoperiostitis
 secondary 731.2
Pachydermoperiostosis
 primary idiopathic 757.39
 secondary 731.2
Pachymeningitis (adhesive) (basal) (brain)
 (cerebral) (cervical) (chronic) (circumscribed)
 (external) (fibrous) (hemorrhagic)
 (hypertrophic) (internal) (purulent) (spinal)
 (suppurative) (*see also* Meningitis) 322.9
 gonococcal 098.82
Pachyonychia (congenital) 757.5
 acquired 703.8
Pachyperiosteodermia
 primary or idiopathic 757.39
 secondary 731.2
Pachyperiostosis
 primary or idiopathic 757.39
 secondary 731.2
Pacinian tumor (M9507/0)—*see* Neoplasm, skin, benign
Pads, knuckle or Garrod's 728.79
Paget's disease (osteitis deformans) 731.0
 with infiltrating duct carcinoma of the breast
  (M8541/3)—*see* Neoplasm, breast, malignant
 bone 731.0
  osteosarcoma in (M9184/3)—*see* Neoplasm, bone, malignant
 breast (M8540/3) 174.0
 extramammary (M8542/3)—*see also* Neoplasm, skin, malignant
  anus 154.3
  skin 173.5
 malignant (M8540/3)
  breast 174.0
  specified site NEC (M8542/3)—*see* Neoplasm, skin, malignant
  unspecified site 174.0
 mammary (M8540/3) 174.0
 necrosis of bone 731.0
 nipple (M8540/3) 174.0
 osteitis deformans 731.0
Paget-Schroetter syndrome (intermittent venous claudication) 453.8
Pain(s) (*see also* Painful) 780.96
 abdominal 789.0
 acute 338.19
  due to trauma 338.11
  postoperative 338.18
   post-thoracotomy 338.12
 adnexa (uteri) 625.9
 alimentary, due to vascular insufficiency 557.9
 anginoid (*see also* Pain, precordial) 786.51
 anus 569.42
 arch 729.5
 arm 729.5
 axillary 729.5

Pain(s)—*continued*
 back (postural) 724.5
  low 724.2
   psychogenic 307.89
 bile duct 576.9
 bladder 788.9
 bone 733.90
 breast 611.71
  psychogenic 307.89
 broad ligament 625.9
 cancer associated 338.3
 cartilage NEC 733.90
 cecum 789.0
 cervicobrachial 723.3
 chest (central) 786.50
  atypical 786.59
  midsternal 786.51
  musculoskeletal 786.59
  noncardiac 786.59
  substernal 786.51
  wall (anterior) 786.52
 chronic 338.29
  associated with significant psychosocial dysfunction 338.4
  due to trauma 338.21
  postoperative 338.28
   post-thoracotomy 338.22
  syndrome 338.4
 coccyx 724.79
 colon 789.0
 common duct 576.9
 coronary—*see* Angina
 costochondral 786.52
 diaphragm 786.52
 due to (presence of) any device, implant, or graft classifiable to 996.0-996.5—*see* Complications, due to (presence of) any device, implant, or graft classified to 996.0-996.5 NEC
 malignancy (primary) (secondary) 338.3
 ear (*see also* Otalgia) 388.70
 epigastric, epigastrium 789.0
 extremity (lower) (upper) 729.5
 eye 379.91
 face, facial 784.0
  atypical 350.2
  nerve 351.8
 false (labor) 644.1
 female genital organ NEC 625.9
  psychogenic 307.89
 finger 729.5
 flank 789.0
 foot 729.5
 gallbladder 575.9
 gas (intestinal) 787.3
 gastric 536.8
 generalized 780.96
 genital organ
  female 625.9
  male 608.9
  psychogenic 307.89
 groin 789.0
 growing 781.99
 hand 729.5
 head (*see also* Headache) 784.0
 heart (*see also* Pain, precordial) 786.51
 infraorbital (*see also* Neuralgia, trigeminal) 350.1

INDEX TO DISEASES

—continued
intermenstrual 625.2
jaw 526.9
joint 719.40
  ankle 719.47
  elbow 719.42
  foot 719.47
  hand 719.44
  hip 719.45
  knee 719.46
  multiple sites 719.49
  pelvic region 719.45
  psychogenic 307.89
  shoulder (region) 719.41
  specified site NEC 719.48
  wrist 719.43
kidney 788.0
labor, false or spurious 644.1
laryngeal 784.1
leg 729.5
limb 729.5
low back 724.2
lumbar region 724.2
mastoid (*see also* Otalgia) 388.70
maxilla 526.9
menstrual 625.3
metacarpophalangeal (joint) 719.44
metatarsophalangeal (joint) 719.47
mouth 528.9
muscle 729.1
  intercostal 786.59
musculoskeletal (*see also* Pain, by site) 729.1
nasal 478.19
nasopharynx 478.29
neck NEC 723.1
  psychogenic 307.89
neoplasm related (acute) (chronic) 338.3
nerve NEC 729.2
neuromuscular 729.1
nose 478.19
ocular 379.91
ophthalmic 379.91
orbital region 379.91
osteocopic 733.90
ovary 625.9
  psychogenic 307.89
over heart (*see also* Pain, precordial) 786.51
ovulation 625.2
pelvic (female) 625.9
  male NEC 789.0
    psychogenic 307.89
  psychogenic 307.89
penis 607.9
  psychogenic 307.89
pericardial (*see also* Pain, precordial) 786.51
perineum
  female 625.9
  male 608.9
pharynx 478.29
pleura, pleural, pleuritic 786.52
post-operative 338.18
  acute 338.18
  chronic 338.28
post-thoracotomy 338.12
  acute 338.12
  chronic 338.22
preauricular 388.70
precordial (region) 786.51
  psychogenic 307.89
premenstrual 625.4
psychogenic 307.80

Pain(s)—*continued*
cardiovascular system 307.89
gastrointestinal system 307.89
genitourinary system 307.89
heart 307.89
musculoskeletal system 307.89
respiratory system 307.89
skin 306.3
radicular (spinal) (*see also* Radiculitis) 729.2
rectum 569.42
respiration 786.52
retrosternal 786.51
rheumatic NEC 729.0
  muscular 729.1
rib 786.50
root (spinal) (*see also* Radiculitis) 729.2
round ligament (stretch) 625.9
sacroiliac 724.6
sciatic 724.3
scrotum 608.9
  psychogenic 307.89
seminal vesicle 608.9
sinus 478.19
skin 782.0
spermatic cord 608.9
spinal root (*see also* Radiculitis) 729.2
stomach 536.8
  psychogenic 307.89
substernal 786.51
temporomandibular (joint) 524.62
temporomaxillary joint 524.62
testis 608.9
  psychogenic 307.89
thoracic spine 724.1
  with radicular and visceral pain 724.4
throat 784.1
tibia 733.90
toe 729.5
tongue 529.6
tooth 525.9
total hip replacement 996.77
total knee replacement 996.77
trigeminal (*see also* Neuralgia, trigeminal) 350.1
tumor associated 338.3
umbilicus 789.0
ureter 788.0
urinary (organ) (system) 788.0
uterus 625.9
  psychogenic 307.89
vagina 625.9
vertebrogenic (syndrome) 724.5
vesical 788.9
vulva 625.9
xiphoid 733.90
Painful —*see also* Pain
arc syndrome 726.19
coitus
  female 625.0
  male 608.89
  psychogenic 302.76
ejaculation (semen) 608.89
  psychogenic 302.79
erection 607.3
feet syndrome 266.2
menstruation 625.3
  psychogenic 306.52
micturition 788.1
ophthalmoplegia 378.55
respiration 786.52
scar NEC 709.2
urination 788.1
wire sutures 998.89

INDEX TO DISEASES   **Pancytopenia**

Painters' colic 984.9
  specified type of lead—*see* Table of drugs and chemicals
Palate —*see* condition
Palatoplegia 528.9
Palatoschisis (*see also* Cleft, palate) 749.00
Palilalia 784.69
Palindromic arthritis (*see also* Rheumatism, palindromic) 719.3
Palliative care V66.7
Pallor 782.61
  temporal, optic disc 377.15
Palmar —*see also* condition
  fascia—*see* condition
Palpable
  cecum 569.89
  kidney 593.89
  liver 573.9
  lymph nodes 785.6
  ovary 620.8
  prostate 602.9
  spleen (*see also* Splenomegaly) 789.2
  uterus 625.8
Palpitation (heart) 785.1
  psychogenic 306.2
Palsy (*see also* Paralysis) 344.9
  atrophic diffuse 335.20
  Bell's 351.0
    newborn 767.5
  birth 767.7
  brachial plexus 353.0
    fetus or newborn 767.6
  brain—*see also* Palsy, cerebral
    noncongenital or noninfantile 344.89
      due to vascular lesion—*see* category 438
      late effect—*see* Late effect(s) (of) cerebrovascular disease
    syphilitic 094.89
      congenital 090.49
  bulbar (chronic) (progressive) 335.22
    pseudo NEC 335.23
    supranuclear NEC 344.89
  cerebral (congenital) (infantile) (spastic) 343.9
    athetoid 333.71
    diplegic 343.0
      mue to prevhous vascular lesion—*see* category 438
      late effect—*see* Late effect(s) (of) cerebrovascular disease
    hemiplegic 343.1
    monoplegic 343.3
    noncongenital or noninfantile 437.8
      mue to prevhous vascular lesion—*see* category 438
      late effect—*see* Late effect(s) (of) cerebrovascular disease
    paraplegic 343.0
    quadriplegic 343.2
    spastic, not congenital or infantile 344.89
    syphilitic 094.89
      congenital 090.49
    tetraplegic 343.2
  cranial nerve—*see also* Disorder, nerve, cranial
    multiple 352.6
  creeping 335.21
  divers' 993.3
  Erb's (birth injury) 767.6
  facial 351.0
    newborn 767.5
  glossopharyngeal 352.2
  Klumpke (-Déjérine) 767.6

Palsy—*continued*
  lead 984.9
    specified type of lead—*see* Table of drugs and chemicals
  median nerve (tardy) 354.0
  peroneal nerve (acute) (tardy) 355.3
  progressive supranuclear 333.0
  pseudobulbar NEC 335.23
  radial nerve (acute) 354.3
  seventh nerve 351.0
    newborn 767.5
  shaking (*see also* Parkinsonism) 332.0
  spastic (cerebral) (spinal) 343.9
    hemiplegic 343.1
  specified nerve NEC—*see* Disorder, nerve
  supranuclear NEC 356.8
    progressive 333.0
  ulnar nerve (tardy) 354.2
  wasting 335.21
Paltauf-Sternberg disease 201.9
Paludism —*see* Malaria
Panama fever 084.0
Panaris (with lymphangitis) 681.9
  finger 681.02
  toe 681.11
Panaritium (with lymphangitis) 681.9
  finger 681.02
  toe 681.11
Panarteritis (nodosa) 446.0
  brain or cerebral 437.4
Pancake heart 793.2
  with cor pulmonale (chronic) 416.9
Pancarditis (acute) (chronic) 429.89
  with
    rheumatic fever (active) (acute) (chronic) (subacute) 391.8
      inactive or quiescent 398.99
  rheumatic, acute 391.8
    chronic or inactive 398.99
Pancoast's syndrome or tumor (carcinoma, pulmonary apex) (M8010/3) 162.3
Pancoast-Tobias syndrome (M8010/3) (carcinoma, pulmonary apex) 162.3
Pancolitis 556.6
Pancreas, pancreatic —*see* condition
Pancreatitis 577.0
  acute (edematous) (hemorrhagic) (recurrent) 577.0
  annular 577.0
  apoplectic 577.0
  calcereous 577.0
  chronic (infectious) 577.1
    recurrent 577.1
  cystic 577.2
  fibrous 577.8
  gangrenous 577.0
  hemorrhagic (acute) 577.0
  interstitial (chronic) 577.1
    acute 577.0
  malignant 577.0
  mumps 072.3
  painless 577.1
  recurrent 577.1
  relapsing 577.1
  subacute 577.0
  suppurative 577.0
  syphilitic 095.8
Pancreatolithiasis 577.8
Pancytolysis 289.9
Pancytopenia (acquired) 284.1
  with malformations 284.09
  congenital 284.09

Panencephalitis —*see also* Encephalitis
   subacute, sclerosing 046.2
Panhematopenia 284.81
   congenital 284.09
   constitutional 284.09
   splenic, primary 289.4
Panhemocytopenia 284.81
   congenital 284.09
   constitutional 284.09
Panhypogonadism 257.2
Panhypopituitarism 253.2
   prepubertal 253.3
Panic (attack) (state) 300.01
   reaction to exceptional stress (transient) 308.0
Panmyelopathy, familial constitutional 284.09
Panmyelophthisis 284.2
   acquired (secondary) 284.81
   congenital 284.2
   idiopathic 284.9
Panmyelosis (acute) (M9951/1) 238.79
Panner's disease 732.3
   capitellum humeri 732.3
   head of humerus 732.3
   tarsal navicular (bone) (osteochondrosis) 732.5
Panneuritis endemica 265.0 *[357.4]*
Panniculitis 729.30
   back 724.8
   knee 729.31
   mesenteric 567.82
   neck 723.6
   nodular, nonsuppurative 729.30
   sacral 724.8
   specified site NEC 729.39
Panniculus adiposus (abdominal) 278.1
Pannus (corneal) 370.62
   abdominal (symptomatic) 278.1
   allergic eczematous 370.62
   degenerativus 370.62
   keratic 370.62
   rheumatoid—*see* Arthritis, rheumatoid
   trachomatosus, trachomatous (active) 076.1 *[370.62]*
      late effect 139.1
Panophthalmitis 360.02
Panotitis —*see* Otitis media
Pansinusitis (chronic) (hyperplastic) (nonpurulent) (purulent) 473.8
   acute 461.8
   due to fungus NEC 117.9
   tuberculous (*see also* Tuberculosis) 012.8
Panuveitis 360.12
   sympathetic 360.11
Panvalvular disease —*see* Endocarditis, mitral
Papageienkrankheit 073.9
Papanicolaou smear
   cervix (screening test) V76.2
   as part of gynecological examination V72.31
   for suspected malignant neoplasm V76.2
      no disease found V71.1
   inadequate sample 795.08
   nonspecific abnormal finding 795.00
      with
         atypical squamous cells—changes of undetermined significance
            cannot exclude high grade squamous intraepithelial lesion (ASC-H) 795.02
            of undetermined significance (ASC-US) 795.01
         cytologic evidence of malignancy 795.06

Papanicolaou smear—*continued*
         high grade squamous intraepithelial lesion (HGSIL) 795.04
         low grade squamous intraepithelial lesion (LGSIL) 795.03
         nonspecific finding NEC 795.09
         to confirm findings of recent normal smear following initial abnormal smear V72.32
   unsatisfactory 795.08
   other specified site—*see also* Screening, malignant neoplasm
      for suspected malignant neoplasm—*see also* Screening, malignant neoplasm
         no disease found V71.1
   nonspecific abnormal finding 795.1
   vagina V76.47
      following hysterectomy for malignant condition V67.01
Papilledema 377.00
   associated with
      decreased ocular pressure 377.02
      increased intracranial pressure 377.01
      retinal disorder 377.03
   choked disc 377.00
   infectional 377.00
Papillitis 377.31
   anus 569.49
   chronic lingual 529.4
   necrotizing, kidney 584.7
   optic 377.31
   rectum 569.49
   renal, necrotizing 584.7
   tongue 529.0
Papilloma (M8050/0)—*see also* Neoplasm, by site, benign

> *Note*—Except where otherwise indicated, the morphological varieties of papilloma in the list below should be coded by site as for "Neoplasm, benign."

   acuminatum (female) (male) 078.11
   bladder (urinary) (transitional cell) (M8120/1) 236.7
      benign (M8120/0) 223.3
   choroid plexus (M9390/0) 225.0
      anaplastic type (M9390/3) 191.5
      malignant (M9390/3) 191.5
   ductal (M8503/0)
   dyskeratotic (M8052/0)
   epidermoid (M8052/0)
   hyperkeratotic (M8052/0)
   intracystic (M8504/0)
   intraductal (M8503/0)
   inverted (M8053/0)
   keratotic (M8052/0)
   parakeratotic (M8052/0)
   pinta (primary) 103.0
   renal pelvis (transitional cell) (M8120/1) 236.99
      benign (M8120/0) 223.1
   Schneiderian (M8121/0)
      specified site—*see* Neoplasm, by site, benign
      unspecified site 212.0
   serous surface (M8461/0)
      borderline malignancy (M8461/1)
         specified site—*see* Neoplasm, by site, uncertain behavior
         unspecified site 236.2
      specified site—*see* Neoplasm, by site, benign
      unspecified site 220
   squamous (cell) (M8052/0)

INDEX TO DISEASES   **Paralysis, paralytic**

Papilloma—*continued*
  transitional (cell) (M8120/0)
    bladder (urinary) (M8120/1) 236.7
    inverted type (M8121/1)—*see* Neoplasm, by site, uncertain behavior
    renal pelvis (M8120/1) 236.91
    ureter (M8120/1) 236.91
  ureter (transitional cell) (M8120/1) 236.91
    benign (M8120/0) 223.2
  urothelial (M8120/1)—*see* Neoplasm, by site, uncertain behavior
  verrucous (M8051/0)
  villous (M8261/1)—*see* Neoplasm, by site, uncertain behavior
  yaws, plantar or palmar 102.1
Papillomata, multiple, of yaws 102.1
Papillomatosis (M8060/0)—*see also* Neoplasm, by site, benign
  confluent and reticulate 701.8
  cutaneous 701.8
  ductal, breast 610.1
  Gougerot-Carteaud (confluent reticulate) 701.8
  intraductal (diffuse) (M8505/0)—*see* Neoplasm, by site, benign
  subareolar duct (M8506/0) 217
Papillon-Léage and Psaume syndrome (orodigitofacial dysostosis) 759.89
Papule 709.8
  carate (primary) 103.0
  fibrous, of nose (M8724/0) 216.3
  pinta (primary) 103.0
Papulosis, malignant 447.8
Papyraceous fetus 779.89
  complicating pregnancy 646.0
Paracephalus 759.7
Parachute mitral valve 746.5
Paracoccidioidomycosis 116.1
  mucocutaneous-lymphangitic 116.1
  pulmonary 116.1
  visceral 116.1
Paracoccidiomycosis —*see* Paracoccidioidomycosis
Paracusis 388.40
Paradentosis 523.5
Paradoxical facial movements 374.43
Paraffinoma 999.9
Paraganglioma (M8680/1)
  adrenal (M8700/0) 227.0
    malignant (M8700/3) 194.0
  aortic body (M8691/1) 237.3
    malignant (M8691/3) 194.6
  carotid body (M8692/1) 237.3
    malignant (M8692/3) 194.5
  chromaffin (M8700/0)—*see also* Neoplasm, by site, benign
    malignant (M8700/3)—*see* Neoplasm, by site, malignant
  extra-adrenal (M8693/1)
    malignant (M8693/3)
      specified site—*see* Neoplasm, by site, malignant
      unspecified site 194.6
    specified site—*see* Neoplasm, by site, uncertain behavior
    unspecified site 237.3
  glomus jugulare (M8690/1) 237.3
    malignant (M8690/3) 194.6
  jugular (M8690/1) 237.3
    malignant (M8680/3)
      specified site—*see* Neoplasm, by site, malignant

Paraganglioma—*continued*
      unspecified site 194.6
  nonchromaffin (M8693/1)
    malignant (M8693/3)
      specified site—*see* Neoplasm, by site, malignant
      unspecified site 194.6
    specified site—*see* Neoplasm, by site, uncertain behavior
    unspecified site 237.3
  parasympathetic (M8682/1)
    specified site—*see* Neoplasm, by site, uncertain behavior
    unspecified site 237.3
  specified site—*see* Neoplasm, by site, uncertain behavior
  sympathetic (M8681/1)
    specified site—*see* Neoplasm, by site, uncertain behavior
    unspecified site 237.3
  unspecified site 237.3
Parageusia 781.1
  psychogenic 306.7
Paragonimiasis 121.2
Paragranuloma, Hodgkin's (M9660/3) 201.0
Parahemophilia (*see also* Defect, coagulation) 286.3
Parakeratosis 690.8
  psoriasiformis 696.2
  variegata 696.2
Paralysis, paralytic (complete) (incomplete) 344.9
  with
    broken
      back—*see* Fracture, vertebra, by site, with spinal cord injury
      neck—*see* Fracture, vertebra, cervical, with spinal cord injury
    fracture, vertebra—*see* Fracture, vertebra, by site, with spinal cord injury
    syphilis 094.89
  abdomen and back muscles 355.9
  abdominal muscles 355.9
  abducens (nerve) 378.54
  abductor 355.9
    lower extremity 355.8
    upper extremity 354.9
  accessory nerve 352.4
  accommodation 367.51
    hysterical 300.11
  acoustic nerve 388.5
  agitans 332.0
    arteriosclerotic 332.0
  alternating 344.89
    oculomotor 344.89
  amyotrophic 335.20
  ankle 355.8
  anterior serratus 355.9
  anus (sphincter) 569.49
  apoplectic (current episode) (*see also* Disease, cerebrovascular, acute) 436
    late effect—*see* Late effect(s) (of) cerebrovascular disease category 438
  arm 344.40
    affecting
      dominant side 344.41
      nondominant side 344.42
    both 344.2
    due to old CVA—*see* Category 438
    hysterical 300.11

Paralysis, paralytic—*continued*
late effect—*see* Late effect(s) (of) cerebrovascular disease
psychogenic 306.0
transient 781.4
  traumatic NDC (*see also* Injury, nerve, upper limb) 955.9
arteriosclerotic (current episode) 437.0
  late effect—*see* Late effect(s) (of) cerebrovascular disease
ascending (spinal), acute 357.0
associated, nuclear 344.89
asthenic bulbar 358.00
ataxic NEC 334.9
  general 094.1
athetoid 333.71
atrophic 356.9
  infantile, acute (*see also* Poliomyelitis, with paralysis) 045.1
  muscle NEC 355.9
  progressive 335.21
  spinal (acute) (*see also* Poliomyelitis, with paralysis) 045.1
attack (*see also* Disease, cerebrovascular, acute) 436
axillary 353.0
Babinski-Nageotte's 344.89
Bell's 351.0
  newborn 767.5
Benedikt's 344.89
birth (injury) 767.7
  brain 767.0
  intracranial 767.0
  spinal cord 767.4
bladder (sphincter) 596.53
  neurogenic 596.54
    with cauda equina syndrome 344.61
  puerperal, postpartum, childbirth 665.5
  sensory 596.54
    with cauda equina 344.61
  spastic 596.54
    with cauda equina 344.61
bowel, colon, or intestine (*see also* Ileus) 560.1
brachial plexus 353.0
  due to birth injury 767.6
  newborn 767.6
brain
  congenital—*see* Palsy, cerebral
  current episode 437.8
  diplegia 344.2
  due to previous vascular lesion—*see* category 438
  hemiplegia 342.9
    due to previous vascular lesion—*see* category 438
    late effect—*see* Late effect(s) (of) cerebrovascular disease
  infantile—*see* Palsy, cerebral
  late effect—*see* Late effect(s) (of) cerebrovascular disease
  monoplegia—*see also* Monoplegia
    due to previous vascular lesion—*see* category 438
    late effect—*see* Late effect(s) (of) cerebrovascular disease
  paraplegia 344.1
  quadriplegia —*see* Quadriplegia
  syphilitic, congenital 090.49
  triplegia 344.89
bronchi 519.19
Brown-Séquard's 344.89

Paralysis, paralytic—*continued*
bulbar (chronic) (progressive) 335.22
  infantile (*see also* Poliomyelitis, bulbar) 045.0
  poliomyelitic (*see also* Poliomyelitis, bulbar) 045.0
  pseudo 335.23
  supranuclear 344.89
bulbospinal 358.00
cardiac (*see also* Failure, heart) 428.9
cerebral
  current episode 437.8
  spastic, infantile—*see* Palsy, cerebral
cerebrocerebellar 437.8
  diplegic infantile 343.0
cervical
  plexus 353.2
  sympathetic NEC 337.0
Céstan-Chenais 344.89
Charcot-Marie-Tooth type 356.1
childhood—*see* Palsy, cerebral
Clark's 343.9
colon (*see also* Ileus) 560.1
compressed air 993.3
compression
  arm NEC 354.9
  cerebral—*see* Paralysis, brain
  leg NEC 355.8
  lower extremity NEC 355.8
  upper extremity NEC 354.9
congenital (cerebral) (spastic) (spinal)—*see* Palsy, cerebral
conjugate movement (of eye) 378.81
cortical (nuclear) (supranuclear) 378.81
convergence 378.83
cordis (*see also* Failure, heart) 428.9
cortical (*see also* Paralysis, brain) 437.8
cranial or cerebral nerve (*see also* Disorder, nerve, cranial) 352.9
creeping 335.21
crossed leg 344.89
crutch 953.4
deglutition 784.99
  hysterical 300.11
dementia 094.1
descending (spinal) NEC 335.9
diaphragm (flaccid) 519.4
  due to accidental section of phrenic nerve during procedure 998.2
digestive organs NEC 564.89
diplegic—*see* Diplegia
divergence (nuclear) 378.85
divers' 993.3
Duchenne's 335.22
due to intracranial or spinal birth injury—*see* Palsy, cerebral
embolic (current episode) (*see also* Embolism, brain) 434.1
  late effect —*see* Late effect(s) (of) cerebrovascular disease
enteric (*see also* Ileus) 560.1
  with hernia—*see* Hernia, by site, with obstruction
Erb's syphilitic spastic spinal 094.89
Erb (-Duchenne) (birth) (newborn) 767.6
esophagus 530.89
essential, infancy (*see also* Poliomyelitis) 045.9
extremity
  lower —*see* Paralysis, leg
  spastic (hereditary) 343.3
    noncongenital or noninfantile 344.1
  transient (cause unknown) 781.4
  upper —*see* Paralysis, arm

INDEX TO DISEASES

Paralysis, paralytic

Paralysis, paralytic—*continued*
  eye muscle (extrinsic) 378.55
    intrinsic 367.51
  facial (nerve) 351.0
    birth injury 767.5
    congenital 767.5
    following operation NEC 998.2
    newborn 767.5
  familial 359.3
    periodic 359.3
    spastic 334.1
  fauces 478.29
  finger NEC 354.9
  foot NEC 355.8
  gait 781.2
  gastric nerve 352.3
  gaze 378.81
  general 094.1
    ataxic 094.1
    insane 094.1
    juvenile 090.40
    progressive 094.1
    tabetic 094.1
  glossopharyngeal (nerve) 352.2
  glottis (*see also* Paralysis, vocal cord) 478.30
  gluteal 353.4
  Gubler (-Millard) 344.89
  hand 354.9
    hysterical 300.11
    psychogenic 306.0
  heart (*see also* Failure, heart) 428.9
  hemifacial, progressive 349.89
  hemiplegic—*see* Hemiplegia
  hyperkalemic periodic (familial) 359.3
  hypertensive (current episode) 437.8
  hypoglossal (nerve) 352.5
  hypokalemic periodic 359.3
  Hyrtl's sphincter (rectum) 569.49
  hysterical 300.11
  ileus (*see also* Ileus) 560.1
  infantile (*see also* Poliomyelitis) 045.9
    atrophic acute 045.1
    bulbar 045.0
    cerebral—*see* Palsy, cerebral
    paralytic 045.1
    progressive acute 045.9
    spastic—*see* Palsy, cerebral
    spinal 045.9
  infective (*see also* Poliomyelitis) 045.9
  inferior nuclear 344.9
  insane, general or progressive 094.1
  internuclear 378.86
  interosseous 355.9
  intestine (*see also* Ileus) 560.1
  intracranial (current episode) (*see also* Paralysis, brain) 437.8
    due to birth injury 767.0
  iris 379.49
    due to diphtheria (toxin) 032.81 *[379.49]*
  ischemic, Volkmann's (complicating trauma) 958.6
  isolated sleep, recurrent 327.43
  Jackson's 344.89
  jake 357.7
  Jamaica ginger (jake) 357.7
  juvenile general 090.40
  Klumpke (-Déjérine) (birth) (newborn) 767.6
  labioglossal (laryngeal) (pharyngeal) 335.22
  Landry's 357.0
  laryngeal nerve (recurrent) (superior) (*see also* Paralysis, vocal cord) 478.30
  larynx (*see also* Paralysis, vocal cord) 478.30

Paralysis, paralytic—*continued*
  due to diphtheria (toxin) 032.3
  late effect
    due to
      birth injury, brain or spinal (cord)—*see* Palsy, cerebral
      edema, brain or cerebral—*see* Paralysis, brain
      lesion
        cerebrovascular—*see* category 438
        late effect—*see* Late effect(s) (of) cerebrovascular disease
      spinal (cord)—*see* Paralysis, spinal
  lateral 335.24
  lead 984.9
    specified type of lead—*see* Table of drugs and chemicals
  left side—*see* Hemiplegia
  leg 344.30
    affecting
      dominant side 344.31
      nondominant side 344.32
    both (*see also* Paraplegia) 344.1
    crossed 344.89
    hysterical 300.11
    psychogenic 306.0
    transient or transitory 781.4
      traumatic NEC (*see also* Injury, nerve, lower limb) 956.9
  levator palpebrae superioris 374.31
  limb NEC 344.5
    all four—*see* Quadriplegia
    quadriplegia—*see* Quadriplegia
  lip 528.5
  Lissauer's 094.1
  local 355.9
  lower limb—*see also* Paralysis, leg
    both (*see also* Paraplegia) 344.1
  lung 518.89
    newborn 770.89
  median nerve 354.1
  medullary (tegmental) 344.89
  mesencephalic NEC 344.89
    tegmental 344.89
  middle alternating 344.89
  Millard-Gubler-Foville 344.89
  monoplegic—*see* Monoplegia
  motor NEC 344.9
    cerebral—*see* Paralysis, brain
    spinal—*see* Paralysis, spinal
  multiple
    cerebral—*see* Paralysis, brain
    spinal—*see* Paralysis, spinal
  muscle (flaccid) 359.9
    due to nerve lesion NEC 355.9
    eye (extrinsic) 378.55
      intrinsic 367.51
      oblique 378.51
    iris sphincter 364.89
    ischemic (complicating trauma) (Volkmann's) 958.6
    pseudohypertrophic 359.1
  muscular (atrophic) 359.9
    progressive 335.21
  musculocutaneous nerve 354.9
  musculospiral 354.9
  nerve—*see also* Disorder, nerve
    third or oculomotor (partial) 378.51
      total 378.52
    fourth or trochlear 378.53
    sixth or abducens 378.54

Paralysis, paralytic — INDEX TO DISEASES

Paralysis, paralytic—*continued*
　seventh or facial 351.0
　　birth injury 767.5
　　due to
　　　injection NEC 999.9
　　　operation NEC 997.09
　　newborn 767.5
　accessory 352.4
　auditory 388.5
　birth injury 767.7
　cranial or cerebral (*see also* Disorder, nerve, cranial) 352.9
　facial 351.0
　　birth injury 767.5
　　newborn 767.5
　laryngeal (*see also* Paralysis, vocal cord) 478.30
　newborn 767.7
　phrenic 354.8
　　newborn 767.7
　radial 354.3
　　birth injury 767.6
　　newborn 767.6
　syphilitic 094.89
　traumatic NEC (*see also* Injury, nerve, by site) 957.9
　trigeminal 350.9
　ulnar 354.2
　newborn NEC 767.0
　normokalemic periodic 359.3
　obstetrical, newborn 767.7
　ocular 378.9
　oculofacial, congenital 352.6
　oculomotor (nerve) (partial) 378.51
　　alternating 344.89
　　external bilateral 378.55
　　total 378.52
　olfactory nerve 352.0
　palate 528.9
　palatopharyngolaryngeal 352.6
　paratrigeminal 350.9
　periodic (familial) (hyperkalemic) (hypokalemic) (normokalemic) (potassium sensitive) (secondary) 359.3
　peripheral
　　autonomic nervous system—*see* Neuropathy, peripheral, autonomic
　　nerve NEC 355.9
　peroneal (nerve) 355.3
　pharynx 478.29
　phrenic nerve 354.8
　plantar nerves 355.6
　pneumogastric nerve 352.3
　poliomyelitis (current) (*see also* Poliomyelitis, with paralysis) 045.1
　　bulbar 045.0
　popliteal nerve 355.3
　pressure (*see also* Neuropathy, entrapment) 355.9
　progressive 335.21
　　atrophic 335.21
　　bulbar 335.22
　　general 094.1
　　hemifacial 349.89
　　infantile, acute (*see also* Poliomyelitis) 045.9
　　multiple 335.20
　pseudobulbar 335.23
　pseudohypertrophic 359.1
　　muscle 359.1
　psychogenic 306.0
　pupil, pupillary 379.49
　quadriceps 355.8

Paralysis, paralytic—*continued*
　quadriplegic (*see also* Quadriplegia) 344.0
　radial nerve 354.3
　　birth injury 767.6
　rectum (sphincter) 569.49
　rectus muscle (eye) 378.55
　recurrent
　　isolated sleep 327.43
　　laryngeal nerve (*see also* Paralysis, vocal cord) 478.30
　respiratory (muscle) (system) (tract) 786.09
　　center NEC 344.89
　　　fetus or newborn 770.87
　　congenital 768.9
　　newborn 768.9
　right side—*see* Hemiplegia
　Saturday night 354.3
　saturnine 984.9
　　specified type of lead—*see* Table of drugs and chemicals
　sciatic nerve 355.0
　secondary—*see* Paralysis, late effect
　seizure (cerebral) (current episode) (*see also* Disease, cerebrovascular, acute) 436
　　late effect—*see* Late effect(s) (of) cerebrovascular disease
　senile NEC 344.9
　serratus magnus 355.9
　shaking (*see also* Parkinsonism) 332.0
　shock (*see also* Disease, cerebrovascular, acute) 436
　　late effect—*see* Late effect(s) (of) cerebrovascular disease
　shoulder 354.9
　soft palate 528.9
　spasmodic—*see* Paralysis, spastic
　spastic 344.9
　　cerebral infantile—*see* Palsy, cerebral
　　congenital (cerebral)—*see* Palsy, cerebral
　　familial 334.1
　　hereditary 334.1
　　infantile 343.9
　　noncongenital or noninfantile, cerebral 344.9
　　syphilitic 094.0
　　spinal 094.89
　sphincter, bladder (*see also* Paralysis, bladder) 596.53
　spinal (cord) NEC 344.1
　　accessory nerve 352.4
　　acute (*see also* Poliomyelitis) 045.9
　　ascending acute 357.0
　　atrophic (acute) (*see also* Poliomyelitis, with paralysis) 045.1
　　　spastic, syphilitic 094.89
　　congenital NEC 343.9
　　hemiplegic —*see* Hemiplegia
　　hereditary 336.8
　　infantile (*see also* Poliomyelitis) 045.9
　　late effect NEC 344.89
　　monoplegic—*see* Monoplegia
　　nerve 355.9
　　progressive 335.10
　　quadriplegic —*see* Quadriplegia
　　spastic NEC 343.9
　　traumatic—*see* Injury, spinal, by site
　sternomastoid 352.4
　stomach 536.3
　　nerve (nondiabetic) 352.3
　stroke (current episode) *see* Infarct, brain
　　late effect—*see* Late effect(s) (of) cerebrovascular disease

1246

INDEX TO DISEASES

Paralysis, paralytic—*continued*
  subscapularis 354.8
  superior nuclear NEC 334.9
  supranuclear 356.8
  sympathetic
    cervical NEC 337.0
    nerve NEC (*see also* Neuropathy, peripheral, autonomic) 337.9
    nervous system—*see* Neuropathy, peripheral, autonomic
  syndrome 344.9
    specified NEC 344.89
  syphilitic spastic spinal (Erb's) 094.89
  tabetic general 094.1
  thigh 355.8
  throat 478.29
    diphtheritic 032.0
    muscle 478.29
  thrombotic (current episode) (*see also* Thrombosis, brain) 434.0
    late effect—*see* Late effect(s) (of) cerebrovascular disease
  thumb NEC 354.9
  tick (-bite) 989.5
  Todd's (postepileptic transitory paralysis) 344.89
  toe 355.6
  tongue 529.8
  transient
    arm or leg NEC 781.4
    traumatic NEC (*see also* Injury, nerve, by site) 957.9
  trapezius 352.4
  traumatic, transient NEC (*see also* Injury, nerve, by site) 957.9
  trembling (*see also* Parkinsonism) 332.0
  triceps brachii 354.9
  trigeminal nerve 350.9
  trochlear nerve 378.53
  ulnar nerve 354.2
  upper limb —*see also* Paralysis, arm
    both (*see also* Diplegia) 344.2
  uremic—*see* Uremia
  uveoparotitic 135
  uvula 528.9
    hysterical 300.11
    postdiphtheritic 032.0
  vagus nerve 352.3
  vasomotor NEC 337.9
  velum palati 528.9
  vesical (*see also* Paralysis, bladder) 596.53
  vestibular nerve 388.5
  visual field, psychic 368.16
  vocal cord 478.30
    bilateral (partial) 478.33
      complete 478.34
    complete (bilateral) 478.34
    unilateral (partial) 478.31
      complete 478.32
  Volkmann's (complicating trauma) 958.6
  wasting 335.21
  Weber's 344.89
  wrist NEC 354.9
Paramedial orifice, urethrovesical 753.8
Paramenia 626.9
Parametritis (chronic) (*see also* Disease, pelvis, inflammatory) 614.4
  acute 614.3
  puerperal, postpartum, childbirth 670
Parametrium, parametric —*see* condition
Paramnesia (*see also* Amnesia) 780.93

Paraplegia

Paramolar 520.1
  causing crowding 524.31
Paramyloidosis 277.30
Paramyoclonus multiplex 333.2
Paramyotonia 359.29
  congenita (of von Eulenburg) 359.29
Paraneoplastic syndrome —*see* condition
Parangi (*see also* Yaws) 102.9
Paranoia 297.1
  alcoholic 291.5
  querulans 297.8
  senile 290.20
Paranoid
  dementia (*see also* Schizophrenia) 295.3
    praecox (acute) 295.3
    senile 290.20
  personality 301.0
  psychosis 297.9
    alcoholic 291.5
    climacteric 297.2
    drug-induced 292.11
    involutional 297.2
    menopausal 297.2
    protracted reactive 298.4
    psychogenic 298.4
      acute 298.3
    senile 290.20
  reaction (chronic) 297.9
    acute 298.3
  schizophrenia (acute) (*see also* Schizophrenia) 295.3
  state 297.9
    alcohol-induced 291.5
    climacteric 297.2
    drug-induced 292.11
    due to or associated with
      arteriosclerosis (cerebrovascular) 290.42
      presenile brain disease 290.12
      senile brain disease 290.20
    involutional 297.2
    menopausal 297.2
    senile 290.20
    simple 297.0
    specified type NEC 297.8
  tendencies 301.0
  traits 301.0
  trends 301.0
  type, psychopathic personality 301.0
Paraparesis (*see also* Paraplegia) 344.1
Paraphasia 784.3
Paraphilia (*see also* Deviation, sexual) 302.9
Paraphimosis (congenital) 605
  chancroidal 099.0
Paraphrenia, paraphrenic (late) 297.2
  climacteric 297.2
  dementia (*see also* Schizophrenia) 295.3
  involutional 297.2
  menopausal 297.2
  schizophrenia (acute) (*see also* Schizophrenia) 295.3
Paraplegia 344.1
  with
    broken back—*see* Fracture, vertebra, by site, with spinal cord injury
    fracture, vertebra—*see* Fracture, vertebra, by site, with spinal cord injury
  ataxic—*see* Degeneration, combined, spinal cord
  brain (current episode) (*see also* Paralysis, brain) 437.8

Paraplegia—*continued*
  cerebral (current episode) (*see also* Paralysis, brain) 437.8
  congenital or infantile (cerebral) (spastic) (spinal) 343.0
  cortical—*see* Paralysis, brain
  familial spastic 334.1
  functional (hysterical) 300.11
  hysterical 300.11
  infantile 343.0
  late effect 344.1
  Pott's (*see also* Tuberculosis) 015.0 [730.88]
  psychogenic 306.0
  spastic
    Erb's spinal 094.89
    hereditary 334.1
    not infantile or congenital 344.1
  spinal (cord)
    traumatic NEC—*see* Injury, spinal, by site
  syphilitic (spastic) 094.89
  traumatic NEC—*see* Injury, spinal, by site
Paraproteinemia 273.2
  benign (familial) 273.1
  monoclonal 273.1
  secondary to malignant or inflammatory disease 273.1
Parapsoriasis 696.2
  en plaques 696.2
  guttata 696.2
  lichenoides chronica 696.2
  retiformis 696.2
  varioliformis (acuta) 696.2
Parascarlatina 057.8
Parasitic —*see also* condition
  disease NEC (*see also* Infestation, parasitic) 136.9
    contact V01.89
    exposure to V01.89
    intestinal NEC 129
    skin NEC 134.9
  stomatitis 112.0
  sycosis 110.0
    beard 110.0
    scalp 110.0
  twin 759.4
Parasitism NEC 136.9
  intestinal NEC 129
  skin NEC 134.9
  specified—*see* Infestation
Parasitophobia 300.29
Parasomnia 307.47
  alcohol induced 291.82
  drug induced 292.85
  nonorganic origin 307.47
  organic 327.40
    in conditions classified elsewhere 327.44
    other 327.49
Paraspadias 752.69
Paraspasm facialis 351.8
Parathyroid gland —*see* condition
Parathyroiditis (autoimmune) 252.1
Parathyroprival tetany 252.1
Paratrachoma 077.0
Paratyphilitis (*see also* Appendicitis) 541
Paratyphoid (fever)—*see* Fever, paratyphoid
Paratyphus —*see* Fever, paratyphoid
Paraurethral duct 753.8
Para-urethritis 597.89
  gonococcal (acute) 098.0
    chronic or duration of 2 months or over 098.2

Paravaccinia NEC 051.9
  milkers' node 051.1
Paravaginitis (*see also* Vaginitis) 616.10
Parencephalitis (*see also* Encephalitis) 323.9
  late effect—*see* category 326
Parergasia 298.9
Paresis (*see also* Paralysis) 344.9
  accommodation 367.51
  bladder (spastic) (sphincter) (*see also* Paralysis, bladder) 596.53
    tabetic 094.0
  bowel, colon, or intestine (*see also* Ileus) 560.1
  brain or cerebral—*see* Paralysis, brain
  extrinsic muscle, eye 378.55
  general 094.1
    arrested 094.1
    brain 094.1
    cerebral 094.1
    insane 094.1
    juvenile 090.40
      remission 090.49
    progressive 094.1
    remission (sustained) 094.1
    tabetic 094.1
  heart (*see also* Failure, heart) 428.9
  infantile (*see also* Poliomyelitis) 045.9
  insane 094.1
  juvenile 090.40
  late effect—*see* Paralysis, late effect
  luetic (general) 094.1
  peripheral progressive 356.9
  pseudohypertrophic 359.1
  senile NEC 344.9
  stomach 536.3
  syphilitic (general) 094.1
    congenital 090.40
  transient, limb 781.4
  vesical (sphincter) NEC 596.53
Paresthesia (*see also* Disturbance, sensation) 782.0
  Berger's (paresthesia of lower limb) 782.0
  Bernhardt 355.1
  Magnan's 782.0
Paretic —*see* condition
Parinaud's
  conjunctivitis 372.02
  oculoglandular syndrome 372.02
  ophthalmoplegia 378.81
  syndrome (paralysis of conjugate upward gaze) 378.81
Parkes Weber and Dimitri syndrome (encephalocutaneous angiomatosis) 759.6
Parkinson's disease, syndrome, or tremor —*see* Parkinsonism
Parkinsonism (arteriosclerotic) (idiopathic) (primary) 332.0
  associated with orthostatic hypotension (idiopathic) (symptomatic) 333.0
  due to drugs 332.1
  neuroleptic-induced 332.1
  secondary 332.1
  syphilitic 094.82
Parodontitis 523.40
Parodontosis 523.5
Paronychia (with lymphangitis) 681.9
  candidal (chronic) 112.3
  chronic 681.9
    candidal 112.3
    finger 681.02
    toe 681.11
  finger 681.02

INDEX TO DISEASES   **Pediculosis**

Paronychia—*continued*
   toe 681.11
   tuberculous (primary) (*see also* Tuberculosis) 017.0
Parorexia NEC 307.52
   hysterical 300.11
Parosmia 781.1
   psychogenic 306.7
Parotid gland —*see* condition
Parotiditis (*see also* Parotitis) 527.2
   epidemic 072.9
   infectious 072.9
Parotitis 527.2
   allergic 527.2
   chronic 527.2
   epidemic (*see also* Mumps) 072.9
   infectious (*see also* Mumps) 072.9
   noninfectious 527.2
   nonspecific toxic 527.2
   not mumps 527.2
   postoperative 527.2
   purulent 527.2
   septic 527.2
   suppurative (acute) 527.2
   surgical 527.2
   toxic 527.2
Paroxysmal —*see also* condition
   dyspnea (nocturnal) 786.09
Parrot's disease (syphilitic osteochondritis) 090.0
Parrot fever 073.9
Parry's disease or syndrome (exophthalmic goiter) 242.0
Parry-Romberg syndrome 349.89
Parson's disease (exophthalmic goiter) 242.0
Parsonage-Aldren-Turner syndrome 353.5
Parsonage-Turner syndrome 353.5
Pars planitis 363.21
Particolored infant 757.39
Parturition —*see* Delivery
Parvovirus 079.83
   B19 079.83
   human 079.83
Passage
   false, urethra 599.4
   meconium noted during delivery 763.84
   of sounds or bougies (*see also* Attention to artificial opening) V55.9
Passive —*see* condition
Pasteurella septica 027.2
Pasteurellosis (*see also* Infection, Pasteurella) 027.2
PAT (paroxysmal atrial tachycardia) 427.0
Patau's syndrome (trisomy D_1) 758.1
Patch
   herald 696.3
Patches
   mucous (syphilitic) 091.3
      congenital 090.0
   smokers' (mouth) 528.6
Patellar —*see* condition
Patellofemoral syndrome 719.46
Patent —*see also* Imperfect closure
   atrioventricular ostium 745.69
   canal of Nuck 752.41
   cervix 622.5
      complicating pregnancy 654.5
         affecting fetus or newborn 761.0
   ductus arteriosus or Botalli 747.0

Patent—*continued*
   Eustachian
      tube 381.7
      valve 746.89
   foramen
      Botalli 745.5
      ovale 745.5
   interauricular septum 745.5
   interventricular septum 745.4
   omphalomesenteric duct 751.0
   os (uteri)—*see* Patent, cervix
   ostium secundum 745.5
   urachus 753.7
   vitelline duct 751.0
Paternity testing V70.4
Paterson's syndrome (sideropenic dysphagia) 280.8
Paterson (-Brown) (-Kelly) **syndrome** (sideropenic dysphagia) 280.8
Paterson-Kelly syndrome or web (sideropenic dysphagia) 280.8
Pathologic, pathological —*see also* condition
   asphyxia 799.01
   drunkenness 291.4
   emotionality 301.3
   liar 301.7
   personality 301.9
   resorption, tooth 521.40
      external 521.42
      internal 521.41
      specified NEC 521.49
   sexuality (*see also* Deviation, sexual) 302.9
Pathology (of)—*see also* Disease
   periradicular, associated with previous endodontic treatment 526.69
Patterned motor discharges, idiopathic (*see also* Epilepsy) 345.5
Patulous —*see also* Patent
   anus 569.49
   Eustachian tube 381.7
Pause, sinoatrial 427.81
Pavor nocturnus 307.46
Pavy's disease 593.6
Paxton's disease (white piedra) 111.2
Payr's disease or syndrome (splenic flexure syndrome) 569.89
PBA (pseudobulbar affect) 310.8
Pearls
   Elschnig 366.51
   enamel 520.2
Pearl-workers' disease (chronic osteomyelitis) (*see also* Osteomyelitis) 730.1
Pectenitis 569.49
Pectenosis 569.49
Pectoral —*see* condition
Pectus
   carinatum (congenital) 754.82
      acquired 738.3
      rachitic (*see also* Rickets) 268.0
   excavatum (congenital) 754.81
      acquired 738.3
      rachitic (*see also* Rickets) 268.0
   recurvatum (congenital) 754.81
      acquired 738.3
Pedatrophia 261
Pederosis 302.2
Pediculosis (infestation) 132.9
   capitis (head louse) (any site) 132.0
   corporis (body louse) (any site) 132.1
   eyelid 132.0 *[373.6]*

Pediculosis—*continued*
  mixed (classifiable to more than one category in 132.0-132.2) 132.3
  pubis (pubic louse) (any site) 132.2
  vestimenti 132.1
  vulvae 132.2
Pediculus (infestation)—*see* Pediculosis
Pedophilia 302.2
Peg-shaped teeth 520.2
Pel's crisis 094.0
Pel-Ebstein disease —*see* Disease, Hodgkin's
Pelade 704.01
Pelger-Huët anomaly or syndrome (hereditary hyposegmentation) 288.2
Peliosis (rheumatica) 287.0
Pelizaeus-Merzbacher
  disease 330.0
  sclerosis, diffuse cerebral 330.0
Pellagra (alcoholic or with alcoholism) 265.2
  with polyneuropathy 265.2 *[357.4]*
Pellagra-cerebellar-ataxia-renal aminoaciduria syndrome 270.0
Pellegrini's disease (calcification, knee joint) 726.62
Pellegrini (-Stieda) disease or syndrome (calcification, knee joint) 726.62
Pellizzi's syndrome (pineal) 259.8
Pelvic —*see also* condition
  congestion-fibrosis syndrome 625.5
  kidney 753.3
Pelvioectasis 591
Pelviolithiasis 592.0
Pelviperitonitis
  female (*see also* Peritonitis, pelvic, female) 614.5
  male (*see also* Peritonitis) 567.21
Pelvis, pelvic —*see also* condition or type
  infantile 738.6
  Nägele's 738.6
  obliquity 738.6
  Robert's 755.69
Pemphigoid 694.5
  benign, mucous membrane 694.60
    with ocular involvement 694.61
  bullous 694.5
  cicatricial 694.60
    with ocular involvement 694.61
  juvenile 694.2
Pemphigus 694.4
  benign 694.5
    chronic familial 757.39
  Brazilian 694.4
  circinatus 694.0
  congenital, traumatic 757.39
  conjunctiva 694.61
  contagiosus 684
  erythematodes 694.4
  erythematosus 694.4
  foliaceus 694.4
  frambesiodes 694.4
  gangrenous (*see also* Gangrene) 785.4
  malignant 694.4
  neonatorum, newborn 684
  ocular 694.61
  papillaris 694.4
  seborrheic 694.4
  South American 694.4
  syphilitic (congenital) 090.0
  vegetans 694.4
  vulgaris 694.4
  wildfire 694.4

Pendred's syndrome (familial goiter with deaf-mutism) 243
Pendulous
  abdomen 701.9
    in pregnancy or childbirth 654.4
      affecting fetus or newborn 763.89
  breast 611.8
Penetrating wound —*see also* Wound, open, by site
  with internal injury—*see* Injury, internal, by site, with open wound
  eyeball 871.7
    with foreign body (nonmagnetic) 871.6
      magnetic 871.5
    ocular (*see also* Penetrating wound, eyeball) 871.7
    adnexa 870.3
      with foreign body 870.4
    orbit 870.3
      with foreign body 870.4
Penetration, pregnant uterus by instrument
  with
    abortion—*see* Abortion, by type, with damage to pelvic organs
    ectopic pregnancy (*see also* categories 633.0-633.9) 639.2
    molar pregnancy (*see also* categories 630-632) 639.2
  complication of delivery 665.1
    affecting fetus or newborn 763.89
  following
    abortion 639.2
    ectopic or molar pregnancy 639.2
Penfield's syndrome (*see also* Epilepsy) 345.5
Penicilliosis of lung 117.3
Penis —*see* condition
Penitis 607.2
Penta X syndrome 758.81
Pentalogy (of Fallot) 745.2
Pentosuria (benign) (essential) 271.8
Peptic acid disease 536.8
Peregrinating patient V65.2
Perforated —*see* Perforation
Perforation, perforative (nontraumatic)
  antrum (*see also* Sinusitis, maxillary) 473.0
  appendix 540.0
    with peritoneal abscess 540.1
  atrial septum, multiple 745.5
  attic, ear 384.22
    healed 384.81
  bile duct, except cystic (*see also* Disease, biliary) 576.3
    cystic 575.4
  bladder (urinary) 596.6
    with
      abortion—*see* Abortion, by type, with damage to pelvic organs
      ectopic pregnancy (*see also* categories 633.0-633.9) 639.2
      molar pregnancy (*see also* categories 630-632) 639.2
    following
      abortion 639.2
      ectopic or molar pregnancy 639.2
    obstetrical trauma 665.5
  bowel 569.83
    with
      abortion—*see* Abortion, by type, with damage to pelvic organs
      ectopic pregnancy (*see also* categories 633.0-633.9) 639.2

INDEX TO DISEASES

Perforation, perforative—*continued*
    molar pregnancy (*see also* categories 630-632) 639.2
    fetus or newborn 777.6
    following
        abortion 639.2
        ectopic or molar pregnancy 639.2
    obstetrical trauma 665.5
  broad ligament
    with
        abortion—*see* Abortion, by type, with damage to pelvic organs
        ectopic pregnancy (*see also* categories 633.0-633.9) 639.2
        molar pregnancy (*see also* categories 630-632) 639.2
    following
        abortion 639.2
        ectopic or molar pregnancy 639.2
    obstetrical trauma 665.6
  by
    device, implant, or graft—*see* Complications, mechanical
    foreign body left accidentally in operation wound 998.4
    instrument (any) during a procedure, accidental 998.2
  cecum 540.0
    with peritoneal abscess 540.1
  cervix (uteri)—*see also* Injury, internal, cervix
    with
        abortion—*see* Abortion, by type, with damage to pelvic organs
        ectopic pregnancy (*see also* categories 633.0-633.9) 639.2
        molar pregnancy (*see also* categories 630-632) 639.2
    following
        abortion 639.2
        ectopic or molar pregnancy 639.2
    obstetrical trauma 665.3
  colon 569.83
  common duct (bile) 576.3
  cornea (*see also* Ulcer, cornea) 370.00
    due to ulceration 370.06
  cystic duct 575.4
  diverticulum (*see also* Diverticula) 562.10
    small intestine 562.00
  duodenum, duodenal (ulcer)—*see* Ulcer, duodenum, with perforation
  ear drum—*see* Perforation, tympanum
  enteritis—*see* Enteritis
  esophagus 530.4
  ethmoidal sinus (*see also* Sinusitis, ethmoidal) 473.2
  foreign body (external site)—*see also* Wound, open, by site, complicated
    internal site, by ingested object—*see* Foreign body
  frontal sinus (*see also* Sinusitis, frontal) 473.1
  gallbladder or duct (*see also* Disease, gallbladder) 575.4
  gastric (ulcer)—*see* Ulcer, stomach, with perforation
  heart valve—*see* Endocarditis
  ileum (*see also* Perforation, intestine) 569.83
  instrumental
    external—*see* Wound, open, by site
    pregnant uterus, complicating delivery 665.9
    surgical (accidental) (blood vessel) (nerve) (organ) 998.2

Perforation, perforative—*continued*
  intestine 569.83
    with
        abortion—*see* Abortion, by type, with damage to pelvic organs
        ectopic pregnancy (*see also* categories 633.0-633.9) 639.2
        molar pregnancy (*see also* categories 630-632) 639.2
    fetus or newborn 777.6
    obstetrical trauma 665.5
    ulcerative NEC 569.83
  jejunum, jejunal 569.83
    ulcer—*see* Ulcer, gastrojejunal, with perforation
  mastoid (antrum) (cell) 383.89
  maxillary sinus (*see also* Sinusitis, maxillary) 473.0
  membrana tympani—*see* Perforation, tympanum
  nasal
    septum 478.19
        congenital 748.1
        syphilitic 095.8
    sinus (*see also* Sinusitis) 473.9
        congenital 748.1
  palate (hard) 526.89
    soft 528.9
        syphilitic 095.8
    syphilitic 095.8
  palatine vault 526.89
    syphilitic 095.8
    congenital 090.5
  pelvic
    floor
      with
        abortion—*see* Abortion, by type, with damage to pelvic organs
        ectopic pregnancy (*see also* categories 633.0-633.9) 639.2
        molar pregnancy (*see also* categories 630-632) 639.2
    obstetrical trauma 664.1
    organ
      with
        abortion—*see* Abortion, by type, with damage to pelvic organs
        ectopic pregnancy (*see also* categories 633.0-633.9) 639.2
        molar pregnancy (*see also* categories 630-632) 639.2
      following
        abortion 639.2
        ectopic or molar pregnancy 639.2
      obstetrical trauma 665.5
  perineum—*see* Laceration, perineum
  periurethral tissue
    with
        abortion—*see* Abortion, by type, with damage to pelvic organs
        ectopic pregnancy (*see also* categories 630-632) 639.2
        molar pregnancy (*see also* categories 630-632) 639.2
  pharynx 478.29
  pylorus, pyloric (ulcer)—*see* Ulcer, stomach, with perforation
  rectum 569.49
  root canal space 526.61
  sigmoid 569.83
  sinus (accessory) (chronic) (nasal) (*see also* Sinusitis) 473.9

Perforation, perforative—*continued*
  sphenoidal sinus (*see also* Sinusitis, sphenoidal) 473.3
  stomach (due to ulcer)—*see* Ulcer, stomach, with perforation
  surgical (accidental) (by instrument) (blood vessel) (nerve) (organ) 998.2
  traumatic
    external—*see* Wound, open, by site
    eye (*see also* Penetrating wound, ocular) 871.7
    internal organ—*see* Injury, internal, by site
  tympanum (membrane) (persistent posttraumatic) (postinflammatory) 384.20
    with
      otitis media—*see* Otitis media
    attic 384.22
    central 384.21
    healed 384.81
    marginal NEC 384.23
    multiple 384.24
    pars flaccida 384.22
    total 384.25
    traumatic—*see* Wound, open, ear, drum
  typhoid, gastrointestinal 002.0
  ulcer—*see* Ulcer, by site, with perforation
  ureter 593.89
  urethra
    with
      abortion—*see* Abortion, by type, with damage to pelvic organs
      ectopic pregnancy (*see also* categories 633.0-633.9) 639.2
      molar pregnancy (*see also* categories 630-632) 639.2
    following
      abortion 639.2
      ectopic or molar pregnancy 639.2
    obstetrical trauma 665.5
  uterus—*see also* Injury, internal, uterus
    with
      abortion—*see* Abortion, by type, with damage to pelvic organs
      ectopic pregnancy (*see also* categories 633.0-633.9) 639.2
      molar pregnancy (*see also* categories 630-632) 639.2
    by intrauterine contraceptive device 996.32
    following
      abortion 639.2
      ectopic or molar pregnancy 639.2
    obstetrical trauma—*see* Injury, internal, uterus, obstetrical trauma
  uvula 528.9
    syphilitic 095.8
  vagina—*see* Laceration, vagina
  viscus NEC 799.89
    traumatic 868.00
      with open wound into cavity 868.10
Periadenitis mucosa necrotica recurrens 528.2
Periangiitis 446.0
Periantritis 535.4
Periappendicitis (acute) (*see also* Appendicitis) 541
Periarteritis (disseminated) (infectious) (necrotizing) (nodosa) 446.0
Periarthritis (joint) 726.90
  Duplay's 726.2
  gonococcal 098.50
  humeroscapularis 726.2
  scapulohumeral 726.2
  shoulder 726.2
  wrist 726.4

Periarthrosis (angioneural)—*see* Periarthritis
Peribronchitis 491.9
  tuberculous (*see also* Tuberculosis) 011.3
Pericapsulitis, adhesive (shoulder) 726.0
Pericarditis (granular) (with decompensation) (with effusion) 423.9
  with
    rheumatic fever (conditions classifiable to 390)
      active (*see also* Pericarditis, rheumatic) 391.0
      inactive or quiescent 393
  actinomycotic 039.8 *[420.0]*
  acute (nonrheumatic) 420.90
    with chorea (acute) (rheumatic) (Sydenham's) 392.0
    bacterial 420.99
    benign 420.91
    hemorrhagic 420.90
    idiopathic 420.91
    infective 420.90
    nonspecific 420.91
    rheumatic 391.0
      with chorea (acute) (rheumatic) (Sydenham's) 392.0
    sicca 420.90
    viral 420.91
  adhesive or adherent (external) (internal) 423.1
    acute—*see* Pericarditis, acute
    rheumatic (external) (internal) 393
  amebic 006.8 *[420.0]*
  bacterial (acute) (subacute) (with serous or seropurulent effusion) 420.99
  calcareous 423.2
  cholesterol (chronic) 423.8
    acute 420.90
  chronic (nonrheumatic) 423.8
    rheumatic 393
  constrictive 423.2
  Coxsackie 074.21
  due to
    actinomycosis 039.8 *[420.0]*
    amebiasis 006.8 *[420.0]*
    Coxsackie (virus) 074.21
    histoplasmosis (*see also* Histoplasmosis) 115.93
    nocardiosis 039.8 *[420.0]*
    tuberculosis (*see also* Tuberculosis) 017.9 *[420.0]*
  fibrinocaseous (*see also* Tuberculosis) 017.9 *[420.0]*
  fibrinopurulent 420.99
  fibrinous—*see* Pericarditis, rheumatic
  fibropurulent 420.99
  fibrous 423.1
  gonococcal 098.83
  hemorrhagic 423.0
  idiopathic (acute) 420.91
  infective (acute) 420.90
  meningococcal 036.41
  neoplastic (chronic) 423.8
    acute 420.90
  nonspecific 420.91
  obliterans, obliterating 423.1
  plastic 423.1
  pneumococcal (acute) 420.99
  postinfarction 411.0
  purulent (acute) 420.99
  rheumatic (active) (acute) (with effusion) (with pneumonia) 391.0
    with chorea (acute) (rheumatic) (Sydenham's) 392.0

INDEX TO DISEASES

Pericarditis—*continued*
   chronic or inactive (with chorea) 393
   septic (acute) 420.99
   serofibrinous—*see* Pericarditis, rheumatic
   staphylococcal (acute) 420.99
   streptococcal (acute) 420.99
   suppurative (acute) 420.99
   syphilitic 093.81
   tuberculous (acute) (chronic) (*see also* Tuberculosis) 017.9 *[420.0]*
   uremic 585.9 *[420.0]*
   viral (acute) 420.91
Pericardium, pericardial —*see* condition
Pericellulitis (*see also* Cellulitis) 682.9
Pericementitis 523.40
   acute 523.30
   chronic (suppurative) 523.40
Pericholecystitis (*see also* Cholecystitis) 575.10
Perichondritis
   auricle 380.00
     acute 380.01
     chronic 380.02
   bronchus 491.9
   ear (external) 380.00
     acute 380.01
     chronic 380.02
   larynx 478.71
     syphilitic 095.8
     typhoid 002.0 *[478.71]*
   nose 478.19
   pinna 380.00
     acute 380.01
     chronic 380.02
   trachea 478.9
Periclasia 523.5
Pericolitis 569.89
Pericoronitis (chronic) 523.40
   acute 523.30
Pericystitis (*see also* Cystitis) 595.9
Pericytoma (M9150/1)—*see also* Neoplasm, connective tissue, uncertain behavior
   benign (M9150/0)—*see* Neoplasm, connective tissue, benign
   malignant (M9150/3)—*see* Neoplasm, connective tissue, malignant
Peridacryocystitis, acute 375.32
Peridiverticulitis (*see also* Diverticulitis) 562.11
Periduodenitis 535.6
Periendocarditis (*see also* Endocarditis) 424.90
   acute or subacute 421.9
Periepididymitis (*see also* Epididymitis) 604.90
Perifolliculitis (abscedens) 704.8
   capitis, abscedens et suffodiens 704.8
   dissecting, scalp 704.8
   scalp 704.8
   superficial pustular 704.8
Perigastritis (acute) 535.0
Perigastrojejunitis (acute) 535.0
Perihepatitis (acute) 573.3
   chlamydial 099.56
   gonococcal 098.86
Peri-ileitis (subacute) 569.89
Perilabyrinthitis (acute)—*see* Labyrinthitis
Perimeningitis —*see* Meningitis
Perimetritis (*see also* Endometritis) 615.9
Perimetrosalpingitis (*see also* Salpingo-oophoritis) 614.2
Perineocele 618.05
Perinephric —*see* condition
Perinephritic —*see* condition

Periostitis

Perinephritis (*see also* Infection, kidney) 590.9
   purulent (*see also* Abscess, kidney) 590.2
Perineum, perineal —*see* condition
Perineuritis NEC 729.2
Periodic —*see also* condition
   disease (familial) 277.31
   edema 995.1
     hereditary 277.6
   fever 277.31
   limb movement disorder 327.51
   paralysis (familial) 359.3
   peritonitis 277.31
   polyserositis 277.31
   somnolence (*see also* Narcolepsy) 347.00
Periodontal
   cyst 522.8
   pocket 523.8
Periodontitis (chronic) (complex) (compound) (simplex) 523.40
   acute 523.33
   aggressive 523.30
     generalized 523.32
     localized 523.31
   apical 522.6
     acute (pulpal origin) 522.4
   generalized 523.42
   localized 523.41
Periodontoclasia 523.5
Periodontosis 523.5
Periods —*see also* Menstruation
   heavy 626.2
   irregular 626.4
Perionychia (with lymphangitis) 681.9
   finger 681.02
   toe 681.11
Perioophoritis (*see also* Salpingo-oophoritis) 614.2
Periorchitis (*see also* Orchitis) 604.90
Periosteum, periosteal —*see* condition
Periostitis (circumscribed) (diffuse) (infective) 730.3

> Note—Use the following fifth-digit subclassification with category 730:
> 0 *site unspdcified*
> 1 *shoulder region*
> 2 *upper arm*
> 3 *forearm*
> 4 *hand*
> 5 *pelvic region and thigh*
> 6 *lower leg*
> 7 *ankle and foot*
> 8 *other specified sites*
> 9 *multiple sites*

   with osteomyelitis (*see also* Osteomyelitis) 730.2
     acute or subacute 730.0
     chronic or old 730.1
   albuminosa, albuminosus 730.3
   alveolar 526.5
   alveolodental 526.5
   dental 526.5
   gonorrheal 098.89
   hyperplastica, generalized 731.2
   jaw (lower) (upper) 526.4
   monomelic 733.99
   orbital 376.02
   syphilitic 095.5
     congenital 090.0 *[730.8]*
     secondary 091.61
   tuberculous (*see also* Tuberculosis, bone) 015.9 *[730.8]*
   yaws (early) (hypertrophic) (late) 102.6

Periostosis (*see also* Periostitis) 730.3
  with osteomyelitis (*see also* Osteomyelitis) 730.2
    acute or subacute 730.0
    chronic or old 730.1
  hyperplastic 756.59
Peripartum cardiomyopathy 674.5
Periphlebitis (*see also* Phlebitis) 451.9
  lower extremity 451.2
    deep (vessels) 451.19
    superficial (vessels) 451.0
  portal 572.1
  retina 362.18
  superficial (vessels) 451.0
  tuberculous (*see also* Tuberculosis) 017.9
    retina 017.3 *[362.18]*
Peripneumonia —*see* Pneumonia
Periproctitis 569.49
Periprostatitis (*see also* Prostatitis) 601.9
Perirectal —*see* condition
Perirenal —*see* condition
Perisalpingitis (*see also* Salpingo-oophoritis) 614.2
Perisigmoiditis 569.89
Perisplenitis (infectional) 289.59
Perispondylitis —*see* Spondylitis
Peristalsis reversed or visible 787.4
Peritendinitis (*see also* Tenosynovitis) 726.90
  adhesive (shoulder) 726.0
Perithelioma (M9150/1)—*see* Pericytoma
Peritoneum, peritoneal —*see also* condition
  equilibration test V56.32
Peritonitis (acute) (adhesive) (fibrinous) (hemorrhagic) (idiopathic) (localized) (perforative) (primary) (with adhesions) (with effusion) 567.9
  with or following
    abortion—*see* Abortion, by type, with sepsis
    abscess 567.21
    appendicitis 540.0
      with peritoneal abscess 540.1
    ectopic pregnancy (*see also* categories 633.0-633.9) 639.0
    molar pregnancy (*see also* categories 630-632) 639.0
  aseptic 998.7
  bacterial 567.29
    spontaneous 567.23
  bile, biliary 567.81
  chemical 998.7
  chlamydial 099.56
  chronic proliferative 567.89
  congenital NEC 777.6
  diaphragmatic 567.22
  diffuse NEC 567.29
  diphtheritic 032.83
  disseminated NEC 567.29
  due to
    bile 567.81
    foreign
      body or object accidentally left during a procedure (instrument) (sponge) (swab) 998.4
      substance accidentally left during a procedure (chemical) (powder) (talc) 998.7
    talc 998.7
    urine 567.89
  fibrinopurulent 567.29
  fibrinous 567.29
  fibrocaseous (*see also* Tuberculosis) 014.0
  fibropurulent 567.29
  general, generalized (acute) 567.21

Peritonitis—*continued*
  gonococcal 098.86
  in infective disease NEC 136.9 *[567.0]*
  meconium (newborn) 777.6
  pancreatic 577.8
  paroxysmal, benign 277.31
  pelvic
    female (acute) 614.5
      chronic NEC 614.7
        with adhesions 614.6
      puerperal, postpartum, childbirth 670
    male (acute) 567.21
  periodic (familial) 277.31
  phlegmonous 567.29
  pneumococcal 567.1
  postabortal 639.0
  proliferative, chronic 567.89
  puerperal, postpartum, childbirth 670
  purulent 567.29
  septic 567.29
  spontaneous bacterial 567.23
  staphylococcal 567.29
  streptococcal 567.29
  subdiaphragmatic 567.29
  subphrenic 567.29
  suppurative 567.29
  syphilitic 095.2
    congenital 090.0 *[567.0]*
  talc 998.7
  tuberculous (*see also* Tuberculosis) 014.0
  urine 567.89
Peritonsillar —*see* condition
Peritonsillitis 475
Perityphlitis (*see also* Appendicitis) 541
Periureteritis 593.89
Periurethral —*see* condition
Periurethritis (gangrenous) 597.89
Periuterine —*see* condition
Perivaginitis (*see also* Vaginitis) 616.10
Perivasculitis, retinal 362.18
Perivasitis (chronic) 608.4
Periventricular leukomalacia 779.7
Perivesiculitis (seminal) (*see also* Vesiculitis) 608.0
Perlèche 686.8
  due to
    moniliasis 112.0
    riboflavin deficiency 266.0
Pernicious —*see* condition
Pernio, perniosis 991.5
Persecution
  delusion 297.9
  social V62.4
Perseveration (tonic) 784.69
Persistence, persistent (congenital) 759.89
  anal membrane 751.2
  arteria stapedia 744.04
  atrioventricular canal 745.69
  bloody ejaculate 792.2
  branchial cleft 744.41
  bulbus cordis in left ventricle 745.8
  canal of Cloquet 743.51
  capsule (opaque) 743.51
  cilioretinal artery or vein 743.51
  cloaca 751.5
  communication—*see* Fistula, congenital
  convolutions
    aortic arch 747.21
    fallopian tube 752.19
    oviduct 752.19

INDEX TO DISEASES

Persistence, persistent—*continued*
   uterine tube 752.19
   double aortic arch 747.21
   ductus
      arteriosus 747.0
      Botalli 747.0
   fetal
      circulation 747.83
      form of cervix (uteri) 752.49
      hemoglobin (hereditary) ("Swiss variety") 282.7
      pulmonary hypertension 747.83
   foramen
      Botalli 745.5
      ovale 745.5
   Gartner's duct 752.41
   hemoglobin, fetal (hereditary) (HPFH) 282.7
   hyaloid
      artery (generally incomplete) 743.51
      system 743.51
   hymen (tag)
      in pregnancy or childbirth 654.8
         causing obstructed labor 660.2
   lanugo 757.4
   left
      posterior cardinal vein 747.49
      root with right arch of aorta 747.21
      superior vena cava 747.49
   Meckel's diverticulum 751.0
   mesonephric duct 752.89
      fallopian tube 752.11
   mucosal disease (middle ear) (with posterior or superior marginal perforation of ear drum) 382.2
   nail(s), anomalous 757.5
   occiput, anterior or posterior 660.3
      fetus or newborn 763.1
   omphalomesenteric duct 751.0
   organ or site NEC—*see* Anomaly, specified type NEC
   ostium
      atrioventriculare commune 745.69
      primum 745.61
      secundum 745.5
   ovarian rests in fallopian tube 752.19
   pancreatic tissue in intestinal tract 751.5
   primary (deciduous)
      teeth 520.6
      vitreous hyperplasia 743.51
   pulmonary hypertension 747.83
   pupillary membrane 743.46
      iris 743.46
   Rhesus (Rh) titer 999.7
   right aortic arch 747.21
   sinus
      urogenitalis 752.89
      venosus with imperfect incorporation in right auricle 747.49
   thymus (gland) 254.8
      hyperplasia 254.0
   thyroglossal duct 759.2
   thyrolingual duct 759.2
   truncus arteriosus or communis 745.0
   tunica vasculosa lentis 743.39
   umbilical sinus 753.7
   urachus 753.7
   vegetative state 780.03
   vitelline duct 751.0
   wolffian duct 752.89

Person (with)
   admitted for clinical research, as participant or control subject V70.7
   awaiting admission to adequate facility elsewhere V63.2
      undergoing social agency investigation V63.8
   concern (normal) about sick person in family V61.49
   consulting on behalf of another V65.19
      pediatric pre-birth visit for expectant mother V65.11
   feared
      complaint in whom no diagnosis was made V65.5
      condition not demonstrated V65.5
   feigning illness V65.2
   healthy, accompanying sick person V65.0
   living (in)
      alone V60.3
      boarding school V60.6
      residence remote from hospital or medical care facility V63.0
      residential institution V60.6
      without
         adequate
            financial resources V60.2
            housing (heating) (space) V60.1
            housing (permanent) (temporary) V60.0
            material resources V60.2
         person able to render necessary care V60.4
         shelter V60.0
   medical services in home not available V63.1
   on waiting list V63.2
      undergoing social agency investigation V63.8
   sick or handicapped in family V61.49
   "worried well" V65.5

Personality
   affective 301.10
   aggressive 301.3
   amoral 301.7
   anancastic, anankastic 301.4
   antisocial 301.7
   asocial 301.7
   asthenic 301.6
   avoidant 301.82
   borderline 301.83
   change 310.1
   compulsive 301.4
   cycloid 301.13
   cyclothymic 301.13
   dependent 301.6
   depressive (chronic) 301.12
   disorder, disturbance NEC 301.9
      with
         antisocial disturbance 301.7
         pattern disturbance NEC 301.9
         sociopathic disturbance 301.7
         trait disturbance 301.9
   dual 300.14
   dyssocial 301.7
   eccentric 301.89
      "haltlose" type 301.89
   emotionally unstable 301.59
   epileptoid 301.3
   explosive 301.3
   fanatic 301.0
   histrionic 301.50
   hyperthymic 301.11
   hypomanic 301.11
   hypothymic 301.12
   hysterical 301.50

Personality—*continued*
  immature 301.89
  inadequate 301.6
  labile 301.59
  masochistic 301.89
  morally defective 301.7
  multiple 300.14
  narcissistic 301.81
  obsessional 301.4
  obsessive-compulsive 301.4
  overconscientious 301.4
  paranoid 301.0
  passive (-dependent) 301.6
  passive-aggressive 301.84
  pathologic NEC 301.9
  pattern defect or disturbance 301.9
  pseudosocial 301.7
  psychoinfantile 301.59
  psychoneurotic NEC 301.89
  psychopathic 301.9
    with
      amoral trend 301.7
      antisocial trend 301.7
      asocial trend 301.7
      pathologic sexuality (*see also* Deviation, sexual) 302.9
      mixed types 301.9
    schizoid 301.20
      introverted 301.21
      schizotypal 301.22
    type A 301.4
    unstable (emotional) 301.59
Perthes' disease (capital femoral osteochondrosis) 732.1
Pertussis (*see also* Whooping cough) 033.9
  vaccination, prophylactic (against) V03.6
Peruvian wart 088.0
Perversion, perverted
  appetite 307.52
  hysterical 300.11
  function
    pineal gland 259.8
    pituitary gland 253.9
      anterior lobe
        deficient 253.2
        excessive 253.1
      posterior lobe 253.6
  placenta—*see* Placenta, abnormal
  sense of smell or taste 781.1
    psychogenic 306.7
  sexual (*see also* Deviation, sexual) 302.9
Pervious, congenital —*see also* Imperfect, closure
  ductus arteriosus 747.0
Pes (congenital) (*see also* Talipes) 754.70
  abductus (congenital) 754.60
    acquired 736.79
  acquired NEC 736.79
    planus 734
  adductus (congenital) 754.79
    acquired 736.79
  cavus 754.71
    acquired 736.73
  planovalgus (congenital) 754.69
    acquired 736.79
  planus (acquired) (any degree) 734
    congenital 754.61

Pes —*continued*
  rachitic 268.1
  valgus (congenital) 754.61
    acquired 736.79
  varus (congenital) 754.50
    acquired 736.79
Pest (*see also* Plague) 020.9
Pestis (*see also* Plague) 020.9
  bubonica 020.0
  fulminans 020.0
  minor 020.8
  pneumonica—*see* Plague, pneumonic
Petechia, petechiae 782.7
  fetus or newborn 772.6
Petechial
  fever 036.0
  typhus 081.9
Petges-Cléjat or Petges-Clégat syndrome (poikilodermatomyositis) 710.3
Petit's
  disease (*see also* Hernia, lumbar) 553.8
Petit mal (idiopathic) (*see also* Epilepsy) 345.0
  status 345.2
Petrellidosis 117.6
Petrositis 383.20
  acute 383.21
  chronic 383.22
Peutz-Jeghers disease or syndrome 759.6
Peyronie's disease 607.85
Pfeiffer's disease 075
Phacentocele 379.32
  traumatic 921.3
Phacoanaphylaxis 360.19
Phacocele (old) 379.32
  traumatic 921.3
Phaehyphomycosis 117.8
Phagedena (dry) (moist) (*see also* Gangrene) 785.4
  arteriosclerotic 440.24
  geometric 686.09
  penis 607.89
  senile 440.24
  sloughing 785.4
  tropical (*see also* Ulcer, skin) 707.9
  vulva 616.50
Phagedenic —*see also* condition
  abscess—*see also* Abscess
    chancroid 099.0
  bubo NEC 099.8
  chancre 099.0
  ulcer (tropical) (*see also* Ulcer, skin) 707.9
Phagomania 307.52
Phakoma 362.89
Phantom limb (syndrome) 353.6
Pharyngeal —*see also* condition
  arch remnant 744.41
  pouch syndrome 279.11
Pharyngitis (acute) (catarrhal) (gangrenous) (infective) (malignant) (membranous) (phlegmonous) (pneumococcal) (pseudomembranous) (simple) (staphylococcal) (subacute) (suppurative) (ulcerative) (viral) 462
  with influenza, flu, or grippe 487.1
  aphthous 074.0
  atrophic 472.1
  chlamydial 099.51
  chronic 472.1
  Coxsackie virus 074.0
  diphtheritic (membranous) 032.0

Pharyngitis—*continued*
  follicular 472.1
  fusospirochetal 101
  gonococcal 098.6
  granular (chronic) 472.1
  herpetic 054.79
  hypertrophic 472.1
  infectional, chronic 472.1
  influenzal 487.1
  lymphonodular, acute 074.8
  septic 034.0
  streptococcal 034.0
  tuberculous (*see also* Tuberculosis) 012.8
  vesicular 074.0
Pharyngoconjunctival fever 077.2
Pharyngoconjunctivitis, viral 077.2
Pharyngolaryngitis (acute) 465.0
  chronic 478.9
  septic 034.0
Pharyngoplegia 478.29
Pharyngotonsillitis 465.8
  tuberculous 012.8
Pharyngotracheitis (acute) 465.8
  chronic 478.9
Pharynx, pharyngeal —*see* condition
Phase of life problem NEC V62.89
Phenomenon
  Arthus' 995.21
  flashback (drug) 292.89
  jaw-winking 742.8
  Jod-Basedow 242.8
  L. E. cell 710.0
  lupus erythematosus cell 710.0
  Pelger-Huët (hereditary hyposegmentation) 288.2
  Raynaud's (paroxysmal digital cyanosis) (secondary) 443.0
  Reilly's (*see also* Neuropathy, peripheral, autonomic) 337.9
  vasomotor 780.2
  vasospastic 443.9
  vasovagal 780.2
  Wenckebach's, heart block (second degree) 426.13
Phenylketonuria (PKU) 270.1
Phenylpyruvicaciduria 270.1
Pheochromoblastoma (M8700/3)
  specified site—*see* Neoplasm, by site, malignant
  unspecified site 194.0
Pheochromocytoma (M8700/0)
  malignant (M8700/3)
    specified site—*see* Neoplasm, by site, malignant
    unspecified site 194.0
  specified site—*see* Neoplasm, by site, benign
  unspecified site 227.0
Phimosis (congenital) 605
  chancroidal 099.0
  due to infection 605
Phlebectasia (*see also* Varicose, vein) 454.9
  congenital NEC 747.60
  esophagus (*see also* Varix, esophagus) 456.1
    with hemorrhage (*see also* Varix, esophagus, bleeding) 456.0
Phlebitis (infective) (pyemic) (septic) (suppurative) 451.9
  antecubital vein 451.82
  arm NEC 451.84
    axillary vein 451.89
    basilic vein 451.82
    deep 451.83
    superficial 451.82

Phlebitis—*continued*
  basilic vein 451.82
  blue 451.19
  brachial vein 451.83
  breast, superficial 451.89
  cavernous (venous) sinus—*see* Phlebitis, intracranial sinus
  cephalic vein 451.82
  cerebral (venous) sinus—*see* Phlebitis, intracranial sinus
  chest wall, superficial 451.89
  complicating pregnancy or puerperium 671.9
    affecting fetus or newborn 760.3
  cranial (venous) sinus—*see* Phlebitis, intracranial sinus
  deep (vessels) 451.19
    femoral vein 451.11
    specified vessel NEC 451.19
  due to implanted device—*see* Complications, due to (presence of) any device, implant, or graft classified to 996.0-996.5 NEC
  during or resulting from a procedure 997.2
  femoral vein (deep) (superficial) 451.11
  femoropopliteal 451.19
  following infusion, perfusion, or transfusion 999.2
  gouty 274.89 *[451.9]*
  hepatic veins 451.89
  iliac vein 451.81
  iliofemoral 451.11
  intracranial sinus (any) (venous) 325
    late effect—*see* category 326
    nonpyogenic 437.6
    in pregnancy or puerperium 671.5
  jugular vein 451.89
  lateral (venous) sinus—*see* Phlebitis, intracranial sinus
  leg 451.2
    deep (vessels) 451.19
      femoral vein 451.11
      specified vessel NEC 451.19
    superficial (vessels) 451.0
      femoral vein 451.11
  longitudinal sinus—*see* Phlebitis, intracranial sinus
  lower extremity 451.2
    deep (vessels) 451.19
      femoral vein 451.11
      specified vessel NEC 451.19
    superficial (vessels) 451.0
      femoral vein 451.11
  migrans, migrating (superficial) 453.1
  pelvic
    with
      abortion—*see* Abortion, by type, with sepsis
      ectopic pregnancy (*see also* categories 633.0-633.9) 639.0
      molar pregnancy (*see also* categories 630-632) 639.0
    following
      abortion 639.0
      ectopic or molar pregnancy 639.0
    puerperal, postpartum 671.4
  popliteal vein 451.19
  portal (vein) 572.1
  postoperative 997.2
  pregnancy 671.9
    deep 671.3
    specified type NEC 671.5
    superficial 671.2

Phlebitis—*continued*
  puerperal, postpartum, childbirth 671.9
    deep 671.4
    lower extremities 671.2
    pelvis 671.4
    specified site NEC 671.5
    superficial 671.2
  radial vein 451.83
  retina 362.18
  saphenous (great) (long) 451.0
    accessory or small 451.0
  sinus (meninges)—*see* Phlebitis, intracranial sinus
  specified site NEC 451.89
  subclavian vein 451.89
  syphilitic 093.89
  tibial vein 451.19
  ulcer, ulcerative 451.9
    leg 451.2
      deep (vessels) 451.19
        femoral vein 451.11
        specified vessel NEC 451.19
      superficial (vessels) 451.0
        femoral vein 451.11
    lower extremity 451.2
      deep (vessels) 451.19
        femoral vein 451.11
        specified vessel NEC 451.19
      superficial (vessels) 451.0
  ulnar vein 451.83
  umbilicus 451.89
  upper extremity—*see* Phlebitis, arm
  uterus (septic) (*see also* Endometritis) 615.9
  varicose (leg) (lower extremity) (*see also* Varicose, vein) 454.1
Phlebofibrosis 459.89
Phleboliths 459.89
Phlebosclerosis 459.89
Phlebothrombosis —*see* Thrombosis
Phlebotomus fever 066.0
Phlegm, choked on 933.1
Phlegmasia
  alba dolens (deep vessels) 451.19
    complicating pregnancy 671.3
    nonpuerperal 451.19
    puerperal, postpartum, childbirth 671.4
  cerulea dolens 451.19
Phlegmon (*see also* Abscess) 682.9
  erysipelatous (*see also* Erysipelas) 035
  iliac 682.2
    fossa 540.1
  throat 478.29
Phlegmonous —*see* condition
Phlyctenulosis (allergic) (keratoconjunctivitis) (nontuberculous) 370.31
  cornea 370.31
    with ulcer (*see also* Ulcer, cornea) 370.00
  tuberculous (*see also* Tuberculosis) 017.3 [370.31]
Phobia, phobic (reaction) 300.20
  animal 300.29
  isolated NEC 300.29
  obsessional 300.3
  simple NEC 300.29
  social 300.23
  specified NEC 300.29
  state 300.20
Phocas' disease 610.1
Phocomelia 755.4
  lower limb 755.32
    complete 755.33

Phocomelia—*continued*
    distal 755.35
    proximal 755.34
  upper limb 755.22
    complete 755.23
    distal 755.25
    proximal 755.24
Phoria (*see also* Heterophoria) 378.40
Phosphate-losing tubular disorder 588.0
Phosphatemia 275.3
Phosphaturia 275.3
Photoallergic response 692.72
Photocoproporphyria 277.1
Photodermatitis (sun) 692.72
  light other than sun 692.82
Photokeratitis 370.24
Photo-ophthalmia 370.24
Photophobia 368.13
Photopsia 368.15
Photoretinitis 363.31
Photoretinopathy 363.31
Photosensitiveness (sun) 692.72
  light other than sun 692.82
Photosensitization (sun) skin 692.72
  light other than sun 692.82
Phototoxic response 692.72
Phrenitis 323.9
Phrynoderma 264.8
Phthiriasis (pubis) (any site) 132.2
  with any infestation classifiable to 132.0 and 132.1 132.3
Phthirus infestation —*see* Phthiriasis
Phthisis (*see also* Tuberculosis) 011.9
  bulbi (infectional) 360.41
  colliers' 011.4
  cornea 371.05
  eyeball (due to infection) 360.41
  millstone makers' 011.4
  miners' 011.4
  potters' 011.4
  sandblasters' 011.4
  stonemasons' 011.4
Phycomycosis 117.7
Physalopteriasis 127.7
Physical therapy NEC V57.1
  breathing exercises V57.0
Physiological cup, optic papilla
  borderline, glaucoma suspect 365.00
  enlarged 377.14
  glaucomatous 377.14
Phytobezoar 938
  intestine 936
  stomach 935.2
Pian (*see also* Yaws) 102.9
Pianoma 102.1
Piarhemia, piarrhemia (*see also* Hyperlipemia) 272.4
  bilharziasis 120.9
Pica 307.52
  hysterical 300.11
Pick's
  cerebral atrophy 331.11
    with dementia
      with behavioral disturbance 331.11 [294.11]
      without behavioral disturbance 331.11 [294.10]
  disease
    brain 331.11
      dementia in

INDEX TO DISEASES   Pitted

Pick's—*continued*
   with behavioral disturbance 331.11
     [294.11]
   without behavioral disturbance 331.11
     [294.10]
   lipid histiocytosis 272.7
   liver (pericardial pseudocirrhosis of liver) 423.2
   pericardium (pericardial pseudocirrhosis of liver) 423.2
   polyserositis (pericardial pseudocirrhosis of liver) 423.2
   syndrome
     heart (pericardial pseudocirrhosis of liver) 423.2
     liver (pericardial pseudocirrhosis of liver) 423.2
   tubular adenoma (M8640/0)
     specified site—*see* Neoplasm, by site, benign
     unspecified site
       female 220
       male 222.0
Pick-Herxheimer syndrome (diffuse idiopathic cutaneous atrophy) 701.8
Pick-Niemann disease (lipid histiocytosis) 272.7
Pickwickian syndrome (cardiopulmonary obesity) 278.8
Piebaldism, classic 709.09
Piedra 111.2
   beard 111.2
     black 111.3
     white 111.2
   black 111.3
   scalp 111.3
     black 111.3
     white 111.2
   white 111.2
Pierre Marie's syndrome (pulmonary hypertrophic osteoarthropathy) 731.2
Pierre Marie-Bamberger syndrome (hypertrophic pulmonary osteoarthropathy) 731.2
Pierre Mauriac's syndrome (diabetes-dwarfism-obesity) 258.1
Pierre Robin deformity or syndrome (congenital) 756.0
Pierson's disease or osteochondrosis 732.1
Pigeon
   breast or chest (acquired) 738.3
     congenital 754.82
     rachitic (*see also* Rickets) 268.0
   breeders' disease or lung 495.2
   fanciers' disease or lung 495.2
   toe 735.8
Pigmentation (abnormal) 709.00
   anomaly 709.00
     congenital 757.33
     specified NEC 709.09
   conjunctiva 372.55
   cornea 371.10
     anterior 371.11
     posterior 371.13
     stromal 371.12
   lids (congenital) 757.33
     acquired 374.52
   limbus corneae 371.10
   metals 709.00
   optic papilla, congenital 743.57
   retina (congenital) (grouped) (nevoid) 743.53
     acquired 362.74
   scrotum, congenital 757.33

Piles —*see* Hemorrhoids
Pili
   annulati or torti (congenital) 757.4
   incarnati 704.8
Pill roller hand (intrinsic) 736.09
Pilomatrixoma (M8110/0)—*see* Neoplasm, skin, benign
Pilonidal —*see* condition
Pimple 709.8
PIN I (prostatic intraepithelial neoplasia I) 602.3
PIN II (prostatic intraepithelial neoplasia II) 602.3
PIN III (prostatic intraepithelial neoplasia III) 233.4
Pinched nerve —*see* Neuropathy, entrapment
Pineal body or gland —*see* condition
Pinealoblastoma (M9362/3) 194.4
Pinealoma (M9360/1) 237.1
   malignant (M9360/3) 194.4
Pineoblastoma (M9362/3) 194.4
Pineocytoma (M9361/1) 237.1
Pinguecula 372.51
Pinhole meatus (*see also* Stricture, urethra) 598.9
Pink
   disease 985.0
   eye 372.03
   puffer 492.8
Pinkus' disease (lichen nitidus) 697.1
Pinpoint
   meatus (*see also* Stricture, urethra) 598.9
   os (uteri) (*see also* Stricture, cervix) 622.4
Pinselhaare (congenital) 757.4
Pinta 103.9
   cardiovascular lesions 103.2
   chancre (primary) 103.0
   erythematous plaques 103.1
   hyperchromic lesions 103.1
   hyperkeratosis 103.1
   lesions 103.9
     cardiovascular 103.2
     hyperchromic 103.1
     intermediate 103.1
     late 103.2
     mixed 103.3
     primary 103.0
     skin (achromic) (cicatricial) (dyschromic) 103.2
       hyperchromic 103.1
       mixed (achromic and hyperchromic) 103.3
   papule (primary) 103.0
   skin lesions (achromic) (cicatricial) (dyschromic) 103.2
     hyperchromic 103.1
     mixed (achromic and hyperchromic) 103.3
   vitiligo 103.2
Pintid 103.0
Pinworms (disease) (infection) (infestation) 127.4
Piry fever 066.8
Pistol wound —*see* Gunshot wound
Pit, lip (mucus), congenital 750.25
Pitchers' elbow 718.82
Pithecoid pelvis 755.69
   with disproportion (fetopelvic) 653.2
     affecting fetus or newborn 763.1
     causing obstructed labor 660.1
Pithiatism 300.11
Pitted —*see also* Pitting
   teeth 520.4

Pitting (edema) (*see also* Edema) 782.3
  lip 782.3
  nail 703.8
    congenital 757.5
Pituitary gland —*see* condition
Pituitary snuff-takers' disease 495.8
Pityriasis 696.5
  alba 696.5
  capitis 690.11
  circinata (et maculata) 696.3
  Hebra's (exfoliative dermatitis) 695.89
  lichenoides et varioliformis 696.2
  maculata (et circinata) 696.3
  nigra 111.1
  pilaris 757.39
    acquired 701.1
    Hebra's 696.4
  rosea 696.3
  rotunda 696.3
  rubra (Hebra) 695.89
    pilaris 696.4
  sicca 690.18
  simplex 690.18
  specified type NEC 696.5
  streptogenes 696.5
  versicolor 111.0
    scrotal 111.0
Placenta, placental
  ablatio 641.2
    affecting fetus or newborn 762.1
  abnormal, abnormality 656.7
    with hemorrhage 641.8
      affecting fetus or newborn 762.1
    affecting fetus or newborn 762.2
  abruptio 641.2
    affecting fetus or newborn 762.1
  accessory lobe—*see* Placenta, abnormal
  accreta (without hemorrhage) 667.0
    with hemorrhage 666.0
  adherent (without hemorrhage) 667.0
    with hemorrhage 666.0
  apoplexy—*see* Placenta, separation
  battledore—*see* Placenta, abnormal
  bilobate—*see* Placenta, abnormal
  bipartita—*see* Placenta, abnormal
  carneous mole 631
  centralis—*see* Placenta, previa
  circumvallata—*see* Placenta, abnormal
  cyst (amniotic)—*see* Placenta, abnormal
  deficiency—*see* Placenta insufficiency
  degeneration—*see* Placenta, insufficiency
  detachment (partial) (premature) (with hemorrhage) 641.2
    affecting fetus or newborn 762.1
  dimidiata—*see* Placenta, abnormal
  disease 656.7
    affecting fetus or newborn 762.2
  duplex—*see* Placenta, abnormal
  dysfunction—*see* Placenta, insufficiency
  fenestrata—*see* Placenta, abnormal
  fibrosis—*see* Placenta, abnormal
  fleshy mole 631
  hematoma—*see* Placenta, abnormal
  hemorrhage NEC—*see* Placenta, separation
  hormone disturbance or malfunction—*see* Placenta, abnormal
  hyperplasia—*see* Placenta, abnormal
  increta (without hemorrhage) 667.0
    with hemorrhage 666.0
  infarction 656.7
    affecting fetus or newborn 762.2

Placenta, placental—*continued*
  insertion, vicious—*see* Placenta, previa
  insufficiency
    affecting
      fetus or newborn 762.2
    management of pregnancy 656.5
  lateral—*see* Placenta, previa
  low implantation or insertion—*see* Placenta, previa
  low-lying—*see* Placenta, previa
  malformation—*see* Placenta, abnormal
  malposition—*see* Placenta, previa
  marginalis, marginata—*see* Placenta, previa
  marginal sinus (hemorrhage) (rupture) 641.2
    affecting fetus or newborn 762.1
  membranacea—*see* Placenta, abnormal
  multilobed—*see* Placenta, abnormal
  multipartita—*see* Placenta, abnormal
  necrosis—*see* Placenta, abnormal
  percreta (without hemorrhage) 667.0
    with hemorrhage 666.0
  polyp 674.4
  previa (central) (centralis) (complete) (lateral) (marginal) (marginalis) (partial) (partialis) (total) (with hemorrhage) 641.1
    affecting fetus or newborn 762.0
    noted
      before labor, without hemorrhage (with cesarean delivery) 641.0
      during pregnancy (without hemorrhage) 641.0
    without hemorrhage (before labor and delivery) (during pregnancy) 641.0
  retention (with hemorrhage) 666.0
    fragments, complicating puerperium (delayed hemorrhage) 666.2
    without hemorrhage 667.1
    postpartum, puerperal 666.2
    without hemorrhage 667.0
  separation (normally implanted) (partial) (premature) (with hemorrhage) 641.2
    affecting fetus or newborn 762.1
  septuplex—*see* Placenta, abnormal
  small—*see* Placenta, insufficiency
  softening (premature)—*see* Placenta, abnormal
  spuria—*see* Placenta, abnormal
  succenturiata—*see* Placenta, abnormal
  syphilitic 095.8
  transfusion syndromes 762.3
  transmission of chemical substance—*see* Absorption, chemical, through placenta
  trapped (with hemorrhage) 666.0
    without hemorrhage 667.0
  trilobate—*see* Placenta, abnormal
  tripartita—*see* Placenta, abnormal
  triplex—*see* Placenta, abnormal
  varicose vessel—*see* Placenta, abnormal
  vicious insertion—*see* Placenta, previa
Placentitis
  affecting fetus or newborn 762.7
  complicating pregnancy 658.4
Plagiocephaly (skull) 754.0
Plague 020.9
  abortive 020.8
  ambulatory 020.8
  bubonic 020.0
  cellulocutaneous 020.1
  lymphatic gland 020.0
  pneumonic 020.5
    primary 020.3
    secondary 020.4

INDEX TO DISEASES

Pneumatosis

Plague—*continued*
  pulmonary—*see* Plague, pneumonic
  pulmonic—*see* Plague, pneumonic
  septicemic 020.2
  tonsillar 020.9
    septicemic 020.2
  vaccination, prophylactic (against) V03.3
Planning, family V25.09
  contraception V25.9
  natural
    procreative V26.41
    to avoid pregnancy V25.04
  procreation V26.49
    natural V26.41
Plaque
  artery, arterial—*see* Arteriosclerosis
  calcareous—*see* Calcification
  Hollenhorst's (retinal) 362.33
  tongue 528.6
Plasma cell myeloma 203.0
Plasmacytoma, plasmocytoma (solitary) (M9731/1) 238.6
  benign (M9731/0)—*see* Neoplasm, by site, benign
  malignant (M9731/3) 203.8
Plasmacytopenia 288.59
Plasmacytosis 288.64
Plaster ulcer (*see also* Decubitus) 707.00
Platybasia 756.0
Platyonychia (congenital) 757.5
  acquired 703.8
Platypelloid pelvis 738.6
  with disproportion (fetopelvic) 653.2
    affecting fetus or newborn 763.1
    causing obstructed labor 660.1
      affecting fetus or newborn 763.1
  congenital 755.69
Platyspondylia 756.19
Plethora 782.62
  newborn 776.4
Pleura, pleural —*see* condition
Pleuralgia 786.52
Pleurisy (acute) (adhesive) (chronic) (costal) (diaphragmatic) (double) (dry) (fetid) (fibrinous) (fibrous) (interlobar) (latent) (lung) (old) (plastic) (primary) (residual) (sicca) (sterile) (subacute) (unresolved) (with adherent pleura) 511.0
  with
    effusion (without mention of cause) 511.9
      bacterial, nontuberculous 511.1
      nontuberculous NEC 511.9
        bacterial 511.1
      pneumococcal 511.1
      specified type NEC 511.8
      staphylococcal 511.1
      streptococcal 511.1
      tuberculous (*see also* Tuberculosis, pleura) 012.0
        primary, progressive 010.1
    influenza, flu, or grippe 487.1
    tuberculosis—*see* Pleurisy, tuberculous
  encysted 511.8
  exudative (*see also* Pleurisy, with effusion) 511.9
    bacterial, nontuberculous 511.1
  fibrinopurulent 510.9
    with fistula 510.0
  fibropurulent 510.9
    with fistula 510.0
  hemorrhagic 511.8

Pleurisy—*continued*
  influenzal 487.1
  pneumococcal 511.0
    with effusion 511.1
  purulent 510.9
    with fistula 510.0
  septic 510.9
    with fistula 510.0
  serofibrinous (*see also* Pleurisy, with effusion) 511.9
    bacterial, nontuberculous 511.1
  seropurulent 510.9
    with fistula 510.0
  serous (*see also* Pleurisy, with effusion) 511.9
    bacterial, nontuberculous 511.1
  staphylococcal 511.0
    with effusion 511.1
  streptococcal 511.0
    with effusion 511.1
  suppurative 510.9
    with fistula 510.0
  traumatic (post) (current) 862.29
    with open wound into cavity 862.39
  tuberculous (with effusion) (*see also* Tuberculosis, pleura) 012.0
    primary, progressive 010.1
Pleuritis sicca —*see* Pleurisy
Pleurobronchopneumonia (*see also* Pneumonia, broncho-) 485
Pleurodynia 786.52
  epidemic 074.1
  viral 074.1
Pleurohepatitis 573.8
Pleuropericarditis (*see also* Pericarditis) 423.9
  acute 420.90
Pleuropneumonia (acute) (bilateral) (double) (septic) (*see also* Pneumonia) 486
  chronic (*see also* Fibrosis, lung) 515
Pleurorrhea (*see also* Hydrothorax) 511.8
Plexitis, brachial 353.0
Plica
  knee 727.83
  polonica 132.0
  tonsil 474.8
Plicae dysphonia ventricularis 784.49
Plicated tongue 529.5
  congenital 750.13
Plug
  bronchus NEC 519.19
  meconium (newborn) NEC 777.1
  mucus—*see* Mucus, plug
Plumbism 984.9
  specified type of lead—*see* Table of drugs and chemicals
Plummer's disease (toxic nodular goiter) 242.3
Plummer-Vinson syndrome (sideropenic dysphagia) 280.8
Pluricarential syndrome of infancy 260
Plurideficiency syndrome of infancy 260
Plus (and minus) hand (intrinsic) 736.09
PMDD (premenstrual dysphoric disorder) 625.4
PMS 625.4
Pneumathemia —*see* Air, embolism, by type
Pneumatic drill or hammer disease 994.9
Pneumatocele (lung) 518.89
  intracranial 348.8
  tension 492.0
Pneumatosis
  cystoides intestinalis 569.89
  peritonei 568.89
  pulmonum 492.8

1261

Pneumaturia 599.84
Pneumoblastoma (M8981/3)—*see* Neoplasm, lung, malignant
Pneumocephalus 348.8
Pneumococcemia 038.2
Pneumococcus, pneumococcal —*see* condition
Pneumoconiosis (due to) (inhalation of) 505
  aluminum 503
  asbestos 501
  bagasse 495.1
  bauxite 503
  beryllium 503
  carbon electrode makers' 503
  coal
    miners' (simple) 500
    workers' (simple) 500
  cotton dust 504
  diatomite fibrosis 502
  dust NEC 504
    inorganic 503
    lime 502
    marble 502
    organic NEC 504
  fumes or vapors (from silo) 506.9
  graphite 503
  hard metal 503
  mica 502
  moldy hay 495.0
  rheumatoid 714.81
  silica NEC 502
    and carbon 500
  silicate NEC 502
  talc 502
Pneumocystis carinii pneumonia 136.3
Pneumocystis jiroveci pneumonia 136.3
Pneumocystosis 136.3
  with pneumonia 136.3
Pneumoenteritis 025
Pneumohemopericardium (*see also* Pericarditis) 423.9
Pneumohemothorax (*see also* Hemothorax) 511.8
  traumatic 860.4
    with open wound into thorax 860.5
Pneumohydropericardium (*see also* Pericarditis) 423.9
Pneumohydrothorax (*see also* Hydrothorax) 511.8
Pneumomediastinum 518.1
  congenital 770.2
  fetus or newborn 770.2
Pneumomycosis 117.9
Pneumonia (acute) (Alpenstich) (benign) (bilateral) (brain) (cerebral) (circumscribed) (congestive) (creeping) (delayed resolution) (double) (epidemic) (fever) (flash) (fulminant) (fungoid) (granulomatous) (hemorrhagic) (incipient) (infantile) (infectious) (infiltration) (insular) (intermittent) (latent) (lobe) (migratory) (newborn) (organized) (overwhelming) (primary) (progressive) (pseudolobar) (purulent) (resolved) (secondary) (senile) (septic) (suppurative) (terminal) (true) (unresolved) (vesicular) 486
  with influenza, flu, or grippe 487.0
  adenoviral 480.0
  adynamic 514
  alba 090.0
  allergic 518.3
  alveolar—*see* Pneumonia, lobar
  anaerobes 482.81
  anthrax 022.1 *[484.5]*

Pneumonia—*continued*
  apex, apical—*see* Pneumonia, lobar
  ascaris 127.0 *[484.8]*
  aspiration 507.0
    due to
      aspiration of microorganisms
        bacterial 482.9
          specified type NEC 482.89
        specified organism NEC 483.8
          bacterial NEC 482.89
        viral 480.9
          specified type NEC 480.8
      food (regurgitated) 507.0
      gastric secretions 507.0
      milk 507.0
      oils, essences 507.1
      solids, liquids NEC 507.8
      vomitus 507.0
    fetal 770.18
      due to
        blood 770.16
        clear amniotic fluid 770.14
        meconium 770.12
        postnatal stomach contents 770.86
    newborn 770.18
      due to
        blood 770.16
        clear amniotic fluid 770.14
        meconium 770.12
        postnatal stomach contents 770.86
  asthenic 514
  atypical (disseminated, focal) (primary) 486
    with influenza 487.0
  bacillus 482.9
    specified type NEC 482.89
  bacterial 482.9
    specified type NEC 482.89
  Bacteroides (fragilis) (oralis) (melaninogenicus) 482.81
  basal, basic, basilar—*see* Pneumonia, lobar
  broncho-, bronchial (confluent) (croupous) (diffuse) (disseminated) (hemorrhagic) (involving lobes) (lobar) (terminal) 485
    with influenza 487.0
    allergic 518.3
    aspiration (*see also* Pneumonia, aspiration) 507.0
    bacterial 482.9
      specified type NEC 482.89
    capillary 466.19
      with bronchospasm or obstruction 466.19
    chronic (*see also* Fibrosis, lung) 515
    congenital (infective) 770.0
    diplococcal 481
    Eaton's agent 483.0
    Escherichia coli (E. coli) 482.82
    Friedländer's bacillus 482.0
    Hemophilus influenzae 482.2
    hiberno-vernal 083.0 *[484.8]*
    hypostatic 514
    influenzal 487.0
    inhalation (*see also* Pneumonia, aspiration) 507.0
      due to fumes or vapors (chemical) 506.0
    Klebsiella 482.0
    lipid 507.1
      endogenous 516.8
    Mycoplasma (pneumoniae) 483.0
    ornithosis 073.0
    pleuropneumonia-like organisms (PPLO) 483.0
    pneumococcal 481
    Proteus 482.83

INDEX TO DISEASES — Pneumonia

Pneumonia—*continued*
  pseudomonas 482.1
  specified organism NEC 483.8
    bacterial NEC 482.89
    staphylococcal 482.40
      aureus 482.41
      specified type NEC 482.49
    streptococcal—*see* Pneumonia, streptococcal
    typhoid 002.0 *[484.8]*
    viral, virus (*see also* Pneumonia, viral) 480.9
  Butyrivibrio (fibriosolvens) 482.81
  Candida 112.4
  capillary 466.19
    with bronchospasm or obstruction 466.19
  caseous (*see also* Tuberculosis) 011.6
  catarrhal—*see* Pneumonia, broncho-
  central—*see* Pneumonia, lobar
  Chlamydia, chlamydial 483.1
    pneumoniae 483.1
    psittaci 073.0
    specified type NEC 483.1
    trachomatis 483.1
  cholesterol 516.8
  chronic (*see also* Fibrosis, lung) 515
  cirrhotic (chronic) (*see also* Fibrosis, lung) 515
  Clostridium (haemolyticum) (novyi) NEC 482.81
  confluent—*see* Pneumonia, broncho-
  congenital (infective) 770.0
    aspiration 770.18
  croupous—*see* Pneumonia, lobar
  cytomegalic inclusion 078.5 *[484.1]*
  deglutition (*see also* Pneumonia, aspiration) 507.0
  desquamative interstitial 516.8
  diffuse—*see* Pneumonia, broncho-
  diplococcal, diplococcus (broncho-) (lobar) 481
  disseminated (focal)—*see* Pneumonia, broncho-
  due to
    adenovirus 480.0
    Bacterium anitratum 482.83
    Chlamydia, chlamydial 483.1
      pneumoniae 483.1
      psittaci 073.0
      specified type NEC 483.1
      trachomatis 483.1
    coccidioidomycosis 114.0
    Diplococcus (pneumoniae) 481
    Eaton's agent 483.0
    Escherichia coli (E. coli) 482.82
    Friedländer's bacillus 482.0
    fumes or vapors (chemical) (inhalation) 506.0
    fungus NEC 117.9 *[484.7]*
      coccidioidomycosis 114.0
    Hemophilus influenzae (H. influenzae) 482.2
    Herellea 482.83
    influenza 487.0
    Klebsiella pneumoniae 482.0
    Mycoplasma (pneumoniae) 483.0
    parainfluenza virus 480.2
    pleuropneumonia-like organism (PPLO) 483.0
    Pneumococcus 481
    Pneumocystis carinii 136.3
    Pneumocystis jiroveci 136.3
    Proteus 482.83
    pseudomonas 482.1
    respiratory syncytial virus 480.1
    rickettsia 083.9 *[484.8]*
    SARS-associated coronavirus 480.3
    specified
      bacteria NEC 482.89

Pneumonia—*continued*
  organism NEC 483.8
  virus NEC 480.8
  Staphylococcus 482.40
    aureus 482.41
    specified type NEC 482.49
  Streptococcus—*see also* Pneumonia, streptococcal
    pneumoniae 481
  virus (*see also* Pneumonia, viral) 480.9
  Eaton's agent 483.0
  embolic, embolism (*see also* Embolism, pulmonary) 415.1
  eosinophilic 518.3
  Escherichia coli (E. coli) 482.82
  Eubacterium 482.81
  fibrinous—*see* Pneumonia, lobar
  fibroid (chronic) (*see also* Fibrosis, lung) 515
  fibrous (*see also* Fibrosis, lung) 515
  Friedländer's bacillus 482.0
  Fusobacterium (nucleatum) 482.81
  gangrenous 513.0
  giant cell (*see also* Pneumonia, viral) 480.9
  gram-negative bacteria NEC 482.83
    anaerobic 482.81
  grippal 487.0
  Hemophilus influenzae (bronchial) (lobar) 482.2
  hypostatic (broncho-) (lobar) 514
  in
    actinomycosis 039.1
    anthrax 022.1 *[484.5]*
    aspergillosis 117.3 *[484.6]*
    candidiasis 112.4
    coccidioidomycosis 114.0
    cytomegalic inclusion disease 078.5 *[484.1]*
    histoplasmosis (*see also* Histoplasmosis) 115.95
    infectious disease NEC 136.9 *[484.8]*
    measles 055.1
    mycosis, systemic NEC 117.9 *[484.7]*
    nocardiasis, nocardiosis 039.1
    ornithosis 073.0
    pneumocystosis 136.3
    psittacosis 073.0
    Q fever 083.0 *[484.8]*
    salmonellosis 003.22
    toxoplasmosis 130.4
    tularemia 021.2
    typhoid (fever) 002.0 *[484.8]*
    varicella 052.1
    whooping cough (*see also* Whooping cough) 033.9 *[484.3]*
  infective, acquired prenatally 770.0
  influenzal (broncho) (lobar) (virus) 487.0
  inhalation (*see also* Pneumonia, aspiration) 507.0
    fumes or vapors (chemical) 506.0
  interstitial 516.8
    with influenzal 487.0
    acute 136.3
    chronic (*see also* Fibrosis, lung) 515
    desquamative 516.8
    hypostatic 514
    lipoid 507.1
    lymphoid 516.8
    plasma cell 136.3
    pseudomonas 482.1
  intrauterine (infective) 770.0
    aspiration 770.18
      blood 770.16
      clear amniotic fluid 770.14
      meconium 770.12

1263

Pneumonia—*continued*
    postnatal stomach contents 770.86
  Klebsiella pneumoniae 482.0
  Legionnaires' 482.84
  lipid, lipoid (exogenous) (interstitial) 507.1
    endogenous 516.8
  lobar (diplococcal) (disseminated) (double)
    (interstitial) (pneumococcal, any type) 481
    with influenza 487.0
    bacterial 482.9
      specified type NEC 482.89
    chronic (*see also* Fibrosis, lung) 515
    Escherichia coli (E. coli) 482.82
    Friedländer's bacillus 482.0
    Hemophilus influenzae (H. influenzae) 482.2
    hypostatic 514
    influenzal 487.0
    Klebsiella 482.0
    ornithosis 073.0
    Proteus 482.83
    pseudomonas 482.1
    psittacosis 073.0
    specified organism NEC 483.8
      bacterial NEC 482.89
    staphylococcal 482.40
      aureus 482.41
      specified type NEC 482.49
    streptococcal—*see* Pneumonia, streptococcal
    viral, virus (*see also* Pneumonia, viral) 480.9
  lobular (confluent)—*see* Pneumonia, broncho-
  Löffler's 518.3
  massive—*see* Pneumonia, lobar
  meconium aspiration 770.12
  metastatic NEC 038.8 *[484.8]*
  Mycoplasma (pneumoniae) 483.0
  necrotic 513.0
  nitrogen dioxide 506.9
  orthostatic 514
  parainfluenza virus 480.2
  parenchymatous (*see also* Fibrosis, lung) 515
  passive 514
  patchy—*see* Pneumonia, broncho
  Peptococcus 482.81
  Peptostreptococcus 482.81
  plasma cell 136.3
  pleurolobar—*see* Pneumonia, lobar
  pleuropneumonia-like organism (PPLO) 483.0
  pneumococcal (broncho) (lobar) 481
  Pneumocystis (carinii) (jiroveci) 136.3
  postinfectional NEC 136.9 *[484.8]*
  postmeasles 055.1
  postoperative 997.3
  primary atypical 486
  Proprionibacterium 482.81
  Proteus 482.83
  pseudomonas 482.1
  psittacosis 073.0
  radiation 508.0
  respiratory syncytial virus 480.1
  resulting from a procedure 997.3
  rheumatic 390 *[517.1]*
  Salmonella 003.22
  SARS-associated coronavirus 480.3
  segmented, segmental—*see* Pneumonia,
    broncho-
  Serratia (marcescens) 482.83
  specified
    bacteria NEC 482.89
    organism NEC 483.8
    virus NEC 480.8
  spirochetal 104.8 *[484.8]*

Pneumonia—*continued*
  staphylococcal (broncho) (lobar) 482.40
    aureus 482.41
    specified type NEC 482.49
  static, stasis 514
  streptococcal (broncho) (lobar) NEC 482.30
    Group
      A 482.31
      B 482.32
      specified NEC 482.39
    pneumoniae 481
    specified type NEC 482.39
  Streptococcus pneumoniae 481
  traumatic (complication) (early) (secondary) 958.8
  tuberculous (any) (*see also* Tuberculosis) 011.6
  tularemic 021.2
  TWAR agent 483.1
  varicella 052.1
  Veillonella 482.81
  ventilator associated 999.9
  viral, virus (broncho) (interstitial) (lobar) 480.9
    with influenza, flu, or grippe 487.0
    adenoviral 480.0
    parainfluenza 480.2
    respiratory syncytial 480.1
    SARS-associated coronavirus 480.3
    specified type NEC 480.8
  white (congenital) 090.0
Pneumonic —*see* condition
Pneumonitis (acute) (primary) (*see also*
    Pneumonia) 486
  allergic 495.9
    specified type NEC 495.8
  aspiration 507.0
    due to fumes or gases 506.0
    fetal 770.18
      due to
        blood 770.16
        clear amniotic fluid 770.14
        meconium 770.12
        postnatal stomach contents 770.86
    newborn 770.18
      due to
        blood 770.16
        clear amniotic fluid 770.14
        meconium 770.12
        postnatal stomach contents 770.86
    obstetric 668.0
  chemical 506.0
    due to fumes or gases 506.0
  cholesterol 516.8
  chronic (*see also* Fibrosis, lung) 515
  congenital rubella 771.0
  crack 506.0
  due to
    crack (cocaine) 506.0
    fumes or vapors 506.0
    inhalation
      food (regurgitated), milk, vomitus 507.0
      oils, essences 507.1
      saliva 507.0
      solids, liquids NEC 507.8
    toxoplasmosis (acquired) 130.4
      congenital (active) 771.2 *[484.8]*
  eosinophilic 518.3
  fetal aspiration 770.18
    due to
      blood 770.16
      clear amniotic fluid 770.14
      meconium 770.12
      postnatal stomach contents 770.86
  hypersensitivity 495.9

INDEX TO DISEASES   **Poisoning**

Pneumonitis—*continued*
   interstitial (chronic) (*see also* Fibrosis, lung) 515
      lymphoid 516.8
   lymphoid, interstitial 516.8
   meconium aspiration 770.12
   postanesthetic
      correct substance properly administered 507.0
      obstetric 668.0
      overdose or wrong substance given 968.4
         specified anesthetic—*see* Table of drugs and chemicals
   postoperative 997.3
      obstetric 668.0
   radiation 508.0
   rubella, congenital 771.0
   "ventilation" 495.7
   wood-dust 495.8
Pneumonoconiosis —*see* Pneumoconiosis
Pneumoparotid 527.8
Pneumopathy NEC 518.89
   alveolar 516.9
      specified NEC 516.8
   due to dust NEC 504
   parietoalveolar 516.9
      specified condition NEC 516.8
Pneumopericarditis (*see also* Pericarditis) 423.9
   acute 420.90
Pneumopericardium —*see also* Pericarditis
   congenital 770.2
   fetus or newborn 770.2
   traumatic (post) (*see also* Pneumothorax, traumatic) 860.0
      with open wound into thorax 860.1
Pneumoperitoneum 568.89
   fetus or newborn 770.2
Pneumophagia (psychogenic) 306.4
Pneumopleurisy, pneumopleuritis (*see also* Pneumonia) 486
Pneumopyopericardium 420.99
Pneumopyothorax (*see also* Pyopneumothorax) 510.9
   with fistula 510.0
Pneumorrhagia 786.3
   newborn 770.3
   tuberculous (*see also* Tuberculosis, pulmonary) 011.9
Pneumosiderosis (occupational) 503
Pneumothorax (acute) (chronic) 512.8
   congenital 770.2
   due to operative injury of chest wall or lung 512.1
      accidental puncture or laceration 512.1
   fetus or newborn 770.2
   iatrogenic 512.1
   postoperative 512.1
   spontaneous 512.8
      fetus or newborn 770.2
      tension 512.0
   sucking 512.8
      iatrogenic 512.1
      postoperative 512.1
   tense valvular, infectional 512.0
   tension 512.0
      iatrogenic 512.1
      postoperative 512.1
      spontaneous 512.0
   traumatic 860.0
      with
         hemothorax 860.4
            with open wound into thorax 860.5
         open wound into thorax 860.1
   tuberculous (*see also* Tuberculosis) 011.7

Pocket(s)
   endocardial (*see also* Endocarditis) 424.90
   periodontal 523.8
Podagra 274.9
Podencephalus 759.89
Poikilocytosis 790.09
Poikiloderma 709.09
   Civatte's 709.09
   congenital 757.33
   vasculare atrophicans 696.2
Poikilodermatomyositis 710.3
Pointed ear 744.29
Poise imperfect 729.9
Poisoned —*see* Poisoning
Poisoning (acute)—*see also* Table of Drugs and Chemicals
   Bacillus, B.
      aertrycke (*see also* Infection, Salmonella) 003.9
      botulinus 005.1
      cholerae (suis) (*see also* Infection, Salmonella) 003.9
      paratyphosus (*see also* Infection, Salmonella) 003.9
      suipestifer (*see also* Infection, Salmonella) 003.9
   bacterial toxins NEC 005.9
   berries, noxious 988.2
   blood (general)—*see* Septicemia
   botulism 005.1
   bread, moldy, mouldy—*see* Poisoning, food
   Ciguatera 988.0
   damaged meat—*see* Poisoning, food
   death-cap (Amanita phalloides) (Amanita verna) 988.1
   decomposed food—*see* Poisoning, food
   diseased food—*see* Poisoning, food
   drug—*see* Table of drugs and chemicals
   epidemic, fish, meat, or other food—*see* Poisoning, food
   fava bean 282.2
   fish (bacterial)—*see also* Poisoning, food
      noxious 988.0
   food (acute) (bacterial) (diseased) (infected) NEC 005.9
      due to
         Bacillus
            aertrycke (*see also* Poisoning, food, due to Salmonella) 003.9
            botulinus 005.1
            cereus 005.89
            choleraesuis (*see also* Poisoning, food, due to Salmonella) 003.9
            paratyphosus (*see also* Poisoning, food, due to Salmonella) 003.9
            suipestifer (*see also* Poisoning, food, due to Salmonella) 003.9
         Clostridium 005.3
            botulinum 005.1
            perfringens 005.2
            welchii 005.2
         Salmonella (aertrycke) (callinarum) (choleraesuis) (enteritidis) (paratyphi) (suipestifer) 003.9
            with
               gastroenteritis 003.0
               localized infection(s) (*see also* Infection, Salmonella) 003.20
               septicemia 003.1
               specified manifestation NEC 003.8
         specified bacterium NEC 005.89
         Staphylococcus 005.0

Poisoning—*continued*
    Streptococcus 005.8
    Vibrio parahaemolyticus 005.4
    Vibrio vulnificus 005.81
  noxious or naturally toxic 988.0
    berries 988.2
    fish 988.0
    mushroom 988.1
    plants NEC 988.2
  ice cream—*see* Poisoning, food
  ichthyotoxism (bacterial) 005.9
  kreotoxism, food 005.9
  malarial—*see* Malaria
  meat—*see* Poisoning, food
  mushroom (noxious) 988.1
  mussel—*see also* Poisoning, food
    noxious 988.0
  noxious foodstuffs (*see also* Poisoning, food, noxious) 988.9
    specified type NEC 988.8
  plants, noxious 988.2
  pork—*see also* Poisoning, food
    specified NEC 988.8
    Trichinosis 124
  ptomaine—*see* Poisoning, food
  putrefaction, food—*see* Poisoning, food
  radiation 508.0
  Salmonella (*see also* Infection, Salmonella) 003.9
  sausage—*see also* Poisoning, food
    Trichinosis 124
  saxitoxin 988.0
  shellfish—*see also* Poisoning, food
    noxious (amnesic) (azaspiracid) (diarrheic) (neurotoxic) (paralytic) 988.0
  Staphylococcus, food 005.0
  toxic, from disease NEC 799.89
  truffles—*see* Poisoning, food
  uremic—*see* Uremia
  uric acid 274.9
  water 276.6
Poison ivy, oak, sumac or other plant dermatitis 692.6
Poker spine 720.0
Policeman's disease 729.2
Polioencephalitis (acute) (bulbar) (*see also* Poliomyelitis, bulbar) 045.0
  inferior 335.22
  influenzal 487.8
  superior hemorrhagic (acute) (Wernicke's) 265.1
  Wernicke's (superior hemorrhagic) 265.1
Polioencephalomyelitis (acute) (anterior) (bulbar) (*see also* Poliomyelitis) 045.0
Polioencephalopathy, superior hemorrhagic 265.1
  with
    beriberi 265.0
    pellagra 265.2
Poliomeningoencephalitis —*see* Meningoencephalitis
Poliomyelitis (acute) (anterior) (epidemic) 045.9

> Note—*Use the following fifth-digit subclassification with category 045:*
>
> 0 *poliovirus, unspecified type*
> 1 *poliovirus, type I*
> 2 *poliovirus, type II*
> 3 *poliovirus, type III*

  with
    paralysis 045.1

Poliomyelitis—*continued*
    bulbar 045.0
  abortive 045.2
  ascending 045.9
    progressive 045.9
  bulbar 045.0
  cerebral 045.0
  chronic 335.21
  congenital 771.2
  contact V01.2
  deformities 138
  exposure to V01.2
  late effect 138
  nonepidemic 045.9
  nonparalytic 045.2
  old with deformity 138
  posterior, acute 053.19
  residual 138
  sequelae 138
  spinal, acute 045.9
  syphilitic (chronic) 094.89
  vaccination, prophylactic (against) V04.0
Poliosis (eyebrow) (eyelashes) 704.3
  circumscripta (congenital) 757.4
    acquired 704.3
  congenital 757.4
Pollakiuria 788.41
  psychogenic 306.53
Pollinosis 477.0
Pollitzer's disease (hidradenitis suppurativa) 705.83
Polyadenitis (*see also* Adenitis) 289.3
  malignant 020.0
Polyalgia 729.9
Polyangiitis (essential) 446.0
Polyarteritis (nodosa) (renal) 446.0
Polyarthralgia 719.49
  psychogenic 306.0
Polyarthritis, polyarthropathy NEC 716.59
  due to or associated with other specified conditions—*see* Arthritis, due to or associated with
  endemic (*see also* Disease, Kaschin-Beck) 716.0
  inflammatory 714.9
    specified type NEC 714.89
  juvenile (chronic) 714.30
    acute 714.31
  migratory—*see* Fever, rheumatic
  rheumatic 714.0
    fever (acute)—*see* Fever, rheumatic
Polycarential syndrome of infancy 260
Polychondritis (atrophic) (chronic) (relapsing) 733.99
Polycoria 743.46
Polycystic (congenital) (disease) 759.89
  degeneration, kidney—*see* Polycystic, kidney
  kidney (congenital) 753.12
    adult type (APKD) 753.13
    autosomal dominant 753.13
    autosomal recessive 753.14
    childhood type (CPKD) 753.14
    infantile type 753.14
  liver 751.62
  lung 518.89
    congenital 748.4
  ovary, ovaries 256.4
  spleen 759.0
Polycythemia (primary) (rubra) (vera) (M9950/1) 238.4
  acquired 289.0
  benign 289.0

INDEX TO DISEASES   **Polyp, polypus**

Polycythemia—*continued*
   familial 289.6
   due to
      donor twin 776.4
      fall in plasma volume 289.0
      high altitude 289.0
      maternal-fetal transfusion 776.4
      stress 289.0
   emotional 289.0
   erythropoietin 289.0
   familial (benign) 289.6
   Gaisböck's (hypertonica) 289.0
   high altitude 289.0
   hypertonica 289.0
   hypoxemic 289.0
   neonatorum 776.4
   nephrogenous 289.0
   relative 289.0
   secondary 289.0
   spurious 289.0
   stress 289.0
Polycytosis cryptogenica 289.0
Polydactylism, polydactyly 755.00
   fingers 755.01
   toes 755.02
Polydipsia 783.5
Polydystrophic oligophrenia 277.5
Polyembryoma (M9072/3)—*see* Neoplasm, by site, malignant
Polygalactia 676.6
Polyglandular
   deficiency 258.9
   dyscrasia 258.9
   dysfunction 258.9
   syndrome 258.8
Polyhydramnios (*see also* Hydramnios) 657
Polymastia 757.6
Polymenorrhea 626.2
Polymicrogyria 742.2
Polymyalgia 725
   arteritica 446.5
   rheumatica 725
Polymyositis (acute) (chronic) (hemorrhagic) 710.4
   with involvement of
      lung 710.4 *[517.8]*
      skin 710.3
   ossificans (generalisata) (progressiva) 728.19
   Wagner's (dermatomyositis) 710.3
Polyneuritis, polyneuritic (*see also* Polyneuropathy) 356.9
   alcoholic 357.5
      with psychosis 291.1
   cranialis 352.6
   demyelinating, chronic inflammatory (CIDP) 357.81
   diabetic 250.6 *[357.2]*
   due to lack of vitamin NEC 269.2 *[357.4]*
   endemic 265.0 *[357.4]*
   erythredema 985.0
   febrile 357.0
   hereditary ataxic 356.3
   idiopathic, acute 357.0
   infective (acute) 357.0
   nutritional 269.9 *[357.4]*
   postinfectious 357.0
Polyneuropathy (peripheral) 356.9
   alcoholic 357.5
   amyloid 277.39 *[357.4]*
   arsenical 357.7
   critical illness 357.82

Polyneuropathy—*continued*
   demyelinating, chronic inflammatory (CIDP) 357.81
   diabetic 250.6 *[357.2]*
   due to
      antitetanus serum 357.6
      arsenic 357.7
      drug or medicinal substance 357.6
         correct substance properly administered 357.6
         overdose or wrong substance given or taken 977.9
            specified drug—*see* Table of drugs and chemicals
      lack of vitamin NEC 269.2 *[357.4]*
      lead 357.7
      organophosphate compounds 357.7
      pellagra 265.2 *[357.4]*
      porphyria 277.1 *[357.4]*
      serum 357.6
      toxic agent NEC 357.7
   hereditary 356.0
   idiopathic 356.9
      progressive 356.4
   in
      amyloidosis 277.39 *[357.4]*
      avitaminosis 269.2 *[357.4]*
         specified NEC 269.1 *[357.4]*
      beriberi 265.0 *[357.4]*
      collagen vascular disease NEC 710.9 *[357.1]*
      deficiency
         B-complex NEC 266.2 *[357.4]*
         vitamin B 266.9 *[357.4]*
         vitamin B_6 266.1 *[357.4]*
      diabetes 250.6 *[357.2]*
      diphtheria (*see also* Diphtheria) 032.89 *[357.4]*
      disseminated lupus erythematosus 710.0 *[357.1]*
      herpes zoster 053.13
      hypoglycemia 251.2 *[357.4]*
      malignant neoplasm (M8000/3) NEC 199.1 *[357.3]*
      mumps 072.72
      pellagra 265.2 *[357.4]*
      polyarteritis nodosa 446.0 *[357.1]*
      porphyria 277.1 *[357.4]*
      rheumatoid arthritis 714.0 *[357.1]*
      sarcoidosis 135 *[357.4]*
      uremia 585.9 *[357.4]*
   lead 357.7
   nutritional 269.9 *[357.4]*
      specified NEC 269.8 *[357.4]*
   postherpetic 053.13
   progressive 356.4
   sensory (hereditary) 356.2
   specified NEC 356.8
Polyonychia 757.5
Polyopia 368.2
   refractive 368.15
Polyorchism, polyorchidism (three testes) 752.89
Polyorrhymenitis (peritoneal) (*see also* Polyserositis) 568.82
   pericardial 423.2
Polyostotic fibrous dysplasia 756.54
Polyotia 744.1
Polyp, polypus

> *Note*—Polyps of organs or sites that do not appear in the list below should be coded to the residual category for diseases of the organ or site concerned.

   accessory sinus 471.8

1267

Polyp, polypus—*continued*
  adenoid tissue 471.0
  adenomatous (M8210/0)—*see also* Neoplasm,
      by site, benign
    adenocarcinoma in (M8210/3)—*see*
        Neoplasm, by site, malignant
    carcinoma in (M8210/3)—*see* Neoplasm, by
        site, malignant
    multiple (M8221/0)—*see* Neoplasm, by site,
        benign
  antrum 471.8
  anus, anal (canal) (nonadenomatous) 569.0
    adenomatous 211.4
  Bartholin's gland 624.6
  bladder (M8120/1) 236.7
  broad ligament 620.8
  cervix (uteri) 622.7
    adenomatous 219.0
    in pregnancy or childbirth 654.6
      affecting fetus or newborn 763.89
      causing obstructed labor 660.2
    mucous 622.7
    nonneoplastic 622.7
  choanal 471.0
  cholesterol 575.6
  clitoris 624.6
  colon (M8210/0) (*see also* Polyp, adenomatous)
      211.3
  corpus uteri 621.0
  dental 522.0
  ear (middle) 385.30
  endometrium 621.0
  ethmoidal (sinus) 471.8
  fallopian tube 620.8
  female genital organs NEC 624.8
  frontal (sinus) 471.8
  gallbladder 575.6
  gingiva 523.8
  gum 523.8
  labia 624.6
  larynx (mucous) 478.4
  malignant (M8000/3)—*see* Neoplasm, by site,
      malignant
  maxillary (sinus) 471.8
  middle ear 385.30
  myometrium 621.0
  nares
    anterior 471.9
    posterior 471.0
  nasal (mucous) 471.9
    cavity 471.0
    septum 471.9
  nasopharyngeal 471.0
  neoplastic (M8210/0)—*see* Neoplasm, by site,
      benign
  nose (mucous) 471.9
  oviduct 620.8
  paratubal 620.8
  pharynx 478.29
    congenital 750.29
  placenta, placental 674.4
  prostate 600.20
    with
      other lower urinary tract symptoms (LUTS)
          600.21
      urinary
        obstruction 600.21
        retention 600.21
  pudenda 624.6
  pulp (dental) 522.0
  rectosigmoid 211.4

Polyp, polypus—*continued*
  rectum (nonadenomatous) 569.0
    adenomatous 211.4
  septum (nasal) 471.9
  sinus (accessory) (ethmoidal) (frontal)
      (maxillary) (sphenoidal) 471.8
  sphenoidal (sinus) 471.8
  stomach (M8210/0) 211.1
  tube, fallopian 620.8
  turbinate, mucous membrane 471.8
  ureter 593.89
  urethra 599.3
  uterine
    ligament 620.8
    tube 620.8
  uterus (body) (corpus) (mucous) 621.0
    in pregnancy or childbirth 654.1
      affecting fetus or newborn 763.89
      causing obstructed labor 660.2
  vagina 623.7
  vocal cord (mucous) 478.4
  vulva 624.6
Polyphagia 783.6
Polypoid —*see* condition
Polyposis —*see also* Polyp
  coli (adenomatous) (M8220/0) 211.3
    adenocarcinoma in (M8220/3) 153.9
    carcinoma in (M8220/3) 153.9
  familial (M8220/0) 211.3
  intestinal (adenomatous) (M8220/0) 211.3
  multiple (M8221/0)—*see* Neoplasm, by site,
      benign
Polyradiculitis (acute) 357.0
Polyradiculoneuropathy (acute) (segmentally
      demyelinating) 357.0
Polysarcia 278.00
Polyserositis (peritoneal) 568.82
  due to pericarditis 423.2
  paroxysmal (familial) 277.31
  pericardial 423.2
  periodic (familial) 277.31
  pleural—*see* Pleurisy
  recurrent 277.31
  tuberculous (*see also* Tuberculosis,
      polyserositis) 018.9
Polysialia 527.7
Polysplenia syndrome 759.0
Polythelia 757.6
Polytrichia (*see also* Hypertrichosis) 704.1
Polyunguia (congenital) 757.5
  acquired 703.8
Polyuria 788.42
Pompe's disease (glycogenosis II) 271.0
Pompholyx 705.81
Poncet's disease (tuberculous rheumatism) (*see
      also* Tuberculosis) 015.9
Pond fracture —*see* Fracture, skull, vault
Ponos 085.0
Pons, pontine —*see* condition
Poor
  aesthetics of existing restoration of tooth 525.67
  contractions, labor 661.2
    affecting fetus or newborn 763.7
  fetal growth NEC 764.9
    affecting management of pregnancy 656.5
  incorporation
    artificial skin graft 996.55
    decellularized allodermis graft 996.55
  obstetrical history V13.49
    affecting management of current pregnancy V23.49
      pre-term labor V23.41

Poor —continued
  pre-term labor V13.41
  sucking reflex (newborn) 796.1
  vision NEC 369.9
Poradenitis, nostras 099.1
Porencephaly (congenital) (development) (true) 742.4
  acquired 348.0
  nondevelopmental 348.0
  traumatic (post) 310.2
Porocephaliasis 134.1
Porokeratosis 757.39
  disseminated superficial actinic (DSAP) 692.75
Poroma, eccrine (M8402/0)—see Neoplasm, skin, benign
Porphyria (acute) (congenital) (constitutional) (erythropoietic) (familial) (hepatica) (idiopathic) (idiosyncratic) (intermittent) (latent) (mixed hepatic) (photosensitive) (South African genetic) (Swedish) 277.1
  acquired 277.1
  cutaneatarda
    hereditaria 277.1
    symptomatica 277.1
  due to drugs
    correct substance properly administered 277.1
    overdose or wrong substance given or taken 977.9
      specified drug—see Table of drugs and chemicals
  secondary 277.1
  toxic NEC 277.1
  variegata 277.1
Porphyrinuria (acquired) (congenital) (secondary) 277.1
Porphyruria (acquired) (congenital) 277.1
Portal —see condition
Port wine nevus or mark 757.32
Posadas-Wernicke disease 114.9
Position
  fetus, abnormal (see also Presentation, fetal) 652.9
  teeth, faulty (see also Anomaly, position tooth) 524.30
Positive
  culture (nonspecific) 795.39
    AIDS virus V08
    blood 790.7
    HIV V08
    human immunodeficiency virus V08
    nose 795.39
    skin lesion NEC 795.39
    spinal fluid 792.0
    sputum 795.39
    stool 792.1
    throat 795.39
    urine 791.9
    wound 795.39
  findings, anthrax 795.31
  HIV V08
  human immunodeficiency virus (HIV) V08
  PPD 795.5
  serology
    AIDS virus V08
      inconclusive 795.71
    HIV V08
      inconclusive 795.71
    human immunodeficiency virus V08
      inconclusive 795.71
  syphilis 097.1
    with signs or symptoms—see Syphilis, by site and stage
    false 795.6

Positive—continued
  skin test 795.7
    tuberculin (without active tuberculosis) 795.5
  VDRL 097.1
    with signs or symptoms—see Syphilis, by site and stage
    false 795.6
  Wassermann reaction 097.1
    false 795.6
Postcardiotomy syndrome 429.4
Postcaval ureter 753.4
Postcholecystectomy syndrome 576.0
Postclimacteric bleeding 627.1
Postcommissurotomy syndrome 429.4
Postconcussional syndrome 310.2
Postcontusional syndrome 310.2
Postcricoid region —see condition
Post-dates (pregnancy) —see Pregnancy
Postencephalitic —see also condition syndrome 310.8
Posterior —see condition
Posterolateral sclerosis (spinal cord)—see Degeneration, combined
Postexanthematous —see condition
Postfebrile —see condition
Postgastrectomy dumping syndrome 564.2
Posthemiplegic chorea 344.89
Posthemorrhagic anemia (chronic) 280.0
  acute 285.1
  newborn 776.5
Posthepatitis syndrome 780.79
Postherpetic neuralgia (intercostal) (syndrome) (zoster) 053.19
  geniculate ganglion 053.11
  ophthalmica 053.19
  trigeminal 053.12
Posthitis 607.1
Postimmunization complication or reaction —see Complications, vaccination
Postinfectious —see condition
Postinfluenzal syndrome 780.79
Postlaminectomy syndrome 722.80
  cervical, cervicothoracic 722.81
  kyphosis 737.12
  lumbar, lumbosacral 722.83
  thoracic, thoracolumbar 722.82
Postleukotomy syndrome 310.0
Postlobectomy syndrome 310.0
Postmastectomy lymphedema (syndrome) 457.0
Postmaturity, postmature (fetus or newborn) (gestation period over 42 completed weeks) 766.22
  affecting management of pregnancy
    post-term pregnancy 645.1
    prolonged pregnancy 645.2
  syndrome 766.22
Postmeasles —see also condition
  complication 055.8
    specified NEC 055.79
Postmenopausal
  endometrium (atrophic) 627.8
    suppurative (see also Endometritis) 615.9
  hormone replacement therapy V07.4
  status (age related) (natural) V49.81
Postnasal drip 784.91
Postnatal —see condition
Postoperative —see also condition
  confusion state 293.9
  psychosis 293.9
  status NEC (see also Status (post)) V45.89
Postpancreatectomy hyperglycemia 251.3

Postpartum —*see also* condition
  anemia 648.2
  cardiomyopathy 674.5
  observation
    immediately after delivery V24.0
    routine follow-up V24.2
Postperfusion syndrome NEC 999.8
  bone marrow 996.85
Postpoliomyelitic —*see* condition
Postsurgery status NEC (*see also* Status (post)) V45.89
Post-term (pregnancy) 645.1
  infant (gestation period over 40 completed weeks to 42 completed weeks) 766.21
Posttraumatic —*see* condition
Posttraumatic brain syndrome, nonpsychotic 310.2
Post-Traumatic Stress Disorder (PTSD) 309.81
Post-typhoid abscess 002.0
Postures, hysterical 300.11
Postvaccinal reaction or complication —*see* Complications, vaccination
Postvagotomy syndrome 564.2
Postvalvulotomy syndrome 429.4
Postvasectomy sperm count V25.8
Potain's disease (pulmonary edema) 514
Potain's syndrome (gastrectasis with dyspepsia) 536.1
Pott's
  curvature (spinal) (*see also* Tuberculosis) 015.0 [737.43]
  disease or paraplegia (*see also* Tuberculosis) 015.0 [730.88]
  fracture (closed) 824.4
    open 824.5
  gangrene 440.24
  osteomyelitis (*see also* Tuberculosis) 015.0 [730.88]
  spinal curvature (*see also* Tuberculosis) 015.0 [737.43]
  tumor, puffy (*see also* Osteomyelitis) 730.2
Potter's
  asthma 502
  disease 753.0
  facies 754.0
  lung 502
  syndrome (with renal agenesis) 753.0
Pouch
  bronchus 748.3
  Douglas'—*see* condition
  esophagus, esophageal (congenital) 750.4
    acquired 530.6
  gastric 537.1
  Hartmann's (abnormal sacculation of gallbladder neck) 575.8
    of intestine V44.3
      attention to V55.3
  pharynx, pharyngeal (congenital) 750.27
Poulet's disease 714.2
Poultrymen's itch 133.8
Poverty V60.2
PPE (plamar plantar erythrodysesthesia) 693.0
Prader-Labhart-Willi-Fanconi syndrome (hypogenital dystrophy with diabetic tendency) 759.81
Prader-Willi syndrome (hypogenital dystrophy with diabetic tendency) 759.81
Preachers' voice 784.49
Pre-AIDS —*see* Human immunodeficiency virus (disease) (illness) (infection)
Preauricular appendage 744.1

Prebetalipoproteinemia (acquired) (essential) (familial) (hereditary) (primary) (secondary) 272.1
  with chylomicronemia 272.3
Precipitate labor 661.3
  affecting fetus or newborn 763.6
Preclimacteric bleeding 627.0
  menorrhagia 627.0
Precocious
  adrenarche 259.1
  menarche 259.1
  menstruation 626.8
  pubarche 259.1
  puberty NEC 259.1
  sexual development NEC 259.1
  thelarche 259.1
Precocity, sexual (constitutional) (cryptogenic) (female) (idiopathic) (male) NEC 259.1
  with adrenal hyperplasia 255.2
Precordial pain 786.51
  psychogenic 307.89
Predeciduous teeth 520.2
Prediabetes, prediabetic 790.29
  complicating pregnancy, childbirth, or puerperium 648.8
  fetus or newborn 775.89
Predislocation status of hip, at birth (*see also* Subluxation, congenital, hip) 754.32
Pre-eclampsia (mild) 642.4
  with pre-existing hypertension 642.7
  affecting fetus or newborn 760.0
  severe 642.5
  superimposed on pre-existing hypertensive disease 642.7
Preeruptive color change, teeth, tooth 520.8
Preexcitation 426.7
  atrioventricular conduction 426.7
  ventricular 426.7
Preglaucoma 365.00
Pregnancy (single) (uterine) (without sickness) V22.2

Note—Use the following fifth-digit subclassification with categories 640-648, 651-676:

0 unspecified as to episode of care
1 delivered, with or without mention of antepartum condition
2 delivered, with mention of postpartum complication
3 antepartum condition or complication
4 postpartum condition or complication

---

  abdominal (ectopic) 633.00
    affecting fetus or newborn 761.4
    with intrauterine pregnancy 633.01
  abnormal NEC 646.9
  ampullar—*see* Pregnancy, tubal
  broad ligament—*see* Pregnancy, cornual
  cervical—*see* Pregnancy, cornual
  combined (extrauterine and intrauterine)—*see* Pregnancy, cornual
  complicated (by) 646.9
    abnormal, abnormality NEC 646.9
      cervix 654.6
      cord (umbilical) 663.9
      glucose tolerance (conditions classifiable to 790.21-790.29) 648.8
      pelvic organs or tissues NEC 654.9
      pelvis (bony) 653.0

INDEX TO DISEASES

Pregnancy

Pregnancy—*continued*
  perineum or vulva 654.8
  placenta, placental (vessel) 656.7
  position
    cervix 654.4
    placenta 641.1
      without hemorrhage 641.0
    uterus 654.4
  size, fetus 653.5
  uterus (congenital) 654.0
  abscess or cellulitis
    bladder 646.6
    genitourinary tract (conditions classifiable to 590, 595, 597, 599.0, 614.0-614.5, 614.7-614.9, 615) 646.6
    kidney 646.6
    urinary tract NEC 646.6
  adhesion, pelvic peritoneal 648.9
  air embolism 673.0
  albuminuria 646.2
    with hypertension—*see* Toxemia, of pregnancy
  amnionitis 658.4
  amniotic fluid embolism 673.1
  anemia (conditions classifiable to 280-285) 648.2
  appendicitis 648.9
  atrophy, yellow (acute) (liver) (subacute) 646.7
  bacilluria, asymptomatic 646.5
  bacteriuria, asymptomatic 646.5
  bariatric surgery status 649.2
  bicornis or bicornuate uterus 654.0
  biliary problems 646.8
  bone and joint disorders (conditions classifiable to 720-724 or conditions affecting lower limbs classifiable to 711-719, 725-738) 648.7
  breech presentation 652.2
    with successful version 652.1
  cardiovascular disease (conditions classifiable to 390-398, 410-429) 648.6
    congenital (conditions classifiable to 745-747) 648.5
  cerebrovascular disorders conditions (classifiable to 430-434, 436-437) 674.0
  cervicitis (conditions classifiable to 616.0) 646.6
  chloasma (gravidarum) 646.8
  cholelithiasis 646.8
  chorea (gravidarum)—*see* Eclampsia, pregnancy
  coagulation defect 649.3
  contraction, pelvis (general) 653.1
    inlet 653.2
    outlet 653.3
  convulsions (eclamptic) (uremic) 642.6
    with pre-existing hypertension 642.7
  current disease or condition (nonobstetric)
    abnormal glucose tolerance 648.8
    anemia 648.2
    bone and joint (lower limb) 648.7
    cardiovascular 648.6
      congenital 648.5
    cerebrovascular 674.0
    diabetic 648.0
    drug dependence 648.3
    female genital mutilation 648.9
    genital organ or tract 646.6
    gonorrheal 647.1

Pregnancy—*continued*
    hypertensive 642.2
      chronic kidney 642.2
      renal 642.1
    infectious 647.9
      specified type NEC 647.8
    liver 646.7
    malarial 647.4
    nutritional deficiency 648.9
    parasitic NEC 647.8
    periodontal disease 648.9
    renal 646.2
      hypertensive 642.1
    rubella 647.5
    specified condition NEC 648.9
    syphilitic 647.0
    thyroid 648.1
    tuberculous 647.3
    urinary 646.6
    venereal 647.2
    viral NEC 647.6
  cystitis 646.6
  cystocele 654.4
  death of fetus (near term) 656.4
    early pregnancy (before 22 completed weeks gestation) 632
  deciduitis 646.6
  decreased fetal movements 655.7
  diabetes (mellitus) (conditions classifiable to 250) 648.0
  disorders of liver 646.7
  displacement, uterus NEC 654.4
  disproportion—*see* Disproportion
  double uterus 654.0
  drug dependence (conditions classifiable to 304) 648.3
  dysplasia, cervix 654.6
  early onset of delivery (spontaneous) 644.2
  eclampsia, eclamptic (coma) (convulsions) (delirium) (nephritis) (uremia) 642.6
    with pre-existing hypertension 642.7
  edema 646.1
    with hypertension—*see* Toxemia, of pregnancy
  effusion, amniotic fluid 658.1
    delayed delivery following 658.2
  embolism
    air 673.0
    amniotic fluid 673.1
    blood-clot 673.2
    cerebral 674.0
    pulmonary NEC 673.2
    pyemic 673.3
    septic 673.3
  emesis (gravidarum)—*see* Pregnancy, complicated, vomiting
  endometritis (conditions classifiable to 615.0-615.9) 670
    decidual 646.6
  epilepsy 649.4
  excessive weight gain NEC 646.1
  face presentation 652.4
  failure, fetal head to enter pelvic brim 652.5
  false labor (pains) 644.1
  fatigue 646.8
  fatty metamorphosis of liver 646.7
  female genital mutilation 648.9
  fetal
    death (near term) 656.4
      early (before 22 completed weeks gestation) 632

Pregnancy — *continued*
    deformity 653.7
    distress 656.8
    reduction of multiple fetuses reduced to single fetus 651.7
    fibroid (tumor) (uterus) 654.1
    footling presentation 652.8
        with successful version 652.1
    gallbladder disease 646.8
    gastric banding status 649.2
    gastric bypass status for obesity 649.2
    goiter 648.1
    gonococcal infection (conditions classifiable to 098) 647.1
    gonorrhea (conditions classifiable to 098) 647.1
    hemorrhage 641.9
        accidental 641.2
        before 22 completed weeks gestation NEC 640.9
        cerebrovascular 674.0
        due to
            afibrinogenemia or other coagulation defect (conditions classifiable to 286.0-286.9) 641.3
            leiomyoma, uterine 641.8
            marginal sinus (rupture) 641.2
            premature separation, placenta 641.2
            trauma 641.8
        early (before 22 completed weeks gestation) 640.9
        threatened abortion 640.0
        unavoidable 641.1
    hepatitis (acute) (malignant) (subacute) 646.7
        viral 647.6
    herniation of uterus 654.4
    high head at term 652.5
    hydatidiform mole (delivered) (undelivered) 630
    hydramnios 657
    hydrocephalic fetus 653.6
    hydrops amnii 657
    hydrorrhea 658.1
    hyperemesis (gravidarum) — *see* Hyperemesis, gravidarum
    hypertension — *see* Hypertension, complicating pregnancy
    hypertensive heart and chronic kidney disease 642.2
    hypertensive
        chronic kidney disease 642.2
        heart and chronic kidney disease 642.2
        heart and renal disease 642.2
        heart disease 642.2
        renal disease 642.2
    hyperthyroidism 648.1
    hypothyroidism 648.1
    hysteralgia 646.8
    icterus gravis 646.7
    incarceration, uterus 654.3
    incompetent cervix (os) 654.5
    infection 647.9
        amniotic fluid 658.4
        bladder 646.6
        genital organ (conditions classifiable to 614.0-614.5, 614.7-614.9, 615) 646.6
        kidney (conditions classifiable to 590.0-590.9) 646.6
        urinary (tract) 646.6
            asymptomatic 646.5
    infective and parasitic diseases NEC 647.8

Pregnancy — *continued*
    inflammation
        bladder 646.6
        genital organ (conditions classifiable to 614.0-614.5, 614.7-614.9, 615) 646.6
        urinary tract NEC 646.6
    injury 648.9
        obstetrical NEC 665.9
    insufficient weight gain 646.8
    intrauterine fetal death (near term) NEC 656.4
        early (before 22 completed weeks' gestation) 632
    malaria (conditions classifiable to 084) 647.4
    malformation, uterus (congenital) 654.0
    malnutrition (conditions classifiable to 260-269) 648.9
    malposition
        fetus — *see* Pregnancy, complicated, malpresentation
        uterus or cervix 654.4
    malpresentation 652.9
        with successful version 652.1
        in multiple gestation 652.6
        specified type NEC 652.8
    marginal sinus hemorrhage or rupture 641.2
    maternal obesity syndrome 646.1
    menstruation 640.8
    mental disorders (conditions classifiable to 290-303, 305.0, 305.2-305.9, 306-316, 317-319) 648.4
    mentum presentation 652.4
    missed
        abortion 632
        delivery (at or near term) 656.4
        labor (at or near term) 656.4
    necrosis
        genital organ or tract (conditions classifiable to 614.0-614.5, 614.7-614.9, 615) 646.6
        liver (conditions classifiable to 570) 646.7
        renal, cortical 646.2
    nephritis or nephrosis (conditions classifiable to 580-589) 646.2
        with hypertension 642.1
    nephropathy NEC 646.2
    neuritis (peripheral) 646.4
    nutritional deficiency (conditions classifiable to 260-269) 648.9
    obesity 649.1
        surgery status 649.2
    oblique lie or presentation 652.3
        with successful version 652.1
    obstetrical trauma NEC 665.9
    oligohydramnios NEC 658.0
    onset of contractions before 37 weeks 644.0
    oversize fetus 653.5
    papyraceous fetus 646.0
    patent cervix 654.5
    pelvic inflammatory disease (conditions classifiable to 614.0-614.5, 614.7-614.9, 615) 646.6
    pelvic peritoneal adhesion 648.9
    placenta, placental
        abnormality 656.7
        abruptio or ablatio 641.2
        detachment 641.2
        disease 656.7
        infarct 656.7
        low implantation 641.1
            without hemorrhage 641.0
        malformation 656.7
        malposition 641.1

INDEX TO DISEASES   **Pregnancy**

Pregnancy—*continued*
    without hemorrhage 641.0
    marginal sinus hemorrhage 641.2
    previa 641.1
        without hemorrhage 641.0
    separation (premature) (undelivered) 641.2
  placentitis 658.4
  polyhydramnios 657
  postmaturity
    post-term 645.1
    prolonged 645.2
  prediabetes 648.8
  pre-eclampsia (mild) 642.4
    severe 642.5
    superimposed on pre-existing hypertensive disease 642.7
  premature rupture of membranes 658.1
    with delayed delivery 658.2
  previous
    infertility V23.0
    nonobstetric condition V23.8
    poor obstetrical history V23.49
    premature delivery V23.41
    trophoblastic disease (conditions classifiable to 630) V23.1
  prolapse, uterus 654.4
  proteinuria (gestational) 646.2
    with hypertension—*see* Toxemia, of pregnancy
  pruritus (neurogenic) 646.8
  psychosis or psychoneurosis 648.4
  ptyalism 646.8
  pyelitis (conditions classifiable to 590.0-590.9) 646.6
  renal disease or failure NEC 646.2
    with secondary hypertension 642.1
    hypertensive 642.2
  retention, retained dead ovum 631
  retroversion, uterus 654.3
  Rh immunization, incompatibility, or sensitization 656.1
  rubella (conditions classifiable to 056) 647.5
  rupture
    amnion (premature) 658.1
      with delayed delivery 658.2
    marginal sinus (hemorrhage) 641.2
    membranes (premature) 658.1
      with delayed delivery 658.2
    uterus (before onset of labor) 665.0
  salivation (excessive) 646.8
  salpingo-oophoritis (conditions classifiable to 614.0-614.2) 646.6
  septicemia (conditions classifiable to 038.0-038.9) 647.8
    postpartum 670
    puerperal 670
  smoking 649.0
  spasms, uterus (abnormal) 646.8
  specified condition NEC 646.8
  spotting 649.5
  spurious labor pains 644.1
  status post
    bariatric surgery 649.2
    gastric banding 649.2
    gastric bypass for obesity 649.2
    obesity surgery 649.2
  superfecundation 651.9
  superfetation 651.9
  syphilis (conditions classifiable to 090-097) 647.0

Pregnancy—*continued*
  threatened
    abortion 640.0
    premature delivery 644.2
    premature labor 644.0
  thrombophlebitis (superficial) 671.2
    deep 671.3
  thrombosis 671.9
    venous (superficial) 671.2
      deep 671.3
  thyroid dysfunction (conditions classifiable to 240-246) 648.1
  thyroiditis 648.1
  thyrotoxicosis 648.1
  tobacco use disorder 649.0
  torsion of uterus 654.4
  toxemia—*see* Toxemia, of pregnancy
  transverse lie or presentation 652.3
    with successful version 652.1
  trauma 648.9
    obstetrical 665.9
  tuberculosis (conditions classifiable to 010-018) 647.3
  tumor
    cervix 654.6
    ovary 654.4
    pelvic organs or tissue NEC 654.4
    uterus (body) 654.1
      cervix 654.6
    vagina 654.7
    vulva 654.8
  unstable lie 652.0
  uremia—*see* Pregnancy, complicated, renal disease
  urethritis 646.6
  vaginitis or vulvitis (conditions classifiable to 616.1) 646.6
  varicose
    placental vessels 656.7
    veins (legs) 671.0
      perineum 671.1
      vulva 671.1
  varicosity, labia or vulva 671.1
  venereal disease NEC (conditions classifiable to 099) 647.2
  viral disease NEC (conditions classifiable to 042, 050-055, 057-079) 647.6
  vomiting (incoercible) (pernicious) (persistent) (uncontrollable) (vicious) 643.9
    due to organic disease or other cause 643.8
    early—*see* Hyperemesis, gravidarum
    late (after 22 completed weeks gestation) 643.2
  young maternal age 659.8
complications NEC 646.9
cornual 633.80
  affecting fetus or newborn 761.4
  with intrauterine pregnancy 633.81
death, maternal NEC 646.9
delivered—*see* Delivery
ectopic (ruptured) NEC 633.90
  with intrauterine pregnancy 633.91
  abdominal—*see* Pregnancy, abdominal
  affecting fetus or newborn 761.4
  combined (extrauterine and intrauterine)—*see* Pregnancy, cornual
  ovarian—*see* Pregnancy, ovarian
  specified type NEC 633.80
    affecting fetus or newborn 761.4
    with intrauterine pregnancy 633.81
  tubal—*see* Pregnancy, tubal

Pregnancy—*continued*
  examination, pregnancy
    negative result V72.41
    not confirmed V72.40
    positive result V72.42
  extrauterine—*see* Pregnancy, ectopic
  fallopian—*see* Pregnancy, tubal
  false 300.11
    labor (pains) 644.1
  fatigue 646.8
  illegitimate V61.6
  incidental finding V22.2
  in double uterus 654.0
  interstitial—*see* Pregnancy, cornual
  intraligamentous—*see* Pregnancy, cornual
  intramural—*see* Pregnancy, cornual
  intraperitoneal—*see* Pregnancy, abdominal
  isthmian—*see* Pregnancy, tubal
  management affected by
    abnormal, abnormality
      fetus (suspected) 655.9
        specified NEC 655.8
      placenta 656.7
    advanced maternal age NEC 659.6
      multigravida 659.6
      primigravida 659.5
    antibodies (maternal)
      anti-c 656.1
      anti-d 656.1
      anti-e 656.1
      blood group (ABO) 656.2
        Rh(esus) 656.1
    appendicitis 648.9
    bariatric surgery status 649.2
    coagulation defect 649.3
    elderly multigravida 659.6
    elderly primigravida 659.5
    epilepsy 649.4
    fetal (suspected)
      abnormality 655.9
        acid-base balance 656.8
        heart rate or rhythm 659.7
        specified NEC 655.8
      acidemia 656.3
      anencephaly 655.0
      bradycardia 659.7
      central nervous system malformation 655.0
      chromosomal abnormalities (conditions
        classifiable to 758.0-758.9) 655.1
      damage from
        drugs 655.5
          obstetric, anesthetic, or sedative 655.5
        environmental toxins 655.8
        intrauterine contraceptive device 655.8
        maternal
          alcohol addiction 655.4
          disease NEC 655.4
          drug use 655.5
          listeriosis 655.4
          rubella 655.3
          toxoplasmosis 655.4
          viral infection 655.3
        radiation 655.6
      death (near term) 656.4
        early (before 22 completed weeks
          gestation) 632
      distress 656.8
      excessive growth 656.6
      growth retardation 656.5
      hereditary disease 655.2
      hydrocephalus 655.0

Pregnancy—*continued*
      intrauterine death 656.4
      poor growth 656.5
      spina bifida (with myelomeningocele) 655.0
    fetal-maternal hemorrhage 656.0
    gastric banding status 649.2
    gastric bypass status for obesity 649.2
    hereditary disease in family (possibly)
      affecting fetus 655.2
    incompatibility, blood groups (ABO) 656.2
      rh(esus) 656.1
    insufficient prenatal care V23.7
    intrauterine death 656.4
    isoimmunization (ABO) 656.2
      rh(esus) 656.1
    large-for-dates fetus 656.6
    light-for-dates fetus 656.5
    meconium in liquor 656.8
    mental disorder (conditions classifiable to
      290-303, 305.0, 305.2-305.9, 306-316,
      317-319) 648.4
    multiparity (grand) 659.4
    obesity 649.1
      surgery status 649.2
    poor obstetric history V23.49
      pre-term labor V23.41
    postmaturity
      post-term 645.1
      prolonged 645.2
    post-term pregnancy 645.1
    previous
      abortion V23.2
        habitual 646.3
      cesarean delivery 654.2
      difficult delivery V23.49
      forceps delivery V23.49
      habitual abortions 646.3
      hemorrhage, antepartum or postpartum
        V23.49
      hydatidiform mole V23.1
      infertility V23.0
      malignancy NEC V23.8
      nonobstetrical conditions V23.8
      premature delivery V23.41
      trophoblastic disease (conditions in 630)
        V23.1
      vesicular mole V23.1
    prolonged pregnancy 645.2
    small-for-dates fetus 656.5
    smoking 649.0
    spotting 649.5
    tobacco use disorder 649.0
    young maternal age 659.8
  maternal death NEC 646.9
  mesometric (mural)—*see* Pregnancy, cornual
  molar 631
    hydatidiform (*see also* Hydatidiform mole)
      630
      previous, affecting management of
        pregnancy V23.1
    previous, affecting management of pregnancy
      V23.49
  multiple NEC 651.9
    with fetal loss and retention of one or more
      fetus(es) 651.6
    affecting fetus or newborn 761.5
    following (elective) fetal reduction 651.7
    specified type NEC 651.8
      with fetal loss and retention of one or more
        fetus(es) 651.6
      following (elective) fetal reduction 651.7

Pregnancy—*continued*
 mural—*see* Pregnancy, cornual
 observation NEC V22.1
  first pregnancy V22.0
  high-risk V23.9
   specified problem NEC V23.8
 ovarian 633.20
  affecting fetus or newborn 761.4
  with intrauterine pregnancy 633.21
 possible, not (yet) confirmed V72.40
 postmature
  post-term 645.1
  prolonged 645.2
 post-term 645.1
 prenatal care only V22.1
  first pregnancy V22.0
  high-risk V23.9
   specified problem NEC V23.8
 prolonged 645.2
 quadruplet NEC 651.2
  with fetal loss and retention of one or more fetus(es) 651.5
  affecting fetus or newborn 761.5
  following (elective) fetal reduction 651.7
 quintuplet NEC 651.8
  with fetal loss and retention of one or more fetus(es) 651.6
  affecting fetus or newborn 761.5
  following (elective) fetal reduction 651.7
 sextuplet NEC 651.8
  with fetal loss and retention of one or more fetus(es) 651.6
  affecting fetus or newborn 761.5
  following (elective) fetal reduction 651.7
 spurious 300.11
 superfecundation NEC 651.9
  with fetal loss and retention of one or more fetus(es) 651.6
  following (elective) fetal reduction 651.7
 superfetation NEC 651.9
  with fetal loss and retention of one or more fetus(es) 651.6
  following (elective) fetal reduction 651.7
 supervision (of) (for)—*see also* Pregnancy, management affected by
  elderly
   multigravida V23.82
   primigravida V23.81
  high-risk V23.9
   insufficient prenatal care V23.7
   specified problem NEC V23.8
  multiparity V23.3
  normal NEC V22.1
   first V22.0
  poor
   obstetric history V23.49
    pre-term labor V23.41
   reproductive history V23.5
  previous
   abortion V23.2
   hydatidiform mole V23.1
   infertility V23.0
   neonatal death V23.5
   stillbirth V23.5
   trophoblastic disease V23.1
   vesicular mole V23.1
  specified problem NEC V23.8
  young
   multigravida V23.84
   primigravida V23.83
 triplet NEC 651.1

Pregnancy—*continued*
 with fetal loss and retention of one or more fetus(es) 651.4
 affecting fetus or newborn 761.5
 following (elective) fetal reduction 651.7
 tubal (with rupture) 633.10
  affecting fetus or newborn 761.4
  with intrauterine pregnancy 633.11
 twin NEC 651.0
  with fetal loss and retention of one or more fetus(es) 651.3
  affecting fetus or newborn 761.5
  following (elective) fetal reduction 651.7
 unconfirmed V72.40
 undelivered (no other diagnosis) V22.2
  with false labor 644.1
  high-risk V23.9
   specified problem NEC V23.8
 unwanted NEC V61.7
Pregnant uterus —*see* condition
Preiser's disease (osteoporosis) 733.09
Prekwashiorkor 260
Preleukemia 238.75
Preluxation of hip, congenital (*see also* Subluxation, congenital, hip) 754.32
Premature —*see also* condition
 beats (nodal) 427.60
  atrial 427.61
  auricular 427.61
  postoperative 997.1
  specified type NEC 427.69
  supraventricular 427.61
  ventricular 427.69
 birth NEC 765.1
 closure
  cranial suture 756.0
  fontanel 756.0
  foramen ovale 745.8
 contractions 427.60
  atrial 427.61
  auricular 427.61
  auriculoventricular 427.61
  heart (extrasystole) 427.60
  junctional 427.60
  nodal 427.60
  postoperative 997.1
  ventricular 427.69
 ejaculation 302.75
 infant NEC 765.1
  excessive 765.0
  light-for-dates—*see* Light-for-dates
 labor 644.2
  threatened 644.0
 lungs 770.4
 menopause 256.31
 puberty 259.1
 rupture of membranes or amnion 658.1
  affecting fetus or newborn 761.1
  delayed delivery following 658.2
 senility (syndrome) 259.8
 separation, placenta (partial)—*see* Placenta, separation
 ventricular systole 427.69
Prematurity NEC 765.1
 extreme 765.0
Premenstrual syndrome 625.4
Premenstrual tension 625.4
Premolarization, cuspids 520.2
Premyeloma 273.1

Prenatal
care, normal pregnancy V22.1
  first V22.0
death, cause unknown—*see* Death, fetus
screening—*see* Antenatal, screening
teeth 520.6
Prepartum —*see* condition
Preponderance, left or right ventricular 429.3
Prepuce —*see* condition
PRES (posterior reversible encephalopathy syndrome) 348.39
Presbycardia 797
  hypertensive (*see also* Hypertension, heart) 402.90
Presbycusis 388.01
Presbyesophagus 530.89
Presbyophrenia 310.1
Presbyopia 367.4
Prescription of contraceptives NEC V25.02
  diaphragm V25.02
  oral (pill) V25.01
    emergency V25.03
    postcoital V25.03
    repeat V25.41
  repeat V25.40
    oral (pill) V25.41
Presenile —*see also* condition
  aging 259.8
  dementia (*see also* Dementia, presenile) 290.10
Presenility 259.8
Presentation, fetal
  abnormal 652.9
    with successful version 652.1
    before labor, affecting fetus or newborn 761.7
    causing obstructed labor 660.0
      affecting fetus or newborn, any, except breech 763.1
    in multiple gestation (one or more) 652.6
    specified NEC 652.8
  arm 652.7
    causing obstructed labor 660.0
  breech (buttocks) (complete) (frank) 652.2
    with successful version 652.1
      before labor, affecting fetus or newborn 761.7
    before labor, affecting fetus or newborn 761.7
  brow 652.4
    causing obstructed labor 660.0
  buttocks 652.2
  chin 652.4
  complete 652.2
  compound 652.8
  cord 663.0
  extended head 652.4
  face 652.4
    to pubes 652.8
  footling 652.8
  frank 652.2
  hand, leg, or foot NEC 652.8
  incomplete 652.8
  mentum 652.4
  multiple gestation (one fetus or more) 652.6
  oblique 652.3
    with successful version 652.1
  shoulder 652.8
    affecting fetus or newborn 763.1
  transverse 652.3
    with successful version 652.1
  umbilical cord 663.0
  unstable 652.0
Prespondylolisthesis (congenital) (lumbosacral) 756.11

Pressure
area, skin ulcer (*see also* Decubitus) 707.00
atrophy, spine 733.99
birth, fetus or newborn NEC 767.9
brachial plexus 353.0
brain 348.4
  injury at birth 767.0
cerebral—*see* Pressure, brain
chest 786.59
cone, tentorial 348.4
  injury at birth 767.0
funis—*see* Compression, umbilical cord
hyposystolic (*see also* Hypotension) 458.9
increased
  intracranial 781.99
    due to
      benign intracranial hypertension 348.2
      hydrocephalus—*see* hydrocephalus
      injury at birth 767.8
    intraocular 365.00
lumbosacral plexus 353.1
mediastinum 519.3
necrosis (chronic) (skin) (*see also* Decubitus) 707.00
nerve—*see* Compression, nerve
paralysis (*see also* Neuropathy, entrapment) 355.9
sore (chronic) (*see also* Decubitus) 707.00
spinal cord 336.9
ulcer (chronic) (*see also* Decubitus) 707.00
umbilical cord—*see* Compression, umbilical cord
venous, increased 459.89
Pre-syncope 780.2
Preterm infant NEC 765.1
  extreme 765.0
Priapism (penis) 607.3
Prickling sensation (*see also* Disturbance, sensation) 782.0
Prickly heat 705.1
Primary —*see* condition
Primigravida, elderly
  affecting
    fetus or newborn 763.89
    management of pregnancy, labor, and delivery 659.5
Primipara, old
  affecting
    fetus or newborn 763.89
    management of pregnancy, labor, and delivery 659.5
Primula dermatitis 692.6
Primus varus (bilateral) (metatarsus) 754.52
PRIND (prolonged reversible ischemic neurologic deficit) 434.91
  history of personal V12.54
Pringle's disease (tuberous sclerosis) 759.5
Prinzmetal's angina 413.1
Prinzmetal-Massumi syndrome (anterior chest wall) 786.52
Prizefighter ear 738.7
Problem (with) V49.9
  academic V62.3
  acculturation V62.4
  adopted child V61.29
  aged
    in-law V61.3
    parent V61.3
    person NEC V61.8
  alcoholism in family V61.41
  anger reaction (*see also* Disturbance, conduct) 312.0
  behavior, child 312.9

Problem—*continued*
  behavioral V40.9
    specified NEC V40.3
  betting V69.3
  cardiorespiratory NEC V47.2
  care of sick or handicapped person in family or household V61.49
  career choice V62.2
  communication V40.1
  conscience regarding medical care V62.6
  delinquency (juvenile) 312.9
  diet, inappropriate V69.1
  digestive NEC V47.3
  ear NEC V41.3
  eating habits, inappropriate V69.1
  economic V60.2
    affecting care V60.9
      specified type NEC V60.8
  educational V62.3
  enuresis, child 307.6
  exercise, lack of V69.0
  eye NEC V41.1
  family V61.9
    specified circumstance NEC V61.8
  fear reaction, child 313.0
  feeding (elderly) (infant) 783.3
    newborn 779.3
    nonorganic 307.59
  fetal, affecting management of pregnancy 656.9
    specified type NEC 656.8
  financial V60.2
  foster child V61.29
    specified NEC V41.8
  functional V41.9
    specified type NEC V41.8
  gambling V69.3
  genital NEC V47.5
  head V48.9
    deficiency V48.0
    disfigurement V48.6
    mechanical V48.2
    motor V48.2
    movement of V48.2
    sensory V48.4
    specified condition NEC V48.8
  hearing V41.2
  high-risk sexual behavior V69.2
  identity 313.82
  influencing health status NEC V49.89
  internal organ NEC V47.9
    deficiency V47.0
    mechanical or motor V47.1
  interpersonal NEC V62.81
  jealousy, child 313.3
  learning V40.0
  legal V62.5
  life circumstance NEC V62.89
  lifestyle V69.9
    specified NEC V69.8
  limb V49.9
    deficiency V49.0
    disfigurement V49.4
    mechanical V49.1
    motor V49.2
    movement, involving
      musculoskeletal system V49.1
      nervous system V49.2
    sensory V49.3
    specified condition NEC V49.5
  litigation V62.5
  living alone V60.3

Problem—*continued*
  loneliness NEC V62.89
  marital V61.10
    involving
      divorce V61.0
      estrangement V61.0
      psychosexual disorder 302.9
      sexual function V41.7
    relationship V61.10
  mastication V41.6
  medical care, within family V61.49
  mental V40.9
    specified NEC V40.2
  mental hygiene, adult V40.9
  multiparity V61.5
  nail biting, child 307.9
  neck V48.9
    deficiency V48.1
    disfigurement V48.7
    mechanical V48.3
    motor V48.3
    movement V48.3
    sensory V48.5
    specified condition NEC V48.8
  neurological NEC 781.99
  none (feared complaint unfounded) V65.5
  occupational V62.2
  parent-child V61.20
    relationship V61.20
  partner V61.10
    relationship V61.10
  personal NEC V62.89
    interpersonal conflict NEC V62.81
  personality (*see also* Disorder, personality) 301.9
  phase of life V62.89
  placenta, affecting management of pregnancy 656.9
    specified type NEC 656.8
  poverty V60.2
  presence of sick or handicapped person in family or household V61.49
  psychiatric 300.9
  psychosocial V62.9
    specified type NEC V62.89
  relational NEC V62.81
  relationship, childhood 313.3
  religious or spiritual belief
    other than medical care V62.89
    regarding medical care V62.6
  self-damaging behavior V69.8
  sexual
    behavior, high-risk V69.2
    function NEC V41.7
  sibling
    relational V61.8
    relationship V61.8
  sight V41.0
  sleep disorder, child 307.40
  sleep, lack of V69.4
  smell V41.5
  speech V40.1
  spite reaction, child (*see also* Disturbance, conduct) 312.0
  spoiled child reaction (*see also* Disturbance, conduct) 312.1
  swallowing V41.6
  tantrum, child (*see also* Disturbance, conduct) 312.1
  taste V41.5
  thumb sucking, child 307.9

Problem—*continued*
  tic (child) 307.21
  trunk V48.9
    deficiency V48.1
    disfigurement V48.7
    mechanical V48.3
    motor V48.3
    movement V48.3
    sensory V48.5
    specified condition NEC V48.8
  unemployment V62.0
  urinary NEC V47.4
  voice production V41.4
Procedure (surgical) not done NEC V64.3
  because of
    contraindication V64.1
    patient's decision V64.2
      for reasons of conscience or religion V62.6
    specified reason NEC V64.3
Procidentia
  anus (sphincter) 569.1
  rectum (sphincter) 569.1
  stomach 537.89
  uteri 618.1
Proctalgia 569.42
  fugax 564.6
  spasmodic 564.6
    psychogenic 307.89
Proctitis 569.49
  amebic 006.8
  chlamydial 099.52
  gonococcal 098.7
  granulomatous 555.1
  idiopathic 556.2
    with ulcerative sigmoiditis 556.3
  tuberculous (*see also* Tuberculosis) 014.8
  ulcerative (chronic) (nonspecific) 556.2
    with ulcerative sigmoiditis 556.3
Proctocele
  female (without uterine prolapse) 618.04
    with uterine prolapse 618.4
      complete 618.3
      incomplete 618.2
  male 569.49
Proctocolitis, idiopathic 556.2
  with ulcerative sigmoiditis 556.3
Proctoptosis 569.1
Proctosigmoiditis 569.89
  ulcerative (chronic) 556.3
Proctospasm 564.6
  psychogenic 306.4
Prodromal-AIDS —*see* Human immunodeficiency virus (disease) (illness) (infection)
Profichet's disease or syndrome 729.9
Progeria (adultorum) (syndrome) 259.8
Prognathism (mandibular) (maxillary) 524.00
Progonoma (melanotic) (M9363/0)—*see* Neoplasm, by site, benign
Progressive —*see* condition
Prolapse, prolapsed
  anus, anal (canal) (sphincter) 569.1
  arm or hand, complicating delivery 652.7
    causing obstructed labor 660.0
      affecting fetus or newborn 763.1
    fetus or newborn 763.1
  bladder (acquired) (mucosa) (sphincter)
    congenital (female) (male) 756.71
    female (*see also* Cystocele, female) 618.01
    male 596.8
  breast implant (prosthetic) 996.54

Prolapse, prolapsed—*continued*
  cecostomy 569.69
  cecum 569.89
  cervix, cervical (hypertrophied) 618.1
    anterior lip, obstructing labor 660.2
      affecting fetus or newborn 763.1
    congenital 752.49
    postpartal (old) 618.1
    stump 618.84
  ciliary body 871.1
  colon (pedunculated) 569.89
  colostomy 569.69
  conjunctiva 372.73
  cord—*see* Prolapse, umbilical cord
  disc (intervertebral)—*see* Displacement, intervertebral disc
  duodenum 537.89
  eye implant (orbital) 996.59
    lens (ocular) 996.53
  fallopian tube 620.4
  fetal extremity, complicating delivery 652.8
    causing obstructed labor 660.0
    fetus or newborn 763.1
  funis—*see* Prolapse, umbilical cord
  gastric (mucosa) 537.89
  genital, female 618.9
    specified NEC 618.89
  globe 360 81
  ileostomy bud 569.69
  intervertebral disc—*see* Displacement, intervertebral disc
  intestine (small) 569.89
  iris 364.89
    traumatic 871.1
  kidney (*see also* Disease, renal) 593.0
    congenital 753.3
  laryngeal muscles or ventricle 478.79
  leg, complicating delivery 652.8
    causing obstructed labor 660.0
    fetus or newborn 763.1
  liver 573.8
  meatus urinarius 599.5
  mitral valve 424.0
  ocular lens implant 996.53
  organ or site, congenital NEC—*see* Malposition, congenital
  ovary 620.4
  pelvic (floor), female 618.89
  perineum, female 618.89
  pregnant uterus 654.4
  rectum (mucosa) (sphincter) 569.1
    due to Trichuris trichiuria 127.3
  spleen 289.59
  stomach 537.89
  umbilical cord
    affecting fetus or newborn 762.4
    complicating delivery 663.0
  ureter 593.89
    with obstruction 593.4
  ureterovesical orifice 593.89
  urethra (acquired) (infected) (mucosa) 599.5
    congenital 753.8
  uterovaginal 618.4
    complete 618.3
    incomplete 618.2
    specified NEC 618.89
  uterus (first degree) (second degree) (third degree) (complete) (without vaginal wall prolapse) 618.1
    with mention of vaginal wall prolapse—*see* Prolapse, uterovaginal

INDEX TO DISEASES   **Protein**

Prolapse, prolapsed—*continued*
  congenital 752.3
  in pregnancy or childbirth 654.4
    affecting fetus or newborn 763.1
    causing obstructed labor 660.2
      affecting fetus or newborn 763.1
    postpartal (old) 618.1
  uveal 871.1
  vagina (anterior) (posterior) (vault) (wall) (without uterine prolapse) 618.00
    with uterine prolapse 618.4
      complete 618.3
      incomplete 618.2
    paravaginal 618.02
    posthysterectomy 618.5
    specified NEC 618.09
  vitreous (humor) 379.26
    traumatic 871.1
  womb—*see* Prolapse, uterus
Prolapsus, female 618.9
Proliferative —*see* condition
Prolinemia 270.8
Prolinuria 270.8
Prolonged, prolongation
  bleeding time (*see also* Defect, coagulation) 790.92
    "idiopathic" (in von Willebrand's disease) 286.4
  coagulation time (*see also* Defect, coagulation) 790.92
  gestation syndrome 766.22
  labor 662.1
    affecting fetus or newborn 763.89
    first stage 662.0
    second stage 662.2
  PR interval 426.11
  pregnancy 645.2
  prothrombin time (*see also* Defect, coagulation) 790.92
  QT interval 794.31
    syndrome 426.82
  rupture of membranes (24 hours or more prior to onset of labor) 658.2
  uterine contractions in labor 661.4
    affecting fetus or newborn 763.7
Prominauris 744.29
Prominence
  auricle (ear) (congenital) 744.29
    acquired 380.32
  ischial spine or sacral promontory
    with disproportion (fetopelvic) 653.3
      affecting fetus or newborn 763.1
      causing obstructed labor 660.1
        affecting fetus or newborn 763.1
  nose (congenital) 748.1
    acquired 738.0
PROMM (proximal myotonic myotonia) 359.21
Pronation
  ankle 736.79
  foot 736.79
    congenital 755.67
Prophylactic
  administration of
    antibiotics V07.39
    antitoxin, any V07.2
    antivenin V07.2
    chemotherapeutic agent NEC V07.39
      fluoride V07.31
    diphtheria antitoxin V07.2
    drug V07.39
    gamma globulin V07.2
    immune sera (gamma globulin) V07.2
    RhoGAM V07.2

Prophylactic—*continued*
    tetanus antitoxin V07.2
  chemotherapy NEC V07.39
    fluoride V07.31
  hormone replacement (postmenopausal) V07.4
  immunotherapy V07.2
  measure V07.9
    specified type NEC V07.8
  medication V07.39
  postmenopausal hormone replacement V07.4
  sterilization V25.2
Proptosis (ocular) (*see also* Exophthalmos) 376.30
  thyroid 242.0
Propulsion
  eyeball 360.81
Prosecution, anxiety concerning V62.5
Prostate, prostatic —*see* condition
Prostatism 600.90
  with
    other lower urinary tract symptoms (LUTS) 600.91
    urinary
      obstruction 600.91
      retention 600.91
Prostatitis (congestive) (suppurative) 601.9
  acute 601.0
  cavitary 601.8
  chlamydial 099.54
  chronic 601.1
  diverticular 601.8
  due to Trichomonas (vaginalis) 131.03
  fibrous 600.90
    with
      other lower urinary tract symptoms (LUTS) 600.91
      urinary
        obstruction 600.91
        retention 600.91
  gonococcal (acute) 098.12
    chronic or duration of 2 months or over 098.32
  granulomatous 601.8
  hypertrophic 600.00
    with
      other lower urinary tract symptoms (LUTS) 600.01
      urinary
        obstruction 600.01
        retention 600.01
  specified type NEC 601.8
  subacute 601.1
  trichomonal 131.03
  tuberculous (*see also* Tuberculosis) 016.5 [601.4]
Prostatocystitis 601.3
Prostatorrhea 602.8
Prostatoseminovesiculitis, trichomonal 131.03
Prostration 780.79
  heat 992.5
    anhydrotic 992.3
    due to
      salt (and water) depletion 992.4
      water depletion 992.3
  nervous 300.5
  newborn 779.89
  senile 797
Protanomaly 368.51
Protanopia (anomalous trichromat) (complete) (incomplete) 368.51
Protection (against) (from) —*see* Prophylactic
Protein
  deficiency 260
  malnutrition 260
  sickness (prophylactic) (therapeutic) 999.5

Proteinemia 790.99
Proteinosis
 alveolar, lung or pulmonary 516.0
 lipid 272.8
Proteinosis
 lipoid (of Urbach) 272.8
Proteinuria (*see also* Albuminuria) 791.0
 Bence-Jones NEC 791.0
 gestational 646.2
  with hypertension—*see* Toxemia, of pregnancy
 orthostatic 593.6
 postural 593.6
Proteolysis, pathologic 286.6
Protocoproporphyria 277.1
Protoporphyria (erythrohepatic) (erythropoietic) 277.1
Protrusio acetabuli 718.65
Protrusion
 acetabulum (into pelvis) 718.65
 device, implant, or graft—*see* Complications, mechanical
 ear, congenital 744.29
 intervertebral disc—*see* Displacement, intervertebral disc
 nucleus pulposus—*see* Displacement, intervertebral disc
Proud flesh 701.5
Prune belly (syndrome) 756.71
Prurigo (ferox) (gravis) (Hebra's) (hebrae) (mitis) (simplex) 698.2
 agria 698.3
 asthma syndrome 691.8
 Besnier's (atopic dermatitis) (infantile eczema) 691.8
 eczematodes allergicum 691.8
 estivalis (Hutchinson's) 692.72
 Hutchinson's 692.72
 nodularis 698.3
 psychogenic 306.3
Pruritus, pruritic 698.9
 ani 698.0
  psychogenic 306.3
 conditions NEC 698.9
  psychogenic 306.3
 due to Onchocerca volvulus 125.3
 ear 698.9
 essential 698.9
 genital organ(s) 698.1
  psychogenic 306.3
 gravidarum 646.8
 hiemalis 698.8
 neurogenic (any site) 306.3
 perianal 698.0
 psychogenic (any site) 306.3
 scrotum 698.1
  psychogenic 306.3
 senile, senilis 698.8
 Trichomonas 131.9
 vulva, vulvae 698.1
  psychogenic 306.3
Psammocarcinoma (M8140/3)—*see* Neoplasm, by site, malignant
Pseudarthrosis, pseudoarthrosis (bone) 733.82
 joint following fusion V45.4
Pseudoacanthosis
 nigricans 701.8
Pseudoaneurysm —*see* Aneurysm
Pseudoangina (pectoris)—*see* Angina
Pseudoangioma 452
Pseudo-Argyll-Robertson pupil 379.45

Pseudoarteriosus 747.89
Pseudoarthrosis —*see* Pseudarthrosis
Pseudoataxia 799.89
Pseudobulbar affect (PBA) 310.8
Pseudobursa 727.89
Pseudocholera 025
Pseudochromidrosis 705.89
Pseudocirrhosis, liver, pericardial 423.2
Pseudocoarctation 747.21
Pseudocowpox 051.1
Pseudocoxalgia 732.1
Pseudocroup 478.75
Pseudocyesis 300.11
Pseudocyst
 lung 518.89
 pancreas 577.2
 retina 361.19
Pseudodementia 300.16
Pseudoelephantiasis neuroarthritica 757.0
Pseudoemphysema 518.89
Pseudoencephalitis
 superior (acute) hemorrhagic 265.1
Pseudoerosion cervix, congenital 752.49
Pseudoexfoliation, lens capsule 366.11
Pseudofracture (idiopathic) (multiple) (spontaneous) (symmetrical) 268.2
Pseudoglanders 025
Pseudoglioma 360.44
Pseudogout —*see* Chondrocalcinosis
Pseudohallucination 780.1
Pseudohemianesthesia 782.0
Pseudohemophilia (Bernuth's) (hereditary) (type B) 286.4
 type A 287.8
 vascular 287.8
Pseudohermaphroditism 752.7
 with chromosomal anomaly—*see* Anomaly, chromosomal
 adrenal 255.2
 female (without adrenocortical disorder) 752.7
  with adrenocortical disorder 255.2
   adrenal 255.2
 male (without gonadal disorder) 752.7
  with
   adrenocortical disorder 255.2
   cleft scrotum 752.7
   feminizing testis 259.5
   gonadal disorder 257.9
   adrenal 255.2
Pseudohole, macula 362.54
Pseudo-Hurler's disease (mucolipidosis III) 272.7
Pseudohydrocephalus 348.2
Pseudohypertrophic muscular dystrophy (Erb's) 359.1
Pseudohypertrophy, muscle 359.1
Pseudohypoparathyroidism 275.49
Psuedopseudohypoparathyroidism 275.49
Pseudoinfluenza 487.1
Pseudoinsomnia 307.49
Pseudoleukemia 288.8
 infantile 285.8
Pseudomembranous —*see* condition
Pseudomeningocele (cerebral) (infective) 349.2
 postprocedural 997.01
 spinal 349.2
Pseudomenstruation 626.8
Pseudomucinous
 cyst (ovary) (M8470/0) 220
 peritoneum 568.89
Pseudomyeloma 273.1

INDEX TO DISEASES   Psychosis

Pseudomyxoma peritonei (M8480/6) 197.6
Pseudoneuritis optic (nerve) 377.24
  papilla 377.24
    congenital 743.57
Pseudoneuroma —*see* Injury, nerve, by site
Pseudo-obstruction
  intestine (chronic) (idiopathic) (intermittent secondary) (primary) 564.89
    acute 560.89
Pseudopapilledema 377.24
Pseudoparalysis
  arm or leg 781.4
  atonic, congenital 358.8
Pseudopelade 704.09
Pseudophakia V43.1
Pseudopolycythemia 289.0
Pseudopolyposis, colon 556.4
Pseudoporencephaly 348.0
Pseudopseudohypoparathyroidism 275.49
Pseudopsychosis 300.16
Pseudopterygium 372.52
Pseudoptosis (eyelid) 374.34
Pseudorabies 078.89
Pseudoretinitis, pigmentosa 362.65
Pseudorickets 588.0
  senile (Pozzi's) 731.0
Pseudorubella 057.8
Pseudoscarlatina 057.8
Pseudosclerema 778.1
Pseudosclerosis (brain)
  Jakob's 046.1
  of Westphal (-Strümpell) (hepatolenticular degeneration) 275.1
  spastic 046.1
    with dementia
      with behavioral disturbance 046.1 *[294.11]*
      without behavioral disturbance 046.1 *[294.10]*
Pseudoseizure 780.39
  non-psychiatric 780.39
  psychiatric 300.11
Pseudotabes 799.89
  diabetic 250.6 *[337.1]*
Pseudotetanus (*see also* Convulsions) 780.39
Pseudotetany 781.7
  hysterical 300.11
Pseudothalassemia 285.0
Pseudotrichinosis 710.3
Pseudotruncus arteriosus 747.29
Pseudotuberculosis, pasteurella (infection) 027.2
Pseudotumor
  cerebri 348.2
  orbit (inflammatory) 376.11
Pseudo-Turner's syndrome 759.89
Pseudoxanthoma elasticum 757.39
Psilosis (sprue) (tropical) 579.1
  Monilia 112.89
  nontropical 579.0
  not sprue 704.00
Psittacosis 073.9
Psoitis 728.89
Psora NEC 696.1
Psoriasis 696.1
  any type, except arthropathic 696.1
  arthritic, arthropathic 696.0
  buccal 528.6
  flexural 696.1
  follicularis 696.1
  guttate 696.1
  inverse 696.1
  mouth 528.6

Psoriasis—*continued*
  nummularis 696.1
  psychogenic 316 *[696.1]*
  punctata 696.1
  pustular 696.1
  rupioides 696.1
  vulgaris 696.1
Psorospermiasis 136.4
Psorospermosis 136.4
  follicularis (vegetans) 757.39
Psychalgia 307.80
Psychasthenia 300.89
  compulsive 300.3
  mixed compulsive states 300.3
  obsession 300.3
Psychiatric disorder or problem NEC 300.9
Psychogenic —*see also* condition
  factors associated with physical conditions 316
Psychoneurosis, psychoneurotic (*see also* Neurosis) 300.9
  anxiety (state) 300.00
  climacteric 627.2
  compensation 300.16
  compulsion 300.3
  conversion hysteria 300.11
  depersonalization 300.6
  depressive type 300.4
  dissociative hysteria 300.15
  hypochondriacal 300.7
  hysteria 300.10
    conversion type 300.11
    dissociative type 300.15
  mixed NEC 300.89
  neurasthenic 300.5
  obsessional 300.3
  obsessive-compulsive 300.3
  occupational 300.89
  personality NEC 301.89
  phobia 300.20
  senile NEC 300.89
Psychopathic —*see also* condition
  constitution, posttraumatic 310.2
    with psychosis 293.9
  personality 301.9
    amoral trends 301.7
    antisocial trends 301.7
    asocial trends 301.7
    mixed types 301.7
  state 301.9
Psychopathy, sexual (*see also* Deviation, sexual) 302.9
Psychophysiologic, psychophysiological condition—*see* Reaction, psychophysiologic
Psychose passionelle 297.8
Psychosexual identity disorder 302.6
  adult-life 302.85
  childhood 302.6
Psychosis 298.9
  acute hysterical 298.1
  affecting management of pregnancy, childbirth, or puerperium 648.4
  affective (*see also* Disorder, mood) 296.90
    drug induced 292.84
    due to or associated with physical condition 293.83

1281

Psychosis

Psychosis—*continued*

> Note—Use the following fifth-digit subclassification with categories 296.0-296.6:
>
> 0 unspecified
> 1 mild
> 2 moderate
> 3 severe, without mention of psychotic behavior
> 4 severe, specified as with psychotic behavior
> 5 in partial or unspecified remission
> 6 in full remission

involutional 296.2
  recurrent episode 296.3
  single episode 296.2
manic-depressive 296.80
  circular (alternating) 296.7
    currently depressed 296.5
    currently manic 296.4
  depressed type 296.2
    atypical 296.82
    recurrent episode 296.3
    single episode 296.2
  manic 296.0
    atypical 296.81
    recurrent episode 296.1
    single episode 296.0
  mixed type NEC 296.89
  specified type NEC 296.89
senile 290.21
specified type NEC 296.99
alcoholic 291.9
  with
    anxiety 291.89
    delirium tremens 291.0
    delusions 291.5
    dementia 291.2
    hallucinosis 291.3
    jealousy 291.5
    mood disturbance 291.89
    paranoia 291.5
    persisting amnesia 291.1
    sexual dysfunction 291.89
    sleep disturbance 291.89
  amnestic confabulatory 291.1
  delirium tremens 291.0
  hallucinosis 291.3
  Korsakoff's, Korsakov's, Korsakow's 291.1
  paranoid type 291.5
  pathological intoxication 291.4
  polyneuritic 291.1
  specified type NEC 291.89
alternating (*see also* Psychosis, manic-depressive, circular) 296.7
anergastic (*see also* Psychosis, organic) 294.9
arteriosclerotic 290.40
  with
    acute confusional state 290.41
    delirium 290.41
    delusions 290.42
    depressed mood 290.43
  depressed type 290.43
  paranoid type 290.42
  simple type 290.40
  uncomplicated 290.40
atypical 298.9
  depressive 296.82
  manic 296.81
borderline (schizophrenia) (*see also* Schizophrenia) 295.5

Psychosis—*continued*

of childhood (*see also* Psychosis, childhood) 299.8
  prepubertal 299.8
brief reactive 298.8
childhood, with origin specific to 299.9

> Note—Use the following fifth-digit subclassification with category 299:
>
> 0 current or active state
> 1 residual state

  atypical 299.8
  specified type NEC 299.8
circular (*see also* Psychosis, manic-depressive, circular) 296.7
climacteric (*see also* Psychosis, involutional) 298.8
confusional 298.9
  acute 293.0
  reactive 298.2
  subacute 293.1
depressive (*see also* Psychosis, affective) 296.2
  atypical 296.82
  involutional 296.2
    recurrent episode 296.3
    single episode 296.2
  psychogenic 298.0
  reactive (emotional stress) (psychological trauma) 298.0
  recurrent episode 296.3
    with hypomania (bipolar II) 296.89
  single episode 296.2
disintegrative, childhood (*see also* Psychosis, childhood) 299.1
drug 292.9
  with
    affective syndrome 292.84
    amnestic syndrome 292.83
    anxiety 292.89
    delirium 292.81
      withdrawal 292.0
    delusions 292.11
    dementia 292.82
    depressive state 292.84
    hallucinations 292.12
    hallucinosis 292.12
    mood disorder 292.84
    mood disturbance 292.84
    organic personality syndrome NEC 292.89
    sexual dysfunction 292.89
    sleep disturbance 292.89
    withdrawal syndrome (and delirium) 292.0
  affective syndrome 292.84
  delusions 292.11
  hallucinatory state 292.12
  hallucinosis 292.12
  paranoid state 292.11
  specified type NEC 292.89
  withdrawal syndrome (and delirium) 292.0
due to or associated with physical condition (*see also* Psychosis, organic) 293.9
epileptic NEC 294.8
excitation (psychogenic) (reactive) 298.1
exhaustive (*see also* Reaction, stress, acute) 308.9
hypomanic (*see also* Psychosis, affective) 296.0
  recurrent episode 296.1
  single episode 296.0
hysterical 298.8
  acute 298.1

INDEX TO DISEASES — Psychosis

Psychosis—*continued*
  incipient 298.8
    schizophrenic (*see also* Schizophrenia) 295.5
  induced 297.3
  infantile (*see also* Psychosis, childhood) 299.0
  infective 293.9
    acute 293.0
    subacute 293.1
  in
    conditions classified elsewhere
      with
        delusions 293.81
        hallucinations 293.82
      pregnancy, childbirth, or puerperium 648.4
  interactional (childhood) (*see also* Psychosis, childhood) 299.1
  involutional 298.8
    depressive (*see also* Psychosis, affective) 296.2
      recurrent episode 296.3
      single episode 296.2
    melancholic 296.2
      recurrent episode 296.3
      single episode 296.2
    paranoid state 297.2
    paraphrenia 297.2
  Korsakoff's, Korakov's, Korsakow's (nonalcoholic) 294.0
    alcoholic 291.1
  mania (phase) (*see also* Psychosis, affective) 296.0
    recurrent episode 296.1
    single episode 296.0
  manic (*see also* Psychosis, affective) 296.0
    atypical 296.81
    recurrent episode 296.1
    single episode 296.0
  manic-depressive 296.80
    circular 296.7
      currently
        depressed 296.5
        manic 296.4
        mixed 296.6
    depressive 296.2
      recurrent episode 296.3
        with hypomania (bipolar II) 296.89
      single episode 296.2
    hypomanic 296.0
      recurrent episode 296.1
      single episode 296.0
    manic 296.0
      atypical 296.81
      recurrent episode 296.1
      single episode 296.0
    mixed NEC 296.89
    perplexed 296.89
    stuporous 296.89
  menopausal (*see also* Psychosis, involutional) 298.8
  mixed schizophrenic and affective (*see also* Schizophrenia) 295.7
  multi-infarct (cerebrovascular) (*see also* Psychosis, arteriosclerotic) 290.40
  organic NEC 294.9
    due to or associated with
      addiction
        alcohol (*see also* Psychosis, alcoholic) 291.9
        drug (*see also* Psychosis, drug) 292.9
      alcohol intoxication, acute (*see also* Psychosis, alcoholic) 291.9

Psychosis—*continued*
      alcoholism (*see also* Psychosis, alcoholic) 291.9
      arteriosclerosis (cerebral) (*see also* Psychosis, arteriosclerotic) 290.40
      cerebrovascular disease
        acute (psychosis) 293.0
        arteriosclerotic (*see also* Psychosis, arteriosclerotic) 290.40
      childbirth—*see* Psychosis, puerperal
      dependence
        alcohol (*see also* Psychosis, alcoholic) 291.9
        drug 292.9
      disease
        alcoholic liver (*see also* Psychosis, alcoholic) 291.9
        brain
          arteriosclerotic (*see also* Psychosis, arteriosclerotic) 290.40
          cerebrovascular
            acute (psychosis) 293.0
            arteriosclerotic (*see also* Psychosis, arteriosclerotic) 290.40
          endocrine or metabolic 293.9
            acute (psychosis) 293.0
            subacute (psychosis) 293.1
          Jakob-Creutzfeldt (new variant)
            with behavioral disturbance 046.1 [294.11]
            without behavioral disturbance 046.1 [294.10]
        liver, alcoholic (*see also* Psychosis, alcoholic) 291.9
      disorder
        cerebrovascular
          acute (psychosis) 293.0
        endocrine or metabolic 293.9
          acute (psychosis) 293.0
          subacute (psychosis) 293.1
      epilepsy
        with behavioral disturbance 345.9 [294.11]
        without behavioral disturbance 345.9 [294.10]
        transient (acute) 293.0
      Huntington's chorea
        with behavioral disturbance 333.4 [294.11]
        without behavioral disturbance 333.4 [294.10]
      infection
        brain 293.9
          acute (psychosis) 293.0
          chronic 294.8
          subacute (psychosis) 293.1
        intracranial NEC 293.9
          acute (psychosis) 293.0
          chronic 294.8
          subacute (psychosis) 293.1
      intoxication
        alcoholic (acute) (*see also* Psychosis, alcoholic) 291.9
          pathological 291.4
        drug (*see also* Psychosis, drug) 292.9
      ischemia
        cerebrovascular (generalized) (*see also* Psychosis, arteriosclerotic) 290.40
        Jakob-Creutzfeldt disease (syndrome) (new variant)

Psychosis—*continued*
  with behavioral disturbance 046.1
      [294.11]
  without behavioral disturbance 046.1
      [294.10]
  multiple sclerosis
    with behavioral disturbance 340 *[294.11]*
    without behavioral disturbance 340
      [294.10]
  physical condition NEC 293.9
    with
      delusions 293.81
      hallucinations 293.82
  presenility 290.10
  puerperium—*see* Psychosis, puerperal
  sclerosis, multiple
    with behavioral disturbance 340 *[294.11]*
    without behavioral disturbance 340
      [294.10]
  senility 290.20
  status epilepticus
    with behavioral disturbance 345.3
      [294.11]
    without behavioral disturbance 345.3
      [294.10]
  trauma
    brain (birth) (from electrical current)
        (surgical) 293.9
      acute (psychosis) 293.0
      chronic 294.8
      subacute (psychosis) 293.1
  unspecified physical condition 293.9
    with
      delusions 293.81
      hallucinations 293.82
  infective 293.9
    acute (psychosis) 293.0
    subacute 293.1
  posttraumatic 293.9
    acute 293.0
    subacute 293.1
  specified type NEC 294.8
  transient 293.9
    with
      anxiety 293.84
      delusions 293.81
      depression 293.83
      hallucinations 293.82
    depressive type 293.83
    hallucinatory type 293.82
    paranoid type 293.81
    specified type NEC 293.89
 paranoic 297.1
 paranoid (chronic) 297.9
   alcoholic 291.5
   chronic 297.1
   climacteric 297.2
   involutional 297.2
   menopausal 297.2
   protracted reactive 298.4
   psychogenic 298.4
     acute 298.3
   schizophrenic (*see also* Schizophrenia) 295.3
   senile 290.20
 paroxysmal 298.9
   senile 290.20
 polyneuritic, alcoholic 291.1
 postoperative 293.9
 postpartum—*see* Psychosis, puerperal
 prepsychotic (*see also* Schizophrenia) 295.5
 presbyophrenic (type) 290.8

Psychosis—*continued*
  presenile (*see also* Dementia, presenile) 290.10
  prison 300.16
  psychogenic 298.8
    depressive 298.0
    paranoid 298.4
      acute 298.3
  puerperal
    specified type—*see* categories 295-298
    unspecified type 293.89
      acute 293.0
      chronic 293.89
      subacute 293.1
  reactive (emotional stress) (psychological
      trauma) 298.8
    brief 298.8
    confusion 298.2
    depressive 298.0
    excitation 298.1
  schizo-affective (depressed) (excited) (*see also*
      Schizophrenia) 295.7
  schizophrenia, schizophrenic (*see also*
      Schizophrenia) 295.9
    borderline type 295.5
      of childhood (*see also* Psychosis, childhood)
        299.8
    catatonic (excited) (withdrawn) 295.2
    childhood type (*see also* Psychosis, childhood)
        299.9
    hebephrenic 295.1
    incipient 295.5
    latent 295.5
    paranoid 295.3
    prepsychotic 295.5
    prodromal 295.5
    pseudoneurotic 295.5
    pseudopsychopathic 295.5
    schizophreniform 295.4
    simple 295.0
    undifferentiated type 295.9
  schizophreniform 295.4
  senile NEC 290.20
    with
      delusional features 290.20
      depressive features 290.21
    depressed type 290.21
    paranoid type 290.20
    simple deterioration 290.20
    specified type—*see* categories 295-298
  shared 297.3
  situational (reactive) 298.8
  symbiotic (childhood) (*see also* Psychosis,
      childhood) 299.1
  toxic (acute) 293.9
Psychotic (*see also* condition) 298.9
  episode 298.9
    due to or associated with physical conditions
        (*see also* Psychosis, organic) 293.9
Pterygium (eye) 372.40
  central 372.43
  colli 744.5
  double 372.44
  peripheral (stationary) 372.41
    progressive 372.42
  recurrent 372.45
Ptilosis 374.55
Ptomaine (poisoning) (*see also* Poisoning, food)
    005.9
Ptosis (adiposa) 374.30
  breast 611.8
  cecum 569.89

INDEX TO DISEASES — Puerperal

Ptosis—*continued*
  colon 569.89
  congenital (eyelid) 743.61
    specified site NEC—*see* Anomaly, specified type NEC
  epicanthus syndrome 270.2
  eyelid 374.30
    congenital 743.61
    mechanical 374.33
    myogenic 374.32
    paralytic 374.31
  gastric 537.5
  intestine 569.89
  kidney (*see also* Disease, renal) 593.0
    congenital 753.3
  liver 573.8
  renal (*see also* Disease, renal) 593.0
    congenital 753.3
  splanchnic 569.89
  spleen 289.59
  stomach 537.5
  viscera 569.89
PTSD (Post-Traumatic Stress Disorder) 309.81
Ptyalism 527.7
  hysterical 300.11
  periodic 527.2
  pregnancy 646.8
  psychogenic 306.4
Ptyalolithiasis 527.5
Pubalgia 848.8
Pubarche, precocious 259.1
Pubertas praecox 259.1
Puberty V21.1
  abnormal 259.9
  bleeding 626.3
  delayed 259.0
  precocious (constitutional) (cryptogenic) (idiopathic) NEC 259.1
    due to
      adrenal
        cortical hyperfunction 255.2
        hyperplasia 255.2
      cortical hyperfunction 255.2
      ovarian hyperfunction 256.1
        estrogen 256.0
      pineal tumor 259.8
      testicular hyperfunction 257.0
  premature 259.1
    due to
      adrenal cortical hyperfunction 255.2
      pineal tumor 259.8
      pituitary (anterior) hyperfunction 253.1
Puckering, macula 362.56
Pudenda, pudendum —*see* condition
Puente's disease (simple glandular cheilitis) 528.5
Puerperal
  abscess
    areola 675.1
    Bartholin's gland 646.6
    breast 675.1
    cervix (uteri) 670
    fallopian tube 670
    genital organ 670
    kidney 646.6
    mammary 675.1
    mesosalpinx 670
    nabothian 646.6
    nipple 675.0
    ovary, ovarian 670
    oviduct 670

Puerperal—*continued*
    parametric 670
    para-uterine 670
    pelvic 670
    perimetric 670
    periuterine 670
    retro-uterine 670
    subareolar 675.1
    suprapelvic 670
    tubal (ruptured) 670
    tubo-ovarian 670
    urinary tract NEC 646.6
    uterine, uterus 670
    vagina (wall) 646.6
    vaginorectal 646.6
    vulvovaginal gland 646.6
  accident 674.9
  adnexitis 670
  afibrinogenemia, or other coagulation defect 666.3
  albuminuria (acute) (subacute) 646.2
    pre-eclamptic 642.4
  anemia (conditions classifiable to 280-285) 648.2
  anuria 669.3
  apoplexy 674.0
  asymptomatic bacteriuria 646.5
  atrophy, breast 676.3
  blood dyscrasia 666.3
  caked breast 676.2
  cardiomyopathy 674.5
  cellulitis—*see* Puerperal, abscess
  cerebrovascular disorder (conditions classifiable to 430-434, 436-437) 674.0
  cervicitis (conditions classifiable to 616.0) 646.6
  coagulopathy (any) 666.3
  complications 674.9
    specified type NEC 674.8
  convulsions (eclamptic) (uremic) 642.6
    with pre-existing hypertension 642.7
  cracked nipple 676.1
  cystitis 646.6
  cystopyelitis 646.6
  deciduitis (acute) 670
  delirium NEC 293.9
  diabetes (mellitus) (conditions classifiable to 250) 648.0
  disease 674.9
    breast NEC 676.3
    cerebrovascular (acute) 674.0
    nonobstetric NEC (*see also* Pregnancy, complicated, current disease or condition) 648.9
    pelvis inflammatory 670
    renal NEC 646.2
    tubo-ovarian 670
    Valsuani's (progressive pernicious anemia) 648.2
  disorder
    lactation 676.9
      specified type NEC 676.8
    nonobstetric NEC (*see also* Pregnancy, complicated, current disease or condition) 648.9
  disruption
    cesarean wound 674.1
    episiotomy wound 674.2
    perineal laceration wound 674.2
  drug dependence (conditions classifiable to 304) 648.3
  eclampsia 642.6

Puerperal—*continued*
  with pre-existing hypertension 642.7
  embolism (pulmonary) 673.2
    air 673.0
    amniotic fluid 673.1
    blood-clot 673.2
    brain or cerebral 674.0
    cardiac 674.8
    fat 673.8
    intracranial sinus (venous) 671.5
    pyemic 673.3
    septic 673.3
    spinal cord 671.5
  endometritis (conditions classifiable to 615.0-615.9) 670
  endophlebitis—*see* Puerperal, phlebitis
  endotrachelitis 646.6
  engorgement, breasts 676.2
  erysipelas 670
  failure
    lactation 676.4
    renal, acute 669.3
  fever 670
    meaning pyrexia (of unknown origin) 672
    meaning sepsis 670
  fissure, nipple 676.1
  fistula
    breast 675.1
    mammary gland 675.1
    nipple 675.0
  galactophoritis 675.2
  galactorrhea 676.6
  gangrene
    gas 670
    uterus 670
  gonorrhea (conditions classifiable to 098) 647.1
  hematoma, subdural 674.0
  hematosalpinx, infectional 670
  hemiplegia, cerebral 674.0
  hemorrhage 666.1
    brain 674.0
    bulbar 674.0
    cerebellar 674.0
    cerebral 674.0
    cortical 674.0
    delayed (after 24 hours) (uterine) 666.2
    extradural 674.0
    internal capsule 674.0
    intracranial 674.0
    intrapontine 674.0
    meningeal 674.0
    pontine 674.0
    subarachnoid 674.0
    subcortical 674.0
    subdural 674.0
    uterine, delayed 666.2
    ventricular 674.0
  hemorrhoids 671.8
  hepatorenal syndrome 674.8
  hypertrophy
    breast 676.3
    mammary gland 676.3
  induration breast (fibrous) 676.3
  infarction
    lung—*see* Puerperal, embolism
    pulmonary—*see* Puerperal, embolism
  infection
    Bartholin's gland 646.6
    breast 675.2
      with nipple 675.9
        specified type NEC 675.8

Puerperal—*continued*
    cervix 646.6
    endocervix 646.6
    fallopian tube 670
    generalized 670
    genital tract (major) 670
      minor or localized 646.6
    kidney (bacillus coli) 646.6
    mammary gland 675.2
      with nipple 675.9
        specified type NEC 675.8
    nipple 675.0
      with breast 675.9
        specified type NEC 675.8
    ovary 670
    pelvic 670
    peritoneum 670
    renal 646.6
    tubo-ovarian 670
    urinary (tract) NEC 646.6
      asymptomatic 646.5
    uterus, uterine 670
    vagina 646.6
  inflammation—*see also* Puerperal, infection
    areola 675.1
    Bartholin's gland 646.6
    breast 675.2
    broad ligament 670
    cervix (uteri) 646.6
    fallopian tube 670
    genital organs 670
      localized 646.6
    mammary gland 675.2
    nipple 675.0
    ovary 670
    oviduct 670
    pelvis 670
    periuterine 670
    tubal 670
    vagina 646.6
    vein—*see* Puerperal, phlebitis
  inversion, nipple 676.3
  ischemia, cerebral 674.0
  lymphangitis 670
    breast 675.2
  malaria (conditions classifiable to 084) 647.4
  malnutrition 648.9
  mammillitis 675.0
  mammitis 675.2
  mania 296.0
    recurrent episode 296.1
    single episode 296.0
  mastitis 675.2
    purulent 675.1
    retromammary 675.1
    submammary 675.1
  melancholia 296.2
    recurrent episode 296.3
    single episode 296.2
  mental disorder (conditions classifiable to 290-303, 305.0, 305.2-305.9, 306-316, 317-319) 648.4
  metritis (septic) (suppurative) 670
  metroperitonitis 670
  metrorrhagia 666.2
  metrosalpingitis 670
  metrovaginitis 670
  milk leg 671.4
  monoplegia, cerebral 674.0
  necrosis
    kidney, tubular 669.3

Puerperal—*continued*
  liver (acute) (subacute) (conditions classifiable to 570) 674.8
  ovary 670
  renal cortex 669.3
  nephritis or nephrosis (conditions classifiable to 580-589) 646.2
    with hypertension 642.1
  nutritional deficiency (conditions classifiable to 260-269) 648.9
  occlusion, precerebral artery 674.0
  oliguria 669.3
  oophoritis 670
  ovaritis 670
  paralysis
    bladder (sphincter) 665.5
    cerebral 674.0
  paralytic stroke 674.0
  parametritis 670
  paravaginitis 646.6
  pelviperitonitis 670
  perimetritis 670
  perimetrosalpingitis 670
  perinephritis 646.6
  perioophoritis 670
  periphlebitis—*see* Puerperal, phlebitis
  perisalpingitis 670
  peritoneal infection 670
  peritonitis (pelvic) 670
  perivaginitis 646.6
  phlebitis 671.9
    deep 671.4
    intracranial sinus (venous) 671.5
    pelvic 671.4
    specified site NEC 671.5
    superficial 671.2
  phlegmasia alba dolens 671.4
  placental polyp 674.4
  pneumonia, embolic—*see* Puerperal, embolism
  prediabetes 648.8
  pre-eclampsia (mild) 642.4
    with pre-existing hypertension 642.7
    severe 642.5
  psychosis, unspecified (*see also* Psychosis, puerperal) 293.89
  pyelitis 646.6
  pyelocystitis 646.6
  pyelohydronephrosis 646.6
  pyelonephritis 646.6
  pyelonephrosis 646.6
  pyemia 670
  pyocystitis 646.6
  pyohemia 670
  pyometra 670
  pyonephritis 646.6
  pyonephrosis 646.6
  pyo-oophoritis 670
  pyosalpingitis 670
  pyosalpinx 670
  pyrexia (of unknown origin) 672
  renal
    disease NEC 646.2
    failure, acute 669.3
  retention
    decidua (fragments) (with delayed hemorrhage) 666.2
      without hemorrhage 667.1
    placenta (fragments) (with delayed hemorrhage) 666.2
      without hemorrhage 667.1

Puerperal—*continued*
    secundines (fragments) (with delayed hemorrhage) 666.2
      without hemorrhage 667.1
  retracted nipple 676.0
  rubella (conditions classifiable to 056) 647.5
  salpingitis 670
  salpingo-oophoritis 670
  salpingo-ovaritis 670
  salpingoperitonitis 670
  sapremia 670
  secondary perineal tear 674.2
  sepsis (pelvic) 670
  septicemia 670
  subinvolution (uterus) 674.8
  sudden death (cause unknown) 674.9
  suppuration—*see* Puerperal, abscess
  syphilis (conditions classifiable to 090-097) 647.0
  tetanus 670
  thelitis 675.0
  thrombocytopenia 666.3
  thrombophlebitis (superficial) 671.2
    deep 671.4
    pelvic 671.4
    specified site NEC 671.5
  thrombosis (venous)—*see* Thrombosis, puerperal
  thyroid dysfunction (conditions classifiable to 240-246) 648.1
  toxemia (*see also* Toxemia, of pregnancy) 642.4
    eclamptic 642.6
      with pre-existing hypertension 642.7
    pre-eclamptic (mild) 642.4
      with
        convulsions 642.6
        pre-existing hypertension 642.7
      severe 642.5
  tuberculosis (conditions classifiable to 010-018) 647.3
  uremia 669.3
  vaginitis (conditions classifiable to 616.1) 646.6
  varicose veins (legs) 671.0
    vulva or perineum 671.1
  vulvitis (conditions classifiable to 616.1) 646.6
  vulvovaginitis (conditions classifiable to 616.1) 646.6
  white leg 671.4
Pulled muscle —*see* Sprain, by site
Pulmolithiasis 518.89
Pulmonary —*see* condition
Pulmonitis (unknown etiology) 486
Pulpitis (acute) (anachoretic) (chronic) (hyperplastic) (putrescent) (suppurative) (ulcerative) 522.0
Pulpless tooth 522.9
Pulse
  alternating 427.89
    psychogenic 306.2
  bigeminal 427.89
  fast 785.0
  feeble, rapid, due to shock following injury 958.4
  rapid 785.0
  slow 427.89
  strong 785.9
  trigeminal 427.89
  water-hammer (*see also* Insufficiency, aortic) 424.1
  weak 785.9
Pulseless disease 446.7

Pulsus
  alternans or trigeminy 427.89
    psychogenic 306.2
Punch drunk 310.2
Puncta lacrimalia occlusion 375.52
Punctiform hymen 752.49
Puncture (traumatic)—*see also* Wound, open, by site
  accidental, complicating surgery 998.2
  bladder, nontraumatic 596.6
  by
    device, implant, or graft—*see* Complications, mechanical
    foreign body
      internal organs—*see also* Injury, internal, by site
        by ingested object—*see* Foreign body
    left accidentally in operation wound 998.4
    instrument (any) during a procedure, accidental 998.2
  internal organs, abdomen, chest, or pelvis—*see* Injury, internal, by site
  kidney, nontraumatic 593.89
Pupil —*see* condition
Pupillary membrane 364.74
  persistent 743.46
Pupillotonia 379.46
  pseudotabetic 379.46
Purpura 287.2
  abdominal 287.0
  allergic 287.0
  anaphylactoid 287.0
  annularis telangiectodes 709.1
  arthritic 287.0
  autoerythrocyte sensitization 287.2
  autoimmune 287.0
  bacterial 287.0
  Bateman's (senile) 287.2
  capillary fragility (hereditary) (idiopathic) 287.8
  cryoglobulinemic 273.2
  devil's pinches 287.2
  fibrinolytic (*see also* Fibrinolysis) 286.6
  fulminans, fulminous 286.6
  gangrenous 287.0
  hemorrhagic (*see also* Purpura, thrombocytopenic) 287.39
    nodular 272.7
    nonthrombocytopenic 287.0
    thrombocytopenic 287.39
  Henoch's (purpura nervosa) 287.0
  Henoch-Schönlein (allergic) 287.0
  hypergammaglobulinemic (benign primary) (Waldenström's) 273.0
  idiopathic 287.31
    nonthrombocytopenic 287.0
    thrombocytopenic 287.31
  immune thrombocytopenic 287.31
  infectious 287.0
  malignant 287.0
  neonatorum 772.6
  nervosa 287.0
  newborn NEC 772.6
  nonthrombocytopenic 287.2
    hemorrhagic 287.0
    idiopathic 287.0
  nonthrombopenic 287.2
  peliosis rheumatica 287.0
  pigmentaria, progressiva 709.09
  posttransfusion 287.4
  primary 287.0
  primitive 287.0

Purpura—*continued*
  red cell membrane sensitivity 287.2
  rheumatica 287.0
  Schönlein (-Henoch) (allergic) 287.0
  scorbutic 267
  senile 287.2
  simplex 287.2
  symptomatica 287.0
  telangiectasia annularis 709.1
  thrombocytopenic (*see also* Thrombocytopenia) 287.30
    congenital 287.33
    essential 287.30
    hereditary 287.31
    idiopathic 287.31
    immune 287.31
    neonatal, transitory (*see also* Thrombocytopenia, neonatal transitory) 776.1
    primary 287.30
    puerperal, postpartum 666.3
    thrombotic 446.6
  thrombohemolytic (*see also* Fibrinolysis) 286.6
  thrombopenic (*see also* Thrombocytopenia) 287.30
    congenital 287.33
    essential 287.30
  thrombotic 446.6
    thrombocytic 446.6
    thrombocytopenic 446.6
  toxic 287.0
  variolosa 050.0
  vascular 287.0
  visceral symptoms 287.0
  Werlhof's (*see also* Purpura, thrombocytopenic) 287.39
Purpuric spots 782.7
Purulent —*see* condition
Pus
  absorption, general—*see* Septicemia
  in
    stool 792.1
    urine 791.9
  tube (rupture) (*see also* Salpingo-oophoritis) 614.2
Pustular rash 782.1
Pustule 686.9
  malignant 022.0
  nonmalignant 686.9
Putnam's disease (subacute combined sclerosis with pernicious anemia) 281.0 *[336.2]*
Putnam-Dana syndrome (subacute combined sclerosis with pernicious anemia) 281.0 *[336.2]*
Putrefaction, intestinal 569.89
Putrescent pulp (dental) 522.1
Pyarthritis —*see* Pyarthrosis
Pyarthrosis (*see also* Arthritis, pyogenic) 711.0
  tuberculous—*see* Tuberculosis, joint
Pycnoepilepsy, pycnolepsy (idiopathic) (*see also* Epilepsy) 345.0
Pyelectasia 593.89
Pyelectasis 593.89
Pyelitis (congenital) (uremic) 590.80
  with
    abortion—*see* Abortion, by type, with specified complication NEC
    contracted kidney 590.00
    ectopic pregnancy (*see also* categories 633.0-633.9) 639.8

INDEX TO DISEASES   **Pyrosis**

Pyelitis—*continued*
  molar pregnancy (*see also* categories 630-632) 639.8
  acute 590.10
    with renal medullary necrosis 590.11
  chronic 590.00
    with
      renal medullary necrosis 590.01
  complicating pregnancy, childbirth, or puerperium 646.6
    affecting fetus or newborn 760.1
  cystica 590.3
  following
    abortion 639.8
    ectopic or molar pregnancy 639.8
  gonococcal 098.19
    chronic or duration of 2 months or over 098.39
  tuberculous (*see also* Tuberculosis) 016.0 [590.81]
Pyelocaliectasis 593.89
Pyelocystitis (*see also* Pyelitis) 590.80
Pyelohydronephrosis 591
Pyelonephritis (*see also* Pyelitis) 590.80
  acute 590.10
    with renal medullary necrosis 590.11
  chronic 590.00
  syphilitic (late) 095.4
  tuberculous (*see also* Tuberculosis) 016.0 [590.81]
Pyelonephrosis (*see also* Pyelitis) 590.80
  chronic 590.00
Pyelophlebitis 451.89
Pyelo-ureteritis cystica 590.3
Pyemia, pyemic (purulent) (*see also* Septicemia) 038.9
  abscess—*see* Abscess
  arthritis (*see also* Arthritis, pyogenic) 711.0
  Bacillus coli 038.42
  embolism—(*see also* Septicemia) 415.12
  fever 038.9
  infection 038.9
  joint (*see also* Arthritis, pyogenic) 711.0
  liver 572.1
  meningococcal 036.2
  newborn 771.81
  phlebitis—*see* Phlebitis
  pneumococcal 038.2
  portal 572.1
  postvaccinal 999.39
  specified organism NEC 038.8
  staphylococcal 038.10
    aureus 038.11
    specified organism NEC 038.19
  streptococcal 038.0
  tuberculous—*see* Tuberculosis, miliary
Pygopagus 759.4
Pykno-epilepsy, pyknolepsy (idiopathic) (*see also* Epilepsy) 345.0
Pyle (-Cohn) disease (craniometaphyseal dysplasia) 756.89
Pylephlebitis (suppurative) 572.1
Pylethrombophlebitis 572.1
Pylethrombosis 572.1
Pyloritis (*see also* Gastritis) 535.5
Pylorospasm (reflex) 537.81
  congenital or infantile 750.5
  neurotic 306.4
  newborn 750.5
  psychogenic 306.4
Pylorus, pyloric —*see* condition
Pyoarthrosis —*see* Pyarthrosis

Pyocele
  mastoid 383.00
  sinus (accessory) (nasal) (*see also* Sinusitis) 473.9
  turbinate (bone) 473.9
  urethra (*see also* Urethritis) 597.0
Pyococcal dermatitis 686.00
Pyococcide, skin 686.00
Pyocolpos (*see also* Vaginitis) 616.10
Pyocyaneus dermatitis 686.09
Pyocystitis (*see also* Cystitis) 595.9
Pyoderma, pyodermia NEC 686.00
  gangrenosum 686.01
  specified type NEC 686.09
  vegetans 686.8
Pyodermatitis 686.00
  vegetans 686.8
Pyogenic —*see* condition
Pyohemia —*see* Septicemia
Pyohydronephrosis (*see also* Pyelitis) 590.80
Pyometra 615.9
Pyometritis (*see also* Endometritis) 615.9
Pyometrium (*see also* Endometritis) 615.9
Pyomyositis 728.0
  ossificans 728.19
  tropical (bungpagga) 040.81
Pyonephritis (*see also* Pyelitis) 590.80
  chronic 590.00
Pyonephrosis (congenital) (*see also* Pyelitis) 590.80
  acute 590.10
Pyo-oophoritis (*see also* Salpingo-oophoritis) 614.2
Pyo-ovarium (*see also* Salpingo-oophoritis) 614.2
Pyopericarditis 420.99
Pyopericardium 420.99
Pyophlebitis —*see* Phlebitis
Pyopneumopericardium 420.99
Pyopneumothorax (infectional) 510.9
  with fistula 510.0
  subdiaphragmatic (*see also* Peritonitis) 567.29
  subphrenic (*see also* Peritonitis) 567.29
  tuberculous (*see also* Tuberculosis, pleura) 012.0
Pyorrhea (alveolar) (alveolaris) 523.40
  degenerative 523.5
Pyosalpingitis (*see also* Salpingo-oophoritis) 614.2
Pyosalpinx (*see also* Salpingo-oophoritis) 614.2
Pyosepticemia —*see* Septicemia
Pyosis
  Corlett's (impetigo) 684
  Manson's (pemphigus contagiosus) 684
Pyothorax 510.9
  with fistula 510.0
  tuberculous (*see also* Tuberculosis, pleura) 012.0
Pyoureter 593.89
  tuberculous (*see also* Tuberculosis) 016.2
Pyramidopallidonigral syndrome 332.0
Pyrexia (of unknown origin) (P.U.O.) 780.6
  atmospheric 992.0
  during labor 659.2
  environmentally-induced
    newborn 778.4
  heat 992.0
  newborn, environmentally-induced 778.4
  puerperal 672
Pyroglobulinemia 273.8
Pyromania 312.33
Pyrosis 787.1

Pyrroloporphyria 277.1
Pyuria (bacterial) 791.9

Q

Q fever 083.0
  with pneumonia 083.0 *[484.8]*
Quadricuspid aortic valve 746.89
Quadrilateral fever 083.0
Quadriparesis —*see* Quadriplegia
  meaning muscle weakness 728.87
Quadriplegia 344.00
  with fracture, vertebra (process)—*see* Fracture, vertebra, cervical, with spinal cord injury
  brain (current episode) 437.8
  cerebral (current episode) 437.8
  C1-C4
    complete 344.01
    incomplete 344.02
  C5-C7
    complete 344.03
    incomplete 344.04
  congenital or infantile (cerebral) (spastic) (spinal) 343.2
  cortical 437.8
  embolic (current episode) (*see also* Embolism, brain) 434.1
  infantile (cerebral) (spastic) (spinal) 343.2
  newborn NEC 767.0
  specified NEC 344.09
  thrombotic (current episode) (*see also* Thrombosis, brain) 434.0
  traumatic—*see* Injury, spinal, cervical
Quadruplet
  affected by maternal complications of pregnancy 761.5
  healthy liveborn—*see* Newborn, multiple
  pregnancy (complicating delivery) NEC 651.8
    with fetal loss and retention of one or more fetus(es) 651.5
    following (elective) fetal reduction 651.7
Quarrelsomeness 301.3
Quartan
  fever 084.2
  malaria (fever) 084.2
Queensland fever 083.0
  coastal 083.0
  seven-day 100.89
Quervain's disease 727.04
  thyroid (subacute granulomatous thyroiditis) 245.1
Queyrat's erythroplasia (M8080/2)
  specified site—*see* Neoplasm, skin, in situ
  unspecified site 233.5
Quincke's disease or edema —*see* Edema, angioneurotic
Quinquaud's disease (acne decalvans) 704.09
Quinsy (gangrenous) 475
Quintan fever 083.1
Quintuplet
  affected by maternal complications of pregnancy 761.5
  healthy liveborn—*see* Newborn, multiple
  pregnancy (complicating delivery) NEC 651.2
    with fetal loss and retention of one or more fetus(es) 651.6
    following (elective) fetal reduction 651.7
Quotidian
  fever 084.0
  malaria (fever) 084.0

R

Rabbia 071
Rabbit fever (*see also* Tularemia) 021.9
Rabies 071
  contact V01.5
  exposure to V01.5
  inoculation V04.5
    reaction—*see* Complications, vaccination
  vaccination, prophylactic (against) V04.5
Rachischisis (*see also* Spina bifida) 741.9
Rachitic —*see also* condition
  deformities of spine 268.1
  pelvis 268.1
    with disproportion (fetopelvic) 653.2
      affecting fetus or newborn 763.1
      causing obstructed labor 660.1
        affecting fetus or newborn 763.1
Rachitis, rachitism —*see also* Rickets
  acute 268.0
  fetalis 756.4
  renalis 588.0
  tarda 268.0
Racket nail 757.5
Radial nerve —*see* condition
Radiation effects or sickness —*see also* Effect, adverse, radiation
  cataract 366.46
  dermatitis 692.82
  sunburn (*see also* Sunburn) 692.71
Radiculitis (pressure) (vertebrogenic) 729.2
  accessory nerve 723.4
  anterior crural 724.4
  arm 723.4
  brachial 723.4
  cervical NEC 723.4
  due to displacement of intervertebral disc—*see* Neuritis, due to, displacement intervertebral disc
  leg 724.4
  lumbar NEC 724.4
  lumbosacral 724.4
  rheumatic 729.2
  syphilitic 094.89
  thoracic (with visceral pain) 724.4
Radiculomyelitis 357.0
  toxic, due to
    Clostridium tetani 037
    Corynebacterium diphtheriae 032.89
Radiculopathy (*see also* Radiculitis) 729.2
Radioactive substances, adverse effect —*see* Effect, adverse, radioactive substance
Radiodermal burns (acute) (chronic) (occupational)—*see* Burn, by site
Radiodermatitis 692.82
Radionecrosis —*see* Effect, adverse, radiation
Radiotherapy session V58.0
Radium, adverse effect —*see* Effect, adverse, radioactive substance
Raeder-Harbitz syndrome (pulseless disease) 446.7
Rage (*see also* Disturbance, conduct) 312.0
  meaning rabies 071
Rag sorters' disease 022.1
Raillietiniasis 123.8
Railroad neurosis 300.16
Railway spine 300.16
Raised —*see* Elevation
Raiva 071
Rake teeth, tooth 524.39
Rales 786.7

Ramifying renal pelvis 753.3
Ramsay Hunt syndrome (herpetic geniculate
  ganglionitis) 053.11
  meaning dyssynergia cerebellaris myoclonica
    334.2
Ranke's primary infiltration (*see also*
  Tuberculosis) 010.0
Ranula 527.6
  congenital 750.26
Rape
  adult 995.83
  alleged, observation or examination V71.5
  child 995.53
Rapid
  feeble pulse, due to shock, following injury
    958.4
  heart (beat) 785.0
    psychogenic 306.2
  respiration 786.06
    psychogenic 306.1
  second stage (delivery) 661.3
    affecting fetus or newborn 763.6
  time-zone change syndrome 327.35
Rarefaction, bone 733.99
Rash 782.1
  canker 034.1
  diaper 691.0
  drug (internal use) 693.0
    contact 692.3
  ECHO 9 virus 078.89
  enema 692.89
  food (*see also* Allergy, food) 693.1
  heat 705.1
  napkin 691.0
  nettle 708.8
  pustular 782.1
  rose 782.1
    epidemic 056.9
    of infants 057.8
  scarlet 034.1
  serum (prophylactic) (therapeutic) 999.5
  toxic 782.1
  wandering tongue 529.1
Rasmussen's aneurysm (*see also* Tuberculosis)
  011.2
Rat-bite fever 026.9
  due to Streptobacillus moniliformis 026.1
  spirochetal (morsus muris) 026.0
Rathke's pouch tumor (M9350/1) 237.0
Raymond (-Céstan) syndrome 433.8
Raynaud's
  disease or syndrome (paroxysmal digital
    cyanosis) 443.0
  gangrene (symmetric) 443.0 *[785.4]*
  phenomenon (paroxysmal digital cyanosis)
    (secondary) 443.0
RDS 769
Reaction
  acute situational maladjustment (*see also*
    Reaction, adjustment) 309.9
  adaptation (*see also* Reaction, adjustment) 309.9
  adjustment 309.9
    with
      anxious mood 309.24
        with depressed mood 309.28
      conduct disturbance 309.3
        combined with disturbance of emotions
          309.4
      depressed mood 309.0
        brief 309.0
          with anxious mood 309.28

Reaction—*continued*
      prolonged 309.1
    elective mutism 309.83
    mixed emotions and conduct 309.4
    mutism, elective 309.83
    physical symptoms 309.82
    predominant disturbance (of)
      conduct 309.3
      emotions NEC 309.29
        mixed 309.28
      mixed, emotions and conduct 309.4
      specified type NEC 309.89
    specific academic or work inhibition 309.23
    withdrawal 309.83
  depressive 309.0
    with conduct disturbance 309.4
    brief 309.0
    prolonged 309.1
  specified type NEC 309.89
  adverse food NEC 995.7
  affective (*see also* Psychosis, affective) 296.90
    specified type NEC 296.99
  aggressive 301.3
    unsocialized (*see also* Disturbance, conduct)
      312.0
  allergic (*see also* Allergy) 995.3
    drug, medicinal substance, and
      biological—*see* Allergy, drug
    food—*see* Allergy, food
    serum 999.5
  anaphylactic—*see* Shock, anaphylactic
  anesthesia—*see* Anesthesia, complication
  anger 312.0
  antisocial 301.7
  antitoxin (prophylactic) (therapeutic)—*see*
    Complications, vaccination
  anxiety 300.00
  Arthus 995.21
  asthenic 300.5
  compulsive 300.3
  conversion (anesthetic) (autonomic)
    (hyperkinetic) (mixed paralytic)
    (paresthetic) 300.11
  deoxyribonuclease (DNA) (DNase)
    hypersensitivity NEC 287.2
  depressive 300.4
    acute 309.0
    affective (*see also* Psychosis, affective) 296.2
      recurrent episode 296.3
      single episode 296.2
    brief 309.0
    manic (*see also* Psychosis, affective) 296.80
    neurotic 300.4
    psychoneurotic 300.4
    psychotic 298.0
  dissociative 300.15
  drug NEC (*see also* Table of Drugs and
    Chemicals) 995.20
    allergic—*see also* Allergy, drug 995.27
    correct substance properly administered 995.20
    obstetric anesthetic or analgesic NEC 668.9
      affecting fetus or newborn 763.5
      specified drug—*see* Table of drugs and
        chemicals
    overdose or poisoning 977.9
      specified drug—*see* Table of drugs and
        chemicals
    specific to newborn 779.4
    transmitted via placenta or breast milk—*see*
      Absorption, drug, through placenta
    withdrawal NEC 292.0

INDEX TO DISEASES

Reaction

Reaction—*continued*
    infant of dependent mother 779.5
    wrong substance given or taken in error 977.9
        specified drug—*see* Table of drugs and chemicals
dyssocial 301.7
dystonic, acute, due to drugs 333.72
erysipeloid 027.1
fear 300.20
    child 313.0
fluid loss, cerebrospinal 349.0
food—*see also* Allergy, food
    adverse NEC 995.7
    anaphylactic shock—*see* Anaphylactic shock, due to food
foreign
    body NEC 728.82
        in operative wound (inadvertently left) 998.4
        due to surgical material intentionally left—*see* Complications, due to (presence of) any device, implant, or graft classified to 996.0-996.5 NEC
    substance accidentally left during a procedure (chemical) (powder) (talc) 998.7
        body or object (instrument) (sponge) (swab) 998.4
graft-versus-host (GVH) 996.85
grief (acute) (brief) 309.0
    prolonged 309.1
gross stress (*see also* Reaction, stress, acute) 308.9
group delinquent (*see also* Disturbance, conduct) 312.2
Herxheimer's 995.0
hyperkinetic (*see also* Hyperkinesia) 314.9
hypochondriacal 300.7
hypoglycemic, due to insulin 251.0
    therapeutic misadventure 962.3
hypomanic (*see also* Psychosis, affective) 296.0
    recurrent episode 296.1
    single episode 296.0
hysterical 300.10
    conversion type 300.11
    dissociative 300.15
id (bacterial cause) 692.89
immaturity NEC 301.89
    aggressive 301.3
    emotional instability 301.59
immunization—*see* Complications, vaccination
incompatibility
    blood group (ABO) (infusion) (transfusion) 999.6
    Rh (factor) (infusion) (transfusion) 999.7
inflammatory—*see* Infection
infusion—*see* Complications, infusion
inoculation (immune serum)—*see* Complications, vaccination
insulin 995.23
involutional
    paranoid 297.2
    psychotic (*see also* Psychosis, affective, depressive) 296.2
leukemoid (basophilic) (lymphocytic) (monocytic) (myelocytic) (neutrophilic) 288.62
LSD (*see also* Abuse, drugs, nondependent) 305.3
lumbar puncture 349.0
manic-depressive (*see also* Psychosis, affective) 296.80
    depressed 296.2

Reaction—*continued*
    recurrent episode 296.3
    single episode 296.2
    hypomanic 296.0
neurasthenic 300.5
neurogenic (*see also* Neurosis) 300.9
neurotic NEC 300.9
neurotic-depressive 300.4
nitritoid—*see* Crisis, nitritoid
obsessive-compulsive 300.3
organic 293.9
    acute 293.0
    subacute 293.1
overanxious, child or adolescent 313.0
paranoid (chronic) 297.9
    acute 298.3
    climacteric 297.2
    involutional 297.2
    menopausal 297.2
    senile 290.20
    simple 297.0
passive
    aggressive 301.84
    dependency 301.6
personality (*see also* Disorder, personality) 301.9
phobic 300.20
postradiation—*see* Effect, adverse, radiation
psychogenic NEC 300.9
psychoneurotic (*see also* Neurosis) 300.9
    anxiety 300.00
    compulsive 300.3
    conversion 300.11
    depersonalization 300.6
    depressive 300.4
    dissociative 300.15
    hypochondriacal 300.7
    hysterical 300.10
        conversion type 300.11
        dissociative type 300.15
    neurasthenic 300.5
    obsessive 300.3
    obsessive-compulsive 300.3
    phobic 300.20
    tension state 300.9
psychophysiologic NEC (*see also* Disorder, psychosomatic) 306.9
    cardiovascular 306.2
    digestive 306.4
    endocrine 306.6
    gastrointestinal 306.4
    genitourinary 306.50
    heart 306.2
    hemic 306.8
    intestinal (large) (small) 306.4
    laryngeal 306.1
    lymphatic 306.8
    musculoskeletal 306.0
    pharyngeal 306.1
    respiratory 306.1
    skin 306.3
    special sense organs 306.7
psychosomatic (*see also* Disorder, psychosomatic) 306.9
psychotic (*see also* Psychosis) 298.9
    depressive 298.0
    due to or associated with physical condition (*see also* Psychosis, organic) 293.9
    involutional (*see also* Psychosis, affective) 296.2
        recurrent episode 296.3

Reaction—*continued*
  single episode 296.2
  pupillary (myotonic) (tonic) 379.46
  radiation—*see* Effect, adverse, radiation
  runaway—*see also* Disturbance, conduct
    socialized 312.2
    undersocialized, unsocialized 312.1
  scarlet fever toxin—*see* Complications, vaccination
  schizophrenic (*see also* Schizophrenia) 295.9
    latent 295.5
  serological for syphilis—*see* Serology for syphilis
  serum (prophylactic) (therapeutic) 999.5
    immediate 999.4
  situational (*see also* Reaction, adjustment) 309.9
    acute, to stress 308.3
    adjustment (*see also* Reaction, adjustment) 309.9
  somatization (*see also* Disorder, psychosomatic) 306.9
  spinal puncture 349.0
  spite, child (*see also* Disturbance, conduct) 312.0
  stress, acute 308.9
    bone or cartilage —*see* Fracture, stress
    with predominant disturbance (of)
      consciousness 308.1
      emotions 308.0
      mixed 308.4
      psychomotor 308.2
      specified type NEC 308.3
  surgical procedure—*see* Complications, surgical procedure
  tetanus antitoxin—*see* Complications, vaccination
  toxin-antitoxin—*see* Complications, vaccination
  transfusion (blood) (bone marrow) (lymphocytes) (allergic)—*see* Complications, transfusion
  tuberculin skin test, nonspecific (without active tuberculosis) 795.5
    positive (without active tuberculosis) 795.5
  ultraviolet—*see* Effect, adverse, ultraviolet
  undersocialized, unsocialized—*see also* Disturbance, conduct
    aggressive (type) 312.0
    unaggressive (type) 312.1
  vaccination (any)—*see* Complications, vaccination
  white graft (skin) 996.52
  withdrawing, child or adolescent 313.22
  x-ray—*see* Effect, adverse, x-rays
Reactive depression (*see also* Reaction, depressive) 300.4
  neurotic 300.4
  psychoneurotic 300.4
  psychotic 298.0
Rebound tenderness 789.6
Recalcitrant patient V15.81
Recanalization, thrombus —*see* Thrombosis
Recession, receding
  chamber angle (eye) 364.77
  chin 524.06
  gingival (postinfective) (postoperative) 523.20
    generalized 523.25
    localized 523.24
    minimal 523.21
    moderate 523.22
    servere 523.23
Recklinghausen's disease (M9540/1) 237.71
  bones (osteitis fibrosa cystica) 252.01

Recklinghausen-Applebaum disease (hemochromatosis) 275.0
Reclus' disease (cystic) 610.1
Recrudescent typhus (fever) 081.1
Recruitment, auditory 388.44
Rectalgia 569.42
Rectitis 569.49
Rectocele
  female (without uterine prolapse) 618.04
    with uterine prolapse 618.4
      complete 618.3
      incomplete 618.2
  in pregnancy or childbirth 654.4
    causing obstructed labor 660.2
      affecting fetus or newborn 763.1
  male 569.49
  vagina, vaginal (outlet) 618.04
Rectosigmoiditis 569.89
  ulcerative (chronic) 556.3
Rectosigmoid junction —*see* condition
Rectourethral —*see* condition
Rectovaginal —*see* condition
Rectovesical —*see* condition
Rectum, rectal —*see* condition
Recurrent —*see* condition
Red bugs 133.8
Red cedar asthma 495.8
Redness
  conjunctiva 379.93
  eye 379.93
  nose 478.19
Reduced ventilatory or vital capacity 794.2
Reduction
  function
    kidney (*see also* Disease, renal) 593.9
    liver 573.8
  ventilatory capacity 794.2
  vital capacity 794.2
Redundant, redundancy
  abdomen 701.9
  anus 751.5
  cardia 537.89
  clitoris 624.2
  colon (congenital) 751.5
  foreskin (congenital) 605
  intestine 751.5
  labia 624.3
  organ or site, congenital NEC—*see* Accessory
  panniculus (abdominal) 278.1
  prepuce (congenital) 605
  pylorus 537.89
  rectum 751.5
  scrotum 608.89
  sigmoid 751.5
  skin (of face) 701.9
    eyelids 374.30
  stomach 537.89
  uvula 528.9
  vagina 623.8
Reduplication —*see* Duplication
Referral
  adoption (agency) V68.89
  nursing care V63.8
  patient without examination or treatment V68.81
  social services V63.8
Reflex —*see also* condition
  blink, deficient 374.45
  hyperactive gag 478.29
  neurogenic bladder NEC 596.54
    atonic 596.54
      with cauda equina syndrome 344.61

INDEX TO DISEASES — Remote effect of cancer

Reflex—*continued*
vasoconstriction 443.9
Reflux
vasovagal 780.2
esophageal 530.81
esophagitis 530.11
gastroesophageal 530.81
mitral—*see* Insufficiency, mitral
ureteral —*see* Reflux, vesicoureteral
vesicoureteral 593.70
  with
    reflux nephropathy 593.73
      bilateral 593.72
      unilateral 593.71
Reformed gallbladder 576.0
Reforming, artificial openings (*see also* Attention to, artificial, opening) V55.9
Refractive error (*see also* Error, refractive) 367.9
Refsum's disease or syndrome (heredopathia atactica polyneuritiformis) 356.3
Refusal of
food 307.59
  hysterical 300.11
treatment because of, due to
  patient's decision NEC V64.2
  reason of conscience or religion V62.6
Regaud
tumor (M8082/3)—*see* Neoplasm, nasopharynx, malignant
type carcinoma (M8082/3)—*see* Neoplasm, nasopharynx, malignant
Regional —*see* condition
Regulation feeding (elderly) (infant) 783.3
newborn 779.3
Regurgitated
food, choked on 933.1
stomach contents, choked on 933.1
Regurgitation 787.03
aortic (valve) (*see also* Insufficiency, aortic) 424.1
  congenital 746.4
  syphilitic 093.22
food—*see also* Vomiting
  with reswallowing—*see* Rumination
  newborn 779.3
gastric contents—*see* Vomiting
heart—*see* Endocarditis
mitral (valve)—*see also* Insufficiency, mitral
  congenital 746.6
myocardial—*see* Endocarditis
pulmonary (heart) (valve) (*see also* Endocarditis, pulmonary) 424.3
stomach—*see* Vomiting
tricuspid—*see* Endocarditis, tricuspid
valve, valvular—*see* Endocarditis
vesicoureteral —*see* Reflux, vesicoureteral
Rehabilitation V57.9
multiple types V57.89
occupational V57.21
specified type NEC V57.89
speech V57.3
vocational V57.22
Reichmann's disease or syndrome (gastrosuccorrhea) 536.8
Reifenstein's syndrome (hereditary familial hypogonadism, male) 259.5
Reilly's syndrome or phenomenon (*see also* Neuropathy, peripheral, autonomic) 337.9
Reimann's periodic disease 277.31
Reinsertion, contraceptive device V25.42
Reiter's disease, syndrome, or urethritis 099.3 [711.1]

Rejection
food, hysterical 300.11
transplant 996.80
  bone marrow 996.85
  corneal 996.51
  organ (immune or nonimmune cause) 996.80
    bone marrow 996.85
    heart 996.83
    intestines 996.87
    kidney 996.81
    liver 996.82
    lung 996.84
    pancreas 996.86
    specified NEC 996.89
  skin 996.52
    artificial 996.55
    decellularized allodermis 996.55
Relapsing fever 087.9
Carter's (Asiatic) 087.0
Dutton's (West African) 087.1
Koch's 087.9
louse-borne (epidemic) 087.0
Novy's (American) 087.1
Obermeyer's (European) 087.0
Spirillum 087.9
tick-borne (endemic) 087.1
Relaxation
anus (sphincter) 569.49
  due to hysteria 300.11
arch (foot) 734
  congenital 754.61
back ligaments 728.4
bladder (sphincter) 596.59
cardio-esophageal 530.89
cervix (*see also* Incompetency, cervix) 622.5
diaphragm 519.4
inguinal rings—*see* Hernia, inguinal
joint (capsule) (ligament) (paralytic) (*see also* Derangement, joint) 718.90
  congenital 755.8
lumbosacral joint 724.6
pelvic floor 618.89
pelvis 618.89
perineum 618.89
posture 729.9
rectum (sphincter) 569.49
sacroiliac (joint) 724.6
scrotum 608.89
urethra (sphincter) 599.84
uterus (outlet) 618.89
vagina (outlet) 618.89
vesical 596.59
Remains
canal of Cloquet 743.51
capsule (opaque) 743.51
Remittent fever (malarial) 084.6
Remnant
canal of Cloquet 743.51
capsule (opaque) 743.51
cervix, cervical stump (acquired) (postoperative) 622.8
cystic duct, postcholecystectomy 576.0
fingernail 703.8
  congenital 757.5
meniscus, knee 717.5
thyroglossal duct 759.2
tonsil 474.8
  infected 474.00
urachus 753.7
Remote effect of cancer —*see* Condition

1295

Removal (of)
catheter (urinary) (indwelling) V53.6
  from artificial opening—*see* Attention to, artificial, opening
  non-vascular V58.82
  vascular V58.81
cerebral ventricle (communicating) shunt V53.01
device—*see also* Fitting (of)
  contraceptive V25.42
  fixation
    external V54.89
    internal V54.01
    traction V54.89
drains V58.49
dressing
  wound V58.30
    nonsurgical V58.30
    surgical V58.31
ileostomy V55.2
Kirschner wire V54.89
non-vascular catheter V58.82
pin V54.01
plaster cast V54.89
plate (fracture) V54.01
rod V54.01
screw V54.01
splint, external V54.89
subdermal implantable contraceptive V25.43
staples V58.32
sutures V58.32
traction device, external V54.89
vascular catheter V58.81
wound packing V58.30
  nonsurgical V58.30
  surgical V58.31
Ren
arcuatus 753.3
mobile, mobilis (*see also* Disease, renal) 593.0
  congenital 753.3
unguliformis 753.3
Renal —*see also* condition
glomerulohyalinosis-diabetic syndrome 250.4 [581.81]
Rendu-Osler-Weber disease or syndrome (familial hemorrhagic telangiectasia) 448.0
Reninoma (M8361/1) 236.91
Rénon-Delille syndrome 253.8
Repair
pelvic floor, previous, in pregnancy or childbirth 654.4
  affecting fetus or newborn 763.89
scarred tissue V51
Replacement by artificial or mechanical device or prosthesis of (*see also* Fitting (of))
artificial skin V43.83
bladder V43.5
blood vessel V43.4
breast V43.82
eye globe V43.0
heart
  with
    assist device V43.21
    fully implantable artificial heart V43.22
    valve V43.3
intestine V43.89
joint V43.60
  ankle 43.66
  elbow V43.62
  finger V43.69
  hip (partial) (total) V43.64
  knee V43.65

Replacement—*continued*
  shoulder V43.61
  specified NEC V43.69
  wrist V43.63
kidney V43.89
larynx V43.81
lens V43.1
limb(s) V43.7
liver V43.89
lung V43.89
organ NEC V43.89
pancreas V43.89
skin (artificial) V43.83
tissue NEC V43.89
Reprogramming
cardiac pacemaker V53.31
Request for expert evidence V68.2
Reserve, decreased or low
cardiac—*see* Disease, heart
kidney (*see also* Disease, renal) 593.9
Residual —*see also* condition
bladder 596.8
foreign body—*see* Retention, foreign body
state, schizophrenic (*see also* Schizophrenia) 295.6
urine 788.69
Resistance, resistant (to)

Note—Use the following subclassification for categories V09.5, V09.7, V09.8, V09.9.:

0 without mention of resistance to multiple drugs
1 with resistance to multiple drugs

V09.5 quinolones and fluoroquinolones
V09.7 antimycobacterial agents
V09.8 specified drugs NEC
V09.9 unspecified drugs

9 multiple sites

activated protein C 289.81
drugs by microorganisms V09.90
  Amikacin V09.4
  aminoglycosides V09.4
  Amodiaquine V09.5
  Amoxicillin V09.0
  Ampicillin V09.0
  antimycobacterial agents V09.7
  Azithromycin V09.2
  Azlocillin V09.0
  Aztreonam V09.1
  B-lactam antibiotics V09.1
  Bacampicillin V09.0
  Bacitracin V09.8
  Benznidazole V09.8
  Capreomycin V09.7
  Carbenicillin V09.0
  Cefaclor V09.1
  Cefadroxil V09.1
  Cefamandole V09.1
  Cefatetan V09.1
  Cefazolin V09.1
  Cefixime V09.1
  Cefonicid V09.1
  Cefoperazone V09.1
  Ceforanide V09.1
  Cefotaxime V09.1
  Cefoxitin V09.1
  Ceftazidine V09.1
  Ceftizoxime V09.1

INDEX TO DISEASES

Respiration

Resistance, resistant (to)—*continued*
  Ceftriaxone V09.1
  Cefuroxime V09.1
  Cephalexin V09.1
  Cephaloglycin V09.1
  Cephaloridine V09.1
  cephalosporins V09.1
  Cephalothin V09.1
  Cephapirin V09.1
  Cephradine V09.1
  Chloramphenicol V09.8
  Chloraquine V09.5
  Chlorguanide V09.8
  Chlorproguanil V09.8
  Chlortetracycline V09.3
  Cinoxacin V09.5
  Ciprofloxacin V09.5
  Clarithromycin V09.2
  Clindamycin V09.8
  Clioquinol V09.5
  Clofazimine V09.7
  Cloxacillin V09.0
  Cyclacillin V09.0
  Cycloserine V09.7
  Dapsone [DZ] V09.7
  Demeclocycline V09.3
  Dicloxacillin V09.0
  Doxycycline V09.3
  Enoxacin V09.5
  Erythromycin V09.2
  Ethambutol [EMB] V09.7
  Ethionamide [ETA] V09.7
  fluoroquinolones NEC V09.5
  Gentamicin V09.4
  Halofantrine V09.8
  Imipenem V09.1
  Iodoquinol V09.5
  Isoniazid [INH] V09.7
  Kanamycin V09.4
  macrolides V09.2
  Mafenide V09.6
  MDRO (multiple drug resistant organisms) NOS V09.91
  Mefloquine V09.8
  Melassoprol V09.8
  Methacillin V09.0
  Methacycline V09.3
  Methenamine V09.8
  Methicillin V09.0
  Metronidazole V09.8
  Mezlocillin V09.0
  Minocycline V09.3
  multiple drug resistant organisms NOS V09.91
  Nafcillin V09.0
  Nalidixic Acid V09.5
  Natamycin V09.2
  Neomycin V09.4
  Netilmicin V09.4
  Nimorazole V09.8
  Nitrofurantoin V09.8
  Nitrofurtimox V09.8
  Norfloxacin V09.5
  Nystatin V09.2
  Ofloxacin V09.5
  Oleandomycin V09.2
  Oxacillin V09.0
  Oxytetracycline V09.3
  Para-amino salicylic acid [PAS] V09.7
  Paromomycin V09.4
  Penicillin (G)(V)(VK) V09.0
  penicillins V09.0

Resistance, resistant (to)—*continued*
  Pentamidine V09.8
  Piperacillin V09.0
  Primaquine V09.5
  Proguanil V09.8
  Pyrazinamide [PZA] V09.7
  Pyrimethamine/Sulfalene V09.8
  Pyrimethamine/Sulfodoxine V09.8
  Quinacrine V09.5
  Quinidine V09.8
  Quinine V09.8
  quinolones V09.5
  Rifabutin V09.7
  Rifampin [RIF] V09.7
  Rifamycin V09.7
  Rolitetracycline V09.3
  specified drugs NEC V09.8
  Spectinomycin V09.8
  Spiramycin V09.2
  Streptomycin [SM] V09.4
  Sulfacetamide V09.6
  Sulfacytine V90.6
  Sulfadiazine V09.6
  Sulfadoxine V09.6
  Sulfamethoxazole V09.6
  Sulfapyridine V09.6
  Sulfasalizine V09.6
  Sulfasoxazole V09.6
  sulfonamides V09.6
  Sulfoxone V09.7
  Tetracycline V09.3
  tetracyclines V09.3
  Thiamphenicol V09.8
  Ticarcillin V09.0
  Tinidazole V09.8
  Tobramycin V09.4
  Triamphenicol V09.8
  Trimethoprim V09.8
  Vancomycin V09.8
  insulin 277.7
  thyroid hormone 246.8

Resorption
  biliary 576.8
    purulent or putrid (*see also* Cholecystitis) 576.8
  dental (roots) 521.40
    alveoli 525.8
    pathological
      external 521.42
      internal 521.41
      specified NEC 521.49
  septic—*see* Septicemia
  teeth (roots) 521.40
    pathological
      external 521.42
      internal 521.41
      specified NEC 521.49

Respiration
  asymmetrical 786.09
  bronchial 786.09
  Cheyne-Stokes (periodic respiration) 786.04
  decreased, due to shock following injury 958.4
  disorder of 786.00
    psychogenic 306.1
    specified NEC 786.09
  failure 518.81
    acute 518.81
    acute and chronic 518.84
    chronic 518.83
    newborn 770.84
  insufficiency 786.09

Respiration — *continued*
    acute 518.82
    newborn NEC 770.89
    Kussmaul (air hunger) 786.09
    painful 786.52
    periodic 786.09
        high altitude 327.22
    poor 786.09
        newborn NEC 770.89
    sighing 786.7
        psychogenic 306.1
    wheezing 786.07
Respiratory —*see also* condition
    distress 786.09
        acute 518.82
        fetus or newborn NEC 770.89
        syndrome (newborn) 769
            adult (following shock, surgery, or trauma) 518.5
                specified NEC 518.82
    failure 518.81
        acute 518.81
        acute and chronic 518.84
        chronic 518.83
Respiratory syncytial virus (RSV) 079.6
    bronchiolitis 466.11
    pneumonia 480.1
    vaccination, prophylactic (against) V04.82
Response
    photoallergic 692.72
    phototoxic 692.72
Rest, rests
    mesonephric duct 752.89
        fallopian tube 752.11
    ovarian, in fallopian tubes 752.19
    wolffian duct 752.89
Restless legs syndrome (RLS) 333.94
Restlessness 799.2
Restoration of organ continuity from previous sterilization (tuboplasty) (vasoplasty) V26.0
Restriction of housing space V60.1
Restzustand, schizophrenic (*see also* Schizophrenia) 295.6
Retained —*see* Retention
Retardation
    development, developmental, specific (*see also* Disorder, development, specific) 315.9
        learning, specific 315.2
            arithmetical 315.1
            language (skills) 315.31
                expressive 315.31
                mixed receptive-expressive 315.32
            mathematics 315.1
            reading 315.00
                phonological 315.39
            written expression 315.2
        motor 315.4
    endochondral bone growth 733.91
    growth (physical) in childhood 783.43
        due to malnutrition 263.2
        fetal (intrauterine) 764.9
            affecting management of pregnancy 656.5
    intrauterine growth 764.9
        affecting management of pregnancy 656.5
    mental 319
        borderline V62.89
        mild, IQ 50-70 317
        moderate, IQ 35-49 318.0
        profound, IQ under 20 318.2
        severe, IQ 20-34 318.1
    motor, specific 315.4

Retardation — *continued*
    physical 783.43
        child 783.43
        due to malnutrition 263.2
        fetus (intrauterine) 764.9
            affecting management of pregnancy 656.5
    psychomotor NEC 307.9
    reading 315.00
Retching —*see* Vomiting
Retention, retained
    bladder NEC (*see also* Retention, urine) 788.20
        psychogenic 306.53
    carbon dioxide 276.2
    cyst—*see* Cyst
    dead
        fetus (after 22 completed weeks gestation) 656.4
            early fetal death (before 22 completed weeks gestation) 632
        ovum 631
    decidua (following delivery) (fragments) (with hemorrhage) 666.2
        without hemorrhage 667.1
    deciduous tooth 520.6
    dental root 525.3
    fecal (*see also* Constipation) 564.00
    fluid 276.6
    foreign body—*see also* Foreign body, retained
        bone 733.99
        current trauma—*see* Foreign body, by site or type
        middle ear 385.83
        muscle 729.6
        soft tissue NEC 729.6
    gastric 536.8
    membranes (following delivery) (with hemorrhage) 666.2
        with abortion—*see* Abortion, by type
        without hemorrhage 667.1
    menses 626.8
    milk (puerperal) 676.2
    nitrogen, extrarenal 788.9
    placenta (total) (with hemorrhage) 666.0
        with abortion—*see* Abortion, by type
        portions or fragments 666.2
            without hemorrhage 667.1
        without hemorrhage 667.0
    products of conception
        early pregnancy (fetal death before 22 completed weeks gestation) 632
        following
            abortion—*see* Abortion, by type
            delivery 666.2
                with hemorrhage 666.2
                without hemorrhage 667.1
    secundines (following delivery) (with hemorrhage) 666.2
        with abortion—*see* Abortion, by type
        complicating puerperium (delayed hemorrhage) 666.2
        without hemorrhage 667.1
    smegma, clitoris 624.8
    urine NEC 788.20
        bladder, incomplete emptying 788.21
        due to
            benign prostatic hypertrophy (BPH)—*see* category 600
        due to
            benign prostatic hypertrophy (BPH)—*see* category 600
        psychogenic 306.53
        specified NEC 788.29
    water (in tissue) (*see also* Edema) 782.3

INDEX TO DISEASES   **Retrocecal**

Reticulation, dust (occupational) 504
Reticulocytosis NEC 790.99
Reticuloendotheliosis
   acute infantile (M9722/3) 202.5
   leukemic (M9940/3) 202.4
   malignant (M9720/3) 202.3
   nonlipid (M9722/3) 202.5
Reticulohistiocytoma (giant cell) 277.89
Reticulohistiocytosis, multicentric 272.8
Reticulolymphosarcoma (diffuse) (M9613/3) 200.8
   follicular (M9691/3) 202.0
   nodular (M9691/3) 202.0
Reticulosarcoma (M9640/3) 200.0
   odular (M9642/3) 200.0
   pleomorphic cell type (M9641/3) 200.0
Reticulosis (skin)
   acute of infancy (M9722/3) 202.5
   familial hemophagocytic 288.4
   histiocytic medullary (M9721/3) 202.3
   lipomelanotic 695.89
   malignant (M9720/3) 202.3
   Sézary's (M9701/3) 202.2
Retina, retinal —*see* condition
Retinitis (*see also* Chorioretinitis) 363.20
   albuminurica 585.9 *[363.10]*
   arteriosclerotic 440.8 *[362.13]*
   central angiospastic 362.41
   Coat's 362.12
   diabetic 250.5 *[362.01]*
   disciformis 362.52
   disseminated 363.10
      metastatic 363.14
      neurosyphilitic 094.83
      pigment epitheliopathy 363.15
   exudative 362.12
   focal 363.00
      in histoplasmosis 115.92
         capsulatum 115.02
         duboisii 115.12
      juxtapapillary 363.05
      macular 363.06
      paramacular 363.06
      peripheral 363.08
      posterior pole NEC 363.07
   gravidarum 646.8
   hemorrhagica externa 362.12
   juxtapapillary (Jensen's) 363.05
   luetic—*see* Retinitis, syphilitic
   metastatic 363.14
   pigmentosa 362.74
   proliferans 362.29
   proliferating 362.29
   punctata albescens 362.76
   renal 585.9 *[363.13]*
   syphilitic (secondary) 091.51
      congenital 090.0 *[363.13]*
      early 091.51
      late 095.8 *[363.13]*
   syphilitica, central, recurrent 095.8 *[363.13]*
   tuberculous (*see also* Tuberculous) 017.3 *[363.13]*
Retinoblastoma (M9510/3) 190.5
   differentiated type (M9511/3) 190.5
   undifferentiated type (M9512/3) 190.5
Retinochoroiditis (*see also* Chorioretinitis) 363.20
   central angiospastic 362.41
   disseminated 363.10
      metastatic 363.14
      neurosyphilitic 094.83
      pigment epitheliopathy 363.15
      syphilitic 094.83

Retinochoroiditis—*continued*
   due to toxoplasmosis (acquired) (focal) 130.2
   focal 363.00
      in histoplasmosis 115.92
         capsulatum 115.02
         duboisii 115.12
      juxtapapillary (Jensen's) 363.05
      macular 363.06
      paramacular 363.06
      peripheral 363.08
      posterior pole NEC 363.07
   juxtapapillaris 363.05
   syphilitic (disseminated) 094.83
Retinopathy (background) 362.10
   arteriosclerotic 440.8 *[362.13]*
   atherosclerotic 440.8 *[362.13]*
   central serous 362.41
   circinate 362.10
   Coat's 362.12
   diabetic 250.5 *[362.01]*
      nonproliferative 250.5 *[362.03]*
         mild 250.5 *[362.04]*
         moderate 250.5 *[362.05]*
         severe 250.5 *[362.06]*
      proliferative 250.5 *[362.02]*
   exudative 362.12
   hypertensive 362.11
   of prematurity 362.21
   nonproliferative
      diabetic 250.5 *[362.03]*
         mild 250.5 *[362.04]*
         moderate 250.5 *[362.05]*
         severe 250.5 *[362.06]*
   pigmentary, congenital 362.74
   proliferative 362.29
      diabetic 250.5 *[362.02]*
      sickle-cell 282.60 *[362.29]*
   solar 363.31
Retinoschisis 361.10
   bullous 361.12
   congenital 743.56
   flat 361.11
   juvenile 362.73
Retractile testis 752.52
Retraction
   cervix *see* Retraction, uterus
   drum (membrane) 384.82
   eyelid 374.41
   finger 736.29
   head 781.0
   lid 374.41
   lung 518.89
   mediastinum 519.3
   nipple 611.79
      congenital 757.6
      puerperal, postpartum 676.0
   palmar fascia 728.6
   pleura (*see also* Pleurisy) 511.0
   ring, uterus (Bandl's) (pathological) 661.4
      affecting fetus or newborn 763.7
   sternum (congenital) 756.3
      acquired 738.3
      during respiration 786.9
   substernal 738.3
   supraclavicular 738.8
   syndrome (Duane's) 378.71
   uterus 621.6
   valve (heart)—*see* Endocarditis
Retrobulbar —*see* condition
Retrocaval ureter 753.4
Retrocecal —*see also* condition
   appendix (congenital) 751.5

Retrocession —see Retroversion
Retrodisplacement —see Retroversion
Retroflection, retroflexion —see Retroversion
Retrognathia, retrognathism (mandibular) (maxillary) 524.06
Retrograde
  ejaculation 608.87
  menstruation 626.8
Retroiliac ureter 753.4
Retroperineal —see condition
Retroperitoneal —see condition
Retroperitonitis 567.39
Retropharyngeal —see condition
Retroplacental —see condition
Retroposition —see Retroversion
Retrosternal thyroid (congenital) 759.2
Retroversion, retroverted
  cervix see Retroversion, uterus
  female NEC (see also Retroversion, uterus) 621.6
  iris 364.70
  testis (congenital) 752.51
  uterus, uterine (acquired) (acute) (adherent) (any degree) (asymptomatic) (cervix) (postinfectional) (postpartal, old) 621.6
    congenital 752.3
    in pregnancy or childbirth 654.3
      affecting fetus or newborn 763.89
      causing obstructed labor 660.2
        affecting fetus or newborn 763.1
Retrusion, premaxilla (developmental) 524.04
Rett's syndrome 330.8
Reverse, reversed
  peristalsis 787.4
Reye's syndrome 331.81
Reye-Sheehan syndrome (postpartum pituitary necrosis) 253.2
Rh (factor)
  hemolytic disease 773.0
  incompatibility, immunization, or sensitization
    affecting management of pregnancy 656.1
    fetus or newborn 773.0
    transfusion reaction 999.7
  negative mother, affecting fetus or newborn 773.0
  titer elevated 999.7
  transfusion reaction 999.7
Rhabdomyolysis (idiopathic) 728.88
Rhabdomyoma (M8900/0)—see also Neoplasm, connective tissue, benign
  adult (M8904/0)—see Neoplasm, connective tissue, benign
  fetal (M8903/0)—see Neoplasm, connective tissue, benign
  glycogenic (M8904/0)—see Neoplasm, connective tissue, benign
Rhabdomyosarcoma (M8900/3)—see also Neoplasm connective tissue, malignant
  alveolar (M8920/3)—see Neoplasm, connective tissue, malignant
  embryonal (M8910/3)—see Neoplasm, connective tissue malignant
  mixed type (M8902/3)—see Neoplasm, connective tissue, malignant
  pleomorphic (M8901/3)—see Neoplasm, connective tissue, malignant
Rhabdosarcoma (M8900/3)—see Rhabdomyosarcoma
Rhesus (factor) (Rh) incompatibility—see Rh, incompatibility
Rheumaticosis —see Rheumatism

Rheumatism, rheumatic (acute NEC) 729.0
  adherent pericardium 393
  arthritis
    acute or subacute—see Fever, rheumatic
    chronic 714.0
      spine 720.0
    articular (chronic) NEC (see also Arthritis) 716.9
    acute or subacute—see Fever, rheumatic
  back 724.9
  blennorrhagic 098.59
  carditis—see Disease, heart, rheumatic
  cerebral—see Fever, rheumatic
  chorea (acute)—see Chorea, rheumatic
  chronic NEC 729.0
  coronary arteritis 391.9
    chronic 398.99
  degeneration, myocardium (see also Degeneration, myocardium, with rheumatic fever) 398.0
  desert 114.0
  febrile—see Fever, rheumatic
  fever—see Fever, rheumatic
  gonococcal 098.59
  gout 274.0
  heart
    disease (see also Disease, heart, rheumatic) 398.90
    failure (chronic) (congestive) (inactive) 398.91
  hemopericardium—see Rheumatic, pericarditis
  hydropericardium—see Rheumatic, pericarditis
  inflammatory (acute) (chronic) (subacute)—see Fever, rheumatic
  intercostal 729.0
    meaning Tietze's disease 733.6
  joint (chronic) NEC (see also Arthritis) 716.9
    acute—see Fever, rheumatic
  mediastinopericarditis—see Rheumatic, pericarditis
  muscular 729.0
  myocardial degeneration (see also Degeneration, myocardium, with rheumatic fever) 398.0
  myocarditis (chronic) (inactive) (with chorea) 398.0
    active or acute 391.2
      with chorea (acute) (rheumatic) (Sydenham's) 392.0
  myositis 729.1
  neck 724.9
  neuralgic 729.0
  neuritis (acute) (chronic) 729.2
  neuromuscular 729.0
  nodose—see Arthritis, nodosa
  nonarticular 729.0
  palindromic 719.30
    ankle 719.37
    elbow 719.32
    foot 719.37
    hand 719.34
    hip 719.35
    knee 719.36
    multiple sites 719.39
    pelvic region 719.35
    shoulder (region) 719.31
    specified site NEC 719.38
    wrist 719.33
  pancarditis, acute 391.8
    with chorea (acute) (rheumatic) (Sydenham's) 392.0
    chronic or inactive 398.99

INDEX TO DISEASES   Ridged ear

Rheumatism, rheumatic—*continued*
  pericarditis (active) (acute) (with effusion) (with
    pneumonia) 391.0
    with chorea (acute) (rheumatic) (Sydenham's)
      392.0
    chronic or inactive 393
  pericardium—*see* Rheumatic, pericarditis
  pleuropericarditis—*see* Rheumatic, pericarditis
  pneumonia 390 *[517.1]*
  pneumonitis 390 *[517.1]*
  pneumopericarditis—*see* Rheumatic,
    pericarditis
  polyarthritis
    acute or subacute—*see* Fever, rheumatic
    chronic 714.0
  polyarticular NEC (*see also* Arthritis) 716.9
  psychogenic 306.0
  radiculitis 729.2
  sciatic 724.3
  septic—*see* Fever, rheumatic
  spine 724.9
  subacute NEC 729.0
  torticollis 723.5
  tuberculous NEC (*see also* Tuberculosis) 015.9
  typhoid fever 002.0
Rheumatoid —*see also* condition
  lungs 714.81
Rhinitis (atrophic) (catarrhal) (chronic)
  (croupous) (fibrinous) (hyperplastic)
  (hypertrophic) (membranous) (purulent)
  (suppurative) (ulcerative) 472.0
  with
    hay fever (*see also* Fever, hay) 477.9
      with asthma (bronchial) 493.0
    sore throat—*see* Nasopharyngitis
  acute 460
  allergic (nonseasonal) (seasonal) (*see also*
    Fever, hay) 477.9
    due to food 477.1
    with asthma (*see also* Asthma) 493.0
  granulomatous 472.0
  infective 460
  obstructive 472.0
  pneumococcal 460
  syphilitic 095.8
    congenital 090.0
  tuberculous (*see also* Tuberculosis) 012.8
  vasomotor (*see also* Fever, hay) 477.9
Rhinoantritis (chronic) 473.0
  acute 461.0
Rhinodacryolith 375.57
Rhinolalia (aperta) (clausa) (open) 784.49
Rhinolith 478.19
  nasal sinus (*see also* Sinusitis) 473.9
Rhinomegaly 478.19
Rhinopharyngitis (acute) (subacute) (*see also*
  Nasopharyngitis) 460
  chronic 472.2
  destructive ulcerating 102.5
  mutilans 102.5
Rhinophyma 695.3
Rhinorrhea 478.19
  cerebrospinal (fluid) 349.81
  paroxysmal (*see also* Fever, hay) 477.9
  spasmodic (*see also* Fever, hay) 477.9
Rhinosalpingitis 381.50
  acute 381.51
  chronic 381.52
Rhinoscleroma 040.1
Rhinosporidiosis 117.0
Rhinovirus infection 079.3

Rhizomelic chrondrodysplasia punctata 277.86
Rhizomelique, pseudopolyarthritic 446.5
Rhoads and Bomford anemia (refractory)
  238.72
Rhus
  diversiloba dermatitis 692.6
  radicans dermatitis 692.6
  toxicodendron dermatitis 692.6
  venenata dermatitis 692.6
  verniciflua dermatitis 692.6
Rhythm
  atrioventricular nodal 427.89
  disorder 427.9
    coronary sinus 427.89
    ectopic 427.89
    nodal 427.89
  escape 427.89
  heart, abnormal 427.9
    fetus or newborn—*see* Abnormal, heart rate
  idioventricular 426.89
    accelerated 427.89
  nodal 427.89
  sleep, inversion 327.39
    nonorganic origin 307.45
Rhytidosis facialis 701.8
Rib —*see also* condition
  cervical 756.2
Riboflavin deficiency 266.0
Rice bodies (*see also* Loose, body, joint) 718.1
  knee 717.6
Richter's hernia —*see* Hernia, Richter's
Ricinism 988.2
Rickets (active) (acute) (adolescent) (adult)
  (chest wall) (congenital) (current) (infantile)
  (intestinal) 268.0
  celiac 579.0
  fetal 756.4
  hemorrhagic 267
  hypophosphatemic with nephrotic-glycosuric
    dwarfism 270.0
  kidney 588.0
  late effect 268.1
  renal 588.0
  scurvy 267
  vitamin D-resistant 275.3
Rickettsial disease 083.9
  specified type NEC 083.8
Rickettsialpox 083.2
Rickettsiosis NEC 083.9
  specified type NEC 083.8
  tick-borne 082.9
    specified type NEC 082.8
  vesicular 083.2
Ricord's chancre 091.0
Riddoch's syndrome (visual disorientation) 368.16
Rider's
  bone 733.99
  chancre 091.0
Ridge, alveolus —*see also* condition
  edentulous
    atrophy 525.20
      mandible 525.20
        minimal 525.21
        moderate 525.22
        severe 525.23
      maxilla 525.20
        minimal 525.24
        moderate 525.25
        severe 525.26
    flabby 525.20
Ridged ear 744.29

Riedel's
  disease (ligneous thyroiditis) 245.3
  lobe, liver 751.69
  struma (ligneous thyroiditis) 245.3
  thyroiditis (ligneous) 245.3
Rieger's anomaly or syndrome (mesodermal dysgenesis, anterior ocular segment) 743.44
Riehl's melanosis 709.09
Rietti-Greppi-Micheli anemia or syndrome 282.49
Rieux's hernia —*see* Hernia, Rieux's
Rift Valley fever 066.3
Riga's disease (cachectic aphthae) 529.0
Riga-Fede disease (cachectic aphthae) 529.0
Riggs' disease (compound periodontitis) 523.40
Right middle lobe syndrome 518.0
Rigid, rigidity —*see also* condition
  abdominal 789.4
  articular, multiple congenital 754.89
  back 724.8
  cervix uteri
    in pregnancy or childbirth 654.6
      affecting fetus or newborn 763.89
      causing obstructed labor 660.2
        affecting fetus or newborn 763.1
  hymen (acquired) (congenital) 623.3
  nuchal 781.6
  pelvic floor
    in pregnancy or childbirth 654.4
      affecting fetus or newborn 763.89
      causing obstructed labor 660.2
        affecting fetus or newborn 763.1
  perineum or vulva
    in pregnancy or childbirth 654.8
      affecting fetus or newborn 763.89
      causing obstructed labor 660.2
        affecting fetus or newborn 763.1
  spine 724.8
  vagina
    in pregnancy or childbirth 654.7
      affecting fetus or newborn 763.89
      causing obstructed labor 660.2
        affecting fetus or newborn 763.1
Rigors 780.99
Riley-Day syndrome (familial dysautonomia) 742.8
RIND (reversible ischemic neurological deficit) 434.91
  history of personal V12.54
Ring(s)
  aorta 747.21
  Bandl's, complicating delivery 661.4
    affecting fetus or newborn 763.7
  contraction, complicating delivery 661.4
    affecting fetus or newborn 763.7
  esophageal (congenital) 750.3
  Fleischer (-Kayser) (cornea) 275.1 *[371.14]*
  hymenal, tight (acquired) (congenital) 623.3
  Kayser-Fleischer (cornea) 275.1 *[371.14]*
  retraction, uterus, pathological 661.4
    affecting fetus or newborn 763.7
  Schatzki's (esophagus) (congenital) (lower) 750.3
    acquired 530.3
  Soemmering's 366.51
  trachea, abnormal 748.3
  vascular (congenital) 747.21
  Vossius' 921.3
    late effect 366.21
Ringed hair (congenital) 757.4
Ringing in the ear (*see also* Tinnitus) 388.30
Ringworm 110.9
  beard 110.0
  body 110.5

Ringworm—*continued*
  Burmese 110.9
  corporeal 110.5
  foot 110.4
  groin 110.3
  hand 110.2
  honeycomb 110.0
  nails 110.1
  perianal (area) 110.3
  scalp 110.0
  specified site NEC 110.8
  Tokelau 110.5
Rise, venous pressure 459.89
Risk
  factor —*see* Problem
  falling V15.88
  suicidal 300.9
Ritter's disease (dermatitis exfoliativa neonatorum) 695.81
Rivalry, sibling 313.3
Rivalta's disease (cervicofacial actinomycosis) 039.3
River blindness 125.3 *[360.13]*
Robert's pelvis 755.69
  with disproportion (fetopelvic) 653.0
    affecting fetus or newborn 763.1
    causing obstructed labor 660.1
      affecting fetus or newborn 763.1
Robin's syndrome 756.0
Robinson's (hidrotic) ectodermal dysplasia 757.31
Robles' disease (onchocerciasis) 125.3 *[360.13]*
Rochalimea —*see* Rickettsial disease
Rocky Mountain fever (spotted) 082.0
Rodent ulcer 9M8090/3)—*see also* Neoplasm, skin, malignant
  cornea 370.07
Roentgen ray, adverse effect —*see* Effect, adverse, x-ray
Roetheln 056.9
Roger's disease (congenital interventricular septal defect) 745.4
Rokitansky's
  disease (*see also* Necrosis, liver) 570
  tumor 620.2
Rokitansky-Aschoff sinuses (mucosal outpouching of gallbladder) (*see also* Disease, gallbladder) 575.8
Rokitansky-Kuster-Hauser syndrome (congenital absence vagina) 752.49
Rollet's chancre (syphilitic) 091.0
Rolling of head 781.0
Romano-Ward syndrome (prolonged QT interval syndrome) 426.82
Romanus lesion 720.1
Romberg's disease or syndrome 349.89
Roof, mouth —*see* condition
Rosacea 695.3
  acne 695.3
  keratitis 695.3 *[370.49]*
Rosary, rachitic 268.0
Rose
  cold 477.0
  fever 477.0
  rash 782.1
    epidemic 056.9
    of infants 057.8
Rosen-Castleman-Liebow syndrome (pulmonary proteinosis) 516.0
Rosenbach's erysipelatoid or erysipeloid 027.1
Rosenthal's disease (factor XI deficiency) 286.2

INDEX TO DISEASES

Rupture, ruptured

Roseola 057.8
  infantum, infantilis (*see also* Exanthem subitum) 058.10
Rossbach's disease (hyperchlorhydria) 536.8
  psychogenic 306.4
Rössle-Urbach-Wiethe lipoproteinosis 272.8
Ross river fever 066.3
Rostan's asthma (cardiac) (*see also* Failure, ventricular, left) 428.1
Rot
  Barcoo (*see also* Ulcer, skin) 707.9
  knife-grinders' (*see also* Tuberculosis) 011.4
Rot-Bernhardt disease 355.1
Rotation
  anomalous, incomplete or insufficient—*see* Malrotation
  cecum (congenital) 751.4
  colon (congenital) 751.4
  manual, affecting fetus or newborn 763.89
  spine, incomplete or insufficient 737.8
  tooth, teeth 524.35
  vertebra, incomplete or insufficient 737.8
Röteln 056.9
Roth's disease or meralgia 355.1
Roth-Bernhardt disease or syndrome 355.1
Rothmund (-Thomson) syndrome 757.33
Rotor's disease or syndrome (idiopathic hyperbilirubinemia) 277.4
Rotundum ulcus —*see* Ulcer, stomach
Round
  back (with wedging of vertebrae) 737.10
    late effect of rickets 268.1
  hole, retina 361.31
    with detachment 361.01
  ulcer (stomach)—*see* Ulcer, stomach
  worms (infestation) (large) NEC 127.0
Roussy-Lévy syndrome 334.3
Routine postpartum follow-up V24.2
Roy (-Jutras) syndrome (acropachyderma) 757.39
Rubella (German measles) 056.9
  complicating pregnancy, childbirth, or puerperium 647.5
  complication 056.8
    neurological 056.00
      encephalomyelitis 056.01
      specified type NEC 056.09
    specified type NEC 056.79
  congenital 771.0
  contact V01.4
  exposure to V01.4
  maternal
    with suspected fetal damage affecting management of pregnancy 655.3
    affecting fetus or newborn 760.2
      manifest rubella in infant 771.0
  specified complications NEC 056.79
  vaccination, prophylactic (against) V04.3
Rubeola (measles) (*see also* Measles) 055.9
  complicated 055.8
  meaning rubella (*see also* Rubella) 056.9
  scarlatinosis 057.8
Rubeosis iridis 364.42
  diabetica 250.5 [364.42]
Rubinstein-Taybi's syndrome (brachydactylia, short stature and mental retardation) 759.89
Rud's syndrome (mental deficiency, epilepsy, and infantilism) 759.89
Rudimentary (congenital)—*see also* Agenesis
  arm 755.22
  bone 756.9
  cervix uteri 752.49

Rudimentary—*continued*
  eye (*see also* Microphthalmos) 743.10
  fallopian tube 752.19
  leg 755.32
  lobule of ear 744.21
  patella 755.64
  respiratory organs in thoracopagus 759.4
  tracheal bronchus 748.3
  uterine horn 752.3
  uterus 752.3
    in male 752.7
    solid or with cavity 752.3
  vagina 752.49
Ruiter-Pompen (-Wyers) syndrome (angiokeratoma corporis diffusum) 272.7
Ruled out condition (*see also* Observation, suspected) V71.9
Rumination —*see also* Vomiting
  disorder 307.53
  neurotic 300.3
  obsessional 300.3
  psychogenic 307.53
Runaway reaction —*see also* Disturbance, conduct
  socialized 312.2
  undersocialized, unsocialized 312.1
Runeberg's disease (progressive pernicious anemia) 281.0
Runge's syndrome (postmaturity) 766.22
Runny nose 784.99
Rupia 091.3
  congenital 090.0
  tertiary 095.9
Rupture, ruptured 553.9
  abdominal viscera NEC 799.89
    obstetrical trauma 665.5
  abscess (spontaneous)—*see* Abscess, by site
  amnion—*see* Rupture, membranes
  aneurysm—*see* Aneurysm
  anus (sphincter)—*see* Laceration, anus
  aorta, aortic 441.5
    abdominal 441.3
    arch 441.1
    ascending 441.1
    descending 441.5
      abdominal 441.3
      thoracic 441.1
    syphilitic 093.0
    thoracoabdominal 441.6
    thorax, thoracic 441.1
    transverse 441.1
    traumatic (thoracic) 901.0
      abdominal 902.0
    valve or cusp (*see also* Endocarditis, aortic) 424.1
  appendix (with peritonitis) 540.0
    traumatic—*see* Injury, internal, gastrointestinal tract
    with peritoneal abscess 540.1
  arteriovenous fistula, brain (congenital) 430
  artery 447.2
    brain (*see also* Hemorrhage, brain) 431
    coronary (*see also* Infarct, myocardium) 410.9
    heart (*see also* Infarct, myocardium) 410.9
    pulmonary 417.8
    traumatic (complication) (*see also* Injury, blood vessel, by site) 904.9
  bile duct, except cystic (*see also* Disease, biliary) 576.3
    cystic 575.4
    traumatic—*see* Injury, internal, intra-abdominal

1303

Rupture, ruptured—continued
  bladder (sphincter) 596.6
    with
      abortion—see Abortion, by type, with damage to pelvic organs
      ectopic pregnancy (see also categories 633.0-633.9) 639.2
      molar pregnancy (see also categories 630-632) 639.2
    following
      abortion 639.2
      ectopic or molar pregnancy 639.2
    nontraumatic 596.6
    obstetrical trauma 665.5
    spontaneous 596.6
    traumatic—see Injury, internal, bladder
  blood vessel (see also Hemorrhage) 459.0
    brain (see also Hemorrhage, brain) 431
    heart (see also Infarct, myocardium) 410.9
    traumatic (complication) (see also Injury, blood vessel, by site) 904.9
  bone—see Fracture, by site
  bowel 569.89
    traumatic—see Injury, internal, intestine
  Bowman's membrane 371.31
  brain
    aneurysm (congenital) (see also Hemorrhage, subarachnoid) 430
      late effect—see Late effect(s) (of) cerebrovascular disease
      syphilitic 094.87
    hemorrhagic (see also Hemorrhage, brain) 431
    injury at birth 767.0
    syphilitic 094.89
  capillaries 448.9
  cardiac (see also Infarct, myocardium) 410.9
  cartilage (articular) (current)—see also Sprain, by site
    knee—see Tear, meniscus
    semilunar—see Tear, meniscus
  cecum (with peritonitis) 540.0
    traumatic 863.89
      with open wound into cavity 863.99
    with peritoneal abscess 540.1
  cerebral aneurysm (congenital) (see also Hemorrhage, subarachnoid) 430
    late effect—see Late effect(s) (of) cerebrovascular disease
  cervix (uteri)
    with
      abortion—see Abortion, by type, with damage to pelvic organs
      ectopic pregnancy (see also categories 633.0-633.9) 639.2
      molar pregnancy (see also categories 630-632) 639.2
    following
      abortion 639.2
      ectopic or molar pregnancy 639.2
    obstetrical trauma 665.3
    traumatic—see Injury, internal, cervix
  chordae tendineae 429.5
  choroid (direct) (indirect) (traumatic) 363.63
  circle of Willis (see also Hemorrhage, subarachnoid) 430
    late effect—see Late effect(s) (of) cerebrovascular disease
  colon 569.89
    traumatic—see Injury, internal, colon
  cornea (traumatic)—see also Rupture, eye
    due to ulcer 370.00

Rupture, ruptured—continued
  coronary (artery) (thrombotic) (see also Infarct, myocardium) 410.9
  corpus luteum (infected) (ovary) 620.1
  cyst—see Cyst
  cystic duct (see also Disease, gallbladder) 575.4
  Descemet's membrane 371.33
    traumatic—see Rupture, eye
  diaphragm—see also Hernia, diaphragm
    traumatic—see Injury, internal, diaphragm
  diverticulum
    bladder 596.3
    intestine (large) (see also Diverticula) 562.10
    small 562.00
  duodenal stump 537.89
  duodenum (ulcer)—see Ulcer, duodenum, with perforation
  ear drum (see also Perforation, tympanum) 384.20
    with otitis media—see Otitis media
    traumatic—see Wound, open, ear
  esophagus 530.4
    traumatic 862.22
      with open wound into cavity 862.32
      cervical region—see Wound, open, esophagus
  eye (without prolapse of intraocular tissue) 871.0
    with
      exposure of intraocular tissue 871.1
      partial loss of intraocular tissue 871.2
      prolapse of intraocular tissue 871.1
    due to burn 940.5
  fallopian tube 620.8
    due to pregnancy—see Pregnancy, tubal
    traumatic—see Injury, internal, fallopian tube
  fontanel 767.3
  free wall (ventricle) (see also Infarct, myocardium) 410.9
  gallbladder or duct (see also Disease, gallbladder) 575.4
    traumatic—see Injury, internal, gallbladder
  gastric (see also Rupture, stomach) 537.89
    vessel 459.0
  globe (eye) (traumatic)—see Rupture, eye
  graafian follicle (hematoma) 620.0
  heart (auricle) (ventricle) (see also Infarct, myocardium) 410.9
    infectional 422.90
    traumatic—see Rupture, myocardium, traumatic
  hymen 623.8
  internal
    organ, traumatic—see also Injury, internal, by site
      heart—see Rupture, myocardium, traumatic
      kidney—see Rupture, kidney
      liver—see Rupture, liver
      spleen—see Rupture, spleen, traumatic
    semilunar cartilage—see Tear, meniscus
  intervertebral disc—see Displacement, intervertebral disc
    traumatic (current)—see Dislocation, vertebra
  intestine 569.89
    traumatic—see Injury, internal, intestine
  intracranial, birth injury 767.0
  iris 364.76
    traumatic—see Rupture, eye
  joint capsule—see Sprain, by site
  kidney (traumatic) 866.03
    with open wound into cavity 866.13
    due to birth injury 767.8

INDEX TO DISEASES

Rupture, ruptured

Rupture, ruptured—*continued*
  nontraumatic 593.89
  lacrimal apparatus (traumatic) 870.2
  lens (traumatic) 366.20
  ligament—*see also* Sprain, by site
    with open wound—*see* Wound, open, by site
    old (*see also* Disorder, cartilage, articular) 718.0
  liver (traumatic) 864.04
    with open wound into cavity 864.14
    due to birth injury 767.8
    nontraumatic 573.8
  lymphatic (node) (vessel) 457.8
  marginal sinus (placental) (with hemorrhage) 641.2
    affecting fetus or newborn 762.1
  meaning hernia—*see* Hernia
  membrana tympani (*see also* Perforation, tympanum) 384.20
    with otitis media—*see* Otitis media
    traumatic—*see* Wound, open, ear
  membranes (spontaneous)
    artificial
      delayed delivery following 658.3
        affecting fetus or newborn 761.1
        fetus or newborn 761.1
    delayed delivery following 658.2
      affecting fetus or newborn 761.1
    premature (less than 24 hours prior to onset of labor) 658.1
      affecting fetus or newborn 761.1
    delayed delivery following 658.2
      affecting fetus or newborn 761.1
  meningeal artery (*see also* Hemorrhage, subarachnoid) 430
    late effect—*see* Late effect(s) (of) cerebrovascular disease
  meniscus (knee)—*see also* Tear, meniscus
    old (*see also* Derangement, meniscus) 717.5
    site other than knee—*see* Disorder, cartilage, articular
    site other than knee—*see* Sprain, by site
  mesentery 568.89
    traumatic—*see* Injury, internal, mesentery
  mitral—*see* Insufficiency, mitral
  muscle (traumatic) NEC—*see also* Sprain, by site
    with open wound—*see* Wound, open, by site
    nontraumatic 728.83
  musculotendinous cuff (nontraumatic) (shoulder) 840.4
  mycotic aneurysm, causing cerebral hemorrhage (*see also* Hemorrhage, subarachnoid) 430
    late effect—*see* Late effect(s) (of) cerebrovascular disease
  myocardium, myocardial (*see also* Infarct, myocardium) 410.9
    traumatic 861.03
      with open wound into thorax 861.13
  nontraumatic (meaning hernia) (*see also* Hernia, by site) 553.9
    obstructed (*see also* Hernia, by site, with obstruction) 552.9
    gangrenous (*see also* Hernia, by site, with gangrene) 551.9
  operation wound 998.32
    internal 998.31
  ovary, ovarian 620.8
    corpus luteum 620.1
    follicle (graafian) 620.0
  oviduct 620.8

Rupture, ruptured—*continued*
  due to pregnancy—*see* Pregnancy, tubal
  pancreas 577.8
    traumatic—*see* Injury, internal, pancreas
  papillary muscle (ventricular) 429.6
  pelvic
    floor, complicating delivery 664.1
    organ NEC—*see* Injury, pelvic, organs
  penis (traumatic)—*see* Wound, open, penis
  perineum 624.8
    during delivery (*see also* Laceration, perineum, complicating delivery) 664.4
  pharynx (nontraumatic) (spontaneous) 478.29
  pregnant uterus (before onset of labor) 665.0
  prostate (traumatic)—*see* Injury, internal, prostate
  pulmonary
    artery 417.8
    valve (heart) (*see also* Endocarditis, pulmonary) 424.3
    vein 417.8
    vessel 417.8
  pupil, sphincter 364.75
  pus tube (*see also* Salpingo-oophoritis) 614.2
  pyosalpinx (*see also* Salpingo-oophoritis) 614.2
  rectum 569.49
    traumatic—*see* Injury, internal, rectum
  retina, retinal (traumatic) (without detachment) 361.30
    with detachment (*see also* Detachment, retina, with retinal defect) 361.00
  rotator cuff (capsule) (traumatic) 840.4
    nontraumatic, complete 727.61
  sclera 871.0
  semilunar cartilage, knee (*see also* Tear, meniscus) 836.2
    old (*see also* Derangement, meniscus) 717.5
  septum (cardiac) 410.8
  sigmoid 569.89
    traumatic—*see* Injury, internal, colon, sigmoid
  sinus of Valsalva 747.29
  spinal cord—*see also* Injury, spinal, by site
    due to injury at birth 767.4
    fetus or newborn 767.4
    syphilitic 094.89
    traumatic—*see also* Injury, spinal, by site
      with fracture—*see* Fracture, vertebra, by site, with spinal cord injury
  spleen 289.59
    congenital 767.8
    due to injury at birth 767.8
    malarial 084.9
    nontraumatic 289.59
    spontaneous 289.59
    traumatic 865.04
      with open wound into cavity 865.14
  splenic vein 459.0
  stomach 537.89
    due to injury at birth 767.8
    traumatic—*see* Injury, internal, stomach
    ulcer—*see* Ulcer, stomach, with perforation
  synovium 727.50
    specified site NEC 727.59
  tendon (traumatic)—*see also* Sprain, by site
    with open wound—*see* Wound, open, by site
    Achilles 845.09
      nontraumatic 727.67
    ankle 845.09
      nontraumatic 727.68
    biceps (long bead) 840.8
      nontraumatic 727.62

Rupture, ruptured—*continued*
  foot 845.10
    interphalangeal (joint) 845.13
    metatarsophalangeal (joint) 845.12
    nontraumatic 727.68
    specified site NEC 845.19
    tarsometatarsal (joint) 845.11
  hand 842.10
    carpometacarpal (joint) 842.11
    interphalangeal (joint) 842.13
    metacarpophalangeal (joint) 842.12
    nontraumatic 727.63
      extensors 727.63
      flexors 727.64
    specified site NEC 842.19
  nontraumatic 727.60
    specified site NEC 727.69
  patellar 844.8
    nontraumatic 727.66
  quadriceps 844.8
    nontraumatic 727.65
  rotator cuff (capsule) 840.4
    nontraumatic, complete 727.61
  wrist 842.00
    carpal (joint) 842.01
    nontraumatic 727.63
      extensors 727.63
      flexors 727.64
    radiocarpal (joint) (ligament) 842.02
    radioulnar (joint), distal 842.09
    specified site NEC 842.09
  testis (traumatic) 878.2
    complicated 878.3
    due to syphilis 095.8
  thoracic duct 457.8
  tonsil 474.8
  traumatic
    with open wound—*see* Wound, open, by site
    aorta—*see* Rupture, aorta, traumatic
    ear drum—*see* Wound, open, ear, drum
    external site—*see* Wound, open, by site
    eye 871.2
    globe (eye)—*see* Wound, open, eyeball
    internal organ (abdomen, chest, or
        pelvis)—*see also* Injury, internal, by site
      heart—*see* Rupture, myocardium, traumatic
      kidney—*see* Rupture, kidney
      liver—*see* Rupture, liver
      spleen—*see* Rupture, spleen, traumatic
    ligament, muscle, or tendon—*see also* Sprain, by site
      with open wound—*see* Wound, open, by site
    meaning hernia—*see* Hernia
  tricuspid (heart) (valve)—*see* Endocarditis, tricuspid
  tube, tubal 620.8
    abscess (*see also* Salpingo-oophoritis) 614.2
    due to pregnancy—*see* Pregnancy, tubal
  tympanum, tympanic (membrane) (*see also* Perforation, tympanum) 384.20
    with otitis media—*see* Otitis media
    traumatic—*see* Wound, open, ear, drum
  umbilical cord 663.8
    fetus or newborn 772.0
  ureter (traumatic) (*see also* Injury, internal, ureter) 867.2
    nontraumatic 593.89
  urethra 599.84
    with
      abortion—*see* Abortion, by type, with damage to pelvic organs

Rupture, ruptured—*continued*
    ectopic pregnancy (*see also* categories 633.0-633.9) 639.2
    molar pregnancy (*see also* categories 630-632) 639.2
    following
      abortion 639.2
      ectopic or molar pregnancy 639.2
    obstetrical trauma 665.5
    traumatic—*see* Injury, internal urethra
  uterosacral ligament 620.8
  uterus (traumatic)—*see also* Injury, internal uterus
    affecting fetus or newborn 763.89
    during labor 665.1
    nonpuerperal, nontraumatic 621.8
    nontraumatic 621.8
    pregnant (during labor) 665.1
      before labor 665.0
  vaginal 878.6
    complicated 878.7
    complicating delivery—*see* Laceration, vagina, complicating delivery
  valve, valvular (heart)—*see* Endocarditis
  varicose vein—*see* Varicose, vein
  varix—*see* Varix
  vena cava 459.0
  ventricle (free wall) (left) (*see also* Infarct, myocardium) 410.9
  vesical (urinary) 596.6
    traumatic—*see* Injury, internal, bladder
  vessel (blood) 459.0
    pulmonary 417.8
  viscus 799.89
  vulva 878.4
    complicated 878.5
    complicating delivery 664.0
Russell's dwarf (uterine dwarfism and craniofacial dysostosis) 759.89
Russell's dysentery 004.8
Russell (-Silver) syndrome (congenital hemihypertrophy and short stature) 759.89
Russian spring-summer type encephalitis 063.0
Rust's disease (tuberculous spondylitis) 015.0 *[720.81]*
Rustitskii's disease (multiple myeloma) (M9730/3) 203.0
Ruysch's disease (Hirschsprung's disease) 751.3
Rytand-Lipsitch syndrome (complete atrioventricular block) 426.0

S

Saber
  shin 090.5
  tibia 090.5
Sac, lacrimal —*see* condition
Saccharomyces infection (*see also* Candidiasis) 112.9
Saccharopinuria 270.7
Saccular —*see* condition
Sacculation
  aorta (nonsyphilitic) (*see also* Aneurysm, aorta) 441.9
    ruptured 441.5
    syphilitic 093.0
  bladder 596.3
  colon 569.89
  intralaryngeal (congenital) (ventricular) 748.3
  larynx (congenital) (ventricular) 748.3
  organ or site, congenital—*see* Distortion
  pregnant uterus, complicating delivery 654.4
    affecting fetus or newborn 763.1
    causing obstructed labor 660.2
      affecting fetus or newborn 763.1
  rectosigmoid 569.89
  sigmoid 569.89
  ureter 593.89
  urethra 599.2
  vesical 596.3
Sachs (-Tay) disease (amaurotic familial idiocy) 330.1
Sacks-Libman disease 710.0 *[424.91]*
Sacralgia 724.6
Sacralization
  fifth lumbar vertebra 756.15
  incomplete (vertebra) 756.15
Sacrodynia 724.6
Sacroiliac joint —*see* condition
Sacroiliitis NEC 720.2
Sacrum —*see* condition
Saddle
  back 737.8
  embolus, aorta 444.0
  nose 738.0
    congenital 754.0
    due to syphilis 090.5
Sadism (sexual) 302.84
Saemisch's ulcer 370.04
Saenger's syndrome 379.46
Sago spleen 277.39
Sailors' skin 692.74
Saint
  Anthony's fire (*see also* Erysipelas) 035
  Guy's dance—*see* Chorea
  Louis-type encephalitis 062.3
  triad (*see also* Hernia, diaphragm) 553.3
  Vitus' dance—*see* Chorea
Salicylism
  correct substance properly administered 535.4
  overdose or wrong substance given or taken 965.1
Salivary duct or gland —*see also* condition
  virus disease 078.5
Salivation (excessive) (*see also* Ptyalism) 527.7
Salmonella (aertrycke) (choleraesuis) (enteritidis) (gallinarum) (suipestifer) (typhimurium) (*see also* Infection, Salmonella) 003.9
  arthritis 003.23
  carrier (suspected) of V02.3

Salmonella—*continued*
  meningitis 003.21
  osteomyelitis 003.24
  pneumonia 003.22
  septicemia 003.1
  typhosa 002.0
  carrier (suspected) of V02.1
Salmonellosis 003.0
  with pneumonia 003.22
Salpingitis (catarrhal) (fallopian tube) (nodular) (pseudofollicular) (purulent) (septic) (*see also* Salpingo-oophoritis) 614.2
  ear 381.50
    acute 381.51
    chronic 381.52
  Eustachian (tube) 381.50
    acute 381.51
    chronic 381.52
  follicularis 614.1
  gonococcal (chronic) 098.37
    acute 098.17
  interstitial, chronic 614.1
  isthmica nodosa 614.1
  old—*see* Salpingo-oophoritis, chronic
  puerperal, postpartum, childbirth 670
  specific (chronic) 098.37
    acute 098.17
  tuberculous (acute) (chronic) (*see also* Tuberculosis) 016.6
  venereal (chronic) 098.37
    acute 098.17
Salpingocele 620.4
Salpingo-oophoritis (catarrhal) (purulent) (ruptured) (septic) (suppurative) 614.2
  acute 614.0
  with
    abortion—*see* Abortion, by type, with sepsis
    ectopic pregnancy (*see also* categories 633.0-633.9) 639.0
    molar pregnancy (*see also* categories 630-632) 639.0
    following
      abortion 639.0
      ectopic or molar pregnancy 639.0
    gonococcal 098.17
    puerperal, postpartum, childbirth 670
    tuberculous (*see also* Tuberculosis) 016.6
  chronic 614.1
    gonococcal 098.37
    tuberculous (*see also* Tuberculosis) 016.6
  complicating pregnancy 646.6
    affecting fetus or newborn 760.8
  gonococcal (chronic) 098.37
    acute 098.17
  old—*see* Salpingo-oophoritis, chronic
  puerperal 670
  specific—*see* Salpingo-oophoritis, gonococcal
  subacute (*see also* Salpingo-oophoritis, acute) 614.0
  tuberculous (acute) (chronic) (*see also* Tuberculosis) 016.6
  venereal—*see* Salpingo-oophoritis, gonococcal
Salpingo-ovaritis (*see also* Salpingo-oophoritis) 614.2
Salpingoperitonitis (*see also* Salpingo-oophoritis) 614.2

Salt-losing
  nephritis (*see also* Disease, renal) 593.9
  syndrome (*see also* Disease, renal) 593.9
Salt-rheum (*see also* Eczema) 692.9
Salzmann's nodular dystrophy 371.46
Sampson's cyst or tumor 617.1
Sandblasters'
  asthma 502
  lung 502
Sander's disease (paranoia) 297.1
Sandfly fever 066.0
Sandhoff's disease 330.1
Sanfilippo's syndrome (mucopolysaccharidosis III) 277.5
Sanger-Brown's ataxia 334.2
San Joaquin Valley fever 114.0
São Paulo fever or typhus 082.0
Saponification, mesenteric 567.89
Sapremia —*see* Septicemia
Sarcocele (benign)
  syphilitic 095.8
  congenital 090.5
Sarcoepiplocele (*see also* Hernia) 553.9
Sarcoepiplomphalocele (*see also* Hernia, umbilicus) 553.1
Sarcoid (any site) 135
  with lung involvement 135 *[517.8]*
  Boeck's 135
  Darier-Roussy 135
  Spiegler-Fendt 686.8
Sarcoidosis 135
  cardiac 135 *[425.8]*
  lung 135 *[517.8]*
Sarcoma (M8800/3)—*see also* Neoplasm, connective tissue, malignant
  alveolar soft part (M9581/3)—*see* Neoplasm, connective tissue, malignant
  ameloblastic (M9330/3) 170.1
    upper jaw (bone) 170.0
  botryoid (M8910/3)—*see* Neoplasm, connective tissue, malignant
  botryoides (M8910/3)—*see* Neoplasm, connective tissue, malignant
  cerebellar (M9480/3) 191.6
  circumscribed (arachnoidal) (M9471/3) 191.6
  circumscribed (arachnoidal) cerebellar (M9471/3) 191.6
  clear cell, of tendons and aponeuroses (M9044/3)—*see* Neoplasm, connective tissue, malignant
  embryonal (M8991/3)—*see* Neoplasm, connective tissue, malignant
  endometrial (stromal) (M8930/3) 182.0
    isthmus 182.1
  endothelial (M9130/3)—*see also* Neoplasm, connective tissue, malignant
    bone (M9260/3)—*see* Neoplasm, bone, malignant
  epithelioid cell (M8804/3)—*see* Neoplasm, connective tissue, malignant
  Ewing's (M9260/3)—*see* Neoplasm, bone, malignant
  follicular dendritic cell 202.9
  germinoblastic (diffuse) (M9632/3) 202.8
    follicular (M9697/3) 202.0
  giant cell (M8802/3)—*see also* Neoplasm, connective tissue, malignant
    bone (M9250/3)—*see* Neoplasm, bone, malignant

Sarcoma—*continued*
  glomoid (M8710/3)—*see* Neoplasm, connective tissue, malignant
  granulocytic (M9930/3) 205.3
  hemangioendothelial (M9130/3)—*see* Neoplasm, connective tissue, malignant
  hemorrhagic, multiple (M9140/3)—*see* Kaposi's, sarcoma
  Hodgkin's (M9662/3) 201.2
  immunoblastic (M9612/3) 200.8
  interdigitating dendritic cell 202.9
  Kaposi's (M9140/3)—*see* Kaposi's, sarcoma
  Kupffer cell (M9124/3) 155.0
  Langerhans cell 202.9
  leptomeningeal (M9530/3)—*see* Neoplasm, meninges, malignant
  lymphangioendothelial (M9170/3)—*see* Neoplasm, connective tissue, malignant
  lymphoblastic (M9630/3) 200.1
  lymphocytic (M9620/3) 200.1
  mast cell (M9740/3) 202.6
  melanotic (M8720/3)—*see* Melanoma
  meningeal (M9530/3)—*see* Neoplasm, meninges, malignant
  meningothelial (M9530/3)—*see* Neoplasm, meninges, malignant
  mesenchymal (M8800/3)—*see also* Neoplasm, connective tissue, malignant
  mixed (M8990/3)—*see* Neoplasm, connective tissue, malignant
  mesothelial (M9050/3)—*see* Neoplasm, by site, malignant
  monstrocellular (M9481/3)
    specified site—*see* Neoplasm, by site, malignant
    unspecified site 191.9
  myeloid (M9930/3) 205.3
  neurogenic (M9540/3)—*see* Neoplasm, connective tissue, malignant
  odontogenic (M9270/3) 170.1
    upper jaw (bone) 170.0
  osteoblastic (M9180/3)—*see* Neoplasm, bone, malignant
  osteogenic (M9180/3)—*see also* Neoplasm, bone, malignant
    juxtacortical (M9190/3)—*see* Neoplasm, bone, malignant
    periosteal (M9190/3)—*see* Neoplasm, bone, malignant
  periosteal (M8812/3)—*see also* Neoplasm, bone, malignant
    osteogenic (M9190/3)—*see* Neoplasm, bone, malignant
  plasma cell (M9731/3) 203.8
  pleomorphic cell (M8802/3)—*see* Neoplasm, connective tissue, malignant
  reticuloendothelial (M9720/3) 202.3
  reticulum cell (M9640/3) 200.0
    nodular (M9642/3) 200.0
    pleomorphic cell type (M9641/3) 200.0
  round cell (M8803/3)—*see* Neoplasm, connective tissue, malignant
  small cell (M8803/3)—*see* Neoplasm, connective tissue, malignant
  spindle cell (M8801/3)—*see* Neoplasm, connective tissue, malignant
  stromal (endometrial) (M8930/3) 182.0
    isthmus 182.1
  synovial (M9040/3)—*see also* Neoplasm, connective tissue, malignant
    biphasic type (M9043/3)—*see* Neoplasm, connective tissue, malignant

INDEX TO DISEASES

Sarcoma—*continued*
epithelioid cell type (M9042/3)—*see* Neoplasm, connective tissue, malignant
spindle cell type (M9041/3)—*see* Neoplasm, connective tissue, malignant
Sarcomatosis
meningeal (M9539/3)—*see* Neoplasm, meninges, malignant
specified site NEC (M8800/3)—*see* Neoplasm, connective tissue, malignant
unspecified site (M8800/6) 171.9
Sarcosinemia 270.8
Sarcosporidiosis 136.5
Satiety, early 780.94
Saturnine —*see* condition
Saturnism 984.9
specified type of lead—*see* Table of drugs and chemicals
Satyriasis 302.89
Sauriasis —*see* Ichthyosis
Sauriderma 757.39
Sauriosis —*see* Ichthyosis
Savill's disease (epidemic exfoliative dermatitis) 695.89
SBE (subacute bacterial endocarditis) 421.0
Scabies (any site) 133.0
Scabs 782.8
Scaglietti-Dagnini syndrome (acromegalic macrospondylitis) 253.0
Scald, scalded —*see also* Burn, by site
skin syndrome 695.1
Scalenus anticus (anterior) syndrome 353.0
Scales 782.8
Scalp —*see* condition
Scaphocephaly 756.0
Scaphoiditis, tarsal 732.5
Scapulalgia 733.90
Scapulohumeral myopathy 359.1
Scar, scarring (*see also* Cicatrix) 709.2
adherent 709.2
atrophic 709.2
cervix
in pregnancy or childbirth 654.6
affecting fetus or newborn 763.89
causing obstructed labor 660.2
affecting fetus or newborn 763.1
cheloid 701.4
chorioretinal 363.30
disseminated 363.35
macular 363.32
peripheral 363.34
posterior pole NEC 363.33
choroid (*see also* Scar, chorioretinal) 363.30
compression, pericardial 423.9
congenital 757.39
conjunctiva 372.64
cornea 371.00
xerophthalmic 264.6
due to previous cesarean delivery, complicating pregnancy or childbirth 654.2
affecting fetus or newborn 763.89
duodenal (bulb) (cap) 537.3
hypertrophic 701.4
keloid 701.4
labia 624.4
lung (base) 518.89
macula 363.32
disseminated 363.35
peripheral 363.34
muscle 728.89

Scar, scarring—*continued*
myocardium, myocardial 412
painful 709.2
papillary muscle 429.81
posterior pole NEC 363.33
macular—*see* Scar, macula
postnecrotic (hepatic) (liver) 571.9
psychic V15.49
retina (*see also* Scar, chorioretinal) 363.30
trachea 478.9
uterus 621.8
in pregnancy or childbirth NEC 654.9
affecting fetus or newborn 763.89
due to previous cesarean delivery 654.2
vulva 624.4
Scarabiasis 134.1
Scarlatina 034.1
anginosa 034.1
maligna 034.1
myocarditis, acute 034.1 *[422.0]*
old (*see also* Myocarditis) 429.0
otitis media 034.1 *[382.02]*
ulcerosa 034.1
Scarlatinella 057.8
Scarlet fever (albuminuria) (angina) (convulsions) (lesions of lid) (rash) 034.1
Schamberg's disease, dermatitis, or dermatosis (progressive pigmentary dermatosis) 709.09
Schatzki's ring (esophagus) (lower) (congenital) 750.3
acquired 530.3
Schaufenster krankheit 413.9
Schaumann's
benign lymphogranulomatosis 135
disease (sarcoidosis) 135
syndrome (sarcoidosis) 135
Scheie's syndrome (mucopolysaccharidosis IS) 277.5
Schenck's disease (sporotrichosis) 117.1
Scheuermann's disease or osteochondrosis 732.0
Scheuthauer-Marie-Sainton syndrome (cleidocranialis dysostosis) 755.59
Schilder (-Flatau) disease 341.1
Schilling-type monocytic leukemia (M9890/3) 206.9
Schimmelbusch's disease, cystic mastitis, or hyperplasia 610.1
Schirmer's syndrome (encephalocutaneous angiomatosis) 759.6
Schistocelia 756.79
Schistoglossia 750.13
Schistosoma infestation —*see* Infestation, Schistosoma
Schistosomiasis 120.9
Asiatic 120.2
bladder 120.0
chestermani 120.8
colon 120.1
cutaneous 120.3
due to
S. hematobium 120.0
S. japonicum 120.2
S. mansoni 120.1
S. mattheii 120.8
eastern 120.2
genitourinary tract 120.0
intestinal 120.1
lung 120.2
Manson's (intestinal) 120.1

Schistosomiasis—continued
  Oriental 120.2
  pulmonary 120.2
  specified type NEC 120.8
  vesical 120.0
Schizencephaly 742.4
Schizo-affective psychosis (see also Schizophrenia) 295.7
Schizodontia 520.2
Schizoid personality 301.20
  introverted 301.21
  schizotypal 301.22
Schizophrenia, schizophrenic (reaction) 295.9

Note—Use the following fifth-digit subclassification with category 295:

0 *unspecified*
1 *subchronic*
2 *chronic*
3 *subchronic with acute exacerbation*
4 *chronic with acute exacerbation*
5 *in remission*

  acute (attack) NEC 295.8
    episode 295.4
  atypical form 295.8
  borderline 295.5
  catalepsy 295.2
  catatonic (type) (acute) (excited) (withdrawn) 295.2
  childhood (type) (see also Psychosis, childhood) 299.9
  chronic NEC 295.6
  coenesthesiopathic 295.8
  cyclic (type) 295.7
  disorganized (type) 295.1
  flexibilitas cerea 295.2
  hebephrenic (type) (acute) 295.1
  incipient 295.5
  latent 295.5
  paranoid (type) (acute) 295.3
  paraphrenic (acute) 295.3
  prepsychotic 295.5
  primary (acute) 295.0
  prodromal 295.5
  pseudoneurotic 295.5
  pseudopsychopathic 295.5
  reaction 295.9
  residual type (state) 295.6
  restzustand 295.6
  schizo-affective (type) (depressed) (excited) 295.7
  schizophreniform type 295.4
  simple (type) (acute) 295.0
  simplex (acute) 295.0
  specified type NEC 295.8
  syndrome of childhood NEC (see also Psychosis, childhood) 299.9
  undifferentiated type 295.9
    acute 295.8
    chronic 295.6
Schizothymia 301.20
  introverted 301.21
  schizotypal 301.22
Schlafkrankheit 086.5
Schlatter's tibia (osteochondrosis) 732.4
Schlatter-Osgood disease (osteochondrosis, tibial tubercle) 732.4
Schloffer's tumor (see also Peritonitis) 567.29

Schmidt's syndrome
  sphallo-pharyngo-laryngeal hemiplegia 352.6
  thyroid-adrenocortical insufficiency 258.1
  vagoaccessory 352.6
Schmincke
  carcinoma (M8082/3)—see Neoplasm, nasopharynx, malignant
  tumor (M8082/3)—see Neoplasm, nasopharynx, malignant
Schmitz (-Stutzer) dysentery 004.0
Schmorl's disease or nodes 722.30
  lumbar, lumbosacral 722.32
  specified region NEC 722.39
  thoracic, thoracolumbar 722.31
Schneider's syndrome 047.9
Schneiderian
  carcinoma (M8121/3)
    specified site—see Neoplasm, by site, malignant
    unspecified site 160.0
  papilloma (M8121/0)
    specified site—see Neoplasm, by site, benign
    unspecified site 212.0
Schnitzler syndrome 273.1
Schoffer's tumor (see also Peritonitis) 567.29
Scholte's syndrome (malignant carcinoid) 259.2
Scholz's disease 330.0
Scholz (-Bielschowsky-Henneberg) syndrome 330.0
Schönlein (-Henoch) disease (primary) (purpura) (rheumatic) 287.0
School examination V70.3
Schottmüller's disease (see also Fever, paratyphoid) 002.9
Schroeder's syndrome (endocrine-hypertensive) 255.3
Schüller-Christian disease or syndrome (chronic histiocytosis X) 277.89
Schultz's disease or syndrome (agranulocytosis) 288.09
Schultze's acroparesthesia, simple 443.89
Schwalbe-Ziehen-Oppenheimer disease 333.6
Schwannoma (M9560/0)—see also Neoplasm, connective tissue, benign
  malignant (M9560/3)—see Neoplasm, connective tissue, malignant
Schwartz (-Jampel) syndrome 359.23
Schwartz-Bartter syndrome (inappropriate secretion of antidiuretic hormone) 253.6
Schweninger-Buzzi disease (macular atrophy) 701.3
Sciatic —see condition
Sciatica (infectional) 724.3
  due to
    displacement of intervertebral disc 722.10
    herniation, nucleus pulposus 722.10
  wallet 724.3
Scimitar syndrome (anomalous venous drainage, right lung to inferior vena cava) 747.49
Sclera —see condition
Sclerectasia 379.11
Scleredema
  adultorum 710.1
  Buschke's 710.1
  newborn 778.1
Sclerema
  adiposum (newborn) 778.1
  adultorum 710.1
  edematosum (newborn) 778.1
  neonatorum 778.1
  newborn 778.1

INDEX TO DISEASES

Sclerosis, sclerotic

Scleriasis —*see* Scleroderma
Scleritis 379.00
  with corneal involvement 379.05
  anterior (annular) (localized) 379.03
  brawny 379.06
  granulomatous 379.09
  posterior 379.07
  specified NEC 379.09
  suppurative 379.09
  syphilitic 095.0
  tuberculous (nodular) (*see also* Tuberculosis) 017.3 *[379.09]*
Sclerochoroiditis (*see also* Scleritis) 379.00
Scleroconjunctivitis (*see also* Scleritis) 379.00
Sclerocystic ovary (syndrome) 256.4
Sclerodactylia 701.0
Scleroderma, sclerodermia (acrosclerotic) (diffuse) (generalized) (progressive) (pulmonary) 710.1
  circumscribed 701.0
  linear 701.0
  localized (linear) 701.0
  newborn 778.1
Sclerokeratitis 379.05
  meaning sclerosing keratitis 370.54
  tuberculous (*see also* Tuberculosis) 017.3 *[379.09]*
Scleroma, trachea 040.1
Scleromalacia
  multiple 731.0
  perforans 379.04
Scleromyxedema 701.8
Scleroperikeratitis 379.05
Sclerose en plaques 340
Sclerosis, sclerotic
  adrenal (gland) 255.8
  Alzheimer's 331.0
    with dementia—*see* Alzheimer's, dementia
  amyotrophic (lateral) 335.20
  annularis fibrosi
    aortic 424.1
    mitral 424.0
  aorta, aortic 440.0
    valve (*see also* Endocarditis, aortic) 424.1
  artery, arterial, arteriolar, arteriovascular—*see* Arteriosclerosis
  ascending multiple 340
  Balo's (concentric) 341.1
  basilar—*see* Sclerosis, brain
  bone (localized) NEC 733.99
  brain (general) (lobular) 341.9
    Alzheimer's—*see* Alzheimer's dementia
    artery, arterial 437.0
    atrophic lobar 331.0
      with dementia
        with behavioral disturbance 331.0 *[294.11]*
        without behavioral disturbance 331.0 *[294.10]*
    diffuse 341.1
      familial (chronic) (infantile) 330.0
      infantile (chronic) (familial) 330.0
      Pelizaeus-Merzbacher type 330.0
    disseminated 340
    hereditary 334.2
    infantile, (degenerative) (diffuse) 330.0
    insular 340
    Krabbe's 330.0
    miliary 340

Sclerosis, sclerotic—*continued*
    multiple 340
    Pelizaeus-Merzbacher 330.0
    progressive familial 330.0
    senile 437.0
    tuberous 759.5
  bulbar, progressive 340
  bundle of His 426.50
    left 426.3
    right 426.4
  cardiac —*see* Arteriosclerosis, coronary
  cardiorenal (*see also* Hypertension, cardiorenal) 404.90
  cardiovascular (*see also* Disease, cardiovascular) 429.2
    renal (*see also* Hypertension, cardiorenal) 404.90
  centrolobar, familial 330.0
  cerebellar—*see* Sclerosis, brain
  cerebral—*see* Sclerosis, brain
  cerebrospinal 340
    disseminated 340
    multiple 340
  cerebrovascular 437.0
  choroid 363.40
    diffuse 363.56
  combined (spinal cord)—*see also* Degeneration, combined
    multiple 340
  concentric, Balo's 341.1
  cornea 370.54
  coronary (artery) —*see* Arteriosclerosis, coronary
  corpus cavernosum
    female 624.8
    male 607.89
  Dewitzky's
    aortic 424.1
    mitral 424.0
  diffuse NEC 341.1
  disease, heart —*see* Arteriosclerosis, coronary
  disseminated 340
  dorsal 340
  dorsolateral (spinal cord)—*see* Degeneration, combined
  endometrium 621.8
  extrapyramidal 333.90
  eye, nuclear (senile) 366.16
  Friedreich's (spinal cord) 334.0
  funicular (spermatic cord) 608.89
  gastritis 535.4
  general (vascular)—*see* Arteriosclerosis
  gland (lymphatic) 457.8
  hepatic 571.9
  hereditary
    cerebellar 334.2
    spinal 334.0
  idiopathic cortical (Garré's) (*see also* Osteomyelitis) 730.1
  ilium, piriform 733.5
  insular 340
    pancreas 251.8
  Islands of Langerhans 251.8
  kidney—*see* Sclerosis, renal
  larynx 478.79
  lateral 335.24
    amyotrophic 335.20
    descending 335.24
    primary 335.24
    spinal 335.24
  liver 571.9

Sclerosis, sclerotic—*continued*
  lobar, atrophic (of brain) 331.0
    with dementia
      with behavioral disturbance 331.0 *[294.11]*
      without behavioral disturbance 331.0 *[294.10]*
  lung (*see also* Fibrosis, lung) 515
  mastoid 383.1
  mitral—*see* Endocarditis, mitral
  Mönckeberg's (medial) (*see also*
    Arteriosclerosis, extremities) 440.20
  multiple (brain stem) (cerebral) (generalized)
    (spinal cord) 340
  myocardium, myocardial —*see*
    Arteriosclerosis, coronary
  nuclear (senile), eye 366.16
  ovary 620.8
  pancreas 577.8
  penis 607.89
  peripheral arteries NEC (*see also*
    Arteriosclerosis, extremities) 440.20
  plaques 340
  pluriglandular 258.8
  polyglandular 258.8
  posterior (spinal cord) (syphilitic) 094.0
  posterolateral (spinal cord)—*see* Degeneration,
    combined
  prepuce 607.89
  primary lateral 335.24
  progressive systemic 710.1
  pulmonary (*see also* Fibrosis, lung) 515
    artery 416.0
    valve (heart) (*see also* Endocarditis,
      pulmonary) 424.3
  renal 587
    with
      cystine storage disease 270.0
      hypertension (*see also* Hypertension,
        kidney) 403.90
      hypertensive heart disease (conditions
        classifiable to 402) (*see also*
        Hypertension, cardiorenal) 404.90
      arteriolar (hyaline) (*see also* Hypertension,
        kidney) 403.90
      hyperplastic (*see also* Hypertension, kidney)
        403.90
  retina (senile) (vascular) 362.17
  rheumatic
    aortic valve 395.9
    mitral valve 394.9
  Schilder's 341.1
  senile—*see* Arteriosclerosis
  spinal (cord) (general) (progressive) (transverse)
    336.8
    ascending 357.0
    combined—*see also* Degeneration, combined
      multiple 340
      syphilitic 094.89
    disseminated 340
    dorsolateral—*see* Degeneration, combined
    hereditary (Friedreich's) (mixed form) 334.0
    lateral (amyotrophic) 335.24
    multiple 340
    posterior (syphilitic) 094.0
  stomach 537.89
  subendocardial, congenital 425.3
  systemic (progressive) 710.1
    with lung involvement 710.1 *[517.2]*
  tricuspid (heart) (valve)—*see* Endocarditis,
    tricuspid
  tuberous (brain) 759.5

Sclerosis, sclerotic—*continued*
  tympanic membrane (*see also*
    Tympanosclerosis) 385.00
  valve, valvular (heart)—*see* Endocarditis
  vascular—*see* Arteriosclerosis
  vein 459.89
Sclerotenonitis 379.07
Sclerotitis (*see also* Scleritis) 379.00
  syphilitic 095.0
  tuberculous (*see also* Tuberculosis) 017.3
    [379.09]
Scoliosis (acquired) (postural) 737.30
  congenital 754.2
  due to or associated with
    Charcot-Marie-Tooth disease 356.1 *[737.43]*
    mucopolysaccharidosis 277.5 *[737.43]*
    neurofibromatosis 237.71 *[737.43]*
    osteitis
      deformans 731.0 *[737.43]*
      fibrosa cystica 252.01 *[737.43]*
    osteoporosis (*see also* Osteoporosis) 733.00
      [737.43]
    poliomyelitis 138 *[737.43]*
    radiation 737.33
    tuberculosis (*see also* Tuberculosis) 015.0
      [737.43]
  idiopathic 737.30
    infantile
      progressive 737.32
      resolving 737.31
  paralytic 737.39
  rachitic 268.1
  sciatic 724.3
  specified NEC 737.39
  thoracogenic 737.34
  tuberculous (*see also* Tuberculosis) 015.0 *[737.43]*
Scoliotic pelvis 738.6
  with disproportion (fetopelvic) 653.0
    affecting fetus or newborn 763.1
    causing obstructed labor 660.1
      affecting fetus or newborn 763.1
Scorbutus, scorbutic 267
  anemia 281.8
Scotoma (ring) 368.44
  arcuate 368.43
  Bjerrum 368.43
  blind spot area 368.42
  central 368.41
  centrocecal 368.41
  paracecal 368.42
  paracentral 368.41
  scintillating 368.12
  Seidel 368.43
Scratch —*see* Injury, superficial, by site
Scratchy throat 784.99
Screening (for) V82.9
  alcoholism V79.1
  anemia, deficiency NEC V78.1
    iron V78.0
  anomaly, congenital V82.89
  antenatal, of mother V28.9
    alphafetoprotein levels, raised V28.1
    based on amniocentesis V28.2
      chromosomal anomalies V28.0
      raised alphafetoprotein levels V28.1
    fetal growth retardation using ultrasonics
      V28.4
    isoimmunization V28.5
    malformations using ultrasonics V28.3
    raised alphafetoprotein levels V28.1
    specified condition NEC V28.8

INDEX TO DISEASES — Screening (for)

Screening (for)—*continued*
  Streptococcus B V28.6
  arterial hypertension V81.1
  arthropod-borne viral disease NEC V73.5
  asymptomatic bacteriuria V81.5
  bacterial
    and spirochetal sexually transmitted diseases V74.5
    conjunctivitis V74.4
    disease V74.9
      sexually transmitted V74.5
      specified condition NEC V74.8
  bacteriuria, asymptomatic V81.5
  blood disorder NEC V78.9
    specified type NEC V78.8
  bronchitis, chronic V81.3
  brucellosis V74.8
  cancer—*see* Screening, malignant neoplasm
  cardiovascular disease NEC V81.2
  cataract V80.2
  Chagas' disease V75.3
  chemical poisoning V82.5
  cholera V74.0
  cholesterol level V77.91
  chromosomal
    anomalies
      by amniocentesis, antenatal V28.0
      maternal postnatal V82.4
    athletes V70.3
  condition
    cardiovascular NEC V81.2
    eye NEC V80.2
    genitourinary NEC V81.6
    neurological V80.0
    respiratory NEC V81.4
    skin V82.0
    specified NEC V82.89
  congenital
    anomaly V82.89
      eye V80.2
    dislocation of hip V82.3
    eye condition or disease V80.2
  conjunctivitis, bacterial V74.4
  contamination NEC (*see also* Poisoning) V82.5
  coronary artery disease V81.0
  cystic fibrosis V77.6
  deficiency anemia NEC V78.1
    iron V78.0
  dengue fever V73.5
  depression V79.0
  developmental handicap V79.9
    in early childhood V79.3
    specified type NEC V79.8
  diabetes mellitus V77.1
  diphtheria V74.3
  disease or disorder V82.9
    bacterial V74.9
      specified NEC V74.8
    blood V78.9
      specified type NEC V78.8
    blood-forming organ V78.9
      specified type NEC V78.8
    cardiovascular NEC V81.2
      hypertensive V81.1
      ischemic V81.0
    Chagas' V75.3
    chlamydial V73.98
      specified NEC V73.88
    ear NEC V80.3
    endocrine NEC V77.99
    eye NEC V80.2

Screening (for)—*continued*
    genitourinary NEC V81.6
    heart NEC V81.2
      hypertensive V81.1
      ischemic V81.0
    HPV (human papillomvirus) V73.81
    human papillomavirus (HPV) V73.81
    immunity NEC V77.99
    infectious NEC V75.9
    lipoid NEC V77.91
    mental V79.9
      specified type NEC V79.8
    metabolic NEC V77.99
      inborn NEC V77.7
    neurological V80.0
    nutritional NEC V77.99
    rheumatic NEC V82.2
    rickettsial V75.0
    sexually transmitted V74.5
      bacterial V74.5
      spirochetal V74.5
    sickle-cell V78.2
      trait V78.2
    specified type NEC V82.89
    thyroid V77.0
    vascular NEC V81.2
      ischemic V81.0
    venereal V74.5
    viral V73.99
      arthropod-borne NEC V73.5
      specified type NEC V73.89
  dislocation of hip, congenital V82.3
  drugs in athletes V70.3
  emphysema (chronic) V81.3
  encephalitis, viral (mosquito or tick borne) V73.5
  endocrine disorder NEC V77.99
  eye disorder NEC V80.2
    congenital V80.2
  fever
    dengue V73.5
    hemorrhagic V73.5
    yellow V73.4
  filariasis V75.6
  galactosemia V77.4
  genetic V82.79
    disease carrier status V82.71
  genitourinary condition NEC V81.6
  glaucoma V80.1
  gonorrhea V74.5
  gout V77.5
  Hansen's disease V74.2
  heart disease NEC V81.2
    hypertensive V81.1
    ischemic V81.0
  heavy metal poisoning V82.5
  helminthiasis, intestinal V75.7
  hematopoietic malignancy V76.89
  hemoglobinopathies NEC V78.3
  hemorrhagic fever V73.5
  Hodgkin's disease V76.89
  hormones in athletes V70.3
  HPV (human papillomavirus) V73.81
  human papillomavirus (HPV) V73.81
  hypercholesterolemia V77.91
  hyperlipidemia V77.91
  hypertension V81.1
  immunity disorder NEC V77.99
  inborn errors of metabolism NEC V77.7

Screening (for)—*continued*
  infection
    bacterial V74.9
      specified type NEC V74.8
    mycotic V75.4
    parasitic NEC V75.8
  infectious disease V75.9
    specified type NEC V75.8
  ingestion of radioactive substance V82.5
  intestinal helminthiasis V75.7
  iron deficiency anemia V78.0
  ischemic heart disease V81.0
  lead poisoning V82.5
  leishmaniasis V75.2
  leprosy V74.2
  leptospirosis V74.8
  leukemia V76.89
  lipoid disorder NEC V77.91
  lymphoma V76.89
  malaria V75.1
  malignant neoplasm (of) V76.9
    bladder V76.3
    blood V76.89
    breast V76.10
      mammogram NEC V76.12
        for high-risk patient V76.11
      specified type NEC V76.19
    cervix V76.2
    colon V76.51
    colorectal V76.51
    hematopoietic system V76.89
    intestine V76.50
      colon V76.51
      small V76.52
    lung V76.0
    lymph (glands) V76.89
    nervous system V76.81
    oral cavity V76.42
    other specified neoplasm NEC V76.89
    ovary V76.46
    prostate V76.44
    rectum V76.41
    respiratory organs V76.0
    skin V76.43
    specified sites NEC V76.49
    testis V76.45
    vagina V76.47
      following hysterectomy for malignant condition V67.01
  malnutrition V77.2
  mammogram NEC V76.12
    for high-risk patient V76.11
  maternal postnatal chromosomal anomalies V82.4
  measles V73.2
  mental
    disorder V79.9
      specified type NEC V79.8
    retardation V79.2
  metabolic errors, inborn V77.7
  metabolic disorder NEC V77.99
  mucoviscidosis V77.6
  multiphasic V82.6
  mycosis V75.4
  mycotic infection V75.4
  nephropathy V81.5
  neurological condition V80.0
  nutritional disorder V77.99
    obesity V77.8
  obesity V77.8
  osteoporosis V82.81

Screening (for)—*continued*
  parasitic infection NEC V75.8
  phenylketonuria V77.3
  plague V74.8
  poisoning
    chemical NEC V82.5
    contaminated water supply V82.5
    heavy metal V82.5
  poliomyelitis V73.0
  postnatal chromosomal anomalies, maternal V82.4
  prenatal—*see* Screening, antenatal
  pulmonary tuberculosis V74.1
  radiation exposure V82.5
  renal disease V81.5
  respiratory condition NEC V81.4
  rheumatic disorder NEC V82.2
  rheumatoid arthritis V82.1
  rickettsial disease V75.0
  rubella V73.3
  schistosomiasis V75.5
  senile macular lesions of eye V80.2
  sexually transmitted diseases V74.5
    bacterial V74.5
    spirochetal V74.5
  sickle-cell anemia, disease, or trait V78.2
  skin condition V82.0
  sleeping sickness V75.3
  smallpox V73.1
  special V82.9
    specified condition NEC V82.89
  specified type NEC V82.89
  spirochetal disease V74.9
    sexually transmitted V74.5
    specified type NEC V74.8
  stimulants in athletes V70.3
  syphilis V74.5
  tetanus V74.8
  thyroid disorder V77.0
  trachoma V73.6
  trypanosomiasis V75.3
  tuberculosis, pulmonary V74.1
  venereal disease V74.5
  viral encephalitis
    mosquito-borne V73.5
    tick-borne V73.5
  whooping cough V74.8
  worms, intestinal V75.7
  yaws V74.6
  yellow fever V73.4
Scrofula (*see also* Tuberculosis) 017.2
Scrofulide (primary) (*see also* Tuberculosis) 017.0
Scrofuloderma, scrofulodermia (any site) (primary) (*see also* Tuberculosis) 017.0
Scrofulosis (universal) (*see also* Tuberculosis) 017.2
Scrofulosis lichen (primary) (*see also* Tuberculosis) 017.0
Scrofulous —*see* condition
Scrotal tongue 529.5
  congenital 750.13
Scrotum —*see* condition
Scurvy (gum) (infantile) (rickets) (scorbutic) 267
Sea-blue histiocyte syndrome 272.7
Seabright-Bantam syndrome (pseudohypoparathyroidism) 275.49
Seasickness 994.6
Seatworm 127.4
Sebaceous
  cyst (*see also* Cyst, sebaceous) 706.2
  gland disease NEC 706.9
Sebocystomatosis 706.2

Seborrhea, seborrheic 706.3
  adiposa 706.3
  capitis 690.11
  congestiva 695.4
  corporis 706.3
  dermatitis 690.10
    infantile 690.12
  diathesis in infants 695.89
  eczema 690.18
    infantile 690.12
  keratosis 702.19
    inflamed 702.11
  nigricans 705.89
  sicca 690.18
  wart 702.19
    inflamed 702.11
Seckel's syndrome 759.89
Seclusion pupil 364.74
Seclusiveness, child 313.22
Secondary —*see also* condition
  neoplasm—*see* Neoplasm, by site, malignant, secondary
Secretan's disease or syndrome (posttraumatic edema) 782.3
Secretion
  antidiuretic hormone, inappropriate (syndrome) 253.6
  catecholamine, by pheochromocytoma 255.6
  hormone
    antidiuretic, inappropriate (syndrome) 253.6
    by
      carcinoid tumor 259.2
      pheochromocytoma 255.6
    ectopic NEC 259.3
  urinary
    excessive 788.42
    suppression 788.5
Section
  cesarean
    affecting fetus or newborn 763.4
    post mortem, affecting fetus or newborn 761.6
    previous, in pregnancy or childbirth 654.2
      affecting fetus or newborn 763.89
  nerve, traumatic—*see* Injury, nerve, by site
Seeligmann's syndrome (ichthyosis congenita) 757.1
Segmentation, incomplete (congenital)—*see also* Fusion
  bone NEC 756.9
  lumbosacral (joint) 756.15
  vertebra 756.15
    lumbosacral 756.15
Seizure(s) 780.39
  akinetic (idiopathic) (*see also* Epilepsy) 345.0
    psychomotor 345.4
  apoplexy, apoplectic (*see also* Disease, cerebrovascular, acute) 436
  atonic (*see also* Epilepsy) 345.0
  autonomic 300.11
  brain or cerebral (*see also* Disease, cerebrovascular, acute) 436
  convulsive (*see also* Convulsions) 780.39
  cortical (focal) (motor) (*see also* Epilepsy) 345.5
  due to stroke 438.89
  epilepsy, epileptic (cryptogenic) (*see also* Epilepsy) 345.9
  epileptiform, epileptoid 780.39
    focal (*see also* Epilepsy) 345.5
  febrile (simple) 780.31
    atypical 780.32
    complex 780.32

Seizure(s)—*continued*
  complicated 780.32
  with status epilepticus 345.3
  heart—*see* Disease, heart
  hysterical 300.11
  Jacksonian (focal) (*see also* Epilepsy) 345.5
    motor type 345.5
    sensory type 345.5
  newborn 779.0
  paralysis (*see also* Disease, cerebrovascular, acute) 436
  recurrent 345.9
    epileptic—*see* Epilepsy
  repetitive 780.39
    epileptic—*see* Epilepsy
  salaam (*see also* Epilepsy) 345.6
  uncinate (*see also* Epilepsy) 345.4
Self-mutilation 300.9
Semicoma 780.09
Semiconsciousness 780.09
Seminal
  vesicle—*see* condition
  vesiculitis (*see also* Vesiculitis) 608.0
Seminoma (M9061/3)
  anaplastic type (M9062/3)
    specified site—*see* Neoplasm, by site, malignant
    unspecified site 186.9
  specified site—*see* Neoplasm, by site, malignant
  spermatocytic (M9063/3)
    specified site—*see* Neoplasm, by site, malignant
    unspecified site 186.9
  unspecified site 186.9
Semliki Forest encephalitis 062.8
Senear-Usher disease or syndrome (pemphigus erythematosus) 694.4
Senecio jacobae dermatitis 692.6
Senectus 797
Senescence 797
Senile (*see also* condition) 797
  cervix (atrophic) 622.8
  degenerative atrophy, skin 701.3
  endometrium (atrophic) 621.8
  fallopian tube (atrophic) 620.3
  heart (failure) 797
  lung 492.8
  ovary (atrophic) 620.3
  syndrome 259.8
  vagina, vaginitis (atrophic) 627.3
  wart 702.0
Senility 797
  with
    acute confusional state 290.3
    delirium 290.3
    mental changes 290.9
    psychosis NEC (*see also* Psychosis, senile) 290.20
  premature (syndrome) 259.8
Sensation
  burning (*see also* Disturbance, sensation) 782.0
    tongue 529.6
  choking 784.99
  loss of (*see also* Disturbance, sensation) 782.0
  prickling (*see also* Disturbance, sensation) 782.0
  tingling (*see also* Disturbance, sensation) 782.0
Sense loss (touch) (*see also* Disturbance, sensation) 782.0
  smell 781.1
  taste 781.1

Sensibility disturbance NEC (cortical) (deep) (vibratory) (*see also* Disturbance, sensation) 782.0
Sensitive dentine 521.89
Sensitiver Beziehungswahn 297.8
Sensitivity, sensitization —*see also* Allergy
  autoerythrocyte 287.2
  carotid sinus 337.0
  child (excessive) 313.21
  cold, autoimmune 283.0
  methemoglobin 289.7
  suxamethonium 289.89
  tuberculin, without clinical or radiological symptoms 795.5
Sensory
  extinction 781.8
  neglect 781.8
Separation
  acromioclavicular—see Dislocation, shoulder
  anxiety, abnormal 309.21
  apophysis, traumatic—*see* Fracture, by site
  choroid 363.70
    hemorrhagic 363.72
    serous 363.71
  costochondral (simple) (traumatic)—*see* Dislocation, costochondral
  delayed
    umbilical cord 779.83
  epiphysis, epiphyseal
    nontraumatic 732.9
      upper femoral 732.2
    traumatic—*see* Fracture, by site
  fracture—*see* Fracture, by site
  infundibulum cardiac from right ventricle by a partition 746.83
  joint (current) (traumatic)—*see* Dislocation, by site
  placenta (normally implanted)—*see* Placenta, separation
  pubic bone, obstetrical trauma 665.6
  retina, retinal (*see also* Detachment, retina) 361.9
    layers 362.40
    sensory (*see also* Retinoschisis) 361.10
    pigment epithelium (exudative) 362.42
      hemorrhagic 362.43
  sternoclavicular (traumatic)—*see* Dislocation, sternoclavicular
  symphysis pubis, obstetrical trauma 665.6
  tracheal ring, incomplete (congenital) 748.3
Sepsis (generalized) 995.91
  with
    abortion—*see* Abortion, by type, with sepsis
    acute organ dysfunction 995.92
    ectopic pregnancy (*see also* categories 633.0-633.9) 639.0
    molar pregnancy (*see also* categories 630-632) 639.0
    multiple organ dysfunction (MOD) 995.92
  buccal 528.3
  complicating labor 659.3
  dental (pulpal origin) 522.4
  female genital organ NEC 614.9
  fetus (intrauterine) 771.81
  following
    abortion 639.0
    ectopic or molar pregnancy 639.0
    infusion, perfusion, or transfusion 999.39
  Friedländer's 038.49
  intraocular 360.00

Sepsis—*continued*
  localized
    in operation wound 998.59
    skin (*see also* Abscess) 682.9
  malleus 024
  newborn (organism unspecified) NEC 771.81
  oral 528.3
  puerperal, postpartum, childbirth (pelvic) 670
  resulting from infusion, injection, transfusion, or vaccination 999.39
  severe 995.92
  skin, localized (*see also* Abscess) 682.9
  umbilical (newborn) (organism unspecified) 771.89
  tetanus 771.3
  urinary 599.0
    meaning sepsis 995.91
    meaning urinary tract infection 599.0
Septate —*see also* Septum
Septic —*see also* condition
  adenoids 474.01
    and tonsils 474.02
  arm (with lymphangitis) 682.3
  embolus—*see* Embolism
  finger (with lymphangitis) 681.00
  foot (with lymphangitis) 682.7
  gallbladder (*see also* Cholecystitis) 575.8
  hand (with lymphangitis) 682.4
  joint (*see also* Arthritis, septic) 711.0
  kidney (*see also* Infection, kidney) 590.9
  leg (with lymphangitis) 682.6
  mouth 528.3
  nail 681.9
    finger 681.02
    toe 681.11
  shock (endotoxic) 785.52
  sore (*see also* Abscess) 682.9
  throat 034.0
    milk-borne 034.0
    streptococcal 034.0
  spleen (acute) 289.59
  teeth (pulpal origin) 522.4
  throat 034.0
  thrombus—*see* Thrombosis
  toe (with lymphangitis) 681.10
  tonsils 474.00
    and adenoids 474.02
  umbilical cord (newborn) (organism unspecified) 771.89
  uterus (*see also* Endometritis) 615.9
Septicemia, septicemic (generalized) (suppurative) 038.9
  with
    abortion—*see* Abortion, by type, with sepsis
    ectopic pregnancy (*see also* categories 633.0-633.9) 639.0
    molar pregnancy (*see also* categories 630-632) 639.0
  Aerobacter aerogenes 038.49
  anaerobic 038.3
  anthrax 022.3
  Bacillus coli 038.42
  Bacteroides 038.3
  Clostridium 038.3
  complicating labor 659.3
  cryptogenic 038.9
  enteric gram-negative bacilli 038.40
  Enterobacter aerogenes 038.49
  Erysipelothrix (insidiosa) (rhusiopathiae) 027.1
  Escherichia coli 038.42

INDEX TO DISEASES

Septicemia—*continued*
  following
    abortion 639.0
    ectopic or molar pregnancy 639.0
    infusion, injection, transfusion, or vaccination 999.39
  Friedländer's (bacillus) 038.49
  gangrenous 038.9
  gonococcal 098.89
  gram-negative (organism) 038.40
    anaerobic 038.3
  Hemophilus influenzae 038.41
  herpes (simplex) 054.5
  herpetic 054.5
  Listeria monocytogenes 027.0
  meningeal—*see* Meningitis
  meningococcal (chronic) (fulminating) 036.2
  navel, newborn (organism unspecified) 771.89
  newborn (organism unspecified) 771.81
  plague 020.2
  pneumococcal 038.2
  postabortal 639.0
  postoperative 998.59
  Proteus vulgaris 038.49
  Pseudomonas (aeruginosa) 038.43
  puerperal, postpartum 670
  Salmonella (aertrycke) (callinarum) (choleraesuis) (enteritidis) (suipestifer) 003.1
  Serratia 038.44
  Shigella (*see also* Dysentery, bacillary) 004.9
  specified organism NEC 038.8
  staphylococcal 038.10
    aureus 038.11
    specified organism NEC 038.19
  streptococcal (anaerobic) 038.0
  suipestifer 003.1
  umbilicus, newborn (organism unspecified) 771.89
  viral 079.99
  Yersinia enterocolitica 038.49
Septum, septate (congenital)—*see also* Anomaly, specified type NEC
  anal 751.2
  aqueduct of Sylvius 742.3
    with spina bifida (*see also* Spina bifida) 741.0
  hymen 752.49
  uterus (*see also* Double, uterus) 752.2
  vagina 752.49
    in pregnancy or childbirth 654.7
      affecting fetus or newborn 763.89
      causing obstructed labor 660.2
        affecting fetus or newborn 763.1
Sequestration
  lung (congenital) (extralobar) (intralobar) 748.5
  orbit 376.10
  pulmonary artery (congenital) 747.3
  splenic 289.52
Sequestrum
  bone (*see also* Osteomyelitis) 730.1
    jaw 526.4
  dental 525.8
  jaw bone 526.4
  sinus (accessory) (nasal) (*see also* Sinusitis) 473.9
    maxillary 473.0
Sequoiosis asthma 495.8
Serology for syphilis
  doubtful
    with signs or symptoms—*see* Syphilis, by site and stage
    follow-up of latent syphilis—*see* Syphilis, latent

Serology for syphilis—*continued*
  false positive 795.6
  negative, with signs or symptoms—*see* Syphilis, by site and stage
  positive 097.1
    with signs or symptoms—*see* Syphilis, by site and stage
    false 795.6
    follow-up of latent syphilis—*see* Syphilis, latent
    only finding—*see* Syphilis, latent
  reactivated 097.1
Seroma (postoperative) (non-infected) 998.13
  infected 998.51
Seropurulent —*see* condition
Serositis, multiple 569.89
  pericardial 423.2
  peritoneal 568.82
  pleural—*see* Pleurisy
Serotonin syndrome 333.99
Serous —*see* condition
Sertoli cell
  adenoma (M8640/0)
    specified site—*see* Neoplasm, by site, benign
    unspecified site
      female 220
      male 222.0
  carcinoma (M8640/3)
    specified site—*see* Neoplasm, by site, malignant
    unspecified site 186.9
  syndrome (germinal aplasia) 606.0
  tumor (M8640/0)
    with lipid storage (M8641/0)
      specified site—*see* Neoplasm, by site, benign
      unspecified site
        female 220
        male 222.0
    specified site—*see* Neoplasm, by site, benign
    unspecified site
      female 220
      male 222.0
Sertoli-Leydig cell tumor (M8631/0)
  specified site—*see* Neoplasm, by site, benign
  unspecified site
    female 220
    male 222.0
Serum
  allergy, allergic reaction 999.5
    shock 999.4
  arthritis 999.5 *[713.6]*
  complication or reaction NEC 999.5
  disease NEC 999.5
  hepatitis 070.3
  intoxication 999.5
  jaundice (homologous) *see* Hepatitis, viral
  neuritis 999.5
  poisoning NEC 999.5
  rash NEC 999.5
  reaction NEC 999.5
  sickness NEC 999.5
Sesamoiditis 733.99
Seven-day fever 061
  of
    Japan 100.89
    Queensland 100.89
Sever's disease or osteochondrosis (calcaneum) 732.5
Sex chromosome mosaics 758.81
Sex reassignment surgery status (*see also* Tran-sexualism) 302.50

Sextuplet
affected by maternal complications of pregnancy 761.5
healthy liveborn—*see* Newborn, multiple
pregnancy (complicating delivery) NEC 651.8
  with fetal loss and retention of one or more fetus(es) 651.6
  following (elective) fetal reduction 651.7
Sexual
anesthesia 302.72
deviation (*see also* Deviation, sexual) 302.9
disorder (*see also* Deviation, sexual) 302.9
frigidity (female) 302.72
function, disorder of (psychogenic) 302.70
  specified type NEC 302.79
immaturity (female) (male) 259.0
impotence 607.84
  organic origin NEC 607.84
  psychogenic 302.72
precocity (constitutional) (cryptogenic) (female) (idiopathic) (male) NEC 259.1
  with adrenal hyperplasia 255.2
sadism 302.84
Sexuality, pathological (*see also* Deviation, sexual) 302.9
Sézary's disease, reticulosis, or syndrome (M9701/3) 202.2
Shadow, lung 793.1
Shaken infant syndrome 995.55
Shaking
head (tremor) 781.0
palsy or paralysis (*see also* Parkinsonism) 332.0
Shallowness, acetabulum 736.39
Shaver's disease or syndrome (bauxite pneumoconiosis) 503
Shearing
artificial skin graft 996.55
decellularized allodermis graft 996.55
Sheath (tendon)—*see* condition
Shedding
nail 703.8
teeth, premature, primary (deciduous) 520.6
Sheehan's disease or syndrome (postpartum pituitary necrosis) 253.2
Shelf, rectal 569.49
Shell
shock (current) (*see also* Reaction, stress, acute) 308.9
  lasting state 300.16
teeth 520.5
Shield kidney 753.3
Shift, mediastinal 793.2
Shifting
pacemaker 427.89
sleep-work schedule (affecting sleep) 327.36
Shiga's
bacillus 004.0
dysentery 004.0
Shigella (dysentery) (*see also* Dysentery, bacillary) 004.9
carrier (suspected) of V02.3
Shigellosis (*see also* Dysentery, bacillary) 004.9
Shingles (*see also* Herpes, zoster) 053.9
eye NEC 053.29
Shin splints 844.9
Shipyard eye or disease 077.1
Shirodkar suture, in pregnancy 654.5

Shock 785.50
with
  abortion—*see* Abortion, by type, with shock
  ectopic pregnancy (*see also* categories 633.0-633.9) 639.5
  molar pregnancy (*see also* categories 630-632) 639.5
allergic—*see* Shock, anaphylactic
anaclitic 309.21
anaphylactic 995.0
  chemical—*see* Table of drugs and chemicals
  correct medicinal substance properly administered 995.0
  drug or medicinal substance
    correct substance properly administered 995.0
    overdose or wrong substance given or taken 977.9
      specified drug—*see* Table of drugs and chemicals
  food—*see* Anaphylactic shock, due to, food
  following sting(s) 989.5
  immunization 999.4
  serum 999.4
anaphylactoid—*see* Shock, anaphylactic
anesthetic
  correct substance properly administered 995.4
  overdose or wrong substance given 968.4
    specified anesthetic—*see* Table of drugs and chemicals
birth, fetus or newborn NEC 779.89
cardiogenic 785.51
chemical substance—*see* Table of drugs and chemicals
circulatory 785.59
complicating
  abortion—*see* Abortion, by type, with shock
  ectopic pregnancy (*see also* categories 633.0-633.9) 639.5
  labor and delivery 669.1
  molar pregnancy (*see also* categories 630-632) 639.5
culture 309.29
due to
  drug 995.0
    correct substance properly administered 995.0
    overdose or wrong substance given or taken 977.9
      specified drug—*see* Table of drugs and chemicals
  food—*see* Anaphylactic shock, due to, food
during labor and delivery 669.1
electric 994.8
endotoxic 785.52
  due to surgical procedure 998.0
following
  abortion 639.5
  ectopic or molar pregnancy 639.5
  injury (immediate) (delayed) 958.4
  labor and delivery 669.1
gram-negative 785.52
hematogenic 785.59
hemorrhagic
  due to
    disease 785.59
    surgery (intraoperative) (postoperative) 998.0
    trauma 958.4

INDEX TO DISEASES

Shock—*continued*
- hypovolemic NEC 785.59
  - surgical 998.0
  - traumatic 958.4
- insulin 251.0
  - therapeutic misadventure 962.3
- kidney 584.5
  - traumatic (following crushing) 958.5
- lightning 994.0
- lung 518.5
- nervous (*see also* Reaction, stress, acute) 308.9
- obstetric 669.1
  - with
    - abortion—*see* Abortion, by type, with shock
    - ectopic pregnancy (*see also* categories 633.0-633.9) 639.5
    - molar pregnancy (*see also* categories 630-632) 639.5
  - following
    - abortion 639.5
    - ectopic or molar pregnancy 639.5
- paralysis, paralytic (*see also* Disease, cerebrovascular, acute) 436
  - late effect—*see* Late effect(s) (of) cerebrovascular disease
- pleural (surgical) 998.0
  - due to trauma 958.4
- postoperative 998.0
  - with
    - abortion—*see* Abortion, by type, with shock
    - ectopic pregnancy (*see also* categories 633.0-633.9) 639.5
    - molar pregnancy (*see also* categories 630-632) 639.5
  - following
    - abortion 639.5
    - ectopic or molar pregnancy 639.5
- psychic (*see also* Reaction, stress, acute) 308.9
  - past history (of) V15.49
- psychogenic (*see also* Reaction, stress, acute) 308.9
- septic 785.52
  - with
    - abortion—*see* Abortion, by type, with shock
    - ectopic pregnancy (*see also* categories 633.0-633.9) 639.5
    - molar pregnancy (*see also* categories 630-632) 639.5
  - due to
    - surgical procedure 998.0
    - transfusion NEC 999.8
      - bone marrow 996.85
  - following
    - abortion 639.5
    - ectopic or molar pregnancy 639.5
    - surgical procedure 998.0
    - transfusion NEC 999.8
      - bone marrow 996.85
- spinal—*see also* Injury, spinal, by site
  - with spinal bone injury—*see* Fracture, vertebra, by site, with spinal cord injury
- surgical 998.0
- therapeutic misadventure NEC (*see also* Complications) 998.89
- thyroxin 962.7
- toxic 040.82
- transfusion—*see* Complications, transfusion
- traumatic (immediate) (delayed) 958.4

Shoemakers' chest 738.3

Short, shortening, shortness
- Achilles tendon (acquired) 727.81
- arm 736.89
  - congenital 755.20
- back 737.9
- bowel syndrome 579.3
- breath 786.05
- chain acyl CoA dehydrogenase deficiency (SCAD) 277.85
- common bile duct, congenital 751.69
- cord (umbilical) 663.4
  - affecting fetus or newborn 762.6
- cystic duct, congenital 751.69
- esophagus (congenital) 750.4
- femur (acquired) 736.81
  - congenital 755.34
- frenulum linguae 750.0
- frenum, lingual 750.0
- hamstrings 727.81
- hip (acquired) 736.39
  - congenital 755.63
- leg (acquired) 736.81
  - congenital 755.30
- metatarsus (congenital) 754.79
  - acquired 736.79
- organ or site, congenital NEC—*see* Distortion
- palate (congenital) 750.26
- P-R interval syndrome 426.81
- radius (acquired) 736.09
  - congenital 755.26
- round ligament 629.89
- sleeper 307.49
- stature, constitutional (hereditary) (idiopathic) 783.43
- tendon 727.81
  - Achilles (acquired) 727.81
    - congenital 754.79
  - congenital 756.89
- thigh (acquired) 736.81
  - congenital 755.34
- tibialis anticus 727.81
- umbilical cord 663.4
  - affecting fetus or newborn 762.6
- urethra 599.84
- uvula (congenital) 750.26
- vagina 623.8

Shortsightedness 367.1
Shoshin (acute fulminating beriberi) 265.0
Shoulder —*see* condition
Shovel-shaped incisors 520.2
Shower, thromboembolic —*see* Embolism
Shunt (status)
- aortocoronary bypass V45.81
- arterial-venous (dialysis) V45.1
- arteriovenous, pulmonary (acquired) 417.0
  - congenital 747.3
  - traumatic (complication) 901.40
- cerebral ventricle (communicating) in situ V45.2
- coronary artery bypass V45.81
- surgical, prosthetic, with complications—*see* Complications, shunt
- vascular NEC V45.89

Shutdown, renal 586
- with
  - abortion—*see* Abortion, by type, with renal failure
  - ectopic pregnancy (*see also* categories 633.0-633.9) 639.3
  - molar pregnancy (*see also* categories 630-632) 639.3

1319

Shutdown, renal—*continued*
  complicating
    abortion 639.3
    ectopic or molar pregnancy 639.3
    following labor and delivery 669.3
Shwachman's syndrome 288.02
Shy-Drager syndrome (orthostatic hypotension with multisystem degeneration) 333.0
Sialadenitis (any gland) (chronic) (suppurative) 527.2
  epidemic—*see* Mumps
Sialadenosis, periodic 527.2
Sialaporia 527.7
Sialectasia 527.8
Sialitis 527.2
Sialoadenitis (*see also* Sialadenitis) 527.2
Sialoangitis 527.2
Sialodochitis (fibrinosa) 527.2
Sialodocholithiasis 527.5
Sialolithiasis 527.5
Sialorrhea (*see also* Ptyalism) 527.7
  periodic 527.2
Sialosis 527.8
  rheumatic 710.2
Siamese twin 759.4
Sicard's syndrome 352.6
Sicca syndrome (keratoconjunctivitis) 710.2
Sick 799.9
  cilia syndrome 759.89
  or handicapped person in family V61.49
Sickle-cell
  anemia (*see also* Disease, sickle-cell) 282.60
  disease (*see also* Disease, sickle-cell) 282.60
  hemoglobin
    C disease (without crisis) 282.63
      with
        crisis 282.64
          vaso-occlusive pain 282.64
    D disease (without crisis) 282.68
      with crisis 282.69
    E disease (without crisis) 282.68
      with crisis 282.69
  thalassemia (without crisis) 282.41
    with
      crisis 282.42
        vaso-occlusive pain 282.42
  trait 282.5
Sicklemia (*see also* Disease, sickle-cell) 282.60
  trait 282.5
Sickness
  air (travel) 994.6
  airplane 994.6
  alpine 993.2
  altitude 993.2
  Andes 993.2
  aviators' 993.2
  balloon 993.2
  car 994.6
  compressed air 993.3
  decompression 993.3
  green 280.9
  harvest 100.89
  milk 988.8
  morning 643.0
  motion 994.6
  mountain 993.2
    acute 289.0
  protein (*see also* Complications, vaccination) 999.5
  radiation NEC 990
  roundabout (motion) 994.6
  sea 994.6

Sickness—*continued*
  serum NEC 999.5
  sleeping (African) 086.5
    by Trypanosoma 086.5
      gambiense 086.3
      rhodesiense 086.4
    Gambian 086.3
    late effect 139.8
    Rhodesian 086.4
  sweating 078.2
  swing (motion) 994.6
  train (railway) (travel) 994.6
  travel (any vehicle) 994.6
Sick sinus syndrome 427.81
Sideropenia (*see also* Anemia, iron deficiency) 280.9
Siderosis (lung) (occupational) 503
  cornea 371.15
  eye (bulbi) (vitreous) 360.23
  lens 360.23
Siegal-Cattan-Mamou disease (periodic) 277.31
Siemens' syndrome
  ectodermal dysplasia 757.31
  keratosis follicularis spinulosa (decalvans) 757.39
Sighing respiration 786.7
Sigmoid
  flexure—*see* condition
  kidney 753.3
Sigmoiditis —*see* Enteritis
Silfverskiöld's syndrome 756.50
Silicosis, sillicotic (complicated) (occupational) (simple) 502
  fibrosis, lung (confluent) (massive) (occupational) 502
  non-nodular 503
  pulmonum 502
Silicotuberculosis (*see also* Tuberculosis) 011.4
Silo fillers' disease 506.9
Silver's syndrome (congenital hemihypertrophy and short stature) 759.89
Silver wire arteries, retina 362.13
Silvestroni-Bianco syndrome (thalassemia minima) 282.49
Simian crease 757.2
Simmonds' cachexia or disease (pituitary cachexia) 253.2
Simons' disease or syndrome (progressive lipodystrophy) 272.6
Simple, simplex —*see* condition
Sinding-Larsen disease (juvenile osteopathia patellae) 732.4
Singapore hemorrhagic fever 065.4
Singers' node or nodule 478.5
Single
  atrium 745.69
  coronary artery 746.85
  umbilical artery 747.5
  ventricle 745.3
Singultus 786.8
  epidemicus 078.89
Sinus —*see also* Fistula
  abdominal 569.81
  arrest 426.6
  arrhythmia 427.89
  bradycardia 427.89
    chronic 427.81
  branchial cleft (external) (internal) 744.41
  coccygeal (infected) 685.1
    with abscess 685.0

INDEX TO DISEASES

Sinus—*continued*
  dental 522.7
  dermal (congenital) 685.1
    with abscess 685.0
  draining—*see* Fistula
  infected, skin NEC 686.9
  marginal, ruptured or bleeding 641.2
    affecting fetus or newborn 762.1
  pause 426.6
  pericranii 742.0
  pilonidal (infected) (rectum) 685.1
    with abscess 685.0
  preauricular 744.46
  rectovaginal 619.1
  sacrococcygeal (dermoid) (infected) 685.1
    with abscess 685.0
  skin
    infected NEC 686.9
    noninfected—*see* Ulcer, skin
  tachycardia 427.89
  tarsi syndrome 726.79
  testis 608.89
  tract (postinfectional)—*see* Fistula
  urachus 753.7
Sinuses, Rokitansky-Aschoff (*see also* Disease, gallbladder) 575.8
Sinusitis (accessory) (nasal) (hyperplastic) (nonpurulent) (purulent) (chronic) 473.9
  with influenza, flu, or grippe 487.1
  acute 461.9
    ethmoidal 461.2
    frontal 461.1
    maxillary 461.0
    specified type NEC 461.8
    sphenoidal 461.3
  allergic (*see also* Fever, hay) 477.9
  antrum—*see* Sinusitis, maxillary
  due to
    fungus, any sinus 117.9
    high altitude 993.1
  ethmoidal 473.2
    acute 461.2
  frontal 473.1
    acute 461.1
  influenzal 478.19
  maxillary 473.0
    acute 461.0
  specified site NEC 473.8
  sphenoidal 473.3
    acute 461.3
  syphilitic, any sinus 095.8
  tuberculous, any sinus (*see also* Tuberculosis) 012.8
Sinusitis-bronchiectasis-situs inversus (syndrome) (triad) 759.3
Sipple's syndrome (medullary thyroid carcinoma-pheochromocytoma) 258.02
SIRS (systemic inflammatory response syndrome) 995.90
  due to
    infectious process 995.91
      with acute organ dysfunction 995.92
    non-infectious process 995.93
      with acute organ dysfunction 995.94
Sirenomelia 759.89
Siriasis 992.0
Sirkari's disease 085.0
Siti 104.0
Sitophobia 300.29
Situation, psychiatric 300.9

Situational
  disturbance (transient) (*see also* Reaction, adjustment) 309.9
    acute 308.3
  maladjustment, acute (*see also* Reaction, adjustment) 309.9
  reaction (*see also* Reaction, adjustment) 309.9
    acute 308.3
Situs inversus or transversus 759.3
  abdominalis 759.3
  thoracis 759.3
Sixth disease
  due to
    human herpesvirus 6 058.11
    human herpesvirus 7 058.12
Sjögren (-Gougerot) **syndrome or disease** (keratoconjunctivitis sicca) 710.2
  with lung involvement 710.2 *[517.8]*
Sjögren-Larsson syndrome (ichthyosis congenita) 757.1
Skeletal —*see* condition
Skene's gland —*see* condition
Skenitis (*see also* Urethritis) 597.89
  gonorrheal (acute) 098.0
  chronic or duration of 2 months or over 098.2
Skerljevo 104.0
Skevas-Zerfus disease 989.5
Skin —*see also* condition
  donor V59.1
  hidebound 710.9
SLAP lesion (superior glenoid labrum) 840.7
Slate-dressers' lung 502
Slate-miners' lung 502
Sleep
  deprivation V69.4
  disorder 780.50
    with apnea—*see* Apnea, sleep
    child 307.40
    movement, unspecified 780.58
    nonorganic origin 307.40
      specified type NEC 307.49
  disturbance 780.50
    with apnea—*see* Apnea, sleep
    nonorganic origin 307.40
      specified type NEC 307.49
  drunkenness 307.47
  movement disorder, unspecified 780.58
  paroxysmal (*see also* Narcolepsy) 347.00
  related movement disorder, unspecified 780.58
  rhythm inversion 327.39
    nonorganic origin 307.45
  walking 307.46
    hysterical 300.13
Sleeping sickness 086.5
  late effect 139.8
Sleeplessness (*see also* Insomnia) 780.52
  menopausal 627.2
  nonorganic origin 307.41
Slipped, slipping
  epiphysis (postinfectional) 732.9
    traumatic (old) 732.9
      current—*see* Fracture, by site
    upper femoral (nontraumatic) 732.2
  intervertebral disc—*see* Displacement, intervertebral disc
  ligature, umbilical 772.3
  patella 717.89
  rib 733.99
  sacroiliac joint 724.6
  tendon 727.9

Slipped, slipping—*continued*
  ulnar nerve, nontraumatic 354.2
  vertebra NEC (*see also* Spondylolisthesis) 756.12
Slocumb's syndrome 255.3
Sloughing (multiple) (skin) 686.9
  abscess—*see* Abscess, by site
  appendix 543.9
  bladder 596.8
  fascia 728.9
  graft—*see* Complications, graft
  phagedena (*see also* Gangrene) 785.4
  reattached extremity (*see also* Complications, reattached extremity) 996.90
  rectum 569.49
  scrotum 608.89
  tendon 727.9
  transplanted organ (*see also* Rejection, transplant, organ, by site) 996.80
  ulcer (*see also* Ulcer, skin) 707.9
Slow
  feeding newborn 779.3
  fetal, growth NEC 764.9
    affecting management of pregnancy 656.5
Slowing
  heart 427.89
  urinary stream 788.62
Sluder's neuralgia or syndrome 337.0
Slurred, slurring, speech 784.5
Small, smallness
  cardiac reserve—*see* Disease, heart
  for dates
    fetus or newborn 764.0
      with malnutrition 764.1
        affecting management of pregnancy 656.5
    infant, term 764.0
      with malnutrition 764.1
        affecting management of pregnancy 656.5
  introitus, vagina 623.3
  kidney, unknown cause 589.9
    bilateral 589.1
    unilateral 589.0
  ovary 620.8
  pelvis
    with disproportion (fetopelvic) 653.1
      affecting fetus or newborn 763.1
    causing obstructed labor 660.1
      affecting fetus or newborn 763.1
  placenta—*see* Placenta, insufficiency
  uterus 621.8
  white kidney 582.9
Small-for-dates (*see also* Light-for-dates) 764.0
  affecting management of pregnancy 656.5
Smallpox 050.9
  contact V01.3
  exposure to V01.3
  hemorrhagic (pustular) 050.0
  malignant 050.0
  modified 050.2
  vaccination
    complications—*see* Complications, vaccination
    prophylactic (against) V04.1
Smith's fracture (separation) (closed) 813.41
  open 813.51
Smith-Lemli-Opitz syndrome (cerebrohepatorenal syndrome) 759.89
Smith-Magenis syndrome 758.33
Smith-Strang disease (oasthouse urine) 270.2

Smokers'
  bronchitis 491.0
  cough 491.0
  syndrome (*see also* Abuse, drugs, nondependent) 305.1
  throat 472.1
  tongue 528.6
Smoking complicating pregnancy, childbirth, or the puerperium 649.0
Smothering spells 786.09
Snaggle teeth, tooth 524.39
Snapping
  finger 727.05
  hip 719.65
  jaw 524.69
    temporomandibular joint sounds on opening or closing 524.64
  knee 717.9
  thumb 727.05
Sneddon-Wilkinson disease or syndrome (subcorneal pustular dermatosis) 694.1
Sneezing 784.99
  intractable 478.19
Sniffing
  cocaine (*see also* Dependence) 304.2
  ether (*see also* Dependence) 304.6
  glue (airplane) (*see also* Dependence) 304.6
Snoring 786.09
Snow blindness 370.24
Snuffles (nonsyphilitic) 460
  syphilitic (infant) 090.0
Social migrant V60.0
Sodoku 026.0
Soemmering's ring 366.51
Soft —*see also* condition
  enlarged prostate 600.00
    with
      other lower urinary tract symptoms (LUTS) 600.01
      urinary
        obstruction 600.01
        retention 600.01
  nails 703.8
Softening
  bone 268.2
  brain (necrotic) (progressive) 434.9
    arteriosclerotic 437.0
    congenital 742.4
    embolic (*see also* Embolism, brain) 434.1
    hemorrhagic (*see also* Hemorrhage, brain) 431
    occlusive 434.9
    thrombotic (*see also* Thrombosis, brain) 434.0
  cartilage 733.92
  cerebellar—*see* Softening, brain
  cerebral—*see* Softening, brain
  cerebrospinal—*see* Softening, brain
  myocardial, heart (*see also* Degeneration, myocardial) 429.1
  nails 703.8
  spinal cord 336.8
  stomach 537.89
Solar fever 061
Soldier's
  heart 306.2
  patches 423.1
Solitary
  cyst
    bone 733.21
    kidney 593.2
  kidney (congenital) 753.0
  tubercle, brain (*see also* Tuberculosis, brain) 013.2
  ulcer, bladder 596.8

INDEX TO DISEASES

Somatization reaction, somatic reaction (*see also* Disorder, psychosomatic) 306.9
    disorder 300.81
Somatoform disorder 300.82
    atypical 300.82
    severe 300.81
    undifferentiated 300.82
Somnambulism 307.46
    hysterical 300.13
Somnolence 780.09
    nonorganic origin 307.43
    periodic 349.89
Sonne dysentery 004.3
Soor 112.0
Sore
    Delhi 085.1
    desert (*see also* Ulcer, skin) 707.9
    eye 379.99
    Lahore 085.1
    mouth 528.9
        canker 528.2
        due to dentures 528.9
    muscle 729.1
    Naga (*see also* Ulcer, skin) 707.9
    oriental 085.1
    pressure (*see also* Decubitus) 707.00
        with gangrene (*see also* Decubitus) 707.00 [785.4]
    skin NEC 709.9
    soft 099.0
    throat 462
        with influenza, flu, or grippe 487.1
        acute 462
        chronic 472.1
        clergyman's 784.49
        coxsackie (virus) 074.0
        diphtheritic 032.0
        epidemic 034.0
        gangrenous 462
        herpetic 054.79
        influenzal 487.1
        malignant 462
        purulent 462
        putrid 462
        septic 034.0
        streptococcal (ulcerative) 034.0
        ulcerated 462
        viral NEC 462
            Coxsackie 074.0
    tropical (*see also* Ulcer, skin) 707.9
    veldt (*see also* Ulcer, skin) 707.9
Sotos' syndrome (cerebral gigantism) 253.0
Sounds
    friction, pleural 786.7
    succussion, chest 786.7
    temporomandibular joint
        on opening or closing 524.64
South African cardiomyopathy syndrome 425.2
South American
    blastomycosis 116.1
    trypanosomiasis—*see* Trypanosomiasis
Southeast Asian hemorrhagic fever 065.4
Spacing, teeth, abnormal 524.30
    excessive 524.32
Spade-like hand (congenital) 754.89
Spading nail 703.8
    congenital 757.5
Spanemia 285.9
Spanish collar 605
Sparganosis 123.5

Spasm, spastic, spasticity (*see also* condition) 781.0
    accommodation 367.53
    ampulla of Vater (*see also* Disease, gallbladder) 576.8
    anus, ani (sphincter) (reflex) 564.6
        psychogenic 306.4
    artery NEC 443.9
        basilar 435.0
        carotid 435.8
        cerebral 435.9
            specified artery NEC 435.8
        retinal (*see also* Occlusion, retinal, artery) 362.30
        vertebral 435.1
        vertebrobasilar 435.3
    Bell's 351.0
    bladder (sphincter, external or internal) 596.8
    bowel 564.9
        psychogenic 306.4
    bronchus, bronchiole 519.11
    cardia 530.0
    cardiac—*see* Angina
    carpopedal (*see also* Tetany) 781.7
    cecum 564.9
        psychogenic 306.4
    cerebral (arteries) (vascular) 435.9
        specified artery NEC 435.8
    cerebrovascular 435.9
    cervix, complicating delivery 661.4
        affecting fetus or newborn 763.7
    ciliary body (of accommodation) 367.53
    colon 564.1
        psychogenic 306.4
    common duct (*see also* Disease, biliary) 576.8
    compulsive 307.22
    conjugate 378.82
    convergence 378.84
    coronary (artery)—*see* Angina
    diaphragm (reflex) 786.8
        psychogenic 306.1
    duodenum, duodenal (bulb) 564.89
    esophagus (diffuse) 530.5
        psychogenic 306.4
    facial 351.8
    fallopian tube 620.8
    gait 781.2
    gastrointestinal (tract) 536.8
        psychogenic 306.4
    glottis 478.75
        hysterical 300.11
        psychogenic 306.1
            specified as conversion reaction 300.11
        reflex through recurrent laryngeal nerve 478.75
    habit 307.20
        chronic 307.22
        transient (of childhood) 307.21
    heart—*see* Angina
    hourglass—*see* Contraction, hourglass
    hysterical 300.11
    infantile (*see also* Epilepsy) 345.6
    internal oblique, eye 378.51
    intestinal 564.9
        psychogenic 306.4
    larynx, laryngeal 478.75
        hysterical 300.11
        psychogenic 306.1
            specified as conversion reaction 300.11
    levator palpebrae superioris 333.81
    lightning (*see also* Epilepsy) 345.6

Spasm, spastic, spasticity—*continued*
 mobile 781.0
 muscle 728.85
  back 724.8
  psychogenic 306.0
 nerve, trigeminal 350.1
 nervous 306.0
 nodding 307.3
  infantile (*see also* Epilepsy) 345.6
 occupational 300.89
 oculogyric 378.87
 ophthalmic artery 362.30
 orbicularis 781.0
 perineal 625.8
 peroneo-extensor (*see also* Flat, foot) 734
 pharynx (reflex) 478.29
  hysterical 300.11
  psychogenic 306.1
   specified as conversion reaction 300.11
 pregnant uterus, complicating delivery 661.4
 psychogenic 306.0
 pylorus 537.81
  adult hypertrophic 537.0
  congenital or infantile 750.5
  psychogenic 306.4
 rectum (sphincter) 564.6
  psychogenic 306.4
 retinal artery NEC (*see also* Occlusion, retina, artery) 362.30
 sacroiliac 724.6
 salaam (infantile) (*see also* Epilepsy) 345.6
 saltatory 781.0
 sigmoid 564.9
  psychogenic 306.4
 sphincter of Oddi (*see also* Disease, gallbladder) 576.5
 stomach 536.8
  neurotic 306.4
 throat 478.29
  hysterical 300.11
  psychogenic 306.1
   specified as conversion reaction 300.11
 tic 307.20
  chronic 307.22
  transient (of childhood) 307.21
 tongue 529.8
 torsion 333.6
 trigeminal nerve 350.1
  postherpetic 053.12
 ureter 593.89
 urethra (sphincter) 599.84
 uterus 625.8
  complicating labor 661.4
   affecting fetus or newborn 763.7
 vagina 625.1
  psychogenic 306.51
 vascular NEC 443.9
 vasomotor NEC 443.9
 vein NEC 459.89
 vesical (sphincter, external or internal) 596.8
 viscera 789.0
Spasmodic —*see* condition
Spasmophilia (*see also* Tetany) 781.7
Spasmus nutans 307.3
Spastic —*see also* Spasm
 child 343.9
Spasticity —*see also* Spasm
 cerebral, child 343.9
Speakers' throat 784.49
Specific, specified —*see* condition

Speech
 defect, disorder, disturbance, impediment NEC 784.5
  psychogenic 307.9
 therapy V57.3
Spells 780.39
 breath-holding 786.9
Spencer's disease (epidemic vomiting) 078.82
Spens' syndrome (syncope with heart block) 426.9
Spermatic cord —*see* condition
Spermatocele 608.1
 congenital 752.89
Spermatocystitis 608.4
Spermatocytoma (M9063/3)
 specified site—*see* Neoplasm, by site, malignant
 unspecified site 186.9
Spermatorrhea 608.89
Sperm counts
 fertility testing V26.21
 following sterilization reversal V26.22
 postvasectomy V25.8
Sphacelus (*see also* Gangrene) 785.4
Sphenoidal —*see* condition
Sphenoiditis (chronic) (*see also* Sinusitis, sphenoidal) 473.3
Sphenopalatine ganglion neuralgia 337.0
Sphericity, increased, lens 743.36
Spherocytosis (congenital) (familial) (hereditary) 282.0
 hemoglobin disease 287.7
 sickle-cell (disease) 282.60
Spherophakia 743.36
Sphincter —*see* condition
Sphincteritis, sphincter of Oddi (*see also* Cholecystitis) 576.8
Sphingolipidosis 272.7
Sphingolipodystrophy 272.7
Sphingomyelinosis 272.7
Spicule tooth 520.2
Spider
 finger 755.59
 nevus 448.1
 vascular 448.1
Spiegler-Fendt sarcoid 686.8
Spielmeyer-Stock disease 330.1
Spielmeyer-Vogt disease 330.1
Spina bifida (aperta) 741.9

> Note—Use the following fifth-digit subclassification with category 741:
>
> 0 *unspecified region*
> 1 *cervical region*
> 2 *dorsal [thoracic] region*
> 3 *lumbar region*

 with hydrocephalus 741.0
 fetal (suspected), affecting management of pregnancy 655.0
 occulta 756.17
Spindle, Krukenberg's 371.13
Spine, spinal —*see* condition
Spiradenoma (eccrine) (M8403/0)—*see* Neoplasm, skin, benign
Spirillosis NEC (*see also* Fever, relapsing) 087.9
Spirillum minus 026.0
Spirillum obermeieri infection 087.0
Spirochetal —*see* condition

INDEX TO DISEASES

Spirochetosis 104.9
  arthritic, arthritica 104.9 *[711.8]*
  bronchopulmonary 104.8
  icterohemorrhagica 100.0
  lung 104.8
Spitting blood *(see also* Hemoptysis) 786.3
Splanchnomegaly 569.89
Splanchnoptosis 569.89
Spleen, splenic —*see also* condition
  agenesis 759.0
  flexure syndrome 569.89
  neutropenia syndrome 289.53
  sequestration syndrome 289.52
Splenectasis *(see also* Splenomegaly) 789.2
Splenitis (interstitial) (malignant) (nonspecific) 289.59
  malarial *(see also* Malaria) 084.6
  tuberculous *(see also* Tuberculosis) 017.7
Splenocele 289.59
Splenomegalia —*see* Splenomegaly
Splenomegalic —*see* condition
Splenomegaly 789.2
  Bengal 789.2
  cirrhotic 289.51
  congenital 759.0
  congestive, chronic 289.51
  cryptogenic 789.2
  Egyptian 120.1
  Gaucher's (cerebroside lipidosis) 272.7
  idiopathic 789.2
  malarial *(see also* Malaria) 084.6
  neutropenic 289.53
  Niemann-Pick (lipid histiocytosis) 272.7
  siderotic 289.51
  syphilitic 095.8
    congenital 090.0
  tropical (Bengal) (idiopathic) 789.2
Splenopathy 289.50
Splenopneumonia —*see* Pneumonia
Splenoptosis 289.59
Splinter —*see* Injury, superficial, by site
Split, splitting
  heart sounds 427.89
  lip, congenital *(see also* Cleft, lip) 749.10
  nails 703.8
  urinary stream 788.61
Spoiled child reaction *(see also* Disturbance, conduct) 312.1
Spondylarthritis *(see also* Spondylosis) 721.90
Spondylarthrosis *(see also* Spondylosis) 721.90
Spondylitis 720.9
  ankylopoietica 720.0
  ankylosing (chronic) 720.0
  atrophic 720.9
    ligamentous 720.9
  chronic (traumatic) *(see also* Spondylosis) 721.90
  deformans (chronic) *(see also* Spondylosis) 721.90
  gonococcal 098.53
  gouty 274.0
  hypertrophic *(see also* Spondylosis) 721.90
  infectious NEC 720.9
  juvenile (adolescent) 720.0
  Kümmell's 721.7
  Marie-Strümpell (ankylosing) 720.0
  muscularis 720.9
  ossificans ligamentosa 721.6
  osteoarthritica *(see also* Spondylosis) 721.90
  posttraumatic 721.7
  proliferative 720.0
  rheumatoid 720.0
  rhizomelica 720.0

Spondylitis—*continued*
  sacroiliac NEC 720.2
  senescent *(see also* Spondylosis) 721.90
  senile *(see also* Spondylosis) 721.90
  static *(see also* Spondylosis) 721.90
  traumatic (chronic) *(see also* Spondylosis) 721.90
  tuberculous *(see also* Tuberculosis) 015.0 *[720.81]*
  typhosa 002.0 *[720.81]*
Spondyloarthrosis *(see also* Spondylosis) 721.90
Spondylolisthesis (congenital) (lumbosacral) 756.12
  with disproportion (fetopelvic) 653.3
    affecting fetus or newborn 763.1
    causing obstructed labor 660.1
      affecting fetus or newborn 763.1
  acquired 738.4
  degenerative 738.4
  traumatic 738.4
    acute (lumbar)—*see* Fracture, vertebra, lumbar
    site other than lumbosacral—*see* Fracture, vertebra, by site
Spondylolysis (congenital) 756.11
  acquired 738.4
  cervical 756.19
  lumbosacral region 756.11
    with disproportion (fetopelvic) 653.3
      affecting fetus or newborn 763.1
      causing obstructed labor 660.1
        affecting fetus or newborn 763.1
Spondylopathy
  inflammatory 720.9
    specified type NEC 720.89
  traumatic 721.7
Spondylose rhizomelique 720.0
Spondylosis 721.90
  with
    disproportion 653.3
      affecting fetus or newborn 763.1
      causing obstructed labor 660.1
        affecting fetus or newborn 763.1
    myelopathy NEC 721.91
  cervical, cervicodorsal 721.0
    with myelopathy 721.1
  inflammatory 720.9
  lumbar, lumbosacral 721.3
    with myelopathy 721.42
  sacral 721.3
    with myelopathy 721.42
  thoracic 721.2
    with myelopathy 721.41
  traumatic 721.7
Sponge
  divers' disease 989.5
  inadvertently left in operation wound 998.4
  kidney (medullary) 753.17
Spongioblastoma (M9422/3)
  multiforme (M9440/3)
    specified site—*see* Neoplasm, by site, malignant
    unspecified site 191.9
  polare (M9423/3)
    specified site—*see* Neoplasm, by site, malignant
    unspecified site 191.9
  primitive polar (M9443/3)
    specified site—*see* Neoplasm, by site, malignant
    unspecified site 191.9
  specified site—*see* Neoplasm, by site, malignant
  unspecified site 191.9

Spongiocytoma (M9400/3)
 specified site—*see* Neoplasm, by site, malignant
 unspecified site 191.9
Spongioneuroblastoma (M9504/3)—*see*
 Neoplasm, by site, malignant
Spontaneous —*see also* condition
 fracture—*see* Fracture, pathologic
Spoon nail 703.8
 congenital 757.5
Sporadic —*see* condition
Sporotrichosis (bones) (cutaneous)
 (disseminated) (epidermal) (lymphatic)
 (lymphocutaneous) (mucous membranes)
 (pulmonary) (skeletal) (visceral) 117.1
Sporotrichum schenckii infection 117.1
Spots, spotting
 atrophic (skin) 701.3
 Bitôt's (in the young child) 264.1
 café au lait 709.09
 cayenne pepper 448.1
 complicating pregnancy 649.5
 cotton wool (retina) 362.83
 de Morgan's (senile angiomas) 448.1
 Fúchs' black (myopic) 360.21
 intermenstrual
  irregular 626.6
  regular 626.5
 interpalpebral 372.53
 Koplik's 055.9
 liver 709.09
 Mongolian (pigmented) 757.33
 of pregnancy 641.9
 purpuric 782.7
 ruby 448.1
Spotted fever —*see* Fever, spotted
Sprain, strain (joint) (ligament) (muscle)
 (tendon) 848.9
 abdominal wall (muscle) 848.8
 Achilles tendon 845.09
 acromioclavicular 840.0
 ankle 845.00
  and foot 845.00
 anterior longitudinal, cervical 847.0
 arm 840.9
  upper 840.9
   and shoulder 840.9
 astragalus 845.00
 atlanto-axial 847.0
 atlanto-occipital 847.0
 atlas 847.0
 axis 847.0
 back (*see also* Sprain, spine) 847.9
 breast bone 848.40
 broad ligament—*see* Injury, internal, broad
   ligament
 calcaneofibular 845.02
 carpal 842.01
 carpometacarpal 842.11
 cartilage
  costal, without mention of injury to sternum
    848.3
   involving sternum 848.42
  ear 848.8
  knee 844.9
   with current tear (*see also* Tear, meniscus)
     836.2
  semilunar (knee) 844.8
   with current tear (*see also* Tear, meniscus)
     836.2
  septal, nose 848.0
  thyroid region 848.2

Sprain, strain—*continued*
 xiphoid 848.49
 cervical, cervicodorsal, cervicothoracic 847.0
 chondrocostal, without mention of injury to
   sternum 848.3
  involving sternum 848.42
 chondrosternal 848.42
 chronic (joint)—*see* Derangement, joint
 clavicle 840.9
 coccyx 847.4
 collar bone 840.9
 collateral, knee (medial) (tibial) 844.1
  lateral (fibular) 844.0
  recurrent or old 717.89
   lateral 717.81
   medial 717.82
 coracoacromial 840.8
 coracoclavicular 840.1
 coracohumeral 840.2
 coracoid (process) 840.9
 coronary, knee 844.8
 costal cartilage, without mention of injury to
   sternum 848.3
  involving sternum 848.42
 cricoarytenoid articulation 848.2
 cricothyroid articulation 848.2
 cruciate
  knee 844.2
  old 717.89
   anterior 717.83
   posterior 717.84
 deltoid
  ankle 845.01
  shoulder 840.8
 dorsal (spine) 847.1
 ear cartilage 848.8
 elbow 841.9
  and forearm 841.9
  specified site NEC 841.8
 femur (proximal end) 843.9
  distal end 844.9
 fibula (proximal end) 844.9
  distal end 845.00
 fibulocalcaneal 845.02
 finger(s) 842.10
 foot 845.10
  and ankle 845.00
 forearm 841.9
  and elbow 841.9
  specified site NEC 841.8
 glenoid (shoulder) (*see also* SLAP lesion) 840.8
 hand 842.10
 hip 843.9
  and thigh 843.9
 humerus (proximal end) 840.9
  distal end 841.9
 iliofemoral 843.0
 infraspinatus 840.3
 innominate
  acetabulum 843.9
  pubic junction 848.5
  sacral junction 846.1
 internal
  collateral, ankle 845.01
  semilunar cartilage 844.8
   with current tear (*see also* Tear, meniscus)
     836.2
  old 717.5
 interphalangeal
  finger 842.13
  toe 845.13

INDEX TO DISEASES

Sprain, strain

Sprain, strain—*continued*
  ischiocapsular 843.1
  jaw (cartilage) (meniscus) 848.1
    old 524.69
  knee 844.9
    and leg 844.9
    old 717.5
      collateral
        lateral 717.81
        medial 717.82
      cruciate
        anterior 717.83
        posterior 717.84
  late effect—*see* Late, effects (of), sprain
  lateral collateral, knee 844.0
    old 717.81
  leg 844.9
    and knee 844.9
  ligamentum teres femoris 843.8
  low back 846.9
  lumbar (spine) 847.2
  lumbosacral 846.0
    chronic or old 724.6
  mandible 848.1
    old 524.69
  maxilla 848.1
  medial collateral, knee 844.1
    old 717.82
  meniscus
    jaw 848.1
      old 524.69
    knee 844.8
      with current tear (*see also* Tear, meniscus) 836.2
      old 717.5
    mandible 848.1
      old 524.69
    specified site NEC 848.8
  metacarpal 842.10
    distal 842.12
    proximal 842.11
  metacarpophalangeal 842.12
  metatarsal 845.10
  metatarsophalangeal 845.12
  midcarpal 842.19
  midtarsal 845.19
  multiple sites, except fingers alone or toes alone 848.8
  neck 847.0
  nose (septal cartilage) 848.0
  occiput from atlas 847.0
  old—*see* Derangement, joint
  orbicular, hip 843.8
  patella(r) 844.8
    old 717.89
  pelvis 848.5
  phalanx
    finger 842.10
    toe 845.10
  radiocarpal 842.02
  radiohumeral 841.2
  radioulnar 841.9
    distal 842.09
  radius, radial (proximal end) 841.9
    and ulna 841.9
      distal 842.09
    collateral 841.0
    distal end 842.00
  recurrent—*see* Sprain, by site
  rib (cage), without mention of injury to sternum 848.3

Sprain, strain—*continued*
  involving sternum 848.42
  rotator cuff (capsule) 840.4
  round ligament—*see also* Injury, internal, round ligament
    femur 843.8
  sacral (spine) 847.3
  sacrococcygeal 847.3
  sacroiliac (region) 846.9
    chronic or old 724.6
    ligament 846.1
    specified site NEC 846.8
  sacrospinatus 846.2
  sacrospinous 846.2
  sacrotuberous 846.3
  scaphoid bone, ankle 845.00
  scapula(r) 840.9
  semilunar cartilage (knee) 844.8
    with current tear (*see also* Tear, meniscus) 836.2
    old 717.5
  septal cartilage (nose) 848.0
  shoulder 840.9
    and arm, upper 840.9
    blade 840.9
  specified site NEC 848.8
  spine 847.9
    cervical 847.0
    coccyx 847.4
    dorsal 847.1
    lumbar 847.2
    lumbosacral 846.0
      chronic or old 724.6
    sacral 847.3
    sacroiliac (*see also* Sprain, sacroiliac) 846.9
      chronic or old 724.6
    thoracic 847.1
  sternoclavicular 848.41
  sternum 848.40
  subglenoid (*see also* SLAP lesion) 840.8
  subscapularis 840.5
  supraspinatus 840.6
  symphysis
    jaw 848.1
      old 524.69
    mandibular 848.1
      old 524.69
    pubis 848.5
  talofibular 845.09
  tarsal 845.10
  tarsometatarsal 845.11
  temporomandibular 848.1
    old 524.69
  teres
    ligamentum femoris 843.8
    major or minor 840.8
  thigh (proximal end) 843.9
    and hip 843.9
    distal end 844.9
  thoracic (spine) 847.1
  thorax 848.8
  thumb 842.10
  thyroid cartilage or region 848.2
  tibia (proximal end) 844.9
    distal end 845.00
  tibiofibular
    distal 845.03
    superior 844.3
  toe(s) 845.10
  trachea 848.8
  trapezoid 840.8

Sprain, strain—*continued*
  ulna, ulnar (proximal end) 841.9
    collateral 841.1
    distal end 842.00
  ulnohumeral 841.3
  vertebrae (*see also* Sprain, spine) 847.9
    cervical, cervicodorsal, cervicothoracic 847.0
  wrist (cuneiform) (scaphoid) (semilunar) 842.00
  xiphoid cartilage 848.49
Sprengel's deformity (congenital) 755.52
Spring fever 309.23
Sprue 579.1
  celiac 579.0
  idiopathic 579.0
  meaning thrush 112.0
  nontropical 579.0
  tropical 579.1
Spur —*see also* Exostosis
  bone 726.91
    calcaneal 726.73
  calcaneal 726.73
  iliac crest 726.5
  nose (septum) 478.19
    bone 726.91
  septal 478.19
Spuria placenta —*see* Placenta, abnormal
Spurway's syndrome (brittle bones and blue sclera) 756.51
Sputum, abnormal (amount) (color) (excessive) (odor) (purulent) 786.4
  bloody 786.3
Squamous —*see also* condition
  cell metaplasia
    bladder 596.8
    cervix—*see* condition
  epithelium in
    cervical canal (congenital) 752.49
    uterine mucosa (congenital) 752.3
  metaplasia
    bladder 596.8
    cervix—*see* condition
Squashed nose 738.0
  congenital 754.0
Squeeze, divers' 993.3
Squint (*see also* Strabismus) 378.9
  accommodative (*see also* Esotropia) 378.00
  concomitant (*see also* Heterotropia) 378.30
Stab —*see also* Wound, open, by site
  internal organs—*see* Injury, internal, by site, with open wound
Staggering gait 781.2
  hysterical 300.11
Staghorn calculus 592.0
Stähl's
  ear 744.29
  pigment line (cornea) 371.11
Stähli's pigment lines (cornea) 371.11
Stain, staining
  meconium 779.84
  port wine 757.32
  tooth, teeth (hard tissues) 521.7
    due to
      accretions 523.6
      deposits (betel) (black) (green) (materia alba) (orange) (tobacco) 523.6
      metals (copper) (silver) 521.7
      nicotine 523.6
      pulpal bleeding 521.7
      tobacco 523.6
Stammering 307.0

Standstill
  atrial 426.6
  auricular 426.6
  cardiac (*see also* Arrest, cardiac) 427.5
  sinoatrial 426.6
  sinus 426.6
  ventricular (*see also* Arrest, cardiac) 427.5
Stannosis 503
Stanton's disease (melioidosis) 025
Staphylitis (acute) (catarrhal) (chronic) (gangrenous) (membranous) (suppurative) (ulcerative) 528.3
Staphylococcemia 038.10
  aureus 038.11
  specified organism NEC 038.19
Staphylococcus, staphylococcal —*see* condition
Staphyloderma (skin) 686.00
Staphyloma 379.11
  anterior, localized 379.14
  ciliary 379.11
  cornea 371.73
  equatorial 379.13
  posterior 379.12
  posticum 379.12
  ring 379.15
  sclera NEC 379.11
Starch eating 307.52
Stargardt's disease 362.75
Starvation (inanition) (due to lack of food) 994.2
  edema 262
  voluntary NEC 307.1
Stasis
  bile (duct) (*see also* Disease, biliary) 576.8
  bronchus (*see also* Bronchitis) 490
  cardiac (*see also* Failure, heart) 428.0
  cecum 564.89
  colon 564.89
  dermatitis (*see also* Varix, with stasis dermatitis) 454.1
  duodenal 536.8
  eczema (*see also* Varix, with stasis dermatitis) 454.1
  edema (*see also* Hypertension, venous) 459.30
  foot 991.4
  gastric 536.3
  ileocecal coil 564.89
  ileum 564.89
  intestinal 564.89
  jejunum 564.89
  kidney 586
  liver 571.9
    cirrhotic—*see* Cirrhosis, liver
  lymphatic 457.8
  pneumonia 514
  portal 571.9
  pulmonary 514
  rectal 564.89
  renal 586
    tubular 584.5
  stomach 536.3
  ulcer
    with varicose veins 454.0
    without varicose veins 459.81
  urine NEC (*see also* Retention, urine) 788.20
  venous 459.81
State
  affective and paranoid, mixed, organic psychotic 294.8
  agitated 307.9
    acute reaction to stress 308.2

State—*continued*
  anxiety (neurotic) (*see also* Anxiety) 300.00
    specified type NEC 300.09
  apprehension (*see also* Anxiety) 300.00
    specified type NEC 300.09
  climacteric, female 627.2
    following induced menopause 627.4
  clouded
    epileptic (*see also* Epilepsy) 345.9
    paroxysmal (idiopathic) (*see also* Epilepsy) 345.9
  compulsive (mixed) (with obsession) 300.3
  confusional 298.9
    acute 293.0
      with
        arteriosclerotic dementia 290.41
        presenile brain disease 290.11
        senility 290.3
        alcoholic 291.0
        drug-induced 292.81
      epileptic 293.0
      postoperative 293.9
      reactive (emotional stress) (psychological trauma) 298.2
      subacute 293.1
  constitutional psychopathic 301.9
  convulsive (*see also* Convulsions) 780.39
  depressive NEC 311
    induced by drug 292.84
    neurotic 300.4
  dissociative 300.15
  hallucinatory 780.1
    induced by drug 292.12
  hypercoagulable (primary) 289.81
    secondary 289.82
  hyperdynamic beta-adrenergic circulatory 429.82
  locked-in 344.81
  menopausal 627.2
    artificial 627.4
    following induced menopause 627.4
  neurotic NEC 300.9
    with depersonalization episode 300.6
  obsessional 300.3
  oneiroid (*see also* Schizophrenia) 295.4
  panic 300.01
  paranoid 297.9
    alcohol-induced 291.5
    arteriosclerotic 290.42
    climacteric 297.2
    drug-induced 292.11
    in
      presenile brain disease 290.12
      senile brain disease 290.20
    involutional 297.2
    menopausal 297.2
    senile 290.20
    simple 297.0
  postleukotomy 310.0
  pregnant (*see also* Pregnancy) V22.2
  psychogenic, twilight 298.2
  psychotic, organic (*see also* Psychosis, organic) 294.9
    mixed paranoid and affective 294.8
    senile or presenile NEC 290.9
    transient NEC 293.9
      with
        anxiety 293.84
        delusions 293.81
        depression 293.83
        hallucinations 293.82

State—*continued*
  residual schizophrenic (*see also* Schizophrenia) 295.6
  tension (*see also* Anxiety) 300.9
  transient organic psychotic 293.9
    anxiety type 293.84
    depressive type 293.83
    hallucinatory type 293.83
    paranoid type 293.81
    specified type NEC 293.89
  twilight
    epileptic 293.0
    psychogenic 298.2
  vegetative (persistent) 780.03
Status (post)
  absence
    epileptic (*see also* Epilepsy) 345.2
    of organ, acquired (postsurgical)—*see* Absence, by site, acquired
  anastomosis of intestine (for bypass) V45.3
  angioplasty, percutaneous transluminal coronary V45.82
  anginosus 413.9
  ankle prosthesis V43.66
  aortocoronary bypass or shunt V45.81
  arthrodesis V45.4
  artificially induced condition NEC V45.89
  artificial opening (of) V44.9
    gastrointestinal tract NEC V44.4
    specified site NEC V44.8
    urinary tract NEC V44.6
    vagina V44.7
  aspirator V46.0
  asthmaticus (*see also* Asthma) 493.9
  awaiting organ transplant V49.83
  bariatric surgery V45.86
    complicating pregnancy, childbirth, or the puerperium 649.2
  bed confinement V49.84
  breast implant removal V45.83
  cardiac
    device (in situ) V45.00
      defibrillator, automatic implantable V45.02
      pacemaker V45.01
        fitting or adjustment V53.3
      carotid sinus V45.09
        fitting or adjustment V53.3
  carotid sinus stimulator V45.09
  cataract extraction V45.61
  chemotherapy V66.2
    current V58.69
  circumcision, female 629.20
  clitorectomy (female genital mutilation type I) 629.21
    with excision of labia minora (female genital mutilation type II) 629.22
  colostomy V44.3
  contraceptive device V45.59
    intrauterine V45.51
    subdermal V45.52
  convulsivus idiopathicus (*see also* Epilepsy) 345.3
  coronary artery bypass or shunt V45.81
  cutting
    female genital 629.20
      specified NEC 629.29
      type I 629.21
      type II 629.22
      type III 629.23
      type IV 629.29

Status

Status—*continued*
  cystostomy V44.50
    appendico-vesicostomy V44.52
    cutaneous-vesicostomy V44.51
    specified type NEC V44.59
  defibrillator, automatic implantable cardiac V45.02
  dental crowns V45.84
  dental fillings V45.84
  dental restoration V45.84
  dental sealant V49.82
  dialysis (hemo) (peritoneal) V45.1
  donor V59.9
  drug therapy or regimen V67.59
    high-risk medication NEC V67.51
  elbow prosthesis V43.62
  enterostomy V44.4
  epileptic, epilepticus (absence) (grand mal) (*see also* Epilepsy) 345.3
    focal motor 345.7
    partial 345.7
    petit mal 345.2
    psychomotor 345.7
    temporal lobe 345.7
  estrogen receptor
    negative [ER-] V86.1
    positive [ER+] V86.0
  eye (adnexa) surgery V45.69
  female genital
    cutting 629.20
      specified NEC 629.29
      type I 629.21
      type II 629.22
      type III 629.23
      type IV 629.29
    mutilation 629.20
      type IV 629.29
  filtering bleb (eye) (postglaucoma) V45.69
    with rupture or complication 997.99
    postcataract extraction (complication) 997.99
  finger joint prosthesis V43.69
  gastric
    banding V45.86
      complicating pregnancy, childbirth, or the puerperium 649.2
    bypass for obesity V45.86
      complicating pregnancy, childbirth, or the puerperium 649.2
  gastrostomy V44.1
  grand mal 345.3
  heart valve prosthesis V43.3
  hemodialysis V45.1
  hip prosthesis (joint) (partial) (total) V43.64
  ileostomy V44.2
  infibulation (female genital mutilation type III) 629.23
  insulin pump V45.85
  intestinal bypass V45.3
  intrauterine contraceptive device V45.51
  jejunostomy V44.4
  knee joint prosthesis V43.65
  lacunaris 437.8
  lacunosis 437.8
  low birth weight V21.30
    less than 500 grams V21.31
    500-999 grams V21.32
    1000-1499 grams V21.33
    1500-1999 grams V21.34
    2000-2500 grams V21.35
  lymphaticus 254.8

Status—*continued*
  malignant neoplasm, ablated or excised—*see* History, malignant neoplasm
  marmoratus 333.79
  mutilation, female 629.20
    type I 629.21
    type II 629.22
    type III 629.23
    type IV 629.29
  nephrostomy V44.6
  neuropacemaker NEC V45.89
    brain V45.89
    carotid sinus V45.09
    neurologic NEC V45.89
  obesity surgery V45.86
    complicating pregnancy, childbirth, or the puerperium 649.2
  organ replacement
    by artificial or mechanical device or prosthesis of
      artery V43.4
      artificial skin V43.83
      bladder V43.5
      blood vessel V43.4
      breast V43.82
      eye globe V43.0
      heart
        assist device V43.21
        fully implantable artificial heart V43.22
        valve V43.3
      intestine V43.89
      joint V43.60
        ankle V43.66
        elbow V43.62
        finger V43.69
        hip (partial) (total) V43.64
        knee V43.65
        shoulder V43.61
        specified NEC 43.69
        wrist V43.63
      kidney V43.89
      larynx V43.81
      lens V43.1
      limb(s) V43.7
      liver V43.89
      lung V43.89
      organ NEC V43.89
      pancreas V43.89
      skin (artificial) V43.83
      tissue NEC V43.89
      vein V43.4
    by organ transplant (heterologous) (homologous)—*see* Status, transplant
  pacemaker
    brain V45.89
    cardiac V45.01
    carotid sinus V45.09
    neurologic NEC V45.89
    specified site NEC V45.89
  percutaneous transluminal coronary angioplasty V45.82
  peritoneal dialysis V45.1
  petit mal 345.2
  postcommotio cerebri 310.2
  postmenopausal (age related) (natural) V49.81
  postoperative NEC V45.89
  postpartum NEC V24.2
    care immediately following delivery V24.0
    routine follow-up V24.2
  postsurgical NEC V45.89
  renal dialysis V45.1

INDEX TO DISEASES — Stenosis

Status—*continued*
  respirator (ventilator) V46.11
    encounter
      during
        mechanical failure V46.14
        power failure V46.12
      for weaning V46.13
  reversed jejunal transposition (for bypass) V45.3
  sex reassignment surgery status (*see also* Tran-sexualism) 302.50
  shoulder prosthesis V43.61
  shunt
    aortocoronary bypass V45.81
    arteriovenous (for dialysis) V45.1
    cerebrospinal fluid V45.2
    vascular NEC V45.89
      aortocoronary (bypass) V45.81
    ventricular (communicating) (for drainage) V45.2
  sterilization
    tubal ligation V26.51
    vasectomy V26.52
  subdermal contraceptive device V45.52
  thymicolymphaticus 254.8
  thymicus 254.8
  thymolymphaticus 254.8
  tooth extraction 525.10
  tracheostomy V44.0
  transplant
    blood vessel V42.89
    bone V42.4
      marrow V42.81
    cornea V42.5
    heart V42.1
      valve V42.2
    intestine V42.84
    kidney V42.0
    liver V42.7
    lung V42.6
    organ V42.9
      specified site NEC V42.89
    pancreas V42.83
    peripheral stem cells V42.82
    skin V42.3
    stem cells, peripheral V42.82
    tissue V42.9
      specified type NEC V42.89
    vessel, blood V42.89
  tubal ligation V26.51
  ureterostomy V44.6
  urethrostomy V44.6
  vagina, artificial V44.7
  vasectomy V26.52
  vascular shunt NEC V45.89
    aortocoronary (bypass) V45.81
  ventilator (respirator) V46.11
    encounter
      during
        mechanical failure V46.14
        power failure V46.12
      for weaning V46.13
  wrist prosthesis V43.63
Stave fracture —*see* Fracture, metacarpus, metacarpal bone(s)
Steal
  subclavian artery 435.2
  vertebral artery 435.1
Stealing, solitary, child problem (*see also* Disturbance, conduct) 312.1
Steam burn —*see* Burn, by site
Steatocystoma multiplex 706.2

Steatoma (infected) 706.2
  eyelid (cystic) 374.84
    infected 373.13
Steatorrhea (chronic) 579.8
  with lacteal obstruction 579.2
  idiopathic 579.0
    adult 579.0
    infantile 579.0
  pancreatic 579.4
  primary 579.0
  secondary 579.8
  specified cause NEC 579.8
  tropical 579.1
Steatosis 272.8
  heart (*see also* Degeneration, myocardial) 429.1
  kidney 593.89
  liver 571.8
Steele-Richardson (-Olszewski) Syndrome 333.0
Stein's syndrome (polycystic ovary) 256.4
Stein-Leventhal syndrome (polycystic ovary) 256.4
Steinbrocker's syndrome (*see also* Neuropathy, peripheral, autonomic) 337.9
Steinert's disease 359.21
STEMI (ST elevation myocardial infarction) (*see also* Infarct, myocardium, ST elevation) 410.9
Stenocardia (*see also* Angina) 413.9
Stenocephaly 756.0
Stenosis (cicatricial)—*see also* Stricture
  ampulla of Vater 576.2
    with calculus, cholelithiasis, or stones—*see* Choledocholithiasis
  anus, anal (canal) (sphincter) 569.2
    congenital 751.2
  aorta (ascending) 747.22
    arch 747.10
    arteriosclerotic 440.0
    calcified 440.0
  aortic (valve) 424.1
    with
      mitral (valve)
        insufficiency or incompetence 396.2
        stenosis or obstruction 396.0
    atypical 396.0
    congenital 746.3
    rheumatic 395.0
      with
        insufficiency, incompetency or regurgitation 395.2
          with mitral (valve) disease 396.8
        mitral (valve)
          disease (stenosis) 396.0
          insufficiency or incompetence 396.2
          stenosis or obstruction 396.0
    specified cause, except rheumatic 424.1
    syphilitic 093.22
  aqueduct of Sylvius (congenital) 742.3
    with spina bifida (*see also* Spina bifida) 741.0
    acquired 331.4
  artery NEC (*see also* Arteriosclerosis) 447.1
    basilar—*see* Narrowing, artery, basilar
    carotid (common) (internal)—*see* Narrowing, artery, carotid
    celiac 447.4
    cerebral 437.0
      due to
        embolism (*see also* Embolism, brain) 434.1
        thrombus (*see also* Thrombosis, brain) 434.0
    extremities 440.20

1331

Stenosis—*continued*
  precerebral—*see* Narrowing, artery, precerebral
  pulmonary (congenital) 747.3
    acquired 417.8
  renal 440.1
  vertebral—*see* Narrowing, artery, vertebral
  bile duct or biliary passage (*see also* Obstruction, biliary) 576.2
    congenital 751.61
  bladder neck (acquired) 596.0
    congenital 753.6
  brain 348.8
  bronchus 519.19
    syphilitic 095.8
  cardia (stomach) 537.89
    congenital 750.7
  cardiovascular (*see also* Disease, cardiovascular) 429.2
  carotid artery—*see* Narrowing, artery, carotid
  cervix, cervical (canal) 622.4
    congenital 752.49
    in pregnancy or childbirth 654.6
      affecting fetus or newborn 763.89
      causing obstructed labor 660.2
        affecting fetus or newborn 763.1
  colon (*see also* Obstruction, intestine) 560.9
    congenital 751.2
  colostomy 569.62
  common bile duct (*see also* Obstruction, biliary) 576.2
    congenital 751.61
  coronary (artery) —*see* Arteriosclerosis, coronary
  cystic duct (*see also* Obstruction, gallbladder) 575.2
    congenital 751.61
  due to (presence of) any device, implant, or graft classifiable to 996.0-996.5—*see* Complications, due to (presence of) any device, implant, or graft classified to 996.0-996.5 NEC
  duodenum 537.3
    congenital 751.1
  ejaculatory duct NEC 608.89
  endocervical os—*see* Stenosis, cervix
  enterostomy 569.62
  esophagostomy 530.87
  esophagus 530.3
    congenital 750.3
    syphilitic 095.8
      congenital 090.5
  external ear canal 380.50
    secondary to
      inflammation 380.53
      surgery 380.52
      trauma 380.51
  gallbladder (*see also* Obstruction, gallbladder) 575.2
  glottis 478.74
  heart valve (acquired)—*see also* Endocarditis
    congenital NEC 746.89
      aortic 746.3
      mitral 746.5
      pulmonary 746.02
      tricuspid 746.1
  hepatic duct (*see also* Obstruction, biliary) 576.2
  hymen 623.3
  hypertrophic subaortic (idiopathic) 425.1
  infundibulum cardiac 746.83

Stenosis—*continued*
  intestine (*see also* Obstruction, intestine) 560.9
    congenital (small) 751.1
      large 751.2
  lacrimal
    canaliculi 375.53
    duct 375.56
      congenital 743.65
    punctum 375.52
      congenital 743.65
    sac 375.54
      congenital 743.65
  lacrimonasal duct 375.56
    congenital 743.65
    neonatal 375.55
  larynx 478.74
    congenital 748.3
    syphilitic 095.8
      congenital 090.5
  mitral (valve) (chronic) (inactive) 394.0
    with
      aortic (valve)
        disease (insufficiency) 396.1
        insufficiency or incompetence 396.1
        stenosis or obstruction 396.0
      incompetency, insufficiency or regurgitation 394.2
        with aortic valve disease 396.8
      active or acute 391.1
        with chorea (acute) (rheumatic) (Sydenham's) 392.0
    congenital 746.5
    specified cause, except rheumatic 424.0
    syphilitic 093.21
  myocardium, myocardial (*see also* Degeneration, myocardial) 429.1
    hypertrophic subaortic (idiopathic) 425.1
  nares (anterior) (posterior) 478.19
    congenital 748.0
  nasal duct 375.56
    congenital 743.65
  nasolacrimal duct 375.56
    congenital 743.65
    neonatal 375.55
  organ or site, congenital NEC—*see* Atresia
  papilla of Vater 576.2
    with calculus, cholelithiasis, or stones—*see* Choledocholithiasis
  pulmonary (artery) (congenital) 747.3
    with ventricular septal defect, dextraposition of aorta and hypertrophy of right ventricle 745.2
    acquired 417.8
    infundibular 746.83
    in tetralogy of Fallot 745.2
    subvalvular 746.83
    valve (*see also* Endocarditis, pulmonary) 424.3
      congenital 746.02
    vein 747.49
      acquired 417.8
    vessel NEC 417.8
  pulmonic (congenital) 746.02
    infundibular 746.83
    subvalvular 746.83
  pylorus (hypertrophic) 537.0
    adult 537.0
    congenital 750.5
    infantile 750.5
  rectum (sphincter) (*see also* Stricture, rectum) 569.2

Stenosis—*continued*
  renal artery 440.1
  salivary duct (any) 527.8
  sphincter of Oddi (*see also* Obstruction, biliary) 576.2
  spinal 724.00
    cervical 723.0
    lumbar, lumbosacral 724.02
    nerve (root) NEC 724.9
    specified region NEC 724.09
    thoracic, thoracolumbar 724.01
  stomach, hourglass 537.6
  subaortic 746.81
    hypertrophic (idiopathic) 425.1
  supra (valvular)-aortic 747.22
  trachea 519.19
    congenital 748.3
    syphilitic 095.8
    tuberculous (*see also* Tuberculosis) 012.8
  tracheostomy 519.02
  tricuspid (valve) (*see also* Endocarditis, tricuspid) 397.0
    congenital 746.1
    nonrheumatic 424.2
  tubal 628.2
  ureter (*see also* Stricture, ureter) 593.3
    congenital 753.29
  urethra (*see also* Stricture, urethra) 598.9
  vagina 623.2
    congenital 752.49
    in pregnancy or childbirth 654.7
      affecting fetus or newborn 763.89
      causing obstructed labor 660.2
        affecting fetus or newborn 763.1
  valve (cardiac) (heart) (*see also* Endocarditis) 424.90
    congenital NEC 746.89
      aortic 746.3
      mitral 746.5
      pulmonary 746.02
      tricuspid 746.1
      urethra 753.6
  valvular (*see also* Endocarditis) 424.90
    congenital NEC 746.89
      urethra 753.6
  vascular graft or shunt 996.1
    atherosclerosis —*see* Arteriosclerosis, extremities
    embolism 996.74
    occlusion NEC 996.74
    thrombus 996.74
  vena cava (inferior) (superior) 459.2
    congenital 747.49
  ventricular shunt 996.2
  vulva 624.8
Stercolith (*see also* Fecalith) 560.39
  appendix 543.9
Stercoraceous, stercoral ulcer 569.82
  anus or rectum 569.41
Stereopsis, defective
  with fusion 368.33
  without fusion 368.32
Stereotypies NEC 307.3
Sterility
  female—*see* Infertility, female
  male (*see also* Infertility, male) 606.9
Sterilization, admission for V25.2
  status
    tubal ligation V26.51
    vasectomy V26.52
Sternalgia (*see also* Angina) 413.9
Sternopagus 759.4

Sternum bifidum 756.3
Sternutation 784.99
Steroid
  effects (adverse) (iatrogenic)
    cushingoid
      correct substance properly administered 255.0
      overdose or wrong substance given or taken 962.0
    diabetes
      correct substance properly administered 251.8
      overdose or wrong substance given or taken 962.0
    due to
      correct substance properly administered 255.8
      overdose or wrong substance given or taken 962.0
    fever
      correct substance properly administered 780.6
      overdose or wrong substance given or taken 962.0
    withdrawal
      correct substance properly administered 255.41
      overdose or wrong substance given or taken 962.0
  responder 365.03
Stevens-Johnson disease or syndrome (erythema multiforme exudativum) 695.1
Stewart-Morel syndrome (hyperostosis frontalis interna) 733.3
Sticker's disease (erythema infectiosum) 057.0
Stickler syndrome 759.89
Sticky eye 372.03
Stieda's disease (calcification, knee joint) 726.62
Stiff
  back 724.8
  neck (*see also* Torticollis) 723.5
Stiff-baby 759.89
Stiff-man syndrome 333.91
Stiffness, joint NEC 719.50
  ankle 719.57
  back 724.8
  elbow 719.52
  finger 719.54
  hip 719.55
  knee 719.56
  multiple sites 719.59
  sacroiliac 724.6
  shoulder 719.51
  specified site NEC 719.58
  spine 724.9
  surgical fusion V45.4
  wrist 719.53
Stigmata, congenital syphilis 090.5
Still's disease or syndrome 714.30
Still-Felty syndrome (rheumatoid arthritis with splenomegaly and leukopenia) 714.1
Stillbirth, stillborn NEC 779.9
Stiller's disease (asthenia) 780.79
Stilling-Türk-Duane syndrome (ocular retraction syndrome) 378.71
Stimulation, ovary 256.1
Sting (animal) (bee) (fish) (insect) (jellyfish) (Portuguese man-o-war) (wasp) (venomous) 989.5
  anaphylactic shock or reaction 989.5
  plant 692.6
Stippled epiphyses 756.59

Stitch
abscess 998.59
burst (in external operation wound) 998.32
  internal 998.31
in back 724.5
Stojano's (subcostal) syndrome 098.86
Stokes' disease (exophthalmic goiter) 242.0
Stokes-Adams syndrome (syncope with heart block) 426.9
Stokvis' (-Talma) disease (enterogenous cyanosis) 289.7
Stomach —see condition
Stoma malfunction
colostomy 569.62
cystostomy 997.5
enterostomy 569.62
esophagostomy 530.87
gastrostomy 536.42
ileostomy 569.62
nephrostomy 997.5
tracheostomy 519.02
ureterostomy 997.5
Stomatitis 528.00
angular 528.5
due to dietary or vitamin deficiency 266.0
aphthous 528.2
candidal 112.0
catarrhal 528.00
denture 528.9
diphtheritic (membranous) 032.0
due to
  dietary deficiency 266.0
  thrush 112.0
  vitamin deficiency 266.0
epidemic 078.4
epizootic 078.4
follicular 528.00
gangrenous 528.1
herpetic 054.2
herpetiformis 528.2
malignant 528.00
membranous acute 528.00
monilial 112.0
mycotic 112.0
necrotic 528.1
  ulcerative 101
necrotizing ulcerative 101
parasitic 112.0
septic 528.00
specified NEC 528.09
spirochetal 101
suppurative (acute) 528.00
ulcerative 528.00
  necrotizing 101
ulceromembranous 101
vesicular 528.00
  with exanthem 074.3
Vincent's 101
Stomatocytosis 282.8
Stomatomycosis 112.0
Stomatorrhagia 528.9
Stone(s) —see also Calculus
bladder 594.1
  diverticulum 594.0
cystine 270.0
heart syndrome (see also Failure, ventricular, left) 428.1
kidney 592.0
prostate 602.0
pulp (dental) 522.2
renal 592.0

Stone(s)—continued
salivary duct or gland (any) 527.5
ureter 592.1
urethra (impacted) 594.2
urinary (duct) (impacted) (passage) 592.9
  bladder 594.1
    diverticulum 594.0
  lower tract NEC 594.9
  specified site 594.8
xanthine 277.2
Stonecutters' lung 502
tuberculous (see also Tuberculosis) 011.4
Stonemasons'
asthma, disease, or lung 502
tuberculous (see also Tuberculosis) 011.4
phthisis (see also Tuberculosis) 011.4
Stoppage
bowel (see also Obstruction, intestine) 560.9
heart (see also Arrest, cardiac) 427.5
intestine (see also Obstruction, intestine) 560.9
urine NEC (see also Retention, urine) 788.20
Storm, thyroid (apathetic) (see also Thyrotoxicosis) 242.9
Strabismus (alternating) (congenital) (nonparalytic) 378.9
concomitant (see also Heterotropia) 378.30
convergent (see also Esotropia) 378.00
divergent (see also Exotropia) 378.10
convergent (see also Esotropia) 378.00
divergent (see also Exotropia) 378.10
due to adhesions, scars—see Strabismus, mechanical
in neuromuscular disorder NEC 378.73
  intermittent 378.20
    vertical 378.31
latent 378.40
  convergent (esophoria) 378.41
  divergent (exophoria) 378.42
  vertical 378.43
mechanical 378.60
  due to
    Brown's tendon sheath syndrome 378.61
    specified musculofascial disorder NEC 378.62
paralytic 378.50
  third or oculomotor nerve (partial) 378.51
    total 378.52
  fourth or trochlear nerve 378.53
  sixth or abducens nerve 378.54
specified type NEC 378.73
vertical (hypertropia) 378.31
Strain —see also Sprain, by site
eye NEC 368.13
heart—see Disease, heart
meaning gonorrhea—see Gonorrhea
on urination 788.65
physical NEC V62.89
postural 729.9
psychological NEC V62.89
Strands
conjunctiva 372.62
vitreous humor 379.25
Strangulation, strangulated 994.7
appendix 543.9
asphyxiation or suffocation by 994.7
bladder neck 596.0
bowel—see Strangulation, intestine
colon—see Strangulation, intestine
cord (umbilical)—see Compression, umbilical cord
due to birth injury 767.8

INDEX TO DISEASES

Strangulation, strangulated—*continued*
  food or foreign body (*see also* Asphyxia, food) 933.1
  hemorrhoids 455.8
    external 455.5
    internal 455.2
  hernia—*see also* Hernia, by site, with obstruction
    gangrenous—*see* Hernia, by site, with gangrene
  intestine (large) (small) 560.2
    with hernia—*see also* Hernia, by site, with obstruction
      gangrenous—*see* Hernia, by site, with gangrene
    congenital (small) 751.1
      large 751.2
  mesentery 560.2
  mucus (*see also* Asphyxia, mucus) 933.1
    newborn 770.18
  omentum 560.2
  organ or site, congenital NEC—*see* Atresia
  ovary 620.8
    due to hernia 620.4
  penis 607.89
    foreign body 939.3
  rupture (*see also* Hernia, by site, with obstruction) 552.9
    gangrenous (*see also* Hernia, by site, with gangrene) 551.9
  stomach, due to hernia (*see also* Hernia, by site, with obstruction) 552.9
    with gangrene (*see also* Hernia, by site, with gangrene) 551.9
  umbilical cord—*see* Compression, umbilical cord
  vesicourethral orifice 596.0

Strangury 788.1

Strawberry
  gallbladder (*see also* Disease, gallbladder) 575.6
  mark 757.32
  tongue (red) (white) 529.3

Straw itch 133.8

Streak, ovarian 752.0

Strephosymbolia 315.01
  secondary to organic lesion 784.69

Streptobacillary fever 026.1

Streptobacillus moniliformis 026.1

Streptococcemia 038.0

Streptococcicosis —*see* Infection, streptococcal

Streptococcus, streptococcal —*see* condition

Streptoderma 686.00

Streptomycosis —*see* Actinomycosis

Streptothricosis —*see* Actinomycosis

Streptothrix —*see* Actinomycosis

Streptotrichosis —*see* Actinomycosis

Stress 308.9
  fracture—*see* Fracture, stress
  polycythemia 289.0
  reaction (gross) (*see also* Reaction, stress, acute) 308.9

Stretching, nerve —*see* Injury, nerve, by site

Striae (albicantes) (atrophicae) (cutis distensae) (distensae) 701.3

Striations of nails 703.8

Stricture (*see also* Stenosis) 799.89
  ampulla of Vater 576.2
    with calculus, cholelithiasis, or stones—*see* Choledocholithiasis

Stricture—*continued*
  anus (sphincter) 569.2
    congenital 751.2
    infantile 751.2
  aorta (ascending) 747.22
    arch 747.10
    arteriosclerotic 440.0
    calcified 440.0
  aortic (valve) (*see also* Stenosis, aortic) 424.1
    congenital 746.3
  aqueduct of Sylvius (congenital) 742.3
    with spina bifida (*see also* Spina bifida) 741.0
    acquired 331.4
  artery 447.1
    basilar—*see* Narrowing, artery, basilar
    carotid (common) (internal)—*see* Narrowing, artery, carotid
    celiac 447.4
    cerebral 437.0
      congenital 747.81
      due to
        embolism (*see also* Embolism, brain) 434.1
        thrombus (*see also* Thrombosis, brain) 434.0
    congenital (peripheral) 747.60
      cerebral 747.81
      coronary 746.85
      gastrointestinal 747.61
      lower limb 747.64
      renal 747.62
      retinal 743.58
      specified NEC 747.69
      spinal 747.82
      umbilical 747.5
      upper limb 747.63
    coronary —*see* Arteriosclerosis, coronary
      congenital 746.85
    precerebral—*see* Narrowing, artery, precerebral NEC
    pulmonary (congenital) 747.3
      acquired 417.8
    renal 440.1
    vertebral—*see* Narrowing, artery, vertebral
  auditory canal (congenital) (external) 744.02
    acquired (*see also* Stricture, ear canal, acquired) 380.50
  bile duct or passage (any) (postoperative) (*see also* Obstruction, biliary) 576.2
    congenital 751.61
  bladder 596.8
    congenital 753.6
    neck 596.0
      congenital 753.6
  bowel (*see also* Obstruction, intestine) 560.9
  brain 348.8
  bronchus 519.19
    syphilitic 095.8
  cardia (stomach) 537.89
    congenital 750.7
  cardiac—*see also* Disease, heart
    orifice (stomach) 537.89
  cardiovascular (*see also* Disease, cardiovascular) 429.2
  carotid artery—*see* Narrowing, artery, carotid
  cecum (*see also* Obstruction, intestine) 560.9
  cervix, cervical (canal) 622.4
    congenital 752.49
    in pregnancy or childbirth 654.6
      affecting fetus or newborn 763.89
      causing obstructed labor 660.2
        affecting fetus or newborn 763.1

Stricture

Stricture—*continued*
  colon (*see also* Obstruction, intestine) 560.9
    congenital 751.2
  colostomy 569.62
  common bile duct (*see also* Obstruction, biliary) 576.2
    congenital 751.61
  coronary (artery) —*see* Arteriosclerosis, coronary
    congenital 746.85
  cystic duct (*see also* Obstruction, gallbladder) 575.2
    congenital 751.61
  cystostomy 997.5
  digestive organs NEC, congenital 751.8
  duodenum 537.3
    congenital 751.1
  ear canal (external) (congenital) 744.02
    acquired 380.50
      secondary to
        inflammation 380.53
        surgery 380.52
        trauma 380.51
  ejaculatory duct 608.85
  enterostomy 569.62
  esophagostomy 530.87
  esophagus (corrosive) (peptic) 530.3
    congenital 750.3
    syphilitic 095.8
      congenital 090.5
  Eustachian tube (*see also* Obstruction, Eustachian tube) 381.60
    congenital 744.24
  fallopian tube 628.2
    gonococcal (chronic) 098.37
      acute 098.17
    tuberculous (*see also* Tuberculosis) 016.6
  gallbladder (*see also* Obstruction, gallbladder) 575.2
    congenital 751.69
  glottis 478.74
  heart—*see also* Disease, heart
    congenital NEC 746.89
    valve—*see also* Endocarditis
      congenital NEC 746.89
        aortic 746.3
        mitral 746.5
        pulmonary 746.02
        tricuspid 746.1
  hepatic duct (*see also* Obstruction, biliary) 576.2
  hourglass, of stomach 537.6
  hymen 623.3
  hypopharynx 478.29
  intestine (*see also* Obstruction, intestine) 560.9
    congenital (small) 751.1
      large 751.2
    ischemic 557.1
  lacrimal
    canaliculi 375.53
      congenital 743.65
    punctum 375.52
      congenital 743.65
    sac 375.54
      congenital 743.65
  lacrimonasal duct 375.56
    congenital 743.65
    neonatal 375.55
  larynx 478.79
    congenital 748.3
    syphilitic 095.8
      congenital 090.5

Stricture—*continued*
  lung 518.89
  meatus
    ear (congenital) 744.02
      acquired (*see also* Stricture, ear canal, acquired) 380.50
    osseous (congenital) (ear) 744.03
      acquired (*see also* Stricture, ear canal, acquired) 380.50
    urinarius (*see also* Stricture, urethra) 598.9
      congenital 753.6
  mitral (valve) (*see also* Stenosis, mitral) 394.0
    congenital 746.5
    specified cause, except rheumatic 424.0
  myocardium, myocardial (*see also* Degeneration, myocardial) 429.1
    hypertrophic subaortic (idiopathic) 425.1
  nares (anterior) (posterior) 478.19
    congenital 748.0
  nasal duct 375.56
    congenital 743.65
    neonatal 375.55
  nasolacrimal duct 375.56
    congenital 743.65
    neonatal 375.55
  nasopharynx 478.29
    syphilitic 095.8
  nephrostomy 997.5
  nose 478.19
    congenital 748.0
  nostril (anterior) (posterior) 478.19
    congenital 748.0
  organ or site, congenital NEC—*see* Atresia
  osseous meatus (congenital) (ear) 744.03
    acquired (*see also* Stricture, ear canal, acquired) 380.50
  os uteri (*see also* Stricture, cervix) 622.4
  oviduct—*see* Stricture, fallopian tube
  pelviureteric junction 593.3
  pharynx (dilation) 478.29
  prostate 602.8
  pulmonary, pulmonic
    artery (congenital) 747.3
      acquired 417.8
      noncongenital 417.8
    infundibulum (congenital) 746.83
    valve (*see also* Endocarditis, pulmonary) 424.3
      congenital 746.02
    vein (congenital) 747.49
      acquired 417.8
    vessel NEC 417.8
  punctum lacrimale 375.52
    congenital 743.65
  pylorus (hypertrophic) 537.0
    adult 537.0
    congenital 750.5
    infantile 750.5
  rectosigmoid 569.89
  rectum (sphincter) 569.2
    congenital 751.2
    due to
      chemical burn 947.3
      irradiation 569.2
      lymphogranuloma venereum 099.1
    gonococcal 098.7
    inflammatory 099.1
    syphilitic 095.8
    tuberculous (*see also* Tuberculosis) 014.8
  renal artery 440.1
  salivary duct or gland (any) 527.8

INDEX TO DISEASES   Struma

Stricture—*continued*
  sigmoid (flexure) (*see also* Obstruction, intestine) 560.9
  spermatic cord 608.85
  stoma (following) (of)
    colostomy 569.62
    cystostomy 997.5
    enterostomy 569.62
    esophagostomy 530.87
    gastrostomy 536.42
    ileostomy 569.62
    nephrostomy 997.5
    tracheostomy 519.02
    ureterostomy 997.5
  stomach 537.89
    congenital 750.7
    hourglass 537.6
  subaortic 746.81
    hypertrophic (acquired) (idiopathic) 425.1
  subglottic 478.74
  syphilitic NEC 095.8
  tendon (sheath) 727.81
  trachea 519.19
    congenital 748.3
    syphilitic 095.8
    tuberculous (*see also* Tuberculosis) 012.8
  tracheostomy 519.02
  tricuspid (valve) (*see also* Endocarditis, tricuspid) 397.0
    congenital 746.1
    nonrheumatic 424.2
  tunica vaginalis 608.85
  ureter (postoperative) 593.3
    congenital 753.29
    tuberculous (*see also* Tuberculosis) 016.2
  ureteropelvic junction 593.3
    congenital 753.21
  ureterovesical orifice 593.3
    congenital 753.22
  urethra (anterior) (meatal) (organic) (posterior) (spasmodic) 598.9
    associated with schistosomiasis (*see also* Schistosomiasis) 120.9 *[598.01]*
    congenital (valvular) 753.6
    due to
      infection 598.00
        syphilis 095.8 *[598.01]*
        trauma 598.1
      gonococcal 098.2 *[598.01]*
      gonorrheal 098.2 *[598.01]*
    infective 598.00
    late effect of injury 598.1
    postcatheterization 598.2
    postobstetric 598.1
    postoperative 598.2
    specified cause NEC 598.8
    syphilitic 095.8 *[598.01]*
    traumatic 598.1
    valvular, congenital 753.6
  urinary meatus (*see also* Stricture, urethra) 598.9
    congenital 753.6
  uterus, uterine 621.5
    os (external) (internal)—see Stricture, cervix
  vagina (outlet) 623.2
    congenital 752.49
  valve (cardiac) (heart) (*see also* Endocarditis) 424.90
    congenital (cardiac) (heart) NEC 746.89
      aortic 746.3
      mitral 746.5

Stricture—*continued*
  pulmonary 746.02
  tricuspid 746.1
  urethra 753.6
  valvular (*see also* Endocarditis) 424.90
  vascular graft or shunt 996.1
    atherosclerosis —*see* Arteriosclerosis, extremities
    embolism 996.74
    occlusion NEC 996.74
    thrombus 996.74
  vas deferens 608.85
    congenital 752.89
  vein 459.2
  vena cava (inferior) (superior) NEC 459.2
    congenital 747.49
  ventricular shunt 996.2
  vesicourethral orifice 596.0
    congenital 753.6
  vulva (acquired) 624.8
Stridor 786.1
  congenital (larynx) 748.3
Stridulous —*see* condition
Strippling of nails 703.8
Stroke 434.91
  apoplectic (*see also* Disease, cerebrovascular, acute) 436
  brain—*see* Infarct, brain
  embolic 434.11
  epileptic—*see* Epilepsy
  healed or old V12.54
  heart—*see* Disease, heart
  heat 992.0
  hemorrhagic—*see* Hemorrhage, brain
  iatrogenic 997.02
  in evolution 434.91
  ischemic 434.91
  late effect—*see* Late effect(s) (of) cerebrovascular disease
  lightning 994.0
  paralytic—*see* Infarct, brain
  postoperative 997.02
  progressive 435.9
  thrombotic 434.01
Stromatosis, endometrial (M8931/1) 236.0
Strong pulse 785.9
Strongyloides stercoralis infestation 127.2
Strongyloidiasis 127.2
Strongyloidosis 127.2
Strongylus (gibsoni) infestation 127.7
Strophulus (newborn) 779.89
  pruriginosus 698.2
Struck by lightning 994.0
Struma (*see also* Goiter) 240.9
  fibrosa 245.3
  Hashimoto (struma lymphomatosa) 245.2
  lymphomatosa 245.2
  nodosa (simplex) 241.9
    endemic 241.9
    multinodular 241.1
    sporadic 241.9
    toxic or with hyperthyroidism 242.3
      multinodular 242.2
      uninodular 242.1
    toxicosa 242.3
      multinodular 242.2
      uninodular 242.1
    uninodular 241.0
  ovarii (M9090/0) 220
    and carcinoid (M9091/1) 236.2
    malignant (M9090/3) 183.0

1337

Struma — *continued*
  Riedel's (ligneous thyroiditis) 245.3
  scrofulous (*see also* Tuberculosis) 017.2
  tuberculous (*see also* Tuberculosis) 017.2
    abscess 017.2
    adenitis 017.2
    lymphangitis 017.2
    ulcer 017.2
Strumipriva cachexia (*see also* Hypothyroidism) 244.9
Strümpell-Marie disease or spine (ankylosing spondylitis) 720.0
Strümpell-Westphal pseudosclerosis (hepatolenticular degeneration) 275.1
Stuart's disease (congenital factor X deficiency) (*see also* Defect, coagulation) 286.3
Stuart-Prower factor deficiency (congenital factor X deficiency) (*see also* Defect, coagulation) 286.3
Students' elbow 727.2
Stuffy nose 478.19
Stump — *see also* Amputation
  cervix, cervical (healed) 622.8
Stupor 780.09
  catatonic (*see also* Schizophrenia) 295.2
  circular (*see also* Psychosis, manic-depressive, circular) 296.7
  manic 296.89
  manic-depressive (*see also* Psychosis, affective) 296.89
  mental (anergic) (delusional) 298.9
  psychogenic 298.8
  reaction to exceptional stress (transient) 308.2
  traumatic NEC — *see also* Injury, intracranial
    with spinal (cord)
      lesion — *see* Injury, spinal, by site
      shock — *see* Injury, spinal, by site
Sturge (-Weber) (-Dimitri) disease or syndrome (encephalocutaneous angiomatosis) 759.6
Sturge-Kalischer-Weber syndrome (encephalocutaneous angiomatosis) 759.6
Stuttering 307.0
Sty, stye 373.11
  external 373.11
  internal 373.12
  meibomian 373.12
Subacidity, gastric 536.8
  psychogenic 306.4
Subacute — *see* condition
Subarachnoid — *see* condition
Subclavian steal syndrome 435.2
Subcortical — *see* condition
Subcostal syndrome 098.86
  nerve compression 354.8
Subcutaneous, subcuticular — *see* condition
Subdelirium 293.1
Subdural — *see* condition
Subendocardium — *see* condition
Subependymoma (M9383/1) 237.5
Suberosis 495.3
Subglossitis — *see* Glossitis
Subhemophilia 286.0
Subinvolution (uterus) 621.1
  breast (postlactational) (postpartum) 611.8
  chronic 621.1
  puerperal, postpartum 674.8
Sublingual — *see* condition
Sublinguitis 527.2

Subluxation — *see also* Dislocation, by site
  congenital NEC — *see also* Malposition, congenital
  hip (unilateral) 754.32
    with dislocation of other hip 754.35
    bilateral 754.33
  joint
    lower limb 755.69
    shoulder 755.59
    upper limb 755.59
  lower limb (joint) 755.69
  shoulder (joint) 755.59
  upper limb (joint) 755.59
  lens 379.32
    anterior 379.33
    posterior 379.34
  rotary, cervical region of spine — *see* Fracture, vertebra, cervical
Submaxillary — *see* condition
Submersion (fatal) (nonfatal) 994.1
Submissiveness (undue), in child 313.0
Submucous — *see* condition
Subnormal, subnormality
  accommodation (*see also* Disorder, accommodation) 367.9
  mental (*see also* Retardation, mental) 319
    mild 317
    moderate 318.0
    profound 318.2
    severe 318.1
  temperature (accidental) 991.6
    not associated with low environmental temperature 780.99
Subphrenic — *see* condition
Subscapular nerve — *see* condition
Subseptus uterus 752.3
Subsiding appendicitis 542
Substernal thyroid (*see also* Goiter) 240.9
  congenital 759.2
Substitution disorder 300.11
Subtentorial — *see* condition
Subtertian
  fever 084.0
  malaria (fever) 084.0
Subthyroidism (acquired) (*see also* Hypothyroidism) 244.9
  congenital 243
Succenturiata placenta — *see* Placenta, abnormal
Succussion sounds, chest 786.7
Sucking thumb, child 307.9
Sudamen 705.1
Sudamina 705.1
Sudanese kala-azar 085.0
Sudden
  death, cause unknown (less than 24 hours) 798.1
    cardiac (SCD)
      family history of V17.41
      personal history of, successfully resuscitated V12.53
    during childbirth 669.9
    infant 798.0
    puerperal, postpartum 674.9
  hearing loss NEC 388.2
  heart failure (*see also* Failure, heart) 428.9
  infant death syndrome 798.0
Sudeck's atrophy, disease, or syndrome 733.7
SUDS (Sudden unexplained death) 798.2

INDEX TO DISEASES   Suppuration, suppurative

Suffocation (see also Asphyxia) 799.01
  by
    bed clothes 994.7
    bunny bag 994.7
    cave-in 994.7
    constriction 994.7
    drowning 994.1
    inhalation
      food or foreign body (see also Asphyxia, food or foreign body) 933.1
      oil or gasoline (see also Asphyxia, food or foreign body) 933.1
    overlying 994.7
    plastic bag 994.7
    pressure 994.7
    strangulation 994.7
  during birth 768.1
  mechanical 994.7
Sugar
  blood
    high 790.29
    low 251.2
  in urine 791.5
Suicide, suicidal (attempted)
  by poisoning—see Table of drugs and chemicals
  ideation V62.84
  risk 300.9
  tendencies 300.9
  trauma NEC (see also nature and site of injury) 959.9
Suipestifer infection (see also Infection, Salmonella) 003.9
Sulfatidosis 330.0
Sulfhemoglobinemia, sulphemoglobinemia (acquired) (congenital) 289.7
Sumatran mite fever 081.2
Summer —see condition
Sunburn 692.71
  dermatitis 692.71
  due to
    other ultraviolet radiation 692.82
    tanning bed 692.82
  first degree 692.71
  second degree 692.76
  third degree 692.77
Sunken
  acetabulum 718.85
  fontanels 756.0
Sunstroke 992.0
Superfecundation 651.9
  with fetal loss and retention of one or more fetus(es) 651.6
  following (elective) fetal reduction 651.7
Superfetation 651.9
  with fetal loss and retention of one or more fetus(es) 651.6
  following (elective) fetal reduction 651.7
Supernumerary (congenital)
  aortic cusps 746.89
  auditory ossicles 744.04
  bone 756.9
  breast 757.6
  carpal bones 755.56
  cusps, heart valve NEC 746.89
    mitral 746.5
    pulmonary 746.09
  digit(s) 755.00
    finger 755.01
    toe 755.02
  ear (lobule) 744.1
  fallopian tube 752.19

Supernumerary—continued
  finger 755.01
  hymen 752.49
  kidney 753.3
  lacrimal glands 743.64
  lacrimonasal duct 743.65
  lobule (ear) 744.1
  mitral cusps 746.5
  muscle 756.82
  nipples 757.6
  organ or site NEC—see Accessory
  ossicles, auditory 744.04
  ovary 752.0
  oviduct 752.19
  pulmonic cusps 746.09
  rib 756.3
    cervical or first 756.2
      syndrome 756.2
  roots (of teeth) 520.2
  spinal vertebra 756.19
  spleen 759.0
  tarsal bones 755.67
  teeth 520.1
    causing crowding 524.31
  testis 752.89
  thumb 755.01
  toe 755.02
  uterus 752.2
  vagina 752.49
  vertebra 756.19
Supervision (of)
  contraceptive method previously prescribed V25.40
    intrauterine device V25.42
    oral contraceptive (pill) V25.41
    specified type NEC V25.49
    subdermal implantable contraceptive V25.43
  dietary (for) V65.3
    allergy (food) V65.3
    colitis V65.3
    diabetes mellitus V65.3
    food allergy intolerance V65.3
    gastritis V65.3
    hypercholesterolemia V65.3
    hypoglycemia V65.3
    intolerance (food) V65.3
    obesity V65.3
    specified NEC V65.3
  lactation V24.1
  pregnancy—see Pregnancy, supervision of
Supplemental teeth 520.1
  causing crowding 524.31
Suppression
  binocular vision 368.31
  lactation 676.5
  menstruation 626.8
  ovarian secretion 256.39
  renal 586
  urinary secretion 788.5
  urine 788.5
Suppuration, suppurative —see also condition
  accessory sinus (chronic) (see also Sinusitis) 473.9
  adrenal gland 255.8
  antrum (chronic) (see also Sinusitis, maxillary) 473.0
  bladder (see also Cystitis) 595.89
  bowel 569.89
  brain 324.0
    late effect 326
  breast 611.0
    puerperal, postpartum 675.1

1339

Suppuration, suppurative—*continued*
  dental periosteum 526.5
  diffuse (skin) 686.00
  ear (middle) (*see also* Otitis media) 382.4
    external (*see also* Otitis, externa) 380.10
    internal 386.33
  ethmoidal (sinus) (chronic) (*see also* Sinusitis,
      ethmoidal) 473.2
  fallopian tube (*see also* Salpingo-oophoritis)
      614.2
  frontal (sinus) (chronic) (*see also* Sinusitis,
      frontal) 473.1
  gallbladder (*see also* Cholecystitis, acute) 575.0
  gum 523.30
  hernial sac—*see* Hernia, by site
  intestine 569.89
  joint (*see also* Arthritis, suppurative) 711.0
  labyrinthine 386.33
  lung 513.0
  mammary gland 611.0
    puerperal, postpartum 675.1
  maxilla, maxillary 526.4
    sinus (chronic) (*see also* Sinusitis, maxillary)
        473.0
  muscle 728.0
  nasal sinus (chronic) (*see also* Sinusitis) 473.9
  pancreas 577.0
  parotid gland 527.2
  pelvis, pelvic
    female (*see also* Disease, pelvis,
        inflammatory) 614.4
      acute 614.3
    male (*see also* Peritonitis) 567.21
  pericranial (*see also* Osteomyelitis) 730.2
  salivary duct or gland (any) 527.2
  sinus (nasal) (*see also* Sinusitis) 473.9
  sphenoidal (sinus) (chronic) (*see also* Sinusitis,
      sphenoidal) 473.3
  thymus (gland) 254.1
  thyroid (gland) 245.0
  tonsil 474.8
  uterus (*see also* Endometritis) 615.9
  vagina 616.10
  wound—*see also* Wound, open, by site,
      complicated
    dislocation—*see* Dislocation, by site,
        compound
    fracture—*see* Fracture, by site, open
    scratch or other superficial injury—*see* Injury,
        superficial, by site
Supraeruption, teeth 524.34
Supraglottitis 464.50
  with obstruction 464.51
Suprapubic drainage 596.8
Suprarenal (gland)—*see* condition
Suprascapular nerve —*see* condition
Suprasellar —*see* condition
Supraspinatus syndrome 726.10
Surfer knots 919.8
  infected 919.9
Surgery
  cosmetic NEC V50.1
    following healed injury or operation V51
    hair transplant V50.0
  elective V50.9
    breast augmentation reduction V50.1
    circumcision, ritual or routine (in absence of
        medical indication) V50.2
    cosmetic NEC V50.1
    ear piercing V50.3
    face-lift V50.1

Surgery—*continued*
    following healed injury or operation V51
    hair transplant V50.0
  not done because of
    contraindication V64.1
    patient's decision V64.2
    specified reason NEC V64.3
  plastic
    breast augmentation or reduction V50.1
    cosmetic V50.1
    face-lift V50.1
    following healed injury or operation V51
    repair of scarred tissue (following healed
        injury or operation) V51
    specified type NEC V50.8
  previous, in pregnancy or childbirth
    cervix 654.6
      affecting fetus or newborn 763.89
      causing obstructed labor 660.2
        affecting fetus or newborn 763.1
    pelvic soft tissues NEC 654.9
      affecting fetus or newborn 763.89
      causing obstructed labor 660.2
        affecting fetus or newborn 763.1
    perineum or vulva 654.8
    uterus NEC 654.9
      affecting fetus or newborn 763.89
      causing obstructed labor 660.2
        affecting fetus or newborn 763.1
      due to previous cesarean delivery 654.2
    vagina 654.7
Surgical
  abortion—*see* Abortion, legal
  emphysema 998.81
  kidney (*see also* Pyelitis) 590.80
  operation NEC 799.9
  procedures, complication or misadventure—*see*
      Complications, surgical procedure
  shock 998.0
Susceptibility
  genetic
    to
      MEN (multiple endocrine neoplasia) V84.81
      neoplasia
        multiple endocrine [MEN] V84.81
      neoplasm
        malignant, of
          breast V84.01
          endometrium V84.04
          other V84.09
          ovary V84.02
          prostate V84.03
      specified disease NEC V84.89
Suspected condition, ruled out (*see also*
    Observation, suspected) V71.9
  specified condition NEC V71.89
Suspended uterus, in pregnancy or childbirth
    654.4
  affecting fetus or newborn 763.89
  causing obstructed labor 660.2
    affecting fetus or newborn 763.1
Sutton's disease 709.09
Sutton and Gull's disease (arteriolar
    nephrosclerosis) (*see also* Hypertension,
    kidney) 403.90
Suture
  burst (in external operation wound) 998.32
    internal 998.31
  inadvertently left in operation wound 998.4
  removal V58.32
  Shirodkar, in pregnancy (with or without
      cervical incompetence) 654.5

INDEX TO DISEASES

Swab inadvertently left in operation wound 998.4
Swallowed, swallowing
  difficulty (*see also* Dysphagia) 787.20
  foreign body NEC (*see also* Foreign body) 938
Swamp fever 100.89
Swan neck hand (intrinsic) 736.09
Sweat (s), sweating
  disease or sickness 078.2
  excessive (*see also* Hyperhidrosis) 780.8
  fetid 705.89
  fever 078.2
  gland disease 705.9
    specified type NEC 705.89
  miliary 078.2
  night 780.8
Sweeley-Klionsky disease (angiokeratoma corporis diffusum) 272.7
Sweet's syndrome (acute febrile neutrophilic dermatosis) 695.89
Swelling 782.3
  abdominal (not referable to specific organ) 789.3
  adrenal gland, cloudy 255.8
  ankle 719.07
  anus 787.99
  arm 729.81
  breast 611.72
  Calabar 125.2
  cervical gland 785.6
  cheek 784.2
  chest 786.6
  ear 388.8
  epigastric 789.3
  extremity (lower) (upper) 729.81
  eye 379.92
  female genital organ 625.8
  finger 729.81
  foot 729.81
  glands 785.6
  gum 784.2
  hand 729.81
  head 784.2
  inflammatory—*see* Inflammation
  joint (*see also* Effusion, joint) 719.0
    tuberculous—*see* Tuberculosis, joint
  kidney, cloudy 593.89
  leg 729.81
  limb 729.81
  liver 573.8
  lung 786.6
  lymph nodes 785.6
  mediastinal 786.6
  mouth 784.2
  muscle (limb) 729.81
  neck 784.2
  nose or sinus 784.2
  palate 784.2
  pelvis 789.3
  penis 607.83
  perineum 625.8
  rectum 787.99
  scrotum 608.86
  skin 782.2
  splenic (*see also* Splenomegaly) 789.2
  substernal 786.6
  superficial, localized (skin) 782.2
  testicle 608.86
  throat 784.2
  toe 729.81
  tongue 784.2

Symptoms, specified

Swelling—*continued*
  tubular (*see also* Disease, renal) 593.9
  umbilicus 789.3
  uterus 625.8
  vagina 625.8
  vulva 625.8
  wandering, due to Gnathostoma (spinigerum) 128.1
  white—*see* Tuberculosis, arthritis
Swift's disease 985.0
Swimmers'
  ear (acute) 380.12
  itch 120.3
Swimming in the head 780.4
Swollen —*see also* Swelling
  glands 785.6
Swyer-James syndrome (unilateral hyperlucent lung) 492.8
Swyer's syndrome (XY pure gonadal dysgenesis) 752.7
Sycosis 704.8
  barbae (not parasitic) 704.8
  contagiosa 110.0
  lupoid 704.8
  mycotic 110.0
  parasitic 110.0
  vulgaris 704.8
Sydenham's chorea —*see* Chorea, Sydenham's
Sylvatic yellow fever 060.0
Sylvest's disease (epidemic pleurodynia) 074.1
Symblepharon 372.63
  congenital 743.62
Symonds' syndrome 348.2
Sympathetic —*see* condition
Sympatheticotonia (*see also* Neuropathy, peripheral, autonomic) 337.9
Sympathicoblastoma (M9500/3)
  specified site—*see* Neoplasm, by site, malignant
  unspecified site 194.0
Sympathicogonioma (M9500/3)—*see* Sympathicoblastoma
Sympathoblastoma (M9500/3)—*see* Sympathicoblastoma
Sympathogonioma (M9500/3)—*see* Sympathicoblastoma
Symphalangy (*see also* Syndactylism) 755.10
Symptoms, specified (general) NEC 780.99
  abdomen NEC 789.9
  bone NEC 733.90
  breast NEC 611.79
  cardiac NEC 785.9
  cardiovascular NEC 785.9
  chest NEC 786.9
  development NEC 783.9
  digestive system NEC 787.99
  eye NEC 379.99
  gastrointestinal tract NEC 787.99
  genital organs NEC
    female 625.9
    male 608.9
  head and neck NEC 784.99
  heart NEC 785.9
  joint NEC 719.60
    ankle 719.67
    elbow 719.62
    foot 719.67
    hand 719.64
    hip 719.65
    knee 719.66
    multiple sites 719.69
    pelvic region 719.65

1341

Symptoms, specified — INDEX TO DISEASES

Symptoms, specified — *continued*
  shoulder (region) 719.61
  specified site NEC 719.68
  wrist 719.63
larynx NEC 784.99
limbs NEC 729.89
lymphatic system NEC 785.9
menopausal 627.2
metabolism NEC 783.9
mouth NEC 528.9
muscle NEC 728.9
musculoskeletal NEC 781.99
  limbs NEC 729.89
nervous system NEC 781.99
neurotic NEC 300.9
nutrition, metabolism, and development NEC 783.9
pelvis NEC 789.9
  female 625.9
peritoneum NEC 789.9
respiratory system NEC 786.9
skin and integument NEC 782.9
subcutaneous tissue NEC 782.9
throat NEC 784.99
tonsil NEC 784.99
urinary system NEC 788.9
vascular NEC 785.9
Sympus 759.89
Synarthrosis 719.80
  ankle 719.87
  elbow 719.82
  foot 719.87
  hand 719.84
  hip 719.85
  knee 719.86
  multiple sites 719.89
  pelvic region 719.85
  shoulder (region) 719.81
  specified site NEC 719.88
  wrist 719.83
Syncephalus 759.4
Synchondrosis 756.9
  abnormal (congenital) 756.9
  ischiopubic (van Neck's) 732.1
Synchysis (senile) (vitreous humor) 379.21
  scintillans 379.22
Syncope (near) (pre-) 780.2
  anginosa 413.9
  bradycardia 427.89
  cardiac 780.2
  carotid sinus 337.0
  complicating delivery 669.2
  due to lumbar puncture 349.0
  fatal 798.1
  heart 780.2
  heat 992.1
  laryngeal 786.2
  tussive 786.2
  vasoconstriction 780.2
  vasodepressor 780.2
  vasomotor 780.2
  vasovagal 780.2
Syncytial infarct —*see* Placenta, abnormal
Syndactylism, syndactyly (multiple sites) 755.10
  fingers (without fusion of bone) 755.11
    with fusion of bone 755.12
  toes (without fusion of bone) 755.13
    with fusion of bone 755.14

Syndrome —*see also* Disease
5q minus 238.74
abdominal
  acute 789.0
  migraine 346.2
  muscle deficiency 756.79
Abercrombie's (amyloid degeneration) 277.39
abnormal innervation 374.43
abstinence
  alcohol 291.81
  drug 292.0
Abt-Letterer-Siwe (acute histiocytosis X) (M9722/3) 202.5
Achard-Thiers (adrenogenital) 255.2
acid pulmonary aspiration 997.3
  obstetric (Mendelson's) 668.0
acquired immune deficiency 042
acquired immunodeficiency 042
acrocephalosyndactylism 755.55
acute abdominal 789.0
acute chest 517.3
acute coronary 411.1
Adair-Dighton (brittle bones and blue sclera, deafness) 756.51
Adams-Stokes (-Morgagni) (syncope with heart block) 426.9
addisonian 255.41
Adie (-Holmes) (pupil) 379.46
adiposogenital 253.8
adrenal
  hemorrhage 036.3
  meningococcic 036.3
adrenocortical 255.3
adrenogenital (acquired) (congenital) 255.2
  feminizing 255.2
  iatrogenic 760.79
  virilism (acquired) (congenital) 255.2
affective organic NEC 293.89
  drug-induced 292.84
afferent loop NEC 537.89
African macroglobulinemia 273.3
Ahumada-Del Castillo (nonpuerperal galactorrhea and amenorrhea) 253.1
air blast concussion—*see* Injury, internal, by site
Alagille 759.89
Albright (-Martin) (pseudohypoparathyroidism) 275.49
Albright-McCune-Sternberg (osteitis fibrosa disseminata) 756.59
alcohol withdrawal 291.81
Alder's (leukocyte granulation anomaly) 288.2
Aldrich (-Wiskott) (eczema-thrombocytopenia) 279.12
Alibert-Bazin (mycosis, fungoides) (M9700/3) 202.1
Alice in Wonderland 293.89
Allen-Masters 620.6
Alligator baby (ichthyosis congenita) 757.1
Alport's (hereditary hematuria-nephropathy-deafness) 759.89
Alvarez (transient cerebral ischemia) 435.9
alveolar capillary block 516.3
Alzheimer's 331.0
  with dementia—*see* Alzheimer's, dementia
amnestic (confabulatory) 294.0
  alcohol-induced persisting 291.1
  drug-induced 292.83
  posttraumatic 294.0
amotivational 292.89
amyostatic 275.1
amyotrophic lateral sclerosis 335.20

1342

INDEX TO DISEASES

Syndrome

Syndrome—*continued*
androgen insensitivity 259.5
Angelman 759.89
angina (*see also* Angina) 413.9
ankyloglossia superior 750.0
anterior
  chest wall 786.52
  compartment (tibial) 958.8
  spinal artery 433.8
    compression 721.1
  tibial (compartment) 958.8
antibody deficiency 279.00
  agammaglobulinemic 279.00
  congenital 279.04
  hypogammaglobulinemic 279.00
anticardiolipin antibody 795.79
antimongolism 758.39
antiphospholipid antibody 795.79
Anton (-Babinski) (hemiasomatognosia) 307.9
anxiety (*see also* Anxiety) 300.00
  organic 293.84
aortic
  arch 446.7
  bifurcation (occlusion) 444.0
  ring 747.21
Apert's (acrocephalosyndactyly) 755.55
Apert-Gallais (adrenogenital) 255.2
aphasia-apraxia-alexia 784.69
apical ballooning 429.83
"approximate answers" 300.16
arcuate ligament (-celiac axis) 447.4
arcus aortae 446.7
arc-welders' 370.24
argentaffin, argintaffinoma 259.2
Argonz-Del Castillo (nonpuerperal galactorrhea and amenorrhea) 253.1
Argyll Robertson's (syphilitic) 094.89
  nonsyphilitic 379.45
arm-shoulder (*see also* Neuropathy, peripheral, autonomic) 337.9
Armenian 277.31
Arnold-Chiari (*see also* Spina bifida) 741.0
  type I 348.4
  type II 741.0
  type III 742.0
  type IV 742.2
Arrillaga-Ayerza (pulmonary artery sclerosis with pulmonary hypertension) 416.0
arteriomesenteric duodenum occlusion 537.89
arteriovenous steal 996.73
arteritis, young female (obliterative brachiocephalic) 446.7
aseptic meningitis—*see* Meningitis, aseptic
Asherman's 621.5
Asperger's 299.8
asphyctic (*see also* Anxiety) 300.00
aspiration, of newborn (massive) 770.18
  meconium 770.12
ataxia-telangiectasia 334.8
Audry's (acropachyderma) 757.39
auriculotemporal 350.8
autosomal—*see also* Abnormal, autosomes NEC
  deletion 758.39
    5p 758.31
    22q11.2 758.32
Avellis' 344.89
Axenfeld's 743.44
Ayerza (-Arrillaga) (pulmonary artery sclerosis with pulmonary hypertension) 416.0

Syndrome—*continued*
Baader's (erythema multiforme exudativum) 695.1
Baastrup's 721.5
Babinski (-Vaquez) (cardiovascular syphilis) 093.89
Babinski-Fröhlich (adiposogenital dystrophy) 253.8
Babinski-Nageotte 344.89
Bagratuni's (temporal arteritis) 446.5
Bakwin-Krida (craniometaphyseal dysplasia) 756.89
Balint's (psychic paralysis of visual disorientation) 368.16
Ballantyne (-Runge) (postmaturity) 766.22
ballooning posterior leaflet 424.0
Banti's—*see* Cirrhosis, liver
Bard-Pic's (carcinoma, head of pancreas) 157.0
Bardet-Biedl (obesity, polydactyly, and mental retardation) 759.89
Barlow's (mitral valve prolapse) 424.0
Barlow (-Möller) (infantile scurvy) 267
Baron Munchausen's 301.51
Barré-Guillain 357.0
Barré-Liéou (posterior cervical sympathetic) 723.2
Barrett's (chronic peptic ulcer of esophagus) 530.85
Bársony-Polgár (corkscrew esophagus) 530.5
Bársony-Teschendorf (corkscrew esophagus) 530.5
Barth 759.89
Bartter's (secondary hyperaldosteronism with juxtaglomerular hyperplasia) 255.13
Basedow's (exophthalmic goiter) 242.0
basilar artery 435.0
basofrontal 377.04
Bassen-Kornzweig (abetalipoproteinemia) 272.5
Batten-Steinert 359.21
battered
  adult 995.81
  baby or child 995.54
  spouse 995.81
Baumgarten-Cruveilhier (cirrhosis of liver) 571.5
Beals 759.82
Bearn-Kunkel (-Slater) (lupoid hepatitis) 571.49
Beau's (*see also* Degeneration, myocardial) 429.1
Bechterew-Strümpell-Marie (ankylosing spondylitis) 720.0
Beck's (anterior spinal artery occlusion) 433.8
Beckwith (-Wiedemann) 759.89
Behçet's 136.1
Bekhterev-Strümpell-Marie (ankylosing spondylitis) 720.0
Benedikt's 344.89
Béquez César (-Steinbrinck-Chédiak-Higashi) (congenital gigantism of peroxidase granules) 288.2
Bernard-Horner (*see also* Neuropathy, peripheral, autonomic) 337.9
Bernard-Sergent (acute adrenocortical insufficiency) 255.41
Bernhardt-Roth 355.1
Bernheim's (*see also* Failure, heart) 428.0
Bertolotti's (sacralization of fifth lumbar vertebra) 756.15
Besnier-Boeck-Schaumann (sarcoidosis) 135
Bianchi's (aphasia-apraxia-alexia syndrome) 784.69

1343

Syndrome—*continued*
Biedl-Bardet (obesity, polydactyly, and mental retardation) 759.89
Biemond's (obesity, polydactyly, and mental retardation) 759.89
big spleen 289.4
bilateral polycystic ovarian 256.4
Bing-Horton's 346.2
Biörck (-Thorson) (malignant carcinoid) 259.2
Blackfan-Diamond (congenital hypoplastic anemia) 284.01
black lung 500
black widow spider bite 989.5
bladder neck (*see also* Incontinence, urine) 788.30
blast (concussion)—*see* Blast, injury
blind loop (postoperative) 579.2
Bloch-Siemens (incontinentia pigmenti) 757.33
Bloch-Sulzberger (incontinentia pigmenti) 757.33
Bloom (-Machacek) (-Torre) 757.39
Blount-Barber (tibia vara) 732.4
blue
 bloater 491.20
  with
   acute bronchitis 491.22
   exacerbation (acute) 491.21
 diaper 270.0
 drum 381.02
 sclera 756.51
 toe 445.02
Boder-Sedgwick (ataxia-telangiectasia) 334.8
Boerhaave's (spontaneous esophageal rupture) 530.4
Bonnevie-Ullrich 758.6
Bonnier's 386.19
Borjeson-Forssman-Lehmann 759.89
Bouillaud's (rheumatic heart disease) 391.9
Bourneville (-Pringle) (tuberous sclerosis) 759.5
Bouveret (-Hoffmann) (paroxysmal tachycardia) 427.2
brachial plexus 353.0
Brachman-de Lange (Amsterdam dwarf, mental retardation, and brachycephaly) 759.89
bradycardia-tachycardia 427.81
Brailsford-Morquio (dystrophy) (mucopolysaccharidosis IV) 277.5
brain (acute) (chronic) (nonpsychotic) (organic) (with behavioral reaction) (with neurotic reaction) 310.9
 with
  presenile brain disease (*see also* Dementia, presenile) 290.10
  psychosis, psychotic reaction (*see also* Psychosis, organic) 294.9
 chronic alcoholic 291.2
 congenital (*see also* Retardation, mental) 319
 postcontusional 310.2
 posttraumatic
  nonpsychotic 310.2
  psychotic 293.9
   acute 293.0
   chronic (*see also* Psychosis, organic) 294.8
   subacute 293.1
 psycho-organic (*see also* Syndrome, psycho-organic) 310.9
 psychotic (*see also* Psychosis, organic) 294.9
 senile (*see also* Dementia, senile) 290.0
branchial arch 744.41
Brandt's (acrodermatitis enteropathica) 686.8
Brennemann's 289.2

Syndrome—*continued*
Briquet's 300.81
Brissaud-Meige (infantile myxedema) 244.9
broad ligament laceration 620.6
Brock's (atelectasis due to enlarged lymph nodes) 518.0
broken heart 429.83
Brown's tendon sheath 378.61
Brown-Séquard 344.89
brown spot 756.59
Brugada 746.89
Brugsch's (acropachyderma) 757.39
bubbly lung 770.7
Buchem's (hyperostosis corticalis) 733.3
Budd-Chiari (hepatic vein thrombosis) 453.0
Büdinger-Ludloff-Läwen 717.89
bulbar 335.22
 lateral (*see also* Disease, cerebrovascular, acute) 436
Bullis fever 082.8
bundle of Kent (anomalous atrioventricular excitation) 426.7
Bürger-Grütz (essential familial hyperlipemia) 272.3
Burke's (pancreatic insufficiency and chronic neutropenia) 577.8
Burnett's (milk-alkali) 275.42
Burnier's (hypophyseal dwarfism) 253.3
burning feet 266.2
Bywaters' 958.5
Caffey's (infantile cortical hyperostosis) 756.59
Calvé-Legg-Perthes (osteochondrosis, femoral capital) 732.1
Caplan (-Colinet) syndrome 714.81
capsular thrombosis (*see also* Thrombosis, brain) 434.0
carbohydrate-deficient glycoprotein (CDGS) 271.8
carcinogenic thrombophlebitis 453.1
carcinoid 259.2
cardiac asthma (*see also* Failure, ventricular, left) 428.1
cardiacos negros 416.0
cardiopulmonary obesity 278.8
cardiorenal (*see also* Hypertension, cardiorenal) 404.90
cardiorespiratory distress (idiopathic), newborn 769
cardiovascular renal (*see also* Hypertension, cardiorenal) 404.90
cardiovasorenal 272.7
Carini's (ichthyosis congenita) 757.1
carotid
 artery (internal) 435.8
 body or sinus 337.0
carpal tunnel 354.0
Carpenter's 759.89
Cassidy (-Scholte) (malignant carcinoid) 259.2
cat-cry 758.31
cauda equina 344.60
causalgia 355.9
 lower limb 355.71
 upper limb 354.4
cavernous sinus 437.6
celiac 579.0
 artery compression 447.4
 axis 447.4
central pain 338.0
cerebellomedullary malformation (*see also* Spina bifida) 741.0
cerebral gigantism 253.0

INDEX TO DISEASES   **Syndrome**

Syndrome—*continued*
cerebrohepatorenal 759.89
cervical (root) (spine) NEC 723.8
   disc 722.71
   posterior, sympathetic 723.2
   rib 353.0
   sympathetic paralysis 337.0
   traumatic (acute) NEC 847.0
cervicobrachial (diffuse) 723.3
cervicocranial 723.2
cervicodorsal outlet 353.2
Céstan's 344.89
Céstan (-Raymond) 433.8
Céstan-Chenais 344.89
chancriform 114.1
Charcot's (intermittent claudication) 443.9
   angina cruris 443.9
   due to atherosclerosis 440.21
Charcot-Marie-Tooth 356.1
Charcot-Weiss-Baker 337.0
CHARGE association 759.89
Cheadle (-Möller) (-Barlow) (infantile scurvy) 267
Chédiak-Higashi (-Steinbrinck) (congenital gigantism of peroxidase granules) 288.2
chest wall 786.52
Chiari's (hepatic vein thrombosis) 453.0
Chiari-Frommel 676.6
chiasmatic 368.41
Chilaiditi's (subphrenic displacement, colon) 751.4
chondroectodermal dysplasia 756.55
chorea-athetosis-agitans 275.1
Christian's (chronic histiocytosis X) 277.89
chromosome 4 short arm deletion 758.39
chronic pain 338.4
Churg-Strauss 446.4
Clarke-Hadfield (pancreatic infantilism) 577.8
Claude's 352.6
Claude Bernard-Horner (*see also* Neuropathy, peripheral, autonomic) 337.9
Clérambault's
   automatism 348.8
   erotomania 297.8
Clifford's (postmaturity) 766.22
climacteric 627.2
Clouston's (hidrotic ectodermal dysplasia) 757.31
clumsiness 315.4
Cockayne's (microencephaly and dwarfism) 759.89
Cockayne-Weber (epidermolysis bullosa) 757.39
Coffin-Lowry 759.89
Cogan's (nonsyphilitic interstitial keratitis) 370.52
cold injury (newborn) 778.2
Collet (-Sicard) 352.6
combined immunity deficiency 279.2
compartment(al) (anterior) (deep) (posterior) 958.8
   nontraumatic
      abdomen 729.73
      arm 729.71
      buttock 729.72
      fingers 729.71
      foot 729.72
      forearm 729.71
      hand 729.71
      hip 729.72
      leg 729.72
      lower extremity 729.72

Syndrome—*continued*
      shoulder 729.71
      specified site NEC 729.79
      thigh 729.72
      toes 729.72
      upper extremity 729.71
      wrist 729.71
   traumatic 958.90
      abdomen 958.93
      arm 958.91
      buttock 958.92
      fingers 958.91
      foot 958.92
      forearm 958.91
      hand 958.91
      hip 958.92
      leg 958.92
      lower extremity 958.92
      shoulder 958.91
      specified site NEC 958.99
      thigh 958.92
      tibial 958.92
      toes 958.92
      upper extremity 958.91
      wrist 958.91
compression 958.5
   cauda equina 344.60
      with neurogenic bladder 344.61
concussion 310.2
congenital
   affecting more than one system 759.7
      specified type NEC 759.89
   congenital central alveolar hypoventilation 327.25
   facial diplegia 352.6
   muscular hypertrophy-cerebral 759.89
congestion-fibrosis (pelvic) 625.5
conjunctivourethrosynovial 099.3
Conn (-Louis) (primary aldosteronism) 255.12
Conradi (-Hünermann) (chondrodysplasia calcificans congenita) 756.59
conus medullaris 336.8
Cooke-Apert-Gallais (adrenogenital) 255.2
Cornelia de Lange's (Amsterdam dwarf, mental retardation, and brachycephaly) 759.8
coronary insufficiency or intermediate 411.1
cor pulmonale 416.9
corticosexual 255.2
Costen's (complex) 524.60
costochondral junction 733.6
costoclavicular 353.0
costovertebral 253.0
Cotard's (paranoia) 297.1
Cowden 759.6
craniovertebral 723.2
Creutzfeldt-Jakob (new variant) 046.1
   with dementia
      with behavioral disturbance 046.1 *[294.11]*
      without behavioral disturbance 046.1 *[294.10]*
crib death 798.0
cricopharyngeal 787.20
cri-du-chat 758.31
Crigler-Najjar (congenital hyperbilirubinemia) 277.4
crocodile tears 351.8
Cronkhite-Canada 211.3
croup 464.4
CRST (cutaneous systemic sclerosis) 710.1
crush 958.5
crushed lung (*see also* Injury, internal, lung) 861.20

1345

Syndrome—*continued*
  Cruveilhier-Baumgarten (cirrhosis of liver) 571.5
  cubital tunnel 354.2
  Cuiffini-Pancoast (M8010/3) (carcinoma, pulmonary apex) 162.3
  Curschmann (-Batten) (-Steinert) 359.21
  Cushing's (iatrogenic) (idiopathic) (pituitary basophilism) (pituitary-dependent) 255.0
    overdose or wrong substance given or taken 962.0
  Cyriax's (slipping rib) 733.99
  cystic duct stump 576.0
  Da Costa's (neurocirculatory asthenia) 306.2
  Dameshek's (erythroblastic anemia) 282.49
  Dana-Putnam (subacute combined sclerosis with pernicious anemia) 281.0 *[336.2]*
  Danbolt (-Closs) (acrodermatitis enteropathica) 686.8
  Dandy-Walker (atresia, foramen of Magendie) 742.3
    with spina bifida (*see also* Spina bifida) 741.0
  Danlos' 756.83
  Davies-Colley (slipping rib) 733.99
  dead fetus 641.3
  defeminization 255.2
  defibrination (*see also* Fibrinolysis) 286.6
  Degos' 447.8
  Deiters' nucleus 386.19
  Déjérine-Roussy 338.0
  Déjérine-Thomas 333.0
  de Lange's (Amsterdam dwarf, mental retardation, and brachycephaly) (Cornelia) 759.89
  Del Castillo's (germinal aplasia) 606.0
  deletion chromosomes 758.39
  delusional
    induced by drug 292.11
  dementia-aphonia, of childhood (*see also* Psychosis, childhood) 299.1
  demyelinating NEC 341.9
  denial visual hallucination 307.9
  depersonalization 300.6
  Dercum's (adiposis dolorosa) 272.8
  de Toni-Fanconi (-Debré) (cystinosis) 270.0
  diabetes-dwarfism-obesity (juvenile) 258.1
  diabetes mellitus-hypertension-nephrosis 250.4 *[581.81]*
  diabetes mellitus in newborn infant 775.1
  diabetes-nephrosis 250.4 *[581.81]*
  diabetic amyotrophy 250.6 *[353.1]*
  Diamond-Blackfan (congenital hypoplastic anemia) 284.01
  Diamond-Gardener (autoerythrocyte sensitization) 287.2
  DIC (diffuse or disseminated intravascular coagulopathy) (*see also* Fibrinolysis) 286.6
  diencephalohypophyseal NEC 253.8
  diffuse cervicobrachial 723.3
  diffuse obstructive pulmonary 496
  DiGeorge's (thymic hypoplasia) 279.11
  Dighton's 756.51
  Di Guglielmo's (erythremic myelosis) (M9841/3) 207.0
  disequilibrium 276.9
  disseminated platelet thrombosis 446.6
  Ditthomska 307.81
  Doan-Wiseman (primary splenic neutropenia) 289.53
  Döhle body-panmyelopathic 288.2
  Donohue's (leprechaunism) 259.8

Syndrome—*continued*
  dorsolateral medullary (*see also* Disease, cerebrovascular, acute) 436
  double athetosis 333.71
  double whammy 360.81
  Down's (mongolism) 758.0
  Dresbach's (elliptocytosis) 282.1
  Dressler's (postmyocardial infarction) 411.0
    hemoglobinuria 283.2
    postcardiotomy 429.4
  drug withdrawal, infant, of dependent mother 779.5
  dry skin 701.1
  eye 375.15
  DSAP (disseminated superficial actinic porokeratosis) 692.75
  Duane's (retraction) 378.71
  Duane-Stilling-Türk (ocular retraction syndrome) 378.71
  Dubin-Johnson (constitutional hyperbilirubinemia) 277.4
  Dubin-Sprinz (constitutional hyperbilirubinemia) 277.4
  Duchenne's 335.22
  due to abnormality
    autosomal NEC (*see also* Abnormal, autosomes NEC) 758.5
      13 758.1
      18 758.2
      21 or 22 758.0
      D_1 758.1
      E_3 758.2
      G 758.0
    chromosomal 758.89
    sex 758.81
  dumping 564.2
    nonsurgical 536.8
  Duplay's 726.2
  Dupré's (meningism) 781.6
  Dyke-Young (acquired macrocytic hemolytic anemia) 283.9
  dyspraxia 315.4
  dystocia, dystrophia 654.9
  Eagle-Barrett 756.71
  Eales' 362.18
  Eaton-Lambert (*see also* Neoplasm, by site, malignant) 199.1 *[358.1]*
  Ebstein's (downward displacement, tricuspid valve into right ventricle) 746.2
  ectopic ACTH secretion 255.0
  eczema-thrombocytopenia 279.12
  Eddowes' (brittle bones and blue sclera) 756.51
  Edwards' 758.2
  efferent loop 537.89
  effort (aviators') (psychogenic) 306.2
  Ehlers-Danlos 756.83
  Eisenmenger's (ventricular septal defect) 745.4
  Ekbom's (restless legs) 333.94
  Ekman's (brittle bones and blue sclera) 756.51
  electric feet 266.2
  Elephant man 237.71
  Ellison-Zollinger (gastric hypersecretion with pancreatic islet cell tumor) 251.5
  Ellis-van Creveld (chondroectodermal dysplasia) 756.55
  embryonic fixation 270.2
  empty sella (turcica) 253.8
  endocrine-hypertensive 255.3
  Engel-von Recklinghausen (osteitis fibrosa cystica) 252.01
  enteroarticular 099.3

INDEX TO DISEASES

Syndrome

Syndrome—*continued*
entrapment—*see* Neuropathy, entrapment
eosinophilia myalgia 710.5
epidemic vomiting 078.82
Epstein's—*see* Nephrosis
Erb (-Oppenheim) -Goldflam 358.00
Erdheim's (acromegalic macrospondylitis) 253.0
Erlacher-Blount (tibia vara) 732.4
erythrocyte fragmentation 283.19
euthyroid sick 790.94
Evans' (thrombocytopenic purpura) 287.32
excess cortisol, iatrogenic 255.0
exhaustion 300.5
extrapyramidal 333.90
eyelid-malar-mandible 756.0
eye retraction 378.71
Faber's (achlorhydric anemia) 280.9
Fabry (-Anderson) (angiokeratoma corporis diffusum) 272.7
facet 724.8
Fallot's 745.2
falx (*see also* Hemorrhage, brain) 431
familial eczema-thrombocytopenia 279.12
Fanconi's (anemia) (congenital pancytopenia) 284.09
Fanconi (-de Toni) (-Debré) (cystinosis) 270.0
Farber (-Uzman) (disseminated lipogranulomatosis) 272.8
fatigue NEC 300.5
   chronic 780.71
faulty bowel habit (idiopathic megacolon) 564.7
FDH (focal dermal hypoplasia) 757.39
fecal reservoir 560.39
Feil-Klippel (brevicollis) 756.16
Felty's (rheumatoid arthritis with splenomegaly and leukopenia) 714.1
fertile eunuch 257.2
fetal alcohol 760.71
   late effect 760.71
fibrillation-flutter 427.32
fibrositis (periarticular) 729.0
Fiedler's (acute isolated myocarditis) 422.91
Fiessinger-Leroy (-Reiter) 099.3
Fiessinger-Rendu (erythema multiforme exudativum) 695.1
first arch 756.0
fish odor 270.8
Fisher's 357.0
Fitz's (acute hemorrhagic pancreatitis) 577.0
Fitz-Hugh and Curtis 098.86
   due to
      Chlamydia trachomatis 099.56
      Neisseria gonorrhoeae (gonococcal peritonitis) 098.86
Flajani (-Basedow) (exophthalmic goiter) 242.0
floppy
   infant 781.99
   iris 364.81
   valve (mitral) 424.0
flush 259.2
Foix-Alajouanine 336.1
Fong's (hereditary osteo-onychodysplasia) 756.89
foramen magnum 348.4
Forbes-Albright (nonpuerperal amenorrhea and lactation associated with pituitary tumor) 253.1
Foster-Kennedy 377.04
Foville's (peduncular) 344.89
Fragile X 759.83

Syndrome—*continued*
Franceschetti's (mandibulofacial dysostosis) 756.0
Fraser's 759.89
Freeman-Sheldon 759.89
Frey's (auriculotemporal) 705.22
Friderichsen-Waterhouse 036.3
Friedrich-Erb-Arnold (acropachyderma) 757.39
Fröhlich's (adiposogenital dystrophy) 253.8
Froin's 336.8
Frommel-Chiari 676.6
frontal lobe 310.0
Fuller Albright's (osteitis fibrosa disseminata) 756.59
Fukuhara 277.87
functional
   bowel 564.9
   prepubertal castrate 752.89
Gaisböck's (polycythemia hypertonica) 289.0
ganglion (basal, brain) 333.90
geniculi 351.1
Ganser's, hysterical 300.16
Gardner-Diamond (autoerythrocyte sensitization) 287.2
gastroesophageal junction 530.0
gastroesophageal laceration-hemorrhage 530.7
gastrojejunal loop obstruction 537.89
Gayet-Wernicke's (superior hemorrhagic polioencephalitis) 265.1
Gee-Herter-Heubner (nontropical sprue) 579.0
Gélineau's (*see also* Narcolepsy) 347.00
genito-anorectal 099.1
Gerhardt's (vocal cord paralysis) 478.30
Gerstmann's (finger agnosia) 784.69
Giannotti Crosti 057.8
   due to known virus—*see* Infection, virus
   due to unknown virus 057.8
Gilbert's 277.4
Gilford (-Hutchinson) (progeria) 259.8
Gilles de la Tourette's 307.23
Gillespie's (dysplasia oculodentodigitalis) 759.89
Glénard's (enteroptosis) 569.89
Glinski-Simmonds (pituitary cachexia) 253.2
glucuronyl transferase 277.4
glue ear 381.20
Goldberg (-Maxwell) (-Morris) (testicular feminization) 259.5
Goldenhar's (oculoauriculovertebral dysplasia) 756.0
Goldflam-Erb 358.00
Goltz-Gorlin (dermal hypoplasia) 757.39
Good's 279.06
Goodpasture's (pneumorenal) 446.21
Gopalan's (burning feet) 266.2
Gorlin-Chaudhry-Moss 759.89
Gougerot (-Houwer) -Sjögren (keratoconjunctivitis sicca) 710.2
Gougerot-Blum (pigmented purpuric lichenoid dermatitis) 709.1
Gougerot-Carteaud (confluent reticulate papillomatosis) 701.8
Gouley's (constrictive pericarditis) 423.2
Gowers' (vasovagal attack) 780.2
Gowers-Paton-Kennedy 377.04
Gradenigo's 383.02
Gray or grey (chloramphenicol) (newborn) 779.4
Greig's (hypertelorism) 756.0
Gubler-Millard 344.89

Syndrome—*continued*
  Guérin-Stern (arthrogryposis multiplex congenita) 754.89
  Guillain-Barré (-Strohl) 357.0
  Gunn's (jaw-winking syndrome) 742.8
  Günther's (congenital erythropoietic porphyria) 277.1
  gustatory sweating 350.8
  H3O 759.81
  Hadfield-Clarke (pancreatic infantilism) 577.8
  Haglund-Läwen-Fründ 717.89
  hairless women 257.8
  hair tourniquet—*see also* Injury, superficial, by site
    finger 915.8
      infected 915.9
    penis 911.8
      infected 911.9
    toe 917.8
      infected 917.9
  Hallermann-Streiff 756.0
  Hallervorden-Spatz 333.0
  Hamman's (spontaneous mediastinal emphysema) 518.1
  Hamman-Rich (diffuse interstitial pulmonary fibrosis) 516.3
  Hand-Schüller-Christian (chronic histiocytosis X) 277.89
  hand-foot 693.0
  Hanot-Chauffard (-Troisier) (bronze diabetes) 275.0
  Harada's 363.22
  Hare's (M8010/3) (carcinoma, pulmonary apex) 162.3
  Harkavy's 446.0
  harlequin color change 779.89
  Harris' (organic hyperinsulinism) 251.1
  Hart's (pellagra-cerebellar ataxia-renal aminoaciduria) 270.0
  Hayem-Faber (achlorhydric anemia) 280.9
  Hayem-Widal (acquired hemolytic jaundice) 283.9
  Heberden's (angina pectoris) 413.9
  Hedinger's (malignant carcinoid) 259.2
  Hegglin's 288.2
  Heller's (infantile psychosis) (*see also* Psychosis, childhood) 299.1
  H.E.L.L.P. 642.5
  hemolytic-uremic (adult) (child) 283.11
  hemophagocytic 288.4
    infection-associated 288.4
  Hench-Rosenberg (palindromic arthritis) (*see also* Rheumatism, palindromic) 719.3
  Henoch-Schönlein (allergic purpura) 287.0
  hepatic flexure 569.89
  hepatorenal 572.4
    due to a procedure 997.4
    following delivery 674.8
  hepatourologic 572.4
  Herrick's (hemoglobin S disease) 282.61
  Herter (-Gee) (nontropical sprue) 579.0
  Heubner-Herter (nontropical sprue) 579.0
  Heyd's (hepatorenal) 572.4
  HHHO 759.81
  high grade myelodysplastic 238.73
    with 5q deletion 238.73
  Hilger's 337.0
  histiocytic 288.4
  Hoffa (-Kastert) (liposynovitis prepatellaris) 272.8
  Hoffmann's 244.9 *[359.5]*

Syndrome—*continued*
  Hoffmann-Bouveret (paroxysmal tachycardia) 427.2
  Hoffmann-Werdnig 335.0
  Holländer-Simons (progressive lipodystrophy) 272.6
  Holmes' (visual disorientation) 368.16
  Holmes-Adie 379.46
  Hoppe-Goldflam 358.00
  Yorner's (sde also Neuropathy, peripheral, autonomic) 337.9
    traumatic—*see* Injury, nerve, cervical sympathetic
  hospital addiction 301.51
  Hunt's (herpetic geniculate ganglionitis) 053.11
    dyssynergia cerebellaris myoclonica 334.2
  Hunter (-Hurler) (mucopolysaccharidosis II) 277.5
  hunterian glossitis 529.4
  Hurler (-Hunter) (mucopolysaccharidosis II) 277.5
  Hutchinson's incisors or teeth 090.5
  Hutchinson-Boeck (sarcoidosis) 135
  Hutchinson-Gilford (progeria) 259.8
  hydralazine
    correct substance properly administered 695.4
    overdose or wrong substance given or taken 972.6
  hydraulic concussion (abdomen) (*see also* Injury, internal, abdomen) 868.00
  hyperabduction 447.8
  hyperactive bowel 564.9
  hyperaldosteronism with hypokalemic alkalosis (Bartter's) 255.13
  hypercalcemic 275.42
  hypercoagulation NEC 289.89
  hypereosinophilic (idiopathic) 288.3
  hyperfusion 997.01
  hyperkalemic 276.7
  hyperkinetic—*see also* Hyperkinesia
    heart 429.82
  hyperlipemia-hemolytic anemia-icterus 571.1
  hypermobility 728.5
  hypernatremia 276.0
  hyperosmolarity 276.0
  hypersomnia-bulimia 349.89
  hypersplenic 289.4
  hypersympathetic (*see also* Neuropathy, peripheral, autonomic) 337.9
  hypertransfusion, newborn 776.4
  hyperventilation, psychogenic 306.1
  hyperviscosity (of serum) NEC 273.3
    polycythemic 289.0
    sclerothymic 282.8
  hypoglycemic (familial) (neonatal) 251.2
    functional 251.1
  hypokalemic 276.8
  hypophyseal 253.8
  hypophyseothalamic 253.8
  hypopituitarism 253.2
  hypoplastic left heart 746.7
  hypopotassemia 276.8
  hyposmolality 276.1
  hypotension, maternal 669.2
  hypothenar hammer 443.89
  hypotonia-hypomentia-hypogonadism-obesity 759.81
  ICF (intravascular coagulation-fibrinolysis) (*see also* Fibrinolysis) 286.6
  idiopathic cardiorespiratory distress, newborn 769

INDEX TO DISEASES

Syndrome—*continued*
idiopathic nephrotic (infantile) 581.9
Imerslund (-Gräsbeck) (anemia due to familial selective vitamin B_{12} malabsorption) 281.1
immobility (paraplegic) 728.3
immunity deficiency, combined 279.2
impending coronary 411.1
impingement
  shoulder 726.2
  vertebral bodies 724.4
inappropriate secretion of antidiuretic hormone (ADH) 253.6
incomplete
  mandibulofacial 756.0
infant
  death, sudden (SIDS) 798.0
  Hercules 255.2
  of diabetic mother 775.0
  shaken 995.55
infantilism 253.3
inferior vena cava 459.2
influenza-like 487.1
inspissated bile, newborn 774.4
insufficient sleep 307.44
intermediate coronary (artery) 411.1
internal carotid artery (*see also* Occlusion, artery, carotid) 433.1
interspinous ligament 724.8
intestinal
  carcinoid 259.2
  gas 787.3
  knot 560.2
intraoperative floppy iris (IFIS) 364.81
intravascular
  coagulation-fibrinolysis (ICF) (*see also* Fibrinolysis) 286.6
  coagulopathy (*see also* Fibrinolysis) 286.6
inverted Marfan's 759.89
IRDS (idiopathic respiratory distress, newborn) 769
irritable
  bowel 564.1
  heart 306.2
  weakness 300.5
ischemic bowel (transient) 557.9
  chronic 557.1
  due to mesenteric artery insufficiency 557.1
Itsenko-Cushing (pituitary basophilism) 255.0
IVC (intravascular coagulopathy) (*see also* Fibrinolysis) 286.6
Ivemark's (asplenia with congenital heart disease) 759.0
Jaccoud's 714.4
Jackson's 344.89
Jadassohn-Lewandowski (pachyonychia congenita) 757.5
Jaffe-Lichtenstein (-Uehlinger) 252.01
Jahnke's (encephalocutaneous angiomatosis) 759.6
Jakob-Creutzfeldt (new variant) 046.1
  with dementia
    with behavioral disturbance 046.1 *[294.11]*
    without behavioral disturbance 046.1 *[294.10]*
Jaksch's (pseudoleukemia infantum) 285.8
Jaksch-Hayem (-Luzet) (pseudoleukemia infantum) 285.8
jaw-winking 742.8
jejunal 564.2
Jervell-Lange-Nielsen 426.82
jet lag 327.35

Syndrome—*continued*
Jeune's (asphyxiating thoracic dystrophy of newborn) 756.4
Job's (chronic granulomatous disease) 288.1
Jordan's 288.2
Joseph-Diamond-Blackfan (congenital hypoplastic anemia) 284.01
Joubert 759.89
jugular foramen 352.6
Kabuki 759.89
Kahler's (multiple myeloma) (M9730/3) 203.0
Kalischer's (encephalocutaneous angiomatosis) 759.6
Kallmann's (hypogonadotropic hypogonadism with anosmia) 253.4
Kanner's (autism) (*see also* Psychosis, childhood) 299.0
Kartagener's (sinusitis, bronchiectasis, situs inversus) 759.3
Kasabach-Merritt (capillary hemangioma associated with thrombocytopenic purpura) 287.39
Kast's (dyschondroplasia with hemangiomas) 756.4
Kaznelson's (congenital hypoplastic anemia) 284.01
Kearns-Sayre 277.87
Kelly's (sideropenic dysphagia) 280.8
Kimmelstiel-Wilson (intercapillary glomerulosclerosis) 250.4 *[581.81]*
Klauder's (erythema multiforme exudativum) 695.1
Klein-Waardenburg (ptosis-epicanthus) 270.2
Kleine-Levin 327.13
Klinefelter's 758.7
Klippel-Feil (brevicollis) 756.16
Klippel-Trenaunay 759.89
Klumpke (-Déjérine) (injury to brachial plexus at birth) 767.6
Klüver-Bucy (-Terzian) 310.0
Köhler-Pellegrini-Stieda (calcification, knee joint) 726.62
König's 564.89
Korsakoff's (nonalcoholic) 294.0
  alcoholic 291.1
Korsakoff (-Wernicke) (nonalcoholic) 294.0
  alcoholic 291.1
Kostmann's (infantile genetic agranulocytosis) 288.01
Krabbe's
  congenital muscle hypoplasia 756.89
  cutaneocerebral angioma 759.6
Kunkel (lupoid hepatitis) 571.49
labyrinthine 386.50
laceration, broad ligament 620.6
Langdon Down (mongolism) 758.0
Larsen's (flattened facies and multiple congenital dislocations) 755.8
lateral
  cutaneous nerve of thigh 355.1
  medullary (*see also* Disease, cerebrovascular acute) 436
Launois' (pituitary gigantism) 253.0
Launois-Cléret (adiposogenital dystrophy) 253.8
Laurence-Moon (-Bardet) -Biedl (obesity, polydactyly, and mental retardation) 759.8
Lawford's (encephalocutaneous angiomatosis) 759.6
lazy
  leukocyte 288.09
  posture 728.3

1349

Syndrome

Syndrome—*continued*
  Lederer-Brill (acquired infectious hemolytic anemia) 283.19
  Legg-Calvé-Perthes (osteochondrosis capital femoral) 732.1
  Lemiere 451.89
  Lennox's (*see also* Epilepsy) 345.0
  Lennox-Gastaut syndrome 345.0
    with tonic seizures 345.1
  lenticular 275.1
  Léopold-Lévi's (paroxysmal thyroid instability) 242.9
  Lepore hemoglobin 282.49
  Léri-Weill 756.59
  Leriche's (aortic bifurcation occlusion) 444.0
  Lermoyez's (*see also* Disease, Ménière's) 386.00
  Lesch-Nyhan (hypoxanthine-guanine-phosphoribosyltransferase deficiency) 277.2
  Lev's (acquired complete heart block) 426.0
  Levi's (pituitary dwarfism) 253.3
  Lévy-Roussy 334.3
  Lichtheim's (subacute combined sclerosis with pernicious anemia) 281.0 *[336.2]*
  Li-Fraumeni V84.01
  Lightwood's (renal tubular acidosis) 588.89
  Lignac (-de Toni) (-Fanconi) (-Debré) (cystinosis) 270.0
  Likoff's (angina in menopausal women) 413.9
  liver-kidney 572.4
  Lloyd's 258.1
  lobotomy 310.0
  Löffler's (eosinophilic pneumonitis) 518.3
  Löfgren's (sarcoidosis) 135
  long arm 18 or 21 deletion 758.39
  Looser (-Debray) -Milkman (osteomalacia with pseudofractures) 268.2
  Lorain-Levi (pituitary dwarfism) 253.3
  Louis-Bar (ataxia-telangiectasia) 334.8
  low
    atmospheric pressure 993.2
    back 724.2
      psychogenic 306.0
    output (cardiac) (*see also* Failure, heart) 428.9
  Lowe's (oculocerebrorenal dystrophy) 270.8
  Lowe-Terrey-MacLachlan (oculocerebrorenal dystrophy) 270.8
  lower radicular, newborn 767.4
  Lown (-Ganong)-Levine (short P-R interval, normal QRS complex, and supraventricular tachycardia) 426.81
  Lucey-Driscoll (jaundice due to delayed conjugation) 774.30
  Luetscher's (dehydration) 276.51
  lumbar vertebral 724.4
  Lutembacher's (atrial septal defect with mitral stenosis) 745.5
  Lyell's (toxic epidermal necrolysis) 695.1
    due to drug
      correct substance properly administered 695.1
      overdose or wrong substance given or taken 977.9
        specified drug—*see* Table of drugs and chemicals
  MacLeod's 492.8
  macrogenitosomia praecox 259.8
  macroglobulinemia 273.3
  macrophage activation 288.4
  Maffucci's (dyschondroplasia with hemangiomas) 756.4

Syndrome—*continued*
  Magenblase 306.4
  magnesium-deficiency 781.7
  Mal de Debarquement 780.4
  malabsorption 579.9
    postsurgical 579.3
    spinal fluid 331.3
  malignant carcinoid 259.2
  Mallory-Weiss 530.7
  mandibulofacial dysostosis 756.0
  manic-depressive (*see also* Psychosis, affective) 296.80
  Mankowsky's (familial dysplastic osteopathy) 731.2
  maple syrup (urine) 270.3
  Marable's (celiac artery compression) 447.4
  Marchesani (-Weill) (brachymorphism and ectopia lentis) 759.89
  Marchiafava-Bignami 341.8
  Marchiafava-Micheli (paroxysmal nocturnal hemoglobinuria) 283.2
  Marcus Gunn's (jaw-winking syndrome) 742.8
  Marfan's (arachnodactyly) 759.82
    meaning congenital syphilis 090.49
      with luxation of lens 090.49 *[379.32]*
  Marie's (acromegaly) 253.0
    primary or idiopathic (acropachyderma) 757.39
    secondary (hypertrophic pulmonary osteoarthropathy) 731.2
  Markus-Adie 379.46
  Maroteaux-Lamy (mucopolysaccharidosis VI) 277.5
  Martin's 715.27
  Martin-Albright (pseudohypoparathyroidism) 275.49
  Martorell-Fabré (pulseless disease) 446.7
  massive aspiration of newborn 770.18
  Masters-Allen 620.6
  mastocytosis 757.33
  maternal hypotension 669.2
  maternal obesity 646.1
  May (-Hegglin) 288.2
  McArdle (-Schmid) (-Pearson) (glycogenosis V) 271.0
  McCune-Albright (osteitis fibrosa disseminata) 756.59
  McQuarrie's (idiopathic familial hypoglycemia) 251.2
  meconium
    aspiration 770.12
    plug (newborn) NEC 777.1
  median arcuate ligament 447.4
  mediastinal fibrosis 519.3
  Meekeren-Ehlers-Danlos 756.83
  Meige (blepharospasm-oromandibular dystonia) 333.82
  -Milroy (chronic hereditary edema) 757.0
  MELAS (mitochondrial encephalopathy, lactic acidosis and stroke-like episodes) 277.87
  Melkersson (-Rosenthal) 351.8
  MEN (multiple endocrine neoplasia)
    type I 258.01
    type IIA 258.02
    type IIB 258.03
  Mende's (ptosis-epicanthus) 270.2
  Mendelson's (resulting from a procedure) 997.3
    during labor 668.0
    obstetric 668.0
  Ménétrier's (hypertrophic gastritis) 535.2
  Ménière's (*see also* Disease, Ménière's) 386.00

INDEX TO DISEASES

Syndrome

Syndrome—*continued*
  meningo-eruptive 047.1
  Menkes' 759.89
    glutamic acid 759.89
    maple syrup (urine) disease 270.3
  menopause 627.2
    postartificial 627.4
  menstruation 625.4
  MERRF (myoclonus with epilepsy and with ragged red fibers) 277.87
  mesenteric
    artery, superior 557.1
    vascular insufficiency (with gangrene) 557.1
  metabolic 277.7
  metastatic carcinoid 259.2
  Meyenburg-Altherr-Uehlinger 733.99
  Meyer-Schwickerath and Weyers (dysplasia oculodentodigitalis) 759.89
  Micheli-Rietti (thalassemia minor) 282.49
  Michotte's 721.5
  micrognathia-glossoptosis 756.0
  microphthalmos (congenital) 759.89
  midbrain 348.8
  middle
    lobe (lung) (right) 518.0
    radicular 353.0
  Miescher's
    familial acanthosis nigricans 701.2
    granulomatosis disciformis 709.3
  Mieten's 759.89
  migraine 346.0
  Mikity-Wilson (pulmonary dysmaturity) 770.7
  Mikulicz's (dryness of mouth, absent or decreased lacrimation) 527.1
  milk alkali (milk drinkers') 275.42
  Milkman (-Looser) (osteomalacia with pseudofractures) 268.2
  Millard-Gubler 344.89
  Miller-Dieker 758.33
  Miller Fisher's 357.0
  Milles' (encephalocutaneous angiomatosis) 759.6
  Minkowski-Chauffard (*see also* Spherocytosis) 282.0
  Mirizzi's (hepatic duct stenosis) 576.2
    with calculus, cholelithiasis, or stones—*see* Choledocholithiasis
  mitochondrial neurogastrointestinal encephalopathy (MNGIE) 277.87
  mitral
    click (-murmur) 785.2
    valve prolapse 424.0
  MNGIE (mitochondrial neurogastrointestinal encephalopathy) 277.87
  Möbius'
    congenital oculofacial paralysis 352.6
    ophthalmoplegic migraine 346.8
  Mohr's (Types I and II) 759.89
  monofixation 378.34
  Moore's (*see also* Epilepsy) 345.5
  Morel-Moore (hyperostosis frontalis interna) 733.3
  Morel-Morgagni (hyperostosis frontalis interna) 733.3
  Morgagni (-Stewart-Morel) (hyperostosis frontalis interna) 733.3
  Morgagni-Adams-Stokes (syncope with heart block) 426.9
  Morquio (-Brailsford) (-Ullrich) (mucopolysaccharidosis IV) 277.5
  Morris (testicular feminization) 259.5

Syndrome—*continued*
  Morton's (foot) (metatarsalgia) (metatarsal neuralgia) (neuralgia) (neuroma) (toe) 355.6
  Moschcowitz (-Singer-Symmers) (thrombotic thrombocytopenic purpura) 446.6
  Mounier-Kuhn 748.3
    with
      acute exacerbation 494.1
      bronchiectasis 494.0
        with (acute) exacerbation 494.1
    acquired 519.19
      with bronchiectasis 494.0
        with (acute) exacerbation 494.1
  Mucha-Haberman (acute parapsoriasis varioliformis) 696.2
  mucocutaneous lymph node (acute) (febrile) (infantile) (MCLS) 446.1
  multiple
    deficiency 260
    endocrine neoplasia [MEN]
      type I 258.01
      type IIA 258.02
      type IIB 258.03
    operations 301.51
  Munchausen's 301.51
  Münchmeyer's (exostosis luxurians) 728.11
  Murchison-Sanderson—*see* Disease, Hodgkin's
  myasthenic—*see* Myasthenia, syndrome
  myelodysplastic 238.75
    with 5q deletion 238.74
    high grade with 5q deletion 238.73
  myeloproliferative (chronic) (M9960/1) 238.79
  myofascial pain NEC 729.1
  Naffziger's 353.0
  Nager-de Reynier (dysostosis mandibularis) 756.0
  nail-patella (hereditary osteo-onychodysplasia) 756.89
  NARP (neuropathy, ataxia and retinitis pigmentosa) 277.87
  Nebécourt's 253.3
  Neill-Dingwall (microencephaly and dwarfism) 759.89
  nephrotic (*see also* Nephrosis) 581.9
    diabetic 250.4 *[581.81]*
  Netherton's (ichthyosiform erythroderma) 757.1
  neurocutaneous 759.6
  neuroleptic malignant 333.92
  Nezelof's (pure alymphocytosis) 279.13
  Niemann-Pick (lipid histiocytosis) 272.7
  Nonne-Milroy-Meige (chronic hereditary edema) 757.0
  nonsense 300.16
  Noonan's 759.89
  Nothnagel's
    ophthalmoplegia-cerebellar ataxia 378.52
    vasomotor acroparesthesia 443.89
  nucleus ambiguous-hypoglossal 352.6
  OAV (oculoauriculovertebral dysplasia) 756.0
  obsessional 300.3
  oculocutaneous 364.24
  oculomotor 378.81
  oculourethroarticular 099.3
  Ogilvie's (sympathicotonic colon obstruction) 560.89
  ophthalmoplegia-cerebellar ataxia 378.52
  Oppenheim-Urbach (necrobiosis lipoidica diabeticorum) 250.8 *[709.3]*
  oral-facial-digital 759.89

Syndrome INDEX TO DISEASES

Syndrome—*continued*
  organic
    affective NEC 293.83
      drug-induced 292.84
    anxiety 293.84
    delusional 293.81
      alcohol-induced 291.5
      drug-induced 292.11
      due to or associated with
        arteriosclerosis 290.42
        presenile brain disease 290.12
        senility 290.20
    depressive 293.83
      drug-induced 292.84
      due to or associated with
        arteriosclerosis 290.43
        presenile brain disease 290.13
        senile brain disease 290.21
    hallucinosis 293.82
      drug-induced 292.84
  organic affective 293.83
    induced by drug 292.84
  organic personality 310.1
    induced by drug 292.89
  Ormond's 593.4
  orodigitofacial 759.89
  orthostatic hypotensive-dysautonomic-dyskinetic 333.0
  Osler-Weber-Rendu (familial hemorrhagic telangiectasia) 448.0
  osteodermopathic hyperostosis 757.39
  osteoporosis-osteomalacia 268.2
  Österreicher-Turner (hereditary osteo-onychodysplasia) 756.89
  Ostrum-Furst 756.59
  otolith 386.19
  otopalatodigital 759.89
  outlet (thoracic) 353.0
  ovarian remnant 620.8
  Owren's (*see also* Defect, coagulation) 286.3
  OX 758.6
  pacemaker 429.4
  Paget-Schroetter (intermittent venous claudication) 453.8
  pain—*see also* Pain
    central 338.0
    chronic 338.4
    myelopathic 338.0
    thalamic (hypersthetic) 338.0
  painful
    apicocostal vertebral (M8010/3) 162.3
    arc 726.19
    bruising 287.2
    feet 266.2
  Pancoast's (carcinoma, pulmonary apex) (M8010/3) 162.3
  panhypopituitary (postpartum) 253.2
  papillary muscle 429.81
    with myocardial infarction 410.8
  Papillon-Léage and Psaume (orodigitofacial dysostosis) 759.89
  parabiotic (transfusion)
    donor (twin) 772.0
    recipient (twin) 776.4
  paralysis agitans 332.0
  paralytic 344.9
    specified type NEC 344.89
  Paraneoplastic —*see* condition
  Parinaud's (paralysis of conjugate upward gaze) 378.81
    oculoglandular 372.02

Syndrome—*continued*
  Parkes Weber and Dimitri (encephalocutaneous angiomatosis) 759.6
  Parkinson's (*see also* Parkinsonism) 332.0
  parkinsonian (*see* also Parkinsonism) 332.0
  Parry's (exophthalmic goiter) 242.0
  Parry-Romberg 349.89
  Parsonage-Aldren-Turner 353.5
  Parsonage-Turner 353.5
  Patau's (trisomy D_1) 758.1
  patella clunk 719.66
  patellofemoral 719.46
  Paterson (-Brown) (-Kelly) (sideropenic dysphagia) 280.8
  Payr's (splenic flexure syndrome) 569.89
  pectoral girdle 447.8
  pectoralis minor 447.8
  Pelger-Huët (hereditary hyposegmentation) 288.2
  pellagra-cerebellar ataxia-renal aminoaciduria 270.0
  Pellegrini-Stieda 726.62
  pellagroid 265.2
  Pellizzi's (pineal) 259.8
  pelvic congestion (-fibrosis) 625.5
  Pendred's (familial goiter with deaf-mutism) 243
  Penfield's (*see also* Epilepsy) 345.5
  Penta X 758.81
  peptic ulcer—*see* Ulcer, peptic 533.9
  perabduction 447.8
  periodic 277.31
  periurethral fibrosis 593.4
  persistent fetal circulation 747.83
  Petges-Cléjat (poikilodermatomyositis) 710.3
  Peutz-Jeghers 759.6
  Pfeiffer (acrocephalosyndactyly) 755.55
  phantom limb 353.6
  pharyngeal pouch 279.11
  Pick's (pericardial pseudocirrhosis of liver) 423.2
    heart 423.2
    liver 423.2
  Pick-Herxheimer (diffuse idiopathic cutaneous atrophy) 701.8
  Pickwickian (cardiopulmonary obesity) 278.8
  PIE (pulmonary infiltration with eosinophilia) 518.3
  Pierre Marie-Bamberger (hypertrophic pulmonary osteoarthropathy) 731.2
  Pierre Mauriac's (diabetes-dwarfism-obesity) 258.1
  Pierre Robin 756.0
  pigment dispersion, iris 364.53
  pineal 259.8
  pink puffer 492.8
  pituitary 253.0
  placental
    dysfunction 762.2
    insufficiency 762.2
    transfusion 762.3
  plantar fascia 728.71
  plica knee 727.83
  Plummer-Vinson (sideropenic dysphagia) 280.8
  pluricarential of infancy 260
  plurideficiency of infancy 260
  pluriglandular (compensatory) 258.8
  polycarential of infancy 260
  polyglandular 258.8
  polysplenia 759.0
  pontine 433.8

INDEX TO DISEASES — Syndrome

Syndrome—*continued*
popliteal
  artery entrapment 447.8
  web 756.89
postartificial menopause 627.4
postcardiac injury
  postcardiotomy 429.4
  postmyocardial infarction 411.0
postcardiotomy 429.4
postcholecystectomy 576.0
postcommissurotomy 429.4
postconcussional 310.2
postcontusional 310.2
postencephalitic 310.8
posterior
  cervical sympathetic 723.2
  fossa compression 348.4
  inferior cerebellar artery (*see also* Disease, cerebrovascular, acute) 436
  reversible encephalopathy (PRES) 348.39
postgastrectomy (dumping) 564.2
post-gastric surgery 564.2
posthepatitis 780.79
postherpetic (neuralgia) (zoster) 053.19
  geniculate ganglion 053.11
  ophthalmica 053.19
postimmunization—*see* Complications, vaccination
postinfarction 411.0
postinfluenza (asthenia) 780.79
postirradiation 990
postlaminectomy 722.80
  cervical, cervicothoracic 722.81
  lumbar, lumbosacral 722.83
  thoracic, thoracolumbar 722.82
postleukotomy 310.0
postlobotomy 310.0
postmastectomy lymphedema 457.0
postmature (of newborn) 766.22
postmyocardial infarction 411.0
postoperative NEC 998.9
  blind loop 579.2
postpartum panhypopituitary 253.2
postperfusion NEC 999.8
  bone marrow 996.85
postpericardiotomy 429.4
postphlebitic (asymptomatic) 459.10
  with
    complications NEC 459.19
    inflammation 459.12
      and ulcer 459.13
    stasis dermatitis 459.12
      with ulcer 459.13
    ulcer 459.11
      with inflammation 459.13
postpolio (myelitis) 138
postvagotomy 564.2
postvalvulotomy 429.4
postviral (asthenia) NEC 780.79
Potain's (gastrectasis with dyspepsia) 536.1
potassium intoxication 276.7
Potter's 753.0
Prader (-Labhart) -Willi (-Fanconi) 759.81
preinfarction 411.1
preleukemic 238.75
premature senility 259.8
premenstrual 625.4
premenstrual tension 625.4
pre ulcer 536.9
Prinzmetal-Massumi (anterior chest wall syndrome) 786.52

Syndrome—*continued*
Profichet's 729.9
progeria 259.8
progressive pallidal degeneration 333.0
prolonged gestation 766.22
Proteus (dermal hypoplasia) 757.39
prune belly 756.71
prurigo-asthma 691.8
pseudocarpal tunnel (sublimis) 354.0
pseudohermaphroditism-virilism-hirsutism 255.2
pseudoparalytica 358.00
pseudo-Turner's 759.89
psycho-organic 293.9
  acute 293.0
  anxiety type 293.84
  depressive type 293.83
  hallucinatory type 293.82
  nonpsychotic severity 310.1
    specified focal (partial) NEC 310.8
  paranoid type 293.81
  specified type NEC 293.89
  subacute 293.1
pterygolymphangiectasia 758.6
ptosis-epicanthus 270.2
pulmonary
  arteriosclerosis 416.0
  hypoperfusion (idiopathic) 769
  renal (hemorrhagic) 446.21
pulseless 446.7
Putnam-Dana (subacute combined sclerosis with pernicious anemia) 281.0 *[336.2]*
pyloroduodenal 537.89
pyramidopallidonigral 332.0
pyriformis 355.0
QT interval prolongation 426.82
radicular NEC 729.2
  lower limbs 724.4
  upper limbs 723.4
  newborn 767.4
Raeder-Harbitz (pulseless disease) 446.7
Ramsay Hunt's
  dyssynergia cerebellaris myoclonica 334.2
  herpetic geniculate ganglionitis 053.11
rapid time-zone change 327.35
Raymond (-Céstan) 433.8
Raynaud's (paroxysmal digital cyanosis) 443.0
RDS (respiratory distress syndrome, newborn) 769
Refsum's (heredopathia atactica polyneuritiformis) 356.3
Reichmann's (gastrosuccorrhea) 536.8
Reifenstein's (hereditary familial hypogonadism, male) 259.5
Reilly's (*see also* Neuropathy, peripheral, autonomic) 337.9
Reiter's 099.3
renal glomerulohyalinosis-diabetic 250.4 *[581.81]*
Rendu-Osler-Weber (familial hemorrhagic telangiectasia) 448.0
renofacial (congenital biliary fibroangiomatosis) 753.0
Rénon-Delille 253.8
respiratory distress (idiopathic) (newborn) 769
  adult (following shock, surgery, or trauma) 518.5
  specified NEC 518.82
  type II 770.6
restless legs (RLS) 333.94
retinoblastoma (familial) 190.5

1353

Syndrome

Syndrome—*continued*
retraction (Duane's) 378.71
retroperitoneal fibrosis 593.4
retroviral seroconversion (acute) V08
Rett's 330.8
Reye's 331.81
Reye-Sheehan (postpartum pituitary necrosis) 253.2
Riddoch's (visual disorientation) 368.16
Ridley's (*see also* Failure, ventricular, left) 428.1
Rieger's (mesodermal dysgenesis, anterior ocular segment) 743.44
Rietti-Greppi-Micheli (thalassemia minor) 282.49
right ventricular obstruction—*see* Failure heart
Riley-Day (familial dysautonomia) 742.8
Robin's 756.0
Rokitansky-Kuster-Hauser (congenital absence, vagina) 752.49
Romano-Ward (prolonged QT interval syndrome) 426.82
Romberg's 349.89
Rosen-Castleman-Liebow (pulmonary proteinosis) 516.0
rotator cuff, shoulder 726.10
Roth's 355.1
Rothmund's (congenital poikiloderma) 757.33
Rotor's (idiopathic hyperbilirubinemia) 277.4
Roussy-Lévy 334.3
Roy (-Jutras) (acropachyderma) 757.39
rubella (congenital) 771.0
Rubinstein-Taybi's (brachydactylia, short stature, and mental retardation) 759.89
Rud's (mental deficiency, epilepsy, and infantilism) 759.89
Ruiter-Pompen (-Wyers) (angiokeratoma corporis diffusum) 272.7
Runge's (postmaturity) 766.22
Russell (-Silver) (congenital hemihypertrophy and short stature) 759.89
Rytand-Lipsitch (complete atrioventricular block) 426.0
sacralization-scoliosis-sciatica 756.15
sacroiliac 724.6
Saenger's 379.46
salt
    depletion (*see also* Disease, renal) 593.9
        due to heat NEC 992.8
            causing heat exhaustion or prostration 992.4
    low (*see also* Disease, renal) 593.9
salt-losing (*see also* Disease, renal) 593.9
Sanfilippo's (mucopolysaccharidosis III) 277.5
Scaglietti-Dagnini (acromegalic macrospondylitis) 253.0
scalded skin 695.1
scalenus anticus (anterior) 353.0
scapulocostal 354.8
scapuloperoneal 359.1
scapulovertebral 723.4
Schaumann's (sarcoidosis) 135
Scheie's (mucopolysaccharidosis IS) 277.5
Scheuthauer-Marie-Sainton (cleidocranialis dysostosis) 755.59
Schirmer's (encephalocutaneous angiomatosis) 759.6
schizophrenic, of childhood NEC (*see also* Psychosis, childhood) 299.9
Schmidt's
    sphallo-pharyngo-laryngeal hemiplegia 352.6

Syndrome—*continued*
thyroid-adrenocortical insufficiency 258.1
vagoaccessory 352.6
Schneider's 047.9
Schnitzler 273.1
Scholte's (malignant carcinoid) 259.2
Scholz (-Bielschowsky-Henneberg) 330.0
Schroeder's (endocrine-hypertensive) 255.3
Schüller-Christian (chronic histiocytosis X) 277.89
Schultz's (agranulocytosis) 288.09
Schwachman's—*see* Syndrome, Shwachman's
Schwartz (-Jampel) 359.23
Schwartz-Bartter (inappropriate secretion of antidiuretic hormone) 253.6
Scimitar (anomalous venous drainage, right lung to inferior vena cave) 747.49
sclerocystic ovary 256.4
sea-blue histiocyte 272.7
Seabright-Bantam (pseudohypoparathyroidism) 275.49
Seckel's 759.89
Secretan's (posttraumatic edema) 782.3
secretoinhibitor (keratoconjunctivitis sicca) 710.2
Seeligmann's (ichthyosis congenita) 757.1
Senear-Usher (pemphigus erythematosus) 694.4
senilism 259.8
seroconversion, retroviral (acute) V08
serotonin 333.99
serous meningitis 348.2
Sertoli cell (germinal aplasia) 606.0
sex chromosome mosaic 758.81
Sézary's (reticulosis) (M9701/3) 202.2
shaken infant 995.55
Shaver's (bauxite pneumoconiosis) 503
Sheehan's (postpartum pituitary necrosis) 253.2
shock (traumatic) 958.4
    kidney 584.5
        following crush injury 958.5
    lung 518.5
    neurogenic 308.9
    psychic 308.9
short
    bowel 579.3
    P-R interval 426.81
shoulder-arm (*see also* Neuropathy, peripheral, autonomic) 337.9
shoulder-girdle 723.4
shoulder-hand (*see also* Neuropathy, peripheral, autonomic) 337.9
Shwachman's 288.02
Shy-Drager (orthostatic hypotension with multisystem degeneration) 333.0
Sicard's 352.6
sicca (keratoconjunctivitis) 710.2
sick
    cell 276.1
    cilia 759.89
    sinus 427.81
sideropenic 280.8
Siemens'
    ectodermal dysplasia 757.31
    keratosis follicularis spinulosa (decalvans) 757.39
Silfverskiöld's (osteochondrodystrophy, extremities) 756.50
Silver's (congenital hemihypertrophy and short stature) 759.89
Silvestroni-Bianco (thalassemia minima) 282.49
Simons' (progressive lipodystrophy) 272.6

INDEX TO DISEASES

Syndrome

Syndrome—*continued*
sinus tarsi 726.79
sinusitis-bronchiectasis-situs inversus 759.3
Sipple's (medullary thyroid
  carcinoma-pheochromocytoma) 258.02
Sjögren (-Gougerot) (keratoconjunctivitis sicca)
  710.2
  with lung involvement 710.2 *[517.8]*
Sjögren-Larsson (ichthyosis congenita) 757.1
Slocumb's 255.3
Sluder's 337.0
Smith-Lemli-Opitz (cerebrohepatorenal
  syndrome) 759.89
Smith-Magenis 758.33
smokers' 305.1
Sneddon-Wilkinson (subcorneal pustular
  dermatosis) 694.1
Sotos' (cerebral gigantism) 253.0
South African cardiomyopathy 425.2
spasmodic
  upward movement, eyes(s) 378.82
  winking 307.20
Spens' (syncope with heart block) 426.9
spherophakia-brachymorphia 759.89
spinal cord injury—*see also* Injury, spinal, by
    site
  with fracture, vertebra—*see* Fracture, vertebra,
    by site, with spinal cord injury
  cervical—*see* Injury, spinal, cervical
  fluid malabsorption (acquired) 331.3
splenic
  agenesis 759.0
  flexure 569.89
  neutropenia 289.53
  sequestration 289.52
Spurway's (brittle bones and blue sclera) 756.51
staphylococcal scalded skin 695.1
Stein's (polycystic ovary) 256.4
Stein-Leventhal (polycystic ovary) 256.4
Steinbrocker's (*see also* Neuropathy, peripheral,
    autonomic) 337.9
Stevens-Johnson (erythema multiforme
    exudativum) 695.1
Stewart-Morel (hyperostosis frontalis interna)
  733.3
Stickler 759.89
stiff-baby 759.89
stiff-man 333.91
Still's (juvenile rheumatoid arthritis) 714.30
Still-Felty (rheumatoid arthritis with
    splenomegaly and leukopenia) 714.1
Stilling-Türk-Duane (ocular retraction
    syndrome) 378.71
Stojano's (subcostal) 098.86
Stokes (-Adams) (syncope with heart block)
  426.9
Stokvis-Talma (enterogenous cyanosis) 289.7
stone heart (*see also* Failure, ventricular, left)
  428.1
straight-back 756.19
stroke (*see also* Disease, cerebrovascular, acute)
  436
  little 435.9
Sturge-Kalischer-Weber (encephalotrigeminal
    angiomatosis) 759.6
Sturge-Weber (-Dimitri) (encephalocutaneous
    angiomatosis) 759.6
subclavian-carotid obstruction (chronic) 446.7
subclavian steal 435.2
subcoracoid-pectoralis minor 447.8

Syndrome—*continued*
subcostal 098.86
  nerve compression 354.8
subperiosteal hematoma 267
subphrenic interposition 751.4
sudden infant death (SIDS) 798.0
Sudeck's 733.7
Sudeck-Leriche 733.7
superior
  cerebellar artery (*see also* Disease,
    cerebrovascular, acute) 436
  mesenteric artery 557.1
  pulmonary sulcus (tumor) (M8010/3) 162.3
  vena cava 459.2
suprarenal cortical 255.3
supraspinatus 726.10
swallowed blood 777.3
sweat retention 705.1
Sweet's (acute febrile neutrophilic dermatosis)
  695.89
Swyer-James (unilateral hyperlucent lung) 492.8
Swyer's (XY pure gonadal dysgenesis) 752.7
Symonds' 348.2
sympathetic
  cervical paralysis 337.0
  pelvic 625.5
syndactylic oxycephaly 755.55
syphilitic-cardiovascular 093.89
systemic
  fibrosclerosing 710.8
  inflammatory response (SIRS) 995.90
    due to
      infectious process 995.91
        with acute organ dysfunction 995.92
      non-infectious process 995.93
        with acute organ dysfunction 995.94
systolic click (-murmur) 785.2
Tabagism 305.1
tachycardia-bradycardia 427.81
Takayasu (-Onishi) (pulseless disease) 446.7
Takotsubo 429.83
Tapia's 352.6
tarsal tunnel 355.5
Taussig-Bing (transposition, aorta and
    overriding pulmonary artery) 745.11
Taybi's (otopalatodigital) 759.89
Taylor's 625.5
teething 520.7
tegmental 344.89
telangiectasis-pigmentation-cataract 757.33
temporal 383.02
  lobectomy behavior 310.0
temporomandibular joint-pain-dysfunction
    [TMJ] NEC 524.60
  specified NEC 524.69
Terry's 362.21
testicular feminization 259.5
testis, nonvirilizing 257.8
tethered (spinal) cord 742.59
thalamic 338.0
Thibierge-Weissenbach (cutaneous systemic
    sclerosis) 710.1
Thiele 724.6
thoracic outlet (compression) 353.0
thoracogenous rheumatic (hypertrophic
    pulmonary osteoarthropathy) 731.2
Thorn's (*see also* Disease, renal) 593.9
Thorson-Biörck (malignant carcinoid) 259.2
thrombopenia-hemangioma 287.39
thyroid-adrenocortical insufficiency 258.1
Tietze's 733.6

1355

Syndrome   INDEX TO DISEASES

Syndrome—*continued*
- time-zone (rapid) 327.35
- Tobias' (carcinoma, pulmonary apex) (M8010/3) 162.3
- toilet seat 926.0
- Tolosa-Hunt 378.55
- Toni-Fanconi (cystinosis) 270.0
- Touraine's (hereditary osteo-onychodysplasia) 756.89
- Touraine-Solente-Golé (acropachyderma) 757.39
- toxic
  - oil 710.5
  - shock 040.82
- transfusion
  - fetal-maternal 772.0
  - twin
    - donor (infant) 772.0
    - recipient (infant) 776.4
- transient left ventricular apical ballooning 429.83
- Treacher Collins' (incomplete mandibulofacial dysostosis) 756.0
- trigeminal plate 259.8
- triple X female 758.81
- trisomy NEC 758.5
  - 13 or D₁ 758.1
  - 16-18 or E 758.2
  - 18 or E₃ 758.2
  - 20 758.5
  - 21 or G (mongolism) 758.0
  - 22 or G (mongolism) 758.0
  - G 758.0
- Troisier-Hanot-Chauffard (bronze diabetes) 275.0
- tropical wet feet 991.4
- Trousseau's (thrombophlebitis migrans visceral cancer) 453.1
- Türk's (ocular retraction syndrome) 378.71
- Turner's 758.6
- Turner-Varny 758.6
- twin-to-twin transfusion 762.3
  - recipient twin 776.4
- Uehlinger's (acropachyderma) 757.39
- Ullrich (-Bonnevie) (-Turner) 758.6
- Ullrich-Feichtiger 759.89
- underwater blast injury (abdominal) (*see also* Injury, internal, abdomen) 868.00
- universal joint, cervix 620.6
- Unverricht (-Lundborg) 333.2
- Unverricht-Wagner (dermatomyositis) 710.3
- upward gaze 378.81
- Urbach-Oppenheim (necrobiosis lipoidica diabeticorum) 250.8 *[709.3]*
- Urbach-Wiethe (lipoid proteinosis) 272.8
- uremia, chronic 585.9
- urethral 597.81
- urethro-oculoarticular 099.3
- urethro-oculosynovial 099.3
- urohepatic 572.4
- uveocutaneous 364.24
- uveomeningeal, uveomeningitis 363.22
- vagohypoglossal 352.6
- vagovagal 780.2
- van Buchem's (hyperostosis corticalis) 733.3
- van der Hoeve's (brittle bones and blue sclera, deafness) 756.51
- van der Hoeve-Halbertsma-Waardenburg (ptosis-epicanthus) 270.2
- van der Hoeve-Waardenburg-Gualdi (ptosis-epicanthus) 270.2

Syndrome—*continued*
- van Neck-Odelberg (juvenile osteochondrosis) 732.1
- vanishing twin 651.33
- vascular splanchnic 557.0
- vasomotor 443.9
- vasovagal 780.2
- VATER 759.89
- Velo-cardio-facial 758.32
- vena cava (inferior) (superior) (obstruction) 459.2
- Verbiest's (claudicatio intermittens spinalis) 435.1
- Vernet's 352.6
- vertebral
  - artery 435.1
    - compression 721.1
  - lumbar 724.4
  - steal 435.1
- vertebrogenic (pain) 724.5
- vertiginous NEC 386.9
- video display tube 723.8
- Villaret's 352.6
- Vinson-Plummer (sideropenic dysphagia) 280.8
- virilizing adrenocortical hyperplasia, congenital 255.2
- virus, viral 079.99
- visceral larval migrans 128.0
- visual disorientation 368.16
- vitamin B₆ deficiency 266.1
- vitreous touch 997.99
- Vogt's (corpus striatum) 333.71
- Vogt-Koyanagi 364.24
- Volkmann's 958.6
- von Bechterew-Strümpell (ankylosing spondylitis) 720.0
- von Graefe's 378.72
- von Hippel-Lindau (angiomatosis retinocerebellosa) 759.6
- von Schroetter's (intermittent venous claudication) 453.8
- von Willebrand (-Jürgens) (angiohemophilia) 286.4
- Waardenburg-Klein (ptosis epicanthus) 270.2
- Wagner (-Unverricht) (dermatomyositis) 710.3
- Waldenström's (macroglobulinemia) 273.3
- Waldenström-Kjellberg (sideropenic dysphagia) 280.8
- Wallenberg's (posterior inferior cerebellar artery) (*see also* Disease, cerebrovascular, acute) 436
- Waterhouse (-Friderichsen) 036.3
- water retention 276.6
- Weber's 344.89
- Weber-Christian (nodular nonsuppurative panniculitis) 729.30
- Weber-Cockayne (epidermolysis bullosa) 757.39
- Weber-Dimitri (encephalocutaneous angiomatosis) 759.6
- Weber-Gubler 344.89
- Weber-Leyden 344.89
- Weber-Osler (familial hemorrhagic telangiectasia) 448.0
- Wegener's (necrotizing respiratory granulomatosis) 446.4
- Weill-Marchesani (brachymorphism and ectopia lentis) 759.89
- Weingarten's (tropical eosinophilia) 518.3
- Weiss-Baker (carotid sinus syncope) 337.0

INDEX TO DISEASES   **Syphilis, syphilitic**

Syndrome—*continued*
  Weissenbach-Thibierge (cutaneous systemic sclerosis) 710.1
  Werdnig-Hoffmann 335.0
  Werlhof-Wichmann (*see also* Purpura, thrombocytopenic) 287.39
  Wermer's (polyendocrine adenomatosis) 258.01
  Werner's (progeria adultorum) 259.8
  Wernicke's (nonalcoholic) (superior hemorrhagic polioencephalitis) 265.1
  Wernicke-Korsakoff (nonalcoholic) 294.0
    alcoholic 291.1
  Westphal-Strümpell (hepatolenticular degeneration) 275.1
  wet
    brain (alcoholic) 303.9
    feet (maceration) (tropical) 991.4
    lung
      adult 518.5
      newborn 770.6
  whiplash 847.0
  Whipple's (intestinal lipodystrophy) 040.2
  "whistling face" (craniocarpotarsal dystrophy) 759.89
  Widal (-Abrami) (acquired hemolytic jaundice) 283.9
  Wilkie's 557.1
  Wilkinson-Sneddon (subcorneal pustular dermatosis) 694.1
  Willan-Plumbe (psoriasis) 696.1
  Willebrand (-Jürgens) (angiohemophilia) 286.4
  Willi-Prader (hypogenital dystrophy with diabetic tendency) 759.81
  Wilson's (hepatolenticular degeneration) 275.1
  Wilson-Mikity 770.7
  Wiskott-Aldrich (eczema-thrombocytopenia) 279.12
  withdrawal
    alcohol 291.81
    drug 292.0
      infant of dependent mother 779.5
  Woakes' (ethmoiditis) 471.1
  Wolff-Parkinson-White (anomalous atrioventricular excitation) 426.7
  Wright's (hyperabduction) 447.8
  X
    cardiac 413.9
    dysmetabolic 277.7
  xiphoidalgia 733.99
  XO 758.6
  XXX 758.81
  XXXXY 758.81
  XXY 758.7
  yellow vernix (placental dysfunction) 762.2
  Zahorsky's 074.0
  Zellweger 277.86
  Zieve's (jaundice, hyperlipemia and hemolytic anemia) 571.1
  Zollinger-Ellison (gastric hypersecretion with pancreatic islet cell tumor) 251.5
  Zuelzer-Ogden (nutritional megaloblastic anemia) 281.2
Synechia (iris) (pupil) 364.70
  anterior 364.72
    peripheral 364.73
  intrauterine (traumatic) 621.5
  posterior 364.71
  vulvae, congenital 752.49
Synesthesia (*see also* Disturbance, sensation) 782.0
Synodontia 520.2
Synophthalmus 759.89

Synorchidism 752.89
Synorchism 752.89
Synostosis (congenital) 756.59
  astragaloscaphoid 755.67
  radioulnar 755.53
  talonavicular (bar) 755.67
  tarsal 755.67
Synovial —*see* condition
Synovioma (M9040/3)—*see also* Neoplasm, connective tissue, malignant
  benign (M9040/3)—*see* Neoplasm, connective tissue, benign
Synoviosarcoma (M9040/3)—*see* Neoplasm, connective tissue, malignant
Synovitis 727.00
  chronic crepitant, wrist 727.2
  due to crystals—*see* Arthritis, due to crystals
  gonococcal 098.51
  gouty 274.0
  syphilitic 095.7
    congenital 090.0
  traumatic, current—*see* Sprain, by site
  tuberculous—*see* Tuberculosis, synovitis
  villonodular 719.20
    ankle 719.27
    elbow 719.22
    foot 719.27
    hand 719.24
    hip 719.25
    knee 719.26
    multiple sites 719.29
    pelvic region 719.25
    shoulder (region) 719.21
    specified site NEC 719.28
    wrist 719.23
Syphilide 091.3
  congenital 090.0
  newborn 090.0
  tubercular 095.8
    congenital 090.0
Syphilis, syphilitic (acquired) 097.9
  with lung involvement 095.1
  abdomen (late) 095.2
  acoustic nerve 094.86
  adenopathy (secondary) 091.4
  adrenal (gland) 095.8
    with cortical hypofunction 095.8
  age under 2 years NEC (*see also* Syphilis, congenital) 090.9
    acquired 097.9
  alopecia (secondary) 091.82
  anemia 095.8
  aneurysm (artery) (ruptured) 093.89
    aorta 093.0
    central nervous system 094.89
    congenital 090.5
  anus 095.8
    primary 091.1
    secondary 091.3
  aorta, aortic (arch) (abdominal) (insufficiency) (pulmonary) (regurgitation) (stenosis) (thoracic) 093.89
    aneurysm 093.0
  arachnoid (adhesive) 094.2
  artery 093.89
    cerebral 094.89
    spinal 094.89
  arthropathy (neurogenic) (tabetic) 094.0 *[713.5]*
  asymptomatic—*see* Syphilis, latent
  ataxia, locomotor (progressive) 094.0
  atrophoderma maculatum 091.3

Syphilis, syphilitic—*continued*
  auricular fibrillation 093.89
  Bell's palsy 094.89
  bladder 095.8
  bone 095.5
    secondary 091.61
  brain 094.89
  breast 095.8
  bronchus 095.8
  bubo 091.0
  bulbar palsy 094.89
  bursa (late) 095.7
  cardiac decompensation 093.89
  cardiovascular (early) (late) (primary)
      (secondary) (tertiary) 093.9
    specified type and site NEC 093.89
  causing death under 2 years of age (*see also*
      Syphilis, congenital) 090.9
    stated to be acquired NEC 097.9
  central nervous system (any site) (early) (late)
      (latent) (primary) (recurrent) (relapse)
      (secondary) (tertiary) 094.9
    with
      ataxia 094.0
      paralysis, general 094.1
        juvenile 090.40
      paresis (general) 094.1
        juvenile 090.40
      tabes (dorsalis) 094.0
        juvenile 090.40
      taboparesis 094.1
        juvenile 090.40
    aneurysm (ruptured) 094.87
    congenital 090.40
    juvenile 090.40
    remission in (sustained) 094.9
    serology doubtful, negative, or positive 094.9
    specified nature or site NEC 094.89
    vascular 094.89
  cerebral 094.89
    meningovascular 094.2
    nerves 094.89
    sclerosis 094.89
    thrombosis 094.89
  cerebrospinal 094.89
    tabetic 094.0
  cerebrovascular 094.89
  cervix 095.8
  chancre (multiple) 091.0
    extragenital 091.2
    Rollet's 091.0
  Charcot's joint 094.0 *[713.5]*
  choked disc 094.89 *[377.00]*
  chorioretinitis 091.51
    congenital 090.0 *[363.13]*
    late 094.83
  choroiditis 091.51
    congenital 090.0 *[363.13]*
    late 094.83
    prenatal 090.0 *[363.13]*
  choroidoretinitis (secondary) 091.51
    congenital 090.0 *[363.13]*
    late 094.83
  ciliary body (secondary) 091.52
    late 095.8 *[364.11]*
  colon (late) 095.8
  combined sclerosis 094.89

Syphilis, syphilitic—*continued*
  complicating pregnancy, childbirth or
      puerperium 647.0
    affecting fetus or newborn 760.2
  condyloma (latum) 091.3
  congenital 090.9
    with
      encephalitis 090.41
      paresis (general) 090.40
      tabes (dorsalis) 090.40
      taboparesis 090.40
    chorioretinitis, choroiditis 090.0 *[363.13]*
    early or less than 2 years after birth NEC 090.2
      with manifestations 090.0
      latent (without manifestations) 090.1
        negative spinal fluid test 090.1
        serology, positive 090.1
      symptomatic 090.0
    interstitial keratitis 090.3
    juvenile neurosyphilis 090.40
    late or 2 years or more after birth NEC 090.7
      chorioretinitis, choroiditis 090.5 *[363.13]*
      interstitial keratitis 090.3
      juvenile neurosyphilis NEC 090.40
      latent (without manifestations) 090.6
        negative spinal fluid test 090.6
        serology, positive 090.6
      symptomatic or with manifestations NEC
          090.5
        interstitial keratitis 090.3
  conjugal 097.9
    tabes 094.0
  conjunctiva 095.8 *[372.10]*
  contact V01.6
  cord, bladder 094.0
  cornea, late 095.8 *[370.59]*
  coronary (artery) 093.89
    sclerosis 093.89
  coryza 095.8
    congenital 090.0
  cranial nerve 094.89
  cutaneous—*see* Syphilis, skin
  dacryocystitis 095.8
  degeneration, spinal cord 094.89
  d'emblée 095.8
  dementia 094.1
    paralytica 094.1
      juvenilis 090.40
  destruction of bone 095.5
  dilatation, aorta 093.0
  due to blood transfusion 097.9
  dura mater 094.89
  ear 095.8
    inner 095.8
      nerve (eighth) 094.86
      neurorecurrence 094.86
  early NEC 091.0
    cardiovascular 093.9
    central nervous system 094.9
      paresis 094.1
      tabes 094.0
    latent (without manifestations) (less than 2
        years after infection) 092.9
      negative spinal fluid test 092.9
      serological relapse following treatment
          092.0
      serology positive 092.9

1358

INDEX TO DISEASES

Syphilis, syphilitic

Syphilis, syphilitic—*continued*
  paresis 094.1
  relapse (treated, untreated) 091.7
  skin 091.3
    symptomatic NEC 091.89
      extragenital chancre 091.2
      primary, except extragenital chancre 091.0
      secondary (*see also* Syphilis, secondary) 091.3
        relapse (treated, untreated) 091.7
    tabes 094.0
    ulcer 091.3
  eighth nerve 094.86
  endemic, nonvenereal 104.0
  endocarditis 093.20
    aortic 093.22
    mitral 093.21
    pulmonary 093.24
    tricuspid 093.23
  epididymis (late) 095.8
  epiglottis 095.8
  epiphysitis (congenital) 090.0
  esophagus 095.8
  Eustachian tube 095.8
  exposure to V01.6
  eye 095.8 *[363.13]*
    neuromuscular mechanism 094.85
  eyelid 095.8 *[373.5]*
    with gumma 095.8 *[373.5]*
    ptosis 094.89
  fallopian tube 095.8
  fracture 095.5
  gallbladder (late) 095.8
  gastric 095.8
    crisis 094.0
    polyposis 095.8
  general 097.9
    paralysis 094.1
      juvenile 090.40
  genital (primary) 091.0
  glaucoma 095.8
  gumma (late) NEC 095.9
    cardiovascular system 093.9
    central nervous system 094.9
    congenital 090.5
    heart or artery 093.89
  heart 093.89
    block 093.89
    decompensation 093.89
    disease 093.89
    failure 093.89
    valve (*see also* Syphilis, endocarditis) 093.20
  hemianesthesia 094.89
  hemianopsia 095.8
  hemiparesis 094.89
  hemiplegia 094.89
  hepatic artery 093.89
  hepatitis 095.3
  hepatomegaly 095.3
    congenital 090.0
  hereditaria tarda (*see also* Syphilis, congenital, late) 090.7
  hereditary (*see also* Syphilis, congenital) 090.9
    interstitial keratitis 090.3
  Hutchinson's teeth 090.5
  hyalitis 095.8
  inactive—*see* Syphilis, latent
  infantum NEC (*see also* Syphilis, congenital) 090.9
  inherited—*see* Syphilis, congenital
  internal ear 095.8

Syphilis, syphilitic—*continued*
  intestine (late) 095.8
  iris, iritis (secondary) 091.52
    late 095.8 *[364.11]*
  joint (late) 095.8
  keratitis (congenital) (early) (interstitial) (late) (parenchymatous) (punctata profunda) 090.3
  kidney 095.4
  lacrimal apparatus 095.8
  laryngeal paralysis 095.8
  larynx 095.8
  late 097.0
    cardiovascular 093.9
    central nervous system 094.9
    latent or 2 years or more after infection (without manifestations) 096
      negative spinal fluid test 096
      serology positive 096
    paresis 094.1
    specified site NEC 095.8
    symptomatic or with symptoms 095.9
    tabes 094.0
  latent 097.1
    central nervous system 094.9
    date of infection unspecified 097.1
    early or less than 2 years after infection 092.9
    late or 2 years or more after infection 096
    serology
      doubtful
        follow-up of latent syphilis 097.1
          central nervous system 094.9
          date of infection unspecified 097.1
          early or less than 2 years after infection 092.9
          late or 2 years or more after infection 096
      positive, only finding 097.1
        date of infection unspecified 097.1
        early or less than 2 years after infection 097.1
        late or 2 years or more after infection 097.1
  lens 095.8
  leukoderma 091.3
    late 095.8
  lienis 095.8
  lip 091.3
    chancre 091.2
    late 095.8
    primary 091.2
  Lissauer's paralysis 094.1
  liver 095.3
    secondary 091.62
  locomotor ataxia 094.0
  lung 095.1
  lymphadenitis (secondary) 091.4
  lymph gland (early) (secondary) 091.4
    late 095.8
  macular atrophy of skin 091.3
    striated 095.8
  maternal, affecting fetus or newborn 760.2
    manifest syphilis in newborn—*see* Syphilis, congenital
  mediastinum (late) 095.8
  meninges (adhesive) (basilar) (brain) (spinal cord) 094.2
  meningitis 094.2
    acute 091.81
    congenital 090.42
  meningoencephalitis 094.2
  meningovascular 094.2
    congenital 090.49

Syphilis, syphilitic—*continued*
mesarteritis 093.89
 brain 094.89
 spine 094.89
middle ear 095.8
mitral stenosis 093.21
monoplegia 094.89
mouth (secondary) 091.3
 late 095.8
mucocutaneous 091.3
 late 095.8
mucous
 membrane 091.3
  late 095.8
 patches 091.3
  congenital 090.0
mulberry molars 090.5
muscle 095.6
myocardium 093.82
myositis 095.6
nasal sinus 095.8
neonatorum NEC (*see also* Syphilis, congenital) 090.9
nerve palsy (any cranial nerve) 094.89
nervous system, central 094.9
neuritis 095.8
 acoustic nerve 094.86
neurorecidive of retina 094.83
neuroretinitis 094.85
newborn (*see also* Syphilis, congenital) 090.9
nodular superficial 095.8
nonvenereal, endemic 104.0
nose 095.8
 saddle back deformity 090.5
 septum 095.8
  perforated 095.8
occlusive arterial disease 093.89
ophthalmic 095.8 *[363.13]*
ophthalmoplegia 094.89
optic nerve (atrophy) (neuritis) (papilla) 094.84
orbit (late) 095.8
orchitis 095.8
organic 097.9
osseous (late) 095.5
osteochondritis (congenital) 090.0
osteoporosis 095.5
ovary 095.8
oviduct 095.8
palate 095.8
 gumma 095.8
 perforated 090.5
pancreas (late) 095.8
pancreatitis 095.8
paralysis 094.89
 general 094.1
 juvenile 090.40
paraplegia 094.89
paresis (general) 094.1
 juvenile 090.40
paresthesia 094.89
Parkinson's disease or syndrome 094.82
paroxysmal tachycardia 093.89
pemphigus (congenital) 090.0
penis 091.0
 chancre 091.0
 late 095.8
pericardium 093.81
perichondritis, larynx 095.8
periosteum 095.5
 congenital 090.0
 early 091.61

Syphilis, syphilitic—*continued*
 secondary 091.61
peripheral nerve 095.8
petrous bone (late) 095.5
pharynx 095.8
 secondary 091.3
pituitary (gland) 095.8
placenta 095.8
pleura (late) 095.8
pneumonia, white 090.0
pontine (lesion) 094.89
portal vein 093.89
primary NEC 091.2
 anal 091.1
 and secondary (*see also* Syphilis, secondary) 091.9
 cardiovascular 093.9
 central nervous system 094.9
 extragenital chancre NEC 091.2
 fingers 091.2
 genital 091.0
 lip 091.2
 specified site NEC 091.2
 tonsils 091.2
prostate 095.8
psychosis (intracranial gumma) 094.89
ptosis (eyelid) 094.89
pulmonary (late) 095.1
 artery 093.89
pulmonum 095.1
pyelonephritis 095.4
recently acquired, symptomatic NEC 091.89
rectum 095.8
respiratory tract 095.8
retina
 late 094.83
 neurorecidive 094.83
retrobulbar neuritis 094.85
salpingitis 095.8
sclera (late) 095.0
sclerosis
 cerebral 094.89
 coronary 093.89
 multiple 094.89
 subacute 094.89
scotoma (central) 095.8
scrotum 095.8
secondary (and primary) 091.9
 adenopathy 091.4
 anus 091.3
 bone 091.61
 cardiovascular 093.9
 central nervous system 094.9
 chorioretinitis, choroiditis 091.51
 hepatitis 091.62
 liver 091.62
 lymphadenitis 091.4
 meningitis, acute 091.81
 mouth 091.3
 mucous membranes 091.3
 periosteum 091.61
 periostitis 091.61
 pharynx 091.3
 relapse (treated) (untreated) 091.7
 skin 091.3
 specified form NEC 091.89
 tonsil 091.3
 ulcer 091.3
 viscera 091.69
 vulva 091.3
seminal vesicle (late) 095.8

INDEX TO DISEASES — **System, systemic**

Syphilis, syphilitic—*continued*
  seronegative
    with signs or symptoms—*see* Syphilis, by site and stage
  seropositive
    with signs or symptoms—*see* Syphilis, by site and stage
    follow-up of latent syphilis—*see* Syphilis, latent
    only finding—*see* Syphilis, latent
  seventh nerve (paralysis) 094.89
  sinus 095.8
  sinusitis 095.8
  skeletal system 095.5
  skin (early) (secondary) (with ulceration) 091.3
    late or tertiary 095.8
  small intestine 095.8
  spastic spinal paralysis 094.0
  spermatic cord (late) 095.8
  spinal (cord) 094.89
    with
      paresis 094.1
      tabes 094.0
  spleen 095.8
  splenomegaly 095.8
  spondylitis 095.5
  staphyloma 095.8
  stigmata (congenital) 090.5
  stomach 095.8
  synovium (late) 095.7
  tabes dorsalis (early) (late) 094.0
    juvenile 090.40
  tabetic type 094.0
    juvenile 090.40
  taboparesis 094.1
    juvenile 090.40
  tachycardia 093.89
  tendon (late) 095.7
  tertiary 097.0
    with symptoms 095.8
    cardiovascular 093.9
    central nervous system 094.9
    multiple NEC 095.8
    specified site NEC 095.8
  testis 095.8
  thorax 095.8
  throat 095.8
  thymus (gland) 095.8
  thyroid (late) 095.8
  tongue 095.8
  tonsil (lingual) 095.8
    primary 091.2
    secondary 091.3
  trachea 095.8
  tricuspid valve 093.23
  tumor, brain 094.89
  tunica vaginalis (late) 095.8
  ulcer (any site) (early) (secondary) 091.3
    late 095.9
    perforating 095.9
      foot 094.0
  urethra (stricture) 095.8
  urogenital 095.8
  uterus 095.8
  uveal tract (secondary) 091.50
    late 095.8 *[363.13]*
  uveitis (secondary) 091.50
    late 095.8 *[363.13]*
  uvula (late) 095.8
    perforated 095.8
  vagina 091.0

Syphilis, syphilitic—*continued*
  late 095.8
  valvulitis NEC 093.20
  vascular 093.89
    brain or cerebral 094.89
  vein 093.89
    cerebral 094.89
  ventriculi 095.8
  vesicae urinariae 095.8
  viscera (abdominal) 095.2
    secondary 091.69
  vitreous (hemorrhage) (opacities) 095.8
  vulva 091.0
    late 095.8
    secondary 091.3
Syphiloma 095.9
  cardiovascular system 093.9
  central nervous system 094.9
  circulatory system 093.9
  congenital 090.5
Syphilophobia 300.29
Syringadenoma (M8400/0)—*see also* Neoplasm, skin, benign
  papillary (M8406/0)—*see* Neoplasm, skin, benign
Syringobulbia 336.0
Syringocarcinoma (M8400/3)—*see* Neoplasm, skin, malignant
Syringocystadenoma (M8400/0)—*see also* Neoplasm, skin, benign
  papillary (M8406/0)—*see* Neoplasm, skin, benign
Syringocystoma (M8407/0)—*see* Neoplasm, skin, benign
Syringoma (M8407/0)—*see also* Neoplasm, skin, benign
  chondroid (M8940/0)—*see* Neoplasm, by site, benign
Syringomyelia 336.0
Syringomyelitis 323.9
  late effect—*see* category 326
Syringomyelocele (*see also* Spina bifida) 741.9
Syringopontia 336.0
System, systemic —*see also* condition
  disease, combined—*see* Degeneration, combined
  fibrosclerosing syndrome 710.8
  inflammatory response syndrome (SIRS) 995.90
    due to
      infectious process 995.91
        with acute organ dysfunction 995.92
      non-infectious process 995.93
        with acute organ dysfunction 995.94
  lupus erythematosus 710.0
    inhibitor 286.5

T

Tab —*see* Tag
Tabacism 989.8
Tabacosis 989.8
Tabardillo 080
  flea-borne 081.0
  louse-borne 080
Tabes, tabetic
  with
    central nervous system syphilis 094.0
    Charcot's joint 094.0 *[713.5]*
    cord bladder 094.0
    crisis, viscera (any) 094.0
    paralysis, general 094.1
    paresis (general) 094.1
    perforating ulcer 094.0
  arthropathy 094.0 *[713.5]*
  bladder 094.0
  bone 094.0
  cerebrospinal 094.0
  congenital 090.40
  conjugal 094.0
  dorsalis 094.0
    neurosyphilis 094.0
  early 094.0
  juvenile 090.40
  latent 094.0
  mesenterica (*see also* Tuberculosis) 014.8
  paralysis insane, general 094.1
  peripheral (nonsyphilitic) 799.89
  spasmodic 094.0
    not dorsal or dorsalis 343.9
  syphilis (cerebrospinal) 094.0
Taboparalysis 094.1
Taboparesis (remission) 094.1
  with
    Charcot's joint 094.1 *[713.5]*
    cord bladder 094.1
    perforating ulcer 094.1
  juvenile 090.40
Tache noir 923.20
Tachyalimentation 579.3
Tachyarrhythmia, tachyrhythmia —*see also*
    Tachycardia
  paroxysmal with sinus bradycardia 427.81
Tachycardia 785.0
  atrial 427.89
  auricular 427.89
  AV nodal re-entry (re-entrant) 427.89
  newborn 779.82
  nodal 427.89
    nonparoxysmal atrioventricular 426.89
    nonparoxysmal atrioventricular (nodal) 426.89
  paroxysmal 427.2
    with sinus bradycardia 427.81
    atrial (PAT) 427.0
      psychogenic 316 *[427.0]*
    atrioventricular (AV) 427.0
      psychogenic 316 *[427.0]*
    essential 427.2
    junctional ectopic 427.0
    nodal 427.0
    psychogenic 316 *[427.2]*
      atrial 316 *[427.0]*
      supraventricular 316 *[427.0]*
      ventricular 316 *[427.1]*
    supraventricular 427.0
      psychogenic 316 *[427.0]*
    ventricular 427.1

Tachycardia—*continued*
    psychogenic 316 *[427.1]*
  postoperative 997.1
  psychogenic 306.2
  sick sinus 427.81
  sinoauricular 427.89
  sinus 427.89
  supraventricular 427.89
  ventricular (paroxysmal) 427.1
    psychogenic 316 *[427.1]*
Tachygastria 536.8
Tachypnea 786.06
  hysterical 300.11
  newborn (idiopathic) (transitory) 770.6
  psychogenic 306.1
  transitory, of newborn 770.6
Taenia (infection) (infestation) (*see also*
    Infestation, taenia) 123.3
  diminuta 123.6
  echinococcal infestation (*see also*
    Echinococcus) 122.9
  nana 123.6
  saginata infestation 123.2
  solium (intestinal form) 123.0
    larval form 123.1
Taeniasis (intestine) (*see also* Infestation, Taenia)
    123.3
  saginata 123.2
  solium 123.0
Taenzer's disease 757.4
Tag (hypertrophied skin) (infected) 701.9
  adenoid 474.8
  anus 455.9
  endocardial (*see also* Endocarditis) 424.90
  hemorrhoidal 455.9
  hymen 623.8
  perineal 624.8
  preauricular 744.1
  rectum 455.9
  sentinel 455.9
  skin 701.9
    accessory 757.39
    anus 455.9
    congenital 757.39
    preauricular 744.1
    rectum 455.9
  tonsil 474.8
  urethra, urethral 599.84
  vulva 624.8
Tahyna fever 062.5
Takayasu (-Onishi) disease or syndrome
    (pulseless disease) 446.7
Takotsubo syndrome 429.83
Talc granuloma 728.82
  in operation wound 998.7
Talcosis 502
Talipes (congenital) 754.70
  acquired NEC 736.79
    planus 734
  asymmetric 754.79
    acquired 736.79
  calcaneovalgus 754.62
    acquired 736.76
  calcaneovarus 754.59
    acquired 736.76
  calcaneus 754.79
    acquired 736.76

Talipes — *continued*
  cavovarus 754.59
    acquired 736.75
  cavus 754.71
    acquired 736.73
  equinovalgus 754.69
    acquired 736.72
  equinovarus 754.51
    acquired 736.71
  equinus 754.79
    acquired, NEC 736.72
  percavus 754.71
    acquired 736.73
  planovalgus 754.69
    acquired 736.79
  planus (acquired) (any degree) 734
    congenital 754.61
    due to rickets 268.1
  valgus 754.60
    acquired 736.79
  varus 754.50
    acquired 736.79
Talma's disease 728.85
Talon noir 924.20
  hand 923.20
  heel 924.20
  toe 924.3
Tamponade heart (Rose's) (*see also* Pericarditis) 423.3
Tanapox 078.89
Tangier disease (familial high-density lipoprotein deficiency) 272.5
Tank ear 380.12
Tantrum (childhood) (*see also* Disturbance, conduct) 312.1
Tapeworm (infection) (infestation) (*see also* Infestation, tapeworm) 123.9
Tapia's syndrome 352.6
Tarantism 297.8
Target-oval cell anemia 282.49
Tarlov's cyst 355.9
Tarral-Besnier disease (pityriasis rubra pilaris) 696.4
Tarsalgia 729.2
Tarsal tunnel syndrome 355.5
Tarsitis (eyelid) 373.00
  syphilitic 095.8 *[373.00]*
  tuberculous (*see also* Tuberculosis) 017.0 *[373.4]*
Tartar (teeth) 523.6
Tattoo (mark) 709.09
Taurodontism 520.2
Taussig-Bing defect, heart, or syndrome (transposition, aorta and overriding pulmonary artery) 745.11
Tay's choroiditis 363.41
Tay-Sachs
  amaurotic familial idiocy 330.1
  disease 330.1
Taybi's syndrome (otopalatodigital) 759.89
Taylor's
  disease (diffuse idiopathic cutaneous atrophy) 701.8
  syndrome 625.5
Tear, torn (traumatic) — *see also* Wound, open, by site
  anus, anal (sphincter) 863.89
    with open wound in cavity 863.99
    complicating delivery (healed) (old) 654.8
      with mucosa 664.3

Tear, torn — *continued*
    not associated with third-degree perineal laceration 664.6
  nontraumatic, nonpuerperal (healed) (old) 569.43
  articular cartilage, old (*see also* Disorder, cartilage, articular) 718.0
  bladder
    with
      abortion — *see* Abortion, by type, with damage to pelvic organs
      ectopic pregnancy (*see also* categories 633.0-633.9) 639.2
      molar pregnancy (*see also* categories 630-632) 639.2
    following
      abortion 639.2
      ectopic or molar pregnancy 639.2
    obstetrical trauma 665.5
  bowel
    with
      abortion — *see* Abortion, by type, with damage to pelvic organs
      ectopic pregnancy (*see also* categories 633.0-633.9) 639.2
      molar pregnancy (*see also* categories 630-632) 639.2
    following
      abortion 639.2
      ectopic or molar pregnancy 639.2
    obstetrical trauma 665.5
  broad ligament
    with
      abortion — *see* Abortion, by type, with damage to pelvic organs
      ectopic pregnancy (*see also* categories 633.0-633.9) 639.2
      molar pregnancy (*see also* categories 630-632) 639.2
    following
      abortion 639.2
      ectopic or molar pregnancy 639.2
    obstetrical trauma 665.6
  bucket handle (knee) (meniscus) — *see* Tear, meniscus
  capsule
    joint — *see* Sprain, by site
    spleen — *see* Laceration, spleen, capsule
  cartilage — *see also* Sprain, by site
    articular, old (*see also* Disorder, cartilage, articular) 718.0
    knee — *see* Tear, meniscus
    semilunar (knee) (current injury) — *see* Tear, meniscus
  cervix
    with
      abortion — *see* Abortion, by type, with damage to pelvic organs
      ectopic pregnancy (*see also* categories 633.0-633.9) 639.2
      molar pregnancy (*see also* categories 630-632) 639.2
    following
      abortion 639.2
      ectopic or molar pregnancy 639.2
    obstetrical trauma (current) 665.3
    old 622.3
  dural 998.2
  internal organ (abdomen, chest, or pelvis) — *see* Injury, internal, by site

INDEX TO DISEASES

Tear, torn—*continued*
  ligament—*see also* Sprain, by site
    with open wound—*see* Wound, open by site
  meniscus (knee) (current injury) 836.2
    bucket handle 836.0
      old 717.0
    lateral 836.1
      anterior horn 836.1
        old 717.42
      bucket handle 836.1
        old 717.41
      old 717.40
      posterior horn 836.1
        old 717.43
      specified site NEC 836.1
        old 717.49
    medial 836.0
      anterior horn 836.0
        old 717.1
      bucket handle 836.0
        old 717.0
      old 717.3
      posterior horn 836.0
        old 717.2
    old NEC 717.5
    site other than knee—*see* Sprain, by site
  muscle—*see also* Sprain, by site
    with open wound—*see* Wound, open by site
  pelvic
    floor, complicating delivery 664.1
    organ NEC
      with
        abortion—*see* Abortion, by type, with damage to pelvic organs
        ectopic pregnancy (*see also* categories 633.0-633.9) 639.2
        molar pregnancy (*see also* categories 630-632) 639.2
      following
        abortion 639.2
        ectopic or molar pregnancy 639.2
      obstetrical trauma 665.5
  perineum—*see also* Laceration, perineum
    obstetrical trauma 665.5
  periurethral tissue
    with
      abortion—*see* Abortion, by type, with damage to pelvic organs
      ectopic pregnancy (*see also* categories 633.0-633.9) 639.2
      molar pregnancy (*see also* categories 630-632) 639.2
    following
      abortion 639.2
      ectopic or molar pregnancy 639.2
    obstetrical trauma 665.5
  rectovaginal septum—*see* Laceration, rectovaginal septum
  retina, retinal (recent) (with detachment) 361.00
    without detachment 361.30
    dialysis (juvenile) (with detachment) 361.04
    giant (with detachment) 361.03
    horseshoe (without detachment) 361.32
    multiple (with detachment) 361.02
      without detachment 361.33
    old
      delimited (partial) 361.06
      partial 361.06
      total or subtotal 361.07
    partial (without detachment)
      giant 361.03

Temporal

Tear, torn—*continued*
    multiple defects 361.02
    old (delimited) 361.06
    single defect 361.01
    round hole (without detachment) 361.31
    single defect (with detachment) 361.01
    total or subtotal (recent) 361.05
      old 361.07
  rotator cuff (traumatic) 840.4
    current injury 840.4
    degenerative 726.10
    nontraumatic 727.61
  semilunar cartilage, knee (*see also* Tear, meniscus) 836.2
    old 717.5
  tendon—*see also* Sprain, by site
    with open wound—*see* Wound, open by site
  tentorial, at birth 767.0
  umbilical cord
    affecting fetus or newborn 772.0
    complicating delivery 663.8
  urethra
    with
      abortion—*see* Abortion, by type, with damage to pelvic organs
      ectopic pregnancy (*see also* categories 633.0-633.9) 639.2
      molar pregnancy (*see also* categories 630-632) 639.2
    following
      abortion 639.2
      ectopic or molar pregnancy 639.2
    obstetrical trauma 665.5
  uterus—*see* Injury, internal, uterus
  vagina—*see* Laceration, vagina
  vessel, from catheter 998.2
  vulva, complicating delivery 664.0
Tear stone 375.57
Teeth, tooth —*see also* condition
  grinding 306.8
  prenatal 520.6
Teething 520.7
  syndrome 520.7
Tegmental syndrome 344.89
Telangiectasia, telangiectasis (verrucous) 448.9
  ataxic (cerebellar) 334.8
  familial 448.0
  hemorrhagic, hereditary (congenital) (senile) 448.0
  hereditary hemorrhagic 448.0
  retina 362.15
  spider 448.1
Telecanthus (congenital) 743.63
Telescoped bowel or intestine (*see also* Intussusception) 560.0
Teletherapy, adverse effect NEC 990
Telogen effluvium 704.02
Temperature
  body, high (of unknown origin) (*see also* Pyrexia) 780.6
  cold, trauma from 991.9
    newborn 778.2
    specified effect NEC 991.8
  high
    body (of unknown origin) (*see also* Pyrexia) 780.6
    trauma from—*see* Heat
Temper tantrum (childhood) (*see also* Disturbance, conduct) 312.1
Temple —*see* condition
Temporal —*see also* condition
  lobe syndrome 310.0

1365

**Temporomandibular joint-pain-dysfunction
  syndrome** 524.60
Temporosphenoidal —*see* condition
Tendency
  bleeding (*see also* Defect, coagulation) 286.9
  homosexual, ego-dystonic 302.0
  paranoid 301.0
  suicide 300.9
Tenderness
  abdominal (generalized) (localized) 789.6
  rebound 789.6
  skin 782.0
Tendinitis, tendonitis (*see also* Tenosynovitis) 726.90
  Achilles 726.71
  adhesive 726.90
    shoulder 726.0
  calcific 727.82
    shoulder 726.11
  gluteal 726.5
  patellar 726.64
  peroneal 726.79
  pes anserinus 726.61
  psoas 726.5
  tibialis (anterior) (posterior) 726.72
  trochanteric 726.5
Tendon —*see* condition
Tendosynovitis —*see* Tenosynovitis
Tendovaginitis —*see* Tenosynovitis
Tenesmus 787.99
  rectal 787.99
  vesical 788.9
Tenia —*see* Taenia
Teniasis —*see* Taeniasis
Tennis elbow 726.32
Tenonitis —*see also* Tenosynovitis
  eye (capsule) 376.04
Tenontosynovitis —*see* Tenosynovitis
Tenontothecitis —*see* Tenosynovitis
Tenophyte 727.9
Tenosynovitis 727.00
  adhesive 726.90
    shoulder 726.0
  ankle 727.06
  bicipital (calcifying) 726.12
  buttock 727.09
  due to crystals—*see* Arthritis, due to crystals
  elbow 727.09
  finger 727.05
  foot 727.06
  gonococcal 098.51
  hand 727.05
  hip 727.09
  knee 727.09
  radial styloid 727.04
  shoulder 726.10
    adhesive 726.0
  spine 720.1
  supraspinatus 726.10
  toe 727.06
  tuberculous—*see* Tuberculosis, tenosynovitis
  wrist 727.05
Tenovaginitis —*see* Tenosynovitis
Tension
  arterial, high (*see also* Hypertension) 401.9
    without diagnosis of hypertension 796.2
  headache 307.81
  intraocular (elevated) 365.00
  nervous 799.2
  ocular (elevated) 365.00

Tension—*continued*
  pneumothorax 512.0
    iatrogenic 512.1
    postoperative 512.1
    spontaneous 512.0
  premenstrual 625.4
  state 300.9
Tentorium —*see* condition
Teratencephalus 759.89
Teratism 759.7
Teratoblastoma (malignant) (M9080/3)—*see* Neoplasm, by site, malignant
Teratocarcinoma (M9081/3)—*see also* Neoplasm, by site, malignant
  liver 155.0
Teratoma (solid) (M9080/1)—*see also* Neoplasm, by site, uncertain behavior
  adult (cystic) (M9080/0)—*see* Neoplasm, by site, benign
  and embryonal carcinoma, mixed (M9081/3)—*see* Neoplasm, by site, malignant
  benign (M9080/0)—*see* Neoplasm, by site, benign
  combined with choriocarcinoma (M9101/3)—*see* Neoplasm, by site, malignant
  cystic (adult) (M9080/0)—*see* Neoplasm, by site, benign
  differentiated type (M9080/0)—*see* Neoplasm, by site, benign
  embryonal (M9080/3)—*see also* Neoplasm, by site, malignant
    liver 155.0
  fetal
    sacral, causing fetopelvic disproportion 653.7
  immature (M9080/3)—*see* Neoplasm, by site, malignant
  liver (M9080/3) 155.0
    adult, benign, cystic, differentiated type or mature (M9080/0) 211.5
  malignant (M9080/3)—*see also* Neoplasm, by site, malignant
    anaplastic type (M9082/3)—*see* Neoplasm, by site, malignant
    intermediate type (M9083/3)—*see* Neoplasm, by site, malignant
    liver (M9080/3) 155.0
    trophoblastic (M9102/3)
      specified site—*see* Neoplasm, by site, malignant
      unspecified site 186.9
    undifferentiated type (M9082/3)—*see* Neoplasm, by site, malignant
  mature (M9080/0)—*see* Neoplasm, by site, benign
  malignant (M9080/3) —*see* Neoplasm, by site, malignant
  ovary (M9080/0) 220
    embryonal, immature, or malignant (M9080/3) 183.0
  suprasellar (M9080/3)—*see* Neoplasm, by site, malignant
  testis (M9080/3) 186.9
    adult, benign, cystic, differentiated type or mature (M9080/0) 222.0
    undescended 186.0
Terminal care V66.7
Termination
  anomalous—*see also* Malposition, congenital
    portal vein 747.49
    right pulmonary vein 747.42

INDEX TO DISEASES   **Thalassemia**

Termination—*continued*
  pregnancy (legal) (therapeutic) (*see* Abortion, legal) 635.9
    fetus NEC 779.6
    illegal (*see also* Abortion, illegal) 636.9
Ternidens diminutus infestation 127.7
Terrors, night (child) 307.46
Terry's syndrome 362.21
Tertiary —*see* condition
Tessellated fundus, retina (tigroid) 362.89
Test(s)
  adequacy
    hemodialysis V56.31
    peritoneal dialysis V56.32
  AIDS virus V72.6
  allergen V72.7
  bacterial disease NEC (*see also* Screening, by name of disease) V74.9
  basal metabolic rate V72.6
  blood-alcohol V70.4
  blood-drug V70.4
    for therapeutic drug monitoring V58.83
  blood typing V72.86
    Rh typing V72.86
  developmental, infant or child V20.2
  Dick V74.8
  fertility V26.21
  genetic
    female V26.32
    for genetic disease carrier status
      female V26.31
      male V26.34
    male V26.39
  hearing V72.19
    following failed hearing screening V72.11
  HIV V72.6
  human immunodeficiency virus V72.6
  Kveim V82.89
  laboratory V72.6
    for medicolegal reason V70.4
  male partner of habitual aborter V26.35
  Mantoux (for tuberculosis) V74.1
  mycotic organism V75.4
  parasitic agent NEC V75.8
  paternity V70.4
  peritoneal equilibration V56.32
  pregnancy
    negative result V72.41
    positive result V72.42
      first pregnancy V72.42
    unconfirmed V72.40
  preoperative V72.84
    cardiovascular V72.81
    respiratory V72.82
    specified NEC V72.83
  procreative management NEC V26.29
    genetic disease carrier status
      female V26.31
      male V26.34
  Rh typing V72.86
  sarcoidosis V82.89
  Schick V74.3
  Schultz-Charlton V74.8
  skin, diagnostic
    allergy V72.7
    bacterial agent NEC (*see also* Screening, by name of disease) V74.9
    Dick V74.8
    hypersensitivity V72.7
    Kveim V82.89
    Mantoux V74.1

Test(s)—*continued*
  mycotic organism V75.4
  parasitic agent NEC V75.8
  sarcoidosis V82.89
  Schick V74.3
  Schultz-Charlton V74.8
  tuberculin V74.1
  specified type NEC V72.85
  tuberculin V74.1
  vision V72.0
  Wassermann
    positive (*see also* Serology for syphilis, positive) 097.1
    false 795.6
Testicle, testicular, testis —*see also* condition
  feminization (syndrome) 259.5
Tetanus, tetanic (cephalic) (convulsions) 037
  with
    abortion—*see* Abortion, by type, with sepsis
    ectopic pregnancy (*see also* categories 633.0-633.9) 639.0
    molar pregnancy (*see* categories 630-632) 639.0
  following
    abortion 639.0
    ectopic or molar pregnancy 639.0
  inoculation V03.7
    reaction (due to serum)—*see* Complications, vaccination
  neonatorum 771.3
  puerperal, postpartum, childbirth 670
Tetany, tetanic 781.7
  alkalosis 276.3
  associated with rickets 268.0
  convulsions 781.7
    hysterical 300.11
  functional (hysterical) 300.11
  hyperkinetic 781.7
    hysterical 300.11
  hyperpnea 786.01
    hysterical 300.11
    psychogenic 306.1
  hyperventilation 786.01
    hysterical 300.11
    psychogenic 306.1
  hypocalcemic, neonatal 775.4
    hysterical 300.11
  neonatal 775.4
  parathyroid (gland) 252.1
  parathyroprival 252.1
  postoperative 252.1
  postthyroidectomy 252.1
  pseudotetany 781.7
    hysterical 300.11
  psychogenic 306.1
  specified as conversion reaction 300.11
Tetralogy of Fallot 745.2
Tetraplegia —*see* Quadriplegia
Thailand hemorrhagic fever 065.4
Thalassanemia 282.49
Thalassemia (alpha) (beta) (disease) (Hb-C) (Hb-D) (Hb-E) (Hb-H) (Hb-I) (high fetal gene) (high fetal hemoglobin) (intermedia) (major) (minima) (minor) (mixed) (trait) (with other hemoglobinopathy) 282.49
  Hb-S (without crisis) 282.41
    with
      crisis 282.42
        vaso-occlusive pain 282.42
    sickle-cell (without crisis) 282.41
      with
        crisis 282.42
          vaso-occlusive pain 282.42

1367

Thalassemic variants 282.49
Thaysen-Gee disease (nontropical sprue) 579.0
Thecoma (M8600/0) 220
  malignant (M8600/3) 183.0
Thelarche, precocious 259.1
Thelitis 611.0
  puerperal, postpartum 675.0
Therapeutic —*see* condition
Therapy V57.9
  blood transfusion, without reported diagnosis V58.2
  breathing V57.0
  chemotherapy, antineoplastic V58.11
    fluoride V07.31
    prophylactic NEC V07.39
  dialysis (intermittent) (treatment)
    extracorporeal V56.0
    peritoneal V56.8
    renal V56.0
    specified type NEC V56.8
  exercise NEC V57.1
    breathing V57.0
  extracorporeal dialysis (renal) V56.0
  fluoride prophylaxis V07.31
  hemodialysis V56.0
  hormone replacement (postmenopausal) V07.4
  immunotherapy, antineoplastic V58.12
  long term oxygen therapy V46.2
  occupational V57.21
  orthoptic V57.4
  orthotic V57.81
  peritoneal dialysis V56.8
  physical NEC V57.1
  postmenopausal hormone replacement V07.4
  radiation V58.0
  speech V57.3
  vocational V57.22
Thermalgesia 782.0
Thermalgia 782.0
Thermanalgesia 782.0
Thermanesthesia 782.0
Thermic —*see* condition
Thermography (abnormal) 793.99
  breast 793.89
Thermoplegia 992.0
Thesaurismosis
  amyloid 277.39
  bilirubin 277.4
  calcium 275.40
  cystine 270.0
  glycogen (*see also* Disease, glycogen storage) 271.0
  kerasin 272.7
  lipoid 272.7
  melanin 255.41
  phosphatide 272.7
  urate 274.9
Thiaminic deficiency 265.1
  with beriberi 265.0
Thibierge-Weissenbach syndrome (cutaneous systemic sclerosis) 710.1
Thickened endometrium 793.5
Thickening
  bone 733.99
    extremity 733.99
  breast 611.79
  hymen 623.3
  larynx 478.79
  nail 703.8
    congenital 757.5
  periosteal 733.99

Thickening—*continued*
  pleura (*see also* Pleurisy) 511.0
  skin 782.8
  subepiglottic 478.79
  tongue 529.8
  valve, heart—*see* Endocarditis
Thiele syndrome 724.6
Thigh —*see* condition
Thinning vertebra (*see also* Osteoporosis) 733.00
Thirst, excessive 783.5
  due to deprivation of water 994.3
Thomsen's disease 359.22
Thomson's disease (congenital poikiloderma) 757.33
Thoracic —*see also* condition
  kidney 753.3
  outlet syndrome 353.0
  stomach—*see* Hernia, diaphragm
Thoracogastroschisis (congenital) 759.89
Thoracopagus 759.4
Thoracoschisis 756.3
Thorax —*see* condition
Thorn's syndrome (*see also* Disease, renal) 593.9
Thornwaldt's, Tornwaldt's
  bursitis (pharyngeal) 478.29
  cyst 478.26
  disease (pharyngeal bursitis) 478.29
Thoracoscopic surgical procedure converted to open procedure V64.42
Thorson-Biörck syndrome (malignant carcinoid) 259.2
Threadworm (infection) (infestation) 127.4
Threatened
  abortion or miscarriage 640.0
    with subsequent abortion (*see also* Abortion, spontaneous) 634.9
    affecting fetus 762.1
  labor 644.1
    affecting fetus or newborn 761.8
    premature 644.0
  miscarriage 640.0
    affecting fetus 762.1
  premature
    delivery 644.2
      affecting fetus or newborn 761.8
    labor 644.0
      before 22 completed weeks gestation 640.0
Three-day fever 066.0
Threshers' lung 495.0
Thrix annulata (congenital) 757.4
Throat —*see* condition
Thrombasthenia (Glanzmann's) (hemorrhagic) (hereditary) 287.1
Thromboangiitis 443.1
  obliterans (general) 443.1
    cerebral 437.1
    vessels
      brain 437.1
      spinal cord 437.1
Thromboarteritis —*see* Arteritis
Thromboasthenia (Glanzmann's) (hemorrhagic) (hereditary) 287.1
Thrombocytasthenia (Glanzmann's) 287.1
Thrombocythemia (primary) (M9962/1) 238.71
  essential 238.71
  hemorrhagic 238.71
  idiopathic (hemorrhagic) (M9962/1) 238.71
Thrombocytopathy (dystrophic) (granulopenic) 287.1

INDEX TO DISEASES

Thrombocytopenia, thrombocytopenic 287.5
  with
    absent radii (TAR) syndrome 287.33
    giant hemangioma 287.39
  amegakaryocytic, congenital 287.33
  congenital 287.33
  cyclic 287.39
  dilutional 287.4
  due to
    drugs 287.4
    extracorporeal circulation of blood 287.4
    massive blood transfusion 287.4
    platelet alloimmunization 287.4
  essential 287.30
  hereditary 287.33
  Kasabach-Merritt 287.39
  neonatal, transitory 776.1
    due to
      exchange transfusion 776.1
      idiopathic maternal thrombocytopenia 776.1
      isoimmunization 776.1
  primary 287.30
  puerperal, postpartum 666.3
  purpura (*see also* Purpura, thrombocytopenic) 287.30
    thrombotic 446.6
  secondary 287.4
  sex-linked 287.39
Thrombocytosis 238.71
  essential 238.71
  primary 238.71
Thromboembolism —*see* Embolism
Thrombopathy (Bernard-Soulier) 287.1
  constitutional 286.4
  Willebrand-Jürgens (angiohemophilia) 286.4
Thrombopenia (*see also* Thrombocytopenia) 287.5
Thrombophlebitis 451.9
  antecubital vein 451.82
  antepartum (superficial) 671.2
    affecting fetus or newborn 760.3
    deep 671.3
  arm 451.89
    deep 451.83
    superficial 451.82
  breast, superficial 451.89
  cavernous (venous) sinus—*see*
    Thrombophlebitis, intracranial venous sinus
  cephalic vein 451.82
  cerebral (sinus) (vein) 325
    late effect—*see* category 326
    nonpyogenic 437.6
      in pregnancy or puerperium 671.5
    late effect—*see* Late effect(s) (of) cerebrovascular disease
  due to implanted device—*see* Complications, due to (presence of) any device, implant, or graft classified to 996.0-996.5 NEC
  during or resulting from a procedure NEC 997.2
  femoral 451.11
  femoropopliteal 451.19
  following infusion, perfusion, or transfusion 999.2
  hepatic (vein) 451.89
  idiopathic, recurrent 453.1
  iliac vein 451.81
  iliofemoral 451.11
  intracranial venous sinus (any) 325
    late effect—*see* category 326
    nonpyogenic 437.6
      in pregnancy or puerperium 671.5

Thrombosis, thrombotic

Thrombophlebitis—*continued*
    late effect—*see* Late effect(s) (of) cerebrovascular disease
  jugular vein 451.89
  lateral (venous) sinus—*see* Thrombophlebitis, intracranial venous sinus
  leg 451.2
    deep (vessels) 451.19
      femoral vein 451.11
      specified vessel NEC 451.19
    superficial (vessels) 451.0
      femoral vein 451.11
  longitudinal (venous) sinus—*see* Thrombophlebitis, intracranial venous sinus
  lower extremity 451.2
    deep (vessels) 451.19
      femoral vein 451.11
      specified vessel NEC 451.19
    superficial (vessels) 451.0
  migrans, migrating 453.1
  pelvic
    with
      abortion—*see* Abortion, by type, with sepsis
      ectopic pregnancy (*see also* categories 633.0-633.9) 639.0
      molar pregnancy (*see also* categories 630-632) 639.0
    following
      abortion 639.0
      ectopic or molar pregnancy 639.0
    puerperal 671.4
  popliteal vein 451.19
  portal (vein) 572.1
  postoperative 997.2
  pregnancy (superficial) 671.2
    affecting fetus or newborn 760.3
    deep 671.3
  puerperal, postpartum, childbirth (extremities) (superficial) 671.2
    deep 671.4
    pelvic 671.4
    specified site NEC 671.5
  radial vein 451.83
  saphenous (greater) (lesser) 451.0
  sinus (intracranial)—*see* Thrombophlebitis, intracranial venous sinus
  specified site NEC 451.89
  tibial vein 451.19
Thrombosis, thrombotic (marantic) (multiple) (progressive) (vein) (vessel) 453.9
  with childbirth or during the puerperium—*see* Thrombosis, puerperal, postpartum
  antepartum—*see* Thrombosis, pregnancy
  aorta, aortic 444.1
    abdominal 444.0
    bifurcation 444.0
    saddle 444.0
    terminal 444.0
    thoracic 444.1
    valve—*see* Endocarditis, aortic
  apoplexy (*see also* Thrombosis, brain) 434.0
    late effect—*see* Late effect(s) (of) cerebrovascular disease
  appendix, septic—*see* Appendicitis, acute
  arteriolar-capillary platelet, disseminated 446.6
  artery, arteries (postinfectional) 444.9
    auditory, internal 433.8
    basilar (*see also* Occlusion, artery, basilar) 433.0
    carotid (common) (internal) (*see also* Occlusion, artery, carotid) 433.1

Thrombosis, thrombotic—*continued*
   with other precerebral artery 433.3
   cerebellar (anterior inferior) (posterior
      inferior) (superior) 433.8
   cerebral (*see also* Thrombosis, brain) 434.0
   choroidal (anterior) 433.8
   communicating posterior 433.8
   coronary (*see also* Infarct, myocardium) 410.9
      due to syphilis 093.89
      healed or specified as old 412
      without myocardial infarction 411.81
   extremities 444.22
      lower 444.22
      upper 444.21
   femoral 444.22
   hepatic 444.89
   hypophyseal 433.8
   meningeal, anterior or posterior 433.8
   mesenteric (with gangrene) 557.0
   ophthalmic (*see also* Occlusion, retina) 362.30
   pontine 433.8
   popliteal 444.22
   precerebral—*see* Occlusion, artery,
      precerebral NEC
   pulmonary 415.19
      iatrogenic 415.11
      postoperative 415.11
      septic 415.12
   renal 593.81
   retinal (*see also* Occlusion, retina) 362.30
   specified site NEC 444.89
   spinal, anterior or posterior 433.8
   traumatic (complication) (early) (*see also*
      Injury, blood vessel, by site) 904.9
   vertebral (*see also* Occlusion, artery,
      vertebral) 433.2
      with other precerebral artery 433.3
  atrial (endocardial) 424.90
   due to syphilis 093.89
   without endocarditis 429.89
  auricular (*see also* Infarct, myocardium) 410.9
  axillary (vein) 453.8
  basilar (artery) (*see also* Occlusion, artery,
     basilar) 433.0
  bland NEC 453.9
  brain (artery) (stem) 434.0
   due to syphilis 094.89
   iatrogenic 997.02
   late effect—*see* Late effect(s) (of)
      cerebrovascular disease
   postoperative 997.02
   puerperal, postpartum, childbirth 674.0
   sinus (*see also* Thrombosis, intracranial
      venous sinus) 325
  capillary 448.9
   arteriolar, generalized 446.6
  cardiac (*see also* Infarct, myocardium) 410.9
   due to syphilis 093.89
   healed or specified as old 412
   valve—*see* Endocarditis
  carotid (artery) (common) (internal) (*see also*
     Occlusion, artery, carotid) 433.1
   with other precerebral artery 433.3
  cavernous sinus (venous)—*see* Thrombosis,
     intracranial venous sinus
  cerebellar artery (anterior inferior) (posterior
     inferior) (superior) 433.8
   late effect—*see* Late effect(s) (of)
      cerebrovascular disease
  cerebral (arteries) (*see also* Thrombosis, brain)
     434.0

Thrombosis, thrombotic—*continued*
   late effect—*see* Late effect(s) (of)
      cerebrovascular disease
  coronary (artery) (*see also* Infarct, myocardium)
     410.9
   due to syphilis 093.89
   healed or specified as old 412
   without myocardial infarction 411.81
  corpus cavernosum 607.82
  cortical (*see also* Thrombosis, brain) 434.0
  due to (presence of) any device, implant, or graft
     classifiable to 996.0-996.5—*see*
     Complications, due to (presence of) any
     device, implant, or graft classified to
     996.0-996.5 NEC
  effort 453.8
  endocardial—*see* Infarct, myocardium
  eye (*see also* Occlusion, retina) 362.30
  femoral (vein) 453.8
   with inflammation or phlebitis 451.11
   artery 444.22
   deep 453.41
  genital organ, male 608.83
  heart (chamber) (*see also* Infarct, myocardium)
     410.9
  hepatic (vein) 453.0
   artery 444.89
   infectional or septic 572.1
  iliac (vein) 453.8
   with inflammation or phlebitis 451.81
   artery (common) (external) (internal) 444.81
  inflammation, vein—*see* Thrombophlebitis
  internal carotid artery (*see also* Occlusion,
     artery, carotid) 433.1
   with other precerebral artery 433.3
  intestine (with gangrene) 557.0
  intracranial (*see also* Thrombosis, brain) 434.0
   venous sinus (any) 325
     nonpyogenic origin 437.6
       in pregnancy or puerperium 671.5
  intramural (*see also* Infarct, myocardium) 410.9
   without
     cardiac condition 429.89
     coronary artery disease 429.89
     myocardial infarction 429.89
   healed or specified as old 412
  jugular (bulb) 453.8
  kidney 593.81
   artery 593.81
  lateral sinus (venous)—*see* Thrombosis,
     intracranial venous sinus
  leg 453.8
   with inflammation or phlebitis—*see*
     Thrombophlebitis
   deep (vessels) 453.40
     lower (distal) 453.42
     upper (proximal) 453.41
   superficial (vessels) 453.8
  liver (venous) 453.0
   artery 444.89
   infectional or septic 572.1
   portal vein 452
  longitudinal sinus (venous)—*see* Thrombosis,
     intracranial venous sinus
  lower extremity 453.8
   deep vessels 453.40
     calf 453.42
     distal (lower leg) 453.42
     femoral 453.41
     iliac 453.41
     lower leg 453.42

INDEX TO DISEASES   Thyroiditis

Thrombosis, thrombotic—*continued*
    peroneal 453.42
    popliteal 453.41
    proximal (upper leg) 453.41
    thigh 453.41
    tibial 453.42
  lung 415.19
    iatrogenic 415.11
    postoperative 415.11
    septic 415.12
  marantic, dural sinus 437.6
  meninges (brain) (*see also* Thrombosis, brain) 434.0
  mesenteric (artery) (with gangrene) 557.0
    vein (inferior) (superior) 557.0
  mitral—*see* Insufficiency, mitral
  mural (heart chamber) (*see also* Infarct, myocardium) 410.9
    without
      cardiac condition 429.89
      coronary artery disease 429.89
      myocardial infarction 429.89
    due to syphilis 093.89
    following myocardial infarction 429.79
    healed or specified as old 412
  omentum (with gangrene) 557.0
  ophthalmic (artery) (*see also* Occlusion, retina) 362.30
  pampiniform plexus (male) 608.83
    female 620.8
  parietal (*see also* Infarct, myocardium) 410.9
  penis, penile 607.82
  peripheral arteries 444.22
    lower 444.22
    upper 444.21
  platelet 446.6
  portal 452
    due to syphilis 093.89
    infectional or septic 572.1
  precerebral artery—*see also* Occlusion, artery, precerebral NEC
  pregnancy 671.9
    deep (vein) 671.3
    superficial (vein) 671.2
  puerperal, postpartum, childbirth 671.9
    brain (artery) 674.0
      venous 671.5
    cardiac 674.8
    cerebral (artery) 674.0
      venous 671.5
    deep (vein) 671.4
    intracranial sinus (nonpyogenic) (venous) 671.5
    pelvic 671.4
    pulmonary (artery) 673.2
    specified site NEC 671.5
    superficial 671.2
  pulmonary (artery) (vein) 415.19
    iatrogenic 415.11
    postoperative 415.11
    septic 415.12
  radial vein 451.83
  renal (artery) 593.81
    vein 453.3
  resulting from presence of shunt or other internal prosthetic device—*see* Complications, due to (presence of) any device, implant, or graft classified to 996.0-996.5 NEC
  retina, retinal (artery) 362.30
    arterial branch 362.32

Thrombosis, thrombotic—*continued*
    central 362.31
    partial 362.33
    vein
      central 362.35
      tributary (branch) 362.36
  scrotum 608.83
  seminal vesicle 608.83
  sigmoid (venous) sinus (*see* Thrombosis, intracranial venous sinus) 325
  silent NEC 453.9
  sinus, intracranial (venous) (any) (*see also* Thrombosis, intracranial venous sinus) 325
  softening, brain (*see also* Thrombosis, brain) 434.0
  specified site NEC 453.8
  spermatic cord 608.83
  spinal cord 336.1
    due to syphilis 094.89
    in pregnancy or puerperium 671.5
    pyogenic origin 324.1
      late effect—*see* category 326
  spleen, splenic 289.59
    artery 444.89
  testis 608.83
  traumatic (complication) (early) (*see also* Injury, blood vessel, by site) 904.9
  tricuspid—*see* Endocarditis, tricuspid
  tumor—*see* Neoplasm, by site
  tunica vaginalis 608.83
  umbilical cord (vessels) 663.6
    affecting fetus or newborn 762.6
  vas deferens 608.83
  vein
    deep 453.40
    lower extremity—*see* Thrombosis, lower extremity
  vena cava (inferior) (superior) 453.2
Thrombus —*see* Thrombosis
Thrush 112.0
  newborn 771.7
Thumb —*see also* condition
  gamekeeper's 842.12
  sucking (child problem) 307.9
Thygeson's superficial punctate keratitis 370.21
Thymergasia (*see also* Psychosis, affective) 296.80
Thymitis 254.8
Thymoma (benign) (M8580/0) 212.6
  malignant (M8580/3) 164.0
Thymus, thymic (gland)—*see* condition
Thyrocele (*see also* Goiter) 240.9
Thyroglossal —*see also* condition
  cyst 759.2
  duct, persistent 759.2
Thyroid (body) (gland)—*see also* condition
  hormone resistance 246.8
  lingual 759.2
Thyroiditis 245.9
  acute (pyogenic) (suppurative) 245.0
    nonsuppurative 245.0
  autoimmune 245.2
  chronic (nonspecific) (sclerosing) 245.8
    fibrous 245.3
    lymphadenoid 245.2
    lymphocytic 245.2
    lymphoid 245.2
  complicating pregnancy, childbirth, or puerperium 648.1
  de Quervain's (subacute granulomatous) 245.1

Thyroiditis—*continued*
  fibrous (chronic) 245.3
  giant (cell) (follicular) 245.1
  granulomatous (de Quervain's) (subacute) 245.1
  Hashimoto's (struma lymphomatosa) 245.2
  iatrogenic 245.4
  invasive (fibrous) 245.3
  ligneous 245.3
  lymphocytic (chronic) 245.2
  lymphoid 245.2
  lymphomatous 245.2
  pseudotuberculous 245.1
  pyogenic 245.0
  radiation 245.4
  Riedel's (ligneous) 245.3
  subacute 245.1
  suppurative 245.0
  tuberculous (*see also* Tuberculosis) 017.5
  viral 245.1
  woody 245.3
Thyrolingual duct, persistent 759.2
Thyromegaly 240.9
Thyrotoxic
  crisis or storm (*see also* Thyrotoxicosis) 242.9
  heart failure (*see also* Thyrotoxicosis) 242.9 *[425.7]*
Thyrotoxicosis 242.9

Note—Use the following fifth-digit subclassification with category 242:

0 *without mention of thyrotoxic crisis or storm*
1 *with mention of thyrotoxic crisis or storm*

  with
    goiter (diffuse) 242.0
      adenomatous 242.3
        multinodular 242.2
        uninodular 242.1
      nodular 242.3
        multinodular 242.2
        uninodular 242.1
      infiltrative
        dermopathy 242.0
        ophthalmopathy 242.0
      thyroid acropachy 242.0
  complicating pregnancy, childbirth, or puerperium 648.1
  due to
    ectopic thyroid nodule 242.4
    ingestion of (excessive) thyroid material 242.8
    specified cause NEC 242.8
  factitia 242.8
  heart 242.9 *[425.7]*
  neonatal (transient) 775.3
TIA (transient ischemic attack) 435.9
  with transient neurologic deficit 435.9
  late effect—*see* Late effect(s) (of) cerebrovascular disease
Tibia vara 732.4
Tic 307.20
  breathing 307.20
  child problem 307.21
  compulsive 307.22
  convulsive 307.20
  degenerative (generalized) (localized) 333.3
    facial 351.8
  douloureux (*see also* Neuralgia, trigeminal) 350.1
    atypical 350.2
  habit 307.20
    chronic (motor or vocal) 307.22
    transient (of childhood) 307.21

Tic —*continued*
  lid 307.20
    transient (of childhood) 307.21
  motor-verbal 307.23
  occupational 300.89
  orbicularis 307.20
    transient (of childhood) 307.21
  organic origin 333.3
  postchoreic—*see* Chorea
  psychogenic 307.20
    compulsive 307.22
  salaam 781.0
  spasm 307.20
    chronic (motor or vocal) 307.22
    transient (of childhood) 307.21
Tick (-borne) fever NEC 066.1
  American mountain 066.1
  Colorado 066.1
  hemorrhagic NEC 065.3
    Crimean 065.0
    Kyasanur Forest 065.2
    Omsk 065.1
  mountain 066.1
  nonexanthematous 066.1
Tick-bite fever NEC 066.1
  African 087.1
  Colorado (virus) 066.1
  Rocky Mountain 082.0
Tick paralysis 989.5
Tics and spasms, compulsive 307.22
Tietze's disease or syndrome 733.6
Tight, tightness
  anus 564.89
  chest 786.59
  fascia (lata) 728.9
  foreskin (congenital) 605
  hymen 623.3
  introitus (acquired) (congenital) 623.3
  rectal sphincter 564.89
  tendon 727.81
    Achilles (heel) 727.81
  urethral sphincter 598.9
Tilting vertebra 737.9
Timidity, child 313.21
Tinea (intersecta) (tarsi) 110.9
  amiantacea 110.0
  asbestina 110.0
  barbae 110.0
  beard 110.0
  black dot 110.0
  blanca 111.2
  capitis 110.0
  corporis 110.5
  cruris 110.3
  decalvans 704.09
  flava 111.0
  foot 110.4
  furfuracea 111.0
  imbricata (Tokelau) 110.5
  lepothrix 039.0
  manuum 110.2
  microsporic (*see also* Dermatophytosis) 110.9
  nigra 111.1
  nodosa 111.2
  pedis 110.4
  scalp 110.0
  specified site NEC 110.8
  sycosis 110.0
  tonsurans 110.0
  trichophytic (*see also* Dermatophytosis) 110.9
  unguium 110.1
  versicolor 111.0

INDEX TO DISEASES

Tingling sensation (*see also* Disturbance, sensation) 782.0
Tin-miners' lung 503
Tinnitus (aurium) 388.30
  audible 388.32
  objective 388.32
  subjective 388.31
Tipped, teeth 524.33
Tipping
  pelvis 738.6
    with disproportion (fetopelvic) 653.0
      affecting fetus or newborn 763.1
      causing obstructed labor 660.1
        affecting fetus or newborn 763.1
  teeth 524.33
Tiredness 780.79
Tissue —*see* condition
Tobacco
  abuse (affecting health) NEC (*see also* Abuse, drugs, nondependent) 305.1
  heart 989.8
  use disorder complicating pregnancy, childbirth, or the puerperium 649.0
Tobias' syndrome (carcinoma, pulmonary apex) (M8010/3) 162.3
Tocopherol deficiency 269.1
Todd's
  cirrhosis—*see* Cirrhosis, biliary
  paralysis (postepileptic transitory paralysis) 344.89
Toe —*see* condition
Toilet, artificial opening (*see also* Attention to, artificial, opening) V55.9
Tokelau ringworm 110.5
Tollwut 071
Tolosa-Hunt syndrome 378.55
Tommaselli's disease
  correct substance properly administered 599.7
  overdose or wrong substance given or taken 961.4
Tongue —*see also* condition
  worms 134.1
Tongue tie 750.0
Toni-Fanconi syndrome (cystinosis) 270.0
Tonic pupil 379.46
Tonsil —*see* condition
Tonsillitis (acute) (catarrhal) (croupous) (follicular) (gangrenous) (infective) (lacunar) (lingual) (malignant) (membranous) (phlegmonous) (pneumococcal) (pseudomembranous) (purulent) (septic) (staphylococcal) (subacute) (suppurative) (toxic) (ulcerative) (vesicular) (viral) 463
  with influenza, flu, or grippe 487.1
  chronic 474.00
  diphtheritic (membranous) 032.0
  hypertrophic 474.00
  influenzal 487.1
  parenchymatous 475
  streptococcal 034.0
  tuberculous (*see also* Tuberculosis) 012.8
  Vincent's 101
Tonsillopharyngitis 465.8
Tooth, teeth —*see* condition
Toothache 525.9
Topagnosis 782.0
Tophi (gouty) 274.0
  ear 274.81
  heart 274.82
  specified site NEC 274.82
Torn —*see* Tear, torn

Tornwaldt's bursitis (disease) (pharyngeal bursitis) 478.29
  cyst 478.26
Torpid liver 573.9
Torsion
  accessory tube 620.5
  adnexa (female) 620.5
  aorta (congenital) 747.29
    acquired 447.1
  appendix
    epididymis 608.24
    testis 608.23
  bile duct 576.8
    with calculus, choledocholithiasis or stones—*see* Choledocholithiasis
    congenital 751.69
  bowel, colon, or intestine 560.2
  cervix (*see* Malposition, uterus)
  duodenum 537.3
  dystonia—*see* Dystonia, torsion
  epididymis 608.24
    appendix 608.24
  fallopian tube 620.5
  gallbladder (*see also* Disease, gallbladder) 575.8
    congenital 751.69
  gastric 537.89
  hydatid of Morgagni (female) 620.5
  kidney (pedicle) 593.89
  Meckel's diverticulum (congenital) 751.0
  mesentery 560.2
  omentum 560.2
  organ or site, congenital NEC—*see* Anomaly, specified type NEC
  ovary (pedicle) 620.5
    congenital 752.0
  oviduct 620.5
  penis 607.89
    congenital 752.69
  renal 593.89
  spasm—*see* Dystonia, torsion
  spermatic cord 608.22
    extravaginal 608.21
    intravaginal 608.22
  spleen 289.59
  testicle, testis 608.20
    appendix 608.23
  tibia 736.89
  umbilical cord—*see* Compression, umbilical cord
  uterus (*see also* Malposition, uterus) 621.6
Torticollis (intermittent) (spastic) 723.5
  congenital 754.1
    sternomastoid 754.1
  due to birth injury 767.8
  hysterical 300.11
  ocular 781.93
  psychogenic 306.0
    specified as conversion reaction 300.11
  rheumatic 723.5
  rheumatoid 714.0
  spasmodic 333.83
  traumatic, current NEC 847.0
Tortuous
  artery 447.1
  fallopian tube 752.19
  organ or site, congenital NEC—*see* Distortion
  renal vessel, congenital 747.62
  retina vessel (congenital) 743.58
    acquired 362.17
  ureter 593.4
  urethra 599.84
  vein—*see* Varicose, vein

Torula, torular (infection) 117.5
  histolytica 117.5
  lung 117.5
Torulosis 117.5
Torus
  fracture
    fibula 823.41
      with tibia 823.42
    radius 813.45
    tibia 823.40
      with fibula 823.42
  mandibularis 526.81
  palatinus 526.81
Touch, vitreous 997.99
Touraine's syndrome (hereditary osteo-onychodysplasia) 756.89
Touraine-Solente-Golé syndrome (acropachyderma) 757.39
Tourette's disease (motor-verbal tic) 307.23
Tower skull 756.0
  with exophthalmos 756.0
Toxemia 799.89
  with abortion—*see* Abortion, by type, with toxemia
  bacterial—*see* Septicemia
  biliary (*see also* Disease, biliary) 576.8
  burn—*see* Burn, by site
  congenital NEC 779.89
  eclamptic 642.6
    with pre-existing hypertension 642.7
  erysipelatous (*see also* Erysipelas) 035
  fatigue 799.89
  fetus or newborn NEC 779.89
  food (*see also* Poisoning, food) 005.9
  gastric 537.89
  gastrointestinal 558.2
  intestinal 558.2
  kidney (*see also* Disease, renal) 593.9
  lung 518.89
  malarial NEC (*see also* Malaria) 084.6
  maternal (of pregnancy), affecting fetus or newborn 760.0
  myocardial—*see* Myocarditis, toxic
  of pregnancy (mild) (pre-eclamptic) 642.4
    with
      convulsions 642.6
      pre-existing hypertension 642.7
    affecting fetus or newborn 760.0
    severe 642.5
  pre-eclamptic—*see* Toxemia, of pregnancy
  puerperal, postpartum—*see* Toxemia, of pregnancy
  pulmonary 518.89
  renal (*see also* Disease, renal) 593.9
  septic (*see also* Septicemia) 038.9
  small intestine 558.2
  staphylococcal 038.10
    aureus 038.11
    due to food 005.0
    specified organism NEC 038.19
  stasis 799.89
  stomach 537.89
  uremic (*see also* Uremia) 586
  urinary 586
Toxemica cerebropathia psychica
  (nonalcoholic) 294.0
  alcoholic 291.1
Toxic (poisoning)—*see also* condition
  from drug or poison—*see* Table of drugs and chemicals
  oil syndrome 710.5
  shock syndrome 040.82
  thyroid (gland) (*see also* Thyrotoxicosis) 242.9

Toxicemia —*see* Toxemia
Toxicity
  dilantin
    asymptomatic 796.0
    symptomatic—*see* Table of Drugs and Chemicals
  drug
    asymptomatic 796.0
    symptomatic—*see* Table of Drugs and Chemicals
  fava bean 282.2
  from drug or poison
    asymptomatic 796.0
    symptomatic—*see* Table of Drugs and Chemicals
Toxicosis (*see also* Toxemia) 799.89
  capillary, hemorrhagic 287.0
Toxinfection 799.89
  gastrointestinal 558.2
Toxocariasis 128.0
Toxoplasma infection, generalized 130.9
Toxoplasmosis (acquired) 130.9
  with pneumonia 130.4
  congenital, active 771.2
  disseminated (multisystemic) 130.8
  maternal
    with suspected damage to fetus affecting management of pregnancy 655.4
    affecting fetus or newborn 760.2
      manifest toxoplasmosis in fetus or newborn 771.2
  multiple sites 130.8
  multisystemic disseminated 130.8
  specified site NEC 130.7
Trabeculation, bladder 596.8
Trachea —*see* condition
Tracheitis (acute)(catarrhal)(infantile) (membranous) (plastic) (pneumococcal) (septic) (suppurative) (viral) 464.10
  with
    bronchitis 490
      acute or subacute 466.0
      chronic 491.8
      tuberculosis—*see* Tuberculosis, pulmonary
    laryngitis (acute) 464.20
      with obstruction 464.21
      chronic 476.1
      tuberculous (*see also* Tuberculosis, larynx) 012.3
    obstruction 464.11
  chronic 491.8
    with
      bronchitis (chronic) 491.8
      laryngitis (chronic) 476.1
    due to external agent—*see* Condition, respiratory, chronic, due to
  diphtheritic (membranous) 032.3
    due to external agent—*see* Inflammation, respiratory, upper, due to
  edematous 464.11
  influenzal 487.1
  streptococcal 034.0
  syphilitic 095.8
  tuberculous (*see also* Tuberculosis) 012.8
Trachelitis (nonvenereal) (*see also* Cervicitis) 616.0
  trichomonal 131.09
Tracheobronchial —*see* condition
Tracheobronchitis (*see also* Bronchitis) 490
  acute or subacute 466.0
    with bronchospasm or obstruction 466.0
  chronic 491.8
  influenzal 487.1
  senile 491.8

INDEX TO DISEASES

Transplant(ed)

Tracheobronchomegaly (congenital) 748.3
  with bronchiectasis 494.0
    with (acute) exacerbation 494.1
  acquired 519.19
    with bronchiectasis 494.0
      with (acute) exacerbation 494.1
Tracheobronchopneumonitis —*see* Pneumonia, broncho
Tracheocele (external) (internal) 519.19
  congenital 748.3
Tracheomalacia 519.19
  congenital 748.3
Tracheopharyngitis (acute) 465.8
  chronic 478.9
    due to external agent—*see* Condition, respiratory, chronic, due to
    due to external agent—*see* Inflammation, respiratory, upper, due to
Tracheostenosis 519.19
  congenital 748.3
Tracheostomy
  attention to V55.0
  complication 519.00
  granuloma 519.09
  hemorrhage 519.09
  infection 519.01
  malfunctioning 519.02
  obstruction 519.09
  sepsis 519.01
  status V44.0
  stenosis 519.02
Trachoma, trachomatous 076.9
  active (stage) 076.1
  contraction of conjunctiva 076.1
  dubium 076.0
  healed or late effect 139.1
  initial (stage) 076.0
  Türck's (chronic catarrhal laryngitis) 476.0
Trachyphonia 784.49
Training
  insulin pump V65.46
  orthoptic V57.4
  orthotic V57.81
Train sickness 994.6
Trait
  hemoglobin
    abnormal NEC 282.7
      with thalassemia 282.49
    C (*see also* Disease, hemoglobin, C) 282.7
      with elliptocytosis 282.7
    S (Hb-S) 282.5
    Lepore 282.49
      with other abnormal hemoglobin NEC 282.49
  paranoid 301.0
  sickle-cell 282.5
    with
      elliptocytosis 282.5
      spherocytosis 282.5
Traits, paranoid 301.0
Tramp V60.0
Trance 780.09
  hysterical 300.13
Transaminasemia 790.4
Transfusion, blood
  donor V59.01
    stem cells V59.02
  incompatible 999.6
  reaction or complication—*see* Complications, transfusion
  related acute lung injury (TRALI) 518.7

Transfusion, blood—*continued*
  syndrome
    fetomaternal 772.0
    twin-to-twin
      blood loss (donor twin) 772.0
      recipient twin 776.4
  without reported diagnosis V58.2
Transient —*see also* condition
  alteration of awareness 780.02
  blindness 368.12
  deafness (ischemic) 388.02
  global amnesia 437.7
  person (homeless) NEC V60.0
Transitional, lumbosacral joint of vertebra 756.19
Translocation
  autosomes NEC 758.5
    13-15 758.1
    16-18 758.2
    21 or 22 758.0
  balanced in normal individual 758.4
  D_1 758.1
  E_3 758.2
  G 758.0
  balanced autosomal in normal individual 758.4
  chromosomes NEC 758.89
  Down's syndrome 758.0
Translucency, iris 364.53
Transmission of chemical substances through the placenta
  (affecting fetus or newborn) 760.70
  alcohol 760.71
  anticonvulsants 760.77
  antifungals 760.74
  anti-infective agents 760.74
  antimetabolics 760.78
  cocaine 760.75
  "crack" 760.75
  diethylstilbestrol [DES] 760.76
  hallucinogenic agents 760.73
  medicinal agents NEC 760.79
  narcotics 760.72
  obstetric anesthetic or analgesic drug 763.5
  specified agent NEC 760.79
  suspected, affecting management of pregnancy 655.5
Transplant(ed)
  bone V42.4
    marrow V42.81
  complication—*see also* Complications, due to (presence of) any device, implant, or graft classified to 996.0-996.5 NEC
    bone marrow 996.85
    corneal graft NEC 996.79
      infection or inflammation 996.69
      reaction 996.51
      rejection 996.51
    organ (failure) (immune or nonimmune cause) (infection) (rejection) 996.80
      bone marrow 996.85
      heart 996.83
      intestines 996.87
      kidney 996.81
      liver 996.82
      lung 996.84
      pancreas 996.86
      specified NEC 996.89
    skin NEC 996.79
      infection or inflammation 996.69
      rejection 996.52
        artificial 996.55

1375

Transplant(ed)—*continued*
    decellularized allodermis 996.55
    cornea V42.5
    hair V50.0
    heart V42.1
        valve V42.2
    intestine V42.84
    kidney V42.0
    liver V42.7
    lung V42.6
    organ V42.9
        specified NEC V42.89
    pancreas V42.83
    peripheral stem cells V42.82
    skin V42.3
    stem cells, peripheral V42.82
    tissue V42.9
        specified NEC V42.89
Transplants, ovarian, endometrial 617.1
Transposed —*see* Transposition
Transposition (congenital)—*see also* Malposition, congenital
    abdominal viscera 759.3
    aorta (dextra) 745.11
    appendix 751.5
    arterial trunk 745.10
    colon 751.5
    great vessels (complete) 745.10
        both originating from right ventricle 745.11
        corrected 745.12
        double outlet right ventricle 745.11
        incomplete 745.11
        partial 745.11
        specified type NEC 745.19
    heart 746.87
        with complete transposition of viscera 759.3
    intestine (large) (small) 751.5
    pulmonary veins 747.49
    reversed jejunal (for bypass) (status) V45.3
    scrotal 752.81
    stomach 750.7
        with general transposition of viscera 759.3
    teeth, tooth 524.30
    vessels (complete) 745.10
        partial 745.11
    viscera (abdominal) (thoracic) 759.3
Trans-sexualism 302.50
    with
        asexual history 302.51
        heterosexual history 302.53
        homosexual history 302.52
Transverse —*see also* condition
    arrest (deep), in labor 660.3
        affecting fetus or newborn 763.1
    lie 652.3
        before labor, affecting fetus or newborn 761.7
        causing obstructed labor 660.0
            affecting fetus or newborn 763.1
        during labor, affecting fetus or newborn 763.1
Transvestism, transvestitism (transvestic fetishism) 302.3
Trapped placenta (with hemorrhage) 666.0
    without hemorrhage 667.0
Trauma, traumatism (*see also* Injury, by site) 959.9
    birth—*see* Birth, injury NEC
    causing hemorrhage of pregnancy or delivery 641.8
    complicating
        abortion—*see* Abortion, by type, with damage to pelvic organs

Trauma, traumatism—*continued*
    ectopic pregnancy (*see also* categories 633.0-633.9) 639.2
    molar pregnancy (*see also* categories 630-632) 639.2
    during delivery NEC 665.9
    following
        abortion 639.2
        ectopic or molar pregnancy 639.2
    maternal, during pregnancy, affecting fetus or newborn 760.5
    neuroma—*see* Injury, nerve, by site
    previous major, affecting management of pregnancy, childbirth, or puerperium V23.8
    psychic (current)—*see also* Reaction, adjustment
        previous (history) V15.49
    psychologic, previous (affecting health) V15.49
    transient paralysis—*see* Injury, nerve, by site
Traumatic —*see* condition
Treacher Collins' syndrome (incomplete facial dysostosis) 756.0
Treitz's hernia —*see* Hernia, Treitz's
Trematode infestation NEC 121.9
Trematodiasis NEC 121.9
Trembles 988.8
Trembling paralysis (*see also* Parkinsonism) 332.0
Tremor 781.0
    essential (benign) 333.1
    familial 333.1
    flapping (liver) 572.8
    hereditary 333.1
    hysterical 300.11
    intention 333.1
    medication-induced postural 333.1
    mercurial 985.0
    muscle 728.85
    Parkinson's (*see also* Parkinsonism) 332.0
    psychogenic 306.0
        specified as conversion reaction 300.11
    senilis 797
    specified type NEC 333.1
Trench
    fever 083.1
    foot 991.4
    mouth 101
    nephritis—*see* Nephritis, acute
Treponema pallidum infection (*see also* Syphilis) 097.9
Treponematosis 102.9
    due to
        T. pallidum—*see* Syphilis
        T. pertenue (yaws) (*see also* Yaws) 102.9
Triad
    Kartagener's 759.3
    Reiter's (complete) (incomplete) 099.3
    Saint's (*see also* Hernia, diaphragm) 553.3
Trichiasis 704.2
    cicatricial 704.2
    eyelid 374.05
        with entropion (*see also* Entropion) 374.00
Trichinella spiralis (infection) (infestation) 124
Trichinelliasis 124
Trichinellosis 124
Trichiniasis 124
Trichinosis 124
Trichobezoar 938
    intestine 936
    stomach 935.2
Trichocephaliasis 127.3

INDEX TO DISEASES — Truancy, childhood

Trichocephalosis 127.3
Trichocephalus infestation 127.3
Trichoclasis 704.2
Trichoepithelioma (M8100/0)—*see also* Neoplasm, skin, benign
 breast 217
 genital organ NEC—*see* Neoplasm, by site, benign
 malignant (M8100/3)—*see* Neoplasm, skin, malignant
Trichofolliculoma (M8101/0)—*see* Neoplasm, skin, benign
Tricholemmoma (M8102/0)—*see* Neoplasm, skin, benign
Trichomatosis 704.2
Trichomoniasis 131.9
 bladder 131.09
 cervix 131.09
 intestinal 007.3
 prostate 131.03
 seminal vesicle 131.09
 specified site NEC 131.8
 urethra 131.02
 urogenitalis 131.00
 vagina 131.01
 vulva 131.01
 vulvovaginal 131.01
Trichomycosis 039.0
 axillaris 039.0
 nodosa 111.2
 nodularis 111.2
 rubra 039.0
Trichonocardiosis (axillaris) (palmellina) 039.0
Trichonodosis 704.2
Trichophytid, trichophyton infection (*see also* Dermatophytosis) 110.9
Trichophytide —*see* Dermatophytosis
Trichophytobezoar 938
 intestine 936
 stomach 935.2
Trichophytosis —*see* Dermatophytosis
Trichoptilosis 704.2
Trichorrhexis (nodosa) 704.2
Trichosporosis nodosa 111.2
Trichostasis spinulosa (congenital) 757.4
Trichostrongyliasis (small intestine) 127.6
Trichostrongylosis 127.6
Trichostrongylus (instabilis) infection 127.6
Trichotillomania 312.39
Trichromat, anomalous (congenital) 368.59
Trichromatopsia, anomalous (congenital) 368.59
Trichuriasis 127.3
Trichuris trichiuria (any site) (infection) (infestation) 127.3
Tricuspid (valve)—*see* condition
Trifid —*see also* Accessory
 kidney (pelvis) 753.3
 tongue 750.13
Trigeminal neuralgia (*see also* Neuralgia, trigeminal) 350.1
Trigeminoencephaloangiomatosis 759.6
Trigeminy 427.89
 postoperative 997.1
Trigger finger (acquired) 727.03
 congenital 756.89
Trigonitis (bladder) (chronic) (pseudomembranous) 595.3
 tuberculous (*see also* Tuberculosis) 016.1
Trigonocephaly 756.0
Trihexosidosis 272.7

Trilobate placenta —*see* Placenta, abnormal
Trilocular heart 745.8
Trimethylaminuria 270.8
Tripartita placenta —*see* Placenta, abnormal
Triple —*see also* Accessory
 kidneys 753.3
 uteri 752.2
 X female 758.81
Triplegia 344.89
 congenital or infantile 343.8
Triplet
 affected by maternal complications of pregnancy 761.5
 healthy liveborn—*see* Newborn, multiple
 pregnancy (complicating delivery) NEC 651.1
  with fetal loss and retention of one or more fetus(es) 651.4
  following (elective) fetal reduction 651.7
Triplex placenta —*see* Placenta, abnormal
Triplication —*see* Accessory
Trismus 781.0
 neonatorum 771.3
 newborn 771.3
Trisomy (syndrome) NEC 758.5
 13 (partial) 758.1
 16-18 758.2
 18 (partial) 758.2
 21 (partial) 758.0
 22 758.0
 autosomes NEC 758.5
 D_1 758.1
 E_3 758.2
 G (group) 758.0
 group D_1 758.1
 group E 758.2
 group G 758.0
Tritanomaly 368.53
Tritanopia 368.53
Troisier-Hanot-Chauffard syndrome (bronze diabetes) 275.0
Trombidiosis 133.8
Trophedema (hereditary) 757.0
 congenital 757.0
Trophoblastic disease (*see also* Hydatidiform mole) 630
 previous, affecting management of pregnancy V23.1
Tropholymphedema 757.0
Trophoneurosis NEC 356.9
 arm NEC 354.9
 disseminated 710.1
 facial 349.89
 leg NEC 355.8
 lower extremity NEC 355.8
 upper extremity NEC 354.9
Tropical —*see also* condition
 maceration feet (syndrome) 991.4
 wet foot (syndrome) 991.4
Trouble —*see also* Disease
 bowel 569.9
 heart—*see* Disease, heart
 intestine 569.9
 kidney (*see also* Disease, renal) 593.9
 nervous 799.2
 sinus (*see also* Sinusitis) 473.9
Trousseau's syndrome (thrombophlebitis migrans) 453.1
Truancy, childhood —*see also* Disturbance, conduct
 socialized 312.2
 undersocialized, unsocialized 312.1

1377

Truncus
  arteriosus (persistent) 745.0
  common 745.0
  communis 745.0
Trunk —*see* condition
Trychophytide —*see* Dermatophytosis
Trypanosoma infestation —*see* Trypanosomiasis
Trypanosomiasis 086.9
  with meningoencephalitis 086.9 *[323.2]*
  African 086.5
    due to Trypanosoma 086.5
      gambiense 086.3
      rhodesiense 086.4
  American 086.2
    with
      heart involvement 086.0
      other organ involvement 086.1
    without mention of organ involvement 086.2
  Brazilian—*see* Trypanosomiasis, American
  Chagas'—*see* Trypanosomiasis, American
  due to Trypanosoma
    cruzi—*see* Trypanosomiasis, American
    gambiense 086.3
    rhodesiense 086.4
  gambiensis, Gambian 086.3
  North American—*see* Trypanosomiasis, American
  rhodesiensis, Rhodesian 086.4
  South American—*see* Trypanosomiasis, American
T-shaped incisors 520.2
Tsutsugamushi fever 081.2
Tube, tubal, tubular —*see also* condition
  ligation, admission for V25.2
Tubercle —*see also* Tuberculosis
  brain, solitary 013.2
  Darwin's 744.29
  epithelioid noncaseating 135
  Ghon, primary infection 010.0
Tuberculid, tuberculide (indurating) (lichenoid) (miliary) (papulonecrotic) (primary) (skin) (subcutaneous) (*see also* Tuberculosis) 017.0
Tuberculoma —*see also* Tuberculosis
  brain (any part) 013.2
  meninges (cerebral) (spinal) 013.1
  spinal cord 013.4

Tuberculosis, tubercular, tuberculous
  (calcification) (calcified) (caseous) (chromogenic acid-fast bacilli) (congenital) (degeneration) (disease) (fibrocaseous) (fistula) (gangrene) (interstitial) (isolated circumscribed lesions) (necrosis) (parenchymatous) (ulcerative) 011.9

> Note—Use the following fifth-digit subclassification with categories 010-018:
>
> 0 unspecified
> 1 bacteriological or histological examination not done
> 2 bacteriological or histological examination unknown (at present)
> 3 tubercle bacilli found (in sputum) by microscopy
> 4 tubercle bacilli not found (in sputum) by microscopy, but found by bacterial culture
> 5 tubercle bacilli not found by bacteriological examination, but tuberculosis confirmed histologically
> 6 tubercle bacilli not found by bacteriological or histological examination, but tuberculosis confirmed by other methods [inoculation of animals]
>
> For tuberculous conditions specified as late effects or sequelae, see category 137.

  abdomen 014.8
    lymph gland 014.8
  abscess 011.9
    arm 017.9
    bone (*see also* Osteomyelitis, due to, tuberculosis) 015.9 *[730.8]*
      hip 015.1 *[730.85]*
      knee 015.2 *[730.86]*
      sacrum 015.0 *[730.88]*
      specified site NEC 015.7 *[730.88]*
      spinal 015.0 *[730.88]*
      vertebra 015.0 *[730.88]*
    brain 013.3
    breast 017.9
    Cowper's gland 016.5
    dura (mater) 013.8
      brain 013.3
      spinal cord 013.5
    epidural 013.8
      brain 013.3
      spinal cord 013.5
    frontal sinus—*see* Tuberculosis, sinus
    genital organs NEC 016.9
      female 016.7
      male 016.5
    genitourinary NEC 016.9
    gland (lymphatic)—*see* Tuberculosis, lymph gland
    hip 015.1
    iliopsoas 015.0 *[730.88]*
    intestine 014.8
    ischiorectal 014.8
    joint 015.9
      hip 015.1
      knee 015.2
      specified joint NEC 015.8
      vertebral 015.0 *[730.88]*
    kidney 016.0 *[590.81]*
    knee 015.2
    lumbar 015.0 *[730.88]*
    lung 011.2

INDEX TO DISEASES   **Tuberculosis, tubercular**

Tuberculosis, tubercular—*continued*
  primary, progressive 010.8
  meninges (cerebral) (spinal) 013.0
  pelvic 016.9
    female 016.7
    male 016.5
  perianal 014.8
    fistula 014.8
  perinephritic 016.0 *[590.81]*
  perineum 017.9
  perirectal 014.8
  psoas 015.0 *[730.88]*
  rectum 014.8
  retropharyngeal 012.8
  sacrum 015.0 *[730.88]*
  scrofulous 017.2
  scrotum 016.5
  skin 017.0
    primary 017.0
  spinal cord 013.5
  spine or vertebra (column) 015.0 *[730.88]*
  strumous 017.2
  subdiaphragmatic 014.8
  testis 016.5
  thigh 017.9
  urinary 016.3
    kidney 016.0 *[590.81]*
  uterus 016.7
accessory sinus—*see* Tuberculosis, sinus
Addison's disease 017.6
adenitis (*see also* Tuberculosis, lymph gland) 017.2
adenoids 012.8
adenopathy (*see also* Tuberculosis, lymph gland) 017.2
  tracheobronchial 012.1
    primary progressive 010.8
adherent pericardium 017.9 *[420.0]*
adnexa (uteri) 016.7
adrenal (capsule) (gland) 017.6
air passage NEC 012.8
alimentary canal 014.8
anemia 017.9
ankle (joint) 015.8
  bone 015.5 *[730.87]*
anus 014.8
apex (*see also* Tuberculosis, pulmonary) 011.9
apical (*see also* Tuberculosis, pulmonary) 011.9
appendicitis 014.8
appendix 014.8
arachnoid 013.0
artery 017.9
arthritis (chronic) (synovial) 015.9 *[711.40]*
  ankle 015.8 *[730.87]*
  hip 015.1 *[711.45]*
  knee 015.2 *[711.46]*
  specified site NEC 015.8 *[711.48]*
  spine or vertebra (column) 015.0 *[720.81]*
  wrist 015.8 *[730.83]*
articular—*see* Tuberculosis, joint
ascites 014.0
asthma (*see also* Tuberculosis, pulmonary) 011.9
axilla, axillary 017.2
  gland 017.2
bilateral (*see also* Tuberculosis, pulmonary) 011.9
bladder 016.1
bone (*see also* Osteomyelitis, due to, tuberculosis) 015.9 *[730.8]*
  hip 015.1 *[730.85]*

Tuberculosis, tubercular—*continued*
  knee 015.2 *[730.86]*
  limb NEC 015.5 *[730.88]*
  sacrum 015.0 *[730.88]*
  specified site NEC 015.7 *[730.88]*
  spinal or vertebral column 015.0 *[730.88]*
bowel 014.8
  miliary 018.9
brain 013.2
breast 017.9
broad ligament 016.7
bronchi, bronchial, bronchus 011.3
  ectasia, ectasis 011.5
  fistula 011.3
    primary, progressive 010.8
  gland 012.1
    primary, progressive 010.8
  isolated 012.2
  lymph gland or node 012.1
    primary, progressive 010.8
bronchiectasis 011.5
bronchitis 011.3
bronchopleural 012.0
bronchopneumonia, bronchopneumonic 011.6
bronchorrhagia 011.3
bronchotracheal 011.3
  isolated 012.2
bronchus—*see* Tuberculosis, bronchi
bronze disease (Addison's) 017.6
buccal cavity 017.9
bulbourethral gland 016.5
bursa (*see also* Tuberculosis, joint) 015.9
cachexia NEC (*see also* Tuberculosis, pulmonary) 011.9
cardiomyopathy 017.9 *[425.8]*
caries (*see also* Tuberculosis, bone) 015.9 *[730.8]*
cartilage (*see also* Tuberculosis, bone) 015.9 *[730.8]*
  intervertebral 015.0 *[730.88]*
catarrhal (*see also* Tuberculosis, pulmonary) 011.9
cecum 014.8
cellular tissue (primary) 017.0
cellulitis (primary) 017.0
central nervous system 013.9
  specified site NEC 013.8
cerebellum (current) 013.2
cerebral (current) 013.2
  meninges 013.0
cerebrospinal 013.6
  meninges 013.0
cerebrum (current) 013.2
cervical 017.2
  gland 017.2
  lymph nodes 017.2
cervicitis (uteri) 016.7
cervix 016.7
chest (*see also* Tuberculosis, pulmonary) 011.9
childhood type or first infection 010.0
choroid 017.3 *[363.13]*
choroiditis 017.3 *[363.13]*
ciliary body 017.3 *[364.11]*
colitis 014.8
colliers' 011.4
colliquativa (primary) 017.0
colon 014.8
  ulceration 014.8
complex, primary 010.0
complicating pregnancy, childbirth, or puerperium 647.3

1379

Tuberculosis, tubercular—*continued*
    affecting fetus or newborn 760.2
    congenital 771.2
    conjunctiva 017.3 *[370.31]*
    connective tissue 017.9
      bone—*see* Tuberculosis, bone
    contact V01.1
    converter (tuberculin skin test) (without disease) 795.5
    cornea (ulcer) 017.3 *[370.31]*
    Cowper's gland 016.5
    coxae 015.1 *[730.85]*
    coxalgia 015.1 *[730.85]*
    cul-de-sac of Douglas 014.8
    curvature, spine 015.0 *[737.40]*
    cutis (colliquativa) (primary) 017.0
    cyst, ovary 016.6
    cystitis 016.1
    dacryocystitis 017.3 *[375.32]*
    dactylitis 015.5
    diarrhea 014.8
    diffuse (*see also* Tuberculosis, miliary) 018.9
      lung—*see* Tuberculosis, pulmonary
      meninges 013.0
    digestive tract 014.8
    disseminated (*see also* Tuberculosis, miliary) 018.9
      meninges 013.0
    duodenum 014.8
    dura (mater) 013.9
      abscess 013.8
        cerebral 013.3
        spinal 013.5
    dysentery 014.8
    ear (inner) (middle) 017.4
      bone 015.6
      external (primary) 017.0
      skin (primary) 017.0
    elbow 015.8
    emphysema—*see* Tuberculosis, pulmonary
    empyema 012.0
    encephalitis 013.6
    endarteritis 017.9
    endocarditis (any valve) 017.9 *[424.91]*
    endocardium (any valve) 017.9 *[424.91]*
    endocrine glands NEC 017.9
    endometrium 016.7
    enteric, enterica 014.8
    enteritis 014.8
    enterocolitis 014.8
    epididymis 016.4
    epididymitis 016.4
    epidural abscess 013.8
      brain 013.3
      spinal cord 013.5
    epiglottis 012.3
    episcleritis 017.3 *[379.00]*
    erythema (induratum) (nodosum) (primary) 017.1
    esophagus 017.8
    Eustachian tube 017.4
    exposure to V01.1
    exudative 012.0
      primary, progressive 010.1
    eye 017.3
      glaucoma 017.3 *[365.62]*
    eyelid (primary) 017.0
      lupus 017.0 *[373.4]*
    fallopian tube 016.6
    fascia 017.9
    fauces 012.8

Tuberculosis, tubercular—*continued*
    finger 017.9
    first infection 010.0
    fistula, perirectal 014.8
    Florida 011.6
    foot 017.9
    funnel pelvis 137.3
    gallbladder 017.9
    galloping (*see also* Tuberculosis, pulmonary) 011.9
    ganglionic 015.9
    gastritis 017.9
    gastrocolic fistula 014.8
    gastroenteritis 014.8
    gastrointestinal tract 014.8
    general, generalized 018.9
      acute 018.0
      chronic 018.8
    genital organs NEC 016.9
      female 016.7
      male 016.5
    genitourinary NEC 016.9
    genu 015.2
    glandulae suprarenalis 017.6
    glandular, general 017.2
    glottis 012.3
    grinders' 011.4
    groin 017.2
    gum 017.9
    hand 017.9
    heart 017.9 *[425.8]*
    hematogenous—*see* Tuberculosis, miliary
    hemoptysis (*see also* Tuberculosis, pulmonary) 011.9
    hemorrhage NEC (*see also* Tuberculosis, pulmonary) 011.9
    hemothorax 012.0
    hepatitis 017.9
    hilar lymph nodes 012.1
      primary, progressive 010.8
    hip (disease) (joint) 015.1
      bone 015.1 *[730.85]*
    hydrocephalus 013.8
    hydropneumothorax 012.0
    hydrothorax 012.0
    hypoadrenalism 017.6
    hypopharynx 012.8
    ileocecal (hyperplastic) 014.8
    ileocolitis 014.8
    ileum 014.8
    iliac spine (superior) 015.0 *[730.88]*
    incipient NEC (*see also* Tuberculosis, pulmonary) 011.9
    indurativa (primary) 017.1
    infantile 010.0
    infection NEC 011.9
      without clinical manifestation 010.0
    infraclavicular gland 017.2
    inguinal gland 017.2
    inguinalis 017.2
    intestine (any part) 014.8
    iris 017.3 *[364.11]*
    iritis 017.3 *[364.11]*
    ischiorectal 014.8
    jaw 015.7 *[730.88]*
    jejunum 014.8
    joint 015.9
      hip 015.1
      knee 015.2
      specified site NEC 015.8
      vertebral 015.0 *[730.88]*

INDEX TO DISEASES

Tuberculosis, tubercular

Tuberculosis, tubercular—*continued*
keratitis 017.3 *[370.31]*
  interstitial 017.3 *[370.59]*
keratoconjunctivitis 017.3 *[370.31]*
kidney 016.0
knee (joint) 015.2
kyphoscoliosis 015.0 *[737.43]*
kyphosis 015.0 *[737.41]*
lacrimal apparatus, gland 017.3
laryngitis 012.3
larynx 012.3
leptomeninges, leptomeningitis (cerebral)
  (spinal) 013.0
lichenoides (primary) 017.0
linguae 017.9
lip 017.9
liver 017.9
lordosis 015.0 *[737.42]*
lung—*see* Tuberculosis, pulmonary
luposa 017.0
  eyelid 017.0 *[373.4]*
lymphadenitis—*see* Tuberculosis, lymph gland
lymphangitis—*see* Tuberculosis, lymph gland
lymphatic (gland) (vessel)—*see* Tuberculosis, lymph gland
lymph gland or node (peripheral) 017.2
  abdomen 014.8
  bronchial 012.1
    primary, progressive 010.8
  cervical 017.2
  hilar 012.1
    primary, progressive 010.8
  intrathoracic 012.1
    primary, progressive 010.8
  mediastinal 012.1
    primary, progressive 010.8
  mesenteric 014.8
  peripheral 017.2
  retroperitoneal 014.8
  tracheobronchial 012.1
    primary, progressive 010.8
malignant NEC (*see also* Tuberculosis, pulmonary) 011.9
mammary gland 017.9
marasmus NEC (*see also* Tuberculosis, pulmonary) 011.9
mastoiditis 015.6
maternal, affecting fetus or newborn 760.2
mediastinal (lymph) gland or node 012.1
  primary, progressive 010.8
mediastinitis 012.8
  primary, progressive 010.8
mediastinopericarditis 017.9 *[420.0]*
mediastinum 012.8
  primary, progressive 010.8
medulla 013.9
  brain 013.2
  spinal cord 013.4
melanosis, Addisonian 017.6
membrane, brain 013.0
meninges (cerebral) (spinal) 013.0
meningitis (basilar) (brain) (cerebral)
  (cerebrospinal) (spinal) 013.0
meningoencephalitis 013.0
mesentery, mesenteric 014.8
  lymph gland or node 014.8
miliary (any site) 018.9
  acute 018.0
  chronic 018.8
  specified type NEC 018.8
millstone makers' 011.4

Tuberculosis, tubercular—*continued*
miners' 011.4
moulders' 011.4
mouth 017.9
multiple 018.9
  acute 018.0
  chronic 018.8
muscle 017.9
myelitis 013.6
myocarditis 017.9 *[422.0]*
myocardium 017.9 *[422.0]*
nasal (passage) (sinus) 012.8
nasopharynx 012.8
neck gland 017.2
nephritis 016.0 *[583.81]*
nerve 017.9
nose (septum) 012.8
ocular 017.3
old NEC 137.0
  without residuals V12.01
omentum 014.8
oophoritis (acute) (chronic) 016.6
optic 017.3 *[377.39]*
  nerve trunk 017.3 *[377.39]*
  papilla, papillae 017.3 *[377.39]*
orbit 017.3
orchitis 016.5 *[608.81]*
organ, specified NEC 017.9
orificialis (primary) 017.0
osseous (*see also* Tuberculosis, bone) 015.9 *[730.8]*
osteitis (*see also* Tuberculosis, bone) 015.9 *[730.8]*
osteomyelitis (*see also* Tuberculosis, bone) 015.9 *[730.8]*
otitis (media) 017.4
ovaritis (acute) (chronic) 016.6
ovary (acute) (chronic) 016.6
oviducts (acute) (chronic) 016.6
pachymeningitis 013.0
palate (soft) 017.9
pancreas 017.9
papulonecrotic (primary) 017.0
parathyroid glands 017.9
paronychia (primary) 017.0
parotid gland or region 017.9
pelvic organ NEC 016.9
  female 016.7
  male 016.5
pelvis (bony) 015.7 *[730.85]*
penis 016.5
peribronchitis 011.3
pericarditis 017.9 *[420.0]*
pericardium 017.9 *[420.0]*
perichondritis, larynx 012.3
perineum 017.9
periostitis (*see also* Tuberculosis, bone) 015.9 *[730.8]*
periphlebitis 017.9
  eye vessel 017.3 *[362.18]*
  retina 017.3 *[362.18]*
perirectal fistula 014.8
peritoneal gland 014.8
peritoneum 014.0
peritonitis 014.0
pernicious NEC (*see also* Tuberculosis, pulmonary) 011.9
pharyngitis 012.8
pharynx 012.8
phlyctenulosis (conjunctiva) 017.3 *[370.31]*

1381

Tuberculosis, tubercular—*continued*
  phthisis NEC (*see also* Tuberculosis,
    pulmonary) 011.9
  pituitary gland 017.9
  placenta 016.7
  pleura, pleural, pleurisy, pleuritis (fibrinous)
    (obliterative) (purulent) (simple plastic)
    (with effusion) 012.0
    primary, progressive 010.1
  pneumonia, pneumonic 011.6
  pneumothorax 011.7
  polyserositis 018.9
    acute 018.0
    chronic 018.8
  potters' 011.4
  prepuce 016.5
  primary 010.9
    complex 010.0
    complicated 010.8
      with pleurisy or effusion 010.1
    progressive 010.8
      with pleurisy or effusion 010.1
    skin 017.0
  proctitis 014.8
  prostate 016.5 *[601.4]*
  prostatitis 016.5 *[601.4]*
  pulmonaris (*see also* Tuberculosis, pulmonary)
    011.9
  pulmonary (artery) (incipient) (malignant)
    (multiple round foci) (pernicious)
    (reinfection stage) 011.9
    cavitated or with cavitation 011.2
      primary, progressive 010.8
    childhood type or first infection 010.0
    chromogenic acid-fast bacilli 795.39
    fibrosis or fibrotic 011.4
    infiltrative 011.0
      primary, progressive 010.9
    nodular 011.1
    specified NEC 011.8
    sputum positive only 795.39
    status following surgical collapse of lung NEC
      011.9
  pyelitis 016.0 *[590.81]*
  pyelonephritis 016.0 *[590.81]*
  pyemia—*see* Tuberculosis, miliary
  pyonephrosis 016.0
  pyopneumothorax 012.0
  pyothorax 012.0
  rectum (with abscess) 014.8
    fistula 014.8
  reinfection stage (*see also* Tuberculosis,
    pulmonary) 011.9
  renal 016.0
  renis 016.0
  reproductive organ 016.7
  respiratory NEC (*see also* Tuberculosis,
    pulmonary) 011.9
    specified site NEC 012.8
  retina 017.3 *[363.13]*
  retroperitoneal (lymph gland or node) 014.8
    gland 014.8
  retropharyngeal abscess 012.8
  rheumatism 015.9
  rhinitis 012.8
  sacroiliac (joint) 015.8
  sacrum 015.0 *[730.88]*
  salivary gland 017.9
  salpingitis (acute) (chronic) 016.6
  sandblasters' 011.4
  sclera 017.3 *[379.09]*

Tuberculosis, tubercular—*continued*
  scoliosis 015.0 *[737.43]*
  scrofulous 017.2
  scrotum 016.5
  seminal tract or vesicle 016.5 *[608.81]*
  senile NEC (*see also* Tuberculosis, pulmonary)
    011.9
  septic NEC (*see also* Tuberculosis, miliary)
    018.9
  shoulder 015.8
    blade 015.7 *[730.8]*
  sigmoid 014.8
  sinus (accessory) (nasal) 012.8
    bone 015.7 *[730.88]*
    epididymis 016.4
  skeletal NEC (*see also* Osteomyelitis, due to
    tuberculosis) 015.9 *[730.8]*
  skin (any site) (primary) 017.0
  small intestine 014.8
  soft palate 017.9
  spermatic cord 016.5
  spinal
    column 015.0 *[730.88]*
    cord 013.4
    disease 015.0 *[730.88]*
    medulla 013.4
    membrane 013.0
    meninges 013.0
  spine 015.0 *[730.88]*
  spleen 017.7
  splenitis 017.7
  spondylitis 015.0 *[720.81]*
  spontaneous pneumothorax—*see* Tuberculosis,
    pulmonary
  sternoclavicular joint 015.8
  stomach 017.9
  stonemasons' 011.4
  struma 017.2
  subcutaneous tissue (cellular) (primary) 017.0
  subcutis (primary) 017.0
  subdeltoid bursa 017.9
  submaxillary 017.9
    region 017.9
  supraclavicular gland 017.2
  suprarenal (capsule) (gland) 017.6
  swelling, joint (*see also* Tuberculosis, joint)
    015.9
  symphysis pubis 015.7 *[730.88]*
  synovitis 015.9 *[727.01]*
    hip 015.1 *[727.01]*
    knee 015.2 *[727.01]*
    specified site NEC 015.8 *[727.01]*
    spine or vertebra 015.0 *[727.01]*
  systemic—*see* Tuberculosis, miliary
  tarsitis (eyelid) 017.0 *[373.4]*
    ankle (bone) 015.5 *[730.87]*
  tendon (sheath)—*see* Tuberculosis,
    tenosynovitis
  tenosynovitis 015.9 *[727.01]*
    hip 015.1 *[727.01]*
    knee 015.2 *[727.01]*
    specified site NEC 015.8 *[727.01]*
    spine or vertebra 015.0 *[727.01]*
  testis 016.5 *[608.81]*
  throat 012.8
  thymus gland 017.9
  thyroid gland 017.5
  toe 017.9
  tongue 017.9
  tonsil (lingual) 012.8
  tonsillitis 012.8

INDEX TO DISEASES — Tumor

Tuberculosis, tubercular—*continued*
 trachea, tracheal 012.8
  gland 012.1
   primary, progressive 010.8
   isolated 012.2
 tracheobronchial 011.3
  glandular 012.1
   primary, progressive 010.8
   isolated 012.2
  lymph gland or node 012.1
   primary, progressive 010.8
 tubal 016.6
 tunica vaginalis 016.5
 typhlitis 014.8
 ulcer (primary) (skin) 017.0
  bowel or intestine 014.8
  specified site NEC—*see* Tuberculosis, by site
 unspecified site—*see* Tuberculosis, pulmonary
 ureter 016.2
 urethra, urethral 016.3
 urinary organ or tract 016.3
  kidney 016.0
 uterus 016.7
 uveal tract 017.3 *[363.13]*
 uvula 017.9
 vaccination, prophylactic (against) V03.2
 vagina 016.7
 vas deferens 016.5
 vein 017.9
 verruca (primary) 017.0
 verrucosa (cutis) (primary) 017.0
 vertebra (column) 015.0 *[730.88]*
 vesiculitis 016.5 *[608.81]*
 viscera NEC 014.8
 vulva 016.7 *[616.51]*
 wrist (joint) 015.8
  bone 015.5 *[730.83]*
Tuberculum
 auriculae 744.29
 occlusal 520.2
 paramolare 520.2
Tuberosity
 jaw, excessive 524.07
 maxillary, entire 524.07
Tuberous sclerosis (brain) 759.5
Tubo-ovarian —*see* condition
Tuboplasty, after previous sterilization V26.0
Tubotympanitis 381.10
Tularemia 021.9
 with
  conjunctivitis 021.3
  pneumonia 021.2
 bronchopneumonic 021.2
 conjunctivitis 021.3
 cryptogenic 021.1
 disseminated 021.8
 enteric 021.1
 generalized 021.8
 glandular 021.8
 intestinal 021.1
 oculoglandular 021.3
 ophthalmic 021.3
 pneumonia 021.2
 pulmonary 021.2
 specified NEC 021.8
 typhoidal 021.1
 ulceroglandular 021.0
 vaccination, prophylactic (against) V03.4
Tularensis conjunctivitis 021.3
Tumefaction —*see also* Swelling
 liver (*see also* Hypertrophy, liver) 789.1

Tumor (M8000/1)—*see also* Neoplasm, by site, unspecified nature
 Abrikossov's (M9580/0)—*see also* Neoplasm, connective tissue, benign
  malignant (M9580/3)—*see* Neoplasm, connective tissue, malignant
 acinar cell (M8550/1)—*see* Neoplasm, by site, uncertain behavior
 acinic cell (M8550/1)—*see* Neoplasm, by site, uncertain behavior
 adenomatoid (M9054/0)—*see also* Neoplasm, by site, benign
  odontogenic (M9300/0) 213.1
   upper jaw (bone) 213.0
 adnexal (skin) (M8390/0)—*see* Neoplasm, skin, benign
 adrenal
  cortical (benign) (M8370/0) 227.0
   malignant (M8370/3) 194.0
  rest (M8671/0)—*see* Neoplasm, by site, benign
 alpha cell (M8152/0)
  malignant (M8152/3)
   pancreas 157.4
   specified site NEC—*see* Neoplasm, by site, malignant
   unspecified site 157.4
  pancreas 211.7
  specified site NEC—*see* Neoplasm, by site, benign
  unspecified site 211.7
 aneurysmal (*see also* Aneurysm) 442.9
 aortic body (M8691/1) 237.3
  malignant (M8691/3) 194.6
 argentaffin (M8241/1)—*see* Neoplasm, by site, uncertain behavior
 basal cell (M8090/1)—*see also* Neoplasm, skin, uncertain behavior
 benign (M8000/0)—*see* Neoplasm, by site, benign
 beta cell (M8151/0)
  malignant (M8151/3)
   pancreas 157.4
   specified site—*see* Neoplasm, by site, malignant
   unspecified site 157.4
  pancreas 211.7
  specified site NEC—*see* Neoplasm, by site, benign
  unspecified site 211.7
 blood—*see* Hematoma
 brenner (M9000/0) 220
  borderline malignancy (M9000/1) 236.2
  malignant (M9000/3) 183.0
  proliferating (M9000/1) 236.2
 Brooke's (M8100/0)—*see* Neoplasm, skin, benign
 brown fat (M8880/0)—*see* Lipoma, by site
 Burkitt's (M9750/3) 200.2
 calcifying epithelial odontogenic (M9340/0) 213.1
  upper jaw (bone) 213.0
 carcinoid (M8240/1)—*see* Carcinoid
 carotid body (M8692/1) 237.3
  malignant (M8692/3) 194.5
 Castleman's (mediastinal lymph node hyperplasia) 785.6
 cells (M8001/1)—*see also* Neoplasm, by site, unspecified nature
  benign (M8001/0)—*see* Neoplasm, by site, benign

1383

Tumor—*continued*
  malignant (M8001/3)—*see* Neoplasm, by site, malignant
  uncertain whether benign or malignant (M8001/1)—*see* Neoplasm, by site, uncertain nature
  cervix
    in pregnancy or childbirth 654.6
      affecting fetus or newborn 763.89
      causing obstructed labor 660.2
        affecting fetus or newborn 763.1
  chondromatous giant cell (M9230/0)—*see* Neoplasm, bone, benign
  chromaffin (M8700/0)—*see also* Neoplasm, by site, benign
    malignant (M8700/3)—*see* Neoplasm, by site, malignant
  Cock's peculiar 706.2
  Codman's (benign chondroblastoma) (M9230/0)—*see* Neoplasm, bone, benign
  dentigerous, mixed (M9282/0) 213.1
    upper jaw (bone) 213.0
  dermoid (M9084/0)—*see* Neoplasm, by site, benign
    with malignant transformation (M9084/3) 183.0
  desmoid (extra-abdominal) (M8821/1)—*see also* Neoplasm, connective tissue, uncertain behavior
    abdominal (M8822/1)—*see* Neoplasm, connective tissue, uncertain behavior
  embryonal (mixed) (M9080/1)—*see also* Neoplasm, by site, uncertain behavior
    liver (M9080/3) 155.0
  endodermal sinus (M9071/3)
    specified site—*see* Neoplasm, by site, malignant
    unspecified site
      female 183.0
      male 186.9
  epithelial
    benign (M8010/0)—*see* Neoplasm, by site, benign
    malignant (M8010/3)—*see* Neoplasm, by site, malignant
  Ewing's (M9260/3)—*see* Neoplasm, bone, malignant
  fatty—*see* Lipoma
  fetal, causing disproportion 653.7
    causing obstructed labor 660.1
  fibroid (M8890/0)—*see* Leiomyoma
  G cell (M8153/1)
    malignant (M8153/3)
      pancreas 157.4
      specified site NEC—*see* Neoplasm, by site, malignant
      unspecified site 157.4
    specified site—*see* Neoplasm, by site, uncertain behavior
    unspecified site 235.5
  giant cell (type) (M8003/1)—*see also* Neoplasm, by site, unspecified nature
    bone (M9250/1) 238.0
      malignant (M9250/3)—*see* Neoplasm, bone, malignant
    chondromatous (M9230/0)—*see* Neoplasm, bone, benign
    malignant (M8003/3)—*see* Neoplasm, by site, malignant
    peripheral (gingiva) 523.8

Tumor—*continued*
  soft parts (M9251/1)—*see also* Neoplasm, connective tissue, uncertain behavior
    malignant (M9251/3)—*see* Neoplasm, connective tissue, malignant
  tendon sheath 727.02
  glomus (M8711/0)—*see also* Hemangioma, by site
    jugulare (M8690/1) 237.3
    malignant (M8690/3) 194.6
  gonadal stromal (M8590/1)—*see* Neoplasm, by site, uncertain behavior
  granular cell (M9580/0)—*see also* Neoplasm, connective tissue, benign
    malignant (M9580/3)—*see* Neoplasm, connective tissue, malignant
  granulosa cell (M8620/1) 236.2
    malignant (M8620/3) 183.0
  granulosa cell-theca cell (M8621/1) 236.2
    malignant (M8621/3) 183.0
  Grawitz's (hypernephroma) (M8312/3) 189.0
  hazard-crile (M8350/3) 193
  hemorrhoidal—*see* Hemorrhoids
  hilar cell (M8660/0) 220
  hurthle cell (benign) (M8290/0) 226
    malignant (M8290/3) 193
  hydatid (*see also* Echinococcus) 122.9
  hypernephroid (M8311/1)—*see also* Neoplasm, by site, uncertain behavior
  interstitial cell (M8650/1)—*see also* Neoplasm, by site, uncertain behavior
    benign (M8650/0)—*see* Neoplasm, by site, benign
    malignant (M8650/3)—*see* Neoplasm, by site, malignant
  islet cell (M8150/0)
    malignant (M8150/3)
      pancreas 157.4
      specified site—*see* Neoplasm, by site, malignant
      unspecified site 157.4
    pancreas 211.7
    specified site NEC—*see* Neoplasm, by site, benign
    unspecified site 211.7
  juxtaglomerular (M8361/1) 236.91
  Krukenberg's (M8490/6) 198.6
  Leydig cell (M8650/1)
    benign (M8650/0)
      specified site—*see* Neoplasm, by site, benign
      unspecified site
        female 220
        male 220.0
    malignant (M8650/3)
      specified site—*see* Neoplasm, by site, malignant
      unspecified site
        female 183.0
        male 186.9
    specified site—*see* Neoplasm, by site, uncertain behavior
    unspecified site
      female 236.2
      male 236.4
  lipid cell, ovary (M8670/0) 220
  lipoid cell, ovary (M8670/0) 220
  lymphomatous, benign (M9590/0)—*see also* Neoplasm, by site, benign
  Malherbe's (M8110/0)—*see* Neoplasm, skin, benign

INDEX TO DISEASES — Tumor

Tumor—*continued*
  malignant (M8000/3)—*see also* Neoplasm, by site, malignant
    fusiform cell (type) (M8004/3)—*see* Neoplasm, by site, malignant
    giant cell (type) (M8003/3)—*see* Neoplasm, by site, malignant
    mixed NEC (M8940/3)—*see* Neoplasm, by site, malignant
    small cell (type) (M8002/3)—*see* Neoplasm, by site, malignant
    spindle cell (type) (M8004/3)—*see* Neoplasm, by site, malignant
  mast cell (M9740/1) 238.5
    malignant (M9740/3) 202.6
  melanotic, neuroectodermal (M9363/0)—*see* Neoplasm, by site, benign
  Merkel cell—*see* Neoplasm, by site, malignant
  mesenchymal
    malignant (M8800/3)—*see* Neoplasm, connective tissue, malignant
    mixed (M8990/1)—*see* Neoplasm, connective tissue, uncertain behavior
  mesodermal, mixed (M8951/3)—*see also* Neoplasm, by site, malignant
    liver 155.0
  mesonephric (M9110/1)—*see also* Neoplasm, by site, uncertain behavior
    malignant (M9110/3)—*see* Neoplasm, by site, malignant
  metastatic
    from specified site (M8000/3)—*see* Neoplasm, by site, malignant
    to specified site (M8000/6)—*see* Neoplasm, by site, malignant, secondary
  mixed NEC (M8940/0)—*see also* Neoplasm, by site, benign
    malignant (M8940/3)—*see* Neoplasm, by site, malignant
  mucocarcinoid, malignant (M8243/3)—*see* Neoplasm, by site, malignant
  mucoepidermoid (M8430/1)—*see* Neoplasm, by site, uncertain behavior
  Mullerian, mixed (M8950/3)—*see* Neoplasm, by site, malignant
  myoepithelial (M8982/0)—*see* Neoplasm, by site, benign
  neurogenic olfactory (M9520/3) 160.0
  nonencapsulated sclerosing (M8350/3) 193
  odontogenic (M9270/1) 238.0
    adenomatoid (M9300/0) 213.1
      upper jaw (bone) 213.0
    benign (M9270/0) 213.1
      upper jaw (bone) 213.0
    calcifying epithelial (M9340/0) 213.1
      upper jaw (bone) 213.0
    malignant (M9270/3) 170.1
      upper jaw (bone) 170.0
    squamous (M9312/0) 213.1
      upper jaw (bone) 213.0
  ovarian stromal (M8590/1) 236.2
  ovary
    in pregnancy or childbirth 654.4
      affecting fetus or newborn 763.89
      causing obstructed labor 660.2
        affecting fetus or newborn 763.1
  pacinian (M9507/0)—*see* Neoplasm, skin, benign
  Pancoast's (M8010/3) 162.3
  papillary—*see* Papilloma
  pelvic, in pregnancy or childbirth 654.9

Tumor—*continued*
    affecting fetus or newborn 763.89
    causing obstructed labor 660.2
      affecting fetus or newborn 763.1
  phantom 300.11
  plasma cell (M9731/1) 238.6
    benign (M9731/0)—*see* Neoplasm, by site, benign
    malignant (M9731/3) 203.8
  polyvesicular vitelline (M9071/3)
    specified site—*see* Neoplasm, by site, malignant
    unspecified site
      female 183.0
      male 186.9
  Pott's puffy (*see also* Osteomyelitis) 730.2
  Rathke's pouch (M9350/1) 237.0
  regaud's (M8082/3)—*see* Neoplasm, nasopharynx, malignant
  rete cell (M8140/0) 222.0
  retinal anlage (M9363/0)—*see* Neoplasm, by site, benign
  Rokitansky's 620.2
  salivary gland type, mixed (M8940/0)—*see also* Neoplasm, by site, benign
    malignant (M8940/3)—*see* Neoplasm, by site, malignant
  Sampson's 617.1
  Schloffer's (*see also* Peritonitis) 567.29
  Schmincke (M8082/3)—*see* Neoplasm, nasopharynx, malignant
  sebaceous (*see also* Cyst, sebaceous) 706.2
  secondary (M8000/6)—*see* Neoplasm, by site, secondary
  Sertoli cell (M8640/0)
    with lipid storage (M8641/0)
      specified site—*see* Neoplasm, by site, benign
      unspecified site
        female 220
        male 222.0
    specified site—*see* Neoplasm, by site, benign
    unspecified site
      female 220
      male 222.0
  Sertoli-Leydig cell (M8631/0)
    specified site—*see* Neoplasm, by site, benign
    unspecified site
      female 220
      male 222.0
  sex cord (-stromal) (M8590/1)—*see* Neoplasm, by site, uncertain behavior
  skin appendage (M8390/0)—*see* Neoplasm, skin, benign
  soft tissue
    benign (M8800/0)—*see* Neoplasm, connective tissue, benign
    malignant (M8800/3)—*see* Neoplasm, connective tissue, malignant
  sternomastoid 754.1
  stromal
    abdomen
      benign 215.5
      malignant 171.5
      uncertain behavior 238.1
    digestive system 238.1
      benign 215.5
      malignant 171.5
      uncertain behavior 238.1
    gastric 238.1
      benign 215.5

Tumor—*continued*
>malignant 171.5
>uncertain behavior 238.1
>gastrointestinal 238.1
>>benign 215.5
>>malignant 171.5
>>uncertain behavior 238.1
>intestine (small) (large) 238.1
>>benign 215.5
>>malignant 171.5
>>uncertain behavior 238.1
>stomach 238.1
>>benign 215.5
>>malignant 171.5
>>uncertain behavior 238.1
>superior sulcus (lung) (pulmonary) (syndrome) (M8010/3) 162.3
>suprasulcus (M8010/3) 162.3
>sweat gland (M8400/1)—*see also* Neoplasm, skin, uncertain behavior
>>benign (M8400/0)—*see* Neoplasm, skin, benign
>>malignant (M8400/3)—*see* Neoplasm, skin, malignant
>syphilitic brain 094.89
>>congenital 090.49
>testicular stromal (M8590/1) 236.4
>theca cell (M8600/0) 220
>theca cell-granulosa cell (M8621/1) 236.2
>theca-lutein (M8610/0) 220
>turban (M8200/0) 216.4
>uterus
>>in pregnancy or childbirth 654.1
>>>affecting fetus or newborn 763.89
>>>causing obstructed labor 660.2
>>>>affecting fetus or newborn 763.1
>vagina
>>in pregnancy or childbirth 654.7
>>>affecting fetus or newborn 763.89
>>>causing obstructed labor 660.2
>>>>affecting fetus or newborn 763.1
>varicose (*see also* Varicose, vein) 454.9
>von Recklinghausen's (M9540/1) 237.71
>vulva
>>in pregnancy or childbirth 654.8
>>>affecting fetus or newborn 763.89
>>>causing obstructed labor 660.2
>>>>affecting fetus or newborn 763.1
>Warthin's (salivary gland) (M8561/0) 210.2
>white—*see also* Tuberculosis, arthritis
>White-Darier 757.39
>Wilms' (nephroblastoma) (M8960/3) 189.0
>yolk sac (M9071/3)
>>specified site—*see* Neoplasm, by site, malignant
>>unspecified site
>>>female 183.0
>>>male 186.9

Tumorlet (M8040/1)—*see* Neoplasm, by site, uncertain behavior
Tungiasis 134.1
Tunica vasculosa lentis 743.39
Tunnel vision 368.45
Turban tumor (M8200/0) 216.4
Türck's trachoma (chronic catarrhal laryngitis) 476.0
Türk's syndrome (ocular retraction syndrome) 378.71
Turner's
>hypoplasia (tooth) 520.4
>syndrome 758.6
>tooth 520.4

Turner-Kieser syndrome (hereditary osteo-onychodysplasia) 756.89
Turner-Varny syndrome 758.6
Turricephaly 756.0
Tussis convulsiva (*see also* Whooping cough) 033.9
Twin
>affected by maternal complications of pregnancy 761.5
>conjoined 759.4
>healthy liveborn—*see* Newborn, twin
>pregnancy (complicating delivery) NEC 651.0
>>with fetal loss and retention of one fetus 651.3
>>following (elective) fetal reduction 651.7

Twinning, teeth 520.2
Twist, twisted
>bowel, colon, or intestine 560.2
>hair (congenital) 757.4
>mesentery 560.2
>omentum 560.2
>organ or site, congenital NEC—*see* Anomaly, specified type NEC
>ovarian pedicle 620.5
>>congenital 752.0
>umbilical cord—*see* Compression, umbilical cord

Twitch 781.0
Tylosis 700
>buccalis 528.6
>gingiva 523.8
>linguae 528.6
>palmaris et plantaris 757.39

Tympanism 787.3
Tympanites (abdominal) (intestine) 787.3
Tympanitis —*see* Myringitis
Tympanosclerosis 385.00
>involving
>>combined sites NEC 385.09
>>>with tympanic membrane 385.03
>>tympanic membrane 385.01
>>>with ossicles 385.02
>>>>and middle ear 385.03

Tympanum —*see* condition
Tympany
>abdomen 787.3
>chest 786.7

Typhlitis (*see also* Appendicitis) 541
Typhoenteritis 002.0
Typhogastric fever 002.0
Typhoid (abortive) (ambulant) (any site) (fever) (hemorrhagic) (infection) (intermittent) (malignant) (rheumatic) 002.0
>with pneumonia 002.0 *[484.8]*
>abdominal 002.0
>carrier (suspected) of V02.1
>cholecystitis (current) 002.0
>clinical (Widal and blood test negative) 002.0
>endocarditis 002.0 *[421.1]*
>inoculation reaction—*see* Complications, vaccination
>meningitis 002.0 *[320.7]*
>mesenteric lymph nodes 002.0
>myocarditis 002.0 *[422.0]*
>osteomyelitis (*see also* Osteomyelitis, due to, typhoid) 002.0 *[730.8]*
>perichondritis, larynx 002.0 *[478.71]*
>pneumonia 002.0 *[484.8]*
>spine 002.0 *[720.81]*
>ulcer (perforating) 002.0
>vaccination, prophylactic (against) V03.1
>Widal negative 002.0

INDEX TO DISEASES

Typhomalaria (fever) (*see also* Malaria) 084.6
Typhomania 002.0
Typhoperitonitis 002.0
Typhus (fever) 081.9
  abdominal, abdominalis 002.0
  African tick 082.1
  amarillic (*see also* Fever, Yellow) 060.9
  brain 081.9
  cerebral 081.9
  classical 080
  endemic (flea-borne) 081.0
  epidemic (louse-borne) 080
  exanthematic NEC 080
  exanthematicus SAI 080
    brillii SAI 081.1
    Mexicanus SAI 081.0
    pediculo vestimenti causa 080
    typhus murinus 081.0
  flea-borne 081.0
  Indian tick 082.1
  Kenya tick 082.1
  louse-borne 080
  Mexican 081.0
    flea-borne 081.0
    louse-borne 080
    tabardillo 080
  mite-borne 081.2
  murine 081.0
  North Asian tick-borne 082.2
  petechial 081.9
  Queensland tick 082.3
  rat 081.0
  recrudescent 081.1
  recurrent (*see also* Fever, relapsing) 087.9
  São Paulo 082.0
  scrub (China) (India) (Malaya) (New Guinea) 081.2
  shop (of Malaya) 081.0
  Siberian tick 082.2
  tick-borne NEC 082.9
  tropical 081.2
  vaccination, prophylactic (against) V05.8
Tyrosinemia 270.2
  neonatal 775.89
Tyrosinosis (Medes) (Sakai) 270.2
Tyrosinuria 270.2
Tyrosyluria 270.2

INDEX TO DISEASES   Ulcer, ulcerated, ulcerating

U

Uehlinger's syndrome (acropachyderma) 757.39
Uhl's anomaly or disease (hypoplasia of myocardium, right ventricle) 746.84
Ulcer, ulcerated, ulcerating, ulceration, ulcerative 707.9
  with gangrene 707.9 *[785.4]*
  abdomen (wall) (*see also* Ulcer, skin) 707.8
  ala, nose 478.19
  alveolar process 526.5
  amebic (intestine) 006.9
    skin 006.6
  anastomotic—*see* Ulcer, gastrojejunal
  anorectal 569.41
  antral—*see* Ulcer, stomach
  anus (sphincter) (solitary) 569.41
    varicose—*see* Varicose, ulcer, anus
  aorta —*see* Aneurysm
  aphthous (oral) (recurrent) 528.2
    genital organ(s)
      female 616.50
      male 608.89
    mouth 528.2
  arm (*see also* Ulcer, skin) 707.8
  arteriosclerotic plaque—*see* Arteriosclerosis, by site
  artery NEC 447.2
    without rupture 447.8
  atrophic NEC—*see* Ulcer, skin
  Barrett's (chronic peptic ulcer of esophagus) 530.85
  bile duct 576.8
  bladder (solitary) (sphincter) 596.8
    bilharzial (*see also* Schistosomiasis) 120.9 *[595.4]*
    submucosal (*see also* Cystitis) 595.1
    tuberculous (*see also* Tuberculosis) 016.1
  bleeding NEC—*see* Ulcer, peptic, with hemorrhage
  bone 730.9
  bowel (*see also* Ulcer, intestine) 569.82
  breast 611.0
  bronchitis 491.8
  bronchus 519.19
  buccal (cavity) (traumatic) 528.9
  burn (acute)—*see* Ulcer, duodenum
  Buruli 031.1
  buttock (*see also* Ulcer, skin) 707.8
    decubitus (*see also* Ulcer, decubitus) 707.00
  cancerous (M8000/3)—*see* Neoplasm, by site, malignant
  cardia—*see* Ulcer, stomach
  cardio-esophageal (peptic) 530.20
    with bleeding 530.21
  cecum (*see also* Ulcer, intestine) 569.82
  cervix (uteri) (trophic) 622.0
    with mention of cervicitis 616.0
  chancroidal 099.0
  chest (wall) (*see also* Ulcer, skin) 707.8
  Chiclero 085.4
  chin (pyogenic) (*see also* Ulcer, skin) 707.8
  chronic (cause unknown)—*see also* Ulcer, skin
    penis 607.89
  Cochin-China 085.1
  colitis —*see* Colitis, ulcerative
  colon (*see also* Ulcer, intestine) 569.82
  conjunctiva (acute) (postinfectional) 372.00

Ulcer, ulcerated, ulcerating—*continued*
  cornea (infectional) 370.00
    with perforation 370.06
    annular 370.02
    catarrhal 370.01
    central 370.03
    dendritic 054.42
    marginal 370.01
    mycotic 370.05
    phlyctenular, tuberculous (*see also* Tuberculosis) 017.3 *[370.31]*
    ring 370.02
    rodent 370.07
    serpent, serpiginous 370.04
    superficial marginal 370.01
    tuberculous (*see also* Tuberculosis) 017.3 *[370.31]*
  corpus cavernosum (chronic) 607.89
  crural—*see* Ulcer, lower extremity
  Curling's—*see* Ulcer, duodenum
  Cushing's—*see* Ulcer, peptic
  cystitis (interstitial) 595.1
  decubitus (unspecified site) 707.00
    with gangrene 707.00 *[785.4]*
    ankle 707.06
    back
      lower 707.03
      upper 707.02
    buttock 707.05
    elbow 707.01
    head 707.09
    heel 707.07
    hip 707.04
    other site 707.09
    sacrum 707.03
    shoulder blades 707.02
  dendritic 054.42
  diabetes, diabetic (mellitus) 250.8 *[707.9]*
    lower limb 250.8 *[707.10]*
      ankle 250.8 *[707.13]*
      calf 250.8 *[707.12]*
      foot 250.8 *[707.15]*
      heel 250.8 *[707.14]*
      knee 250.8 *[707.19]*
      specified site NEC 250.8 *[707.19]*
      thigh 250.8 *[707.11]*
      toes 250.8 *[707.15]*
    specified site NEC 250.8 *[707.8]*
  Dieulafoy—*see* Lesion, Dieulafoy
  due to
    infection NEC—*see* Ulcer, skin
    radiation, radium—*see* Ulcer, by site
    trophic disturbance (any region)—*see* Ulcer, skin
    x-ray—*see* Ulcer, by site
  duodenum, duodenal (eroded) (peptic) 532.9

Note—Use the following fifth-digit subclassification with categories 531-534:

0 *without mention of obstruction*
1 *with obstruction*

---

    with
      hemorrhage (chronic) 532.4
        and perforation 532.6
      perforation (chronic) 532.5
        and hemorrhage 532.6

Ulcer, ulcerated, ulcerating—*continued*
    acute 532.3
        with
            hemorrhage 532.0
                and perforation 532.2
            perforation 532.1
                and hemorrhage 532.2
    bleeding (recurrent)—*see* Ulcer, duodenum, with hemorrhage
    chronic 532.7
        with
            hemorrhage 532.4
                and perforation 532.6
            perforation 532.5
                and hemorrhage 532.6
    penetrating—*see* Ulcer, duodenum, with perforation
    perforating—*see* Ulcer, duodenum, with perforation
    dysenteric NEC 009.0
    elusive 595.1
    endocarditis (any valve) (acute) (chronic) (subacute) 421.0
    enteritis —*see* Colitis, ulcerative
    enterocolitis 556.0
    epiglottis 478.79
    esophagus (peptic) 530.20
        with bleeding 530.21
        due to ingestion
            aspirin 530.20
            chemicals 530.20
            medicinal agents 530.20
        fungal 530.20
        infectional 530.20
        varicose (*see also* Varix, esophagus) 456.1
            bleeding (*see also* Varix, esophagus, bleeding) 456.0
    eye NEC 360.00
        dendritic 054.42
    eyelid (region) 373.01
    face (*see also* Ulcer, skin) 707.8
    fauces 478.29
    Fenwick (-Hunner) (solitary) (*see also* Cystitis) 595.1
    fistulous NEC—*see* Ulcer, skin
    foot (indolent) (*see also* Ulcer, lower extremity) 707.15
        perforating 707.15
            leprous 030.1
            syphilitic 094.0
        trophic 707.15
        varicose 454.0
            inflamed or infected 454.2
    frambesial, initial or primary 102.0
    gallbladder or duct 575.8
    gall duct 576.8
    gangrenous (*see also* Gangrene) 785.4
    gastric—*see* Ulcer, stomach
    gastrocolic—*see* Ulcer, gastrojejunal
    gastroduodenal—*see* Ulcer, peptic
    gastroesophageal—*see* Ulcer, stomach
    gastrohepatic—*see* Ulcer, stomach
    gastrointestinal—*see* Ulcer, gastrojejunal
    gastrojejunal (eroded) (peptic) 534.9

Note—*Use the following fifth-digit subclassification with categories 531-534:*

0 *without mention of obstruction*
1 *with obstruction*

Ulcer, ulcerated, ulcerating—*continued*
    with
        hemorrhage (chronic) 534.4
            and perforation 534.6
        perforation 534.5
            and hemorrhage 534.6
    acute 534.3
        with
            hemorrhage 534.0
                and perforation 534.2
            perforation 534.1
                and hemorrhage 534.2
    bleeding (recurrent)—*see* Ulcer, gastrojejunal, with hemorrhage
    chronic 534.7
        with
            hemorrhage 534.4
                and perforation 534.6
            perforation 534.5
                and hemorrhage 534.6
    penetrating—*see* Ulcer, gastrojejunal, with perforation
    perforating—*see* Ulcer, gastrojejunal, with perforation
    gastrojejunocolic—*see* Ulcer, gastrojejunal
    genital organ
        female 629.89
        male 608.89
    gingiva 523.8
    gingivitis 523.10
    glottis 478.79
    granuloma of pudenda 099.2
    groin (*see also* Ulcer, skin) 707.8
    gum 523.8
    gumma, due to yaws 102.4
    hand (*see also* Ulcer, skin) 707.8
    hard palate 528.9
    heel (*see also* Ulcer, lower extremity) 707.14
        decubitus (*see also* Ulcer, decubitus) 707.07
    hemorrhoids 455.8
        external 455.5
        internal 455.2
    hip (*see also* Ulcer, skin) 707.8
        decubitus (*see also* Ulcer, decubitus) 707.04
    Hunner's 595.1
    hypopharynx 478.29
    hypopyon (chronic) (subacute) 370.04
    hypostaticum—*see* Ulcer, varicose
    ileocolitis 556.1
    ileum (*see also* Ulcer, intestine) 569.82
    intestine, intestinal 569.82
        with perforation 569.83
        amebic 006.9
        duodenal—*see* Ulcer, duodenum
        granulocytopenic (with hemorrhage) 288.09
        marginal 569.82
        perforating 569.83
        small, primary 569.82
        stercoraceous 569.82
        stercoral 569.82
        tuberculous (*see also* Tuberculosis) 014.8
        typhoid (fever) 002.0
        varicose 456.8
    ischemic 707.9
        lower extremity (*see also* Ulcer, lower extremity) 707.10
            ankle 707.13
            calf 707.12
            foot 707.15
            heel 707.14
            knee 707.19

INDEX TO DISEASES

Ulcer, ulcerated, ulcerating—*continued*
    specified site NEC 707.19
        thigh 707.11
        toes 707.15
    jejunum, jejunal—*see* Ulcer, gastrojejunal
    keratitis (*see also* Ulcer, cornea) 370.00
    knee—*see* Ulcer, lower extremity
    labium (majus) (minus) 616.50
    laryngitis (*see also* Laryngitis) 464.00
        with obstruction 464.01
    larynx (aphthous) (contact) 478.79
        diphtheritic 032.3
    leg—*see* Ulcer, lower extremity
    lip 528.5
    Lipschütz's 616.50
    lower extremity (atrophic) (chronic)
        (neurogenic) (perforating) (pyogenic)
        (trophic) (tropical) 707.10
        with gangrene (*see also* Ulcer, lower
            extremity) 707.10 *[785.4]*
            arteriosclerotic 440.24
        ankle 707.13
            arteriosclerotic 440.23
                with gangrene 440.24
        calf 707.12
        decubitus 707.00
            with gangrene 707.00 *[785.4]*
            ankle 707.06
            buttock 707.05
            heel 707.07
            hip 707.04
        foot 707.15
        heel 707.14
        knee 707.19
        specified site NEC 707.19
        thigh 707.11
        toes 707.15
        varicose 454.0
            inflamed or infected 454.2
    luetic—*see* Ulcer, syphilitic
    lung 518.89
        tuberculous (*see also* Tuberculosis) 011.2
    malignant (M8000/3)—*see* Neoplasm, by site,
        malignant
    marginal NEC—*see* Ulcer, gastrojejunal
    meatus (urinarius) 597.89
    Meckel's diverticulum 751.0
    Meleney's (chronic undermining) 686.09
    Mooren's (cornea) 370.07
    mouth (traumatic) 528.9
    mycobacterial (skin) 031.1
    nasopharynx 478.29
    navel cord (newborn) 771.4
    neck (*see also* Ulcer, skin) 707.8
        uterus 622.0
    neurogenic NEC—*see* Ulcer, skin
    nose, nasal (infectional) (passage) 478.19
        septum 478.19
            varicose 456.8
        skin—*see* Ulcer, skin
        spirochetal NEC 104.8
    oral mucosa (traumatic) 528.9
    palate (soft) 528.9
    penetrating NEC—*see* Ulcer, peptic, with
        perforation
    penis (chronic) 607.89
    peptic (site unspecified) 533.9

Ulcer, ulcerated, ulcerating—*continued*

Note—*Use the following fifth-digit subclassification with categories 531-534:*

  0 without mention of obstruction
  1 with obstruction

    with
        hemorrhage 533.4
            and perforation 533.6
        perforation (chronic) 533.5
            and hemorrhage 533.6
    acute 533.3
        with
            hemorrhage 533.0
                and perforation 533.2
            perforation 533.1
                and hemorrhage 533.2
    bleeding (recurrent)—*see* Ulcer, peptic, with
        hemorrhage
    chronic 533.7
        with
            hemorrhage 533.4
                and perforation 533.6
            perforation 533.5
                and hemorrhage 533.6
    penetrating—*see* Ulcer, peptic, with
        perforation
    perforating NEC (*see also* Ulcer, peptic, with
        perforation) 533.5
        skin 707.9
    perineum (*see also* Ulcer, skin) 707.8
    peritonsillar 474.8
    phagedenic (tropical) NEC—*see* Ulcer, skin
    pharynx 478.29
    phlebitis—*see* Phlebitis
    plaster (*see also* Ulcer, decubitus) 707.00
    popliteal space—*see* Ulcer, lower extremity
    postpyloric—*see* Ulcer, duodenum
    prepuce 607.89
    prepyloric—*see* Ulcer, stomach
    pressure (*see also* Ulcer, decubitus) 707.00
    primary of intestine 569.82
        with perforation 569.83
    proctitis 556.2
        with ulcerative sigmoiditis 556.3
    prostate 601.8
    pseudopeptic—*see* Ulcer, peptic
    pyloric—*see* Ulcer, stomach
    rectosigmoid 569.82
        with perforation 569.83
    rectum (sphincter) (solitary) 569.41
        stercoraceous, stercoral 569.41
        varicose—*see* Varicose, ulcer, anus
    retina (*see also* Chorioretinitis) 363.20
    rodent (M8090/3)—*see also* Neoplasm, skin,
        malignant
        cornea 370.07
    round—*see* Ulcer, stomach
    sacrum (region) (*see also* Ulcer, skin) 707.8
    Saemisch's 370.04
    scalp (*see also* Ulcer, skin) 707.8
    sclera 379.09
    scrofulous (*see also* Tuberculosis) 017.2
    scrotum 608.89
        tuberculous (*see also* Tuberculosis) 016.5
        varicose 456.4
    seminal vesicle 608.89
    sigmoid 569.82
        with perforation 569.83

Ulcer, ulcerated, ulcerating — *continued*
- skin (atrophic) (chronic) (neurogenic) (non-healing) (perforating) (pyogenic) (trophic) 707.9
  - with gangrene 707.9 *[785.4]*
  - amebic 006.6
  - decubitus (*see also* Ulcer, decubitus) 707.00
    - with gangrene 707.00 *[785.4]*
  - in granulocytopenia 288.09
  - lower extremity (*see also* Ulcer, lower extremity) 707.10
    - with gangrene 707.10 *[785.4]*
      - arteriosclerotic 440.24
    - ankle 707.13
    - arteriosclerotic 440.23
      - with gangrene 440.24
    - calf 707.12
    - foot 707.15
    - heel 707.14
    - knee 707.19
    - specified site NEC 707.19
    - thigh 707.11
    - toes 707.15
  - mycobacterial 031.1
  - syphilitic (early) (secondary) 091.3
  - tuberculous (primary) (*see also* Tuberculosis) 017.0
  - varicose—*see* Ulcer, varicose
- sloughing NEC—*see* Ulcer, skin
- soft palate 528.9
- solitary, anus or rectum (sphincter) 569.41
- sore throat 462
  - streptococcal 034.0
- spermatic cord 608.89
- spine (tuberculous) 015.0 *[730.88]*
- stasis (leg) (venous) 454.0
  - with varicose veins 454.0
  - inflamed or infected 454.2
  - without varicose veins 459.81
- stercoral, stercoraceous 569.82
  - with perforation 569.83
  - anus or rectum 569.41
- stoma, stomal—*see* Ulcer, gastrojejunal
- stomach (eroded) (peptic) (round) 531.9

Note—*Use the following fifth-digit subclassification with categories 531-534:*

0 *without mention of obstruction*
1 *with obstruction*

  - with
    - hemorrhage 531.4
      - and perforation 531.6
    - perforation (chronic) 531.5
      - and hemorrhage 531.6
  - acute 531.3
    - with
      - hemorrhage 531.0
        - and perforation 531.2
      - perforation 531.1
        - and hemorrhage 531.2
  - bleeding (recurrent)—*see* Ulcer, stomach, with hemorrhage
  - chronic 531.7
    - with
      - hemorrhage 531.4
        - and perforation 531.6
      - perforation 531.5
        - and hemorrhage 531.6
  - penetrating—*see* Ulcer, stomach, with perforation

Ulcer, ulcerated, ulcerating — *continued*
- perforating—*see* Ulcer, stomach, with perforation
- stomatitis 528.00
- stress—*see* Ulcer, peptic
- strumous (tuberculous) (*see also* Tuberculosis) 017.2
- submental (*see also* Ulcer, skin) 707.8
- submucosal, bladder 595.1
- syphilitic (any site) (early) (secondary) 091.3
  - late 095.9
  - perforating 095.9
    - foot 094.0
- testis 608.89
- thigh—*see* Ulcer, lower extremity
- throat 478.29
  - diphtheritic 032.0
- toe—*see* Ulcer, lower extremity
- tongue (traumatic) 529.0
- tonsil 474.8
  - diphtheritic 032.0
- trachea 519.19
- trophic—*see* Ulcer, skin
- tropical NEC (*see also* Ulcer, skin) 707.9
- tuberculous—*see* Tuberculosis, ulcer
- tunica vaginalis 608.89
- turbinate 730.9
- typhoid (fever) 002.0
  - perforating 002.0
- umbilicus (newborn) 771.4
- unspecified site NEC—*see* Ulcer, skin
- urethra (meatus) (*see also* Urethritis) 597.89
- uterus 621.8
  - cervix 622.0
    - with mention of cervicitis 616.0
  - neck 622.0
    - with mention of cervicitis 616.0
- vagina 616.89
- valve, heart 421.0
- varicose (lower extremity, any part) 454.0
  - anus—*see* Varicose, ulcer, anus
  - broad ligament 456.5
  - esophagus (*see also* Varix, esophagus) 456.1
    - bleeding (*see also* Varix, esophagus, bleeding) 456.0
  - inflamed or infected 454.2
  - nasal septum 456.8
  - perineum 456.6
  - rectum—*see* Varicose, ulcer, anus
  - scrotum 456.4
  - specified site NEC 456.8
  - sublingual 456.3
  - vulva 456.6
- vas deferens 608.89
- vesical (*see also* Ulcer, bladder) 596.8
- vulva (acute) (infectional) 616.50
  - Behçet's syndrome 136.1 *[616.51]*
  - herpetic 054.12
  - tuberculous 016.7 *[616.51]*
- vulvobuccal, recurring 616.50
- x-ray—*see* Ulcer, by site
- yaws 102.4

Ulcerosa scarlatina 034.1
Ulcus —*see also* Ulcer
- cutis tuberculosum (*see also* Tuberculosis) 017.0
- duodeni—*see* Ulcer, duodenum
- durum 091.0
  - extragenital 091.2
- gastrojejunale—*see* Ulcer, gastrojejunal
- hypostaticum—*see* Ulcer, varicose

Ulcus—*continued*
  molle (cutis) (skin) 099.0
  serpens cornea (pneumococcal) 370.04
  ventriculi—*see* Ulcer, stomach
Ulegyria 742.4
Ulerythema
  acneiforma 701.8
  centrifugum 695.4
  ophryogenes 757.4
Ullrich (-Bonnevie) (-Turner) syndrome 758.6
Ullrich-Feichtiger syndrome 759.89
Ulnar —*see* condition
Ulorrhagia 523.8
Ulorrhea 523.8
Umbilicus, umbilical —*see also* condition
  cord necrosis, affecting fetus or newborn 762.6
Unacceptable
  existing dental restoration
    contours 525.65
    morphology 525.65
Unavailability of medical facilities (at) V63.9
  due to
    investigation by social service agency V63.8
    lack of services at home V63.1
    remoteness from facility V63.0
    waiting list V63.2
  home V63.1
  outpatient clinic V63.0
  specified reason NEC V63.8
Uncinaria americana infestation 126.1
Uncinariasis (*see also* Ancylostomiasis) 126.9
Unconscious, unconsciousness 780.09
Underdevelopment —*see also* Undeveloped
  sexual 259.0
Underfill, endodontic 526.63
Undernourishment 269.9
Undernutrition 269.9
Under observation —*see* Observation
Underweight 783.22
  for gestational age—*see* Light-for-dates
Underwood's disease (sclerema neonatorum) 778.1
Undescended —*see also* Malposition, congenital
  cecum 751.4
  colon 751.4
  testis 752.51
Undetermined diagnosis or cause 799.9
Undeveloped, undevelopment —*see also* Hypoplasia
  brain (congenital) 742.1
  cerebral (congenital) 742.1
  fetus or newborn 764.9
  heart 746.89
  lung 748.5
  testis 257.2
  uterus 259.0
Undiagnosed (disease) 799.9
Undulant fever (*see also* Brucellosis) 023.9
Unemployment, anxiety concerning V62.0
Unequal leg (acquired) (length) 736.81
  congenital 755.30
Unerupted teeth, tooth 520.6
Unextracted dental root 525.3
Unguis incarnatus 703.0
Unicornis uterus 752.3
Unicorporeus uterus 752.3
Uniformis uterus 752.3

Unilateral —*see also* condition
  development, breast 611.8
  organ or site, congenital NEC—*see* Agenesis
  vagina 752.49
Unilateralis uterus 752.3
Unilocular heart 745.8
Uninhibited (neurogenic) bladder 596.54
  with cauda equina syndrome 344.61
  neurogenic—*see* Neurogenic, bladder 596.54
Union, abnormal —*see also* Fusion
  divided tendon 727.89
  larynx and trachea 748.3
Universal
  joint, cervix 620.6
  mesentery 751.4
Unknown
  cause of death 799.9
  diagnosis 799.9
Unna's disease (seborrheic dermatitis) 690.10
Unresponsiveness, adrenocorticotropin (ACTH) 255.41
Unsoundness of mind (*see also* Psychosis) 298.9
Unspecified cause of death 799.9
Unsatisfactory
  restoration, tooth (existing) 525.60
    specified NEC 525.69
  smear 795.08
Unstable
  back NEC 724.9
  colon 569.89
  joint—*see* Instability, joint
  lie 652.0
    affecting fetus or newborn (before labor) 761.7
    causing obstructed labor 660.0
      affecting fetus or newborn 763.1
  lumbosacral joint (congenital) 756.19
    acquired 724.6
  sacroiliac 724.6
  spine NEC 724.9
Untruthfulness, child problem (*see also* Disturbance, conduct) 312.0
Unverricht (-Lundborg) disease, syndrome, or epilepsy 333.2
Unverricht-Wagner syndrome (dermatomyositis) 710.3
Upper respiratory —*see* condition
Upset
  gastric 536.8
    psychogenic 306.4
  gastrointestinal 536.8
    psychogenic 306.4
  virus (*see also* Enteritis, viral) 008.8
  intestinal (large) (small) 564.9
    psychogenic 306.4
  menstruation 626.9
  mental 300.9
  stomach 536.8
    psychogenic 306.4
Urachus —*see also* condition
  patent 753.7
  persistent 753.7
Uratic arthritis 274.0
Urbach's lipoid proteinosis 272.8
Urbach-Oppenheim disease or syndrome (necrobiosis lipoidica diabeticorum) 250.8 [709.3]
Urbach-Wiethe disease or syndrome (lipoid proteinosis) 272.8
Urban yellow fever 060.1
Urea, blood, high —*see* Uremia

Uremia, uremic (absorption) (amaurosis) (amblyopia) (aphasia) (apoplexy) (coma) (delirium) (dementia) (dropsy) (dyspnea) (fever) (intoxication) (mania) (paralysis) (poisoning) (toxemia) (vomiting) 586
  with
    abortion—*see* Abortion, by type, with renal failure
    ectopic pregnancy (*see also* categories 633.0-633.9) 639.3
    hypertension (*see also* Hypertension, kidney) 403.91
    molar pregnancy (*see also* categories 630-632) 639.3
  chronic 585.9
  complicating
    abortion 639.3
    ectopic or molar pregnancy 639.3
    hypertension (*see also* Hypertension, kidney) 403.91
    labor and delivery 669.3
  congenital 779.89
  extrarenal 788.9
  hypertensive (chronic) (*see also* Hypertension, kidney) 403.91
  maternal NEC, affecting fetus or newborn 760.1
  neuropathy 585.9 *[357.4]*
  pericarditis 585.9 *[420.0]*
  prerenal 788.9
  pyelitic (*see also* Pyelitis) 590.80
Ureter, ureteral —*see* condition
Ureteralgia 788.0
Ureterectasis 593.89
Ureteritis 593.89
  cystica 590.3
  due to calculus 592.1
  gonococcal (acute) 098.19
    chronic or duration of 2 months or over 098.39
  nonspecific 593.89
Ureterocele (acquired) 593.89
  congenital 753.23
Ureterolith 592.1
Ureterolithiasis 592.1
Ureterostomy status V44.6
  with complication 997.5
Urethra, urethral —*see* condition
Urethralgia 788.9
Urethritis (abacterial) (acute) (allergic) (anterior) (chronic) (nonvenereal) (posterior) (recurrent) (simple) (subacute) (ulcerative) (undifferentiated) 597.80
  diplococcal (acute) 098.0
    chronic or duration of 2 months or over 098.2
  due to Trichomonas (vaginalis) 131.02
  gonococcal (acute) 098.0
    chronic or duration of 2 months or over 098.2
  nongonococcal (sexually transmitted) 099.40
    Chlamydia trachomatis 099.41
    Reiter's 099.3
    specified organism NEC 099.49
  nonspecific (sexually transmitted) (*see also* Urethritis, nongonococcal) 099.40
  not sexually transmitted 597.80
  Reiter's 099.3
  trichomonal or due to Trichomonas (vaginalis) 131.02
  tuberculous (*see also* Tuberculosis) 016.3
  venereal NEC (*see also* Urethritis, nongonococcal) 099.40

Urethrocele
  female 618.03
    with uterine prolapse 618.4
      complete 618.3
      incomplete 618.2
  male 599.5
Urethrolithiasis 594.2
Urethro-oculoarticular syndrome 099.3
Urethro-oculosynovial syndrome 099.3
Urethrorectal —*see* condition
Urethrorrhagia 599.84
Urethrorrhea 788.7
Urethrostomy status V44.6
  with complication 997.5
Urethrotrigonitis 595.3
Urethrovaginal —*see* condition
Urhidrosis, uridrosis 705.89
Uric acid
  diathesis 274.9
  in blood 790.6
Uricacidemia 790.6
Uricemia 790.6
Uricosuria 791.9
Urination
  frequent 788.41
  painful 788.1
  urgency 788.63
Urine, urinary —*see also* condition
  abnormality NEC 788.69
  blood in (*see also* Hematuria) 599.7
  discharge, excessive 788.42
  enuresis 788.30
    nonorganic origin 307.6
  extravasation 788.8
  frequency 788.41
  hesitancy 788.64
  incontinence 788.30
    active 788.30
    female 788.30
      stress 625.6
        and urge 788.33
    male 788.30
      stress 788.32
        and urge 788.33
    mixed (stress and urge) 788.33
    neurogenic 788.39
    nonorganic origin 307.6
    overflow 788.38
    stress (female) 625.6
      male NEC 788.32
  intermittent stream 788.61
  pus in 791.9
  retention or stasis NEC 788.20
    bladder, incomplete emptying 788.21
    psychogenic 306.53
    specified NEC 788.29
  secretion
    deficient 788.5
    excessive 788.42
    frequency 788.41
  strain 788.65
  stream
    intermittent 788.61
    slowing 788.62
    splitting 788.61
    weak 788.62
  urgency 788.63
Urinemia —*see* Uremia

INDEX TO DISEASES

Urinoma NEC 599.9
  bladder 596.8
  kidney 593.89
  renal 593.89
  ureter 593.89
  urethra 599.84
Uroarthritis, infectious 099.3
Urodialysis 788.5
Urolithiasis 592.9
Uronephrosis 593.89
Uropathy 599.9
  obstructive 599.60
Urosepsis 599.0
  meaning sepsis 995.91
  meaning urinary tract infection 599.0
Urticaria 708.9
  with angioneurotic edema 995.1
    hereditary 277.6
  allergic 708.0
  cholinergic 708.5
  chronic 708.8
  cold, familial 708.2
  dermatographic 708.3
  due to
    cold or heat 708.2
    drugs 708.0
    food 708.0
    inhalants 708.0
    plants 708.8
    serum 999.5
  factitial 708.3
  giant 995.1
    hereditary 277.6
  gigantea 995.1
    hereditary 277.6
  idiopathic 708.1
  larynx 995.1
    hereditary 277.6
  neonatorum 778.8
  nonallergic 708.1
  papulosa (Hebra) 698.2
  perstans hemorrhagica 757.39
  pigmentosa 757.33
  recurrent periodic 708.8
  serum 999.5
  solare 692.72
  specified type NEC 708.8
  thermal (cold) (heat) 708.2
  vibratory 708.4
Urticarioides acarodermatitis 133.9
Use of
  nonprescribed drugs (*see also* Abuse, drugs, nondependent) 305.9
  patent medicines (*see also* Abuse, drugs, nondependent) 305.9
Usher-Senear disease (pemphigus erythematosus) 694.4
Uta 085.5
Uterine size-date discrepancy 649.6
Uteromegaly 621.2
Uterovaginal —*see* condition
Uterovesical —*see* condition
Uterus —*see* condition
Utriculitis (utriculus prostaticus) 597.89
Uveal —*see* condition

Uveitis (anterior) (*see also* Iridocyclitis) 364.3
  acute or subacute 364.00
    due to or associated with
      gonococcal infection 098.41
      herpes (simplex) 054.44
        zoster 053.22
    primary 364.01
    recurrent 364.02
    secondary (noninfectious) 364.04
      infectious 364.03
  allergic 360.11
  chronic 364.10
    due to or associated with
      sarcoidosis 135 *[364.11]*
      tuberculosis (*see also* Tuberculosis) 017.3 *[364.11]*
  due to
    operation 360.11
    toxoplasmosis (acquired) 130.2
      congenital (active) 771.2
  granulomatous 364.10
  heterochromic 364.21
  lens-induced 364.23
  nongranulomatous 364.00
  posterior 363.20
    disseminated—*see* Chorioretinitis, disseminated
    focal—*see* Chorioretinitis, focal
  recurrent 364.02
  sympathetic 360.11
  syphilitic (secondary) 091.50
    congenital 090.0 *[363.13]*
    late 095.8 *[363.13]*
  tuberculous (*see also* Tuberculosis) 017.3 *[364.11]*
Uveoencephalitis 363.22
Uveokeratitis (*see also* Iridocyclitis) 364.3
Uveoparotid fever 135
Uveoparotitis 135
Uvula —*see* condition
Uvulitis (acute) (catarrhal) (chronic) (gangrenous) (membranous) (suppurative) (ulcerative) 528.3

V

Vaccination
  complication or reaction—*see* Complications, vaccination
  not carried out V64.00
    because of
      acute illness V64.01
      allergy to vaccine or component V64.04
      caregiver refusal V64.05
      chronic illness V64.02
      guardian refusal V64.05
      immune compromised state V64.03
      parent refusal V64.05
      patient had disease being vaccinated against V64.08
      patient refusal V64.06
      reason NEC V64.09
      religious reasons V64.07
  prophylactic (against) V05.9
    arthropod-borne viral
      disease NEC V05.1
      encephalitis V05.0
    chickenpox V05.4
    cholera (alone) V03.0
      with typhoid-paratyphoid (cholera + TAB) V06.0
    common cold V04.7
    diphtheria (alone) V03.5
      with
        poliomyelitis (DTP + polio) V06.3
        tetanus V06.5
          pertussis combined [DTP] [DTaP] V06.1
        typhoid-paratyphoid (DTP + TAB) V06.2
    disease (single) NEC V05.9
      bacterial NEC V03.9
        specified type NEC V03.89
      combinations NEC V06.9
        specified type NEC V06.8
      specified type NEC V05.8
    encephalitis, viral, arthropod-borne V05.0
    Hemophilus influenzae, type B [Hib] V03.81
    hepatitis, viral V05.3
    influenza V04.81
      with
        Streptococcus pneumoniae [pneumococcus] V06.6
    leishmaniasis V05.2
    measles (alone) V04.2
      with mumps-rubella (MMR) V06.4
    mumps (alone) V04.6
      with measles and rubella (MMR) V06.4
    pertussis alone V03.6
    plague V03.3
    poliomyelitis V04.0
      with diphtheria-tetanus-pertussis (DTP + polio) V06.3
    rabies V04.5
    respiratory syncytial virus (RSV) V04.82
    rubella (alone) V04.3
      with measles and mumps (MMR) V06.4
    smallpox V04.1
    Streptococcus pneumoniae [pneumococcus] V03.82
      with
        influenza V06.6
    tetanus toxoid (alone) V03.7
      with diphtheria [Td] [DT] V06.5
        with
          pertussis [DTP] [DTaP] V06.1

Vaccination—*continued*
      with poliomyelitis (DTP + polio) V06.3
    tuberculosis (BCG) V03.2
    tularemia V03.4
    typhoid-paratyphoid (TAB) (alone) V03.1
      with diphtheria-tetanus-pertussis (TAB + DTP) V06.2
    varicella V05.4
    viral
      disease NEC V04.89
      encephalitis, arthropod-borne V05.0
      hepatitis V05.3
    yellow fever V04.4
Vaccinia (generalized) 999.0
  congenital 771.2
  conjunctiva 999.39
  eyelids 999.0 *[373.5]*
  localized 999.39
  nose 999.39
  not from vaccination 051.0
    eyelid 051.0 *[373.5]*
  sine vaccinatione 051.0
  without vaccination 051.0
Vacuum
  extraction of fetus or newborn 763.3
  in sinus (accessory) (nasal) (*see also* Sinusitis) 473.9
Vagabond V60.0
Vagabondage V60.0
Vagabonds' disease 132.1
Vagina, vaginal —*see* condition
Vaginalitis (tunica) 608.4
Vaginismus (reflex) 625.1
  functional 306.51
  hysterical 300.11
  psychogenic 306.51
Vaginitis (acute) (chronic) (circumscribed) (diffuse) (emphysematous) (Hemophilus vaginalis) (nonspecific) (nonvenereal) (ulcerative) 616.10
  with
    abortion—*see* Abortion, by type, with sepsis
    ectopic pregnancy (*see also* categories 633.0-633.9) 639.0
    molar pregnancy (*see also* categories 630-632) 639.0
  adhesive, congenital 752.49
  atrophic, postmenopausal 627.3
  bacterial 616.10
  blennorrhagic (acute) 098.0
    chronic or duration of 2 months or over 098.2
  candidal 112.1
  chlamydial 099.53
  complicating pregnancy or puerperium 646.6
    affecting fetus or newborn 760.8
  congenital (adhesive) 752.49
  due to
    C. albicans 112.1
    Trichomonas (vaginalis) 131.01
  following
    abortion 639.0
    ectopic or molar pregnancy 639.0
  gonococcal (acute) 098.0
    chronic or duration of 2 months or over 098.2
  granuloma 099.2
  Monilia 112.1
  mycotic 112.1

Vaginitis—*continued*
  pinworm 127.4 *[616.11]*
  postirradiation 616.10
  postmenopausal atrophic 627.3
  senile (atrophic) 627.3
  syphilitic (early) 091.0
    late 095.8
  trichomonal 131.01
  tuberculous (*see also* Tuberculosis) 016.7
  venereal NEC 099.8
Vaginosis —*see* Vaginitis
Vagotonia 352.3
Vagrancy V60.0
VAIN I (vaginal intraepithelial neoplasia I) 623.0
VAIN II (vaginal intraepithelial neoplasia II) 623.0
VAIN III (vaginal intraepithelial neoplasia III) 233.31
Vallecula —*see* condition
Valley fever 114.0
Valsuani's disease (progressive pernicious anemia, puerperal) 648.2
Valve, valvular (formation)—*see also* condition
  cerebral ventricle (communicating) in situ V45.2
  cervix, internal os 752.49
  colon 751.5
  congenital NEC—*see* Atresia
  formation, congenital NEC—*see* Atresia
  heart defect—*see* Anomaly, heart, valve
  ureter 753.29
    pelvic junction 753.21
    vesical orifice 753.22
  urethra 753.6
Valvulitis (chronic) (*see also* Endocarditis) 424.90
  rheumatic (chronic) (inactive) (with chorea) 397.9
    active or acute (aortic) (mitral) (pulmonary) (tricuspid) 391.1
  syphilitic NEC 093.20
    aortic 093.22
    mitral 093.21
    pulmonary 093.24
    tricuspid 093.23
Valvulopathy —*see* Endocarditis
van Bogaert's leukoencephalitis (sclerosing) (subacute) 046.2
van Bogaert-Nijssen (-Peiffer) disease 330.0
van Buchem's syndrome (hyperostosis corticalis) 733.3
Vancomycin (glycopeptide)
  intermediate staphylococcus aureus (VISA/GISA) V09.8
  resistant
    enterococcus (VRE) V09.8
    staphylococcus aureus (VRSA/GRSA) V09.8
van Creveld-von Gierke disease (glycogenosis I) 271.0
van den Bergh's disease (enterogenous cyanosis) 289.7
van der Hoeve's syndrome (brittle bones and blue sclera, deafness) 756.51
van der Hoeve-Halbertsma-Waardenburg syndrome (ptosis-epicanthus) 270.2
van der Hoeve-Waardenburg-Gualdi syndrome (ptosis epicanthus) 270.2
Vanillism 692.89
Vanishing lung 492.0
Vanishing twin 651.33

van Neck (-Odelberg) disease or syndrome (juvenile osteochondrosis) 732.1
Vapor asphyxia or suffocation NEC 987.9
  specified agent—*see* Table of drugs and chemicals
Vaquez's disease (M9950/1) 238.4
Vaquez-Osler disease (polycythemia vera) (M9950/1) 238.4
Variance, lethal ball, prosthetic heart valve 996.02
Variants, thalassemic 282.49
Variations in hair color 704.3
Varicella 052.9
  with
    complication 052.8
      specified NEC 052.7
    pneumonia 052.1
  exposure to V01.71
  vaccination and inoculation (prophylactic) V05.4
Varices —*see* Varix
Varicocele (scrotum) (thrombosed) 456.4
  ovary 456.5
  perineum 456.6
  spermatic cord (ulcerated) 456.4
Varicose
  aneurysm (ruptured) (*see also* Aneurysm) 442.9
  dermatitis (lower extremity)—*see* Varicose, vein, inflamed or infected
  eczema—*see* Varicose, vein
  phlebitis—*see* Varicose, vein, inflamed or infected
  placental vessel—*see* Placenta, abnormal
  tumor—*see* Varicose, vein
  ulcer (lower extremity, any part) 454.0
    anus 455.8
    external 455.5
    internal 455.2
    esophagus (*see also* Varix, esophagus) 456.1
      bleeding (*see also* Varix, esophagus, bleeding) 456.0
    inflamed or infected 454.2
    nasal septum 456.8
    perineum 456.6
    rectum—*see* Varicose, ulcer, anus
    scrotum 456.4
    specified site NEC 456.8
  vein (lower extremity) (ruptured) (*see also* Varix) 454.9
    with
      complications NEC 454.8
      edema 454.8
      inflammation or infection 454.1
        ulcerated 454.2
      pain 454.8
      stasis dermatitis 454.1
        with ulcer 454.2
      swelling 454.8
      ulcer 454.0
        inflamed or infected 454.2
    anus—*see* Hemorrhoids
    broad ligament 456.5
    congenital (peripheral) NEC 747.60
      gastrointestinal 747.61
      lower limb 747.64
      renal 747.62
      specified NEC 747.69
      upper limb 747.63
    esophagus (ulcerated) (*see also* Varix, esophagus) 456.1

INDEX TO DISEASES

Vasitis

Varicose—*continued*
  bleeding (*see also* Varix, esophagus, bleeding) 456.0
  inflamed or infected 454.1
    with ulcer 454.2
  in pregnancy or puerperium 671.0
    vulva or perineum 671.1
  nasal septum (with ulcer) 456.8
  pelvis 456.5
  perineum 456.6
    in pregnancy, childbirth, or puerperium 671.1
  rectum—*see* Hemorrhoids
  scrotum (ulcerated) 456.4
  specified site NEC 456.8
  sublingual 456.3
  ulcerated 454.0
    inflamed or infected 454.2
  umbilical cord, affecting fetus or newborn 762.6
  urethra 456.8
  vulva 456.6
    in pregnancy, childbirth, or puerperium 671.1
  vessel—*see also* Varix
  placenta—*see* Placenta, abnormal
Varicosis, varicosities, varicosity (*see also* Varix) 454.9
Variola 050.9
  hemorrhagic (pustular) 050.0
  major 050.0
  minor 050.1
  modified 050.2
Varioloid 050.2
Variolosa, purpura 050.0
Varix (lower extremity) (ruptured) 454.9
  with
    complications NEC 454.8
    edema 454.8
    inflammation or infection 454.1
      with ulcer 454.2
    pain 454.8
    stasis dermatitis 454.1
      with ulcer 454.2
    swelling 454.8
    ulcer 454.0
      with inflammation or infection 454.2
  aneurysmal (*see also* Aneurysm) 442.9
  anus—*see* Hemorrhoids
  arteriovenous (congenital) (peripheral) NEC 747.60
    gastrointestinal 747.61
    lower limb 747.64
    renal 747.62
    specified NEC 747.69
    spinal 747.82
    upper limb 747.63
  bladder 456.5
  broad ligament 456.5
  congenital (peripheral) NEC 747.60
  esophagus (ulcerated) 456.1
    bleeding 456.0
      in
        cirrhosis of liver 571.5 *[456.20]*
        portal hypertension 572.3 *[456.20]*
    congenital 747.69
    in
      cirrhosis of liver 571.5 *[456.21]*
        with bleeding 571.5 *[456.20]*
      portal hypertension 572.3 *[456.21]*
        with bleeding 572.3 *[456.20]*

Varix—*continued*
  gastric 456.8
  inflamed or infected 454.1
    ulcerated 454.2
  in pregnancy or puerperium 671.0
    perineum 671.1
    vulva 671.1
  labia (majora) 456.6
  orbit 456.8
    congenital 747.69
  ovary 456.5
  papillary 448.1
  pelvis 456.5
  perineum 456.6
    in pregnancy or puerperium 671.1
  pharynx 456.8
  placenta—*see* Placenta, abnormal
  prostate 456.8
  rectum—*see* Hemorrhoids
  renal papilla 456.8
  retina 362.17
  scrotum (ulcerated) 456.4
  sigmoid colon 456.8
  specified site NEC 456.8
  spinal (cord) (vessels) 456.8
  spleen, splenic (vein) (with phlebolith) 456.8
  sublingual 456.3
  ulcerated 454.0
    inflamed or infected 454.2
  umbilical cord, affecting fetus or newborn 762.6
  uterine ligament 456.5
  vocal cord 456.8
  vulva 456.6
    in pregnancy, childbirth, or puerperium 671.1
Vasa previa 663.5
  affecting fetus or newborn 762.6
  hemorrhage from, affecting fetus or newborn 772.0
Vascular —*see also* condition
  loop on papilla (optic) 743.57
  sheathing, retina 362.13
  spasm 443.9
  spider 448.1
Vascularity, pulmonary, congenital 747.3
Vascularization
  choroid 362.16
  cornea 370.60
    deep 370.63
    localized 370.61
  retina 362.16
  subretinal 362.16
Vasculitis 447.6
  allergic 287.0
  cryoglobulinemic 273.2
  disseminated 447.6
  kidney 447.8
  leukocytoclastic 446.29
  nodular 695.2
  retinal 362.18
  rheumatic—*see* Fever, rheumatic
Vasculopathy
  cardiac allograft 996.83
Vas deferens —*see* condition
Vas deferentitis 608.4
Vasectomy, admission for V25.2
Vasitis 608.4
  nodosa 608.4
  scrotum 608.4
  spermatic cord 608.4
  testis 608.4
  tuberculous (*see also* Tuberculosis) 016.5
  tunica vaginalis 608.4
  vas deferens 608.4

1399

Vasodilation

Vasodilation 443.9
Vasomotor —*see* condition
Vasoplasty, after previous sterilization V26.0
Vasoplegia, splanchnic (*see also* Neuropathy, peripheral, autonomic) 337.9
Vasospasm 443.9
   cerebral (artery) 435.9
      with transient neurologic deficit 435.9
   coronary 413.1
   nerve
      arm NEC 354.9
      autonomic 337.9
      brachial plexus 353.0
      cervical plexus 353.2
      leg NEC 355.8
      lower extremity NEC 355.8
      peripheral NEC 355.9
      spinal NEC 355.9
      sympathetic 337.9
      upper extremity NEC 354.9
   peripheral NEC 443.9
   retina (artery) (*see also* Occlusion, retinal, artery) 362.30
Vasospastic —*see* condition
Vasovagal attack (paroxysmal) 780.2
   psychogenic 306.2
Vater's ampulla —*see* condition
VATER syndrome 759.89
Vegetation, vegetative
   adenoid (nasal fossa) 474.2
   consciousness (persistent) 780.03
   endocarditis (acute) (any valve) (chronic) (subacute) 421.0
   heart (mycotic) (valve) 421.0
   state (persistent) 780.03
Veil
   Jackson's 751.4
   over face (causing asphyxia) 768.9
Vein, venous —*see* condition
Veldt sore (*see also* Ulcer, skin) 707.9
Velo-cardio-facial syndrome 758.32
Velpeau's hernia —*see* Hernia, femoral
Venereal
   balanitis NEC 099.8
   bubo 099.1
   disease 099.9
      specified nature or type NEC 099.8
   granuloma inguinale 099.2
   lymphogranuloma (Durand-Nicolas-Favre), any site 099.1
   salpingitis 098.37
   urethritis (*see also* Urethritis, nongonococcal) 099.40
   vaginitis NEC 099.8
   warts 078.19
Vengefulness, in child (*see also* Disturbance, conduct) 312.0
Venofibrosis 459.89
Venom, venomous
   bite or sting (animal or insect) 989.5
   poisoning 989.5
Venous —*see* condition
Ventouse delivery NEC 669.5
   affecting fetus or newborn 763.3
Ventral —*see* condition
Ventricle, ventricular —*see also* condition
   escape 427.69
   standstill (*see also* Arrest, cardiac) 427.5
Ventriculitis, cerebral (*see also* Meningitis) 322.9
Ventriculostomy status V45.2

INDEX TO DISEASES

Verbiest's syndrome (claudicatio intermittens spinalis) 435.1
Vernet's syndrome 352.6
Verneuil's disease (syphilitic bursitis) 095.7
Verruca (filiformis) 078.10
   acuminata (any site) 078.11
   necrogenica (primary) (*see also* Tuberculosis) 017.0
   peruana 088.0
   peruviana 088.0
   plana (juvenilis) 078.19
   plantaris 078.19
   seborrheica 702.19
      inflamed 702.11
   senilis 702.0
   tuberculosa (primary) (*see also* Tuberculosis) 017.0
   venereal 078.19
   viral NEC 078.10
Verrucosities (*see also* Verruca) 078.10
Verrucous endocarditis (acute) (any valve) (chronic) (subacute) 710.0 *[424.91]*
   nonbacterial 710.0 *[424.91]*
Verruga
   peruana 088.0
   peruviana 088.0
Verse's disease (calcinosis intervertebralis) 275.49 *[722.90]*
Version
   before labor, affecting fetus or newborn 761.7
   cephalic (correcting previous malposition) 652.1
      affecting fetus or newborn 763.1
   cervix (*see* Version, uterus)
   uterus (postinfectional) (postpartal, old) (*see also* Malposition, uterus) 621.6
      forward—*see* Anteversion, uterus
      lateral—*see* Lateroversion, uterus
Vertebra, vertebral —*see* condition
Vertigo 780.4
   auditory 386.19
   aural 386.19
   benign paroxysmal positional 386.11
   central origin 386.2
   cerebral 386.2
   Dix and Hallpike (epidemic) 386.12
   endemic paralytic 078.81
   epidemic 078.81
      Dix and Hallpike 386.12
      Gerlier's 078.81
      Pedersen's 386.12
      vestibular neuronitis 386.12
   epileptic—*see* Epilepsy
   Gerlier's (epidemic) 078.81
   hysterical 300.11
   labyrinthine 386.10
   laryngeal 786.2
   malignant positional 386.2
   Ménière's (*see also* Disease, Ménière's) 386.00
   menopausal 627.2
   otogenic 386.19
   paralytic 078.81
   paroxysmal positional, benign 386.11
   Pedersen's (epidemic) 386.12
   peripheral 386.10
      specified type NEC 386.19
   positional
      benign paroxysmal 386.11
      malignant 386.2
Verumontanitis (chronic) (*see also* Urethritis) 597.89
Vesania (*see also* Psychosis) 298.9
Vesical —*see* condition

INDEX TO DISEASES

Vesicle
  cutaneous 709.8
  seminal—*see* condition
  skin 709.8
Vesicocolic —*see* condition
Vesicoperineal —*see* condition
Vesicorectal —*see* condition
Vesicourethrorectal —*see* condition
Vesicovaginal —*see* condition
Vesicular —*see* condition
Vesiculitis (seminal) 608.0
  amebic 006.8
  gonorrheal (acute) 098.14
    chronic or duration of 2 months or over 098.34
  trichomonal 131.09
  tuberculous (*see also* Tuberculosis) 016.5 [608.81]
Vestibulitis (ear) (*see also* Labyrinthitis) 386.30
  nose (external) 478.19
  vulvar 616.10
Vestibulopathy, acute peripheral (recurrent) 386.12
Vestige, vestigial —*see also* Persistence
  branchial 744.41
  structures in vitreous 743.51
Vibriosis NEC 027.9
Vidal's disease (lichen simplex chronicus) 698.3
Video display tube syndrome 723.8
Vienna type encephalitis 049.8
Villaret's syndrome 352.6
Villous —*see* condition
VIN I (vulvar intraepithelial neoplasia I) 624.01
VIN II (vulvar intraepithelial neoplasia II) 624.02
VIN III (vulvar intraepithelial neoplasia III) 233.32
Vincent's
  angina 101
  bronchitis 101
  disease 101
  gingivitis 101
  infection (any site) 101
  laryngitis 101
  stomatitis 101
  tonsillitis 101
Vinson-Plummer syndrome (sideropenic dysphagia) 280.8
Viosterol deficiency (*see also* Deficiency, calciferol) 268.9
Virchow's disease 733.99
Viremia 790.8
Virilism (adrenal) (female) NEC 255.2
  with
    3-beta-hydroxysteroid dehydrogenase defect 255.2
    11-hydroxylase defect 255.2
    21-hydroxylase defect 255.2
    adrenal
      hyperplasia 255.2
      insufficiency (congenital) 255.2
      cortical hyperfunction 255.2
Virilization (female) (suprarenal) (*see also* Virilism) 255.2
  isosexual 256.4
Virulent bubo 099.0
Virus, viral —*see also* condition
  infection NEC (*see also* Infection, viral) 079.99
  septicemia 079.99
VISA (vancomycin intermediate staphylococcus aureus) V09.8
Viscera, visceral —*see* condition
Visceroptosis 569.89

Volvulus

Visible peristalsis 787.4
Vision, visual
  binocular, suppression 368.31
  blurred, blurring 368.8
    hysterical 300.11
  defect, defective (*see also* Impaired, vision) 369.9
  disorientation (syndrome) 368.16
  disturbance NEC (*see also* Disturbance, vision) 368.9
  hysterical 300.11
  examination V72.0
  field, limitation 368.40
  fusion, with defective steropsis 368.33
  hallucinations 368.16
  halos 368.16
  loss 369.9
    both eyes (*see also* Blindness, both eyes) 369.3
    complete (*see also* Blindness, both eyes) 369.00
    one eye 369.8
    sudden 368.16
  low (both eyes) 369.20
    one eye (other eye normal) (*see also* Impaired, vision) 369.70
      blindness, other eye 369.10
  perception, simultaneous without fusion 368.32
  tunnel 368.45
Vitality, lack or want of 780.79
  newborn 779.89
Vitamin deficiency NEC (*see also* Deficiency, vitamin) 269.2
Vitelline duct, persistent 751.0
Vitiligo 709.01
  due to pinta (carate) 103.2
  eyelid 374.53
  vulva 624.8
Vitium cordis —*see* Disease, heart
Vitreous —*see also* condition
  touch syndrome 997.99
VLCAD (long chain/very long chain acyl CoA dehydrogenase deficiency, LCAD) 277.85
Vocal cord —*see* condition
Vocational rehabilitation V57.22
Vogt's (Cecile) disease or syndrome 333.7
Vogt-Koyanagi syndrome 364.24
Vogt-Spielmeyer disease (amaurotic familial idiocy) 330.1
Voice
  change (*see also* Dysphonia) 784.49
  loss (*see also* Aphonia) 784.41
Volhard-Fahr disease (malignant nephrosclerosis) 403.00
Volhynian fever 083.1
Volkmann's ischemic contracture or paralysis (complicating trauma) 958.6
Voluntary starvation 307.1
Volvulus (bowel) (colon) (intestine) 560.2
  with
    hernia—*see also* Hernia, by site, with obstruction
      gangrenous—*see* Hernia, by site, with gangrene
    perforation 560.2
  congenital 751.5
  duodenum 537.3
  fallopian tube 620.5
  oviduct 620.5
  stomach (due to absence of gastrocolic ligament) 537.89

Vomiting 787.03
  with nausea 787.01
  allergic 535.4
  asphyxia 933.1
  bilious (cause unknown) 787.0
    following gastrointestinal surgery 564.3
  blood (*see also* Hematemesis) 578.0
  causing asphyxia, choking, or suffocation (*see also* Asphyxia, food) 933.1
  cyclical 536.2
    psychogenic 306.4
  epidemic 078.82
  fecal matter 569.89
  following gastrointestinal surgery 564.3
  functional 536.8
    psychogenic 306.4
  habit 536.2
  hysterical 300.11
  nervous 306.4
  neurotic 306.4
  newborn 779.3
  of or complicating pregnancy 643.9
    due to
      organic disease 643.8
      specific cause NEC 643.8
    early—*see* Hyperemesis, gravidarum
    late (after 22 completed weeks of gestation) 643.2
  pernicious or persistent 536.2
    complicating pregnancy—*see* Hyperemesis, gravidarum
    psychogenic 306.4
  physiological 787.0
  psychic 306.4
  psychogenic 307.54
  stercoral 569.89
  uncontrollable 536.2
    psychogenic 306.4
  uremic—*see* Uremia
  winter 078.82
von Bechterew (-Strumpell) disease or syndrome (ankylosing spondylitis) 720.0
von Bezold's abscess 383.01
von Economo's disease (encephalitis lethargica) 049.8
von Eulenburg's disease (congenital paramyotonia) 359.29
von Gierke's disease (glycogenosis I) 271.0
von Gies' joint 095.8
von Graefe's disease or syndrome 378.72
von Hippel (-Lindau) disease or syndrome (retinocerebral angiomatosis) 759.6
von Jaksch's anemia or disease (pseudoleukemia infantum) 285.8
von Recklinghausen's
  disease or syndrome (nerves) (skin) (M9540/1) 237.71
    bones (osteitis fibrosa cystica) 252.01
  tumor (M9540/1) 237.71
von Recklinghausen-Applebaum disease (hemochromatosis) 275.0
von Schroetter's syndrome (intermittent venous claudication) 453.8
von Willebrand (-Jürgens) (-Minot) disease or syndrome (angiohemophilia) 286.4
von Zambusch's disease (lichen sclerosus et atrophicus) 701.0
Voorhoeve's disease or dyschondroplasia 756.4
Vossius' ring 921.3
  late effect 366.21
Voyeurism 302.82

VRE (vancomycin resistant enterococcus) V09.8
Vrolik's disease (osteogenesis imperfecta) 756.51
VRSA (vancomycin resistant staphylococcus aureus) V09.8
Vulva —*see* condition
Vulvismus 625.1
Vulvitis (acute) (allergic) (chronic) (gangrenous) (hypertrophic) (intertriginous) 616.10
  with
    abortion—*see* Abortion, by type, with sepsis
    ectopic pregnancy (*see also* categories 633.0-633.9) 639.0
    molar pregnancy (*see also* categories 630-632) 639.0
  adhesive, congenital 752.49
  blennorrhagic (acute) 098.0
    chronic or duration of 2 months or over 098.2
  chlamydial 099.53
  complicating pregnancy or puerperium 646.6
  due to Ducrey's bacillus 099.0
  following
    abortion 639.0
    ectopic or molar pregnancy 639.0
  gonococcal (acute) 098.0
    chronic or duration of 2 months or over 098.2
  herpetic 054.11
  leukoplakic 624.09
  monilial 112.1
  puerperal, postpartum, childbirth 646.6
  syphilitic (early) 091.0
    late 095.8
  trichomonal 131.01
Vulvodynia 625.8
Vulvorectal —*see* condition
Vulvovaginitis (*see also* Vulvitis) 616.10
  amebic 006.8
  chlamydial 099.53
  gonococcal (acute) 098.0
    chronic or duration of 2 months or over 098.2
  herpetic 054.11
  monilial 112.1
  trichomonal (Trichomonas vaginalis) 131.01

W

Waardenburg's syndrome 756.89
  meaning ptosis-epicanthus 270.2
Waardenburg-Klein syndrome
  (ptosis-epicanthus) 270.2
Wagner's disease (colloid milium) 709.3
Wagner (-Unverricht) syndrome
  (dermatomyositis) 710.3
Waiting list, person on V63.2
  undergoing social agency investigation V63.8
Wakefulness disorder (*see also* Hypersomnia) 780.54
  nonorganic origin 307.43
Waldenström's
  disease (osteochondrosis, capital femoral) 732.1
  hepatitis (lupoid hepatitis) 571.49
  hypergammaglobulinemia 273.0
  macroglobulinemia 273.3
  purpura, hypergammaglobulinemic 273.0
  syndrome (macroglobulinemia) 273.3
Waldenström-Kjellberg syndrome (sideropenic dysphagia) 280.8
Walking
  difficulty 719.7
    psychogenic 307.9
  sleep 307.46
    hysterical 300.13
Wall, abdominal —*see* condition
Wallenberg's syndrome (posterior inferior cerebellar artery) (*see also* Disease, cerebrovascular, acute) 436
Wallgren's
  disease (obstruction of splenic vein with collateral circulation) 459.89
  meningitis (*see also* Meningitis, aseptic) 047.9
Wandering
  acetabulum 736.39
  gallbladder 751.69
  kidney, congenital 753.3
  organ or site, congenital NEC—*see* Malposition, congenital
  pacemaker (atrial) (heart) 427.89
  spleen 289.59
Wardrop's disease (with lymphangitis) 681.9
  finger 681.02
  toe 681.11
War neurosis 300.16
Wart (common) (digitate) (filiform) (infectious) (juvenile) (plantar) (viral) 078.10
  external genital organs (venereal) 078.19
  fig 078.19
  Hassall-Henle's (of cornea) 371.41
  Henle's (of cornea) 371.41
  juvenile 078.19
  moist 078.10
  Peruvian 088.0
  plantar 078.19
  prosector (*see also* Tuberculosis) 017.0
  seborrheic 702.19
    inflamed 702.11
  senile 702.0
  specified NEC 078.19
  syphilitic 091.3
  tuberculous (*see also* Tuberculosis) 017.0
  venereal (female) (male) 078.19
Warthin's tumor (salivary gland) (M8561/0) 210.2
Washerwoman's itch 692.4
Wassilieff's disease (leptospiral jaundice) 100.0

Wasting
  disease 799.4
    due to malnutrition 261
    extreme (due to malnutrition) 261
  muscular NEC 728.2
  palsy, paralysis 335.21
  pelvic muscle 618.83
Water
  clefts 366.12
  deprivation of 994.3
  in joint (*see also* Effusion, joint) 719.0
  intoxication 276.6
  itch 120.3
  lack of 994.3
  loading 276.6
  on
    brain—*see* Hydrocephalus
    chest 511.8
  poisoning 276.6
Waterbrash 787.1
Water-hammer pulse (*see also* Insufficiency, aortic) 424.1
Waterhouse (-Friderichsen) disease or syndrome 036.3
Water-losing nephritis 588.89
Watermelon stomach 537.82
  with hemorrhage 537.83
  without hemorrhage 537.82
Wax in ear 380.4
Waxy
  degeneration, any site 277.39
  disease 277.39
  kidney 277.39 *[583.81]*
  liver (large) 277.39
  spleen 277.39
Weak, weakness (generalized) 780.79
  arches (acquired) 734
    congenital 754.61
  bladder sphincter 596.59
  congenital 779.89
  eye muscle—*see* Strabismus
  facial 781.94
  foot (double)—*see* Weak, arches
  heart, cardiac (*see also* Failure, heart) 428.9
    congenital 746.9
  mind 317
  muscle (generalized) 728.87
  myocardium (*see also* Failure, heart) 428.9
  newborn 779.89
  pelvic fundus
    pubocervical tissue 618.81
    rectovaginal tissue 618.82
  pulse 785.9
  senile 797
  valvular—*see* Endocarditis
Wear, worn, tooth, teeth (approximal) (hard tissues) (interproximal) (occlusal)—*see also* Attrition, teeth 521.10
Weather, weathered
  effects of
    cold NEC 991.9
      specified effect NEC 991.8
    hot (*see also* Heat) 992.9
  skin 692.74
Web, webbed (congenital)—*see also* Anomaly, specified type NEC
  canthus 743.63
  digits (*see also* Syndactylism) 755.10

Web, webbed

Web, webbed—*continued*
  duodenal 751.5
  esophagus 750.3
  fingers (*see also* Syndactylism, fingers) 755.11
  larynx (glottic) (subglottic) 748.2
  neck (pterygium colli) 744.5
  Paterson-Kelly (sideropenic dysphagia) 280.8
  popliteal syndrome 756.89
  toes (*see also* Syndactylism, toes) 755.13
Weber's paralysis or syndrome 344.89
Weber-Christian disease or syndrome (nodular nonsuppurative panniculitis) 729.30
Weber-Cockayne syndrome (epidermolysis bullosa) 757.39
Weber-Dimitri syndrome 759.6
Weber-Gubler syndrome 344.89
Weber-Leyden syndrome 344.89
Weber-Osler syndrome (familial hemorrhagic telangiectasia) 448.0
Wedge-shaped or wedging vertebra (*see also* Osteoporosis) 733.00
Wegener's granulomatosis or syndrome 446.4
Wegner's disease (syphilitic osteochondritis) 090.0
Weight
  gain (abnormal) (excessive) 783.1
    during pregnancy 646.1
      insufficient 646.8
  less than 1000 grams at birth 765.0
  loss (cause unknown) 783.21
Weightlessness 994.9
Weil's disease (leptospiral jaundice) 100.00
Weill-Marchesani syndrome (brachymorphism and ectopia lentis) 759.89
Weingarten's syndrome (tropical eosinophilia) 518.3
Weir Mitchell's disease (erythromelalgia) 443.82
Weiss-Baker syndrome (carotid sinus syncope) 337.0
Weissenbach-Thibierge syndrome (cutaneous systemic sclerosis) 710.1
Wen (*see also* Cyst, sebaceous) 706.2
Wenckebach's phenomenon, heart block (second degree) 426.13
Werdnig-Hoffmann syndrome (muscular atrophy) 335.0
Werlhof's disease (*see also* Purpura, thrombocytopenic) 287.39
Werlhof-Wichmann syndrome (*see also* Purpura, thrombocytopenic) 287.39
Wermer's syndrome or disease (polyendocrine adenomatosis) 258.01
Werner's disease or syndrome (progeria adultorum) 259.8
Werner-His disease (trench fever) 083.1
Werner-Schultz disease (agranulocytosis) 288.09
Wernicke's encephalopathy, disease or syndrome (superior hemorrhagic polioencephalitis) 265.1
Wernicke-Korsakoff syndrome or psychosis (nonalcoholic) 294.0
  alcoholic 291.1
Wernicke-Posadas disease (*see also* Coccidioidomycosis) 114.9
Wesselsbron fever 066.3
West African fever 084.8

West Nile
  encephalitis 066.41
  encephalomyelitis 066.41
  fever 066.40
    with
      cranial nerve disorders 066.42
      encephalitis 066.41
      optic neuritis 066.42
      other complications 066.49
      other neurologic manifestations 066.42
      polyradiculitis 066.42
  virus 066.40
Westphal-Strümpell syndrome (hepatolenticular degeneration) 275.1
Wet
  brain (alcoholic) (*see also* Alcoholism) 303.9
  feet, tropical (syndrome) (maceration) 991.4
  lung (syndrome)
    adult 518.5
    newborn 770.6
Wharton's duct —*see* condition
Wheal 709.8
Wheezing 786.07
Whiplash injury or syndrome 847.0
Whipple's disease or syndrome (intestinal lipodystrophy) 040.2
Whipworm 127.3
"Whistling face" syndrome (craniocarpotarsal dystrophy) 759.89
White —*see also* condition
  kidney
    large—*see* Nephrosis
    small 582.9
  leg, puerperal, postpartum, childbirth 671.4
    nonpuerperal 451.19
  mouth 112.0
  patches of mouth 528.6
  sponge nevus of oral mucosa 750.26
  spot lesions, teeth 521.01
White's disease (congenital) (keratosis follicularis) 757.39
Whitehead 706.2
Whitlow (with lymphangitis) 681.01
  herpetic 054.6
Whitmore's disease or fever (melioidosis) 025
Whooping cough 033.9
  with pneumonia 033.9 *[484.3]*
  due to
    Bordetella
      bronchoseptica 033.8
        with pneumonia 033.8 *[484.3]*
      parapertussis 033.1
        with pneumonia 033.1 *[484.3]*
      pertussis 033.0
        with pneumonia 033.0 *[484.3]*
    specified organism NEC 033.8
      with pneumonia 033.8 *[484.3]*
  vaccination, prophylactic (against) V03.6
Wichmann's asthma (laryngismus stridulus) 478.75
Widal (-Abrami) syndrome (acquired hemolytic jaundice) 283.9
Widening aorta (*see also* Aneurysm, aorta) 441.9
  ruptured 441.5
Wilkie's disease or syndrome 557.1
Wilkinson-Sneddon disease or syndrome (subcorneal pustular dermatosis) 694.1
Willan's lepra 696.1
Willan-Plumbe syndrome (psoriasis) 696.1

INDEX TO DISEASES

Wound, open

Willebrand (-Jürgens) syndrome or thrombopathy (angiohemophilia) 286.4
Willi-Prader syndrome (hypogenital dystrophy with diabetic tendency) 759.81
Willis' disease (diabetes mellitus) (*see also* Diabetes) 250.0
Wilms' tumor or neoplasm (nephroblastoma) (M8960/3) 189.0
Wilson's
  disease or syndrome (hepatolenticular degeneration) 275.1
  hepatolenticular degeneration 275.1
  lichen ruber 697.0
Wilson-Brocq disease (dermatitis exfoliativa) 695.89
Wilson-Mikity syndrome 770.7
Window —*see also* Imperfect, closure
  aorticopulmonary 745.0
Winged scapula 736.89
Winter —*see also* condition
  vomiting disease 078.82
Wise's disease 696.2
Wiskott-Aldrich syndrome (eczema-thrombocytopenia) 279.12
Withdrawal symptoms, syndrome
  alcohol 291.81
    delirium (acute) 291.0
      chronic 291.1
      newborn 760.71
  drug or narcotic 292.0
  newborn, infant of dependent mother 779.5
  steroid NEC
    correct substance properly administered 255.41
    overdose or wrong substance given or taken 962.0
Withdrawing reaction, child or adolescent 313.22
Witts' anemia (achlorhydric anemia) 280.9
Witzelsucht 301.9
Woakes' syndrome (ethmoiditis) 471.1
Wohlfart-Kugelberg-Welander disease 335.11
Woillez's disease (acute idiopathic pulmonary congestion) 518.5
Wolff-Parkinson-White syndrome (anomalous atrioventricular excitation) 426.7
Wolhynian fever 083.1
Wolman's disease (primary familial xanthomatosis) 272.7
Wood asthma 495.8
Woolly, wooly hair (congenital) (nevus) 757.4
Wool-sorters' disease 022.1
Word
  blindness (congenital) (developmental) 315.01
    secondary to organic lesion 784.61
  deafness (secondary to organic lesion) 784.69
    developmental 315.31
Worm (s) (colic) (fever) (infection) (infestation) (*see also* Infestation) 128.9
  guinea 125.7
  in intestine NEC 127.9
Worm-eaten soles 102.3
Worn out (*see also* Exhaustion) 780.79
"Worried well" V65.5
Wound, open (by cutting or piercing instrument) (by firearms) (cut) (dissection) (incised) (laceration) (penetration) (perforating) (puncture) (with initial hemorrhage, not internal) 879.8

Wound, open—*continued*

> *Note*—*For fracture with open wound, see Fracture. For laceration, traumatic rupture, tear or penetrating wound of internal organs, such as heart, lung, liver, kidney, pelvic organs, etc., whether or not accompanied by open wound or fracture in the same region, see Injury, internal. For contused wound, see Contusion. For crush injury, see Crush. For abrasion, insect bite (nonvenomous), blister, or scratch, see Injury, superficial.*
>
> *Complicated includes wounds with:*
>   *delayed healing*
>   *delayed treatment*
>   *foreign body*
>   *primary infection*
>
> *For late effect of open wound, see Late, effect, wound, open, by site.*

  abdomen, abdominal (external) (muscle) 879.2
    complicated 879.3
    wall (anterior) 879.2
      complicated 879.3
      lateral 879.4
        complicated 879.5
  alveolar (process) 873.62
    complicated 873.72
  ankle 891.0
    with tendon involvement 891.2
    complicated 891.1
  anterior chamber, eye (*see also* Wound, open, intraocular) 871.9
  anus 879.6
    complicated 879.7
  arm 884.0
    with tendon involvement 884.2
    complicated 884.1
    forearm 881.00
      with tendon involvement 881.20
      complicated 881.10
    multiple sites—*see* Wound, open, multiple, upper limb
    upper 880.03
      with tendon involvement 880.23
      complicated 880.13
      multiple sites (with axillary or shoulder regions) 880.09
        with tendon involvement 880.29
        complicated 880.19
  artery—*see* Injury, blood vessel, by site
  auditory
    canal (external) (meatus) 872.02
      complicated 872.12
    ossicles (incus) (malleus) (stapes) 872.62
      complicated 872.72
  auricle, ear 872.01
    complicated 872.11
  axilla 880.02
    with tendon involvement 880.22
    complicated 880.12
    with tendon involvement 880.29
    involving other sites of upper arm 880.09
      complicated 880.19
  back 876.0
    complicated 876.1
  bladder—*see* Injury, internal, bladder
  blood vessel—*see* Injury, blood vessel, by site
  brain—*see* Injury, intracranial, with open intracranial wound

1405

Wound, open—*continued*
  breast 879.0
    complicated 879.1
  brow 873.42
    complicated 873.52
  buccal mucosa 873.61
    complicated 873.71
  buttock 877.0
    complicated 877.1
  calf 891.0
    with tendon involvement 891.2
    complicated 891.1
  canaliculus lacrimalis 870.8
    with laceration of eyelid 870.2
  canthus, eye 870.8
    laceration—*see* Laceration, eyelid
  cavernous sinus—*see* Injury, intracranial
  cerebellum—*see* Injury, intracranial
  cervical esophagus 874.4
    complicated 874.5
  cervix—*see* Injury, internal, cervix
  cheek(s) (external) 873.41
    complicated 873.51
    internal 873.61
      complicated 873.71
  chest (wall) (external) 875.0
    complicated 875.1
  chin 873.44
    complicated 873.54
  choroid 363.63
  ciliary body (eye) (*see also* Wound, open, intraocular) 871.9
  clitoris 878.8
    complicated 878.9
  cochlea 872.64
    complicated 872.74
  complicated 879.9
  conjunctiva—*see* Wound, open, intraocular
  cornea (nonpenetrating) (*see also* Wound, open, intraocular) 871.9
  costal region 875.0
    complicated 875.1
  Descemet's membrane (*see also* Wound, open, intraocular) 871.9
  digit(s)
    foot 893.0
      with tendon involvement 893.2
      complicated 893.1
    hand 883.0
      with tendon involvement 883.2
      complicated 883.1
  drumhead, ear 872.61
    complicated 872.71
  ear 872.8
    canal 872.02
      complicated 872.12
    complicated 872.9
    drum 872.61
      complicated 872.71
    external 872.00
      complicated 872.10
    multiple sites 872.69
      complicated 872.79
    ossicles (incus) (malleus) (stapes) 872.62
      complicated 872.72
    specified part NEC 872.69
      complicated 872.79
  elbow 881.01
    with tendon involvement 881.21
    complicated 881.11
  epididymis 878.2

Wound, open—*continued*
    complicated 878.3
  epigastric region 879.2
    complicated 879.3
  epiglottis 874.01
    complicated 874.11
  esophagus (cervical) 874.4
    complicated 874.5
    thoracic—*see* Injury, internal, esophagus
  Eustachian tube 872.63
    complicated 872.73
  extremity
    lower (multiple) NEC 894.0
      with tendon involvement 894.2
      complicated 894.1
    upper (multiple) NEC 884.0
      with tendon involvement 884.2
      complicated 884.1
  eye(s) (globe)—*see* Wound, open, intraocular
  eyeball NEC 871.9
    laceration (*see also* Laceration, eyeball) 871.4
    penetrating (*see also* Penetrating wound, eyeball) 871.7
  eyebrow 873.42
    complicated 873.52
  eyelid NEC 870.8
    laceration—*see* Laceration, eyelid
  face 873.40
    complicated 873.50
    multiple sites 873.49
      complicated 873.59
    specified part NEC 873.49
      complicated 873.59
  fallopian tube—*see* Injury, internal, fallopian tube
  finger(s) (nail) (subungual) 883.0
    with tendon involvement 883.2
    complicated 883.1
  flank 879.4
    complicated 879.5
  foot (any part except toe(s) alone) 892.0
    with tendon involvement 892.2
    complicated 892.1
  forearm 881.00
    with tendon involvement 881.20
    complicated 881.10
  forehead 873.42
    complicated 873.52
  genital organs (external) NEC 878.8
    complicated 878.9
    internal—*see* Injury, internal, by site
  globe (eye) (*see also* Wound, open, eyeball) 871.9
  groin 879.4
    complicated 879.5
  gum(s) 873.62
    complicated 873.72
  hand (except finger(s) alone) 882.0
    with tendon involvement 882.2
    complicated 882.1
  head NEC 873.8
    with intracranial injury—*see* Injury, intracranial
      due to or associated with skull fracture—*see* Fracture, skull
    complicated 873.9
    scalp—*see* Wound, open, scalp
  heel 892.0
    with tendon involvement 892.2
    complicated 892.1

INDEX TO DISEASES   **Wound, open**

Wound, open—*continued*
  high-velocity (grease gun)—*see* Wound, open, complicated, by site
  hip 890.0
    with tendon involvement 890.2
    complicated 890.1
  hymen 878.6
    complicated 878.7
  hypochondrium 879.4
    complicated 879.5
  hypogastric region 879.2
    complicated 879.3
  iliac (region) 879.4
    complicated 879.5
  incidental to
    dislocation—*see* Dislocation, open, by site
    fracture—*see* Fracture, open, by site
    intracranial injury—*see* Injury, intracranial, with open intracranial wound
    nerve injury—*see* Injury, nerve, by site
  inguinal region 879.4
    complicated 879.5
  instep 892.0
    with tendon involvement 892.2
    complicated 892.1
  interscapular region 876.0
    complicated 876.1
  intracranial—*see* Injury, intracranial, with open intracranial wound
  intraocular 871.9
    with
      partial loss (of intraocular tissue) 871.2
      prolapse or exposure (of intraocular tissue) 871.1
    laceration (*see also* Laceration, eyeball) 871.4
    penetrating 871.7
      with foreign body (nonmagnetic) 871.6
        magnetic 871.5
    without prolapse (of intraocular tissue) 871.0
  iris (*see also* Wound, open, eyeball) 871.9
  jaw (fracture not involved) 873.44
    with fracture—*see* Fracture, jaw
    complicated 873.54
  knee 891.0
    with tendon involvement 891.2
    complicated 891.1
  labium (majus) (minus) 878.4
    complicated 878.5
  lacrimal apparatus, gland, or sac 870.8
    with laceration of eyelid 870.2
  larynx 874.01
    with trachea 874.00
      complicated 874.10
    complicated 874.11
  leg (multiple) 891.0
    with tendon involvement 891.2
    complicated 891.1
    lower 891.0
      with tendon involvement 891.2
      complicated 891.1
    thigh 890.0
      with tendon involvement 890.2
      complicated 890.1
    upper 890.0
      with tendon involvement 890.2
      complicated 890.1
  lens (eye) (alone) (*see also* Cataract, traumatic) 366.20
    with involvement of other eye structures—*see* Wound, open, eyeball

Wound, open—*continued*
  limb
    lower (multiple) NEC 894.0
      with tendon involvement 894.2
      complicated 894.1
    upper (multiple) NEC 884.0
      with tendon involvement 884.2
      complicated 884.1
  lip 873.43
    complicated 873.53
  loin 876.0
    complicated 876.1
  lumbar region 876.0
    complicated 876.1
  malar region 873.41
    complicated 873.51
  mastoid region 873.49
    complicated 873.59
  mediastinum—*see* Injury, internal, mediastinum
  midthoracic region 875.0
    complicated 875.1
  mouth 873.60
    complicated 873.70
    floor 873.64
      complicated 873.74
    multiple sites 873.69
      complicated 873.79
    specified site NEC 873.69
      complicated 873.79
  multiple, unspecified site(s) 879.8

> *Note—Multiple open wounds of sites classifiable to the same four-digit category should be classified to that category unless they are in different limbs.*
>
> *Multiple open wounds of sites classifiable to different four-digit categories, or to different limbs, should be coded separately.*

    complicated 879.9
    lower limb(s) (one or both) (sites classifiable to more than one three-digit category in 890 to 893) 894.0
      with tendon involvement 894.2
      complicated 894.1
    upper limb(s) (one or both) (sites classifiable to more than one three-digit category in 880 to 883) 884.0
      with tendon involvement 884.2
      complicated 884.1
  muscle—*see* Sprain, by site
  nail
    finger(s) 883.0
      complicated 883.1
    thumb 883.0
      complicated 883.1
    toe(s) 893.0
      complicated 893.1
  nape (neck) 874.8
    complicated 874.9
    specified part NEC 874.8
      complicated 874.9
  nasal—*see also* Wound, open, nose
    cavity 873.22
      complicated 873.32
    septum 873.21
      complicated 873.31
    sinuses 873.23
      complicated 873.33
  nasopharynx 873.22

Wound, open—*continued*
    complicated 873.32
  neck 874.8
    complicated 874.9
    nape 874.8
      complicated 874.9
    specified part NEC 874.8
      complicated 874.9
  nerve—*see* Injury, nerve, by site
  non-healing surgical 998.83
  nose 873.20
    complicated 873.30
    multiple sites 873.29
      complicated 873.39
    septum 873.21
      complicated 873.31
    sinuses 873.23
      complicated 873.33
  occipital region—*see* Wound, open, scalp
  ocular NEC 871.9
    adnexa 870.9
      specified region NEC 870.8
    laceration (*see also* Laceration, ocular) 871.4
    muscle (extraocular) 870.3
      with foreign body 870.4
      eyelid 870.1
      intraocular—*see* Wound, open, eyeball
    penetrating (*see also* Penetrating wound, ocular) 871.7
  orbit 870.8
    penetrating 870.3
      with foreign body 870.4
  orbital region 870.9
  ovary—*see* Injury, internal, pelvic organs
  palate 873.65
    complicated 873.75
  palm 882.0
    with tendon involvement 882.2
    complicated 882.1
  parathyroid (gland) 874.2
    complicated 874.3
  parietal region—*see* Wound, open, scalp
  pelvic floor or region 879.6
    complicated 879.7
  penis 878.0
    complicated 878.1
  perineum 879.6
    complicated 879.7
  periocular area 870.8
    laceration of skin 870.0
  pharynx 874.4
    complicated 874.5
  pinna 872.01
    complicated 872.11
  popliteal space 891.0
    with tendon involvement 891.2
    complicated 891.1
  prepuce 878.0
    complicated 878.1
  pubic region 879.2
    complicated 879.3
  pudenda 878.8
    complicated 878.9
  rectovaginal septum 878.8
    complicated 878.9
  sacral region 877.0
    complicated 877.1
  sacroiliac region 877.0
    complicated 877.1
  salivary (ducts) (glands) 873.69
    complicated 873.79

Wound, open—*continued*
  scalp 873.0
    complicated 873.1
  scalpel, fetus or newborn 767.8
  scapular region 880.01
    with tendon involvement 880.21
    complicated 880.11
    involving other sites of upper arm 880.09
      with tendon involvement 880.29
      complicated 880.19
  sclera (*see also* Wound, open, intraocular) 871.9
  scrotum 878.2
    complicated 878.3
  seminal vesicle—*see* Injury, internal, pelvic organs
  shin 891.0
    with tendon involvement 891.2
    complicated 891.1
  shoulder 880.00
    with tendon involvement 880.20
    complicated 880.10
    involving other sites of upper arm 880.09
      with tendon involvement 880.29
      complicated 880.19
  skin NEC 879.8
    complicated 879.9
  skull—*see also* Injury, intracranial, with open intracranial wound
    with skull fracture—*see* Fracture, skull
  spermatic cord (scrotal) 878.2
    complicated 878.3
    pelvic region—*see* Injury, internal, spermatic cord
  spinal cord—*see* Injury, spinal
  sternal region 875.0
    complicated 875.1
  subconjunctival—*see* Wound, open, intraocular
  subcutaneous NEC 879.8
    complicated 879.9
  submaxillary region 873.44
    complicated 873.54
  submental region 873.44
    complicated 873.54
  subungual
    finger(s) (thumb)—*see* Wound, open, finger
    toe(s)—*see* Wound, open, toe
  supraclavicular region 874.8
    complicated 874.9
  supraorbital 873.42
    complicated 873.52
  surgical, non-healing 998.83
  temple 873.49
    complicated 873.59
  temporal region 873.49
    complicated 873.59
  testis 878.2
    complicated 878.3
  thigh 890.0
    with tendon involvement 890.2
    complicated 890.1
  thorax, thoracic (external) 875.0
    complicated 875.1
  throat 874.8
    complicated 874.9
  thumb (nail) (subungual) 883.0
    with tendon involvement 883.2
    complicated 883.1
  thyroid (gland) 874.2
    complicated 874.3
  toe(s) (nail) (subungual) 893.0
    with tendon involvement 893.2

INDEX TO DISEASES

Wound, open—*continued*
   complicated 893.1
  tongue 873.64
   complicated 873.74
  tonsil—*see* Wound, open, neck
  trachea (cervical region) 874.02
   with larynx 874.00
    complicated 874.10
   complicated 874.12
   intrathoracic—*see* Injury, internal, trachea
  trunk (multiple) NEC 879.6
   complicated 879.7
   specified site NEC 879.6
    complicated 879.7
  tunica vaginalis 878.2
   complicated 878.3
  tympanic membrane 872.61
   complicated 872.71
  tympanum 872.61
   complicated 872.71
  umbilical region 879.2
   complicated 879.3
  ureter—*see* Injury, internal, ureter
  urethra—*see* Injury, internal, urethra
  uterus—*see* Injury, internal, uterus
  uvula 873.69
   complicated 873.79
  vagina 878.6
   complicated 878.7
  vas deferens—*see* Injury, internal, vas deferens
  vitreous (humor) 871.2
  vulva 878.4
   complicated 878.5
  wrist 881.02
   with tendon involvement 881.22
   complicated 881.12
Wright's syndrome (hyperabduction) 447.8
  pneumonia 390 *[517.1]*
Wringer injury —*see* Crush injury, by site
Wrinkling of skin 701.8
Wrist —*see also* condition
  drop (acquired) 736.05
Wrong drug (given in error) NEC 977.9
  specified drug or substance—*see* Table of drugs and chemicals
Wry neck —*see also* Torticollis
  congenital 754.1
Wuchereria infestation 125.0
  bancrofti 125.0
  Brugia malayi 125.1
  malayi 125.1
Wuchereriasis 125.0
Wuchereriosis 125.0
Wuchernde struma langhans (M8332/3) 193

INDEX TO DISEASES

X

Xanthelasma 272.2
  eyelid 272.2 *[374.51]*
  palpebrarum 272.2 *[374.51]*
Xanthelasmatosis (essential) 272.2
Xanthelasmoidea 757.33
Xanthine stones 277.2
Xanthinuria 277.2
Xanthofibroma (M8831/0)—*see* Neoplasm, connective tissue, benign
Xanthoma(s), xanthomatosis 272.2
  with
    hyperlipoproteinemia
      type I 272.3
      type III 272.2
      type IV 272.1
      type V 272.3
  bone 272.7
  craniohypophyseal 277.89
  cutaneotendinous 272.7
  diabeticorum 250.8 *[272.2]*
  disseminatum 272.7
  eruptive 272.2
  eyelid 272.2 *[374.51]*
  familial 272.7
  hereditary 272.7
  hypercholesterinemic 272.0
  hypercholesterolemic 272.0
  hyperlipemic 272.4
  hyperlipidemic 272.4
  infantile 272.7
  joint 272.7
  juvenile 272.7
  multiple 272.7
  multiplex 272.7
  primary familial 272.7
  tendon (sheath) 272.7
  tuberosum 272.2
  tuberous 272.2
  tubo-eruptive 272.2
Xanthosis 709.09
  surgical 998.81
Xenophobia 300.29
Xeroderma (congenital) 757.39
  acquired 701.1
    eyelid 373.33
  eyelid 373.33
  pigmentosum 757.33
  vitamin A deficiency 264.8
Xerophthalmia 372.53
  vitamin A deficiency 264.7
Xerosis
  conjunctiva 372.53
    with Bitôt's spot 372.53
      vitamin A deficiency 264.1
    vitamin A deficiency 264.0
  cornea 371.40
    with corneal ulceration 370.00
      vitamin A deficiency 264.3
    vitamin A deficiency 264.2
  cutis 706.8
  skin 706.8
Xerostomia 527.7
Xiphodynia 733.90
Xiphoidalgia 733.90
Xiphoiditis 733.99
Xiphopagus 759.4
XO syndrome 758.6

X-ray
  effects, adverse, NEC 990
  of chest
    for suspected tuberculosis V71.2
    routine V72.5
XXX syndrome 758.81
XXXXY syndrome 758.81
XXY syndrome 758.7
Xyloketosuria 271.8
Xylosuria 271.8
Xylulosuria 271.8
XYY syndrome 758.81

INDEX TO DISEASES

Y

Yawning 786.09
   psychogenic 306.1
Yaws 102.9
   bone or joint lesions 102.6
   butter 102.1
   chancre 102.0
   cutaneous, less than five years after infection 102.2
   early (cutaneous) (macular) (maculopapular) (micropapular) (papular) 102.2
      frambeside 102.2
      skin lesions NEC 102.2
   eyelid 102.9 *[373.4]*
   ganglion 102.6
   gangosis, gangosa 102.5
   gumma, gummata 102.4
      bone 102.6
   gummatous
      frambeside 102.4
      osteitis 102.6
      periostitis 102.6
   hydrarthrosis 102.6
   hyperkeratosis (early) (late) (palmar) (plantar) 102.3
   initial lesions 102.0
   joint lesions 102.6
   juxta-articular nodules 102.7
   late nodular (ulcerated) 102.4
   latent (without clinical manifestations) (with positive serology) 102.8
   mother 102.0
   mucosal 102.7
   multiple papillomata 102.1
   nodular, late (ulcerated) 102.4
   osteitis 102.6
   papilloma, papillomata (palmar) (plantar) 102.1
   periostitis (hypertrophic) 102.6
   ulcers 102.4
   wet crab 102.1
Yeast infection (*see also* Candidiasis) 112.9
Yellow
   atrophy (liver) 570
      chronic 571.8
      resulting from administration of blood, plasma, serum, or other biological substance (within 8 months of administration)—*see* Hepatitis, viral
   fever—*see* Fever, yellow
   jack (*see also* Fever, yellow) 060.9
   jaundice (*see also* Jaundice) 782.4
Yersinia septica 027.8

Z

Zagari's disease (xerostomia) 527.7
Zahorsky's disease (exanthema subitum) (*see also* Exanthem subitum) 058.10
   syndrome (herpangina) 074.0
Zellweger syndrome 277.86
Zenker's diverticulum (esophagus) 530.6
Ziehen-Oppenheim disease 333.6
Zieve's syndrome (jaundice, hyperlipemia, and hemolytic anemia) 571.1
Zika fever 066.3
Zollinger-Ellison syndrome (gastric hypersecretion with pancreatic islet cell tumor) 251.5
Zona (*see also* Herpes, zoster) 053.9
Zoophilia (erotica) 302.1
Zoophobia 300.29
Zoster (herpes) (*see also* Herpes, zoster) 053.9
Zuelzer (-Ogden) anemia or syndrome (nutritional megaloblastic anemia) 281.2
Zygodactyly (*see also* Syndactylism) 755.10
Zygomycosis 117.7
Zymotic —*see* condition

SECTION 2

ALPHABETIC INDEX TO POISONING AND EXTERNAL CAUSES OF ADVERSE EFFECTS OF DRUGS AND OTHER CHEMICAL SUBSTANCES

TABLE OF DRUGS AND CHEMICALS

This table contains a classification of drugs and other chemical substances to identify poisoning states and external causes of adverse effects.

Each of the listed substances in the table is assigned a code according to the poisoning classification (960–989). These codes are used when there is a statement of poisoning, overdose, wrong substance given or taken, or intoxication.

The table also contains a listing of external causes of adverse effects. An adverse effect is a pathologic manifestation due to ingestion or exposure to drugs or other chemical substances (e.g., dermatitis, hypersensitivity reaction, aspirin gastritis). The adverse effect is to be identified by the appropriate code found in Section 1, Index to Diseases and Injuries. An external cause code can then be used to identify the circumstances involved. The table headings pertaining to external causes are defined below:

Accidental poisoning (E850–E869)—accidental overdose of drug, wrong substance given or taken, drug taken inadvertently, accidents in the usage of drugs and biologicals in medical and surgical procedures, and to show external causes of poisonings classifiable to 980–989.

Therapeutic use (E930–E949)—a correct substance properly administered in therapeutic or prophylactic dosage as the external cause of adverse effects.

Suicide attempt (E950–E952)—instances in which self-inflicted injuries or poisonings are involved.

Assault (E961–E962)—injury or poisoning inflicted by another person with the intent to injure or kill.

Undetermined (E980–E982)—to be used when the intent of the poisoning or injury cannot be determined whether it was intentional or accidental.

The American Hospital Formulary Service list numbers are included in the table to help classify new drugs not identified in the table by name. The AHFS list numbers are keyed to the continually revised American Hospital Formulary Service (AHFS).* These listings are found in the table under the main term **Drug**.

Excluded from the table are radium and other radioactive substances. The classification of adverse effects and complications pertaining to these substances will be found in Section 1, Index to Diseases and Injuries, and Section 3, Index to External Causes of Injuries.

Although certain substances are indexed with one or more subentries, the majority are listed according to one use or state. It is recognized that many substances may be used in various ways, in medicine and in industry, and may cause adverse effects whatever the state of the agent (solid, liquid, or fumes arising from a liquid). In cases in which the reported data indicates a use or state not in the table, or which is clearly different from the one listed, an attempt should be made to classify the substance in the form which most nearly expresses the reported facts.

*American Hospital Formulary Service, 2 vol. (Washington, DC: American Society of Hospital Pharmacists, 1959)

TABLE OF DRUGS AND CHEMICALS

Substance	Poisoning	Accident	Therapeutic Use	Suicide Attempt	Assault	Undetermined
			External Cause (E-Code)			
1–propanol	980.3	E860.4	—	E950.9	E962.1	E980.9
2–propanol	980.2	E860.3	—	E950.9	E962.1	E980.9
2, 4–D (dichlorophenoxyacetic acid)	989.4	E863.5	—	E950.6	E962.1	E980.7
2, 4–toluene diisocyanate	983.0	E864.0	—	E950.7	E962.1	E980.6
2, 4, 5–T (trichlorophenoxyacetic acid)	989.2	E863.5	—	E950.6	E962.1	E980.7
14–hydroxydihydromorphinone	965.09	E850.2	E935.2	E950.0	E962.0	E980.0
ABOB	961.7	E857	E931.7	E950.4	E962.0	E980.4
Abrus (seed)	988.2	E865.3	—	E950.9	E962.1	E980.9
Absinthe	980.0	E860.1	—	E950.9	E962.1	E980.9
beverage	980.0	E860.0	—	E950.9	E962.1	E980.9
Acenocoumarin, acenocoumarol	964.2	E858.2	E934.2	E950.4	E962.0	E980.4
Acepromazine	969.1	E853.0	E939.1	E950.3	E962.0	E980.3
Acetal	982.8	E862.4	—	E950.9	E962.1	E980.9
Acetaldehyde (vapor)	987.8	E869.8	—	E952.8	E962.2	E982.8
liquid	989.89	E866.8	—	E950.9	E962.1	E980.9
Acetaminophen	965.4	E850.4	E935.4	E950.0	E962.0	E980.0
Acetaminosalol	965.1	E850.3	E935.3	E950.0	E962.0	E980.0
Acetanilid(e)	965.4	E850.4	E935.4	E950.0	E962.0	E980.0
Acetarsol, acetarsone	961.1	E857	E931.1	E950.4	E962.0	E980.4
Acetazolamide	974.2	E858.5	E944.2	E950.4	E962.0	E980.4
Acetic						
acid	983.1	E864.1	—	E950.7	E962.1	E980.6
with sodium acetate (ointment)	976.3	E858.7	E946.3	E950.4	E962.0	E980.4
irrigating solution	974.5	E858.5	E944.5	E950.4	E962.0	E980.4
lotion	976.2	E858.7	E946.2	E950.4	E962.0	E980.4
anhydride	983.1	E864.1	—	E950.7	E962.1	E980.6
ether (vapor)	982.8	E862.4	—	E950.9	E962.1	E980.9
Acetohexamide	962.3	E858.0	E932.3	E950.4	E962.0	E980.4
Acetomenaphthone	964.3	E858.2	E934.3	E950.4	E962.0	E980.4
Acetomorphine	965.01	E850.0	E935.0	E950.0	E962.0	E980.0
Acetone (oils) (vapor)	982.8	E862.4	—	E950.9	E962.1	E980.9
Acetophenazine (maleate)	969.1	E853.0	E939.1	E950.3	E962.0	E980.3
Acetophenetidin	965.4	E850.4	E935.4	E950.0	E962.0	E980.0
Acetophenone	982.0	E862.4	—	E950.9	E962.1	E980.9
Acetorphine	965.09	E850.2	E935.2	E950.0	E962.0	E980.0
Acetosulfone (sodium)	961.8	E857	E931.8	E950.4	E962.0	E980.4
Acetrizoate (sodium)	977.8	E858.8	E947.8	E950.4	E962.0	E980.4
Acetylcarbromal	967.3	E852.2	E937.3	E950.2	E962.0	E980.2
Acetylcholine (chloride)	971.0	E855.3	E941.0	E950.4	E962.0	E980.4
Acetylcysteine	975.5	E858.6	E945.5	E950.4	E962.0	E980.4
Acetyldigitoxin	972.1	E858.3	E942.1	E950.4	E962.0	E980.4
Acetyldihydrocodeine	965.09	E850.2	E935.2	E950.0	E962.0	E980.0
Acetyldihydrocodeinone	965.09	E850.2	E935.2	E950.0	E962.0	E980.0
Acetylene (gas) (industrial)	987.1	E868.1	—	E951.8	E962.2	E981.8
incomplete combustion of — see Carbon monoxide, fuel, utility						
tetrachloride (vapor)	982.3	E862.4	—	E950.9	E962.1	E980.9
Acetyliodosalicylic acid	965.1	E850.3	E935.3	E950.0	E962.0	E980.0
Acetylphenylhydrazine	965.8	E850.8	E935.8	E950.0	E962.0	E980.0
Acetylsalicylic acid	965.1	E850.3	E935.3	E950.0	E962.0	E980.0
Achromycin	960.4	E856	E930.4	E950.4	E962.0	E980.4
ophthalmic preparation	976.5	E858.7	E946.5	E950.4	E962.0	E980.4
topical NEC	976.0	E858.7	E946.0	E950.4	E962.0	E980.4
Acidifying agents	963.2	E858.1	E933.2	E950.4	E962.0	E980.4
Acids (corrosive) NEC	983.1	E864.1	—	E950.7	E962.1	E980.6
Aconite (wild)	988.2	E865.4	—	E950.9	E962.1	E980.9
Aconitine (liniment)	976.8	E858.7	E946.8	E950.4	E962.0	E980.4
Aconitum ferox	988.2	E865.4	—	E950.9	E962.1	E980.9
Acridine	983.0	E864.0	—	E950.7	E962.1	E980.6
vapor	987.8	E869.8	—	E952.8	E962.2	E982.8

TABLE OF DRUGS AND CHEMICALS

Substance	Poisoning	Accident	Therapeutic Use	Suicide Attempt	Assault	Undetermined
		\multicolumn{5}{c}{External Cause (E-Code)}				

Substance	Poisoning	Accident	Therapeutic Use	Suicide Attempt	Assault	Undetermined
Acriflavine	961.9	E857	E931.9	E950.4	E962.0	E980.4
Acrisorcin	976.0	E858.7	E946.0	E950.4	E962.0	E980.4
Acrolein (gas)	987.8	E869.8	—	E952.8	E962.2	E982.8
liquid	989.89	E866.8	—	E950.9	E962.1	E980.9
Actaea spicata	988.2	E865.4	—	E950.9	E962.1	E980.9
Acterol	961.5	E857	E931.5	E950.4	E962.0	E980.4
ACTH	962.4	E858.0	E932.4	E950.4	E962.0	E980.4
Acthar	962.4	E858.0	E932.4	E950.4	E962.0	E980.4
Actinomycin (C) (D)	960.7	E856	E930.7	E950.4	E962.0	E980.4
Adalin (acetyl)	967.3	E852.2	E937.3	E950.2	E962.0	E980.2
Adenosine (phosphate)	977.8	E858.8	E947.8	E950.4	E962.0	E980.4
Adhesives	989.89	E866.6	—	E950.9	E962.1	E980.9
ADH	962.5	E858.0	E932.5	E950.4	E962.0	E980.4
Adicillin	960.0	E856	E930.0	E950.4	E962.0	E980.4
Adiphenine	975.1	E855.6	E945.1	E950.4	E962.0	E980.4
Adjunct, pharmaceutical	977.4	E858.8	E947.4	E950.4	E962.0	E980.4
Adrenal (extract, cortex or medulla) (glucocorticoids) (hormones) (mineralocorticoids)	962.0	E858.0	E932.0	E950.4	E962.0	E980.4
ENT agent	976.6	E858.7	E946.6	E950.4	E962.0	E980.4
ophthalmic preparation	976.5	E858.7	E946.5	E950.4	E962.0	E980.4
topical NEC	976.0	E858.7	E946.0	E950.4	E962.0	E980.4
Adrenalin	971.2	E855.5	E941.2	E950.4	E962.0	E980.4
Adrenergic blocking agents	971.3	E855.6	E941.3	E950.4	E962.0	E980.4
Adrenergics	971.2	E855.5	E941.2	E950.4	E962.0	E980.4
Adrenochrome (derivatives)	972.8	E858.3	E942.8	E950.4	E962.0	E980.4
Adrenocorticotropic hormone	962.4	E858.0	E932.4	E950.4	E962.0	E980.4
Adrenocorticotropin	962.4	E858.0	E932.4	E950.4	E962.0	E980.4
Adriamycin	960.7	E856	E930.7	E950.4	E962.0	E980.4
Aerosol spray — see Sprays						
Aerosporin	960.8	E856	E930.8	E950.4	E962.0	E980.4
ENT agent	976.6	E858.7	E946.6	E950.4	E962.0	E980.4
ophthalmic preparation	976.5	E858.7	E946.5	E950.4	E962.0	E980.4
topical NEC	976.0	E858.7	E946.0	E950.4	E962.0	E980.4
Aethusa cynapium	988.2	E865.4	—	E950.9	E962.1	E980.9
Afghanistan black	969.6	E854.1	E939.6	E950.3	E962.0	E980.3
Aflatoxin	989.7	E865.9	—	E950.9	E962.1	E980.9
African boxwood	988.2	E865.4	—	E950.9	E962.1	E980.9
Agar (–agar)	973.3	E858.4	E943.3	E950.4	E962.0	E980.4
Agricultural agent NEC	989.89	E863.9	—	E950.6	E962.1	E980.7
Agrypnal	967.0	E851	E937.0	E950.1	E962.0	E980.1
Air contaminant(s), source or type						
not specified	987.9	E869.9	—	E952.9	E962.2	E982.9
specified type — see specific substance						
Akee	988.2	E865.4	—	E950.9	E962.1	E980.9
Akrinol	976.0	E858.7	E946.0	E950.4	E962.0	E980.4
Alantolactone	961.6	E857	E931.6	E950.4	E962.0	E980.4
Albamycin	960.8	E856	E930.8	E950.4	E962.0	E980.4
Albumin (normal human serum)	964.7	E858.2	E934.7	E950.4	E962.0	E980.4
Albuterol	975.7	E858.6	E945.7	E950.4	E962.0	E980.4
Alcohol	980.9	E860.9	—	E950.9	E962.1	E980.9
absolute	980.0	E860.1	—	E950.9	E962.1	E980.9
beverage	980.0	E860.0	E947.8	E950.9	E962.1	E980.9
amyl	980.3	E860.4	—	E950.9	E962.1	E980.9
antifreeze	980.1	E860.2	—	E950.9	E962.1	E980.9
butyl	980.3	E860.4	—	E950.9	E962.1	E980.9
dehydrated	980.0	E860.1	—	E950.9	E862.1	E980.9
beverage	980.0	E860.0	E947.8	E950.9	E962.1	E980.9
denatured	980.0	E860.1	—	E950.9	E962.1	E980.9
deterrents	977.3	E858.8	E947.3	E950.4	E962.0	E980.4
diagnostic (gastric function)	977.8	E858.8	E947.8	E950.4	E962.0	E980.4

1417

TABLE OF DRUGS AND CHEMICALS

Substance	Poisoning	Accident	Therapeutic Use	Suicide Attempt	Assault	Undetermined
		External Cause (E-Code)				
ethyl	980.0	E860.1	—	E950.9	E962.1	E980.9
beverage	980.0	E860.0	E947.8	E950.9	E962.1	E980.9
grain	980.0	E860.1	—	E950.9	E962.1	E980.9
beverage	980.0	E860.0	E947.8	E950.9	E962.1	E980.9
industrial	980.9	E860.9	—	E950.9	E962.1	E980.9
isopropyl	980.2	E860.3	—	E950.9	E962.1	E980.9
methyl	980.1	E860.2	—	E950.9	E962.1	E980.9
preparation for consumption	980.0	E860.0	E947.8	E950.9	E962.1	E980.9
propyl	980.3	E860.4	—	E950.9	E962.1	E980.9
secondary	980.2	E860.3	—	E950.9	E962.1	E980.9
radiator	980.1	E860.2	—	E950.9	E962.1	E980.9
rubbing	980.2	E860.3	—	E950.9	E962.1	E980.9
specified type NEC	980.8	E860.8	—	E950.9	E962.1	E980.9
surgical	980.9	E860.9	—	E950.9	E962.1	E980.9
vapor (from any type of alcohol)	987.8	E869.8	—	E952.8	E962.2	E982.8
wood	980.1	E860.2	—	E950.9	E962.1	E980.9
Alcuronium chloride	975.2	E858.6	E945.2	E950.4	E962.0	E980.4
Aldactone	974.4	E858.5	E944.4	E950.4	E962.0	E980.4
Aldicarb	989.3	E863.2	—	E950.6	E962.1	E980.7
Aldomet	972.6	E858.3	E942.6	E950.4	E962.0	E980.4
Aldosterone	962.0	E858.0	E932.0	E950.4	E962.0	E980.4
Aldrin (dust)	989.2	E863.0	—	E950.6	E962.1	E980.7
Algeldrate	973.0	E858.4	E943.0	E950.4	E962.0	E980.4
Alidase	963.4	E858.1	E933.4	E950.4	E962.0	E980.4
Aliphatic thiocyanates	989.0	E866.8	—	E950.9	E962.1	E980.9
Alkaline antiseptic solution (aromatic)	976.6	E858.7	E946.6	E950.4	E962.0	E980.4
Alkalinizing agents (medicinal)	963.3	E858.1	E933.3	E950.4	E962.0	E980.4
Alkalis, caustic	983.2	E864.2	—	E950.7	E962.1	E980.6
Alkalizing agents (medicinal)	963.3	E858.1	E933.3	E950.4	E962.0	E980.4
Alka–seltzer	965.1	E850.3	E935.3	E950.0	E962.0	E980.0
Alkavervir	972.6	E858.3	E942.6	E950.4	E962.0	E980.4
Allegron	969.0	E854.0	E939.0	E950.3	E962.0	E980.3
Alleve see Naproxen						
Allobarbital, allobarbitone	967.0	E851	E937.0	E950.1	E962.0	E980.1
Allopurinol	974.7	E858.5	E944.7	E950.4	E962.0	E980.4
Allylestrenol	962.2	E858.0	E932.2	E950.4	E962.0	E980.4
Allylisopropylacetylurea	967.8	E852.8	E937.8	E950.2	E962.0	E980.2
Allylisopropylmalonylurea	967.0	E851	E937.0	E950.1	E962.0	E980.1
Allyltribromide	967.3	E852.2	E937.3	E950.2	E962.0	E980.2
Aloe, aloes, aloin	973.1	E858.4	E943.1	E950.4	E962.0	E980.4
Alosetron	973.8	E858.4	E943.8	E950.4	E962.0	E980.4
Aloxidone	966.0	E855.0	E936.0	E950.4	E962.0	E980.4
Aloxiprin	965.1	E850.3	E935.3	E950.0	E962.0	E980.0
Alpha amylase	963.4	E858.1	E933.4	E950.4	E962.0	E980.4
Alpha-1 blockers	971.3	E855.6	E941.3	E950.4	E962.0	E980.4
Alpha tocopherol	963.5	E858.1	E933.5	E950.4	E962.0	E980.4
Alphaprodine (hydrochloride)	965.09	E850.2	E935.2	E950.0	E962.0	E980.0
Alseroxylon	972.6	E858.3	E942.6	E950.4	E962.0	E980.4
Alum (ammonium) (potassium)	983.2	E864.2	—	E950.7	E962.1	E980.6
medicinal (astringent) NEC	976.2	E858.7	E946.2	E950.4	E962.0	E980.4
Aluminium, aluminum (gel) (hydroxide)	973.0	E858.4	E943.0	E950.4	E962.0	E980.4
acetate solution	976.2	E858.7	E946.2	E950.4	E962.0	E980.4
aspirin	965.1	E850.3	E935.3	E950.0	E962.0	E980.0
carbonate	973.0	E858.4	E943.0	E950.4	E962.0	E980.4
glycinate	973.0	E858.4	E943.0	E950.4	E962.0	E980.4
nicotinate	972.2	E858.3	E942.2	E950.4	E962.0	E980.4
ointment (surgical) (topical)	976.3	E858.7	E946.3	E950.4	E962.0	E980.4
phosphate	973.0	E858.4	E943.0	E950.4	E962.0	E980.4
subacetate	976.2	E858.7	E946.2	E950.4	E962.0	E980.4
topical NEC	976.3	E858.7	E946.3	E950.4	E962.0	E980.4

TABLE OF DRUGS AND CHEMICALS

Substance	Poisoning	Accident	Therapeutic Use	Suicide Attempt	Assault	Undetermined
			External Cause (E-Code)			
Alurate 967.0	E851	E937.0	E950.1	E962.0	E980.1
Alverine (citrate) 975.1	E858.6	E945.1	E950.4	E962.0	E980.4
Alvodine 965.09	E850.2	E935.2	E950.0	E962.0	E980.0
Amanita phalloides 988.1	E865.5	—	E950.9	E962.1	E980.9
Amantadine (hydrochloride) 966.4	E855.0	E936.4	E950.4	E962.0	E980.4
Ambazone 961.9	E857	E931.9	E950.4	E962.0	E980.4
Ambenonium 971.0	E855.3	E941.0	E950.4	E962.0	E980.4
Ambutonium bromide 971.1	E855.4	E941.1	E950.4	E962.0	E980.4
Ametazole 977.8	E858.8	E947.8	E950.4	E962.0	E980.4
Amethocaine (infiltration) (topical) 968.5	E855.2	E938.5	E950.4	E962.0	E980.4
nerve block (peripheral) (plexus) 968.6	E855.2	E938.6	E950.4	E962.0	E980.4
spinal 968.7	E855.2	E938.7	E950.4	E962.0	E980.4
Amethopterin 963.1	E858.1	E933.1	E950.4	E962.0	E980.4
Amfepramone 977.0	E858.8	E947.0	E950.4	E962.0	E980.4
Amidon 965.02	E850.1	E935.1	E950.0	E962.0	E980.0
Amidopyrine 965.5	E850.5	E935.5	E950.0	E962.0	E980.0
Aminacrine 976.0	E858.7	E946.0	E950.4	E962.0	E980.4
Aminitrozole 961.5	E857	E931.5	E950.4	E962.0	E980.4
Aminoacetic acid 974.5	E858.5	E944.5	E950.4	E962.0	E980.4
Amino acids 974.5	E858.5	E944.5	E950.4	E962.0	E980.4
Aminocaproic acid 964.4	E858.2	E934.4	E950.4	E962.0	E980.4
Aminoethylisothiourium 963.8	E858.1	E933.8	E950.4	E962.0	E980.4
Aminoglutethimide 966.3	E855.0	E936.3	E950.4	E962.0	E980.4
Aminometradine 974.3	E858.5	E944.3	E950.4	E962.0	E980.4
Aminopentamide 971.1	E855.4	E941.1	E950.4	E962.0	E980.4
Aminophenazone 965.5	E850.5	E935.5	E950.0	E962.0	E980.0
Aminophenol 983.0	E864.0	—	E950.7	E962.1	E980.6
Aminophenylpyridone 969.5	E853.8	E939.5	E950.3	E962.0	E980.3
Aminophyllin 975.7	E858.6	E945.7	E950.4	E962.0	E980.4
Aminopterin 963.1	E858.1	E933.1	E950.4	E962.0	E980.4
Aminopyrine 965.5	E850.5	E935.5	E950.0	E962.0	E980.0
Aminosalicylic acid 961.8	E857	E931.8	E950.4	E962.0	E980.4
Amiphenazole 970.1	E854.3	E940.1	E950.4	E962.0	E980.4
Amiquinsin 972.6	E858.3	E942.6	E950.4	E962.0	E980.4
Amisometradine 974.3	E858.5	E944.3	E950.4	E962.0	E980.4
Amitriptyline 969.0	E854.0	E939.0	E950.3	E962.0	E980.3
Ammonia (fumes) (gas) (vapor) 987.8	E869.8	—	E952.8	E962.2	E982.8
liquid (household) NEC 983.2	E861.4	—	E950.7	E962.1	E980.6
spirit, aromatic 970.8	E854.3	E940.8	E950.4	E962.0	E980.4
Ammoniated mercury 976.0	E858.7	E946.0	E950.4	E962.0	E980.4
Ammonium					
carbonate 983.2	E864.2	—	E950.7	E962.1	E980.6
chloride (acidifying agent) 963.2	E858.1	E933.2	E950.4	E962.0	E980.4
expectorant 975.5	E858.6	E945.5	E950.4	E962.0	E980.4
compounds (household) NEC 983.2	E861.4	—	E950.7	E962.1	E980.6
fumes (any usage) 987.8	E869.8	—	E952.8	E962.2	E982.8
industrial 983.2	E864.2	—	E950.7	E962.1	E980.6
ichthyosulfonate 976.4	E858.7	E946.4	E950.4	E962.0	E980.4
mandelate 961.9	E857	E931.9	E950.4	E962.0	E980.4
Amobarbital 967.0	E851	E937.0	E950.1	E962.0	E980.1
Amodiaquin(e) 961.4	E857	E931.4	E950.4	E962.0	E980.4
Amopyroquin(e) 961.4	E857	E931.4	E950.4	E962.0	E980.4
Amphenidone 969.5	E853.8	E939.5	E950.3	E962.0	E980.3
Amphetamine 969.7	E854.2	E939.7	E950.3	E962.0	E980.3
Amphomycin 960.8	E856	E930.8	E950.4	E962.0	E980.4
Amphotericin B 960.1	E856	E930.1	E950.4	E962.0	E980.4
topical 976.0	E858.7	E946.0	E950.4	E962.0	E980.4
Ampicillin 960.0	E856	E930.0	E950.4	E962.0	E980.4
Amprotropine 971.1	E855.4	E941.1	E950.4	E962.0	E980.4
Amygdalin 977.8	E858.8	E947.8	E950.4	E962.0	E980.4
Amyl					

1419

TABLE OF DRUGS AND CHEMICALS

Substance	Poisoning	Accident	Therapeutic Use	Suicide Attempt	Assault	Undetermined
		\multicolumn{5}{c}{External Cause (E-Code)}

Substance	Poisoning	Accident	Therapeutic Use	Suicide Attempt	Assault	Undetermined
acetate (vapor)	982.8	E862.4	—	E950.9	E962.1	E980.9
alcohol	980.3	E860.4	—	E950.9	E962.1	E980.9
nitrite (medicinal)	972.4	E858.3	E942.4	E950.4	E962.0	E980.4
Amylase (alpha)	963.4	E858.1	E933.4	E950.4	E962.0	E980.4
Amylene hydrate	980.8	E860.8	—	E950.9	E962.1	E980.9
Amylobarbitone	967.0	E851	E937.0	E950.1	E962.0	E980.1
Amylocaine	968.9	E855.2	E938.9	E950.4	E962.0	E980.4
infiltration (subcutaneous)	968.5	E855.2	E938.5	E950.4	E962.0	E980.4
nerve block (peripheral) (plexus)	968.6	E855.2	E938.6	E950.4	E962.0	E980.4
spinal	968.7	E855.2	E938.7	E950.4	E962.0	E980.4
topical (surface)	968.5	E855.2	E938.5	E950.4	E962.0	E980.4
Amytal (sodium)	967.0	E851	E937.0	E950.1	E962.0	E980.1
Analeptics	970.0	E854.3	E940.0	E950.4	E962.0	E980.4
Analgesics	965.9	E850.9	E935.9	E950.0	E962.0	E980.0
aromatic NEC	965.4	E850.4	E935.4	E950.0	E962.0	E980.0
non–narcotic NEC	965.7	E850.7	E935.7	E950.0	E962.0	E980.0
specified NEC	965.8	E850.8	E935.8	E950.0	E962.0	E980.0
Anamirta cocculus	988.2	E865.3	—	E950.9	E962.1	E980.9
Ancillin	960.0	E856	E930.0	E950.4	E962.0	E980.4
Androgens (anabolic congeners)	962.1	E858.0	E932.1	E950.4	E962.0	E980.4
Androstalone	962.1	E858.0	E932.1	E950.4	E962.0	E980.4
Androsterone	962.1	E858.0	E932.1	E950.4	E962.0	E980.4
Anemone pulsatilla	988.2	E865.4	—	E950.9	E962.1	E980.9
Anesthesia, anesthetic (general) NEC	968.4	E855.1	E938.4	E950.4	E962.0	E980.4
block (nerve) (plexus)	968.6	E855.2	E938.6	E950.4	E962.0	E980.4
gaseous NEC	968.2	E855.1	E938.2	E950.4	E962.0	E980.4
halogenated hydrocarbon derivatives NEC	968.2	E855.1	E938.2	E950.4	E962.0	E980.4
infiltration (intradermal) (subcutaneous) (submucosal)	968.5	E855.2	E938.5	E950.4	E962.0	E980.4
intravenous	968.3	E855.1	E938.3	E950.4	E962.0	E980.4
local NEC	968.9	E855.2	E938.9	E950.4	E962.0	E980.4
nerve blocking (peripheral) (plexus)	968.6	E855.2	E938.6	E950.4	E962.0	E980.4
rectal NEC	968.3	E855.1	E938.3	E950.4	E962.0	E980.4
spinal	968.7	E855.2	E938.7	E950.4	E962.0	E980.4
surface	968.5	E855.2	E938.5	E950.4	E962.0	E980.4
topical	968.5	E855.2	E938.5	E950.4	E962.0	E980.4
Aneurine	963.5	E858.1	E933.5	E950.4	E962.0	E980.4
Angio–Conray	977.8	E858.8	E947.8	E950.4	E962.0	E980.4
Anginine *see* Glyceryl trinitrate						
Angiotensin	971.2	E855.5	E941.2	E950.4	E962.0	E980.4
Anhydrohydroxyprogesterone	962.2	E858.0	E932.2	E950.4	E962.0	E980.4
Anhydron	974.3	E858.5	E944.3	E950.4	E962.0	E980.4
Anileridine	965.09	E850.2	E935.2	E950.0	E962.0	E980.0
Aniline (dye) (liquid)	983.0	E864.0	—	E950.7	E962.1	E980.6
analgesic	965.4	E850.4	E935.4	E950.0	E962.0	E980.0
derivatives, therapeutic NEC	965.4	E850.4	E935.4	E950.0	E962.0	E980.0
vapor	987.8	E869.8	—	E952.8	E962.2	E982.8
Anisindione	964.2	E858.2	E934.2	E950.4	E962.0	E980.4
Anisotropine	971.1	E855.4	E941.1	E950.4	E962.0	E980.4
Anorexic agents	977.0	E858.8	E947.0	E950.4	E962.0	E980.4
Ant (bite) (sting)	989.5	E905.5	—	E950.9	E962.1	E980.9
Antabuse	977.3	E858.8	E947.3	E950.4	E962.0	E980.4
Antacids	973.0	E858.4	E943.0	E950.4	E962.0	E980.4
Antazoline	963.0	E858.1	E933.0	E950.4	E962.0	E980.4
Anthelmintics	961.6	E857	E931.6	E950.4	E962.0	E980.4
Anthralin	976.4	E858.7	E946.4	E950.4	E962.0	E980.4
Anthramycin	960.7	E856	E930.7	E950.4	E962.0	E980.4
Antiadrenergics	971.3	E855.6	E941.3	E950.4	E962.0	E980.4
Antiallergic agents	963.0	E858.1	E933.0	E950.4	E962.0	E980.4

1420

TABLE OF DRUGS AND CHEMICALS

Substance	Poisoning	Accident	Therapeutic Use	Suicide Attempt	Assault	Undetermined
			External Cause (E-Code)			
Antianemic agents NEC	964.1	E858.2	E934.1	E950.4	E962.0	E980.4
Antiaris toxicaria	988.2	E865.4	—	E950.9	E962.1	E980.9
Antiarteriosclerotic agents	972.2	E858.3	E942.2	E950.4	E962.0	E980.4
Antiasthmatics	975.7	E858.6	E945.7	E950.4	E962.0	E980.4
Antibiotics	960.9	E856	E930.9	E950.4	E962.0	E980.4
antifungal	960.1	E856	E930.1	E950.4	E962.0	E980.4
antimycobacterial	960.6	E856	E930.6	E950.4	E962.0	E980.4
antineoplastic	960.7	E856	E930.7	E950.4	E962.0	E980.4
cephalosporin (group)	960.5	E856	E930.5	E950.4	E962.0	E980.4
chloramphenicol (group)	960.2	E856	E930.2	E950.4	E962.0	E980.4
macrolides	960.3	E856	E930.3	E950.4	E962.0	E980.4
specified NEC	960.8	E856	E930.8	E950.4	E962.0	E980.4
tetracycline (group)	960.4	E856	E930.4	E950.4	E962.0	E980.4
Anticancer agents NEC	963.1	E858.1	E933.1	E950.4	E962.0	E980.4
antibiotics	960.7	E856	E930.7	E950.4	E962.0	E980.4
Anticholinergics	971.1	E855.4	E941.1	E950.4	E962.0	E980.4
Anticholinesterase (organophosphorus)						
(reversible)	971.0	E855.3	E941.0	E950.4	E962.0	E980.4
Anticoagulants	964.2	E858.2	E934.2	E950.4	E962.0	E980.4
antagonists	964.5	E858.2	E934.5	E950.4	E962.0	E980.4
Anti–common cold agents NEC	975.6	E858.6	E945.6	E950.4	E962.0	E980.4
Anticonvulsants NEC	966.3	E855.0	E936.3	E950.4	E962.0	E980.4
Antidepressants	969.0	E854.0	E939.0	E950.3	E962.0	E980.3
Antidiabetic agents	962.3	E858.0	E932.3	E950.4	E962.0	E980.4
Antidiarrheal agents	973.5	E858.4	E943.5	E950.4	E962.0	E980.4
Antidiuretic hormone	962.5	E858.0	E932.5	E950.4	E962.0	E980.4
Antidotes NEC	977.2	E858.8	E947.2	E950.4	E962.0	E980.4
Antiemetic agents	963.0	E858.1	E933.0	E950.4	E962.0	E980.4
Antiepilepsy agent NEC	966.3	E855.0	E936.3	E950.4	E962.0	E980.4
Antifertility pills	962.2	E858.0	E932.2	E950.4	E962.0	E980.4
Antiflatulents	973.8	E858.4	E943.8	E950.4	E962.0	E980.4
Antifreeze	989.89	E866.8	—	E950.9	E962.1	E980.9
alcohol	980.1	E860.2	—	E950.9	E962.1	E980.9
ethylene glycol	982.8	E862.4	—	E950.9	E962.1	E980.9
Antifungals (nonmedicinal) (sprays) . . .	989.4	E863.6	—	E950.6	E962.1	E980.7
medicinal NEC	961.9	E857	E931.9	E950.4	E962.0	E980.4
antibiotic	960.1	E856	E930.1	E950.4	E962.0	E980.4
topical	976.0	E858.7	E946.0	E950.4	E962.0	E980.4
Antigastric secretion agents	973.0	E858.4	E943.0	E950.4	E962.0	E980.4
Antihelmintics	961.6	E857	E931.6	E950.4	E962.0	E980.4
Antihemophilic factor (human)	964.7	E858.2	E934.7	E950.4	E962.0	E980.4
Antihistamine	963.0	E858.1	E933.0	E950.4	E962.0	E980.4
Antihypertensive agents NEC	972.6	E858.3	E942.6	E950.4	E962.0	E980.4
Anti–infectives NEC	961.9	E857	E931.9	E950.4	E962.0	E980.4
antibiotics	960.9	E856	E930.9	E950.4	E962.0	E980.4
specified NEC	960.8	E856	E930.8	E950.4	E962.0	E980.4
antihelmintic	961.6	E857	E931.6	E950.4	E962.0	E980.4
antimalarial	961.4	E857	E931.4	E950.4	E962.0	E980.4
antimycobacterial NEC	961.8	E857	E931.8	E950.4	E962.0	E980.4
antibiotics	960.6	E856	E930.6	E950.4	E962.0	E980.4
antiprotozoal NEC	961.5	E857	E931.5	E950.4	E962.0	E980.4
blood	961.4	E857	E931.4	E950.4	E962.0	E980.4
antiviral	961.7	E857	E931.7	E950.4	E962.0	E980.4
arsenical	961.1	E857	E931.1	E950.4	E962.0	E980.4
ENT agents	976.6	E858.7	E946.6	E950.4	E962.0	E980.4
heavy metals NEC	961.2	E857	E931.2	E950.4	E962.0	E980.4
local	976.0	E858.7	E946.0	E950.4	E962.0	E980.4
ophthalmic preparation	976.5	E858.7	E946.5	E950.4	E962.0	E980.4
topical NEC	976.0	E858.7	E946.0	E950.4	E962.0	E980.4
Anti–inflammatory agents (topical) . . .	976.0	E858.7	E946.0	E950.4	E962.0	E980.4
Antiknock (tetraethyl lead)	984.1	E862.1	—	E950.9	E962.1	E980.9

1421

TABLE OF DRUGS AND CHEMICALS

Substance	Poisoning	Accident	Therapeutic Use	Suicide Attempt	Assault	Undetermined
			External Cause (E-Code)			

Antilipemics	972.2	E858.3	E942.2	E950.4	E962.0	E980.4
Antimalarials	961.4	E857	E931.4	E950.4	E962.0	E980.4
Antimony (compounds) (vapor) NEC	985.4	E866.2	—	E950.9	E962.1	E980.9
anti–infectives	961.2	E857	E931.2	E950.4	E962.0	E980.4
pesticides (vapor)	985.4	E863.4	—	E950.6	E962.2	E980.7
potassium tartrate	961.2	E857	E931.2	E950.4	E962.0	E980.4
tartrated	961.2	E857	E931.2	E950.4	E962.0	E980.4
Antimuscarinic agents	971.1	E855.4	E941.1	E950.4	E962.0	E980.4
Antimycobacterials NEC	961.8	E857	E931.8	E950.4	E962.0	E980.4
antibiotics	960.6	E856	E930.6	E950.4	E962.0	E980.4
Antineoplastic agents	963.1	E858.1	E933.1	E950.4	E962.0	E980.4
antibiotics	960.7	E856	E930.7	E950.4	E962.0	E980.4
Anti–Parkinsonism agents	966.4	E855.0	E936.4	E950.4	E962.0	E980.4
Antiphlogistics	965.69	E850.6	E935.6	E950.0	E962.0	E980.0
Antiprotozoals NEC	961.5	E857	E931.5	E950.4	E962.0	E980.4
blood	961.4	E857	E931.4	E950.4	E962.0	E980.4
Antipruritics (local)	976.1	E858.7	E946.1	E950.4	E962.0	E980.4
Antipsychotic agents NEC	969.3	E853.8	E939.3	E950.3	E962.0	E980.3
Antipyretics	965.9	E850.9	E935.9	E950.0	E962.0	E980.0
specified NEC	965.8	E850.8	E935.8	E950.0	E962.0	E980.0
Antipyrine	965.5	E850.5	E935.5	E950.0	E962.0	E980.0
Antirabies serum (equine)	979.9	E858.8	E949.9	E950.4	E962.0	E980.4
Antirheumatics	965.69	E850.6	E935.6	E950.0	E962.0	E980.0
Antiseborrheics	976.4	E858.7	E946.4	E950.4	E962.0	E980.4
Antiseptics (external) (medicinal)	976.0	E858.7	E946.0	E950.4	E962.0	E980.4
Antistine	963.0	E858.1	E933.0	E950.4	E962.0	E980.4
Antithyroid agents	962.8	E858.0	E932.8	E950.4	E962.0	E980.4
Antitoxin, any	979.9	E858.8	E949.9	E950.4	E962.0	E980.4
Antituberculars	961.8	E857	E931.8	E950.4	E962.0	E980.4
antibiotics	960.6	E856	E930.6	E950.4	E962.0	E980.4
Antitussives	975.4	E858.6	E945.5	E950.4	E962.0	E980.4
Antivaricose agents (sclerosing)	972.7	E858.3	E942.7	E950.4	E962.0	E980.4
Antivenin (crotaline) (spider–bite)	979.9	E858.8	E949.9	E950.4	E962.0	E980.4
Antivert	963.0	E858.1	E933.0	E950.4	E962.0	E980.4
Antivirals NEC	961.7	E857	E931.7	E950.4	E962.0	E980.4
Ant poisons — see Pesticides						
Antrol	989.4	E863.4	—	E950.6	E962.1	E980.7
fungicide	989.4	E863.6	—	E950.6	E962.1	E980.7
Apomorphine hydrochloride (emetic)	973.6	E858.4	E943.6	E950.4	E962.0	E980.4
Appetite depressants, central	977.0	E858.8	E947.0	E950.4	E962.0	E980.4
Apresoline	972.6	E858.3	E942.6	E950.4	E962.0	E980.4
Aprobarbital, aprobarbitone	967.0	E851	E937.0	E950.1	E962.0	E980.1
Apronalide	967.8	E852.8	E937.8	E950.2	E962.0	E980.2
Aqua fortis	983.1	E864.1	—	E950.7	E962.1	E980.6
Arachis oil (topical)	976.3	E858.7	E946.3	E950.4	E962.0	E980.4
cathartic	973.2	E858.4	E943.2	E950.4	E962.0	E980.4
Aralen	961.4	E857	E931.4	E950.4	E962.0	E980.4
Arginine salts	974.5	E858.5	E944.5	E950.4	E962.0	E980.4
Argyrol	976.0	E858.7	E946.0	E950.4	E962.0	E980.4
ENT agent	976.6	E858.7	E946.6	E950.4	E962.0	E980.4
ophthalmic preparation	976.5	E858.7	E946.5	E950.4	E962.0	E980.4
Aristocort	962.0	E858.0	E932.0	E950.4	E962.0	E980.4
ENT agent	976.6	E858.7	E946.6	E950.4	E962.0	E980.4
ophthalmic preparation	976.5	E858.7	E946.5	E950.4	E962.0	E980.4
topical NEC	976.0	E858.7	E946.0	E950.4	E962.0	E980.4
Aromatics, corrosive	983.0	E864.0	—	E950.7	E962.1	E980.6
disinfectants	983.0	E861.4	—	E950.7	E962.1	E980.6
Arsenate of lead (insecticide)	985.1	E863.4	—	E950.8	E962.1	E980.8
herbicide	985.1	E863.5	—	E950.8	E962.1	E980.8

1422

TABLE OF DRUGS AND CHEMICALS

Substance	Poisoning	Accident	Therapeutic Use	Suicide Attempt	Assault	Undetermined
		\multicolumn{5}{c}{External Cause (E-Code)}

Substance	Poisoning	Accident	Therapeutic Use	Suicide Attempt	Assault	Undetermined
Arsenic, arsenicals (compounds) (dust) (fumes) (vapor) NEC	985.1	E866.3	—	E950.8	E962.1	E980.8
anti–infectives	961.1	E857	E931.1	E950.4	E962.0	E980.4
pesticide (dust) (fumes)	985.1	E863.4	—	E950.8	E962.1	E980.8
Arsine (gas)	985.1	E866.3	—	E950.8	E962.1	E980.8
Arsphenamine (silver)	961.1	E857	E931.1	E950.4	E962.0	E980.4
Arsthinol	961.1	E857	E931.1	E950.4	E962.0	E980.4
Artane	971.1	E855.4	E941.1	E950.4	E962.0	E980.4
Arthropod (venomous) NEC	989.5	E905.5	—	E950.9	E962.1	E980.9
Asbestos	989.81	E866.8	—	E950.9	E962.1	E980.9
Ascaridole	961.6	E857	E931.6	E950.4	E962.0	E980.4
Ascorbic acid	963.5	E858.1	E933.5	E950.4	E962.0	E980.4
Asiaticoside	976.0	E858.7	E946.0	E950.4	E962.0	E980.4
Aspidium (oleoresin)	961.6	E857	E931.6	E950.4	E962.0	E980.4
Aspirin	965.1	E850.3	E935.3	E950.0	E962.0	E980.0
Astringents (local)	976.2	E858.7	E946.2	E950.4	E962.0	E980.4
Atabrine	961.3	E857	E931.3	E950.4	E962.0	E980.4
Ataractics	969.5	E853.8	E939.5	E950.3	E962.0	E980.3
Atonia drug, intestinal	973.3	E858.4	E943.3	E950.4	E962.0	E980.4
Atophan	974.7	E858.5	E944.7	E950.4	E962.0	E980.4
Atropine	971.1	E855.4	E941.1	E950.4	E962.0	E980.4
Attapulgite	973.5	E858.4	E943.5	E950.4	E962.0	E980.4
Attenuvax	979.4	E858.8	E949.4	E950.4	E962.0	E980.4
Aureomycin	960.4	E856	E930.4	E950.4	E962.0	E980.4
ophthalmic preparation	976.5	E858.7	E946.5	E950.4	E962.0	E980.4
topical NEC	976.0	E858.7	E946.0	E950.4	E962.0	E980.4
Aurothioglucose	965.69	E850.6	E935.6	E950.0	E962.0	E980.0
Aurothioglycanide	965.69	E850.6	E935.6	E950.0	E962.0	E980.0
Aurothiomalate	965.69	E850.6	E935.6	E950.0	E962.0	E980.0
Automobile fuel	981	E862.1	—	E950.9	E962.1	E980.9
Autonomic nervous system agents NEC	971.9	E855.9	E941.9	E950.4	E962.0	E980.4
Avlosulfon	961.8	E857	E931.8	E950.4	E962.0	E980.4
Avomine	967.8	E852.8	E937.8	E950.2	E962.0	E980.2
Azacyclonol	969.5	E853.8	E939.5	E950.3	E962.0	E980.3
Azapetine	971.3	E855.6	E941.3	E950.4	E962.0	E980.4
Azaribine	963.1	E858.1	E933.1	E950.4	E962.0	E980.4
Azaserine	960.7	E856	E930.7	E950.4	E962.0	E980.4
Azathioprine	963.1	E858.1	E933.1	E950.4	E962.0	E980.4
Azosulfamide	961.0	E857	E931.0	E950.4	E962.0	E980.4
Azulfidine	961.0	E857	E931.0	E950.4	E962.0	E980.4
Azuresin	977.8	E858.8	E947.8	E950.4	E962.0	E980.4
Bacimycin	976.0	E858.7	E946.0	E950.4	E962.0	E980.4
ophthalmic preparation	976.5	E858.7	E946.5	E950.4	E962.0	E980.4
Bacitracin	960.8	E856	E930.8	E950.4	E962.0	E980.4
ENT agent	976.6	E858.7	E946.6	E950.4	E962.0	E980.4
ophthalmic preparation	976.5	E858.7	E946.5	E950.4	E962.0	E980.4
topical NEC	976.0	E858.7	E946.0	E950.4	E962.0	E980.4
Baking soda	963.3	E858.1	E933.3	E950.4	E962.0	E980.4
BAL	963.8	E858.1	E933.8	E950.4	E962.0	E980.4
Bamethan (sulfate)	972.5	E858.3	E942.5	E950.4	E962.0	E980.4
Bamipine	963.0	E858.1	E933.0	E950.4	E962.0	E980.4
Baneberry	988.2	E865.4	—	E950.9	E962.1	E980.9
Banewort	988.2	E865.4	—	E950.9	E962.1	E980.9
Barbenyl	967.0	E851	E937.0	E950.1	E962.0	E980.1
Barbital, barbitone	967.0	E851	E937.0	E950.1	E962.0	E980.1
Barbiturates, barbituric acid	967.0	E851	E937.0	E950.1	E962.0	E980.1
anesthetic (intravenous)	968.3	E855.1	E938.3	E950.4	E962.0	E980.4
Barium (carbonate) (chloride) (sulfate)	985.8	E866.4	—	E950.9	E962.1	E980.9
diagnostic agent	977.8	E858.8	E947.8	E950.4	E962.0	E980.4
pesticide	985.8	E863.4	—	E950.6	E962.1	E980.7
rodenticide	985.8	E863.7	—	E950.6	E962.1	E980.7

1423

TABLE OF DRUGS AND CHEMICALS

Substance	Poisoning	Accident	Therapeutic Use	Suicide Attempt	Assault	Undetermined
		\multicolumn{5}{c}{External Cause (E-Code)}

Substance	Poisoning	Accident	Therapeutic Use	Suicide Attempt	Assault	Undetermined
Barrier cream	976.3	E858.7	E946.3	E950.4	E962.0	E980.4
Battery acid or fluid	983.1	E864.1	—	E950.7	E962.1	E980.6
Bay rum	980.8	E860.8	—	E950.9	E962.1	E980.9
BCG vaccine	978.0	E858.8	E948.0	E950.4	E962.0	E980.4
Bearsfoot	988.2	E865.4	—	E950.9	E962.1	E980.9
Beclamide	966.3	E855.0	E936.3	E950.4	E962.0	E980.4
Bee (sting) (venom)	989.5	E905.3	—	E950.9	E962.1	E980.9
Belladonna (alkaloids)	971.1	E855.4	E941.1	E950.4	E962.0	E980.4
Bemegride	970.0	E854.3	E940.0	E950.4	E962.0	E980.4
Benactyzine	969.8	E855.8	E939.8	E950.3	E962.0	E980.3
Benadryl	963.0	E858.1	E933.0	E950.4	E962.0	E980.4
Bendrofluazide	974.3	E858.5	E944.3	E950.4	E962.0	E980.4
Bendroflumethiazide	974.3	E858.5	E944.3	E950.4	E962.0	E980.4
Benemid	974.7	E858.5	E944.7	E950.4	E962.0	E980.4
Benethamine penicillin G	960.0	E856	E930.0	E950.4	E962.0	E980.4
Benisone	976.0	E858.7	E946.0	E950.4	E962.0	E980.4
Benoquin	976.8	E858.7	E946.8	E950.4	E962.0	E980.4
Benoxinate	968.5	E855.2	E938.5	E950.4	E962.0	E980.4
Bentonite	976.3	E858.7	E946.3	E950.4	E962.0	E980.4
Benzalkonium (chloride)	976.0	E858.7	E946.0	E950.4	E962.0	E980.4
ophthalmic preparation	976.5	E858.7	E946.5	E950.4	E962.0	E980.4
Benzamidosalicylate (calcium)	961.8	E857	E931.8	E950.4	E962.0	E980.4
Benzathine penicillin	960.0	E856	E930.0	E950.4	E962.0	E980.4
Benzcarbimine	963.1	E858.1	E933.1	E950.4	E962.0	E980.4
Benzedrex	971.2	E855.5	E941.2	E950.4	E962.0	E980.4
Benzedrine (amphetamine)	969.7	E854.2	E939.7	E950.3	E962.0	E980.3
Benzene (acetyl) (dimethyl) (methyl) (solvent) (vapor)	982.0	E862.4	—	E950.9	E962.1	E980.9
hexachloride (gamma) (insecticide) (vapor)	989.2	E863.0	—	E950.6	E962.1	E980.7
Benzethonium	976.0	E858.7	E946.0	E950.4	E962.0	E980.4
Benzhexol (chloride)	966.4	E855.0	E936.4	E950.4	E962.0	E980.4
Benzilonium	971.1	E855.4	E941.1	E950.4	E962.0	E980.4
Benzin(e) — see Ligroin						
Benziodarone	972.4	E858.3	E942.4	E950.4	E962.0	E980.4
Benzocaine	968.5	E855.2	E938.5	E950.4	E962.0	E980.4
Benzodiapin	969.4	E853.2	E939.4	E950.3	E962.0	E980.3
Benzodiazepines (tranquilizers) NEC	969.4	E853.2	E939.4	E950.3	E962.0	E980.3
Benzoic acid (with salicylic acid) (anti–infective)	976.0	E858.7	E946.0	E950.4	E962.0	E980.4
Benzoin	976.3	E858.7	E946.3	E950.4	E962.0	E980.4
Benzol (vapor)	982.0	E862.4	—	E950.9	E962.1	E980.9
Benzomorphan	965.09	E850.2	E935.2	E950.0	E962.0	E980.0
Benzonatate	975.4	E858.6	E945.4	E950.4	E962.0	E980.4
Benzothiadiazides	974.3	E858.5	E944.3	E950.4	E962.0	E980.4
Benzoylpas	961.8	E857	E931.8	E950.4	E962.0	E980.4
Benzperidol	969.5	E853.8	E939.5	E950.3	E962.0	E980.3
Benzphetamine	977.0	E858.8	E947.0	E950.4	E962.0	E980.4
Benzpyrinium	971.0	E855.3	E941.0	E950.4	E962.0	E980.4
Benzquinamide	963.0	E858.1	E933.0	E950.4	E962.0	E980.4
Benzthiazide	974.3	E858.5	E944.3	E950.4	E962.0	E980.4
Benztropine	971.1	E855.4	E941.1	E950.4	E962.0	E980.4
Benzyl						
acetate	982.8	E862.4	—	E950.9	E962.1	E980.9
benzoate (anti–infective)	976.0	E858.7	E946.0	E950.4	E962.0	E980.4
morphine	965.09	E850.2	E935.2	E950.0	E962.0	E980.0
penicillin	960.0	E856	E930.0	E950.4	E962.0	E980.4
Bephenium hydroxynapthoate	961.6	E857	E931.6	E950.4	E962.0	E980.4
Bergamot oil	989.89	E866.8	—	E950.9	E962.1	E980.9
Berries, poisonous	988.2	E865.3	—	E950.9	E962.1	E980.9

1424

TABLE OF DRUGS AND CHEMICALS

Substance	Poisoning	Accident	Therapeutic Use	Suicide Attempt	Assault	Undetermined
		\multicolumn{5}{c}{External Cause (E-Code)}				
Beryllium (compounds) (fumes)	985.3	E866.4	—	E950.9	E962.1	E980.9
Beta–carotene	976.3	E858.7	E946.3	E950.4	E962.0	E980.4
Beta–Chlor	967.1	E852.0	E937.1	E950.2	E962.0	E980.2
Betamethasone	962.0	E858.0	E932.0	E950.4	E962.0	E980.4
topical	976.0	E858.7	E946.0	E950.4	E962.0	E980.4
Betazole	977.8	E858.8	E947.8	E950.4	E962.0	E980.4
Bethanechol	971.0	E855.3	E941.0	E950.4	E962.0	E980.4
Bethanidine	972.6	E858.3	E942.6	E950.4	E962.0	E980.4
Betula oil	976.3	E858.7	E946.3	E950.4	E962.0	E980.4
Bhang	969.6	E854.1	E939.6	E950.3	E962.0	E980.3
Bialamicol	961.5	E857	E931.5	E950.4	E962.0	E980.4
Bichloride of mercury — *see* Mercury, chloride						
Bichromates (calcium) (crystals) (potassium) (sodium)	983.9	E864.3	—	E950.7	E962.1	E980.6
fumes	987.8	E869.8	—	E952.8	E962.2	E982.8
Biguanide derivatives, oral	962.3	E858.0	E932.3	E950.4	E962.0	E980.4
Biligrafin	977.8	E858.8	E947.8	E950.4	E962.0	E980.4
Bilopaque	977.8	E858.8	E947.8	E950.4	E962.0	E980.4
Bioflavonoids	972.8	E858.3	E942.8	E950.4	E962.0	E980.4
Biological substance NEC	979.9	E858.8	E949.9	E950.4	E962.0	E980.4
Biperiden	966.4	E855.0	E936.4	E950.4	E962.0	E980.4
Bisacodyl	973.1	E858.4	E943.1	E950.4	E962.0	E980.4
Bishydroxycoumarin	964.2	E858.2	E934.2	E950.4	E962.0	E980.4
Bismarsen	961.1	E857	E931.1	E950.4	E962.0	E980.4
Bismuth (compounds) NEC	985.8	E866.4	—	E950.9	E962.1	E980.9
anti–infectives	961.2	E857	E931.2	E950.4	E962.0	E980.4
subcarbonate	973.5	E858.4	E943.5	E950.4	E962.0	E980.4
sulfarsphenamine	961.1	E857	E931.1	E950.4	E962.0	E980.4
Bisphosphonates						
intravenous	963.1	E858.1	E933.7	E950.4	E962.0	E980.4
oral	963.1	E858.1	E933.6	E950.4	E962.0	E980.4
Bithionol	961.6	E857	E931.6	E950.4	E962.0	E980.4
Bitter almond oil	989.0	E866.8	—	E950.9	E962.1	E980.9
Bittersweet	988.2	E865.4	—	E950.9	E962.1	E980.9
Black						
flag	989.4	E863.4	—	E950.6	E962.1	E980.7
henbane	988.2	E865.4	—	E950.9	E962.1	E980.9
leaf (40)	989.4	E863.4	—	E950.6	E962.1	E980.7
widow spider (bite)	989.5	E905.1	—	E950.9	E962.1	E980.9
antivenin	979.9	E858.8	E949.9	E950.4	E962.0	E980.4
Blast furnace gas (carbon monoxide from)	986	E868.8	—	E952.1	E962.2	E982.1
Bleach NEC	983.9	E864.3	—	E950.7	E962.1	E980.6
Bleaching solutions	983.9	E864.3	—	E950.7	E962.1	E980.6
Bleomycin (sulfate)	960.7	E856	E930.7	E950.4	E962.0	E980.4
Blockain	968.9	E855.2	E938.9	E950.4	E962.0	E980.4
infiltration (subcutaneous)	968.5	E855.2	E938.5	E950.4	E962.0	E980.4
nerve block (peripheral) (plexus)	968.6	E855.2	E938.6	E950.4	E962.0	E980.4
topical (surface)	968.5	E855.2	E938.5	E950.4	E962.0	E980.4
Blood (derivatives) (natural) (plasma) (whole)	964.7	E858.2	E934.7	E950.4	E962.0	E980.4
affecting agent	964.9	E858.2	E934.9	E950.4	E962.0	E980.4
specified NEC	964.8	E858.2	E934.8	E950.4	E962.0	E980.4
substitute (macromolecular)	964.8	E858.2	E934.8	E950.4	E962.0	E980.4
Blue velvet	965.09	E850.2	E935.2	E950.0	E962.0	E980.0
Bone meal	989.89	E866.5	—	E950.9	E962.1	E980.9
Bonine	963.0	E858.1	E933.0	E950.4	E962.0	E980.4
Boracic acid	976.0	E858.7	E946.0	E950.4	E962.0	E980.4
ENT agent	976.6	E858.7	E946.6	E950.4	E962.0	E980.4
ophthalmic preparation	976.5	E858.7	E946.5	E950.4	E962.0	E980.4
Borate (cleanser) (sodium)	989.6	E861.3	—	E950.9	E962.1	E980.9

TABLE OF DRUGS AND CHEMICALS

Substance	Poisoning	Accident	Therapeutic Use	Suicide Attempt	Assault	Undetermined
		External Cause (E-Code)				
Borax (cleanser) 989.6		E861.3	—	E950.9	E962.1	E980.9
Boric acid. 976.0		E858.7	E946.0	E950.4	E962.0	E980.4
ENT agent. 976.6		E858.7	E946.6	E950.4	E962.0	E980.4
ophthalmic preparation 976.5		E858.7	E946.5	E950.4	E962.0	E980.4
Boron hydride NEC. 989.89		E866.8	—	E950.9	E962.1	E980.9
fumes or gas. 987.8		E869.8	—	E952.8	E962.2	E982.8
Botox 975.3		E858.6	E945.3	E950.4	E962.0	E980.4
Brake fluid vapor. 987.8		E869.8	—	E952.8	E962.2	E982.8
Brass (compounds) (fumes). 985.8		E866.4	—	E950.9	E962.1	E980.9
Brasso 981		E861.3	—	E950.9	E962.1	E980.9
Bretylium (tosylate). 972.6		E858.3	E942.6	E950.4	E962.0	E980.4
Brevital (sodium). 968.3		E855.1	E938.3	E950.4	E962.0	E980.4
British antilewisite 963.8		E858.1	E933.8	E950.4	E962.0	E980.4
Bromal (hydrate) 967.3		E852.2	E937.3	E950.2	E962.0	E980.2
Bromelains 963.4		E858.1	E933.4	E950.4	E962.0	E980.4
Bromides NEC. 967.3		E852.2	E937.3	E950.2	E962.0	E980.2
Bromine (vapor) 987.8		E869.8	—	E952.8	E962.2	E982.8
compounds (medicinal). 967.3		E852.2	E937.3	E950.2	E962.0	E980.2
Bromisovalum 967.3		E852.2	E937.3	E950.2	E962.0	E980.2
Bromobenzyl cyanide 987.5		E869.3	—	E952.8	E962.2	E982.8
Bromodiphenhydramine 963.0		E858.1	E933.0	E950.4	E962.0	E980.4
Bromoform 967.3		E852.2	E937.3	E950.2	E962.0	E980.2
Bromophenol blue reagent 977.8		E858.8	E947.8	E950.4	E962.0	E980.4
Bromosalicylhydroxamic acid. 961.8		E857	E931.8	E950.4	E962.0	E980.4
Bromo–seltzer 965.4		E850.4	E935.4	E950.0	E962.0	E980.0
Brompheniramine 963.0		E858.1	E933.0	E950.4	E962.0	E980.4
Bromural 967.3		E852.2	E937.3	E950.2	E962.0	E980.2
Brown spider (bite) (venom) 989.5		E905.1	—	E950.9	E962.1	E980.9
Brucia 988.2		E865.3	—	E950.9	E962.1	E980.9
Brucine 989.1		E863.7	—	E950.6	E962.1	E980.7
Brunswick green — see Copper						
Bruten — see Ibuprofen						
Bryonia (alba) (dioica) 988.2		E865.4	—	E950.9	E962.1	E980.9
Buclizine 969.5		E853.8	E939.5	E950.3	E962.0	E980.3
Bufferin. 965.1		E850.3	E935.3	E950.0	E962.0	E980.0
Bufotenine 969.6		E854.1	E939.6	E950.3	E962.0	E980.3
Buphenine 971.2		E855.5	E941.2	E950.4	E962.0	E980.4
Bupivacaine 968.9		E855.2	E938.9	E950.4	E962.0	E980.4
infiltration (subcutaneous) 968.5		E855.2	E938.5	E950.4	E962.0	E980.4
nerve block (peripheral) (plexus) . . . 968.6		E855.2	E938.6	E950.4	E962.0	E980.4
Busulfan 963.1		E858.1	E933.1	E950.4	E962.0	E980.4
Butabarbital (sodium) 967.0		E851	E937.0	E950.1	E962.0	E980.1
Butabarbitone 967.0		E851	E937.0	E950.1	E962.0	E980.1
Butabarpal 967.0		E851	E937.0	E950.1	E962.0	E980.1
Butacaine 968.5		E855.2	E938.5	E950.4	E962.0	E980.4
Butallylonal 967.0		E851	E937.0	E950.1	E962.0	E980.1
Butane (distributed in mobile container) . . . 987.0		E868.0	—	E951.1	E962.2	E981.1
distributed through pipes 987.0		E867	—	E951.0	E962.2	E981.0
incomplete combustion of — see Carbon monoxide, butane						
Butanol 980.3		E860.4	—	E950.9	E962.1	E980.9
Butanone 982.8		E862.4	—	E950.9	E962.1	E980.9
Butaperazine 969.1		E853.0	E939.1	E950.3	E962.0	E980.3
Butazolidin 965.5		E850.5	E935.5	E950.0	E962.0	E980.0
Butethal 967.0		E851	E937.0	E950.1	E962.0	E980.1
Butethamate 971.1		E855.5	E941.1	E950.4	E962.0	E980.4
Buthalitone (sodium) 968.3		E855.1	E938.3	E950.4	E962.0	E980.4
Butisol (sodium) 967.0		E851	E937.0	E950.1	E962.0	E980.1
Butobarbital, butobarbitone 967.0		E851	E937.0	E950.1	E962.0	E980.1
Butriptyline 969.0		E854.0	E939.0	E950.3	E962.0	E980.3

TABLE OF DRUGS AND CHEMICALS

Substance	Poisoning	Accident	Therapeutic Use	Suicide Attempt	Assault	Undetermined
			External Cause (E-Code)			
Buttercups	988.2	E865.4	—	E950.9	E962.1	E980.9
Butter of antimony — *see* Antimony						
Butyl						
acetate (secondary)	982.8	E862.4	—	E950.9	E962.1	E980.9
alcohol	980.3	E860.4	—	E950.9	E962.1	E980.9
carbinol	980.8	E860.8	—	E950.9	E962.1	E980.9
carbitol	982.8	E862.4	—	E950.9	E962.1	E980.9
cellosolve	982.8	E862.4	—	E950.9	E962.1	E980.9
chloral (hydrate)	967.1	E852.0	E937.1	E950.2	E962.0	E980.2
formate	982.8	E862.4	—	E950.9	E962.1	E980.9
scopolammonium bromide	971.1	E855.4	E941.1	E950.4	E962.0	E980.4
Butyn	968.5	E855.2	E938.5	E950.4	E962.0	E980.4
Butyrophenone (–based tranquilizers)	969.2	E853.1	E939.2	E950.3	E962.0	E980.3
Cacodyl, cacodylic acid — *see* Arsenic						
Cactinomycin	960.7	E856	E930.7	E950.4	E962.0	E980.4
Cade oil	976.4	E858.7	E946.4	E950.4	E962.0	E980.4
Cadmium (chloride) (compounds) (dust)						
(fumes) (oxide)	985.5	E866.4	—	E950.9	E962.1	E980.9
sulfide (medicinal) NEC	976.4	E858.7	E946.4	E950.4	E962.0	E980.4
Caffeine	969.7	E854.2	E939.7	E950.3	E962.0	E980.3
Calabar bean	988.2	E865.4	—	E950.9	E962.1	E980.9
Caladium seguinium	988.2	E865.4	—	E950.9	E962.1	E980.9
Calamine (liniment) (lotion)	976.3	E858.7	E946.3	E950.4	E962.0	E980.4
Calciferol	963.5	E858.1	E933.5	E950.4	E962.0	E980.4
Calcium (salts) NEC	974.5	E858.5	E944.5	E950.4	E962.0	E980.4
acetylsalicylate	965.1	E850.3	E935.3	E950.0	E962.0	E980.0
benzamidosalicylate	961.8	E857	E931.8	E950.4	E962.0	E980.4
carbaspirin	965.1	E850.3	E935.3	E950.0	E962.0	E980.0
carbamide (citrated)	977.3	E858.8	E947.3	E950.4	E962.0	E980.4
carbonate (antacid)	973.0	E858.4	E943.0	E950.4	E962.0	E980.4
cyanide (citrated)	977.3	E858.8	E947.3	E950.4	E962.0	E980.4
dioctyl sulfosuccinate	973.2	E858.4	E943.2	E950.4	E962.0	E980.4
disodium edathamil	963.8	E858.1	E933.8	E950.4	E962.0	E980.4
disodium edetate	963.8	E858.1	E933.8	E950.4	E962.0	E980.4
EDTA	963.8	E858.1	E933.8	E950.4	E962.0	E980.4
hydrate, hydroxide	983.2	E864.2	—	E950.7	E962.1	E980.6
mandelate	961.9	E857	E931.9	E950.4	E962.0	E980.4
oxide	983.2	E864.2	—	E950.7	E962.1	E980.6
Calomel — *see* Mercury, chloride						
Caloric agents NEC	974.5	E858.5	E944.5	E950.4	E962.0	E980.4
Calusterone	963.1	E858.1	E933.1	E950.4	E962.0	E980.4
Camoquin	961.4	E857	E931.4	E950.4	E962.0	E980.4
Camphor (oil)	976.1	E858.7	E946.1	E950.4	E962.0	E980.4
Candeptin	976.0	E858.7	E946.0	E950.4	E962.0	E980.4
Candicidin	976.0	E858.7	E946.0	E950.4	E962.0	E980.4
Cannabinols	969.6	E854.1	E939.6	E950.3	E962.0	E980.3
Cannabis (derivatives) (indica) (sativa)	969.6	E854.1	E939.6	E950.3	E962.0	E980.3
Canned heat	980.1	E860.2	—	E950.9	E962.1	E980.9
Cantharides, cantharidin, cantharis	976.8	E858.7	E946.8	E950.4	E962.0	E980.4
Capillary agents	972.8	E858.3	E942.8	E950.4	E962.0	E980.4
Capreomycin	960.6	E856	E930.6	E950.4	E962.0	E980.4
Captodiame, captodiamine	969.5	E853.8	E939.5	E950.3	E962.0	E980.3
Caramiphen (hydrochloride)	971.1	E855.4	E941.1	E950.4	E962.0	E980.4
Carbachol	971.0	E855.3	E941.0	E950.4	E962.0	E980.4
Carbacrylamine resins	974.5	E858.5	E944.5	E950.4	E962.0	E980.4
Carbamate (sedative)	967.8	E852.8	E937.8	E950.2	E962.0	E980.2
herbicide	989.3	E863.5	—	E950.6	E962.1	E980.7
insecticide	989.3	E863.2	—	E950.6	E962.1	E980.7
Carbamazepine	966.3	E855.0	E936.3	E950.4	E962.0	E980.4
Carbamic esters	967.8	E852.8	E937.8	E950.2	E962.0	E980.2
Carbamide	974.4	E858.5	E944.4	E950.4	E962.0	E980.4

1427

TABLE OF DRUGS AND CHEMICALS

Substance	Poisoning	Accident	Therapeutic Use	Suicide Attempt	Assault	Undetermined
			External Cause (E-Code)			
topical	976.8	E858.7	E946.8	E950.4	E962.0	E980.4
Carbamylcholine chloride	971.0	E855.3	E941.0	E950.4	E962.0	E980.4
Carbarsone	961.1	E857	E931.1	E950.4	E962.0	E980.4
Carbaryl	989.3	E863.2	—	E950.6	E962.1	E980.7
Carbaspirin	965.1	E850.3	E935.3	E950.0	E962.0	E980.0
Carbazochrome	972.8	E858.3	E942.8	E950.4	E962.0	E980.4
Carbenicillin	960.0	E856	E930.0	E950.4	E962.0	E980.4
Carbenoxolone	973.8	E858.4	E943.8	E950.4	E962.0	E980.4
Carbetapentane	975.4	E858.6	E945.4	E950.4	E962.0	E980.4
Carbimazole	962.8	E858.0	E932.8	E950.4	E962.0	E980.4
Carbinol	980.1	E860.2	—	E950.9	E962.1	E980.9
Carbinoxamine	963.0	E858.1	E933.0	E950.4	E962.0	E980.4
Carbitol	982.8	E862.4	—	E950.9	E962.1	E980.9
Carbocaine	968.9	E855.2	E938.9	E950.4	E962.0	E980.4
infiltration (subcutaneous)	968.5	E855.2	E938.5	E950.4	E962.0	E980.4
nerve block (peripheral) (plexus)	968.6	E855.2	E938.6	E950.4	E962.0	E980.4
topical (surface)	968.5	E855.2	E938.5	E950.4	E962.0	E980.4
Carbol–fuchsin solution	976.0	E858.7	E946.0	E950.4	E962.0	E980.4
Carbolic acid (*see also* Phenol)	983.0	E864.0	—	E950.7	E962.1	E980.6
Carbomycin	960.8	E856	E930.8	E950.4	E962.0	E980.4
Carbon						
bisulfide (liquid) (vapor)	982.2	E862.4	—	E950.9	E962.1	E980.9
dioxide (gas)	987.8	E869.8	—	E952.8	E962.2	E982.8
disulfide (liquid) (vapor)	982.2	E862.4	—	E950.9	E962.1	E980.9
monoxide (from incomplete combustion of) (in) NEC	986	E868.9	—	E952.1	E962.2	E982.1
blast furnace gas	986	E868.8	—	E952.1	E962.2	E982.1
butane (distributed in mobile container)	986	E868.0	—	E951.1	E962.2	E981.1
distributed through pipes	986	E867	—	E951.0	E962.2	E981.0
charcoal fumes	986	E868.3	—	E952.1	E962.2	E982.1
coal						
gas (piped)	986	E867	—	E951.0	E962.2	E981.0
solid (in domestic stoves, fireplaces)	986	E868.3	—	E952.1	E962.2	E982.1
coke (in domestic stoves, fireplaces)	986	E868.3	—	E952.1	E962.2	E982.1
exhaust gas (motor) not in transit	986	E868.2	—	E952.0	E962.2	E982.0
combustion engine, any not in watercraft	986	E868.2	—	E952.0	E962.2	E982.0
farm tractor, not in transit	986	E868.2	—	E952.0	E962.2	E982.0
gas engine	986	E868.2	—	E952.0	E962.2	E982.0
motor pump	986	E868.2	—	E952.0	E962.2	E982.0
motor vehicle, not in transit	986	E868.2	—	E952.0	E962.2	E982.0
fuel (in domestic use)	986	E868.3	—	E952.1	E962.2	E982.1
gas (piped)	986	E867	—	E951.0	E962.2	E981.0
in mobile container	986	E868.0	—	E951.1	E962.2	E981.1
utility	986	E868.1	—	E951.8	E962.2	E981.1
in mobile container	986	E868.0	—	E951.1	E962.2	E981.1
piped (natural)	986	E867	—	E951.0	E962.2	E981.0
illuminating gas	986	E868.1	—	E951.8	E962.2	E981.8
industrial fuels or gases, any	986	E868.8	—	E952.1	E962.2	E982.1
kerosene (in domestic stoves, fireplaces)	986	E868.3	—	E952.1	E962.2	E982.1
kiln gas or vapor	986	E868.8	—	E952.1	E962.2	E982.1
motor exhaust gas, not in transit	986	E868.2	—	E952.0	E962.2	E982.0
piped gas (manufactured) (natural)	986	E867	—	E951.0	E962.2	E981.0
producer gas	986	E868.8	—	E952.1	E962.2	E982.1
propane (distributed in mobile container)	986	E868.0	—	E951.1	E962.2	E981.1
distributed through pipes	986	E867	—	E951.0	E962.2	E981.0

TABLE OF DRUGS AND CHEMICALS

Substance	Poisoning	Accident	Therapeutic Use	Suicide Attempt	Assault	Undetermined
		\multicolumn{5}{c|}{External Cause (E-Code)}				
specified source NEC	986	E868.8	—	E952.1	E962.2	E982.1
stove gas	986	E868.1	—	E951.8	E962.2	E981.8
piped	986	E867	—	E951.0	E962.2	E981.0
utility gas	986	E868.1	—	E951.8	E962.2	E981.8
piped	986	E867	—	E951.0	E962.2	E981.0
water gas	986	E868.1	—	E951.8	E962.2	E981.8
wood (in domestic stoves, fireplaces)	986	E868.3	—	E952.1	E962.2	E982.1
tetrachloride (vapor) NEC	987.8	E869.8	—	E952.8	E962.2	E982.8
liquid (cleansing agent) NEC	982.1	E861.3	—	E950.9	E962.1	E980.9
solvent	982.1	E862.4	—	E950.9	E962.1	E980.9
Carbonic acid (gas)	987.8	E869.8	—	E952.8	E962.2	E982.8
anhydrase inhibitors	974.2	E858.5	E944.2	E950.4	E962.0	E980.4
Carbowax	976.3	E858.7	E946.3	E950.4	E962.0	E980.4
Carbrital	967.0	E851	E937.0	E950.1	E962.0	E980.1
Carbromal (derivatives)	967.3	E852.2	E937.3	E950.2	E962.0	E980.2
Cardiac						
depressants	972.0	E858.3	E942.0	E950.4	E962.0	E980.4
rhythm regulators	972.0	E858.3	E942.0	E950.4	E962.0	E980.4
Cardiografin	977.8	E858.8	E947.8	E950.4	E962.0	E980.4
Cardio–green	977.8	E858.8	E947.8	E950.4	E962.0	E980.4
Cardiotonic glycosides	972.1	E858.3	E942.1	E950.4	E962.0	E980.4
Cardiovascular agents NEC	972.9	E858.3	E942.9	E950.4	E962.0	E980.4
Cardrase	974.2	E858.5	E944.2	E950.4	E962.0	E980.4
Carfusin	976.0	E858.7	E946.0	E950.4	E962.0	E980.4
Carisoprodol	968.0	E855.1	E938.0	E950.4	E962.0	E980.4
Carmustine	963.1	E858.1	E933.1	E950.4	E962.0	E980.4
Carotene	963.5	E858.1	E933.5	E950.4	E962.0	E980.4
Carphenazine (maleate)	969.1	E853.0	E939.1	E950.3	E962.0	E980.3
Carter's Little Pills	973.1	E858.4	E943.1	E950.4	E962.0	E980.4
Cascara (sagrada)	973.1	E858.4	E943.1	E950.4	E962.0	E980.4
Cassava	988.2	E865.4	—	E950.9	E962.1	E980.9
Castellani's paint	976.0	E858.7	E946.0	E950.4	E962.0	E980.4
Castor						
bean	988.2	E865.3	—	E950.9	E962.1	E980.9
oil	973.1	E858.4	E943.1	E950.4	E962.0	E980.4
Caterpillar (sting)	989.5	E905.5	—	E950.9	E962.1	E980.9
Catha (edulis)	970.8	E854.3	E940.8	E950.4	E962.0	E980.4
Cathartics NEC	973.3	E858.4	E943.3	E950.4	E962.0	E980.4
contact	973.1	E858.4	E943.1	E950.4	E962.0	E980.4
emollient	973.2	E858.4	E943.2	E950.4	E962.0	E980.4
intestinal irritants	973.1	E858.4	E943.1	E950.4	E962.0	E980.4
saline	973.3	E858.4	E943.3	E950.4	E962.0	E980.4
Cathomycin	960.8	E856	E930.8	E950.4	E962.0	E980.4
Caustic(s)	983.9	E864.4	—	E950.7	E962.1	E980.6
alkali	983.2	E864.2	—	E950.7	E962.1	E980.6
hydroxide	983.2	E864.2	—	E950.7	E962.1	E980.6
potash	983.2	E864.2	—	E950.7	E962.1	E980.6
soda	983.2	E864.2	—	E950.7	E962.1	E980.6
specified NEC	983.9	E864.3	—	E950.7	E962.1	E980.6
Ceepryn	976.0	E858.7	E946.0	E950.4	E962.0	E980.4
ENT agent	976.6	E858.7	E946.6	E950.4	E962.0	E980.4
lozenges	976.6	E858.7	E946.6	E950.4	E962.0	E980.4
Celestone	962.0	E858.0	E932.0	E950.4	E962.0	E980.4
topical	976.0	E858.7	E946.0	E950.4	E962.0	E980.4
Cellosolve	982.8	E862.4	—	E950.9	E962.1	E980.9
Cell stimulants and proliferants	976.8	E858.7	E946.8	E950.4	E962.0	E980.4
Cellulose derivatives, cathartic	973.3	E858.4	E943.3	E950.4	E962.0	E980.4
nitrates (topical)	976.3	E858.7	E946.3	E950.4	E962.0	E980.4
Centipede (bite)	989.5	E905.4	—	E950.9	E962.1	E980.9
Central nervous system						
depressants	968.4	E855.1	E938.4	E950.4	E962.0	E980.4

1429

TABLE OF DRUGS AND CHEMICALS

Substance	Poisoning	Accident	Therapeutic Use	Suicide Attempt	Assault	Undetermined
		\multicolumn{5}{c}{External Cause (E-Code)}				
anesthetic (general) NEC	968.4	E855.1	E938.4	E950.4	E962.0	E980.4
gases NEC	968.2	E855.1	E938.2	E950.4	E962.0	E980.4
intravenous	968.3	E855.1	E938.3	E950.4	E962.0	E980.4
barbiturates	967.0	E851	E937.0	E950.1	E962.0	E980.1
bromides	967.3	E852.2	E937.3	E950.2	E962.0	E980.2
cannabis sativa	969.6	E854.1	E939.6	E950.3	E962.0	E980.3
chloral hydrate	967.1	E852.0	E937.1	E950.2	E962.0	E980.2
hallucinogenics	969.6	E854.1	E939.6	E950.3	E962.0	E980.3
hypnotics	967.9	E852.9	E937.9	E950.2	E962.0	E980.2
specified NEC	967.8	E852.8	E937.8	E950.2	E962.0	E980.2
muscle relaxants	968.0	E855.1	E938.0	E950.4	E962.0	E980.4
paraldehyde	967.2	E852.1	E937.2	E950.2	E962.0	E980.2
sedatives	967.9	E852.9	E937.9	E950.2	E962.0	E980.2
mixed NEC	967.6	E852.5	E937.6	E950.2	E962.0	E980.2
specified NEC	967.8	E852.8	E937.8	E950.2	E962.0	E980.2
muscle–tone depressants	968.0	E855.1	E938.0	E950.4	E962.0	E980.4
stimulants	970.9	E854.3	E940.9	E950.4	E962.0	E980.4
amphetamines	969.7	E854.2	E939.7	E950.3	E962.0	E980.3
analeptics	970.0	E854.3	E940.0	E950.4	E962.0	E980.4
antidepressants	969.0	E854.0	E939.0	E950.3	E962.0	E980.3
opiate antagonists	970.1	E854.3	E940.0	E950.4	E962.0	E980.4
specified NEC	970.8	E854.3	E940.8	E950.4	E962.0	E980.4
Cephalexin	960.5	E856	E930.5	E950.4	E962.0	E980.4
Cephaloglycin	960.5	E856	E930.5	E950.4	E962.0	E980.4
Cephaloridine	960.5	E856	E930.5	E950.4	E962.0	E980.4
Cephalosporins NEC	960.5	E856	E930.5	E950.4	E962.0	E980.4
N (adicillin)	960.0	E856	E930.0	E950.4	E962.0	E980.4
Cephalothin (sodium)	960.5	E856	E930.5	E950.4	E962.0	E980.4
Cerbera (odallam)	988.2	E865.4	—	E950.9	E962.1	E980.9
Cerberin	972.1	E858.3	E942.1	E950.4	E962.0	E980.4
Cerebral stimulants	970.9	E854.3	E940.9	E950.4	E962.0	E980.4
psychotherapeutic	969.7	E854.2	E939.7	E950.3	E962.0	E980.3
specified NEC	970.8	E854.3	E940.8	E950.4	E962.0	E980.4
Cetalkonium (chloride)	976.0	E858.7	E946.0	E950.4	E962.0	E980.4
Cetoxime	963.0	E858.1	E933.0	E950.4	E962.0	E980.4
Cetrimide	976.2	E858.7	E946.2	E950.4	E962.0	E980.4
Cetylpyridinium	976.0	E858.7	E946.0	E950.4	E962.0	E980.4
ENT agent	976.6	E858.7	E946.6	E950.4	E962.0	E980.4
lozenges	976.6	E858.7	E946.6	E950.4	E962.0	E980.4
Cevadilla — see Sabadilla						
Cevitamic acid	963.5	E858.1	E933.5	E950.4	E962.0	E980.4
Chalk, precipitated	973.0	E858.4	E943.0	E950.4	E962.0	E980.4
Charcoal						
fumes (carbon monoxide)	986	E868.3	—	E952.1	E962.2	E982.1
industrial	986	E868.8	—	E952.1	E962.2	E982.1
medicinal (activated)	973.0	E858.4	E943.0	E950.4	E962.0	E980.4
Chelating agents NEC	977.2	E858.8	E947.2	E950.4	E962.0	E980.4
Chelidonium majus	988.2	E865.4	—	E950.9	E962.1	E980.9
Chemical substance	989.9	E866.9	—	E950.9	E962.1	E980.9
specified NEC	989.89	E866.8	—	E950.9	E962.1	E980.9
Chemotherapy, antineoplastic	963.1	E858.1	E933.1	E950.4	E962.0	E980.4
Chenopodium (oil)	961.6	E857	E931.6	E950.4	E962.0	E980.4
Cherry laurel	988.2	E865.4	—	E950.9	E962.1	E980.9
Chiniofon	961.3	E857	E931.3	E950.4	E962.0	E980.4
Chlophedianol	975.4	E858.6	E945.4	E950.4	E962.0	E980.4
Chloral (betaine) (formamide) (hydrate)	967.1	E852.0	E937.1	E950.2	E962.0	E980.2
Chloralamide	967.1	E852.0	E937.1	E950.2	E962.0	E980.2
Chlorambucil	963.1	E858.1	E933.1	E950.4	E962.0	E980.4
Chloramphenicol	960.2	E856	E930.2	E950.4	E962.0	E980.4
ENT agent	976.6	E858.7	E946.6	E950.4	E962.0	E980.4

TABLE OF DRUGS AND CHEMICALS

Substance	Poisoning	Accident	Therapeutic Use	Suicide Attempt	Assault	Undetermined
		\multicolumn{5}{c|}{External Cause (E-Code)}				

Substance	Poisoning	Accident	Therapeutic Use	Suicide Attempt	Assault	Undetermined
ophthalmic preparation	976.5	E858.7	E946.5	E950.4	E962.0	E980.4
topical NEC	976.0	E858.7	E946.0	E950.4	E962.0	E980.4
Chlorate(s) (potassium) (sodium) NEC	983.9	E864.3	—	E950.7	E962.1	E980.6
herbicides	989.4	E863.5	—	E950.6	E962.1	E980.7
Chlorcyclizine	963.0	E858.1	E933.0	E950.4	E962.0	E980.4
Chlordan(e) (dust)	989.2	E863.0	—	E950.6	E962.1	E980.7
Chlordantoin	976.0	E858.7	E946.0	E950.4	E962.0	E980.4
Chlordiazepoxide	969.4	E853.2	E939.4	E950.3	E962.0	E980.3
Chloresium	976.8	E858.7	E946.8	E950.4	E962.0	E980.4
Chlorethiazol	967.1	E852.0	E937.1	E950.2	E962.0	E980.2
Chlorethyl — see Ethyl, chloride						
Chloretone	967.1	E852.0	E937.1	E950.2	E962.0	E980.2
Chlorex	982.3	E862.4	—	E950.9	E962.1	E980.9
Chlorhexadol	967.1	E852.0	E937.1	E950.2	E962.0	E980.2
Chlorhexidine (hydrochloride)	976.0	E858.7	E946.0	E950.4	E962.0	E980.4
Chlorhydroxyquinolin	976.0	E858.7	E946.0	E950.4	E962.0	E980.4
Chloride of lime (bleach)	983.9	E864.3	—	E950.7	E962.1	E980.6
Chlorinated						
camphene	989.2	E863.0	—	E950.6	E962.1	E980.7
diphenyl	989.89	E866.8	—	E950.9	E962.1	E980.9
hydrocarbons NEC	989.2	E863.0	—	E950.6	E962.1	E980.7
solvent	982.3	E862.4	—	E950.9	E962.1	E980.9
lime (bleach)	983.9	E864.3	—	E950.7	E962.1	E980.6
naphthalene — see Naphthalene						
pesticides NEC	989.2	E863.0	—	E950.6	E962.1	E980.7
soda — see Sodium, hypochlorite						
Chlorine (fumes) (gas)	987.6	E869.8	—	E952.8	E962.2	E982.8
bleach	983.9	E864.3	—	E950.7	E962.1	E980.6
compounds NEC	983.9	E864.3	—	E950.7	E962.1	E980.6
disinfectant	983.9	E861.4	—	E950.7	E962.1	E980.6
releasing agents NEC	983.9	E864.3	—	E950.7	E962.1	E980.6
Chlorisondamine	972.3	E858.3	E942.3	E950.4	E962.0	E980.4
Chlormadinone	962.2	E858.0	E932.2	E950.4	E962.0	E980.4
Chlormerodrin	974.0	E858.5	E944.0	E950.4	E962.0	E980.4
Chlormethiazole	967.1	E852.0	E937.1	E950.2	E962.0	E980.2
Chlormethylenecycline	960.4	E856	E930.4	E950.4	E962.0	E980.4
Chlormezanone	969.5	E853.8	E939.5	E950.3	E962.0	E980.3
Chloroacetophenone	987.5	E869.3	—	E952.8	E962.2	E982.8
Chloroaniline	983.0	E864.0	—	E950.7	E962.1	E980.6
Chlorobenzene, chlorobenzol	982.0	E862.4	—	E950.9	E962.1	E980.9
Chlorobutanol	967.1	E852.0	E937.1	E950.2	E962.0	E980.2
Chlorodinitrobenzene	983.0	E864.0	—	E950.7	E962.1	E980.6
dust or vapor	987.8	E869.8	—	E952.8	E962.2	E982.8
Chloroethane — see Ethyl, chloride						
Chloroform (fumes) (vapor)	987.8	E869.8	—	E952.8	E962.2	E982.8
anesthetic (gas)	968.2	E855.1	E938.2	E950.4	E962.0	E980.4
liquid NEC	968.4	E855.1	E938.4	E950.4	E962.0	E980.4
solvent	982.3	E862.4	—	E950.9	E962.1	E980.9
Chloroguanide	961.4	E857	E931.4	E950.4	E962.0	E980.4
Chloromycetin	960.2	E856	E930.2	E950.4	E962.0	E980.4
ENT agent	976.6	E858.7	E946.6	E950.4	E962.0	E980.4
ophthalmic preparation	976.5	E858.7	E946.5	E950.4	E962.0	E980.4
otic solution	976.6	E858.7	E946.6	E950.4	E962.0	E980.4
topical NEC	976.0	E858.7	E946.0	E950.4	E962.0	E980.4
Chloronitrobenzene	983.0	E864.0	—	E950.7	E962.1	E980.6
dust or vapor	987.8	E869.8	—	E952.8	E962.2	E982.8
Chlorophenol	983.0	E864.0	—	E950.7	E962.1	E980.6
Chlorophenothane	989.2	E863.0	—	E950.6	E962.1	E980.7
Chlorophyll (derivatives)	976.8	E858.7	E946.8	E950.4	E962.0	E980.4
Chloropicrin (fumes)	987.8	E869.8	—	E952.8	E962.2	E982.8
fumigant	989.4	E863.8	—	E950.6	E962.1	E980.7

TABLE OF DRUGS AND CHEMICALS

Substance	Poisoning	Accident	Therapeutic Use	Suicide Attempt	Assault	Undetermined
		\multicolumn{5}{c}{External Cause (E-Code)}

Substance	Poisoning	Accident	Therapeutic Use	Suicide Attempt	Assault	Undetermined
fungicide	989.4	E863.6	—	E950.6	E962.1	E980.7
pesticide (fumes)	989.4	E863.4	—	E950.6	E962.1	E980.7
Chloroprocaine	968.9	E855.2	E938.9	E950.4	E962.0	E980.4
infiltration (subcutaneous)	968.5	E855.2	E938.5	E950.4	E962.0	E980.4
nerve block (peripheral) (plexus)	968.6	E855.2	E938.6	E950.4	E962.0	E980.4
Chloroptic	976.5	E858.7	E946.5	E950.4	E962.0	E980.4
Chloropurine	963.1	E858.1	E933.1	E950.4	E962.0	E980.4
Chloroquine (hydrochloride) (phosphate)	961.4	E857	E931.4	E950.4	E962.0	E980.4
Chlorothen	963.0	E858.1	E933.0	E950.4	E962.0	E980.4
Chlorothiazide	974.3	E858.5	E944.3	E950.4	E962.0	E980.4
Chlorotrianisene	962.2	E858.0	E932.2	E950.4	E962.0	E980.4
Chlorovinyldichloroarsine	985.1	E866.3	—	E950.8	E962.1	E980.8
Chloroxylenol	976.0	E858.7	E946.0	E950.4	E962.0	E980.4
Chlorphenesin (carbamate)	968.0	E855.1	E938.0	E950.4	E962.0	E980.4
topical (antifungal)	976.0	E858.7	E946.0	E950.4	E962.0	E980.4
Chlorpheniramine	963.0	E858.1	E933.0	E950.4	E962.0	E980.4
Chlorophenoxamine	966.4	E855.0	E936.4	E950.4	E962.0	E980.4
Chlorophentermine	977.0	E858.8	E947.0	E950.4	E962.0	E980.4
Chlorproguanil	961.4	E857	E931.4	E950.4	E962.0	E980.4
Chlorpromazine	969.1	E853.0	E939.1	E950.3	E962.0	E980.3
Chlorpropamide	962.3	E858.0	E932.3	E950.4	E962.0	E980.4
Chlorprothixene	969.3	E853.8	E939.3	E950.3	E962.0	E980.3
Chlorquinaldol	976.0	E858.7	E946.0	E950.4	E962.0	E980.4
Chlortetracycline	960.4	E856	E930.4	E950.4	E962.0	E980.4
Chlorthalidone	974.4	E858.5	E944.4	E950.4	E962.0	E980.4
Chlortrianisene	962.2	E858.0	E932.2	E950.4	E962.0	E980.4
Chlor–Trimeton	963.0	E858.1	E933.0	E950.4	E962.0	E980.4
Chlorzoxazone	968.0	E855.1	E938.0	E950.4	E962.0	E980.4
Choke damp	987.8	E869.8	—	E952.8	E962.2	E982.8
Cholebrine	977.8	E858.8	E947.8	E950.4	E962.0	E980.4
Cholera vaccine	978.2	E858.8	E948.2	E950.4	E962.0	E980.4
Cholesterol–lowering agents	972.2	E858.3	E942.2	E950.4	E962.0	E980.4
Cholestyramine (resin)	972.2	E858.3	E942.2	E950.4	E962.0	E980.4
Cholic acid	973.4	E858.4	E943.4	E950.4	E962.0	E980.4
Choline						
dihydrogen citrate	977.1	E858.8	E947.1	E950.4	E962.0	E980.4
salicylate	965.1	E850.3	E935.3	E950.0	E962.0	E980.0
theophyllinate	974.1	E858.5	E944.1	E950.4	E962.0	E980.4
Cholinergics	971.0	E855.3	E941.0	E950.4	E962.0	E980.4
Cholografin	977.8	E858.8	E947.8	E950.4	E962.0	E980.4
Chorionic gonadotropin	962.4	E858.0	E932.4	E950.4	E962.0	E980.4
Chromates	983.9	E864.3	—	E950.7	E962.1	E980.6
dust or mist	987.8	E869.8	—	E952.8	E962.2	E982.8
lead	984.0	E866.0	—	E950.9	E962.1	E980.9
paint	984.0	E861.5	—	E950.9	E962.1	E980.9
Chromic acid	983.9	E864.3	—	E950.7	E962.1	E980.6
dust or mist	987.8	E869.8	—	E952.8	E962.2	E982.8
Chromium	985.6	E866.4	—	E950.9	E962.1	E980.9
compounds — see Chromates						
Chromonar	972.4	E858.3	E942.4	E950.4	E962.0	E980.4
Chromyl chloride	983.9	E864.3	—	E950.7	E962.1	E980.6
Chrysarobin (ointment)	976.4	E858.7	E946.4	E950.4	E962.0	E980.4
Chrysazin	973.1	E858.4	E943.1	E950.4	E962.0	E980.4
Chymar	963.4	E858.1	E933.4	E950.4	E962.0	E980.4
ophthalmic preparation	976.5	E858.7	E946.5	E950.4	E962.0	E980.4
Chymotrypsin	963.4	E858.1	E933.4	E950.4	E962.0	E980.4
ophthalmic preparation	976.5	E858.7	E946.5	E950.4	E962.0	E980.4
Cicuta maculata or virosa	988.2	E865.4	—	E950.9	E962.1	E980.9
Cigarette lighter fluid	981	E862.1	—	E950.9	E962.1	E980.9
Cinchocaine (spinal)	968.7	E855.2	E938.7	E950.4	E962.0	E980.4

TABLE OF DRUGS AND CHEMICALS

Substance	Poisoning	Accident	Therapeutic Use	Suicide Attempt	Assault	Undetermined
		\multicolumn{5}{c}{External Cause (E-Code)}				
topical (surface)	968.5	E855.2	E938.5	E950.4	E962.0	E980.4
Cinchona	961.4	E857	E931.4	E950.4	E962.0	E980.4
Cinchonine alkaloids	961.4	E857	E931.4	E950.4	E962.0	E980.4
Cinchophen	974.7	E858.5	E944.7	E950.4	E962.0	E980.4
Cinnarizine	963.0	E858.1	E933.0	E950.4	E962.0	E980.4
Citanest	968.9	E855.2	E938.9	E950.4	E962.0	E980.4
infiltration (subcutaneous)	968.5	E855.2	E938.5	E950.4	E962.0	E980.4
nerve block (peripheral) (plexus)	968.6	E855.2	E938.6	E950.4	E962.0	E980.4
Citric acid	989.89	E866.8	—	E950.9	E962.1	E980.9
Citrovorum factor	964.1	E858.2	E934.1	E950.4	E962.0	E980.4
Claviceps purpurea	988.2	E865.4	—	E950.9	E962.1	E980.9
Cleaner, cleansing agent NEC	989.89	E861.3	—	E950.9	E962.1	E980.9
of paint or varnish	982.8	E862.9	—	E950.9	E962.1	E980.9
Clematis vitalba	988.2	E865.4	—	E950.9	E962.1	E980.9
Clemizole	963.0	E858.1	E933.0	E950.4	E962.0	E980.4
penicillin	960.0	E856	E930.0	E950.4	E962.0	E980.4
Clidinium	971.1	E855.4	E941.1	E950.4	E962.0	E980.4
Clindamycin	960.8	E856	E930.8	E950.4	E962.0	E980.4
Cliradon	965.09	E850.2	E935.2	E950	E962.0	E980.0
Clocortolone	962.0	E858.0	E932.0	E950.4	E962.0	E980.4
Clofedanol	975.4	E858.6	E945.4	E950.4	E962.0	E980.4
Clofibrate	972.2	E858.3	E942.2	E950.4	E962.0	E980.4
Clomethiazole	967.1	E852.0	E937.1	E950.2	E962.0	E980.2
Clomiphene	977.8	E858.8	E947.8	E950.4	E962.0	E980.4
Clonazepam	969.4	E853.2	E939.4	E950.3	E962.0	E980.3
Clonidine	972.6	E858.3	E942.6	E950.4	E962.0	E980.4
Clopamide	974.3	E858.5	E944.3	E950.4	E962.0	E980.4
Clorazepate	969.4	E853.2	E939.4	E950.3	E962.0	E980.3
Clorexolone	974.4	E858.5	E944.4	E950.4	E962.0	E980.4
Clorox (bleach)	983.9	E864.3	—	E950.7	E962.1	E980.6
Clortermine	977.0	E858.8	E947.0	E950.4	E962.0	E980.4
Clotrimazole	976.0	E858.7	E946.0	E950.4	E962.0	E980.4
Cloxacillin	960.0	E856	E930.0	E950.4	E962.0	E980.4
Coagulants NEC	964.5	E858.2	E934.5	E950.4	E962.0	E980.4
Coal (carbon monoxide from) — *see also* Carbon, monoxide, coal						
oil — *see* Kerosene						
tar NEC	983.0	E864.0	—	E950.7	E962.1	E980.6
fumes	987.8	E869.8	—	E952.8	E962.2	E982.8
medicinal (ointment)	976.4	E858.7	E946.4	E950.4	E962.0	E980.4
analgesics NEC	965.5	E850.5	E935.5	E950	E962.0	E980.0
naphtha (solvent)	981	E862.0	—	E950.9	E962.1	E980.9
Cobalt (fumes) (industrial)	985.8	E866.4	—	E950.9	E962.1	E980.9
Cobra (venom)	989.5	E905.0	—	E950.9	E962.1	E980.9
Coca (leaf)	970.8	E854.3	E940.8	E950.4	E962.0	E980.4
Cocaine (hydrochloride) (salt)	970.8	E854.3	E940.8	E950.4	E962.0	E980.4
topical anesthetic	968.5	E855.2	E938.5	E950.4	E962.0	E980.4
Coccidioidin	977.8	E858.8	E947.8	E950.4	E962.0	E980.4
Cocculus indicus	988.2	E865.3	—	E950.9	E962.1	E980.9
Cochineal	989.89	E866.8	—	E950.9	E962.1	E980.9
medicinal products	977.4	E858.8	E947.4	E950.4	E962.0	E980.4
Codeine	965.09	E850.2	E935.2	E950	E962.0	E980.0
Coffee	989.89	E866.8	—	E950.9	E962.1	E980.9
Cogentin	971.1	E855.4	E941.1	E950.4	E962.0	E980.4
Coke fumes or gas (carbon monoxide)	986	E868.3	—	E952.1	E962.2	E982.1
industrial use	986	E868.8	—	E952.1	E962.2	E982.1
Colace	973.2	E858.4	E943.2	E950.4	E962.0	E980.4
Colchicine	974.7	E858.5	E944.7	E950.4	E962.0	E980.4
Colchicum	988.2	E865.3	—	E950.9	E962.1	E980.9
Cold cream	976.3	E858.7	E946.3	E950.4	E962.0	E980.4
Colestipol	972.2	E858.3	E942.2	E950.4	E962.0	E980.4

1433

TABLE OF DRUGS AND CHEMICALS

Substance	Poisoning	Accident	Therapeutic Use	Suicide Attempt	Assault	Undetermined
		\multicolumn{5}{c}{External Cause (E-Code)}				

Substance	Poisoning	Accident	Therapeutic Use	Suicide Attempt	Assault	Undetermined
Colistimethate	960.8	E856	E930.8	E950.4	E962.0	E980.4
Colistin	960.8	E856	E930.8	E950.4	E962.0	E980.4
Collagen	977.8	E866.8	E947.8	E950.9	E962.1	E980.9
Collagenase	976.8	E858.7	E946.8	E950.4	E962.0	E980.4
Collodion (flexible)	976.3	E858.7	E946.3	E950.4	E962.0	E980.4
Colocynth	973.1	E858.4	E943.1	E950.4	E962.0	E980.4
Coloring matter — see Dye(s)						
Combustion gas — see Carbon, monoxide						
Compazine	969.1	E853.0	E939.1	E950.3	E962.0	E980.3
Compound						
42 (warfarin)	989.4	E863.7	—	E950.6	E962.1	E980.7
269 (endrin)	989.2	E863.0	—	E950.6	E962.1	E980.7
497 (dieldrin)	989.2	E863.0	—	E950.6	E962.1	E980.7
1080 (sodium fluoroacetate)	989.4	E863.7	—	E950.6	E962.1	E980.7
3422 (parathion)	989.3	E863.1	—	E950.6	E962.1	E980.7
3911 (phorate)	989.3	E863.1	—	E950.6	E962.1	E980.7
3956 (toxaphene)	989.2	E863.0	—	E950.6	E962.1	E980.7
4049 (malathion)	989.3	E863.1	—	E950.6	E962.1	E980.7
4124 (dicapthon)	989.4	E863.4	—	E950.6	E962.1	E980.7
E (cortisone)	962.0	E858.0	E932.0	E950.4	E962.0	E980.4
F (hydrocortisone)	962.0	E858.0	E932.0	E950.4	E962.0	E980.4
Congo red	977.8	E858.8	E947.8	E950.4	E962.0	E980.4
Coniine, conine	965.7	E850.7	E935.7	E950.0	E962.0	E980
Conium (maculatum)	988.2	E865.4	—	E950.9	E962.1	E980.9
Conjugated estrogens (equine)	962.2	E858.0	E932.2	E950.4	E962.0	E980.4
Contac	975.6	E858.6	E945.6	E950.4	E962.0	E980.4
Contact lens solution	976.5	E858.7	E946.5	E950.4	E962.0	E980.4
Contraceptives (oral)	962.2	E858.0	E932.2	E950.4	E962.0	E980.4
vaginal	976.8	E858.7	E946.8	E950.4	E962.0	E980.4
Contrast media (roentgenographic)	977.8	E858.8	E947.8	E950.4	E962.0	E980.4
Convallaria majalis	988.2	E865.4	—	E950.9	E962.1	E980.9
Copper (dust) (fumes) (salts) NEC	985.8	E866.4	—	E950.9	E962.1	E980.9
arsenate, arsenite	985.1	E866.3	—	E950.8	E962.1	E980.8
insecticide	985.1	E863.4	—	E950.6	E962.1	E980.8
emetic	973.6	E858.4	E943.6	E950.4	E962.0	E980.4
fungicide	985.8	E863.6	—	E950.6	E962.1	E980.7
insecticide	985.8	E863.4	—	E950.6	E962.1	E980.7
oleate	976.0	E858.7	E946.0	E950.4	E962.0	E980.4
sulfate	983.9	E864.3	—	E950.7	E962.1	E980.6
fungicide	983.9	E863.6	—	E950.7	E962.1	E980.6
cupric	973.6	E858.4	E943.6	E950.4	E962.0	E980.4
cuprous	983.9	E864.3	—	E950.7	E962.1	E980.6
Copperhead snake (bite) (venom)	989.5	E905.0	—	E950.9	E962.1	E980.9
Coral (sting)	989.5	E905.6	—	E950.9	E962.1	E980.9
snake (bite) (venom)	989.5	E905.0	—	E950.9	E962.1	E980.9
Cordran	976.0	E858.7	E946.0	E950.4	E962.0	E980.4
Corn cures	976.4	E858.7	E946.4	E950.4	E962.0	E980.4
Cornhusker's lotion	976.3	E858.7	E946.3	E950.4	E962.0	E980.4
Corn starch	976.3	E858.7	E946.3	E950.4	E962.0	E980.4
Corrosive	983.9	E864.4	—	E950.7	E962.1	E980.6
acids NEC	983.1	E864.1	—	E950.7	E962.1	E980.6
aromatics	983.0	E864.0	—	E950.7	E962.1	E980.6
disinfectant	983.0	E861.4	—	E950.7	E962.1	E980.6
fumes NEC	987.9	E869.9	—	E952.9	E962.2	E982.9
specified NEC	983.9	E864.3	—	E950.7	E962.1	E980.6
sublimate — see Mercury, chloride						
Cortate	962.0	E858.0	E932.0	E950.4	E962.0	E980.4
Cort–Dome	962.0	E858.0	E932.0	E950.4	E962.0	E980.4
ENT agent	976.6	E858.7	E946.6	E950.4	E962.0	E980.4
ophthalmic preparation	976.5	E858.7	E946.5	E950.4	E962.0	E980.4

TABLE OF DRUGS AND CHEMICALS

Substance	Poisoning	Accident	Therapeutic Use	Suicide Attempt	Assault	Undetermined
		\multicolumn{5}{c}{External Cause (E-Code)}
topical NEC	976.0	E858.7	E946.0	E950.4	E962.0	E980.4
Cortef	962.0	E858.0	E932.0	E950.4	E962.0	E980.4
ENT agent	976.6	E858.7	E946.6	E950.4	E962.0	E980.4
ophthalmic preparation	976.5	E858.7	E946.5	E950.4	E962.0	E980.4
topical NEC	976.0	E858.7	E946.0	E950.4	E962.0	E980.4
Corticosteroids (fluorinated)	962.0	E858.0	E932.0	E950.4	E962.0	E980.4
ENT agent	976.6	E858.7	E946.6	E950.4	E962.0	E980.4
ophthalmic preparation	976.5	E858.7	E946.5	E950.4	E962.0	E980.4
topical NEC	976.0	E858.7	E946.0	E950.4	E962.0	E980.4
Corticotropin	962.4	E858.0	E932.4	E950.4	E962.0	E980.4
Cortisol	962.0	E858.0	E932.0	E950.4	E962.0	E980.4
ENT agent	976.6	E858.7	E946.6	E950.4	E962.0	E980.4
ophthalmic preparation	976.5	E858.7	E946.5	E950.4	E962.0	E980.4
topical NEC	976.0	E858.7	E946.0	E950.4	E962.0	E980.4
Cortisone derivatives (acetate)	962.0	E858.0	E932.0	E950.4	E962.0	E980.4
ENT agent	976.6	E858.7	E946.6	E950.4	E962.0	E980.4
ophthalmic preparation	976.5	E858.7	E946.5	E950.4	E962.0	E980.4
topical NEC	976.0	E858.7	E946.0	E950.4	E962.0	E980.4
Cortogen	962.0	E858.0	E932.0	E950.4	E962.0	E980.4
ENT agent	976.6	E858.7	E946.6	E950.4	E962.0	E980.4
ophthalmic preparation	976.5	E858.7	E946.5	E950.4	E962.0	E980.4
Cortone	962.0	E858.0	E932.0	E950.4	E962.0	E980.4
ENT agent	976.6	E858.7	E946.6	E950.4	E962.0	E980.4
ophthalmic preparation	976.5	E858.7	E946.5	E950.4	E962.0	E980.4
Cortril	962.0	E858.0	E932.0	E950.4	E962.0	E980.4
ENT agent	976.6	E858.7	E946.6	E950.4	E962.0	E980.4
ophthalmic preparation	976.5	E858.7	E946.5	E950.4	E962.0	E980.4
topical NEC	976.0	E858.7	E946.0	E950.4	E962.0	E980.4
Cosmetics	989.89	E866.7	—	E950.9	E962.1	E980.9
Cosyntropin	977.8	E858.8	E947.8	E950.4	E962.0	E980.4
Cotarnine	964.5	E858.2	E934.5	E950.4	E962.0	E980.4
Cottonseed oil	976.3	E858.7	E946.3	E950.4	E962.0	E980.4
Cough mixtures (antitussives)	975.4	E858.6	E945.4	E950.4	E962.0	E980.4
containing opiates	965.09	E850.2	E935.2	E950.0	E962.0	E980.0
expectorants	975.5	E858.6	E945.5	E950.4	E962.0	E980.4
Coumadin	964.2	E858.2	E934.2	E950.4	E962.0	E980.4
rodenticide	989.4	E863.7	—	E950.6	E962.1	E980.7
Coumarin	964.2	E858.2	E934.2	E950.4	E962.0	E980.4
Coumetarol	964.2	E858.2	E934.2	E950.4	E962.0	E980.4
Cowbane	988.2	E865.4	—	E950.9	E962.1	E980.9
Cozyme	963.5	E858.1	E933.5	E950.4	E962.0	E980.4
Crack	970.8	E854.3	E940.8	E950.4	E962.0	E980.4
Creolin	983.0	E864.0	—	E950.7	E962.1	E980.6
disinfectant	983.0	E861.4	—	E950.7	E962.1	E980.6
Creosol (compound)	983.0	E864.0	—	E950.7	E962.1	E980.6
Creosote (beechwood) (coal tar)	983.0	E864.0	—	E950.7	E962.1	E980.6
medicinal (expectorant)	975.5	E858.6	E945.5	E950.4	E962.0	E980.4
syrup	975.5	E858.6	E945.5	E950.4	E962.0	E980.4
Cresol	983.0	E864.0	—	E950.7	E962.1	E980.6
disinfectant	983.0	E861.4	—	E950.7	E962.1	E980.6
Cresylic acid	983.0	E864.0	—	E950.7	E962.1	E980.6
Cropropamide	965.7	E850.7	E935.7	E950.0	E962.0	E980.0
with crotethamide	970.0	E854.3	E940.0	E950.4	E962.0	E980.4
Crotamiton	976.0	E858.7	E946.0	E950.4	E962.0	E980.4
Crotethamide	965.7	E850.7	E935.7	E950.0	E962.0	E980.0
with cropropamide	970.0	E854.3	E940.0	E950.4	E962.0	E980.4
Croton (oil)	973.1	E858.4	E943.1	E950.4	E962.0	E980.4
chloral	967.1	E852.0	E937.1	E950.2	E962.0	E980.2
Crude oil	981	E862.1	—	E950.9	E962.1	E980.9
Cryogenine	965.8	E850.8	E935.8	E950.0	E962.0	E980.0
Cryolite (pesticide)	989.4	E863.4	—	E950.6	E962.1	E980.7

1435

TABLE OF DRUGS AND CHEMICALS

Substance	Poisoning	Accident	Therapeutic Use	Suicide Attempt	Assault	Undetermined
			External Cause (E-Code)			
Cryptenamine	972.6	E858.3	E942.6	E950.4	E962.0	E980.4
Crystal violet	976.0	E858.7	E946.0	E950.4	E962.0	E980.4
Cuckoopint	988.2	E865.4	—	E950.9	E962.1	E980.9
Cumetharol	964.2	E858.2	E934.2	E950.4	E962.0	E980.4
Cupric sulfate	973.6	E858.4	E943.6	E950.4	E962.0	E980.4
Cuprous sulfate	983.9	E864.3	—	E950.7	E962.1	E980.6
Curare, curarine	975.2	E858.6	E945.2	E950.4	E962.0	E980.4
Cyanic acid — *see* Cyanide(s)						
Cyanide(s) (compounds) (hydrogen)						
(potassium) (sodium) NEC	989.0	E866.8	—	E950.9	E962.1	E980.9
dust or gas (inhalation) NEC	987.7	E869.8	—	E952.8	E962.2	E982.8
fumigant	989.0	E863.8	—	E950.6	E962.1	E980.7
mercuric — *see* Mercury						
pesticide (dust) (fumes)	989.0	E863.4	—	E950.6	E962.1	E980.7
Cyanocobalamin	964.1	E858.2	E934.1	E950.4	E962.0	E980.4
Cyanogen (chloride) (gas) NEC	987.8	E869.8	—	E952.8	E962.2	E982.8
Cyclaine	968.5	E855.2	E938.5	E950.4	E962.0	E980.4
Cyclamen europaeum	988.2	E865.4	—	E950.9	E962.1	E980.9
Cyclandelate	972.5	E858.3	E942.5	E950.4	E962.0	E980.4
Cyclazocine	965.09	E850.2	E935.2	E950.0	E962.0	E980.0
Cyclizine	963.0	E858.1	E933.0	E950.4	E962.0	E980.4
Cyclobarbital, cyclobarbitone	967.0	E851	E937.0	E950.1	E962.0	E980.1
Cycloguanil	961.4	E857	E931.4	E950.4	E962.0	E980.4
Cyclohexane	982.0	E862.4	—	E950.9	E962.1	E980.9
Cyclohexanol	980.8	E860.8	—	E950.9	E962.1	E980.9
Cyclohexanone	982.8	E862.4	—	E950.9	E962.1	E980.9
Cyclomethycaine	968.5	E855.2	E938.5	E950.4	E962.0	E980.4
Cyclopentamine	971.2	E855.5	E941.2	E950.4	E962.0	E980.4
Cyclopenthiazide	974.3	E858.5	E944.3	E950.4	E962.0	E980.4
Cyclopentolate	971.1	E855.4	E941.1	E950.4	E962.0	E980.4
Cyclophosphamide	963.1	E858.1	E933.1	E950.4	E962.0	E980.4
Cyclopropane	968.2	E855.1	E938.2	E950.4	E962.0	E980.4
Cycloserine	960.6	E856	E930.6	E950.4	E962.0	E980.4
Cyclothiazide	974.3	E858.5	E944.3	E950.4	E962.0	E980.4
Cycrimine	966.4	E855.0	E936.4	E950.4	E962.0	E980.4
Cymarin	972.1	E858.3	E942.1	E950.4	E962.0	E980.4
Cyproheptadine	963.0	E858.1	E933.0	E950.4	E962.0	E980.4
Cyprolidol	969.0	E854.0	E939.0	E950.3	E962.0	E980.3
Cytarabine	963.1	E858.1	E933.1	E950.4	E962.0	E980.4
Cytisus						
laburnum	988.2	E865.4	—	E950.9	E962.1	E980.9
scoparius	988.2	E865.4	—	E950.9	E962.1	E980.9
Cytomel	962.7	E858.0	E932.7	E950.4	E962.0	E980.4
Cytosine (antineoplastic)	963.1	E858.1	E933.1	E950.4	E962.0	E980.4
Cytoxan	963.1	E858.1	E933.1	E950.4	E962.0	E980.4
Dacarbazine	963.1	E858.1	E933.1	E950.4	E962.0	E980.4
Dactinomycin	960.7	E856	E930.7	E950.4	E962.0	E980.4
DADPS	961.8	E857	E931.8	E950.4	E962.0	E980.4
Dakin's solution (external)	976.0	E858.7	E946.0	E950.4	E962.0	E980.4
Dalmane	969.4	E853.2	E939.4	E950.3	E962.0	E980.3
DAM	977.2	E858.8	E947.2	E950.4	E962.0	E980.4
Danilone	964.2	E858.2	E934.2	E950.4	E962.0	E980.4
Danthron	973.1	E858.4	E943.1	E950.4	E962.0	E980.4
Dantrolene	975.2	E858.6	E945.2	E950.4	E962.0	E980.4
Daphne (gnidium) (mezereum)	988.2	E865.4	—	E950.9	E962.1	E980.9
berry	988.2	E865.3	—	E950.9	E962.1	E980.9
Dapsone	961.8	E857	E931.8	E950.4	E962.0	E980.4
Daraprim	961.4	E857	E931.4	E950.4	E962.0	E980.4
Darnel	988.2	E865.3	—	E950.9	E962.1	E980.9
Darvon	965.8	E850.8	E935.8	E950.0	E962.0	E980.0

TABLE OF DRUGS AND CHEMICALS

Substance	Poisoning	Accident	Therapeutic Use	Suicide Attempt	Assault	Undetermined
		\multicolumn{5}{c}{External Cause (E-Code)}

Substance	Poisoning	Accident	Therapeutic Use	Suicide Attempt	Assault	Undetermined
Daunorubicin	960.7	E856	E930.7	E950.4	E962.0	E980.4
DBI	962.3	E858.0	E932.3	E950.4	E962.0	E980.4
D–Con (rodenticide)	989.4	E863.7	—	E950.6	E962.1	E980.7
DDS	961.8	E857	E931.8	E950.4	E962.0	E980.4
DDT	989.2	E863.0	—	E950.6	E962.1	E980.7
Deadly nightshade	988.2	E865.4	—	E950.9	E962.1	E980.9
berry	988.2	E865.3	—	E950.9	E962.1	E980.9
Deanol	969.7	E854.2	E939.7	E950.3	E962.0	E980.3
Debrisoquine	972.6	E858.3	E942.6	E950.4	E962.0	E980.4
Decaborane	989.89	E866.8	—	E950.9	E962.1	E980.9
fumes	987.8	E869.8	—	E952.8	E962.2	E982.8
Decadron	962.0	E858.0	E932.0	E950.4	E962.0	E980.4
ENT agent	976.6	E858.7	E946.6	E950.4	E962.0	E980.4
ophthalmic preparation	976.5	E858.7	E946.5	E950.4	E962.0	E980.4
topical NEC	976.0	E858.7	E946.0	E950.4	E962.0	E980.4
Decahydronaphthalene	982.0	E862.4	—	E950.9	E962.1	E980.9
Decalin	982.0	E862.4	—	E950.9	E962.1	E980.9
Decamethonium	975.2	E858.6	E945.2	E950.4	E962.0	E980.4
Decholin	973.4	E858.4	E943.4	E950.4	E962.0	E980.4
sodium (diagnostic)	977.8	E858.8	E947.8	E950.4	E962.0	E980.4
Declomycin	960.4	E856	E930.4	E950.4	E962.0	E980.4
Deferoxamine	963.8	E858.1	E933.8	E950.4	E962.0	E980.4
Dehydrocholic acid	973.4	E858.4	E943.4	E950.4	E962.0	E980.4
DeKalin	982.0	E862.4	—	E950.9	E962.1	E980.9
Delalutin	962.2	E858.0	E932.2	E950.4	E962.0	E980.4
Delphinium	988.2	E865.3	—	E950.9	E962.1	E980.9
Deltasone	962.0	E858.0	E932.0	E950.4	E962.0	E980.4
Deltra	962.0	E858.0	E932.0	E950.4	E962.0	E980.4
Delvinal	967.0	E851	E937.0	E950.1	E962.0	E980.1
Demecarium (bromide)	971.0	E855.3	E941.0	E950.4	E962.0	E980.4
Demeclocycline	960.4	E856	E930.4	E950.4	E962.0	E980.4
Demecolcine	963.1	E858.1	E933.1	E950.4	E962.0	E980.4
Demelanizing agents	976.8	E858.7	E946.8	E950.4	E962.0	E980.4
Demerol	965.09	E850.2	E935.2	E950.0	E962.0	E980.0
Demethylchlortetracycline	960.4	E856	E930.4	E950.4	E962.0	E980.4
Demethyltetracycline	960.4	E856	E930.4	E950.4	E962.0	E980.4
Demeton	989.3	E863.1	—	E950.6	E962.1	E980.7
Demulcents	976.3	E858.7	E946.3	E950.4	E962.0	E980.4
Demulen	962.2	E858.0	E932.2	E950.4	E962.0	E980.4
Denatured alcohol	980.0	E860.1	—	E950.9	E962.1	E980.9
Dendrid	976.5	E858.7	E946.5	E950.4	E962.0	E980.4
Dental agents, topical	976.7	E858.7	E946.7	E950.4	E962.0	E980.4
Deodorant spray (feminine hygiene)	976.8	E858.7	E946.8	E950.4	E962.0	E980.4
Deoxyribonuclease	963.4	E858.1	E933.4	E950.4	E962.0	E980.4
Depressants						
appetite, central	977.0	E858.8	E947.0	E950.4	E962.0	E980.4
cardiac	972.0	E858.3	E942.0	E950.4	E962.0	E980.4
central nervous system (anesthetic)	968.4	E855.1	E938.4	E950.4	E962.0	E980.4
psychotherapeutic	969.5	E853.9	E939.5	E950.3	E962.0	E980.3
Dequalinium	976.0	E858.7	E946.0	E950.4	E962.0	E980.4
Dermolate	976.2	E858.7	E946.2	E950.4	E962.0	E980.4
DES	962.2	E858.0	E932.2	E950.4	E962.0	E980.4
Desenex	976.0	E858.7	E946.0	E950.4	E962.0	E980.4
Deserpidine	972.6	E858.3	E942.6	E950.4	E962.0	E980.4
Desipramine	969.0	E854.0	E939.0	E950.3	E962.0	E980.3
Deslanoside	972.1	E858.3	E942.1	E950.4	E962.0	E980.4
Desocodeine	965.09	E850.2	E935.2	E950.0	E962.0	E980.0
Desomorphine	965.09	E850.2	E935.2	E950.0	E962.0	E980.0
Desonide	976.0	E858.7	E946.0	E950.4	E962.0	E980.4
Desoxycorticosterone derivatives	962.0	E858.0	E932.0	E950.4	E962.0	E980.4
Desoxyephedrine	969.7	E854.2	E939.7	E950.3	E962.0	E980.3

1437

TABLE OF DRUGS AND CHEMICALS

Substance	Poisoning	Accident	Therapeutic Use	Suicide Attempt	Assault	Undetermined
			External Cause (E-Code)			
DET	969.6	E854.1	E939.6	E950.3	E962.0	E980.3
Detergents (ingested) (synthetic)	989.6	E861.0	—	E950.9	E962.1	E980.9
external medication	976.2	E858.7	E946.2	E950.4	E962.0	E980.4
Deterrent, alcohol	977.3	E858.8	E947.3	E950.4	E962.0	E980.4
Detrothyronine	962.7	E858.0	E932.7	E950.4	E962.0	E980.4
Dettol (external medication)	976.0	E858.7	E946.0	E950.4	E962.0	E980.4
Dexamethasone	962.0	E858.0	E932.0	E950.4	E962.0	E980.4
ENT agent	976.6	E858.7	E946.6	E950.4	E962.0	E980.4
ophthalmic preparation	976.5	E858.7	E946.5	E950.4	E962.0	E980.4
topical NEC	976.0	E858.7	E946.0	E950.4	E962.0	E980.4
Dexamphetamine	969.7	E854.2	E939.7	E950.3	E962.0	E980.3
Dexedrine	969.7	E854.2	E939.7	E950.3	E962.0	E980.3
Dexpanthenol	963.5	E858.1	E933.5	E950.4	E962.0	E980.4
Dextran	964.8	E858.2	E934.8	E950.4	E962.0	E980.4
Dextriferron	964.0	E858.2	E934.0	E950.4	E962.0	E980.4
Dextroamphetamine	969.7	E854.2	E939.7	E950.3	E962.0	E980.3
Dextro calcium pantothenate	963.5	E858.1	E933.5	E950.4	E962.0	E980.4
Dextromethorphan	975.4	E858.6	E945.4	E950.4	E962.0	E980.4
Dextromoramide	965.09	E850.2	E935.2	E950.0	E962.0	E980.0
Dextro pantothenyl alcohol	963.5	E858.1	E933.5	E950.4	E962.0	E980.4
topical	976.8	E858.7	E946.8	E950.4	E962.0	E980.4
Dextropropoxyphene (hydrochloride)	965.8	E850.8	E935.8	E950.0	E962.0	E980.0
Dextrorphan	965.09	E850.2	E935.2	E950.0	E962.0	E980.0
Dextrose NEC	974.5	E858.5	E944.5	E950.4	E962.0	E980.4
Dextrothyroxin	962.7	E858.0	E932.7	E950.4	E962.0	E980.4
DFP	971.0	E855.3	E941.0	E950.4	E962.0	E980.4
DHE–45	972.9	E858.3	E942.9	E950.4	E962.0	E980.4
Diabinese	962.3	E858.0	E932.3	E950.4	E962.0	E980.4
Diacetyl monoxime	977.2	E858.8	E947.2	E950.4	E962.0	E980.4
Diacetylmorphine	965.01	E850.0	E935.0	E950.0	E962.0	E980.0
Diagnostic agents	977.8	E858.8	E947.8	E950.4	E962.0	E980.4
Dial (soap)	976.2	E858.7	E946.2	E950.4	E962.0	E980.4
sedative	967.0	E851	E937.0	E950.1	E962.0	E980.1
Diallylbarbituric acid	967.0	E851	E937.0	E950.1	E962.0	E980.1
Diaminodiphenylsulfone	961.8	E857	E931.8	E950.4	E962.0	E980.4
Diamorphine	965.01	E850.0	E935.0	E950.0	E962.0	E980.0
Diamox	974.2	E858.5	E944.2	E950.4	E962.0	E980.4
Diamthazole	976.0	E858.7	E946.0	E950.4	E962.0	E980.4
Diaphenylsulfone	961.8	E857	E931.8	E950.4	E962.0	E980.4
Diasone (sodium)	961.8	E857	E931.8	E950.4	E962.0	E980.4
Diazepam	969.4	E853.2	E939.4	E950.3	E962.0	E980.3
Diazinon	989.3	E863.1	—	E950.6	E962.1	E980.7
Diazomethane (gas)	987.8	E869.8	—	E952.8	E962.2	E982.8
Diazoxide	972.5	E858.3	E942.5	E950.4	E962.0	E980.4
Dibenamine	971.3	E855.6	E941.3	E950.4	E962.0	E980.4
Dibenzheptropine	963.0	E858.1	E933.0	E950.4	E962.0	E980.4
Dibenzyline	971.3	E855.6	E941.3	E950.4	E962.0	E980.4
Diborane (gas)	987.8	E869.8	—	E952.8	E962.2	E982.8
Dibromomannitol	963.1	E858.1	E933.1	E950.4	E962.0	E980.4
Dibucaine (spinal)	968.7	E855.2	E938.7	E950.4	E962.0	E980.4
topical (surface)	968.5	E855.2	E938.5	E950.4	E962.0	E980.4
Dibunate sodium	975.4	E858.6	E945.4	E950.4	E962.0	E980.4
Dibutoline	971.1	E855.4	E941.1	E950.4	E962.0	E980.4
Dicapthon	989.4	E863.4	—	E950.6	E962.1	E980.7
Dichloralphenazone	967.1	E852.0	E937.1	E950.2	E962.0	E980.2
Dichlorodifluoromethane	987.4	E869.2	—	E952.8	E962.2	E982.8
Dichloroethane	982.3	E862.4	—	E950.9	E962.1	E980.9
Dichloroethylene	982.3	E862.4	—	E950.9	E962.1	E980.9
Dichloroethyl sulfide	987.8	E869.8	—	E952.8	E962.2	E982.8
Dichlorohydrin	982.3	E862.4	—	E950.9	E962.1	E980.9

TABLE OF DRUGS AND CHEMICALS

Substance	Poisoning	Accident	Therapeutic Use	Suicide Attempt	Assault	Undetermined
			External Cause (E-Code)			
Dichloromethane (solvent) (vapor)	982.3	E862.4	—	E950.9	E962.1	E980.9
Dichlorophen(e)	961.6	E857	E931.6	E950.4	E962.0	E980.4
Dichlorphenamide	974.2	E858.5	E944.2	E950.4	E962.0	E980.4
Dichlorvos	989.3	E863.1	—	E950.6	E962.1	E980.7
Diclofenac sodium	965.69	E850.6	E935.6	E950.0	E962.0	E980.0
Dicoumarin, dicumarol	964.2	E858.2	E934.2	E950.4	E962.0	E980.4
Dicyanogen (gas)	987.8	E869.8	—	E952.8	E962.2	E982.8
Dicyclomine	971.1	E855.4	E941.1	E950.4	E962.0	E980.4
Dieldrin (vapor)	989.2	E863.0	—	E950.6	E962.1	E980.7
Dienestrol	962.2	E858.0	E932.2	E950.4	E962.0	E980.4
Dietetics	977.0	E858.8	E947.0	E950.4	E962.0	E980.4
Diethazine	966.4	E855.0	E936.4	E950.4	E962.0	E980.4
Diethyl						
barbituric acid	967.0	E851	E937.0	E950.1	E962.0	E980.1
carbamazene	961.6	E857	E931.6	E950.4	E962.0	E980.4
carbinol	980.8	E860.8	—	E950.9	E962.1	E980.9
carbonate	982.8	E862.4	—	E950.9	E962.1	E980.9
ether (vapor) — see Ether(s)						
propion	977.0	E858.8	E947.0	E950.4	E962.0	E980.4
stilbestrol	962.2	E858.0	E932.2	E950.4	E962.0	E980.4
Diethylene						
dioxide	982.8	E862.4	—	E950.9	E962.1	E980.9
glycol (monoacetate) (monoethyl ether)	982.8	E862.4	—	E950.9	E962.1	E980.9
Diethylsulfone–diethylmethane	967.8	E852.8	E937.8	E950.2	E962.0	E980.2
Difencloxazine	965.09	E850.2	E935.2	E950.0	E962.0	E980.0
Diffusin	963.4	E858.1	E933.4	E950.4	E962.0	E980.4
Diflos	971.0	E855.3	E941.0	E950.4	E962.0	E980.4
Digestants	973.4	E858.4	E943.4	E950.4	E962.0	E980.4
Digitalin(e)	972.1	E858.3	E942.1	E950.4	E962.0	E980.4
Digitalis glycosides	972.1	E858.3	E942.1	E950.4	E962.0	E980.4
Digitoxin	972.1	E858.3	E942.1	E950.4	E962.0	E980.4
Digoxin	972.1	E858.3	E942.1	E950.4	E962.0	E980.4
Dihydrocodeine	965.09	E850.2	E935.2	E950.0	E962.0	E980.0
Dihydrocodeinone	965.09	E850.2	E935.2	E950.0	E962.0	E980.0
Dihydroergocristine	972.9	E858.3	E942.9	E950.4	E962.0	E980.4
Dihydroergotamine	972.9	E858.3	E942.9	E950.4	E962.0	E980.4
Dihydroergotoxine	972.9	E858.3	E942.9	E950.4	E962.0	E980.4
Dihydrohydroxycodeinone	965.09	E850.2	E935.2	E950.0	E962.0	E980.0
Dihydrohydroxymorphinone	965.09	E850.2	E935.2	E950.0	E962.0	E980.0
Dihydroisocodeine	965.09	E850.2	E935.2	E950.0	E962.0	E980.0
Dihydromorphine	965.09	E850.2	E935.2	E950.0	E962.0	E980.0
Dihydromorphinone	965.09	E850.2	E935.2	E950.0	E962.0	E980.0
Dihydrostreptomycin	960.6	E856	E930.6	E950.4	E962.0	E980.4
Dihydrotachysterol	962.6	E858.0	E932.6	E950.4	E962.0	E980.4
Dihydroxyanthraquinone	973.1	E858.4	E943.1	E950.4	E962.0	E980.4
Dihydroxycodeinone	965.09	E850.2	E935.2	E950.0	E962.0	E980.0
Diiodohydroxyquin	961.3	E857	E931.3	E950.4	E962.0	E980.4
topical	976.0	E858.7	E946.0	E950.4	E962.0	E980.4
Diiodohydroxyquinoline	961.3	E857	E931.3	E950.4	E962.0	E980.4
Dilantin	966.1	E855.0	E936.1	E950.4	E962.0	E980.4
Dilaudid	965.09	E850.2	E935.2	E950.0	E962.0	E980.0
Diloxanide	961.5	E857	E931.5	E950.4	E962.0	E980.4
Dimefline	970.0	E854.3	E940.0	E950.4	E962.0	E980.4
Dimenhydrinate	963.0	E858.1	E933.0	E950.4	E962.0	E980.4
Dimercaprol	963.8	E858.1	E933.8	E950.4	E962.0	E980.4
Dimercaptopropanol	963.8	E858.1	E933.8	E950.4	E962.0	E980.4
Dimetane	963.0	E858.1	E933.0	E950.4	E962.0	E980.4
Dimethicone	976.3	E858.7	E946.3	E950.4	E962.0	E980.4
Dimethindene	963.0	E858.1	E933.0	E950.4	E962.0	E980.4
Dimethisoquin	968.5	E855.2	E938.5	E950.4	E962.0	E980.4
Dimethisterone	962.2	E858.0	E932.2	E950.4	E962.0	E980.4

TABLE OF DRUGS AND CHEMICALS

Substance	Poisoning	Accident	Therapeutic Use	Suicide Attempt	Assault	Undetermined
		\multicolumn{5}{c}{External Cause (E-Code)}				

Substance	Poisoning	Accident	Therapeutic Use	Suicide Attempt	Assault	Undetermined
Dimethoxanate	975.4	E858.6	E945.4	E950.4	E962.0	E980.4
Dimethyl						
arsine, arsinic acid — see Arsenic						
carbinol	980.2	E860.3	—	E950.9	E962.1	E980.9
diguanide	962.3	E858.0	E932.3	E950.4	E962.0	E980.4
ketone	982.8	E862.4	—	E950.9	E962.1	E980.9
vapor	987.8	E869.8	—	E952.8	E962.2	E982.8
meperidine	965.09	E850.2	E935.2	E950.0	E962.0	E980.0
parathion	989.3	E863.1	—	E950.6	E962.1	E980.7
polysiloxane	973.8	E858.4	E943.8	E950.4	E962.0	E980.4
sulfate (fumes)	987.8	E869.8	—	E952.8	E962.2	E982.8
liquid	983.9	E864.3	—	E950.7	E962.1	E980.6
sulfoxide NEC	982.8	E862.4	—	E950.9	E962.1	E980.9
medicinal	976.4	E858.7	E946.4	E950.4	E962.0	E980.4
triptamine	969.6	E854.1	E939.6	E950.3	E962.0	E980.3
tubocurarine	975.2	E858.6	E945.2	E950.4	E962.0	E980.4
Dindevan	964.2	E858.2	E934.2	E950.4	E962.0	E980.4
Dinitro (–ortho–) cresol (herbicide) (spray)	989.4	E863.5	—	E950.6	E962.1	E980.7
insecticide	989.4	E863.4	—	E950.6	E962.1	E980.7
Dinitrobenzene	983.0	E864.0	—	E950.7	E962.1	E980.6
vapor	987.8	E869.8	—	E952.8	E962.2	E982.8
Dinitro–orthocresol (herbicide)	989.4	E863.5	—	E950.6	E962.1	E980.7
insecticide	989.4	E863.4	—	E950.6	E962.1	E980.7
Dinitrophenol (herbicide) (spray)	989.4	E863.5	—	E950.6	E962.1	E980.7
insecticide	989.4	E863.4	—	E950.6	E962.1	E980.7
Dinoprost	975.0	E858.6	E945.0	E950.4	E962.0	E980.4
Dioctyl sulfosuccinate (calcium) (sodium)	973.2	E858.4	E943.2	E950.4	E962.0	E980.4
Diodoquin	961.3	E857	E931.3	E950.4	E962.0	E980.4
Dione derivatives NEC	966.3	E855.0	E936.3	E950.4	E962.0	E980.4
Dionin	965.09	E850.2	E935.2	E950.0	E962.0	E980.0
Dioxane	982.8	E862.4	—	E950.9	E962.1	E980.9
Dioxin — see herbicide						
Dioxyline	972.5	E858.3	E942.5	E950.4	E962.0	E980.4
Dipentene	982.8	E862.4	—	E950.9	E962.1	E980.9
Diphemanil	971.1	E855.4	E941.1	E950.4	E962.0	E980.4
Diphenadione	964.2	E858.2	E934.2	E950.4	E962.0	E980.4
Diphenhydramine	963.0	E858.1	E933.0	E950.4	E962.0	E980.4
Diphenidol	963.0	E858.1	E933.0	E950.4	E962.0	E980.4
Diphenoxylate	973.5	E858.4	E943.5	E950.4	E962.0	E980.4
Diphenylchloroarsine	985.1	E866.3	—	E950.8	E962.1	E980.8
Diphenylhydantoin (sodium)	966.1	E855.0	E936.1	E950.4	E962.0	E980.4
Diphenylpyraline	963.0	E858.1	E933.0	E950.4	E962.0	E980.4
Diphtheria						
antitoxin	979.9	E858.8	E949.9	E950.4	E962.0	E980.4
toxoid	978.5	E858.8	E948.5	E950.4	E962.0	E980.4
with tetanus toxoid	978.9	E858.8	E948.9	E950.4	E962.0	E980.4
with pertussis component	978.6	E858.8	E948.6	E950.4	E962.0	E980.4
vaccine	978.5	E858.8	E948.5	E950.4	E962.0	E980.4
Dipipanone	965.09	E850.2	E935.2	E950.0	E962.0	E980.0
Diplovax	979.5	E858.8	E949.5	E950.4	E962.0	E980.4
Diprophylline	975.1	E858.6	E945.1	E950.4	E962.0	E980.4
Dipyridamole	972.4	E858.3	E942.4	E950.4	E962.0	E980.4
Dipyrone	965.5	E850.5	E935.5	E950.0	E962.0	E980.0
Diquat	989.4	E863.5	—	E950.6	E962.1	E980.7
Disinfectant NEC	983.9	E861.4	—	E950.7	E962.1	E980.6
alkaline	983.2	E861.4	—	E950.7	E962.1	E980.6
aromatic	983.0	E861.4	—	E950.7	E962.1	E980.6
Disipal	966.4	E855.0	E936.4	E950.4	E962.0	E980.4
Disodium edetate	963.8	E858.1	E933.8	E950.4	E962.0	E980.4
Disulfamide	974.4	E858.5	E944.4	E950.4	E962.0	E980.4

TABLE OF DRUGS AND CHEMICALS

Substance	Poisoning	Accident	Therapeutic Use	Suicide Attempt	Assault	Undetermined
		\multicolumn{5}{c|}{External Cause (E-Code)}				

Substance	Poisoning	Accident	Therapeutic Use	Suicide Attempt	Assault	Undetermined
Disulfanilamide	961.0	E857	E931.0	E950.4	E962.0	E980.4
Disulfiram	977.3	E858.8	E947.3	E950.4	E962.0	E980.4
Dithiazanine	961.6	E857	E931.6	E950.4	E962.0	E980.4
Dithioglycerol	963.8	E858.1	E933.8	E950.4	E962.0	E980.4
Dithranol	976.4	E858.7	E946.4	E950.4	E962.0	E980.4
Diucardin	974.3	E858.5	E944.3	E950.4	E962.0	E980.4
Diupres	974.3	E858.5	E944.3	E950.4	E962.0	E980.4
Diuretics NEC	974.4	E858.5	E944.4	E950.4	E962.0	E980.4
carbonic acid anhydrase inhibitors	974.2	E858.5	E944.2	E950.4	E962.0	E980.4
mercurial	974.0	E858.5	E944.0	E950.4	E962.0	E980.4
osmotic	974.4	E858.5	E944.4	E950.4	E962.0	E980.4
purine derivatives	974.1	E858.5	E944.1	E950.4	E962.0	E980.4
saluretic	974.3	E858.5	E944.3	E950.4	E962.0	E980.4
Diuril	974.3	E858.5	E944.3	E950.4	E962.0	E980.4
Divinyl ether	968.2	E855.1	E938.2	E950.4	E962.0	E980.4
D–lysergic acid diethylamide	969.6	E854.1	E939.6	E950.3	E962.0	E980.3
DMCT	960.4	E856	E930.4	E950.4	E962.0	E980.4
DMSO	982.8	E862.4	—	E950.9	E962.1	E980.9
DMT	969.6	E854.1	E939.6	E950.3	E962.0	E980.3
DNOC	989.4	E863.5	—	E950.6	E962.1	E980.7
DOCA	962.0	E858.0	E932.0	E950.4	E962.0	E980.4
Dolophine	965.02	E850.1	E935.1	E950.0	E962.0	E980.0
Doloxene	965.8	E850.8	E935.8	E950.0	E962.0	E980.0
DOM	969.6	E854.1	E939.6	E950.3	E962.0	E980.3
Domestic gas — see Gas, utility						
Domiphen (bromide) (lozenges)	976.6	E858.7	E946.6	E950.4	E962.0	E980.4
Dopa (levo)	966.4	E855.0	E936.4	E950.4	E962.0	E980.4
Dopamine	971.2	E855.5	E941.2	E950.4	E962.0	E980.4
Doriden	967.5	E852.4	E937.5	E950.2	E962.0	E980.2
Dormiral	967.0	E851	E937.0	E950.1	E962.0	E980.1
Dormison	967.8	E852.8	E937.8	E950.2	E962.0	E980.2
Dornase	963.4	E858.1	E933.4	E950.4	E962.0	E980.4
Dorsacaine	968.5	E855.2	E938.5	E950.4	E962.0	E980.4
Dothiepin hydrochloride	969.0	E854.0	E939.0	E950.3	E962.0	E980.3
Doxapram	970.0	E854.3	E940.0	E950.4	E962.0	E980.4
Doxepin	969.0	E854.0	E939.0	E950.3	E962.0	E980.3
Doxorubicin	960.7	E856	E930.7	E950.4	E962.0	E980.4
Doxycycline	960.4	E856	E930.4	E950.4	E962.0	E980.4
Doxylamine	963.0	E858.1	E933.0	E950.4	E962.0	E980.4
Dramamine	963.0	E858.1	E933.0	E950.4	E962.0	E980.4
Drano (drain cleaner)	983.2	E864.2	—	E950.7	E962.1	E980.6
Dromoran	965.09	E850.2	E935.2	E950.0	E962.0	E980.0
Dromostanolone	962.1	E858.0	E932.1	E950.4	E962.0	E980.4
Droperidol	969.2	E853.1	E939.2	E950.3	E962.0	E980.3
Drotrecogin alfa	964.2	E858.2	E934.2	E950.4	E962.0	E980.4
Drug	977.9	E858.9	E947.9	E950.5	E962.0	E980.5
specified NEC	977.8	E858.8	E947.8	E950.4	E962.0	E980.4
AHFS List						
4:00 antihistamine drugs	963.0	E858.1	E933.0	E950.4	E962.0	E980.4
8:04 amebacides	961.5	E857	E931.5	E950.4	E962.0	E980.4
arsenical anti–infectives	961.1	E857	E931.1	E950.4	E962.0	E980.4
quinoline derivatives	961.3	E857	E931.3	E950.4	E962.0	E980.4
8:08 anthelmintics	961.6	E857	E931.6	E950.4	E962.0	E980.4
quinoline derivatives	961.3	E857	E931.3	E950.4	E962.0	E980.4
8:12.04 antifungal antibiotics	960.1	E856	E930.1	E950.4	E962.0	E980.4
8:12.06 cephalosporins	960.5	E856	E930.5	E950.4	E962.0	E980.4
8:12.08 chloramphenicol	960.2	E856	E930.2	E950.4	E962.0	E980.4
8:12.12 erythromycins	960.3	E856	E930.3	E950.4	E962.0	E980.4
8:12.16 penicillins	960.0	E856	E930.0	E950.4	E962.0	E980.4
8:12.20 streptomycins	960.6	E856	E930.6	E950.4	E962.0	E980.4
8:12.24 tetracyclines	960.4	E856	E930.4	E950.4	E962.0	E980.4

TABLE OF DRUGS AND CHEMICALS

Substance	Poisoning	Accident	Therapeutic Use	Suicide Attempt	Assault	Undetermined
			External Cause (E-Code)			
8:12.28 other antibiotics	960.8	E856	E930.8	E950.4	E962.0	E980.4
antimycobacterial	960.6	E856	E930.6	E950.4	E962.0	E980.4
macrolides	960.3	E856	E930.3	E950.4	E962.0	E980.4
8:16 antituberculars	961.8	E857	E931.8	E950.4	E962.0	E980.4
antibiotics	960.6	E856	E930.6	E950.4	E962.0	E980.4
8:18 antivirals	961.7	E857	E931.7	E950.4	E962.0	E980.4
8:20 plasmodicides (antimalarials)	961.4	E857	E931.4	E950.4	E962.0	E980.4
8:24 sulfonamides	961.0	E857	E931.0	E950.4	E962.0	E980.4
8:26 sulfones	961.8	E857	E931.8	E950.4	E962.0	E980.4
8:28 treponemicides	961.2	E857	E931.2	E950.4	E962.0	E980.4
8:32 trichomonacides	961.5	E857	E931.5	E950.4	E962.0	E980.4
quinoline derivatives	961.3	E857	E931.3	E950.4	E962.0	E980.4
nitrofuran derivatives	961.9	E857	E931.9	E950.4	E962.0	E980.4
8:36 urinary germicides	961.9	E857	E931.9	E950.4	E962.0	E980.4
quinoline derivatives	961.3	E857	E931.3	E950.4	E962.0	E980.4
8:40 other anti-infectives	961.9	E857	E931.9	E950.4	E962.0	E980.4
10:00 antineoplastic agents	963.1	E858.1	E933.1	E950.4	E962.0	E980.4
antibiotics	960.7	E856	E930.7	E950.4	E962.0	E980.4
progestogens	962.2	E858.0	E932.2	E950.4	E962.0	E980.4
12:04 parasympathomimetic (cholinergic) agents	971.0	E855.3	E941.0	E950.4	E962.0	E980.4
12:08 parasympatholytic (cholinergic –blocking) agents	971.1	E855.4	E941.1	E950.4	E962.0	E980.4
12:12 Sympathomimetic (adrenergic) agents	971.2	E855.5	E941.2	E950.4	E962.0	E980.4
12:16 sympatholytic (adrenergic– blocking) agents	971.3	E855.6	E941.3	E950.4	E962.0	E980.4
12:20 skeletal muscle relaxants central nervous system muscle-tone depressants	968.0	E855.1	E938.0	E950.4	E962.0	E980.4
myoneural blocking agents	975.2	E858.6	E945.2	E950.4	E962.0	E980.4
16:00 blood derivatives	964.7	E858.2	E934.7	E950.4	E962.0	E980.4
20:04 antianemia drugs	964.1	E858.2	E934.1	E950.4	E962.0	E980.4
20:04.04 iron preparations	964.0	E858.2	E934.0	E950.4	E962.0	E980.4
20:04.08 liver and stomach preparations	964.1	E858.2	E934.1	E950.4	E962.0	E980.4
20:12.04 anticoagulants	964.2	E858.2	E934.2	E950.4	E962.0	E980.4
20:12.08 antiheparin agents	964.5	E858.2	E934.5	E950.4	E962.0	E980.4
20:12.12 coagulants	964.5	E858.2	E934.5	E950.4	E962.0	E980.4
20:12.16 hemostatics NEC	964.5	E858.2	E934.5	E950.4	E962.0	E980.4
capillary active drugs	972.8	E858.3	E942.8	E950.4	E962.0	E980.4
24:04 cardiac drugs	972.9	E858.3	E942.9	E950.4	E962.0	E980.4
cardiotonic agents	972.1	E858.3	E942.1	E950.4	E962.0	E980.4
rhythm regulators	972.0	E858.3	E942.0	E950.4	E962.0	E980.4
24:06 antilipemic agents	972.2	E858.3	E942.2	E950.4	E962.0	E980.4
thyroid derivatives	962.7	E858.0	E932.7	E950.4	E962.0	E980.4
24:08 hypotensive agents	972.6	E858.3	E942.6	E950.4	E962.0	E980.4
adrenergic blocking agents	971.3	E855.6	E941.3	E950.4	E962.0	E980.4
ganglion blocking agents	972.3	E858.3	E942.3	E950.4	E962.0	E980.4
vasodilators	972.5	E858.3	E942.5	E950.4	E962.0	E980.4
24:12 vasodilating agents NEC	972.5	E858.3	E942.5	E950.4	E962.0	E980.4
coronary	972.4	E858.3	E942.4	E950.4	E962.0	E980.4
nicotinic acid derivatives	972.2	E858.3	E942.2	E950.4	E962.0	E980.4
24:16 sclerosing agents	972.7	E858.3	E942.7	E950.4	E962.0	E980.4
28:04 general anesthetics	968.4	E855.1	E938.4	E950.4	E962.0	E980.4
gaseous anesthetics	968.2	E855.1	E938.2	E950.4	E962.0	E980.4
halothane	968.1	E855.1	E938.1	E950.4	E962.0	E980.4
intravenous anesthetics	968.3	E855.1	E938.3	E950.4	E962.0	E980.4
28:08 analgesics and antipyretics	965.9	E850.9	E935.9	E950.0	E962.0	E980.0
antirheumatics	965.69	E850.6	E935.6	E950.0	E962.0	E980.0
aromatic analgesics	965.4	E850.4	E935.4	E950.0	E962.0	E980.0

TABLE OF DRUGS AND CHEMICALS

Substance	Poisoning	Accident	Therapeutic Use	Suicide Attempt	Assault	Undetermined
			External Cause (E-Code)			
non–narcotic NEC	965.7	E850.7	E935.7	E950.0	E962.0	E980.0
opium alkaloids	965.00	E850.2	E935.2	E950.0	E962.0	E980.0
heroin	965.01	E850.0	E935.0	E950.0	E962.0	E980.0
methadone	965.02	E850.1	E935.1	E950.0	E962.0	E980.0
specified type NEC	965.09	E850.2	E935.2	E950.0	E962.0	E980.0
pyrazole derivatives	965.5	E850.5	E935.5	E950.0	E962.0	E980.0
salicylates	965.1	E850.3	E935.3	E950.0	E962.0	E980.0
specified NEC	965.8	E850.8	E935.8	E950.0	E962.0	E980.0
28:10 narcotic antagonists	970.1	E854.3	E940.1	E950.4	E962.0	E980.4
28:12 anticonvulsants	966.3	E855.0	E936.3	E950.4	E962.0	E980.4
barbiturates	967.0	E851	E937.0	E950.1	E962.0	E980.1
benzodiazepine–based tranquilizers	969.4	E853.2	E939.4	E950.3	E962.0	E980.3
bromides	967.3	E852.2	E937.3	E950.2	E962.0	E980.2
hydantoin derivatives	966.1	E855.0	E936.1	E950.4	E962.0	E980.4
oxazolidine (derivatives)	966.0	E855.0	E936.0	E950.4	E962.0	E980.4
succinimides	966.2	E855.0	E936.2	E950.4	E962.0	E980.4
28:16.04 antidepressants	969.0	E854.0	E939.0	E950.3	E962.0	E980.3
28:16.08 tranquilizers	969.5	E853.9	E939.5	E950.3	E962.0	E980.3
benzodiazepine–based	969.4	E853.2	E939.4	E950.3	E962.0	E980.3
butyrophenone–based	969.2	E853.1	E939.2	E950.3	E962.0	E980.3
major NEC	969.3	E853.8	E939.3	E950.3	E962.0	E980.3
phenothiazine–based	969.1	E853.0	E939.1	E950.3	E962.0	E980.3
28:16.12 other psychotherapeutic agents	969.8	E855.8	E939.8	E950.3	E962.0	E980.3
28:20 respiratory and cerebral stimulants	970.9	E854.3	E940.9	E950.4	E962.0	E980.4
analeptics	970.0	E854.3	E940.0	E950.4	E962.0	E980.4
anorexigenic agents	977.0	E858.8	E947.0	E950.4	E962.0	E980.4
psychostimulants	969.7	E854.2	E939.7	E950.3	E962.0	E980.3
specified NEC	970.8	E854.3	E940.8	E950.4	E962.0	E980.4
28:24 sedatives and hypnotics	967.9	E852.9	E937.9	E950.2	E962.0	E980.2
barbiturates	967.0	E851	E937.0	E950.1	E962.0	E980.1
benzodiazepine–based tranquilizers	969.4	E853.2	E939.4	E950.3	E962.0	E980.3
chloral hydrate (group)	967.1	E852.0	E937.1	E950.2	E962.0	E980.2
glutethamide group	967.5	E852.4	E937.5	E950.2	E962.0	E980.2
intravenous anesthetics	968.3	E855.1	E938.3	E950.4	E962.0	E980.4
methaqualone (compounds)	967.4	E852.3	E937.4	E950.2	E962.0	E980.2
paraldehyde	967.2	E852.1	E937.2	E950.2	E962.0	E980.2
phenothiazine–based tranquilizers	969.1	E853.0	E939.1	E950.3	E962.0	E980.3
specified NEC	967.8	E852.8	E937.8	E950.2	E962.0	E980.2
thiobarbiturates	968.3	E855.1	E938.3	E950.4	E962.0	E980.4
tranquilizer NEC	969.5	E853.9	E939.5	E950.3	E962.0	E980.3
36:04 to 36:88 diagnostic agents	977.8	E858.8	E947.8	E950.4	E962.0	E980.4
40:00 electrolyte, caloric, and water balance agents NEC	974.5	E858.5	E944.5	E950.4	E962.0	E980.4
40:04 acidifying agents	963.2	E858.1	E933.2	E950.4	E962.0	E980.4
40:08 alkalinizing agents	963.3	E858.1	E933.3	E950.4	E962.0	E980.4
40:10 ammonia detoxicants	974.5	E858.5	E944.5	E950.4	E962.0	E980.4
40:12 replacement solutions	974.5	E858.5	E944.5	E950.4	E962.0	E980.4
plasma expanders	964.8	E858.2	E934.8	E950.4	E962.0	E980.4
40:16 sodium–removing resins	974.5	E858.5	E944.5	E950.4	E962.0	E980.4
40:18 potassium–removing resins	974.5	E858.5	E944.5	E950.4	E962.0	E980.4
40:20 caloric agents	974.5	E858.5	E944.5	E950.4	E962.0	E980.4
40:24 salt and sugar substitutes	974.5	E858.5	E944.5	E950.4	E962.0	E980.4
40:28 diuretics NEC	974.4	E858.5	E944.4	E950.4	E962.0	E980.4
carbonic acid anhydrase inhibitors	974.2	E858.5	E944.2	E950.4	E962.0	E980.4
mercurials	974.0	E858.5	E944.0	E950.4	E962.0	E980.4
purine derivatives	974.1	E858.5	E944.1	E950.4	E962.0	E980.4
saluretics	974.3	E858.5	E944.3	E950.4	E962.0	E980.4
thiazides	974.3	E858.5	E944.3	E950.4	E962.1	E980.4
40:36 irrigating solutions	974.5	E858.5	E944.5	E950.4	E962.0	E980.4
40:40 uricosuric agents	974.7	E858.5	E944.7	E950.4	E962.0	E980.4

TABLE OF DRUGS AND CHEMICALS

Substance	Poisoning	Accident	Therapeutic Use	Suicide Attempt	Assault	Undetermined
		\multicolumn{5}{c}{External Cause (E-Code)}				

Substance	Poisoning	Accident	Therapeutic Use	Suicide Attempt	Assault	Undetermined
44:00 enzymes	963.4	E858.1	E933.4	E950.4	E962.0	E980.4
fibrinolysis–affecting agents	964.4	E858.2	E934.4	E950.4	E962.0	E980.4
gastric agents	973.4	E858.4	E943.4	E950.4	E962.0	E980.4
48:00 expectorants and cough preparations						
antihistamine agents	963.0	E858.1	E933.0	E950.4	E962.0	E980.4
antitussives	975.4	E858.6	E945.4	E950.4	E962.0	E980.4
codeine derivatives	965.09	E850.2	E935.2	E950.0	E962.0	E980.0
expectorants	975.5	E858.6	E945.5	E950.4	E962.0	E980.4
narcotic agents NEC	965.09	E850.2	E935.2	E950.0	E962.0	E980.0
52:04 anti–infectives (EENT)						
ENT agent	976.6	E858.7	E946.6	E950.4	E962.0	E980.4
ophthalmic preparation	976.5	E858.7	E946.5	E950.4	E962.0	E980.4
52:04.04 antibiotics (EENT)						
ENT agent	976.6	E858.7	E946.6	E950.4	E962.0	E980.4
ophthalmic preparation	976.5	E858.7	E946.5	E950.4	E962.0	E980.4
52:04.06 antivirals (EENT)						
ENT agent	976.6	E858.7	E946.6	E950.4	E962.0	E980.4
ophthalmic preparation	976.5	E858.7	E946.5	E950.4	E962.0	E980.4
52:04.08 sulfonamides (EENT)						
ENT agent	976.6	E858.7	E946.6	E950.4	E962.0	E980.4
ophthalmic preparation	976.5	E858.7	E946.5	E950.4	E962.0	E980.4
52:04.12 miscellaneous anti–infectives (EENT)						
ENT agent	976.6	E858.7	E946.6	E950.4	E962.0	E980.4
ophthalmic preparation	976.5	E858.7	E946.5	E950.4	E962.0	E980.4
52:08 anti–inflammatory agents (EENT)						
ENT agent	976.6	E858.7	E946.6	E950.4	E962.0	E980.4
ophthalmic preparation	976.5	E858.7	E946.5	E950.4	E962.0	E980.4
52:10 carbonic anhydrase inhibitors	974.2	E858.5	E944.2	E950.4	E962.0	E980.4
52:12 contact lens solutions	976.5	E858.7	E946.5	E950.4	E962.0	E980.4
52:16 local anesthetics (EENT)	968.5	E855.2	E938.5	E950.4	E962.0	E980.4
52:20 miotics	971.0	E855.3	E941.0	E950.4	E962.0	E980.4
52:24 mydriatics						
adrenergics	971.2	E855.5	E941.2	E950.4	E962.0	E980.4
anticholinergics	971.1	E855.4	E941.1	E950.4	E962.0	E980.4
antimuscarinics	971.1	E855.4	E941.1	E950.4	E962.0	E980.4
parasympatholytics	971.1	E855.4	E941.1	E950.4	E962.0	E980.4
spasmolytics	971.1	E855.4	E941.1	E950.4	E962.0	E980.4
sympathomimetics	971.2	E855.5	E941.2	E950.4	E962.0	E980.4
52:28 mouth washes and gargles	976.6	E858.7	E946.6	E950.4	E962.0	E980.4
52:32 vasoconstrictors (EENT)	971.2	E855.5	E941.2	E950.4	E962.0	E980.4
52:36 unclassified agents (EENT)						
ENT agent	976.6	E858.7	E946.6	E950.4	E962.0	E980.4
ophthalmic preparation	976.5	E858.7	E946.5	E950.4	E962.0	E980.4
56:04 antacids and adsorbents	973.0	E858.4	E943.0	E950.4	E962.0	E980.4
56:08 antidiarrhea agents	973.5	E858.4	E943.5	E950.4	E962.0	E980.4
56:10 antiflatulents	973.8	E858.4	E943.8	E950.4	E962.0	E980.4
56:12 cathartics NEC	973.3	E858.4	E943.3	E950.4	E962.0	E980.4
emollients	973.2	E858.4	E943.2	E950.4	E962.0	E980.4
irritants	973.1	E858.4	E943.1	E950.4	E962.0	E980.4
56:16 digestants	973.4	E858.4	E943.4	E950.4	E962.0	E980.4
56:20 emetics and antiemetics						
antiemetics	963.0	E858.1	E933.0	E950.4	E962.0	E980.4
emetics	973.6	E858.4	E943.6	E950.4	E962.0	E980.4
56:24 lipotropic agents	977.1	E858.8	E947.1	E950.4	E962.0	E980.4
56:40 miscellaneous G.I. drugs	973.8	E858.4	E943.8	E950.4	E962.0	E980.4
60:00 gold compounds	965.69	E850.6	E935.6	E950.0	E962.0	E980.0
64:00 heavy metal antagonists	963.8	E858.1	E933.8	E950.4	E962.0	E980.4
68:04 adrenals	962.0	E858.0	E932.0	E950.4	E962.0	E980.4
68:08 androgens	962.1	E858.0	E932.1	E950.4	E962.0	E980.4
68:12 contraceptives, oral	962.2	E858.0	E932.2	E950.4	E962.0	E980.4

TABLE OF DRUGS AND CHEMICALS

Substance	Poisoning	Accident	Therapeutic Use	Suicide Attempt	Assault	Undetermined
		\multicolumn{5}{c}{External Cause (E-Code)}				

Substance	Poisoning	Accident	Therapeutic Use	Suicide Attempt	Assault	Undetermined
68:16 estrogens	962.2	E858.0	E932.2	E950.4	E962.0	E980.4
68:18 gonadotropins	962.4	E858.0	E932.4	E950.4	E962.0	E980.4
68:20 insulins and antidiabetic agents	962.3	E858.0	E932.3	E950.4	E962.0	E980.4
68:20.08 insulins	962.3	E858.0	E932.3	E950.4	E962.0	E980.4
68:24 parathyroid	962.6	E858.0	E932.6	E950.4	E962.0	E980.4
68:28 pituitary (posterior)	962.5	E858.0	E932.5	E950.4	E962.0	E980.4
anterior	962.4	E858.0	E932.4	E950.4	E962.0	E980.4
68:32 progestogens	962.2	E858.0	E932.2	E950.4	E962.0	E980.4
68:34 other corpus luteum hormones NEC	962.2	E858.0	E932.2	E950.4	E962.0	E980.4
68:36 thyroid and antithyroid antithyroid	962.8	E858.0	E932.8	E950.4	E962.0	E980.4
thyroid (derivatives)	962.7	E858.0	E932.7	E950.4	E962.0	E980.4
72:00 local anesthetics NEC	968.9	E855.2	E938.9	E950.4	E962.0	E980.4
topical (surface)	968.5	E855.2	E938.5	E950.4	E962.0	E980.4
infiltration (intradermal) (subcutaneous) (submucosal)	968.5	E855.2	E938.5	E950.4	E962.0	E980.4
nerve blocking (peripheral) (plexus) (regional)	968.6	E855.2	E938.6	E950.4	E962.0	E980.4
spinal	968.7	E855.2	E938.7	E950.4	E962.0	E980.4
76:00 oxytocics	975.0	E858.6	E945.0	E950.4	E962.0	E980.4
78:00 radioactive agents	990	—	—	—	—	—
80:04 serums NEC	979.9	E858.8	E949.9	E950.4	E962.0	E980.4
immune gamma globulin (human)	964.6	E858.2	E934.6	E950.4	E962.0	E980.4
80:08 toxoids NEC	978.8	E858.8	E948.8	E950.4	E962.0	E980.4
diphtheria	978.5	E858.8	E948.5	E950.4	E962.0	E980.4
and tetanus	978.9	E858.8	E948.9	E950.4	E962.0	E980.4
with pertussis component	978.6	E858.8	E948.6	E950.4	E962.0	E980.4
tetanus	978.4	E858.8	E948.4	E950.4	E962.0	E980.4
and diphtheria	978.9	E858.8	E948.9	E950.4	E962.0	E980.4
with pertussis component	978.6	E858.8	E948.6	E950.4	E962.0	E980.4
80:12 vaccines	979.9	E858.8	E949.9	E950.4	E962.0	E980.4
bacterial NEC	978.8	E858.8	E948.8	E950.4	E962.0	E980.4
with other bacterial components	978.9	E858.8	E948.9	E950.4	E962.0	E980.4
pertussis component	978.6	E858.8	E948.6	E950.4	E962.0	E980.4
viral and rickettsial components	979.7	E858.8	E949.7	E950.4	E962.0	E980.4
rickettsial NEC	979.6	E858.8	E949.6	E950.4	E962.0	E980.4
with bacterial component	979.7	E858.8	E949.7	E950.4	E962.0	E980.4
pertussis component	978.6	E858.8	E948.6	E950.4	E962.0	E980.4
viral component	979.7	E858.8	E949.7	E950.4	E962.0	E980.4
viral NEC	979.6	E858.8	E949.6	E950.4	E962.0	E980.4
with bacterial component	979.7	E858.8	E949.7	E950.4	E962.0	E980.4
pertussis component	978.6	E858.8	E948.6	E950.4	E962.0	E980.4
rickettsial component	979.7	E858.8	E949.7	E950.4	E962.0	E980.4
84:04.04 antibiotics (skin and mucous membrane)	976.0	E858.7	E946.0	E950.4	E962.0	E980.4
84:04.08 fungicides (skin and mucous membrane)	976.0	E858.7	E946.0	E950.4	E962.0	E980.4
84:04.12 scabicides and pediculicides (skin and mucous membrane)	976.0	E858.7	E946.0	E950.4	E962.0	E980.4
84:04.16 miscellaneous local anti-infectives (skin and mucous membrane)	976.0	E858.7	E946.0	E950.4	E962.0	E980.4
84:06 anti–inflammatory agents (skin and mucous membrane)	976.0	E858.7	E946.0	E950.4	E962.0	E980.4
84:08 antipruritics and local anesthetics antipruritics	976.1	E858.7	E946.1	E950.4	E962.0	E980.4

1445

TABLE OF DRUGS AND CHEMICALS

Substance	Poisoning	Accident	Therapeutic Use	Suicide Attempt	Assault	Undetermined
		\multicolumn{5}{c}{External Cause (E-Code)}				

Substance	Poisoning	Accident	Therapeutic Use	Suicide Attempt	Assault	Undetermined
local anesthetics	968.5	E855.2	E938.5	E950.4	E962.0	E980.4
84:12 astringents	976.2	E858.7	E946.2	E950.4	E962.0	E980.4
84:16 cell stimulants and proliferants	976.8	E858.7	E946.8	E950.4	E962.0	E980.4
84:20 detergents	976.2	E858.7	E946.2	E950.4	E962.0	E980.4
84:24 emollients, demulcents, and protectants	976.3	E858.7	E946.3	E950.4	E962.0	E980.4
84:28 keratolytic agents	976.4	E858.7	E946.4	E950.4	E962.0	E980.4
84:32 keratoplastic agents	976.4	E858.7	E946.4	E950.4	E962.0	E980.4
84:36 miscellaneous agents (skin and mucous membrane)	976.8	E858.7	E946.8	E950.4	E962.0	E980.4
86:00 spasmolytic agents	975.1	E858.6	E945.1	E950.4	E962.0	E980.4
antiasthmatics	975.7	E858.6	E945.7	E950.4	E962.0	E980.4
papaverine	972.5	E858.3	E942.5	E950.4	E962.0	E980.4
theophylline	974.1	E858.5	E944.1	E950.4	E962.0	E980.4
88:04 vitamin A	963.5	E858.1	E933.5	E950.4	E962.0	E980.4
88:08 vitamin B complex	963.5	E858.1	E933.5	E950.4	E962.0	E980.4
hematopoietic vitamin	964.1	E858.2	E934.1	E950.4	E962.0	E980.4
nicotinic acid derivatives	972.2	E858.3	E942.2	E950.4	E962.0	E980.4
88:12 vitamin C	963.5	E858.1	E933.5	E950.4	E962.0	E980.4
88:16 vitamin D	963.5	E858.1	E933.5	E950.4	E962.0	E980.4
88:20 vitamin E	963.5	E858.1	E933.5	E950.4	E962.0	E980.4
88:24 vitamin K activity	964.3	E858.2	E934.3	E950.4	E962.0	E980.4
88:28 multivitamin preparations	963.5	E858.1	E933.5	E950.4	E962.0	E980.4
92:00 unclassified therapeutic agents	977.8	E858.8	E947.8	E950.4	E962.0	E980.4
Duboisine	971.1	E855.4	E941.1	E950.4	E962.0	E980.4
Dulcolax	973.1	E858.4	E943.1	E950.4	E962.0	E980.4
Duponol (C) (EP)	976.2	E858.7	E946.2	E950.4	E962.0	E980.4
Durabolin	962.1	E858.0	E932.1	E950.4	E962.0	E980.4
Dyclone	968.5	E855.2	E938.5	E950.4	E962.0	E980.4
Dyclonine	968.5	E855.2	E938.5	E950.4	E962.0	E980.4
Dydrogesterone	962.2	E858.0	E932.2	E950.4	E962.0	E980.4
Dyes NEC	989.89	E866.8	—	E950.9	E962.1	E980.9
diagnostic agents	977.8	E858.8	E947.8	E950.4	E962.0	E980.4
pharmaceutical NEC	977.4	E858.8	E947.4	E950.4	E962.0	E980.4
Dyfols	971.0	E855.3	E941.0	E950.4	E962.0	E980.4
Dymelor	962.3	E858.0	E932.3	E950.4	E962.0	E980.4
Dynamite	989.89	E866.8	—	E950.9	E962.1	E980.9
fumes	987.8	E869.8	—	E952.8	E962.2	E982.8
Dyphylline	975.1	E858.6	E945.1	E950.4	E962.0	E980.4
Ear preparations	976.6	E858.7	E946.6	E950.4	E962.0	E980.4
Echothiopate, ecothiopate	971.0	E855.3	E941.0	E950.4	E962.0	E980.4
Ecstasy	969.7	E854.2	E939.7	E950.3	E962.0	E980.3
Ectylurea	967.8	E852.8	E937.8	E950.2	E962.0	E980.2
Edathamil disodium	963.8	E858.1	E933.8	E950.4	E962.0	E980.4
Edecrin	974.4	E858.5	E944.4	E950.4	E962.0	E980.4
Edetate, disodium (calcium)	963.8	E858.1	E933.8	E950.4	E962.0	E980.4
Edrophonium	971.0	E855.3	E941.0	E950.4	E962.0	E980.4
Elase	976.8	E858.7	E946.8	E950.4	E962.0	E980.4
Elaterium	973.1	E858.4	E943.1	E950.4	E962.0	E980.4
Elder	988.2	E865.4	—	E950.9	E962.1	E980.9
berry (unripe)	988.2	E865.3	—	E950.9	E962.1	E980.9
Electrolytes NEC	974.5	E858.5	E944.5	E950.4	E962.0	E980.4
Electrolytic agent NEC	974.5	E858.5	E944.5	E950.4	E962.0	E980.4
Embramine	963.0	E858.1	E933.0	E950.4	E962.0	E980.4
Emetics	973.6	E858.4	E943.6	E950.4	E962.0	E980.4
Emetine (hydrochloride)	961.5	E857	E931.5	E950.4	E962.0	E980.4
Emollients	976.3	E858.7	E946.3	E950.4	E962.0	E980.4
Emylcamate	969.5	E853.8	E939.5	E950.3	E962.0	E980.3
Encyprate	969.0	E854.0	E939.0	E950.3	E962.0	E980.3
Endocaine	968.5	E855.2	E938.5	E950.4	E962.0	E980.4

TABLE OF DRUGS AND CHEMICALS

Substance	Poisoning	Accident	Therapeutic Use	Suicide Attempt	Assault	Undetermined
		\multicolumn{5}{c}{External Cause (E-Code)}				

Substance	Poisoning	Accident	Therapeutic Use	Suicide Attempt	Assault	Undetermined
Endrin	989.2	E863.0	—	E950.6	E962.1	E980.7
Enflurane	968.2	E855.1	E938.2	E950.4	E962.0	E980.4
Enovid	962.2	E858.0	E932.2	E950.4	E962.0	E980.4
ENT preparations (anti–infectives)	976.6	E858.7	E946.6	E950.4	E962.0	E980.4
Enzodase	963.4	E858.1	E933.4	E950.4	E962.0	E980.4
Enzymes NEC	963.4	E858.1	E933.4	E950.4	E962.0	E980.4
Epanutin	966.1	E855.0	E936.1	E950.4	E962.0	E980.4
Ephedra (tincture)	971.2	E855.5	E941.2	E950.4	E962.0	E980.4
Ephedrine	971.2	E855.5	E941.2	E950.4	E962.0	E980.4
Epiestriol	962.2	E858.0	E932.2	E950.4	E962.0	E980.4
Epilim — *see* Sodium valproate						
Epinephrine	971.2	E855.5	E941.2	E950.4	E962.0	E980.4
Epsom salt	973.3	E858.4	E943.3	E950.4	E962.0	E980.4
Equanil	969.5	E853.8	E939.5	E950.3	E962.0	E980.3
Equisetum (diuretic)	974.4	E858.5	E944.4	E950.4	E962.0	E980.4
Ergometrine	975.0	E858.6	E945.0	E950.4	E962.0	E980.4
Ergonovine	975.0	E858.6	E945.0	E950.4	E962.0	E980.4
Ergot NEC	988.2	E865.4	—	E950.9	E962.1	E980.9
medicinal (alkaloids)	975.0	E858.6	E945.0	E950.4	E962.0	E980.4
Ergotamine (tartrate) (for migraine) NEC	972.9	E858.3	E942.9	E950.4	E962.0	E980.4
Ergotrate	975.0	E858.6	E945.0	E950.4	E962.0	E980.4
Erythrityl tetranitrate	972.4	E858.3	E942.4	E950.4	E962.0	E980.4
Erythrol tetranitrate	972.4	E858.3	E942.4	E950.4	E962.0	E980.4
Erythromycin	960.3	E856	E930.3	E950.4	E962.0	E980.4
ophthalmic preparation	976.5	E858.7	E946.5	E950.4	E962.0	E980.4
topical NEC	976.0	E858.7	E946.0	E950.4	E962.0	E980.4
Eserine	971.0	E855.3	E941.0	E950.4	E962.0	E980.4
Eskabarb	967.0	E851	E937.0	E950.1	E962.0	E980.1
Eskalith	969.8	E855.8	E939.8	E950.3	E962.0	E980.3
Estradiol (cypionate) (dipropionate) (valerate)	962.2	E858.0	E932.2	E950.4	E962.0	E980.4
Estriol	962.2	E858.0	E932.2	E950.4	E962.0	E980.4
Estrogens (with progestogens)	962.2	E858.0	E932.2	E950.4	E962.0	E980.4
Estrone	962.2	E858.0	E932.2	E950.4	E962.0	E980.4
Etafedrine	971.2	E855.5	E941.2	E950.4	E962.0	E980.4
Ethacrynate sodium	974.4	E858.5	E944.4	E950.4	E962.0	E980.4
Ethacrynic acid	974.4	E858.5	E944.4	E950.4	E962.0	E980.4
Ethambutol	961.8	E857	E931.8	E950.4	E962.0	E980.4
Ethamide	974.2	E858.5	E944.2	E950.4	E962.0	E980.4
Ethamivan	970.0	E854.3	E940.0	E950.4	E962.0	E980.4
Ethamsylate	964.5	E858.2	E934.5	E950.4	E962.0	E980.4
Ethanol	980.0	E860.1	—	E950.9	E962.1	E980.9
beverage	980.0	E860.0	—	E950.9	E962.1	E980.9
Etchlorvynol	967.8	E852.8	E937.8	E950.2	E962.0	E980.2
Ethebenecid	974.7	E858.5	E944.7	E950.4	E962.0	E980.4
Ether(s) (diethyl) (ethyl) (vapor)	987.8	E869.8	—	E952.8	E962.2	E982.8
anesthetic	968.2	E855.1	E938.2	E950.4	E962.0	E980.4
petroleum — *see* Ligroin						
solvent	982.8	E862.4	—	E950.9	E962.1	E980.9
Ethidine chloride (vapor)	987.8	E869.8	—	E952.8	E962.2	E982.8
liquid (solvent)	982.3	E862.4	—	E950.9	E962.1	E980.9
Ethinamate	967.8	E852.8	E937.8	E950.2	E962.0	E980.2
Ethinylestradiol	962.2	E858.0	E932.2	E950.4	E962.0	E980.4
Ethionamide	961.8	E857	E931.8	E950.4	E962.0	E980.4
Ethisterone	962.2	E858.0	E932.2	E950.4	E962.0	E980.4
Ethobral	967.0	E851	E937.0	E950.1	E962.0	E980.1
Ethocaine (infiltration) (topical)	968.5	E855.2	E938.5	E950.4	E962.0	E980.4
nerve block (peripheral) (plexus)	968.6	E855.2	E938.6	E950.4	E962.0	E980.4
spinal	968.7	E855.2	E938.7	E950.4	E962.0	E980.4
Ethoheptazine (citrate)	965.7	E850.7	E935.7	E950.0	E962.0	E980.0
Ethopropazine	966.4	E855.0	E936.4	E950.4	E962.0	E980.4

1447

TABLE OF DRUGS AND CHEMICALS

Substance	Poisoning	Accident	Therapeutic Use	Suicide Attempt	Assault	Undetermined
			External Cause (E-Code)			
Ethosuximide	966.2	E855.0	E936.2	E950.4	E962.0	E980.4
Ethotoin	966.1	E855.0	E936.1	E950.4	E962.0	E980.4
Ethoxazene	961.9	E857	E931.9	E950.4	E962.0	E980.4
Ethoxzolamide	974.2	E858.5	E944.2	E950.4	E962.0	E980.4
Ethyl						
acetate (vapor)	982.8	E862.4	—	E950.9	E962.1	E980.9
alcohol	980.0	E860.1	—	E950.9	E962.1	E980.9
beverage	980.0	E860.0	—	E950.9	E962.1	E980.9
aldehyde (vapor)	987.8	E869.8	—	E952.8	E962.2	E982.8
liquid	989.89	E866.8	—	E950.9	E962.1	E980.9
aminobenzoate	968.5	E855.2	E938.5	E950.4	E962.0	E980.4
biscoumacetate	964.2	E858.2	E934.2	E950.4	E962.0	E980.4
bromide (anesthetic)	968.2	E855.1	E938.2	E950.4	E962.0	E980.4
carbamate (antineoplastic)	963.1	E858.1	E933.1	E950.4	E962.0	E980.4
carbinol	980.3	E860.4	—	E950.9	E962.1	E980.9
chaulmoograte	961.8	E857	E931.8	E950.4	E962.0	E980.4
chloride (vapor)	987.8	E869.8	—	E952.8	E962.2	E982.8
anesthetic (local)	968.5	E855.2	E938.5	E950.4	E962.0	E980.4
inhaled	968.2	E855.1	E938.2	E950.4	E962.0	E980.4
solvent	982.3	E862.4	—	E950.9	E962.1	E980.9
estranol	962.1	E858.0	E932.1	E950.4	E962.0	E980.4
ether — *see* Ether(s)						
formate (solvent) NEC	982.8	E862.4	—	E950.9	E962.1	E980.9
iodoacetate	987.5	E869.3	—	E952.8	E962.2	E982.8
lactate (solvent) NEC	982.8	E862.4	—	E950.9	E962.1	E980.9
methylcarbinol	980.8	E860.8	—	E950.9	E962.1	E980.9
morphine	965.09	E850.2	E935.2	E950.0	E962.0	E980.0
Ethylene (gas)	987.1	E869.8	—	E952.8	E962.2	E982.8
anesthetic (general)	968.2	E855.1	E938.2	E950.4	E962.0	E980.4
chlorohydrin (vapor)	982.3	E862.4	—	E950.9	E962.1	E980.9
dichloride (vapor)	982.3	E862.4	—	E950.9	E962.1	E980.9
glycol(s) (any) (vapor)	982.8	E862.4	—	E950.9	E962.1	E980.9
Ethylidene						
chloride NEC	982.3	E862.4	—	E950.9	E962.1	E980.9
diethyl ether	982.8	E862.4	—	E950.9	E962.1	E980.9
Ethynodiol	962.2	E858.0	E932.2	E950.4	E962.0	E980.4
Etidocaine	968.9	E855.2	E938.9	E950.4	E962.0	E980.4
infiltration (subcutaneous)	968.5	E855.2	E938.5	E950.4	E962.0	E980.4
nerve (peripheral) (plexus)	968.6	E855.2	E938.6	E950.4	E962.0	E980.4
Etilfen	967.0	E851	E937.0	E950.1	E962.0	E980.1
Etomide	965.7	E850.7	E935.7	E950.0	E962.0	E980.0
Etorphine	965.09	E850.2	E935.2	E950.0	E962.0	E980.0
Etoval	967.0	E851	E937.0	E950.1	E962.0	E980.1
Etryptamine	969.0	E854.0	E939.0	E950.3	E962.0	E980.3
Eucaine	968.5	E855.2	E938.5	E950.4	E962.0	E980.4
Eucalyptus (oil) NEC	975.5	E858.6	E945.5	E950.4	E962.0	E980.4
Eucatropine	971.1	E855.4	E941.1	E950.4	E962.0	E980.4
Eucodal	965.09	E850.2	E935.2	E950.0	E962.0	E980.0
Euneryl	967.0	E851	E937.0	E950.1	E962.0	E980.1
Euphthalmine	971.1	E855.4	E941.1	E950.4	E962.0	E980.4
Eurax	976.0	E858.7	E946.0	E950.4	E962.0	E980.4
Euresol	976.4	E858.7	E946.4	E950.4	E962.0	E980.4
Euthroid	962.7	E858.0	E932.7	E950.4	E962.0	E980.4
Evans blue	977.8	E858.8	E947.8	E950.4	E962.0	E980.4
Evipal	967.0	E851	E937.0	E950.1	E962.0	E980.1
sodium	968.3	E855.1	E938.3	E950.4	E962.0	E980.4
Evipan	967.0	E851	E937.0	E950.1	E962.0	E980.1
sodium	968.3	E855.1	E938.3	E950.4	E962.0	E980.4
Exalgin	965.4	E850.4	E935.4	E950.0	E962.0	E980.0
Excipients, pharmaceutical	977.4	E858.8	E947.4	E950.4	E962.0	E980.4

TABLE OF DRUGS AND CHEMICALS

Substance	Poisoning	Accident	Therapeutic Use	Suicide Attempt	Assault	Undetermined
		\multicolumn{5}{c}{External Cause (E-Code)}				

Substance	Poisoning	Accident	Therapeutic Use	Suicide Attempt	Assault	Undetermined
Exhaust gas — *see* Carbon, monoxide						
Ex–Lax (phenolphthalein)	973.1	E858.4	E943.1	E950.4	E962.0	E980.4
Expectorants	975.5	E858.6	E945.5	E950.4	E962.0	E980.4
External medications (skin) (mucous membrane)	976.9	E858.7	E946.9	E950.4	E962.0	E980.4
dental agent	976.7	E858.7	E946.7	E950.4	E962.0	E980.4
ENT agent	976.6	E858.7	E946.6	E950.4	E962.0	E980.4
ophthalmic preparation	976.5	E858.7	E946.5	E950.4	E962.0	E980.4
specified NEC	976.8	E858.7	E946.8	E950.4	E962.0	E980.4
Eye agents (anti–infective)	976.5	E858.7	E946.5	E950.4	E962.0	E980.4
Factor IX complex (human)	964.5	E858.2	E934.5	E950.4	E962.0	E980.4
Fecal softeners	973.2	E858.4	E943.2	E950.4	E962.0	E980.4
Fenbutrazate	977.0	E858.8	E947.0	E950.4	E962.0	E980.4
Fencamfamin	970.8	E854.3	E940.8	E950.4	E962.0	E980.4
Fenfluramine	977.0	E858.8	E947.0	E950.4	E962.0	E980.4
Fenoprofen	965.61	E850.6	E935.6	E950.0	E962.0	E980.0
Fentanyl	965.09	E850.2	E935.2	E950.0	E962.0	E980.0
Fentazin	969.1	E853.0	E939.1	E950.3	E962.0	E980.3
Fenticlor, fentichlor	976.0	E858.7	E946.0	E950.4	E962.0	E980.4
Fer de lance (bite) (venom)	989.5	E905.0	—	E950.9	E962.1	E980.9
Ferric — *see* Iron						
Ferrocholinate	964.0	E858.2	E934.0	E950.4	E962.0	E980.4
Ferrous fumarate, gluconate, lactate, salt NEC, sulfate (medicinal)	964.0	E858.2	E934.0	E950.4	E962.0	E980.4
Ferrum — *see* Iron						
Fertilizers NEC	989.89	E866.5	—	E950.9	E962.1	E980.4
with herbicide mixture	989.4	E863.5	—	E950.6	E962.1	E980.7
Fibrinogen (human)	964.7	E858.2	E934.7	E950.4	E962.0	E980.4
Fibrinolysin	964.4	E858.2	E934.4	E950.4	E962.0	E980.4
Fibrinolysis–affecting agents	964.4	E858.2	E934.4	E950.4	E962.0	E980.4
Filix mas	961.6	E857	E931.6	E950.4	E962.0	E980.4
Fiorinal	965.1	E850.3	E935.3	E950.0	E962.0	E980.0
Fire damp	987.1	E869.8	—	E952.8	E962.2	E982.8
Fish, nonbacterial or noxious	988.0	E865.2	—	E950.9	E962.1	E980.9
shell	988.0	E865.1	—	E950.9	E962.1	E980.9
Flagyl	961.5	E857	E931.5	E950.4	E962.0	E980.4
Flavoxate	975.1	E858.6	E945.1	E950.4	E962.0	E980.4
Flaxedil	975.2	E858.6	E945.2	E950.4	E962.0	E980.4
Flaxseed (medicinal)	976.3	E858.7	E946.3	E950.4	E962.0	E980.4
Flomax	971.3	E855.6	E941.3	E950.4	E962.0	E980.4
Florantyrone	973.4	E858.4	E943.4	E950.4	E962.0	E980.4
Floraquin	961.3	E857	E931.3	E950.4	E962.0	E980.4
Florinef	962.0	E858.0	E932.0	E950.4	E962.0	E980.4
ENT agent	976.6	E858.7	E946.6	E950.4	E962.0	E980.4
ophthalmic preparation	976.5	E858.7	E946.5	E950.4	E962.0	E980.4
topical NEC	976.0	E858.7	E946.0	E950.4	E962.0	E980.4
Flowers of sulfur	976.4	E858.7	E946.4	E950.4	E962.0	E980.4
Floxuridine	963.1	E858.1	E933.1	E950.4	E962.0	E980.4
Flucytosine	961.9	E857	E931.9	E950.4	E962.0	E980.4
Fludrocortisone	962.0	E858.0	E932.0	E950.4	E962.0	E980.4
ENT agent	976.6	E858.7	E946.6	E950.4	E962.0	E980.4
ophthalmic preparation	976.5	E858.7	E946.5	E950.4	E962.0	E980.4
topical NEC	976.0	E858.7	E946.0	E950.4	E962.0	E980.4
Flumethasone	976.0	E858.7	E946.0	E950.4	E962.0	E980.4
Flumethiazide	974.3	E858.5	E944.3	E950.4	E962.0	E980.4
Flumidin	961.7	E857	E931.7	E950.4	E962.0	E980.4
Flunitrazepam	969.4	E853.2	E939.4	E950.3	E962.0	E980.3
Fluocinolone	976.0	E858.7	E946.0	E950.4	E962.0	E980.4
Fluocortolone	962.0	E858.0	E932.0	E950.4	E962.0	E980.4
Fluohydrocortisone	962.0	E858.0	E932.0	E950.4	E962.0	E980.4
ENT agent	976.6	E858.7	E946.6	E950.4	E962.0	E980.4

TABLE OF DRUGS AND CHEMICALS

Substance	Poisoning	Accident	Therapeutic Use	Suicide Attempt	Assault	Undetermined
			External Cause (E-Code)			
ophthalmic preparation	976.5	E858.7	E946.5	E950.4	E962.0	E980.4
topical NEC	976.0	E858.7	E946.0	E950.4	E962.0	E980.4
Fluonid	976.0	E858.7	E946.0	E950.4	E962.0	E980.4
Fluopromazine	969.1	E853.0	E939.1	E950.3	E962.0	E980.3
Fluoracetate	989.4	E863.7	—	E950.6	E962.1	E980.7
Fluorescein (sodium)	977.8	E858.8	E947.8	E950.4	E962.0	E980.4
Fluoride(s) (pesticides) (sodium) NEC	989.4	E863.4	—	E950.6	E962.1	E980.7
hydrogen — *see* Hydrofluoric acid						
medicinal	976.7	E858.7	E946.7	E950.4	E962.0	E980.4
not pesticide NEC	983.9	E864.4	—	E950.7	E962.1	E980.6
stannous	976.7	E858.7	E946.7	E950.4	E962.0	E980.4
Fluorinated corticosteroids	962.0	E858.0	E932.0	E950.4	E962.0	E980.4
Fluorine (compounds) (gas)	987.8	E869.8	—	E952.8	E962.2	E982.8
salt — *see* Fluoride(s)						
Fluoristan	976.7	E858.7	E946.7	E950.4	E962.0	E980.4
Fluoroacetate	989.4	E863.7	—	E950.6	E962.1	E980.7
Fluorodeoxyuridine	963.1	E858.1	E933.1	E950.4	E962.0	E980.4
Fluorometholone (topical) NEC	976.0	E858.7	E946.0	E950.4	E962.0	E980.4
ophthalmic preparation	976.5	E858.7	E946.5	E950.4	E962.0	E980.4
Fluorouracil	963.1	E858.1	E933.1	E950.4	E962.0	E980.4
Fluothane	968.1	E855.1	E938.1	E950.4	E962.0	E980.4
Fluoxetine hydrochloride	969.0	E854.0	E939.0	E950.3	E962.0	E980.3
Fluoxymesterone	962.1	E858.0	E932.1	E950.4	E962.0	E980.4
Fluphenazine	969.1	E853.0	E939.1	E950.3	E962.0	E980.3
Fluprednisolone	962.0	E858.0	E932.0	E950.4	E962.0	E980.4
Flurandrenolide	976.0	E858.7	E946.0	E950.4	E962.0	E980.4
Flurazepam (hydrochloride)	969.4	E853.2	E939.4	E950.3	E962.0	E980.3
Flurbiprofen	965.61	E850.6	E935.6	E950.0	E962.0	E980.0
Flurobate	976.0	E858.7	E946.0	E950.4	E962.0	E980.4
Flurothyl	969.8	E855.8	E939.8	E950.3	E962.0	E980.3
Fluroxene	968.2	E855.1	E938.2	E950.4	E962.0	E980.4
Folacin	964.1	E858.2	E934.1	E950.4	E962.0	E980.4
Folic acid	964.1	E858.2	E934.1	E950.4	E962.0	E980.4
Follicle stimulating hormone	962.4	E858.0	E932.4	E950.4	E962.0	E980.4
Food, foodstuffs, nonbacterial or noxious	988.9	E865.9	—	E950.9	E962.1	E980.9
berries, seeds	988.2	E865.3	—	E950.9	E962.1	E980.9
fish	988.0	E865.2	—	E950.9	E962.1	E980.9
mushrooms	988.1	E865.5	—	E950.9	E962.1	E980.9
plants	988.2	E865.9	—	E950.9	E962.1	E980.9
specified type NEC	988.2	E865.4	—	E950.9	E962.1	E980.9
shellfish	988.0	E865.1	—	E950.9	E962.1	E980.9
specified NEC	988.8	E865.8	—	E950.9	E962.1	E980.9
Fool's parsley	988.2	E865.4	—	E950.9	E962.1	E980.9
Formaldehyde (solution)	989.89	E861.4	—	E950.9	E962.1	E980.9
fungicide	989.4	E863.6	—	E950.6	E962.1	E980.7
gas or vapor	987.8	E869.8	—	E952.8	E962.2	E982.8
Formalin	989.89	E861.4	—	E950.9	E962.1	E980.9
fungicide	989.4	E863.6	—	E950.6	E962.1	E980.7
vapor	987.8	E869.8	—	E952.8	E962.2	E982.8
Formic acid	983.1	E864.1	—	E950.7	E962.1	E980.6
vapor	987.8	E869.8	—	E952.8	E962.2	E982.8
Fowler's solution	985.1	E866.3	—	E950.8	E962.1	E980.8
Foxglove	988.2	E865.4	—	E950.9	E962.1	E980.9
Fox green	977.8	E858.8	E947.8	E950.4	E962.0	E980.4
Framycetin	960.8	E856	E930.8	E950.4	E962.0	E980.4
Frangula (extract)	973.1	E858.4	E943.1	E950.4	E962.0	E980.4
Frei antigen	977.8	E858.8	E947.8	E950.4	E962.0	E980.4
Freons	987.4	E869.2	—	E952.8	E962.2	E982.8
Fructose	974.5	E858.5	E944.5	E950.4	E962.0	E980.4
Frusemide	974.4	E858.5	E944.4	E950.4	E962.0	E980.4

1450

TABLE OF DRUGS AND CHEMICALS

Substance	Poisoning	Accident	Therapeutic Use	Suicide Attempt	Assault	Undetermined
		\multicolumn{5}{c}{External Cause (E-Code)}				

Substance	Poisoning	Accident	Therapeutic Use	Suicide Attempt	Assault	Undetermined
FSH	962.4	E858.0	E932.4	E950.4	E962.0	E980.4
Fuel						
automobile	981	E862.1	—	E950.9	E962.1	E980.9
exhaust gas, not in transit	986	E868.2	—	E952.0	E962.2	E982.0
vapor NEC	987.1	E869.8	—	E952.8	E962.2	E982.8
gas (domestic use) — see also Carbon, monoxide, fuel						
utility	987.1	E868.1	—	E951.8	E962.2	E981.8
incomplete combustion of — see Carbon, monoxide, fuel, utility						
in mobile container	987.0	E868.0	—	E951.1	E962.2	E981.1
piped (natural)	987.1	E867	—	E951.0	E962.2	E981.0
industrial, incomplete combustion	986	E868.3	—	E952.1	E962.2	E982.1
Fugillin	960.8	E856	E930.8	E950.4	E962.0	E980.4
Fulminate of mercury	985.0	E866.1	—	E950.9	E962.1	E980.9
Fulvicin	960.1	E856	E930.1	E950.4	E962.0	E980.4
Fumadil	960.8	E856	E930.8	E950.4	E962.0	E980.4
Fumagillin	960.8	E856	E930.8	E950.4	E962.0	E980.4
Fumes (from)	987.9	E869.9	—	E952.9	E962.2	E982.9
carbon monoxide — see Carbon, monoxide						
charcoal (domestic use)	986	E868.3	—	E952.1	E962.2	E982.1
chloroform — see Chloroform						
coke (in domestic stoves, fireplaces)	986	E868.3	—	E952.1	E962.2	E982.1
corrosive NEC	987.8	E869.8	—	E952.8	E962.2	E982.8
ether — see Ether(s)						
freons	987.4	E869.2	—	E952.8	E962.2	E982.8
hydrocarbons	987.1	E869.8	—	E952.8	E962.2	E982.8
petroleum (liquefied)	987.0	E868.0	—	E951.1	E962.2	E981.1
distributed through pipes (pure or mixed with air)	987.0	E867	—	E951.0	E962.2	E981.0
lead — see Lead						
metals — see specified metal						
nitrogen dioxide	987.2	E869.0	—	E952.8	E962.2	E982.8
pesticides — see Pesticides						
petroleum (liquefied)	987.0	E868.0	—	E951.1	E962.2	E981.1
distributed through pipes (pure or mixed with air)	987.0	E867	—	E951.0	E962.2	E981.0
polyester	987.8	E869.8	—	E952.8	E962.2	E982.8
specified source, other (see also substance specified)	987.8	E869.8	—	E952.8	E962.2	E982.8
sulfur dioxide	987.3	E869.1	—	E952.8	E962.2	E982.8
Fumigants	989.4	E863.8	—	E950.6	E962.1	E980.7
Fungi, noxious, used as food	988.1	E865.5	—	E950.9	E962.1	E980.9
Fungicides (see also Antifungals)	989.4	E863.6	—	E950.6	E962.1	E980.7
Fungizone	960.1	E856	E930.1	E950.4	E962.0	E980.4
topical	976.0	E858.7	E946.0	E950.4	E962.0	E980.4
Furacin	976.0	E858.7	E946.0	E950.4	E962.0	E980.4
Furadantin	961.9	E857	E931.9	E950.4	E962.0	E980.4
Furazolidone	961.9	E857	E931.9	E950.4	E962.0	E980.4
Furnace (coal burning) (domestic), gas from	986	E868.3	—	E952.1	E962.2	E982.1
industrial	986	E868.8	—	E952.1	E962.2	E982.1
Furniture polish	989.89	E861.2	—	E950.9	E962.1	E980.9
Furosemide	974.4	E858.5	E944.4	E950.4	E962.0	E980.4
Furoxone	961.9	E857	E931.9	E950.4	E962.0	E980.4
Fusel oil (amyl) (butyl) (propyl)	980.3	E860.4	—	E950.9	E962.1	E980.9
Fusidic acid	960.8	E856	E930.8	E950.4	E962.0	E980.4
Gallamine	975.2	E858.6	E945.2	E950.4	E962.0	E980.4
Gallotannic acid	976.2	E858.7	E946.2	E950.4	E962.0	E980.4
Gamboge	973.1	E858.4	E943.1	E950.4	E962.0	E980.4
Gamimune	964.6	E858.2	E934.6	E950.4	E962.0	E980.4

TABLE OF DRUGS AND CHEMICALS

Substance	Poisoning	Accident	Therapeutic Use	Suicide Attempt	Assault	Undetermined
			External Cause (E-Code)			
Gamma–benzene hexachloride (vapor)	989.2	E863.0	—	E950.6	E962.1	E980.7
Gamma globulin	964.6	E858.2	E934.6	E950.4	E962.0	E980.4
Gamma Hydroxy Butyrate (GHB)	968.4	E855.1	E938.4	E950.4	E962.0	E980.4
Gamulin	964.6	E858.2	E934.6	E950.4	E962.0	E980.4
Ganglionic blocking agents	972.3	E858.3	E942.3	E950.4	E962.0	E980.4
Ganja	969.6	E854.1	E939.6	E950.3	E962.0	E980.3
Garamycin	960.8	E856	E930.8	E950.4	E962.0	E980.4
ophthalmic preparation	976.5	E858.7	E946.5	E950.4	E962.0	E980.4
topical NEC	976.0	E858.7	E946.0	E950.4	E962.0	E980.4
Gardenal	967.0	E851	E937.0	E950.1	E962.0	E980.1
Gardepanyl	967.0	E851	E937.0	E950.1	E962.0	E980.1
Gas	987.9	E869.9	—	E952.9	E962.2	E982.9
acetylene	987.1	E868.1	—	E951.8	E962.2	E981.8
incomplete combustion of — see Carbon, monoxide, fuel, utility						
air contaminants, source or type not specified	987.9	E869.9	—	E952.9	E962.2	E982.9
anesthetic (general) NEC	968.2	E855.1	E938.2	E950.4	E962.0	E980.4
blast furnace	986	E868.8	—	E952.1	E962.2	E982.1
butane — see Butane						
carbon monoxide — see Carbon, monoxide						
chlorine	987.6	E869.8	—	E952.8	E962.2	E982.8
coal — see Carbon, monoxide, coal						
cyanide	987.7	E869.8	—	E952.8	E962.2	E982.8
dicyanogen	987.8	E869.8	—	E952.8	E962.2	E982.8
domestic — see Gas, utility						
exhaust — see Carbon, monoxide, exhaust gas						
from wood– or coal–burning stove or fireplace	986	E868.3	—	E952.1	E962.2	E982.1
fuel (domestic use) — see also Carbon, monoxide, fuel						
industrial use	986	E868.8	—	E952.1	E962.2	E982.1
utility	987.1	E868.1	—	E951.8	E962.2	E981.8
incomplete combustion of — see Carbon, monoxide, fuel, utility						
in mobile container	987.0	E868.0	—	E951.1	E962.2	E981.1
piped (natural)	987.1	E867	—	E951.0	E962.2	E981.0
garage	986	E868.2	—	E952.0	E962.2	E982.0
hydrocarbon NEC	987.1	E869.8	—	E952.8	E962.2	E982.8
incomplete combustion of — see Carbon, monoxide, fuel, utility						
liquefied (mobile container)	987.0	E868.0	—	E951.1	E962.2	E981.1
piped	987.0	E867	—	E951.0	E962.2	E981.0
hydrocyanic acid	987.7	E869.8	—	E952.8	E962.2	E982.8
illuminating — see Gas, utility						
incomplete combustion, any — see Carbon, monoxide						
kiln	986	E868.8	—	E952.1	E962.2	E982.1
lacrimogenic	987.5	E869.3	—	E952.8	E962.2	E982.8
marsh	987.1	E869.8	—	E952.8	E962.2	E982.8
motor exhaust, not in transit	986	E868.8	—	E952.1	E962.2	E982.1
mustard — see Mustard, gas						
natural	987.1	E867	—	E951.0	E962.2	E981.0
nerve (war)	987.9	E869.9	—	E952.9	E962.2	E982.9
oils	981	E862.1	—	E950.9	E962.1	E980.9
petroleum (liquefied) (distributed in mobile containers)	987.0	E868.0	—	E951.1	E962.2	E981.1
piped (pure or mixed with air)	987.0	E867	—	E951.1	E962.2	E981.1
piped (manufactured) (natural) NEC	987.1	E867	—	E951.0	E962.2	E981.0
producer	986	E868.8	—	E952.1	E962.2	E982.1

TABLE OF DRUGS AND CHEMICALS

Substance	Poisoning	Accident	Therapeutic Use	Suicide Attempt	Assault	Undetermined
		\multicolumn{5}{c}{External Cause (E-Code)}				

Substance	Poisoning	Accident	Therapeutic Use	Suicide Attempt	Assault	Undetermined
propane — *see* Propane						
refrigerant (freon)	987.4	E869.2	—	E952.8	E962.2	E982.8
not freon	987.9	E869.9	—	E952.9	E962.2	E982.9
sewer	987.8	E869.8	—	E952.8	E962.2	E982.8
specified source NEC (*see also* substance specified)	987.8	E869.8	—	E952.8	E962.2	E982.8
stove — *see* Gas, utility						
tear	987.5	E869.3	—	E952.8	E962.2	E982.8
utility (for cooking, heating, or lighting) (piped) NEC	987.1	E868.1	—	E951.8	E962.2	E981.8
incomplete combustion of — *see* Carbon, monoxide, fuel, utility						
in mobile container	987.0	E868.0	—	E951.1	E962.2	E981.1
piped (natural)	987.1	E867	—	E951.0	E962.2	E981.0
water	987.1	E868.1	—	E951.8	E962.2	E981.8
incomplete combustion of — *see* Carbon, monoxide, fuel, utility						
Gaseous substance — *see* Gas						
Gasoline, gasolene	981	E862.1	—	E950.9	E962.1	E980.9
vapor	987.1	E869.8	—	E952.8	E962.2	E982.8
Gastric enzymes	973.4	E858.4	E943.4	E950.4	E962.0	E980.4
Gastrografin	977.8	E858.8	E947.8	E950.4	E962.0	E980.4
Gastrointestinal agents	973.9	E858.4	E943.9	E950.4	E962.0	E980.4
specified NEC	973.8	E858.4	E943.8	E950.4	E962.0	E980.4
Gaultheria procumbens	988.2	E865.4	—	E950.9	E962.1	E980.9
Gelatin (intravenous)	964.8	E858.2	E934.8	E950.4	E962.0	E980.4
absorbable (sponge)	964.5	E858.2	E934.5	E950.4	E962.0	E980.4
Gelfilm	976.8	E858.7	E946.8	E950.4	E962.0	E980.4
Gelfoam	964.5	E858.2	E934.5	E950.4	E962.0	E980.4
Gelsemine	970.8	E854.3	E940.8	E950.4	E962.0	E980.4
Gelsemium (sempervirens)	988.2	E865.4	—	E950.9	E962.1	E980.9
Gemonil	967.0	E851	E937.0	E950.1	E962.0	E980.1
Gentamicin	960.8	E856	E930.8	E950.4	E962.0	E980.4
ophthalmic preparation	976.5	E858.7	E946.5	E950.4	E962.0	E980.4
topical NEC	976.0	E858.7	E946.0	E950.4	E962.0	E980.4
Gentian violet	976.0	E858.7	E946.0	E950.4	E962.0	E980.4
Gexane	976.0	E858.7	E946.0	E950.4	E962.0	E980.4
Gila monster (venom)	989.5	E905.0	—	E950.9	E962.1	E980.9
Ginger, Jamaica	989.89	E866.8	—	E950.9	E962.1	E980.9
Gitalin	972.1	E858.3	E942.1	E950.4	E962.0	E980.4
Gitoxin	972.1	E858.3	E942.1	E950.4	E962.0	E980.4
Glandular extract (medicinal) NEC	977.9	E858.9	E947.9	E950.5	E962.0	E980.5
Glaucarubin	961.5	E857	E931.5	E950.4	E962.0	E980.4
Globin zinc insulin	962.3	E858.0	E932.3	E950.4	E962.0	E980.4
Glucagon	962.3	E858.0	E932.3	E950.4	E962.0	E980.4
Glucochloral	967.1	E852.0	E937.1	E950.2	E962.0	E980.2
Glucocorticoids	962.0	E858.0	E932.0	E950.4	E962.0	E980.4
Glucose	974.5	E858.5	E944.5	E950.4	E962.0	E980.4
oxidase reagent	977.8	E858.8	E947.8	E950.4	E962.0	E980.4
Glucosulfone sodium	961.8	E857	E931.8	E950.4	E962.0	E980.4
Glue(s)	989.89	E866.6	—	E950.9	E962.1	E980.9
Glutamic acid (hydrochloride)	973.4	E858.4	E943.4	E950.4	E962.0	E980.4
Glutaraldehyde	989.89	E861.4	—	E950.9	E962.1	E980.9
Glutathione	963.8	E858.1	E933.8	E950.4	E962.0	E980.4
Glutethimide (group)	967.5	E852.4	E937.5	E950.2	E962.0	E980.2
Glycerin (lotion)	976.3	E858.7	E946.3	E950.4	E962.0	E980.4
Glycerol (topical)	976.3	E858.7	E946.3	E950.4	E962.0	E980.4
Glyceryl						
guaiacolate	975.5	E858.6	E945.5	E950.4	E962.0	E980.4
triacetate (topical)	976.0	E858.7	E946.0	E950.4	E962.0	E980.4
trinitrate	972.4	E858.3	E942.4	E950.4	E962.0	E980.4

TABLE OF DRUGS AND CHEMICALS

Substance	Poisoning	Accident	Therapeutic Use	Suicide Attempt	Assault	Undetermined
		\multicolumn{5}{c	}{External Cause (E-Code)}

Substance	Poisoning	Accident	Therapeutic Use	Suicide Attempt	Assault	Undetermined
Glycine	974.5	E858.5	E944.5	E950.4	E962.0	E980.4
Glycobiarsol	961.1	E857	E931.1	E950.4	E962.0	E980.4
Glycols (ether)	982.8	E862.4	—	E950.9	E962.1	E980.9
Glycopyrrolate	971.1	E855.4	E941.1	E950.4	E962.0	E980.4
Glymidine	962.3	E858.0	E932.3	E950.4	E962.0	E980.4
Gold (compounds) (salts)	965.69	E850.6	E935.6	E950.0	E962.0	E980.0
Golden sulfide of antimony	985.4	E866.2	—	E950.9	E962.1	E980.9
Goldylocks	988.2	E865.4	—	E950.9	E962.1	E980.9
Gonadal tissue extract	962.9	E858.0	E932.9	E950.4	E962.0	E980.4
female	962.2	E858.0	E932.2	E950.4	E962.0	E980.4
male	962.1	E858.0	E932.1	E950.4	E962.0	E980.4
Gonadotropin	962.4	E858.0	E932.4	E950.4	E962.0	E980.4
Grain alcohol	980.0	E860.1	—	E950.9	E962.1	E980.9
beverage	980.0	E860.0	—	E950.9	E962.1	E980.9
Gramicidin	960.8	E856	E930.8	E950.4	E962.0	E980.4
Gratiola officinalis	988.2	E865.4	—	E950.9	E962.1	E980.9
Grease	989.89	E866.8	—	E950.9	E962.1	E980.9
Green hellebore	988.2	E865.4	—	E950.9	E962.1	E980.9
Green soap	976.2	E858.7	E946.2	E950.4	E962.0	E980.4
Grifulvin	960.1	E856	E930.1	E950.4	E962.0	E980.4
Griseofulvin	960.1	E856	E930.1	E950.4	E962.0	E980.4
Growth hormone	962.4	E858.0	E932.4	E950.4	E962.0	E980.4
Guaiacol	975.5	E858.6	E945.5	E950.4	E962.0	E980.4
Guaiac reagent	977.8	E858.8	E947.8	E950.4	E962.0	E980.4
Guaifenesin	975.5	E858.6	E945.5	E950.4	E962.0	E980.4
Guaiphenesin	975.5	E858.6	E945.5	E950.4	E962.0	E980.4
Guanatol	961.4	E857	E931.4	E950.4	E962.0	E980.4
Guanethidine	972.6	E858.3	E942.6	E950.4	E962.0	E980.4
Guano	989.89	E866.5	—	E950.9	E962.1	E980.9
Guanochlor	972.6	E858.3	E942.6	E950.4	E962.0	E980.4
Guanoctine	972.6	E858.3	E942.6	E950.4	E962.0	E980.4
Guanoxan	972.6	E858.3	E942.6	E950.4	E962.0	E980.4
Hair treatment agent NEC	976.4	E858.7	E946.4	E950.4	E962.0	E980.4
Halcinonide	976.0	E858.7	E946.0	E950.4	E962.0	E980.4
Halethazole	976.0	E858.7	E946.0	E950.4	E962.0	E980.4
Hallucinogens	969.6	E854.1	E939.6	E950.3	E962.0	E980.3
Haloperidol	969.2	E853.1	E939.2	E950.3	E962.0	E980.3
Haloprogin	976.0	E858.7	E946.0	E950.4	E962.0	E980.4
Halotex	976.0	E858.7	E946.0	E950.4	E962.0	E980.4
Halothane	968.1	E855.1	E938.1	E950.4	E962.0	E980.4
Halquinols	976.0	E858.7	E946.0	E950.4	E962.0	E980.4
Harmonyl	972.6	E858.3	E942.6	E950.4	E962.0	E980.4
Hartmann's solution	974.5	E858.5	E944.5	E950.4	E962.0	E980.4
Hashish	969.6	E854.1	E939.6	E950.3	E962.0	E980.3
Hawaiian wood rose seeds	969.6	E854.1	E939.6	E950.3	E962.0	E980.3
Headache cures, drugs, powders NEC	977.9	E858.9	E947.9	E950.5	E962.0	E980.9
Heavenly Blue (morning glory)	969.6	E854.1	E939.6	E950.3	E962.0	E980.3
Heavy metal						
antagonists	963.8	E858.1	E933.8	E950.4	E962.0	E980.4
anti-infectives	961.2	E857	E931.2	E950.4	E962.0	E980.4
Hedaquinium	976.0	E858.7	E946.0	E950.4	E962.0	E980.4
Hedge hyssop	988.2	E865.4	—	E950.9	E962.1	E980.9
Heet	976.8	E858.7	E946.8	E950.4	E962.0	E980.4
Helenin	961.6	E857	E931.6	E950.4	E962.0	E980.4
Hellebore (black) (green) (white)	988.2	E865.4	—	E950.9	E962.1	E980.9
Hemlock	988.2	E865.4	—	E950.9	E962.1	E980.9
Hemostatics	964.5	E858.2	E934.5	E950.4	E962.0	E980.4
capillary active drugs	972.8	E858.3	E942.8	E950.4	E962.0	E980.4
Henbane	988.2	E865.4	—	E950.9	E962.1	E980.9
Heparin (sodium)	964.2	E858.2	E934.2	E950.4	E962.0	E980.4

TABLE OF DRUGS AND CHEMICALS

Substance	Poisoning	Accident	Therapeutic Use	Suicide Attempt	Assault	Undetermined
			External Cause (E-Code)			
Heptabarbital, heptabarbitone	967.0	E851	E937.0	E950.1	E962.0	E980.1
Heptachlor	989.2	E863.0	—	E950.6	E962.1	E980.7
Heptalgin	965.09	E850.2	E935.2	E950.0	E962.0	E980.0
Herbicides	989.4	E863.5	—	E950.6	E962.1	E980.7
Heroin	965.01	E850.0	E935.0	E950.0	E962.0	E980.0
Herplex	976.5	E858.7	E946.5	E950.4	E962.0	E980.4
HES	964.8	E858.2	E934.8	E950.4	E962.0	E980.4
Hetastarch	964.8	E858.2	E934.8	E950.4	E962.0	E980.4
Hexachlorocyclohexane	989.2	E863.0	—	E950.6	E962.1	E980.7
Hexachlorophene	976.2	E858.7	E946.2	E950.4	E962.0	E980.4
Hexadimethrine (bromide)	964.5	E858.2	E934.5	E950.4	E962.0	E980.4
Hexafluorenium	975.2	E858.6	E945.2	E950.4	E962.0	E980.4
Hexa–germ	976.2	E858.7	E946.2	E950.4	E962.0	E980.4
Hexahydrophenol	980.8	E860.8	—	E950.9	E962.1	E980.9
Hexalin	980.8	E860.8	—	E950.9	E962.1	E980.9
Hexamethonium	972.3	E858.3	E942.3	E950.4	E962.0	E980.4
Hexamethyleneamine	961.9	E857	E931.9	E950.4	E962.0	E980.4
Hexamine	961.9	E857	E931.9	E950.4	E962.0	E980.4
Hexanone	982.8	E862.4	—	E950.9	E962.1	E980.9
Hexapropymate	967.8	E852.8	E937.8	E950.2	E962.0	E980.2
Hexestrol	962.2	E858.0	E932.2	E950.4	E962.0	E980.4
Hexethal (sodium)	967.0	E851	E937.0	E950.1	E962.0	E980.1
Hexetidine	976.0	E858.7	E946.0	E950.4	E962.0	E980.4
Hexobarbital, hexobarbitone	967.0	E851	E937.0	E950.1	E962.0	E980.1
sodium (anesthetic)	968.3	E855.1	E938.3	E950.4	E962.0	E980.4
soluble	968.3	E855.1	E938.3	E950.4	E962.0	E980.4
Hexocyclium	971.1	E855.4	E941.1	E950.4	E962.0	E980.4
Hexoestrol	962.2	E858.0	E932.2	E950.4	E962.0	E980.4
Hexone	982.8	E862.4	—	E950.9	E962.1	E980.9
Hexylcaine	968.5	E855.2	E938.5	E950.4	E962.0	E980.4
Hexylresorcinol	961.6	E857	E931.6	E950.4	E962.0	E980.4
Hinkle's pills	973.1	E858.4	E943.1	E950.4	E962.0	E980.4
Histalog	977.8	E858.8	E947.8	E950.4	E962.0	E980.4
Histamine (phosphate)	972.5	E858.3	E942.5	E950.4	E962.0	E980.4
Histoplasmin	977.8	E858.8	E947.8	E950.4	E962.0	E980.4
Holly berries	988.2	E865.3	—	E950.9	E962.1	E980.9
Homatropine	971.1	E855.4	E941.1	E950.4	E962.0	E980.4
Homo–tet	964.6	E858.2	E934.6	E950.4	E962.0	E980.4
Hormones (synthetic substitute) NEC	962.9	E858.0	E932.9	E950.4	E962.0	E980.4
adrenal cortical steroids	962.0	E858.0	E932.0	E950.4	E962.0	E980.4
antidiabetic agents	962.3	E858.0	E932.3	E950.4	E962.0	E980.4
follicle stimulating	962.4	E858.0	E932.4	E950.4	E962.0	E980.4
gonadotropic	962.4	E858.0	E932.4	E950.4	E962.0	E980.4
growth	962.4	E858.0	E932.4	E950.4	E962.0	E980.4
ovarian (substitutes)	962.2	E858.0	E932.2	E950.4	E962.0	E980.4
parathyroid (derivatives)	962.6	E858.0	E932.6	E950.4	E962.0	E980.4
pituitary (posterior)	962.5	E858.0	E932.5	E950.4	E962.0	E980.4
anterior	962.4	E858.0	E932.4	E950.4	E962.0	E980.4
thyroid (derivative)	962.7	E858.0	E932.7	E950.4	E962.0	E980.4
Hornet (sting)	989.5	E905.3	—	E950.9	E962.1	E980.9
Horticulture agent NEC	989.4	E863.9	—	E950.6	E962.1	E980.7
Hyaluronidase	963.4	E858.1	E933.4	E950.4	E962.0	E980.4
Hyazyme	963.4	E858.1	E933.4	E950.4	E962.0	E980.4
Hycodan	965.09	E850.2	E935.2	E950.0	E962.0	E980.0
Hydantoin derivatives	966.1	E855.0	E936.1	E950.4	E962.0	E980.4
Hydeltra	962.0	E858.0	E932.0	E950.4	E962.0	E980.4
Hydergine	971.3	E855.6	E941.3	E950.4	E962.0	E980.4
Hydrabamine penicillin	960.0	E856	E930.0	E950.4	E962.0	E980.4
Hydralazine, hydrallazine	972.6	E858.3	E942.6	E950.4	E962.0	E980.4
Hydrargaphen	976.0	E858.7	E946.0	E950.4	E962.0	E980.4
Hydrazine	983.9	E864.3	—	E950.7	E962.1	E980.6

TABLE OF DRUGS AND CHEMICALS

Substance	Poisoning	Accident	Therapeutic Use	Suicide Attempt	Assault	Undetermined
		\multicolumn{5}{c}{External Cause (E-Code)}				

Substance	Poisoning	Accident	Therapeutic Use	Suicide Attempt	Assault	Undetermined
Hydriodic acid	975.5	E858.6	E945.5	E950.4	E962.0	E980.4
Hydrocarbon gas	987.1	E869.8	—	E952.8	E962.2	E982.8
incomplete combustion of — *see* Carbon, monoxide, fuel, utility						
liquefied (mobile container)	987.0	E868.0	—	E951.1	E962.2	E981.1
piped (natural)	987.0	E867	—	E951.0	E962.2	E981.0
Hydrochloric acid (liquid)	983.1	E864.1	—	E950.7	E962.1	E980.6
medicinal	973.4	E858.4	E943.4	E950.4	E962.0	E980.4
vapor	987.8	E869.8	—	E952.8	E962.2	E982.8
Hydrochlorothiazide	974.3	E858.5	E944.3	E950.4	E962.0	E980.4
Hydrocodone	965.09	E850.2	E935.2	E950.0	E962.0	E980.0
Hydrocortisone	962.0	E858.0	E932.0	E950.4	E962.0	E980.4
ENT agent	976.6	E858.7	E946.6	E950.4	E962.0	E980.4
ophthalmic preparation	976.5	E858.7	E946.5	E950.4	E962.0	E980.4
topical NEC	976.0	E858.7	E946.0	E950.4	E962.0	E980.4
Hydrocortone	962.0	E858.0	E932.0	E950.4	E962.0	E980.4
ENT agent	976.6	E858.7	E946.6	E950.4	E962.0	E980.4
ophthalmic preparation	976.5	E858.7	E946.5	E950.4	E962.0	E980.4
topical NEC	976.0	E858.7	E946.0	E950.4	E962.0	E980.4
Hydrocyanic acid — *see* Cyanide(s)						
Hydroflumethiazide	974.3	E858.5	E944.3	E950.4	E962.0	E980.4
Hydrofluoric acid (liquid)	983.1	E864.1	—	E950.7	E962.1	E980.6
vapor	987.8	E869.8	—	E952.8	E962.2	E982.8
Hydrogen	987.8	E869.8	—	E952.8	E962.2	E982.8
arsenide	985.1	E866.3	—	E950.8	E962.1	E980.8
arseniureted	985.1	E866.3	—	E950.8	E962.1	E980.8
cyanide (salts)	989.0	E866.8	—	E950.9	E962.1	E980.9
gas	987.7	E869.8	—	E952.8	E962.2	E982.8
fluoride (liquid)	983.1	E864.1	—	E950.7	E962.1	E980.6
vapor	987.8	E869.8	—	E952.8	E962.2	E982.8
peroxide (solution)	976.6	E858.7	E946.6	E950.4	E962.0	E980.4
phosphureted	987.8	E869.8	—	E952.8	E962.2	E982.8
sulfide (gas)	987.8	E869.8	—	E952.8	E962.2	E982.8
arseniureted	985.1	E866.3	—	E950.8	E962.1	E980.8
sulfureted	987.8	E869.8	—	E952.8	E962.2	E982.8
Hydromorphinol	965.09	E850.2	E935.2	E950.0	E962.0	E980.0
Hydromorphinone	965.09	E850.2	E935.2	E950.0	E962.0	E980.0
Hydromorphone	965.09	E850.2	E935.2	E950.0	E962.0	E980.0
Hydromox	974.3	E858.5	E944.3	E950.4	E962.0	E980.4
Hydrophilic lotion	976.3	E858.7	E946.3	E950.4	E962.0	E980.4
Hydroquinone	983.0	E864.0	—	E950.7	E962.1	E980.6
vapor	987.8	E869.8	—	E952.8	E962.2	E982.8
Hydrosulfuric acid (gas)	987.8	E869.8	—	E952.8	E962.2	E982.8
Hydrous wool fat (lotion)	976.3	E858.7	E946.3	E950.4	E962.0	E980.4
Hydroxide, caustic	983.2	E864.2	—	E950.7	E962.1	E980.6
Hydroxocobalamin	964.1	E858.2	E934.1	E950.4	E962.0	E980.4
Hydroxyamphetamine	971.2	E855.5	E941.2	E950.4	E962.0	E980.4
Hydroxychloroquine	961.4	E857	E931.4	E950.4	E962.0	E980.4
Hydroxydihydrocodeinone	965.09	E850.2	E935.2	E950.0	E962.0	E980.0
Hydroxyethyl starch	964.8	E858.2	E934.8	E950.4	E962.0	E980.4
Hydroxyphenamate	969.5	E853.8	E939.5	E950.3	E962.0	E980.3
Hydroxyphenylbutazone	965.5	E850.5	E935.5	E950.0	E962.0	E980.0
Hydroxyprogesterone	962.2	E858.0	E932.2	E950.4	E962.0	E980.4
Hydroxyquinoline derivatives	961.3	E857	E931.3	E950.4	E962.0	E980.4
Hydroxystilbamidine	961.5	E857	E931.5	E950.4	E962.0	E980.4
Hydroxyurea	963.1	E858.1	E933.1	E950.4	E962.0	E980.4
Hydroxyzine	969.5	E853.8	E939.5	E950.3	E962.0	E980.3
Hyoscine (hydrobromide)	971.1	E855.4	E941.1	E950.4	E962.0	E980.4
Hyoscyamine	971.1	E855.4	E941.1	E950.4	E962.0	E980.4
Hyoscyamus (albus) (niger)	988.2	E865.4	—	E950.9	E962.1	E980.9

TABLE OF DRUGS AND CHEMICALS

Substance	Poisoning	Accident	Therapeutic Use	Suicide Attempt	Assault	Undetermined
		\multicolumn{5}{c}{External Cause (E-Code)}				

Substance	Poisoning	Accident	Therapeutic Use	Suicide Attempt	Assault	Undetermined
Hypaque	977.8	E858.8	E947.8	E950.4	E962.0	E980.4
Hypertussis	964.6	E858.2	E934.6	E950.4	E962.0	E980.4
Hypnotics NEC	967.9	E852.9	E937.9	E950.2	E962.0	E980.2
Hypochlorites — see Sodium, hypochlorite						
Hypotensive agents NEC	972.6	E858.3	E942.6	E950.4	E962.0	E980.4
Ibufenac	965.69	E850.6	E935.6	E950.0	E962.0	E980.0
ibuprofen	965.61	E850.6	E935.6	E950.0	E962.0	E980.0
ICG	977.8	E858.8	E947.8	E950.4	E962.0	E980.4
Ichthammol	976.4	E858.7	E946.4	E950.4	E962.0	E980.4
Ichthyol	976.4	E858.7	E946.4	E950.4	E962.0	E980.4
Idoxuridine	976.5	E858.7	E946.5	E950.4	E962.0	E980.4
IDU	976.5	E858.7	E946.5	E950.4	E962.0	E980.4
Iletin	962.3	E858.0	E932.3	E950.4	E962.0	E980.4
Ilex	988.2	E865.4	—	E950.9	E962.1	E980.9
Illuminating gas — see Gas, utility						
Ilopan	963.5	E858.1	E933.5	E950.4	E962.0	E980.4
Ilotycin	960.3	E856	E930.3	E950.4	E962.0	E980.4
ophthalmic preparation	976.5	E858.7	E946.5	E950.4	E962.0	E980.4
topical NEC	976.0	E858.7	E946.0	E950.4	E962.0	E980.4
Imipramine	969.0	E854.0	E939.0	E950.3	E962.0	E980.3
Immu–G	964.6	E858.2	E934.6	E950.4	E962.0	E980.4
Immuglobin	964.6	E858.2	E934.6	E950.4	E962.0	E980.4
Immune serum globulin	964.6	E858.2	E934.6	E950.4	E962.0	E980.4
Immunosuppressive agents	963.1	E858.1	E933.1	E950.4	E962.0	E980.4
Immu–tetanus	964.6	E858.2	E934.6	E950.4	E962.0	E980.4
Indandione (derivatives)	964.2	E858.2	E934.2	E950.4	E962.0	E980.4
Inderal	972.0	E858.3	E942.0	E950.4	E962.0	E980.4
Indian						
hemp	969.6	E854.1	E939.6	E950.3	E962.0	E980.3
tobacco	988.2	E865.4	—	E950.9	E962.1	E980.9
Indigo carmine	977.8	E858.8	E947.8	E950.4	E962.0	E980.4
Indocin	965.69	E850.6	E935.6	E950.0	E962.0	E980.0
Indocyanine green	977.8	E858.8	E947.8	E950.4	E962.0	E980.4
Indomethacin	965.69	E850.6	E935.6	E950.0	E962.0	E980.0
Industrial						
alcohol	980.9	E860.9	—	E950.9	E962.1	E980.9
fumes	987.8	E869.8	—	E952.8	E962.2	E982.8
solvents (fumes) (vapors)	982.8	E862.9	—	E950.9	E962.1	E980.9
Influenza vaccine	979.6	E858.8	E949.6	E950.4	E962.0	E982.8
Ingested substances NEC	989.9	E866.9	—	E950.9	E962.1	E980.9
INH (isoniazid)	961.8	E857	E931.8	E950.4	E962.0	E980.4
Inhalation, gas (noxious) — see Gas						
Ink	989.89	E866.8	—	E950.9	E962.1	E980.9
Innovar	967.6	E852.5	E937.6	E950.2	E962.0	E980.2
Inositol niacinate	972.2	E858.3	E942.2	E950.4	E962.0	E980.4
Inproquone	963.1	E858.1	E933.1	E950.4	E962.0	E980.4
Insect (sting), venomous	989.5	E905.5	—	E950.9	E962.1	E980.9
Insecticides (see also Pesticides)	989.4	E863.4	—	E950.6	E962.1	E980.7
chlorinated	989.2	E863.0	—	E950.6	E962.1	E980.7
mixtures	989.4	E863.3	—	E950.6	E962.1	E980.7
organochlorine (compounds)	989.2	E863.0	—	E950.6	E962.1	E980.7
organophosphorus (compounds)	989.3	E863.1	—	E950.6	E962.1	E980.7
Insular tissue extract	962.3	E858.0	E932.3	E950.4	E962.0	E980.4
Insulin (amorphous) (globin) (isophane) (Lente) (NPH) (protamine) (Semilente) (Ultralente) (zinc)	962.3	E858.0	E932.3	E950.4	E962.0	E980.4
Intranarcon	968.3	E855.1	E938.3	E950.4	E962.0	E980.4
Inulin	977.8	E858.8	E947.8	E950.4	E962.0	E980.4
Invert sugar	974.5	E858.5	E944.5	E950.4	E962.0	E980.4
Inza — see Naproxen						
Iodide NEC (see also Iodine)	976.0	E858.7	E946.0	E950.4	E962.0	E980.4

1457

TABLE OF DRUGS AND CHEMICALS

Substance	Poisoning	Accident	Therapeutic Use	Suicide Attempt	Assault	Undetermined
		\multicolumn{5}{c}{External Cause (E-Code)}				

Substance	Poisoning	Accident	Therapeutic Use	Suicide Attempt	Assault	Undetermined
mercury (ointment)	976.0	E858.7	E946.0	E950.4	E962.0	E980.4
methylate	976.0	E858.7	E946.0	E950.4	E962.0	E980.4
potassium (expectorant) NEC	975.5	E858.6	E945.5	E950.4	E962.0	E980.4
Iodinated glycerol	975.5	E858.6	E945.5	E950.4	E962.0	E980.4
Iodine (antiseptic, external) (tincture) NEC	976.0	E858.7	E946.0	E950.4	E962.0	E980.4
diagnostic	977.8	E858.8	E947.8	E950.4	E962.0	E980.4
for thyroid conditions (antithyroid)	962.8	E858.0	E932.8	E950.4	E962.0	E980.4
vapor	987.8	E869.8	—	E952.8	E962.2	E982.8
Iodized oil	977.8	E858.8	E947.8	E950.4	E962.0	E980.4
Iodobismitol	961.2	E857	E931.2	E950.4	E962.0	E980.4
Iodochlorhydroxyquin	961.3	E857	E931.3	E950.4	E962.0	E980.4
topical	976.0	E858.7	E946.0	E950.4	E962.0	E980.4
Iodoform	976.0	E858.7	E946.0	E950.4	E962.0	E980.4
Iodopanoic acid	977.8	E858.8	E947.8	E950.4	E962.0	E980.4
Iodophthalein	977.8	E858.8	E947.8	E950.4	E962.0	E980.4
Ion exchange resins	974.5	E858.5	E944.5	E950.4	E962.0	E980.4
Iopanoic acid	977.8	E858.8	E947.8	E950.4	E962.0	E980.4
Iophendylate	977.8	E858.8	E947.8	E950.4	E962.0	E980.4
Iothiouracil	962.8	E858.0	E932.8	E950.4	E962.0	E980.4
Ipecac	973.6	E858.4	E943.6	E950.4	E962.0	E980.4
Ipecacuanha	973.6	E858.4	E943.6	E950.4	E962.0	E980.4
Ipodate	977.8	E858.8	E947.8	E950.4	E962.0	E980.4
Ipral	967.0	E851	E937.0	E950.1	E962.0	E980.1
Ipratropium	975.1	E858.6	E945.1	E950.4	E962.0	E980.4
Iproniazid	969.0	E854.0	E939.0	E950.3	E962.0	E980.3
Iron (compounds) (medicinal) (preparations)	964.0	E858.2	E934.0	E950.4	E962.0	E980.4
dextran	964.0	E858.2	E934.0	E950.4	E962.0	E980.4
nonmedicinal (dust) (fumes) NEC	985.8	E866.4	—	E950.9	E962.1	E980.9
Irritant drug	977.9	E858.9	E947.9	E950.5	E962.0	E980.5
Ismelin	972.6	E858.3	E942.6	E950.4	E962.0	E980.4
Isoamyl nitrite	972.4	E858.3	E942.4	E950.4	E962.0	E980.4
Isobutyl acetate	982.8	E862.4	—	E950.9	E962.1	E980.9
Isocarboxazid	969.0	E854.0	E939.0	E950.3	E962.0	E980.3
Isoephedrine	971.2	E855.5	E941.2	E950.4	E962.0	E980.4
Isoetharine	971.2	E855.5	E941.2	E950.4	E962.0	E980.4
Isofluorophate	971.0	E855.3	E941.0	E950.4	E962.0	E980.4
Isoniazid (INH)	961.8	E857	E931.8	E950.4	E962.0	E980.4
Isopentaquine	961.4	E857	E931.4	E950.4	E962.0	E980.4
Isophane insulin	962.3	E858.0	E932.3	E950.4	E962.0	E980.4
Isopregnenone	962.2	E858.0	E932.2	E950.4	E962.0	E980.4
Isoprenaline	971.2	E855.5	E941.2	E950.4	E962.0	E980.4
Isopropamide	971.1	E855.4	E941.1	E950.4	E962.0	E980.4
Isopropanol	980.2	E860.3	—	E950.9	E962.1	E980.9
topical (germicide)	976.0	E858.7	E946.0	E950.4	E962.0	E980.4
Isopropyl acetate	982.8	E862.4	—	E950.9	E962.1	E980.9
alcohol	980.2	E860.3	—	E950.9	E962.1	E980.9
topical (germicide)	976.0	E858.7	E946.0	E950.4	E962.0	E980.4
ether	982.8	E862.4	—	E950.9	E962.1	E980.9
Isoproterenol	971.2	E855.5	E941.2	E950.4	E962.0	E980.4
Isosorbide dinitrate	972.4	E858.3	E942.4	E950.4	E962.0	E980.4
Isothipendyl	963.0	E858.1	E933.0	E950.4	E962.0	E980.4
Isoxazolyl penicillin	960.0	E856	E930.0	E950.4	E962.0	E980.4
Isoxsuprine hydrochloride	972.5	E858.3	E942.5	E950.4	E962.0	E980.4
l–thyroxine sodium	962.7	E858.0	E932.7	E950.4	E962.0	E980.4
Jaborandi (pilocarpus) (extract)	971.0	E855.3	E941.0	E950.4	E962.0	E980.4
Jalap	973.1	E858.4	E943.1	E950.4	E962.0	E980.4
Jamaica						

1458

TABLE OF DRUGS AND CHEMICALS

Substance	Poisoning	Accident	Therapeutic Use	Suicide Attempt	Assault	Undetermined
			External Cause (E-Code)			
dogwood (bark)	965.7	E850.7	E935.7	E950.0	E962.0	E980.0
ginger	989.89	E866.8	—	E950.9	E962.1	E980.9
Jatropha	988.2	E865.4	—	E950.9	E962.1	E980.9
curcas	988.2	E865.3	—	E950.9	E962.1	E980.9
Jectofer	964.0	E858.2	E934.0	E950.4	E962.0	E980.4
Jellyfish (sting)	989.5	E905.6	—	E950.9	E962.1	E980.9
Jequirity (bean)	988.2	E865.3	—	E950.9	E962.1	E980.9
Jimson weed	988.2	E865.4	—	E950.9	E962.1	E980.9
seeds	988.2	E865.3	—	E950.9	E962.1	E980.9
Juniper tar (oil) (ointment)	976.4	E858.7	E946.4	E950.4	E962.0	E980.4
Kallikrein	972.5	E858.3	E942.5	E950.4	E962.0	E980.4
Kanamycin	960.6	E856	E930.6	E950.4	E962.0	E980.4
Kantrex	960.6	E856	E930.6	E950.4	E962.0	E980.4
Kaolin	973.5	E858.4	E943.5	E950.4	E962.0	E980.4
Karaya (gum)	973.3	E858.4	E943.3	E950.4	E962.0	E980.4
Kemithal	968.3	E855.1	E938.3	E950.4	E962.0	E980.4
Kenacort	962.0	E858.0	E932.0	E950.4	E962.0	E980.4
Keratolytics	976.4	E858.7	E946.4	E950.4	E962.0	E980.4
Keratoplastics	976.4	E858.7	E946.4	E950.4	E962.0	E980.4
Kerosene, kerosine (fuel) (solvent) NEC	981	E862.1	—	E950.9	E962.1	E980.9
insecticide	981	E863.4	—	E950.6	E962.1	E980.7
vapor	987.1	E869.8	—	E952.8	E962.2	E982.8
Ketamine	968.3	E855.1	E938.3	E950.4	E962.0	E980.4
Ketobemidone	965.09	E850.2	E935.2	E950.0	E962.0	E980.0
Ketols	982.8	E862.4	—	E950.9	E962.1	E980.9
Ketone oils	982.8	E862.4	—	E950.9	E962.1	E980.9
Ketoprofen	965.61	E850.6	E935.6	E950.0	E962.0	E980.0
Kiln gas or vapor (carbon monoxide)	986	E868.8	—	E952.1	E962.2	E982.1
Konsyl	973.3	E858.4	E943.3	E950.4	E962.0	E980.4
Kosam seed	988.2	E865.3	—	E950.9	E962.1	E980.9
Krait (venom)	989.5	E905.0	—	E950.9	E962.1	E980.9
Kwell (insecticide)	989.2	E863.0	—	E950.6	E962.1	E980.7
anti–infective (topical)	976.0	E858.7	E946.0	E950.4	E962.0	E980.4
Laburnum (flowers) (seeds)	988.2	E865.3	—	E950.9	E962.1	E980.9
leaves	988.2	E865.4	—	E950.9	E962.1	E980.9
Lacquers	989.89	E861.6	—	E950.9	E962.1	E980.9
Lacrimogenic gas	987.5	E869.3	—	E952.8	E962.2	E982.8
Lactic acid	983.1	E864.1	—	E950.7	E962.1	E980.6
Lactobacillus acidophilus	973.5	E858.4	E943.5	E950.4	E962.0	E980.4
Lactoflavin	963.5	E858.1	E933.5	E950.4	E962.0	E980.4
Lactuca (virosa) (extract)	967.8	E852.8	E937.8	E950.2	E962.0	E980.2
Lactucarium	967.8	E852.8	E937.8	E950.2	E962.0	E980.2
Laevulose	974.5	E858.5	E944.5	E950.4	E962.0	E980.4
Lanatoside(C)	972.1	E858.3	E942.1	E950.4	E962.0	E980.4
Lanolin (lotion)	976.3	E858.7	E946.3	E950.4	E962.0	E980.4
Largactil	969.1	E853.0	E939.1	E950.3	E962.0	E980.3
Larkspur	988.2	E865.3	—	E950.9	E962.1	E980.9
Laroxyl	969.0	E854.0	E939.0	E950.3	E962.0	E980.3
Lasix	974.4	E858.5	E944.4	E950.4	E962.0	E980.4
Latex	989.82	E866.8	—	E950.9	E962.1	E980.9
Lathyrus (seed)	988.2	E865.3	—	E950.9	E962.1	E980.9
Laudanum	965.09	E850.2	E935.2	E950.0	E962.0	E980.0
Laudexium	975.2	E858.6	E945.2	E950.4	E962.0	E980.4
Laurel, black or cherry	988.2	E865.4	—	E950.9	E962.1	E980.9
Laurolinium	976.0	E858.7	E946.0	E950.4	E962.0	E980.4
Lauryl sulfoacetate	976.2	E858.7	E946.2	E950.4	E962.0	E980.4
Laxatives NEC	973.3	E858.4	E943.3	E950.4	E962.0	E980.4
emollient	973.2	E858.4	E943.2	E950.4	E962.0	E980.4
L–dopa	966.4	E855.0	E936.4	E950.4	E962.0	E980.4
L Tryptophan—*see* amino acid						
Lead (dust) (fumes) (vapor) NEC	984.9	E866.0	—	E950.9	E962.1	E980.9

1459

TABLE OF DRUGS AND CHEMICALS

Substance	Poisoning	Accident	Therapeutic Use	Suicide Attempt	Assault	Undetermined
		\multicolumn{5}{c}{External Cause (E-Code)}				
acetate (dust)	984.1	E866.0	—	E950.9	E962.1	E980.9
anti–infectives	961.2	E857	E931.2	E950.4	E962.0	E980.4
antiknock compound (tetraethyl)	984.1	E862.1	—	E950.9	E962.1	E980.9
arsenate, arsenite (dust) (insecticide) (vapor)	985.1	E863.4	—	E950.8	E962.1	E980.8
herbicide	985.1	E863.5	—	E950.8	E962.1	E980.8
carbonate	984.0	E866.0	—	E950.9	E962.1	E980.9
paint	984.0	E861.5	—	E950.9	E962.1	E980.9
chromate	984.0	E866.0	—	E950.9	E962.1	E980.9
paint	984.0	E861.5	—	E950.9	E962.1	E980.9
dioxide	984.0	E866.0	—	E950.9	E962.1	E980.9
inorganic (compound)	984.0	E866.0	—	E950.9	E962.1	E980.9
paint	984.0	E861.5	—	E950.9	E962.1	E980.9
iodine	984.0	E866.0	—	E950.9	E962.1	E980.9
pigment (paint)	984.0	E861.5	—	E950.9	E962.1	E980.9
monoxide (dust)	984.0	E866.0	—	E950.9	E962.1	E980.9
paint	984.0	E861.5	—	E950.9	E962.1	E980.9
organic	984.1	E866.0	—	E950.9	E962.1	E980.9
oxide	984.0	E866.0	—	E950.9	E962.1	E980.9
paint	984.0	E861.5	—	E950.9	E962.1	E980.9
paint	984.0	E861.5	—	E950.9	E962.1	E980.9
salts	984.0	E866.0	—	E950.9	E962.1	E980.9
specified compound NEC	984.8	E866.0	—	E950.9	E962.1	E980.9
tetra–ethyl	984.1	E862.1	—	E950.9	E962.1	E980.9
Lebanese red	969.6	E854.1	E939.6	E950.3	E962.0	E980.3
Lente Iletin (insulin)	962.3	E858.0	E932.3	E950.4	E962.0	E980.4
Leptazol	970.0	E854.3	E940.0	E950.4	E962.0	E980.4
Leritine	965.09	E850.2	E935.2	E950.4	E962.0	E980.0
Letter	962.7	E858.0	E932.7	E950.4	E962.0	E980.4
Lettuce opium	967.8	E852.8	E937.8	E950.2	E962.0	E980.2
Leucovorin (factor)	964.1	E858.2	E934.1	E950.4	E962.0	E980.4
Leukeran	963.1	E858.1	E933.1	E950.4	E962.0	E980.4
Levalbuterol	975.7	E858.6	E945.7	E950.4	E962.0	E980.4
Levallorphan	970.1	E854.3	E940.1	E950.4	E962.0	E980.4
Levanil	967.8	E852.8	E937.8	E950.2	E962.0	E980.2
Levarterenol	971.2	E855.5	E941.2	E950.4	E962.0	E980.4
Levodopa	966.4	E855.0	E936.4	E950.4	E962.0	E980.4
Levo–dromoran	965.09	E850.2	E935.2	E950.0	E962.0	E980.0
Levoid	962.7	E858.0	E932.7	E950.4	E962.0	E980.4
Levo–iso–methadone	965.02	E850.1	E935.1	E950.0	E962.0	E980.0
Levomepromazine	967.8	E852.8	E937.8	E950.2	E962.0	E980.2
Levoprome	967.8	E852.8	E937.8	E950.2	E962.0	E980.2
Levopropoxyphene	975.4	E858.6	E945.4	E950.4	E962.0	E980.4
Levorphan, levophanol	965.09	E850.2	E935.2	E950.0	E962.0	E980.0
Levothyroxine (sodium)	962.7	E858.0	E932.7	E950.4	E962.0	E980.4
Levsin	971.1	E855.4	E941.1	E950.4	E962.0	E980.4
Levulose	974.5	E858.5	E944.5	E950.4	E962.0	E980.4
Lewisite (gas)	985.1	E866.3	—	E950.8	E962.1	E980.8
Librium	969.4	E853.2	E939.4	E950.3	E962.0	E980.3
Lidex	976.0	E858.7	E946.0	E950.4	E962.0	E980.4
Lidocaine (infiltration) (topical)	968.5	E855.2	E938.5	E950.4	E962.0	E980.4
nerve block (peripheral) (plexus)	968.6	E855.2	E938.6	E950.4	E962.0	E980.4
spinal	968.7	E855.2	E938.7	E950.4	E962.0	E980.4
Lighter fluid	981	E862.1	—	E950.9	E962.1	E980.9
Lignocaine (infiltration) (topical)	968.5	E855.2	E938.5	E950.4	E962.0	E980.4
nerve block (peripheral) (plexus)	968.6	E855.2	E938.6	E950.4	E962.0	E980.4
spinal	968.7	E855.2	E938.7	E950.4	E962.0	E980.4
Ligroin(e) (solvent)	981	E862.0	—	E950.9	E962.1	E980.9
vapor	987.1	E869.8	—	E952.8	E962.2	E982.8
Ligustrum vulgare	988.2	E865.3	—	E950.9	E962.1	E980.9

1460

TABLE OF DRUGS AND CHEMICALS

Substance	Poisoning	Accident	Therapeutic Use	Suicide Attempt	Assault	Undetermined
		\multicolumn{5}{c}{External Cause (E-Code)}				
Lily of the valley.	988.2	E865.4	—	E950.9	E962.1	E980.9
Lime (chloride)	983.2	E864.2	—	E950.7	E962.1	E980.6
solution, sulferated	976.4	E858.7	E946.4	E950.4	E962.0	E980.4
Limonene.	982.8	E862.4	—	E950.9	E962.1	E980.9
Lincomycin	960.8	E856	E930.8	E950.4	E962.0	E980.4
Lindane (insecticide) (vapor)	989.2	E863.0	—	E950.6	E962.1	E980.7
anti–infective (topical)	976.0	E858.7	E946.0	E950.4	E962.0	E980.4
Liniments NEC	976.9	E858.7	E946.9	E950.4	E962.0	E980.4
Linoleic acid.	972.2	E858.3	E942.2	E950.4	E962.0	E980.4
Liothyronine	962.7	E858.0	E932.7	E950.4	E962.0	E980.4
Liotrix	962.7	E858.0	E932.7	E950.4	E962.0	E980.4
Lipancreatin	973.4	E858.4	E943.4	E950.4	E962.0	E980.4
Lipo–Lutin	962.2	E858.0	E932.2	E950.4	E962.0	E980.4
Lipotropic agents	977.1	E858.8	E947.1	E950.4	E962.0	E980.4
Liquefied petroleum gases	987.0	E868.0	—	E951.1	E962.2	E981.1
piped (pure or mixed with air)	987.0	E867	—	E951.0	E962.2	E981.0
Liquid petrolatum.	973.2	E858.4	E943.2	E950.4	E962.0	E980.4
substance	989.9	E866.9	—	E950.9	E962.1	E980.9
specified NEC	989.89	E866.8	—	E950.9	E962.1	E980.9
Lirugen	979.4	E858.8	E949.4	E950.4	E962.0	E980.4
Lithane	969.8	E855.8	E939.8	E950.3	E962.0	E980.3
Lithium	985.8	E866.4	—	E950.9	E962.1	E980.9
carbonate	969.8	E855.8	E939.8	E950.3	E962.0	E980.3
Lithonate	969.8	E855.8	E939.8	E950.3	E962.0	E980.3
Liver (extract) (injection) (preparations) . . .	964.1	E858.2	E934.1	E950.4	E962.0	E980.4
Lizard (bite) (venom)	989.5	E905.0	—	E950.9	E962.1	E980.9
LMD	964.8	E858.2	E934.8	E950.4	E962.0	E980.4
Lobelia	988.2	E865.4	—	E950.9	E962.1	E980.9
Lobeline	970.0	E854.3	E940.0	E950.4	E962.0	E980.4
Locorten	976.0	E858.7	E946.0	E950.4	E962.0	E980.4
Lolium temulentum	988.2	E865.3	—	E950.9	E962.1	E980.9
Lomotil	973.5	E858.4	E943.5	E950.4	E962.0	E980.4
Lomustine	963.1	E858.1	E933.1	E950.4	E962.0	E980.4
Lophophora williamsii	969.6	E854.1	E939.6	E950.3	E962.0	E980.3
Lorazepam	969.4	E853.2	E939.4	E950.3	E962.0	E980.3
Lotions NEC	976.9	E858.7	E946.9	E950.4	E962.0	E980.4
Lotronex	973.8	E858.4	E943.8	E950.4	E962.0	E980.4
Lotusate	967.0	E851	E937.0	E950.1	E962.0	E980.1
Lowila	976.2	E858.7	E946.2	E950.4	E962.0	E980.4
Loxapine	969.3	E853.8	E939.3	E950.3	E962.0	E980.3
Lozenges (throat)	976.6	E858.7	E946.6	E950.4	E962.0	E980.4
LSD (25)	969.6	E854.1	E939.6	E950.3	E962.0	E980.3
Lubricating oil NEC	981	E862.2	—	E950.9	E962.1	E980.9
Lucanthone	961.6	E857	E931.6	E950.4	E962.0	E980.4
Luminal	967.0	E851	E937.0	E950.1	E962.0	E980.1
Lung irritant (gas) NEC	987.9	E869.9	—	E952.9	E962.2	E982.9
Lutocylol	962.2	E858.0	E932.2	E950.4	E962.0	E980.4
Lutromone	962.2	E858.0	E932.2	E950.4	E962.0	E980.4
Lututrin	975.0	E858.6	E945.0	E950.4	E962.0	E980.4
Lye (concentrated)	983.2	E864.2	—	E950.7	E962.1	E980.6
Lygranum (skin test)	977.8	E858.8	E947.8	E950.4	E962.0	E980.4
Lymecycline	960.4	E856	E930.4	E950.4	E962.0	E980.4
Lymphogranuloma venereum antigen . . .	977.8	E858.8	E947.8	E950.4	E962.0	E980.4
Lynestrenol	962.2	E858.0	E932.2	E950.4	E962.0	E980.4
Lyovac Sodium Edecrin	974.4	E858.5	E944.4	E950.4	E962.0	E980.4
Lypressin	962.5	E858.0	E932.5	E950.4	E962.0	E980.4
Lysergic acid (amide) (diethylamide)	969.6	E854.1	E939.6	E950.3	E962.0	E980.3
Lysergide	969.6	E854.1	E939.6	E950.3	E962.0	E980.3
Lysine vasopressin	962.5	E858.0	E932.5	E950.4	E962.0	E980.4
Lysol	983.0	E864.0	—	E950.7	E962.1	E980.6
Lytta (vitatta)	976.8	E858.7	E946.8	E950.4	E962.0	E980.4

TABLE OF DRUGS AND CHEMICALS

Substance	Poisoning	Accident	Therapeutic Use	Suicide Attempt	Assault	Undetermined
			External Cause (E-Code)			
Mace	987.5	E869.3	—	E952.8	E962.2	E982.8
Macrolides (antibiotics)	960.3	E856	E930.3	E950.4	E962.0	E980.4
Mafenide	976.0	E858.7	E946.0	E950.4	E962.0	E980.4
Magaldrate	973.0	E858.4	E943.0	E950.4	E962.0	E980.4
Magic mushroom	969.6	E854.1	E939.6	E950.3	E962.0	E980.3
Magnamycin	960.8	E856	E930.8	E950.4	E962.0	E980.4
Magnesia magma	973.0	E858.4	E943.0	E950.4	E962.0	E980.4
Magnesium (compounds) (fumes) NEC	985.8	E866.4	—	E950.9	E962.1	E980.9
antacid	973.0	E858.4	E943.0	E950.4	E962.0	E980.4
carbonate	973.0	E858.4	E943.0	E950.4	E962.0	E980.4
cathartic	973.3	E858.4	E943.3	E950.4	E962.0	E980.4
citrate	973.3	E858.4	E943.3	E950.4	E962.0	E980.4
hydroxide	973.0	E858.4	E943.0	E950.4	E962.0	E980.4
oxide	973.0	E858.4	E943.0	E950.4	E962.0	E980.4
sulfate (oral)	973.3	E858.4	E943.3	E950.4	E962.0	E980.4
intravenous	966.3	E855.0	E936.3	E950.4	E962.0	E980.4
trisilicate	973.0	E858.4	E943.0	E950.4	E962.0	E980.4
Malathion (insecticide)	989.3	E863.1	—	E950.6	E962.1	E980.7
Male fern (oleoresin)	961.6	E857	E931.6	E950.4	E962.0	E980.4
Mandelic acid	961.9	E857	E931.9	E950.4	E962.0	E980.4
Manganese compounds (fumes) NEC	985.2	E866.4	—	E950.9	E962.1	E980.9
Mannitol (diuretic) (medicinal) NEC	974.4	E858.5	E944.4	E950.4	E962.0	E980.4
hexanitrate	972.4	E858.3	E942.4	E950.4	E962.0	E980.4
mustard	963.1	E858.1	E933.1	E950.4	E962.0	E980.4
Mannomustine	963.1	E858.1	E933.1	E950.4	E962.0	E980.4
MAO inhibitors	969.0	E854.0	E939.0	E950.3	E962.0	E980.3
Mapharsen	961.1	E857	E931.1	E950.4	E962.0	E980.4
Marcaine	968.9	E855.2	E938.9	E950.4	E962.0	E980.4
infiltration (subcutaneous)	968.5	E855.2	E938.5	E950.4	E962.0	E980.4
nerve block (peripheral) (plexus)	968.6	E855.2	E938.6	E950.4	E962.0	E980.4
Marezine	963.0	E858.1	E933.0	E950.4	E962.0	E980.4
Marihuana, marijuana (derivatives)	969.6	E854.1	E939.6	E950.3	E962.0	E980.3
Marine animals or plants (sting)	989.5	E905.6	—	E950.9	E962.1	E980.9
Marplan	969.0	E854.0	E939.0	E950.3	E962.0	E980.3
Marsh gas	987.1	E869.8	—	E952.8	E962.2	E982.8
Marsilid	969.0	E854.0	E939.0	E950.3	E962.0	E980.3
Matulane	963.1	E858.1	E933.1	E950.4	E962.0	E980.4
Mazindol	977.0	E858.8	E947.0	E950.4	E962.0	E980.4
MDMA	969.7	E854.2	E939.7	E950.3	E962.0	E980.3
Meadow saffron	988.2	E865.3	—	E950.9	E962.1	E980.9
Measles vaccine	979.4	E858.8	E949.4	E950.4	E962.0	E980.4
Meat, noxious or nonbacterial	988.8	E865.0	—	E950.9	E962.1	E980.9
Mebanazine	969.0	E854.0	E939.0	E950.3	E962.0	E980.3
Mebaral	967.0	E851	E937.0	E950.1	E962.0	E980.1
Mebendazole	961.6	E857	E931.6	E950.4	E962.0	E980.4
Mebeverine	975.1	E858.6	E945.1	E950.4	E962.0	E980.4
Mebhydroline	963.0	E858.1	E933.0	E950.4	E962.0	E980.4
Mebrophenhydramine	963.0	E858.1	E933.0	E950.4	E962.0	E980.4
Mebutamate	969.5	E853.8	E939.5	E950.3	E962.0	E980.3
Mecamylamine (chloride)	972.3	E858.3	E942.3	E950.4	E962.0	E980.4
Mechlorethamine hydrochloride	963.1	E858.1	E933.1	E950.4	E962.0	E980.4
Meclizene (hydrochloride)	963.0	E858.1	E933.0	E950.4	E962.0	E980.4
Meclofenoxate	970.0	E854.3	E940.0	E950.4	E962.0	E980.4
Meclozine (hydrochloride)	963.0	E858.1	E933.0	E950.4	E962.0	E980.4
Medazepam	969.4	E853.2	E939.4	E950.3	E962.0	E980.3
Medicine, medicinal substance	977.9	E858.9	E947.9	E950.5	E962.0	E980.5
specified NEC	977.8	E858.8	E947.8	E950.4	E962.0	E980.4
Medinal	967.0	E851	E937.0	E950.1	E962.0	E980.1
Medomin	967.0	E851	E937.0	E950.1	E962.0	E980.1
Medroxyprogesterone	962.2	E858.0	E932.2	E950.4	E962.0	E980.4

TABLE OF DRUGS AND CHEMICALS

Substance	Poisoning	Accident	Therapeutic Use	Suicide Attempt	Assault	Undetermined
		\multicolumn{5}{c}{External Cause (E-Code)}				
Medrysone	976.5	E858.7	E946.5	E950.4	E962.0	E980.4
Mefenamic acid	965.7	E850.7	E935.7	E950.0	E962.0	E980.0
Megahallucinogen	969.6	E854.1	E939.6	E950.3	E962.0	E980.3
Megestrol	962.2	E858.0	E932.2	E950.4	E962.0	E980.4
Meglumine	977.8	E858.8	E947.8	E950.4	E962.0	E980.4
Meladinin	976.3	E858.7	E946.3	E950.4	E962.0	E980.4
Melanizing agents	976.3	E858.7	E946.3	E950.4	E962.0	E980.4
Melarsoprol	961.1	E857	E931.1	E950.4	E962.0	E980.4
Melia azedarach	988.2	E865.3	—	E950.9	E962.1	E980.9
Mellaril	969.1	E853.0	E939.1	E950.3	E962.0	E980.3
Meloxine	976.3	E858.7	E946.3	E950.4	E962.0	E980.4
Melphalan	963.1	E858.1	E933.1	E950.4	E962.0	E980.4
Menadiol sodium diphosphate	964.3	E858.2	E934.3	E950.4	E962.0	E980.4
Menadione (sodium bisulfate)	964.3	E858.2	E934.3	E950.4	E962.0	E980.4
Menaphthone	964.3	E858.2	E934.3	E950.4	E962.0	E980.4
Meningococcal vaccine	978.8	E858.8	E948.8	E950.4	E962.0	E980.4
Menningovax–C	978.8	E858.8	E948.8	E950.4	E962.0	E980.4
Menotropins	962.4	E858.0	E932.4	E950.4	E962.0	E980.4
Menthol NEC	976.1	E858.7	E946.1	E950.4	E962.0	E980.4
Mepacrine	961.3	E857	E931.3	E950.4	E962.0	E980.4
Meparfynol	967.8	E852.8	E937.8	E950.2	E962.0	E980.2
Mepazine	969.1	E853.0	E939.1	E950.3	E962.0	E980.3
Mepenzolate	971.1	E855.4	E941.1	E950.4	E962.0	E980.4
Meperidine	965.09	E850.2	E935.2	E950.0	E962.0	E980.0
Mephenamin(e)	966.4	E855.0	E936.4	E950.4	E962.0	E980.4
Mephenesin (carbamate)	968.0	E855.1	E938.0	E950.4	E962.0	E980.4
Mephenoxalone	969.5	E853.8	E939.5	E950.3	E962.0	E980.3
Mephentermine	971.2	E855.5	E941.2	E950.4	E962.0	E980.4
Mephenytoin	966.1	E855.0	E936.1	E950.4	E962.0	E980.4
Mephobarbital	967.0	E851	E937.0	E950.1	E962.0	E980.1
Mepiperphenidol	971.1	E855.4	E941.1	E950.4	E962.0	E980.4
Mepivacaine	968.9	E855.2	E938.9	E950.4	E962.0	E980.4
infiltration (subcutaneous)	968.5	E855.2	E938.5	E950.4	E962.0	E980.4
nerve block (peripheral) (plexus)	968.6	E855.2	E938.6	E950.4	E962.0	E980.4
topical (surface)	968.5	E855.2	E938.5	E950.4	E962.0	E980.4
Meprednisone	962.0	E858.0	E932.0	E950.4	E962.0	E980.4
Meprobam	969.5	E853.8	E939.5	E950.3	E962.0	E980.3
Meprobamate	969.5	E853.8	E939.5	E950.3	E962.0	E980.3
Mepyramine (maleate)	963.0	E858.1	E933.0	E950.4	E962.0	E980.4
Meralluride	974.0	E858.5	E944.0	E950.4	E962.0	E980.4
Merbaphen	974.0	E858.5	E944.0	E950.4	E962.0	E980.4
Merbromin	976.0	E858.7	E946.0	E950.4	E962.0	E980.4
Mercaptomerin	974.0	E858.5	E944.0	E950.4	E962.0	E980.4
Mercaptopurine	963.1	E858.1	E933.1	E950.4	E962.0	E980.4
Mercumatilin	974.0	E858.5	E944.0	E950.4	E962.0	E980.4
Mercuramide	974.0	E858.5	E944.0	E950.4	E962.0	E980.4
Mercuranin	976.0	E858.7	E946.0	E950.4	E962.0	E980.4
Mercurochrome	976.0	E858.7	E946.0	E950.4	E962.0	E980.4
Mercury, mercuric, mercurous (compounds) (cyanide) (fumes) (nonmedicinal) (vapor) NEC	985.0	E866.1	—	E950.9	E962.1	E980.9
ammoniated	976.0	E858.7	E946.0	E950.4	E962.0	E980.4
anti–infective	961.2	E857	E931.2	E950.4	E962.0	E980.4
topical	976.0	E858.7	E946.0	E950.4	E962.0	E980.4
chloride (antiseptic) NEC	976.0	E858.7	E946.0	E950.4	E962.0	E980.4
fungicide	985.0	E863.6	—	E950.6	E962.1	E980.7
diuretic compounds	974.0	E858.5	E944.0	E950.4	E962.0	E980.4
fungicide	985.0	E863.6	—	E950.6	E962.1	E980.7
organic (fungicide)	985.0	E863.6	—	E950.6	E962.1	E980.7
Merethoxylline	974.0	E858.5	E944.0	E950.4	E962.0	E980.4
Mersalyl	974.0	E858.5	E944.0	E950.4	E962.0	E980.4

TABLE OF DRUGS AND CHEMICALS

Substance	Poisoning	Accident	Therapeutic Use	Suicide Attempt	Assault	Undetermined
			External Cause (E-Code)			
Merthiolate (topical)	976.0	E858.7	E946.0	E950.4	E962.0	E980.4
ophthalmic preparation	976.5	E858.7	E946.5	E950.4	E962.0	E980.4
Meruvax	979.4	E858.8	E949.4	E950.4	E962.0	E980.4
Mescal buttons	969.6	E854.1	E939.6	E950.3	E962.0	E980.3
Mescaline (salts)	969.6	E854.1	E939.6	E950.3	E962.0	E980.3
Mesoridazine besylate	969.1	E853.0	E939.1	E950.3	E962.0	E980.3
Mestanolone	962.1	E858.0	E932.1	E950.4	E962.0	E980.4
Mestranol	962.2	E858.0	E932.2	E950.4	E962.0	E980.4
Metacresylacetate	976.0	E858.7	E946.0	E950.4	E962.0	E980.4
Metaldehyde (snail killer) NEC	989.4	E863.4	—	E950.6	E962.1	E980.7
Metals (heavy) (nonmedicinal) NEC	985.9	E866.4	—	E950.9	E962.1	E980.9
dust, fumes, or vapor NEC	985.9	E866.4	—	E950.9	E962.1	E980.9
light NEC	985.9	E866.4	—	E950.9	E962.1	E980.9
dust, fumes, or vapor NEC	985.9	E866.4	—	E950.9	E962.1	E980.9
pesticides (dust) (vapor)	985.9	E863.4	—	E950.6	E962.1	E980.7
Metamucil	973.3	E858.4	E943.3	E950.4	E962.0	E980.4
Metaphen	976.0	E858.7	E946.0	E950.4	E962.0	E980.4
Metaproterenol	975.1	E858.6	E945.1	E950.4	E962.0	E980.4
Metaraminol	972.8	E858.3	E942.8	E950.4	E962.0	E980.4
Metaxalone	968.0	E855.1	E938.0	E950.4	E962.0	E980.4
Metformin	962.3	E858.0	E932.3	E950.4	E962.0	E980.4
Methacycline	960.4	E856	E930.4	E950.4	E962.0	E980.4
Methadone	965.02	E850.1	E935.1	E950.0	E962.0	E980.0
Methallenestril	962.2	E858.0	E932.2	E950.4	E962.0	E980.4
Methamphetamine	969.7	E854.2	E939.7	E950.3	E962.0	E980.3
Methandienone	962.1	E858.0	E932.1	E950.4	E962.0	E980.4
Methandriol	962.1	E858.0	E932.1	E950.4	E962.0	E980.4
Methandrostenolone	962.1	E858.0	E932.1	E950.4	E962.0	E980.4
Methane gas	987.1	E869.8	—	E952.8	E962.2	E982.8
Methanol	980.1	E860.2	—	E950.9	E962.1	E980.9
vapor	987.8	E869.8	—	E952.8	E962.2	E982.8
Methantheline	971.1	E855.4	E941.1	E950.4	E962.0	E980.4
Methaphenilene	963.0	E858.1	E933.0	E950.4	E962.0	E980.4
Methapyrilene	963.0	E858.1	E933.0	E950.4	E962.0	E980.4
Methaqualone (compounds)	967.4	E852.3	E937.4	E950.2	E962.0	E980.2
Metharbital, metharbitone	967.0	E851	E937.0	E950.1	E962.0	E980.1
Methazolamide	974.2	E858.5	E944.2	E950.4	E962.0	E980.4
Methdilazine	963.0	E858.1	E933.0	E950.4	E962.0	E980.4
Methedrine	969.7	E854.2	E939.7	E950.3	E962.0	E980.3
Methenamine (mandelate)	961.9	E857	E931.9	E950.4	E962.0	E980.4
Methenolone	962.1	E858.0	E932.1	E950.4	E962.0	E980.4
Methergine	975.0	E858.6	E945.0	E950.4	E962.0	E980.4
Methiacil	962.8	E858.0	E932.8	E950.4	E962.0	E980.4
Methicillin (sodium)	960.0	E856	E930.0	E950.4	E962.0	E980.4
Methimazole	962.8	E858.0	E932.8	E950.4	E962.0	E980.4
Methionine	977.1	E858.8	E947.1	E950.4	E962.0	E980.4
Methisazone	961.7	E857	E931.7	E950.4	E962.0	E980.4
Methitural	967.0	E851	E937.0	E950.1	E962.0	E980.1
Methixene	971.1	E855.4	E941.1	E950.4	E962.0	E980.4
Methobarbital, methobarbitone	967.0	E851	E937.0	E950.1	E962.0	E980.1
Methocarbamol	968.0	E855.1	E938.0	E950.4	E962.0	E980.4
Methohexital, methohexitone (sodium)	968.3	E855.1	E938.3	E950.4	E962.0	E980.4
Methoin	966.1	E855.0	E936.1	E950.4	E962.0	E980.4
Methopholine	965.7	E850.7	E935.7	E950.0	E962.0	E980.0
Methorate	975.4	E858.6	E945.4	E950.4	E962.0	E980.4
Methoserpidine	972.6	E858.3	E942.6	E950.4	E962.0	E980.4
Methotrexate	963.1	E858.1	E933.1	E950.4	E962.0	E980.4
Methotrimeprazine	967.8	E852.8	E937.8	E950.2	E962.0	E980.2
Methoxa–Dome	976.3	E858.7	E946.3	E950.4	E962.0	E980.4
Methoxamine	971.2	E855.5	E941.2	E950.4	E962.0	E980.4

TABLE OF DRUGS AND CHEMICALS

Substance	Poisoning	Accident	Therapeutic Use	Suicide Attempt	Assault	Undetermined
		\multicolumn{5}{c}{External Cause (E-Code)}				
Methoxsalen	976.3	E858.7	E946.3	E950.4	E962.0	E980.4
Methoxybenzyl penicillin	960.0	E856	E930.0	E950.4	E962.0	E980.4
Methoxychlor	989.2	E863.0	—	E950.6	E962.1	E980.7
Methoxyflurane	968.2	E855.1	E938.2	E950.4	E962.0	E980.4
Methoxyphenamine	971.2	E855.5	E941.2	E950.4	E962.0	E980.4
Methoxypromazine	969.1	E853.0	E939.1	E950.3	E962.0	E980.3
Methoxypsoralen	976.3	E858.7	E946.3	E950.4	E962.0	E980.4
Methscopolamine (bromide)	971.1	E855.4	E941.1	E950.4	E962.0	E980.4
Methsuximide	966.2	E855.0	E936.2	E950.4	E962.0	E980.4
Methyclothiazide	974.3	E858.5	E944.3	E950.4	E962.0	E980.4
Methyl						
acetate	982.8	E862.4	—	E950.9	E962.1	E980.9
acetone	982.8	E862.4	—	E950.9	E962.1	E980.9
alcohol	980.1	E860.2	—	E950.9	E962.1	E980.9
amphetamine	969.7	E854.2	E939.7	E950.3	E962.0	E980.3
androstanolone	962.1	E858.0	E932.1	E950.4	E962.0	E980.4
atropine	971.1	E855.4	E941.1	E950.4	E962.0	E980.4
benzene	982.0	E862.4	—	E950.9	E962.1	E980.9
bromide (gas)	987.8	E869.8	—	E952.8	E962.2	E982.8
fumigant	987.8	E863.8	—	E950.6	E962.2	E980.7
butanol	980.8	E860.8	—	E950.9	E962.1	E980.9
carbinol	980.1	E860.2	—	E950.9	E962.1	E980.9
cellosolve	982.8	E862.4	—	E950.9	E962.1	E980.9
cellulose	973.3	E858.4	E943.3	E950.4	E962.0	E980.4
chloride (gas)	987.8	E869.8	—	E952.8	E962.2	E982.8
cyclohexane	982.8	E862.4	—	E950.9	E962.1	E980.9
cyclohexanone	982.8	E862.4	—	E950.9	E962.1	E980.9
dihydromorphinone	965.09	E850.2	E935.2	E950.0	E962.0	E980.0
ergometrine	975.0	E858.6	E945.0	E950.4	E962.0	E980.4
ergonovine	975.0	E858.6	E945.0	E950.4	E962.0	E980.4
ethyl ketone	982.8	E862.4	—	E950.9	E962.1	E980.9
hydrazine	983.9	E864.3	—	E950.7	E962.1	E980.6
isobutyl ketone	982.8	E862.4	—	E950.9	E962.1	E980.9
morphine NEC	965.09	E850.2	E935.2	E950.0	E962.0	E980.0
parafynol	967.8	E852.8	E937.8	E950.2	E962.0	E980.2
parathion	989.3	E863.1	—	E950.6	E962.1	E980.7
pentynol NEC	967.8	E852.8	E937.8	E950.2	E962.0	E980.2
peridol	969.2	E853.1	E939.2	E950.3	E962.0	E980.3
phenidate	969.7	E854.2	E939.7	E950.3	E962.0	E980.3
prednisolone	962.0	E858.0	E932.0	E950.4	E962.0	E980.4
ENT agent	976.6	E858.7	E946.6	E950.4	E962.0	E980.4
ophthalmic preparation	976.5	E858.7	E946.5	E950.4	E962.0	E980.4
topical NEC	976.0	E858.7	E946.0	E950.4	E962.0	E980.4
propylcarbinol	980.8	E860.8	—	E950.9	E962.1	E980.9
rosaniline NEC	976.0	E858.7	E946.0	E950.4	E962.0	E980.4
salicylate NEC	976.3	E858.7	E946.3	E950.4	E962.0	E980.4
sulfate (fumes)	987.8	E869.8	—	E952.8	E962.2	E982.8
liquid	983.9	E864.3	—	E950.7	E962.1	E980.6
sulfonal	967.8	E852.8	E937.8	E950.2	E962.0	E980.2
testosterone	962.1	E858.0	E932.1	E950.4	E962.0	E980.4
thiouracil	962.8	E858.0	E932.8	E950.4	E962.0	E980.4
Methylated spirit	980.0	E860.1	—	E950.9	E962.1	E980.9
Methyldopa	972.6	E858.3	E942.6	E950.4	E962.0	E980.4
Methylene						
blue	961.9	E857	E931.9	E950.4	E962.0	E980.4
chloride or dichloride (solvent) NEC	982.3	E862.4	—	E950.9	E962.1	E980.9
Methylhexabital	967.0	E851	E937.0	E950.1	E962.0	E980.1
Methylparaben (ophthalmic)	976.5	E858.7	E946.5	E950.4	E962.0	E980.4
Methyprylon	967.5	E852.4	E937.5	E950.2	E962.0	E980.2
Methysergide	971.3	E855.6	E941.3	E950.4	E962.0	E980.4
Metoclopramide	963.0	E858.1	E933.0	E950.4	E962.0	E980.4

TABLE OF DRUGS AND CHEMICALS

Substance	Poisoning	Accident	Therapeutic Use	Suicide Attempt	Assault	Undetermined
			External Cause (E-Code)			

Metofoline	965.7	E850.7	E935.7	E950.0	E962.0	E980.0
Metopon	965.09	E850.2	E935.2	E950.0	E962.0	E980.0
Metronidazole	961.5	E857	E931.5	E950.4	E962.0	E980.4
Metycaine	968.9	E855.2	E938.9	E950.4	E962.0	E980.4
infiltration (subcutaneous)	968.5	E855.2	E938.5	E950.4	E962.0	E980.4
nerve block (peripheral) (plexus)	968.6	E855.2	E938.6	E950.4	E962.0	E980.4
topical (surface)	968.5	E855.2	E938.5	E950.4	E962.0	E980.4
Metyrapone	977.8	E858.8	E947.8	E950.4	E962.0	E980.4
Mevinphos	989.3	E863.1	—	E950.6	E962.1	E980.7
Mezereon (berries)	988.2	E865.3	—	E950.9	E962.1	E980.9
Micatin	976.0	E858.7	E946.0	E950.4	E962.0	E980.4
Miconazole	976.0	E858.7	E946.0	E950.4	E962.0	E980.4
Midol	965.1	E850.3	E935.3	E950.0	E962.0	E980.0
Mifepristone	962.9	E858.0	E932.9	E950.4	E962.0	E980.4
Milk of magnesia	973.0	E858.4	E943.0	E950.4	E962.0	E980.4
Millipede (tropical) (venomous)	989.5	E905.4	—	E950.9	E962.1	E980.9
Miltown	969.5	E853.8	E939.5	E950.3	E962.0	E980.3
Mineral						
oil (medicinal)	973.2	E858.4	E943.2	E950.4	E962.0	E980.4
nonmedicinal	981	E862.1	—	E950.9	E962.1	E980.9
topical	976.3	E858.7	E946.3	E950.4	E962.0	E980.4
salts NEC	974.6	E858.5	E944.6	E950.4	E962.0	E980.4
spirits	981	E862.0	—	E950.9	E962.1	E980.9
Minocycline	960.4	E856	E930.4	E950.4	E962.0	E980.4
Mithramycin (antineoplastic)	960.7	E856	E930.7	E950.4	E962.0	E980.4
Mitobronitol	963.1	E858.1	E933.1	E950.4	E962.0	E980.4
Mitomycin (antineoplastic)	960.7	E856	E930.7	E950.4	E962.0	E980.4
Mitotane	963.1	E858.1	E933.1	E950.4	E962.0	E980.4
Moderil	972.6	E858.3	E942.6	E950.4	E962.0	E980.4
Mogadon—*see* Nitrazepam						
Molindone	969.3	E853.8	E939.3	E950.3	E962.0	E980.3
Monistat	976.0	E858.7	E946.0	E950.4	E962.0	E980.4
Monkshood	988.2	E865.4	—	E950.9	E962.1	E980.9
Monoamine oxidase inhibitors	969.0	E854.0	E939.0	E950.3	E962.0	E980.3
Monochlorobenzene	982.0	E862.4	—	E950.9	E962.1	E980.9
Monosodium glutamate	989.89	E866.8	—	E950.9	E962.1	E980.9
Monoxide, carbon — *see* Carbon, monoxide						
Moperone	969.2	E853.1	E939.2	E950.3	E962.0	E980.3
Morning glory seeds	969.6	E854.1	E939.6	E950.3	E962.0	E980.3
Moroxydine (hydrochloride)	961.7	E857	E931.7	E950.4	E962.0	E980.4
Morphazinamide	961.8	E857	E931.8	E950.4	E962.0	E980.4
Morphinans	965.09	E850.2	E935.2	E950.0	E962.0	E980.0
Morphine NEC	965.09	E850.2	E935.2	E950.0	E962.0	E980.0
antagonists	970.1	E854.3	E940.1	E950.4	E962.0	E980.4
Morpholinylethylmorphine	965.09	E850.2	E935.2	E950.0	E962.0	E980.0
Morrhuate sodium	972.7	E858.3	E942.7	E950.4	E962.0	E980.4
Moth balls (*see also* Pesticides)	989.4	E863.4	—	E950.6	E962.1	E980.7
naphthalene	983.0	E863.4	—	E950.7	E962.1	E980.6
Motor exhaust gas — *see* Carbon, monoxide, exhaust gas						
Mouth wash	976.6	E858.7	E946.6	E950.4	E962.0	E980.4
Mucolytic agent	975.5	E858.6	E945.5	E950.4	E962.0	E980.4
Mucomyst	975.5	E858.6	E945.5	E950.4	E962.0	E980.4
Mucous membrane agents (external)	976.9	E858.7	E946.9	E950.4	E962.0	E980.4
specified NEC	976.8	E858.7	E946.8	E950.4	E962.0	E980.4
Mumps						
immune globulin (human)	964.6	E858.2	E934.6	E950.4	E962.0	E980.4
skin test antigen	977.8	E858.8	E947.8	E950.4	E962.0	E980.4
vaccine	979.6	E858.8	E949.6	E950.4	E962.0	E980.4
Mumpsvax	979.6	E858.8	E949.6	E950.4	E962.0	E980.4

TABLE OF DRUGS AND CHEMICALS

Substance	Poisoning	Accident	Therapeutic Use	Suicide Attempt	Assault	Undetermined
			External Cause (E-Code)			
Muriatic acid — *see* Hydrochloric acid						
Muscarine	971.0	E855.3	E941.0	E950.4	E962.0	E980.4
Muscle affecting agents NEC	975.3	E858.6	E945.3	E950.4	E962.0	E980.4
oxytocic	975.0	E858.6	E945.0	E950.4	E962.0	E980.4
relaxants	975.3	E858.6	E945.3	E950.4	E962.0	E980.4
central nervous system	968.0	E855.1	E938.0	E950.4	E962.0	E980.4
skeletal	975.2	E858.6	E945.2	E950.4	E962.0	E980.4
smooth	975.1	E858.6	E945.1	E950.4	E962.0	E980.4
Mushrooms, noxious	988.1	E865.5	—	E950.9	E962.1	E980.9
Mussel, noxious	988.0	E865.1	—	E950.9	E962.1	E980.9
Mustard (emetic)	973.6	E858.4	E943.6	E950.4	E962.0	E980.4
gas	987.8	E869.8	—	E952.8	E962.2	E982.8
nitrogen	963.1	E858.1	E933.1	E950.4	E962.0	E980.4
Mustine	963.1	E858.1	E933.1	E950.4	E962.0	E980.4
M–vac	979.4	E858.8	E949.4	E950.4	E962.0	E980.4
Mycifradin	960.8	E856	E930.8	E950.4	E962.0	E980.4
topical	976.0	E858.7	E946.0	E950.4	E962.0	E980.4
Mycitracin	960.8	E856	E930.8	E950.4	E962.0	E980.4
ophthalmic preparation	976.5	E858.7	E946.5	E950.4	E962.0	E980.4
Mycostatin	960.1	E856	E930.1	E950.4	E962.0	E980.4
topical	976.0	E858.7	E946.0	E950.4	E962.0	E980.4
Mydriacyl	971.1	E855.4	E941.1	E950.4	E962.0	E980.4
Myelobromal	963.1	E858.1	E933.1	E950.4	E962.0	E980.4
Myleran	963.1	E858.1	E933.1	E950.4	E962.0	E980.4
Myochrysin(e)	965.69	E850.6	E935.6	E950.0	E962.0	E980.0
Myoneural blocking agents	975.2	E858.6	E945.2	E950.4	E962.0	E980.4
Myristica fragrans	988.2	E865.3	—	E950.9	E962.1	E980.9
Myristicin	988.2	E865.3	—	E950.9	E962.1	E980.9
Mysoline	966.3	E855.0	E936.3	E950.4	E962.0	E980.4
Nafcillin (sodium)	960.0	E856	E930.0	E950.4	E962.0	E980.4
Nail polish remover	982.8	E862.4	—	E950.9	E962.1	E980.9
Nalidixic acid	961.9	E857	E931.9	E950.4	E962.0	E980.4
Nalorphine	970.1	E854.3	E940.1	E950.4	E962.0	E980.4
Naloxone	970.1	E854.3	E940.1	E950.4	E962.0	E980.4
Nandrolone (decanoate) (phenproprioate)	962.1	E858.0	E932.1	E950.4	E962.0	E980.4
Naphazoline	971.2	E855.5	E941.2	E950.4	E962.0	E980.4
Naphtha (painter's) (petroleum)	981	E862.0	—	E950.9	E962.1	E980.9
solvent	981	E862.0	—	E950.9	E962.1	E980.9
vapor	987.1	E869.8	—	E952.8	E962.2	E982.8
Naphthalene (chlorinated)	983.0	E864.0	—	E950.7	E962.1	E980.6
insecticide or moth repellent	983.0	E863.4	—	E950.7	E962.1	E980.6
vapor	987.8	E869.8	—	E952.8	E962.2	E982.8
Naphthol	983.0	E864.0	—	E950.7	E962.1	E980.6
Naphthylamine	983.0	E864.0	—	E950.7	E962.1	E980.6
Naprosyn—*see* Naproxen						
Naproxen	965.61	E850.6	E935.6	E950.0	E962.0	E980.0
Narcotic (drug)	967.9	E852.9	E937.9	E950.2	E962.0	E980.2
analgesic NEC	965.8	E850.8	E935.8	E950.0	E962.0	E980.0
antagonist	970.1	E854.3	E940.1	E950.4	E962.0	E980.4
specified NEC	967.8	E852.8	E937.8	E950.2	E962.0	E980.2
Narcotine	975.4	E858.6	E945.4	E950.4	E962.0	E980.4
Nardil	969.0	E854.0	E939.0	E950.3	E962.0	E980.3
Natrium cyanide — *see* Cyanide(s)						
Natural						
blood (product)	964.7	E858.2	E934.7	E950.4	E962.0	E980.4
gas (piped)	987.1	E867	—	E951.0	E962.2	E981.0
incomplete combustion	986	E867	—	E951.0	E962.2	E981.0
Nealbarbital, nealbarbitone	967.0	E851	E937.0	E950.1	E962.0	E980.1
Nectadon	975.4	E858.6	E945.4	E950.4	E962.0	E980.4
Nematocyst (sting)	989.5	E905.6	—	E950.9	E962.1	E980.9
Nembutal	967.0	E851	E937.0	E950.1	E962.0	E980.1

1467

TABLE OF DRUGS AND CHEMICALS

Substance	Poisoning	Accident	Therapeutic Use	Suicide Attempt	Assault	Undetermined
		\multicolumn{5}{c}{External Cause (E-Code)}				
Neoarsphenamine	961.1	E857	E931.1	E950.4	E962.0	E980.4
Neocinchophen	974.7	E858.5	E944.7	E950.4	E962.0	E980.4
Neomycin	960.8	E856	E930.8	E950.4	E962.0	E980.4
ENT agent	976.6	E858.7	E946.6	E950.4	E962.0	E980.4
ophthalmic preparation	976.5	E858.7	E946.5	E950.4	E962.0	E980.4
topical NEC	976.0	E858.7	E946.0	E950.4	E962.0	E980.4
Neonal	967.0	E851	E937.0	E950.1	E962.0	E980.1
Neoprontosil	961.0	E857	E931.0	E950.4	E962.0	E980.4
Neosalvarsan	961.1	E857	E931.1	E950.4	E962.0	E980.4
Neosilversalvarsan	961.1	E857	E931.1	E950.4	E962.0	E980.4
Neosporin	960.8	E856	E930.8	E950.4	E962.0	E980.4
ENT agent	976.6	E858.7	E946.6	E950.4	E962.0	E980.4
ophthalmic preparation	976.5	E858.7	E946.5	E950.4	E962.0	E980.4
topical NEC	976.0	E858.7	E946.0	E950.4	E962.0	E980.4
Neostigmine	971.0	E855.3	E941.0	E950.4	E962.0	E980.4
Neraval	967.0	E851	E937.0	E950.1	E962.0	E980.1
Neravan	967.0	E851	E937.0	E950.1	E962.0	E980.1
Nerium oleander	988.2	E865.4	—	E950.9	E962.1	E980.9
Nerve gases (war)	987.9	E869.9	—	E952.9	E962.2	E982.9
Nesacaine	968.9	E855.2	E938.9	E950.4	E962.0	E980.4
infiltration (subcutaneous)	968.5	E855.2	E938.5	E950.4	E962.0	E980.4
nerve block (peripheral) (plexus) . .	968.6	E855.2	E938.6	E950.4	E962.0	E980.4
Neurobarb	967.0	E851	E937.0	E950.1	E962.0	E980.1
Neuroleptics NEC	969.3	E853.8	E939.3	E950.3	E962.0	E980.3
Neuroprotective agent	977.8	E858.8	E947.8	E950.4	E962.0	E980.4
Neutral spirits	980.0	E860.1	—	E950.9	E962.1	E980.9
beverage	980.0	E860.0	—	E950.9	E962.1	E980.9
Niacin, niacinamide	972.2	E858.3	E942.2	E950.4	E962.0	E980.4
Nialamide	969.0	E854.0	E939.0	E950.3	E962.0	E980.3
Nickle (carbonyl) (compounds) (fumes) (tetracarbonyl) (vapor)	985.8	E866.4	—	E950.9	E962.1	E980.9
Niclosamide	961.6	E857	E931.6	E950.4	E962.0	E980.4
Nicomorphine	965.09	E850.2	E935.2	E950.0	E962.0	E980.0
Nicotinamide	972.2	E858.3	E942.2	E950.4	E962.0	E980.4
Nicotine (insecticide) (spray) (sulfate) NEC . .	989.4	E863.4	—	E950.6	E962.1	E980.7
not insecticide	989.89	E866.8	—	E950.9	E962.1	E980.9
Nicotinic acid (derivatives)	972.2	E858.3	E942.2	E950.4	E962.0	E980.4
Nicotinyl alcohol	972.2	E858.3	E942.2	E950.4	E962.0	E980.4
Nicoumalone	964.2	E858.2	E934.2	E950.4	E962.0	E980.4
Nifenazone	965.5	E850.5	E935.5	E950.0	E962.0	E980.0
Nifuraldezone	961.9	E857	E931.9	E950.4	E962.0	E980.4
Nightshade (deadly)	988.2	E865.4	—	E950.9	E962.1	E980.9
Nikethamide	970.0	E854.3	E940.0	E950.4	E962.0	E980.4
Nilstat	960.1	E856	E930.1	E950.4	E962.0	E980.4
topical	976.0	E858.7	E946.0	E950.4	E962.0	E980.4
Nimodipine	977.8	E858.8	E947.8	E950.4	E962.0	E980.4
Niridazole	961.6	E857	E931.6	E950.4	E962.0	E980.4
Nisentil	965.09	E850.2	E935.2	E950.0	E962.0	E980.0
Nitrates	972.4	E858.3	E942.4	E950.4	E962.0	E980.4
Nitrazepam	969.4	E853.2	E939.4	E950.3	E962.0	E980.3
Nitric						
acid (liquid)	983.1	E864.1	—	E950.7	E962.1	E980.6
vapor	987.8	E869.8	—	E952.8	E962.2	E982.8
oxide (gas)	987.2	E869.0	—	E952.8	E962.2	E982.8
Nitrite, amyl (medicinal) (vapor) . . .	972.4	E858.3	E942.4	E950.4	E962.0	E980.4
Nitroaniline	983.0	E864.0	—	E950.7	E962.1	E980.6
vapor	987.8	E869.8	—	E952.8	E962.2	E982.8
Nitrobenzene, nitrobenzol	983.0	E864.0	—	E950.7	E962.1	E980.6
vapor	987.8	E869.8	—	E952.8	E962.2	E982.8
Nitrocellulose	976.3	E858.7	E946.3	E950.4	E962.0	E980.4

TABLE OF DRUGS AND CHEMICALS

Substance	Poisoning	Accident	Therapeutic Use	Suicide Attempt	Assault	Undetermined
		\multicolumn{5}{c}{External Cause (E-Code)}				
Nitrofuran derivatives	961.9	E857	E931.9	E950.4	E962.0	E980.4
Nitrofurantoin	961.9	E857	E931.9	E950.4	E962.0	E980.4
Nitrofurazone	976.0	E858.7	E946.0	E950.4	E962.0	E980.4
Nitrogen (dioxide) (gas) (oxide)	987.2	E869.0	—	E952.8	E962.2	E982.8
mustard (antineoplastic)	963.1	E858.1	E933.1	E950.4	E962.0	E980.4
Nitroglycerin, nitroglycerol (medicinal)	972.4	E858.3	E942.4	E950.4	E962.0	E980.4
nonmedicinal	989.89	E866.8	—	E950.9	E962.1	E980.9
fumes	987.8	E869.8	—	E952.8	E962.2	E982.8
Nitrohydrochloric acid	983.1	E864.1	—	E950.7	E962.1	E980.6
Nitromersol	976.0	E858.7	E946.0	E950.4	E962.0	E980.4
Nitronaphthalene	983.0	E864.0	—	E950.7	E962.2	E980.6
Nitrophenol	983.0	E864.0	—	E950.7	E962.2	E980.6
Nitrothiazol	961.6	E857	E931.6	E950.4	E962.0	E980.4
Nitrotoluene, nitrotoluol	983.0	E864.0	—	E950.7	E962.1	E980.6
vapor	987.8	E869.8	—	E952.8	E962.2	E982.8
Nitrous	968.2	E855.1	E938.2	E950.4	E962.0	E980.4
acid (liquid)	983.1	E864.1	—	E950.7	E962.1	E980.6
fumes	987.2	E869.0	—	E952.8	E962.2	E982.8
oxide (anesthetic) NEC	968.2	E855.1	E938.2	E950.4	E962.0	E980.4
Nitrozone	976.0	E858.7	E946.0	E950.4	E962.0	E980.4
Noctec	967.1	E852.0	E937.1	E950.2	E962.0	E980.2
Noludar	967.5	E852.4	E937.5	E950.2	E962.0	E980.2
Noptil	967.0	E851	E937.0	E950.1	E962.0	E980.1
Noradrenalin	971.2	E855.5	E941.2	E950.4	E962.0	E980.4
Noramidopyrine	965.5	E850.5	E935.5	E950.0	E962.0	E980.0
Norepinephrine	971.2	E855.5	E941.2	E950.4	E962.0	E980.4
Norethandrolone	962.1	E858.0	E932.1	E950.4	E962.0	E980.4
Norethindrone	962.2	E858.0	E932.2	E950.4	E962.0	E980.4
Norethisterone	962.2	E858.0	E932.2	E950.4	E962.0	E980.4
Norethynodrel	962.2	E858.0	E932.2	E950.4	E962.0	E980.4
Norlestrin	962.2	E858.0	E932.2	E950.4	E962.0	E980.4
Norlutin	962.2	E858.0	E932.2	E950.4	E962.0	E980.4
Normison—*see* Benzodiazepines						
Normorphine	965.09	E850.2	E935.2	E950.0	E962.0	E980.0
Nortriptyline	969.0	E854.0	E939.0	E950.3	E962.0	E980.3
Noscapine	975.4	E858.6	E945.4	E950.4	E962.0	E980.4
Nose preparations	976.6	E858.7	E946.6	E950.4	E962.0	E980.4
Novobiocin	960.8	E856	E930.8	E950.4	E962.0	E980.4
Novocain (infiltration) (topical)	968.5	E855.2	E938.5	E950.4	E962.0	E980.4
nerve block (peripheral) (plexus)	968.6	E855.2	E938.6	E950.4	E962.0	E980.4
spinal	968.7	E855.2	E938.7	E950.4	E962.0	E980.4
Noxythiolin	961.9	E857	E931.9	E950.4	E962.0	E980.4
NPH Iletin (insulin)	962.3	E858.0	E932.3	E950.4	E962.0	E980.4
Numorphan	965.09	E850.2	E935.2	E950.0	E962.0	E980.0
Nunol	967.0	E851	E937.0	E950.1	E962.0	E980.1
Nupercaine (spinal anesthetic)	968.7	E855.2	E938.7	E950.4	E962.0	E980.4
topical (surface)	968.5	E855.2	E938.5	E950.4	E962.0	E980.4
Nutmeg oil (liniment)	976.3	E858.7	E946.3	E950.4	E962.0	E980.4
Nux vomica	989.1	E863.7	—	E950.6	E962.1	E980.7
Nydrazid	961.8	E857	E931.8	E950.4	E962.0	E980.4
Nylidrin	971.2	E855.5	E941.2	E950.4	E962.0	E980.4
Nystatin	960.1	E856	E930.1	E950.4	E962.0	E980.4
topical	976.0	E858.7	E946.0	E950.4	E962.0	E980.4
Nytol	963.0	E858.1	E933.0	E950.4	E962.0	E980.4
Oblivion	967.8	E852.8	E937.8	E950.2	E962.0	E980.2
Octyl nitrite	972.4	E858.3	E942.4	E950.4	E962.0	E980.4
Oestradiol (cypionate) (dipropionate) (valerate)	962.2	E858.0	E932.2	E950.4	E962.0	E980.4
Oestriol	962.2	E858.0	E932.2	E950.4	E962.0	E980.4
Oestrone	962.2	E858.0	E932.2	E950.4	E962.0	E980.4
Oil (of) NEC	989.89	E866.8	—	E950.9	E962.1	E980.9

1469

TABLE OF DRUGS AND CHEMICALS

Substance	Poisoning	Accident	Therapeutic Use	Suicide Attempt	Assault	Undetermined
			External Cause (E-Code)			
bitter almond	989.0	E866.8	—	E950.9	E962.1	E980.9
camphor	976.1	E858.7	E946.1	E950.4	E962.0	E980.4
colors	989.89	E861.6	—	E950.9	E962.1	E980.9
fumes	987.8	E869.8	—	E952.8	E962.2	E982.8
lubricating	981	E862.2	—	E950.9	E962.1	E980.9
specified source, other — see substance specified						
vitriol (liquid)	983.1	E864.1	—	E950.7	E962.1	E980.6
fumes	987.8	E869.8	—	E952.8	E962.2	E982.8
wintergreen (bitter) NEC	976.3	E858.7	E946.3	E950.4	E962.0	E980.4
Ointments NEC	976.9	E858.7	E946.9	E950.4	E962.0	E980.4
Oleander	988.2	E865.4	—	E950.9	E962.1	E980.9
Oleandomycin	960.3	E856	E930.3	E950.4	E962.0	E980.4
Oleovitamin A	963.5	E858.1	E933.5	E950.4	E962.0	E980.4
Oleum ricini	973.1	E858.4	E943.1	E950.4	E962.0	E980.4
Olive oil (medicinal) NEC	973.2	E858.4	E943.2	E950.4	E962.0	E980.4
OMPA	989.3	E863.1	—	E950.6	E962.1	E980.7
Oncovin	963.1	E858.1	E933.1	E950.4	E962.0	E980.4
Ophthaine	968.5	E855.2	E938.5	E950.4	E962.0	E980.4
Ophthetic	968.5	E855.2	E938.5	E950.4	E962.0	E980.4
Opiates, opioids, opium NEC	965.00	E850.2	E935.2	E950.0	E962.1	E980.0
antagonists	970.1	E854.3	E940.1	E950.4	E962.0	E980.4
Oracon	962.2	E858.0	E932.2	E950.4	E962.0	E980.4
Oragrafin	977.8	E858.8	E947.8	E950.4	E962.0	E980.4
Oral contraceptives	962.2	E858.0	E932.2	E950.4	E962.0	E980.4
Orciprenaline	975.1	E858.6	E945.1	E950.4	E962.0	E980.4
Organidin	975.5	E858.6	E945.5	E950.4	E962.0	E980.4
Organophosphates	989.3	E863.1	—	E950.6	E962.1	E980.7
Orimune	979.5	E858.8	E949.5	E950.4	E962.0	E980.4
Orinase	962.3	E858.0	E932.3	E950.4	E962.0	E980.4
Orphenadrine	966.4	E855.0	E936.4	E950.4	E962.0	E980.4
Ortal (sodium)	967.0	E851	E937.0	E950.1	E962.0	E980.1
Orthoboric acid	976.0	E858.7	E946.0	E950.4	E962.0	E980.4
ENT agent	976.6	E858.7	E946.6	E950.4	E962.0	E980.4
ophthalmic preparation	976.5	E858.7	E946.5	E950.4	E962.0	E980.4
Orthocaine	968.5	E855.2	E938.5	E950.4	E962.0	E980.4
Ortho–Novum	962.2	E858.0	E932.2	E950.4	E962.0	E980.4
Orthotolidine (reagent)	977.8	E858.8	E947.8	E950.4	E962.0	E980.4
Osmic acid (liquid)	983.1	E864.1	—	E950.7	E962.1	E980.6
fumes	987.8	E869.8	—	E952.8	E962.2	E982.8
Osmotic diuretics	974.4	E858.5	E944.4	E950.4	E962.0	E980.4
Ouabain	972.1	E858.3	E942.1	E950.4	E962.0	E980.4
Ovarian hormones (synthetic substitutes)	962.2	E858.0	E932.2	E950.4	E962.0	E980.4
Ovral	962.2	E858.0	E932.2	E950.4	E962.0	E980.4
Ovulation suppressants	962.2	E858.0	E932.2	E950.4	E962.0	E980.4
Ovulen	962.2	E858.0	E932.2	E950.4	E962.0	E980.4
Oxacillin (sodium)	960.0	E856	E930.0	E950.4	E962.0	E980.4
Oxalic acid	983.1	E864.1	—	E950.7	E962.1	E980.6
Oxanamide	969.5	E853.8	E939.5	E950.3	E962.0	E980.3
Oxandrolone	962.1	E858.0	E932.1	E950.4	E962.0	E980.4
Oxaprozin	965.61	E850.6	E935.6	E950.0	E962.0	E980.0
Oxazepam	969.4	E853.2	E939.4	E950.3	E962.0	E980.3
Oxazolidine derivatives	966.0	E855.0	E936.0	E950.4	E962.0	E980.4
Ox bile extract	973.4	E858.4	E943.4	E950.4	E962.0	E980.4
Oxedrine	971.2	E855.5	E941.2	E950.4	E962.0	E980.4
Oxeladin	975.4	E858.6	E945.4	E950.4	E962.0	E980.4
Oxethazaine NEC	968.5	E855.2	E938.5	E950.4	E962.0	E980.4
Oxidizing agents NEC	983.9	E864.3	—	E950.7	E962.1	E980.6
Oxolinic acid	961.3	E857	E931.3	E950.4	E962.0	E980.4
Oxophenarsine	961.1	E857	E931.1	E950.4	E962.0	E980.4

TABLE OF DRUGS AND CHEMICALS

Substance	Poisoning	Accident	Therapeutic Use	Suicide Attempt	Assault	Undetermined
		\multicolumn{5}{c}{External Cause (E-Code)}				
Oxsoralen	976.3	E858.7	E946.3	E950.4	E962.0	E980.4
Oxtriphylline	975.7	E858.6	E945.7	E950.4	E962.0	E980.4
Oxybuprocaine	968.5	E855.2	E938.5	E950.4	E962.0	E980.4
Oxybutynin	975.1	E858.6	E945.1	E950.4	E962.0	E980.4
Oxycodone	965.09	E850.2	E935.2	E950.0	E962.0	E980.0
Oxygen	987.8	E869.8	—	E952.8	E962.2	E982.8
Oxylone	976.0	E858.7	E946.0	E950.4	E962.0	E980.4
ophthalmic preparation	976.5	E858.7	E946.5	E950.4	E962.0	E980.4
Oxymesterone	962.1	E858.0	E932.1	E950.4	E962.0	E980.4
Oxymetazoline	971.2	E855.5	E941.2	E950.4	E962.0	E980.4
Oxymetholone	962.1	E858.0	E932.1	E950.4	E962.0	E980.4
Oxymorphone	965.09	E850.2	E935.2	E950.0	E962.0	E980.0
Oxypertine	969.0	E854.0	E939.0	E950.3	E962.0	E980.3
Oxyphenbutazone	965.5	E850.5	E935.5	E950.0	E962.0	E980.0
Oxyphencyclimine	971.1	E855.4	E941.1	E950.4	E962.0	E980.4
Oxyphenisatin	973.1	E858.4	E943.1	E950.4	E962.0	E980.4
Oxyphenonium	971.1	E855.4	E941.1	E950.4	E962.0	E980.4
Oxyquinoline	961.3	E857	E931.3	E950.4	E962.0	E980.4
Oxytetracycline	960.4	E856	E930.4	E950.4	E962.0	E980.4
Oxytocics	975.0	E858.6	E945.0	E950.4	E962.0	E980.4
Oxytocin	975.0	E858.6	E945.0	E950.4	E962.0	E980.4
Ozone	987.8	E869.8	—	E952.8	E962.2	E982.8
PABA	976.3	E858.7	E946.3	E950.4	E962.0	E980.4
Packed red cells	964.7	E858.2	E934.7	E950.4	E962.0	E980.4
Paint NEC	989.89	E861.6	—	E950.9	E962.1	E980.9
cleaner	982.8	E862.9	—	E950.9	E962.1	E980.9
fumes NEC	987.8	E869.8	—	E952.8	E962.1	E982.8
lead (fumes)	984.0	E861.5	—	E950.9	E962.1	E980.9
solvent NEC	982.8	E862.9	—	E950.9	E962.1	E980.9
stripper	982.8	E862.9	—	E950.9	E962.1	E980.9
Palfium	965.09	E850.2	E935.2	E950.0	E962.0	E980.0
Palivizumab	979.9	E858.8	E949.6	E950.4	E962.0	E980.4
Paludrine	961.4	E857	E931.4	E950.4	E962.0	E980.4
PAM	977.2	E855.8	E947.2	E950.4	E962.0	E980.4
Pamaquine (naphthoate)	961.4	E857	E931.4	E950.4	E962.0	E980.4
Pamprin	965.1	E850.3	E935.3	E950.0	E962.0	E980.0
Panadol	965.4	E850.4	E935.4	E950.0	E962.0	E980.0
Pancreatic dornase (mucolytic)	963.4	E858.1	E933.4	E950.4	E962.0	E980.4
Pancreatin	973.4	E858.4	E943.4	E950.4	E962.0	E980.4
Pancrelipase	973.4	E858.4	E943.4	E950.4	E962.0	E980.4
Pangamic acid	963.5	E858.1	E933.5	E950.4	E962.0	E980.4
Panthenol	963.5	E858.1	E933.5	E950.4	E962.0	E980.4
topical	976.8	E858.7	E946.8	E950.4	E962.0	E980.4
Pantopaque	977.8	E858.8	E947.8	E950.4	E962.0	E980.4
Pantopon	965.00	E850.2	E935.2	E950.0	E962.0	E980.0
Pantothenic acid	963.5	E858.1	E933.5	E950.4	E962.0	E980.4
Panwarfin	964.2	E858.2	E934.2	E950.4	E962.0	E980.4
Papain	973.4	E858.4	E943.4	E950.4	E962.0	E980.4
Papaverine	972.5	E858.3	E942.5	E950.4	E962.0	E980.4
Para–aminobenzoic acid	976.3	E858.7	E946.3	E950.4	E962.0	E980.4
Para–aminophenol derivatives	965.4	E850.4	E935.4	E950.0	E962.0	E980.0
Para–aminosalicylic acid (derivatives)	961.8	E857	E931.8	E950.4	E962.0	E980.4
Paracetaldehyde (medicinal)	967.2	E852.1	E937.2	E950.2	E962.0	E980.2
Paracetamol	965.4	E850.4	E935.4	E950.0	E962.0	E980.0
Paracodin	965.09	E850.2	E935.2	E950.0	E962.0	E980.0
Paradione	966.0	E855.0	E936.0	E950.4	E962.0	E980.4
Paraffin(s) (wax)	981	E862.3	—	E950.9	E962.1	E980.9
liquid (medicinal)	973.2	E858.4	E943.2	E950.4	E962.0	E980.4
nonmedicinal (oil)	981	E962.1	—	E950.9	E962.1	E980.9
Paraldehyde (medicinal)	967.2	E852.1	E937.2	E950.2	E962.0	E980.2
Paramethadione	966.0	E855.0	E936.0	E950.4	E962.0	E980.4

TABLE OF DRUGS AND CHEMICALS

Substance	Poisoning	Accident	Therapeutic Use	Suicide Attempt	Assault	Undetermined
			External Cause (E-Code)			
Paramethasone	962.0	E858.0	E932.0	E950.4	E962.0	E980.4
Paraquat	989.4	E863.5	—	E950.6	E962.1	E980.7
Parasympatholytics	971.1	E855.4	E941.1	E950.4	E962.0	E980.4
Parasympathomimetics	971.0	E855.3	E941.0	E950.4	E962.0	E980.4
Parathion	989.3	E863.1	—	E950.6	E962.1	E980.7
Parathormone	962.6	E858.0	E932.6	E950.4	E962.0	E980.4
Parathyroid (derivatives)	962.6	E858.0	E932.6	E950.4	E962.0	E980.4
Paratyphoid vaccine	978.1	E858.8	E948.1	E950.4	E962.0	E980.4
Paredrine	971.2	E855.5	E941.2	E950.4	E962.0	E980.4
Paregoric	965.00	E850.2	E935.2	E950.0	E962.0	E980.0
Pargyline	972.3	E858.3	E942.3	E950.4	E962.0	E980.4
Paris green	985.1	E866.3	—	E950.8	E962.1	E980.8
insecticide	985.1	E863.4	—	E950.8	E962.1	E980.8
Parnate	969.0	E854.0	E939.0	E950.3	E962.0	E980.3
Paromomycin	960.8	E856	E930.8	E950.4	E962.0	E980.4
Paroxypropione	963.1	E858.1	E933.1	E950.4	E962.0	E980.4
Parzone	965.09	E850.2	E935.2	E950.0	E962.0	E980.0
PAS	961.8	E857	E931.8	E950.4	E962.0	E980.4
PCBs	981	E862.3	—	E950.9	E962.1	E980.9
PCP (pentachlorophenol)	989.4	E863.6	—	E950.6	E962.1	E980.7
herbicide	989.4	E863.5	—	E950.6	E962.1	E980.7
insecticide	989.4	E863.4	—	E950.6	E962.1	E980.7
phencyclidine	968.3	E855.1	E938.3	E950.4	E962.0	E980.4
Peach kernel oil (emulsion)	973.2	E858.4	E943.2	E950.4	E962.0	E980.4
Peanut oil (emulsion) NEC	973.2	E858.4	E943.2	E950.4	E962.0	E980.4
topical	976.3	E858.7	E946.3	E950.4	E962.0	E980.4
Pearly Gates (morning glory seeds)	969.6	E854.1	E939.6	E950.3	E962.0	E980.3
Pecazine	969.1	E853.0	E939.1	E950.3	E962.0	E980.3
Pecilocin	960.1	E856	E930.1	E950.4	E962.0	E980.4
Pectin (with kaolin) NEC	973.5	E858.4	E943.5	E950.4	E962.0	E980.4
Pelletierine tannate	961.6	E857	E931.6	E950.4	E962.0	E980.4
Pemoline	969.7	E854.2	E939.7	E950.3	E962.0	E980.3
Pempidine	972.3	E858.3	E942.3	E950.4	E962.0	E980.4
Penamecillin	960.0	E856	E930.0	E950.4	E962.0	E980.4
Penethamate hydriodide	960.0	E856	E930.0	E950.4	E962.0	E980.4
Penicillamine	963.8	E858.1	E933.8	E950.4	E962.0	E980.4
Penicillin (any type)	960.0	E856	E930.0	E950.4	E962.0	E980.4
Penicillinase	963.4	E858.1	E933.4	E950.4	E962.0	E980.4
Pentachlorophenol (fungicide)	989.4	E863.6	—	E950.6	E962.1	E980.7
herbicide	989.4	E863.5	—	E950.6	E962.1	E980.7
insecticide	989.4	E863.4	—	E950.6	E962.1	E980.7
Pentaerythritol	972.4	E858.3	E942.4	E950.4	E962.0	E980.4
chloral	967.1	E852.0	E937.1	E950.2	E962.0	E980.2
tetranitrate NEC	972.4	E858.3	E942.4	E950.4	E962.0	E980.4
Pentagastrin	977.8	E858.8	E947.8	E950.4	E962.0	E980.4
Pentalin	982.3	E862.4	—	E950.9	E962.1	E980.9
Pentamethonium (bromide)	972.3	E858.3	E942.3	E950.4	E962.0	E980.4
Pentamidine	961.5	E857	E931.5	E950.4	E962.0	E980.4
Pentanol	980.8	E860.8	—	E950.9	E962.1	E980.9
Pentaquine	961.4	E857	E931.4	E950.4	E962.0	E980.4
Pentazocine	965.8	E850.8	E935.8	E950.0	E962.0	E980.0
Penthienate	971.1	E855.4	E941.1	E950.4	E962.0	E980.4
Pentobarbital, pentobarbitone (sodium)	967.0	E851	E937.0	E950.1	E962.0	E980.1
Pentolinium (tartrate)	972.3	E858.3	E942.3	E950.4	E962.0	E980.4
Pentothal	968.3	E855.1	E938.3	E950.4	E962.0	E980.4
Pentylenetetrazol	970.0	E854.3	E940.0	E950.4	E962.0	E980.4
Pentylsalicylamide	961.8	E857	E931.8	E950.4	E962.0	E980.4
Pepsin	973.4	E858.4	E943.4	E950.4	E962.0	E980.4
Peptavlon	977.8	E858.8	E947.8	E950.4	E962.0	E980.4
Percaine (spinal)	968.7	E855.2	E938.7	E950.4	E962.0	E980.4

TABLE OF DRUGS AND CHEMICALS

Substance	Poisoning	Accident	Therapeutic Use	Suicide Attempt	Assault	Undetermined
			External Cause (E-Code)			
topical (surface)	968.5	E855.2	E938.5	E950.4	E962.0	E980.4
Perchloroethylene (vapor)	982.3	E862.4	—	E950.9	E962.1	E980.9
medicinal	961.6	E857	E931.6	E950.4	E962.0	E980.4
Percodan	965.09	E850.2	E935.2	E950.0	E962.0	E980.0
Percogesic	965.09	E850.2	E935.2	E950.0	E962.0	E980.0
Percorten	962.0	E858.0	E932.0	E950.4	E962.0	E980.4
Pergonal	962.4	E858.0	E932.4	E950.4	E962.0	E980.4
Perhexiline	972.4	E858.3	E942.4	E950.4	E962.0	E980.4
Periactin	963.0	E858.1	E933.0	E950.4	E962.0	E980.4
Periclor	967.1	E852.0	E937.1	E950.2	E962.0	E980.2
Pericyazine	969.1	E853.0	E939.1	E950.3	E962.0	E980.3
Peritrate	972.4	E858.3	E942.4	E950.4	E962.0	E980.4
Permanganates NEC	983.9	E864.3	—	E950.7	E962.1	E980.6
potassium (topical)	976.0	E858.7	E946.0	E950.4	E962.0	E980.4
Pernocton	967.0	E851	E937.0	E950.1	E962.0	E980.1
Pernoston	967.0	E851	E937.0	E950.1	E962.0	E980.1
Peronin(e)	965.09	E850.2	E935.2	E950.0	E962.0	E980.0
Perphenazine	969.1	E853.0	E939.1	E950.3	E962.0	E980.3
Pertofrane	969.0	E854	E939.0	E950.3	E962.0	E980.3
Pertussis						
immune serum (human)	964.6	E858.2	E934.6	E950.4	E962.0	E980.4
vaccine (with diphtheria toxoid) (with tetanus toxoid)	978.6	E858.8	E948.6	E950.4	E962.0	E980.4
Peruvian balsam	976.8	E858.7	E946.8	E950.4	E962.0	E980.4
Pesticides (dust) (fumes) (vapor)	989.4	E863.4	—	E950.6	E962.1	E980.7
arsenic	985.1	E863.4	—	E950.8	E962.1	E980.8
chlorinated	989.2	E863.0	—	E950.6	E962.1	E980.7
cyanide	989.0	E863.4	—	E950.6	E962.1	E980.7
kerosene	981	E863.4	—	E950.6	E962.1	E980.7
mixture (of compounds)	989.4	E863.3	—	E950.6	E962.1	E980.7
naphthalene	983.0	E863.4	—	E950.7	E962.1	E980.6
organochlorine (compounds)	989.2	E863.0	—	E950.6	E962.1	E980.7
petroleum (distillate) (products) NEC	981	E863.4	—	E950.6	E962.1	E980.7
specified ingredient NEC	989.4	E863.4	—	E950.6	E962.1	E980.7
strychnine	989.1	E863.4	—	E950.6	E962.1	E980.7
thallium	985.8	E863.7	—	E950.6	E962.1	E980.7
Pethidine (hydrochloride)	965.09	E850.2	E935.2	E950.0	E962.0	E980.0
Petrichloral	967.1	E852.0	E937.1	E950.2	E962.0	E980.2
Petrol	981	E862.1	—	E950.9	E962.1	E980.9
vapor	987.1	E869.8	—	E952.8	E962.2	E982.8
Petrolatum (jelly) (ointment)	976.3	E858.7	E946.3	E950.4	E962.0	E980.4
hydrophilic	976.3	E858.7	E946.3	E950.4	E962.0	E980.4
liquid	973.2	E858.4	E943.2	E950.4	E962.0	E980.4
topical	976.3	E858.7	E946.3	E950.4	E962.0	E980.4
nonmedicinal	981	E862.1	—	E950.9	E962.1	E980.9
Petroleum (cleaners) (fuels) (products) NEC	981	E862.1	—	E950.9	E962.1	E980.9
benzin(e) — see Ligroin						
ether — see Ligroin						
jelly — see Petrolatum						
naphtha — see Ligroin						
pesticide	981	E863.4	—	E950.6	E962.1	E980.7
solids	981	E862.3	—	E950.9	E962.1	E980.9
solvents	981	E862.0	—	E950.9	E962.1	E980.9
vapor	987.1	E869.8	—	E952.8	E962.2	E982.8
Peyote	969.6	E854.1	E939.6	E950.3	E962.0	E980.3
Phanodorm, phanodorn	967.0	E851	E937.0	E950.1	E962.0	E980.1
Phanquinone, phanquone	961.5	E857	E931.5	E950.4	E962.0	E980.4
Pharmaceutical excipient or adjunct	977.4	E858.8	E947.4	E950.4	E962.0	E980.4
Phenacemide	966.3	E855.0	E936.3	E950.4	E962.0	E980.4

1473

TABLE OF DRUGS AND CHEMICALS

Substance	Poisoning	Accident	Therapeutic Use	Suicide Attempt	Assault	Undetermined
		\multicolumn{5}{c}{External Cause (E-Code)}

Substance	Poisoning	Accident	Therapeutic Use	Suicide Attempt	Assault	Undetermined
Phenacetin	965.4	E850.4	E935.4	E950.0	E962.0	E980.0
Phenadoxone	965.09	E850.2	E935.2	E950.0	E962.0	E980.0
Phenaglycodol	969.5	E853.8	E939.5	E950.3	E962.0	E980.3
Phenantoin	966.1	E855.0	E936.1	E950.4	E962.0	E980.4
Phenaphthazine reagent	977.8	E858.8	E947.8	E950.4	E962.0	E980.4
Phenazocine	965.09	E850.2	E935.2	E950.0	E962.0	E980.0
Phenazone	965.5	E850.5	E935.5	E950.0	E962.0	E980.0
Phenazopyridine	976.1	E858.7	E946.1	E950.4	E962.0	E980.4
Phenbenicillin	960.0	E856	E930.0	E950.4	E962.0	E980.4
Phenbutrazate	977.0	E858.8	E947.0	E950.4	E962.0	E980.4
Phencyclidine	968.3	E855.1	E938.3	E950.4	E962.0	E980.4
Phendimetrazine	977.0	E858.8	E947.0	E950.4	E962.0	E980.4
Phenelzine	969.0	E854.0	E939.0	E950.3	E962.0	E980.3
Phenergan	967.8	E852.8	E937.8	E950.2	E962.0	E980.2
Phenethicillin (potassium)	960.0	E856	E930.0	E950.4	E962.0	E980.4
Phenetsal	965.1	E850.3	E935.3	E950.0	E962.0	E980.0
Pheneturide	966.3	E855.0	E936.3	E950.4	E962.0	E980.4
Phenformin	962.3	E858.0	E932.3	E950.4	E962.0	E980.4
Phenglutarimide	971.1	E855.4	E941.1	E950.4	E962.0	E980.4
Phenicarbazide	965.8	E850.8	E935.8	E950.0	E962.0	E980.0
Phenindamine (tartrate)	963.0	E858.1	E933.0	E950.4	E962.0	E980.4
Phenindione	964.2	E858.2	E934.2	E950.4	E962.0	E980.4
Pheniprazine	969.0	E854.0	E939.0	E950.3	E962.0	E980.3
Pheniramine (maleate)	963.0	E858.1	E933.0	E950.4	E962.0	E980.4
Phenmetrazine	977.0	E858.8	E947.0	E950.4	E962.0	E980.4
Phenobal	967.0	E851	E937.0	E950.1	E962.0	E980.1
Phenobarbital	967.0	E851	E937.0	E950.1	E962.0	E980.1
Phenobarbitone	967.0	E851	E937.0	E950.1	E962.0	E980.1
Phenoctide	976.0	E858.7	E946.0	E950.4	E962.0	E980.4
Phenol (derivatives) NEC	983.0	E864.0	—	E950.7	E962.1	E980.6
disinfectant	983.0	E864.0	—	E950.7	E962.1	E980.6
pesticide	989.4	E863.4	—	E950.6	E962.1	E980.7
red	977.8	E858.8	E947.8	E950.4	E962.0	E980.4
Phenolphthalein	973.1	E858.4	E943.1	E950.4	E962.0	E980.4
Phenolsulfonphthalein	977.8	E858.8	E947.8	E950.4	E962.0	E980.4
Phenomorphan	965.09	E850.2	E935.2	E950.0	E962.0	E980.0
Phenonyl	967.0	E851	E937.0	E950.1	E962.0	E980.1
Phenoperidine	965.09	E850.2	E935.2	E950.0	E962.0	E980.0
Phenoquin	974.7	E858.5	E944.7	E950.4	E962.0	E980.4
Phenothiazines (tranquilizers) NEC	969.1	E853.0	E939.1	E950.3	E962.0	E980.3
insecticide	989.3	E863.4	—	E950.6	E962.1	E980.7
Phenoxybenzamine	971.3	E855.6	E941.3	E950.4	E962.0	E980.4
Phenoxymethyl penicillin	960.0	E856	E930.0	E950.4	E962.0	E980.4
Phenprocoumon	964.2	E858.2	E934.2	E950.4	E962.0	E980.4
Phensuximide	966.2	E855.0	E936.2	E950.4	E962.0	E980.4
Phentermine	977.0	E858.8	E947.0	E950.4	E962.0	E980.4
Phentolamine	971.3	E855.6	E941.3	E950.4	E962.0	E980.4
Phenyl						
butazone	965.5	E850.5	E935.5	E950.0	E962.0	E980.0
enediamine	983.0	E864.0	—	E950.7	E962.1	E980.6
hydrazine	983.0	E864.0	—	E950.7	E962.1	E980.6
antineoplastic	963.1	E858.1	E933.1	E950.4	E962.0	E980.4
mercuric compounds — see Mercury						
salicylate	976.3	E858.7	E946.3	E950.4	E962.0	E980.4
Phenylephrin	971.2	E855.5	E941.2	E950.4	E962.0	E980.4
Phenylethybiguanide	962.3	E858.0	E932.3	E950.4	E962.0	E980.4
Phenylpropanolamine	971.2	E855.5	E941.2	E950.4	E962.0	E980.4
Phenylsulfthion	989.3	E863.1	—	E950.6	E962.1	E980.7
Phenyramidol, phenyramidon	965.7	E850.7	E935.7	E950.0	E962.0	E980.0
Phenytoin	966.1	E855.0	E936.1	E950.4	E962.0	E980.4

TABLE OF DRUGS AND CHEMICALS

Substance	Poisoning	Accident	Therapeutic Use	Suicide Attempt	Assault	Undetermined
		\multicolumn{5}{c}{External Cause (E-Code)}

Substance	Poisoning	Accident	Therapeutic Use	Suicide Attempt	Assault	Undetermined
pHisoHex	976.2	E858.7	E946.2	E950.4	E962.0	E980.4
Pholcodine	965.09	E850.2	E935.2	E950.0	E962.0	E980.0
Phorate	989.3	E863.1	—	E950.6	E962.1	E980.7
Phosdrin	989.3	E863.1	—	E950.6	E962.1	E980.7
Phosgene (gas)	987.8	E869.8	—	E952.8	E962.2	E982.8
Phosphate (tricresyl)	989.89	E866.8	—	E950.9	E962.1	E980.9
organic	989.3	E863.1	—	E950.6	E962.1	E980.7
solvent	982.8	E862.4	—	E950.9	E926.1	E980.9
Phosphine	987.8	E869.8	—	E952.8	E962.2	E982.8
fumigant	987.8	E863.8	—	E950.6	E962.2	E980.7
Phospholine	971.0	E855.3	E941.0	E950.4	E962.0	E980.4
Phosphoric acid	983.1	E864.1	—	E950.7	E962.1	E980.6
Phosphorus (compounds) NEC	983.9	E864.3	—	E950.7	E962.1	E980.6
rodenticide	983.9	E863.7	—	E950.7	E962.1	E980.6
Phthalimidogluarimide	967.8	E852.8	E937.8	E950.2	E962.0	E980.2
Phthalylsulfathiazole	961.0	E857	E931.0	E950.4	E962.0	E980.4
Phylloquinone	964.3	E858.2	E934.3	E950.4	E962.0	E980.4
Physeptone	965.02	E850.1	E935.1	E950.0	E962.0	E980.0
Physostigma venenosum	988.2	E865.4	—	E950.9	E962.1	E980.9
Physostigmine	971.0	E855.3	E941.0	E950.4	E962.0	E980.4
Phytolacca decandra	988.2	E865.4	—	E950.9	E962.1	E980.9
Phytomenadione	964.3	E858.2	E934.3	E950.4	E962.0	E980.4
Phytonadione	964.3	E858.2	E934.3	E950.4	E962.0	E980.4
Picric (acid)	983.0	E864.0	—	E950.7	E962.1	E980.6
Picrotoxin	970.0	E854.3	E940.0	E950.4	E962.0	E980.4
Pilocarpine	971.0	E855.3	E941.0	E950.4	E962.0	E980.4
Pilocarpus (jaborandi) extract	971.0	E855.3	E941.0	E950.4	E962.0	E980.4
Pimaricin	960.1	E856	E930.1	E950.4	E962.0	E980.4
Piminodine	965.09	E850.2	E935.2	E950.0	E962.0	E980.0
Pine oil, pinesol (disinfectant)	983.9	E861.4	—	E950.7	E962.1	E980.6
Pinkroot	961.6	E857	E931.6	E950.4	E962.0	E980.4
Pipadone	965.09	E850.2	E935.2	E950.0	E962.0	E980.0
Pipamazine	963.0	E858.1	E933.0	E950.4	E962.0	E980.4
Pipazethate	975.4	E858.6	E945.4	E950.4	E962.0	E980.4
Pipenzolate	971.1	E855.4	E941.1	E950.4	E962.0	E980.4
Piperacetazine	969.1	E853.0	E939.1	E950.3	E962.0	E980.3
Piperazine NEC	961.6	E857	E931.6	E950.4	E962.0	E980.4
estrone sulfate	962.2	E858.0	E932.2	E950.4	E962.0	E980.4
Piper cubeba	988.2	E865.4	—	E950.9	E962.1	E980.9
Piperidione	975.4	E858.6	E945.4	E950.4	E962.0	E980.4
Piperidolate	971.1	E855.4	E941.1	E950.4	E962.0	E980.4
Piperocaine	968.9	E855.2	E938.9	E950.4	E962.0	E980.4
infiltration (subcutaneous)	968.5	E855.2	E938.5	E950.4	E962.0	E980.4
nerve block (peripheral) (plexus)	968.6	E855.2	E938.6	E950.4	E962.0	E980.4
topical (surface)	968.5	E855.2	E938.5	E950.4	E962.0	E980.4
Pipobroman	963.1	E858.1	E933.1	E950.4	E962.0	E980.4
Pipradrol	970.8	E854.3	E940.8	E950.4	E962.0	E980.4
Piscidia (bark) (erythrina)	965.7	E850.7	E935.7	E950.0	E962.0	E980.0
Pitch	983.0	E864.0	—	E950.7	E962.1	E980.6
Pitkin's solution	968.7	E855.2	E938.7	E950.4	E962.0	E980.4
Pitocin	975.0	E858.6	E945.0	E950.4	E962.0	E980.4
Pitressin (tannate)	962.5	E858.0	E932.5	E950.4	E962.0	E980.4
Pituitary extracts (posterior)	962.5	E858.0	E932.5	E950.4	E962.0	E980.4
anterior	962.4	E858.0	E932.4	E950.4	E962.0	E980.4
Pituitrin	962.5	E858.0	E932.5	E950.4	E962.0	E980.4
Placental extract	962.9	E858.0	E932.9	E950.4	E962.0	E980.4
Placidyl	967.8	E852.8	E937.8	E950.2	E962.0	E980.2
Plague vaccine	978.3	E858.8	E948.3	E950.4	E962.0	E980.4
Plant foods or fertilizers NEC	989.89	E866.5	—	E950.9	E962.1	E980.9
mixed with herbicides	989.4	E863.5	—	E950.6	E962.1	E980.7
Plants, noxious, used as food	988.2	E865.9	—	E950.9	E962.1	E980.9

TABLE OF DRUGS AND CHEMICALS

Substance	Poisoning	Accident	Therapeutic Use	Suicide Attempt	Assault	Undetermined
		\multicolumn{5}{c}{External Cause (E-Code)}

Substance	Poisoning	Accident	Therapeutic Use	Suicide Attempt	Assault	Undetermined
berries and seeds	988.2	E865.3	—	E950.9	E962.1	E980.9
specified type NEC	988.2	E865.4	—	E950.9	E962.1	E980.9
Plasma (blood)	964.7	E858.2	E934.7	E950.4	E962.0	E980.4
expanders	964.8	E858.2	E934.8	E950.4	E962.0	E980.4
Plasmanate	964.7	E858.2	E934.7	E950.4	E962.0	E980.4
Plegicil	969.1	E853.0	E939.1	E950.3	E962.0	E980.3
Podophyllin	976.4	E858.7	E946.4	E950.4	E962.0	E980.4
Podophyllum resin	976.4	E858.7	E946.4	E950.4	E962.0	E980.4
Poison NEC	989.9	E866.9	—	E950.9	E962.1	E980.9
Poisonous berries	988.2	E865.3	—	E950.9	E962.1	E980.9
Pokeweed (any part)	988.2	E865.4	—	E950.9	E962.1	E980.9
Poldine	971.1	E855.4	E941.1	E950.4	E962.0	E980.4
Poliomyelitis vaccine	979.5	E858.8	E949.5	E950.4	E962.0	E980.4
Poliovirus vaccine	979.5	E858.8	E949.5	E950.4	E962.0	E980.4
Polish (car) (floor) (furniture) (metal) (silver)	989.89	E861.2	—	E950.9	E962.1	E980.9
abrasive	989.89	E861.3	—	E950.9	E962.1	E980.9
porcelain	989.89	E861.3	—	E950.9	E962.1	E980.9
Poloxalkol	973.2	E858.4	E943.2	E950.4	E962.0	E980.4
Polyaminostyrene resins	974.5	E858.5	E944.5	E950.4	E962.0	E980.4
Polychlorinated biphenyl—see PCBs						
Polycycline	960.4	E856	E930.4	E950.4	E962.0	E980.4
Polyester resin hardener	982.8	E862.4	—	E950.9	E962.1	E980.9
fumes	987.8	E869.8	—	E952.8	E962.2	E982.8
Polyestradiol (phosphate)	962.2	E858.0	E932.2	E950.4	E962.0	E980.4
Polyethanolamine alkyl sulfate	976.2	E858.7	E946.2	E950.4	E962.0	E980.4
Polyethylene glycol	976.3	E858.7	E946.3	E950.4	E962.0	E980.4
Polyferose	964.0	E858.2	E934.0	E950.4	E962.0	E980.4
Polymyxin B	960.8	E856	E930.8	E950.4	E962.0	E980.4
ENT agent	976.6	E858.7	E946.6	E950.4	E962.0	E980.4
ophthalmic preparation	976.5	E858.7	E946.5	E950.4	E962.0	E980.4
topical NEC	976.0	E858.7	E946.0	E950.4	E962.0	E980.4
Polynoxylin(e)	976.0	E858.7	E946.0	E950.4	E962.0	E980.4
Polyoxymethyleneurea	976.0	E858.7	E946.0	E950.4	E962.0	E980.4
Polytetrafluoroethylene (inhaled)	987.8	E869.8	—	E952.8	E962.2	E982.8
Polythiazide	974.3	E858.5	E944.3	E950.4	E962.0	E980.4
Polyvinylpyrrolidone	964.8	E858.2	E934.8	E950.4	E962.0	E980.4
Pontocaine (hydrochloride) (infiltration) (topical)	968.5	E855.2	E938.5	E950.4	E962.0	E980.4
nerve block (peripheral) (plexus)	968.6	E855.2	E938.6	E950.4	E962.0	E980.4
spinal	968.7	E855.2	E938.7	E950.4	E962.0	E980.4
Pot	969.6	E854.1	E939.6	E950.3	E962.0	E980.3
Potash (caustic)	983.2	E864.2	—	E950.7	E962.1	E980.6
Potassic saline injection (lactated)	974.5	E858.5	E944.5	E950.4	E962.0	E980.4
Potassium (salts) NEC	974.5	E858.5	E944.5	E950.4	E962.0	E980.4
aminosalicylate	961.8	E857	E931.8	E950.4	E962.0	E980.4
arsenite (solution)	985.1	E866.3	—	E950.8	E962.1	E980.8
bichromate	983.9	E864.3	—	E950.7	E962.1	E980.6
bisulfate	983.9	E864.3	—	E950.7	E962.1	E980.6
bromide (medicinal) NEC	967.3	E852.2	E937.3	E950.2	E962.0	E980.2
carbonate	983.2	E864.2	—	E950.7	E962.1	E980.6
chlorate NEC	983.9	E864.3	—	E950.7	E962.1	E980.6
cyanide — see Cyanide						
hydroxide	983.2	E864.2	—	E950.7	E962.1	E980.6
iodide (expectorant) NEC	975.5	E858.6	E945.5	E950.4	E962.0	E980.4
nitrate	989.89	E866.8	—	E950.9	E962.1	E980.9
oxalate	983.9	E864.3	—	E950.7	E962.1	E980.6
perchlorate NEC	977.8	E858.8	E947.8	E950.4	E962.0	E980.4
antithyroid	962.8	E858.0	E932.8	E950.4	E962.0	E980.4
permanganate	976.0	E858.7	E946.0	E950.4	E962.0	E980.4

TABLE OF DRUGS AND CHEMICALS

Substance	Poisoning	Accident	Therapeutic Use	Suicide Attempt	Assault	Undetermined
			External Cause (E-Code)			
nonmedicinal	983.9	E864.3	—	E950.7	E962.1	E980.6
Povidone–iodine (anti–infective) NEC	976.0	E858.7	E946.0	E950.4	E962.0	E980.4
Practolol	972.0	E858.3	E942.0	E950.4	E962.0	E980.4
Pralidoxime (chloride)	977.2	E858.8	E947.2	E950.4	E962.0	E980.4
Pramoxine	968.5	E855.2	E938.5	E950.4	E962.0	E980.4
Prazosin	972.6	E858.3	E942.6	E950.4	E962.0	E980.4
Prednisolone	962.0	E858.0	E932.0	E950.4	E962.0	E980.4
ENT agent	976.6	E858.7	E946.6	E950.4	E962.0	E980.4
ophthalmic preparation	976.5	E858.7	E946.5	E950.4	E962.0	E980.4
topical NEC	976.0	E858.7	E946.0	E950.4	E962.0	E980.4
Prednisone	962.0	E858.0	E932.0	E950.4	E962.0	E980.4
Pregnanediol	962.2	E858.0	E932.2	E950.4	E962.0	E980.4
Pregneninolone	962.2	E858.0	E932.2	E950.4	E962.0	E980.4
Preludin	977.0	E858.8	E947.0	E950.4	E962.0	E980.4
Premarin	962.2	E858.0	E932.2	E950.4	E962.0	E980.4
Prenylamine	972.4	E858.3	E942.4	E950.4	E962.0	E980.4
Preparation H	976.8	E858.7	E946.8	E950.4	E962.0	E980.4
Preservatives	989.89	E866.8	—	E950.9	E962.1	E980.9
Pride of China	988.2	E865.3	—	E950.9	E962.1	E980.9
Prilocaine	968.9	E855.2	E938.9	E950.4	E962.0	E980.4
infiltration (subcutaneous)	968.5	E855.2	E938.5	E950.4	E962.0	E980.4
nerve block (peripheral) (plexus)	968.6	E855.2	E938.6	E950.4	E962.0	E980.4
Primaquine	961.4	E857	E931.4	E950.4	E962.0	E980.4
Primidone	966.3	E855.0	E936.3	E950.4	E962.0	E980.4
Primula (veris)	988.2	E865.4	—	E950.9	E962.1	E980.9
Prinadol	965.09	E850.2	E935.2	E950.0	E962.0	E980.0
Priscol, Priscoline	971.3	E855.6	E941.3	E950.4	E962.0	E980.4
Privet	988.2	E865.4	—	E950.9	E962.1	E980.9
Privine	971.2	E855.5	E941.2	E950.4	E962.0	E980.4
Pro–Banthine	971.1	E855.4	E941.1	E950.4	E962.0	E980.4
Probarbital	967.0	E851	E937.0	E950.1	E962.0	E980.1
Probenecid	974.7	E858.5	E944.7	E950.4	E962.0	E980.4
Procainamide (hydrochloride)	972.0	E858.3	E942.0	E950.4	E962.0	E980.4
Procaine (hydrochloride) (infiltration) (topical)	968.5	E855.2	E938.5	E950.4	E962.0	E980.4
nerve block (peripheral) (plexus)	968.6	E855.2	E938.6	E950.4	E962.0	E980.4
penicillin G	960.0	E856	E930.0	E950.4	E962.0	E980.4
spinal	968.7	E855.2	E938.7	E950.4	E962.0	E980.4
Procalmidol	969.5	E853.8	E939.5	E950.3	E962.0	E980.3
Procarbazine	963.1	E858.1	E933.1	E950.4	E962.0	E980.4
Prochlorperazine	969.1	E853.0	E939.1	E950.3	E962.0	E980.3
Procyclidine	966.4	E855.0	E936.4	E950.4	E962.0	E980.4
Producer gas	986	E868.8	—	E952.1	E962.2	E982.1
Profenamine	966.4	E855.0	E936.4	E950.4	E962.0	E980.4
Profenil	975.1	E858.6	E945.1	E950.4	E962.0	E980.4
Progesterones	962.2	E858.0	E932.2	E950.4	E962.0	E980.4
Progestin	962.2	E858.0	E932.2	E950.4	E962.0	E980.4
Progestogens (with estrogens)	962.2	E858.0	E932.2	E950.4	E962.0	E980.4
Progestone	962.2	E858.0	E932.2	E950.4	E962.0	E980.4
Proguanil	961.4	E857	E931.4	E950.4	E962.0	E980.4
Prolactin	962.4	E858.0	E932.4	E950.4	E962.0	E980.4
Proloid	962.7	E858.0	E932.7	E950.4	E962.0	E980.4
Proluton	962.2	E858.0	E932.2	E950.4	E962.0	E980.4
Promacetin	961.8	E857	E931.8	E950.4	E962.0	E980.4
Promazine	969.1	E853.0	E939.1	E950.3	E962.0	E980.3
Promedol	965.09	E850.2	E935.2	E950.0	E962.0	E980.0
Promethazine	967.8	E852.8	E937.8	E950.2	E962.0	E980.2
Promin	961.8	E857	E931.8	E950.4	E962.0	E980.4
Pronestyl (hydrochloride)	972.0	E858.3	E942.0	E950.4	E962.0	E980.4
Pronetalol, pronethalol	972.0	E858.3	E942.0	E950.4	E962.0	E980.4
Prontosil	961.0	E857	E931.0	E950.4	E962.0	E980.4

TABLE OF DRUGS AND CHEMICALS

Substance	Poisoning	Accident	Therapeutic Use	Suicide Attempt	Assault	Undetermined
			External Cause (E-Code)			

Substance	Poisoning	Accident	Therapeutic Use	Suicide Attempt	Assault	Undetermined
Propamidine isethionate	961.5	E857	E931.5	E950.4	E962.0	E980.4
Propanal (medicinal)	967.8	E852.8	E937.8	E950.2	E962.0	E980.2
Propane (gas) (distributed in mobile container)	987.0	E868.0	—	E951.1	E962.2	E981.1
distributed through pipes	987.0	E867	—	E951.0	E962.2	E981.0
incomplete combustion of – see Carbon monoxide, Propane						
Propanidid	968.3	E855.1	E938.3	E950.4	E962.0	E980.4
Propanol	980.3	E860.4	—	E950.9	E962.1	E980.9
Propantheline	971.1	E855.4	E941.1	E950.4	E962.0	E980.4
Proparacaine	968.5	E855.2	E938.5	E950.4	E962.0	E980.4
Propatyl nitrate	972.4	E858.3	E942.4	E950.4	E962.0	E980.4
Propicillin	960.0	E856	E930.0	E950.4	E962.0	E980.4
Propiolactone (vapor)	987.8	E869.8	—	E952.8	E962.2	E982.8
Propiomazine	967.8	E852.8	E937.8	E950.2	E962.0	E980.2
Propionaldehyde (medicinal)	967.8	E852.8	E937.8	E950.2	E962.0	E980.2
Propionate compound	976.0	E858.7	E946.0	E950.4	E962.0	E980.4
Propion gel	976.0	E858.7	E946.0	E950.4	E962.0	E980.4
Propitocaine	968.9	E855.2	E938.9	E950.4	E962.0	E980.4
infiltration (subcutaneous)	968.5	E855.2	E938.5	E950.4	E962.0	E980.4
nerve block (peripheral) (plexus)	968.6	E855.2	E938.6	E950.4	E962.0	E980.4
Propoxur	989.3	E863.2	—	E950.6	E962.1	E980.7
Propoxycaine	968.9	E855.2	E938.9	E950.4	E962.0	E980.4
infiltration (subcutaneous)	968.5	E855.2	E938.5	E950.4	E962.0	E980.4
nerve block (peripheral) (plexus)	968.6	E855.2	E938.6	E950.4	E962.0	E980.4
topical (surface)	968.5	E855.2	E938.5	E950.4	E962.0	E980.4
Propoxyphene (hydrochloride)	965.8	E850.8	E935.8	E950.0	E962.0	E980.0
Propranolol	972.0	E858.3	E942.0	E950.4	E962.0	E980.4
Propyl						
alcohol	980.3	E860.4	—	E950.9	E962.1	E980.9
carbinol	980.3	E860.4	—	E950.9	E962.1	E980.9
hexadrine	971.2	E855.5	E941.2	E950.4	E962.0	E980.4
iodone	977.8	E858.8	E947.8	E950.4	E962.0	E980.4
thiouracil	962.8	E858.0	E932.8	E950.4	E962.0	E980.4
Propylene	987.1	E869.8	—	E952.8	E962.2	E982.8
Propylparaben (ophthalmic)	976.5	E858.7	E946.5	E950.4	E962.0	E980.4
Proscillaridin	972.1	E858.3	E942.1	E950.4	E962.0	E980.4
Prostaglandins	975.0	E858.6	E945.0	E950.4	E962.0	E980.4
Prostigmin	971.0	E855.3	E941.0	E950.4	E962.0	E980.4
Protamine (sulfate)	964.5	E858.2	E934.5	E950.4	E962.0	E980.4
zinc insulin	962.3	E858.0	E932.3	E950.4	E962.0	E980.4
Protectants (topical)	976.3	E858.7	E946.3	E950.4	E962.0	E980.4
Protein hydrolysate	974.5	E858.5	E944.5	E950.4	E962.0	E980.4
Prothiaden—see Dothiepin hydrochloride						
Prothionamide	961.8	E857	E931.8	E950.4	E962.0	E980.4
Prothipendyl	969.5	E853.8	E939.5	E950.3	E962.0	E980.3
Protokylol	971.2	E855.5	E941.2	E950.4	E962.0	E980.4
Protopam	977.2	E858.8	E947.2	E950.4	E962.0	E980.4
Protoveratrine(s) (A) (B)	972.6	E858.3	E942.6	E950.4	E962.0	E980.4
Protriptyline	969.0	E854.0	E939.0	E950.3	E962.0	E980.3
Provera	962.2	E858.0	E932.2	E950.4	E962.0	E980.4
Provitamin A	963.5	E858.1	E933.5	E950.4	E962.0	E980.4
Proxymetacaine	968.5	E855.2	E938.5	E950.4	E962.0	E980.4
Proxyphylline	975.1	E858.6	E945.1	E950.4	E962.0	E980.4
Prozac—see Fluoxetine hydrochloride						
Prunus						
laurocerasus	988.2	E865.4	—	E950.9	E962.1	E980.9
virginiana	988.2	E865.4	—	E950.9	E962.1	E980.9
Prussic acid	989.0	E866.8	—	E950.9	E962.1	E980.9
vapor	987.7	E869.8	—	E952.8	E962.2	E982.8

1478

TABLE OF DRUGS AND CHEMICALS

Substance	Poisoning	Accident	Therapeutic Use	Suicide Attempt	Assault	Undetermined
			External Cause (E-Code)			
Pseudoephedrine	971.2	E855.5	E941.2	E950.4	E962.0	E980.4
Psilocin	969.6	E854.1	E939.6	E950.3	E962.0	E980.3
Psilocybin	969.6	E854.1	E939.6	E950.3	E962.0	E980.3
PSP	977.8	E858.8	E947.8	E950.4	E962.0	E980.4
Psychedelic agents	969.6	E854.1	E939.6	E950.3	E962.0	E980.3
Psychodysleptics	969.6	E854.1	E939.6	E950.3	E962.0	E980.3
Psychostimulants	969.7	E854.2	E939.7	E950.3	E962.0	E980.3
Psychotherapeutic agents	969.9	E855.9	E939.9	E950.3	E962.0	E980.3
antidepressants	969.0	E854.0	E939.0	E950.3	E962.0	E980.3
specified NEC	969.8	E855.8	E939.8	E950.3	E962.0	E980.3
tranquilizers NEC	969.5	E853.9	E939.5	E950.3	E962.0	E980.3
Psychotomimetic agents	969.6	E854.1	E939.6	E950.3	E962.0	E980.3
Psychotropic agents	969.9	E854.8	E939.9	E950.3	E962.0	E980.3
specified NEC	969.8	E854.8	E939.8	E950.3	E962.0	E980.3
Psyllium	973.3	E858.4	E943.3	E950.4	E962.0	E980.4
Pteroylglutamic acid	964.1	E858.2	E934.1	E950.4	E962.0	E980.4
Pteroyltriglutamate	963.1	E858.1	E933.1	E950.4	E962.0	E980.4
PTFE	987.8	E869.8	—	E952.8	E962.2	E982.8
Pulsatilla	988.2	E865.4	—	E950.9	E962.1	E980.9
Purex (bleach)	983.9	E864.3	—	E950.7	E962.1	E980.6
Purine diuretics	974.1	E858.5	E944.1	E950.4	E962.0	E980.4
Purinethol	963.1	E858.1	E933.1	E950.4	E962.0	E980.4
PVP	964.8	E858.2	E934.8	E950.4	E962.0	E980.4
Pyrabital	965.7	E850.7	E935.7	E950.0	E962.0	E980.0
Pyramidon	965.5	E850.5	E935.5	E950.0	E962.0	E980.0
Pyrantel (pamoate)	961.6	E857	E931.6	E950.4	E962.0	E980.4
Pyrathiazine	963.0	E858.1	E933.0	E950.4	E962.0	E980.4
Pyrazinamide	961.8	E857	E931.8	E950.4	E962.0	E980.4
Pyrazinoic acid (amide)	961.8	E857	E931.8	E950.4	E962.0	E980.4
Pyrazole (derivatives)	965.5	E850.5	E935.5	E950.0	E962.0	E980.0
Pyrazolone (analgesics)	965.5	E850.5	E935.5	E950.0	E962.0	E980.0
Pyrethrins, pyrethrum	989.4	E863.4	—	E950.6	E962.1	E980.7
Pyribenzamine	963.0	E858.1	E933.0	E950.4	E962.0	E980.4
Pyridine (liquid) (vapor)	982.0	E862.4	—	E950.9	E962.1	E980.9
aldoxime chloride	977.2	E858.8	E947.2	E950.4	E962.0	E980.4
Pyridium	976.1	E858.7	E946.1	E950.4	E962.0	E980.4
Pyridostigmine	971.0	E855.3	E941.0	E950.4	E962.0	E980.4
Pyridoxine	963.5	E858.1	E933.5	E950.4	E962.0	E980.4
Pyrilamine	963.0	E858.1	E933.0	E950.4	E962.0	E980.4
Pyrimethamine	961.4	E857	E931.4	E950.4	E962.0	E980.4
Pyrogallic acid	983.0	E864.0	—	E950.7	E962.1	E980.6
Pyroxylin	976.3	E858.7	E946.3	E950.4	E962.0	E980.4
Pyrrobutamine	963.0	E858.1	E933.0	E950.4	E962.0	E980.4
Pyrrocaine	968.5	E855.2	E938.5	E950.4	E962.0	E980.4
Pyrvinium (pamoate)	961.6	E857	E931.6	E950.4	E962.0	E980.4
PZI	962.3	E858.0	E932.3	E950.4	E962.0	E980.4
Quaalude	967.4	E852.3	E937.4	E950.2	E962.0	E980.2
Quaternary ammonium derivatives	971.1	E855.4	E941.1	E950.4	E962.0	E980.4
Quicklime	983.2	E864.2	—	E950.7	E962.1	E980.6
Quinacrine	961.3	E857	E931.3	E950.4	E962.0	E980.4
Quinaglute	972.0	E858.3	E942.0	E950.4	E962.0	E980.4
Quinalbarbitone	967.0	E851	E937.0	E950.1	E962.0	E980.1
Quinestradiol	962.2	E858.0	E932.2	E950.4	E962.0	E980.4
Quinethazone	974.3	E858.5	E944.3	E950.4	E962.0	E980.4
Quinidine (gluconate) (polygalacturonate) (salts) (sulfate)	972.0	E858.3	E942.0	E950.4	E962.0	E980.4
Quinine	961.4	E857	E931.4	E950.4	E962.0	E980.4
Quiniobine	961.3	E857	E931.3	E950.4	E962.0	E980.4
Quinolines	961.3	E857	E931.3	E950.4	E962.0	E980.4
Quotane	968.5	E855.2	E938.5	E950.4	E962.0	E980.4
Rabies						

TABLE OF DRUGS AND CHEMICALS

Substance	Poisoning	Accident	Therapeutic Use	Suicide Attempt	Assault	Undetermined
			External Cause (E-Code)			
immune globulin (human)	964.6	E858.2	E934.6	E950.4	E962.0	E980.4
vaccine	979.1	E858.8	E949.1	E950.4	E962.0	E980.4
Racemoramide	965.09	E850.2	E935.2	E950.0	E962.0	E980.0
Racemorphan	965.09	E850.2	E935.2	E950.0	E962.0	E980.0
Radiator alcohol	980.1	E860.2	—	E950.9	E962.1	E980.9
Radio–opaque (drugs) (materials)	977.8	E858.8	E947.8	E950.4	E962.0	E980.4
Ranunculus	988.2	E865.4	—	E950.9	E962.1	E980.9
Rat poison	989.4	E863.7	—	E950.6	E962.1	E980.7
Rattlesnake (venom)	989.5	E905.0	—	E950.9	E962.1	E980.9
Raudixin	972.6	E858.3	E942.6	E950.4	E962.0	E980.4
Rautensin	972.6	E858.3	E942.6	E950.4	E962.0	E980.4
Rautina	972.6	E858.3	E942.6	E950.4	E962.0	E980.4
Rautotal	972.6	E858.3	E942.6	E950.4	E962.0	E980.4
Rauwiloid	972.6	E858.3	E942.6	E950.4	E962.0	E980.4
Rauwoldin	972.6	E858.3	E942.6	E950.4	E962.0	E980.4
Rauwolfia (alkaloids)	972.6	E858.3	E942.6	E950.4	E962.0	E980.4
Realgar	985.1	E866.3	—	E950.8	E962.1	E980.8
Red cells, packed	964.7	E858.2	E934.7	E950.4	E962.0	E980.4
Reducing agents, industrial NEC	983.9	E864.3	—	E950.7	E962.1	E980.6
Refrigerant gas (freon)	987.4	E869.2	—	E952.8	E962.2	E982.8
not freon	987.9	E869.9	—	E952.9	E962.2	E982.9
Regroton	974.4	E858.5	E944.4	E950.4	E962.0	E980.4
Rela	968.0	E855.1	E938.0	E950.4	E962.0	E980.4
Relaxants, skeletal muscle (autonomic)	975.2	E858.6	E945.2	E950.4	E962.0	E980.4
central nervous system	968.0	E855.1	E938.0	E950.4	E962.0	E980.4
Renese	974.3	E858.5	E944.3	E950.4	E962.0	E980.4
Renografin	977.8	E858.8	E947.8	E950.4	E962.0	E980.4
Replacement solutions	974.5	E858.5	E944.5	E950.4	E962.0	E980.4
Rescinnamine	972.6	E858.3	E942.6	E950.4	E962.0	E980.4
Reserpine	972.6	E858.3	E942.6	E950.4	E962.0	E980.4
Resorcin, resorcinol	976.4	E858.7	E946.4	E950.4	E962.0	E980.4
Respaire	975.5	E858.6	E945.5	E950.4	E962.0	E980.4
Respiratory agents NEC	975.8	E858.6	E945.8	E950.4	E962.0	E980.4
Retinoic acid	976.8	E858.7	E946.8	E950.4	E962.0	E980.4
Retinol	963.5	E858.1	E933.5	E950.4	E962.0	E980.4
Rh$_0$ (D) immune globulin (human)	964.6	E858.2	E934.6	E950.4	E962.0	E980.4
Rhodine	965.1	E850.3	E935.3	E950.0	E962.0	E980.0
RhoGAM	964.6	E858.2	E934.6	E950.4	E962.0	E980.4
Riboflavin	963.5	E858.1	E933.5	E950.4	E962.0	E980.4
Ricin	989.89	E866.8	—	E950.9	E962.1	E980.9
Ricinus communis	988.2	E865.3	—	E950.9	E962.1	E980.9
Rickettsial vaccine NEC	979.6	E858.8	E949.6	E950.4	E962.0	E980.4
with viral and bacterial vaccine	979.7	E858.8	E949.7	E950.4	E962.0	E980.4
Rifampin	960.6	E856	E930.6	E950.4	E962.0	E980.4
Rimifon	961.8	E857	E931.8	E950.4	E962.0	E980.4
Ringer's injection (lactated)	974.5	E858.5	E944.5	E950.4	E962.0	E980.4
Ristocetin	960.8	E856	E930.8	E950.4	E962.0	E980.4
Ritalin	969.7	E854.2	E939.7	E950.3	E962.0	E980.3
Roach killers — see Pesticides						
Rocky Mountain spotted fever vaccine	979.6	E858.8	E949.6	E950.4	E962.0	E980.4
Rodenticides	989.4	E863.7	—	E950.6	E962.1	E980.7
Rohypnol	969.4	E853.2	E939.4	E950.3	E962.0	E980.3
Rolaids	973.0	E858.4	E943.0	E950.4	E962.0	E980.4
Rolitetracycline	960.4	E856	E930.4	E950.4	E962.0	E980.4
Romilar	975.4	E858.6	E945.4	E950.4	E962.0	E980.4
Rose water ointment	976.3	E858.7	E946.3	E950.4	E962.0	E980.4
Rotenone	989.4	E863.7	—	E950.6	E962.1	E980.7
Rotoxamine	963.0	E858.1	E933.0	E950.4	E962.0	E980.4
Rough–on–rats	989.4	E863.7	—	E950.6	E962.1	E980.7
Rubbing alcohol	980.2	E860.3	—	E950.9	E962.1	E980.9

TABLE OF DRUGS AND CHEMICALS

Substance	Poisoning	Accident	Therapeutic Use	Suicide Attempt	Assault	Undetermined
			External Cause (E-Code)			
Rubella virus vaccine	979.4	E858.8	E949.4	E950.4	E962.0	E980.4
Rubelogen	979.4	E858.8	E949.4	E950.4	E962.0	E980.4
Rubeovax	979.4	E858.8	E949.4	E950.4	E962.0	E980.4
Rubidomycin	960.7	E856	E930.7	E950.4	E962.0	E980.4
Rue	988.2	E965.4	—	E950.9	E962.1	E980.9
RU486	962.9	E858.0	E932.9	E950.4	E962.0	E980.4
Ruta	988.2	E865.4	—	E950.9	E962.1	E980.9
Sabadilla (medicinal)	976.0	E858.7	E946.0	E950.4	E962.0	E980.4
pesticide	989.4	E863.4	—	E950.6	E962.1	E980.7
Sabin oral vaccine	979.5	E858.8	E949.5	E950.4	E962.0	E980.4
Saccharated iron oxide	964.0	E858.2	E934.0	E950.4	E962.0	E980.4
Saccharin	974.5	E858.5	E944.5	E950.4	E962.0	E980.4
Safflower oil	972.2	E858.3	E942.2	E950.4	E962.0	E980.4
Salbutamol sulfate	975.7	E858.6	E945.7	E950.4	E962.0	E980.4
Salicylamide	965.1	E850.3	E935.3	E950.0	E962.0	E980.0
Salicylate(s)	965.1	E850.3	E935.3	E950.0	E962.0	E980.0
methyl	976.3	E858.7	E946.3	E950.4	E962.0	E980.4
theobromine calcium	974.1	E858.5	E944.1	E950.4	E962.0	E980.4
Salicylazosulfapyridine	961.0	E857	E931.0	E950.4	E962.0	E980.4
Salicylhydroxamic acid	976.0	E858.7	E946.0	E950.4	E962.0	E980.4
Salicylic acid (keratolytic) NEC	976.4	E858.7	E946.4	E950.4	E962.0	E980.4
congeners	965.1	E850.3	E935.3	E950.0	E962.0	E980.0
salts	965.1	E850.3	E935.3	E950.0	E962.0	E980.0
Saliniazid	961.8	E857	E931.8	E950.4	E962.0	E980.4
Salol	976.3	E858.7	E946.3	E950.4	E962.0	E980.4
Salt (substitute) NEC	974.5	E858.5	E944.5	E950.4	E962.0	E980.4
Saluretics	974.3	E858.5	E944.3	E950.4	E962.0	E980.4
Saluron	974.3	E858.5	E944.3	E950.4	E962.0	E980.4
Salvarsan 606 (neosilver) (silver)	961.1	E857	E931.1	E950.4	E962.0	E980.4
Sambucus canadensis	988.2	E865.4	—	E950.9	E962.1	E980.9
berry	988.2	E865.3	—	E950.9	E962.1	E980.9
Sandril	972.6	E858.3	E942.6	E950.4	E962.0	E980.4
Sanguinaria canadensis	988.2	E865.4	—	E950.9	E962.1	E980.9
Saniflush (cleaner)	983.9	E861.3	—	E950.7	E962.1	E980.6
Santonin	961.6	E857	E931.6	E950.4	E962.0	E980.4
Santyl	976.8	E858.7	E946.8	E950.4	E962.0	E980.4
Sarkomycin	960.7	E856	E930.7	E950.4	E962.0	E980.4
Saroten	969.0	E854.0	E939.0	E950.3	E962.0	E980.3
Saturnine – see Lead						
Savin (oil)	976.4	E858.7	E946.4	E950.4	E962.0	E980.4
Scammony	973.1	E858.4	E943.1	E950.4	E962.0	E980.4
Scarlet red	976.8	E858.7	E946.8	E950.4	E962.0	E980.4
Scheele's green	985.1	E866.3	—	E950.8	E962.1	E980.8
insecticide	985.1	E863.4	—	E950.8	E962.1	E980.8
Schradan	989.3	E863.1	—	E950.6	E962.1	E980.7
Schweinfurt (h) green	985.1	E866.3	—	E950.8	E962.1	E980.8
insecticide	985.1	E863.4	—	E950.8	E962.1	E980.8
Scilla — see Squill						
Sclerosing agents	972.7	E858.3	E942.7	E950.4	E962.0	E980.4
Scopolamine	971.1	E855.4	E941.1	E950.4	E962.0	E980.4
Scouring powder	989.89	E861.3	—	E950.9	E962.1	E980.9
Sea						
anemone (sting)	989.5	E905.6	—	E950.9	E962.1	E980.9
cucumber (sting)	989.5	E905.6	—	E950.9	E962.1	E980.9
snake (bite) (venom)	989.5	E905.0	—	E950.9	E962.1	E980.9
urchin spine (puncture)	989.5	E905.6	—	E950.9	E962.1	E980.9
Secbutabarbital	967.0	E851	E937.0	E950.1	E962.0	E980.1
Secbutabaritone	967.0	E851	E937.0	E950.1	E962.0	E980.1
Secobarbital	967.0	E851	E937.0	E950.1	E962.0	E980.1
Seconal	967.0	E851	E937.0	E950.1	E962.0	E980.1
Secretin	977.8	E858.8	E947.8	E950.4	E962.0	E980.4

TABLE OF DRUGS AND CHEMICALS

Substance	Poisoning	Accident	Therapeutic Use	Suicide Attempt	Assault	Undetermined
			External Cause (E-Code)			

Sedatives, nonbarbiturate	967.9	E852.9	E937.9	E950.2	E962.0	E980.2
specified NEC	967.8	E852.8	E937.8	E950.2	E962.0	E980.2
Sedormid	967.8	E852.8	E937.8	E950.2	E962.0	E980.2
Seed (plant)	988.2	E865.3	—	E950.9	E962.1	E980.9
disinfectant or dressing	989.89	E866.5	—	E950.9	E962.1	E980.9
Selenium (fumes) NEC	985.8	E866.4	—	E950.9	E962.1	E980.9
disulfide or sulfide	976.4	E858.7	E946.4	E950.4	E962.0	E980.4
Selsun	976.4	E858.7	E946.4	E950.4	E962.0	E980.4
Senna	973.1	E858.4	E943.1	E950.4	E962.0	E980.4
Septisol	976.2	E858.7	E946.2	E950.4	E962.0	E980.4
Serax	969.4	E853.2	E939.4	E950.3	E962.0	E980.3
Serenesil	967.8	E852.8	E937.8	E950.2	E962.0	E980.2
Serenium (hydrochloride)	961.9	E857	E931.9	E950.4	E962.0	E980.4
Serepax—see Oxazepam						
Sernyl	968.3	E855.1	E938.3	E950.4	E962.0	E980.4
Serotonin	977.8	E858.8	E947.8	E950.4	E962.0	E980.4
Serpasil	972.6	E858.3	E942.6	E950.4	E962.0	E980.4
Sewer gas	987.8	E869.8	—	E952.8	E962.2	E982.8
Shampoo	989.6	E861.0	—	E950.9	E962.1	E980.9
Shellfish, nonbacterial or noxious	988.0	E865.1	—	E950.9	E962.1	E980.9
Silicones NEC	989.83	E866.8	E947.8	E950.9	E962.1	E980.9
Silvadene	976.0	E858.7	E946.0	E950.4	E962.0	E980.4
Silver (compound) (medicinal) NEC	976.0	E858.7	E946.0	E950.4	E962.0	E980.4
anti-infectives	976.0	E858.7	E946.0	E950.4	E962.0	E980.4
arsphenamine	961.1	E857	E931.1	E950.4	E962.0	E980.4
nitrate	976.0	E858.7	E946.0	E950.4	E962.0	E980.4
ophthalmic preparation	976.5	E858.7	E946.5	E950.4	E962.0	E980.4
toughened (keratolytic)	976.4	E858.7	E946.4	E950.4	E962.0	E980.4
nonmedicinal (dust)	985.8	E866.4	—	E950.9	E962.1	E980.9
protein (mild) (strong)	976.0	E858.7	E946.0	E950.4	E962.0	E980.4
salvarsan	961.1	E857	E931.1	E950.4	E962.0	E980.4
Simethicone	973.8	E858.4	E943.8	E950.4	E962.0	E980.4
Sinequan	969.0	E854.0	E939.0	E950.3	E962.0	E980.3
Singoserp	972.6	E858.3	E942.6	E950.4	E962.0	E980.4
Sintrom	964.2	E858.2	E934.2	E950.4	E962.0	E980.4
Sitosterols	972.2	E858.3	E942.2	E950.4	E962.0	E980.4
Skeletal muscle relaxants	975.2	E858.6	E945.2	E950.4	E962.0	E980.4
Skin						
agents (external)	976.9	E858.7	E946.9	E950.4	E962.0	E980.4
specified NEC	976.8	E858.7	E946.8	E950.4	E962.0	E980.4
test antigen	977.8	E858.8	E947.8	E950.4	E962.0	E980.4
Sleep–eze	963.0	E858.1	E933.0	E950.4	E962.0	E980.4
Sleeping draught (drug) (pill) (tablet)	967.9	E852.9	E937.9	E950.2	E962.0	E980.2
Smallpox vaccine	979.0	E858.8	E949.0	E950.4	E962.0	E980.4
Smelter fumes NEC	985.9	E866.4	—	E950.9	E962.1	E980.9
Smog	987.3	E869.1	—	E952.8	E962.2	E982.8
Smoke NEC	987.9	E869.9	—	E952.9	E962.2	E982.9
Smooth muscle relaxant	975.1	E858.6	E945.1	E950.4	E962.0	E980.4
Snail killer	989.4	E863.4	—	E950.6	E962.1	E980.7
Snake (bite) (venom)	989.5	E905.0	—	E950.9	E962.1	E980.9
Snuff	989.89	E866.8	—	E950.9	E962.1	E980.9
Soap (powder) (product)	989.6	E861.1	—	E950.9	E962.1	E980.9
medicinal, soft	976.2	E858.7	E946.2	E950.4	E962.0	E980.4
Soda (caustic)	983.2	E864.2	—	E950.7	E962.1	E980.6
bicarb	963.3	E858.1	E933.3	E950.4	E962.0	E980.4
chlorinated — Sodium, hypochlorite						
Sodium						
acetosulfone	961.8	E857	E931.8	E950.4	E962.0	E980.4
acetrizoate	977.8	E858.8	E947.8	E950.4	E962.0	E980.4
amytal	967.0	E851	E937.0	E950.1	E962.0	E980.1

1482

TABLE OF DRUGS AND CHEMICALS

Substance	Poisoning	Accident	Therapeutic Use	Suicide Attempt	Assault	Undetermined
		\multicolumn{5}{c}{External Cause (E-Code)}				

Substance	Poisoning	Accident	Therapeutic Use	Suicide Attempt	Assault	Undetermined
arsenate — see Arsenic						
bicarbonate	963.3	E858.1	E933.3	E950.4	E962.0	E980.4
bichromate	983.9	E864.3	—	E950.7	E962.1	E980.6
biphosphate	963.2	E858.1	E933.2	E950.4	E962.0	E980.4
bisulfate	983.9	E864.3	—	E950.7	E962.1	E980.6
borate (cleanser)	989.6	E861.3	—	E950.9	E962.1	E980.9
bromide NEC	967.3	E852.2	E937.3	E950.2	E962.0	E980.2
cacodylate (nonmedicinal) NEC	978.8	E858.8	E948.8	E950.4	E962.0	E980.4
anti-infective	961.1	E857	E931.1	E950.4	E962.0	E980.4
herbicide	989.4	E863.5	—	E950.6	E962.1	E980.7
calcium edetate	963.8	E858.1	E933.8	E950.4	E962.0	E980.4
carbonate NEC	983.2	E864.2	—	E950.7	E962.1	E980.6
chlorate NEC	983.9	E864.3	—	E950.7	E962.1	E980.6
herbicide	983.9	E863.5	—	E950.7	E962.1	E980.6
chloride NEC	974.5	E858.5	E944.5	E950.4	E962.0	E980.4
chromate	983.9	E864.3	—	E950.7	E962.1	E980.6
citrate	963.3	E858.1	E933.3	E950.4	E962.0	E980.4
cyanide — see Cyanide(s)						
cyclamate	974.5	E858.5	E944.5	E950.4	E962.0	E980.4
diatrizoate	977.8	E858.8	E947.8	E950.4	E962.0	E980.4
dibunate	975.4	E858.6	E945.4	E950.4	E962.0	E980.4
dioctyl sulfosuccinate	973.2	E858.4	E943.2	E950.4	E962.0	E980.4
edetate	963.8	E858.1	E933.8	E950.4	E962.0	E980.4
ethacrynate	974.4	E858.5	E944.4	E950.4	E962.0	E980.4
fluoracetate (dust) (rodenticide)	989.4	E863.7	—	E950.6	E962.1	E980.7
fluoride — see Fluoride(s)						
free salt	974.5	E858.5	E944.5	E950.4	E962.0	E980.4
glucosulfone	961.8	E857	E931.8	E950.4	E962.0	E980.4
hydroxide	983.2	E864.2	—	E950.7	E962.1	E980.6
hypochlorite (bleach) NEC	983.9	E864.3	—	E950.7	E962.1	E980.6
disinfectant	983.9	E861.4	—	E950.7	E962.1	E980.6
medicinal (anti-infective) (external)	976.0	E858.7	E946.0	E950.4	E962.0	E980.4
vapor	987.8	E869.8	—	E952.8	E962.2	E982.8
hyposulfite	976.0	E858.7	E946.0	E950.4	E962.0	E980.4
indigotindisulfonate	977.8	E858.8	E947.8	E950.4	E962.0	E980.4
iodide	977.8	E858.8	E947.8	E950.4	E962.0	E980.4
iothalamate	977.8	E858.8	E947.8	E950.4	E962.0	E980.4
iron edetate	964.0	E858.2	E934.0	E950.4	E962.0	E980.4
lactate	963.3	E858.1	E933.3	E950.4	E962.0	E980.4
lauryl sulfate	976.2	E858.7	E946.2	E950.4	E962.0	E980.4
L–triiodothyronine	962.7	E858.0	E932.7	E950.4	E962.0	E980.4
metrizoate	977.8	E858.8	E947.8	E950.4	E962.0	E980.4
monofluoracetate (dust) (rodenticide)	989.4	E863.7	—	E950.6	E962.1	E980.7
morrhuate	972.7	E858.3	E942.7	E950.4	E962.0	E980.4
nafcillin	960.0	E856	E930.0	E950.4	E962.0	E980.4
nitrate (oxidizing agent)	983.9	E864.3	—	E950.7	E962.1	E980.6
nitrite (medicinal)	972.4	E858.3	E942.4	E950.4	E962.0	E980.4
nitroferricyanide	972.6	E858.3	E942.6	E950.4	E962.0	E980.4
nitroprusside	972.6	E858.3	E942.6	E950.4	E962.0	E980.4
para–aminohippurate	977.8	E858.8	E947.8	E950.4	E962.0	E980.4
perborate (non-medicinal) NEC	989.89	E866.8	—	E950.9	E962.1	E980.9
medicinal	976.6	E858.7	E946.6	E950.4	E962.0	E980.4
soap	989.6	E861.1	—	E950.9	E962.1	E980.9
percarbonate — *see* Sodium, perborate						
phosphate	973.3	E858.4	E943.3	E950.4	E962.0	E980.4
polystyrene sulfonate	974.5	E858.5	E944.5	E950.4	E962.0	E980.4
propionate	976.0	E858.7	E946.0	E950.4	E962.0	E980.4
psylliate	972.7	E858.3	E942.7	E950.4	E962.0	E980.4
removing resins	974.5	E858.5	E944.5	E950.4	E962.0	E980.4
salicylate	965.1	E850.3	E935.3	E950.0	E962.0	E980.0
sulfate	973.3	E858.4	E943.3	E950.4	E962.0	E980.4

TABLE OF DRUGS AND CHEMICALS

Substance	Poisoning	Accident	Therapeutic Use	Suicide Attempt	Assault	Undetermined
		\multicolumn{5}{c}{External Cause (E-Code)}				
sulfoxone	961.8	E857	E931.8	E950.4	E962.0	E980.4
tetradecyl sulfate	972.7	E858.3	E942.7	E950.4	E962.0	E980.4
thiopental	968.3	E855.1	E938.3	E950.4	E962.0	E980.4
thiosalicylate	965.1	E850.3	E935.3	E950.0	E962.0	E980.0
thiosulfate	976.0	E858.7	E946.0	E950.4	E962.0	E980.4
tolbutamide	977.8	E858.8	E947.8	E950.4	E962.0	E980.4
tyropanoate	977.8	E858.8	E947.8	E950.4	E962.0	E980.4
valproate	966.3	E855.0	E936.3	E950.4	E962.0	E980.4
Solanine	977.8	E858.8	E947.8	E950.4	E962.0	E980.4
Solanum dulcamara	988.2	E865.4	—	E950.9	E962.1	E980.9
Solapsone	961.8	E857	E931.8	E950.4	E962.0	E980.4
Solasulfone	961.8	E857	E931.8	E950.4	E962.0	E980.4
Soldering fluid	983.1	E864.1	—	E950.7	E962.1	E980.6
Solid substance	989.9	E866.9	—	E950.9	E962.1	E980.9
specified NEC	989.9	E866.8	—	E950.9	E962.1	E980.9
Solvents, industrial	982.8	E862.9	—	E950.9	E962.1	E980.9
naphtha	981	E862.0	—	E950.9	E962.1	E980.9
petroleum	981	E862.0	—	E950.9	E962.1	E980.9
specified NEC	982.8	E862.4	—	E950.9	E962.1	E980.9
Soma	968.0	E855.1	E938.0	E950.4	E962.0	E980.4
Somatotropin	962.4	E858.0	E932.4	E950.4	E962.0	E980.4
Sominex	963.0	E858.1	E933.0	E950.4	E962.0	E980.4
Somnos	967.1	E852.0	E937.1	E950.2	E962.0	E980.2
Somonal	967.0	E851	E937.0	E950.1	E962.0	E980.1
Soneryl	967.0	E851	E937.0	E950.1	E962.0	E980.1
Soothing syrup	977.9	E858.9	E947.9	E950.5	E962.0	E980.5
Sopor	967.4	E852.2	E937.4	E950.2	E962.0	E980.2
Soporific drug	967.9	E852.9	E937.9	E950.2	E962.0	E980.2
specified type NEC	967.8	E852.8	E937.8	E950.2	E962.0	E980.2
Sorbitol NEC	977.4	E858.8	E947.4	E950.4	E962.0	E980.4
Sotradecol	972.7	E858.3	E942.7	E950.4	E962.0	E980.4
Spacoline	975.1	E858.6	E945.1	E950.4	E962.0	E980.4
Spanish fly	976.8	E858.7	E946.8	E950.4	E962.0	E980.4
Sparine	969.1	E853.0	E939.1	E950.3	E962.0	E980.3
Sparteine	975.0	E858.6	E945.0	E950.4	E962.0	E980.4
Spasmolytics	975.1	E858.6	E945.1	E950.4	E962.0	E980.4
anticholinergics	971.1	E855.4	E941.1	E950.4	E962.0	E980.4
Spectinomycin	960.8	E856	E930.8	E950.4	E962.0	E980.4
Speed	969.7	E854.2	E939.7	E950.3	E962.0	E980.3
Spermicides	976.8	E858.7	E946.8	E950.4	E962.0	E980.4
Spider (bite) (venom)	989.5	E905.1	—	E950.9	E962.1	E980.9
antivenin	979.9	E858.8	E949.9	E950.4	E962.0	E980.4
Spigelia (root)	961.6	E857	E931.6	E950.4	E962.0	E980.4
Spiperone	969.2	E853.1	E939.2	E950.3	E962.0	E980.3
Spiramycin	960.3	E856	E930.3	E950.4	E962.0	E980.4
Spirilene	969.5	E853.8	E939.5	E950.3	E962.0	E980.3
Spirit(s) (neutral) NEC	980.0	E860.1	—	E950.9	E962.1	E980.9
beverage	980.0	E860.0	—	E950.9	E962.1	E980.9
industrial	980.9	E860.9	—	E950.9	E962.1	E980.9
mineral	981	E862.0	—	E950.9	E962.1	E980.9
of salt — see Hydrochloric acid						
surgical	980.9	E860.9	—	E950.9	E962.1	E980.9
Spironolactone	974.5	E858.5	E944.4	E950.4	E962.0	E980.4
Sponge, absorbable (gelatin)	964.5	E858.2	E934.5	E950.4	E962.0	E980.4
Sporostacin	976.0	E858.7	E946.0	E950.4	E962.0	E980.4
Sprays (aerosol)	989.89	E866.8	—	E950.9	E962.1	E980.9
cosmetic	989.89	E866.7	—	E950.9	E962.1	E980.9
medicinal NEC	977.9	E858.9	E947.9	E950.5	E962.0	E980.5
pesticides — see Pesticides						
specified content — see substance						

TABLE OF DRUGS AND CHEMICALS

Substance	Poisoning	Accident	Therapeutic Use	Suicide Attempt	Assault	Undetermined
		\multicolumn{5}{c|}{External Cause (E-Code)}				

Substance	Poisoning	Accident	Therapeutic Use	Suicide Attempt	Assault	Undetermined
specified Spurge flax	988.2	E865.4	—	E950.9	E962.1	E980.9
Spurges	988.2	E865.4	—	E950.9	E962.1	E980.9
Squill (expectorant) NEC	975.5	E858.6	E945.5	E950.4	E962.0	E980.4
rat poison	989.4	E863.7	—	E950.6	E962.1	E980.7
Squirting cucumber (cathartic)	973.1	E858.4	E943.1	E950.4	E962.0	E980.4
Stains	989.89	E866.8	—	E950.9	E962.1	E980.9
Stannous — see also Tin						
fluoride	976.7	E858.7	E946.7	E950.4	E962.0	E980.4
Stanolone	962.1	E858.0	E932.0	E950.4	E962.0	E980.4
Stanozolol	962.1	E853.0	E932.1	E950.4	E962.0	E980.4
Staphisagria or stavesacre (pediculicide)	976.0	E858.7	E946.0	E950.4	E962.0	E980.4
Stelazine	969.1	E853.0	E939.1	E950.3	E962.0	E980.3
Stemetil	969.1	E853.0	E939.1	E950.3	E962.0	E980.3
Sterculia (cathartic) (gum)	973.3	E858.4	E943.3	E950.4	E962.0	E980.4
Sternutator gas	987.8	E869.8	—	E952.8	E962.2	E982.8
Steroids NEC	962.0	E858.0	E932.0	E950.4	E962.0	E980.4
ENT agent	976.6	E858.7	E946.6	E950.4	E962.0	E980.4
ophthalmic preparation	976.5	E858.7	E946.5	E950.4	E962.0	E980.4
topical NEC	976.0	E858.7	E946.0	E950.4	E962.0	E980.4
Stibine	985.8	E866.4	—	E950.9	E962.1	E980.9
Stibophen	961.2	E857	E931.2	E950.4	E962.0	E980.4
Stilbamide, stilbamidine	961.5	E857	E931.5	E950.4	E962.0	E980.4
Stilbestrol	962.2	E858.0	E932.2	E950.4	E962.0	E980.4
Stimulants (central nervous system)	970.9	E854.3	E940.9	E950.4	E962.0	E980.4
analeptics	970.0	E854.3	E940.0	E950.4	E962.0	E980.4
opiate antagonist	970.1	E854.3	E940.1	E950.4	E962.0	E980.4
psychotherapeutic NEC	969.0	E854.0	E939.0	E950.3	E962.0	E980.3
specified NEC	970.8	E854.3	E940.8	E950.4	E962.0	E980.4
Storage batteries (acid) (cells)	983.1	E864.1	—	E950.7	E962.1	E980.6
Stovaine	968.9	E855.2	E938.9	E950.4	E962.0	E980.4
infiltration (subcutaneous)	968.5	E855.2	E938.5	E950.4	E962.0	E980.4
nerve block (peripheral) (plexus)	968.6	E855.2	E938.6	E950.5	E962.0	E980.4
spinal	968.7	E855.2	E938.7	E950.4	E962.0	E980.4
topical (surface)	968.5	E855.2	E938.5	E950.4	E962.0	E980.4
Stovarsal	961.1	E857	E931.1	E950.4	E962.0	E980.4
Stove gas — see Gas, utility						
Stoxil	976.5	E858.7	E946.5	E950.4	E962.0	E980.4
STP	969.6	E854.1	E939.6	E950.3	E962.0	E980.3
Stramonium (medicinal) NEC	971.1	E855.4	E941.1	E950.4	E962.0	E980.4
natural state	988.2	E865.4	—	E950.9	E962.1	E980.9
Streptodornase	964.4	E858.2	E934.4	E950.4	E962.0	E980.4
Streptoduocin	960.6	E856	E930.6	E950.4	E962.0	E980.4
Streptokinase	964.4	E858.2	E934.4	E950.4	E962.0	E980.4
Streptomycin	960.6	E856	E930.6	E950.4	E962.0	E980.4
Streptozocin	960.7	E856	E930.7	E950.4	E962.0	E980.4
Stripper (paint) (solvent)	982.8	E862.9	—	E950.9	E962.1	E980.9
Strobane	989.2	E863.0	—	E950.6	E962.1	E980.7
Strophanthin	972.1	E858.3	E942.1	E950.4	E962.0	E980.4
Strophanthus hispidus or kombe	988.2	E865.4	—	E950.9	E962.1	E980.9
Strychnine (rodenticide) (salts)	989.1	E863.7	—	E950.6	E962.1	E980.7
medicinal NEC	970.8	E854.3	E940.8	E950.4	E962.0	E980.4
Strychnos (ignatii) — see Strychnine						
Styramate	968.0	E855.1	E938.0	E950.4	E962.0	E980.4
Styrene	983.0	E864.0	—	E950.7	E962.1	E980.6
Succinimide (anticonvulsant)	966.2	E855.0	E936.2	E950.4	E962.0	E980.4
mercuric — see Mercury						
Succinylcholine	975.2	E858.6	E945.2	E950.4	E962.0	E980.4
Succinylsulfathiazole	961.0	E857	E931.0	E950.4	E962.0	E980.4
Sucrose	974.5	E858.5	E944.5	E950.4	E962.0	E980.4
Sulfacetamide	961.0	E857	E931.0	E950.4	E962.0	E980.4

TABLE OF DRUGS AND CHEMICALS

Substance	Poisoning	Accident	Therapeutic Use	Suicide Attempt	Assault	Undetermined
			External Cause (E-Code)			
ophthalmic preparation	976.5	E858.7	E946.5	E950.4	E962.0	E980.4
Sulfachlorpyridazine	961.0	E857	E931.0	E950.4	E962.0	E980.4
Sulfacytine	961.0	E857	E931.0	E950.4	E962.0	E980.4
Sulfadiazine	961.0	E857	E931.0	E950.4	E962.0	E980.4
silver (topical)	976.0	E858.7	E946.0	E950.4	E962.0	E980.4
Sulfadimethoxine	961.0	E857	E931.0	E950.4	E962.0	E980.4
Sulfadimidine	961.0	E857	E931.0	E950.4	E962.0	E980.4
Sulfaethidole	961.0	E857	E931.0	E950.4	E962.0	E980.4
Sulfafurazole	961.0	E857	E931.0	E950.4	E962.0	E980.4
Sulfaguanidine	961.0	E857	E931.0	E950.4	E962.0	E980.4
Sulfamerazine	961.0	E857	E931.0	E950.4	E962.0	E980.4
Sulfameter	961.0	E857	E931.0	E950.4	E962.0	E980.4
Sulfamethizole	961.0	E857	E931.0	E950.4	E962.0	E980.4
Sulfamethoxazole	961.0	E857	E931.0	E950.4	E962.0	E980.4
Sulfamethoxydiazine	961.0	E857	E931.0	E950.4	E962.0	E980.4
Sulfamethoxypyridazine	961.0	E857	E931.0	E950.4	E962.0	E980.4
Sulfamethylthiazole	961.0	E857	E931.0	E950.4	E962.0	E980.4
Sulfamylon	976.0	E858.7	E946.0	E950.4	E962.0	E980.4
Sulfan blue (diagnostic dye)	977.8	E858.8	E947.8	E950.4	E962.0	E980.4
Sulfanilamide	961.0	E857	E931.0	E950.4	E962.0	E980.4
Sulfanilylguanidine	961.0	E857	E931.0	E950.4	E962.0	E980.4
Sulfaphenazole	961.0	E857	E931.0	E950.4	E962.0	E980.4
Sulfaphenylthiazole	961.0	E857	E931.0	E950.4	E962.0	E980.4
Sulfaproxyline	961.0	E857	E931.0	E950.4	E962.0	E980.4
Sulfapyridine	961.0	E857	E931.0	E950.4	E962.0	E980.4
Sulfapyrimidine	961.0	E857	E931.0	E950.4	E962.0	E980.4
Sulfarsphenamine	961.1	E857	E931.1	E950.4	E962.0	E980.4
Sulfasalazine	961.0	E857	E931.0	E950.4	E962.0	E980.4
Sulfasomizole	961.0	E857	E931.0	E950.4	E962.0	E980.4
Sulfasuxidine	961.0	E857	E931.0	E950.4	E962.0	E980.4
Sulfinpyrazone	974.7	E858.5	E944.7	E950.4	E962.0	E980.4
Sulfisoxazole	961.0	E857	E931.0	E950.4	E962.0	E980.4
ophthalmic preparation	976.5	E858.7	E946.5	E950.4	E962.0	E980.4
Sulfomyxin	960.8	E856	E930.8	E950.4	E962.0	E980.4
Sulfonal	967.8	E852.8	E937.8	E950.2	E962.0	E980.2
Sulfonamides (mixtures)	961.0	E857	E931.0	E950.4	E962.0	E980.4
Sulfones	961.8	E857	E931.8	E950.4	E962.0	E980.4
Sulfonethylmethane	967.8	E852.8	E937.8	E950.2	E962.0	E980.2
Sulfonmethane	967.8	E852.8	E937.8	E950.2	E962.0	E980.2
Sulfonphthal, sulfonphthol	977.8	E858.8	E947.8	E950.4	E962.0	E980.4
Sulfonylurea derivatives, oral	962.3	E858.0	E932.3	E950.4	E962.0	E980.4
Sulfoxone	961.8	E857	E931.8	E950.4	E962.0	E980.4
Sulfur, sulfureted, sulfuric, sulfurous, sulfuryl (compounds) NEC	989.89	E866.8	—	E950.9	E962.1	E980.9
acid	983.1	E864.1	—	E950.7	E962.1	E980.6
dioxide	987.3	E869.1	—	E952.8	E962.2	E982.8
ether — see Ether(s)						
hydrogen	987.8	E869.8	—	E952.8	E962.2	E982.8
medicinal (keratolytic) (ointment) NEC	976.4	E858.7	E946.4	E950.4	E962.0	E980.4
pesticide (vapor)	989.4	E863.4	—	E950.6	E962.1	E980.7
vapor NEC	987.8	E869.8	—	E952.8	E962.2	E982.8
Sulkowitch's reagent	977.8	E858.8	E947.8	E950.4	E962.0	E980.4
Sulph — see also Sulf–						
Sulphadione	961.8	E857	E931.8	E950.4	E962.0	E980.4
Sulthiame, sultiame	966.3	E855.0	E936.3	E950.4	E962.0	E980.4
Superinone	975.5	E858.6	E945.5	E950.4	E962.0	E980.4
Suramin	961.5	E857	E931.5	E950.4	E962.0	E980.4
Surfacaine	968.5	E855.2	E938.5	E950.4	E962.0	E980.4
Surital	968.3	E855.1	E938.3	E950.4	E962.0	E980.4
Sutilains	976.8	E858.7	E946.8	E950.4	E962.0	E980.4

TABLE OF DRUGS AND CHEMICALS

Substance	Poisoning	Accident	Therapeutic Use	Suicide Attempt	Assault	Undetermined
			External Cause (E-Code)			
Suxamethoniam (bromide) (chloride) (iodide)	975.2	E858.6	E945.2	E950.4	E962.0	E980.4
Suxethonium (bromide)	975.2	E858.6	E945.2	E950.4	E962.0	E980.4
Sweet oil (birch)	976.3	E858.7	E946.3	E950.4	E962.0	E980.4
Sym–dichloroethyl ether	982.3	E862.4	—	E950.9	E962.1	E980.9
Sympatholytics	971.3	E855.6	E941.3	E950.4	E962.0	E980.4
Sympathomimetics	971.2	E855.5	E941.2	E950.4	E962.0	E980.4
Synagis	979.6	E858.8	E949.6	E950.4	E962.0	E980.4
Synalar	976.0	E858.7	E946.0	E950.4	E962.0	E980.4
Synthroid	962.7	E858.0	E932.7	E950.4	E962.0	E980.4
Syntocinon	975.0	E858.6	E945.0	E950.4	E962.0	E950.4
Syrosingopine	972.6	E858.3	E942.6	E950.4	E962.0	E980.4
Systemic agents (primarily)	963.9	E858.1	E933.9	E950.4	E962.0	E980.4
specified NEC	963.8	E858.1	E933.8	E950.4	E962.0	E980.4
Tablets (see also specified substance)	977.9	E858.9	E947.9	E950.5	E962.0	E980.5
Tace	962.2	E858.0	E932.2	E950.4	E962.0	E980.4
Tacrine	971.0	E855.3	E941.0	E950.4	E962.0	E980.4
Talbutal	967.0	E851	E937.0	E950.1	E962.0	E980.1
Talc	976.3	E858.7	E946.3	E950.4	E962.0	E980.4
Talcum	976.3	E858.7	E946.3	E950.4	E962.0	E980.4
Tamsulosin	971.3	E855.6	E941.3	E950.4	E962.0	E980.4
Tandearil, tanderil	965.5	E850.5	E935.5	E950.0	E962.0	E980.0
Tannic acid	983.1	E864.1	—	E950.7	E962.1	E980.6
medicinal (astringent)	976.2	E858.7	E946.2	E950.4	E962.0	E980.4
Tannin — see Tannic acid						
Tansy	988.2	E865.4	—	E950.9	E962.1	E980.9
TAO	960.3	E856	E930.3	E950.4	E962.0	E980.4
Tapazole	962.8	E858.0	E932.8	E950.4	E962.0	E980.4
Tar NEC	983.0	E864.0	—	E950.7	E962.1	E980.6
camphor — see Naphthalene						
fumes	987.8	E869.8	—	E952.8	E962.2	E982.8
Taractan	969.3	E853.8	E939.3	E950.3	E962.0	E980.3
Tarantula (venomous)	989.5	E905.1	—	E950.9	E962.1	E980.9
Tartar emetic (anti–infective)	961.2	E857	E931.2	E950.4	E962.0	E980.4
Tartaric acid	983.1	E864.1	—	E950.7	E962.1	E980.6
Tartrated antimony (anti–infective)	961.2	E857	E931.2	E950.4	E962.0	E980.4
TCA — see Trichloroacetic acid						
TDI	983.0	E864.0	—	E950.7	E962.1	E980.6
vapor	987.8	E869.8	—	E952.8	E962.2	E982.8
Tear gas	987.5	E869.3	—	E952.8	E962.2	E982.8
Teclothiazide	974.3	E858.5	E944.3	E950.4	E962.0	E980.4
Tegretol	966.3	E855.0	E936.3	E950.4	E962.0	E980.4
Telepaque	977.8	E858.8	E947.8	E950.4	E962.0	E980.4
Tellurium	985.8	E866.4	—	E950.9	E962.1	E980.9
fumes	985.8	E866.4	—	E950.9	E962.1	E980.9
TEM	963.1	E858.1	E933.1	E950.4	E962.0	E980.4
Temazepan—see Benzodiazepines						
TEPA	963.1	E858.1	E933.1	E950.4	E962.0	E980.4
TEPP	989.3	E863.1	—	E950.6	E962.1	E980.7
Terbutaline	971.2	E855.5	E941.2	E950.4	E962.0	E980.4
Teroxalene	961.6	E857	E931.6	E950.4	E962.0	E980.4
Terpin hydrate	975.5	E858.6	E945.5	E950.4	E962.0	E980.4
Terramycin	960.4	E856	E930.4	E950.4	E962.0	E980.4
Tessalon	975.4	E858.6	E945.4	E950.4	E962.0	E980.4
Testosterone	962.1	E858.0	E932.1	E950.4	E962.0	E980.4
Tetanus (vaccine)	978.4	E858.8	E948.4	E950.4	E962.0	E980.4
antitoxin	979.9	E858.8	E949.9	E950.4	E962.0	E980.4
immune globulin (human)	964.6	E858.2	E934.6	E950.4	E962.0	E980.4
toxoid	978.4	E858.8	E948.4	E950.4	E962.0	E980.4
with diphtheria toxoid	978.9	E858.8	E948.9	E950.4	E962.0	E980.4
with pertussis	978.6	E858.8	E948.6	E950.4	E962.0	E980.4

TABLE OF DRUGS AND CHEMICALS

Substance	Poisoning	Accident	Therapeutic Use	Suicide Attempt	Assault	Undetermined
		\multicolumn{5}{c}{External Cause (E-Code)}				

Substance	Poisoning	Accident	Therapeutic Use	Suicide Attempt	Assault	Undetermined
Tetrabenazine	969.5	E853.8	E939.5	E950.3	E962.0	E980.3
Tetracaine (infiltration) (topical)	968.5	E855.2	E938.5	E950.4	E962.0	E980.4
nerve block (peripheral) (plexus)	968.6	E855.2	E938.6	E950.4	E962.0	E980.4
spinal	968.7	E855.2	E938.7	E950.4	E962.0	E980.4
Tetrachlorethylene—see Tetrachloroethylene						
Tetrachlormethiazide	974.3	E858.5	E944.3	E950.4	E962.0	E980.4
Tetrachloroethane (liquid) (vapor)	982.3	E862.4	—	E950.9	E962.1	E980.9
paint or varnish	982.3	E861.6	—	E950.9	E962.1	E980.9
Tetrachloroethylene (liquid) (vapor)	982.3	E862.4	—	E950.9	E962.1	E980.9
medicinal	961.6	E857	E931.6	E950.4	E962.0	E980.4
Tetrachloromethane — see Carbon, tetrachloride						
Tetracycline	960.4	E856	E930.4	E950.4	E962.0	E980.4
ophthalmic preparation	976.5	E858.7	E946.5	E950.4	E962.0	E980.4
topical NEC	976.0	E858.7	E946.0	E950.4	E962.0	E980.4
Tetraethylammonium chloride	972.3	E858.3	E942.3	E950.4	E962.0	E980.4
Tetraethyl lead (antiknock compound)	984.1	E862.1	—	E950.9	E962.1	E980.9
Tetraethyl pyrophosphate	989.3	E863.1	—	E950.6	E962.1	E980.7
Tetraethylthiuram disulfide	977.3	E858.8	E947.3	E950.4	E962.0	E980.4
Tetrahydroaminoacridine	971.0	E855.3	E941.0	E950.4	E962.0	E980.4
Tetrahydrocannabinol	969.6	E854.1	E939.6	E950.3	E962.0	E980.3
Tetrahydronaphthalene	982.0	E862.4	—	E950.9	E962.1	E980.9
Tetrahydrozoline	971.2	E855.5	E941.2	E950.4	E962.0	E980.4
Tetralin	982.0	E862.4	—	E950.9	E962.1	E980.9
Tetramethylthiuram (disulfide) NEC	989.4	E863.6	—	E950.6	E962.1	E980.7
medicinal	976.2	E858.7	E946.2	E950.4	E962.0	E980.4
Tetronal	967.8	E852.8	E937.8	E950.2	E962.0	E980.2
Tetryl	983.0	E864.0	—	E950.7	E962.1	E980.6
Thalidomide	967.8	E852.8	E937.8	E950.2	E962.0	E980.2
Thallium (compounds) (dust) NEC	985.8	E866.4	—	E950.9	E962.1	E980.9
pesticide (rodenticide)	985.8	E863.7	—	E950.6	E962.1	E980.7
THC	969.6	E854.1	E939.6	E950.3	E962.0	E980.3
Thebacon	965.09	E850.2	E935.2	E950.0	E962.0	E980.0
Thebaine	965.09	E850.2	E935.2	E950.0	E962.0	E980.0
Theobromine (calcium salicylate)	974.1	E858.5	E944.1	E950.4	E962.0	E980.4
Theophylline (diuretic)	974.1	E858.5	E944.1	E950.4	E962.0	E980.4
ethylenediamine	975.7	E858.6	E945.7	E950.4	E962.0	E980.4
Thiabendazole	961.6	E857	E931.6	E950.4	E962.0	E980.4
Thialbarbital, thialbarbitone	968.3	E855.1	E938.3	E950.4	E962.0	E980.4
Thiamine	963.5	E858.1	E933.5	E950.4	E962.0	E980.4
Thiamylal (sodium)	968.3	E855.1	E938.3	E950.4	E962.0	E980.4
Thiazesim	969.0	E854.0	E939.0	E950.3	E962.0	E980.3
Thiazides (diuretics)	974.3	E858.5	E944.3	E950.4	E962.0	E980.4
Thiethylperazine	963.0	E858.1	E933.0	E950.4	E962.0	E980.4
Thimerosal (topical)	976.0	E858.7	E946.0	E950.4	E962.0	E980.4
ophthalmic preparation	976.5	E858.7	E946.5	E950.4	E962.0	E980.4
Thioacetazone	961.8	E857	E931.8	E950.4	E962.0	E980.4
Thiobarbiturates	968.3	E855.1	E938.3	E950.4	E962.0	E980.4
Thiobismol	961.2	E857	E931.2	E950.4	E962.0	E980.4
Thiocarbamide	962.8	E858.0	E932.8	E950.4	E962.0	E980.4
Thiocarbarsone	961.1	E857	E931.1	E950.4	E962.0	E980.4
Thiocarlide	961.8	E857	E931.8	E950.4	E962.0	E980.4
Thioguanine	963.1	E858.1	E933.1	E950.4	E962.0	E980.4
Thiomercaptomerin	974.0	E858.5	E944.0	E950.4	E962.0	E980.4
Thiomerin	974.0	E858.5	E944.0	E950.4	E962.0	E980.4
Thiopental, thiopentone (sodium)	968.3	E855.1	E938.3	E950.4	E962.0	E980.4
Thiopropazate	969.1	E853.0	E939.1	E950.3	E962.0	E980.3
Thioproperazine	969.1	E853.0	E939.1	E950.3	E962.0	E980.3
Thioridazine	969.1	E853.0	E939.1	E950.3	E962.0	E980.3
Thio–TEPA, thiotepa	963.1	E858.1	E933.1	E950.4	E962.0	E980.4

TABLE OF DRUGS AND CHEMICALS

Substance	Poisoning	Accident	Therapeutic Use	Suicide Attempt	Assault	Undetermined
			External Cause (E-Code)			
Thiothixene	969.3	E853.8	E939.3	E950.3	E962.0	E980.3
Thiouracil	962.8	E858.0	E932.8	E950.4	E962.0	E980.4
Thiourea	962.8	E858.0	E932.8	E950.4	E962.0	E980.4
Thiphenamil	971.1	E855.4	E941.1	E950.4	E962.0	E980.4
Thiram NEC	989.4	E863.6	—	E950.6	E962.1	E980.7
medicinal	976.2	E858.7	E946.2	E950.4	E962.0	E980.4
Thonzylamine	963.0	E858.1	E933.0	E950.4	E962.0	E980.4
Thorazine	969.1	E853.0	E939.1	E950.3	E962.0	E980.3
Thornapple	988.2	E865.4	—	E950.9	E962.1	E980.9
Throat preparation (lozenges) NEC	976.6	E858.7	E946.6	E950.4	E962.0	E980.4
Thrombin	964.5	E858.2	E934.5	E950.4	E962.0	E980.4
Thrombolysin	964.4	E858.2	E934.4	E950.4	E962.0	E980.4
Thymol	983.0	E864.0	—	E950.7	E962.1	E980.6
Thymus extract	962.9	E858.0	E932.9	E950.4	E962.0	E980.4
Thyroglobulin	962.7	E858.0	E932.7	E950.4	E962.0	E980.4
Thyroid (derivatives) (extract)	962.7	E858.0	E932.7	E950.4	E962.0	E980.4
Thyrolar	962.7	E858.0	E932.7	E950.4	E962.0	E980.4
Thyrothrophin, thyrotropin	977.8	E858.8	E947.8	E950.4	E962.0	E980.4
Thyroxin(e)	962.7	E858.0	E932.7	E950.4	E962.0	E980.4
Tigan	963.0	E858.1	E933.0	E950.4	E962.0	E980.4
Tigloidine	968.0	E855.1	E938.0	E950.4	E962.0	E980.4
Tin (chloride) (dust) (oxide) NEC	985.8	E866.4	—	E950.9	E962.1	E980.9
anti–infectives	961.2	E857	E931.2	E950.4	E962.0	E980.4
Tinactin	976.0	E858.7	E946.0	E950.4	E962.0	E980.4
Tincture, iodine — see Iodine						
Tindal	969.1	E853.0	E939.1	E950.3	E962.0	E980.3
Titanium (compounds) (vapor)	985.8	E866.4	—	E950.9	E962.1	E980.9
ointment	976.3	E858.7	E946.3	E950.4	E962.0	E980.4
Titroid	962.7	E858.0	E932.7	E950.4	E962.0	E980.4
TMTD — see Tetramethylthiuram disulfide						
TNT	989.89	E866.8	—	E950.9	E962.1	E980.9
fumes	987.8	E869.8	—	E952.8	E962.2	E982.8
Toadstool	988.1	E865.5	—	E950.9	E962.1	E980.9
Tobacco NEC	989.84	E866.8	—	E950.9	E962.1	E980.9
Indian	988.2	E865.4	—	E950.9	E962.1	E980.9
smoke, second-hand	987.8	E869.4	—	—	—	—
Tocopherol	963.5	E858.1	E933.5	E950.4	E962.0	E980.4
Tocosamine	975.0	E858.6	E945.0	E950.4	E962.0	E980.4
Tofranil	969.0	E854.0	E939.0	E950.3	E962.0	E980.3
Toilet deodorizer	989.8	E866.8	—	E950.9	E962.1	E980.9
Tolazamide	962.3	E858.0	E932.3	E950.4	E962.0	E980.4
Tolazoline	971.3	E855.6	E941.3	E950.4	E962.0	E980.4
Tolbutamide	962.3	E858.0	E932.3	E950.4	E962.0	E980.4
sodium	977.8	E858.8	E947.8	E950.4	E962.0	E980.4
Tolmetin	965.69	E850.6	E935.6	E950.0	E962.0	E980.0
Tolnaftate	976.0	E858.7	E946.0	E950.4	E962.0	E980.4
Tolpropamine	976.1	E858.7	E946.1	E950.4	E962.0	E980.4
Tolserol	968.0	E855.1	E938.0	E950.4	E962.0	E980.4
Toluene (liquid) (vapor)	982.0	E862.4	—	E950.9	E962.1	E980.9
diisocyanate	983.0	E864.0	—	E950.7	E962.1	E980.6
Toluidine	983.0	E864.0	—	E950.7	E962.1	E980.6
vapor	987.8	E869.8	—	E952.8	E962.2	E982.8
Toluol (liquid) (vapor)	982.0	E862.4	—	E950.9	E962.1	E980.9
Tolylene–2,4–diisocyanate	983.0	E864.0	—	E950.7	E962.1	E980.6
Tonics, cardiac	972.1	E858.3	E942.1	E950.4	E962.0	E980.4
Toxaphene (dust) (spray)	989.2	E863.0	—	E950.6	E962.1	E980.7
Toxoids NEC	978.8	E858.8	E948.8	E950.4	E962.0	E980.4
Tractor fuel NEC	981	E862.1	—	E950.9	E962.1	E980.9
Tragacanth	973.3	E858.4	E943.3	E950.4	E962.0	E980.4
Tramazoline	971.2	E855.5	E941.2	E950.4	E962.0	E980.4
Tranquilizers	969.5	E853.9	E939.5	E950.3	E962.0	E980.3

TABLE OF DRUGS AND CHEMICALS

Substance	Poisoning	Accident	Therapeutic Use	Suicide Attempt	Assault	Undetermined
			External Cause (E-Code)			
benzodiazepine–based	969.4	E853.2	E939.4	E950.3	E962.0	E980.3
butyrophenone–based	969.2	E853.1	E939.2	E950.3	E962.0	E980.3
major NEC	969.3	E853.8	E939.3	E950.3	E962.0	E980.3
phenothiazine–based	969.1	E853.0	E939.1	E950.3	E962.0	E980.3
specified NEC	969.5	E853.8	E939.5	E950.3	E962.0	E980.3
Trantoin	961.9	E857	E931.9	E950.4	E962.0	E980.4
Tranxene	969.4	E853.2	E939.4	E950.3	E962.0	E980.3
Tranylcypromine (sulfate)	969.0	E854.0	E939.0	E950.3	E962.0	E980.3
Trasentine	975.1	E858.6	E945.1	E950.4	E962.0	E980.4
Travert	974.5	E858.5	E944.5	E950.4	E962.0	E980.4
Trecator	961.8	E857	E931.8	E950.4	E962.0	E980.4
Tretinoin	976.8	E858.7	E946.8	E950.4	E962.0	E980.4
Triacetin	976.0	E858.7	E946.0	E950.4	E962.0	E980.4
Triacetyloleandomycin	960.3	E856	E930.3	E950.4	E962.0	E980.4
Triamcinolone	962.0	E858.0	E932.0	E950.4	E962.0	E980.4
ENT agent	976.6	E858.7	E946.6	E950.4	E962.0	E980.4
ophthalmic preparation	976.5	E858.7	E946.5	E950.4	E962.0	E980.4
topical NEC	976.0	E858.7	E946.0	E950.4	E962.0	E980.4
Triamterene	974.4	E858.5	E944.4	E950.4	E962.0	E980.4
Triaziquone	963.1	E858.1	E933.1	E950.4	E962.0	E980.4
Tribromacetaldehyde	967.3	E852.2	E937.3	E950.2	E962.0	E980.2
Tribromoethanol	968.2	E855.1	E938.2	E950.4	E962.0	E980.4
Tribromomethane	967.3	E852.2	E937.3	E950.2	E962.0	E980.2
Trichlorethane	982.3	E862.4	—	E950.9	E962.1	E980.9
Trichlormethiazide	974.3	E858.5	E944.3	E950.4	E962.0	E980.4
Trichloroacetic acid	983.1	E864.1	—	E950.7	E962.1	E980.6
medicinal (keratolytic)	976.4	E858.7	E946.4	E950.4	E962.0	E980.4
Trichloroethanol	967.1	E852.0	E937.1	E950.2	E962.0	E980.2
Trichloroethylene (liquid) (vapor)	982.3	E862.4	—	E950.9	E962.1	E980.9
anesthetic (gas)	968.2	E855.1	E938.2	E950.4	E962.0	E980.4
Trichloroethyl phosphate	967.1	E852.0	E937.1	E950.2	E962.0	E980.2
Trichlorofluoromethane NEC	987.4	E869.2	—	E952.8	E962.2	E982.8
Trichlorotriethylamine	963.1	E858.1	E933.1	E950.4	E962.0	E980.4
Trichomonacides NEC	961.5	E857	E931.5	E950.4	E962.0	E980.4
Trichomycin	960.1	E856	E930.1	E950.4	E962.0	E980.4
Triclofos	967.1	E852.0	E937.1	E950.2	E962.0	E980.2
Tricresyl phosphate	989.89	E866.8	—	E950.9	E962.1	E980.9
solvent	982.8	E862.4	—	E950.9	E962.1	E980.9
Tricyclamol	966.4	E855.0	E936.4	E950.4	E962.0	E980.4
Tridesilon	976.0	E858.7	E946.0	E950.4	E962.0	E980.4
Tridihexethyl	971.1	E855.4	E941.1	E950.4	E962.0	E980.4
Tridione	966.0	E855.0	E936.0	E950.4	E962.0	E980.4
Triethanolamine NEC	983.2	E864.2	—	E950.7	E962.1	E980.6
detergent	983.2	E861.0	—	E950.7	E962.1	E980.6
trinitrate	972.4	E858.3	E942.4	E950.4	E962.0	E980.4
Triethanomelamine	963.1	E858.1	E933.1	E950.4	E962.0	E980.4
Triethylene melamine	963.1	E858.1	E933.1	E950.4	E962.0	E980.4
Triethylenephosphoramide	963.1	E858.1	E933.1	E950.4	E962.0	E980.4
Triethylenethiophosphoramide	963.1	E858.1	E933.1	E950.4	E962.0	E980.4
Trifluoperazine	969.1	E853.0	E939.1	E950.3	E962.0	E980.3
Trifluperidol	969.2	E853.1	E939.2	E950.3	E962.0	E980.3
Triflupromazine	969.1	E853.0	E939.1	E950.3	E962.0	E980.3
Trihexyphenidyl	971.1	E855.4	E941.1	E950.4	E962.0	E980.4
Triiodothyronine	962.7	E858.0	E932.7	E950.4	E962.0	E980.4
Trilene	968.2	E855.1	E938.2	E950.4	E962.0	E980.4
Trimeprazine	963.0	E858.1	E933.0	E950.4	E962.0	E980.4
Trimetazidine	972.4	E858.3	E942.4	E950.4	E962.0	E980.4
Trimethadione	966.0	E855.0	E936.0	E950.4	E962.0	E980.4
Trimethaphan	972.3	E858.3	E942.3	E950.4	E962.0	E980.4
Trimethidinium	972.3	E858.3	E942.3	E950.4	E962.0	E980.4

TABLE OF DRUGS AND CHEMICALS

Substance	Poisoning	Accident	Therapeutic Use	Suicide Attempt	Assault	Undetermined
			External Cause (E-Code)			
Trimethobenzamide	963.0	E858.1	E933.0	E950.4	E962.0	E980.4
Trimethylcarbinol	980.8	E860.8	—	E950.9	E962.1	E980.9
Trimethylpsoralen	976.3	E858.7	E946.3	E950.4	E962.0	E980.4
Trimeton	963.0	E858.1	E933.0	E950.4	E962.0	E980.4
Trimipramine	969.0	E854.0	E939.0	E950.3	E962.0	E980.3
Trimustine	963.1	E858.1	E933.1	E950.4	E962.0	E980.4
Trinitrin	972.4	E858.3	E942.4	E950.4	E962.0	E980.4
Trinitrophenol	983.0	E864.0	—	E950.7	E962.1	E980.6
Trinitrotoluene	989.89	E866.8	—	E950.9	E962.1	E980.9
fumes	987.8	E869.8	—	E952.8	E962.2	E982.8
Trional	967.8	E852.8	E937.8	E950.2	E962.0	E980.2
Trioxide of arsenic — see Arsenic						
Trioxsalen	976.3	E858.7	E946.3	E950.4	E962.0	E980.4
Tripelennamine	963.0	E858.1	E933.0	E950.4	E962.0	E980.4
Triperidol	969.2	E853.1	E939.2	E950.3	E962.0	E980.3
Triprolidine	963.0	E858.1	E933.0	E950.4	E962.0	E980.4
Trisoralen	976.3	E858.7	E946.3	E950.4	E962.0	E980.4
Troleandomycin	960.3	E856	E930.3	E950.4	E962.0	E980.4
Trolnitrate (phosphate)	972.4	E858.3	E942.4	E950.4	E962.0	E980.4
Trometamol	963.3	E858.1	E933.3	E950.4	E962.0	E980.4
Tromethamine	963.3	E858.1	E933.3	E950.4	E962.0	E980.4
Tronothane	968.5	E855.2	E938.5	E950.4	E962.0	E980.4
Tropicamide	971.1	E855.4	E941.1	E950.4	E962.0	E980.4
Troxidone	966.0	E855.0	E936.0	E950.4	E962.0	E980.4
Tryparsamide	961.1	E857	E931.1	E950.4	E962.0	E980.4
Trypsin	963.4	E858.1	E933.4	E950.4	E962.0	E980.4
Tryptizol	969.0	E854.0	E939.0	E950.3	E962.0	E980.3
Tuaminoheptane	971.2	E855.5	E941.2	E950.4	E962.0	E980.4
Tuberculin (old)	977.8	E858.8	E947.8	E950.4	E962.0	E980.4
Tubocurare	975.2	E858.6	E945.2	E950.4	E962.0	E980.4
Tubocurarine	975.2	E858.6	E945.2	E950.4	E962.0	E980.4
Turkish green	969.6	E854.1	E939.6	E950.3	E962.0	E980.3
Turpentine (spirits of) (liquid) (vapor)	982.8	E862.4	—	E950.9	E962.1	E980.9
Tybamate	969.5	E853.8	E939.5	E950.3	E962.0	E980.3
Tyloxapol	975.5	E858.6	E945.5	E950.4	E962.0	E980.4
Tymazoline	971.2	E855.5	E941.2	E950.4	E962.0	E980.4
Typhoid vaccine	978.1	E858.8	E948.1	E950.4	E962.0	E980.4
Typhus vaccine	979.2	E858.8	E949.2	E950.4	E962.0	E980.4
Tyrothricin	976.0	E858.7	E946.0	E950.4	E962.0	E980.4
ENT agent	976.6	E858.7	E946.6	E950.4	E962.0	E980.4
ophthalmic preparation	976.5	E858.7	E946.5	E950.4	E962.0	E980.4
Undecenoic acid	976.0	E858.7	E946.0	E950.4	E962.0	E980.4
Undecylenic acid	976.0	E858.7	E946.0	E950.4	E962.0	E980.4
Unna's boot	976.3	E858.7	E946.3	E950.4	E962.0	E980.4
Uracil mustard	963.1	E858.1	E933.1	E950.4	E962.0	E980.4
Uramustine	963.1	E858.1	E933.1	E950.4	E962.0	E980.4
Urari	975.2	E858.6	E945.2	E950.4	E962.0	E980.4
Urea	974.4	E858.5	E944.4	E950.4	E962.0	E980.4
topical	976.8	E858.7	E946.8	E950.4	E962.0	E980.4
Urethan(e) (antineoplastic)	963.1	E858.1	E933.1	E950.4	E962.0	E980.4
Urginea (maritima) (scilla) — see Squill						
Uric acid metabolism agents NEC	974.7	E858.5	E944.7	E950.4	E962.0	E980.4
Urokinase	964.4	E858.2	E934.4	E950.4	E962.0	E980.4
Urokon	977.8	E858.8	E947.8	E950.4	E962.0	E980.4
Urotropin	961.9	E857	E931.9	E950.4	E962.0	E980.4
Urtica	988.2	E865.4	—	E950.9	E962.1	E980.9
Utility gas — see Gas, utility						
Vaccine NEC	979.9	E858.8	E949.9	E950.4	E962.0	E980.4
bacterial NEC	978.8	E858.8	E948.8	E950.4	E962.0	E980.4
with						
other bacterial component	978.9	E858.8	E948.9	E950.4	E962.0	E980.4

TABLE OF DRUGS AND CHEMICALS

Substance	Poisoning	Accident	Therapeutic Use	Suicide Attempt	Assault	Undetermined
		\multicolumn{5}{c|}{External Cause (E-Code)}				

Substance	Poisoning	Accident	Therapeutic Use	Suicide Attempt	Assault	Undetermined
pertussis component	978.6	E858.8	E948.6	E950.4	E962.0	E980.4
viral–rickettsial component	979.7	E858.8	E949.7	E950.4	E962.0	E980.4
mixed NEC	978.9	E858.8	E948.9	E950.4	E962.0	E980.4
BCG	978.0	E858.8	E948.0	E950.4	E962.0	E980.4
cholera	978.2	E858.8	E948.2	E950.4	E962.0	E980.4
diphtheria	978.5	E858.8	E948.5	E950.4	E962.0	E980.4
influenza	979.6	E858.8	E949.6	E950.4	E962.0	E980.4
measles	979.4	E858.8	E949.4	E950.4	E962.0	E980.4
meningococcal	978.8	E858.8	E948.8	E950.4	E962.0	E980.4
mumps	979.6	E858.8	E949.6	E950.4	E962.0	E980.4
paratyphoid	978.1	E858.8	E948.1	E950.4	E962.0	E980.4
pertussis (with diphtheria toxoid) (with tetanus toxoid)	978.6	E858.8	E948.6	E950.4	E962.0	E980.4
plague	978.3	E858.8	E948.3	E950.4	E962.0	E980.4
poliomyelitis	979.5	E858.8	E949.5	E950.4	E962.0	E980.4
poliovirus	979.5	E858.8	E949.5	E950.4	E962.0	E980.4
rabies	979.1	E858.8	E949.1	E950.4	E962.0	E980.4
respiratory syncytial virus	979.6	E858.8	E949.6	E950.4	E962.0	E980.4
rickettsial NEC	979.6	E858.8	E949.6	E950.4	E962.0	E980.4
with						
bacterial component	979.7	E858.8	E949.7	E950.4	E962.0	E980.4
pertussis component	978.6	E858.8	E948.6	E950.4	E962.0	E980.4
viral component	979.7	E858.8	E949.7	E950.4	E962.0	E980.4
Rocky Mountain spotted fever	979.6	E858.8	E949.6	E950.4	E962.0	E980.4
rotavirus	979.6	E858.8	E949.6	E950.4	E962.0	E980.4
rubella virus	979.4	E858.8	E949.4	E950.4	E962.0	E980.4
sabin oral	979.5	E858.8	E949.5	E950.4	E962.0	E980.4
smallpox	979.0	E858.8	E949.0	E950.4	E962.0	E980.4
tetanus	978.4	E858.8	E948.4	E950.4	E962.0	E980.4
typhoid	978.1	E858.8	E948.1	E950.4	E962.0	E980.4
typhus	979.2	E858.8	E949.2	E950.4	E962.0	E980.4
viral NEC	979.6	E858.8	E949.6	E950.4	E962.0	E980.4
with						
bacterial component	979.7	E858.8	E949.7	E950.4	E962.0	E980.4
pertussis component	978.6	E858.8	E948.6	E950.4	E962.0	E980.4
rickettsial component	979.7	E858.8	E949.7	E950.4	E962.0	E980.4
yellow fever	979.3	E858.8	E949.3	E950.4	E962.0	E980.4
Vaccinia immune globulin (human)	964.6	E858.2	E934.6	E950.4	E962.0	E980.4
Vaginal contraceptives	976.8	E858.7	E946.8	E950.4	E962.0	E980.4
Valethamate	971.1	E855.4	E941.1	E950.4	E962.0	E980.4
Valisone	976.0	E858.7	E946.0	E950.4	E962.0	E980.4
Valium	969.4	E853.2	E939.4	E950.3	E962.0	E980.3
Valmid	967.8	E852.8	E937.8	E950.2	E962.0	E980.2
Vanadium	985.8	E866.4	—	E950.9	E962.1	E980.9
Vancomycin	960.8	E856	E930.8	E950.4	E962.0	E980.4
Vapor (see also Gas)	987.9	E869.9	—	E952.9	E962.2	E982.9
kiln (carbon monoxide)	986	E868.8	—	E952.1	E962.2	E982.1
lead — see Lead						
specified source NEC (see also specific substance)	987.8	E869.8	—	E952.8	E962.2	E982.8
Varidase	964.4	E858.2	E934.4	E950.4	E962.0	E980.4
Varnish	989.89	E861.6	—	E950.9	E962.1	E980.9
cleaner	982.8	E862.9	—	E950.9	E962.1	E980.9
Vaseline	976.3	E858.7	E946.3	E950.4	E962.0	E980.4
Vasodilan	972.5	E858.3	E942.5	E950.4	E962.0	E980.4
Vasodilators NEC	972.5	E858.3	E942.5	E950.4	E962.0	E980.0
coronary	972.4	E858.3	E942.4	E950.4	E962.0	E980.4
Vasopressin	962.5	E858.0	E932.5	E950.4	E962.0	E980.4
Vasopressor drugs	962.5	E858.0	E932.5	E950.4	E962.0	E980.4
Venom, venomous (bite) (sting)	989.5	E905.9	—	E950.9	E962.1	E980.9

TABLE OF DRUGS AND CHEMICALS

Substance	Poisoning	Accident	Therapeutic Use	Suicide Attempt	Assault	Undetermined
			External Cause (E-Code)			
arthropod NEC	989.5	E905.5	—	E950.9	E962.1	E980.9
bee	989.5	E905.3	—	E950.9	E962.1	E980.9
centipede	989.5	E905.4	—	E950.9	E962.1	E980.9
hornet	989.5	E905.3	—	E950.9	E962.1	E980.9
lizard	989.5	E905.0	—	E950.9	E962.1	E980.9
marine animals or plants	989.5	E905.6	—	E950.9	E962.1	E980.9
millipede (topical)	989.5	E905.4	—	E950.9	E962.1	E980.9
plant NEC	989.5	E905.7	—	E950.9	E962.1	E980.9
marine	989.5	E905.6	—	E950.9	E962.1	E980.9
scorpion	989.5	E905.2	—	E950.9	E962.1	E980.9
snake	989.5	E905.0	—	E950.9	E962.1	E980.9
specified NEC	989.5	E905.8	—	E950.9	E962.1	E980.9
spider	989.5	E905.1	—	E950.9	E962.1	E980.9
wasp	989.5	E905.3	—	E950.9	E962.1	E980.9
Ventolin—see Salbutamol sulfate						
Veramon	967.0	E851	E937.0	E950.1	E962.0	E980.1
Veratrum						
album	988.2	E865.4	—	E950.9	E962.1	E980.9
alkaloids	972.6	E858.3	E942.6	E950.4	E962.0	E980.4
viride	988.2	E865.4	—	E950.9	E962.1	E980.9
Verdigris (see also Copper)	985.8	E866.4	—	E950.9	E962.1	E980.9
Veronal	967.0	E851	E937.0	E950.1	E962.0	E980.1
Veroxil	961.6	E857	E931.6	E950.4	E962.0	E980.4
Versidyne	965.7	E850.7	E935.7	E950.0	E962.0	E980.0
Viagra	972.5	E858.3	E942.5	E950.4	E962.0	E980.4
Vienna						
green	985.1	E866.3	—	E950.8	E962.1	E980.8
insecticide	985.1	E863.4	—	E950.6	E962.1	E980.7
red	989.89	E866.8	—	E950.9	E962.1	E980.9
pharmaceutical dye	977.4	E858.8	E947.4	E950.4	E962.0	E980.4
Vinbarbital, vinbarbitone	967.0	E851	E937.0	E950.1	E962.0	E980.1
Vinblastine	963.1	E858.1	E933.1	E950.4	E962.0	E980.4
Vincristine	963.1	E858.1	E933.1	E950.4	E962.0	E980.4
Vinesthene, vinethene	968.2	E855.1	E938.2	E950.4	E962.0	E980.4
Vinyl						
bital	967.0	E851	E937.0	E950.1	E962.0	E980.1
ether	968.2	E855.1	E938.2	E950.4	E962.0	E980.4
Vioform	961.3	E857	E931.3	E950.4	E962.0	E980.4
topical	976.0	E858.7	E946.0	E950.4	E962.0	E980.4
Viomycin	960.6	E856	E930.6	E950.4	E962.0	E980.4
Viosterol	963.5	E858.1	E933.5	E950.4	E962.0	E980.4
Viper (venom)	989.5	E905.0	—	E950.9	E962.1	E980.9
Viprynium (embonate)	961.6	E857	E931.6	E950.4	E962.0	E980.4
Virugon	961.7	E857	E931.7	E950.4	E962.0	E980.4
Visine	976.5	E858.7	E946.5	E950.4	E962.0	E980.4
Vitamins NEC	963.5	E858.1	E933.5	E950.4	E962.0	E980.4
B_{12}	964.1	E858.2	E934.1	E950.4	E962.0	E980.4
hematopoietic	964.1	E858.2	E934.1	E950.4	E962.0	E980.4
K	964.3	E858.2	E934.3	E950.4	E962.0	E980.4
Vleminckx's solution	976.4	E858.7	E946.4	E950.4	E962.0	E980.4
Voltaren—see Diclofenac sodium						
Warfarin (potassium) (sodium)	964.2	E858.2	E934.2	E950.4	E962.0	E980.4
rodenticide	989.4	E863.7	—	E950.6	E962.1	E980.7
Wasp (sting)	989.5	E905.3	—	E950.9	E962.1	E980.9
Water						
balance agents NEC	974.5	E858.5	E944.5	E950.4	E962.0	E980.4
gas	987.1	E868.1	—	E951.8	E962.2	E981.8
incomplete combustion of — see Carbon, monoxide, fuel, utility						
hemlock	988.2	E865.4	—	E950.9	E962.1	E980.9
moccasin (venom)	989.5	E905.0	—	E950.9	E962.1	E980.9

1493

TABLE OF DRUGS AND CHEMICALS

Substance	Poisoning	Accident	Therapeutic Use	Suicide Attempt	Assault	Undetermined
		\multicolumn{5}{c|}{External Cause (E-Code)}				

Substance	Poisoning	Accident	Therapeutic Use	Suicide Attempt	Assault	Undetermined
Wax (paraffin) (petroleum)	981	E862.3	—	E950.9	E962.1	E980.9
automobile	989.89	E861.2	—	E950.9	E962.1	E980.9
floor	981	E862.0	—	E950.9	E962.1	E980.9
Weed killers NEC	989.4	E863.5	—	E950.6	E962.1	E980.7
Welldorm	967.1	E852.0	E937.1	E950.2	E962.0	E980.2
White						
arsenic — see Arsenic						
hellebore	988.2	E865.4	—	E950.9	E962.1	E980.9
lotion (keratolytic)	976.4	E858.7	E946.4	E950.4	E962.0	E980.4
spirit	981	E862.0	—	E950.9	E962.1	E980.9
Whitewashes	989.89	E861.6	—	E950.9	E962.1	E980.9
Whole blood	964.7	E858.2	E934.7	E950.4	E962.0	E980.4
Wild						
black cherry	988.2	E865.4	—	E950.9	E962.1	E980.9
poisonous plants NEC	988.2	E865.4	—	E950.9	E962.1	E980.9
Window cleaning fluid	989.89	E861.3	—	E950.9	E962.1	E980.9
Wintergreen (oil)	976.3	E858.7	E946.3	E950.4	E962.0	E980.4
Witch hazel	976.2	E858.7	E946.2	E950.4	E962.0	E980.4
Wood						
alcohol	980.1	E860.2	—	E950.9	E962.1	E980.9
spirit	980.1	E860.2	—	E950.9	E962.1	E980.9
Woorali	975.2	E858.6	E945.2	E950.4	E962.0	E980.4
Wormseed, American	961.6	E857	E931.6	E950.4	E962.0	E980.4
Xanthine diuretics	974.1	E858.5	E944.1	E950.4	E962.0	E980.4
Xanthocillin	960.0	E856	E930.0	E950.4	E962.0	E980.4
Xanthotoxin	976.3	E858.7	E946.3	E950.4	E962.0	E980.4
Xigris	964.2	E858.2	E934.2	E950.4	E962.0	E980.4
Xylene (liquid) (vapor)	982.0	E862.4	—	E950.9	E962.1	E980.9
Xylocaine (infiltration) (topical)	968.5	E855.2	E938.5	E950.4	E962.0	E980.4
nerve block (peripheral) (plexus)	968.6	E855.2	E938.6	E950.4	E962.0	E980.4
spinal	968.7	E855.2	E938.7	E950.4	E962.0	E980.4
Xylol (liquid) (vapor)	982.0	E862.4	—	E950.9	E962.1	E980.9
Xylometazoline	971.2	E855.5	E941.2	E950.4	E962.0	E980.4
Yellow						
fever vaccine	979.3	E858.8	E949.3	E950.4	E962.0	E980.4
jasmine	988.2	E865.4	—	E950.9	E962.1	E980.9
Yew	988.2	E865.4	—	E950.9	E962.1	E980.9
Zactane	965.7	E850.7	E935.7	E950.0	E962.0	E980.0
Zaroxolyn	974.3	E858.5	E944.3	E950.4	E962.0	E980.4
Zephiran (topical)	976.0	E858.7	E946.0	E950.4	E962.0	E980.4
ophthalmic preparation	976.5	E858.7	E946.5	E950.4	E962.0	E980.4
Zerone	980.1	E860.2	—	E950.9	E962.1	E980.9
Zinc (compounds) (fumes) (salts) (vapor) NEC	985.8	E866.4	—	E950.9	E962.1	E980.9
anti–infectives	976.0	E858.7	E946.0	E950.4	E962.0	E980.4
antivaricose	972.7	E858.3	E942.7	E950.4	E962.0	E980.4
bacitracin	976.0	E858.7	E946.0	E950.4	E962.0	E980.4
chloride	976.2	E858.7	E946.2	E950.4	E962.0	E980.4
gelatin	976.3	E858.7	E946.3	E950.4	E962.0	E980.4
oxide	976.3	E858.7	E946.3	E950.4	E962.0	E980.4
peroxide	976.0	E858.7	E946.0	E950.4	E962.0	E980.4
pesticides	985.8	E863.4	—	E950.6	E962.1	E980.7
phosphide (rodenticide)	985.8	E863.7	—	E950.6	E962.1	E980.7
stearate	976.3	E858.7	E946.3	E950.4	E962.0	E980.4
sulfate (antivaricose)	972.7	E858.3	E942.7	E950.4	E962.0	E980.4
ENT agent	976.6	E858.7	E946.6	E950.4	E962.0	E980.4
ophthalmic solution	976.5	E858.7	E946.5	E950.4	E962.0	E980.4
topical NEC	976.0	E858.7	E946.0	E950.4	E962.0	E980.4
undecylenate	976.0	E858.7	E946.0	E950.4	E962.0	E980.4
Zovant	964.2	E858.2	E934.2	E950.4	E962.0	E980.4

TABLE OF DRUGS AND CHEMICALS

Substance	Poisoning	Accident	Therapeutic Use	Suicide Attempt	Assault	Undetermined
		\multicolumn{5}{c}{External Cause (E-Code)}

Substance	Poisoning	Accident	Therapeutic Use	Suicide Attempt	Assault	Undetermined
Zoxazolamine	968.0	E855.1	E938.0	E950.4	E962.0	E980.4
Zygadenus (venenosus)	988.2	E865.4	—	E950.9	E962.1	E980.9

TABLE OF DRUGS AND CHEMICALS

Substance	Poisoning	Accident	Therapeutic Use	Suicide Attempt	Assault	Undetermined
		\multicolumn{5}{c	}{External Cause (E-Code)}

SECTION 3

ALPHABETIC INDEX TO EXTERNAL CAUSES OF INJURY AND POISONING (E CODE)

This section contains the index to the codes which classify environmental events, circumstances, and other conditions as the cause of injury and other adverse effects. Where a code from the section Supplementary Classification of External Causes of Injury and Poisoning (E800-E998) is applicable, it is intended that the E code shall be used in addition to a code from the main body of the classification, Chapters 1-17.

The alphabetic index to the E codes is organized by main terms which describe the *accident, circumstance, event,* or specific *agent* which caused the injury or other adverse effect.

>   *Note—Transport accidents (E800-E848) include accidents involving:*
>   *aircraft and space craft (E840-E845)*
>   *watercraft (E830-E838)*
>   *motor vehicle (E810-E825)*
>   *railway (E800-E807)*
>   *other road vehicles (E826-E829)*

>   *For definitions and examples related to transport accidents—see Volume 1, pages 571-585.*

>   *The fourth-digit subdivisions for use with categories E800-E848 to identify the injured person are found on pages 1447-1451.*

>   *For identifying the place in which an accident or poisoning occurred (circumstances classifiable to categories E850-E869 and E880-E928)— see the listing in this section under "Accident, occurring."*

See the Table of Drugs and Chemicals (Section 2 of this volume) for identifying the specific agent involved in drug overdose or a wrong substance given or taken in error, and for intoxication or poisoning by a drug or other chemical substance.

The specific adverse effect, reaction, or localized toxic effect to a correct drug or substance properly administered in therapeutic or prophylactic dosage should be classified according to the nature of the adverse effect (e.g.: allergy, dermatitis, tachycardia) listed in Section 1 of this volume.

A

Abandonment
  causing exposure to weather conditions—*see* Exposure
  child, with intent to injure or kill E968.4
  helpless person, infant, newborn E904.0
    with intent to injure or kill E968.4
Abortion, criminal, injury to child E968.8
Abuse, (alleged) (suspected)
  adult
    by
      child E967.4
      ex-partner E967.3
      ex-spouse E967.3
      father E967.0
      grandchild E967.7
      grandparent E967.6
      mother E967.2
      non-related caregiver E967.8
      other relative E967.7
      other specified person(s) E967.1
      partner E967.3
      sibling E967.5
      spouse E967.3
      stepfather E967.0
      stepmother E967.2
      unspecified person E967.9
  child
    by
      boyfriend of parent or guardian E967.0
      child E967.4
      father E967.0
      female partner of parent or guardian E967.2
      girlfriend of parent or guardian E967.2
      grandchild E967.7
      grandparent E967.6
      male partner of parent or guardian E967.0
      mother E967.2
      non-related caregiver E967.8
      other relative E967.7
      other specified person(s) E967.1
      sibling E967.5
      stepfather E967.0
      stepmother E967.2
      unspecified person E967.9
Accident (to) E928.9
  aircraft (in transit) (powered) E841
    at landing, take-off E840
    due to, caused by cataclysm—*see* categories E908, E909
    late effect of E929.1
    unpowered (*see also* Collision, aircraft, unpowered) E842
    while alighting, boarding E843
  amphibious vehicle
    on
      land—*see* Accident, motor vehicle
      water—*see* Accident, watercraft
  animal, ridden NEC E828
  animal-drawn vehicle NEC E827
  balloon (*see also* Collision, aircraft, unpowered) E842
  caused by, due to
    abrasive wheel (metalworking) E919.3
    animal NEC E906.9
      being ridden (in sport or transport) E828
    avalanche NEC E909.2
    band saw E919.4
    bench saw E919.4

Accident—*continued*
    bore, earth-drilling or mining (land) (seabed) E919.1
    bulldozer E919.7
    cataclysmic
      earth surface movement or eruption E909.9
      storm E908.9
    chain
      hoist E919.2
        agricultural operations E919.0
        mining operations E919.1
      saw E920.1
    circular saw E919.4
    cold (excessive) (*see also* Cold, exposure to) E901.9
    combine E919.0
    conflagration—*see* Conflagration
    corrosive liquid, substance NEC E924.1
    cotton gin E919.8
    crane E919.2
      agricultural operations E919.0
      mining operations E919.1
    cutting or piercing instrument (*see also* Cut) E920.9
    dairy equipment E919.8
    derrick E919.2
      agricultural operations E919.0
      mining operations E919.1
    drill E920.1
      earth (land) (seabed) E919.1
      hand (powered) E920.1
        not powered E920.4
      metalworking E919.3
      woodworking E919.4
    earth(-)
      drilling machine E919.1
      moving machine E919.7
      scraping machine E919.7
    electric
      current (*see also* Electric shock) E925.9
      motor—*see also* Accident, machine, by type of machine
        current (of)—*see* Electric shock
    elevator (building) (grain) E919.2
      agricultural operations E919.0
      mining operations E919.1
    environmental factors NEC E928.9
    excavating machine E919.7
    explosive material (*see also* Explosion) E923.9
    farm machine E919.0
    fire, flames—*see also* Fire
      conflagration—*see* Conflagration
    firearm missile—*see* Shooting
    forging (metalworking) machine E919.3
    forklift (truck) E919.2
      agricultural operations E919.0
      mining operations E919.1
    gas turbine E919.5
    harvester E919.0
    hay derrick, mower, or rake E919.0
    heat (excessive) (*see also* Heat) E900.9
    hoist (*see also* Accident, caused by, due to, lift) E919.2
      chain—*see* Accident, caused by, due to, chain
      shaft E919.1

INDEX TO EXTERNAL CAUSES   **Accident**

Accident—*continued*
  hot
    liquid E924.0
      caustic or corrosive E924.1
    object (not producing fire or flames)
      E924.8
    substance E924.9
      caustic or corrosive E924.1
      liquid (metal) NEC E924.0
      specified type NEC E924.8
  human bite E928.3
  ignition—*see* Ignition
  internal combustion engine E919.5
  landslide NEC E909.2
  lathe (metalworking) E919.3
    turnings E920.8
    woodworking E919.4
  lift, lifting (appliances) E919.2
    agricultural operations E919.0
    mining operations E919.1
    shaft E919.1
  lightning NEC E907
  machine, machinery—*see also* Accident,
      machine
    drilling, metal E919.3
    manufacturing, for manufacture of
      beverages E919.8
      clothing E919.8
      foodstuffs E919.8
      paper E919.8
      textiles E919.8
    milling, metal E919.3
    moulding E919.4
    power press, metal E919.3
    printing E919.8
    rolling mill, metal E919.3
    sawing, metal E919.3
    specified type NEC E919.8
    spinning E919.8
    weaving E919.8
  natural factor NEC E928.9
  overhead plane E919.4
  plane E920.4
    overhead E919.4
  powered
    hand tool NEC E920.1
    saw E919.4
      hand E920.1
  printing machine E919.8
  pulley (block) E919.2
    agricultural operations E919.0
    mining operations E919.1
    transmission E919.6
  radial saw E919.4
  radiation—*see* Radiation
  reaper E919.0
  road scraper E919.7
    when in transport under its own
      power—*see* categories E810—E825
  roller coaster E919.8
  sander E919.4
  saw E920.4
    band E919.4
    bench E919.4
    chain E920.1
    circular E919.4
    hand E920.4
      powered E920.1
    powered, except hand E919.4
    radial E919.4
  sawing machine, metal E919.3

Accident—*continued*
  shaft
    hoist E919.1
    lift E919.1
    transmission E919.6
  shears E920.4
    hand E920.4
      powered E920.1
    mechanical E919.3
  shovel E920.4
    steam E919.7
  spinning machine E919.8
  steam—*see also* Burning, steam
    engine E919.5
    shovel E919.7
  thresher E919.0
  thunderbolt NEC E907
  tractor E919.0
    when in transport under its own
      power—*see* categories E810-E825
  transmission belt, cable, chain, gear, pinion,
    pulley, shaft E919.6
  turbine (gas) (water driven) E919.5
  under-cutter E919.1
  weaving machine E919.8
  winch E919.2
    agricultural operations E919.0
    mining operations E919.1
  diving E883.0
    with insufficient air supply E913.2
  glider (hang) (*see also* Collision, aircraft,
    unpowered) E842
  hovercraft
    on
      land—*see* Accident, motor vehicle
      water—*see* Accident, watercraft
  ice yacht (*see also* Accident, vehicle NEC)
    E848
  in
    medical, surgical procedure
      as, or due to misadventure—*see*
        Misadventure
      causing an abnormal reaction or later
        complication without mention of
        misadventure—*see* Reaction, abnormal
  kite carrying a person (*see also* Collision,
    aircraft, unpowered) E842
  land yacht (*see also* Accident, vehicle NEC)
    E848
  late effect of—*see* Late effect
  launching pad E845
  machine, machinery (*see also* Accident,
    caused by, due to, by specific type of
    machine) E919.9
    agricultural including animal-powered
      E919.0
    earth-drilling E919.1
    earth moving or scraping E919.7
    excavating E919.7
    involving transport under own power on
      highway or transport vehicle—*see*
        categories E810-E825, E840-E845
    lifting (appliances) E919.2
    metalworking E919.3
    mining E919.1
    prime movers, except electric motors E919.5
      electric motors—*see* Accident, machine, by
        specific type of machine
    recreational E919.8
    specified type NEC E919.8

Accident   INDEX TO EXTERNAL CAUSES

Accident—*continued*
  transmission E919.6
  watercraft (deck) (engine room) (galley)
    (laundry) (loading) E836
  woodworking or forming E919.4
  motor vehicle (on public highway) (traffic)
    E819
    due to cataclysm—*see* categories E908,
      E909
    involving
      collision (*see also* Collision, motor
        vehicle) E812
      nontraffic, not on public highway—*see*
        categories E820-E825
      not involving collision—*see* categories
        E816-E819
  nonmotor vehicle NEC E829
    nonroad—*see* Accident, vehicle NEC
    road, except pedal cycle, animal-drawn
      vehicle, or animal being ridden E829
  nonroad vehicle NEC—*see* Accident, vehicle
    NEC
  not elsewhere classifiable involving
    cable car (not on rails) E847
      on rails E829
    coal car in mine E846
    hand truck—*see* Accident, vehicle NEC
    logging car E846
    sled(ge), meaning snow or ice vehicle E848
    tram, mine or quarry E846
    truck
      mine or quarry E846
      self-propelled, industrial E846
      station baggage E846
    tub, mine or quarry E846
    vehicle NEC E848
      snow and ice E848
      used only on industrial premises E846
    wheelbarrow E848
  occurring (at) (in)
    apartment E849.0
    baseball field, diamond E849.4
    construction site, any E849.3
    dock E849.8
      yard E849.3
    dormitory E849.7
    factory (building) (premises) E849.3
    farm E849.1
      buildings E849.1
      house E849.0
    football field E849.4
    forest E849.8
    garage (place of work) E849.3
      private (home) E849.0
    gravel pit E849.2
    gymnasium E849.4
    highway E849.5
    home (private) (residential) E849.0
      institutional E849.7
    hospital E849.7
    hotel E849.6
    house (private) (residential) E849.0
      movie E849.6
      public E849.6
    institution, residential E849.7
    jail E849.7
    mine E849.2
    motel E849.6
    movie house E849.6
    office (building) E849.6

Accident—*continued*
    orphanage E849.7
    park (public) E849.4
      mobile home E849.8
      trailer E849.8
    parking lot or place E849.8
    place
      industrial NEC E849.3
      parking E849.8
      public E849.8
        specified place NEC E849.5
      recreational NEC E849.4
      sport NEC E849.4
    playground (park) (school) E849.4
    prison E849.6
    public building NEC E849.6
    quarry E849.2
    railway
      line NEC E849.8
      yard E849.3
    residence
      home (private) E849.0
    resort (beach) (lake) (mountain) (seashore)
      (vacation) E849.4
    restaurant E849.6
    sand pit E849.2
    school (building) (private) (public) (state)
      E849.6
      reform E849.7
      riding E849.4
    seashore E849.8
      resort E849.4
    shop (place of work) E849.3
      commercial E849.6
    skating rink E849.4
    sports palace E849.4
    stadium E849.4
    store E849.6
    street E849.5
    swimming pool (public) E849.4
      private home or garden E849.0
    tennis court E849.4
    theatre, theater E849.6
    trailer court E849.8
    tunnel E849.8
      under construction E849.2
    warehouse E849.3
    yard
      dock E849.3
      industrial E849.3
      private (home) E849.0
      railway E849.3
  off-road type motor vehicle (not on public
    highway) NEC E821
  on public highway—*see* categories
    E810-E819
  pedal cycle E826
  railway E807
    due to cataclysm—*see* categories E908,
      E909
    involving
      avalanche E909.2
      burning by engine, locomotive, train (*see
        also* Explosion, railway engine) E803
      collision (*see also* Collision, railway) E800
      derailment (*see also* Derailment, railway)
        E802
      explosion (*see also* Explosion, railway
        engine) E803
      fall (*see also* Fall, from, railway rolling
        stock) E804

1500

Accident—*continued*
  fire (*see also* Explosion, railway engine) E803
  hitting by, being struck by
    object falling in, on, from, rolling stock, train, vehicle E806
    rolling stock, train, vehicle E805
    overturning, railway rolling stock, train, vehicle (*see also* Derailment, railway) E802
    running off rails, railway (*see also* Derailment, railway) E802
    specified circumstances NEC E806
    train or vehicle hit by
      avalanche E909
      falling object (earth, rock, tree) E806
        due to cataclysm—*see* categories E908, E909
      landslide E909
  roller skate E885.1
  scooter (nonmotorized) E885.0
  skateboard E885.2
  ski(ing) E885.3
    jump E884.9
    lift or tow (with chair or gondola) E847
  snowboard E885.4
  snow vehicle, motor driven (not on public highway) E820
    on public highway—*see* categories E810-E819
  spacecraft E845
  specified cause NEC E928.8
  street car E829
  traffic NEC E819
  vehicle NEC (with pedestrian) E848
    battery powered
      airport passenger vehicle E846
      truck (baggage) (mail) E846
    powered commercial or industrial (with other vehicle or object within commercial or industrial premises) E846
  watercraft E838
    with
      drowning or submersion resulting from
        accident other than to watercraft E832
        accident to watercraft E830
      injury, except drowning or submersion, resulting from
        accident other than to watercraft—*see* categories E833-E838
        accident to watercraft E831
    due to, caused by cataclysm—*see* categories E908, E909
    machinery E836
Acid throwing E961
Acosta syndrome E902.0
Aeroneurosis E902.1
Aero-otitis media —*see* Effects of, air pressure
Aerosinusitis —*see* Effects of, air pressure
After-effect, late —*see* Late effect
Air
  blast
    in
      terrorism E979.2
      war operations E993
  embolism (traumatic) NEC E928.9
    in
      infusion or transfusion E874.1
      perfusion E874.2
  sickness E903
Alpine sickness E902.0

Altitude sickness —*see* Effects of, air pressure
Anaphylactic shock, anaphylaxis (*see also* Table of drugs and chemicals) E947.9
  due to bite or sting (venomous)—*see* Bite, venomous
Andes disease E902.0
Apoplexy heat—*see* Heat
Arachnidism E905.1
Arson E968.0
Asphyxia, asphyxiation
  by
    chemical
      in
        terrorism E979.7
        war operations E997.2
    explosion—*see* Explosion
    food (bone) (regurgitated food) (seed) E911
    foreign object, except food E912
    fumes
      in
        terrorism (chemical weapons) E979.7
        war operations E997.2
    gas—*see also* Table of drugs and chemicals
      in
        terrorism E979.7
        war operations E997.2
      legal
        execution E978
        intervention (tear) E972
      tear E972
    mechanical means (*see also* Suffocation) E913.9
  from
    conflagration—*see* Conflagration
    fire—*see also* Fire E899
      in
        terrorism E979.3
        war operations E990.9
    ignition—*see* Ignition
Aspiration
  foreign body—*see* Foreign body, aspiration
  mucus, not of newborn (with asphyxia, obstruction respiratory passage, suffocation) E912
  phlegm (with asphyxia, obstruction respiratory passage, suffocation) E912
  vomitus (with asphyxia, obstruction respiratory passage, suffocation) (*see also* Foreign body, aspiration, food) E911
Assassination (attempt) (*see also* Assault) E968.9
Assault (homicidal) (by) (in) E968.9
  acid E961
    swallowed E962.1
  air gun E968.6
  BB gun E968.6
  bite NEC E968.8
    of human being E968.7
  bomb ((placed in) car or house) E965.8
    antipersonnel E965.5
    letter E965.7
    petrol E965.7
  brawl (hand) (fists) (foot) E960.0
  burning, burns (by fire) E968.0
    acid E961
      swallowed E962.1
    caustic, corrosive substance E961
      swallowed E962.1
    chemical from swallowing caustic, corrosive substance NEC E962.1
    hot liquid E968.3

Assault—*continued*
    scalding E968.3
    vitriol E961
        swallowed E962.1
  caustic, corrosive substance E961
    swallowed E962.1
  cut, any part of body E966
  dagger E966
  drowning E964
  explosive(s) E965.9
    bomb (*see also* Assault, bomb) E965.8
    dynamite E965.8
  fight (hand) (fists) (foot) E960.0
    with weapon E968.9
      blunt or thrown E968.2
      cutting or piercing E966
      firearm—*see* Shooting, homicide
  fire E968.0
  firearm(s)—*see* Shooting, homicide
  garrotting E963
  gunshot (wound)—*see* Shooting, homicide
  hanging E963
  injury NEC E968.9
  knife E966
  late effect of E969
  ligature E963
  poisoning E962.9
    drugs or medicinals E962.0
    gas(es) or vapors, except drugs and medicinals E962.2
    solid or liquid substances, except drugs and medicinals E962.1
  puncture, any part of body E966
  pushing
    before moving object, train, vehicle E968.5
    from high place E968.1
  rape E960.1
  scalding E968.3
  shooting—*see* Shooting, homicide
  sodomy E960.1
  stab, any part of body E966
  strangulation E963
  submersion E964
  suffocation E963
  transport vehicle E968.5
  violence NEC E968.9
  vitriol E961
    swallowed E962.1
  weapon E968.9
    blunt or thrown E968.2
    cutting or piercing E966
    firearm—*see* Shooting, homicide
  wound E968.9
    cutting E966
    gunshot—*see* Shooting, homicide
    knife E966
    piercing E966
    puncture E966
    stab E966
Attack by animal NEC E906.9
Avalanche E909.2
  falling on or hitting
    motor vehicle (in motion) (on public highway) E909.2
    railway train E909.2
Aviators' disease E902.1

B

Barotitis, barodontalgia, barosinusitis, barotrauma (otitic) (sinus)—*see* Effects of, air pressure
Battered
  baby or child (syndrome)—*see* Abuse, child; category E967
  person other than baby or child—*see* Assault
Bayonet wound (*see also* Cut, by bayonet) E920.3
  in
    legal intervention E974
    terrorism E979.8
    war operations E995
Bean in nose E912
Bed set on fire NEC E898.0
Beheading (by guillotine)
  homicide E966
  legal execution E978
Bending, injury in E927
Bends E902.0
Bite
  animal (nonvenomous) NEC E906.5
    venomous NEC E905.9
  arthropod (nonvenomous) NEC E906.4
    venomous—*see* Sting
  black widow spider E905.1
  cat E906.3
  centipede E905.4
  cobra E905.0
  copperhead snake E905.0
  coral snake E905.0
  dog E906.0
  fer de lance E905.0
  gila monster E905.0
  human being
    accidental E928.3
    assault E968.7
  insect (nonvenomous) E906.4
    venomous—*see* Sting
  krait E905.0
  late effect of—*see* Late effect
  lizard E906.2
    venomous E905.0
  mamba E905.0
  marine animal
    nonvenomous E906.3
      snake E906.2
    venomous E905.6
      snake E905.0
  millipede E906.4
    venomous E905.4
  moray eel E906.3
  rat E906.1
  rattlesnake E905.0
  rodent, except rat E906.3
  serpent—*see* Bite, snake
  shark E906.3
  snake (venomous) E905.0
    nonvenomous E906.2
    sea E905.0
  spider E905.1
    nonvenomous E906.4
  tarantula (venomous) E905.1
  venomous NEC E905.9
    by specific animal—*see* category E905
  viper E905.0
  water moccasin E905.0

INDEX TO EXTERNAL CAUSES

Blast (air)
  from nuclear explosion E996
  in
    terrorism E979.2
      from nuclear explosion E979.5
      underwater E979.0
    war operations E993
      from nuclear explosion E996
      underwater E992
  underwater E992
Blizzard E908.3
Blow E928.9
  by law-enforcing agent, police (on duty) E975
    with blunt object (baton) (nightstick) (stave) (truncheon) E973
Blowing up (*see also* Explosion) E923.9
Brawl (hand) (fists) (foot) E960.0
Breakage (accidental)
  cable of cable car not on rails E847
  ladder (causing fall) E881.0
  part (any) of
    animal-drawn vehicle E827
    ladder (causing fall) E881.0
    motor vehicle
      in motion (on public highway) E818
      not on public highway E825
    nonmotor road vehicle, except animal-drawn vehicle or pedal cycle E829
    off-road type motor vehicle (not on public highway) NEC E821
      on public highway E818
    pedal cycle E826
    scaffolding (causing fall) E881.1
    snow vehicle, motor-driven (not on public highway) E820
      on public highway E818
  vehicle NEC—*see* Accident, vehicle
Broken
  glass
    fall on E888.0
    injury by E920.8
  power line (causing electric shock) E925.1
Bumping against, into (accidentally)
  object (moving) E917.9
    caused by crowd E917.1
      with subsequent fall E917.6
    furniture E917.3
      with subsequent fall E917.7
    in
      running water E917.2
      sports E917.0
        with subsequent fall E917.5
      stationary E917.4
        with subsequent fall E917.8
  person(s) E917.9
    with fall E886.9
      in sports E886.0
    as, or caused by, a crowd E917.1
      with subsequent fall E917.6
      in sports E917.0
        with fall E886.0
Burning, burns (accidental) (by) (from) (on) E899
  acid (any kind) E924.1
    swallowed—*see* Table of drugs and chemicals
  bedclothes (*see also* Fire, specified NEC) E898.0
  blowlamp (*see also* Fire, specified NEC) E898.1

Burning, burns—*continued*
  blowtorch (*see also* Fire, specified NEC) E898.1
  boat, ship, watercraft—*see* categories E830, E831, E837
  bonfire (controlled) E897
    uncontrolled E892
  candle (*see also* Fire, specified NEC) E898.1
  caustic liquid, substance E924.1
    swallowed—*see* Table of drugs and chemicals
  chemical E924.1
    from swallowing caustic, corrosive substance—*see* Table of drugs and chemicals
  in
    terrorism E979.7
    war operations E997.2
  cigar(s) or cigarette(s) (*see also* Fire, specified NEC) E898.1
  clothes, clothing, nightdress—*see* Ignition, clothes
    with conflagration—*see* Conflagration
  conflagration—*see* Conflagration
  corrosive liquid, substance E924.1
    swallowed—*see* Table of drugs and chemicals
  electric current (*see also* Electric shock) E925.9
  fire, flames (*see also* Fire) E899
  flare, Verey pistol E922.8
  heat
    from appliance (electrical) E924.8
    in local application or packing during medical or surgical procedure E873.5
  homicide (attempt) (*see also* Assault, burning) E968.0
  hot
    liquid E924.0
      caustic or corrosive E924.1
    object (not producing fire or flames) E924.8
    substance E924.9
      caustic or corrosive E924.1
      liquid (metal) NEC E924.0
      specified type NEC E924.8
    tap water E924.2
  ignition—*see also* Ignition
    clothes, clothing, nightdress—*see also* Ignition, clothes
      with conflagration—*see* Conflagration
    highly inflammable material (benzine) (fat) (gasoline) (kerosine) (paraffin) (petrol) E894
  inflicted by other person
    stated as
      homicidal, intentional (*see also* Assault, burning) E968.0
      undetermined whether accidental or intentional (*see also* Burn, stated as undetermined whether accidental or intentional) E988.1
  internal, from swallowed caustic, corrosive liquid, substance—*see* Table of drugs and chemicals
  in
    from nuclear explosion E996
    petrol bomb E990.0
    terrorism E979.3
      from nuclear explosion E979.5
      petrol bomb E979.3

1503

Burning, burns—*continued*
    war operations (from fire-producing device or conventional weapon) E990.9
        from nuclear explosion E996
        petrol bomb E990.0
  lamp (*see also* Fire, specified NEC) E898.1
  late effect of NEC E929.4
  lighter (cigar) (cigarette) (*see also* Fire, specified NEC) E898.1
  lightning E907
  liquid (boiling) (hot) (molten) E924.0
    caustic, corrosive (external) E924.1
        swallowed—*see* Table of drugs and chemicals
  local application of externally applied substance in medical or surgical care E873.5
  machinery—*see* Accident, machine
  matches (*see also* Fire, specified NEC) E898.1
  medicament, externally applied E873.5
  metal, molten E924.0
  object (hot) E924.8
    producing fire or flames—*see* Fire
  oven (electric) (gas) E924.8
  pipe (smoking) (*see also* Fire, specified NEC) E898.1
  radiation—*see* Radiation
  railway engine, locomotive, train (*see also* Explosion, railway engine) E803
  self-inflicted (unspecified whether accidental or intentional) E988.1
    caustic or corrosive substance NEC E988.7
    stated as intentional, purposeful E958.1
        caustic or corrosive substance NEC E958.7
    stated as undetermined whether accidental or intentional E988.1
        caustic or corrosive substance NEC E988.7
  steam E924.0
    pipe E924.8
  substance (hot) E924.9
    boiling or molten E924.0
    caustic, corrosive (external) E924.1
        swallowed—*see* Table of drugs and chemicals
  suicidal (attempt) NEC E958.1
    caustic substance E958.7
    late effect of E959
  tanning bed E926.2
  therapeutic misadventure
    overdose of radiation E873.2
  torch, welding (*see also* Fire, specified NEC) E898.1
  trash fire (*see also* Burning, bonfire) E897
  vapor E924.0
  vitriol E924.1
  x-rays E926.3
    in medical, surgical procedure—*see* Misadventure, failure, in dosage, radiation
Butted by animal E906.8

C

Cachexia, lead or saturnine E866.0
  from pesticide NEC (*see also* Table of drugs and chemicals) E863.4
Caisson disease E902.2
Capital punishment (any means) E978
Car sickness E903
Casualty (not due to war) NEC E928.9
  terrorism E979.8
  war (*see also* War operations) E995
Cat
  bite E906.3
  scratch E906.8
Cataclysmic (any injury)
  earth surface movement or eruption E909.9
    specified type NEC E909.8
  storm or flood resulting from storm E908.9
    specified type NEC E909.8
Catching fire —*see* Ignition
Caught
  between
    objects (moving) (stationary and moving) E918
    and machinery—*see* Accident, machine
  by cable car, not on rails E847
  in
    machinery (moving parts of)—*see* Accident, machine
    object E918
Cave-in (causing asphyxia, suffocation (by pressure)) (*see also* Suffocation, due to, cave-in) E913.3
Cave-in—*continued*
  with injury other than asphyxia or suffocation E916
    with asphyxia or suffocation (*see also* Suffocation, due to, cave-in) E913.3
  struck or crushed by E916
    with asphyxia or suffocation (*see also* Suffocation, due to, cave-in) E913.3
Change(s) in air pressure—*see also* Effects of, air pressure
  sudden, in aircraft (ascent) (descent) (causing aeroneurosis or aviators' disease) E902.1
Chilblains E901.0
  due to manmade conditions E901.1
Choking (on) (any object except food or vomitus) E912
  apple E911
  bone E911
  food, any type (regurgitated) E911
  mucus or phlegm E912
  seed E911
Civil insurrection —*see* War operations
Cloudburst E908.8
Cold, exposure to (accidental) (excessive) (extreme) (place) E901.9
  causing chilblains or immersion foot E901.0
  due to
    manmade conditions E901.1
    specified cause NEC E901.8
    weather (conditions) E901.0
  late effect of NEC E929.5
  self-inflicted (undetermined whether accidental or intentional) E988.3
    suicidal E958.3
  suicide E958.3
Colic, lead, painters', or saturnine —*see* category E866

INDEX TO EXTERNAL CAUSES

Collision

Collapse
 building E916
  burning (uncontrolled fire) E891.8
   in terrorism E979.3
  private E890.8
 dam E909.3
 due to heat—*see* Heat
 machinery—*see* Accident, machine
 man-made structure E909.3
 postoperative NEC E878.9
 structure, burning NEC E891.8
  burning (uncontrolled fire)
   in terrorism E979.3

Collision (accidental)

Note—In the case of collisions between different types of vehicles, persons and objects, priority in classification is in the following order:

 Aircraft
 Watercraft
 Motor vehicle
 Railway vehicle
 Pedal Cycle
 Animal-drawn vehicle
 Animal being ridden
 Streetcar or other nonmotor road vehicle
 Other vehicle
 Pedestrian or person using pedestrian conveyance
 Object (except where falling from or set in motion by vehicle etc. listed above)

In the listing below, the combinations are listed only under the vehicle etc. having priority. For definitions, *see* E code introduction.

 aircraft (with object or vehicle) (fixed) (movable) (moving) E841
  with
   person (while landing, taking off) (without accident to aircraft) E844
   powered (in transit) (with unpowered aircraft) E841
    while landing, taking off E840
   unpowered E842
    while landing, taking off E840
 animal being ridden (in sport or transport) E828
  and
   animal (being ridden) (herded) (unattended) E828
   nonmotor road vehicle, except pedal cycle or animal-drawn vehicle E828
   object (fallen) (fixed) (movable) (moving)
    not falling from or set in motion by vehicle of higher priority E828
   pedestrian (conveyance or vehicle) E828
 animal-drawn vehicle E827
  and
   animal (being ridden) (herded) (unattended) E827
   nonmotor road vehicle, except pedal cycle E827
   object (fallen) (fixed) (movable) (moving)
    not falling from or set in motion by vehicle of higher priority E827
   pedestrian (conveyance or vehicle) E827
   streetcar E827
 motor vehicle (on public highway) (traffic accident) E812

Collision—*continued*
 after leaving, running off, public highway (without antecedent collision) (without re-entry) E816
  with antecedent collision on public highway—*see* categories E810-E815
  with re-entrance collision with another motor vehicle E811
 and
  abutment (bridge) (overpass) E815
  animal (herded) (unattended) E815
   carrying person, property E813
  animal-drawn vehicle E813
  another motor vehicle (abandoned) (disabled) (parked) (stalled) (stopped) E812
   with, involving re-entrance (on same roadway) (across median strip) E811
  any object, person, or vehicle off the public highway resulting from a noncollision motor vehicle nontraffic accident E816
  avalanche, fallen or not moving E815
   falling E909
  boundary fence E815
  culvert E815
  fallen
   stone E815
   tree E815
  falling E909.2
  guard post or guard rail E815
  inter-highway divider E815
  landslide, fallen or not moving E815
   moving E909
  machinery (road) E815
  moving E909.2
  nonmotor road vehicle NEC E813
  object (any object, person, or vehicle off the public highway resulting from a noncollision motor vehicle nontraffic accident) E815
   off, normally not on, public highway resulting from a noncollision motor vehicle traffic accident E816
  pedal cycle E813
  pedestrian (conveyance) E814
  person (using pedestrian conveyance) E814
  post or pole (lamp) (light) (signal) (telephone) (utility) E815
  railway rolling stock, train, vehicle E810
  safety island E815
  street car E813
  traffic signal, sign, or marker (temporary) E815
  tree E815
  tricycle E813
  wall of cut made for road E815
 due to cataclysm—*see* categories E908, E909
 not on public highway, nontraffic accident E822
  and
   animal (carrying person, property) (herded) (unattended) E822
   animal-drawn vehicle E822
   another motor vehicle (moving), except off-road motor vehicle E822
    stationary E823
   avalanche, fallen, not moving E823
    moving E909
   landslide, fallen, not moving E823

1505

Collision | **INDEX TO EXTERNAL CAUSES**

Collision—*continued*
    moving E909
    nonmotor vehicle (moving) E822
        stationary E823
    object (fallen) (normally) (fixed) (movable but not in motion) (stationary) E823
        moving, except when falling from, set in motion by, aircraft or cataclysm E822
    pedal cycle (moving) E822
        stationary E823
    pedestrian (conveyance) E822
    person (using pedestrian conveyance) E822
    railway rolling stock, train, vehicle (moving) E822
        stationary E823
    road vehicle (any) (moving) E822
        stationary E823
    tricycle (moving) E822
        stationary E823
    moving E909.2
  off-road type motor vehicle (not on public highway) E821
  and
    animal (being ridden) (-drawn vehicle) E821
    another off-road motor vehicle, except snow vehicle E821
    other motor vehicle, not on public highway E821
    other object or vehicle NEC, fixed or movable, not set in motion by aircraft, motor vehicle on highway, or snow vehicle, motor-driven E821
    pedal cycle E821
    pedestrian (conveyance) E821
    railway train E821
  on public highway—*see* Collision, motor vehicle
  pedal cycle E826
  and
    animal (carrying person, property) (herded) (unherded) E826
    animal-drawn vehicle E826
    another pedal cycle E826
    nonmotor road vehicle E826
    object (fallen) (fixed) (movable) (moving) not falling from or set in motion by aircraft, motor vehicle, or railway train NEC E826
    pedestrian (conveyance) E826
    person (using pedestrian conveyance) E826
    street car E826
  pedestrian(s) (conveyance) E917.9
    with fall E886.9
    in sports E886.0
    and
      crowd, human stampede E917.1
        with subsequent fall E917.6
      furniture E917.3
        with subsequent fall E917.7
      machinery—*see* Accident, machine
      object (fallen) (moving) not falling from or set in motion by any vehicle classifiable to E800-E848, E917.9
        caused by a crowd E917.1
          with subsequent fall E917.6
        furniture E917.3
          with subsequent fall E917.7

Collision—*continued*
  in
    running water E917.2
      with drowning or submersion—*see* Submersion
    sports E917.0
      with subsequent fall E917.5
    stationary E917.4
      with subsequent fall E917.8
  vehicle, nonmotor, nonroad E848
  in
    running water E917.2
      with drowning or submersion—*see* Submersion
    sports E917.0
      with fall E886.0
  person(s) (using pedestrian conveyance) (*see also* Collision, pedestrian) E917.9
  railway (rolling stock) (train) (vehicle) (with (subsequent) derailment, explosion, fall or fire) E800
    with antecedent derailment E802
    and
      animal (carrying person) (herded) (unattended) E801
      another railway train or vehicle E800
      buffers E801
      fallen tree on railway E801
      farm machinery, nonmotor (in transport) (stationary) E801
      gates E801
      nonmotor vehicle E801
      object (fallen) (fixed) (movable) (moving) not falling from, set in motion by, aircraft or motor vehicle NEC E801
      pedal cycle E801
      pedestrian (conveyance) E805
      person (using pedestrian conveyance) E805
      platform E801
      rock on railway E801
      street car E801
  snow vehicle, motor-driven (not on public highway) E820
  and
    animal (being ridden) (-drawn vehicle) E820
    another off-road motor vehicle E820
    other motor vehicle, not on public highway E820
    other object or vehicle NEC, fixed or movable, not set in motion by aircraft or motor vehicle on highway E820
    pedal cycle E820
    pedestrian (conveyance) E820
    railway train E820
  on public highway—*see* Collision, motor vehicle
  street car(s) E829
  and
    animal, herded, not being ridden, unattended E829
    nonmotor road vehicle NEC E829
    object (fallen) (fixed) (movable) (moving) not falling from or set in motion by aircraft, animal-drawn vehicle, animal being ridden, motor vehicle, pedal cycle, or railway train E829
    pedestrian (conveyance) E829
    person (using pedestrian conveyance) E829

INDEX TO EXTERNAL CAUSES — Crushed

Collision—*continued*
vehicle
  animal-drawn—*see* Collision, animal-drawn vehicle
  motor—*see* Collision, motor vehicle
  nonmotor
    nonroad E848
      and
        another nonmotor, nonroad vehicle E848
        object (fallen) (fixed) (movable) (moving) not falling from or set in motion by aircraft, animal-drawn vehicle, animal being ridden, motor vehicle, nonmotor road vehicle, pedal cycle, railway train, or streetcar E848
    road, except animal being ridden, animal-drawn vehicle, or pedal cycle E829
      and
        animal, herded, not being ridden, unattended E829
        another nonmotor road vehicle, except animal being ridden, animal-drawn vehicle, or pedal cycle E829
        object (fallen) (fixed) (movable) (moving) not falling from or set in motion by, aircraft, animal-drawn vehicle, animal being ridden, motor vehicle, pedal cycle, or railway train E829
        pedestrian (conveyance) E829
        person (using pedestrian conveyance) E829
        vehicle, nonmotor, nonroad E829
  watercraft E838
    and
      person swimming or water skiing E838
    causing
      drowning, submersion E830
      injury except drowning, submersion E831
Combustion, spontaneous —*see* Ignition
Complication of medical or surgical procedure or treatment
  as an abnormal reaction—*see* Reaction, abnormal
  delayed, without mention of misadventure—*see* Reaction, abnormal
  due to misadventure—*see* Misadventure
Compression
  divers' squeeze E902.2
  trachea by
    food E911
    foreign body, except food E912
Conflagration
  building or structure, except private dwelling (barn) (church) (convalescent or residential home) (factory) (farm outbuilding) (hospital) (hotel) (institution) (educational) (dormitory) (residential) (school) (shop) (store) (theatre) E891.9
    with or causing (injury due to)
      accident or injury NEC E891.9
        specified circumstance NEC E891.8
      burns, burning E891.3
      carbon monoxide E891.2
      fumes E891.2
        polyvinylchloride (PVC) or similar material E891.1
      smoke E891.2

Conflagration—*continued*
  causing explosion E891.0
  in terrorism E979.3
  not in building or structure E892
  private dwelling (apartment) (boarding house) (camping place) (caravan) (farmhouse) (home (private)) (house) (lodging house) (private garage) (rooming house) (tenement) E890.9
    with or causing (injury due to)
      accident or injury NEC E890.9
        specified circumstance NEC E890.8
      burns, burning E890.3
      carbon monoxide E890.2
      fumes E890.2
        polyvinylchloride (PVC) or similar material E890.1
      smoke E890.2
    causing explosion E890.0
Constriction, external
  caused by
    hair E928.4
    other object E928.5
Contact with
  dry ice E901.1
  liquid air, hydrogen, nitrogen E901.1
Cramp(s)
  Heat—*see* Heat
  swimmers (*see also* category E910) E910.2
    not in recreation or sport E910.3
Cranking (car) (truck) (bus) (engine), injury by E917.9
Crash
  aircraft (in transit) (powered) E841
    at landing, take-off E840
    in
      terrorism E979.1
      war operations E994
    on runway NEC E840
    stated as
      homicidal E968.8
      suicidal E958.6
      undetermined whether accidental or intentional E988.6
    unpowered E842
  glider E842
  motor vehicle—*see also* Accident, motor vehicle
    homicidal E968.5
    suicidal E958.5
    undetermined whether accidental or intentional E988.5
Crushed (accidentally) E928.9
  between
    boat(s), ship(s), watercraft (and dock or pier) (without accident to watercraft) E838
      after accident to, or collision, watercraft E831
    objects (moving) (stationary and moving) E918
  by
    avalanche NEC E909.2
    boat, ship, watercraft after accident to, collision, watercraft E831
    cave-in E916
      with asphyxiation or suffocation (*see also* Suffocation, due to, cave-in) E913.3
    crowd, human stampede E917.1
    falling
      aircraft (*see also* Accident, aircraft) E841

1507

Crushed—*continued*
    in
        terrorism E979.1
        war operations E994
    earth, material E916
    with asphyxiation or suffocation (*see also* Suffocation, due to, cave-in) E913.3
    object E916
        on ship, watercraft E838
        while loading, unloading watercraft E838
    landslide NEC E909.2
    lifeboat after abandoning ship E831
    machinery—*see* Accident, machine
    railway rolling stock, train, vehicle (part of) E805
    street car E829
    vehicle NEC—*see* Accident, vehicle NEC
in
    machinery—*see* Accident, machine
    object E918
    transport accident—*see* categories E800-E848
late effect of NEC E929.9
Cut, cutting (any part of body) (accidental) E920.9
by
    arrow E920.8
    axe E920.4
    bayonet (*see also* Bayonet wound) E920.3
    blender E920.2
    broken glass E920.8
        following fall E888.0
    can opener E920.4
        powered E920.2
    chisel E920.4
    circular saw E919.4
    cutting or piercing instrument—*see also* category E920
        following fall E888.0
        late effect of E929.8
    dagger E920.3
    dart E920.8
    drill—*see* Accident, caused by drill
    edge of stiff paper E920.8
    electric
        beater E920.2
        fan E920.2
        knife E920.2
        mixer E920.2
    fork E920.4
    garden fork E920.4
    hand saw or tool (not powered) E920.4
        powered E920.1
    hedge clipper E920.4
        powered E920.1
    hoe E920.4
    ice pick E920.4
    knife E920.3
        electric E920.2
    lathe turnings E920.8
    lawn mower E920.4
        powered E920.0
        riding E919.8
    machine—*see* Accident, machine
    meat
        grinder E919.8
        slicer E919.8
    nails E920.8
    needle E920.4
        hypodermic E920.5

Cut, cutting—*continued*
    object, edged, pointed, sharp—*see* category E920
    following fall E888.0
    paper cutter E920.4
    piercing instrument—*see also* category E920
        late effect of E929.8
    pitchfork E920.4
    powered
        can opener E920.2
        garden cultivator E920.1
            riding E919.8
        hand saw E920.1
        hand tool NEC E920.1
        hedge clipper E920.1
        household appliance or implement E920.2
        lawn mower (hand) E920.0
            riding E919.8
        rivet gun E920.1
        staple gun E920.1
    rake E920.4
    saw
        circular E919.4
        hand E920.4
    scissors E920.4
    screwdriver E920.4
    sewing machine (electric) (powered) E920.2
        not powered E920.4
    shears E920.4
    shovel E920.4
    spade E920.4
    splinters E920.8
    sword E920.3
    tin can lid E920.8
    wood slivers E920.8
homicide (attempt) E966
inflicted by other person
    stated as
        intentional, homicidal E966
        undetermined whether accidental or intentional E986
late effect of NEC E929.8
legal
    execution E978
    intervention E974
self-inflicted (unspecified whether accidental or intentional) E986
    stated as intentional, purposeful E956
    stated as undetermined whether accidental or intentional E986
    suicidal (attempt) E956
war operations E995
terrorism E979.8
Cyclone E908.1

D

Death due to injury occurring one year or more previous —*see* Late effect
Decapitation (accidental circumstances) NEC E928.9
    homicidal E966
    legal execution (by guillotine) E978
Deprivation —*see also* Privation
    homicidal intent E968.4
Derailment (accidental)
    railway (rolling stock) (train) (vehicle) (with subsequent collision) E802
    with
        collision (antecedent) (*see also* Collision, railway) E800

INDEX TO EXTERNAL CAUSES   Execution, legal

Derailment (accidental)—*continued*
    explosion (subsequent) (without antecedent
        collision) E802
        antecedent collision E803
    fall (without collision (antecedent)) E802
    fire (without collision (antecedent)) E802
    street car E829
Descent
    parachute (voluntary) (without accident to
        aircraft) E844
    due to accident to aircraft—*see* categories
        E840-E842
Desertion
    child, with intent to injure or kill E968.4
    helpless person, infant, newborn E904.0
    with intent to injure or kill E968.4
Destitution —*see* Privation
Disability, late effect or sequela of injury
    —*see* Late effect
Disease
    Andes E902.0
    aviators' E902.1
    caisson E902.2
    range E902.0
Divers' disease, palsy, paralysis, squeeze
    E902.0
Dog bite E906.0
Dragged by
    cable car (not on rails) E847
        on rails E829
    motor vehicle (on highway) E814
        not on highway, nontraffic accident E825
    street car E829
Drinking poison (accidental) —*see* Table of
    drugs and chemicals
Drowning —*see* Submersion
Dust in eye E914

E

Earth falling (on) (with asphyxia or suffocation
    (by pressure)) (*see also* Suffocation, due to,
    cave-in) E913.3
    as, or due to, a cataclysm (involving any
        transport vehicle)—*see* categories E908,
        E909
    not due to cataclysmic action E913.3
        motor vehicle (in motion) (on public
            highway) E818
            not on public highway E825
        nonmotor road vehicle NEC E829
        pedal cycle E826
        railway rolling stock, train, vehicle E806
        street car E829
        struck or crushed by E916
            with asphyxiation or suffocation E913.3
            with injury other than asphyxia,
                suffocation E916
Earthquake (any injury) E909.0
Effect(s) (adverse) of
    air pressure E902.9
        at high altitude E902.9
            in aircraft E902.1
            residence or prolonged visit (causing
                conditions classifiable to E902.0)
                E902.0
        due to
            diving E902.2
            specified cause NEC E902.8
        in aircraft E902.1

Effect(s) (adverse) of—*continued*
    cold, excessive (exposure to) (*see also* Cold,
        exposure to) E901.9
    heat (excessive) (*see also* Heat) E900.9
    hot
        place—*see* Heat
        weather E900.0
    insulation—*see* Heat
    late—*see* Late effect of
    motion E903
    nuclear explosion or weapon
        in
            terrorism E979.5
            war operations (blast) (fireball) (heat)
                (radiation) (direct) (secondary) E996
    radiation—*see* Radiation
    terrorism, secondary E979.9
    travel E903
Electric shock, electrocution (accidental) (from
    exposed wire, faulty appliance, high voltage
    cable, live rail, open socket) (by) (in) E925.9
    appliance or wiring
        domestic E925.0
        factory E925.2
        farm (building) E925.8
            house E925.0
        home E925.0
        industrial (conductor) (control apparatus)
            (transformer) E925.2
        outdoors E925.8
        public building E925.8
        residential institution E925.8
        school E925.8
        specified place NEC E925.8
    caused by other person
        stated as
            intentional, homicidal E968.8
            undetermined whether accidental or
                intentional E988.4
    electric power generating plant, distribution
        station E925.1
    homicidal (attempt) E968.8
    legal execution E978
    lightning E907
    machinery E925.9
        domestic E925.0
        factory E925.2
        farm E925.8
        home E925.0
    misadventure in medical or surgical procedure
        in electroshock therapy E873.4
    self-inflicted (undetermined whether accidental
        or intentional) E988.4
        stated as intentional E958.4
    stated as undetermined whether accidental or
        intentional E988.4
    suicidal (attempt) E958.4
    transmission line E925.1
Electrocution —*see* Electric shock
Embolism
    air (traumatic) NEC—*see* Air, embolism
Encephalitis
    lead or saturnine E866.0
        from pesticide NEC E863.4
Entanglement
    in
        bedclothes, causing suffocation E913.0
        wheel of pedal cycle E826
Entry of foreign body, material, any —*see*
    Foreign body
Execution, legal (any method) E978

1509

Exhaustion
  cold—*see* Cold, exposure to
  due to excessive exertion E927
  heat—*see* Heat
Explosion (accidental) (in) (of) (on) E923.9
  acetylene E923.2
  aerosol can E921.8
  aircraft (in transit) (powered) E841
    at landing, take-off E840
    in
      terrorism E979.1
      war operations E994
    unpowered E842
  air tank (compressed) (in machinery) E921.1
  anesthetic gas in operating theatre E923.2
  automobile tire NEC E921.8
    causing transport accident—*see* categories E810-E825
  blasting (cap) (materials) E923.1
  boiler (machinery), not on transport vehicle E921.0
    steamship—*see* Explosion, watercraft
  bomb E923.8
    in
      terrorism E979.2
      war operations E993
        after cessation of hostilities E998
        atom, hydrogen or nuclear E996
        injury by fragments from E991.9
          antipersonnel bomb E991.3
  butane E923.2
  caused by
    other person
      stated as
        intentional, homicidal—*see* Assault, explosive
        undetermined whether accidental or homicidal E985.5
  coal gas E923.2
  detonator E923.1
  dynamite E923.1
  explosive (material) NEC E923.9
    gas(es) E923.2
    missile E923.8
      in
        terrorism E979.2
        war operations E993
          injury by fragments from E991.9
            antipersonnel bomb E991.3
    used in blasting operations E923.1
  fire-damp E923.2
  fireworks E923.0
  gas E923.2
    cylinder (in machinery) E921.1
    pressure tank (in machinery) E921.1
  gasoline (fumes) (tank) not in moving motor vehicle E923.2
  grain store (military) (munitions) E923.8
  grenade E923.8
    in
      terrorism E979.2
      war operations E993
        injury by fragments from E991.9
  homicide (attempt)—*see* Assault, explosive
  hot water heater, tank (in machinery) E921.0
  in mine (of explosive gases) NEC E923.2
  late effect of NEC E929.8
  machinery—*see also* Accident, machine
    pressure vessel—*see* Explosion, pressure vessel
  methane E923.2

Explosion—*continued*
  missile E923.8
    in
      terrorism E979.2
      war operations E993
        injury by fragments from E991.9
  motor vehicle (part of)
    in motion (on public highway) E818
    not on public highway E825
  munitions (dump) (factory) E923.8
    in
      terrorism E979.2
      war operations E993
  of mine E923.8
    in
      terrorism
        at sea or in harbor E979.0
        land E979.2
        marine E979.0
      war operations
        after cessation of hostilities E998
        at sea or in harbor E992
        land E993
          after cessation of hostilities E998
          injury by fragments from E991.9
        marine E992
  own weapons
    in
      terrorism (*see also* Suicide) E979.2
      war operations E993
        injury by fragments from E991.9
          antipersonnel bomb E991.3
  pressure
    cooker E921.8
    gas tank (in machinery) E921.1
    vessel (in machinery) E921.9
      on transport vehicle—*see* categories E800-E848
      specified type NEC E921.8
  propane E923.2
  railway engine, locomotive, train (boiler) (with subsequent collision, derailment, fall) E803
    with
      collision (antecedent) (*see also* Collision, railway) E800
      derailment (antecedent) E802
      fire (without antecedent collision or derailment) E803
  secondary fire resulting from—*see* Fire
  self-inflicted (unspecified whether accidental or intentional) E985.5
    stated as intentional, purposeful E955.5
  shell (artillery) E923.8
    in
      terrorism E979.2
      war operations E993
        injury by fragments from E991.9
  stated as undetermined whether caused accidentally or purposely inflicted E985.5
  steam or water lines (in machinery) E921.0
  suicide (attempted) E955.5
  terrorism—*see* Terrorism, explosion
  torpedo E923.8
    in
      terrorism E979.0
      war operations E992
  transport accident—*see* categories E800-E848
  war operations—*see* War operations, explosion
  watercraft (boiler) E837
    causing drowning, submersion (after jumping from watercraft) E830

INDEX TO EXTERNAL CAUSES

Fall, falling

Exposure (weather) (conditions) (rain) (wind) E904.3
  with homicidal intent E968.4
  environmental
    to
      algae bloom E928.6
      blue-green algae bloom E928.6
      brown tide E928.6
      cyanobacteria bloom E928.6
      Florida red tide E928.6
      harmful algae
        and toxins E928.6
        bloom E928.6
      pfisteria piscicida E928.6
      red tide E928.6
  excessive E904.3
    cold (*see also* Cold, exposure to) E901.9
      self-inflicted—*see* Cold, exposure to, self-inflicted
    heat (*see also* Heat) E900.9
  fire—*see* Fire
  helpless person, infant, newborn due to abandonment or neglect E904.0
  noise E928.1
  prolonged in deep-freeze unit or refrigerator E901.1
  radiation—*see* Radiation
  resulting from transport accident—*see* categories E800-E848
  smoke from, due to
    fire—*see* Fire
  tobacco, second-hand E869.4
  vibration E928.2

F

Fall, falling (accidental) E888.9
  building E916
    burning E891.8
      private E890.8
  down
    escalator E880.0
    ladder E881.0
      in boat, ship, watercraft E833
    staircase E880.9
    stairs, steps—*see* Fall, from, stairs
  earth (with asphyxia or suffocation (by pressure)) (*see also* Earth, falling) E913.3
  from, off
    aircraft (at landing, take-off) (in-transit) (while alighting, boarding) E843
      resulting from accident to aircraft—*see* categories E840-E842
    animal (in sport or transport) E828
    animal-drawn vehicle E827
    balcony E882
    bed E884.4
    bicycle E826
    boat, ship, watercraft (into water) E832
      after accident to, collision, fire on E830
        and subsequently struck by (part of) boat E831
      and subsequently struck by (part of) boat E838
      burning, crushed, sinking E830
        and subsequently struck by (part of) boat E831
    bridge E882
    building E882
      burning (uncontrolled fire) E891.8
        in terrorism E979.3

Fall, falling—*continued*
    private E890.8
    bunk in boat, ship, watercraft E834
      due to accident to watercraft E831
    cable car (not on rails) E847
      on rails E829
    car—*see* Fall from motor vehicle
    chair E884.2
    cliff E884.1
    commode E884.6
    curb (sidewalk) E880.1
    elevation aboard ship E834
      due to accident to ship E831
    embankment E884.9
    escalator E880.0
    fire escape E882
    flagpole E882
    furniture NEC E884.5
    gangplank (into water) (*see also* Fall, from, boat) E832
      to deck, dock E834
    hammock on ship E834
      due to accident to watercraft E831
    haystack E884.9
    high place NEC E884.9
      stated as undetermined whether accidental or intentional—*see* Jumping, from, high place
    horse (in sport or transport) E828
    in-line skates E885.1
    ladder E881.0
      in boat, ship, watercraft E833
        due to accident to watercraft E831
    machinery—*see also* accident, machine
      not in operation E884.9
    motor vehicle (in motion) (on public highway) E818
      not on public highway E825
        stationary, except while alighting, boarding, entering, leaving E884.9
        while alighting, boarding, entering, leaving E824
      stationary, except while alighting, boarding, entering, leaving E884.9
      while alighting, boarding, entering, leaving, except off-road type motor vehicle E817
      off-road type—*see* Fall, from, off-road type motor vehicle
    nonmotor road vehicle (while alighting, boarding) NEC E829
      stationary, except while alighting, boarding, entering, leaving E884.9
    off road type motor vehicle (not on public highway) NEC E821
      on public highway E818
        while alighting, boarding, entering, leaving E817
    snow vehicle—*see* Fall from snow vehicle, motor-driven
    one
      deck to another on ship E834
        due to accident to ship E831
      level to another NEC E884.9
        boat, ship, or watercraft E834
          due to accident to watercraft E831
    pedal cycle E826
    playground equipment E884.0
    railway rolling stock, train, vehicle (while alighting, boarding) E804
      with

1511

Fall, falling

Fall, falling—*continued*
    collision (*see also* Collision, railway) E800
    derailment (*see also* Derailment, railway) E802
    explosion (*see also* Explosion, railway engine) E803
  rigging (aboard ship) E834
    due to accident to watercraft E831
  roller skates E885.1
  scaffolding E881.1
  scooter (nonmotorized) E885.0
  sidewalk (curb) E880.1
    moving E885.9
  skateboard E885.2
  skis E885.3
  snowboard E885.4
  snow vehicle, motor-driven (not on public highway) E820
    on public highway E818
      while alighting, boarding, entering, leaving E817
  stairs, steps E880.9
    boat, ship, watercraft E833
      due to accident to watercraft E831
    motor bus, motor vehicle—*see* Fall, from, motor vehicle, while alighting, boarding
    street car E829
  stationary vehicle NEC E884.9
  stepladder E881.0
  street car (while boarding, alighting) E829
    stationary, except while boarding or alighting E884.9
  structure NEC E882
    burning (uncontrolled fire) E891.8
      in terrorism E979.3
  table E884.9
  toilet E884.6
  tower E882
  tree E884.9
  turret E882
  vehicle NEC—*see also* Accident, vehicle NEC
    stationary E884.9
  viaduct E882
  wall E882
  wheelchair E884.3
  window E882
  in, on
    aircraft (at landing, take-off) (in-transit) E843
      resulting from accident to aircraft—*see* categories E840-E842
    boat, ship, watercraft E835
      due to accident to watercraft E831
      one level to another NEC E834
      on ladder, stairs E833
    cutting or piercing instrument or machine E888.0
    deck (of boat, ship, watercraft) E835
      due to accident to watercraft E831
    escalator E880.0
    gangplank E835
    glass, broken E888.0
    knife E888.0
    ladder E881.0
      in boat, ship, watercraft E833
        due to accident to watercraft E831
    object
      edged, pointed or sharp E888.0

INDEX TO EXTERNAL CAUSES

Fall, falling—*continued*
    other E888.1
  pitchfork E888.0
  railway rolling stock, train, vehicle (while alighting, boarding) E804
    with
      collision (*see also* Collision, railway) E800
      derailment (*see also* Derailment, railway) E802
      explosion (*see also* Explosion, railway engine) E803
  scaffolding E881.1
  scissors E888.0
  staircase, stairs, steps (*see also* Fall, from, stairs) E880.9
  street car E829
  water transport (*see also* Fall, in, boat) E835
  into
    cavity E883.9
    dock E883.9
      from boat, ship, watercraft (*see also* Fall, from, boat) E832
    hold (of ship) E834
      due to accident to watercraft E831
    hole E883.9
    manhole E883.2
    moving part of machinery—*see* Accident, machine
    opening in surface NEC E883.9
    pit E883.9
    quarry E883.9
    shaft E883.9
    storm drain E883.2
    tank E883.9
    water (with drowning or submersion) E910.9
    well E883.1
  late effect of NEC E929.3
  object (*see also* Hit by, object, falling) E916
  other E888.8
  over
    animal E885.9
    cliff E884.1
    embankment E884.9
    small object E885.9
  overboard (*see also* Fall, from, boat) E832
  resulting in striking against object E888.1
    sharp E888.0
  rock E916
  same level NEC E888.9
    aircraft (any kind) E843
      resulting from accident to aircraft—*see* categories E840-E842
    boat, ship, watercraft E835
      due to accident to, collision, watercraft E831
    from
      collision, pushing, shoving, by or with other person(s) E886.9
        as, or caused by, a crowd E917.6
          in sports E886.0
      in-line skates E885.1
      roller skates E885.1
      scooter (nonmotorized) E885.0
      skateboard E885.2
      skis E885.3
      slipping, stumbling, tripping E885.9
      snowboard E885.4
  snowslide E916
    as avalanche E909.2
  stone E916

INDEX TO EXTERNAL CAUSES   Forced landing

Fall, falling—*continued*
  through
    hatch (on ship) E834
      due to accident to watercraft E831
    roof E882
    window E882
  timber E916
  while alighting from, boarding, entering,
      leaving
    aircraft (any kind) E843
    motor bus, motor vehicle—*see* Fall, from,
      motor vehicle, while alighting, boarding
    nonmotor road vehicle NEC E829
    railway train E804
    street car E829
Fallen on by
  animal (horse) (not being ridden) E906.8
  being ridden (in sport or transport) E828
Fell or jumped from high place, so stated
  —*see* Jumping, from, high place
Felo-de-se (*see also* Suicide) E958.9
Fever
  heat—*see* Heat
  thermic—*see* Heat
Fight (hand) (fist) (foot) (*see also* Assault,
    fight) E960.0
Fire (accidental) (caused by great heat from
    appliance (electrical), hot object or hot
    substance) (secondary, resulting from
    explosion) E899
  conflagration—*see* Conflagration
  controlled, normal (in brazier, fireplace,
    furnace, or stove) (charcoal) (coal) (coke)
    (electric) (gas) (wood)
    bonfire E897
    brazier, not in building or structure E897
    in building or structure, except private
      dwelling (barn) (church) (convalescent or
      residential home) (factory) (farm
      outbuilding) (hospital) (hotel) (institution
      (educational) (dormitory) (residential))
      (private garage) (school) (shop) (store)
      (theatre) E896
    in private dwelling (apartment) (boarding
      house) (camping place) (caravan)
      (farmhouse) (home (private)) (house)
      (lodging house) (rooming house)
      (tenement) E895
    not in building or structure E897
    trash E897
  forest (uncontrolled) E892
  grass (uncontrolled) E892
  hay (uncontrolled) E892
  homicide (attempt) E968.0
    late effect of E969
  in, of, on, starting in E892
    aircraft (in transit) (powered) E841
      at landing, take-off E840
      stationary E892
      unpowered (balloon) (glider) E842
    balloon E842
    boat, ship, watercraft—*see* categories E830,
      E831, E837
    building or structure, except private dwelling
      (barn) (church) (convalescent or
      residential home) (factory) (farm
      outbuilding) (hospital) (hotel) (institution
      (educational) (dormitory) (residential))
      (school) (shop) (store) (theatre) (*see also*
      Conflagration, building or structure,
      except private dwelling) E891.9

Fire—*continued*
  forest (uncontrolled) E892
  glider E842
  grass (uncontrolled) E892
  hay (uncontrolled) E892
  lumber (uncontrolled) E892
  machinery—*see* Accident, machine
  mine (uncontrolled) E892
  motor vehicle (in motion) (on public
    highway) E818
    not on public highway E825
    stationary E892
  prairie (uncontrolled) E892
  private dwelling (apartment) (boarding
    house) (camping place) (caravan)
    (farmhouse) (home (private)) (house)
    (lodging house) (private garage) (rooming
    house) (tenement) (*see also*
    Conflagration, private dwelling) E890.9
  railway rolling stock, train, vehicle (*see also*
    Explosion, railway engine) E803
    stationary E892
  room NEC E898.1
  street car (in motion) E829
    stationary E892
  terrorism (by fire-producing device) E979.3
    fittings or furniture (burning building)
      (uncontrolled fire) E979.3
    from nuclear explosion E979.5
  transport vehicle, stationary NEC E892
  tunnel (uncontrolled) E892
  war operations (by fire-producing device or
    conventional weapon) E990.9
    from nuclear explosion E996
    petrol bomb E990.0
  late effect of NEC E929.4
  lumber (uncontrolled) E892
  mine (uncontrolled) E892
  prairie (uncontrolled) E892
  self-inflicted (unspecified whether accidental
    or intentional) E988.1
    stated as intentional, purposeful E958.1
  specified NEC E898.1
    with
      conflagration—*see* Conflagration
      ignition (of)
        clothing—*see* Ignition, clothes
        highly inflammable material (benzine)
          (fat) (gasoline) (kerosene) (paraffin)
          (petrol) E894
  started by other person
    stated as
      with intent to injure or kill E968.0
      undetermined whether or not with intent to
        injure or kill E988.1
  suicide (attempted) E958.1
    late effect of E959
  tunnel (uncontrolled) E892
Fireball effects from nuclear explosion
  in
    terrorism E979.5
    war operations E996
Fireworks (explosion) E923.0
Flash burns from explosion (*see also*
    Explosion) E923.9
Flood (any injury) (resulting from storm)
    E908.2
  caused by collapse of dam or manmade
    structure E909.3
Forced landing (aircraft) E840

1513

Foreign body, object or material

Foreign body, object or material (entrance into (accidental))
  air passage (causing injury) E915
    with asphyxia, obstruction, suffocation E912
      food or vomitus E911
    nose (with asphyxia, obstruction, suffocation) E912
      causing injury without asphyxia, obstruction, suffocation E915
  alimentary canal (causing injury) (with obstruction) E915
    with asphyxia, obstruction respiratory passage, suffocation E912
      food E911
    mouth E915
      with asphyxia, obstruction, suffocation E912
        food E911
    pharynx E915
      with asphyxia, obstruction, suffocation E912
        food E911
  aspiration (with asphyxia, obstruction respiratory passage, suffocation) E912
    causing injury without asphyxia, obstruction respiratory passage, suffocation E915
    food (regurgitated) (vomited) E911
      causing injury without asphyxia, obstruction respiratory passage, suffocation E915
    mucus (not of newborn) E912
    phlegm E912
  bladder (causing injury or obstruction) E915
  bronchus, bronchi—*see* Foreign body, air passages
  conjunctival sac E914
  digestive system—*see* Foreign body, alimentary canal
  ear (causing injury or obstruction) E915
  esophagus (causing injury or obstruction) (*see also* Foreign body, alimentary canal) E915
  eye (any part) E914
  eyelid E914
  hairball (stomach) (with obstruction) E915
  ingestion—*see* Foreign body, alimentary canal
  inhalation—*see* Foreign body, aspiration
  intestine (causing injury or obstruction) E915
  iris E914
  lacrimal apparatus E914
  larynx—*see* Foreign body, air passage
  late effect of NEC E929.8
  lung—*see* Foreign body, air passage
  mouth—*see* Foreign body, alimentary canal, mouth
  nasal passage—*see* Foreign body, air passage, nose
  nose—*see* Foreign body, air passage, nose
  ocular muscle E914
  operation wound (left in)—*see* Misadventure, foreign object
  orbit E914
  pharynx—*see* Foreign body, alimentary canal, pharynx
  rectum (causing injury or obstruction) E915
  stomach (hairball) (causing injury or obstruction) E915
  tear ducts or glands E914
  trachea—*see* Foreign body, air passage
  urethra (causing injury or obstruction) E915
  vagina (causing injury or obstruction) E915

INDEX TO EXTERNAL CAUSES

Found dead, injured
  from exposure (to)—*see* Exposure
  on
    public highway E819
    railway right of way E807
Fracture (circumstances unknown or unspecified) E887
  due to specified external means—*see* manner of accident
  late effect of NEC E929.3
  occurring in water transport NEC E835
Freezing —*see* Cold, exposure to
Frostbite E901.0
  due to manmade conditions E901.1
Frozen —*see* Cold, exposure to

G

Garrotting, homicidal (attempted) E963
Gored E906.8
Gunshot wound (*see also* Shooting) E922.9

H

Hailstones, injury by E904.3
Hairball (stomach) (with obstruction) E915
Hanged himself (*see also* Hanging, self-inflicted) E983.0
Hang gliding E842
Hanging (accidental) E913.8
  caused by other person
    in accidental circumstances E913.8
    stated as
      intentional, homicidal E963
      undetermined whether accidental or intentional E983.0
  homicide (attempt) E963
  in bed or cradle E913.0
  legal execution E978
  self-inflicted (unspecified whether accidental or intentional) E983.0
    in accidental circumstances E913.8
    stated as intentional, purposeful E953.0
  stated as undetermined whether accidental or intentional E983.0
  suicidal (attempt) E953.0
Heat (apoplexy) (collapse) (cramps) (effects of) (excessive) (exhaustion) (fever) (prostration) (stroke) E900.9
  due to
    manmade conditions (listed in E900.1, except boat, ship, watercraft) E900.1
    weather (conditions) E900.0
  from
    electric heating apparatus causing burning E924.8
    nuclear explosion
      in
        terrorism E979.5
        war operations E996
  generated in, boiler, engine, evaporator, fire room of boat, ship, watercraft E838
  inappropriate in local application or packing in medical or surgical procedure E873.5
  late effect of NEC E989
Hemorrhage
  delayed following medical or surgical treatment without mention of misadventure—*see* Reaction, abnormal
  during medical or surgical treatment as misadventure—*see* Misadventure, cut

1514

INDEX TO EXTERNAL CAUSES — Hypothermia

High
  altitude, effects E902.9
  level of radioactivity, effects—*see* Radiation
  pressure effects—*see also* Effects of, air pressure
    from rapid descent in water (causing caisson or divers' disease, palsy, or paralysis) E902.2
  temperature, effects—*see* Heat

Hit, hitting (accidental) by
  aircraft (propeller) (without accident to aircraft) E844
    unpowered E842
  avalanche E909.2
  being thrown against object in or part of
    motor vehicle (in motion) (on public highway) E818
      not on public highway E825
    nonmotor road vehicle NEC E829
    street car E829
  boat, ship, watercraft
    after fall from watercraft E838
      damaged, involved in accident E831
      while swimming, water skiing E838
  bullet (*see also* Shooting) E922.9
    from air gun E922.4
    in
      terrorism E979.4
      war operations E991.2
        rubber E991.0
  flare, Very pistol (*see also* Shooting) E922.8
  hailstones E904.3
  landslide E909.2
  law-enforcing agent (on duty) E975
    with blunt object (baton) (night stick) (stave) (truncheon) E973
  machine—*see* Accident, machine
  missile
    firearm (*see also* Shooting) E922.9
    in
      terrorism—*see* Terrorism, missle
      war operations—*see* War operations, missile
  motor vehicle (on public highway) (traffic accident) E814
    not on public highway, nontraffic accident E822
  nonmotor road vehicle NEC E829
  object
    falling E916
      from, in, on
        aircraft E844
          due to accident to aircraft—*see* categories E840-E842
          unpowered E842
        boat, ship, watercraft E838
          due to accident to watercraft E831
        building E916
          burning E891.8
            in terrorism E979.3
            private E890.8
        cataclysmic
          earth surface movement or eruption E909.9
          storm E908.9
        cave-in E916
          with asphyxiation or suffocation (*see also* Suffocation, due to, cave-in) E913.3
        earthquake E909.0

Hit, hitting—*continued*
    motor vehicle (in motion) (on public highway) E818
      not on public highway E825
      stationary E916
    nonmotor road vehicle NEC E829
    pedal cycle E826
    railway rolling stock, train, vehicle E806
    street car E829
    structure, burning NEC E891.8
    vehicle, stationary E916
  moving NEC—*see* Striking against, object
  projected NEC—*see* Striking against, object
  set in motion by
    compressed air or gas, spring, striking, throwing—*see* Striking against, object
    explosion—*see* Explosion
  thrown into, on, or towards
    motor vehicle (in motion) (on public highway) E818
      not on public highway E825
    nonmotor road vehicle NEC E829
    pedal cycle E826
    street car E829
  off-road type motor vehicle (not on public highway) E821
    on public highway E814
  other person(s) E917.9
    with blunt or thrown object E917.9
      in sports E917.0
        with subsequent fall E917.5
      intentionally, homicidal E968.2
    as, or caused by, a crowd E917.1
      with subsequent fall E917.6
    in sports E917.0
  pedal cycle E826
  police (on duty) E975
    with blunt object (baton) (nightstick) (stave) (truncheon) E973
  railway, rolling stock, train, vehicle (part of) E805
  shot—*see* Shooting
  snow vehicle, motor-driven (not on public highway) E820
    on public highway E814
  street car E829
  vehicle NEC—*see* Accident, vehicle NEC

Homicide, homicidal (attempt) (justifiable) (*see also* Assault) E968.9

Hot
  liquid, object, substance, accident caused by—*see also* Accident, caused by, hot, by type of substance
    late effect of E929.8
  place, effects—*see* Heat
  weather, effects E900.0

Humidity, causing problem E904.3

Hunger E904.1
  resulting from
    abandonment or neglect E904.0
    transport accident—*see* categories E800-E848

Hurricane (any injury) E908.0

Hypobarism, hypobaropathy —*see* Effects of, air pressure

Hypothermia —*see* Cold, exposure to

I

Ictus
  caloris—*see* Heat
  solaris E900.0
Ignition (accidental)
  anesthetic gas in operating theatre E923.2
  bedclothes
    with
      conflagration—*see* Conflagration
      ignition (of)
        clothing—*see* Ignition, clothes
        highly inflammable material (benzine)
          (fat) (gasoline) (kerosene) (paraffin)
          (petrol) E894
  benzine E894
  clothes, clothing (from controlled fire) (in
      building) E893.9
    with conflagration—*see* Conflagration
    from
      bonfire E893.2
      highly inflammable material E894
      sources or material as listed in E893.8
      trash fire E893.2
      uncontrolled fire—*see* Conflagration
    in
      private dwelling E893.0
      specified building or structure, except
          private dwelling E893.1
    not in building or structure E893.2
  explosive material—*see* Explosion
  fat E894
  gasoline E894
  kerosene E894
  material
    explosive—*see* Explosion
    highly inflammable E894
      with conflagration—*see* Conflagration
      with explosion E923.2
  nightdress—*see* Ignition, clothes
  paraffin E894
  petrol E894
Immersion —*see* Submersion
Implantation of quills of porcupine E906.8
Inanition (from) E904.9
  hunger—*see* Lack of, food
  resulting from homicidal intent E968.4
  thirst—*see* Lack of, water
Inattention after, at birth E904.0
  homicidal, infanticidal intent E968.4
Infanticide (*see also* Assault)
Ingestion
  foreign body (causing injury) (with
      obstruction)—*see* Foreign body, alimentary
      canal
  poisonous substance NEC—*see* Table of drugs
      and chemicals
Inhalation
  excessively cold substance, manmade E901.1
  foreign body—*see* Foreign body, aspiration
  liquid air, hydrogen, nitrogen E901.1
  mucus, not of newborn (with asphyxia,
      obstruction respiratory passage,
      suffocation) E912
  phlegm (with asphyxia, obstruction respiratory
      passage, suffocation) E912
  poisonous gas—*see* Table of drugs and chemicals
  smoke from, due to
    fire —*see* Fire
    tobacco, second-hand E869.4
  vomitus (with asphyxia, obstruction respiratory
      passage, suffocation) E911

Injury, injured (accidental(ly)) NEC E928.9
  by, caused by, from
    air rifle (B-B gun) E922.4
    animal (not being ridden) NEC E906.9
      being ridden (in sport or transport) E828
    assault (*see also* Assault) E968.9
    avalanche E909.2
    bayonet (*see also* Bayonet wound) E920.3
    being thrown against some part of, or object
        in
      motor vehicle (in motion) (on public
          highway) E818
        not on public highway E825
      nonmotor road vehicle NEC E829
      off-road motor vehicle NEC E821
      railway train E806
      snow vehicle, motor-driven E820
      street car E829
    bending E927
    bite, human E928.3
    broken glass E920.8
    bullet—*see* Shooting
    cave-in (*see also* Suffocation, due to,
        cave-in) E913.3
      without asphyxiation or suffocation E916
    cloudburst E908.8
    cutting or piercing instrument (*see also* Cut)
        E920.9
    cyclone E908.1
    earth surface movement or eruption E909.9
    earthquake E909.0
    electric current (*see also* Electric shock)
        E925.9
    explosion (*see also* Explosion) E923.9
    fire—*see* Fire
    flare, Very pistol E922.8
    flood E908.2
    foreign body—*see* Foreign body
    hailstones E904.3
    hurricane E908.0
    landslide E909.2
    law-enforcing agent, police, in course of
        legal intervention—*see* Legal intervention
    lightning E907
    live rail or live wire—*see* Electric shock
    machinery—*see also* Accident, machine
      aircraft, without accident to aircraft E844
      boat, ship, watercraft (deck) (engine room)
          (galley) (laundry) (loading) E836
    missile
      explosive E923.8
      firearm—*see* Shooting
      in
        terrorism—*see* Terrorism, missile
        war operations—*see* War operations,
            missile
    moving part of motor vehicle (in motion)
        (on public highway) E818
      not on public highway, nontraffic accident
          E825
      while alighting, boarding, entering,
          leaving—*see* Fall, from, motor vehicle,
          while alighting, boarding
    nail E920.8
    needle (sewing) E920.4
      hypodermic E920.5
    noise E928.1
    object
      fallen on

INDEX TO EXTERNAL CAUSES — Jumping

Injury, injured—*continued*
    motor vehicle (in motion) (on public highway) E818
      not on public highway E825
    falling—*see* Hit by, object, falling
    paintball gun E922.5
    radiation—*see* Radiation
    railway rolling stock, train, vehicle (part of) E805
      door or window E806
    rotating propeller, aircraft E844
    rough landing of off-road type motor vehicle (after leaving ground or rough terrain) E821
      snow vehicle E820
    saber (*see also* Wound, saber) E920.3
    shot—*see* Shooting
    sound waves E928.1
    splinter or sliver, wood E920.8
    storm E908.9
    straining E927
    street car (door) E829
    suicide (attempt) E958.9
    sword E920.3
    terrorism—*see* Terrorism
    third rail—*see* Electric shock
    thunderbolt E907
    tidal wave E909.4
      caused by storm E908.0
    tornado E908.1
    torrential rain E908.2
    twisting E927
    vehicle NEC—*see* Accident, vehicle NEC
    vibration E928.2
    volcanic eruption E909.1
    weapon burst, in war operations E993
    weightlessness (in spacecraft, real or simulated) E928.0
    wood splinter or sliver E920.8
  due to
    civil insurrection—*see* War operations
      occurring after cessation of hostilities E998
    terrorism—*see* Terrorism
    war operations—*see* War operations
      occurring after cessation of hostilities E998
  homicidal (*see also* Assault) E968.9
  in, on
    civil insurrection—*see* War operations
    fight E960.0
    parachute descent (voluntary) (without accident to aircraft) E844
      with accident to aircraft—*see* categories E840-E842
    public highway E819
    railway right of way E807
    terrorism—*see* Terrorism
    war operations—*see* War operations
  inflicted (by)
    in course of arrest (attempted), suppression of disturbance, maintenance of order, by law-enforcing agents—*see* Legal intervention
    law-enforcing agent (on duty)—*see* Legal intervention
    other person
      stated as
        accidental E928.9
        homicidal, intentional—*see* Assault

Injury, injured—*continued*
        undetermined whether accidental or intentional—*see* Injury, stated as undetermined
    police (on duty)—*see* Legal intervention
  late effect of E929.9
  purposely (inflicted) by other person(s)—*see* Assault
  self-inflicted (unspecified whether accidental or intentional) E988.9
    stated as
      accidental E928.9
      intentionally, purposely E958.9
  specified cause NEC E928.8
  stated as
    undetermined whether accidentally or purposely inflicted (by) E988.9
      cut (any part of body) E986
      cutting or piercing instrument (classifiable to E920) E986
      drowning E984
      explosive(s) (missile) E985.5
      falling from high place E987.9
        manmade structure, except residential E987.1
        natural site E987.2
        residential premises E987.0
      hanging E983.0
      knife E986
      late effect of E989
      puncture (any part of body) E986
      shooting—*see* Shooting, stated as undetermined whether accidental or intentional
      specified means NEC E988.8
      stab (any part of body) E986
      strangulation—*see* Suffocation, stated as undetermined whether accidental or intentional
      submersion E984
      suffocation—*see* Suffocation, stated as undetermined whether accidental or intentional
  to child due to criminal abortion E968.8
Insufficient nourishment —*see also* Lack of, food
  homicidal intent E968.4
Insulation, effects —*see* Heat
Interruption of respiration by
  food lodged in esophagus E911
  foreign body, except food, in esophagus E912
Intervention, legal —*see* Legal intervention
Intoxication, drug or poison —*see* Table of drugs and chemicals
Irradiation —*see* Radiation

J

Jammed (accidentally)
  between objects (moving) (stationary and moving) E918
  in object E918
Jumped or fell from high place, so stated
  —*see Jumping, from, high place, stated as in undetermined circumstances*
Jumping
  before train, vehicle or other moving object (unspecified whether accidental or intentional) E988.0
    stated as

1517

Jumping—*continued*
- intentional, purposeful E958.0
- suicidal (attempt) E958.0
- from
  - aircraft
    - by parachute (voluntarily) (without accident to aircraft) E844
    - due to accident to aircraft—*see* categories E840-E842
  - boat, ship, watercraft (into water)
    - after accident to, fire on, watercraft E830
      - and subsequently struck by (part of) boat E831
    - burning, crushed, sinking E830
      - and subsequently struck by (part of) boat E831
    - voluntarily, without accident (to boat) with injury other than drowning or submersion E883.0
  - building—*see also* Jumping, from, high place
    - burning (uncontrolled fire) E891.8
    - in terrorism E979.3
    - private E890.8
  - cable car (not on rails) E847
    - on rails E829
  - high place
    - in accidental circumstances or in sport—*see* categories E880-E884
    - stated as
      - with intent to injure self E957.9
        - man-made structures NEC E957.1
        - natural sites E957.2
        - residential premises E957.0
      - in undetermined circumstances E987.9
        - man-made structures NEC E987.1
        - natural sites E987.2
        - residential premises E987.0
      - suicidal (attempt) E957.9
        - man-made structures NEC E957.1
        - natural sites E957.2
        - residential premises E957.0
  - motor vehicle (in motion) (on public highway)—*see* Fall, from, motor vehicle
  - nonmotor road vehicle NEC E829
  - street car E829
  - structure—*see also* Jumping, from, high place
    - burning NEC (uncontrolled fire) E891.8
    - in terrorism E979.3
  - into water
    - with injury other than drowning or submersion E883.0
    - drowning or submersion—*see* Submersion
  - from, off, watercraft—*see* Jumping, from, boat

Justifiable homicide —*see* Assault

K

Kicked by
- animal E906.8
- person(s) (accidentally) E917.9
  - with intent to injure or kill E960.0
  - as, or caused by a crowd E917.1
    - with subsequent fall E917.6
  - in fight E960.0
  - in sports E917.0
    - with subsequent fall E917.5

Kicking against
- object (moving) E917.9
  - in sports E917.0
    - with subsequent fall E917.5
  - stationary E917.4
    - with subsequent fall E917.8
- person—*see* Striking against, person

Killed, killing (accidentally) NEC (*see also* Injury) E928.9
- in
  - action—*see* War operations
  - brawl, fight (hand) (fists) (foot) E960.0
    - by weapon—*see also* Assault
      - cutting, piercing E966
      - firearm—*see* Shooting, homicide
- self
  - stated as
    - accident E928.9
    - suicide—*see* Suicide
  - unspecified whether accidental or suicidal E988.9

Knocked down (accidentally) (by) NEC E928.9
- animal (not being ridden) E906.8
  - being ridden (in sport or transport) E828
- blast from explosion (*see also* Explosion) E923.9
- crowd, human stampede E917.6
- late effect of—*see* Late effect
- person (accidentally) E917.9
  - in brawl, fight E960.0
  - in sports E917.5
- transport vehicle—*see* vehicle involved under Hit by
- while boxing E917.5

L

Laceration NEC E928.9
Lack of
- air (refrigerator or closed place), suffocation by E913.2
- care (helpless person) (infant) (newborn) E904.0
  - homicidal intent E968.4
- food except as result of transport accident E904.1
  - helpless person, infant, newborn due to abandonment or neglect E904.0
- water except as result of transport accident E904.2
  - helpless person, infant, newborn due to abandonment or neglect E904.0

Landslide E909.2
- falling on, hitting
  - motor vehicle (any) (in motion) (on or off public highway) E909.2
  - railway rolling stock, train, vehicle E909.2

Late effect of
- accident NEC (accident classifiable to E928.9) E929.9
  - specified NEC (accident classifiable to E910-E928.8) E929.8
- assault E969
- fall, accidental (accident classifiable to E880-E888) E929.3
- fire, accident caused by (accident classifiable to E890-E899) E929.4
- homicide, attempt (any means) E969
- injury due to terrorism E999.1

INDEX TO EXTERNAL CAUSES   Misadventure(s)

Late effect of—*continued*
  injury undetermined whether accidentally or purposely inflicted (injury classifiable to E980-E988) E989
  legal intervention (injury classifiable to E970-E976) E977
  medical or surgical procedure, test or therapy as, or resulting in, or from
    abnormal or delayed reaction or complication—*see* Reaction, abnormal
    misadventure—*see* Misadventure
  motor vehicle accident (accident classifiable to E810-E825) E929.0
  natural or environmental factor, accident due to (accident classifiable to E900-E909) E929.5
  poisoning, accidental (accident classifiable to E850-E858, E860-E869) E929.2
  suicide, attempt (any means) E959
  transport accident NEC (accident classifiable to E800-E807, E826-E838, E840-E848) E929.1
  war operations, injury due to (injury classifiable to E990-E998) E999.0
Launching pad accident E845
Legal
  execution, any method E978
  intervention (by) (injury from) E976
    baton E973
    bayonet E974
    blow E975
    blunt object (baton) (nightstick) (stave) (truncheon) E973
    cutting or piercing instrument E974
    dynamite E971
    execution, any method E973
    explosive(s) (shell) E971
    firearms(s) E970
    gas (asphyxiation) (poisoning) (tear) E972
    grenade E971
    late effect of E977
    machine gun E970
    manhandling E975
    mortar bomb E971
    nightstick E973
    revolver E970
    rifle E970
    specified means NEC E975
    stabbing E974
    stave E973
    truncheon E973
Lifting, injury in E927
Lightning (shock) (stroke) (struck by) E907
Liquid (noncorrosive) in eye E914
  corrosive E924.1
Loss of control
  motor vehicle (on public highway) (without antecedent collision) E816
    with
      antecedent collision on public highway—*see* Collision, motor vehicle
      involving any object, person or vehicle not on public highway E816
        on public highway—*see* Collision, motor vehicle
    not on public highway, nontraffic accident E825
      with antecedent collision—*see* Collision, motor vehicle, not on public highway
  off-road type motor vehicle (not on public highway) E821

Loss of control—*continued*
  on public highway—*see* Loss of control, motor vehicle
  snow vehicle, motor-driven (not on public highway) E820
    on public highway—*see* Loss of control, motor vehicle
Lost at sea E832
  with accident to watercraft E830
  in war operations E995
Low
  pressure, effects—*see* Effects of, air pressure
  temperature, effects—*see* Cold, exposure to
Lying before train, vehicle or other moving object (unspecified whether accidental or intentional) E988.0
  stated as intentional, purposeful, suicidal (attempt) E958.0
Lynching (*see also* Assault) E968.9

M

Malfunction, atomic power plant in water transport E838
Mangled (accidentally) NEC E928.9
Manhandling (in brawl, fight) E960.0
  legal intervention E975
Manslaughter (nonaccidental)—*see* Assault
Marble in nose E912
Mauled by animal E906.8
Medical procedure, complication of
  delayed or as an abnormal reaction without mention of misadventure—*see* Reaction, abnormal
  due to or as a result of misadventure—*see* Misadventure
Melting of fittings and furniture in burning
  in terrorism E979.3
Minamata disease E865.2
Misadventure(s) to patient(s) during surgical or medical care E876.9
  contaminated blood, fluid, drug or biological substance (presence of agents and toxins as listed in E875) E875.9
    administered (by) NEC E875.9
      infusion E875.0
      injection E875.1
      specified means NEC E875.2
      transfusion E875.0
      vaccination E875.1
  cut, cutting, puncture, perforation or hemorrhage (accidental) (inadvertent) (inappropriate) (during) E870.9
    aspiration of fluid or tissue (by puncture or catheterization, except heart) E870.5
    biopsy E870.8
      needle (aspirating) E870.5
    blood sampling E870.5
    catheterization E870.5
      heart E870.6
    dialysis (kidney) E870.2
    endoscopic examination E870.4
    enema E870.7
    infusion E870.1
    injection E870.3
    lumbar puncture E870.5
    needle biopsy E870.5
    paracentesis, abdominal E870.5
    perfusion E870.2
    specified procedure NEC E870.8

1519

Misadventure(s)

INDEX TO EXTERNAL CAUSES

Misadventure(s)—*continued*
- surgical operation E870.0
- thoracentesis E870.5
- transfusion E870.1
- vaccination E870.3
- excessive amount of blood or other fluid during transfusion or infusion E873.0
- failure
  - in dosage E873.9
    - electroshock therapy E873.4
    - inappropriate temperature (too hot or too cold) in local application and packing E873.5
  - infusion
    - excessive amount of fluid E873.0
    - incorrect dilution of fluid E873.1
  - insulin-shock therapy E873.4
  - nonadministration of necessary drug or medicinal E873.6
  - overdose—*see also* Overdose
    - radiation, in therapy E873.2
  - radiation
    - inadvertent exposure of patient (receiving radiation for test or therapy) E873.3
    - not receiving radiation for test or therapy—*see* Radiation
    - overdose E873.2
  - specified procedure NEC 873.8
  - transfusion
    - excessive amount of blood E873.0
  - mechanical, of instrument or apparatus (during procedure) E874.9
    - aspiration of fluid or tissue (by puncture or catheterization, except of heart) E874.4
    - biopsy E874.8
      - needle (aspirating) E874.4
    - blood sampling E874.4
    - catheterization E874.4
      - heart E874.5
    - dialysis (kidney) E874.2
    - endoscopic examination E874.3
    - enema E874.8
    - infusion E874.1
    - injection E874.8
    - lumbar puncture E874.4
    - needle biopsy E874.4
    - paracentesis, abdominal E874.4
    - perfusion E874.2
    - specified procedure NEC E874.8
    - surgical operation E874.0
    - thoracentesis E874.4
    - transfusion E874.1
    - vaccination E874.8
  - sterile precautions (during procedure) E872.9
    - aspiration of fluid or tissue (by puncture or catheterization, except heart) E872.5
    - biopsy E872.8
      - needle (aspirating) E872.5
    - blood sampling E872.5
    - catheterization E872.5
      - heart E872.6
    - dialysis (kidney) E872.2
    - endoscopic examination E872.4
    - enema E872.8
    - infusion E872.1
    - injection E872.3
    - lumbar puncture E872.5
    - needle biopsy E872.5
    - paracentesis, abdominal E872.5
    - perfusion E872.2

Misadventure(s)—*continued*
- removal of catheter or packing E872.8
- specified procedure NEC E872.8
- surgical operation E872.0
- thoracentesis E872.5
- transfusion E872.1
- vaccination E872.3
- suture or ligature during surgical procedure E876.2
- to introduce or to remove tube or instrument E876.4
- foreign object left in body—*see* Misadventure, foreign object
- foreign object left in body (during procedure) E871.9
  - aspiration of fluid or tissue (by puncture or catheterization, except heart) E871.5
  - biopsy E871.8
    - needle (aspirating) E871.5
  - blood sampling E871.5
  - catheterization E871.5
    - heart E871.6
  - dialysis (kidney) E871.2
  - endoscopic examination E871.4
  - enema E871.8
  - infusion E871.1
  - injection E871.3
  - lumbar puncture E871.5
  - needle biopsy E871.5
  - paracentesis, abdominal E871.5
  - perfusion E871.2
  - removal of catheter or packing E871.7
  - specified procedure NEC E871.8
  - surgical operation E871.0
  - thoracentesis E871.5
  - transfusion E871.1
  - vaccination E871.3
- hemorrhage—*see* Misadventure, cut
- inadvertent exposure of patient to radiation (being received for test or therapy) E873.3
- inappropriate
  - operation performed E876.5
  - temperature (too hot or too cold) in local application or packing E873.5
- infusion—*see also* Misadventure, by specific type, infusion
  - excessive amount of fluid E873.0
  - incorrect dilution of fluid E873.1
  - wrong fluid E876.1
- mismatched blood in transfusion E876.0
- nonadministration of necessary drug or medicinal E873.6
- overdose—*see also* Overdose
  - radiation, in therapy E873.2
- perforation—*see* Misadventure, cut
- performance of inappropriate operation E876.5
- puncture—*see* Misadventure, cut
- specified type NEC E876.8
  - failure
    - suture or ligature during surgical operation E876.2
    - to introduce or to remove tube or instrument E876.4
      - foreign object left in body E871.9
  - infusion of wrong fluid E876.1
  - performance of inappropriate operation E876.5
- transfusion of mismatched blood E876.0
- wrong
  - fluid in infusion E876.1

1520

INDEX TO EXTERNAL CAUSES   Overturning

Misadventure(s)—*continued*
   placement of endotracheal tube during
      anesthetic procedure E876.3
   transfusion—*see also* Misadventure, by
      specific type, transfusion
     excessive amount of blood E873.0
     mismatched blood E876.0
   wrong
     drug given in error—*see* Table of drugs and
       chemicals
     fluid in infusion E876.1
     placement of endotracheal tube during
       anesthetic procedure E876.3
Motion (effects) E903
   sickness E903
Mountain sickness E902.0
**Mucus aspiration or inhalation, not of
   newborn** (with asphyxia, obstruction
   respiratory passage, suffocation) E912
Mudslide of cataclysmic nature E909.2
Murder (attempt) (*see also* Assault) E968.9

N

Nail, injury by E920.8
Needlestick (sewing needle) E920.4
   hypodermic E920.5
Neglect —*see also* Privation
   criminal E968.4
   homicidal intent E968.4
Noise (causing injury) (pollution) E928.1

O

Object
   falling
     from, in, on, hitting
      aircraft E844
       due to accident to aircraft—*see*
        categories E840-E842
      machinery—*see also* Accident, machine
       not in operation E916
      motor vehicle (in motion) (on public
       highway) E818
       not on public highway E825
       stationary E916
      nonmotor road vehicle NEC E829
      pedal cycle E826
      person E916
      railway rolling stock, train, vehicle E806
      street car E829
      watercraft E838
       due to accident to watercraft E831
   set in motion by
     accidental explosion of pressure vessel—*see*
       category E921
     firearm—*see* category E922
     machine(ry)—*see* Accident, machine
     transport vehicle—*see* categories E800-E848
   thrown from, in, on, towards
     aircraft E844
     cable car (not on rails) E847
       on rails E829
     motor vehicle (in motion) (on public
       highway) E818
       not on public highway E825
     nonmotor road vehicle NEC E829
     pedal cycle E826
     street car E829
     vehicle NEC—*see* Accident, vehicle NEC

Obstruction
   air passages, larynx, respiratory passages
     by
      external means NEC—*see* Suffocation
      food, any type (regurgitated) (vomited)
       E911
      material or object, except food E912
      mucus E912
      phlegm E912
      vomitus E911
   digestive tract, except mouth or pharynx
     by
      food, any type E915
      foreign body (any) E915
   esophagus
     food E911
     foreign body, except food E912
     without asphyxia or obstruction of
       respiratory passage E915
   mouth or pharynx
     by
      food, any type E911
      material or object, except food E912
   respiration—*see* Obstruction, air passages
Oil in eye E914
Overdose
   anesthetic (drug)—*see* Table of drugs and
     chemicals
   drug—*see* Table of drugs and chemicals
Overexertion (lifting) (pulling) (pushing) E927
Overexposure (accidental) (to)
   cold (*see also* Cold, exposure to) E901.9
     due to manmade conditions E901.1
   heat (*see also* Heat) E900.9
   radiation—*see* Radiation
   radioactivity—*see* Radiation
   sun, except sunburn E900.0
   weather—*see* Exposure
   wind—*see* Exposure
Overheated (*see also* Heat) E900.9
Overlaid E913.0
Overturning (accidental)
   animal-drawn vehicle E827
   boat, ship, watercraft
     causing
      drowning, submersion E830
      injury except drowning, submersion E831
   machinery—*see* Accident, machine
   motor vehicle (*see also* Loss of control, motor
     vehicle) E816
     with antecedent collision on public
       highway—*see* Collision, motor vehicle
     not on public highway, nontraffic accident
      E825
      with antecedent collision—*see* Collision,
       motor vehicle, not on public highway
   nonmotor road vehicle NEC E829
   off-road type motor vehicle—*see* Loss of
     control, off-road type motor vehicle
   pedal cycle E826
   railway rolling stock, train, vehicle (*see also*
     Derailment, railway) E802
   street car E829
   vehicle NEC—*see* Accident, vehicle NEC

P

Palsy, divers' E902.2
Parachuting (voluntary) (without accident to aircraft) E844
  due to accident to aircraft—*see* categories E840-E842
Paralysis
  divers' E902.2
  lead or saturnine E866.0
  from pesticide NEC E863.4
Pecked by bird E906.8
Phlegm aspiration or inhalation (with asphyxia, obstruction respiratory passage, suffocation) E912
Piercing (*see also* Cut) E920.9
Pinched
  between objects (moving) (stationary and moving) E918
  in object E918
Pinned under
  machine(ry)—*see* Accident, machine
Place of occurrence of accident —*see* Accident (to), occurring (at) (in)
Plumbism E866.0
  from insecticide NEC E863.4
Poisoning (accidental) (by)—*see also* Table of drugs and chemicals
  carbon monoxide
    generated by
      aircraft in transit E844
      motor vehicle
        in motion (on public highway) E818
        not on public highway E825
      watercraft (in transit) (not in transit) E838
  caused by injection of poisons or toxins into or through skin by plant thorns, spines, or other mechanism E905.7
  marine or sea plants E905.6
  fumes or smoke due to
    conflagration—*see* Conflagration
    explosion or fire—*see* Fire
    ignition—*see* Ignition
  gas
    in legal intervention E972
    legal execution, by E978
    on watercraft E838
    used as anesthetic—*see* Table of drugs and chemicals
  in
    terrorism (chemical weapons) E979.7
    war operations E997.2
  late effect of—*see* Late effect
  legal
    execution E978
    intervention
      by gas E972
Pressure, external, causing asphyxia, suffocation (*see also* Suffocation) E913.9
Privation E904.9
  food (*see also* Lack of, food) E904.1
  helpless person, infant, newborn due to abandonment or neglect E904.0
  late effect of NEC E929.5
  resulting from transport accident—*see* categories E800-E848
  water (*see also* Lack of, water) E904.2
Projected objects, striking against or struck by —*see* Striking against, object

Prolonged stay in
  high altitude (causing conditions as listed in E902.0) E902.0
  weightless environment E928.0
Prostration
  heat—*see* Heat
Pulling, injury in E927
Puncture, puncturing (*see also* Cut) E920.9
  by
    plant thorns or spines E920.8
      toxic reaction E905.7
        marine or sea plants E905.6
    sea-urchin spine E905.6
Pushing (injury in) (overexertion) E927
  by other person(s) (accidental) E917.9
    as, or caused by, a crowd, human stampede E917.1
      with subsequent fall E917.6
    before moving vehicle or object
      stated as
        intentional, homicidal E968.5
        undetermined whether accidental or intentional E988.8
  from
    high place
      in accidental circumstances—*see* categories E880-E884
      stated as
        intentional, homicidal E968.1
        undetermined whether accidental or intentional E987.9
        man-made structure, except residential E987.1
        natural site E987.2
        residential E987.0
    motor vehicle (*see also* Fall, from, motor vehicle) E818
      stated as
        intentional, homicidal E968.5
        undetermined whether accidental or intentional E988.8
  in sports E917.0
    with fall E886.0
  with fall E886.9
    in sports E886.0

R

Radiation (exposure to) E926.9
  abnormal reaction to medical test or therapy E879.2
  arc lamps E926.2
  atomic power plant (malfunction) NEC E926.9
    in water transport E838
  electromagnetic, ionizing E926.3
  gamma rays E926.3
  in
    terrorism (from or following nuclear explosion) (direct) (secondary) E979.5
      laser E979.8
    war operations (from or following nuclear explosion) (direct) (secondary) E996
      laser(s) E997.0
    water transport E838
  inadvertent exposure of patient (receiving test or therapy) E873.3
  infrared (heaters and lamps) E926.1
    excessive heat E900.1
  ionized, ionizing (particles, artificially accelerated) E926.8
    electromagnetic E926.3

INDEX TO EXTERNAL CAUSES   Residual

Radiation—*continued*
  isotopes, radioactive—*see* Radiation,
    radioactive isotopes
  laser(s) E926.4
    in
      terrorism E979.8
      war operations E997.0
  misadventure in medical care—*see*
    Misadventure, failure, in dosage,
    radiation
  late effect of NEC E929.8
    excessive heat from—*see* Heat
  light sources (visible) (ultraviolet) E926.2
  misadventure in medical or surgical
    procedure—*see* Misadventure, failure, in
    dosage, radiation
  overdose (in medical or surgical procedure)
    E873.2
  radar E926.0
  radioactive isotopes E926.5
    atomic power plant malfunction E926.5
      in water transport E838
    misadventure in medical or surgical
      treatment—*see* Misadventure, failure, in
      dosage, radiation
  radiobiologicals—*see* Radiation, radioactive
    isotopes
  radiofrequency E926.0
  radiopharmaceuticals—*see* Radiation,
    radioactive isotopes
  radium NEC E926.9
  sun E926.2
    excessive heat from E900.0
  tanning bed E926.2
  welding arc or torch E926.2
    excessive heat from E900.1
  x-rays (hard) (soft) E926.3
    misadventure in medical or surgical
      treatment—*see* Misadventure, failure, in
      dosage, radiation
Rape E960.1
Reaction —abnormal to or following(medical or
  surgical procedure) E879.9
  amputation (of limbs) E878.5
  anastomosis (arteriovenous) (blood vessel)
    (gastrojejunal) (skin) (tendon) (natural,
    artificial material, tissue) E878.2
    external stoma, creation of E878.3
  aspiration (of fluid) E879.4
    tissue E879.8
  biopsy E879.8
  blood
    sampling E879.7
    transfusion
      procedure E879.8
  bypass—*see* Reaction, abnormal, anastomosis
  catheterization
    cardiac E879.0
    urinary E879.6
  colostomy E878.3
  cystostomy E878.3
  dialysis (kidney) E879.1
  drugs or biologicals—*see* Table of drugs and
    chemicals
  duodenostomy E878.3
  electroshock therapy E879.3
  formation of external stoma E878.3
  gastrostomy E878.3
  graft—*see* Reaction, abnormal, anastomosis
  hypothermia E879.8

Reaction—*continued*
  implant, implantation (of)
    artificial
      internal device (cardiac pacemaker)
        (electrodes in brain) (heart valve
        prosthesis) (orthopedic) E878.1
      material or tissue (for anastomosis or
        bypass) E878.2
        with creation of external stoma E878.3
    natural tissues (for anastomosis or bypass)
      E878.2
      as transplantion—*see* Reaction, abnormal,
        transplant
      with creation of external stoma E878.3
  infusion
    procedure E879.8
  injection
    procedure E879.8
  insertion of gastric or duodenal sound E879.5
  insulin-shock therapy E879.3
  lumbar puncture E879.4
  perfusion E879.1
  procedures other than surgical operation (*see
    also* Reaction, abnormal, by specific type
    of procedure) E879.9
    specified procedure NEC E879.8
  radiological procedure or therapy E879.2
  removal of organ (partial) (total) NEC E878.6
    with
      anastomosis, bypass or graft E878.2
      formation of external stoma E878.3
      implant of artificial internal device E878.1
      transplant(ation)
        partial organ E878.4
        whole organ E878.0
  sampling
    blood E879.7
    fluid NEC E879.4
    tissue E879.8
  shock therapy E879.3
  surgical operation (*see also* Reaction,
    abnormal, by specified type of operation)
    E878.9
    restorative NEC E878.4
      with
        anastomosis, bypass or graft E878.2
        formation of external stoma E878.3
        implant(ation)—*see* Reaction, abnormal,
          implant
        transplant(ation)—*see* Reaction,
          abnormal, transplant
    specified operation NEC E878.8
  thoracentesis E879.4
  transfusion
    procedure E879.8
  transplant, transplantation (heart) (kidney)
    (liver) E878.0
    partial organ E878.4
  ureterostomy E878.3
  vaccination E879.8
Reduction in
  atmospheric pressure—*see also* Effects of, air
    pressure
    while surfacing from
      deep water diving causing caisson or
        divers' disease, palsy or paralysis
        E902.2
      underground E902.8
Residual (effect)—*see* Late effect

Rock falling on or hitting (accidentally)
  motor vehicle (in motion) (on public highway) E818
  not on public highway E825
  nonmotor road vehicle NEC E829
  pedal cycle E826
  person E916
  railway rolling stock, train, vehicle E806
Running off, away
  animal (being ridden) (in sport or transport) E828
    not being ridden E906.8
  animal-drawn vehicle E827
  rails, railway (*see also* Derailment) E802
  roadway
    motor vehicle (without antecedent collision) E816
      nontraffic accident E825
        with antecedent collision—*see* Collision, motor vehicle, not on public highway
    with
      antecedent collision—*see* Collision motor vehicle
      subsequent collision
        involving any object, person or vehicle
          not on public highway E816
          on public highway E811
    nonmotor road vehicle NEC E829
    pedal cycle E826
Run over (accidentally) (by)
  animal (not being ridden) E906.8
    being ridden (in sport or transport) E828
  animal-drawn vehicle E827
  machinery—*see* Accident, machine
  motor vehicle (on public highway)—*see* Hit by, motor vehicle
  nonmotor road vehicle NEC E829
  railway train E805
  street car E829
  vehicle NEC E848

S

Saturnism E866.0
  from insecticide NEC E863.4
Scald, scalding (accidental) (by) (from) (in) E924.0
  acid—*see* Scald, caustic
  boiling tap water E924.2
  caustic or corrosive liquid, substance E924.1
    swallowed—*see* Table of drugs and chemicals
  homicide (attempt)—*see* Assault, burning
  inflicted by other person
    stated as
      intentional or homicidal E968.3
      undetermined whether accidental or intentional E988.2
  late effect of NEC E929.8
  liquid (boiling) (hot) E924.0
  local application of externally applied substance in medical or surgical care E873.5
  molten metal E924.0
  self-inflicted (unspecified whether accidental or intentional) E988.2
    stated as intentional, purposeful E958.2
    stated as undetermined whether accidental or intentional E988.2

Scald, scalding—*continued*
  steam E924.0
  tap water (boiling) E924.2
  transport accident—*see* categories E800-E848
  vapor E924.0
Scratch, cat E906.8
Sea
  sickness E903
Self-mutilation —*see* Suicide
Sequelai (of)
  in
    terrorism E999.1
    war operations E999.0
Shock
  anaphylactic (*see also* Table of drugs and chemicals) E947.9
  due to
    bite (venomous)—*see* Bite, venomous NEC
    sting—*see* Sting
  electric (*see also* Electric shock) E925.9
    from electric appliance or current (*see also* Electric shock) E925.9
Shooting, shot (accidental(ly)) E922.9
  air gun E922.4
  BB gun E922.4
  hand gun (pistol) (revolver) E922.0
  himself (*see also* Shooting, self-inflicted) E985.4
    hand gun (pistol) (revolver) E985.0
    military firearm, except hand gun E985.3
      hand gun (pistol) (revolver) E985.0
    rifle (hunting) E985.2
      military E985.3
    shotgun (automatic) E985.1
    specified firearm NEC E985.4
    Verey pistol E985.4
  homicide (attempt) E965.4
    air gun E968.6
    BB gun E968.6
    hand gun (pistol) (revolver) E965.0
    military firearm, except hand gun E965.3
      hand gun (pistol) (revolver) E965.0
    paintball gun E965.4
    rifle (hunting) E965.2
      military E965.3
    shotgun (automatic) E965.1
    specified firearm NEC E965.4
    Verey pistol E965.4
  inflicted by other person
    in accidental circumstances E922.9
      hand gun (pistol) (revolver) E922.0
      military firearm, except hand gun E922.3
        hand gun (pistol) (revolver) E922.0
      rifle (hunting) E922.2
        military E922.3
      shotgun (automatic) E922.1
      specified firearm NEC E922.8
      Verey pistol E922.8
    stated as
      intentional, homicidal E965.4
        hand gun (pistol) (revolver) E965.0
        military firearm, except hand gun E965.3
          hand gun (pistol) (revolver) E965.0
        paintball gun E965.4
        rifle (hunting) E965.2
          military E965.3
        shotgun (automatic) E965.1
        specified firearm E965.4
        Verey pistol E965.4

INDEX TO EXTERNAL CAUSES — Starvation

Shooting, shot—*continued*
  undetermined whether accidental or
    intentional E985.4
    air gun E985.6
    BB gun E985.6
    hand gun (pistol) (revolver) E985.0
    military firearm, except hand gun E985.3
      hand gun (pistol) (revolver) E985.0
    paintball gun E985.7
    rifle (hunting) E985.2
    shotgun (automatic) E985.1
    specified firearm NEC E985.4
    Verey pistol E985.4
  in
    terrorism—*see* Terrorism, shooting
    war operations—*see* War operations,
      shooting
  legal
    execution E978
    intervention E970
  military firearm, except hand gun E922.3
    hand gun (pistol) (revolver) E922.0
  paintball gun E922.5
  rifle (hunting) 922.2
    military E922.3
  self-inflicted (unspecified whether accidental
    or intentional) E985.4
    air gun E985.6
    BB gun E985.6
    hand gun (pistol) (revolver) E985.0
    military firearm, except hand gun E985.3
      hand gun (pistol) (revolver) E985.0
    paintball gun E985.7
    rifle (hunting) E985.2
      military E985.3
    shotgun (automatic) E985.1
    specified firearm NEC E985.4
  stated as
    accidental E922.9
      hand gun (pistol) (revolver) E922.0
      military firearm, except hand gun E922.3
        hand gun (pistol) (revolver) E922.0
      paintball gun E922.5
      rifle (hunting) E922.2
        military E922.3
      shotgun (automatic) E922.1
      specified firearm NEC E922.8
      Verey pistol E922.8
    intentional, purposeful E955.4
      hand gun (pistol) (revolver) E955.0
      military firearm, except hand gun E955.3
        hand gun (pistol) (revolver) E955.0
      paintball gun E955.7
      rifle (hunting) E955.2
        military E955.3
      shotgun (automatic) E955.1
      specified firearm NEC E955.4
      Verey pistol E955.4
  shotgun (automatic) E922.1
  specified firearm NEC E922.8
  stated as undetermined whether accidental or
    intentional E985.4
    hand gun (pistol) (revolver) E985.0
    military firearm, except hand gun E985.3
      hand gun (pistol) (revolver) E985.0
    paintball gun E985.7
    rifle (hunting) E985.2
      military E985.3
    shotgun (automatic) E985.1
    specified firearm NEC E985.4
    Verey pistol E985.4

Shooting, shot—*continued*
  suicidal (attempt) E955.4
    air gun E955.6
    BB gun E955.6
    hand gun (pistol) (revolver) E955.0
    military firearm, except hand gun E955.3
      hand gun (pistol) (revolver) E955.0
    paintball gun E955.7
    rifle (hunting) E955.2
      military E955.3
    shotgun (automatic) E955.1
    specified firearm NEC E955.4
    Verey pistol E955.4
  Verey pistol E922.8
Shoving (accidentally) by other person (*see also* Pushing by other person) E917.9
Sickness
  air E903
  alpine E902.0
  car E903
  motion E903
  mountain E902.0
  sea E903
  travel E903
Sinking (accidental)
  boat, ship, watercraft (causing drowning, submersion) E830
    causing injury except drowning, submersion E831
Siriasis E900.0
Skydiving E844
Slashed wrists (*see also* Cut, self-inflicted) E986
Slipping (accidental)
  on
    deck (of boat, ship, watercraft) (icy) (oily) (wet) E835
    ice E885.9
    ladder of ship E833
      due to accident to watercraft E831
    mud E885.9
    oil E885.9
    snow E885.9
    stairs of ship E833
      due to accident to watercraft E831
    surface
      slippery E885.9
      wet E885.9
Sliver, wood, injury by E920.8
Smothering, smothered (*see also* Suffocation) E913.9
Smouldering building or structure in terrorism E979.3
Sodomy (assault) E960.1
Solid substance in eye (any part) or adnexa E914
Sound waves (causing injury) E928.1
Splinter, injury by E920.8
Stab, stabbing E966
  accidental—*see* Cut
Starvation E904.1
  helpless person, infant, newborn—*see* Lack of food
  homicidal intent E968.4
  late effect of NEC E929.5
  resulting from accident connected with transport—*see* categories E800-E848

Stepped on
by
  animal (not being ridden) E906.8
    being ridden (in sport or transport) E828
  crowd E917.1
  person E917.9
    in sports E917.0
  in sports E917.0
Stepping on
  object (moving) E917.9
    in sports E917.0
      with subsequent fall E917.5
    stationary E917.4
      with subsequent fall E917.8
  person E917.9
    as, or caused by a crowd E917.1
      with subsequent fall E917.6
    in sports E917.0
Sting E905.9
  ant E905.5
  bee E905.3
  caterpillar E905.5
  coral E905.6
  hornet E905.3
  insect NEC E905.5
  jelly fish E905.6
  marine animal or plant E905.6
  nematocysts E905.6
  scorpion E905.2
  sea anemone E905.6
  sea cucumber E905.6
  wasp E905.3
  yellow jacket E905.3
Storm E908.9
  specified type NEC E908.8
Straining, injury in E927
Strangling —*see* Suffocation
Strangulation —*see* Suffocation
Strenuous movements (in recreational or other activities) E927
Striking against
  bottom (when jumping or diving into water) E883.0
  object (moving) E917.9
    caused by crowd E917.1
      with subsequent fall E917.6
    furniture E917.3
      with subsequent fall E917.7
    in
      running water E917.2
        with drowning or submersion—*see* Submersion
      sports E917.0
        with subsequent fall E917.5
    stationary E917.4
      with subsequent fall E917.8
  person(s) E917.9
    with fall E886.9
      in sports E886.0
    as, or caused by, a crowd E917.1
      with subsequent fall E917.6
    in sports E917.0
      with fall E886.0
Stroke
  heat—*see* Heat
  lightning E907
Struck by —*see also* Hit by
  bullet
    in
      terrorism E979.4
      war operation E991.2
        rubber E991.0

Struck by—*continued*
  lightning E907
  missile
    in terrorism—*see* Terrorism, missile
  object
    falling
      from, in, on
        building
          burning (uncontrolled fire)
            in terrorism E979.3
    thunderbolt E907
Stumbling over animal, carpet, curb, rug or (small) object (with fall) E885.9
  without fall—*see* Striking against, object
Submersion (accidental) E910.8
  boat, ship, watercraft (causing drowning, submersion) E830
    causing injury except drowning, submersion E831
  by other person
    in accidental circumstances—*see* category E910
    intentional, homicidal E964
    stated as undetermined whether accidental or intentional E984
  due to
    accident
      machinery—*see* Accident, machine
      to boat, ship, watercraft E830
      transport—*see* categories E800-E848
    avalanche E909.2
    cataclysmic
      earth surface movement or eruption E909.9
      storm E908.9
    cloudburst E908.8
    cyclone E908.1
    fall
      from
        boat, ship, watercraft (not involved in accident) E832
          burning, crushed E830
          involved in accident, collision E830
        gangplank (into water) E832
      overboard NEC E832
    flood E908.2
    hurricane E908.0
    jumping into water E910.8
      from boat, ship, watercraft
        burning, crushed, sinking E830
        involved in accident, collision E830
        not involved in accident, for swim E910.2
      in recreational activity (without diving equipment) E910.2
        with or using diving equipment E910.1
      to rescue another person E910.3
    homicide (attempt) E964
  in
    bathtub E910.4
    specified activity, not sport, transport or recreational E910.3
    sport or recreational activity (without diving equipment) E910.2
      with or using diving equipment E910.1
      water skiing E910.0
    swimming pool NEC E910.8
    terrorism E979.8
    war operations E995
    water transport E832

INDEX TO EXTERNAL CAUSES

Suicide, suicidal

Submersion—*continued*
    due to accident to boat, ship, watercraft E830
  landslide E909.2
    overturning boat, ship, watercraft E909.2
    sinking boat, ship, watercraft E909.2
    submersion boat, ship, watercraft E909.2
    tidal wave E909.4
      caused by storm E908.0
    torrential rain E908.2
  late effect of NEC E929.8
  quenching tank E910.8
  self-inflicted (unspecified whether accidental or intentional) E984
    in accidental circumstances—*see* category E910
    stated as intentional, purposeful E954
    stated as undetermined whether accidental or intentional E984
  suicidal (attempted) E954
  while
    attempting rescue of another person E910.3
    engaged in
      marine salvage E910.3
      underwater construction or repairs E910.3
    fishing, not from boat E910.2
    hunting, not from boat E910.2
    ice skating E910.2
    pearl diving E910.3
    placing fishing nets E910.3
    playing in water E910.2
    scuba diving E910.1
      nonrecreational E910.3
    skin diving E910.1
    snorkel diving E910.2
    spear fishing underwater E910.1
    surfboarding E910.2
    swimming (swimming pool) E910.2
    wading (in water) E910.2
    water skiing E910.0

Sucked
  into
    jet (aircraft) E844

Suffocation (accidental) (by external means) (by pressure) (mechanical) E913.9
  caused by other person
    in accidental circumstances—*see* category E913
    stated as
      intentional, homicidal E963
      undetermined whether accidental or intentional E983.9
        by, in
          hanging E983.0
          plastic bag E983.1
          specified means NEC E983.3
  due to, by
    avalanche E909.2
    bedclothes E913.0
    bib E913.0
    blanket E913.0
    cave-in E913.3
      caused by cataclysmic earth surface movement or eruption E909.9
    conflagration—*see* Conflagration
    explosion—*see* Explosion
    falling earth, other substance E913.3
    fire—*see* Fire
    food, any type (ingestion) (inhalation) (regurgitated) (vomited) E911

Suffocation—*continued*
    foreign body, except food (ingestion) (inhalation) E912
    ignition—*see* Ignition
    landslide E909.2
    machine(ry)—*see* Accident, machine
    material, object except food entering by nose or mouth, ingested, inhaled E912
    mucus (aspiration) (inhalation), not of newborn E912
    phlegm (aspiration) (inhalation) E912
    pillow E913.0
    plastic bag—*see* Suffocation, in, plastic bag
    sheet (plastic) E913.0
    specified means NEC E913.8
    vomitus (aspiration) (inhalation) E911
  homicidal (attempt) E963
  in
    airtight enclosed place E913.2
    baby carriage E913.0
    bed E913.0
    closed place E913.2
    cot, cradle E913.0
    perambulator E913.0
    plastic bag (in accidental circumstances) E913.1
      homicidal, purposely inflicted by other person E963
      self-inflicted (unspecified whether accidental or intentional) E983.1
      in accidental circumstances E913.1
      intentional, suicidal E953.1
      stated as undetermined whether accidentally or purposely inflicted E983.1
      suicidal, purposely self-inflicted E953.1
    refrigerator E913.2
  self-inflicted—*see also* Suffocation, stated as undetermined whether accidental or intentional E953.9
    in accidental circumstances—*see* category E913
    stated as intentional, purposeful—*see* Suicide, suffocation
  stated as undetermined whether accidental or intentional E983.9
    by, in
      hanging E983.0
      plastic bag E983.1
      specified means NEC E983.8
  suicidal—*see* Suicide, suffocation

Suicide, suicidal (attempted) (by) E958.9
  burning, burns E958.1
  caustic substance E958.7
    poisoning E950.7
    swallowed E950.7
  cold, extreme E958.3
  cut (any part of body) E956
  cutting or piercing instrument (classifiable to E920) E956
  drowning E954
  electrocution E958.4
  explosive(s) (classifiable to E923) E955.5
  fire E958.1
  firearm (classifiable to E922)—*see* Shooting, suicidal
  hanging E953.0
  jumping
    before moving object, train, vehicle E958.0
    from high place—*see* Jumping, from, high place, stated as, suicidal

Suicide, suicidal—*continued*
  knife E956
  late effect of E959
  motor vehicle, crashing of E958.5
  poisoning—*see* Table of drugs and chemicals
  puncture (any part of body) E956
  scald E958.2
  shooting—*see* Shooting, suicidal
  specified means NEC E958.8
  stab (any part of body) E956
  strangulation—*see* Suicide, suffocation
  submersion E954
  suffocation E953.9
    by, in
      hanging E953.0
      plastic bag E953.1
      specified means NEC E953.8
  wound NEC E958.9
Sunburn E926.2
Sunstroke E900.0
Supersonic waves (causing injury) E928.1
Surgical procedure, complication of
  delayed or as an abnormal reaction without mention of misadventure—*see* Reaction, abnormal
  due to or as a result of misadventure—*see* Misadventure
Swallowed, swallowing
  foreign body—*see* Foreign body, alimentary canal
  poison—*see* Table of drugs and chemicals
  substance
    caustic—*see* Table of drugs and chemicals
    corrosive—*see* Table of drugs and chemicals
    poisonous—*see* Table of drugs and chemicals
Swimmers cramp (*see also* category E910) E910.2
  not in recreation or sport E910.3
Syndrome, battered
  baby or child—*see* Abuse, child
  wife—*see* Assault

T

Tackle in sport E886.0
Terrorism (injury) (by) (in) E979.8
  air blast E979.2
  aircraft burned, destroyed, exploded, shot down E979.1
    used as a weapon E979.1
  anthrax E979.6
  asphyxia from
    chemical (weapons) E979.7
    fire, conflagration (caused by fire-producing device) E979.3
    from nuclear explosion E979.5
    gas or fumes E979.7
  bayonet E979.8
  biological agents E979.6
  blast (air) (effects) E979.2
    from nuclear explosion E979.5
    underwater E979.0
  bomb (antipersonnel) (mortor) (explosion) (fragments) E979.2
  bullet(s) (from carbine, machine gun, pistol, rifle, shotgun) E979.4
  burn from
    chemical E979.7

Terrorism—*continued*
    fire, conflagration (caused by fire-producing device) E979.3
    from nuclear explosion E979.5
    gas E979.7
  burning aircraft E979.1
  chemical E979.7
  cholera E979.6
  conflagration E979.3
  crushed by falling aircraft E979.1
  depth charge E979.0
  destruction of aircraft E979.1
  disability, as seqelae one year or more after injury E999.1
  drowning E979.8
  effect
    of nuclear weapon (direct) (secondary) E979.5
    secondary NEC E979.9
  sequelae E999.1
  explosion (artillery shell) (breech-block) (cannon block) E979.2
    aircraft E979.1
    bomb (antipersonnel) (mortar) E979.2
    nuclear (atom) (hydrogen) E979.5
    depth-charge E979.0
    grenade E979.2
    injury by fragments from E979.2
    land-mine E979.2
    marine weapon E979.0
    mine (land) E979.2
      at sea or in harbor E979.0
      marine E979.0
    missile (explosive) NEC E979.2
    munitions (dump) (factory) E979.2
    nuclear (weapon) E979.5
    other direct and secondary effects of E979.5
    sea-based artillery shell E979.0
    torpedo E979.0
  exposure to ionizing radiation from nuclear explosion E979.5
  falling aircraft E979.1
  fire or fire-producing device E979.3
  firearms E979.4
  fireball effects from nuclear explosion E979.5
  fragments from artillery shell, bomb NEC, grenade, guided missile, land-mine, rocket, shell, shrapnel E979.2
  gas or fumes E979.7
  grenade (explosion) (fragments) E979.2
  guided missile (explosion) (fragments) E979.2
    nuclear E979.5
  heat from nuclear explosion E979.5
  hot substances E979.3
  hydrogen cyanide E979.7
  land-mine (explosion) (fragments) E979.2
  laser(s) E979.8
  late effect of E999.1
  lewisite E979.7
  lung irritant (chemical) (fumes) (gas) E979.7
  marine mine E979.0
  mine E979.2
    at sea E979.0
    in harbor E979.0
    land (explosion) (fragments) E979.2
    marine E979.0
  missile (explosion) (fragments) (guided) E979.2
    marine E979.0
    nuclear E979.5

INDEX TO EXTERNAL CAUSES

Terrorism—*continued*
  mortar bomb (explosion) (fragments) E979.2
  mustard gas E979.7
  nerve gas E979.7
  nuclear weapons E979.5
  pellets (shotgun) E979.4
  petrol bomb E979.3
  piercing object E979.8
  phosgene E979.7
  poisoning (chemical) (fumes) (gas) E979.7
  radiation, ionizing from nuclear explosion E979.5
  rocket (explosion) (fragments) E979.2
  saber, sabre E979.8
  sarin E979.7
  screening smoke E979.7
  sequelae effect (of) E999.1
  shell (aircraft) (artillery) (cannon) (land-based) (explosion) (fragments) E979.2
    sea-based E979.0
  shooting E979.4
    bullet(s) E979.4
    pellet(s) (rifle) (shotgun) E979.4
  shrapnel E979.2
  smallpox E979.7
  stabbing object(s) E979.8
  submersion E979.8
  torpedo E979.0
  underwater blast E979.0
  vesicant (chemical) (fumes) (gas) E979.7
  weapon burst E979.2
Thermic fever E900.9
Thermoplegia E900.9
Thirst —*see also* Lack of water
  resulting from accident connected with transport—*see* categories E800-E848
Thrown (accidentally)
  against object in or part of vehicle
    by motion of vehicle
      aircraft E844
      boat, ship, watercraft E838
      motor vehicle (on public highway) E818
        not on public highway E825
        off-road type (not on public highway) E821
          on public highway E818
        snow vehicle E820
          on public highway E818
      nonmotor road vehicle NEC E829
      railway rolling stock, train, vehicle E806
      street car E829
  from
    animal (being ridden) (in sport or transport) E828
    high place, homicide (attempt) E968.1
    machinery—*see* Accident, machine
    vehicle NEC—*see* Accident, vehicle NEC
  off—*see* Thrown, from
  overboard (by motion of boat, ship, watercraft) E832
    by accident to boat, ship, watercraft E830
Thunderbolt NEC E907
Tidal wave (any injury) E909.4
  caused by storm E908.0
Took
  overdose of drug—*see* Table of drugs and chemicals
  poison—*see* Table of drugs and chemicals
Tornado (any injury) E908.1
Torrential rain (any injury) E908.2
Traffic accident NEC E819

War operations

Trampled by animal E906.8
  being ridden (in sport or transport) E828
Trapped (accidentally)
  between
    objects (moving) (stationary and moving) E918
  by
    door of
      elevator E918
      motor vehicle (on public highway) (while alighting, boarding)—*see* Fall, from, motor vehicle, while alighting
      railway train (underground) E806
      street car E829
      subway train E806
  in object E918
Travel (effects) E903
  sickness E903
Tree
  falling on or hitting E916
    motor vehicle (in motion) (on public highway) E818
      not on public highway E825
    nonmotor road vehicle NEC E829
    pedal cycle E826
    person E916
    railway rolling stock, train, vehicle E806
    street car E829
Trench foot E901.0
Tripping over animal, carpet, curb, rug, or small object (with fall) E885.9
  without fall—*see* Striking against, object
Tsunami E909.4
Twisting, injury in E927

V

Violence, nonaccidental (*see also* Assault) E968.9
Volcanic eruption (any injury) E909.1
Vomitus in air passages (with asphyxia, obstruction or suffocation) E911

W

War operations (during hostilities) (injury) (by) (in) E995
  after cessation of hostilities, injury due to E998
  air blast E993
  aircraft burned, destroyed, exploded, shot down E994
  asphyxia from
    chemical E997.2
    fire, conflagration (caused by fire-producing device or conventional weapon) E990.9
      from nuclear explosion E996
      petrol bomb E990.0
    fumes E997.2
    gas E997.2
  battle wound NEC E995
  bayonet E995
  biological warfare agents E997.1
  blast (air) (effects) E993
    from nuclear explosion E996
    underwater E992
  bomb (mortar) (explosion) E993
    after cessation of hostilities E998
    fragments, injury by E991.9

War operations — INDEX TO EXTERNAL CAUSES

War operations—*continued*
    antipersonnel E991.3
    bullet(s) (from carbine, machine gun, pistol, rifle, shotgun) E991.2
      rubber E991.0
    burn from
      chemical E997.2
      fire, conflagration (caused by fire-producing device or conventional weapon) E990.9
        from nuclear explosion E996
        petrol bomb E990.0
      gas E997.2
    burning aircraft E994
    chemical E997.2
    chlorine E997.2
    conventional warfare, specified form NEC E995
    crushing by falling aircraft E994
    depth charge E992
    destruction of aircraft E994
    disability as sequela one year or more after injury E999.0
    drowning E995
    effect (direct) (secondary) nuclear weapon E996
    explosion (artillery shell) (breech block) (cannon shell) E993
      after cessation of hostilities of bomb, mine placed in war E998
      aircraft E994
      bomb (mortar) E993
        atom E996
        hydrogen E996
        injury by fragments from E991.9
          antipersonnel E991.3
        nuclear E996
      depth charge E992
      injury by fragments from E991.9
        antipersonnel E991.3
      marine weapon E992
      mine
        at sea or in harbor E992
        land E993
          injury by fragments from E991.9
        marine E992
      munitions (accidental) (being used in war) (dump) (factory) E993
      nuclear (weapon) E996
      own weapons (accidental) E993
        injury by fragments from E991.9
          antipersonnel E991.3
      sea-based artillery shell E992
      torpedo E992
    exposure to ionizing radiation from nuclear explosion E996
    falling aircraft E994
    fire or fire-producing device E990.9
      petrol bomb E990.0
    fireball effects from nuclear explosion E996
    fragments from
      antipersonnel bomb E991.3
      artillery shell, bomb NEC, grenade, guided missile, land mine, rocket, shell, shrapnel E991.9
    fumes E997.2
    gas E997.2
    grenade (explosion) E993
      fragments, injury by E991.9
    guided missile (explosion) E993
      fragments, injury by E991.9
      nuclear E996

War operations—*continued*
    heat from nuclear explosion E996
    injury due to, but occurring after cessation of hostilities E998
    lacrimator (gas) (chemical) E997.2
    land mine (explosion) E993
      after cessation of hostilities E998
      fragments, injury by E991.9
    laser(s) E997.0
    late effect of E999.0
    lewisite E997.2
    lung irritant (chemical) (fumes) (gas) E997.2
    marine mine E992
    mine
      after cessation of hostilities E998
      at sea E992
      in harbor E992
      land (explosion) E993
        fragments, injury by E991.9
      marine E992
    missile (guided) (explosion) E993
      fragments, injury by E991.9
      marine E992
      nuclear E996
    mortar bomb (explosion) E993
      fragments, injury by E991.9
    mustard gas E997.2
    nerve gas E997.2
    phosgene E997.2
    poisoning (chemical) (fumes) (gas) E997.2
    radiation, ionizing from nuclear explosion E996
    rocket (explosion) E993
      fragments, injury by E991.9
    saber, sabre E995
    screening smoke E997.8
    shell (aircraft) (artillery) (cannon) (land based) (explosion) E993
      fragments, injury by E991.9
      sea-based E992
    shooting E991.2
      after cessation of hostilities E998
      bullet(s) E991.2
        rubber E991.0
      pellet(s) (rifle) E991.1
    shrapnel E991.9
    submersion E995
    torpedo E992
    unconventional warfare, except by nuclear weapon E997.9
      biological (warfare) E997.1
      gas, fumes, chemicals E997.2
      laser(s) E997.0
      specified type NEC E997.8
    underwater blast E992
    vesicant (chemical) (fumes) (gas) E997.2
    weapon burst E993

Washed
    away by flood—*see* Flood
    away by tidal wave—*see* Tidal wave
    off road by storm (transport vehicle) E908.9
    overboard E832

Weather exposure —*see also* Exposure
    cold E901.0
    hot E900.0

Weightlessness (causing injury) (effects of) (in spacecraft, real or simulated) E928.0

Wound (accidental) NEC (*see also* Injury) E928.9
    battle (*see also* War operation) E995
    bayonet E920.3
    in

INDEX TO EXTERNAL CAUSES

Wound—*continued*
  legal intervention E974
  war operations E995
gunshot—*see* Shooting
incised—*see* Cut
saber, sabre E920.3
  in war operations E995

INDEX TO EXTERNAL CAUSES

RAILWAY ACCIDENTS (E800–E807)

The following fourth-digit subdivisions are for use with categories E800-E807 to identify the injured person.

.0 Railway employee

Any person who by virtue of his employment in connection with a railway, whether by the railway company or not, is at increased risk of involvement in a railway accident, such as:

catering staff on train	postal staff on train
driver	railway fireman
guard	shunter
porter	sleeping car attendant

.1 Passenger on railway

Any authorized person traveling on a train, except a railway employee

Excludes: intending passenger waiting at station (.8)
unauthorized rider on railway vehicle (.8)

.2 Pedestrian

See definition (r), Vol. 1, E code introduction

.3 Pedal cyclist

See definition (p), Vol. 1, E code introduction

.8 Other specified person

Intending passenger waiting at station

Unauthorized rider on railway vehicle

.9 Unspecified person

INDEX TO EXTERNAL CAUSES

MOTOR VEHICLE TRAFFIC AND NONTRAFFIC ACCIDENTS (E810–825)

The following fourth–digit subdivisions are for use with categories E810–E819 and E820–E825 to identify the injured person:

.0 Driver of motor vehicle other than motorcycle

See definition (l), Vol. 1, E code introduction

.1 Passenger in motor vehicle other than motorcycle

See definition (l), Vol. 1, E code introduction

.2 Motorcyclist

See definition (l), Vol. 1, E code introduction

.3 Passenger on motorcycle

See definition (l), Vol. 1, E code introduction

.4 Occupant of streetcar

.5 Rider of animal; occupant of animal–drawn vehicle

.6 Pedal cyclist

See definition (p), Vol. 1, E code introduction

.7 Pedestrian

See definition (r), Vol. 1, E code introduction

.8 Other specified person

Occupant of vehicle other than above

Person in railway train involved in accident

Unauthorized rider of motor vehicle

.9 Unspecified person

OTHER ROAD VEHICLE ACCIDENTS (E826–E829)

(animal–drawn vehicle, streetcar, pedal cycle, and other nonmotor road vehicle accidents)

The following fourth–digit subdivisions are for use with categories E826–E829 to identify the injured person:

.0 Pedestrian

    See definition (r), Vol. 1, E code introduction

.1 Pedal cyclist (does not apply to codes E827, E828, E829)

    See definition (p), Vol. 1, E code introduction

.2 Rider of animal (does not apply to code E829)

.3 Occupant of animal–drawn vehicle (does not apply to codes E828, E829)

.4 Occupant of streetcar

.8 Other specified person

.9 Unspecified person

WATER TRANSPORT ACCIDENTS (E830–E838)

The following fourth-digit subdivisions are for use with categories E830–E838 to identify the injured person:

.0 Occupant of small boat, unpowered

.1 Occupant of small boat, powered

    See definition (t), Vol. 1, E code introduction

    Excludes: water skier (.4)

.2 Occupant of other watercraft — crew

    Persons:

        engaged in operation of watercraft

        providing passenger services [cabin attendants, ship's physician, catering personnel]

        working on ship during voyage in other capacity [musician in band, operators of shops and beauty parlors]

.3 Occupant of other watercraft — other than crew

    Passenger

    Occupant of lifeboat, other than crew, after abandoning ship

.4 Water skier

.5 Swimmer

.6 Dockers, stevedores

    Longshoreman employed on the dock in loading and unloading ships

.8 Other specified person

    Immigration and custom officials on board ship

    Person:
        accompanying passenger or member of crew
        visiting boat

    Pilot (guiding ship into port)

.9 Unspecified person

INDEX TO EXTERNAL CAUSES

AIR AND SPACE TRANSPORT ACCIDENTS (E840–E845)

The following fourth–digit subdivisions are for use with categories E840–E845 to identify the injured person:

.0 Occupant of spacecraft

.1 Occupant of military aircraft, any

> Crew in military aircraft [air force] [army] [national guard] [navy]
>
> Passenger (civilian) (military) in military aircraft [air force] [army] [national guard] [navy]
>
> Troops in military aircraft [air force] [army] [national guard] [navy]
>
> *Excludes:* occupants of aircraft operated under jurisdiction of police departments (.5)
> parachutist (.7).

.2 Crew of commercial aircraft (powered) in surface to surface transport

.3 Other occupant of commercial aircraft (powered) in surface to surface transport

> Flight personnel:
> > not part of crew
> > on familiarization flight
>
> Passenger on aircraft (powered) NOS

.4 Occupant of commercial aircraft (powered) in surface to air transport

> Occupant [crew] [passenger] of aircraft (powered) engaged in activities, such as:
> > aerial spraying (crops) (fire retardants)
> > air drops of emergency supplies
> > air drops of parachutists, except from military craft
> > crop dusting
> > lowering of construction material [bridge or telephone pole]
> > sky writing

.5 Occupant of other powered aircraft

> Occupant [crew] [passenger] of aircraft (powered) engaged in activities, such as:
> > aerobatic flying
> > aircraft racing
> > rescue operation
> > storm surveillance
> > traffic surveillance
>
> Occupant of private plane NOS

.6 Occupant of unpowered aircraft, except parachutist

> Occupant of aircraft classifiable to E842

.7 Parachutist (military) (other)

> Person making voluntary descent
>
> *Excludes:* person making descent after accident to aircraft (.1–.6)

.8 Ground crew, airline employee

> Persons employed at airfields (civil) (military) or launching pads, not occupants of aircraft

.9 Other person

INDEX TO EXTERNAL CAUSES

SUMMARY OF ADDITIONS, DELETIONS AND REVISIONS TO VOLUME 1 IN 2008

Code	Description
005.1	Botulism food poisoning Code revised; add description and exclusion terms
040.4	Other specified botulism New subcategory
040.41	Infant botulism New code
040.42	Wound botulism New code
041	Bacterial infection in conditions classified elsewhere and of unspecified site Revise exclusion term
049.8	Other specified non-arthropod-borne viral diseases of central nervous system Add exclusion terms
054.3	Herpetic meningoencephalitis Add exclusion terms
057.8	Other specified viral exanthemata Delete description terms, add exclusion terms
058	Other human herpesvirus New category
058.1	Roseola infantum New subcategory
058.10	Roseola infantum, unspecified New code
058.11	Roseola infantum due to human herpesvirus 6 New code
058.12	Roseola infantum due to human herpesvirus 7 New code
058.2	Other human herpesvirus encephalitis New subcategory
058.21	Human herpesvirus 6 encephalitis New code
058.29	Other human herpesvirus encephalitis New code
058.8	Other human herpesvirus infections New subcategory
058.81	Human herpesvirus 6 infection New code
058.82	Human herpesvirus 7 infection New code
058.89	Other human herpesvirus infection New code
079.83	Parvovirus B19 New code
184	Malignant neoplasm of other and unspecified female genital organs Revise exclusion term
193	Malignant neoplasm of thyroid gland Delete description
200	Lymphosarcoma and reticulosarcoma and other specified malignant tumors of lymphatic tissue Revise category
200.3	Marginal zone lymphoma New code
200.4	Mantle cell lymphoma New code
200.5	Primary central nervous system lymphoma New code
200.6	Anaplastic large cell lymphoma New code
200.7	Large cell lymphoma New code
202.7	Peripheral T-cell lymphoma New code
232.5	Skin of trunk, except scrotum Revise exclusion term
233.1	Cervix uteri Add description
233.30	Unspecified female genital organ New code
233.31	Vagina New code
233.32	Vulva New code
233.39	Other female genital organ New code
250	Diabetes mellitus Revise exclusion
250.6	Diabetes with neurological manifestations Revise "Use additional code" note
255.4	Corticoadrenal insufficiency Delete description
255.41	Glucocorticoid deficiency New code
255.42	Mineralocorticoid deficiency New code
258.0	Polyglandular activity in multiple endocrine adenomatosis Delete description term, add description term, add "Use additional" note
258.01	Multiple endocrine neoplasia [MEN] type I New code
258.02	Multiple endocrine neoplasia [MEN] type IIA New code
258.03	Multiple endocrine neoplasia [MEN] type IIB New code
268.1	Rickets, late effect Revise "Code first" note
276.6	Fluid overload Revise exclusion term
284.1	Pancytopenia Revise exclusion term
284.8	Other specified aplastic anemias Delete description
284.81	Red cell aplasia (acquired) (adult) (with thymoma) New code
284.89	Other specified aplastic anemias New code
288.0	Neutropenia Revise "Use additional" note

SUMMARY OF ADDITIONS, DELETIONS AND REVISIONS TO VOLUME 1

288.66	**Bandemia** New code		389.05	**Conductive hearing loss, unilateral** New code
302.5	**Tran-sexualism** Add description		389.06	**Conductive hearing loss, bilateral** New code
302.85	**Gender identity disorder in adolescents or adults** Add "Use additional code" note		389.1	**Sensorineural hearing loss** Add exclusion term
			389.13	**Neural hearing loss, unilateral** New code
315.32	**Mixed receptive-expressive language disorder** Add description and exclusion term		389.14	**Central hearing loss** Revise code
315.34	**Speech and language developmental delay due to hearing loss** New code		389.17	**Sensory hearing loss, unilateral** New code
			389.18	**Sensorineural hearing loss, bilateral** Revise code
331	**Other cerebral degenerations** Add "Use additional code" note		389.2	**Mixed conductive and sensorineural hearing loss** Revise description
331.1	**Frontotemporal dementia** Delete "Use additional code" note			
331.3	**Communicating hydrocephalus** Add description and exclusion terms		389.20	**Mixed hearing loss, unspecified** New code
331.4	**Obstructive hydrocephalus** Add exclusion terms		389.21	**Mixed hearing loss, unilateral** New code
331.5	**Idiopathic normal pressure hydrocephalus (INPH)** New code		389.22	**Mixed hearing loss, bilateral** New code
			389.7	**Deaf nonspeaking, not elsewhere classifiable** Revise code, delete description term
331.82	**Dementia with Lewy bodies** Delete "Use additional code" note			
353.1	**Lumbosacral plexus lesions** Add "Code first" note		414.0	**Coronary atherosclerosis** Add "Use additional code" note
358.1	**Myasthenic syndromes in diseases classified elsewhere** Delete descriptive term and "Code first" term		414.2	**Chronic total occlusion of coronary artery** New code
			415.12	**Septic pulmonary embolism** New code
359.2	**Myotonic disorders** Delete description, add exclusion		423.3	**Cardiac tamponade** New code
359.21	**Myotonic muscular dystrophy** New code		425.8	**Cardiomyopathy in other diseases classified elsewhere** Revise "Code first" note
359.22	**Myotonia congenita** New code		438	**Late effects of cerebrovascular disease** Add exclusions
359.23	**Myotonic chondrodystrophy** New code		438.82	**Dysphagia** Add "Use additional code" note
359.24	**Drug-induced myotonia** New code		438.89	**Other late effects of cerebrovascular disease** Revise code
359.29	**Other specified myotonic disorder** New code			
359.3	**Periodic paralysis** Revise subcategory, add description and exclusion terms		440.2	**Of native arteries of the extremities** Add "Use additional code" note
			440.4	**Chronic total occlusion of artery of the extremities** New code
359.5	**Myopathy in endocrine diseases classified elsewhere** Revise "Code first" note			
364.8	**Other disorders of iris and ciliary body** Delete description and exclusion terms		444	**Arterial embolism and thrombosis** Add exclusion term
			449	**Septic arterial embolism** New code
364.81	**Floppy iris syndrome** New code		487	**Influenza** Add exclusion term
364.89	**Other disorders of iris and ciliary body** New code		488	**Influenza due to identified avian influenza virus** New code
366.43	**Myotonic cataract** Revise "Code first" note		525.7	**Endosseous dental implant failure** New subcategory
388.45	**Acquired auditory processing disorder** New code		525.71	**Osseointegration failure of dental implant** New code
389.0	**Conductive hearing loss** Add exclusion term			

1540

SUMMARY OF ADDITIONS, DELETIONS AND REVISIONS TO VOLUME 1

525.72	**Post-osseointegration biological failure of dental implant** New code		756.4	**Chondrodystrophy** Add exclusion term
525.73	**Post-osseointegration mechanical failure of dental implant** New code		771	**Infections specific to the perinatal period** Add exclusion term
525.79	**Other endosseous dental implant failure** New code		780.39	**Other convulsions** Add description term
526.4	**Inflammatory conditions** Add exclusion		782.3	**Edema** Revise exclusion term
528.7	**Other disturbances of oral epithelium, including tongue** Revise exclusion		784.1	**Throat pain** Revise exclusion term
536.3	**Gastroparesis** Add "Code first" note		784.99	**Other symptoms involving head and neck** Add description and exclusion terms
565.0	**Anal fissure** Delete description, add exclusion		787.2	**Dysphagia** Delete description, add "Code first" note
568.82	**Peritoneal effusion (chronic)** Revise exclusion		787.20	**Dysphagia, unspecified** New code
569.43	**Anal sphincter tear (healed) (old)** New code		787.21	**Dysphagia, oral phase** New code
572.2	**Hepatic coma** Add exclusion		787.22	**Dysphagia, oropharyngeal phase** New code
585	**Chronic kidney disease (CKD)** Revise "Code first" note		787.23	**Dysphagia, pharyngeal phase** New code
608.22	**Intravaginal torsion of spermatic cord** Add description		787.24	**Dysphagia, pharyngoesophageal phase** New code
622.1	**Dysplasia of cervix (uteri)** Revise exclusion		787.29	**Other dysphagia** New code
623.0	**Dysplasia of vagina** Add description, revise exclusion		789.3	**Abdominal or pelvic swelling, mass, or lump** Revise exclusion term
624.0	**Dystrophy of vulva** Delete description, revise exclusion		789.51	**Malignant ascites** New code
624.01	**Vulvar intraepithelial neoplasia I [VIN I]** New code		789.59	**Other ascites** New code
624.02	**Vulvar intraepithelial neoplasia II [VIN II]** New code		996	**Complications peculiar to certain specified procedures** Add exclusion terms
624.09	**Other dystrophy of vulva** New code		996.62	**Due to vascular device, implant and graft** Revise description, add exclusion terms
646.3	**Habitual aborter** Revise exclusion term		996.77	**Due to internal joint prosthesis** Add "Use additional code" note
654	**Abnormality of organs and soft tissues of pelvis** Add exclusion term		998.5	**Postoperative infections** Revise exclusion term
654.8	**Congenital or acquired abnormality of vulva** Add description and exclusion terms		999	**Complications of medical care, not elsewhere classified** Add "Use additional code" note
661.2	**Other and unspecified uterine inertia** Add description and exclusion terms		999.3	**Other infection** Add "Use additional code" note
664.2	**Third-degree perineal laceration** Add exclusion term		999.31	**Infection due to central venous catheter** New code
664.6	**Anal sphincter tear complicating delivery, not associated with third-degree perineal laceration** New code		999.39	**Infection following other infusion, injection, transfusion, or vaccination** New code
666.1	**Other immediate postpartum hemorrhage** Add description, revise exclusion		V12.53	**Sudden cardiac arrest** New code
731.3	**Major osseous defects** Revise "Code first" note		V12.54	**Transient ischemic attack (TIA), and cerebral infarction without residual deficits** New code
733.45	**Jaw** New code		V13.2	**Other genital system and obstetric disorders** Revise exclusion term

SUMMARY OF ADDITIONS, DELETIONS AND REVISIONS TO VOLUME 1

V13.22	**Personal history of cervical dysplasia** New code	V80.3	**Ear diseases** Revise exclusion term
V16.5	**Urinary organs** Revise description	V82.7	**Genetic screening** Revise exclusion term
V16.52	**Bladder** New code	V84.81	**Genetic susceptibility to multiple endocrine neoplasia [MEN]** New code
V17.41	**Family history of sudden cardiac death (SCD)** New code	V84.89	**Genetic susceptibility to other disease** New code
V17.49	**Family history of other cardiovascular diseases** New code	E928.6	**Environmental exposure to harmful algae and toxins** New code
V18.11	**Multiple endocrine neoplasia [MEN] syndrome** New code	E933.6	**Oral bisphosphonates** New code
V18.19	**Other endocrine and metabolic diseases** New code	E933.7	**Intravenous bisphosphonates** New code
V23.2	**Pregnancy with history of abortion** Revise exclusion term		
V25.04	**Counseling and instruction in natural family planning to avoid pregnancy** New code		
V26.41	**Procreative counseling and advice using natural family planning** New code		
V26.49	**Other procreative management counseling and advice** New code		
V26.81	**Encounter for assisted reproductive fertility procedure cycle** New code		
V26.89	**Other specified procreative management** New code		
V49.85	**Dual sensory impairment** New code		
V58.69	**Long-term (current) use of other medications** Revise description		
V58.78	**Aftercare following surgery of the musculoskeletal system NEC** Add exclusion term		
V64.05	**Vaccination not carried out because of caregiver refusal** Add description		
V65.4	**Other counseling, not elsewhere classified** Revise exclusion term		
V68.0	**Issue of medical certificates** Delete description terms		
V68.01	**Disability examination** New code		
V68.09	**Other issue of medical certificates** New code		
V72.12	**Encounter for hearing conservation and treatment** New code		
V72.31	**Routine gynecological examination** Revise "Use additional code" note		
V73.81	**Human papillomavirus (HPV)** New code		
V74.5	**Venereal disease** Add description and exclusion terms		
V76.2	**Cervix** Add exclusion term		